Consultative Hemostasis and Thrombosis

Consultative Hemostasis and Thrombosis

SECOND EDITION

Craig S. Kitchens, MD, MACP

Professor of Medicine
University of Florida
Associate Chief of Staff (Education)
Malcom Randall Veterans Administration Medical Center
Gainesville, Florida

Barbara M. Alving, MD, MACP

Bethesda, Maryland

Craig M. Kessler, MD, MACP

Professor of Medicine and Pathology
Georgetown University School of Medicine
Director, Coagulation Laboratory
Lombardi Comprehensive Cancer Center
Washington, DC

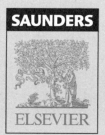

SAUNDERS

ELSEVIER

SAUNDERS
ELSEVIER

1600 John F. Kennedy Blvd.
Ste 1800
Philadelphia, PA 19103-2899

CONSULTATIVE HEMOSTASIS AND THROMBOSIS   ISBN: 978-1-4160-2401-9

Notice

Knowledge and best practice in this field are constantly changing. As new research and experience broaden our knowledge, changes in practice, treatment, and drug therapy may become necessary or appropriate. Readers are advised to check the most current information provided (i) on procedures featured or (ii) by the manufacturer of each product to be administered, to verify the recommended dose or formula, the method and duration of administration, and contraindications. It is the responsibility of the practitioner, relying on his or her experience and knowledge of the patient, to make diagnoses, to determine dosages and the best treatment for each individual patient, and to take all appropriate safety precautions. To the fullest extent of the law, neither the Publisher nor the Editors assume any liability for any injury and/or damage to persons or property arising out of or related to any use of the material contained in this book.

The Publisher

Library of Congress Cataloging-in-Publication Data

Consultative hemostasis and thrombosis / [edited by] Craig S. Kitchens, Barbara M. Alving, Craig M. Kessler.—2nd ed.
    p. ; cm.
    Includes bibliographical references and index.
    ISBN 978-1-4160-2401-9
    1. Blood coagulation disorders.   2. Hemostasis.   I. Kitchens, Craig S.   II. Alving, Barbara M.
III. Kessler, Craig M.
    [DNLM: 1. Blood Coagulation Disorders.   2. Anticoagulants—therapeutic use.
3. Blood Platelet Disorders.   4. Fibrinolytic Agents—therapeutic use.   5. Hemostasis—physiology.
6. Thrombosis.   WH 322 C758 2007]
RC647.C55C655 2007   616.1′57—dc22

                                      2007007888

Acquisitions Editor: Dolores Meloni
Developmental Editor: Kim DePaul
Publishing Services Manager: Frank Polizzano
Project Manager: Jeff Gunning

Printed in the United States of America

Last digit is the print number: 9 8 7 6 5 4 3 2 1

Working together to grow
libraries in developing countries

www.elsevier.com | www.bookaid.org | www.sabre.org

ELSEVIER   BOOK AID International   Sabre Foundation

DEDICATION

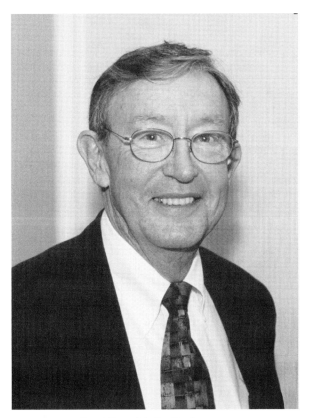

Dr. Harold R. Roberts

The editors dedicate the second edition of *Consultative Hemostasis and Thrombosis* to Dr. Harold R. Roberts, Professor of Pathology and Medicine at the University of North Carolina (UNC) at Chapel Hill, in recognition of the enduring contributions he has made to the diagnosis and treatment of persons with inherited and acquired disorders of hemostasis and thrombosis. His accomplishments are the result of a long and distinguished career as a laboratory investigator, clinical researcher, and practicing physician.

A native of North Carolina, Dr. Roberts received both his undergraduate training and his medical degree from UNC. His postgraduate training included an internship, residency, and subspecialty training at the Vanderbilt School of Medicine in Nashville, Tennessee, and a year as a Fulbright Scholar in experimental pathology in Copenhagen, Denmark, where he worked in the area of fibrinolysis in the laboratory of Professor Tage Astrup. He then entered

a fellowship in the Department of Pathology at UNC under the direction of Dr. Kenneth Brinkhous. After completing his fellowship, Dr. Roberts became a research associate at UNC; seven years later he was named Chief of the Division of Hematology.

While exploring genetic alterations resulting in factor IX deficiency (hemophilia B), Dr. Roberts and his laboratory investigators were the first to recognize that persons with hemophilia B could have any one of numerous point mutations or deletions in the gene coding for factor IX. The gene alterations could result either in no expression of protein or in the expression of a protein that was recognized by immunologic methods but had little or no functional activity. Dr. Roberts' laboratory also was the first to discover that a patient who presented with deficiencies of factors II, VII, IX, and X had a congenital deficiency of the enzymes regulating the vitamin K–γ-carboxylase system.

As a clinical researcher, Dr Roberts focused on new and improved biologics for the treatment of bleeding disorders. His team was the first to test commercially prepared (large-scale) plasma fractions for the treatment of factor VIII deficiency (hemophilia A). These studies resulted in the development of purified concentrates of factor VIII, marking the beginning of a new era for the treatment of hemophilia. In a natural evolution of this work, Dr. Roberts and his team conducted some of the first clinical trials with recombinant factor VIII. His group also has been actively engaged in gene therapy as a next step in improving treatment for patients with hemophilia.

Dr. Roberts has played a seminal role in defining the mechanism of action of recombinant factor VIIa (rFVIIa), as well as in the commercial development of this agent for the treatment of hemophilia in patients who have inhibitors.

Throughout his career, Dr. Roberts has held leadership positions in professional societies nationally and internationally and has served on editorial boards or as editor of multiple journals. He has worked tirelessly with the International Society on Thrombosis and Haemostasis, the American Society of Hematology, the World Federation of Hemophilia, the College of American Pathologists, and the National Hemophilia Foundation. He has chaired study sections and served on councils for the National Institutes of Health, and he has been an invited guest lecturer throughout North Carolina, the nation, and the world.

Numerous societies and governments have honored Dr. Roberts for his laboratory and clinical research, as well as for the establishment of centers for the treatment of disorders of thrombosis or hemostasis. Dr. Roberts was the 2001 recipient of the Henry M. Stratton Medal presented by the American Society of Hematology. As a tribute to the outstanding care and advances in treatment that Dr. Roberts has provided for patients at the former UNC Hemophilia Treatment Center, university officials have renamed the Center as the Harold R. Roberts Comprehensive Hemophilia Diagnostic and Treatment Center.

The outstanding academic work of Dr. Roberts is evident in the more than 300 articles that he has authored during his career. However, the publications do not begin to document completely all of the successes of the numerous students, fellows, and faculty whom he has trained and mentored. Those who have been privileged to work with him recount stories that reveal his warmth, humility, and wonderfully dry sense of humor. Dr. Roberts' ability to nurture and sustain long-lasting relationships with patients, health care providers, public advocacy groups, and government officials across multiple countries ensures that the advances in clinical care that he has developed are available to patients throughout the nation and the world.

Contributors

Victoria Afshani, MD
Hematologist/Medical Oncologist, Georgia Cancer Specialists, Atlanta, Georgia

Management of Bleeding Disorders in Pregnancy

William C. Aird, MD
Associate Professor of Medicine, Harvard Medical School; Attending Physician and Chief, Division of Molecular and Vascular Medicine, Beth Israel Deaconess Medical Center, Boston, Massachusetts

Endothelium

Barbara M. Alving, MD
Bethesda, Maryland

The Antiphospholipid Syndrome: Clinical Presentation, Diagnosis, and Patient Management; Risk Factors for Cardiovascular Disease and Arterial Thrombosis; Management of Thrombophilia and Antiphospholipid Syndrome During Pregnancy

Jack E. Ansell, MD
Professor of Medicine, Boston University School of Medicine; Vice Chairman, Department of Medicine, Boston Medical Center, Boston, Massachusetts

Outpatient Anticoagulant Therapy

Kenneth Ataga, MD
Assistant Professor, University of North Carolina at Chapel Hill School of Medicine; Attending Physician, University of North Carolina Hospitals, Chapel Hill, North Carolina

Hemostatic Aspects of Sickle Cell Disease

Richard C. Becker, MD
Professor of Medicine, Divisions of Cardiology and Hematology, Duke University School of Medicine; Director, Cardiovascular Thrombosis Center, Duke Clinical Research Institute, Durham, North Carolina

Hemostatic Aspects of Cardiovascular Medicine

Peter C. Block, MD
Professor of Medicine, Emory University School of Medicine; Attending Physician, Emory University Hospitals and Grady Hospital, Atlanta, Georgia

Atrial Septal Abnormalities and Cryptogenic Stroke

Lisa N. Boggio, MS, MD
Assistant Professor of Medicine and Pediatrics, Rush University Medical Center, Chicago, Illinois

Hemophilia A and B

Charles D. Bolan, MD
Associate Professor of Medicine, Uniformed Services University of the Health Sciences F. Edward Hébert School of Medicine; Staff Clinician and Hematology Fellowship Program Director, Hematology Branch, National Heart, Lung, and Blood Institute, National Institutes of Health, Bethesda, Maryland

Blood Component and Pharmacologic Therapy of Hemostatic Disorders

Andrew K. Burroughs, MD
Professor of Hepatology, Royal Free and University College School of Medicine; Consultant Physician and Hepatologist, Royal Free Hospital, London, United Kingdom

Hemostatic Alterations in Liver Disease and Liver Transplantation

Hugo ten Cate, MD
Department of Internal Medicine, University of Maastricht Medical School, Maastricht, The Netherlands

The Cross-Talk of Inflammation and Coagulation in Infectious Disease and Their Roles in Disseminated Intravascular Coagulation

Richard Chang, MD
Chief, Special Procedures, Department of Radiology, W. G. Magnuson Clinical Center, National Institutes of Health, Bethesda, Maryland

Thrombosis Related to Venous Access Devices

Mary Cushman, MD, MSc
Associate Professor of Medicine, University of Vermont College of Medicine; Director, Thrombosis and Hemostasis Program, Division of Hematology & Oncology, Fletcher Allen Health Care, Burlington, Vermont

Risk Factors for Cardiovascular Disease and Arterial Thrombosis

Thomas G. DeLoughery, MD
Professor of Medicine and Pathology, Divisions of Hematology/Oncology and Laboratory Medicine, Oregon Health and Science University, Portland, Oregon

Anticoagulation for Atrial Fibrillation and Prosthetic Cardiac Valves

Jorge Di Paola, MD
Associate Professor of Pediatrics; Director, Hemophilia Treatment Center, Carver College of Medicine, University of Iowa, Iowa City, Iowa

Congenital and Acquired Disorders of Platelet Function and Number

Tieraona Low Dog, MD
Clinical Assistant Professor, Department of Medicine, University of Arizona College of Medicine; Director of Education, Program in Integrative Medicine, University of Arizona Health Sciences Center, Tucson, Arizona

Dietary Supplements and Hemostasis

Miguel A. Escobar, MD
Assistant Professor of Medicine and Pediatrics, University of Texas Medical School at Houston; Associate Medical Director, Gulf States Hemophilia & Thrombophilia Center, Houston, Texas

Less Common Congenital Disorders of Hemostasis

Bruce M. Ewenstein, MD, PhD
Global Medical Director, Baxter BioScience, Westlake Village, California

Nonhemophilic Inhibitors of Coagulation

Andres Fernandez, MD
Postdoctoral Research Fellow, Neurology Department, Columbia University College of Physicians and Surgeons, New York, New York

Hematologic Interventions for Acute Central Nervous System Disease

Charles W. Francis, MD
Professor of Medicine and Pathology and Laboratory Medicine, University of Rochester School of Medicine and Dentistry, Rochester, New York

Antithrombotic Agents

James N. George, MD
George Lynn Cross Professor, Department of Medicine, University of Oklahoma College of Medicine, Oklahoma City, Oklahoma

Immune Thrombocytopenic Purpura

David L. Gillespie, MD
Professor of Surgery, Uniformed Services University of the Health Sciences F. Edward Hébert School of Medicine, Bethesda, Maryland; Chief and Program Director, Vascular Surgery, Walter Reed Army Medical Center, Washington, DC

Prevention, Diagnosis, and Treatment of the Postphlebitic Syndrome

Samuel Z. Goldhaber, MD
Professor of Medicine, Harvard Medical School; Director, Venous Thromboembolism Research Group; Director, Anticoagulation Service; and Staff Cardiologist, Brigham and Women's Hospital, Boston, Massachusetts

Deep Vein Thrombosis and Pulmonary Embolism

David Green, MD, PhD
Professor of Medicine, Northwestern University Feinberg School of Medicine; Attending Physician, Northwestern Memorial Hospital; Physician, Northwestern Medical Faculty Foundation, Chicago, Illinois

Prevention and Treatment of Venous Thromboembolism in Neurologic and Neurosurgical Patients

Christine L. Hann, MD, PhD
Clinical Fellow, Department of Medical Oncology, Johns Hopkins University School of Medicine, Baltimore, Maryland

Vena Caval Filters

John A. Heit, MD
Professor of Medicine, Mayo Clinic College of Medicine; Director, Coagulation Laboratories and Clinic, and Consultant, Division of Cardiovascular Diseases, Mayo Clinic, Rochester, Minnesota

Thrombophilia: Clinical and Laboratory Assessment and Management

John R. Hess, MD
Professor of Pathology and Medicine, University of Maryland School of Medicine, Baltimore, Maryland

Hemorrhage Control and Thrombosis Following Severe Injury

William R. Hiatt, MD
Professor of Medicine, University of Colorado School of Medicine, Denver, Colorado

Peripheral Arterial Disease

Christopher D. Hillyer, MD
Professor, Department of Pathology and Laboratory Medicine, and Director, Transfusion Medicine, Emory University School of Medicine; Director, Medical, Blood Bank, Emory University Hospital, Atlanta, Georgia

Therapeutic Apheresis

John B. Holcomb, MD
Adjunct Professor of Surgery, University of Texas School of Medicine at San Antonio, San Antonio; Trauma Consultant for the Surgeon General and Commander, U.S. Army Institute of Surgical Research, Fort Sam Houston, Texas

Hemorrhage Control and Thrombosis Following Severe Injury

McDonald K. Horne, III, MD
Senior Clinical Investigator, Hematology Service, W. G. Magnuson Clinical Center, National Institutes of Health, Bethesda, Maryland

Thrombosis Related to Venous Access Devices

Mark R. Jackson, MD
Assistant Clinical Professor, Department of Surgery, Columbia University College of Physicians and Surgeons, New York, New York; Vascular Surgeon, St. Francis Hospital, Greenville, South Carolina

Topical Hemostatic Agents for Localized Bleeding

Shawn Jobe, MD, PhD
Fellow, Pediatric Hematology Oncology, Carver College of Medicine, University of Iowa, Iowa City, Iowa

Congenital and Acquired Disorders of Platelet Function and Number

Eefje Jong, MD
Resident, Department of Internal Medicine, University of Amsterdam Academic Medical Center, Amsterdam, The Netherlands

The Cross-Talk of Inflammation and Coagulation in Infectious Disease and Their Roles in Disseminated Intravascular Coagulation

Craig M. Kessler, MD
Professor of Medicine and Pathology, Georgetown University School of Medicine; Chief, Coagulation Laboratory, Lombardi Comprehensive Cancer Center, Washington, DC

A Systematic Approach to the Bleeding Patient: Correlation of Clinical Symptoms and Signs with Laboratory Testing; Hemophilia A and B; Thrombocytosis: Essential Thrombocythemia and Reactive Causes

Nushmia Khokhar, MD
Department of Internal Medicine, Washington Hospital Center/Georgetown University Hospital, Washington, DC

A Systematic Approach to the Bleeding Patient: Correlation of Clinical Symptoms and Signs with Laboratory Testing

Craig S. Kitchens, MD
Professor of Medicine, University of Florida; Associate Chief of Staff, Malcom Randall Veterans Administration Medical Center, Gainesville, Florida

The Consultative Process; Purpura and Other Hematovascular Disorders; Disseminated Intravascular Coagulation; Venous Thromboses at Unusual Sites; Surgery and Hemostasis

Harvey G. Klein, MD
Adjunct Professor of Medicine and Pathology, Johns Hopkins, University School of Medicine; Chief, Department of Transfusion Medicine, W. G. Magnuson Clinical Center, National Institutes of Health, Bethesda, Maryland

Blood Component and Pharmacologic Therapy of Hemostatic Disorders

Kiarash Kojouri, MD, MPH
Assistant Professor of Medicine, University of Oklahoma College of Medicine, Oklahoma City, Oklahoma

Immune Thrombocytopenic Purpura

Barbara A. Konkle, MD
Professor of Medicine; Director, Penn Comprehensive Hemophilia and Thrombosis Program, University of Pennsylvania, Philadelphia, Pennsylvania

Thrombotic Risk of Contraceptives and Other Hormonal Therapies

Kendra Kubiak, MD
Clinical Instructor in Medicine, University of Virginia School of Medicine, Charlottesville, Virginia

Point-of-Care Testing for Hemostatic Disorders

Jody L. Kujovich, MD
Clinical Assistant Professor of Medicine, Oregon Health & Science University School of Medicine; Physician, Northwest Cancer Specialists, Portland, Oregon

Management of Thrombophilia and Antiphospholipid Syndrome During Pregnancy

David J. Kuter, MD, DPhil
Assistant Professor of Medicine, Harvard Medical School, Boston; Associate Professor of Medicine, Health Sciences and Technology, Massachusetts Institute of Technology, Cambridge; Director of Clinical Hematology, Massachusetts General Hospital, Boston, Massachusetts

General Aspects of Thrombocytopenia, Platelet Transfusions, and Thrombopoietic Growth Factors

Carrie LaBelle, MD
Medical Director, Compensation and Pension Service, Veterans Health System, Malcom Randall VA Medical Center, Gainesville, Florida

Disseminated Intravascular Coagulation

Marcel Levi, MD
Professor of Medicine, University of Amsterdam School of Medicine; Chairman, Department of Medicine, University of Amsterdam Academic Medical Center, Amsterdam, The Netherlands

The Cross-Talk of Inflammation and Coagulation in Infectious Disease and Their Roles in Disseminated Intravascular Coagulation

Miles B. Levin, MD
Chief Resident in Pathology, Montefiore Medical Center, Bronx, New York

The Antiphospholipid Syndrome: Clinical Presentation, Diagnosis, and Patient Management

Mark Levine, MD, MSc
Professor of Clinical Epidemiology and Biostatistics and Medicine and Buffet Taylor Chair of Breast Cancer Research, Michael G. DeGroote School of Medicine, McMaster University Faculty of Health Sciences, Hamilton, Ontario, Canada

Thrombosis and Cancer

Minetta Liu, MD
Assistant Professor of Medicine and Oncology, Lombardi Comprehensive Cancer Center, Georgetown University Hospital, Washington, DC

A Systematic Approach to the Bleeding Patient: Correlation of Clinical Symptoms and Signs with Laboratory Testing

Richard Lottenberg, MD
Professor of Medicine, Division of Hematology/Oncology, University of Florida College of Medicine, Gainesville, Florida

Hemostatic Aspects of Sickle Cell Disease

B. Gail Macik, MD
Associate Clinical Professor of Medicine and Pathology, University of Virginia School of Medicine, Charlottesville, Virginia

Point-of-Care Testing for Hemostatic Disorders

Victor J. Marder, MD
Professor of Medicine, Division of Hematology/Medical Oncology, David Geffen School of Medicine at UCLA, Los Angeles, California

Thrombolytic Therapy

Merry Jennifer Markham, MD
Fellow, Division of Hematology/Oncology, University of Florida Department of Medicine, Gainesville, Florida

Dietary Supplements and Hemostasis

Stephan A. Mayer, MD
Associate Professor of Clinical Neurology and Neurosurgery, Columbia University College of Physicians and Surgeons; Director, Neuro-ICU, NewYork–Presbyterian Hospital, New York, New York

Hematologic Interventions for Acute Central Nervous System Disease

Jan Jacques Michiels, MD, PhD
Professor, Department of Hematology, Blood Coagulation and Vascular Research, University of Antwerp Faculty of Medicine/University Hospital Antwerp, Antwerp, Belgium; Director, Department of Hematology, Hemostasis and Thrombosis Research, Hemostasis and Thrombosis Science Center, Goodheart Institute and Foundation, Rotterdam; Scientific Medical Advisor, Medical Diagnostic Center, Rotterdam; and Project Leader, Deep Vein Thrombosis and the Post-thrombotic Syndrome, Erasmus Medical Center, Rotterdam, The Netherlands

Thrombocytosis: Essential Thrombocythemia and Reactive Causes

Joel L. Moake, MD
Professor of Medicine, Baylor College of Medicine; Associate Director, Biomedical Engineering Laboratory, Rice University, Houston, Texas

Thrombotic Thrombocytopenic Purpura

Thomas L. Ortel, MD, PhD
Associate Professor of Medicine and Pathology, Duke University School of Medicine, Durham, North Carolina

Anticoagulation in the Perioperative Period

Reagan W. Quan, MD
Fellow, Vascular Surgery, Uniformed Services University of the Health Sciences F. Edward Hébert School of Medicine, Bethesda, Maryland, and Walter Reed Army Medical Center, Washington, DC

Prevention, Diagnosis, and Treatment of the Postphlebitic Syndrome

Jacob H. Rand, MD
Professor of Pathology and Medicine, Albert Einstein College of Medicine of Yeshiva University; Director of Hematology Laboratories, Montefiore Medical Center, Bronx, New York

The Antiphospholipid Syndrome: Clinical Presentation, Diagnosis, and Patient Management

Margaret E. Rick, MD
Assistant Chief, Hematology Service, W. G. Magnuson Clinical Center, National Institutes of Health, Bethesda, Maryland

von Willebrand Disease

Frederick R. Rickles, MD, FACP
Professor of Medicine, Pediatrics, and Pharmacology and Physiology, George Washington University School of Medicine and Health Sciences, Washington, DC; Fellow, Center for Science and Technology, Noblis, Falls Church, Virginia

Thrombosis and Cancer

Fred Rincon, MD
Clinical Assistant in Neurology and Post-Doctoral Clinical Fellow, Columbia University Medical Center, New York, New York

Hematologic Interventions for Acute Central Nervous System Disease

Harold R. Roberts, MD
Sarah Graham Kenan Distinguished Professor of Medicine and Pathology, Department of Medicine, Division of Hematology and Oncology, and Carolina Cardiovascular Biology Center, University of North Carolina at Chapel Hill School of Medicine; Director, Comprehensive Hemophilia Treatment Center, University of North Carolina Hospitals, Chapel Hill, North Carolina

Less Common Congenital Disorders of Hemostasis

Lewis J. Rubin, MD
Professor of Medicine, University of California, San Diego, School of Medicine, La Jolla, California

Pulmonary Hypertension: Thrombotic and Nonthrombotic in Origin

Marco Senzolo, MD
Consultant Gastroenterologist/Hepatologist, Gastroenterology Unit, Department of Surgical and Gastroenterological Sciences, University Hospital of Padua, Padua, Italy

Hemostatic Alterations in Liver Disease and Liver Transplanatation

Stephanie Seremetis, MD
Global Medical Director, Hemostasis, NovoNordisk A/S, Bagsvaerd, Denmark

Management of Bleeding Disorders in Pregnancy

Chelsea A. Sheppard, MD
Transfusion Medicine Fellow, Department of Pathology and Laboratory Medicine, Emory University School of Medicine/Emory University Hospital, Atlanta, Georgia

Therapeutic Apheresis

Suman Sood, MD
Instructor in Medicine, Division of Hematology-Oncology, University of Pennsylvania School of Medicine; Penn Comprehensive Hemophilia and Thrombosis Program, University of Pennsylvania Health System, Philadelphia, Pennsylvania

Thrombotic Risk of Contraceptives and Other Hormonal Therapies

Steven Stein, MD
Adjunct Assistant Professor, Hemophilia and Thrombosis Program, University of Pennsylvania School of Medicine, Philadelphia, Pennsylvania

Thrombotic Risk of Contraceptives and Other Hormonal Therapies

Michael B. Streiff, MD
Assistant Professor of Medicine, Johns Hopkins University School of Medicine; Medical Director, Anticoagulation Management Service, Johns Hopkins Medical Institutions, Baltimore, Maryland

Vena Caval Filters

Bundarika Suwanawiboon, MD
Instructor, Division of Hematology, Department of Medicine, Faculty of Medicine, Mahidal University/Siriraj Hospital, Bangkok, Thailand

Anticoagulation in the Perioperative Period

Eric C.M. van Gorp, MD
Staff Physician, Department of Internal Medicine, Slotervaart Hospital, Amsterdam, The Netherlands

The Cross-Talk of Inflammation and Coagulation in Infectious Disease and Their Roles in Disseminated Intravascular Coagulation

Theodore E. Warkentin, MD
Professor, Department of Pathology and Molecular Medicine and Department of Medicine, Michael G. DeGroote School of Medicine, McMaster University Faculty of Health Sciences; Associate Head, Transfusion Medicine, Hamilton Regional Laboratory Medicine Program; Hematologist, Service of Clinical Hematology, Hamilton Health Sciences, Hamilton General Hospital, Hamilton, Ontario, Canada

Heparin-Induced Thrombocytopenia

Ann B. Zimrin, MD
Assistant Professor of Medicine, University of Maryland School of Medicine/Marlene and Stewart Greenebaum Cancer Center, Baltimore, Maryland

Hemorrhage Control and Thrombosis Following Severe Injury

Marc Zumberg, MD
Associate Professor of Medicine, University of Florida College of Medicine, Gainesville, Florida

Purpura and Other Hematovascular Disorders; Venous Thromboses at Unusual Sites

Preface

We editors were pleased by the enthusiasm and success with which the first edition of *Consultative Hemostasis and Thrombosis* was met. Clearly, there is a niche for a mid-sized textbook on hemostasis and thrombosis that can authoritatively assist the busy consultant; thus, we are presenting an updated second edition.

Much has happened since the first edition appeared in early 2002. For example, the discovery of ADAMTS-13 and the elucidation of its role in thrombotic thrombocytopenic purpura were just being accomplished when the first edition was published.

The use of recombinant activated factor VII (rFVIIa) has expanded greatly beyond the original indication for which it was licensed. This is reviewed in detail in this new edition. We are now seeing the increased use of thrombin-specific inhibitors, and initial studies of the pentasaccharide fondaparinux in the treatment of heparin-induced thrombocytopenia are promising.

As editors of the book, we have focused on two primary goals. One was to provide updates on the "core material" for hemostasis and thrombosis, with internationally renowned experts writing chapters on deep vein thrombosis, pulmonary embolus, hypercoagulability, thrombocytopenia, von Willebrand disease, and heparin-induced thrombocytopenia, as well as thrombotic thrombocytopenia purpura and other disorders. Our second goal was to ensure a very strong integration among the specialties that deal with clinical issues in thrombosis and hemostasis; these include cardiology, neurology, oncology, obstetrics, and vascular surgery. Accordingly, we tapped internationally renowned authors writing on hemostatic and thrombotic complications associated with such conditions as a patent foraman ovale, pulmonary hypertension, malignancy, indwelling catheters, trauma, and pregnancy.

We are deeply grateful to our contributing authors, and we appreciate the colleagues who have given us support and constructive criticism for this second edition. We hope that this book will serve as an improved and useful guide for all who are involved in providing consultation and care for patients with hemostatic or thrombotic disorders.

Craig S. Kitchens, MD

Barbara M. Alving, MD

Craig M. Kessler, MD

Contents

Color Plates follow pages xxiv and 168.

Part IV
THERAPEUTIC MEASURES, 447

Part V
ISSUES SPECIFIC TO WOMEN, 567

Consultative
Hemostasis
and Thrombosis

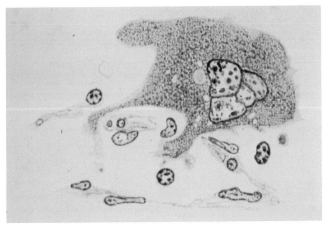

Color Plate 8-1 Megakaryocyte protruding into the bone marrow sinusoid and producing platelets. Camera lucida drawing by James Homer Wright.

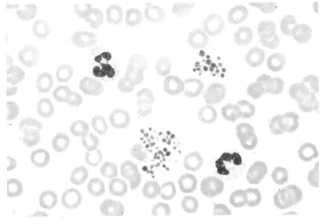

Color Plate 9-3 Platelet clumping. Note that several platelets clump to one another on the peripheral blood smear. This clumping is independent of the nearby neutrophils.

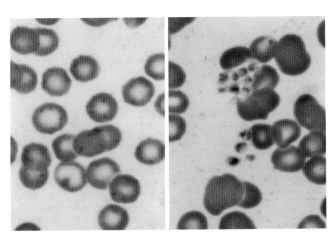

Color Plate 8-2 Platelet clumping (pseudothrombocytopenia). Peripheral blood smear of patient shows no platelets in one field *(left panel)* but large platelet clumps in another field *(right panel)*.

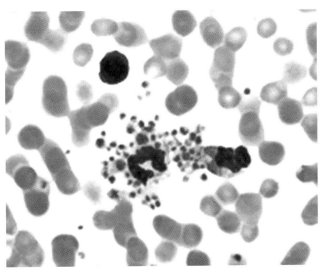

Color Plate 9-4 Platelet satellitism. Platelets adhere in a necklace-like pattern around two neutrophils yet do not clump together.

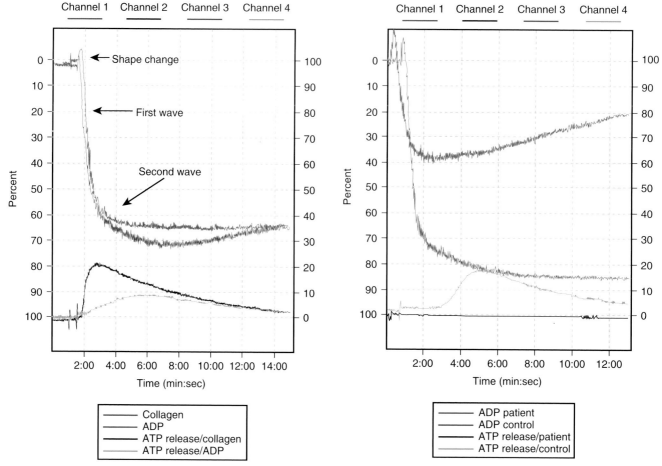

Collagen
ADP
ATP release/collagen
ATP release/ADP

Color Plate 10-2 Normal aggregation pattern. Adenosine diphosphate (ADP) and collagen were used as agonists. The curve reflects percentage of aggregation as a function of time. The arrows indicate the different steps observed during platelet aggregation. The first wave of aggregation is caused by exogenous agonists, in this case, collagen and ADP; the second wave is due to endogenous release of dense granular content. Curves in green and black indicate adenosine triphosphate (ATP) release.

ADP patient
ADP control
ATP release/patient
ATP release/control

Color Plate 10-3 Abnormal aggregation pattern. Adenosine diphosphate (ADP) was used as an agonist. The first wave of aggregation (due to the exogenous agonist) is conserved in the patient and the normal control subject. However, the second wave of aggregation and adenosine triphosphate (ATP) release are absent in this patient, indicating an intrinsic defect in platelet activation. A similar pattern of aggregation and desaggregation is observed when platelets are inhibited by aspirin or nonsteroidal anti-inflammatory drugs (NSAIDs).

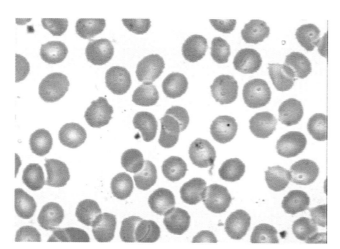

Color Plate 10-6 Wiskott-Aldrich syndrome. There are three platelets on this blood smear. Notice their small size. Department of Haematological Pathology, Tygerberg Hospital and University of Stellenbosch, South Africa, with permission.

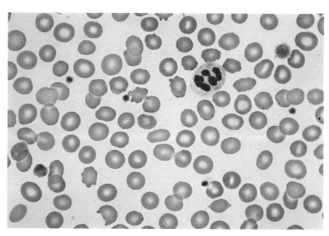

Color Plate 10-7 Bernard-Soulier syndrome. There are six platelets on this blood smear. Notice that two platelets are very large.

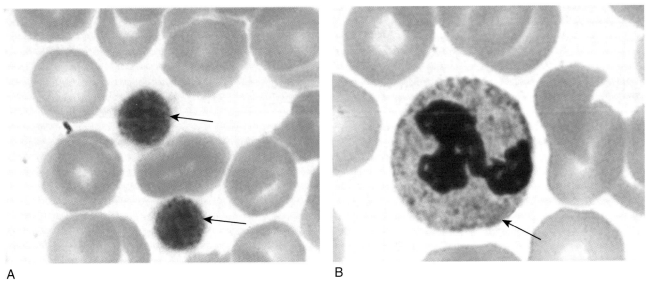

A

B

Color Plate 10-10 May-Hegglin syndrome. In panel **A,** notice the two large platelets. In panel **B,** the neutrophil contains a pale blue inclusion body.

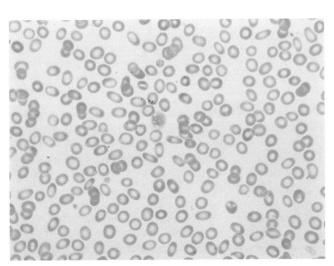

Color Plate 10-11 Gray platelet syndrome. There is a large ghost-like platelet near the middle. Its pale color is due to lack of stainable granules.

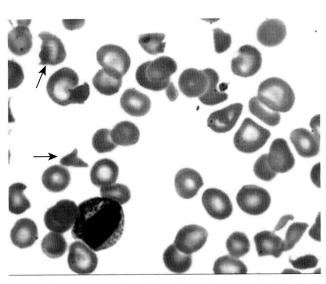

Color Plate 24-1 Peripheral blood smear from a patient with TTP. Notice that several red blood cells are schistocytes, which result from mechanical hemolysis. Some resemble apples from which a large bite has been taken.

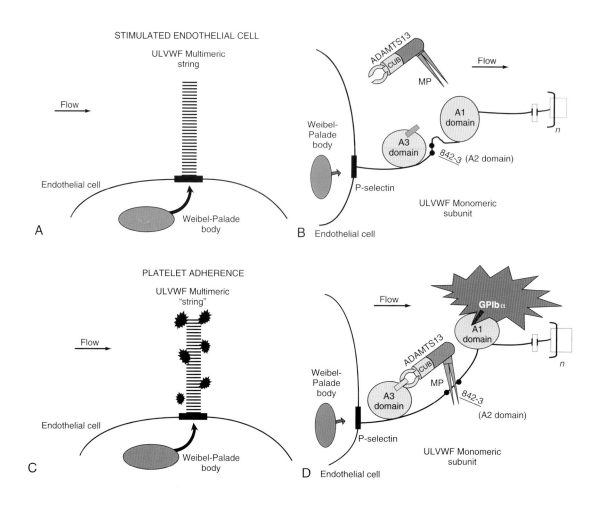

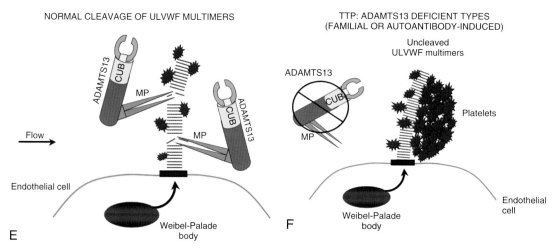

Color Plate 24-3 Proposed mechanism of ultra-large von Willebrand factor (ULVWF) multimeric string cleavage by ADAMTS13 (*a d*isintegrin *and m*etalloproteinase with *t*hrombospondin components). **A,** Stimulation of endothelial cells causes secretion of long ULVWF multimeric strings. **B,** "Close-up" of one of the many monomeric subunits that make up a ULVWF multimeric string. ULVWF multimeric strings may be anchored in the endothelial cell membrane to P-selectin molecules that are secreted concurrently with ULVWF multimers from Weibel-Palade bodies. The A1, A2 (with the 842Tyr-843Met ADAMTS13 proteolytic cleavage site), and A3 domains are shown. Adequate quantities of ADAMTS13 enzymes are present in the plasma of normal individuals. The carboxylterminal CUB region (two nonidentical domains that contain peptide segments similar to complement components, C1r/C1s, a sea *u*rchin protein, and a *b*one morphogenic protein) is indicated, and the proteolytic metalloprotease domain (MP) is drawn as a pincer-like structure on the aminoterminal portion of the enzyme. **C,** Platelets from flowing blood adhere to the long ULVWF multimeric strings immediately after string secretion. **D,** Platelet adherence (via platelet glycoprotein [GP]-Ib) to the A1 domain of ULVWF monomeric subunits increases the exposure of neighboring A2 842Tyr-843Met peptide bonds in ULVWF multimeric strings. ADAMTS13 molecules attach via one of their CUB domains to the A3 domain of ULVWF monomeric subunits, and then cleave the adjacent (and now exposed) 842Tyr-843Met bond. **E,** ADAMTS13 cleavage through this mechanism occurs in various monomers along the length of ULVWF multimeric strings. The smaller VWF forms that circulate after cleavage do not induce the adhesion and aggregation of platelets during normal blood flow. **F,** Absent or severely reduced activity of ADAMTS13 in the plasma of patients with TTP prevents the timely cleavage of ULVWF multimeric strings as they are secreted from endothelial cells. Uncleaved ULVWF multimers induce the adhesion and subsequent aggregation of platelets in flowing blood. TTP may be caused by familial deficiencies of ADAMTS13 secretion or activity caused by ADAMTS13 gene mutations, or they may result from acquired autoantibody-induced defects of ADAMTS13 activity (or survival).

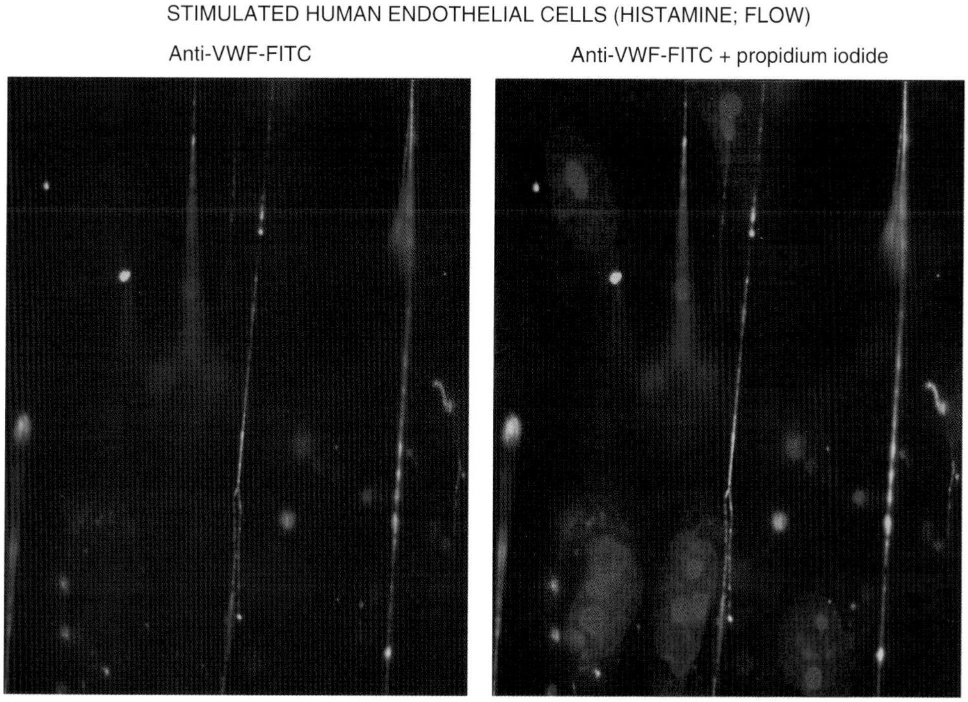

STIMULATED HUMAN ENDOTHELIAL CELLS (HISTAMINE; FLOW)

Anti-VWF-FITC   Anti-VWF-FITC + propidium iodide

Color Plate 24-4   Unusually large (UL) VWF multimeric strings, secreted by human umbilical vein endothelial cells stimulated by histamine under flowing conditions, were stained green by rabbit anti-human VWF IgG + goat anti-rabbit-fluorescein isothyocyanate (FITC) in the absence *(left)* or presence *(right)* of the red nuclear stain, propidium iodide.

Part I

General Information

Chapter 1

The Consultative Process

Craig S. Kitchens, MD

Life is short, and the art long, the occasion fleeting, experience fallacious, and judgment difficult.

—Hippocrates[a]

As long as medicine is an art, its chief and characteristic instrument must be the human faculty. We come therefore to the very practical question of what aspects of human faculty it is necessary for the good doctor to cultivate. The first to be named must always be the power of attention, of giving one's whole mind to the patient without the interposition of oneself. It sounds simple but only the very greatest doctors ever fully attain it. It is an active process and not either mere resigned listening or even politely waiting until you can interrupt. Disease often tells its secret in the casual parentheses.

—Wilfred Trotter[b]

As a specialist, the hematologist is frequently asked to consult on a patient in order to clarify or solidify the diagnosis, prognosis, or treatment plan of another physician. Consultation is done in either the inpatient or the outpatient setting and can in turn be requested on a stat, urgent, subacute, or leisurely basis. By inference, the referring physician remains the physician in control of the patient's care, but the consultant's expertise, experience, judgment, wisdom, and even approval are sought in order to assist the referring physician's concept of the case in its entirety. In this era of cost containment and managed care, expert evaluation is cost-effective because it may curtail the diagnostic process, limit unnecessary or even ill-directed testing, and shorten overall hospital time as well as minimize patient suffering. A well-directed consultation is the best bargain for all stakeholders.

Several papers have discussed the mechanics and elements of a proper consultation and have suggested that just so many items are necessary in the review of systems or family history in order to justify a certain billing code. This chapter does not attempt to address such impermanent or regional matters but focuses instead on foundations allied with the precepts of internal medicine

The diagnostic procedure is a fascinating exercise. It involves the most acute use of our senses and the accurate recording of our observations. It requires a logical synthesis of the central nervous system of the responsible doctor, of information from the patient and his family, from other doctors who have cared for the patient in the past, from colleagues in various specialties who are helping with the immediate problem, and from the laboratory. Prognosis and correct therapy depend upon the correct use of the diagnostic process.

—Eugene A. Stead, Jr.[c]

[The] oldest and most effective act of doctors [is] touching. Some people don't like being handled by others, but not, or almost never, sick people. They need being touched, and part of the dismay in being very sick is the lack of close human contact. Ordinary people, even close friends, even family members, tend to stay away from the very sick, touching them as infrequently as possible for fear of interfering, or catching the illness, of just for fear of bad luck. The doctor's oldest skill in trade was to place his hands on the patient.

Over the centuries, the skill became more specialized and refined, the hands learned other things to do beyond mere contact. They probed to feel the pulse at the wrist, the tip of the spleen, or the edge of the liver, thumped to elicit resonant or dull sounds over the lungs, spread ointments over the skin, nicked veins for bleeding, but the same time touched, caressed, and at the end held on to the patient's fingers.

Touching with the naked ear was one of the great advances in the history of medicine. Once it was learned that the heart and lungs made sounds of their own, and that the sounds

---

[a] Hippocrates (460–370 B.C.) is considered to be the founder of European medicine. He lived in Greece during the Classic Period and was a contemporary of Socrates, Plato, Herodotus, and others. He is credited with three advances in medicine: the separation of medicine as an art and science from magic, the development of the written detailed study of disease, and the promulgation of the highest of moral standards that characterize the profession. Descriptive bedside medicine was his forte. His writings showed him to be humble, containing frequent admissions of errors in his thinking in order that others might not stumble in the same manner. This timeless aphorism contains all the essential elements of clinical practice in a concise statement.

[b] Wilfred Batten Trotter (1872–1939) was an English sociologist and neurosurgeon who was very interested in the sociologic aspects of medicine. He is credited with originating the term *herd instinct*. He was also a surgeon to King George V. This quote is taken from the chapter entitled "The Art of Being a Physician" by Lloyd H. Smith, Jr., in the 19th edition of the *Cecil Textbook of Medicine* (W. B. Saunders, Philadelphia, 1992).

---

[c] Eugene A. Stead, Jr., (1908–2005) is a primary pillar of American internal medicine. He was born and educated in Atlanta and then went to Harvard University in Boston, where he was strongly influenced by Soma Weiss. He was a pioneer in clinical investigation of the human circulatory system. At 34 years of age, he returned to Emory University as the Chairman of Medicine in 1943 but was recruited to the new Duke Medical School in Durham, North Carolina, in 1947, where he was Chairman for 20 years, founding and elevating that department of medicine to one of the greatest in the nation. He trained innumerable professors and chairs of medicine. Dr. Stead was a master of clinical thought and piercing observations and had a keen wit bettered by none. The two quotes are from E. A. Stead, Jr., *What this Patient Needs is a Doctor*, edited by Wagner, Cebe, and Rozer (Carolina Academic Press, Durham, North Carolina, 1978).

were sometimes useful for diagnosis, physicians placed an ear over the heart, and over areas on the front and back of the chest, and listened. It is hard to imagine a friendlier human gesture, a more intimate signal of personal concern and affection, than these close bowed heads affixed to the skin. The stethoscope was invented in the nineteenth century, vastly enhancing the acoustics of the thorax, but removing the physician a certain distance from his patient. It was the earliest device of many still to come, one new technology after another, designed to increase that distance.

—*Lewis Thomas*[d]

There are many facets of the consultative process, ranging from the extent and reason for the consultation to the nature of recommendations and outcomes expected. These are listed in Table 1-1.

EXTENT OF THE CONSULTATION

It is essential that both the referring physician and the consultant have in mind the extent of consultation requested, which will in turn govern the aim and comprehensiveness of the consultation.

Confirmatory Consultation

In this situation the referring physician is quite comfortable with the diagnosis, prognosis, and treatment. He or she generally wishes the consultant to focus on efforts already made and to corroborate those findings. This type is frequent in the second opinion consultation or one in which the referring physician needs encouragement as well as perhaps some advice garnered from the consultant's experience. These consultations are therefore focused, often brief, yet may involve reviewing substantial previously collected data. In general, the consultant does not need to request extra tests.

A subtype of the confirmatory consultation exists when the referring physician does not think the services of the consultant are indicated but, because of uncertainty or pressure from family members, wishes the consultant to document such in the chart. The most common reason for not using specific services is severe illness in the patient, which would make the consultant's services worthless, futile, or even contraindicated by unnecessarily extending the dying process. Examples in hematology might include evaluation for mild thrombocytopenia in an intensive care unit (ICU) patient with multiorgan dysfunction syndrome or whether a "hypercoagulable workup" is indicated in an elderly patient dying of carcinomatosis yet presenting with new

---

[d] Lewis Thomas (1913–1993) was a native New Yorker and a graduate of Harvard Medical School. He was on the faculty of the University of Minnesota, and then became Dean of New York University Medical Center, followed by his appointment as Dean at Yale Medical School. He became president of Memorial Sloan-Kettering Cancer Center in New York City. He was a member of the National Academy of Sciences. His ability to translate with both clarity and intense interest things scientific, biologic, and medical into prose readable and enjoyable to the average reader was unparalleled. Three of his major works were *The Lives of A Cell*, *The Medusa and the Snail*, and *The Youngest Science: Notes of Medicine Watcher*, all of which received broad recognition and multiple prizes. The first citation comes from a short piece entitled "Leech Leech, et cetera," and the second from "Housecalls."

Table 1-1   The Consultative Process
Extent of the consultation
Confirmatory consultation
Brief consultation
Comprehensive consultation
Urgent consultation on a catastrophically ill patient
"Undiagnosing" consultation
Telemedicine consultation
The curbside consultation
Reason for consultation
Helping another physician
Second opinion requested by the primary physician
Second opinion requested by the patient
Second opinion requested by a third-party payor
Other third parties
The disgruntled patient or family
Inappropriate consultations
Consultant's point of view
Duties of the referring physician and consultant
Timing
How to do the consultation
Role of the clinical laboratory
Recommendations
Concerns
Outcomes
Total agreement
Supporting consultation
Finding another physician for the patient
Consultant assumes primary care of the patient
Serious troubles
Redirecting thrust of a workup
Major disagreements between physicians
Duration of consultation
Noncompliant patients
End-of-life issues
Family members
When a diagnosis is not forthcoming
When should a consultant request a consultation?

deep venous thrombosis. The referring physician should indicate to the consultant that services may not be indicated. The consultant should not be reluctant to see such patients.

Brief Consultation

In this consultation, the questions are more broad based and in an appropriately diagnosed and managed patient commonly involve long-term questions such as length of therapy with glucocorticosteroids in a patient with immune thrombocytopenia purpura before one proceeds to splenectomy or the duration of anticoagulant therapy in a patient with hypercoagulability who has developed a major thrombosis. The consultant's long-term experience with many similar patients and knowledge of the literature are often more important than his or her diagnostic or therapeutic acumen.

Comprehensive Consultation

In a comprehensive consultation, the referring practitioner may not be a subspecialist but an internist or possibly another physician who needs comprehensive assistance regarding the diagnosis, prognosis, and therapy. This consultation often is generated by surgeons or obstetricians/gynecologists attending a patient with thrombosis who needs thorough evaluation for hypercoagulability. In these situations the consultant more often than not is the manager of laboratory testing and can do so in a cost-effective manner based on his or her expertise. Key decisions are often made by the consultant with the approval of the referring physician. Occasionally, the referring physician will ask the consultant to manage entirely hematologic aspects of the patient's care, which can be easily done conjointly with the referring physician. A common example is consulting with an obstetrician attending a woman with antiphospholipid syndrome. Together they can discuss preconception issues, anticoagulant therapy throughout gestation, and anticoagulant management during and after delivery of the child with the patient and her family.

Urgent Consultation on a Catastrophically Ill Patient

Catastrophically ill patients are often hospitalized in an ICU and may be seen by multiple experts attempting to assist the attending physician in a diagnosis. These consultations require subspecialty expertise and a solid knowledge of general internal medicine. Anyone may make the single unifying diagnosis that underpins all manifestations in such extremely ill patients. The consultant hematologist may be the first to recognize that thrombocytopenia in a febrile, confused, azotemic patient supports an overall diagnosis of Rocky Mountain spotted fever, thus corroborating all findings made by all previous consultants.

"Undiagnosing" Consultation

Sometimes patients may be incorrectly diagnosed and thus inappropriately sent to the hematologist. In these situations one must be rather careful to exclude explicitly the diagnosis that the referring physician made. It is both professional and cost-effective to rule out the diagnosis that was being entertained. One must carefully garner laboratory data that justify the negation of the working diagnosis and compile corroborating evidence, such as historical and physical examination findings, that may be incompatible with that diagnosis. It is easier to diagnose a patient incorrectly than to undo a diagnosis. One could argue that higher standards are required for undiagnosing an illness than diagnosing that illness. An example is a physician who seeks your endorsement of his or her diagnosis of protein C deficiency only to learn the protein C level was low because of concurrent warfarin therapy. The incorrect diagnosis not only is wrong but has financial, familial, and insurability ramifications. A forthright consultation will steer the referring physician away from the incorrect diagnosis so that the diagnostic process may be redirected.

Telemedicine Consultations

In an increasingly electronic world, telemedicine (telephone, video, and electronic transmissions [e-mail]) of medical information) is a reality. The accelerating use of telemedicine has left in its wake numerous unanswered legal, ethical, financial, and medical questions.

It is clear that such modern modalities are useful if for no other reasons than the rapidity of correspondence and the availability of consultative expertise in more remote and underserved areas. Because of uncertainty of its standing,

one must be cautious and expect rapid changes in resolutions of these questions from government, professional societies, and insurance carriers. Legal issues will arise, and precedents will be established.

In 2002 the American Medical Association (AMA) officially endorsed on-line consultation and billing of these services. A CPT code, 0074T, has been established. In a 2003 policy paper, the American College of Physicians (ACP), further urged the Center for Medicare and Medicaid Services (CMS) to reimburse for such services. Some third-party payors will reimburse fees whereas others have yet to decide. Several other related unresolved issues exist but are beyond the scope of this chapter. Most of these other issues have yet to be addressed, let alone solved:[1]

1. Confidentiality, because telemedicine is not as secure as hoped. Encryption is recommended at a minimum.
2. Because confidentiality is not certain, issues will arise regarding the Health Insurance Portability and Accountability Act (HIPAA).
3. Because the consultant and consultee may reside in different localities, issues of licensure and jurisdiction are inevitable.
4. Differing from typical "curbside" consultation, a durable, retrievable, and probably discoverable written record exists, which could impact questions of establishment of a doctor–patient relationship.
5. Ethics and quality of care issues. One study reported 50% of physicians will respond to unsolicited e-mail consultations, and of these, 84% offer diagnostic and therapeutic advice.[2]

Traditional medicine requires face-to-face interactions and appropriate examination and testing prior to diagnostic and therapeutic considerations. If there exists a previous doctor–patient relationship then the traditional face-to-face evaluation has been established, so that this issue may be moot in most cases.

In this rapidly evolving and effervescent climate one should consult expert advice. The website eRisk Working Group for Healthcare (www.medem.com/phy/phy_eriskguidelines.cfm) provides frequent updates.

The Curbside Consultation

Although many condemn "curbside consultations," they are a fact of professional life. These consults occur serendipitously in the doctors' lounge, in the hallway, or occasionally by telephone. They are unofficial, and both the "consultant" and the requesting physician must realize any suggestions arising from this act are not based on a real doctor–patient relationship because there is no traditional history, physical examination, or counseling of the patient; therefore a doctor (consultant)–patient relationship is not established. Accordingly, no fee is generated.

Liability for injury arising from one's unofficial advice can always be claimed. Considerable case law exists supporting that failure to have an established doctor–patient relationship is key to such a challenge. No duty is owed to a patient without creation of a doctor–patient relationship.[3]

A recent federal case (Newborn v USA) supported that even considerable and repetitious e-mail consultation between a Walter Reed Medical Center hematologist and pediatricians at an Army medical facility in Germany did not establish "close management and control" in a disputed wrongful death case. The deciding judge noted that encroachment on such informal consultation would negatively impact accessibility of practitioners to consultation, resulting in grave public policy implications.[4] That decision was upheld in the U.S. Court of Appeals.[5]

Rather, the requesting physician is inquiring in an unofficial broad manner about generalities that may well apply for a group of patients (e.g., those with mild thrombocytopenia undergoing colonoscopy) yet might not apply to a specific patient (e.g., as above but in a Jehovah's Witness). Giving of one's professional advice, even without compensation, is part of professionalism. Practitioners should not abuse this precept either by repeatedly taking advantage of this courtesy or by using the general unofficial advice in a specific official capacity.

A name provides an illusion of clarity where there was mystery and gives illness a tangibility which makes it seem more likely to be overcome. This applies not only to the patient but also to the doctor.

—*Richard Asher*[e]

While a doctor's knowledge may be extraordinarily precise for predicting what would happen to a thousand patients with a given condition, as the denominator becomes smaller, accuracy in prediction attenuates exponentially. It nearly disappears when the sample size recedes to unity, namely, when the doctor is called to prophesy outcome for a single individual. It is difficult to apply statistics to an individual patient. The unique challenge in doctoring is to determine where, if anywhere, a particular patient fits on the Gaussian distribution curve derived from a larger population. The decisive factor is the physician's breadth of clinical experience.

—*Bernard Lown*[f]

REASON FOR CONSULTATION

At first glance it seems intuitive that the reason to consult is to help another physician's management of a patient.

---

[e] Richard Asher (1911–1969) was a keen English clinician and consummate wordsmith. His writings and lecture style clearly showed that he liked what he did. He excelled especially at the interface of internal medicine and psychiatry. He coined the terms *Munchausen syndrome* and *myxedema madness*. His writings and lectures demonstrate that he made cogent observations from the simplest of medical situations and wrote about them in an economic style. This quote comes from a collection of his best essays on how doctors should use words, *Talking Sense* (University Park Press, Baltimore, 1972).

[f] Bernard Lown (b. 1921) graduated from Johns Hopkins Medical School in 1942 and spent his clinical years in Boston. He was a cardiologist of the old school, giving most of his credit as a clinician to Dr. Samuel Levine. Dr. Lown taught a whole generation of clinical cardiologists not only cardiology but also the art of being a physician, with particular reference to listening to the patient and making a strong, empathetic connection. Dr. Lown's contributions are numerous and include seminal observations on digitalis intoxication, use of lidocaine in arrhythmias, the establishment of DC cardioversion, and the establishment of what would become the modern coronary care unit. He won the Nobel Peace Prize in 1985 for his work in prevention of nuclear war. These quotations are taken from his 1996 book *The Lost Art of Healing* (Houghton, Mifflin, Boston, 1996), which is highly recommended to any physician cherishing aspects we may well be losing as the burden of the technological approach to medicine increases.

Although this view is fundamental, it is not all inclusive. Several reasons exist for the consultation and cover the entire spectrum of the consultant–patient interaction.

Helping Another Physician

This is still the most common reason for the consult to be requested. In these situations, the primary physician requests assistance in the patient's diagnosis, prognosis, or treatment while he or she maintains overall care of the patient.

Second Opinion Requested by the Primary Physician

In this situation the primary physician has made a diagnosis and plan, but because of his or her unfamiliarity with the process or because of the seriousness of the illness, he or she requests a second corroborating opinion. In nearly all cases, the patient's care remains with the referring physician.

Second Opinion Requested by the Patient

In this situation the patient either has pressed for a second opinion or may have secured the consultation without informing the primary physician. This circumstance should be elucidated early in the consultative process and is probably best done by asking to whom the report should be sent. The patient and family may vary in reasons for pursuing a second opinion, but more often than not it is the result of a benign motivation. They generally wish the report to go back to the referring physician. That should be done with an opening sentence in the consultation letter stating that the patient sought the second opinion and that your information is being transmitted to the primary physician.

Second Opinion Sought by a Third-Party Payor

Increasingly, third-party payors are requesting second opinions, especially if a new diagnosis or planned procedure has significant financial implications. These consultations are worthwhile financially to the payor but also especially to the patient because the correct diagnosis and treatment are always best for the patient. These second opinions should be honored and are part of good modern medicine.

Other Third Parties

Occasionally, because of disputes regarding quality of care, causation, injury, prognostication, and workers' compensation, an independent medical evaluation (IME) is requested. This is one of the few situations in which a consulting physician should remain an uninvolved neutral party; the goal of this type of consultation is to remain objective and try to find facts to assist the mediation process while serving as an advocate for neither side. It is of great importance for the consultant to project this neutrality to the patient, his or her family, and both parties of a dispute and to document in the report that he or she is not and will not be a provider of care and thus no traditional doctor–patient relationship has been established. Therefore, treatment will not be instituted (unless absolutely emergently so) but rather is described in the report, which should be an objective statement of findings. Some consultants do not do IME or workers' compensation consults, and this should be clearly stated to those who are requesting such consultation. Recently, Baum has described liability issues that can arise from IMEs.[6]

A physician shall, in the provision of appropriate patient care, except in emergencies, be free to choose whom to serve, with whom to associate, and the environment in which to provide medical service.

—*AMA Code of Medical Ethics*[g]

The Disgruntled Patient or Family

Occasionally a patient has lost confidence in a practitioner for either a real or perceived cause. These patients and especially their families may rail against a physician for missing or delaying a diagnosis, for treating too rapidly or too slowly, or for a less-than-perfect outcome. It is generally best to allow some degree of emotional venting by such parties during the consultation visit, but the consultant should make it clear soon thereafter that even if the patient is not to return to that initial practitioner, the patient's well-being remains dependent on records, reports, and tests from the other physician. At this time, the consultant should discuss with the patient the importance of the background work collected by the primary physician because it serves as the foundation for the consultation. All previous information is useful. Information from the first physician should be requested by the consulting physician (not by the patient) in a nonthreatening but honest manner, preferably face-to-face or by telephone rather than the mail; such direct discourse between the two physicians greatly facilitates the initial practitioner's efforts to elaborate his or her side of the story, to diminish concerns that the patient and consultant may be conspiring against the primary physician, and finally, in fact, to expedite patient care. The new consultant may assume primary care of the patient, find another qualified practitioner appropriate for the patient, or facilitate continued care of the patient by the original physician, especially if there have been only minor misunderstandings between these two parties.

In explaining to patients the failure of other physicians to have reached the correct diagnosis in the past, it should be pointed out that one cannot judge the past by the present. It often takes time for changes to occur to the point where a correct diagnosis is possible.

—*Philip A. Tumulty*[h]

Acknowledged mistakes provide potent learning experiences. Admitting them helps ensure that they will not be repeated. The humbling avowal of error prevents doctors from confusing their mission with a divine one. We possess no omniscient powers, only intuition, experience, and a patina of knowledge. These are most effective when one is constantly probing to advance the interest of an ailing human being.

—*Bernard Lown*[f]

Inappropriate Consultations

Occasionally consultations are requested that may be inappropriate. Although a consultant should always be at the service of a physician calling for a consultation, the consultant must be on guard against any consultation that reflects adversely on the patient, cost containment, or the profession. Physicians must minimize inappropriate consultations and identify abuses.

One such inappropriate consultation involves what the author refers to as "institutional elitism." This may occur when a patient with an existing chronic condition is admitted to a hospital for an acute hematologic problem. Unless proved otherwise, assume that chronic problems that are managed by other physicians are adequately treated; new consultations for these problems need not be generated. For example, if a patient with bipolar disorder is admitted with acute idiopathic thrombocytopenia (ITP), assume that the patient's chronic bipolar disorder has been appropriately treated for many years by a physician who is regarded as an expert and with whom the patient and family are perfectly happy; it is inappropriate to ask one's own institutional psychiatrist to see the patient unless one can conceive of some situation in which the bipolarism or its treatment may have something to do with the acute ITP. If the bipolar disorder or its treatment has nothing to do with ITP, it is best to continue the patient's pharmacologic management and then send a copy of the discharge summary to the psychiatrist for his or her office file.

A second, more pervasive form of inappropriate consultation is often referred to as "churning." In this situation, a patient is admitted, and each and every system or organ that is abnormal is immediately and with little forethought consulted on by experts. Basic internal medicine expertise should eliminate the notion that every murmur requires an immediate visit from a cardiologist, every wheeze requires a pulmonologist, and every arthritic joint requires a rheumatologist. This thesis is especially true with the very brief length of hospitalizations we currently endure. A consultation should be carefully chosen, and the question regarding the management should be focused toward any problem that is relevant to the current clinical setting.

A British study showed that 75 percent of the information leading to a correct diagnosis comes from a detailed history, 10 percent from the physical examination, 5 percent from simple routine tests, 5 percent from all the costly invasive tests; in 5 percent, no answer is forthcoming. Some of the most challenging medical problems I have encountered could be solved only through information provided by the patient. The time invested in obtaining a meticulous history is never ill spent. Careful history-taking actually saves time. The history provides the road map; without it the journey is merely

---

[g] American Medical Association Code of Medical Ethics, 1997, a compilation of medical ethics with its supporting case law, opinions, and foundations is extremely concise and well written. Unfortunately, it is not regarded by enough physicians as a foundation for a most important part of modern medical practice.

[h] Philip A. Tumulty (1912–1989) was the master consulting physician at Johns Hopkins Hospital and a professor of medicine for many decades. The three editors of this book were fortunate to have worked with Dr. Tumulty as house officers. Dr. Tumulty was the quintessential diagnostician and curator of the art of medicine exemplifying the highest attributes of an internist. His quotes in this chapter are taken from his book *The Effective Clinician* (W.B. Saunders, Philadelphia, 1973).

a shopping around at numerous garages for technological fixes.

—Bernard Lown[f]

CONSULTANT'S POINT OF VIEW

As a general rule, the consultant should approach each case from the point of view of having a degree of training more specialized than the referring practitioner. If the referring physician is another hematologist/oncologist, one can more likely than not appropriately review the case as a subspecialist (e.g., coagulationist) for that hematology/oncology referring physician. The consultation will thus be quite focused. When another internist refers the patient to the subspecialist, the consultant should regard the patient from the position of a hematologist/oncologist and therefore approach the patient in a more general manner. Therefore, other hematologic matters such as anemia, elevated white count, or splenomegaly can and should be addressed if they are found by the consultant. When consultation is originated by a noninternist such as a surgeon, obstetrician/gynecologist, or psychiatrist, approach the patient from the point of view of a general internist. In these situations one might also want to address elevated blood glucose, hypertension, or a dermatologic process not previously appreciated by the referring doctor. Although it is not necessary to address each of these problems oneself, the fact that one has found them when they had not been previously appreciated warrants consideration. The consultant may evaluate these personally or may wish to refer these patients to a diabetologist, hypertension specialist, or dermatologist, respectively. However, the fact remains that the consultant as an internist has found these items that are of medical importance and clearly parts of the overall consultation process. Increasingly patients are being referred to subspecialists by nonphysicians such as dentists, physician assistants, advanced registered nurse practitioners, and even third-party payors. In these situations, the consultant must look at the patient from a physician's perspective as well as from a specialist's perspective unless this has clearly been done by someone else. The consultant serving as physician *and* specialist must often ascertain that a patient has had appropriate preventive care (e.g., Papanicoulaou [Pap] smears and mammograms) or at least make sure that those very important points have been addressed in addition to addressing the question that is being directly asked by the referring health care provider.

I do not know a better training for a writer than to spend some years in the medical profession. I suppose that you can learn a good deal about human nature in a solicitor's office; but there on the whole you have to deal with men in full control of themselves. They lie perhaps as much as they lie to the doctor, but they lie more consistently, and it may be that for the solicitor it is not so necessary to know the truth. The interests he deals with, besides, are usually material. He sees human nature from a specialized standpoint. But the doctor, especially the hospital doctor, sees it bare. Reticences can generally be undermined; very often there are none. Fear for the most part will shatter every defense; even vanity is unnerved by it. Most people have a furious itch to talk about themselves and are restrained only by the disinclination of others to

listen. Reserve is an artificial quality that is developed in most of us but is the result of innumerable rebuffs. The doctor is discreet. It is his business to listen and no details are too intimate for his ears.

—W. Somerset Maugham[i]

DUTIES OF THE REFERRING PHYSICIAN AND THE CONSULTANT

The consultant should focus as directly, efficiently, and cost effectively as possible on the precise question that the referring physician has formulated. This, of course, depends on the accuracy of the referring physician's question as well as the possibility that the referring physician may have missed some important points. In all cases, the consultant should provide that level of consultation that is best for the patient.

Consultants are increasingly working along with physician extenders such as physician assistants or advanced registered nurse practitioners. Such professionals are usually highly knowledgeable in their areas and clearly enhance the efficiency of the busy consultant. However, it must remain absolutely clear to the referring physician and the patient that the extender is working with the consultant and not independently. If the extender dictates the report, it is wise and reassuring to have joint signatures on the correspondence.

Too little has been made of the duties of the referring practitioner. In this era of brief visits in which time is at a premium, the referring physician cannot simply ask a consultant to go in depth into a patient's multiyear history of present illness with multiple hospitalizations, innumerable radiographs, biopsies, and sheaves of laboratory data just to "figure it all out" in a 45-minute consultation. Rather, the referring physician must prepare a brief (one-page) summary of what has happened and construct a chief question that is to be asked of the consultant. If radiographs, biopsies, or other special tests are of importance and pertinent, they must come with the patient, preferably hand-delivered by the patient directly to the consultant. Mailing important material that will be delivered a week after the consultation is perfunctory and disrespectful. On the other hand, if these previous records are not important, they are best left with the referring physician because they will only clutter the diagnostic process and further encroach on effective consultation time.

If I failed to send a letter along with a new referral, which I more often did than not, this man would call me before he saw the patient and bluntly ask, "Dr. Sams, what do you want me to do for this patient?" The first time this happened I was taken aback, for specialists are not usually that open or that direct, and I am afraid I stammered a little with confusion and surprise. Then I learned just as bluntly to reply, "Prove to me he does not have a brain tumor," or, "Tell me she is having migraines," or, "I am worried about multiple

[i] W. Somerset Maugham (1874–1965) was trained at St. Thomas' Hospital in London and used his medical background in his more famous career as a novelist, short-story writer, and playwright. He wrote more than 60 books. Of special interest to physicians is *Of Human Bondage*. This quote comes from his autobiography, *The Summing Up* (Bantam, Doubleday Dell Publishing Group, New York).

sclerosis and need you to confirm or deny it," or even, "She is a crock and forgive me for dumping on you."

—*Ferrol Sams*[j]

We sometimes forget that the fifth Oslerian essential skill of an internist (and the most important) after observation, palpation, percussion and auscultation, was contemplation.

I had a patient once with multisystem complaints who carried with her folders full of lab results, reports of endoscopies and multiple imaging studies, and a variety of other test records. I set it aside. "Aren't you going to look at this?" she asked. "If the answer to your problem was in there somewhere, you wouldn't be here." I said.

After a detailed history and physical examination I had some ideas but no answers. I wanted to read more about some possibilities that had come to mind. "I'll call you in a couple of days," I told her.

"No tests?"

"You've had plenty," I said.

"Then what are you going to do?" she asked.

"I'm going to think." I answered.

"Oh!" she said, "Nobody's ever done that before."

I believe that an internist's expertise, annealed to experience and analytical thought process, and the time to fully engage these most powerful tools are not only the core of our craft, but assure the patient the most cost-effective and humane medicine possible.

—*Faith Fitzgerald*[k]

TIMING

The timing of the consultation plays an important part in determining the tempo and depth of the consultant's evaluation of a patient. For instance, for a coagulation evaluation, it is important to know whether the patient is being considered for impending surgery. In this situation the consultation would usually be more exhaustive because the hemostatic challenge of surgery is imminent. On the other hand, one may be asked to see a patient with postoperative hemorrhage in whom another operation is not currently planned. It is characteristically difficult to make sense out of postoperative intrahemorrhagic coagulation tests because most diagnostic hemostatic testing is designed to ferret out problems in stable situations. Hemostatic studies from a patient who has been stressed by operation and hemorrhage, and is in the midst of receiving a variety of therapeutic agents and blood products, are difficult to interpret. Another situation involves patients who seek

hemostatic evaluation as part of a kindred analysis when another family member, often a first-degree relative, has been found to have a genetic disease such as the factor V Leiden mutation.

*Accurate diagnosis and knowledge of the prognosis, both with and without various modes of therapy, should guide the physician in answering three major questions of therapy: **Whether** to treat, **When** to treat, and with **Which** modality.*

—*Maxwell M. Wintrobe*[l]

HOW TO DO THE CONSULTATION

A consultation is fundamentally similar to an admission evaluation of a patient but can be and usually is more focused, because the consultant is answering specific questions posed by the referring physician. Nonetheless, a careful history and physical examination are still in order and should be in depth, particularly in the area of expertise of the consultant. If the question posed is clearly focused and the encounter is a simple confirmatory or second opinion consultation, the consultation can be brief and therefore very circumscribed with respect to laboratory tests. Stumbling blocks, particularly in the areas of coagulation and thrombosis, regard not only *what* laboratory studies are reviewed but also *when* the tests were drawn. Every hematologist has had the problem of finding low and then normal protein C and protein S activity levels randomly spread throughout a patient's chart without clear indication whether the patient was receiving warfarin therapy at the time of testing. Similarly, a prolonged partial thromboplastin time may be the result of a traumatic venipuncture, contaminating heparin, or a true underlying process such as disseminated intravascular coagulation. One cannot simply look at raw laboratory data without knowing what the clinical circumstances were at that time in order to interpret those data. The obverse of this is that when the consultant performs laboratory tests, he or she is expected to state explicitly in the chart the ongoing events at the time those laboratory specimens were collected. It is important to know whether warfarin therapy or heparin therapy was concurrent, whether liver disease was manifest, or if there was a recent massive thrombosis. Otherwise one is unable to convert data into information useful to the patient and the physician.

ROLE OF THE CLINICAL LABORATORY

The traditional relationship between clinical hemostasis and the coagulation laboratory is longstanding, time-honored, and intertwined. At one time, diagnostic and investigational

---

[j] Ferrol Sams (b. 1922) was educated at Emory University School of Medicine and still practices in southern Georgia. He is a master storyteller and has written several novels, including *Run with the Horsemen* and *Whisper of the River*. The quotation used comes from *The Widow's Mite* (Peachtree Publishers, Atlanta, 1987).

[k] Faith Fitzgerald (b. 1943) was born in Massachusetts and received her M.D. degree from the University of California, San Francisco, where she was also an intern and resident. She was then Chief Resident in Medicine at San Francisco General Hospital. She currently is Assistant Dean of Humanities and Bioethics at the University of California, Davis School of Medicine. Her bright intellect, quick wit, and sagacious personality make her a most popular medical speaker. This citation originated in an American College of Physicians chat room for Governors and Regents on February 24, 2003, and is too priceless to exist only in cyberspace, and so, with Dr. Fitzgerald's permission, it is included.

[l] Maxwell M. Wintrobe (1901–1986) is considered the father of American hematology. Born and trained in Canada, he joined the faculty at Johns Hopkins in 1929 and in 1943 became the founding icon at the new medical school in Salt Lake City, where he helped build that service into one of preeminence. A host of American hematologists can trace their academic lineage directly or indirectly to Dr. Wintrobe. His quotation is taken from the introduction to his textbook, *Clinical Hematology*, first published in 1942. It has been wisely retained by the current editors of the 10th edition (Williams & Wilkins, Baltimore, 1998).

laboratories were managed by clinicians, which significantly contributed to the clinicians' ability to unravel and understand the intricate complexities of physiologic and pathophysiologic events. Unfortunately, through modern regulations, laboratories are no longer supervised by clinicians. Residents in clinical training have considerably less exposure to even basic coagulation testing. It is strongly encouraged that residents in training seek out experience (hands-on if possible) in a diagnostic laboratory in order to understand the vagaries and underpinning of this craft. Effective consultative diagnostics requires that the laboratory not be viewed as an incomprehensible yet unquestioned "black-box" into which samples are placed and from which data emerge. What the chest x-ray is to the pulmonologist and the electrocardiogram is to the cardiologist, the coagulation laboratory is to the hematologist.

The weight of laboratory results in the diagnostic process varies considerably. On one extreme, no clinician, no matter how talented, can distinguish between congenital factor VIII deficiency and factor IX deficiency, given the identical manifestations and genetics, clinical expressions, and courses of these two disorders. The laboratory can promptly and easily distinguish these, a matter of considerable importance considering the key differences in treatment. On the other hand, the preponderance of diagnostic evidence is clinically derived with the laboratory serving primarily to confirm one's clinical diagnosis. Common clinical diagnoses include thrombotic thrombocytopenic purpura, immune thrombocytopenic purpura, disseminated intravascular coagulation, and heparin-induced thrombocytopenia. The more facile one becomes in laboratory methods, to consider its prelaboratory variables (e.g., wrong sample, wrong patient, heparin contamination) and false-positive and false-negative results, the more correctly the diagnostic laboratory will be viewed. The diagnostically naive clinician tends to rely inordinately and inflexibly on the laboratory.

RECOMMENDATIONS

A consultant's recommendations should be clearly stated and easily found. In urgent cases or especially if information is pivotal in patient management, the referring physician should be called as soon as feasible to discuss the events of the consultation. This rapid communication is then followed up with a more formal consultation note.

In preparing the final report, the consultant should state in the first sentence or two the reason for the consultation. An example may be "Thank you very much for sending this 37-year-old white man with clear-cut ITP in for consultation for my opinion regarding length of prednisone treatment prior to possible splenectomy." This first sentence thus makes clear at least what your expectations were of the consultation, and, if such expectations prove to be wrong, the consultation can be refocused. For inpatient consultation, particularly when the patient is not on an internal medicine service, one's diagnoses and recommendations are probably best tabulated in a numeric fashion, because the entire history, physical examination results, and recounting of laboratory data more likely than not will not be read by the busy referring doctor.

Genetic counseling also may be an aspect of the consultation. For example, when patients are found to have heritable diseases, such as hemophilia or thrombophilia, it is wise to tell both the family and the referring physician that at least first-degree relatives might be screened for the presence or absence of the genetic disease. It is useful for first-degree relatives to know whether they do or do not have the defect, regardless of prior symptomatology, because future therapeutic plans are impacted by either positive or negative diagnoses of such illnesses.

One should be perfectly clear about to whom to send the consultation report. In inpatient work, the report is usually left on the chart for all appropriate persons to see.

In outpatient consultations, the initial copy is sent to that practitioner who referred the patient. Frequently patients wish to have copies of the consultation, and this should be honored in almost all respects. In rare situations in which the consultant feels uncomfortable, he or she should inform the patient that it is his or her obligation to send the consultation report back to the referring physician and let the referring physician and patient discuss those matters between themselves. Keep in mind, however, that any report is rightfully discoverable, so if a patient wishes to have a report, such inevitably will be accomplished.

More often than not patients will have seen other physicians who may have a stake in the patient's overall care, so it is pertinent to ask the patient whether he or she wishes to have a copy of the report sent to other health care practitioners who have cared for the patient or may in the near future.

In the special circumstances of IME and workers' compensation cases, the report is sent to the party who requested and paid for the consultation. Here it is not advisable to send copies to other practitioners without the explicit permission of the patient or the parties requesting the IME or workers' compensation evaluation.

Time after time I have gone out into my office in the evening feeling as if I couldn't keep my eyes open a moment longer. I would start out on my morning calls after only a few hours' sleep, sit in front of some house waiting to get the courage to climb the steps and push the front door bell. But once I saw the patient all that would disappear. In a flash the details of the case would begin to formulate themselves into a recognizable outline, the diagnosis would unravel itself, or would refuse to make itself plain, and the hunt was on.
—William Carlos Williams[m]

CONCERNS

Sometimes circumstances develop during the consultation that place the consultant in an unenviable position. Maturity and professionalism will serve to direct the correct course of action even if initially it seems totally impossible. The fundamental commandment should be to do that which is best for the patient rather than one's own emotional comfort. These dilemmas usually involve the relationship between the referring physician and the patient.

[m] The American physician William Carlos Williams (1883–1963) translated his hard work as a practitioner into everyday-life scenarios that characterized his enormous production of poetry and short stories. The quotation comes from a short story called "The Practice" from the *Autobiography of William Carlos Williams* (New Directions Publishing Company, New York, NY, 1951).

A patient or his or her family may be disgruntled with the original physician. Diagnoses are missed by all practitioners, and therapy provided can be incorrect. Bad outcomes should be clearly separated from deviation in standard of care. Tact with honesty and forthrightness should be employed. Often diagnoses that are perfectly clear in retrospect are in fact initiated and validated by prior efforts made on behalf of the patient. Treatments can be controversial, and even bizarre treatments have their vocal advocates. One should never openly fault another practitioner without knowing all the facts involved. It is best to limit oneself to what is known and carefully document such in the record because the stated facts may change if and when more data are collected. It is usually wise to refer such cases to a third practitioner or assume the care oneself rather than force the patient and physician back together if care does appear in fact to be suboptimal. One should find a way to discuss this matter with the other physician because it will eventually be revealed in some manner regardless. Early communication will allow the other practitioner to voice facts of which the consultant may not be aware. As mentioned previously, it is often possible to reconcile the patient's and the referring physician's problems. Early communication also allows the initial physician, if he or she indeed has practiced below the standard of care, to make amends with the patient or, if appropriate, for the physician to contact his or her risk management personnel sooner rather than later.

Some practitioners initially may be curt, hurried, or disrespectful or do not offer enough of their time to their patients, but nonetheless, are practicing within the medical-legal standard of care. If reparations cannot be made, the patient is best served by finding an equally intelligent but more humanistic physician.

Some patients are habitually malcontent; this can be determined by both discussion with the practitioner and discovery that the patient is persistently unable to establish and maintain profitable relationships with any health care provider. This category may include patients with personality disorders, drug-seekers, and persons with self-induced or factitious illnesses. These patients are most difficult because their problems are far deeper than just those that apply to one's subspecialty.

What the scalpel is to the surgeon, words are to the clinician. When he uses them effectively, his patients do well. If not, the results may be disastrous.

—*Philip A. Tumulty*[h]

OUTCOMES

Total Agreement

In this situation the consultant totally agrees with the evaluation of the referring physician and consultation serves primarily to add a layer of understanding and confidence to the patient and his or her family. Almost always one can make some minor suggestions, the thrust of the consultation is clearly to agree with and support the diagnosis, prognosis, and treatment plan of the referring physician. In almost all cases, the referring physician will continue with the assumption of care of the patient.

Supporting Consultation

Occasionally a physician will refer a noncompliant or doubtful patient to a consultant in order to have the latter reinforce a point with which the referring physician is having difficulty because of poor patient acceptance or compliance. Common examples of this type of consultation include the acceptance of certain diagnoses and especially cessation of smoking. Surprisingly, some patients refuse to accept the determination that they are normal despite all the supporting evidence. They continue to hang on to mildly abnormal laboratory data or minor findings such as normal bruising as evidence for some underlying pathologic process. Wisely, the referring physician usually communicates this informally with the consulting physician prior to the consultation. When it is clear that the referring physician will continue to assume care of the patient, the consultation is an opportune time for the consulting physician to strongly reinforce the stance of the referring physician (assuming that it is correct). Inappropriate behavior on the part of the patient can be addressed. This may occasionally generate some degree of resentment on the part of the patient, who may report such resentment to the referring physician or even distort details of the consultation. The strong advocacy role played by the consultant physician rightfully justifies the benevolent attempt of the consultant to positively modify the patient's understanding or behavior. One should promptly alert the referring physician of these events by telephone so that the referring physician will be forewarned regarding possible negative opinions of the consulting physician voiced by the patient.

Finding Another Physician for the Patient

It may become clear to the consultant that the referring physician has not made the correct diagnosis, prognostication, or treatment and that perhaps another primary physician should assume care of the patient. The consultant must be prepared to relate this opinion to the referring physician, especially if the patient or his or her family is obviously upset with the referring physician. The consultant, as a neutral third party, can sometimes improve patient care, but it is always still advisable as well as truthful to acknowledge to all parties the foundation work prepared and gathered by the original physician.

Consultant Assumes Primary Care of the Patient

Very rarely the consultant will assume primary care of the patient; this is not an advisable practice because if this does occur the relationship between the referring physician and consultant may be eroded. Transference of care is clearly understood whenever a patient moves from an area where he or she was previously attended by the referring physician to the consultant's geographic area. One may occasionally have a patient and his or her family so positively impressed by the attention and clinical sophistication of the consultant that they ask the consultant to assume their care. Flattering though it may be, it is advisable not to do this unless there is absolute agreement from all parties, and to include third-party payors. It is not intrinsically unethical but generally should be held to an absolute minimum.

It is not unethical to enter into a patient–physician relationship with a patient who has been receiving care from another physician. By accepting second-opinion patients for treatment, physicians affirm the right of patients to have a free choice in the selection of their physicians.

—*AMA Code of Ethics*[g]

Serious Troubles

Rarely, a patient's case has been so mismanaged that there is clear and immediate danger to the patient. If this occurs, the consultant is helping the patient and also potentially the referring physician by extracting the patient from continued mismanagement. If the patient's care is severely compromised and immediate care is necessary, prompt hospitalization at the consultant's facility is a way to address the problem and defuse potential ill will with the referring physician. In this manner, diagnostic and therapeutic procedures can be initiated promptly and the consultant allowed time and data to justify this aggressive maneuver to the referring physician. Whether the patient should be returned to the referring physician may be a matter of the preference for the patient, the referring physician, or both, and the decision must take into consideration the referring physician's abilities to continue the correct treatment. Jones and colleagues outlined various communication options when discussing prior practitioners' mismanagement with patients and family.[7]

The best way to get a difficult job done is face-to-face or ear-to-ear. Sending notes is never satisfactory.

—*Eugene A. Stead, Jr.*[c]

Redirecting the Thrust of a Workup

The consultant has the benefit of having more time, laboratory data, and response to therapy than the original physician. Occasionally the consultant may suddenly visualize the correct diagnosis, which, while explaining all the findings in the case, is far different from that of the referring physician. At this juncture the diagnostic and therapeutic thrusts must be changed from one direction to another. A example would be a patient who is being evaluated for anemia and is referred for a bone marrow examination because a myriad of tests have been negative. If the consultant recognizes that a history of fatigue, chills, fevers, weight loss, and night sweats has been overlooked and detects a new cardiac murmur, it is clear that the evaluation should be focused more toward infectious endocarditis than anemia of unknown etiology. Rarely do any parties become upset with this new direction, especially when the new diagnosis proves to be correct. Credit again must be given to the foundation of material gathered by the original physicians.

Major Disagreements between Physicians

This most unfortunate but rare situation usually occurs in the inpatient rather than the outpatient setting. Not all the

recommendations that a consultant makes need be carried out by any referring physician, and the decision to follow the recommendations is certainly the prerogative of the attending physician. No code holds that the attending physician must execute each and every recommendation made by the consulting physician. Lo and colleagues explored variables for and against adherence and lack of adherence to suggestions made by infectious disease consultants.[8]

On some occasions, however, the consultant's feelings are so strong and so clear that for the primary physician to continue to ignore the recommendations may well fall below the standard of care in the consultant's opinion. In this situation, frank face-to-face discussion with the attending physician is mandatory. This is particularly true in teaching institutions, where there are several buffers of communication between the consultant faculty member and the attending physician of record. If these matters cannot be resolved, it may be wisest to sign off a case in writing in the chart. Admittedly this should be a very rare event, but it does occur perhaps a few times in a decade among consultants in a very busy consultation service. The note need not be long or give reasons but simply state that one as the consultant is signing off this case but availability can be reestablished by reconsultation. The consultant might name other consultants who may be contacted on this case.

From the day you begin practice never under any circumstances listen to a tale told to the detriment of a brother practitioner. And when any dispute or trouble does arise, go frankly, ere sunset, and talk the matter over, in which way you may gain a brother and a friend.

—*William Osler*[n]

Duration of Consultation

There is often question about how long one should be involved as a consultant in the outpatient setting and in the inpatient setting. This question may be more pertinent on an inpatient basis. Some focused questions are effectively answered by an equally focused single note. In other situations, those questions are quickly and efficiently answered with one or two brief follow-up visits to ascertain results of certain requested laboratory data or the response to therapy after which the consultation can be terminated. It is advisable to sign off in writing in the medical record so that it is clear to all parties that one has ceased closely following the patient yet is still available if another question emerges or if things do not go as planned.

Some consultations involve "clearing a patient for surgery." All parties should understand that the term *cleared for surgery* implies clearance *at that time*. Therefore, any events that happen later cannot have been considered; a patient is not cleared for surgery in perpetuity. This often must be expressly written in the outpatient consultation as facts can change between the consultation and the actual surgery. For instance, a patient

---

[n] William Osler (1849–1919) received his M.D. degree from McGill University and was the founding physician of the new Johns Hopkins University. While helping to establish the preeminence of Johns Hopkins, he wrote his *Principles and Practice of Medicine* and subsequently became the Regis Professor of Medicine at Oxford University, the chair presently held by Dr. Weatherall, who was kind enough to write the preface to the first edition of this text. Dr. Osler wrote prolifically on medical and nonmedical subjects. The quotation used is one of his *Aphorisms.*

with chronic thrombocytopenia who has a platelet count of 60,000/µL may be currently cleared for nearly any surgery, but that clearance does not hold true forever. If the patient returns in a year for another operation, and the platelet count is 20,000/µL, the situation has clearly changed. It is wise to signify the limits of the clearance in the body of the consultation. Clearance is not to be confused with a guarantee of success but implies that the risk:benefit ratio is made as favorable as possible for the patient and that parties acknowledge the risk and agree that the perceived benefit is worth that risk.

In general the consultant should follow the case for as long as the expertise is needed. If one is consulted for preparing an individual with hemophilia for surgery, it would be wise for the consultant to see the patient several visits postoperatively because bleeding can be immediate, intermediate, or sometimes delayed.

Noncompliant Patients

We cannot assume that a course of treatment advised for a patient will be followed. Patients may have a variety of reasons to be noncompliant. This author found that approximately one half of prescriptions written for outpatient low-molecular-weight heparin are not filled when the patient leaves the hospital, primarily because of financial considerations. Some patients may have no faith in our suggestions, whereas others will deny they have any problem and therefore believe no nostrum is needed. Self-determination is held extremely highly in the United States. We do owe the patient a duty to fully explain our treatment and its best-estimated risk:benefit ratio. Often more disturbing is failure to address behavior that is unhealthy. It is important to continue to support the patient even (or specially) if one does not agree with the patient and their behavior.

Some physicians dismiss patients from their practice if they do not adhere to recommended treatment plans or correct harmful habits. Many more of us try to maintain a patient-doctor relationship even when our advice seems to be discounted. Perhaps we believe that we will eventually prevail in our advocacy for changed life-styles. More likely, we see within our patients certain characteristics that we also share and hence cannot honestly condemn. I never gave up the quest to convince [a particular patient] to care for his diabetes. Would it have made a difference in the coming collapse of his health? I do not know. Sometimes diabetes, and most other illnesses as well, behave in totally unpredictable fashions. Sometimes the most carefully followed treatment plan will not slow a disease at all. Sometimes a patient may ignore an illness and for many years seem none the worse. These instances force humility upon us. Our word is not law. It is to be considered advice in the light of an uncertain science that races ahead of us.

—Clif Cleaveland[o]

End of Life Issues

It is all too common that major illnesses, including fatal illnesses, are encountered in consultative hematology. This is the nature of our work. At some point, the patient and the physician (i.e., those comprising the doctor–patient relationship) will elect to forgo further treatments, tests, and hospitalizations. This point in time will vary from patient to patient and may differ from a physician's own experience, beliefs and value systems, and views on quality of life. That these are variable and hard to define does not detract from their existence and importance. Palliative care is, appropriately, a rapidly developing area. Changing direction in a patient's care is not giving up.

Being an agent of healing for another human at the end of life confers a personal richness that is difficult to find elsewhere in medicine. It is not just the patient who is healed.

—Mary Bretscher[P]

Family Members

No segment of society consumes fewer medical resources than physicians and their immediate families. This may be due in part to the familiarity with informed consent issues or that physicians may not wish to bother other physicians. To the extent that the latter is true, it is ill-advised for a practitioner to get more entwined in family care than anything more involved than the simplest issues. Conflict of interest and prescribing issues aside, it is the clearly recognizable inability of even the most veteran diagnostician to be objective that is the most obvious and concerning. One should get another physician to do this work.

At times of illnesses of our children, I experience almost unbearable conflict. Along with my wife, I need the informed comforting by an empathetic physician. I need the reassurance that all that is reasonable is being done. At the same time the scientist within me seeks insights into the disease process, and that invariably means becoming aware of the worst possible outcomes. Reassurance and fear compete. When one of my family members coughs or runs a fever, my senses sharpen. Am I over-responding, or am I at risk of ignoring something potentially dangerous? Our clinical work keeps us suspicious, observant, and uneasy, making it all but impossible to maintain balanced judgment when the patient is one of our flesh and blood.

—Clif Cleaveland[o]

When a Diagnosis Is Not Forthcoming

Not all diagnoses can be established. The wise consultant should never feel pressed to force a diagnosis, because an

---

[o] Clif Cleaveland (b. 1936) grew up in Georgia and South Carolina and attended Duke University. He was a Rhodes Scholar and received his M.D. from Johns Hopkins Medical School. He completed his residency in internal medicine at Vanderbilt University Hospital. He has been practicing medicine in Chattanooga, Tennessee, for over 30 years. In 1995, he was President of the American College of Physicians. Dr. Cleaveland is a gifted writer who is able to translate day-to-day clinical experiences into prose that is humanistic, interesting, and poignant. He has penned two excellent books, *Sacred Space* in 1998 and *Healers and Heroes* in 2004.

Dr. Cleaveland began the exceedingly popular Tennessee Literature and Medicine Reading Retreat in 1988 in which he leads discussions regarding medicine and its practitioners as portrayed in literature. His Reading Retreat has been emulated but never equaled. His first excerpt is from *Healers and Heroes*, and the second one from *Sacred Space*.

[P] Mary E. Bretscher (b. 1959) is in the private practice of hematology and oncology in Springfield, Illinois. She received her medical degree from Southern Illinois University, where she also performed her residency and served as Chief Resident. She followed this with a fellowship at the Mayo Graduate School of Medicine in Minnesota. Her practice is hematology/oncology, but her passion is palliative care.

incorrect diagnosis is worse than no diagnosis. In making an incorrect diagnosis, one shuts the window of opportunity to pursue the correct diagnosis. It is wisest to realize and state that one affirmatively knows he or she does not know the answer rather than to force a diagnosis. It often is the responsibility of the consultant to energize the referring physician to continue observation in a conservative course. Failure to do so frequently results in erratic testing and troublesome indecisive therapeutics. If a therapeutic course is taken, it must be maintained sufficiently long enough to either succeed or fail on its own merits while one constantly reevaluates for signs of success or failure as well as entertains another diagnosis. Often the remaining and most important procedure in such cases is observation. Therapies that are not effective should be neither initiated nor maintained.[9] With observation, some diagnoses become clear while other cases spontaneously improve.

The essential and wise thing to do is not to force a diagnosis when the answer is not evident, but rather to follow a conservative program of support and periodic reexamination, retaining an open mind as to the basis of the patient's complaints.

—*Philip A. Tumulty*[h]

[My father] carried his prescription pad everywhere and wrote voluminous prescriptions for all his patients. These were fantastic formulations, containing five or six different vegetable ingredients, each one requiring careful measuring and weighing by the druggist, who pounded the powder, dissolved it in alcohol, and bottled it with a label giving only the patient's name, the date, and the instructions about dosage. The contents were a deep mystery, and intended to be a mystery. The prescriptions were always written in Latin, to heighten the mystery. The purpose of this kind of therapy was essentially reassurance. A skilled, experienced physician might have dozens of different formulations in his memory, ready for writing out in flawless detail at a moment's notice, but all he could have predicted about them with any certainty were the variations in the degree of bitterness of taste, the color, the smell, and the likely effects of the concentrations of alcohol used as solvent. They were placebos, and they had been the principal mainstay of medicine, the sole technology, for so long a time—millennia—that they had the incantatory power of religious ritual. My father had little faith in the effectiveness of any of them, but he used them daily in his practice. They were expected by his patients; a doctor who did not provide such prescriptions would soon have no practice at all; they did no harm, so far as he could see; if nothing else, they gave the patient something to do while the illness, whatever, was working its way through its appointed course.

—*Lewis Thomas*[d]

Once a particular therapeutic program has been launched, give the patient's response to it time to mature and produce clear-cut answers before it is stopped or altered.

—*Philip A. Tumulty*[h]

You can observe a lot just by watching.

—*Yogi Berra*[q]

WHEN SHOULD A CONSULTANT REQUEST CONSULTATION?

Sometimes consultations can be extremely difficult, and a well-trained, experienced consultant may find that he or she needs a special laboratory test or special consultation with other experienced experts. These facts are clearly understandable, and often for geographic reasons such discussions are made telephonically. It is appropriate to enter such a secondary consultation in the body of the report, but one should recall that the secondary consultant has not had the benefit of seeing the patient first-hand and therefore is relying on the primary consultant's presentation, perception, and understanding of the case. Should blood or biopsy material be referred to yet another consultant, it is best to have the understanding and permission of the patient for reasons of confidentiality as well as the potential for fees generated for services.

There is always a strong impulse to do something to help a sick person, but no action is better than the wrong action.

—*Philip A. Tumulty*[h]

Everyone is ignorant, only on different subjects.

—*Will Rogers*[r]

In order to enhance this chapter, the editor has borrowed the thoughts and words of several highly regarded medical teachers and medical philosophers as well as five physician-writers of renown and two American icons of wit.

Students continue to enroll in medical school, coming to the profession for timeless reasons—because of a physician they admire, or because they want to serve, or because they have suffered or witnessed suffering. Perhaps some lucky ones even today have been called to medicine through the medium of a book. If they have a love for literature, reading might well help them to discover a way to understand and identify with the ambitions, sorrows, and joys of the people whose lives are put in their hands. In medicine, we often separate life events from their meaning for those who live them. In literature, the two are united. That is reason enough to keep reading. And writing.

—*Abraham Verghese*[s]

---

[r] Will Rogers (1879–1935) was one of our great American humorists. He was also a showman of great repute. His wit was usually sharp and at times critical. His favorite target was politics and any type of pretension. The quote is from *Will Rogers: Wise and Witty Sayings of a Great American Humorist* (Hallmark, Claremore, Oklahoma, 1969).

[s] Abraham Verghese (b. 1955) was born in India and graduated with his medical degree from Madras University in 1979. He came to the United States as a resident in medicine to East Tennessee State University, and later served at that institution as Chief Resident. He was a Fellow in Infectious Diseases at Boston University. He has also received a Master of Fine Arts from the University of Iowa. Dr. Verghese's style is fluid, haunting, and piercing, as though he writes directly to one's subconscious. Two books, *My Own Country* (1994) and *The Tennis Partner* (1998), have been widely acclaimed and outstandingly reviewed, with both designated in the top ten books published during their respective years. Dr. Verghese is currently director for the Center of Medical Humanities and Ethics at the University of Texas, San Antonio, where he is the Forland Distinguished Professor of Medical Ethics and Professor of Medicine. The excerpt included is extracted from "The Calling," which appeared in the *New England Journal of Medicine* (2005; 352:1844–1847).

---

[q] Yogi Berra (b. 1925) was born in St. Louis, Missouri, and became one of the greatest catchers in baseball history. He is well known for his malapropisms, usually now referred to as "Yogi-isms." These have been richly collected in *The Wit and Wisdom of Yogi Berra* by Phil Pepe (Meckler Boos, Westport, Conn., 1988), from which this Yogi-ism was taken.

REFERENCES

1. Weiss N: E-mail consultation: Clinical, financial, legal, and ethical implications. Surg Neurol 2004; 61:455–459.
2. Eysenbach G, Diepgan TL: Responses to unsolicited patient email requests for medical advice on the World Wide Web. JAMA 1998; 280:1333–1335.
3. Howard ML: Physician-patient relationship. In: Sanbar SS, Fivestone MH, Buckner F, et al (eds): Legal Medicine, 6th ed. Philadelphia, Mosby, 2004, p 334.
4. Newborn V: United States of America, 238 F. Supp. 2d (U.S. District Court, DC, 2002).
5. Newborn V: United States of America, 84 Fed Appx (U.S. Court of Appeals, DC, 2003).
6. Baum K: Independent medical examinations: An expanding source of physician liability. Ann Intern Med 2005; 142:974–978.
7. Jones JW, McCullough LB, Richman BW: What to tell patients harmed by other physicians. J Vasc Surg 2003; 38:866–867.
8. Lo E, Rezai K, Evans AT, et al: Why don't they listen? Adherence to recommendations of infectious disease consultations. Clin Infect Dis 2004; 38:1212–1218.
9. Doust J, Del Mar C: Why do doctors use treatments that do not work? Br Med J 2004; 328:474–475.

Chapter 2

A Systematic Approach to the Bleeding Patient: Correlation of Clinical Symptoms and Signs With Laboratory Testing

Craig M. Kessler, MD • Nushmia Khokhar, MD • Minetta Liu, MD

INTRODUCTION

In the current medical climate of laboratory automation, highly detailed radiographic techniques, and time/economic constraints on physicians in general and the hematologist specifically, the value of the comprehensive patient interview and medical history has been minimized. Furthermore, examination of the peripheral blood smear and bone marrow aspirate to establish a diagnosis based on visual and morphologic criteria has been supplanted by considerably more accurate and sensitive immunohistochemical, cytogenetic, and flow cytometric analyses with monoclonal antibodies. Perhaps more unique to the bleeding patient than to other categories of illness, the patient interview provides the foundation for making the diagnosis, determining which laboratory tests are most appropriate to order, and formulating treatment strategies. Careful attention to these elements of patient assessment substantially reduces morbidity, mortality, and the cost of care while minimizing the medical-legal exposure of the physician.

This chapter offers a systematic approach to the patient with a clinically significant risk of bleeding or an immediate history of spontaneous, excessive hemorrhage. Approaches to laboratory confirmation of the causes of bleeding are also presented because interpretation of data from the coagulation laboratory requires an understanding and appreciation of the vagaries of the techniques employed to generate them. In addition, this chapter discusses how the coagulation laboratory can provide insight into the pathophysiology of the patient's condition and presents a rationale for treatment.

The evaluation of patients with hemorrhagic complications is a multistep process that involves a complete history, a detailed physical examination, and a directed laboratory evaluation. The relative emphasis placed on each of these components varies according to each unique clinical situation, but all factors must be considered. Important points of differentiation include localized defects versus systemic defects, acquired defects versus inherited defects, and disorders of primary hemostasis (i.e., those related to platelet abnormalities) versus disorders of secondary hemostasis (i.e., those related to coagulation factor, fibrinogen, or connective tissue abnormalities).

It is important for the clinician to understand that some clinical situations do not allow for a comprehensive evaluation and may therefore require a more streamlined approach. Intubated patients who develop brisk bleeding during the immediate postoperative period, for example, will not be able to provide any information about their personal or family history; a determination of these patients' most likely cause for bleeding will therefore rest on the pertinent physical and laboratory findings. Of primary importance for all consulting hematologists is the realization that the management of coagulation abnormalities—which are often epiphenomena or complications of other medical illnesses—is often empirical and cannot always be approached through a standard algorithm.

THE CLINICAL EVALUATION

Each component of the clinical assessment provides critical information that supports or refutes the possibility that a true hemorrhagic disorder actually exists. The information garnered from the history and physical examination ultimately guides the direction and extent of the laboratory evaluation and helps the clinician to determine how future bleeding complications can be managed and/or prevented. This multifactorial approach is necessary because the likelihood of false-positive and false-negative diagnoses is high when the decision rests on one component alone. Consider, for example, the process required to obtain an accurate medical history. Patients' perception of their own bleeding tendency is often exaggerated or understated. In one study conducted in the Åland Islands, where von Willebrand disease (VWD) was originally detected in 1928, 65% of women and 35% of men from families with no history of bleeding and no personal laboratory evidence of a bleeding disorder answered a self-administered binary questionnaire with responses indicative of a symptomatic bleeding diathesis. In contrast, 38% of the women and 54% of the men with documented laboratory evidence of a coagulation defect and a positive family history of symptomatic VWD or qualitative platelet disorders answered the same questionnaire as if they were completely unaware of their bleeding diathesis.[1]

Obtaining a Detailed History

Several authors have formulated basic comprehensive questionnaires in an effort to simplify and standardize the evaluation of individuals with easy bruising or bleeding.[1–3] Standardized questionnaire bleeding score systems have recently been devised to evaluate patient hemorrhagic symptoms and the potential to bleed for VWD (http://www.euvwd.group.shef.ac.uk/files/scoremar04revision),[4] factor XI deficiency,[5] Quebec thrombasthenia,[6] and autoimmune thrombocytopenic purpura.[7] The format of these questionnaires generally involves the use of binary (i.e., yes or no) questions that elicit immediate, unambiguous responses from patients; quantitative and qualitative qualifiers are used where appropriate. Examples of questions effectively applied to the present history are presented in the following sections.

Have you ever experienced a serious hemorrhagic complication during or after a surgical procedure?

The initial assessment of postoperative bleeding complications should differentiate between incomplete surgical ligation or cauterization of blood vessels and the presence of an underlying defect in hemostasis. Clinical suspicion of a bleeding diathesis should be substantiated with objective evidence from the case in question: a description of all wounds and venipuncture sites, an evaluation of all laboratory abnormalities (e.g., worsening anemia, thrombocytopenia, alterations in prothrombin time [PT] or partial thromboplastin time [PTT]), calculations of the estimated blood loss and subsequent transfusion requirements, knowledge of the means required to stop the bleeding, and documentation of a prolonged hospital stay. In addition, the timing of the hemorrhagic complication in relation to the procedure (i.e., immediate vs delayed) may provide important clues. Intraoperative and immediate postoperative bleeding at the surgical site is often due to defects in primary hemostasis, that is, abnormalities of platelet number, adhesion, and/or aggregation (Table 2-1). In contrast, delayed postoperative bleeding at the surgical site is typically due to coagulation factor deficiencies, qualitative or quantitative disorders of fibrinogen, or vascular abnormalities related to defects in collagen structure (Table 2-2); notably, factor XIII deficiency, fibrinogen deficiency, and several of the collagen disorders are often marked by poor wound healing and subsequent wound dehiscence as well. Furthermore, excessive bleeding from the umbilical cord stump at birth or bleeding from the circumcision site is strongly indicative of a severe inherited disorder, whereas bleeding related to abdominal or cardiothoracic surgery in a previously "normal" adult is not. Nevertheless, a number of cases of factor XI deficiency, mild VWD, and mild Ehlers-Danlos syndrome have escaped diagnosis until later in life when the defect in hemostasis is manifested as mucosal surface bleeding during or after routine surgery.

Have you ever experienced excessive vaginal bleeding during pregnancy or immediately after childbirth or perineal bleeding from an episiotomy?

Multiparous women should be questioned about each pregnancy in detail with regard to complications and outcomes.

Table 2-1 Disorders of Primary Hemostasis*

Hereditary Disease States
von Willebrand disease
Glanzmann thrombasthenia
Bernard-Soulier syndrome
Platelet storage pool disease
Gray platelet syndrome
Wiskott-Aldrich syndrome
May-Hegglin anomaly

Iatrogenic Disease States
Posttransfusion purpura
Drug-induced immunologic thrombocytopenia (e.g., quinine, heparin, sulfonamide antibiotics)
Drug-induced qualitative platelet disorders (e.g., aspirin, nonsteroidal anti-inflammatory drugs [NSAIDs], ticlopidine, abciximab, mithramycin)

Acquired Disease States
Autoimmune thrombocytopenic purpura
Disseminated intravascular coagulation
Systemic amyloidosis
Hypersplenism
Aplastic anemia
Uremia
Mechanical platelet destruction from turbulent circulation (e.g., cardiac bypass, severe aortic stenosis)

*Primary hemostasis involves formation of the platelet plug. The above is a representative list of potential causes of abnormalities in platelet number, adhesion, or aggregation.

Table 2-2 Disorders of Secondary Hemostasis*

Coagulation Factor Abnormalities
Hemophilia A (factor VIII deficiency)
Hemophilia B (factor IX deficiency)
Deficiencies in factor II, V, VII, or X
Acquired inhibitors to specific coagulation factors (e.g., factor VIII or factor V inhibitors)
Factor XIII deficiency

Contact Factor Abnormalities
Factor XI deficiency

Fibrinogen Abnormalities
Afibrinogenemia
Hypofibrinogenemia
Inherited dysfibrinogenemias
Hyperfibrinolysis

Connective Tissue Disorders
Ehlers-Danlos syndrome
Osler-Weber-Rendu syndrome (hereditary hemorrhagic telangiectasia)
Scurvy (vitamin C deficiency)

*Secondary hemostasis involves humoral coagulation subsequent to formation of the platelet plug. The above is a representative list of potential causes of abnormalities in coagulation factors, contact factors, fibrinogen, or connective tissues.

Obstetric histories are particularly important because multiple spontaneous miscarriages and infertility may be associated with congenital maternal coagulopathies (e.g., factor XIII deficiency, the dysfibrinogenemias) and some acquired syndromes (e.g., anticardiolipin/antiphospholipid syndrome). Bleeding before 20 weeks gestation may be due to miscarriage, ectopic pregnancy, or gestational trophoblastic disease. Bleeding after the 20th week of pregnancy usually results in placental abruption and placenta previa. Hemorrhage during delivery most commonly reflects evolving placental abruption, uterine rupture, or placenta accreta. The most common causes of postpartum hemorrhage are uterine atony, laceration, and retained placenta. Postpartum hemorrhage is defined as blood loss greater than 500 mL in a vaginal delivery or 1000 mL in a caesarean birth.[8]

In general, disseminated intravascular coagulation (DIC) is the most common cause of abnormal bleeding during the puerperium and is most frequently the result of abruptio placentae, eclampsia, retention of a dead fetus, amniotic fluid embolism, placental retention, or bacterial sepsis.[9] It is interesting to note that women who have mild or moderate VWD or who are carriers of hemophilia A typically do not experience easy bruising or bleeding manifestations during pregnancy, during the delivery, or when they are taking such estrogen-containing compounds as oral contraceptives or hormone replacement therapy. This is most likely related to the increased synthesis of von Willebrand factor (VWF) and factor VIII as acute phase reactant proteins in response to high-estrogen states; the activity levels of these factors begin to fall immediately postpartum and do not reach baseline levels for weeks (or even longer in women who are nursing). In addition, acquired autoantibodies directed against factor VIII may occur within the first year postpartum after an otherwise normal delivery; this acquired postpartum hemophilia is marked by pronounced bleeding and bruising and by spontaneous remissions and rare recurrences with subsequent pregnancies.[10]

Have you experienced persistent menorrhagia in the absence of fibroids or other uterine abnormalities?

Menstrual histories often provide useful clues for an underlying hemostatic defect, particularly in those women with persistent menorrhagia and/or a microcytic anemia despite adequate iron supplementation. A history of severe iron deficiency in a young woman, the use of packed red blood cell transfusions for an anemia of unknown cause, the need for a dilation and curettage procedure for persistent uterine bleeding, or the need for a hysterectomy to treat menorrhagia should increase the suspicion for an underlying defect in hemostasis. Recent surveys suggest that a significant number of hysterectomies for menorrhagia are performed in women with VWD.[11] Unfortunately, each woman's definition of menorrhagia can be somewhat vague, rendering menorrhagia a relatively poor indicator of an underlying coagulation disorder. The poor specificity of menorrhagia as a bleeding symptom is further underscored by the fact that 23% to 44% of healthy, noncoagulopathic women claim to experience this symptom.[12] Numerous bleeding scales have been devised to circumvent this variability, but these may be very cumbersome to use. They all attempt to quantitate menstrual blood loss according to the duration of heavy flow (i.e., longer than 3 days), the duration of each menstrual cycle (i.e., longer than 7 days total), and the number of pads or tampons used. The accuracy of this latter factor, however, may vary as it depends on the individual patient's hygienic habits and fastidiousness. The recent addition of menstrual symptometric devices, such as pictorial blood assessment charts,[13,14] has improved the accuracy of quantifying excessive blood loss, which would be useful in diagnosing underlying coagulopathy. These tools appear to have a high level of patient acceptability and can provide instant feedback to the physician. Finally, the need for oral contraceptives to control excessive menstrual bleeding should be noted, because this may also serve as an indicator of the degree of menorrhagia that is present but may confound the clinician's ability to diagnose VWD, secondary to the acute phase reactivity of factor VIII and VWF.

Do you experience brisk or prolonged bleeding after epistaxis or minor cuts or exaggerated bruising after minor trauma?

Excessive and persistent bleeding or oozing from a relatively minor superficial injury and the appearance of ecchymoses or purpura (especially true hematomas) after minimal trauma may be indicative of an underlying congenital or acquired hemostatic defect. For example, profuse bleeding and the need for prolonged times of direct pressure for a small paper cut or razor nick are unusual; this crude bleeding time may be a manifestation of qualitative or quantitative platelet defects, or of VWD. The loss of deciduous teeth and extractions of molar teeth are also inadvertent but accurate tests of hemostasis; again, immediate bleeding after the initial event is consistent with a vascular or platelet abnormality, and delayed bleeding and/or rebleeding is more consistent with a coagulation factor deficiency. Finally, poor or delayed wound healing is uncharacteristic of platelet disorders but may be associated with factor XIII deficiency, hereditary dysfibrinogenemia, and Ehlers-Danlos syndrome.

Habitual non–trauma-induced epistaxis, particularly those episodes that occur in postpubertal individuals that last longer than 5 minutes and require medical attention, should raise suspicion for an underlying bleeding disorder. Symptom-specific assessment and severity grading tools for epistaxis are available to supplement clinical acumen.[15,16]

Epistaxis is reported as a bleeding problem in 5% to 39% of healthy individuals,[12] but only approximately 27% of habitual nose-bleeders have hereditary coagulation defects, predominantly involving components of primary hemostasis (e.g., VWF protein).[17]

Inherited vascular abnormalities of the nasal mucosa, such as the observed angiodysplasia associated with hereditary hemorrhagic telangiectasia and VWD, should also be considered in the differential diagnosis of recurrent epistaxis. In fact, these two diseases have been reported to coexist within families.

Have you ever developed hemarthrosis, retroperitoneal hematoma, or soft tissue hematoma in the absence of major trauma?

These clinical events are typical manifestations of defects in secondary hemostasis, that is, problems of humoral coagulation subsequent to platelet adhesion and formation of the platelet plug. The hemophilias are good examples of this type of delayed but severe bleeding, which may persist until the involved compartment has achieved self-tamponade. Of note, individuals who develop acquired neutralizing autoantibodies against specific coagulation factors are clinically similar but not identical to those with classic hemophilia; although both patient populations usually present with extensive spontaneous bleeds in critical areas, spontaneous hemarthrosis is remarkably rare in those with acquired coagulation factor autoantibodies but is very common among those with classic hemophilia.

Have you ever experienced spontaneous bleeding, poor wound healing, or dehiscence of a surgical wound?

A spontaneous hemorrhage is one that occurs in the absence of any identifiable trauma other than the stress of weight bearing. Bleeding that spontaneously originates from the mucous membranes (e.g., epistaxis, melena, menorrhagia) is more commonly associated with severe thrombocytopenia (defined as a platelet count <10,000/μL), qualitative platelet dysfunction, or VWD. Spontaneous cutaneous bruising in the form of purpura is often a feature of prolonged corticosteroid administration, Ehlers-Danlos syndrome, or the senile purpura syndrome. Dramatic ecchymoses frequently are observed in individuals who develop acquired autoantibodies that target factor VIII (acquired hemophilia A). Poor wound healing is a nonspecific indicator of an underlying coagulation defect; however, when it occurs around 7 to 10 days postoperatively at any age, and particularly after circumcision or loss of the umbilical cord in the infant, the clinician should consider the possibility of hypo(dys)fibrinogenemia, factor XIII deficiency, zinc deficiency, or hereditary connective tissue diseases such as Ehlers-Danlos syndrome and Marfan syndrome. Diabetes mellitus and Cushing syndrome may also be associated with delayed wound healing.

Spontaneous hemarthroses and intramuscular bleeds, on the other hand, are more characteristic of certain severe coagulation factor deficiencies. If bleeding is multifocal, an underlying acquired bleeding diathesis, such as DIC, should be suspected. As in all other bleeding situations, an objective clinical and laboratory assessment is critical to determine the need for and type of appropriate medical intervention. In addition, hematemesis, hematochezia, melena, hemoptysis, and hematuria may occur spontaneously in confirmed hemorrhagic disorders, but a thorough investigation should be pursued in an effort to identify a critical anatomic lesion as the source of bleeding.

Has any member of your family experienced severe bleeding complications, perhaps requiring transfusion of packed red blood cells?

The most common congenital hemorrhagic diatheses and qualitative thrombocytopathies follow distinct patterns of inheritance (Table 2-3). One must keep in mind, however, that a negative family history does not necessarily preclude the presence of a familial disorder; patients may not be aware of their family members' medical histories, the genetic defect may be characterized by variable penetrance, the coagulation disorder may lead to a mild bleeding diathesis that is not always manifested clinically, or the mutation may have occurred spontaneously. Nonetheless, a careful review of the patient's pedigree may reveal the underlying inheritance pattern to be one of the following: (1) sex-linked recessive, including hemophilia A, hemophilia B, and Wiskott-Aldrich syndrome; (2) autosomal dominant, including VWD, Osler-Weber-Rendu syndrome

---

Table 2-3 Congenital Coagulopathies and Qualitative Thrombocytopathies
Sex-Linked Recessive Disorders
Hemophilia A (factor VIII deficiency)
Hemophilia B (factor IX deficiency)
Wiskott-Aldrich syndrome
Autosomal Dominant Disorders
von Willebrand disease
Osler-Weber-Rendu syndrome (hereditary hemorrhagic telangiectasia)
Dysfibrinogenemias
Autosomal Recessive Disorders
Deficiencies in factor II, V, VII, X, XI, or XIII
α_2-Plasmin inhibitor deficiency
Bernard-Soulier syndrome
Glanzmann thrombasthenia
Gray platelet syndrome
Afibrinogenemia
Hypofibrinogenemia
Type 3 von Willebrand disease

(hereditary hemorrhagic telangiectasia), and hereditary dysfibrinogenemia; or (3) autosomal recessive, including factor II deficiency, factor VII deficiency, and Bernard-Soulier syndrome.

Do you have any known medical problems?

A number of medical conditions are associated with the development of acquired defects in coagulation and/or hemostasis. One of the best documented associations is that between the lupus-type anticoagulants and systemic lupus erythematosus, other autoimmune disorders, medications (including phenothiazines and tricyclic antidepressants), acute infections, and some lymphoproliferative disorders. Although the lupus-type anticoagulants do prolong in vitro coagulation assays, the major risk is for thrombosis as opposed to bleeding. Hemorrhagic manifestations may occur, however, in those patients with the lupus anticoagulant who concurrently develop autoantibodies to prothrombin (resulting in a true decrease in the circulating half-life of factor II) or to platelet membrane glycoproteins (resulting in thrombocytopenia or platelet dysfunction).

Other medical conditions associated with a potential for bleeding complications warrant mention as well. For example, catastrophic and life-threatening hemorrhagic events may occur in cases of acute promyelocytic leukemia as a result of the secondary DIC that is induced by the release of tissue factor from the malignant promyelocytes. Uremia secondary to renal failure, on the other hand, is associated with qualitative as opposed to quantitative platelet defects. This is in contrast to severe end-stage hepatic dysfunction, which may lead to defects in primary and secondary hemostasis; thrombocytopenia caused by portal hypertension and hypersplenism; deficient synthesis and postribosomal modification of the vitamin K–dependent clotting factors; low-grade DIC resulting from decreased clearance of activated procoagulant proteins and decreased synthesis and clearance of such fibrinolytic modulatory proteins as α_2-plasmin inhibitor, the primary inhibitor of plasmin; and acquired dysfibrinogenemia of liver disease, in which increased susceptibility to fibrinolytic enzyme degradation may play a key role.[18] In addition, systemic amyloidosis is associated with the development of factor X deficiency, which may result from the specific adsorption of the factor X protein by amyloid fibrils[19]; amyloid-induced gastrointestinal malabsorption syndromes may exacerbate this coagulation defect through vitamin K deficiency. Finally, associations between Gaucher disease and factor IX deficiency and between hypothyroidism, right-to-left cardiac shunts, and Wilms tumors and VWD have been reported, each with a different underlying cause.

Do you take any prescription medications, over-the-counter medications, or homeopathic remedies on a regular basis?

The use of warfarin or any of the heparin or heparinoid products poses obvious bleeding risks. Antiplatelet agents such as aspirin, cilostazol, clopidogrel, dipyridamole, ticlopidine, the traditional nonsteroidal anti-inflammatory drugs (NSAIDs), and the monoclonal antibody inhibitors directed against the platelet glycoprotein (GP)-IIb/IIIa complex, are of concern as well. Various "alternative medicines," including the Chinese black tree fungus and large quantities of garlic, vitamin E, vitamin C, and ginger, have also been associated with abnormalities of platelet function as manifested by a prolonged bleeding time and an increased risk for clinically significant bleeding.[20] Physicians and patients alike should be aware that certain antibiotics are notorious for their ability to affect the synthesis of the vitamin K–dependent clotting factors; cephazolin, levofloxacin, and trimethoprim/sulfamethoxazole are just a few examples of these. In addition, the penicillins, sulfonamides, and tricyclic antidepressants are among the medications associated with the development of factor VIII autoantibody inhibitors and the lupus-type anticoagulants. Finally, the use of iron supplements should be noted, as this may be related to a previous diagnosis of iron deficiency anemia produced by severe or chronic blood loss.

Have you noticed any unusual rashes or easy bruisability?

Petechiae, purpura, ecchymoses, and telangiectasias are often indicative of an underlying coagulopathy or vasculitis. The definition of "easy bruisability" is entirely subjective; both terms should therefore be qualified with and substantiated by objective physical findings (see Chapter 11). Suspicious lesions include those that develop spontaneously or with minimal trauma and those that are located over the torso rather than on the extensor surfaces of the extremities. If a patient develops a painful eschar while on warfarin, the possibility of warfarin-induced skin necrosis, a prothrombotic disorder associated with warfarin-induced deficiencies of protein C or protein S, should be considered. Of note, heparin-induced thrombocytopenia with resultant thrombosis may also be associated with severe skin manifestations, although these are typically more variable in nature.

Objective Findings on the Physical Examination

The physical examination of individuals with suspected coagulation disorders should concentrate on detecting gross evidence of bleeding and bruising. This evidence may be seen as petechiae, purpura, ecchymoses, sites of previous or active hemorrhage, or signs of hemarthrosis or hematoma. Table 2-4 summarizes the major clinical manifestations and correlative laboratory data for some of the more common acquired causes of bleeding, particularly in patients without a previous history of hemorrhagic complications. In addition, characteristic cutaneous findings may provide clues to an underlying defect in hemostasis. Examples of these include the following: the joint laxity, skin hyperelasticity, and "tissue paper-thin" scars typical of patients with Ehlers-Danlos syndrome; the follicular keratoses, perifollicular purpura with associated

---

Table 2-4 Acquired Causes of Bleeding in Ambulatory Patients

Diagnosis	Manifestation	Confirmation
Thrombocytopenia	Petechial bleeding	Platelet count <20,000/μL
Scurvy	Subcutaneous bleeding, especially in confluent sheets	Normal platelet count, dietary history
Acquired hemophilia	Soft tissue hemorrhage	Low factor VIII activity with factor VIII antibody; rarely, antibodies to factor V, XI, or XIII
Antibodies against factor II and/or V after use of "fibrin glue"	Soft tissue hemorrhage	History of recent use of "fibrin glue" prepared from bovine products; low levels of factors II and V with antibodies
Hyperfibrinolysis from acute promyelocytic leukemia (APL)	Multiple ecchymoses	Normal PT, PTT; often prolonged TT; low fibrinogen and plasminogen with elevated FSP; APL in marrow.
Amyloidosis	Soft tissue hemorrhage	Variable factor levels; fat pad biopsy for amyloid
Vitamin K deficiency	Soft tissue hemorrhage, hematuria	Dietary history; low factors II, VII, IX, and X levels; long PT, PTT; normal TT
Warfarin ingestion*†	Soft tissue hemorrhage, hematuria	Drug history; low factors II, VII, IX, and X levels; long PT, PTT; normal TT
Heparin administration*‡	Soft tissue hemorrhage	Long PTT; very long TT, heparin level
Factitious purpura	Bizarre pattern of lesions	Normal studies; psychological studies

*Inadvertent or surreptitious.
†Also caused by "superwarfarin" rodenticide exposure.
‡Rare cases of heparin production in systemic mastocytosis.
PT, prothrombin time; PTT, partial thromboplastin time; TT, thrombin time; FSP, fibrin split products.

"corkscrew hairs," and diffuse petechiae characteristic of patients with vitamin C deficiency and scurvy; the subcutaneous extravasation of blood, "loose-fitting skin," and loss of the subcutaneous fat pad seen in patients with senile purpura; the skin fragility and purplish striae (usually located on the flexor and extensor surfaces of the upper and lower extremities and on the torso) typical of patients with Cushing syndrome; and the macroglossia and non-thrombocytopenic purpura often seen in patients with systemic amyloidosis (see Chapter 11).

Petechiae measure less than 3 mm in diameter; purpura and ecchymoses are generally larger than 3 mm in diameter. These cutaneous lesions result from the rupture of venules, capillaries, or arterioles in the skin and may be related to a qualitative or quantitative platelet abnormality or vasculitis. Nonetheless, some bruising may occur in the absence of an increased risk of hemorrhage. Purpura simplex, a common and predominantly female phenomenon marked by excessive bruising in relation to menses; senile purpura, marked by the development of irregular, reddish-purple ecchymoses on the extensor surfaces of the upper extremities that result from decreased elasticity of blood vessels and subcutaneous fat with age; and psychogenic purpura, marked by bruises that repeatedly occur in areas accessible to the patient persist for months with denial of repeated trauma; they resolve only after the affected limb has been casted.

Telangiectasias, on the other hand, are blanching lesions that are frequently detected under the tongue and on the face, oral and nasal mucosa, vermilion borders of the lips, chest wall, shoulders, legs, and nail beds. These lesions may occur in association with (1) the normal aging process, (2) estrogen surges related to pregnancy or to the use of oral contraceptives or estrogen replacement therapy, (3) underlying liver disease, and (4) some of the collagen vascular diseases (e.g., the CREST syndrome, which is characterized by *c*alcinosis, *R*aynaud phenomenon, *e*sophageal disease, *s*clerodactyly, and *t*elangiectasias). Mucosal and visceral telangiectasias, on the other hand, are the hallmarks of Osler-Weber-Rendu syndrome (hereditary hemorrhagic telangiectasia) and serve as potential sources of bleeding, arteriovenous malformation, or aneurysm.

INTEGRATING PATIENT HISTORY AND PHYSICAL EXAMINATION FINDINGS WITH LABORATORY RESULTS

Basic Laboratory Evaluation of Coagulation and Hemostasis

No matter how comprehensive and careful the clinical assessment is in patients with bleeding manifestations, the findings are nonspecific. Furthermore, many disorders of coagulation are asymptomatic until the individual is surgically or traumatically challenged. Thus, information derived from the history and physical examination may increase clinical suspicion for a particular hemorrhagic disorder, but laboratory confirmation is required to define the specific defect and to develop a logical treatment or prophylactic strategy. Laboratory testing can also provide a risk assessment for potential bleeding tendencies and may offer insight into the pathophysiology of the clinical bleeding problem. Unfortunately, no validated assay is available to

Table 2-5 Basic Screening Tests for Patients with Hemorrhagic Complications

Automated complete blood cell count (with platelet count and mean platelet volume)
Peripheral blood smear review
Bleeding time or platelet function assay
Prothrombin time (PT)
Partial thromboplastin time (PTT)
Plasma clot solubility assay
Fibrin clot retraction assay

assess global hemostasis, which necessitates the performance of nonspecific test panels to examine each generic phase of hemostasis and coagulation (Table 2-5). These screening laboratory tests are readily available and typically are automated, so that results are provided in real time, which is critical for decision making. These tests can usually distinguish between the broad categories of primary hemostatic defects (i.e., platelet disorders) and humoral coagulation disorders (see Table 2-5). Subsequently, more specialized and esoteric assays may be selected to establish the definitive diagnosis (Table 2-6). Initial testing requires some combination of the following: a complete blood cell count (CBC) with platelet count; examination of the peripheral blood smear for platelet and erythrocyte morphology and platelet number and clumping; a bleeding time; PT; PTT; thrombin time; and fibrinogen concentration. Examples of laboratory profiles for some of the more frequently encountered hemorrhagic disorders are provided in Table 2-7.

Clinicians should bear in mind that proper sample acquisition and technique are critical to attaining valid results. Erroneous findings may result from simple avoidable mistakes, such as inadequate filling or mixing of the collection tubes. Most assays require a precise final ratio of whole blood (from which plasma for testing will be separated) to anticoagulant, and this relationship is imperative for accurate results. The plasma:anticoagulant ratio is also disturbed in polycythemia vera, where a markedly elevated red cell volume in the citrated collection tube concentrates the anticoagulant in a decreased plasma volume. This results in spuriously prolonged clot-based assays because the amount of citrate present in the plasma cannot be overcome and/or neutralized by the usual amounts of calcium contained in the standardized commercial recalcification

Table 2-6 Specific Laboratory Assays for Patients with Hemorrhagic Complications

For Suspected Platelet Disorders
Platelet aggregation studies
Bone marrow aspirate and biopsy
Platelet-associated immunoglobulin levels
Electron microscopy for platelet morphology

For Suspected Coagulation Factor Abnormalities
Mixing studies
Fibrinogen levels, D-dimer levels
Specific clotting factor levels
Bethesda assay (for coagulation factor inhibitors)
Thrombin time
Reptilase time
Euglobulin clot lysis assay
Molecular and immunologic fibrinogen assays

Table 2-7 Laboratory Profiles for Selected Disorders Associated with a Defect in Hemostasis

	Platelet Count	Platelet Size or Morphology	Bleeding Time	PT/INR	PTT	Plasma Clot Solubility Assay	Standard Platelet Aggregation Studies	Mixing Studies	Fibrinogen Levels	Thrombin Time	Euglobulin Clot Lysis Assay
Disseminated intravascular coagulation	↓	NL	(↑)	(↑)	(↑)	acc	N/I	(+)	(↓)	(↑)	(acc)
Idiopathic thrombocytopenic purpura	↓	abnl	(↑)	NL	NL	NL	N/I	N/I	NL	NL	NL
von Willebrand disease, type 2B	V	abnl	↑	NL	(↑)	NL	abnl*	+	NL	NL	N/I
von Willebrand disease, other	NL	NL	(↑)	NL	(↑)	NL	abnl*	+	NL	NL	N/I
Glanzmann thrombasthenia	NL	NL	↑	NL	NL	NL	abnl	N/I	NL	NL	N/I
Wiskott-Aldrich syndrome	↓	abnl	(↑)	NL	NL	NL	(abnl)	N/I	NL	NL	N/I
Bernard-Soulier syndrome	↓	abnl	↑	NL	NL	NL	abnl*	N/I	NL	NL	N/I
Gray platelet syndrome	↓	abnl	↑	NL	NL	NL	V	N/I	NL	NL	N/I
Afibrinogenemia/ hypofibrinogenemia	NL	NL	(↑)	↑	↑	NL	(abnl)	(+)	↓	↑	(acc)
Congenital dysfibrinogenemia	NL	NL	NL	(↑)	(↑)	NL	(NL)	−	(↓)	↑	acc
Ehlers-Danlos syndrome	NL	NL	(↑)	NL	NL	NL	(abnl)	N/I	NL	NL	NL

*Deficient platelet aggregation by ristocetin only, with normal aggregation to adenosine diphosphate, epinephrine, and collagen.
↑, increased; ↓, decreased; NL, normal laboratory value; abnl, abnormal laboratory test results in favor of the abnormality; V, results are variable; ( ), usually but not always; N/I, not indicated; acc, accelerated; +, corrects on mixing; −, does not correct on mixing.

reagents required to activate the coagulation process in vitro. This testing artefact may be circumvented by reducing the volume of citrate in the collecting tube by one half so that the whole blood/citrate ratio is approximately 19:1 (instead of 9:1). Another very common mistake in blood collection for coagulation testing occurs when whole blood is withdrawn from heparinized indwelling venous access devices and arterial catheters or from extremities in which intravenous fluids are actively running. Finally, for accurate results, the integrity of the blood specimen must be fastidiously maintained for coagulation testing. This includes constant low temperatures to prevent activation of the serine proteases, which can inactivate coagulation proteins, and reduced time of plasma contact with platelets in whole blood and with the wall of the siliconized collection tubes, because factor XII can be activated in vitro which subsequently may result in spuriously activated downstream clotting factors on screening and specific clotting factor assays. Similarly, the phospholipid proteins, which are made up of lupus anticoagulants, may become adsorbed to platelets over time and yield falsely normal PTTs. These artefacts are extremely problematic in today's climate of "send outs" for laboratory testing, instead of rapid processing of plasma and testing on fresh plasma in a specialized coagulation laboratory within a few hours. If the clinician is skeptical about the results from "send out" samples, particularly when they do not support clinical suspicions, these should be repeated in a specialized coagulation laboratory that can maintain the integrity of the specimen.

Basic Laboratory Tests to Distinguish Between Platelet and Coagulation Defects

Physiologic hemostasis is initiated when platelets encounter a breach in the microvasculature at the site of injury. Circulating platelets come into contact with VWF protein bound to collagen exposed in the subendothelial matrix, first through rheologically sensitive, high-affinity interactions of the platelet surface membrane GP-Ib-IX (integrin $\alpha_2\beta_1$) to VWF, and then by a low-affinity interaction with collagen itself that is mediated by GP-VI. These events trigger a series of cytoplasmic reactions that ultimately result in platelet activation with thromboxane A_2 generation and the transformation of platelet surface membrane GP-IIb/IIIa into an active receptor for VWF and fibrinogen (see Chapter 7). Subsequently, these activated platelets aggregate and recruit other circulating platelets in the environment to form a platelet plug that is mediated by fibrinogen and VWF crosslinking. Humoral coagulation can then proceed with the use of exposed phospholipids on the surfaces of activated platelets as a stable template. Thus, coagulation is localized at sites of vessel injury.

A platelet abnormality should be suspected in patients with a history of intraoperative or immediate postoperative hemorrhagic complications, frequent mucosal bleeds in the absence of known trauma, and/or frequent petechiae. Quantitative platelet abnormalities are immediately apparent once an automated blood cell count has been performed and the patient's peripheral blood smear has been reviewed. Platelet concentration is measured electronically with the use of instruments that detect cells through their effects on electrical impedance or light scatter. Thrombocytopenia, defined as a platelet count of less than 150,000/μL,

should be confirmed by direct observation to exclude the laboratory phenomenon of pseudothrombocytopenia, in which platelet clumping occurs in vitro in a temperature- and time-dependent manner in the presence of ethylenediaminetetraacetic acid (EDTA); the mean platelet volume (MPV) is therefore increased because the clumps of platelets are "sized" as single platelets as they pass through the apertures of automated cell counters. Repeat platelet counts in freshly collected, citrate-anticoagulated whole blood should provide substantially higher, more accurate values because platelet agglutination in pseudothrombocytopenia typically results from the chelation of calcium ions by the standard EDTA anticoagulant. Phase or manual platelet counts should also reveal more accurate platelet counts because the actual platelet count may be ascertained visually, whether or not clumping is present.

Finally, platelet size and morphology may help to differentiate between peripheral platelet destruction (which is marked by a higher MPV and an increase in platelet size) and decreased bone marrow production. Morphologic evaluation of the peripheral smear is critical when platelet counts are decreased or increased. For instance, thrombocytopenia in the presence of so-called helmet cells or schistocytes may alert the clinician to the possibility of a microangiopathic hemolytic process and thrombotic thrombocytopenic purpura (TTP) (see Chapter 24). Bleeding associated with marked thrombocytosis characterized by giant forms may suggest essential thrombocythemia with acquired VWD. Morphologic examination may also distinguish between various congenital causes of thrombocytopenia: the gray, vacuolated platelets seen in α-granule deficiency; the basophilic cytoplasmic inclusion bodies (Döhle bodies) found in the granulocytes of patients with the May-Hegglin anomaly; the microplatelets characteristic of Wiskott-Aldrich syndrome; and the massively giant circulating platelets associated with Mediterranean megathrombocytopenia are only a few examples (see Chapter 10).

Platelet counts may be obtained through manual methods, on the basis of direct visualization of platelets under phase contrast microscopy and a stained peripheral smear, or by automated multiparameter systems, which provide quantitative and qualitative information on all circulating cellular elements. Although direct visualization methods may also be helpful for the morphologic evaluation of platelets, they are most often reserved for assessment after abnormal platelet counts have been generated by automated, rapid, high-throughput screening methods. Automated platelet counting has traditionally been based on electrical impedance principles and is accurate for most clinical samples; however, impedance techniques may yield spurious results in severe thrombocytopenia or thrombocytosis. The former is illustrated by such pathologic states as TTP, idiopathic thrombocytopenic purpura (ITP), and hemolytic disease with considerable erythrocyte fragmentation. Essentially, cellular debris and fragments may be counted as platelets, resulting in overestimation of the platelet count. In contrast, impedance counting may exclude very large platelets (e.g., Bernard-Soulier syndrome, Mediterranean megathrombocytopenia syndrome, myeloproliferative diseases) and may yield spuriously low counts. The problems of counting imprecision in the low thrombocytopenic range appear to be minimized by the use of direct or indirect immunologic counting methods with monoclonal antibodies such as CD61 (GP-IIIa) in an automated hematology blood-analyzer system (Cell-Dyn 4000; Abbott Diagnostics, Maidenhead, Berkshire, UK), or integrated into a flow cytometry–based counting method with or without a platelet-specific monoclonal antibody such as CD41a (GP-IIb).

If concomitant macrocytic anemia is noted, red blood cell folate levels and serum vitamin B_{12} levels should be checked to exclude the possibility of megaloblastic anemia. If evidence of intravascular hemolysis (e.g., clinical icterus, low serum haptoglobin, reticulocytosis, hemoglobinuria, detection of urinary hemosiderin) accompanies thrombocytopenia, paroxysmal nocturnal hemoglobinuria (PNH) should be considered with or without evidence of systemic hypercoagulability. The sucrose hemolysis test and the Ham test have been supplanted by the more specific and sensitive flow cytometry of peripheral blood to assess for specific erythrocyte membrane protein deficiencies in CD59 (the membrane inhibitor of reactive lysis [MIRL]) and CD55 (the *decay accelerating factor* [DAF]).

If a patient's clinical picture is consistent with a defect in primary hemostasis, and platelet count is within normal limits, a qualitative platelet abnormality should be excluded. The severity of bleeding complications among patients with qualitative disorders typically is out of proportion to the platelet count. Congenital thrombasthenias are very rare in the absence of a family history. Acquired defects in platelet function are considerably more common and frequently are medication induced (e.g., aspirin, NSAIDs, selective serotonin reuptake inhibitors [SSRIs]).

Bleeding time (BT) is the traditional initial test for detecting and evaluating primary hemostasis. In general, it allows for a gross indication of overall platelet function and of the activity of those plasma proteins involved in the interaction between platelets and the subendothelial matrix (e.g., collagen and VWF). Since its initial development, the BT has been purported as a clinically useful tool for diagnosing qualitative platelet disorders, predicting significant bleeding propensity due to platelet dysfunction, and evaluating the adequacy of treatment modalities to reverse the bleeding potential. Unfortunately, the BT has exhibited shortcomings in all of these aspects of its use because it is affected by a large number of diseases, drugs, physiologic factors, test conditions, and therapeutic actions—not all of them platelet related.[21] For example, BTs increased significantly after the removal of 2 U of red blood cells (RBCs) from normal individuals who had not taken medications that would affect platelet function; their prolonged BTs decreased significantly after RBCs were reinfused.[22] In patients with VWD who underwent surgical procedures, the extent of decrease in prolonged BT after VWF replacement therapy frequently did not correlate with achieving or maintaining normal hemostasis or with the amount of bleeding observed during surgery.[23] Furthermore, serial measurement of BTs in patients with VWD may yield considerable intraindividual variability. In any case, the BT remains a widely used screening test for the diagnosis of VWD. BT measurements in individuals with VWD and thrombasthenia are not necessary or helpful after the diagnosis has been established.

BT is usually normal when platelet counts are higher than 100,000/μL, and it is usually prolonged proportionately as platelet counts decrease from 100,000/μL to 10,000/μL. In autoimmune thrombocytopenic purpura, however, BT may remain normal despite a significant quantitative deficiency. This may reflect the fact that younger platelets are larger, contain a higher concentration of procoagulant proteins within their cytoplasmic granules, and are "more active" in their capacity to adhere to areas of damaged endothelium and to aggregate with other platelets to form a localized platelet plug.

BT is most frequently performed with the Ivy or Simplate II (BioControl, Bellevue, Wash, USA) method. With a blood pressure cuff inflated on the upper arm to maintain a consistent pressure of 40 mm Hg, the Ivy BT is determined after three puncture wounds are made with a sterile mechanical lancet (blade depth, 2.5 mm) on the ventral surface of the forearm, versus two incisions for the Simplate II technique with a standardized spring-loaded razor blade device (blade depth, 1 mm). Randomized, controlled studies show no significant differences between BT methods or results produced by incisions made horizontal to the antecubital crease and those made vertical/perpendicular to it, although better scar formation may be associated with the latter direction.[24] Filter paper is used to blot the blood at 15- to 30-second intervals, with care taken not to disturb the wounds. A stopwatch records the time taken to reach the end point, defined as the average time for bleeding to cease from all wounds, which presumably corresponds to the time required for formation of a hemostatic platelet plug. "Normal" bleeding time ranges between 2 and 9 minutes, depending on the technique used. The reproducibility and validity of BT results are determined most often by operator-dependent variables, such as depth of the puncture wounds made, the ability to maintain a constant venous blood pressure throughout the procedure, and the fastidiousness of filter paper blotting. The Duke bleeding time, first described in 1910, involves a prick or incision of the earlobe.[25] Because of its comparative imprecision and poor reproducibility, it is rarely used. Attempts to increase the sensitivity of BTs have proved impractical. An example of this was a technique called hemorrhagometry, which measured bleeding intensity and blood volume lost from a small standardized BT skin wound.[26]

Because of the vagaries associated with BT techniques, standardized, automated techniques have been designed to examine and simulate the platelet contribution to primary hemostasis in a more specific manner. The Platelet Function Analyzer (PFA)-100 (Dade-Behring, Marburg, Germany) has been developed as an automated, rapid technique designed to assess platelet adhesion and aggregation. In many hospitals, it has replaced BT as the predominant assessment tool used to screen patients for their bleeding potential. The PFA-100 measures the ability of platelets activated in a high-shear environment to occlude an aperture in a membrane treated with collagen and epinephrine (CEPI) or collagen and adenosine diphosphate (CADP). The time taken for flow across the membrane to stop (closure time) is recorded.[27] Data from a small selected cohort revealed that BTs and PFA-100 were in agreement in 74.3% of patients, and that the PFA-100 was particularly more sensitive than the BT to aspirin-induced platelet dysfunction.[28] The sensitivity of the PFA-100 for identification of VWD appears significantly better ($P < .01$) than that of BT, with similar specificity. In contrast, the PFA-100 was comparable but not superior to BT in detecting congenital or acquired platelet hypofunction.[29]

In a prospective attempt to identify individuals with documented hereditary mucocutaneous hemorrhagic disorders, the BT and PFA-100 assays were equally insensitive (BT prolonged in 35.8% of all patients vs 29.7% for PFA-100 [$P = .23$]).[30] In patients with VWD, the PFA-100 performed slightly better (BT increased in 42% vs 61.5% for PFA-100 [$P = .18$]), whereas the opposite was observed for platelet secretion defects (BT increased in 42% vs 24% [$P = .11$]). In the group with undefined qualitative platelet defects, both tests lost sensitivity, but the BT detected 1.8 times more patients than were identified with the PFA-100 (BT increased in 27.5% vs 15% [$P = .06$]). On the basis of the published literature, the Platelet Physiology Subcommittee of the Scientific and Standardization Committee of the International Society on Thrombosis and Haemostasis determined that the PFA-100 does not have sufficient sensitivity or specificity to be used as a routine screening tool to detect platelet disorders or to monitor the efficacy of any therapeutic strategy.[31]

Platelet aggregation assays are the in vitro approaches most commonly used to assess platelet function. They focus on the later aspects of primary hemostasis, when platelets are stimulated to generate thromboxane A_2, and they release their α granule and dense body constituents to recruit other platelets to "plug up" the bleeding site within a blood vessel (Fig. 2-1). This platelet plug serves as the template on which humoral coagulation can proceed. Although readily accessible in most comprehensive coagulation laboratories, aggregometry is very time consuming and labor intensive, and preanalytical preparation, choice of anticoagulant, and agonists have not been standardized. Agonists are added to platelet-rich plasma isolated from the patient's whole blood under controlled conditions of temperature and constant agitation. Platelets are stimulated to aggregate in vitro, and the extent of aggregation is quantitated as the increase in light transmission through a cuvette containing the originally turbid, untreated platelet-rich plasma. By convention, platelet-rich plasma has 0% light transmission and platelet-free plasma has 100% light transmission when compared with normal controls. The agonists typically used in platelet aggregation studies include ADP, epinephrine, and collagen (Fig. 2-2); arachidonic acid may be used to exclude the surreptitious ingestion of aspirin or NSAIDs as the underlying cause of abnormal, suboptimal platelet aggregation responses to standard agonists. High and low concentrations of ristocetin induce platelet agglutination (RIPA), as opposed to platelet aggregation, and help to differentiate among the classic type and variants of VWD (see Chapter 7). Bernard-Soulier syndrome, which is characterized by a suboptimal agglutination response to ristocetin, may also be diagnosed (see Chapter 10).

Normal responses in standard platelet aggregation assays will exclude most qualitative platelet defects as the primary cause of easy bruisability or abnormal bleeding, but mild VWD can remain a possibility. Platelet aggregation studies may be performed in the absence of an in vitro agonist to determine whether any evidence of spontaneous platelet hyperaggregability is present; this is apparent in some cases of essential thrombocythemia[32] and in Kawasaki disease.[33]

Other modifications of routine platelet aggregation techniques are intended to enhance the sensitivity of the assay. For instance, radiolabeled ^{14}C-serotonin–"loaded" donor platelets isolated from normal platelet-rich plasma may be activated by various agonists, and the release of the isotope

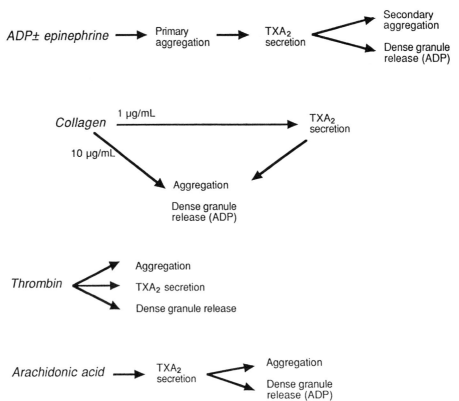

Figure 2-1 Platelet reaction in response to commonly used agonists. TXA$_2$, thromboxane A$_2$.

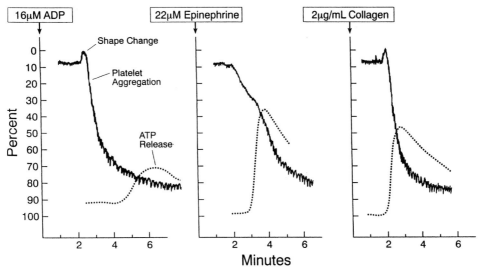

Figure 2-2 Platelet aggregation and adenosine triphosphate (ATP) release in response to adenosine diphosphate (ADP), epinephrine, and collagen. Primary and secondary waves of ADP-induced aggregation *(left panel)* are merged, but the secondary wave can be recognized by the ATP release. Two waves are distinguishable with epinephrine *(middle panel)*; ATP release coincides with the second wave. With collagen *(right panel)*, only one wave of aggregation occurs, and this appears simultaneously with ATP release. Shape change is induced by ADP and collagen but not by epinephrine.

from dense granules can be quantitated. Heparin-induced thrombocytopenia (HIT) may be diagnosed by the detection of >20% release of ^{14}C-serotonin from "loaded" platelets incubated with patient heat-treated serum in the presence of unfractionated heparin. Whole blood impedance lumi-aggregometry, which measures chemiluminescence-based platelet activation, aggregation, and adenosine triphosphate (ATP) release from dense granules, remains to be validated in its ability to predict clinical bleeding or thrombotic propensity (see Chapter 10).

Similarly, methods used to assess the vague clinical condition referred to as "aspirin resistance" remain to be correlated with the occurrence of myocardial infarction, stroke, or death from vascular events. Three assays have been approved by the U.S. Food and Drug Administration to specifically detect aspirin resistance; these are based on assessment of platelet cyclo-oxygenase enzyme pathway activity. Increased urinary excretion of 11-dehydro-thromboxane B_2 (indirect measurement of thromboxane A_2 activity in vivo) (AspirinWorks; Corgenix, Broomfield, Colo, USA) has been associated with increased cardiovascular event rates in a retrospective case-controlled study.[34] Aspirin resistance measured by the PFA-100 apparatus, with the use of CEPI cartridge closure time, has not gained favor because of its weak correlation with the occurrence of clinical cardiovascular and cerebrovascular events.[35] The VerifyNow Aspirin Assay (Accumetrics, San Diego, Calif, USA) detects aspirin resistance in terms of increased whole blood platelet agglutination on fibrinogen-coated beads after addition of an arachidonic acid agonist. Assay results correlated with significantly increased levels of serum cardiac enzymes as surrogate markers of cardiovascular events after percutaneous coronary interventions in the context of aspirin therapy.[36] Additional studies are needed to validate these assays in randomized, prospectively controlled studies of treatment strategies designed to reverse aspirin resistance.

Laboratory Assessment of the Procoagulant System

PT is an ex vivo coagulation assay performed by adding a commercial source of tissue factor (TF) and calcium to patient citrate-anticoagulated plasma. Time to clot formation reflects the activities of the coagulation factor proteins involved in the common and extrinsic pathways of coagulation factors II, V, VII, and X, as well as fibrinogen. Prolongation of PT correlates with the degree of deficiency of one or more of these procoagulant proteins, or with the extent of neutralization of their function, by circulating inhibitors in a specific (alloantibodies) or nonspecific (e.g., lupus anticoagulant, heparin, argatroban, hirudin) manner. Commercially available agents most often used to activate the clotting process in PT consist of standardized mixtures of tissue factor/thromboplastin (extracted from rabbit brain) and calcium chloride; however, preparations of recombinant human tissue factor mixed with synthetic phospholipids are becoming more popular because they are free of the contaminating coagulation factor proteins present in tissue factor extracts. This increases the sensitivity of the PT assay for factor deficiencies. Ox brain extracts of tissue factor/thromboplastin may be particularly useful in the detection of the rare congenital coagulopathy, variant factor VII Padua.[37]

Because numerous tissue factor/thromboplastin reagents possess various procoagulant properties, PT results may vary widely from one laboratory to another—even for the same plasma specimen. Thus, PTs are reported as an international normalized ratio (INR), which was developed to minimize these differences when patients are anticoagulated with warfarin. This conversion allows for warfarin dosing to be reliably adjusted, regardless of where the PT assay is performed. Each thromboplastin reagent has an assigned international sensitivity index (ISI) that is derived by comparing its prothrombotic potential against an international reference standard thromboplastin (with an ISI defined as 1.0) from the World Health Organization. The INR is calculated as the ratio of the patient's PT to the mean normal PT obtained from pooled normal plasma, which is then raised to the ISI as an exponential power: INR = (patient's PT/mean normal PT)^{ISI}. The ISI of recombinant tissue factor–activating reagents is approximately 1.0. Low-ISI thromboplastins improve the sensitivity of the PT assay. Although the INR is employed in the safety monitoring and efficacy evaluations of anticoagulation with warfarin, it has *not* been a useful predictor of potential bleeding complications in patients with liver disease or congenital coagulopathy in the common or extrinsic pathways. In the presence of lupus anticoagulants, or when direct thrombin inhibitor (DTI) anticoagulants (such as argatroban and hirudin) are administered, PT may be increased but does not accurately reflect the actual degree of anticoagulation. In these situations, chromogenic measurements of factors X and II may be more predictive of hemorrhagic potential.

The PTT estimates the activities of the coagulation factor proteins involved in the common and intrinsic pathways of coagulation—factors V, X, II, VIII, IX, XI, and XII, along with fibrinogen, prekallikrein, and high molecular weight kininogen. The addition of phospholipids (variable ratios of phosphatidylserine and phosphatidylinositol), a phospholipid surface activator (kaolin, silica, or ellagic acid), and calcium to citrate-anticoagulated plasma triggers clot formation. Clotting factor activity levels must be decreased to at least 40% of normal if the PTT is to become prolonged. In addition, a deficiency of prekallikrein, which is one of the components of the contact phase of coagulation, results in a prolonged PTT that can be corrected with the extended incubation of the patient's plasma with an exogenous source of phospholipid and contact activator at 37°C prior to recalcification. Of note, deficiencies of factor XII, prekallikrein, and/or high molecular weight kininogen are not associated with a bleeding diathesis, despite the fact that they are associated with extreme prolongations of the PTT. Lupus anticoagulants, unfractionated (but not low molecular weight) heparin, long-term warfarin therapy, DTIs, and specific (alloantibodies or autoantibodies) neutralizing inhibitors of coagulation proteins prolong the PTT. The ability to correct prolonged PTT by mixing equal volumes of patient plasma with pooled normal plasma over 1 to 2 hours at 37°C indicates a clotting factor deficiency, which can then be identified with the use of assays and specific clotting factor–deficient substrates. If the prolonged PTT does not correct with mixing studies, then an acquired inhibitor—pharmacologic or immunologic in origin—must be considered. Alloantibodies or antibodies against factor VIII require 1 to 2 hours incubation at 37°C before they are maximally expressed in mixing studies; thus, the time 0 PTT mixing study may be normal. In contrast, the lupus anticoagulant mixing study will produce a prolonged PTT, which does not substantially increase with incubation. This distinction is critical to proper diagnosis and treatment of prolonged PTTs.

When 1:1 mixing studies of patient and normal plasma show normalization of prolonged PT and/or PTT in patient plasma specimens after 0, 60, and 120 minutes of incubation at 37°C, the presence of one or more coagulation factor deficiency(ies) is the most likely cause and should be confirmed by quantitation of specific clotting

factor protein activities. The choice as to which specific clotting factor assays should be performed is determined by whether one or both of these screening assays is prolonged, and whether the deficiency lies in the extrinsic (abnormal PT and normal PTT: measure factor VII), intrinsic (prolonged PTT and normal PT: measure factors XII, XI, IX, and VIII), or common pathways (prolonged PTT and PT: measure fibrinogen and factors II, V, X initially, and then, because of the possibility of multiple factor deficiencies, measure other vitamin K–dependent factors VII and IX, and subsequently factors XI and XII) (see Chapter 5).

Accordingly, many causes of prolongation of the PTT have been proposed. Some of these causes are of hemostatic importance, and others are not. No correlation has been made between the degree of prolongation of the PTT and hemorrhagic potential; rather, it is the cause of the prolongation that determines the risk. A prolongation of 20 seconds due to lupus anticoagulant (LA) is of no hemorrhagic risk, but an 8-second prolongation due to mild hemophilia A with 8% factor VIII activity represents extreme risk for bleeding with a surgical procedure. The PTT is frequently ordered so clinicians can prognosticate about whether a given patient will bleed or not—a question the PTT was never designed to do.[38]

Specific clotting factor assays are performed by mixing patient plasma with "substrate" plasma that is deficient in the specific clotting factor to be measured. This substrate plasma may be obtained directly from individuals with a severe deficiency of that particular clotting factor, or it can be prepared commercially by rendering normal plasma deficient of a particular clotting factor through immunodepletion techniques. Specific assays performed to quantitate factors VIII, IX, XI, and XII are one-stage PTT-based assays; those for factors VII, X, and II are PT based. The activity of the specific clotting factor protein in patient plasma is determined on a standard curve in which the times (in seconds) required for various dilutions of normal plasma (presumed by convention to contain 100% activity of the specific clotting factor in question prior to dilution with physiologic buffer) to clot are plotted against the actual clotting factor activity levels of diluted normal plasma.

Specific clotting factor assays can also be measured with the use of chromogenic factor assays and immunoassays (antigen assays). Chromogenic assays are based on the principle that the thrombin or factor Xa generated after activation of the specific clotting factors in question can be measured directly by the ability of thrombin or Xa to proteolyze specific commercially available chromogenic substrates. The chromogenic substrates are complexed to a dye (p-nitroaniline) via an amide bond. When thrombin or factor Xa proteolyzes the substrate, the dye is released (amidolytic reaction) and is measured spectrophotometrically. These assays are more sensitive than clotting time–based assays and are not interfered with by LAs. Because of their increased cost per assay, they have not yet pervaded most of the coagulation laboratories in the United States.

Shortened PTTs and PTs have little clinical significance and probably reflect elevated FVIII activity levels or other clotting factors activated as a result of DIC or the presence of pregnancy (and its complications), use of estrogen hormones, active or occult thrombosis, carcinoma, or infection. The risk of developing venous thromboembolic complications is increased by high levels of factors II, VIII, and XI, which are often determined by genetic polymorphisms (see Chapter 14). The use of prophylactic anticoagulants is not routinely recommended for those individuals with shortened PTs and PTTs in the absence of active or previous thrombosis.

Thrombin time (TT) (also known as thrombin clotting time [TCT]) is a very simple, underused, yet instructive assay that measures only the rate of conversion of fibrinogen to polymerized fibrin after the addition of a known amount of thrombin to platelet-poor plasma. A prolonged TT suggests the presence of heparin or pharmacologic DTIs (e.g., argatroban or lepirudin); greatly decreased fibrinogen levels, hypofibrinogenemia, or dysfibrinogenemias; high concentrations of immunoglobulins, particularly large monoclonal gammopathies, such as those seen in Waldenström macroglobulinemia; and the generation of fibrin degradation products. Because of its extreme sensitivity to even small amounts of unfractionated heparin, the TT is a useful screening test for excluding the presence of contaminating heparin in blood samples obtained from central venous access devices, which may spuriously alter PTT results. Rarely, but more and more often, acquired specific thrombin inhibitors (with or without concurrent factor V inhibitors) may develop in patients who have been exposed to topical bovine thrombin, particularly during cardiac or spinal surgery (see Chapter 6).

Fibrinogen concentrations are routinely measured in platelet-poor plasma to ascertain sufficient substrate for generated thrombin to form the fibrin clot end point necessary for chronometric clotting assays used for PT, PTT, TT, and specific clotting factor assays. Decreased fibrinogen concentrations should be complemented by the measurement of fibrinogen mass performed through an immunologic or chemical method. When a discrepancy of greater than 25% to 30% is detected between the lower fibrinogen concentration when measured as functional protein and the higher fibrinogen concentration when measured as immunologically detectable protein, a dysfibrinogenemia should be suspected. The definitive diagnosis is based on the identification of a specific structural or molecular defect: (1) confirmation of the abnormal fibrinogen structure using sodium dodecyl sulfate (SDS) polyacrylimide gel electrophoresis; (2) evaluation of abnormal fibrinopeptide cleavage and release, as well as of abnormal fibrin polymerization; and (3) detailed analysis of the mutation site in the fibrinogen DNA and the fibrinogen gene product. It is important to note that structure/function relationships in the congenital dysfibrinogenemias remain unclear and have no established means by which to predict whether or not the abnormal fibrinogen protein will be associated with hypercoagulability or with a bleeding diathesis, poor wound healing, and/or recurrent spontaneous miscarriages (see Chapter 5).

Tests for Lupus Anticoagulants (LA)

When mixing studies indicate the persistence of a prolonged PTT, the presence of an LA should be confirmed with assays that show that the antibody is directed against the phospholipid component of coagulation. Because PTT is routinely performed on platelet-free plasma, phospholipids (in the form of platelets) to accelerate the clotting system are extremely limiting, so that LA antibodies are rather easily detected. This is illustrated by the platelet neutralization assay, in which a lysate of normal platelets, serving as a copious source of phospholipids, is incubated with patient plasma to determine whether the initially prolonged PTT will be normalized. If this correction occurs, it is presumed that the LA antibody has been absorbed out of the test plasma. Other inhibitors of coagulation, such as heparin or acquired autoantibodies directed against specific clotting factors, would not be absorbed from plasma by phospholipids. A simplified commercial modification of the platelet neutralization assay involves incubating hexagonal phase phospholipids with patient plasma and showing decreased prolongation of the PTT toward normal—characteristic of the interaction between an LA and lipid.

In many coagulation laboratories, LA are diagnosed in patient plasma specimens with the use of clotting assays that detect interference with formation of the prothrombinase complex. The dilute Russell's viper venom test (DRVVT) is based on the activation of factor X to Xa to initiate coagulation without contributions from any of the other coagulation factor proteins proximal to the tenase complex. This is accomplished by the highly lapidated proteolytic venom extracted from the *Vipera russelli pulchella* and *Vipera russelli siamensis* snakes found along the Indian-Pakistani border, peninsular India, Sri Lanka, Myanmar, and Taiwan. When lipidated venom is diluted to yield a clotting time of 23 to 27 seconds, the assay becomes extremely sensitive to antibodies directed against the diluted phospholipid concentration. A prolonged DRVVT in patient plasma suggests the presence of LA, which should be confirmed through one of the other LA assays. The DRVVT test is considered more sensitive than the PTT for the detection of LA.

Kaolin is a negatively charged particulate activator of the intrinsic clotting pathway. The kaolin clotting time (KCT) is sensitive to LA because clotting is activated in the absence of exogenously added phospholipids to the patient plasma test system. A prolonged KCT is considered sensitive but nonspecifically indicative of an LA.

The diagnosis of LA requires at least two confirmatory tests. In addition, because of LA interaction with phospholipids, freshly obtained citrated whole blood specimens should be double-centrifuged and fastidiously handled before freezing; thawed plasma may contain enough platelets/platelet fragments with phospholipids to adsorb and squelch the lipophilic antibody, resulting in a false-negative test for LA and a normal PTT screening assay.

The possibility of factor XIII (FXIII) deficiency or α_2-plasmin inhibitor (α_2-PI) (also known as α_2-antiplasmin [α_2-AP]) deficiency should be excluded when all of the basic screening tests are unremarkable and clinical suspicion for a bleeding diathesis still remains. Factor XIII is a fibrin-stabilizing factor that functions through the covalent cross-linking of fibrin strands in the presence of calcium and thrombin. α_2-PI, on the other hand, functions by controlling lysis of the fibrin plug through the regulation of plasmin activity. As such, neither qualitative nor quantitative defects in factor XIII or α_2-PI may be detected by the standard assays used to evaluate clot formation, including PT and PTT (see Chapter 5).

The plasma clot solubility assay serves as a screening assay for factor XIII deficiency. Under normal conditions, the addition of 1% monochloracetic acid or 5M urea does not result in dissolution of a formed clot. If factor XIII activity level is less than 1%, the fibrin clot rapidly dissolves in the presence of monochloracetic acid, or 5M urea. Because α_2-PI deficiency may also be associated with increased urea clot solubility, α_2-PI activity and antigen levels should be directly assessed to confirm the cause of the increased clot solubility, particularly given that both inherited deficiencies are exceedingly rare. In contrast, acquired decreases in α_2-PI activity levels may develop as the result of consumptive hypercoagulable states, such as DIC. Activity levels below 30% of normal have been predictive of bleeding complications in patients with acute promyelocytic leukemia (APL). The propensity toward increased bleeding and the laboratory evidence of hyperfibrinolysis in APL may be reversed by administration of inhibitors of fibrinolysis, such as ε-aminocaproic acid.[39]

Increased levels of plasmin:antiplasmin complexes (PAP), measured in patient plasma by commercially available enzyme-linked sandwich immunoassay kits, are surrogate indicators of hypercoagulability and reflect the effects of increased thrombin generation/fibrin formation and associated increased reactive plasminemia and endogenous fibrinolytic activity.

Euglobulin clot lysis time (ECLT) assay, a global measurement of fibrinolytic activity, is the net result of interaction between plasminogen and plasminogen activator inhibitor (PAI)-1 in whole blood or plasma. Clot lysis in this assay system is usually completed within 2 to 6 hours, and accelerated lysis (< 2 hours; i.e., one of the few examples of a shortened time on a coagulation test that indicates hemorrhagic potential) is indicative of increased fibrinolysis, such as occurs in the rare condition of primary hyperfibrinolysis. ECLT is usually normal in early DIC; it becomes accelerated when endogenous plasminogen activator inhibitor type 1, α_2-PI, or fibrinogen has been consumed. Other disease states associated with accelerated ECLT include cirrhosis, prostate cancer, and thrombotic states (e.g., acute myocardial infarction) that have been treated with thrombolytic agents, such as urokinase and recombinant tissue plasminogen activator. Vigorous exercise and increasing age are also associated with increased fibrinolysis and reduced ECLT. Reduced ECLT may precipitate or exacerbate clinical bleeding. Clinical states characterized by impaired fibrinolysis prolong the ECLT assay and include arterial (transient ischemic attack [TIA], cerebrovascular accident [CVA], and myocardial infarction [MI]) and venous thrombotic events (e.g., superficial and deep venous thrombosis, pulmonary embolism [PE]), advanced atherosclerosis, acute coronary syndrome, diabetes mellitus, and hypertriglyceridemia. Impaired fibrinolysis and prolonged ECLT assays reflect the presence of increased levels of plasminogen activator inhibitor type 1 and α_2-PI or decreased levels of tissue plasminogen activator or plasminogen. Dysfibrinogens have been associated with both accelerated and prolonged ECLT assays, depending on their effects on plasminogen activation, their susceptibility to plasmin degradation, and their propensity to impair fibrin assembly and factor XIII–mediated crosslinking. Traditional ECLT is a time and labor intensive assay that is not performed widely. Newer automated assays may overcome the resistance of coagulation laboratories to make this test available.[40]

Measurement of D-dimers detects the plasmin-degraded by-product of crosslinked fibrin that is indicative of thrombin generation, factor XIII activation and crosslinking of the fibrin clot, and reactive fibrinolysis. Because fibrinogen does not contain any crosslinked entities, this assay is useful in discriminating between fibrinolysis and fibrinogenolysis. Specific monoclonal antibodies are commercially available for use in measuring D-dimers in patient citrated plasma samples; these have been included in latex agglutination, immunoturbidimetric, and enzyme-linked immunosorbent assay (ELISA) assays. Latex agglutination assays are less sensitive than other assays techniques for detecting D-dimers in critical clinical situations, such as deep venous thrombosis and PE. These latter assays have a sensitivity greater than 90%, and a negative test for D-dimers carries a negative predictive value greater than 90% for the existence of venous thromboembolism (VTE). D-Dimers may be positive in a number of clinical conditions associated with inflammation and activation of the coagulation system; however, in this context, a positive value may be too nonspecific to establish clinical diagnoses. For example, D-dimers may be elevated in association with malignancies, obstetric catastrophes (e.g., HELLP [Hemolysis, Elevated Liver function tests, and Low Platelets syndrome], preeclampsia), DIC, sickle cell crisis, rheumatoid arthritis, subarachnoid hemorrhage, acute aortic dissection, and cirrhosis (www.pathology.vcu.edu/clinical/coag/D-Dimer.pdf).

The "holy grail" of the future for laboratory diagnoses of bleeding and thrombophilic disorders is the development of a single assay that could discern each of the elements of coagulation and could predict whether abnormalities detected by the assay would produce clinical bleeding or thrombotic complications. Furthermore, these assays should be useful for monitoring the effects of pharmacologic interventions and showing the reversal of thrombotic or hemorrhagic tendencies. To date, no automated system fulfills these desires or prerequisites. We have already described assays that have been developed to substitute for current techniques to assess platelet function. The thromboelastogram (TEG) and its modifications provide an automated measurement of interactive dynamic coagulation processes, starting with initial hemostasis and proceeding through humoral coagulation, clot crosslinking, and fibrinolysis.[41] TEG has been particularly helpful in monitoring liver transplantation–related bleeding problems and has been used to minimize transfusion requirements in cardiovascular surgeries. Numerous investigations are under way to determine whether TEG would be useful in monitoring therapeutic interventions, such as ensuring the adequacy of dosing of recombinant factor VIIa concentrate for bleeding problems or determining the adequacy of low molecular weight heparin dosing for preventing hypercoagulable complications. Although study results show class effects and epidemiologic effects, TEG remains too insensitive for use in predicting the occurrence of bleeding or clotting events in an individual patient. The technique does, however, provide valuable insight into the pathophysiology of bleeding and clotting complications observed in a variety of clinical situations. Thus far, TEG has yet to be accepted as part of a routine hematologic evaluation of coagulation status in a variety of perioperative and critical care settings.[41]

Similarly, automated fluorogenic substrate–based techniques designed to measure endogenous thrombin potential

(ETP) are currently being developed. These assays quantify the enzymatic "work" that thrombin can accomplish over time[42] and await clinical validation for the individual patient rather than for clinical disease scenarios in general. For example, all anticoagulants and antiplatelet aggregation medications reduce ETP; however, various individuals with reduced ETP continue to develop thromboses. Such assays have also been used to predict the likelihood of recurrence of VTE in high-risk populations. After 4 years, the probability of recurrent VTE was 6.5% among individuals with a thrombin generation of less than 400 nM compared with 20% recurrence among patients with higher values ($P < .001$). Conversely, those with thrombin generation of less than 400 nM had a 60% lower relative risk of recurrence than did those with higher levels ($P < .001$). Nevertheless, prediction of which individual was susceptible to recurrent VTE was not possible.[43]

The coagulation laboratory can perform many esoteric assays to establish the causes of coagulation disorders. In today's environment, many of these are so time and labor intensive that they are "send outs" that are usually not necessary or available for immediate diagnosis and initiation of treatment. These assays are discussed in greater detail in other specific disease–orientated chapters; they include techniques such as measurement of serum thrombopoietin to diagnose the causes of thrombocytopenia and thrombocytosis; flow cytometric evaluation of platelets to document storage pool deficiency and the presence of platelet membrane glycoproteins that may contribute to platelet dysfunction; and assays to measure functional ADAMTS13 (a *d*isintegrin *a*nd *m*etalloproteinase with *t*hrombo*s*pondin motifs) activity for the appropriate diagnosis and treatment of TTP.

FORMULATION OF TREATMENT STRATEGIES FOR THE MANAGEMENT OF ACUTE HEMORRHAGIC EPISODES: HOW TO USE DATA FROM THE COAGULATION LABORATORY

It is not always possible to adhere to an algorithmic approach to the bleeding patient. This is especially true in cases of unexpected intraoperative or postoperative bleeding in which immediate intervention is required (see Chapter 37). Time may not allow for the completion of basic laboratory screening tests prior to initiation of therapy, so the clinician is often forced to treat the patient empirically. The first priority is to exclude the possibility of incomplete surgical ligation or incomplete cauterization of blood vessels. Surgeons usually consider this cause of bleeding to be a diagnosis of exclusion of acquired hematologic conditions; however, results of the coagulation assays are not likely to be available until after a therapeutic decision has been made or the acute situation has resolved. Nevertheless, blood should be collected prior to any intervention because that intervention may affect test results and may delay confirmation of the ultimate diagnosis.

One crude but helpful bedside screening test is the fibrin clot retraction assay. This assay is performed by collecting an aliquot of the patient's blood into a plain glass tube that does not contain any anticoagulant (e.g., a serum "red-top" tube). The blood is carefully observed over time for clot formation at room temperature. A normal response is characterized by clot retraction from one wall of the glass tube, whereas altered clot structure secondary to impeded fibrin formation or impaired platelet aggregation is marked by gelatinous clot formation without evidence of clot retraction. The fibrin clot retraction assay is therefore a "quick and dirty" test for hyperfibrinolysis, hypofibrinogenemia, dysfibrinogenemia, the presence of fibrin degradation products, thrombocytopenia, and qualitative platelet disorders. It can also be affected by an elevated hematocrit level, and results of this assay should be interpreted accordingly. It is interesting to note that normal clot retraction may occur despite the absence of factor XIII.

Empirical therapy in these acute bleeding situations typically begins with the administration of standard blood products—platelets, fresh frozen plasma, and, less often recently, cryoprecipitate. Single-donor or pooled random-donor platelets should be transfused, regardless of preoperative laboratory values, because infusion of normal unaffected platelets will transiently compensate for any undiagnosed platelet dysfunction that may be contributing to the bleeding diathesis. This type of scenario has been associated particularly with surgical procedures that involve cardiopulmonary bypass, in which both thrombocytopenia and platelet dysfunction can occur immediately after surgery and may last for several days into the postoperative period.

Fresh frozen plasma (FFP) contains physiologic levels of labile and stable components of the coagulation system and is indicated for the replacement of deficient coagulation factors. It may also be administered in cases of massive blood loss in which the transfusion of more than one blood volume is required over 24 hours; this occurs with a dilutional or "washout" phenomenon of coagulation factors and as the result of factor consumption through bleeding (see Chapters 12 and 46). In general, 3 to 5 U of FFP are needed for coagulation factors to be adequately replaced in an average-sized adult (10 to 20 mL per kilogram of body weight). Viral attenuated plasma-derived prothrombin complex concentrates (PCCs) may be considered in lieu of FFP when deficiencies of vitamin K–dependent clotting factors are contributing to active or potential bleeding complications (e.g., end-stage liver disease [see Chapter 39]). These products are useful because of their small volumes and rapid action in reversing coagulation defects, and because of their enhanced viral safety profile over FFP. PCCs are more expensive than single-donor units of FFP and may precipitate a thrombogenic state if used repeatedly and in large quantities. PCCs may also be used to reverse bleeding precipitated by the use of warfarin anticoagulation. No prospective, randomized, controlled studies have been conducted to determine whether PCCs are more efficient, safer, or more effective than FFP or rFVIIa concentrate in reversing warfarin-induced bleeding complications. Once PCCs have been administered, accurate coagulation testing cannot be performed because PCCs contain activated clotting factors that confound in vitro screening and specific clotting factor assays.

In the future, FFP, which has been used with solvent detergents, psoralen, or methylene blue, may become available commercially to improve the viral safety profile of FFP, because lipid-enveloped pathogenic blood-borne viruses—including human immunodeficiency virus, hepatitis B virus, and hepatitis C virus—are virtually eliminated in the preparative process. Unfortunately, no FFP treatment method to date has been consistently successful in the removal of prions responsible for variant Creutzfeldt-Jakob disease (vCJD). In experimental animal models, prions appear to be transmissible in blood fractions; however, no cases of vCJD have been reported to occur in transfusion-dependent individuals given contaminated blood products, including packed RBCs, platelets, FFP, or pooled plasma–derived clotting factor concentrates in patients with hemophilia or VWD. Large government-funded surveillance projects in North America and the United Kingdom continue to monitor blood recipients for evidence of vCJD transmission. If specific deficiencies of factor VIII or IX are known to exist preoperatively, the corresponding recombinant factor concentrate should be administered (in the absence of high-titer inhibitors to the clotting factor protein) to eliminate the potential for transmitting infectious blood-borne pathogens associated with plasma.

Cryoprecipitate, on the other hand, is primarily used to correct quantitative or qualitative fibrinogen abnormalities. It is prepared by thawing FFP at 4°C and removing the supernatant. The remaining precipitate is rich in factor VIII, VWF multimers of various sizes, fibrinogen, fibronectin, and factor XIII. As a rough rule of thumb, 1 U of cryoprecipitate per 7 kg of body weight is necessary to increase the plasma fibrinogen level by 75 mg/dL. Formerly, cryoprecipitate was also administered as a source of VWF protein in individuals with VWD; because of its inferior viral safety profile, however, it should be used only in emergency life- and limb-threatening situations when viral attenuated factor VIII concentrates of intermediate purity are not available.

Recombinant factor VIIa concentrate (rFVIIa) (NovoSeven; NovoNordisk, Inc., Princeton, NJ, USA) has been used to reverse or prevent bleeding complications in individuals with severe FVII deficiency and in FVIII, FIX, or VWF protein-deficient states complicated by alloantibodies or autoantibodies that target the clotting factor and neutralize its coagulation function (see Chapter 6). Anecdotal data indicate that rFVIIa can also be used safely and effectively to reverse warfarin bleeding complications, although randomized, controlled trials with FFP or PCCs are lacking. rFVIIa has been used to limit acute intracranial hemorrhages not induced by anticoagulation (see Chapter 43). Despite the "pancoagulant" properties attributed to this new replacement therapy, its administration must be approached with extreme caution because thrombogenic complications have occurred with its use. These have predominated in nonhemophilia bleeding states and in older populations. Patient selection and subsequent monitoring are critical to its careful use. It is evident that outside of the hemophilia bleeding scenario, smaller doses (e.g., 20 to 30 μg per kilogram) administered at one time may be safer than much larger doses yet equally effective.

Plasma-derived FXIII concentrate is undergoing clinical trials, and a recombinant FXIII concentrate is in development. FXI concentrate is available in Canada and the United Kingdom but not in the United States, because of vCJD issues related to plasma pools used to manufacture the concentrate. A fibrinogen concentrate is available in Europe but not in the United States.

If transfusion of platelets, FFP, and/or cryoprecipitate cannot reverse or prevent active bleeding not due to hemophilia A or B or VWD in cases where specific replacement therapy is indicated, the administration of DDAVP (1-deamino-8-D-arginine vasopressin), ε-aminocaproic acid, tranexamic acid, or topical fibrin sealants should be considered. DDAVP is a useful therapy for the qualitative platelet defects associated with uremia or with ingestion of aspirin, for mild or moderately severe hemophilia A, and for VWD (especially type 1). This agent is infused at a dose of 0.3 μg/kg of body weight intravenously over 15 to 30 minutes in 50 mL normal saline, to a maximum total dose of 20–25 μg. Although its exact mechanism of action remains unknown, DDAVP ultimately produces transient increases in levels of VWF antigen, factor VIII activity, ristocetin cofactor activity, tissue plasminogen activator, and PAI-1. It also increases the circulating concentrations of the highest molecular weight VWF protein multimers. Because of its antidiuretic effects, DDAVP is associated with a definite risk of water retention, which may lead to dilutional hyponatremia and seizures, particularly in infants and the elderly; free water intake should be minimized and sodium concentrations followed to monitor for this risk. Angina pectoris and thrombotic stroke have also been reported as potential complications in older, susceptible patients. The peak drug effect occurs within 30 minutes of administration and usually lasts for at least several hours. Of note, intranasal preparations of DDAVP do exist, but their use is usually reserved for situations of long-term administration and/or prophylaxis for simple surgical procedures in patients with mild hemophilia A or VWD.

ε-Aminocaproic acid (Amicar; Wyeth Pharmaceuticals, Madison, NJ, USA) and tranexamic acid (Cyclokapron; Pharmacia, Mississauga, Canada) are antifibrinolytic agents that are often used in the treatment of acute, severe mucosal hemorrhage associated with systemic hyperfibrinolysis. They are particularly useful adjunctive therapies in the management of mucosal bleeding, in that they modulate the effects of the tPA that is released when DDAVP is administered. These antifibrinolytic agents are generally well tolerated, although nausea, vomiting, diarrhea, dizziness, malaise, fever, rash, and transient hypotension or cardiac arrhythmias may occur. ε-Aminocaproic acid may also rarely cause rhabdomyolysis, particularly with prolonged use, in which cases appropriate laboratory monitoring is in order. It is important to note that neither drug should be administered to individuals who also have evidence of hypercoagulability. Finally, fibrin sealants are commercially available as topical procoagulants for active bleeding on surfaces; these are derived from plasma, are virally inactivated, and can be applied easily in the operative setting to sites of active bleeding and anastomosis (see Chapter 29).

In summary, effective diagnosis and treatment of bleeding disorders depend on the physician's expertise in eliciting specific answers to probing questions, in recognizing clinical signs and symptoms on physical examination, and in properly ordering and interpreting laboratory tests to confirm clinical suspicions. Each of these components by itself is too nonspecific and insensitive to be useful; however, when they are combined, high-quality, cost-effective medical care can be rendered and lives and limbs may be saved.

REFERENCES

1. Wahlberg T, Blomback M, Hall P, Axelsson G: Applications of indicators, predictors and diagnostic indices in coagulation disorders. I. Evaluation of a self-administered questionnaire with binary questions. Methods Inf Med 19:194–200, 1980.

2. Coller B, Schneiderman PI: Clinical evaluation of hemorrhagic disorders: Bleeding history and differential diagnosis of purpura. In Hoffman R, Benz EJ, and Shattil SJ, et al (eds): Hematology: Basic Principles and Practice, 2nd ed. New York, Churchill Livingstone, 1995, pp 1606–1622.

3. Miller C, Graham JB, Goldin LR, Elston RC: Genetics of classic von Willebrand's disease. II. Optimal assignment of the heterozygous genotype (diagnosis) by discriminant analysis. Blood 54:137–145, 1979.

4. Rodeghiero F, Castaman G, Tosetto A, et al: The discriminant power of bleeding history for the diagnosis of type I von Willebrand disease: An international, multicenter study. J Thromb Haemost 3:2619–2626, 2005.

5. Bolton-Maggs PH, Patterson DA, Wensley RT, Tuddenham EG: Definition of the bleeding tendency in factor XI—Deficient kindreds: A clinical and laboratory study. Thromb Haemost 73:194–202, 1995.

6. McKay H, Derome F, Haq MA, et al: Bleeding risks associated with inheritance of the Quebec platelet disorder. Blood 104:159–165, 2004.

7. Buchanan GR, Adix L: Grading of hemorrhage in children with idiopathic thrombocytopenic purpura. J Pediatr 141:683–688, 2002.

8. MacMullen NJ, Dulski LA, Meagher B: Red alert: Perinatal hemorrhage. MCN Am J Matern Child Nurs 30:46–51, 2005.

9. Alamia V, Meyer BA: Peripartum hemorrhage. Obstet Gynecol Clin North Am 26:385–398, 1999.

10. Michiels JJ: Acquired hemophilia A in women postpartum: Clinical manifestations, diagnosis, and treatment. Clin Appl Thromb Hemost 6:82–86, 2000.

11. Kadir R, Economides DL, Sabin CA, et al: Assessment of menstrual blood loss and gynaecological problems in patients with inherited bleeding disorders. Haemophilia 5:40–48, 1999.

12. Sadler JE: Von Willebrand disease type 1: A diagnosis in search of a disease. Blood 101:2089–2093, 2003.

13. Kulkarni A, Lee CA, Griffeon A, Kadir RA: Disorders of menstruation and their effect on the quality of life in women with congenital factor VII deficiency. Haemophilia 12:248–252, 2006.

14. Wyatt KM, Dimmock PW, Hayes-Gill B, et al: Menstrual symptometrics: A simple computer-aided method to quantify menstrual cycle disorders. Fertil Steril 78:96–101, 2002.

15. Katsanis E, Luke KH, Hsu E, et al: Prevalence and significance of mild bleeding disorders in children with recurrent epistaxis. J Pediatr 113 (Part 1): 73–76, 1988.

16. Kiley V, Stuart JJ, Johnson CA: Coagulation studies in children with isolated recurrent epistaxis. J Pediatr 100:579–581, 1982.

17. Beran M, Stigendal L, Petruson B: Haemostatic disorders in habitual nose-bleeders. J Laryngol Otol 101:1020–1028, 1987.

18. Violi F, Basili S, Ferro D, et al: Association between high values of D-dimer and tissue-plasminogen activator activity and first gastrointestinal bleeding in cirrhotic patients. CALC Group. Thromb Haemost 76:177–183, 1996.

19. Furie B, Voo L, McAdam K, Furie BC: Mechanism of factor X deficiency in systemic amyloidosis. N Engl J Med 304:827–830, 1981.

20. George JN, Shattil SJ: The clinical importance of acquired abnormalities of platelet function. N Engl J Med 324:27–39, 1991.

21. Rodgers RP, Levin J: A critical reappraisal of the bleeding time. Semin Thromb Hemost 16:1–20, 1990.

22. Robert VC, Ragno G: In vitro testing of platelets using the thromboelastogram, platelet function analyzer, and the clot signature analyzer to predict the bleeding time. Transfus Apher Sci 35:33–41, 2006.

23. Mannucci PM, Chediak J, Hanna W, et al: Treatment of von Willebrand disease with a high purity factor VIII/von Willebrand factor concentrate: A prospective, multicenter study. Blood 99:450–456, 2002.

24. Sramek R, Sramek A, Koster K, et al: A randomized and blinded comparison of three bleeding time techniques: The Ivy method and the Simplate II® method in two directions. Thromb Haemost 67:514–518, 1992.

25. Duke WW: The relation of blood platelets to hemorrhagic disease: Description of a method for determining the bleeding time and coagulation time and report of three cases of hemorrhagic disease relieved by transfusion. JAMA 55:1185–1192, 1910.

26. Sutor AH, Bowie EJ, Owen CA: Quantitative bleeding time (hemorrhagometry): A review. Mayo Clin Proc 52:238–240, 1977.

27. Kratzer MAA, Kretschmer V: Platelet function analyzer (PFA)-100® closure time in the evaluation of platelet disorders and platelet function—A rebuttal. J Thromb Haemost 4:1429–1431, 2006.

28. Anonymous: Can the platelet function analyzer (PFA)-100 test substitute for the template bleeding time in routine clinical practice? Platelets 10:132–136, 1999.

29. Posan E, McBane RD, Grill DE, et al: Comparison of PFA-100 testing and bleeding time for detecting platelet hypofunction and von Willebrand disease in clinical practice. Thromb Haemost 90:483–490, 2003.

30. Quiroga T, Goycoolea M, Munoz B, et al: Template bleeding time and PFA-100 have low sensitivity to screen patients with hereditary mucocutaneous hemorrhages: Comparative study in 148 patients. J Thromb Haemost 2:892–898, 2004.

31. Hayward CP, Harrison P, Cattaneo M, et al: Platelet function analyzer (PFA)-100 closure time in the evaluation of platelet disorders and platelet function. J Thromb Haemost 4:312–319, 2006.

32. Legrand C, Bellucci S, Disdier M, et al: Platelet thrombospondin and glycoprotein IV abnormalities in patients with essential thrombocythemia: Effect of alpha interferon treatment. Am J Hematol 38:307–313, 1991.

33. Taki M, Kobayashi M, Ohi C, et al: Spontaneous platelet aggregation in Kawasaki disease using the particle counting method. Pediatr Int 45:649–652, 2003.

34. Eikelboom JW, Hirsh J, Weitz JI, et al: Aspirin-resistant thromboxane biosynthesis and the risk of myocardial infarction, stroke, or cardiovascular death in patients at high risk for cardiovascular events. Circulation 105:1850–1855, 2002.

35. Grundman K, Jaschonek K, Kleine B, et al: Aspirin non-responder status in patients with recurrent cerebral ischemic attacks. J Neurol 250:63–66, 2003.

36. Chen WH, Lee P, Ng W, et al: Aspirin resistance is associated with a high incidence of myonecrosis after non-urgent percutaneous coronary intervention despite clopidogrel pretreatment. J Am Coll Cardiol 43:1122–1126, 2004.

37. Girolami A, Cattarozzi G, Dal Bo Zanon R, Troffanin F: Factor VII Padua 2: Another factor VII abnormality with defective ox brain thromboplastin activity and a complex hereditary pattern. Blood 54:46–53, 1979.

38. Kitchens CS: To bleed or not to bleed? Is that the question for the PTT? J Thromb Haemost 3:2607–2611, 2005.

39. Schwartz BS, Williams EC, Conlan MG, Mosher DF: Epsilon aminocaproic acid in the treatment of patients with acute promyelocytic leukemia and acquired alpha-2-plasmin inhibitor deficiency. Ann Intern Med 105:873–877, 1986.

40. Boudjeltia KZ, Cauchie P, Remacle C, et al: A new device for measurement of fibrin clot lysis: Application to the euglobulin clot lysis time. BMC Biotechnol 2:8–13, 2001.

41. Srinivasa V, Gilbertson LI, Bhavani-Shankar K: Thromboelastography: Where is it and where is it heading? Int Anesthesiol Clin 39:35–49, 2001.

42. Hemker HC, Al Dieri R, Beguin S: Thrombin generation assays: Accruing clinical relevance. Curr Opin Hematol 11:170–175, 2004.

43. Hron G, Kollars M, Binder BR, et al: Identification of patients at low risk for recurrent venous thromboembolism by measuring thrombin generation. JAMA 296:397–402, 2006.

Chapter 3

Endothelium

William C. Aird, MD

The endothelium, which forms the inner cell lining of all blood vessels in the body, is a spatially distributed organ. The endothelium weighs approximately 1 kg in the average patient and covers a total surface area of 4000 to 7000 square meters. The endothelium is underappreciated as a clinically relevant organ. Indeed, the bench-to-bedside gap in endothelial biomedicine is wide.[1] The importance of closing this gap is highlighted by the fact that the endothelium is involved in most if not all disease states, either as a primary determinant of pathophysiology or as a victim of collateral damage. Moreover, the endothelium has a remarkable, yet largely untapped diagnostic and therapeutic potential. The overall goal of this chapter is to promote a better awareness of the endothelium as an organizing principle in health and disease. Given the current pace of basic and translational discoveries, it is likely that over the next two decades, the endothelium will gain recognition in the clinic as a bona fide organ system.

HISTORICAL OVERVIEW

Early descriptions of the cardiovascular system during the times of Hippocrates and Galen depicted the veins and arteries as separate, unconnected systems. Without the benefit of microscopy, these early investigators observed arteries as deeply situated, thick, pulsating vessels that contain red blood, and veins as superficial, distended, thin-walled, nonpulsating vessels that carry blue blood. The notion that veins and arteries constitute distinct systems would hold sway until William Harvey's discovery of the closed circulation in 1628. Harvey did not see the capillaries that connect arteries with veins but rather surmised their existence through a series of elegant physiologic studies. Marcello Malpighi was the first to actually observe the capillaries under light microscopy in 1659. The term *endothelium* was coined by Wilhelm His in 1865 to distinguish the inner lining of blood vessels from outer epithelial layers. In the early 20th century, most research in endothelial biology focused on physiologic assays of fluid transport across the endothelium. In the 1950s and 1960s, electron microscopy provided an exciting new window into the endothelium, revealing evidence for the existence of specialized organelles, such as Weibel-Palade bodies; unique junctional complexes; and remarkable structural heterogeneity between different segments of the vascular tree. The first successful, reproducible isolation and propagation of endothelial cells in the 1970s revolutionized the field of endothelial cell biology.[2,3] Cell culture provided a means of carefully dissecting—under controlled conditions—fundamental aspects of endothelial

cell structure and function, leading to breathtaking advances in our understanding of this cell type, as well as an exponential increase in the number of publications related to endothelial cells and the endothelium.[4] In vitro and in vivo studies in the 1980s led to the introduction of the descriptors, endothelial cell activation and endothelial cell dysfunction. The evolving definitions of these terms are discussed later in the chapter.

Over the past 40 years, there has been an increasing appreciation that endothelial cells behave very differently in vivo than they do in vitro, and that any interpretation of in vitro–based assays must be interpreted with caution and validated in the intact organism. Although this principle holds true for all cell types, it seems that endothelial cells, by virtue of their tight coupling to the tissue microenvironment, are particularly prone to phenotypic drift when isolated and cultured. Indeed, the application of novel genomic and proteomic approaches has led to the identification of previously hidden levels of complexity, and has provided important new insights into mechanisms of endothelial heterogeneity.[5,6]

EVOLUTION AND DEVELOPMENT

Phylogeny

Most multicellular animals possess a circulation that provides bulk flow of oxygen to the various tissues of the body. Invertebrates typically possess an open circulation in which a heart pumps blood (called *hemolymph*) through one or more blood vessels into an open body cavity (called a *hematocoele*), where it bathes virtually every tissue in the body.[7] In vertebrates, the cardiovascular system is "closed," meaning that blood is always contained with the vasculature (one exception occurs within the spleen, where blood is permitted to exit from the circulation only to reenter after it has been scrutinized and filtered). The endothelium is present in all living vertebrates and absent in all extant invertebrates. Thus, it may be concluded that the common ancestor to vertebrates and invertebrates lacked an endothelium, and that this cell type evolved 450 million to 500 million years ago. In addition to the closed circulation and the endothelium, several other features of the vertebrate body plan seem to have evolved around the same time, including the formation of three distinct blood lineages (erythroid, myeloid, and megakaryocyte/platelet), the clotting cascade (consisting of serine proteases of the extrinsic and intrinsic pathways, and fibrinogen), and acquired immunity (antibody production). An interesting question is: Which selective pressures were responsible for the evolution of the endothelium? Perhaps most important is that higher blood pressures associated with increasing body size would have required a mechanism for offsetting transmural leakage. If one considers the Starling-Landis equation (Equation 1), it is apparent that the permselective properties of a cellular lining would serve such a purpose; the endothelium is a major determinant of hydraulic conductivity and the reflection coefficient for plasma proteins.

$$J_c = L_pA[(P_c - P_t) - s_p(p_c - p_t)] \qquad \text{(Equation 1)}$$

where J_c = net transcapillary fluid shift, L_p = hydraulic conductivity of capillary wall, A = capillary membrane filtration area, P_c = capillary blood pressure, P_t = tissue fluid pressure, s_p = reflection coefficient for plasma proteins, p_c = capillary blood colloid osmotic pressure, and p_t = tissue fluid colloid osmotic pressure.

An important evolutionary consideration is that the modern human endothelium (similar to other organ systems) was "designed" to maximize fitness in a far earlier era, perhaps some 30,000 years ago. This is the time frame necessary to "filter" the gene pool through natural selection. The hunter-gatherers of the time lived a different lifestyle, that is, in terms of salt intake, fat intake, exercise, and life span. Although we will never know the precise details of the early ancestral environment, we can safely conclude that our endothelium is not optimized to withstand the rigors of high-density living (and resulting epidemics), a high-fat diet, a sedentary lifestyle, a prolonged life span, or artificial life support.

Ontogeny

During embryogenesis, the cardiovascular system is the first organ to develop. Blood vessels form via two mechanisms: vasculogenesis and angiogenesis.[8] These processes are remarkably conserved between zebrafish, xenopus, avian species, and mammals. Vasculogenesis, the process that describes the in situ differentiation of endothelial precursor cells (angioblasts) from embryonic mesoderm (paraxial and lateral plate), results in the formation of the earliest vascular plexus (also called *primary capillary plexus*) in the embryo proper.[9] Within a given embryo, some, but not all, angioblasts are derived from a common precursor of endothelial and hematopoietic cells (the hemangioblast). Later development of the mature vessel system involves angiogenesis, with proliferation and sprouting of new vessels from existing ones.[10] Programmed branching (stereotypic patterning) of new blood vessels is governed by a delicate balance of attractive and repellent guidance cues.[11] It is interesting to note that the endothelium lining arteries and veins demonstrates site-specific properties (venous–arterial) even before blood flow is initiated, suggesting that artery–vein identity is epigenetically programmed.[12] This has important implications for an understanding of the focal nature of vasculopathic disease states in humans, in that the propensity for such diseases may be specified—at least in part—by a fixed program within the vessel. Finally, stabilization or maturation involves the recruitment of mural cells, including smooth muscle cells and pericytes.[13]

ENDOTHELIAL BIOLOGY

Levels of Organization

The cardiovascular system, consisting of the heart and blood vessels, is said to be closed because blood is always maintained within the vascular tree. Arteries have thick walls that consist of an endothelium-lined intima, smooth muscle cell–rich media, and an adventitia. The artery is a conduit vessel whose primary function is to provide bulk flow delivery of blood to the various tissues of the body. Arteries branch into arterioles, which are lined by a thinner layer of vascular smooth muscle cells. Arterioles are resistance vessels that mediate vascular tone and blood flow. The endothelium that lines arteries and arterioles is exposed to high flow rates and a relatively constant blood composition (an exception is the pulmonary artery, in which endothelial cells are bathed by mixed venous blood, and certain vascular beds that contain two arterial beds separated by capillaries [e.g., the glomerulus]). Blood flows from arterioles into capillaries. Capillaries are the "business end" of the circulation, in that they mediate the vast majority of exchanges of gases and nutrients between blood and underlying tissues. In keeping with Fick's law of diffusion (Equation 2), capillaries account for the vast majority of the surface area of the vascular tree.

$$\frac{dQ_g}{dt} = D_gA\frac{dP_g}{dx} \qquad \text{(Equation 2)}$$

where $\frac{dQ_g}{dt}$ = rate of diffusion of gas (g)′, D_g = the Krogh diffusion coefficient; A = surface area; dP = partial pressure gradient; and dx = diffusion distance.

Also consistent with their primary role in diffusion, capillaries are extremely thin (thus minimizing dx). They are essentially three-dimensional tubes of endothelium that consist of little more than a single layer of flattened endothelial cells surrounded to a varying degree by extracellular matrix and occasional pericytes (see Chapter 11, Fig. 11-2). Deoxygenated blood is drained from capillaries into venules and subsequently into veins. The endothelium that lines the veins is exposed to blood with composition that varies according to the net exchange of substances that has taken place in the prevenule capillaries.

Input–Output Device

Each of the human body's 60 trillion endothelial cells is analogous to a miniature adaptive input–output device. Input arises from the extracellular environment and may include any number of biochemical and biomechanical forces. Examples of biochemical mediators include growth factors, cytokines, chemokines, temperature, pH, and oxygenation (Table 3-1). Output, or cellular phenotype, depends on the level of organization. Single endothelial cells may undergo a change in calcium flux or shape, or an alteration in protein or mRNA expression; they may migrate, proliferate, or undergo apoptosis. Monolayers of endothelial cells express barrier properties and may be assayed for leukocyte adhesion and transmigration. Finally, other phenotypes (called *emergent properties*), including endothelium-mediated changes in vasomotor tone, are apparent only at the level of the blood vessel, organ, or whole organism. Input is coupled to output through

Table 3-1   Examples of Endothelial Cell Input and Output

Input
Growth factors
    Vascular endothelial growth factor
    Fibroblast growth factor
    Hepatocyte growth factor
    Epidermal growth factor
    Insulin/insulin-like growth factor (IGF)
Cytokines
    Tumor necrosis factor
Chemokines
    Monocyte chemoattractant protein-1
Nucleotides
Complement
pH
Oxygen
Glucose
Temperature

Output
Level of single cell
    Cell shape
    Calcium flux
    Migration
    Proliferation
    Apoptosis
    Gene expression
    Protein expression
Level of cell monolayers
    Barrier function
    Leukocyte adhesion and transmigration
Level of blood vessel/whole organ
    Vasomotor tone
    Hemostatic balance

a complex array of nonlinear signaling pathways that typically begin at the level of cell surface receptors and end at the level of posttranscriptional modification or gene transcription.

Endothelial Cell Heterogeneity

At any given time, endothelial cells throughout the body are exposed to a myriad of microenvironments. For example, blood–brain barrier endothelium is exposed to a mixture of astroglial-derived paracrine factors that are critical for maintaining blood–brain barrier phenotype.[14] In contrast, the endothelial lining of capillaries in the heart is exposed to regional forces generated by the pumping heart, as well as to paracrine factors derived from surrounding cardiomyocytes.[15,16] As another example, endothelial cells in the vasa recta in the inner medulla of the kidney are exposed to a profoundly hypoxic and hyperosmolar environment. At any given site of the vasculature, the endothelium is exposed to temporal changes in input. For example, the endothelial cells in the portal vein and hepatic sinusoids are exposed to fluctuating concentrations of nutrients during preprandial and postprandial periods. In response to infection, trauma, or surgery, cytokines and other components may be released into the circulation during the innate immune response. Because input varies in time and space, and because endothelial cells are capable of sensing and responding to their extracellular environment, cellular output varies. Indeed, if one could "color code" the phenotype of an endothelial cell—for example, assign each phenotype with a shade of color—the endothelium would display a richly colored palette that might fade in and out or blink on and off over time.

Nature versus Nurture

If the extracellular microenvironment were the sole mediator of endothelial cell heterogeneity, then the endothelium would be considered a "blank slate." According to this model, all endothelial cells are "created equally" (through lineage determination/epigenetic modification), and any differences in phenotype merely reflect variation in the extracellular environment (i.e., spatial differences in net signal input). If one were to remove endothelial cells from various sites of the vasculature—say, from the pulmonary vein and from heart capillaries—and culture them in vitro under identical conditions, then differences in phenotype would "wash out" over time, and cellular phenotypes would ultimately reach identity. However, this is not the case. Evidence suggests that although many site-specific properties are indeed lost with culturing, others are retained during sequential passaging.[17,18] These latter properties are epigenetically programmed and thus mitotically heritable. In the final analysis, both the microenvironment (nurture) and epigenetics (nature) contribute to endothelial cell heterogeneity.

Endothelial Functions

The endothelium plays an important role in physiology (Table 3-2), including barrier function, leukocyte trafficking, innate immunity, and vasomotor tone (discussed later), as well as hemostasis (discussed in a subsequent section).

Endothelial cells form a permselective (i.e., semipermeable) membrane that mediates transfer of ions, solutes, and fluids between the blood and interstitial compartments.[19] As a general rule, gases pass through the endothelium via simple diffusion, whereas ions, solutes, and fluids require convective flow between endothelial cells (paracellular route) or through the endothelial cell (transcellular route). Transcellular flux is mediated by specialized transport processes, including transendothelial channels, caveolae, and vesicular-vacuolar organelles (VVOs). In keeping with the theme of heterogeneity, barrier properties differ significantly between different vascular beds. For example, the blood–brain barrier forms a highly efficient barrier by virtue of its tight junctional complexes (limiting paracellular transport) and paucity of caveolae (limiting transcellular transport). The blood–brain barrier relies on a unique repertoire of receptor-mediated transport systems and channels to deliver nutrients across the endothelium. In contrast, the liver sinusoidal endothelium is fenestrated

Table 3-2   Endothelial Functions

Vasomotor tone
Barrier function
Hemostatic balance
Leukocyte trafficking
Angiogenesis
Cell survival/apoptosis
Antigen presentation
Innate immunity

and possesses a discontinuous basement membrane; it is thus highly permeable.

The endothelium regulates the traffic of leukocytes between blood and underlying tissue. Under normal conditions, constitutive trafficking of lymphocytes from blood to lymph nodes occurs via specialized blood vessels, called *high endothelial venules* (HEVs).[20] In states of inflammation, endothelial cells in postcapillary venules (in nonlymphoid tissue) mediate the adhesion and transendothelial migration of leukocytes to the extravascular space.[21] This process involves a highly orchestrated multistep adhesion cascade that begins with initial attachment, rolling, and arrest, and ends with diapedesis through the endothelium and migration through tissues. Over the past several years, significant advances have been made in our understanding of the molecular basis for leukocyte trafficking. For example, initial attachment is mediated primarily by E-selectin and P-selectin on endothelial cells, which bind to respective ligands on leukocytes, and L-selectin on neutrophils, which binds to endothelial ligands; arrest is mediated by endothelial intercellular adhesion molecule (ICAM)-1–leukocyte β2 integrin interactions. In addition to regulating leukocyte transfer, the endothelium plays other roles in the innate immune response. For example, activated endothelial cells may express and/or release a multitude of inflammatory mediators.

The endothelium plays a key role in mediating vasomotor tone. Endothelial cells express several molecules that influence blood vessel diameter and flow dynamics, most notably nitric oxide (NO). The enzyme responsible for endothelial production of NO is endothelial nitric oxide synthase (eNOS).[22] eNOS was once called a constitutive enzyme, but its expression or activity is now recognized to be modulated by many extracellular signals, including (but not limited to) shear stress and growth factors. Diagnostic flow studies of endothelial function provide indirect measures of NO release from the endothelium. Other vasomotor molecules released by the endothelium include prostaglandins and endothelin-1.

ENDOTHELIUM IN DISEASE

The two most common descriptors used to discuss the role of the endothelium in disease are endothelial cell activation and dysfunction. Both terms were coined in the early 1980s. *Endothelial cell activation* was introduced to describe agonist-induced hyperadhesiveness of cultured endothelial cells to leukocytes.[23–25] Today, the term is used more broadly to characterize the response of endothelial cells to an inflammatory stimulus under in vitro and/or in vivo conditions. Activation is not an all-or-nothing response. Rather, activated endothelial cells display a spectrum of response. This caveat notwithstanding, the activation phenotype typically consists of some combination of increased leukocyte adhesion, a shift in the hemostatic balance toward the procoagulant side, and increased permeability. *Endothelial cell dysfunction* was originally introduced to describe increased platelet adhesion to endothelium.[26] Over the years, the term became synonymous with abnormal endothelium–mediated vasorelaxation in atherosclerotic arteries. However, the endothelium is (1) spatially distributed (endothelial coverage of the conduit vessels

represents a miniscule fraction of the total surface area of the endothelium), (2) involved in multiple functions (over and above regulation of vasomotor tone), and (3) involved in virtually every disease. Thus, the term *endothelial cell dysfunction* should not be restricted to a single function, organ/blood vessel type, or disease state. Indeed, endothelial cell dysfunction may be defined as an endothelial phenotype—whether or not it meets the definition of activation—that poses a net liability to the host, as occurs for example locally in coronary artery disease and systemically in severe sepsis.

ENDOTHELIUM AND HEMOSTASIS

Hemostasis represents a balance between procoagulant and anticoagulant forces. Procoagulant forces include tissue factor (TF), serine proteases of the intrinsic and extrinsic pathways, cofactors, fibrinogen, plasminogen activator inhibitor-1 (PAI-1), and an activated or negatively charged cell surface membrane. Anticoagulant forces include non–protein-specific mechanisms such as blood flow (which removes activated clotting factors and maintains protective flow at the level of the endothelium) and vascular integrity (causes separation of blood from underlying TF-rich adventitia and parenchyma), as well as protein-specific mechanisms such as antithrombin III (ATIII)–heparan (which inhibits the serine proteases of the clotting cascade), thrombomodulin (TM)–endothelial protein C receptor (EPCR)-activated protein C (aPC)–protein S (which inactivates factors Va and VIIIa and inhibits endothelial cell activation), tissue factor pathway inhibitor (TFPI) (which inhibits the extrinsic pathway by forming a ternary complex with TF and factors VIIa and Xa), and plasmin (which degrades fibrin).

A shift in hemostatic balance to one or the other side may result in bleeding or thrombosis. An interesting feature of congenital and acquired hypercoagulable states is that they are invariably associated with local thrombotic lesions. This may seem counterintuitive in conditions in which the abnormality lies in a systemically distributed factor, such as factor V Leiden or congenital deficiency of ATIII. A clue to the focal distribution of clots lies in the endothelium.[16] The endothelium is a mini-factory for procoagulant and anticoagulant molecules. On the procoagulant side, endothelial cells synthesize PAI-1, von Willebrand factor (VWF), protease-activated receptors, and rarely, TF. On the anticoagulant side, endothelial cells express, synthesize, and/or release TFPI, TM, EPCR, tissue plasminogen activator (tPA), and heparan. However, these factors are not expressed uniformly throughout the vasculature. For example, VWF is expressed predominantly in venous endothelium,[27] TFPI in microvascular endothelium,[28] EPCR in large vessel endothelium,[29] TM in vessels of all sizes in all organs with the notable exception of the brain,[30] and tPA in arterioles (particularly in the brain and lungs).[31] The picture that emerges is one of heterogeneity layered on heterogeneity. Indeed, if one were to survey endothelial cells from different sites of the vasculature, one would find that they mediate hemostasis via site-specific "formulas" of procoagulants and anticoagulants (Fig. 3-1).[16,32]

These considerations give rise to a revised model of hemostasis (Fig. 3-2).[33] The liver synthesizes a relatively

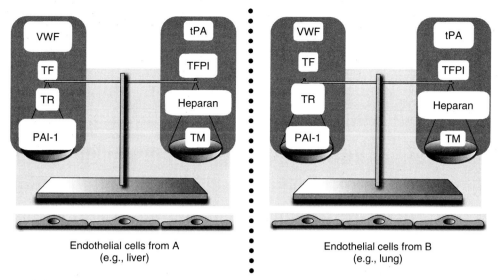

Figure 3-1 Site-specific hemostatic formulas. Each endothelial cell contributes to the hemostatic balance by expressing and/or secreting surface receptors and soluble mediators. Receptors include the protease-activated receptors (or TR [thrombin receptor]), thrombomodulin (TM), tissue factor (TF), and ectoADPase (not shown). Soluble mediators include von Willebrand factor (VWF), plasminogen activator inhibitor-1 (PAI-1), tissue plasminogen activator (tPA), tissue factor pathway inhibitor (TFPI), and heparan. Each of these factors is differentially expressed from one site of the vascular tree to another. Thus, at any point in time, the hemostatic balance is regulated by vascular bed–specific "formulas." Shown is a hypothetical example, in which an endothelial cell from a liver capillary relies more on VWF, PAI-1, and TFPI to balance hemostasis, whereas an endothelial cell from a lung capillary expresses more thrombin receptor, tPA, and heparan. (Adapted with permission from Aird WC: Crit Care Med 29[7 suppl]:S28–S34, 2001.)

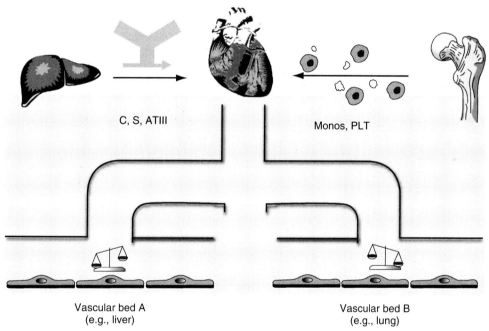

Figure 3-2 Integrated model of hemostasis. The liver *(left)* produces the serine proteases, cofactors, and fibrinogen of the clotting cascade (shown as Y-shape) and many of the circulating natural anticoagulants (shown are protein C [C], protein S [S], and antithrombin III [ATIII]). The bone marrow *(right)* releases monocytes and platelets that are capable of expressing tissue factor and/or an activated cell surface. The liver- and bone marrow–derived proteins and cells are systemically distributed and integrated into the unique hemostatic balance of each vascular bed (shown are balances in two hypothetical vascular beds). Monos, monocytes; PLT, platelets. (Adapted with permission from Aird WC: Crit Care Med 29 (7 suppl):S28–S34, 2001.)

consistent quantity of serine proteases (factors XII, XI, X, IX, VII, and II), cofactors (factors V and VIII), fibrinogen, and anticoagulants (ATIII, protein C, protein S). Under normal conditions, the bone marrow releases a relatively constant quantity of monocytes and platelets, cells that are capable of expressing TF and activated cell surface membrane, respectively. Liver-derived soluble factors and

bone marrow–derived hematopoietic cells are systemically distributed where they are uniquely integrated into the hemostatic balance of each and every vascular bed. When a shift in systemic factors occurs—for example, increased release of hepatocyte proteins during an acute phase response, congenital deficiency of ATIII, or sepsis-mediated efflux and/or activation of monocytes and platelets—the changes influence site-specific hemostatic formulas in ways that differ from one vascular bed to another, resulting in local thrombosis. This model provides several important perspectives, in that it (1) incorporates both the cellular phase (endothelium, platelets, and monocytes) and the soluble phase (circulating procoagulants and anticoagulants) of coagulation; (2) illustrates the various organs that contribute to hemostasis (endothelium, liver, and bone marrow); and (3) emphasizes the vascular bed–specific nature of hemostasis.

The endothelium also contributes in indirect ways to the hemostatic balance. For example, endothelium-mediated vasoregulation plays a key role in maintaining blood flow. Limited expression of cell adhesion molecules and induction of leukocyte adhesion minimizes blockage of vessel lumina and secondary disruption of flow. Endothelial dysfunction in any of these parameters may lead to an increased propensity to form clots.

DIAGNOSIS

Few symptoms are directly referable or specific to the endothelium. The endothelium is hidden from view and is not amenable to traditional physical diagnostic maneuvers such as inspection, percussion, palpation, or auscultation. In contrast to other organs that are difficult to examine at the bedside, such as the pancreas, the endothelium is not spatially confined and therefore is difficult to image with traditional imaging modalities.

The most commonly used diagnostic assays for endothelial function in the clinic are noninvasive flow studies that measure endothelium-mediated vasorelaxation in response to acetylcholine or release of external compression (Table 3-3).[34-37] Abundant studies have shown abnormal endothelium–mediated changes in flow in patients with coronary artery disease or in those with risk factors for coronary artery disease.[38] An important limitation of these assays, as alluded to earlier, is that they provide limited information about other aspects of endothelial function or other sites of the vasculature (e.g., capillaries).

Circulating biomarkers for the endothelium include soluble and cell-based assays. Soluble mediators include endothelium-derived factors involved in hemostasis (e.g., VWF, PAI-1, tPA, sTM, sEPCR), cell adhesion (e.g., sE-selectin, sP-selectin, sICAM-1, soluble vascular cell adhesion molecule-1 [sVCAM-1]), and/or vasomotor tone (e.g., endothelin-1). Although many studies have reported the association of one or another of these mediators in different disease states, few if any markers consistently and reliably predict presence/stage of disease, prognosis, or response to therapy. It seems likely that advances will depend on the use of proteomic technology to simultaneously assay for multiple soluble mediators and the use of bioinformatics to identify the association between patterns of markers and disease. Given that the hemostatic balance is differentially regulated between different vascular beds, it may be possible to correlate changes in hemostatic parameters with the site of dysfunction. As an example, if the brain does in fact express little in the way of TM, then large increases in circulating sTM are unlikely to reflect primary or localized brain disease.

Cell-based assays offer considerable promise. For example, circulating endothelial cells (CECs) are increased in

Table 3-3 Diagnostic Markers for Endothelium

Marker	Comments
Pathology	Not readily available, except for skin biopsies. Results from skin biopsies may not be extrapolatable to other vascular beds
Soluble Mediators	
sICAM-1	Not specific to endothelial cells
sVCAM-1	Not specific to endothelial cells
sP-selectin	Not specific to endothelial cells
sE-selectin	Specific to endothelial cells
sTM	Specific to endothelial cells
tPA	Not specific to endothelial cells
PAI-1	Not specific to endothelial cells
VWF	Not specific to endothelial cells
sEPCR	Specific to endothelial cells
Others	
Cell-Based Mediators	
CECs	May be quantitated and phenotyped; limited by small numbers in the blood
MPs	May be quantitated and phenotyped
EPCs	May be quantitated and phenotyped
Molecular Imaging	Holds tremendous promise for vascular bed–specific diagnosis
Flow Studies	The only diagnostic assays that have reached the clinical mainstream

sICAM, soluble intercellular adhesion molecule; sVCAM, soluble vascular cell adhesion molecule; sTM, soluble thrombomodulin; tPA, tissue plasminogen activator; PAI-1, plasminogen activator inhibitor-1; VWF, von Willebrand factor; sEPCR, soluble endothelial protein C receptor; CEC, circulating endothelial cell; MP, microparticle; EPC, endothelial progenitor cell.

disease states such as sepsis, acute coronary syndromes, and connective tissue disease.[39,40] These cells, which are derived from the blood vessel wall, may be quantified and phenotyped with the use of fluorescence-activated cell sorting (FACS) analysis. Quantitative and qualitative analyses of CECs may ultimately provide information about the health of the endothelium at the site of origin. Circulating microparticles are derived from multiple cell types, including leukocytes, platelets, red blood cells, and endothelial cells. Endothelial microparticles (EMPs) are increased in many disease states.[41] As is the case with CECs, EMPs may be quantified and phenotyped by FACS. Increasing evidence suggests that different diseases are associated with distinct EMP phenotypes. Moreover, EMPs may carry TF and cell adhesion molecules on their surface, thus contributing to underlying pathophysiology. Endothelial progenitor cells (EPCs) are derived from the bone marrow and circulate in the blood. These cells are believed to be mobilized and taken up by newly formed blood vessels (although their role in replacing preexisting endothelium in established blood vessels is less clear). The latter process has been called *adult vasculogenesis* because it mimics the process of vasculogenesis in the embryo, in which angioblasts from the mesoderm differentiate into endothelial cells and form the earliest blood vessels. Data suggest that the number of EPCs correlates inversely with the health of the endothelium and is associated with reparative potential.[42] Because circulating blood cells are in intimate contact with the endothelium, they may carry special signatures related to these interactions. Indeed, studies of sepsis have revealed characteristic changes in monocyte transcriptome, some of which are presumably reflective of endothelial function or dysfunction. Another interesting concept is the use of vascular bed–specific catheters to sample local sites of endothelial dysfunction (hot spots), whose manifestations become "washed out" or diluted in blood from the peripheral vein or artery.

THERAPY

The endothelium is an attractive therapeutic target. Endothelial cells are preferentially and rapidly exposed to systemically delivered agents. Owing to its wide spatial distribution, the endothelium provides a window into each and every tissue of the body. Moreover, endothelial cells are highly malleable and thus modulatable from a therapeutic standpoint. The endothelium should be targeted for two main reasons: (1) to directly modulate endothelial function, and (2) to gain site-specific access to underlying tissue.

Treating the Endothelium

Therapy may be directed toward ameliorating endothelial function. To return to the analogy of the endothelial cell as an input–output device, therapy may be aimed toward cellular output (i.e., phenotype) and/or intracellular coupling mechanisms. Examples of targeting output include using neutralizing antibodies against adhesion molecules such as ICAM-1 or VCAM-1; inducing the expression/synthesis of TM, EPCR, TFPI, or heparan; and increasing barrier function. Examples of modulating intracellular coupling mechanisms include neutralization of cell surface receptors (e.g., antibodies against the vascular endothelial growth factor [VEGF] receptor) and administration of antioxidants or inhibitors of NF-κB signaling. Increasing evidence suggests that certain U.S. Food and Drug Administration (FDA)-approved drugs exert their beneficial effect—at least in part—by attenuating endothelial dysfunction. For example, lipid-lowering statins have been shown to have pleiotropic effects at the level of the endothelium.[43] Recombinant human protein C, which is used to treat patients with severe sepsis,[44] has been shown to promote endothelial barrier function and inhibit endothelial apoptosis.[45–47] It is tempting to speculate that the proved efficacy of tight glucose control[48] and low-dose steroids[49] in critically ill patients serves to attenuate the deleterious effects of high glucose and NF-κB, respectively, on the endothelium. Indeed, given the remarkable capacity of the endothelium to sense and respond to its extracellular environment, it seems likely that most if not all drugs that are systemically administered to patients will alter endothelial phenotypes in one way or another—whether the effect is beneficial, toxic, or neutral.

Targeting the Endothelium as a Means of Gaining Access to Tissue

Most drugs are small lipophilic molecules that readily cross cell membranes and distribute throughout the body. An important goal in therapeutics is to develop strategies for selectively targeting organs of interest. In this regard, the permselective properties of the endothelium present both challenges and opportunities. For example, the blood–brain barrier poses a formidable obstacle to drug therapy in neurologic disease.[50] However, recent advances in the field of endothelial cell biology suggest that the transcytotic machinery (e.g., caveolae) may be exploited to deliver drugs to the extravascular compartment. Moreover, because the endothelium displays remarkable heterogeneity in cell surface receptor expression, it is hoped that these so-called vascular addresses may be selectively targeted to promote vascular bed–specific (hence, organ-specific) delivery of drugs.

CONCLUSIONS

Since 1950, more than 100,000 articles have been published on endothelial cells and the endothelium.[1] In contrast, the endothelium is underrecognized in the clinical setting. Many physicians are cognizant of its role in mediating vasomotor tone and its pathophysiologic involvement in atherosclerosis. However, appreciation for its myriad of functions in other vascular beds is typically divided along traditional "organ lines." For example, neurologists consider the blood–brain barrier; ophthalmologists, the retinal circulation; nephrologists, kidney glomeruli; and urologists, the corpus spongiosum. Given that the endothelium is systemically distributed, is involved in many if not most disease states, and has remarkable diagnostic and therapeutic potential, an urgent need to adopt a more integrative approach to this cell layer has been acknowledged. Bridging the bench-to-bedside gap in endothelial biomedicine will require the dismantling of existing barriers between organ-specific disciplines. Indeed, acceptance of the endothelium as a clinically relevant system (i.e., organ) will provide a necessary foundation for future breakthroughs in the field.

REFERENCES

1. Hwa C, Sebastian A, Aird WC: Endothelial biomedicine: Its status as an interdisciplinary field, its progress as a basic science, and its translational bench-to-bedside gap. Endothelium 12:139–151, 2005.
2. Jaffe EA, Nachman RL, Becker CG, et al: Culture of human endothelial cells derived from umbilical veins: Identification by morphologic and immunologic criteria. J Clin Invest 52:2745–2756, 1973.
3. Gimbrone MA Jr, Cotran RS, Folkman J: Human vascular endothelial cells in culture: Growth and DNA synthesis. J Cell Biol 60:673–684, 1974.
4. Nachman RL, Jaffe EA: Endothelial cell culture: Beginnings of modern vascular biology. J Clin Invest 114:1037–1040, 2004.
5. Arap W, Kolonin MG, Trepel M, et al: Steps toward mapping the human vasculature by phage display. Nat Med 8:121–127, 2002.
6. Oh P, Li Y, Yu J, et al: Subtractive proteomic mapping of the endothelial surface in lung and solid tumours for tissue-specific therapy. Nature 429:629–635, 2004.
7. Munoz-Chapuli R, Carmona R, Guadix JA, et al: The origin of the endothelial cells: An evo-devo approach for the invertebrate/vertebrate transition of the circulatory system. Evol Dev 7:351–358, 2005.

3

8. Patan S: Vasculogenesis and angiogenesis. Cancer Treat Res 117:3–32, 2004.

9. Risau W, Flamme I: Vasculogenesis. Annu Rev Cell Dev Biol 11:73–91, 1995.

10. Risau W: Mechanisms of angiogenesis. Nature 386:671–674, 1997.

11. Autiero M, De Smet F, Claes F, et al: Role of neural guidance signals in blood vessel navigation. Cardiovasc Res 65:629–638, 2005.

12. Torres-Vazquez J, Kamei M, Weinstein BM: Molecular distinction between arteries and veins. Cell Tissue Res 314:43–59, 2003.

13. Jain RK: Molecular regulation of vessel maturation. Nat Med 9:685–693, 2003.

14. Hawkins BT, Davis TP: The blood–brain barrier/neurovascular unit in health and disease. Pharmacol Rev 57:173–185, 2005.

15. Brutsaert DL: Cardiac endothelial-myocardial signaling: Its role in cardiac growth, contractile performance, and rhythmicity. Physiol Rev 83:59–115, 2003.

16. Rosenberg RD, Aird WC: Vascular-bed–specific hemostasis and hypercoagulable states. N Engl J Med 340:1555–1564, 1999.

17. Chi JT, Chang HY, Haraldsen G, et al: Endothelial cell diversity revealed by global expression profiling. Proc Natl Acad Sci U S A 100:10623–10628, 2003.

18. Lacorre DA, Baekkevold ES, Garrido I, et al: Plasticity of endothelial cells: Rapid dedifferentiation of freshly isolated high endothelial venule endothelial cells outside the lymphoid tissue microenvironment. Blood 103:4164–4172, 2004.

19. Mehta D, Malik AB: Signaling mechanisms regulating endothelial permeability. Physiol Rev 86:279–367, 2007.

20. von Andrian UH, Mempel TR: Homing and cellular traffic in lymph nodes. Nat Rev Immunol 3:867–878, 2003.

21. Rao RM, Shaw SK, Kim M, et al: Emerging topics in the regulation of leukocyte transendothelial migration. Microcirculation 12:83–89, 2005.

22. Sessa WC: eNOS at a glance. J Cell Sci 117 (Pt 12): 2427–2429, 2004.

23. Pober JS, Gimbrone MA Jr: Expression of Ia-like antigens by human vascular endothelial cells is inducible in vitro: Demonstration by monoclonal antibody binding and immunoprecipitation. Proc Natl Acad Sci U S A 79:6641–6645, 1982.

24. Gamble JR, Harlan JM, Klebanoff SJ, et al: Stimulation of the adherence of neutrophils to umbilical vein endothelium by human recombinant tumor necrosis factor. Proc Natl Acad Sci U S A 82:8667–8671, 1985.

25. Schleimer RP, Rutledge BK: Cultured human vascular endothelial cells acquire adhesiveness for neutrophils after stimulation with interleukin 1, endotoxin, and tumor-promoting phorbol diesters. J Immunol 136:649–654, 1986.

26. Gimbrone MA Jr (ed): Endothelial Dysfunction and the Pathogenesis of Atherosclerosis. New York, Springer-Verlag, 1980.

27. Yamamoto K, de Waard V, Fearns C, et al: Tissue distribution and regulation of murine von Willebrand factor gene expression in vivo. Blood 92:2791–2801, 1998.

28. Osterud B, Bajaj MS, Bajaj SP: Sites of tissue factor pathway inhibitor (TFPI) and tissue factor expression under physiologic and pathologic conditions. On behalf of the Subcommittee on Tissue Factor Pathway Inhibitor (TFPI) of the Scientific and Standardization Committee of the ISTH. Thromb Haemost 73:873–875, 1995.

29. Laszik Z, Mitro A, Taylor FB Jr, et al: Human protein C receptor is present primarily on endothelium of large blood vessels: Implications for the control of the protein C pathway. Circulation 96:3633–3640, 1997.

30. Ishii H, Salem HH, Bell CE, et al: Thrombomodulin, an endothelial anticoagulant protein, is absent from the human brain. Blood 67:362–365, 1986.

31. Levin EG, Banka CL, Parry GC: Progressive and transient expression of tissue plasminogen activator during fetal development. Arterioscler Thromb Vasc Biol 20:1668–1674, 2000.

32. Aird WC: Vascular bed–specific hemostasis: Role of endothelium in sepsis pathogenesis. Crit Care Med 29:S28–S35, 2001.

33. Aird WC: Spatial and temporal dynamics of the endothelium. J Thromb Haemost 3:1392–1406, 2005.

34. Celermajer DS, Sorensen KE, Gooch VM, et al: Non-invasive detection of endothelial dysfunction in children and adults at risk of atherosclerosis. Lancet 340:1111–1115, 1992.

35. Corretti MC, Anderson TJ, Benjamin EJ, et al: Guidelines for the ultrasound assessment of endothelial-dependent flow-mediated vasodilation of the brachial artery: A report of the International Brachial Artery Reactivity Task Force. J Am Coll Cardiol 39:257–265, 2002.

36. Ludmer PL, Selwyn AP, Shook TL, et al: Paradoxical vasoconstriction induced by acetylcholine in atherosclerotic coronary arteries. N Engl J Med 315:1046–1051, 1986.

37. Edmundowicz D: Noninvasive studies of coronary and peripheral arterial blood-flow. Curr Atheroscler Rep 4:381–385, 2002.

38. Patel SN, Rajaram V, Pandya S, et al: Emerging, noninvasive surrogate markers of atherosclerosis. Curr Atheroscler Rep 6:60–68, 2004.

39. Goon PK, Boos CJ, Lip GY: Circulating endothelial cells: Markers of vascular dysfunction. Clin Lab 51:531–538, 2005.

40. Blann AD, Woywodt A, Bertolini F, et al: Circulating endothelial cells: Biomarker of vascular disease. Thromb Haemost 93:228–235, 2005.

41. Horstman LL, Jy W, Jimenez JJ, et al: Endothelial microparticles as markers of endothelial dysfunction. Front Biosci 9:1118–1135, 2004.

42. Ribatti D, Nico B, Crivellato E, et al: Endothelial progenitor cells in health and disease. Histol Histopathol 20:1351–1358, 2005.

43. Walter DH, Dimmeler S, Zeiher AM: Effects of statins on endothelium and endothelial progenitor cell recruitment. Semin Vasc Med 4:385–393, 2004.

44. Bernard GR, Vincent JL, Laterre PF, et al: Efficacy and safety of recombinant human activated protein C for severe sepsis. N Engl J Med 344:699–709, 2001.

45. Finigan JH, Dudek SM, Singleton PA, et al: Activated protein C mediates novel lung endothelial barrier enhancement: Role of sphingosine 1-phosphate receptor transactivation. J Biol Chem 280:17286–17293, 2005.

46. Feistritzer C, Riewald M: Endothelial barrier protection by activated protein C through PAR1-dependent sphingosine 1-phosphate receptor-1 crossactivation. Blood 105:3178–3184, 2005.

47. Joyce DE, Gelbert L, Ciaccia A, et al: Gene expression profile of antithrombotic protein C defines new mechanisms modulating inflammation and apoptosis. J Biol Chem 276:11199–11203, 2001.

48. van den Berghe G, Wouters P, Weekers F, et al: Intensive insulin therapy in the critically ill patients. N Engl J Med 345:1359–1367, 2001.

49. Annane D, Sebille V, Charpentier C, et al: Effect of treatment with low doses of hydrocortisone and fludrocortisone on mortality in patients with septic shock. JAMA 288:862–871, 2002.

50. Pardridge WM: The blood–brain barrier: Bottleneck in brain drug development. NeuroRx 2:3–14, 2005.

Part II

Hemorrhagic Processes

Chapter 4

Hemophilia A and B

Lisa N. Boggio, MS, MD • Craig M. Kessler, MD

INTRODUCTION/EPIDEMIOLOGY/GENETICS

The hemophilias are the best known of the hereditary bleeding disorders. Hemophilia A arises as the result of congenital deficiency of coagulation factor VIII, and those with hemophilia B lack coagulation factor IX. Both are transmitted genetically as X-linked recessive disorders, almost exclusively affecting males whose daughters and mothers are obligate carriers of the gene defect. Hemophilia A occurs in 1 of every 5000 live male births and accounts for approximately 80% to 85% of hemophilia cases. Hemophilia B is far less common, occurring in 1 of every 30,000 live male births. The incidence of these hemophilias is equal across all ethnic and racial groups.

The factor VIII gene comprises 186,000 base pairs and is considerably larger than the factor IX gene, which consists of 34,000 base pairs. These genes are located on particularly fragile portions of the X chromosome. By virtue of its size alone, the factor VIII gene is more susceptible to mutations; this may explain the greater prevalence of hemophilia A versus hemophilia B (4:1) in the population. The incidence of hemophilia has not changed over the years despite the availability of genetic counseling and prenatal testing of at-risk mothers. Approximately 30% of hemophilias present as spontaneous mutations, with no prior family history of coagulation disorders.

Symptomatic hemophilia A or B rarely affects females but can do so by virtue of any of the following genetic mechanisms: (1) high degree of lyonization of factor VIII or IX alleles in carriers; (2) hemizygosity of the X chromosome in females with Turner syndrome (XO karyotype); or (3) homozygosity in female progeny of hemophilia carriers and affected hemophilic males.[1] Females who are phenotypically hemophilic should undergo diagnostic evaluation for exclusion of von Willebrand disease variant type 2N or type 3, or testicular feminization syndrome.

The most common mutation of the factor VIII gene, responsible for at least 45% of cases of severe hemophilia A, involves the inversion of intron 22 on the X chromosome. This results from the translocation and exchange of DNA between either of 2 "nonfunctional" factor VIII–related genes within intron 22 and areas of homologous DNA within the functional factor VIII gene.[2] A second inversion, involving an inversion of intron 1, has been reported in up to 5% of cases.[3,4] The recombination produces disjointed and inverted DNA sequences, preventing the transcription of a normal full-length factor VIII molecule. The coded protein typically possesses no functional or immunologic factor VIII activity in severe hemophilia A.

Less commonly, severe hemophilia A may be due to large gene deletions involving multiple or single domains, small point mutations resulting in the formation of stop codon sequences, or insertions and/or deletions within the gene. Moderate and mild severity types of hemophilia A are mainly the result of missense mutations; many different point mutations and deletions have been identified in patients with mild or moderate hemophilia A.[5] The incidence of alloantibody inhibitors in individuals with hemophilia A is highest in those with stop mutations in light-chain domains.[6] This is significant in that alloantibodies (and autoantibody inhibitors) are directed against epitopes on the $A_2 > C_2 > A_3$ domains of the factor VIII coagulant protein. The A_2 and A_3 domains normally interact with factor IXa; C_2 interacts with phospholipid and von Willebrand factor protein. These inhibitors block these interactions and interfere with formation of the tenase complex of coagulation (Fig. 4-1). A resource for the known mutations of factor VIII, along with a method for inputting new mutations, is HAMSTeRS (Hemophilia A Mutation, Structure, Test, and Resource Site), which can be found on the Internet at the following address: http://europium.csc.mrc.ac.uk/WebPages/Main/main.htm.

Numerous point mutations and deletions have been identified in individuals with hemophilia B. These frequently result in the production of a defective, nonfunctioning, but immunologically detectable, factor IX protein ("cross-reacting material," or CRM$^+$) in the plasma. Individuals with large gene deletions and nonsense mutations are usually CRM$^-$ and are most susceptible to the development of factor IX alloantibodies.[7] The Hemophilia B Mutation Database, which is an excellent resource for the factor IX gene, may be found on the Internet at the following address: http://www.kcl.ac.uk/ip/petergreen/haemBdatabase.html.

PRENATAL DIAGNOSIS/CARRIER TESTING

Evaluation of carrier status is a critical aspect in the routine medical care of carriers of the hemophilias and in the management of their future pregnancies. Genetic counseling and testing of obligate carriers and at-risk family members of the propositus with hemophilia may be useful in family and peripartum planning. The most common methods for identification of carrier status include direct gene mutation analysis and linkage analysis with the use of DNA

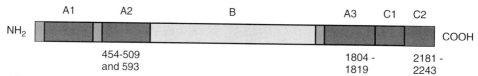

Figure 4-1 Factor VIII gene structure reveals the structural domains and known "hot spots" for antibody formation.

polymorphisms. For patients with severe hemophilia A, first-line testing involves identification of the intron 22 inversion. In individuals in whom the inversion is not detected, or for whom no family members are available for testing, the more cumbersome and labor-intensive method of linkage analysis can be performed with restriction fragment length polymorphism (RFLP) in the search for DNA polymorphisms.[8] Prior to any suggestion of testing, patients may be referred to a genetic counselor, who provides advice and recommends appropriate diagnostic testing. Gene mutations of the factor IX gene are more easily detected because it is one third the size of the factor VIII gene. More than 300 mutations of the factor IX gene have been identified, most common of which are single point mutations.[9] Microarray analysis may provide rapid screening for factor IX gene mutations.[10] The City of Hope National Medical Center has a central laboratory that provides much of this testing. (Contact Steve S. Sommer, MD, PhD, Clinical Molecular Diagnostic Laboratory, City of Hope National Medical Center Fox South, Second Floor, 1500 East Duarte Road, Duarte, CA 91010. Telephone: 888-8-COH-DNA; http://www.cityofhope.org/cmdl.) Other resources for gene testing may be found on the Internet at http://www.genetests.org.

Techniques for detecting hemophilia in the fetus include chorionic villous sampling at 12 weeks gestation or amniocentesis at 16 weeks. The risk of miscarriage from these procedures ranges between 0.5% and 1.0%. If DNA testing is unavailable, fetal blood sampling through fetoscopy can be performed at 20 weeks to measure factor VIII activity; however, this approach is associated with a significant (1% to 6%) risk of fetal demise.[11] This technique is not useful for measurement of factor IX levels because these are routinely reduced in newborns, along with the other vitamin K–dependent clotting factor proteins. The risks of prenatal testing must be balanced against the need for the clinician to know the diagnosis prior to delivery, or if termination is being considered. In a review by Ljung and Tedgård,[12] prenatal diagnosis was found to be more common among women who perceived hemophilia to be a very serious disease, had a positive attitude toward legal abortion, and belonged to a higher social class. Women with a brother or father with hemophilia considered the disease to be serious, but women with a hemophilic child did not.[12] This difference in perception may reflect the enhanced effectiveness of modern day treatment of patients with hemophilia, the reduced joint destruction and contracture formation, the ease of obtaining replacement products, and the use of central venous devices for delivery of treatment.

POSTNATAL DIAGNOSIS

Postnatal recognition and diagnosis of hemophilia A or B are facilitated when other family members are known to have hemophilia. The degree of severity of hemophilia is usually similar in all affected family members. The exception is Heckathorn disease,[13] in which considerable variability of factor VIII levels is noted among family members with hemophilia A.

Frequently, family members and the details of their medical histories are unavailable at the time of patient presentation. Moreover, approximately 30% of all hemophilia is due to spontaneous mutations in families without prior history of coagulation abnormalities. For instance, Queen Victoria of England appears to have spontaneously mutated her factor VIII gene and then spread it throughout European royalty. Measurement of factor VIII or IX activity in the affected individual is necessary to establish the diagnosis. For hemophilia A, factor VIII coagulant activity can be assessed through a direct functional plasma clot-based assay or with a chromogenic substrate-based assay. Factor IX activity levels also are measured with the use of a plasma clot-based assay. Hemophilia A must be differentiated from von Willebrand disease (VWD) by the measurement of von Willebrand factor (VWF) antigen and ristocetin cofactor activity, and by examination of the multimeric composition of the VWF protein with sodium dodecyl sulfate (SDS) gel chromatography, if clinically indicated. VWD variant types 2 Normandy (2N) and 3 may be phenotypically similar to severe hemophilia A, although the autosomally transmitted inheritance pattern of VWD should help to distinguish it from the sex-linked recessive genetic pattern of hemophilia A (see Chapter 7). In addition and in contrast to hemophilia A, replacement therapy with VWF-containing products produces an exaggerated recovery (higher than calculated incremental rise from baseline levels) and a sustained elevation and circulating half-life of factor VIII activity in individuals with VWD, particularly among those with severe type 3 VWD.

When hemophilia is suspected in a male fetus of a known carrier, factor VIII or IX activity (or both) should be measured from a cord blood sample. This avoids the need for venipuncture, which can produce clinically important bruising and/or hemorrhage in the severely affected neonate. The diagnosis of hemophilia B in the neonate may be confounded by the fact that factor IX levels (as well as those of other hepatically synthesized proteins) are significantly reduced at birth and may remain so for up to 6 months. Normal plasma activity levels of coagulation factors VIII and IX in individuals after infancy range between 0.5 and 1.5 IU/mL (50% and 150%). The severity of hemophilia is defined by the measured level of clotting factor activity: Severe hemophilia is defined as factor VIII or IX activity below 1% (<0.01 IU/mL); it occurs in approximately half of affected hemophiliacs. Moderate severity hemophilia occurs in about 10% of hemophiliacs, who have factor VIII or IX levels between 1% and 5% (0.01 and 0.05 IU/mL). Mild hemophilia occurs in 30% to 40% of hemophiliacs, who have factor VIII or IX activity levels above 5% (above 0.05 IU/mL).

Between 2% and 8% of hemophilic infants develop intracranial hemorrhage and scalp hematoma during the perinatal period. These complications are associated with prolonged and difficult labor, the use of vacuum extraction and forceps to facilitate delivery, the presence of cephalo-pelvic disproportion, and precipitous delivery.[14] Caesarean section does not eliminate bleeding risks. The Medical and Scientific Advisory Council (MASAC) of the National Hemophilia Foundation (NHF) recommends that vacuum devices and instrumentation such as fetal scalp samples and internal fetal scalp monitors should not be used because of the risk of bleeding in the infant.[15] Full recommendations may be found at the NHF website: http://www.hemophilia.org/NHFWeb/MainPgs/MainNHF.aspx?menuid=157&contentid=347.

Recently, intrauterine transfusion of clotting factor concentrate immediately before delivery of a male fetus known to have severe hemophilia A has been attempted in an effort to prevent such problems.[16] Unfortunately, this resulted in the formation of a high-titer alloantibody inhibitor in the infant shortly after birth, which suggests that this approach should be avoided because of its potential adverse stimulation of the immature immune system. In general, the most common initial bleeding events in hemophilic children occur in association with circumcision and cord necrosis. Ecchymoses may develop during the first few months of life, but spontaneous hemarthroses, the hallmark of the hemophilias, usually do not occur until approximately 1 year of age with the onset of walking. The development of hematomas at the site of intramuscular injection of routine vaccinations or medications (including the postnatal administration of vitamin K) should increase the suspicion that an abnormality exists. This type of bleeding can be avoided by administering these injections subcutaneously or after pretreatment with clotting factor concentrates. Oral bleeding due to loss of deciduous teeth, tongue biting, and frenulum injury is common in the young child and may require clotting factor replacement and adjunctive use of antifibrinolytic agents, such as tranexamic acid or ε-aminocaproic acid.

Patients with moderately severe hemophilia usually do not experience spontaneous hemorrhagic episodes, but minor trauma or surgery can precipitate bleeding unless clotting factor replacement or 1-deamino-8-D-arginine vasopressin (DDAVP) is provided prophylactically. Mild hemophilia may be detected incidentally during routine preoperative screening of the coagulation mechanism, which reveals a prolonged partial thromboplastin time (PTT).[17] Patients should be screened for VWD type 2N unless a definitive family history of hemophilia A has been established. Bleeding complications in hemophilia of moderate severity may occur after significant trauma or surgery, but spontaneous hemarthroses are rare, and some patients may never experience a bleeding event.

CLINICAL FEATURES OF THE HEMOPHILIAS

Intra-articular Bleeding: Hemarthroses and Hemophilic Arthropathy

The most common sites of spontaneous bleeding in individuals with severe hemophilia A or B involve the joints and muscles. The knees (greater than 50% of all bleeding events), elbows, ankles, shoulders, and wrists are affected in decreasing incidence. It is the recurrent nature of the bleeds into these joints that results in degeneration of the cartilage and progressive destruction of the joint space. The pathophysiology of hemophilic arthropathy can be divided into three phases. After hemorrhage into the joint occurs, iron is deposited into the synovium and chondrocytes of the articular cartilage (the first phase). Subsequently, focal areas of villous hypertrophy develop on the synovial surface, which, because of their vascularity and friability, continue to rebleed with normal joint stresses even with routine weight bearing. This ultimately establishes the "target joint" situation, which is characterized by recurrent, painful, and destructive bleeds into the same joint.[18]

Associated with iron deposition is the release of inflammatory cytokines that recruit macrophages and fibroblasts into the joint space and establish a favorable environment for progression of joint disease. This second phase of hemophilic arthropathy involves the development of chronic synovitis, pain, fibrosis, and progressive joint stiffness with decreased range of motion. Within the joint space can be found hydrolytic and proteolytic enzymes, such as acid phosphatase and cathepsin D.[19] In the final stage of hemophilic arthropathy (phase three), progressive and erosive destruction of the cartilage, narrowing of the joint space, subchondral cyst formation, and eventual collapse and sclerosis of the joint become apparent. Conventional roentgenographs traditionally have been used to monitor the progression of hemophilic arthropathy; however, until bone changes become apparent, the films appear normal and may cause the clinician to underestimate the extent of joint disease. Magnetic resonance imaging (MRI) is more sensitive than conventional radiographic studies for early identification of hemarthrosis, synovial hypertrophy, hemosiderin deposition, and osteochondral changes (cartilage thinning and erosion). Joint scoring systems have been developed for use in evaluating the degree of joint destruction over time.[20]

The predominant clinical manifestations of recurrent joint hemorrhage are pain and swelling. Well before the onset of pain, patients describe prickly sensations and burning within the joint as the first signs of bleeding. If the bleeding is allowed to continue, pain and swelling lead to fixation of the joint in a flexed position until the swelling subsides. Early recognition and prompt treatment of acute bleeding episodes are essential for preventing excessive hemorrhage into the joint space and minimizing subsequent joint destruction. The goal of administration of replacement clotting factor concentrate to treat the acute bleed ("on demand" therapy) is to increase factor VIII or IX activity levels to 30% to 50% of normal. Occasionally, repeat infusions of factor concentrate are necessary to terminate bleeding and reduce pain, especially in target joints. If significant pain and swelling are protracted, a short course of corticosteroids (prednisone 1 mg/kg/day for 4–5 days) may be given. This has proved more beneficial in children than in adults and should probably be avoided in patients with human immunodeficiency virus (HIV) infection. Rarely, joint aspirations are performed for patients with intractable pain despite factor replacement therapy, or for those with fever and in whom septic arthritis

4

is suspected. Prior to joint aspiration, adequate factor replacement therapy should be administered. Aspiration should be avoided in patients with alloantibody inhibitors because of the increased risks of bleeding complications associated with the procedure.

Narcotic analgesics frequently are a necessary therapeutic adjunct for pain control, and application of ice packs and avoidance of weight bearing with the use of crutches reduce the inflammation and pain that accompany the hemarthrosis. Initiation of physical therapy as soon as pain control is achieved reduces the development of muscle atrophy around the affected joint and prevents permanent flexion contractures. Plaster casting of target joints should not be performed.

A secondary prophylaxis regimen of replacement therapy can be of immense benefit to patients with target joints. This consists of administering the appropriate clotting factor concentrate two or three times weekly, to maintain trough clotting factor activity levels of 1% to 3%. When sustained for at least 3 months, this approach can effectively interrupt the cycle of recurrent bleeding.[21,22] In patients who have developed chronic synovitis that is refractory to medical management, surgical debridement and synovectomy should be considered to reduce the bleeding and pain; however, joint destruction may progress, albeit at a much slower pace. This procedure is of greatest benefit in patients with minimal hemarthropathy.

Radioactive and chemical nonsurgical synovectomies have been used to break the vicious cycle of hemarthrosis–chronic synovitis–hemarthrosis. These techniques currently are most commonly used in developing countries, where surgery and the required clotting factor replacement concentrates are not available. Nonsurgical synovectomies may also be beneficial for individuals with high-titer alloantibody inhibitors, in whom surgery is particularly risky and the ability to achieve adequate hemostasis is unpredictable, despite administration of inhibitor "bypassing" clotting factor replacement therapies. Most radionuclide synovectomies in hemophilia have been performed with the β emitter isotopes yttrium-90 (^{90}Y) and phosphorus-32 (^{32}P); these are less likely than γ emitters to be mutagenic and to produce localized inflammatory reactions within the synovium.[23] A greater than 50% reduction in frequency of bleeding events and pain occurs after radionuclide synovectomy, and the range of motion of the joints is stabilized or improved in more than 50% of patients.

Unfortunately, despite this treatment, long-term follow-up studies show that gradual deterioration in range of motion in the affected joint continues. Of concern is that acute lymphocytic leukemia recently was reported in two young hemophiliac patients a few years after they underwent radioactive synovectomy.[24,25] However, since 1988, more than 1000 joint injections of ^{32}P have occurred in more than 563 hemophiliac patients, and because the incidence of acute leukemia in children in the United States is approximately 2.8 per 100,000 persons/year, it is difficult to determine whether these isolated cases of leukemia are due to radioactive synovectomy, or whether they represent coincidental events that occur in accordance with population statistical expectations. Chemical synovectomies with osmic acid or rifampicin reduce the frequency of hemarthroses but produce acute and painful inflammatory reactions, with overall results that are inferior to those of the radionuclides. The best method of preventing progressive joint destruction is to prevent intra-articular bleeding in the first place. Thus, the use of primary prophylaxis regimens (twice or thrice weekly with clotting factor replacement therapy, beginning in infancy after the first bleed and continuing indefinitely thereafter) is being investigated as a means of achieving this goal.

Intramuscular Hemorrhage

Intramuscular hemorrhages, which represent the second most common site of bleeding in individuals with hemophilia, account for 30% of bleeding events. The location of the intramuscular hemorrhage determines the morbidity of the event. Hemorrhage into large muscles, although extensive, generally resolves without complications because it is not into a confined space. Bleeding into a closed fascial compartment may lead to significant compression of vital structures with resultant ischemia, gangrene, flexion contractures, and neuropathy (compartment syndrome). Intramuscular hematomas manifest with localized tenderness and pain and may be associated with low-grade fevers, large ecchymoses, and elevations of serum lactate dehydrogenase (LDH) and creatine kinase. Bleeding into the psoas muscles and retroperitoneal space can produce sudden onset of inguinal pain and decreased range of motion in the ipsilateral hip, which assumes a markedly flexed position, usually with lateral rotation. Hemorrhage may become life threatening if a large volume of blood is lost. In addition, femoral nerve compression can occur with permanent disability if a compartment syndrome develops. The diagnosis can be confirmed by pelvic ultrasonography or computed tomography (CT).[26] Bleeding into this area must be controlled rapidly by raising and maintaining clotting factor activity at 80% to 100% of normal for at least 48 to 72 hours. Surgery is to be strictly avoided in this situation.

Hematuria

Spontaneous gross hematuria occurs frequently in patients with hemophilia and is usually painless unless intraureteral clots develop. Hematuria may be precipitated by the use of nonsteroidal anti-inflammatory drugs, trauma, or exertion. Pelvic clots, obstructive hydronephrosis, compromised collecting systems, and retroperitoneal fibrosis can be demonstrated on intravenous pyelograms. The cause of spontaneous hematuria in individuals with hemophilia is unknown, but it may be due to direct tubular and glomerular damage caused by circulating immune complexes formed after clotting factor replacement therapy. Immune complexes may also mediate the development of anaphylaxis and nephrotic syndrome, which can occur after factor IX replacement therapy in patients with severe hemophilia B and alloantibodies directed against factor IX.[27] Individuals with large deletions in the factor IX gene appear to be at highest risk. This syndrome has been reported to occur with all commercially available factor IX products.[28] Avoidance of any or all sources of coagulation factor IX for replacement therapy is necessary, and recombinant factor VIIa (rFVIIa) concentrate has become the treatment of choice for acute bleeding events in these individuals.

Other causes of hematuria that should be considered include infection, neoplasm, and renal or ureteral stones.

Nephrolithiasis has been seen most commonly in HIV-infected hemophiliac patients who take the HIV protease inhibitor indinavir (Crixivan; Merck & Co., Inc., Whitehouse Station, NJ), which produces crystalluria and calculi consisting of the intact drug.

The generally recommended approach to the management of hematuria depends on the cause; however, the mainstay of treatment initially is hydration. If hematuria persists beyond several days, clotting factor replacement therapy to raise factor activity levels to 50% of normal should be administered. Antifibrinolytic agents generally should be avoided because they may precipitate intraureteral clot formation, which can lead to obstruction of the collecting system and eventual renal failure.

Intracranial Hemorrhage

The most common cause of death from bleeding in patients with the hemophilias is intracranial/intracerebral hemorrhage. Intracranial hemorrhage may occur with minimal trauma, particularly in children, or spontaneously in the absence of identifiable trauma; intracranial hemorrhage is spontaneous 50% of the time in affected adults. HIV-infected hemophilia patients who receive antiretroviral protease inhibitors may have an increased risk of developing spontaneous intracranial (and intramuscular) hemorrhage.[29] Fifty percent of patients with intracranial hemorrhage develop permanent neurologic sequelae, and 30% of events result in death. Presenting clinical symptoms usually include headaches, which can be associated with nausea and vomiting, and occasional seizures. Whenever an intracranial hemorrhage is documented, suspected, or even remotely possible after head trauma, it is imperative that factor VIII or IX concentrate (appropriate to the type of hemophilia) be administered immediately to achieve 100% of normal factor activity. This treatment must precede any diagnostic testing. CT scan of the head may show no evidence of bleeding immediately after the event. In patients who require a lumbar puncture, factor VIII or IX replacement therapy should be given 15 to 30 minutes prior to the procedure to increase the factor activity to 100% of normal. If the patient has not undergone a recent recovery study to assess response to factor infusion, a clotting factor level should be performed after the factor has been infused and prior to the procedure. Because of the serious implications of ignoring an intracranial bleed, even patients with mild hemophilia and factor VIII or IX activity levels below 50% of normal should receive clotting factor replacement therapy for severe head trauma.

Gastrointestinal and Oropharyngeal Bleeding

Gastrointestinal bleeding occurs in approximately 10% to 15% of adult hemophilia patients. Anatomic lesions are more common than is spontaneous hemorrhage. Neoplastic processes, peptic ulcer disease, gastritis, and varices should be excluded as sources of bleeding. In those individuals with chronic hepatitis C and cirrhosis, varices that result from portal hypertension are the leading cause of acute bleeds. Patients with gastrointestinal hemorrhage should be treated with clotting factor replacement to at least 50% of normal activity for several days.

The oropharynx is a highly vascular area, and excessive bleeding may occur from small lacerations, a bitten tongue, and even the appearance of a new tooth. Of particular concern are retropharyngeal bleeds that may lead to upper airway obstruction.[30] This type of hemorrhage is a hematologic emergency and requires clotting factor replacement to levels of 80% to 100% of normal. Bleeding associated with simple dental extractions after local injections of anesthesia can be managed with oral administration of antifibrinolytic agents and topical application of fibrin sealants. If nerve block injections are used for anesthesia in more complex oral surgery, clotting factor concentrate should be administered prior to the procedure to prevent untoward hemorrhage along fascial planes in the neck, which could result in airway compromise. Major oral surgery requires clotting factor replacement to levels of between 25% and 50% of normal, along with administration of antifibrinolytic agents following surgery for 3 to 10 days. Other comments regarding surgical procedures in hemophiliac patients are discussed in Chapter 37.

Pseudotumor Formation in Hemophilia

In 1% to 2% of those with severe hemophilia, hematomas produced by repetitive bleeding episodes continue to enlarge and may encapsulate. These have the appearance of expanding masses on roentgenography and may invade contiguous structures, including bone, muscle, or soft tissue organs. Pseudotumors themselves are composed of old clot and necrotic tissue and arise because of inadequate treatment during bleeding events. Symptoms associated with expanding pseudotumors are related to the size of the encapsulated mass and the degree of compromise of the integrity of the structures they are invading. Noninvasive techniques, such as MRI, ultrasonography, and CT, should be used to diagnose pseudotumor; needle biopsy may produce serious bleeding complications. Operative biopsies and subsequent surgical removal are associated with up to 20% mortality despite adequate coverage with clotting factor concentrates. Improved surgical results may be attained if the pseudotumor is evacuated and the cavity packed with copious amounts of fibrin sealant.[31] Adequate and immediate clotting factor replacement therapy of acute bleeds should minimize the risk of pseudotumor formation.

LABORATORY CHARACTERISTICS

Hemophilia A or B should be suspected in male patients with unusually easy bruisability and abnormal bleeding, accompanied by an isolated prolongation of the PTT. Individuals with any of the hemophilias have normal prothrombin times, platelet counts, and platelet function studies. Usually, bleeding times are normal. Mixing studies performed with equal parts of patient plasma and normal pooled plasma incubated at 37°C should show complete and prompt correction of the prolonged PTT. Correction of the PTT in the mixture at 0 and 120 minutes of incubation essentially excludes the presence of an alloantibody inhibitor directed against a specific clotting factor or the presence of a lupus-like anticoagulant directed against phospholipid in the PTT assay system (see Chapter 6).

Correction of the PTT through the mixing studies conducted at 2 hours incubation eliminates the likelihood that any weak neutralizing inhibitors are present. Factor VIII alloantibody and autoantibody inhibitors interact with the factor VIII coagulant protein in a time- and temperature-dependent manner. If a lupus-like anticoagulant is suspected, a dilute phospholipid-based assay, such as dilute Russell's viper venom time, the tissue thromboplastin inhibition time, or the platelet neutralization procedure, which uses platelets as a source of phospholipid, should be performed to confirm its presence (see Chapter 19). If a clotting factor deficiency is suspected from the mixing study, assays should be performed to determine the activity levels of specific clotting factor proteins in the intrinsic pathway of coagulation, including factors XII, XI, IX, and VIII. Such assays also define the severity of the specific clotting factor deficiency.

In general, specific clotting factor assays are performed through a PTT-based one-stage clotting time. This type of assay assumes that the level of factor VIII is rate limiting, and that all other components of the assay are present at saturating levels. The one-stage PTT assay is the most physiologic of the factor VIII assays.[32] Recently, chromogenic assays for factor VIII activity have been introduced that are based on the quantity of factor Xa generated in the presence of factor VIII:C, factor IX, thrombin, calcium, and phospholipid. Chromogenic assays generally yield about 30% higher levels of factor VIII activity, compared with the standard partial thromboplastin time (PTT)-based factor VIII:C assay, in individuals who have received the B-domain deleted form of recombinant factor VIII concentrate,[33] and to a lesser degree in individuals on recombinant full-length factor VIII concentrates. Discrepancies between the one-stage clotting assay and the chromogenic assay with recombinant B-domain deleted factor VIII concentrate probably reflect differences in phospholipid content between the two assay systems. The use of a B-domain deleted factor VIII specific reference standard has resolved this discrepancy among the clotting assays and has been used to confirm that B-domain deleted factor VIII and plasma-derived factor VIII are bioequivalent.[34] No standardization of inhibitor quantitation (Bethesda unit calculation) uses the chromogenic assay.

In individuals having low levels of factor VIII activity, especially females, VWD type 2N must be considered. These individuals are phenotypic hemophilic patients with normally functioning VWF protein in ristocetin-based assays and their VWF multimeric structure is normal on SDS polyacrylamide gel electrophoresis; however, assays that examine factor VIII binding to VWF protein are abnormal, reflecting the presence of an inherited point mutation in the VWF gene at the specific binding site for factor VIII. This results in a significantly decreased plasma circulation time and decreased plasma concentration for factor VIII. Additionally, the inheritance pattern is autosomal rather than X-linked.

Up to 35% of individuals with severe hemophilia A and 1% to 4% of those with hemophilia B will develop alloantibody inhibitors. These neutralizing alloantibodies should be suspected in hemophilic patients in whom recovery (the percent incremental response to clotting factor concentrate 15 to 30 minutes after administration) of clotting factor activity levels is less than 60% of the expected increase beyond baseline levels. The inhibitor can be quantitated through the Bethesda assay,[35] in which residual clotting factor activity in a mixture of patient plasma and pooled normal plasma (PNP) is determined by means of a one-stage clotting time. One Bethesda unit (BU) is arbitrarily defined as the amount of antibody in a patient's plasma that causes a 50% decrease in factor VIII activity in PNP after incubation at 37°C for 2 hours. Although this assay originally was developed for use in patients with hemophilia A, the same procedure is useful for quantitating inhibitors in patients with hemophilia B and those with autoantibodies directed against clotting factors.

Autoantibody inhibitors directed specifically against factor VIII (acquired hemophilia) and less commonly against factor IX may occur in individuals with previously normal coagulation. In acquired hemophilia, quantitation through the Bethesda assay may not accurately reflect the bleeding tendency because these autoantibodies follow type II pharmacokinetics with a nonlinear neutralization pattern and incomplete inactivation of factor VIII activity, even at the highest concentrations (see Chapter 6).[36]

Low-titer inhibitors (low responders) are defined as patients having less than 5 BU—a level that does not rise after reexposure to the clotting factor protein contained in replacement therapies (anamnestic response). High-titer inhibitors are defined as greater than 10 BU in association with significant anamnesis soon after reexposure to clotting factor concentrate (high responders). Individuals with antibody titers between 5 and 10 BU may be high or low responders, depending on the presence or absence of anamnesis. A modification of the Bethesda assay, the Nijmegen assay, was developed to improve the specificity and reliability of detecting low-titer inhibitors in the range of 0 to 0.8 BU. Both test and control mixtures are buffered with an imidazole buffer to stabilize the pH at 7.4, and the original buffer in the control mixture is replaced by immunodepleted factor VIII–deficient plasma to attain comparable protein concentrations in both mixtures.[37] This assay is generally reserved for clinical research studies in which detection of the presence of low-titer inhibitors is important.

THERAPEUTIC MODALITIES FOR THE HEMOPHILIAS

Hemophilia Treatment Centers

Hemophilia treatment centers (HTCs) provide comprehensive medical and psychosocial services to patients and their families with inherited bleeding disorders. Through a multidisciplinary team of nurses, physicians, psychosocial professionals, and laboratory technologists, state-of-the-art care is provided for patients with hemophilia and its complications. A survival advantage for patients with hemophilia has been shown for those patients followed and treated at an HTC.[38] Additionally, HTCs provide more cost-effective care, can distribute considerably less expensive clotting factor concentrates to patients (through the Public Health Service 340B Drug Pricing Program), and facilitate patient independence by training patients and family members to infuse clotting factor concentrate at the first sign of bleeding, or when prophylaxis against bleeding is desired. In the United States and Canada, HTCs are subsidized by funding from their respective federal governments.

Clotting Factor Replacement Therapy With Coagulation Factor Concentrates

Replacement of factor VIII or IX to hemostatically adequate plasma levels for prevention or treatment of acute bleeding forms the basis of management in hemophilia (Tables 4-1 and 4-2). Treatment should be administered at early onset of symptoms to limit the amount of bleeding and to prevent damage to the surrounding tissues. Replacement therapy should also be administered immediately before surgery to minimize intraoperative bleeding complications, or prophylactically to prevent hemophilic arthropathy.

Factor VIII and factor IX replacement products may be derived from plasma or may be genetically engineered through recombinant technology that uses mammalian cell lines transfected with normal human genes that code for clotting factor proteins (Tables 4-3 and 4-4). Factor replacement products are often classified on the basis of their final purity, defined as specific activity (international units [IU] of clotting factor activity per mg of protein). Intermediate purity products have relatively low specific activities (<50 IU/mg) because they are contaminated by additional plasma proteins, including von Willebrand factor, fibrinogen, fibronectin, and other noncoagulant proteins. High-purity (>50 IU/mg) and ultra-high-purity (>3000 IU/mg for factor VIII concentrates; >160 IU/mg for factor IX concentrates) products contain few or no contaminating plasma proteins other than albumin as a stabilizer. Recently, albumin-free final formulations of recombinant "full-length" and B-domain

Table 4-1 Product Dosing

Type of Bleed	Goal of Therapy (% Clotting Factor Activity Level)
Joint Dental	>30–50
Genitourinary Gastrointestinal	50
Muscle	>80
Intracranial	100

Factor IX dose to be administered = (weight in kg × desired change in clotting factor activity level)*; 1 IU factor IX concentrate per kilogram is estimated to raise the clotting factor IX activity level in plasma by 1%.

Factor VIII dose to be administered = {1/2} factor IX dose; 1 IU factor VIII concentrate per kilogram is estimated to raise the clotting factor VIII activity level in plasma by 2%.

Consider the use of recombinant factor VIII or IX concentrates in those individuals not previously exposed to blood products, or who are human immunodeficiency virus (HIV) and/or hepatitis C seronegative.

For high titer or for refractory bleeding associated with factor VIII or IX alloantibody inhibitors: Recombinant factor VIIa concentrate, 90 μg per kilogram intravenous bolus every 2 to 3 hours until bleeding ceases (larger dosing regimens are experimental but may be useful in refractory bleeding). This product is the treatment of choice for individuals with factor IX alloantibody inhibitors and anaphylaxis and/or renal disease associated with the use of factor IX–containing concentrates.

FEIBA VH: 50 to 100 IU per kilogram intravenous infusion, not to exceed 200 IU/kg/24 hr.

*Need to multiply calculated factor IX dose by 1.2 when factor IX deficiency is replaced with recombinant factor IX concentrate.

Table 4-2 Options for Acute and Chronic Replacement Treatment of Individuals with Alloantibody Inhibitors to Factor VIII or IX

Desmopressin (0.3 μg per kilogram in 50 mL normal saline administered IV over 20 min); may be useful for raising factor VIII activity levels for a short time in individuals with low-titer FVIII alloantibodies and minor bleeds, or in anticipation of minor surgery. Not effective for factor IX.

High doses of FVIII or FIX concentrate (200 IU per kilogram); effective in preventing or treating acute bleeding episodes in low-titer inhibitors (≤5 Bethesda units and absent anamnestic responses); daily dosing may provide an effective approach to suppressing high-titer inhibitors (>5 Bethesda units with anamnestic responses) in immune tolerance induction regimens.

Daily administration of factor concentrates (50–200 IU per kilogram); may be an effective approach to suppressing low-titer inhibitors (≤5 Bethesda units), particularly when immune tolerance induction regimens are initiated within weeks after the alloantibody inhibitor is developed.

Cyclophosphamide, intravenous immune globulin, and daily factor concentrates (50–200 IU per kilogram); may be more effective in suppressing high-titer and high-responding anamnestic inhibitors or refractory low-titer alloantibody inhibitors as part of immune tolerance induction regimens; concern about increased susceptibility to opportunistic infections and potential leukemogenesis of alkylating agent.

Rituximab (375 mg/m^2) to suppress the lymphocyte clone(s) responsible for synthesizing the alloantibody; to be used in conjunction with daily administration of clotting factor concentrates (experimental).

Treatment of bleeding episodes with "bypassing agents"; useful for reversing or preventing hemorrhagic complications in those with high- or low-titer alloantibody inhibitors; in those with factor IX alloantibody inhibitors and prior anaphylactic responses or nephrotic syndrome complications with plasma-derived bypassing agents, recombinant factor VIIa concentrate replacement therapy is considered the treatment of choice for acute bleeding episodes.

deleted factor VIII concentrates and a third-generation "full-length" factor VIII concentrate manufactured in the absence of any added mammalian protein have become available. Monoclonal antibody–purified, plasma-derived factor IX concentrate and recombinant factor IX concentrate are free of albumin.

All coagulation factor concentrates, plasma-derived and recombinant, have been subjected to some method of viral inactivation, attenuation, or elimination. These techniques include high dry heating, pasteurization, and solvent detergent extraction used singly or in combination. Viral safety may be further enhanced by the addition of immunoaffinity chromatography (monoclonal antibody purification) and gel filtration chromatography steps to segregate the desired therapeutic clotting factor protein from contaminating proteins and viruses. Viral attenuated plasma-derived factor concentrates have been eradicated of lipid-enveloped viruses such as HIV, West Nile virus, and hepatitis B and C, and no transmissions of these diseases have been documented since 1985 for factor VIII concentrates, and since 1990 for factor IX concentrates. Non–lipid-enveloped viruses such as hepatitis A and parvovirus B19 are not susceptible to these techniques, and sporadic outbreaks have been reported.[39,40]

All patients who are to receive clotting factor concentrates should be vaccinated against hepatitis A and B during infancy. Recombinant factor concentrates by definition will not

Table 4-3 Clotting Factor Concentrates Available in the United States

Type/Product Name	Manufacturer	Method of Viral Inactivation	Specific Activity (IU/mg Protein, Discounting Albumin)
Ultrapure Recombinant			
Advate rAHF PFM (third-generation full-length rFVIII)	Baxter BioScience (Switzerland)	Solvent detergent (TNBP/polysorbate 80), Triton X 100; immunoaffinity chromatography; ion exchange	4000–10,000 (albumin free; no human or animal protein used in the culture medium or manufacturing process)
Helixate FS (second-generation full-length rFVIII)	CSL Behring (Germany)	Solvent detergent (TNBP/polysorbate 80); immunoaffinity chromatography; ion exchange; ultrafiltration	2600–6800 (human albumin-free final formulation; sucrose as stabilizer)
Kogenate FS (second-generation full-length rFVIII)	Bayer (USA)	Solvent detergent (TNBP/polysorbate 80); immunoaffinity chromatography; ion exchange; ultrafiltration	2600–6800 (human albumin-free final formulation; sucrose as stabilizer)
ReFacto (second-generation rFVIII, B-domain deleted)	Wyeth (Sweden)	Solvent detergent (TNBP/Triton X 100); immunoaffinity chromatography; ion exchange; nanofiltration	13,000 (human albumin-free final formulation)
Recombinate AHF (first-generation full-length rFVIII)	Baxter BioScience	Immunoaffinity, ion exchange chromatography (bovine serum albumin used in culture medium for Chinese hamster ovary cells)	>4000 (human albumin as a stabilizer)
Ultrapure Plasma–Derived (Immunopurified by Monoclonal Antibody Chromatography)			
Monoclate P	CSL Behring	Pasteurization (heated in solution, 60°C, 10 hr); immunoaffinity chromatography	No intact von Willebrand factor protein; >3000
Hemofil M AHF	Baxter BioScience	Solvent detergent (TNBP/octoxynol 9); immunoaffinity chromatography	>3000
Monarc-M	Baxter/American Red Cross (with recovered plasma from the American Red Cross)	Solvent detergent (TNBP/octoxynol 9); immunoaffinity chromatography	>3000
Intermediate-Purity and High-Purity Plasma–Derived			
Alphanate	Grifols (United Kingdom)	Solvent detergent (TNBP/polysorbate 80); affinity chromatography; dry heat (80°C, 72 hr)	140 (contains von Willebrand factor [VWF] protein; >400 IU per milligram after correction for VWF content)
Humate P	CSL Behring	Pasteurization (heating in solution, 60°C, 10 hr)	38 (contains large amount of VWF protein)
Koate DVI	Talecris (USA)	Solvent detergent (TNBP/polysorbate 80) and dry heat (80°C, 72 hr)	50–100 (contains VWF protein)

Table 4-4 Factor IX Concentrates Available in the United States

Type/Product Name	Manufacturer	Method of Viral Inactivation	Specific Activity (IU/mg Protein, Discounting Albumin)
Ultrapure Recombinant Factor IX			
Benefix	Wyeth (Sweden)	Nanofiltration; affinity chromatography	>200 (no albumin added to final product; no animal- or human-derived protein in cell culture)
Very Highly Purified Plasma–Derived Factor IX			
Alphanine	Grifols (United Kingdom)	Solvent/detergent (TNBP/polysorbate 80); dual-affinity chromatography; nanofiltration (viral filter)	>200
Mononine	CSL Behring (Germany)	Sodium thiocyanate and ultrafiltration; monoclonal antibody immunoaffinity chromatography	>190
Low-Purity Plasma–Derived Factor IX/Prothrombin Complex Concentrates (Nonactivated)			
Bebulin VH	Baxter BioScience (Austria)	Vapor heat (60°C, 10 hr, 1190 mbar; then 80°C, 1 hr, 375 mbar)	<50
Profilnine SD	Grifols	Solvent detergent (TNBP/polysorbate 80)	<50
Proplex-T	Baxter BioScience	20% ethanol, dry heat (60°C, 144 hr)	<50

transmit any of the hepatitides, HIV, or parvovirus B19; however, if they contain human albumin as a stabilizer, the theoretical concern has been raised that they could transmit the prion(s) associated with Creutzfeldt-Jakob disease (CJD) or variant CJD. Up until this time, longitudinal epidemiologic surveillance and autopsy studies analyzing postmortem brain tissue from individuals with hemophilia have yielded no evidence for transmission of CJD despite repeated exposure to blood products. However, recent reports from the United Kingdom confirm that variant CJD can be transmitted through blood transfusions, thus justifying longitudinal surveillance for this and other blood-borne pathogens within the hemophilia population.

All commercially available factor VIII replacement concentrates appear to be equally efficacious, with equivalent postadministration recovery levels observed for plasma-derived and recombinant full-length and B-domain deleted factor VIII preparations.[34,41] The dosing of clotting factor replacement therapy in hemophilia is based on the patient's plasma volume, the distribution of the clotting protein between intravascular and extravascular compartments, the circulating half-life of the clotting factor within the plasma, and the level of clotting factor activity required to achieve adequate hemostasis or prophylaxis. Dosage is calculated by assuming that 1 IU per kilogram of body weight of factor VIII concentrate will raise the plasma activity of factor VIII by approximately 0.02 IU per milliliter (2%), and 1 IU per kilogram of factor IX concentrate, which has a larger volume of distribution, will increase plasma factor IX levels by 0.01 IU per milliliter (1%).

Administration of the recombinant factor IX concentrate may yield recoveries that are 80% of expected at 15 to 30 minutes, requiring a correction factor of 1.2 when the dose to be infused is calculated. Not all individuals with hemophilia B exhibit this variation in recovery, necessitating baseline recovery studies before treatment with the product is begun.

The circulating half-life for factor VIII is 8 to 12 hours; for factor IX, it is around 18 hours. Optimal hemostatic plasma levels of factors VIII and IX vary according to the clinical situation. "On-demand" regimens administer factor concentrate at the time of the hemorrhagic event; levels of 30% to 50% of normal clotting factor activity are required to control bleeding of minor to moderate severity, to prevent recurrent hemorrhage, and to support tissue healing. Levels of 50% to 100% clotting factor activity should be achieved and maintained for a minimum of 7 to 10 days to treat or prevent life- and limb-threatening hemorrhage or for major surgical procedures (see Chapter 37). Routinely, clotting factor replacement therapy is delivered by bolus infusion immediately after reconstitution.

The use of continuous infusion regimens for clotting factor replacement has become more common, especially in the postoperative setting. Continuous infusion maintains a stable and continuous therapeutic level of factor activity without a "peaks and troughs" effect. This translates into a decrease in the total amount of factor infused (and therefore decreased cost of care) and easy laboratory monitoring with random blood samples.[42] None of the clotting factor concentrates have been licensed for use as a continuous infusion. Many of the HTCs have developed their own protocols for preparation, infusion, and standards of safety with little risk of infection. These protocols are developed in cooperation with research pharmacists. How much added albumin is necessary to maintain the stability of a particular product is not defined. Currently, infusion pumps have not been licensed for use with clotting factor concentrates.

The choice of which clotting factor concentrate to administer to individuals with hemophilia A or B should be individualized; participation of the patient or family in this decision is essential. Consideration should be given to cost, age of the patient, presence of an alloantibody inhibitor, and HIV and hepatitis C virus (HCV) status. In addition, some practitioners who treat patients with hemophilia believe that the ultra-high-purity factor VIII concentrates (devoid of VWF protein), both plasma-derived and recombinant types, may have a greater tendency to induce alloantibody development.[43] Because of this belief, they will not use these products in previously untreated patients. The literature suggests, however, that the increased incidence of alloantibodies with these factor VIII concentrates actually may be related to increased surveillance testing for alloantibodies with the use of very sensitive assays.[44] Factor VIII concentrates of intermediate purity have been shown to inhibit normal lymphocyte immune responses in vitro, probably through extraneous proteins or the presence of transforming growth factor (TGF)-β within the preparations. Absolute CD4 lymphocyte counts have been shown to decrease more quickly in HIV-seropositive patients with factor VIII concentrates of intermediate purity than in those who use ultra-high-purity products[45]; however, this has not been shown to affect survival in hemophiliacs with acquired immunodeficiency syndrome (AIDS) or with progression of asymptomatic to symptomatic HIV disease. Similar immune effects have been reported with factor IX concentrates.

The choice of which factor IX concentrate to administer should take into account the thrombogenic potential of the intermediate-purity products, which contain some activated factors II, VII, and X, in addition to IX. Prolonged and repeated use of these intermediate products has been associated with the development of disseminated intravascular coagulopathy, stroke, and myocardial infarction; this risk is increased further in patients with hepatic insufficiency. This fact may be related to the cumulative and sustained procoagulant effects of the activated clotting factors Xa and IIa, which have considerably longer circulating half-lives than factor IX. Little or no thrombogenicity has been observed with the ultra-high-purity factor IX plasma-derived or recombinant concentrates; therefore, these products are more appropriate for immune tolerance induction regimens, primary prophylaxis, and surgery. Despite the risk of thrombogenicity, when used appropriately, intermediate-purity factor IX concentrates are safe and effective.

New methods of delivering and producing factor concentrates are being investigated. Clinical trials have begun to study a factor VIII concentrate with a half-life of days rather than hours. A recent report described improved production of factor VIII via the mammary glands of transgenically altered pigs; this may provide a ready source of recombinant factor for developing countries.[46]

DDAVP

1-Deamino-8-D-arginine vasopressin (DDAVP) plays an important role in the management of patients with mild hemophilia A. Intravenous infusion of DDAVP at a dose of 0.3 μg per kilogram of body weight in 50 mL of normal saline over 30 minutes, or intranasal spray of 150 μg per nostril produces a rise in circulating factor VIII and VWF protein levels by two- or threefold over the patient's baseline level through induction of exocytosis of factor VIII/VWF from Weibel-Palade bodies in endothelial cells, and perhaps from α granules in platelets. The peak effect of the intravenous form is seen in 30 to 60 minutes,[47] and the intranasal form peaks 60 to 90 minutes[48] after administration. Thus, DDAVP can be given in advance of dental work and minor surgical procedures or at the time of acute spontaneous or traumatic bleeding events to avoid the need for factor VIII replacement products. DDAVP can be administered every 12 to 24 hours; however, tachyphylaxis often develops because of the depletion of factor VIII/VWF from their storage sites. Common adverse effects associated with the use of DDAVP include flushing, hypertension, and retention of free water. This last effect can induce severe hyponatremia, especially in infants and the elderly, and can precipitate the onset of seizures. Therefore, free-water fluid intake should be restricted and serum sodium levels monitored in these individuals. Of concern in the elderly population is the occurrence of angina pectoris, stroke, and coronary artery thrombosis; DDAVP should be used cautiously in this population. DDAVP releases tissue plasminogen activator from endothelial cells and may stimulate local fibrinolysis, particularly on mucosal surfaces. Therefore, for bleeding in the gastrointestinal or genitourinary tract or in the oropharyngeal area, antifibrinolytic agents (see below) should be administered concurrently with DDAVP.

ANCILLARY TREATMENTS

Antifibrinolytic Agents

Antifibrinolytic agents are a useful but underused form of ancillary therapy in the management of patients with hemophilia A or B. By inhibiting fibrinolysis of the thrombus by plasmin, antifibrinolytics can maintain the integrity of the clot and prevent hemorrhage. They are particularly useful in the management of mucous membrane bleeding from the oropharynx, nose, and genitourinary tract because secretions from these sites naturally contain fibrinolytic enzymes. ε-Aminocaproic acid (EACA) (Amicar; Xanodyne Pharmaceuticals, Inc., Newport, Ky) and tranexamic acid (Cyklokapron) may be administered intravenously, orally, or topically in patients with hemophilia. These medications can be used alone or in conjunction with DDAVP for the prevention or control of bleeding. Optimum dose and duration have not been well defined, but Amicar is usually dosed at 50 mg per kilogram every 6 hours for 3 to 10 days, and Cyklokapron is given at a dose of 1.5 g every 6 hours for 3 to 6 days.

Fibrin Glues or Sealants

Fibrin glues, also known as fibrin sealants or fibrin tissue adhesives, are composed of thrombin, fibrinogen, and sometimes factor XIII and antifibrinolytic agents (see Chapter 29). Major benefits have been attained when fibrin sealants are combined with continuous or bolus infusions of factor concentrate. A "swish and swallow" regimen with tranexamic acid solution daily for 2 weeks can be used after fibrin sealant has been applied topically to sites of oral surgery.[49] Fibrin tissue adhesives have been used very successfully and have reduced bleeding in patients with hemophilia who undergo orthopaedic surgery.[50] The fibrin sealants available in the United States have been virally inactivated.

PROPHYLAXIS/INDWELLING VENOUS ACCESS DEVICE

With the increased safety of coagulation factor replacement products, primary prophylaxis regimens with factor VIII or IX concentrates have become very acceptable. The goal of primary prophylaxis in severe hemophilia is to prevent hemarthroses and the subsequent development of hemophilic arthropathy. Primary prophylaxis is initiated prior to or after the first hemarthrosis, usually around the age of 14 to 18 months, at the time that the child begins to walk. Enough factor replacement therapy is administered to maintain coagulation factor trough levels of only 1% to 3% activity, which reduces the incidence of spontaneous hemarthrosis. In severe hemophilia A, this is usually achieved by infusing factor VIII concentrate on Monday and Wednesday at a dose of 25 to 40 IU per kilogram, and on Friday at a dose of 40 IU per kilogram. For severe hemophilia B, dosing with factor IX concentrate at 25 to 40 IU per kilogram occurs twice weekly, usually on Monday and Thursday. Primary prophylaxis has been shown (1) to decrease the total number and frequency of all bleeding episodes; (2) to decrease the frequency of repetitive joint bleeds; (3) to decrease the rate of deterioration of the joint as observed on x-ray; (4) to reduce the number of days lost from school; and (5) to decrease the number of days spent in the hospital undergoing treatment for severe bleeds.

To administer clotting factor two or three times per week, it may be necessary to implant an indwelling venous access device when peripheral access is unavailable. This is especially true for small children. Venous access devices consist of Port-a-Caths, which do not require daily care by the family, and Hickman or Broviac catheters. These indwelling venous access devices, however, are the cause of most of the complications associated with prophylaxis. Systemic infections complicate the long-term use of venous access devices in 10% to 50% of patients with hemophilia. Catheter-related thromboses in the upper extremities occur up to 50% of the time. To reduce the risk of thrombosis, it is standard procedure to flush the catheters after use with 20 mL of normal saline and 300 to 500 U of unfractionated heparin (3- to 5-mL volume).

The short-term costs of clotting factor replacement in primary prophylaxis are greater than those associated with on-demand therapy; however, the long-term cost savings may be greater with primary prophylaxis if patients' joints are preserved, if their lives are more productive financially and personally, and if expensive surgical interventions can be avoided.[51] Longitudinal randomized controlled studies currently are being conducted to confirm these premises. Secondary prophylaxis can be used in patients with target joints who are experiencing recurrent events. Coagulation factor concentrate is administered similarly to primary prophylaxis but over a limited period of 3 to 6 months.

Dental Care

Routine dental treatment can be a major source of morbidity in individuals with hemophilia. The best dental care is aimed at the prevention of dental caries, gingivitis, and periodontal disease. Caries are prevented by periodic fluoride applications. Sealants can be applied to the biting surfaces of molar teeth to reduce the incidence of caries. Gingival disease can be reduced by controlling the development of dental plaque through effective tooth brushing and the use of antibacterial mouth rinses such as chlorohexidine. Early dental care of children with hemophilia provided by a dental team whose members coordinate their efforts with the hemophilia treatment center is essential. If patients with severe hemophilia require extractions or oral or periodontal surgery, clotting factor replacement therapy may be necessary. For mild hemophilia, DDAVP administration immediately prior to the procedure is sufficient. Antifibrinolytic agents should be used as adjunctive therapy. The dose and duration of EACA therapy are variable but range from as low as 500 mg as a total dose for minor work to as high as 50 mg per kilogram of body weight every 6 hours for 3 to 10 days for extensive procedures.

TREATMENT COMPLICATIONS

Inhibitors

A major complication of treatment with coagulation factor concentrates in hemophilia is the development of alloantibodies directed against factor VIII or IX. The development of these alloantibodies in patients with severe hemophilia A occurs more frequently with the use of ultra-high-purity factor concentrates (plasma derived and recombinant) than with intermediate-purity factor concentrates (occurs in 15% to 35% of patients with hemophilia A and in 1% to 4% of those with severe hemophilia B).[52] Approximately 50% of factor VIII or IX inhibitors are low titer and transient. High-titer, high-responding inhibitors present the major clinical concern. Alloantibody inhibitors occur after at least one infusion of factor concentrate and at a median of 9 to 12 exposure days. They do not occur naturally prior to any factor exposure. Most alloantibody inhibitors occur before the age of 20, are immunoglobulin G (IgG) subclass 4 or 1, and follow type 1 pharmacokinetics (characterized by specific and total neutralization of factor VIII or IX procoagulant activity). Risk factors for the development of these inhibitors include increased severity of hemophilia (patients with severe disease are affected to a much greater degree than are those with moderate or mild disease, probably because they are also more heavily treated), age (younger rather than older), race (blacks and Hispanics are more often affected than whites for factor VIII alloantibodies; Scandinavians are more commonly affected than other ethnicities for factor IX alloantibodies), family incidence of inhibitors (increased incidence among brother pairs and maternal relatives), and extent and type of genetic mutation underlying the hemophilia (intron 22 inversion for factor VIII inhibitor; large gene deletions for factor IX inhibitor).

The development of an alloantibody inhibitor should be suspected when active bleeding does not subside despite the administration of clotting factor concentrate in doses deemed sufficient to raise factor VIII or IX activities to adequate hemostatic levels. Once suspected, the alloantibody inhibitor can be detected and measured in the laboratory with use of the Bethesda assay. By definition, the recovery study, performed by infusing clotting factor concentrate to achieve a level of 100% of normal activity, will yield less than 60% of expected values 15 to 30 minutes after factor infusion. Ideally, this maneuver should be performed after a "washout period" of 72 to 96 hours without factor administration. The immediate management of inhibitors consists of treating the acute bleeding event; long-range management involves the reduction/eradication of the inhibitor. Sources of the specific clotting factor should be withheld indefinitely unless immune tolerance induction is to be attempted. This withholding will allow the inhibitor titer to drop spontaneously over time. Acute bleeding events associated with low-titer factor inhibitors (<5 BU) can be managed by overwhelming the inhibitor with large doses of human clotting factor concentrate (200 IU/kg). For high-titer inhibitors, alternative clotting factor concentrates must be used because human factor concentrates cannot overwhelm the inhibitor (see Table 4-3). Porcine factor VIII concentrate (Hyate C; Ipsen, Maidenhead, UK) is particularly useful in allo– or auto–factor VIII antibody situations because low cross-reactivity is observed between anti–human factor VIII antibodies and the porcine-derived factor VIII coagulant protein. Porcine factor VIII concentrate is the only inhibitor treatment available that allows for the measurement of circulating factor VIII activity levels after infusion. Disadvantages of this product include anamnestic antibody generation against human or porcine factor VIII, episodic thrombocytopenia, and rare anaphylaxis. Although no transmission of blood-borne infectious agents, including parvovirus,[53] has been documented, Hyate C was removed from production in 2004 because of porcine parvovirus contamination. Clinical trials of a recombinant porcine factor VIII product are under way.

Infusions of so-called bypassing agents offer another useful treatment modality for bleeding associated with factor VIII allo- and auto-antibodies. These products include factor IX complex concentrates (also known as prothrombin complex concentrates, or PCCs) of the unactivated and activated varieties and recombinant factor VIIa concentrate. PCCs have an increased risk of thromboembolic events, and repeat dosing is based on clinical response after infusion. Usual doses range from 50 to 100 IU per kilogram given as intravenous boluses every 8 to 12 hours, as needed. Recombinant factor VIIa (rFVIIa) concentrate (NovoSeven; Novo Nordisk, Princeton, NJ) has a low but finite risk of thromboembolic events, particularly in older individuals, and requires repetition of IV bolus infusions every 2 to 3 hours at a dose of 90 µg/kg until bleeding is controlled.[54] No useful laboratory measurement is available; factor VII levels are very high and prothrombin times are substantially reduced yet neither is predictive for adequate hemostasis. The management of acute bleeding events in hemophilia B complicated with high-titer inhibitors also involves the use of PCCs or recombinant rFVIIa (Table 4-5).

Immune tolerance induction (ITI) regimens have been devised to reduce the levels of alloantibodies against factors VIII and IX. ITI is a prolonged desensitization process in which immune system production of inhibitory antibody is suppressed permanently after prolonged daily infusions of clotting factor concentrate. During this induction period, anamnestic antibody responses may occur, necessitating the use of one of the bypassing agents to manage acute bleeding events. Successful ITI can be achieved in approximately 50% of high-titer inhibitors, but ITI has been most successful in low-titer inhibitors, which have been present for less than one year.[55] More than 60% of individuals achieve inhibitor levels lower than 1 BU within 6 months of initiating ITI; by 1 year, 80% have levels lower than 1 BU. By 30 months, 90% have been successfully tolerized according to clotting factor kinetics and recovery data. A variety of protocols for ITI have been developed, including high-dose regimens that infuse up to 200 IU of clotting factor concentrate per kilogram of body weight per day and low-dose regimens of 50 IU clotting factor per kilogram of body weight administered daily. Once the inhibitor resolves, patients are placed on prophylaxis regimens indefinitely, with bolus infusions of factor VIII concentrate thrice weekly or factor IX concentrate twice weekly. Initial immunosuppressive therapy with cyclophosphamide or glucocorticosteroids was included, as were infusions of intravenous immune globulin, in some ITI regimens; however, this approach has fallen out of favor because of its increased potential for resultant infection and malignancy. Because ITI success is better with low-titer inhibitors, occasionally, plasmapheresis is used to acutely decrease a high-titer inhibitor to low titers. This improves the success of clotting factor infusions given to reverse bleeding and facilitates the initiation of ITI.

Table 4-5 Inhibitor Therapy

Type/Product Name	Manufacturer	Method of Viral Attenuation
FEIBA VH (pooled human plasma–derived prothrombin complex concentrates/factor IX complex concentrate–activated)	Baxter BioScience (Switzerland)	Vapor heat (60°C, 10 hr, 1190 mbar; then 80°C, 1 hr 375 mbar)
NovoSeven (recombinant factor VIIa [rFVIIa]) (no albumin added to final formulation; stabilized in mannitol; bovine calf serum used in culture medium)	Novo Nordisk (USA)	Affinity chromatography Solvent/detergent (TNPB/polysorbate 80)

INFECTIOUS COMPLICATIONS OF REPLACEMENT THERAPY IN HEMOPHILIA: HIV, HEPATITIS, AND PARVOVIRUS B19

AIDS was first identified in individuals with hemophilia in 1981, and by 1984, more than 90% of patients with severe hemophilia A and 50% with severe hemophilia B were HIV seropositive. The HIV virus was contracted from repeated infusions of plasma-derived coagulation factor replacement products in this population of obligate recipients. In 1984, high dry heating and pasteurization techniques for viral attentuation were introduced into the manufacturing process of factor VIII concentrates. Shortly thereafter, solvent detergent treatment regimens were developed. All of these processes were added to the manufacture of factor IX concentrates in the late 1980s. Combined with strict donor viral screening protocols and intensive donor self-exclusion programs in the United States, these viral attenuation processes have prevented since the late 1980s any documented HIV or HCV seroconversions produced by the use of plasma-derived clotting factor concentrates. Recombinant factor concentrates would not be expected to transmit these blood-borne pathogenic viruses. Unfortunately, viral attenuation processes are effective only against lipid-enveloped viruses such as HIV, HCV, and hepatitis B virus (HBV), but not against parvovirus B19, hepatitis A virus (HAV), or Creutzfeldt-Jakob prions.

Patients with HIV and hemophilia have benefited from the introduction of anti-HIV protease inhibitor medications. An increase in bleeding severity and frequency with unusual sites of bleeding has been a hallmark complication in some hemophilia patients treated with these medications. The cause remains unclear but may involve the development of qualitative platelet defects.[29]

Prior to the availability of the specific hepatitis B vaccine, hepatitis B was found in as many as 70% to 90% of severe hemophilia patients. HCV seroprevalence is greater than 90% in hemophilia patients treated with plasma-derived factor concentrates prior to 1985. Coinfection of HCV and HIV has resulted in high morbidity, increasing the risk of cirrhosis, hepatocellular carcinoma, and liver failure. Currently, treatment with pegylated interferon-alpha and ribavirin provides the greatest response rate and longest duration of HCV suppression.[56] The best and most durable responses to this therapeutic regimen are observed in those with the lowest HCV RNA viral titers and with HCV genotypes other than type 1. Hemophilia patients most commonly have been infected with HCV genotypes 1 and 3. All those diagnosed with hemophilia should be vaccinated against HBV starting at birth or the time of diagnosis, and against HAV at 2 years of age, or older if found to be seronegative.

The seroprevalence of parvovirus B19 in hemophilia is 80%—significantly higher than the normal population matched for age and socioeconomic status. This non–lipid-enveloped virus, similar to hepatitis A, is not eradicated from plasma-derived clotting factor concentrates through currently used viral attentuation techniques. Acute parvovirus B19 infection usually is asymptomatic when acquired through blood products; however, rarely, it may induce aplastic anemia or pure red cell aplasia, particularly in the presence of HIV. The vertical transmission of parvovirus in pregnant women may cause hydrops fetalis.

Creutzfeldt-Jakob disease (CJD) is a rare, incurable, fatal degenerative disease of the central nervous system that has been described as a spongiform encephalopathy. The cause of CJD has been most recently linked to a disease-causing prion protein.[57] CJD is transmitted usually through direct inoculation (most commonly associated with implants of dura mater from infected individuals) or administration of growth hormone derived from the pituitary glands of infected cadavers, and after transplantation of organs from infected donors. A new variant form of CJD has been described in cattle ("mad cow disease" [bovine spongiform encephalopathy, or BSE]) and has been transmitted to humans via ingestion of contaminated beef. Sporadic cases of human transmission of variant CJD have been reported to result from blood transfusions (none in hemophilia patients). Furthermore, prions have been identified in the buffy coat leukocytes of variant CJD–affected humans and subsequently were transmitted experimentally to rodents after those cells were inoculated into the animals' brains. Because of an incubation time as long as 35 years, the actual potential of human-to-human transmissibility through blood transfusions and components cannot be determined readily. To reduce the theoretical risk of CJD transmission to hemophilia patients through pooled plasma-derived clotting factor concentrates, donor pools have been reduced in number; the use of recombinant replacement products has been encouraged, and albumin-free formulations and mammalian protein–free manufacturing processes for these products have been developed; screening of blood donors for CJD risks has been implemented as well. No prospective studies have been performed to determine the incidence of parvovirus B19 transmission from plasma-derived products. This is an important issue for pregnant female carriers of hemophilia A or B, who may require replacement therapy for active bleeding, for delivery, or for other purposes. Parvovirus B19 transmission is not an issue for recombinant products. No HIV transmission from plasma-derived factor VIII concentrates has been documented since 1985, nor from factor IX concentrates since 1987, when viral attenuation processes were added to replacement product manufacturing. Although sporadic cases of HCV have been reported, this also occurs in the normal population. No epidemics of HCV infection have resulted from virally attenuated factor concentrates.

GENE THERAPY

Gene therapy in the treatment of patients with hemophilia A or B has received increased interest in recent years; results from clinical studies are somewhat disappointing but promising. Plasma factor levels increased to above 1% can make a dramatic difference in clinical outcomes and quality of life for individuals with severe hemophilia A or B. Coagulation factors VIII and IX can be synthesized efficiently in a variety of somatic cell types. Thus, the hemophilias are highly amenable to gene therapy. A number of viral vectors have been used to transfer human factor VIII or IX genes into target cells. These have included retroviral vectors, adenoviral vectors, adeno-associated viral vectors, and lentiviral vectors. Potential complications of gene therapy include the development of inhibitory antibodies,[58] the risk of integration of the transgene into essential genes in the host, and the risk of inadvertent integration of the transgene into the germline with transmission to later generations. Furthermore, strategies for gene therapy in general have been modified since a death occurred in a gene therapy trial for ornithine transcarbamylase deficiency, and because cases of acute T-cell leukemia were reported in patients with X-linked recessive severe combined immunodeficiency (SCID) treated with retroviral vectors, attributable to insertional mutagenesis. To date, the promise of a gene therapy cure for hemophilia A or B has not been realized, primarily because no gene delivery system has been nonimmunogenic enough to permit long-term expression of clotting factor activity. Six gene therapy trials have been conducted in hemophilia patients with minimal and short-lived clinical and/or laboratory improvement. Currently, no gene therapy trials are open for hemophilia, although additional trials are under review.[59-61] Even if future gene therapy clinical trials in both hemophilia A and B are successful, approaches based on current technology will only palliate disease severity (e.g., rendering severe hemophilia into a moderate or mild case), albeit disease morbidity and mortality should be substantially reduced. Safe, effective, and reasonably priced clotting factor concentrates will be needed, even after gene therapy, to provide prophylaxis during the perioperative period; patients with acute traumatic and surgical bleeds will be treated, and ITI will be initiated should these individuals develop alloantibody inhibitors.

Until gene therapy successes are realized, other novel therapeutic approaches may offer alternative benefits, including (1) gene delivery of engineered, secreted, activated FVII; (2) applications of new viral vector technology; (3) use of nanoparticle technology for the delivery of genes to hepatocytes; and (4) gene "pharming." Any of these, if successful, could enhance the quality of life for the individual with hemophilia.[61]

REFERENCES

1. Lusher JM, McMillan CW: Severe factor VIII and factor IX deficiency in females. Am J Med 65:637–648, 1978.
2. Antonarakis SE, Rossiter JP, Young M, et al: Factor VIII gene inversions in severe hemophilia A: results of an international consortium study. Blood 86:2206–2212, 1995.
3. Cumming AM, UK Haemophilia Centre Doctors' Organization Haemophilia Genetics Laboratory Network: The factor VIII gene intron 1 inversion mutation: Prevalence in severe hemophilia A patients in the UK. J Thromb Haemost 2:205–206, 2004.
4. Hill M, Deam S, Gordon B, Dolan G: Mutation analysis in 51 patients with haemophilia A: Report of 10 novel mutations and correlations between genotype and clinical phenotype. Haemophilia 11:133–141, 2005.
5. Kemball-Cook G, Tuddenham EG, Wacey AI: The factor VIII structure and mutation resource site: HAMSTeRS version 4. Nucleic Acid Res 26:216–219, 1998.
6. Goodeve A: The incidence of inhibitor development according to specific mutations—and treatment? Blood Coagul Fibrinolysis 14 (suppl 1): S17–S21, 2003.
7. White GC 2nd, Beebe A, Nielsen B: Recombinant factor IX. Thromb Haemost 78:261–265, 1997.
8. Goodeve AC: Advances in carrier detection in haemophilia. Haemophilia 4:358–364, 1998.
9. Giannelli F, Green PM, Sommer SS, et al: Haemophilia B: Database of point mutations and short additions and deletions, 7th edition. Nucleic Acids Res 25:133–135, 1997.
10. Chan K, Sasanakul W, Mellars G, et al: Detection of known haemophilia B mutations and carrier testing by microarray. Thromb Haemost 94:872–878, 2005.
11. Gustavii B, Cordesius E, Lofberg L, Stromberg P: Fetoscopy. Acta Obstet Gynecol Scand 58:409–410, 1979.
12. Ljung R, Tedgård U: Genetic counseling of hemophilia carriers. Semin Thromb Hemost 29:31–36, 2003.
13. Ratnoff OD, Lewis JH: Heckathorn's disease: Variable functional deficiency of antihemophilic factor (factor VIII). Blood 46:161–173, 1975.
14. Kulkarni R, Lusher J: Perinatal management of newborns with haemophilia. Br J Haematol 112:264–274, 2001.
15. Medical and Scientific Advisory Council (MASAC): MASAC recommendation regarding neonatal intracranial hemorrhage and postpartum hemorrhage. In MASAC Recommendations #77. New York, National Hemophilia Foundation, 1998.
16. Gilchrist GS, Wilke JL, Muehlenbein LR, Danilenko-Dixon D: Intrauterine correction of factor VIII (FVIII) deficiency. Haemophilia 7:497–499, 2001.
17. Kitchens CS: Occult hemophilia. Johns Hopkins Med J 146:255–259, 1980.
18. Rodriguez-Merchan EC: Pathogenesis, early diagnosis, and prophylaxis for chronic hemophilic synovitis. Clin Orthop Rel Res 343:6–11, 1997.
19. Hilgartner MW: Hemophilic arthropathy. Adv Pediatr 21:139–165, 1974.
20. Doria AS, Lundin B, Kilcoyne RF, et al: Reliability of progressive and additive MRI scoring systems for evaluation of haemophilic arthropathy in children: Expert MRI Working Group of the International Prophylaxis Study Group. Haemophilia 11:245–253, 2005.
21. Manco-Johnson MJ, Nuss R, Geraghty S, et al: Results of secondary prophylaxis in children with severe hemophilia. Am J Hematol 47:113–117, 1994.
22. Valentino LA: Secondary prophylaxis therapy: What are the benefits, limitations and unknowns? Haemophilia 10:147–157, 2004.
23. Siegel HJ, Luck JV, Siegel ME, et al: Hemarthrosis and synovitis associated with hemophilia: Clinical use of P-32 chromic phosphate synoviorthesis for treatment. Radiology 190:257–261, 1994.
24. Manco-Johnson MJ, Nuss R, Lear J, et al: 32P Radiosynoviorthesis in children with hemophilia. J Pediatr Hematol Oncol 24:534–539, 2002.
25. Dunn AL, Manco-Johnson M, Busch MT, et al: Leukemia and P32 radionuclide synovectomy for hemophilic arthropathy. J Thromb Haemost 3:1541–1542, 2005.
26. Jones JJ, Kitchens CS: Spontaneous intra-abdominal hemorrhage in hemophilia. Arch Intern Med 144:297–300, 1984.
27. Ewenstein BM, Takemoto C, Warrier I, et al: Nephrotic syndrome as a complication of immune tolerance in hemophilia B. Blood 89:1115–1116, 1997.
28. Warrier I, Ewenstein BM, Koerper MA, et al: Factor IX inhibitors and anaphylaxis in hemophilia B. J Pediatr Hematol Oncol 19:23–27, 1997.
29. Wilde JT: Protease inhibitor therapy and bleeding. Haemophilia 6:487–490, 2000.
30. Kitchens CS: Retropharyngeal hematoma in a hemophiliac. South Med J 70:1421–1422, 1977.
31. Rodriguez Merchan EC: The haemophilic pseudotumour. Int Orthop 19:255–260, 1995.
32. Lundblad RL, Kingdon HS, Mann KG, White GC: Issues with the assay of factor VIII activity in plasma and factor VIII concentrates (see comment). Thromb Haemost 84:942–948, 2000.
33. Ingerslev J, Jankowski MA, Weston SB, Charles LA: Collaborative field study on the utility of a BDD factor VIII concentrate standard in the estimation of BDDr Factor VIII:C activity in hemophilic plasma using one-stage clotting assays. for the ReFacto Field Study ParticipantsJ Thromb Haemost 2:623–628, 2004.
34. Kessler CM, Gill JC, White GC 2nd, et al: B-domain deleted recombinant factor VIII preparations are bioequivalent to a monoclonal antibody purified plasma–derived factor VIII concentrate: A randomized, three-way crossover study. Haemophilia 11:84–91, 2005.
35. Kasper CK, Aledort L, Aronson D, et al: Proceedings: A more uniform measurement of factor VIII inhibitors. Thromb Diath Haemorrh 34:612, 1975.
36. Biggs R, Austen DE, Denson KW, et al: The mode of action of antibodies which destroy factor VIII. I. Antibodies which have second-order concentration graphs. Br J Haematol 23:125–135, 1972.
37. Verbruggen B, Novakova I, Wessels H, et al: The Nijmegen modification of the Bethesda assay for factor VIII:C inhibitors: Improved specificity and reliability. Thromb Haemost 73:247–251, 1995.
38. Soucie JM, Nuss R, Evatt B, et al: Mortality among males with hemophilia: Relations with source of medical care. The Hemophilia Surveillance System Project Investigators. Blood 96:437–442, 2000.
39. Mannucci PM, Gdovin S, Gringeri A, et al: Transmission of hepatitis A to patients with hemophilia by factor VIII concentrates treated with

organic solvent and detergent to inactivate viruses. The Italian Collaborative Group. (see comment) Ann Intern Med 120:1–7, 1994.

40. Wu CG, Mason B, Jong J, et al: Parvovirus B19 transmission by a high-purity factor VIII concentrate. Transfusion 45:1003–1010, 2005.

41. Fijnvandraat K, Berntorp E, ten Cate JW, et al: Recombinant, B-domain deleted factor VIII (r-VIII SQ): Pharmacokinetics and initial safety aspects in hemophilia A patients. Thromb Haemost 77:298–302, 1997.

42. Martinowitz U, Schulman S, Gitel S, et al: Adjusted dose continuous infusion of factor VIII in patients with haemophilia A. Br J Haematol 82:729–734, 1992.

43. Lusher JM: Is the incidence and prevalence of inhibitors greater with recombinant products? No. (see comment) J Thromb Haemost 2:863–865, 2004.

44. Aledort LM: Is the incidence and prevalence of inhibitors greater with recombinant products? Yes. (see comment) J Thromb Haemost 2:861–862, 2004.

45. Seremetis SV, Aledort LM, Bergman GE, et al: Three-year randomised study of high-purity or intermediate-purity factor VIII concentrates in symptom-free HIV-seropositive haemophiliacs: Effects on immune status. (see comment) Lancet 342:700–703, 1993.

46. Pipe SW: The promise and challenges of bioengineered recombinant clotting factors. J Thromb Haemost 3:1692–1701, 2005.

47. de la Fuente B, Kasper CK, Rickles FR, Hoyer LW: Response of patients with mild and moderate hemophilia A and von Willebrand's disease to treatment with desmopressin. Ann Intern Med 103:6–14, 1985.

48. Lethagen S, Harris AS, Nilsson IM: Intranasal desmopressin (DDAVP) by spray in mild hemophilia A and von Willebrand's disease type I. Blut 60:187–191, 1990.

49. Rakocz M, Mazar A, Varon D, et al: Dental extractions in patients with bleeding disorders: The use of fibrin glue. Oral Surg Oral Med Oral Pathol 75:280–282, 1993.

50. Martinowitz U, Schulman S, Horoszowski H, Heim M: Role of fibrin sealants in surgical procedures on patients with hemostatic disorders. Clin Orthop Rel Res 328:65–75, 1996.

51. Miners AH, Lee CA: Setting research priorities to improve cost-effectiveness estimations of primary prophylaxis with clotting factor for people with severe haemophilia. Haemophilia 10 (suppl 1): 58–62, 2004.

52. Oldenburg J, Schroder J, Brackmann HH, et al: Environmental and genetic factors influencing inhibitor development. Semin Hematol 41 (1 suppl 1): 82–88, 2004.

53. Giangrande PL, Kessler CM, Jenkins CE, et al: Viral pharmacovigilance study of haemophiliacs receiving porcine factor VIII. Haemophilia 8:798–801, 2002.

54. Key NS, Aledort LM, Beardsley D, et al: Home treatment of mild to moderate bleeding episodes using recombinant factor VIIa (Novoseven) in haemophiliacs with inhibitors. Thromb Haemost 80:912–918, 1998.

55. Ewing NP, Sanders NL, Dietrich SL, Kasper CK: Induction of immune tolerance to factor VIII in hemophiliacs with inhibitors. JAMA 259:65–68, 1988.

56. McHutchison JG, Gordon SC, Schiff ER, et al: Interferon alfa-2b alone or in combination with ribavirin as initial treatment for chronic hepatitis C. Hepatitis Interventional Therapy Group. (see comment) N Engl J Med 339:1485–1492, 1998.

57. Pablos-Mendez A, Netto EM, Defendini R: Infectious prions or cytotoxic metabolites? Lancet 341:159–161, 1993.

58. Fields PA, Kowalczyk DW, Arruda VR, et al: Role of vector in activation of T cell subsets in immune responses against the secreted transgene product factor IX. Mol Ther 1:225–235, 2000.

59. Manno CS, Chew AJ, Hutchison S, et al: AAV-mediated factor IX gene transfer to skeletal muscle in patients with severe hemophilia B. Blood 101:2963–2972, 2003.

60. Roth DA, Tawa NE Jr, O'Brien JM, et al: Nonviral transfer of the gene encoding coagulation factor VIII in patients with severe hemophilia A. (see comment) N Engl J Med 344:1735–1742, 2001.

61. Kessler C: New perspectives in hemophilia treatment. Hematology 1:429–435, 2005.

4

Chapter 5

Less Common Congenital Disorders of Hemostasis

Harold R. Roberts, MD • Miguel A. Escobar, MD

In this chapter, the less common congenital disorders of hemostasis are discussed. These include disorders of fibrinogen, prothrombin, and factors V, VII, X, and XI. In addition, the nonbleeding disorders associated with deficiencies of factor XII (Hageman factor), prekallikrein (PK), and high molecular weight kininogen (HK) are discussed because these disorders are characterized by prolonged partial thromboplastin times (PTTs) and may be confused with the procoagulant defects associated with bleeding. Furthermore, the rare bleeding syndromes of factor XIII deficiency, α_2-plasmin inhibitor (α_2-PI) deficiency, and α_1-antitrypsin Pittsburgh (α_1-ATP) are described. For the sake of completeness, the potential role of protein Z and the protein Z–dependent protease inhibitor deficiencies is considered. Although protein Z deficiencies were initially believed to be a cause of hemorrhage in humans, recent animal data suggest that defects in protein Z and the protein Z inhibitor are more likely related to thrombotic phenomena.

Certain biologic and laboratory characteristics of these factors are important in determining their clinical consequences; these are depicted in Table 5-1. Clotting factors discussed in this chapter can best be classified as proenzymes, cofactors, structural proteins, or physiologic inhibitors, as shown in Table 5-2. The information in these tables will help the consultant to gain an understanding of the basis for the clinical condition, as well as the diagnosis and treatment options for each deficiency, as summarized in Table 5-3.

As with all hereditary disorders, deficiencies of each of the clotting factors discussed in this chapter are genetically heterogeneous.[1] Selected genetic variants are described here for several clotting factors, but the reader is referred to up-to-date registries of websites because new variants are discovered almost daily. The two registries pertinent to the clotting factor deficiencies discussed herein are www.hgmd.org (Human Gene Mutation Database) and http://193.60.222.13/.

DISORDERS OF FIBRINOGEN

Congenital disorders of fibrinogen can be divided into afibrinogenemia and dysfibrinogenemia.

Afibrinogenemia

Congenital afibrinogenemia is a very rare disorder that occurs in patients who have no detectable circulating fibrinogen in the plasma or blood platelets. It was first described in 1920, and since that time, more than 200 cases have been reported.[2] The heterozygous state of afibrinogenemia results in low circulating levels of normal fibrinogen. These hypofibrinogenemias are discussed in the section on dysfibrinogenemias.

Pathogenesis and Genetics

Three individual genes on the long arm of chromosome 4 encode for the α, β, and γ chains that constitute the fibrinogen molecule. Fibrinogen is a homodimer that consists of two identical pairs of three chains, intertwined to form a trinodular fibrinogen structure. Fibrinogen is converted to a visible fibrin clot by thrombin, which cleaves fibrinopeptides A and B from the α and β chains, respectively. Gene defects in any of the three chains can result in afibrinogenemia. A list of reported mutations resulting in this disorder (FGA, FGB, FGG) can be found on the Internet at www.hgmd.org. The most common mutations resulting in complete absence of fibrinogen occur in the gene that encodes for the α chain.[3,4]

Afibrinogenemia is inherited in an autosomal recessive pattern, and symptomatic individuals are homozygotes. Heterozygous individuals usually have mild hypofibrinogenemia and are asymptomatic unless the fibrinogen level is less than 50 mg/dL. The estimated incidence of congenital afibrinogenemia is approximately 1 to 2 per million of the population, and usually, a history of consanguinity is reported within the family. This disorder occurs in either sex with no known racial predilection. The characteristics of two patients with afibrinogenemia are shown in Table 5-4.

Clinical Manifestations

Individuals with congenital afibrinogenemia have a lifelong bleeding tendency of variable severity. Hemorrhagic manifestations are usually observed in the neonatal period with bleeding from the umbilical cord ($\approx$75%) and after circumcision.[5] In infancy or childhood, intracerebral hemorrhage is a leading cause of death.[6] Easy bruising and mucosal, gastrointestinal, and genitourinary hemorrhages are common. Hemopericardium, hemoperitoneum, and spontaneous splenic rupture have been reported rarely.[7] Hemarthroses occur in up to 20% of patients, but musculoskeletal bleeding that leads to chronic hemophilic arthropathy, as seen in patients with classic hemophilia, is surprisingly uncommon.[8] Spontaneous abortions, which usually occur early in pregnancy, are common in affected women, who are also prone to menometrorrhagia, abruptio

Table 5-1 Summary of Less Common Clotting Factor Deficiencies

Factor Deficiency	Biologic Half-life	Estimated Incidence	Type of Bleeding	Screening Abnormalities	
				Abnormal	*Normal*
I	2–4 days	1:1 million	None to severe	PT, PTT, TCT, BT	None
II	3 days	Very rare	Mild to moderate	PT, PTT	TCT, BT
V	36 hours	1:1 million	Moderate	PT, PTT, BT	TCT
VII	3–6 hours	1:500,000	Mild to severe	PT	PTT, TCT, BT
X	40 hours	1:500,000	Mild to severe	PT, PTT	TCT, BT
XI	80 hours	1:1 million*	Mild to moderate	PTT	PT, TCT, BT
XII	50–70 hours	Unknown	No bleeding	PTT	PT, TCT, BT
XIII	9 days	1:5 million	Moderate to severe	None	PT, PTT, TCT, BT
PK	35 hours	Unknown	None	PTT	PT, TCT, BT
HK	150 hours	Very rare	None	PTT	PT, TCT, BT
α_2-PI	3 days	Unknown	Mild to moderate	None	PT, PTT, TCT, BT
α_1-ATP	–	Very rare	Variable to severe	PT, PTT, TCT, BT	None
Protein Z	2–3 days	Unknown	None	None	PT, PTT, TCT, BT
ZPI	Unknown	Unknown	None	None	PT, PTT, TCT, BT

*More prevalent in countries with a large Jewish population.

α_1-ATP, α_1-antitrypsin Pittsburgh; α_2-PI, α_2-plasmin inhibitor; BT, bleeding time; HK, high molecular weight kininogen; PK, prekallikrein; PT, prothrombin time; PTT, partial thromboplastin time; TCT, thrombin clotting time; ZPI, protein Z–dependent protease inhibitor.

Table 5-2 Classification of Less Common Clotting Factors

	Clotting Factor	Gene	Activator	Product
Structural Protein	Fibrinogen	4q28	Thrombin	Fibrin
Zymogen	Prothrombin	11p11-q12	Xa/Va/Ca/PL	Thrombin
	Factor VII	13q34	? Xa	Factor VIIa
	Factor X	13q34	TF/VIIa or IXa/Ca/PL	Factor Xa
	Factor XI	4q32-q35	Thrombin	Factor XIa
	Factor XII	5q33	Factor XIa	Factor XIIa
	Factor XIII	A: 6p24-p25 B: 1q31-q32	Thrombin	Factor XIIIa
	Prekallikrein	4q35	Factor XIIa	Kallikrein
Cofactor	Factor V	1q21-q25	Xa or thrombin	Factor Va
	HK	3q26	Factor XIIa	Bradykinin
	Protein Z	13q34	?	?
Inhibitors	ZPI		?	Xa inhibitors
	α_2-PI	17p13	–	Plasmin α_2-PI complex
	α_1-ATP		–	Thrombin α_1-ATP complex

α_1-ATP, α_1-antitrypsin Pittsburgh; α_2-PI, α_2-plasmin inhibitor; Ca, calcium; HK, high molecular weight kininogen; PL, phospholipid (activated platelets); TF, tissue factor; Va, activated factor V; ZPI, protein Z–dependent protease inhibitor.

placentae, and postpartum hemorrhage.[9–11] It is surprising that thrombosis has been reported in some patients with afibrinogenemia, even in the absence of replacement therapy, but whether such patients have true afibrinogenemia as opposed to dysfibrinogenemia is not completely clear. Thrombin generation is normal in these patients and platelet aggregation occurs, even though fibrinogen is absent, which may explain why patients with undetectable fibrinogen have fewer long-term effects from repeated hemorrhaging compared with patients with classic hemophilia and similar disorders.

Diagnosis

The diagnosis of afibrinogenemia can be made on the basis of careful history and coagulation screening tests. Patients give a long history of intermittent hemorrhagic episodes, usually in the soft tissues, and all screening tests of coagulation, including prothrombin time (PT), partial thromboplastin time (PTT), and thrombin clotting time (TCT) (also known as thrombin time [TT]), exhibit infinite clotting times. These tests normalize in vitro through 1:1 mixing with normal plasma, thereby excluding an inhibitor.

To confirm the diagnosis of afibrinogenemia, specific fibrinogen assays should be used, including clotting and immunologic methods, both of which will show no detectable fibrinogen. Bleeding time in afibrinogenemic patients is prolonged because of the absence of platelet fibrinogen.[12,13] Mild thrombocytopenia has also been reported in ≈25% of patients with congenital afibrinogenemia, but platelet counts are usually not lower than 100,000/μL.[14]

Table 5-3 Clotting Factor Deficiencies: Treatment

Deficiency	Bleeding Symptoms	Treatment*	Target Hemostatic Level
I	Umbilical stump, joints, mucous membranes, recurrent miscarriages	Cryoprecipitate, fibrinogen concentrate[†]	>50 mg/dL
II	Soft tissue, CNS, menorrhagia	FFP, PCCs	20%–40%
V	Soft tissue, umbilical stump, postpartum, postoperative	FFP	20%–50%
VII	Soft tissue, joints, mucosal membrane	rFVIIa	15%–20%
X	Soft tissue, joints, menorrhagia	FFP, PCCs	10%–15%
XI	Postoperative and after trauma	FFP, rFVIIa, FXI concentrate[†]	30%–40%
XIII	Umbilical stump, soft tissue, CNS	FFP, cryoprecipitate, FXIII concentrate[†]	2%–5%
FCFD-type I	Postoperative and after trauma	FFP and FVIII	30%
FCFD-type III	Umbilical stump, CNS, and after trauma	Vitamin K, PCCs	As needed
α_2-PI	Joints, hematuria, menorrhagia	Antifibrinolytics	See package insert

α_2-PI, α_2-plasmin inhibitor; CNS, central nervous system; EACA, epsilon-aminocaproic acid; FCFD, familial combined factor deficiencies; FFP, fresh frozen plasma; PCCs, prothrombin complex concentrates; rFVIIa, recombinant factor VIIa; TA, tranexamic acid.
*Antifibrinolytic therapy is frequently used for most clotting factor deficiencies.
[†]Not available in the United States.

Table 5-4 Characteristics of Two Patients with Afibrinogenemia

Location Defect	Genetic Defect	Symptoms	Consanguinity
α Chain	Deletion Intron 1	Umbilical cord bleeding	No
β Chain	Missense mutations in exons 7 and 8	Umbilical cord bleeding Circumcisional bleeding Muscle hematoma Hemarthroses	Yes

Delayed-type hypersensitivity skin tests in individuals with afibrinogenemia typically show only erythema and no induration because of the lack of fibrin deposition in the subcutaneous tissue.[15] The erythrocyte sedimentation rate is also very slow in these individuals because fibrinogen is one of the main determinants of this rate.[16]

Differential Diagnosis

Hereditary dysfibrinogenemia, especially in homozygotes or combined heterozygotes, may result in very low to virtually undetectable fibrinogen levels and must be distinguished from true afibrinogenemia. Sensitive tests for fibrinogen always detect some amount of protein in dysfibrinogenemia but not in true afibrinogenemia.

Acquired fibrinogen abnormalities must also be excluded. Severe disseminated intravascular coagulation can result in virtual absence of fibrinogen, but usually, other clotting factors and platelets are also markedly decreased. Acquired hypofibrinogenemia has been reported with liver disease and with the use of certain medications such as sodium valproate[17] and L-asparaginase,[18] both of which impair the hepatic synthesis of fibrinogen. These acquired defects can be excluded easily through a careful history.

Treatment

The treatment of choice for individuals with afibrinogenemia and hypofibrinogenemia is cryoprecipitate, a source rich in fibrinogen. Solvent detergent–treated products are preferred for inactivating the human immunodeficiency virus and hepatitis viruses. In European countries, purified and virally inactivated fibrinogen concentrates are available. Replacement treatment is obviously indicated for episodes of active bleeding, preoperatively and during pregnancy. For achieving hemostasis, maintaining the fibrinogen level at 50 to 100 mg/dL is usually adequate. Prophylactic therapy is always indicated before operations are performed and throughout pregnancy. To avoid miscarriage, a fibrinogen level above 60 mg/dL must be maintained during the entire course of pregnancy.[19]

Each bag of cryoprecipitate, which contains approximately 250 to 300 mg of fibrinogen, will raise the fibrinogen level by about 10 mg/dL with an in vivo half-life of about 2 to 4 days. Thus, 5 to 10 bags of cryoprecipitate are usually adequate for an individual who weighs 70 kg. However, daily monitoring of fibrinogen levels is necessary if the fibrinogen dose is to be determined because fibrinogen levels can vary over time. For major surgical procedures (e.g., knee replacement) or severe trauma, the duration of treatment with daily fibrinogen may be as long as 2 to 3 weeks. For minor trauma, a single dose of fibrinogen sufficient to raise the level to 50 to 100 mg/dL is adequate. Administration of 1-desamino-8-D-arginine-vasopressin (DDAVP) may reduce bleeding time in some patients, but given alone, it is not adequate for hemostasis.

Complications of replacement therapy include risk of allergic reaction, transmission of viral disease, and the development of antifibrinogen antibodies.[20] Thrombotic phenomena have been reported in patients after the fibrinogen level has been normalized. Some episodes have occurred in women who are taking oral contraceptives, suggesting that they may have had an underlying hypercoagulable state.[21–23] Should thrombotic phenomena occur during the perioperative period, appropriate anticoagulation therapy should be used in combination with fibrinogen replacement.[24]

Dysfibrinogenemia

The first case of dysfibrinogenemia was reported in 1964, but since that time, several hundred other cases have been described, and numerous genetic defects leading to abnormal function have been detected.[25] A list of dysfibrinogens (FGA, FGB, FGG) can be found on the Internet at www.hgmd.org.

Pathogenesis and Genetics

Congenital dysfibrinogenemia is characterized by the synthesis of an abnormal fibrinogen molecule that does not function properly in its conversion from fibrinogen to fibrin. Functional defects include (1) abnormal fibrinopeptide release, (2) defects in fibrin polymerization, (3) abnormal fibrin stabilization, and (4) resistance to fibrinolysis. The most common dysfibrinogenemias are those that cause polymerization defects.[26]

In most cases, congenital dysfibrinogenemia is inherited as an autosomal dominant trait with high levels of penetrance, but some patients exhibit an autosomal recessive inheritance pattern. Patients may be homozygous or heterozygous for the defect. Most affected individuals are heterozygous with ≈50% of normal fibrinogen, which is adequate for normal hemostasis, unless the dysfunctional molecule disrupts the function of the normal fibrinogen component. Some individuals with dysfibrinogenemia have fibrinogen levels that are well below normal.

Clinical Manifestations

Clinically, patients with dysfibrinogenemia have one of the following phenotypes: no hemorrhagic manifestations; mild to moderate bleeding, usually after trauma; thromboses; or a combination of thrombotic and hemorrhagic manifestations. Approximately 43% of all individuals with congenital dysfibrinogenemia are asymptomatic, about 20% have bleeding symptoms, and 17% report thrombotic manifestations. About 20% of patients experience a combination of bleeding and thrombosis.[26,27] The bleeding tendency is variable, and most individuals have mild to moderate hemorrhage. Easy bruising, soft tissue bleeding, menorrhagia, and intraoperative and postoperative bleeding are the most common events. Both venous and arterial thromboses, including deep vein thrombosis of the lower extremities, pulmonary embolism, recurrent spontaneous abortion, and thrombosis of the carotid arteries and abdominal aorta, have been associated with congenital dysfibrinogenemia.[26] Dysfibrinogenemias most likely associated with bleeding occur with abnormalities in the amino terminus of the α chain, although exceptions to this generalization have been found. Thrombotic manifestations, on the other hand, are most often associated with fibrinogen variants that have a free cysteine residue that results in a disulfide linkage to albumin. These variants are resistant to lysis by plasmin, which probably accounts for their thrombotic tendency. In many cases, however, thrombotic manifestations may be related to concurrent disorders (e.g., factor V Leiden, protein C deficiency) rather than to the abnormal fibrinogen molecule itself, and clinicians should be aware of these possibilities. Because a normal fibrin clot provides the necessary framework for normal wound healing, it is not surprising that poor healing and dehiscence of wounds are seen in some patients with dysfibrinogenemia.[28] Examples of dysfibrinogenemia in the α, β, and γ chains are shown in Table 5-5.

Diagnosis

In most cases of dysfibrinogenemia, screening tests of coagulation such as PT, PTT, and TCT are prolonged and may or may not correct with 1:1 mixing with normal plasma. This occurs because some dysfibrinogenemias interfere with normal fibrin formation. In some dysfibrinogenemias associated with thrombotic episodes, the TCT may be shorter than normal. Fibrinogen levels are variable and can be relatively normal or low. Through immunologic methods, one may encounter normal levels of fibrinogen; at the same time, reduced levels of fibrinogen can be detected on functional analysis. Other important diagnostic tests include the reptilase time and fibrinogen immunoelectrophoresis. Reptilase, derived from snake venom, cleaves fibrinopeptide A from the α chain, resulting in the formation of visible clot, even in the presence of heparin. Reptilase time is often prolonged and may be more sensitive than the thrombin time. Fibrinogen immunoelectrophoresis sometimes shows an abnormal migration in agarose gel. However, definitive diagnosis depends on biochemical characterization of the fibrinogen defect, which may require amino acid sequencing. More sophisticated diagnosis requires genetic analyses that are not available in most clinical coagulation laboratories.

Table 5-5   Examples of Dysfibrinogenemia Variants*

Variant	Clinical Effect	Functional Defect
Chapel Hill IV	Asymptomatic	Polymerization defect
Fukuoka II	Asymptomatic	Fibrinopeptide B release defect
Chapel Hill I	Bleeding	Polymerization defect
Christchurch II	Bleeding	Fibrinopeptide B release defect
Guarenas I	Bleeding	Fibrinopeptide A release and polymerization defect
Nijmegen	Thrombosis	Associated with disulfide-linked albumin and tPA–binding defect
Naples II	Thrombosis	Fibrinopeptide A and B release defects
Paris V	Thrombosis	Polymerization defect, decreased binding of plasminogen, and decreased tPA–induced fibrinolysis
Marburg	Bleeding/thrombosis	Deletion of 150 aa with linkage to albumin

aa, amino acid; tPA, tissue plasminogen activator.
*See references 26 and 27.

Differential Diagnosis

Dysfibrinogenemias can also be acquired, particularly in patients with liver disease of varying causes. Frequently, the abnormality is due to an increase in sialic acid residues.[29] In dysfibrinogenemia of liver disease, other clotting proteins synthesized by the liver are low. Autoantibodies against fibrinogen in nondeficient individuals should be distinguished from dysfibrinogenemia, in that they interfere with fibrinogen function and mimic the abnormalities seen with dysfibrinogenemia. Antifibrinogen antibodies have been associated with systemic lupus erythematosus, ulcerative colitis, liver cirrhosis, and other disorders. Fibrinogen degradation products seen in many diseases may also interfere with normal fibrinogen function and may produce a condition that resembles dysfibrinogenemia.

Treatment

Therapy is obviously not indicated in patients with congenital dysfibrinogenemia who are asymptomatic. To treat dysfibrinogenemic patients who are known to bleed, fresh frozen plasma, cryoprecipitate, or fibrinogen concentrates should be administered for bleeding episodes or for preoperative procedures. In the United States, cryoprecipitate is the most commonly used replacement therapy. Guidelines provided in the afibrinogenemia section can also be applied to the dysfibrinogenemias. Dysfibrinogenemic patients who have thrombotic episodes require anticoagulation with heparin, followed by oral anticoagulants. Recurrent thrombotic episodes require prophylactic anticoagulation with the use of low molecular weight heparin or oral anticoagulants. Women with recurrent spontaneous abortion and dysfibrinogenemia should be treated with fibrinogen replacement therapy throughout the course of pregnancy, as is stated in the section on afibrinogenemia.

PROTHROMBIN DEFICIENCY (HYPOPROTHROMBINEMIA AND DYSPROTHROMBINEMIA)

Congenital prothrombin deficiency was first described by Quick and colleagues.[30,31] Fewer than 100 cases have been reported; examples are listed in Table 5-6.

Pathogenesis and Genetics

Various mutations in the prothrombin gene have been discovered and are listed on the Internet at www.hgmd.org (F2). These usually are caused by a missense mutation (i.e., the substitution of a single amino acid in regions that affect the function and/or structure of the prothrombin molecule).[32] These mutations result in dysprothrombinemia, in which prothrombin activity is reduced and the prothrombin antigen may be normal or decreased, as is shown in Table 5-6.

Table 5-6 Prothrombin Variants*

Variant	Activity, %	Antigen, %	Bleeding Tendency
Homozygous			
Barcelona/Madrid	5–15	100	Yes
Carora	4	0	Yes
Dharan	5	95	Yes
Frankfurt/Salatka	15	100	Yes/No
Marburg	3	100	Yes
Obihiro	18	100	Yes
Poissy	2	50	Yes
Perija	2	70	Yes
Segovia	7–20	100	Yes
Heterozygous			
Brussels	25–50	84	Yes
Cardeza	30–50	100	No
Clamart	50	100	No
Magdeburg	45	100	Yes
Padua	50	100	Yes
San Antonio	50	100	Yes
Compound Heterozygous			
Corpus Christi	2	25	No
Denver	5	21	Yes
Habana	1–10	50	Yes
Himi I	10	100	No
Himi II	10	100	No
Metz	10	50	Yes
Mexico City	<10	<10	No
Molise	10	45	Yes
Quick	<2	37–40	Yes
Quick II	<1	–	Yes
San Juan I and II	20	93	Yes
Tokushima	12	42	Yes
Uncharacterized genetics			
Gainesville	25	70	Yes
Houston	5–10	50	Yes

*Modified from references 27 and 48.

Prothrombin is normally converted to thrombin, which is necessary for the formation of a normal fibrin clot. Molecular defects in dysprothrombinemia may affect the amino terminal pro-piece of prothrombin or the carboxyl terminal thrombin portion of the molecule. Defects in the pro-piece usually result in delayed thrombin generation, but the thrombin that is generated functions normally. An example of a defect in the pro-piece of the molecule is prothrombin San Juan. Defects in the thrombin end of the molecule result in the generation of an abnormal thrombin, such as that seen in prothrombin Quick II. In some patients, dysprothrombinemia may be homozygous; in others, it may be heterozygous or compound heterozygous.

Dysprothrombinemia is inherited in an autosomal recessive pattern. No predilection for race is known, although many patients are of Southern European ancestry.[33] Complete deficiency of prothrombin has not been reported and is probably incompatible with life. Mice in whom the gene has been knocked out do not survive in utero—a fact that supports the important role of prothrombin in embryogenesis.

Clinical Manifestations

A weak correlation has been found between functional prothrombin levels and the clinical picture of hemorrhage. All reported dysprothrombinemic patients have had measurable prothrombin activity. This is corroborated in knockout mice when complete deficiency of prothrombin results in fatal neonatal hemorrhage.[34,35]

In general, heterozygous patients are asymptomatic or have minor bleeding symptoms, whereas homozygous or compound heterozygous individuals have more severe symptoms. Heterozygous individuals usually have prothrombin activity levels of 50%, along with normal antigen levels.[33] Such patients are usually asymptomatic but may develop bleeding after undergoing surgical procedures. Individuals who are homozygous or compound heterozygous have symptoms of mild to moderate bleeding. These include hemarthroses and intracranial bleeding, but hemorrhage is more likely to occur at these sites when prothrombin levels are in the 4% to 7% range, as was reported in a series of patients from Iran. Other types of hemorrhage include easy bruising, epistaxis, hematoma, and postoperative bleeding. In women, menorrhagia, postpartum hemorrhage, and miscarriage have been reported.[36,37]

Diagnosis

The diagnosis of dysprothrombinemia is suggested by a lifelong history of bleeding in patients with prolonged PT and PTT values that are corrected when mixed 1:1 with normal plasma. Bleeding time and TCT are normal. Definitive diagnosis requires a specific assay for prothrombin functional activity. Immunologic assays of prothrombin may be helpful but are sometimes normal. Patients with type I deficiency have similar levels of prothrombin on functional and immunologic assays; in type II patients, prothrombin antigen levels are normal and functional prothrombin is low.

Differential Diagnosis

Hereditary prothrombin deficiency must be distinguished from other congenital deficiencies that are characterized by prolonged PT and PTT and normal TCT. The most common deficiencies seen with this pattern are factor V and factor X deficiencies; these can be diagnosed with the use of specific assays for factors V and X, respectively. Acquired prothrombin deficiency is commonly seen in patients with liver disease, vitamin K deficiency, or ingestion of vitamin K antagonists such as warfarin or super-warfarins, both of which are found in rodenticides. In all these conditions, all vitamin K–dependent factors, including protein C and protein S, are low. The surreptitious use of warfarin or super-warfarins such as brodificoum should be suspected in individuals with a severe bleeding tendency who are otherwise apparently normal and without liver dysfunction. Such patients often ingest rodenticides and induce bleeding symptoms for secondary gain. Super-warfarins cannot be detected by simple warfarin assays, but specific testing is available at reference laboratories.

Dysprothrombinemias must also be distinguished from other causes of vitamin K deficiency, such as antibiotics that contain the N-methyl-thio-tetrazole side chain present in third-generation cephalosporins. This side chain inhibits the vitamin K–dependent γ-carboxylation of glutamic acid residues required for production of normal prothrombin and other vitamin K–dependent factors.[38]

Antibodies against prothrombin can be seen in patients with the lupus anticoagulant, antiphospholipid syndrome (APLS), and systemic lupus erythematosus and, on rare occasions, in isolated cases.[39,40] These antibodies usually cause a true prothrombin deficiency through accelerated clearance of the antibody–prothrombin complex.[39,41] Patients with this type of acquired prothrombin deficiency report symptoms similar to those in patients with dysprothrombinemia, except that symptoms are not lifelong.

Treatment

Pure prothrombin concentrates are not available for clinical use. Patients with minor bleeding episodes may not need replacement therapy but may respond to infusion of fresh frozen plasma. Those with major hemorrhage can be treated with fresh frozen plasma at a loading dose of 15 to 20 mL per kilogram body weight, followed by 3 mL per kilogram body weight every 12 to 24 hours because the prothrombin half-life is approximately 3 days. Prothrombin levels of 20% to 40% are usually sufficient to maintain adequate hemostasis.[42] In patients with recurrent bleeding episodes, prophylactic plasma infusions can be administered every 3 to 5 weeks.[43]

An alternative treatment for dysprothrombinemia is the use of prothrombin complex concentrate (PCC). Some of these concentrates contain significant quantities of prothrombin and other vitamin K–dependent factors. Care should be taken when PCCs are used because they have been associated with thromboembolic complications, presumably caused by contamination with variable quantities of activated factors VIIa, Xa, and IXa.[44,45] Two PCCs are commercially available on the U.S. market—Bebulin (Baxter Bioscience, Vienna, Austria) and Profilnine (Grifols, Inc.,

Table 5-7	**Prothrombin Complex Concentrates**			
	Relative Amount of Factor			
Product (Manufacturer)	Prothrombin	VII	IX	X
Bebulin VH (Baxter Bioscience)	120	13	100	139
Profilnine SD (Grifols)	120	Trace	100	55–65

All factor levels are expressed relative to 100 U of factor IX.

Los Angeles, Calif, USA); these consist of varying levels of vitamin K–dependent factors. Therefore, before using PCCs for replacement therapy in patients with prothrombin deficiency, one should know the prothrombin level of a particular product, as is shown in Table 5-7. One regimen consists of an initial loading dose of 20 U of prothrombin per kilogram body weight, followed by 5 U of prothrombin per kilogram body weight every 24 hours.[46] Care should be taken to avoid exceeding the 20-U/kg dose because of the risk of dangerous thrombotic phenomena. Patients should be monitored for the development of disseminated intravascular coagulation during and after PCC use.[47] To avoid the use of PCCs in patients who need surgery, plasma exchange can be performed before the time of the operation so that near-normal levels of prothrombin can be achieved.[48]

FACTOR V DEFICIENCY

In 1943, Quick[49] described a "labile factor" present in plasma that was required for normal PT. A few years later, Owren[50] reported a patient with a lifelong history of bleeding who was found to be deficient in a "labile factor." Both were describing an activity that is now known as factor V. Factor V deficiency is an uncommon disorder with an estimated incidence of less than 1 in 1 million of the population.

Pathogenesis and Genetics

Factor V is a glycoprotein that is found in plasma and in the α granules of platelets. The origin of factor V found in platelets is not known for certain. Most secretable platelet-derived factor V is believed to be derived from plasma, although this concept has been challenged.[51,52] Even though hepatocytes synthesize most of the plasma factor V, megakaryocytes have been shown to contain factor V mRNA.[53] Platelet factor V accounts for about 20% of the total body pool of factor V and is released on activation and degranulation of platelets.[54] The relative roles of plasma and platelet factor V in hemostasis are not precisely known, although platelet factor V is known to be fully functional.

Congenital factor V deficiency, which is inherited as an autosomal recessive trait, is characterized by decreased or absent factor V activity in plasma and platelets. Consanguinity is common. Molecular variants that account for factor V deficiency have been increasingly reported and can be found on the Internet at www.hgmd.org (F5).[55,56] Although reports have described factor V deficiency in which neither plasma nor platelet factor V can be detected, there is reason to suspect that minute levels of factor V sufficient to sustain life may be present in vivo. In at least one patient who had no detectable factor V, bleeding symptoms were minor; in other patients, bleeding symptoms have been more severe.

In any discussion of blood clotting factor V, one must remember that in addition to its role in preventing hemorrhage, factor V helps to regulate coagulation reactions, so that mutations that prevent its cleavage by activated protein C (factor V Leiden) predispose the patient to thrombotic rather than hemorrhagic complications.[57]

Clinical Manifestations

Factor V deficiency occurs in mild, moderate, and severe forms. Patients with severe deficiency (<1%) usually develop symptoms within the first 6 years of life and present with umbilical stump bleeding, easy bruising, and epistaxis.[58] Menorrhagia and postpartum and postoperative hemorrhage have also been described. Hemarthroses may occur, but these are usually traumatic in origin. In contrast to patients with less than 1% factor VIII or IX who experience frequent spontaneous hemarthroses, those with less than 1% factor V activity have few joint hemorrhages. This suggests that even severely affected factor V–deficient patients are not completely deficient in the factor. For example, mice that are completely deficient in factor V—a condition derived through gene knockout techniques—suffer neonatal death but may be rescued by the insertion of a minigene that expresses less than 1% normal factor V activity.[59] Clinical evidence suggests that the bleeding tendency correlates to a greater extent with platelet factor V levels than with plasma levels.[60] Mildly affected patients are asymptomatic with factor V plasma levels above 20%, which makes diagnosis difficult; some cases may not be diagnosed until the patient reaches adulthood. Paradoxically, several reports have described patients with congenital factor V deficiency who presented with thrombosis.[61] Inhibitors to factor V are very rare in patients with congenital factor V deficiency.[62]

Diagnosis

Laboratory evaluation reveals prolonged PT and PTT and normal TCT. In severely affected patients who lack platelet factor V, bleeding time is also prolonged—sometimes longer than 20 minutes. Definitive diagnosis of factor V deficiency requires the use of a specific factor V assay.

Differential Diagnosis

Acquired factor V deficiency may be seen in patients with significant liver disease or in those with disseminated intravascular coagulation. A syndrome of combined congenital deficiencies of factors V and VIII may be diagnosed and must be distinguished from simple factor V deficiency (see later).

Spontaneous inhibitors of factor V in patients without factor V deficiency have been frequently reported postoperatively and in association with the use of antibiotics such as aminoglycosides and penicillin. Some inhibitors have been reported with infection (tuberculosis) and certain malignancies. In more than half of patients with acquired inhibitors, antibodies disappear spontaneously within a period of several weeks to months. Some patients develop factor V antibodies after they have been exposed to topical bovine thrombin that contains bovine factor V. Human antibodies to these bovine products may cross-react with human thrombin and human factor V; in some cases, bleeding is severe. The treatment of choice for hemorrhaging patients consists of corticosteroids and exchange transfusion.[63] Frequently, no therapy is required and the event is transient. Platelet factor V deficiency initially reported as factor V Quebec has now been shown to be a platelet disorder caused by proteolysis of factor V, multimerin, and other proteins within platelet α granules.[64,65]

Treatment

No commercial factor V concentrates are available for replacement therapy. Patients with minor bleeds such as those caused by epistaxis or dental extraction can be treated with local measures and antifibrinolytic therapy, including tranexamic acid and ε-aminocaproic acid. Fresh frozen plasma is the treatment of choice when more serious bleeding occurs. Patients with mild to moderate hemorrhagic episodes can be treated with plasma at a loading dose of 15 to 20 mL per kilogram body weight, followed by 3 to 6 mL per kilogram body weight every 24 hours, to achieve a level of approximately 25% of normal. More frequent infusions are not necessary, given the long half-life of factor V ($\approx$36 hr).[66] Higher levels may be achieved through plasma exchange in patients with severe hemorrhage, in preparation for surgery, or when fluid overload is a concern.[67] Platelet transfusions have been reported to correct bleeding in some patients because they are a source of factor V; however, they are not always effective and have the potential for development of antiplatelet alloantibodies[68] (see Chapter 8). Factor VIIa has been used to staunch bleeding in a few patients; it is less likely to be effective in patients with undetectable levels of factor V.[69]

FACTOR VII DEFICIENCY

Alexander and colleagues[70] described the first case of congenital factor VII deficiency in 1951. Over the years, many more cases have been described, and specific genetic defects have been characterized. Factor VII deficiency occurs at an estimated incidence of 1 in 500,000. No race or sex predilection has been observed for this defect.

Pathogenesis and Genetics

Because the factor VIIa/tissue factor complex is essential for the initiation of coagulation in vivo, a deficiency or a structural defect in the factor VII molecule can lead to

significant bleeding symptoms. The gene is located on the long arm of chromosome 13, close to the gene for factor X. About 1% of factor VII circulates in its active form; it has a biologic half-life of about 3.5 hours—very similar to the half-life of the zymogen. More than 50% of patients seem to have low functional activity and antigen levels; others have a dysfunctional molecule (normal antigen and reduced activity). Factor VII deficiency is inherited in an autosomal recessive fashion, with homozygotes and double heterozygotes exhibiting most of the bleeding symptoms. Numerous and various genetic mutations have been described, many with a phenotypic expression leading to mild, moderate, or severe bleeding manifestations.[71] A detailed database of these mutations can be found on the Internet at http://193.60.222.13/ or at www.hgmd.org (F7).

A remarkable difference has been observed between genotype and phenotype in factor VII variants. Some mutations show virtually undetectable factor VII levels through clotting or immunologic assays, and yet the patient suffers little or no bleeding. PT, which is prolonged in factor VII deficiency, is variable according to the source of the tissue factor. Ox brain and other tissue factor preparations of nonhuman origin may yield very different results from those obtained with the use of human tissue factor. Presumably, varying human polymorphisms may respond in variable manners to different tissue factor sources. It is generally agreed that human tissue factor should be used in all clotting assays for factor VII. Variability in the clinical expression of factor VII deficiency has led to confusion regarding treatment of patients with this disorder.

Clinical Manifestations

The clinical manifestation of factor VII deficiency varies widely from patient to patient, and a poor correlation has been found between plasma level of factor VII and bleeding symptoms. As was stated earlier, this may be explained by the fact that in vitro factor VII activity is dependent on the type of tissue factor used in the assay. Assay that uses human tissue factor seems to correlate best with the bleeding diathesis.[72] In some patients, less than 1% factor VII activity is seen when rabbit tissue factor is used in the assay, although measurable factor VII activity is observed when human tissue factor is used.

In general, individuals with factor VII levels lower than 8% of normal are those more likely to exhibit hemorrhagic episodes than are those with higher levels of this factor.[73] Often, bleeding in factor VII–deficient patients involves easy bruising, epistaxis, and soft tissue hemorrhage. Women may present with menorrhagia, menometrorrhagia, and postpartum bleeding. Postoperative bleeding is not rare but almost always occurs in severely affected patients. Patients with factor VII levels lower than 1% may have severe bleeding, equivalent to that seen in hemophilia A or B with hemarthroses, retroperitoneal bleeding, muscle hematomas, and fatal intracranial hemorrhage. Rarely, however, patients with activity levels lower than 1% have no history of bleeding, yet are found by work-up of a prolonged PT. A high incidence of hemarthrosis, which occurs most often with grades 3 and 4 arthropathy, has been described in 40 patients from eight European hemophilia centers.[72] Central nervous system bleeding has been reported most often in infants after vaginal delivery, with an incidence of up to 16%.[74] A few cases of thrombosis have been described in factor VII–deficient patients, but in most cases, other risk factors have been identified.[75] Inhibitory antibodies against exogenously administered factor VII have been reported in very few patients with severe congenital deficiency of factor VII.[75,76]

Diagnosis

Individuals with factor VII deficiency have an isolated, prolonged PT with normal PTT, TCT, and bleeding time. On rare occasions, the PTT may be prolonged—a condition that is usually due to unique genetic defects in the factor VII molecule. A specific factor VII assay that is usually based on the PT is required to confirm the diagnosis; in addition, activity may vary according to the species from which the tissue factor used in the assay was derived. Immunologic assays for factor VII may also be used, but these are not as readily available as clotting tests. Factor VIIa assays are also available and can be helpful when factor VIIa is used for treatment.[77]

Differential Diagnosis

Acquired factor VII deficiency is the most common cause of prolonged PT. Warfarin use, vitamin K deficiency, and liver disease are the main causes of acquired factor VII deficiency. Individuals have low levels not only of factor VII, but of all other vitamin K–dependent factors as well. Other less common causes of factor VII deficiency include familial combined factor deficiencies (types III and IV), acquired factor VII inhibitors,[78] and homocystinuria[79] and aplastic anemia.[80] Seligsohn and colleagues[81] described an association between hereditary factor VII deficiency and the Dubin-Johnson and Rotor syndromes.[81] An association between Gilbert syndrome and factor VII deficiency has also been suggested.[82]

Treatment

For mild hemorrhage, treatment to factor VII levels of 5% to 10% of normal are sufficient to stop bleeding. For individuals undergoing surgery, levels of 15% to 25% of normal are recommended. In the United States, products that are used for treatment include fresh frozen plasma, prothrombin complex concentrates, and recombinant factor VIIa. Given the short half-life of factor VII (3 to 4 hr), it is difficult to administer plasma every 4 to 6 hours to maintain normal levels without producing volume overload. Recombinant factor VIIa (NovoSeven; Novo Nordisk, Inc., Princeton, NJ, USA), which has been approved for use in the United States and other countries for individuals with hemophilia who have inhibitors and congenital factor VII deficiency, has been shown to be efficacious and is clearly the treatment of choice.[83] A dose of 15 to 30 µg per kilogram of body weight is sufficient for hemostasis. Frequency of dosing varies with severity of the bleeding episode. For mild to moderate bleeding, a single dose of factor VIIa may be sufficient. For more severe episodes, factor VIIa administered every 4 to 6 hours for several days may be required. Despite the reported short half-lives of factors VII and VIIa, cumulative experience suggests that the effects of factor VIIa last longer than one would expect,

given the reported short half-life of the product. Virally inactivated purified plasma–derived factor VII is available in some European countries.[84]

FACTOR X DEFICIENCY

In the 1950s, two independent groups of investigators discovered factor X when they showed that two different patients lacked an identical factor that could be distinguished from all other known factor deficiencies.[85,86]

Factor X plays a central role in coagulation and in the presence of its cofactor, factor Va, it converts prothrombin to thrombin. Factor X deficiency occurs worldwide, with an estimated incidence of 1 in 500,000. In countries in which consanguineous marriages are common, the relative frequency may be higher.

Pathogenesis and Genetics

Congenital factor X deficiency, which has been reported in more than 50 kindred, is inherited as an autosomal recessive trait. The gene for factor X is found on chromosome 13, close to the gene for factor VII. Genetic and molecular defects resulting in factor X deficiency include small deletions, missense mutations, and frameshifts.[87] Individuals with factor X deficiency may synthesize abnormal factor X molecules in normal or reduced amounts. One of the original patients had no detectable factor X antigen, and the genetic defect in this patient probably resulted in intracellular destruction of the molecule. An absolute deficiency of factor X may be incompatible with life; in mice in which the factor X gene has been knocked out, embryonic or neonatal death occurs regularly.[88] Genetic variants of factor X can be found on the Internet at www.hgmd.org (F10).

Clinical Manifestations

Hemorrhagic events in factor X–deficient patients may be mild, moderate, or severe, depending on the specific mutation. Bleeding symptoms seem to correlate roughly with level of factor X activity. Individuals with severe deficiency (<1% of normal) have bleeding episodes that are comparable with those experienced by patients with severe classic hemophilia, including hemarthrosis, soft tissue hemorrhage, retroperitoneal bleeding, central nervous system hemorrhage, hematuria, menorrhagia, and pseudotumor. In a study of 32 Iranian individuals with congenital factor X deficiency, 69% developed recurrent hemarthrosis and 16% experienced disabling joint disease.[89] In the same study, bleeding from the umbilical stump was described in 28% of infants. Patients with factor X activity of 15% or greater have fewer spontaneous bleeding episodes, although hemorrhage may occur in association with surgery or trauma. Neutralizing antibodies for factor X rarely occur in patients with hereditary deficiency of this factor.

Diagnosis

In general, the diagnosis of inherited factor X deficiency is suggested by a lifelong history of excessive bleeding and laboratory studies showing prolonged PT and PTT values that correct with 1:1 mixing with normal plasma. TCT and bleeding time are normal. Russell's viper venom time, which measures the direct activation of factor X, is also prolonged. Definitive diagnosis of factor X deficiency requires a specific factor X assay because prolonged PT and PTT are also seen in other factor deficiencies (e.g., factor V, prothrombin).

Differential Diagnosis

Acquired factor X deficiency is most commonly seen in patients with liver disease and vitamin K deficiency. In these patients, levels of other vitamin K–dependent factors are also reduced. Isolated factor X deficiency has been reported in association with respiratory infection,[90,91] acute myeloid leukemia,[92] and other malignancies.[93] Acquired factor X inhibitors in patients without congenital factor X deficiency are rare, although cases have been described in patients with leprosy[94] and after antibiotic and agricultural chemical exposure, among others.[95,96] Factor X deficiency in association with primary amyloidosis, which may be seen in up to ≈14% of patients with amyloidosis, is due to adsorption of factor X onto amyloid fibrils.[97,98] Factor X levels in these patients range from 2% to 50% of normal, and usually, individuals have bleeding symptoms if factor levels drop to below 10% of normal.

Treatment

Replacement therapy should be guided by the severity of bleeding. Factor X levels of 10% to 15% should be sufficient for control of mild hemorrhagic episodes, including hemarthroses and uncomplicated soft tissue bleeds. Given the long half-life of factor X (≈40 hr), plasma replacement therapy can be used with an initial loading dose of 15 to 20 mL per kilogram of fresh frozen plasma, followed by 3 to 6 mL per kilogram every 24 hours. These amounts of plasma may cause congestive heart failure in patients with compromised cardiac and pulmonary function, so care must be taken to evaluate patients carefully before large amounts of plasma are infused.

For major bleeds, trauma, or surgical procedures, those prothrombin complex concentrates containing significant amounts of factor X can be used to maintain a factor X level of about 50% of normal. Factor X levels persistently above 50% of normal are not recommended when PCCs are used because of the risk of thromboembolic events. Administration of "factor X–rich" PCCs in doses of 20 to 30 U per kilogram body weight every 24 hours is sufficient to maintain hemostasis.[89] Patients undergoing surgical procedures may need treatment for several days (5 to 10 days) or until healing of surgical wounds is well under way. Only products that are virally inactivated should be used.

Factor X–deficient patients who develop inhibitors to this factor can be treated with larger than normal doses of factor X (with the use of PCCs) or by exchange transfusion. Long-term treatment of patients with factor X inhibitors consists of immunosuppression with alkylating agents and prednisone. Inhibitors that occur in patients without congenital factor X deficiency are usually transient, and patients should be treated with corticosteroids and intravenous gamma-globulin preparations. In some cases, exchange transfusion and activated PCCs may be useful.[91,95]

Treatment of patients with factor X deficiency due to amyloidosis is difficult because the half-life of factor X is shortened, most likely as a consequence of absorption of factor X by amyloid fibrils. Factor X replacement therapy may thus be virtually useless in some patients.[97] In those with amyloidosis and factor X deficiency, splenectomy, chemotherapy, and plasma exchange have all been tried with varying results.[99–101] Recently, factor VIIa and PCCs have been used for the treatment of those with bleeding in factor X deficiency due to amyloidosis.[102,103] It is important to know that for factor VIIa to be effective, measurable levels of factor X in vivo are needed.[104]

FACTOR XI DEFICIENCY

The first report of congenital factor XI deficiency was published in 1953, when three related individuals were described who developed excessive bleeding after dental extractions.[105] Factor XI deficiency is more prevalent among Ashkenazi Jews, with a gene frequency of 4.3%, but the deficiency also occurs in non-Jewish populations.[106,107]

Pathogenesis and Genetics

Factor XI is a homodimer that consists of two identical polypeptide chains and two active serine sites. The gene is located on the long arm of chromosome 4, a serine protease that is not dependent on vitamin K for synthesis. Factor XI deficiency is inherited in an autosomal recessive fashion, with no sex predilection. Three different common genotypes have been described; two of them (types II and III) occur with a higher frequency in the Ashkenazi Jewish population.[107,108] Type I mutations occur at the intron–exon boundaries (splice junction mutations), type II mutations result from a premature stop codon (nonsense mutations), and type III mutations are caused by missense mutations. A database for factor XI mutations can be found on the Internet at www.hgmd.org (F11). It has been suggested that platelets have factor XI–like activity, but the clinical significance of this finding is unknown.[109]

Clinical Manifestations

Factor XI–deficient individuals have a mild bleeding tendency or, in some cases, no bleeding tendency, even after surgery. However, in those patients who have a bleeding tendency, the most serious hemorrhage is likely to occur after surgical procedures or other trauma. The deficiency can occur in the heterozygous, homozygous, or combined heterozygous form. It is one of the procoagulant deficiencies for which bleeding has been reported in patients heterozygous for the condition. An explanation for why bleeding manifestations in factor XI–deficient patients are never as severe as those seen in severely affected patients with either hemophilia A or B is that the "tenase" and "prothrombinase" complexes that lead to ultimate thrombin generation are intact in patients with factor XI deficiency. Thus, factor XI serves to "boost" thrombin generation in subjects who need boosting, but thrombin generation is never as impeded in factor XI–deficient patients as it is in other factor deficiencies. This does not mean that severe bleeding is never seen in factor XI–deficient patients; bleeding can occur after surgery, such as prostatectomy or other procedures that involve tissues rich in fibrinolytic activity. However, the general rule stands that under basal conditions, bleeding in pure factor XI deficiency is never as severe as that seen in severely affected patients with deficiency of factor VIII or factor IX.

Some patients with factor XI deficiency have close to normal thrombin generation, even when factor XI is virtually undetectable—an observation that explains why many severely affected factor XI–deficient patients exhibit normal hemostasis during surgery. The reason for this is not entirely clear but may be related to the amount of factor XI–like activity that occurs on platelets.

Even though factor XI levels do not always correlate with bleeding tendency, members of an affected family tend to have similar hemorrhagic symptoms. Individuals in whom factor XI activity occurs at less than 20% are most likely homozygotes or compound heterozygotes who can experience excessive bleeding. "Spontaneous" hemorrhagic episodes such as hemarthroses are not features of factor XI deficiency. Increased bleeding may be seen after aspirin ingestion, prostatectomy, and oral cavity surgery; it may also be noted in circumstances in which fibrinolytic activity is increased.[110,111] Common bleeding manifestations include hematoma, epistaxis, menorrhagia, postpartum bleeding, hematuria, and postoperative hemorrhage. As a general rule, the best predictor of whether a factor XI–deficient patient will experience excessive hemorrhage is the presence or absence of a past history of significant bleeding.

Diagnosis

Individuals with factor XI deficiency have a prolonged PTT with normal PT and TT. As opposed to both hemophilia A and B, factor XI deficiency occurs in both males and females. Diagnosis requires a specific factor XI assay. In our experience, factor XI can best be assayed when plasma from patients is collected fresh in plastic containers and is processed rapidly; results may be affected if the plasma is processed in a glass tube or is frozen and thawed before it is assayed.

Differential Diagnosis

Congenital deficiency of factor XI may also be seen in individuals with familial combined factor deficiencies (types V and VI). It has been associated with Noonan syndrome,[112] factor VIII deficiency,[113] factor IX deficiency,[114] and von Willebrand disease,[115] and it occurs in patients with platelet defects.[116] Acquired factor XI inhibitors may be seen in patients with immunologic diseases such as systemic lupus erythematosus.

Treatment

Patients with mild bleeding episodes may not require treatment. A variety of successful surgical procedures have been performed in patients with factor XI deficiency who were receiving adequate replacement therapy,[117,118] even though it is not established what level of factor XI would be ideal for maintaining hemostasis. It seems safe to maintain a minimum level of 45% of normal for major surgery and 30% for minor surgery. Some clinicians have found that lower levels are adequate for hemostasis, but others believe that higher levels may occasionally be necessary. When therapy is required, fresh frozen plasma can be used at a loading dose of 15 to 20 mL per kilogram, followed by 3 to 6 mL per kilogram every 12 hours. The half-life of factor XI is approximately 50 ± 22 hours. On occasion, when bleeding cannot be controlled with plasma alone, plasma exchange may be helpful in maintaining higher levels of factor XI. Patients with factor XI deficiency, even when severe, who have no past history of bleeding after significant trauma or surgery usually do not require replacement therapy.

Antifibrinolytic agents, such as ε-aminocaproic acid or tranexamic acid, can be used alone or in combination with plasma to control bleeding. Berliner and coworkers[119] successfully treated 19 patients with severe factor XI deficiency who underwent dental surgery with tranexamic acid alone without excessive bleeding. Caution should be used in patients with hematuria when antifibrinolytic therapy is administered because ureteral or urethral obstruction from clots that are refractory to lysis can occur. Fibrin glue alone has been used successfully for dental extractions.[120]

Some clinicians now prefer to treat all factor XI–deficient patients with factor VIIa. This product has also been used successfully to control hemorrhage in factor XI–deficient patients, even in those patients who experience severe bleeding after surgery, and in those who have developed high titer inhibitors to factor XI.[121,122] Factor VIIa has not been approved by the U.S. Food and Drug Administration for use in factor XI deficiency. However, we have found it to be an effective alternative to plasma therapy. A factor XI concentrate is available in Europe, but it has been associated with occasional thrombotic adverse effects.[123]

Inhibitors to factor XI have been described in several affected factor XI–deficient patients; these usually consist of immunoglobulin (Ig)G alloantibodies. These inhibitors are rare, but they complicate replacement therapy and can prolong bleeding episodes in susceptible patients.[124,125] The treatment of choice for inhibitors is recombinant factor VIIa. Commonly used doses of factor VIIa range from 90 to 120 μg per kilogram of body weight adjusted every 2 to 4 hours until bleeding stops.[126] Eradication of factor XI inhibitor should be attempted through the administration of cyclophosphamide (100 to 200 mg/day) and prednisone (1 mg/kg/day) until the inhibitor disappears or adverse effects of therapy prohibit further treatment.

DEFICIENCY OF CONTACT FACTORS

The physiologic role of contact factors (factor XII [Hageman factor], PK, and HK) in coagulation is not yet well understood. Individuals with a deficiency of any of these contact factors do not have a bleeding tendency, even during major surgery. Reasonable evidence suggests that these factors may play a role in host defense mechanisms and may contribute to the interaction between coagulation, fibrinolysis, the complement system, and other pathways of the inflammatory response.[127]

Factor XII Deficiency

Ratnoff and Colopy[128] were the first to describe a patient with congenital factor XII deficiency (Mr. Hageman) after he was found to have a prolonged clotting time in a glass tube in a routine preoperative evaluation. He had no personal or family history of excessive bleeding. Since then, hundreds of cases have been described, but in only a few of these cases has the structural defect in factor XII been recognized.

Pathogenesis and Genetics

In general, congenital factor XII deficiency is inherited in an autosomal recessive pattern, although autosomal dominant inheritance has been described in one family.[129] Homozygous individuals usually have undetectable factor XII activity levels, and heterozygotes have factor XII levels between 20% and 60% of normal. Heterozygosity for factor XII deficiency was found in 2% of a series of 300 normal blood donors.[129a] The Asian population seems to have lower factor XII levels when compared with whites.[130]

Clinical Manifestations

Individuals with factor XII deficiency do not experience excessive bleeding, even after major surgical procedures or trauma. Various anecdotal case reports describing an association between factor XII deficiency and spontaneous abortion, premature delivery, arterial and venous thromboses, myocardial infarction, and pulmonary embolism have been published, but a definite cause and effect relationship has not been established. More likely, the decreased factor XII activity as well as these thrombotic symptoms are due to APLS.[130a]

Diagnosis

Severe factor XII deficiency is characterized by a markedly prolonged PTT (>100 sec) with normal PT, TCT, and bleeding time in patients with no personal or family history of excessive bleeding. The PTT corrects with 1:1 mixing with normal plasma. Diagnosis requires a specific factor XII assay.

Differential Diagnosis

Spontaneous autoantibodies (inhibitor) against factor XII occur rarely.[131] Sporadic case reports of inhibitors have been described in patients with autoimmune disorders and in individuals treated with procainamide or chlorpromazine.[132,133] Congenital factor XII deficiency has also been described in association with other coagulation disorders, including von Willebrand disease and factor IX deficiency.[134,135] Low factor XII levels may also be seen in patients with liver disease. Prekallikrein and HK deficiencies must be distinguished from factor XII deficiency by means of specific assays.

Treatment

No treatment is necessary for individuals with factor XII deficiency.

Prekallikrein Deficiency

In 1965, Hathaway and associates[136] described deficiency of prekallikrein (PK; Fletcher factor) in a family with prolonged PTT and no history of excessive bleeding. Prekallikrein deficiency is inherited in an autosomal recessive pattern. Homozygous individuals have less than 1% of activity, whereas heterozygotes have 20% to 60% of normal activity. Rare variants of abnormal prekallikrein molecules have been described. Paradoxically, some reports describe a possible association of prekallikrein deficiency with thromboembolic phenomena, but this seems more likely due

to APLS.[130a,137] Individuals with this disorder have a markedly prolonged PTT that corrects to normal with the addition of normal plasma. PT, bleeding time, and TCT are normal. Prekallikrein deficiency is clinically identical to factor XII and HK deficiency, and diagnosis requires a specific assay. No specific therapy is required for patients with PK deficiency because they do not manifest excessive bleeding. The differential diagnosis includes other contact factor deficiencies. Because prekallikrein is synthesized in the liver, acquired deficiency can occur in liver disease.[138]

High Molecular Weight Kininogen Deficiency

HK, also known as Fitzgerald factor, Williams factor, and Flaujeac factor, was first described in 1979.[139] Its deficiency is an autosomal recessive transmitted disorder. Individuals with HK deficiency have a prolonged PTT with no bleeding abnormalities. The PTT corrects through 1:1 mixing with normal plasma. Diagnosis requires a specific assay. No treatment is required.

Factor XIII Deficiency

In 1960, Duckert and colleagues[140] described the first case of congenital factor XIII deficiency in a patient with severe hemorrhage and poor wound healing. Since then, more than 200 cases of congenital deficiency of this protein have been reported in the literature.

Pathogenesis and Genetics

In vivo, factor XIII acts as a transglutaminase that stabilizes the fibrin clot by crosslinking fibrin fibers through formation of peptide bonds between specific amino acid residues on adjacent α and γ chains of fibrin polymers. In the absence of factor XIII, clots are unstable and are held together by weak hydrogen bonds and electrostatic forces. Such clots are permeable, form a poor framework for wound healing, and are extremely sensitive to fibrinolysis.

Human factor XIII is found in plasma and platelets. In plasma, it circulates as a tetramer consisting of two A chains and two B chains (A_2B_2). The B chains function as carriers for the A chains, which contain the enzymatic component of factor XIII. In platelets, factor XIII is a dimer composed of two A chains (A_2). Platelet factor XIII accounts for about 50% of total body factor XIII activity.[141] Three forms of factor XIII deficiency have been described. In type I deficiency, there is absence of both A and B chains. Type II deficiency is characterized by lack of the A chain; in Type III, the B chain is absent.[142] Most of the reported cases of factor XIII deficiency are due to the lack of A chains. Deficiency of factor XIII is an autosomal recessive disorder, with an estimated incidence of one in several million. Consanguinity is frequently found.

Clinical Manifestations

Symptomatic individuals with factor XIII deficiency have <1% of normal activity. Bleeding manifestations can present as early as the neonatal period with umbilical stump hemorrhage in up to 80% of cases. Hematoma, soft tissue hemorrhage, pseudotumor, and poor wound healing are other manifestations of severely affected individuals. Children can present with severe hemorrhage after circumcision and recurrent gum bleeding while teething.[143] Women have recurrent spontaneous abortions,[144-146] and males manifest oligospermia and infertility.[146] Trauma is usually the triggering factor for most of the bleeding episodes, except for intracranial hemorrhage, which can be spontaneous. Intracranial hemorrhage occurs at an incidence of up to 30% and is the leading cause of death in this disorder.[147] Some patients with congenital factor XIII deficiency develop alloantibodies against the factor after undergoing replacement therapy.

Diagnosis

The hallmark of diagnosis of factor XIII deficiency consists of normal routine coagulation studies (PTT, PT, TCT, bleeding time, and platelet count) in a patient who is clearly a bleeder. Diagnosis can be made through a simple clot solubility test, with the use of 5 M urea or 1% monochloroacetic acid. Plasma clots may be removed from thrombin-treated plasma samples and placed in one of the above solutions. Rapid dissolution of the clot within a few minutes will be noted in affected individuals, whereas normal clots remain insoluble for at least 24 hours. The patient's plasma mixed with normal plasma should also be tested to rule out an inhibitor to factor XIII. Factor XIII inhibitors neutralize factor XIII in normal plasma. Confirmation of the deficiency with the use of a quantitative test should be done if the clot solubility test result is abnormal. Quantitative tests are based on the amine–casein incorporation assay or on ammonia production through the transamidase activity of factor XIII.[148]

Differential Diagnosis

Because inhibitory antibodies develop against factor XIII, acquired factor XIII deficiency may be seen in patients without a congenital deficiency. Such antibodies have been reported in association with isoniazid, penicillin, and phenytoin.[149–151] In some patients, antibodies against factor XIII are idiopathic.[152–154] Decreased levels of factor XIII also have been described in patients with Henoch-Schönlein purpura, Crohn disease, and ulcerative colitis.[155,156]

Treatment

Because only low levels of factor XIII activity ($\approx 5\%$) are needed to completely control bleeding and because its half-life is long (9 to 10 days), prophylactic therapy is indicated, especially if intracranial bleeds are to be prevented.[157] For prophylaxis, fresh frozen plasma can be administered in doses of approximately 2 to 3 mL of plasma per kilogram body weight.[158] Cryoprecipitate is another source of factor XIII and can be given in doses of 1 bag per 10 to 20 kg of body weight every 3 to 4 weeks. Plasma-derived pasteurized factor XIII concentrates are available in Europe (Fibrogammin-P; Aventis Behring Ltd., West Sussex, UK) and can be used prophylactically through intravenous administration every 5 to 6 weeks. Pregnancy in women with a history of spontaneous abortions can be carried to term with the use of fresh frozen plasma every 14 days or with factor XIII concentrates given every 21 days.[145] Complications from replacement therapy include blood-borne infection (hepatitis, HIV, other viruses), allergic reaction to plasma, and the development of antibodies to factor XIII in individuals with congenital deficiency.[159] Patients with factor XIII deficiency who develop antibodies

to exogenous factor XIII can be difficult to treat. Administration of normal platelets containing factor XIII can be tried. Exchange transfusion may be necessary. Combination therapy consisting of exchange transfusion and immunosuppression with intravenous gammaglobulin, cyclophosphamide, and steroids can also be tried.

FAMILIAL COMBINED FACTOR DEFICIENCIES

Multiple combined coagulation factor deficiencies have been described (Table 5-8). Type I (factor V–factor VIII deficiency) and type III deficiencies (combined factors II, VII, IX, and X deficiencies) are well characterized. Familial combined deficiencies may be due to a single genetic defect, resulting in multiple factor deficiencies, or to different genetic defects associated with each deficient factor. The latter situation is usually associated with consanguinity.

Combined Factor V–Factor VIII Deficiency (Type I)

More than 30 affected families have been described in the literature. Affected individuals have factor V and factor VIII levels between 5% and 15% of normal. These patients usually have bleeding symptoms after trauma and during or after surgery.

Pathogenesis and Genetics

Combined factor V–factor VIII deficiency is inherited in an autosomal recessive pattern. Defects in one of two genes appear to account for all cases of combined deficiencies of factors V and VIII. The lectin mannose binding gene (LMAN-1, initially referred to as ERGIC53) is located on the long arm of chromosome 18, and the multiple coagulation factor deficiency gene (MCFD2) is located on the short arm of chromosome 2. These two genes form a protein complex in the endoplasmic reticulum–Golgi apparatus that is necessary for the transport of factors V and VIII from the endoplasmic reticulum (ER) to the Golgi.[160]

Diagnosis

Patients will have a mildly prolonged PT and PTT and a normal TCT. In patients who have lifelong bleeding episodes after undergoing surgery or trauma, and who have a prolonged PT and PTT, combined factors V and VIII deficiencies should be suspected.

Table 5-8 Familial Combined Factor Deficiencies

Type	Deficient Factors	Genetic Defect
I	V and VIII	*LMAN-1* and *MCFD2* genes
II	VIII and IX	Unknown
III	II, VII, IX, X	Vitamin K carboxylase or reductase deficiency
IV	VII and VIII	Unknown
V	VIII, IX, and XI	Unknown
VI	IX and XI	Unknown

Clinical Manifestations

Affected patients will have bleeding after trauma, surgical or otherwise. In patients with the combined disorder, mild factor V deficiency is sometimes misdiagnosed.

Treatment

Therapy consists of fresh frozen plasma (to replace factor V) and factor VIII concentrates. Whereas factor VIII levels can be made normal with the use of factor VIII concentrates, it is difficult to raise factor V levels to much above 30% of normal with plasma infusions, especially in patients with heart disease who may develop congestive heart failure from hypervolemia. For major surgery, it may be necessary to raise factor V to near-normal levels through plasma exchange. Platelet transfusions can be used to functionally elevate factor V levels. Factor levels can then be maintained with infusions of plasma and factor VIII concentrates.

Combined Factors II, VII, IX, and X, Proteins C and S Deficiencies (Type III)

Pathogenesis and Genetics

The combined deficiency of the vitamin K–dependent factors was first described by McMillan and Roberts in 1966.[161] It is a very rare autosomal recessive disorder that has been described in fewer than 15 families.[162] The combined deficiency of the vitamin K–dependent factors appears to be due to defects in the vitamin K carboxylase or reductase genes. These genes have already been characterized and identified in at least three individuals.[163–166] Consanguinity has been described in some individuals.

Clinical Manifestations

Bleeding in individuals with combined deficiency of the vitamin K–dependent factors can on occasions be severe. Umbilical stump bleeding and intracerebral hemorrhage may occur when factor levels are severely low.[167]

Diagnosis

Patients present with marked prolongation of the PTT and PT and a normal TCT. The PT and PTT correct with 1:1 mixing with normal plasma. Assays for proteins S and C are also low.

Treatment

In some patients with a congenital deficiency of vitamin K–dependent clotting factors, the use of high doses of oral vitamin K may be beneficial.[161,168] In one patient, 50 mg of vitamin K daily partially corrected the markedly prolonged PT, although complete correction was never achieved. When excessive bleeding occurs, fresh frozen plasma or PCCs can be used to correct the clotting abnormality. PCCs should be used with caution in view of scattered reports of thrombotic complications with these products. Some investigators recommend that factor IX levels should not be raised more than 50% from baseline.

Differential Diagnosis

Hemorrhagic disease of the newborn may resemble the congenital deficiency syndrome and was once common. However, in recent times, most gravid women are given prophylactic vitamin K as well as their newborns, so this condition is now rarely reported. When present, it can be easily treated with vitamin K, and symptoms do not return. Malabsorption can also cause vitamin K deficiency in children, but again, symptoms of malabsorption are evident, and the clotting defect is rapidly corrected by administration of vitamin K. Liver disease may cause a decrease in vitamin K–dependent factors, and this cause can be suspected on the basis of abnormal liver function test results.

Care must be taken to exclude the possibility of accidental or furtive administration of warfarin or "super-warfarin," both of which may cause a deficiency of the same factors as those seen in a congenital deficiency syndrome. The difference is that congenital deficiency of vitamin K–dependent factors may cause bleeding at birth, but warfarin poisoning can produce an acquired deficiency of K-dependent clotting factors.

Special consideration must be given to a class of warfarins now referred to as "super-warfarins." These were developed to overcome resistance of rats to warfarin-containing rodenticides. In contrast to warfarin, super-warfarins have an extremely long half-life and, when ingested, are stored in the liver and have a high affinity for lipids. Once ingested by humans, they may remain in the body for months and can closely resemble the congenital deficiency syndrome, unless one takes a careful history and determines that the bleeding symptoms were acquired. Poisoning with super-warfarin may result from accidental administration (most commonly seen in children), psychiatric conditions, industrial exposure, surreptitious ingestion, or deliberate self-poisoning with denial (Munchausen syndrome). Many cases of surreptitious ingestion of brodifacoum are seen in medical or paramedical personnel, who take the compound for secondary gain, for example, a spouse may ingest the substance to punish or get sympathy from the partner. The potency of super-warfarin is 100 times that of warfarin, and the half-life is between 16 and 69 days, compared with 37 hours for warfarin.[169] Three types of super-warfarins are available: (1) hydroxycoumarin derivatives with a 4-bromo (1-1 biphenyl) side chain, (2) coumatetryls, and (3) indanediones. Brodifacoum, a 4-hydroxycoumarin derivative, is the most commonly used super-warfarin and is primarily absorbed from the gastrointestinal tract, although skin absorbency is also possible. Super-warfarins block the carboxylation of vitamin K–dependent factors by inhibiting the vitamin K 2,3-epoxide reductase enzyme in the liver. Bleeding is the most common manifestation and may occur from any mucosal site, soft tissue, or organ. Coagulation studies show prolonged PT and PTT that are corrected with 1:1 mixing with normal plasma. TCT is normal. Decreased levels of vitamin K–dependent factors are the hallmark of this condition. Special assays are needed to detect the presence of warfarin or super-warfarin in blood. Assays for brodifacoum and other super-warfarins are not usually readily available in most clinical laboratories; thus, samples must be sent to special centers for measurement. Treatment of patients with super-warfarin poisoning requires the administration of fresh frozen plasma or PCCs if the patient is actively bleeding; in addition, large doses of vitamin K must be administered. The latter can be given orally or parenterally at a daily maintenance dose that can range from 20 mg to more than 100 mg, depending on the severity of the coagulopathy. Intravenous administration of vitamin K requires that the appropriate dose be given in a dilute solution that is administered slowly with caution and constant observation. It is important to remember that because of the long half-life of the substance and its affinity for lipids, long-term treatment with vitamin K is necessary, requiring that the vitamin be given over a long period, sometimes for several months to a year.[170] In adult patients who surreptitiously take the drug or who have Munchausen syndrome, psychiatric counseling may help, but repeated ingestion of brodifacoum has been reported, even after counseling was provided. This clinical picture was recently discussed in a clinicopathology conference forum.[170a]

Other Combined Familial Deficiencies

Other combined familial factor deficiencies (see Table 5-8) occur less often than those discussed previously. The genetic nature of these defects is largely unknown. When bleeding occurs, plasma or specific factor concentrates may be used for treatment.

α_2-PLASMIN INHIBITOR DEFICIENCY

α_2-Plasmin inhibitor deficiency was first described in 1976. Occasionally, it has been referred to as α_2-antiplasmin deficiency. Since its discovery, more than 10 families have been identified who have this disorder.[171] These patients may be "missed" unless a high index of suspicion is present, because routine test results of coagulation may be only slightly prolonged.

Pathogenesis and Genetics

Individuals with α_2-plasmin inhibitor deficiency exhibit a hemorrhagic tendency caused by reduced inhibition of plasmin, accompanied by resultant increased fibrinolytic activity. Deficiency is inherited in an autosomal recessive pattern, with no predilection for sex or race. The gene is located on chromosome 17, and a variety of genetic defects, including additions, small deletions, and specific nucleotide substitutions, have been reported.

Clinical Manifestations

Bleeding manifestations are more pronounced in homozygous individuals and are characterized by easy bruising, epistaxis, hematuria, menorrhagia, and hemarthrosis. Bleeding after trauma or surgery may be severe and often is delayed. Heterozygous individuals usually have hemorrhagic symptoms only in association with trauma.

Differential Diagnosis

α_2-Plasmin inhibitor deficiency may also be acquired and has been reported in individuals with liver failure, amyloidosis, solid tumor, acute promyelocytic leukemia, and disseminated intravascular coagulation.[172] Decreased levels of α_2-plasmin inhibitor have also been described in patients who received thrombolytic therapy and in those with other conditions associated with a hyperfibrinolytic state.[173]

Diagnosis

Diagnosis of α_2-plasmin inhibitor deficiency requires a high degree of suspicion because laboratory evaluation may reveal completely normal PT, PTT, TCT, and bleeding time. Clots that are formed are not rapidly soluble in 5-molar urea as normal factor XIII activity is retained. However, whole blood and euglobulin lysis times are markedly accelerated. Definite diagnosis requires a specific α_2-plasmin inhibitor assay.

Treatment

Antifibrinolytics are the mainstay of treatment. During bleeding situations, ϵ-aminocaproic acid may be used orally or intravenously at a dose of 2 to 3 g every 6 hours. Continuous intravenous infusion can also be provided at a dose of 1 g per hour. The maximum recommended dose is 30 g a day in patients with normal renal function. Some clinicians find that lower doses, for example, 4 to 6 g every 4 to 6 hours, are equally efficacious. Myolysis has been reported with long-term antifibrinolytic therapy.

α_1-ANTITRYPSIN PITTSBURGH (ANTITHROMBIN III PITTSBURGH)

To date, only two individuals with this defect have been described.[174,175] Both patients had the same genetic mutation, even though the hemorrhagic manifestations were different. Bleeding manifestations occurred after trauma, which induced an increase in the level of the mutant enzyme that is an acute phase reactant. The mutation observed in α_1-antitrypsin Pittsburgh is characterized by the substitution of methionine for arginine at position 358 of the α_1-antitrypsin AT (α_1-AT) molecule. This substitution essentially converts α_1-antitrypsin into an antithrombin with both antithrombin and antifactor Xa activity. One individual had severe bleeding episodes with soft tissue hematoma, hematuria, and melena. He died of massive hemorrhage. Another individual had only mild bleeding symptoms. PT, PTT, TCT, and bleeding time were prolonged in both individuals. Low protein C (13%) was also seen in the second individual, but its cause and role are not clear.

PROTEIN Z DEFICIENCY

Protein Z is a vitamin K–dependent protein that was first described in bovine plasma.[176] Human protein Z was discovered and purified by Broze and Miletich in 1984.[177] The plasma half-life is estimated to be 2 to 3 days. No correlation has been found between age and sex. Protein Z plasma concentration is variable. Because it is a vitamin K–dependent factor, its level is exquisitely sensitive to warfarin.[178] Protein Z is mentioned in this chapter because early studies suggested that patients with low protein Z levels have a mild bleeding tendency.[179] More recent reports, however, indicate that protein Z is a cofactor for a protein Z–dependent protease inhibitor (ZPI), a member of the serpin family of inhibitors.[180,181] ZPI, with protein Z as a cofactor, inhibits factor Xa (a serine protease) on phospholipid surfaces. Thus, deficiency of protein Z has been shown to predispose protein Z–deficient mice to thrombosis rather than hemorrhage. This suggests that protein Z deficiency in humans may be prothrombotic.[182] Reports suggesting that protein Z deficiency is associated with excessive bleeding may be inaccurate.

CONSULTATION CONSIDERATIONS

Although some factor deficiencies occur rarely, patients with these conditions are exactly the type of patient for whom the hematologist will be consulted. The consultant should be aware that mild prolongation on any of the screening tests of coagulation should be investigated. If such abnormalities appear to be lifelong, the patient most likely has a congenital bleeding disorder. However, it should be emphasized that the most important diagnostic information to be sought regarding a hereditary bleeding disease is a personal or family history of bleeding spontaneously or after trauma or surgery.[183] Mildly affected patients may have normal screening tests of coagulation; prolonged tests do not always denote a bleeding abnormality. Some mildly affected patients may have no bleeding until late in life, and the consultant will have to carefully assess the family history to rule out other acquired causes of a hemorrhagic disorder. Because many diseases are recessive in inheritance, a high degree of consideration must be given to consanguinity. Finally, the consultant should remember the importance of genetic counseling for affected patients and their families.

MEDICAL-LEGAL ISSUES

A firmly established diagnosis is important. It was not uncommon to see patients given a misdiagnosis of lupus anticoagulant or factor VIII or IX deficiency followed by treatment with concentrates that were dubious, expensive, and perhaps dangerous, when they had an acquired inhibitor to a specific coagulation protein (i.e., factor VIII). On the other hand, many patients receive fresh frozen plasma indiscriminately in the hope that "a missing factor" would be replaced and result in improvement in symptoms. Potential adverse effects of therapy, including possible allergic reactions and any specific adverse effects associated with therapeutic products, should always be explained to the patient.

When an unusual diagnosis is made in a family member, consideration should be given to notifying and possibly testing other members of the family. Genetic counseling should always be part of the consultation, when indicated.

COST CONTAINMENT ISSUES

Once the correct diagnosis has been established, patients should be treated with the most effective and safest material available. Cost consideration should not be the deciding factor in treatment but should always be considered. For example, recombinant products, although they often are more expensive than plasma-derived clotting factor concentrates, are preferred because they are less likely to be contaminated by potentially transmissible agents that are not susceptible to currently used eradication techniques. Specific therapy is preferred when available.

REFERENCES

1. Bolton-Maggs PHB, Perry DJ, Chalmers A, et al: The rare coagulation disorders—Review with guidelines for management from the United Kingdom Haemophilia Centre Doctor's Organization. Haemophilia 10:593–628, 2004.
2. Rabe F, Salomon E: Uber Faserstoffmangel im Blut bei einem Falle von Hamophilie. Dtsch Arch Klin Med 132:240–244, 1920.
3. Neerman-Arbez M, Honsberger A, Antonarakis SE, Morris MA: Deletion of the fibrinogen alpha-chain gene (FGA) causes congenital afibrogenemia. J Clin Invest 103:215–218, 1999.
4. Duga S, Asselta R, Santagostino E, et al: Missense mutations in the human beta fibrinogen gene cause congenital afibrogenemia by impairing fibrinogen secretion. Blood 95:343–347, 2000.
5. Al-Mondhiry H, Ehmann WC: Congenital afibrinogenemia. Am J Hematol 46:343–347, 1994.
6. Menache D: Congenital fibrinogen abnormalities. Ann NY Acad Sci 408:121–130, 1983.
7. Ehmann WC, al-Mondhiry H: Congenital afibrinogenemia and splenic rupture. Am J Hematol 46:343–347, 1994.
8. Mammen EF: Fibrinogen abnormalities. Semin Thromb Hemost 9:1–72, 1983.
9. Evron S, Anteby SO, Brzezinsky A, et al: Congenital afibrinogenemia and recurrent early abortion: A case report. Eur J Obstet Gynecol Reprod Biol 19:307–311, 1985.
10. Goodwin TM: Congenital hypofibrinogenemia in pregnancy. Obstet Gynecol Surv 44:157–161, 1989.
11. Ness PM, Budzynski AZ, Olexa SA, Rodvien R: Congenital hypofibrinogenemia and recurrent placental abruption. Obstet Gynecol 61:519–523, 1983.
12. Weiss HJ, Rodgers J: Fibrinogen and platelets in the primary arrest of bleeding: Studies in two patients with congenital afibrinogenemia. N Engl J Med 285:369–374, 1971.
13. Soria J, Soria C, Borg JY, et al: Platelet aggregation occurs in congenital afibrinogenemia despite the absence of fibrinogen or its fragments in plasma and platelets, as demonstrated by immunoenzymology. Br Med Bull 33:253–259, 1977.
14. Flute PT: Disorders of plasma fibrinogen synthesis. Br Med Bull 33:253–259, 1977.
15. Colvin RB, Mosesson MW, Dvorak HF: Delayed-type hypersensitivity skin reactions in congenital afibrinogenemia lack fibrin deposition and induration. J Clin Invest 63:1302–1306, 1979.
16. Bithell TC: Hereditary coagulation disorders. In Lee GR, Bithell TC, Foerster J, et al (eds): Wintrobe's Clinical Hematology, 9th ed vol 2. Philadelphia, Lea and Febiger, 1993, p 1439.
17. Dale BM, Purdie GH, Rischbieth RH: Fibrinogen depletion with sodium valproate [letter]. Lancet 1:1316–1317, 1978.
18. Gralnick HR, Henderson E: Hypofibrogenemia and coagulation factor deficiencies with L-asparaginase treatment. Cancer 27:1313–1320, 1971.
19. Inanmoto Y, Terao T: First report of a case of congenital afibrinogenemia with successful delivery. Am J Obstet Gynecol 153:803–804, 1985.
20. DeVries A, Rosenberg T, Kochwa S, Boss JH: Precipitating antifibrinogen antibody appears after fibrinogen infusions in a patient with congenital afibrinogenemia. Am J Med 30:486–494, 1961.
21. Ingram GI, McBrien DJ, Spencer H: Fatal pulmonary embolus in congenital fibrinopenia: Report of two cases. Acta Haematol 35:56–62, 1966.
22. MacKinnon HH, Fekete JF: Congenital afibrinogenemia: Vascular changes and multiple thromboses induced by fibrinogen infusions and contraceptive medication. Can Med Assoc J 104:597–599, 1971.
23. Cronin C, Fitzpatrick D, Temperley I: Multiple pulmonary emboli in a patient with afibrinogenemia. Acta Haematol 79:53–54, 1988.
24. Calenda E, Bor JY, Peillon C, et al: Perioperative management of a patient with congenital hypofibrinogenemia [letter]. Anesthesiology 71:622–623, 1989.
25. Martinez J, Ferber A: Disorders of fibrinogen. In Hoffman R, Benz EJ, Shattil SJ, et al (eds): Hematology: Basic Principles and Practice, 4th ed. New York, Churchill Livingstone, 2005, pp 2097–2109.
26. Lord ST: Fibrinogen. In High KA and Roberts HR (eds): Molecular Basis of Thrombosis and Hemostasis, New York, Marcel Dekker, Inc., 1995, pp 51–74.
27. Roberts HR, Escobar MA: Other coagulation deficiencies. In Loscalzo J, Schafer AI (eds): Thrombosis and Hemorrhage, 3rd ed. Baltimore, Williams & Wilkins, 2003, pp 575–598.
28. Forman WB, Ratnoff OD, Boyer MH: An inherited qualitative abnormality in plasma fibrinogen: Fibrinogen Cleveland. J Lab Clin Med 72:455–472, 1968.
29. Martinez J, Palascak JE, Kwasniak D: Abnormal sialic acid content of the dysfibrinogenemia associated with liver disease. J Clin Invest 61:535–538, 1978.

30. Quick AJ: Congenital hypoprothrombinemia and pseudo-hypoprothrombinemia. Lancet 2:379–382, 1947.
31. Quick AJ, Pisciotta AV, Hussey CV: Congenital hypoprothrombinemic states. Arch Intern Med 95:2–14, 1955.
32. Degen SJF: Prothrombin. In High KA, Roberts HR (eds): Molecular Basis of Thrombosis and Hemostasis. New York, Marcel Dekker, 1995, pp 75–99.
33. Girolami A, Scarano L, Saggiorato G, et al: Congenital deficiencies and abnormalities of prothrombin. Blood Coagul Fibrinolysis 9:7603–7607, 1998.
34. Xue J, Wu Q, Westfield LA, et al: Incomplete embryonic lethality and fatal neonatal hemorrhage caused by prothrombin deficiency in mice. Proc Natl Acad Sci USA 95:7603–7607, 1998.
35. Sun WY, Witte DP, Degen JL, et al: Incomplete embryonic lethality and fatal neonatal hemorrhage caused by prothrombin deficiency in mice. Proc Natl Acad Sci USA 95:7597–7602, 1998.
36. Catanzarite VA, Novotny WF, Cousins LM, Schneider JM: Pregnancies in a patient with congenital absence of prothrombin activity: Case report. Am J Perinatol 14:135–138, 1997.
37. Acharya SS, Coughlin A, Dimichele DM, et al: Rare bleeding disorder registry: Deficiencies of factors II, V, VII, X, XII, fibrinogen and dysfibrinogenemias. J Thromb Haemost 2:248–256, 2004.
38. Roberts HR, Liles D: Deficiencies of the vitamin K–dependent clotting factors. In Brain MC, Carbone PP (eds): Current Therapy in Hematology-Oncology, 5th ed. St. Louis, Mosby, 1995, pp 171–176.
39. Bajaj SP, Rapaport SI, Barclay S, Herbst KD: Acquired hypoprothrombinemia due to non-neutralizing antibodies to prothrombin: Mechanism and management. Blood 65:1538–1543, 1985.
40. Vivaldi P, Rossetti G, Galli M, Finazzi G: Severe bleeding due to acquired hypoprothrombinemia–lupus anticoagulant syndrome: Case report and review of literature. Haematologica 82:345–347, 1997.
41. Cote HC, Huntsman DG, Wu J, et al: A new method for characterization and epitope determination of a lupus anticoagulant–associated neutralizing antiprothrombin antibody. Am J Clin Pathol 107:197–205, 1997.
42. Gill FM, Shapiro SS, Schwartz E: Severe congenital hypoprothrombinemia. J Pediatr 93:264–266, 1978.
43. Owen CA Jr, Hendriksen RA, McDduffie FC Mann KG: Prothrombin Quick: A newly identified dysprothombinemia. Mayo Clin 53:29–33, 1978.
44. White GC, Roberts HR, Kingdon HS, Lundblad RL: Prothrombin complex concentrates: Potentially thrombogenic materials and clues to the mechanism of thrombosis in vivo. Blood 49:159–170, 1977.
45. Philippou H, Adami A, Lane DA, et al: High purity factor IX and prothrombin complex concentrate (PCC): Pharmacokinetics and evidence that factor IXa is the thromogenic trigger in PCC. Thromb Haemost 76:23–28, 1996.
46. Lechler E: Use of prothrombin complex concentrates for prophylaxis and treatment of bleeding episodes in patients with hereditary deficiency of prothrombin, factor VII, factor X, protein C, protein S, or protein Z. Thromb Res 95 (4 suppl 1):S39–S50, 1999.
47. Halbmayer WM: Rational, high quality laboratory monitoring before, during, and after infusion of prothrombin complex concentrates. Thromb Res 95 (4 suppl 1):S25–S30, 1999.
48. Roberts HR, Escobar MA: Other clotting factor deficiencies. In Hoffman R, Benz EJ, Shattil EJ, et al (eds): Hematology: Basic Principles and Practice, 4th ed. New York, Churchill Livingstone, 2005, pp 2081–2095.
49. Quick AJ: On the constitution of prothrombin. Am J Physiol 140:212, 1943.
50. Owren PA: The coagulation of blood: Investigations on a new clotting factor. Acta Med Scand 194:11–41, 1947.
51. Camire RM, Pottak ES, Kaushansky K, Tracy PB: Secretable human platelet–derived factor V originates from the plasma pool. Blood 92:3035–3041, 1998.
52. Colman RW: Where does platelet factor V originate? [letter]. Blood 93:3152–3153, 1999.
53. Gewirtz AM, Shapiro C, Shen YM, et al: Cellular and molecular regulation of factor V expression in human megakaryocytes. J Cell Physiol 153:277–287, 1992.
54. Breederveld K, Giddings JC, ten Cate JW, Bloom AL: The localization of factor V within normal human platelets and the demonstration of a platelet–factor antigen in congenital factor V deficiency. Br J Haematol 293:405–412, 1975.
55. Tracy PB, Mann KG: Abnormal formation of the prothrombinase complex: Factor V deficiency and related disorders. Hum Pathol 18:162–169, 1987.
56. Chiu HC, Whitaker E, Colman RW: Heterogeneity of human factor V deficiency: Evidence for the existence of antigen-positive variants. J Clin Invest 72:493–503, 1983.
57. Vos HL: Inherited defects of coagulation factor V: The thrombotic side. J Thromb Haemost 4:35–40, 2006.
58. Asselta R, Tenchini ML, Duga S: Inherited defects of coagulation factor V: The hemorrhagic side. J Thromb Haemost 4:26–34, 2006.
59. Yang TL, Cui J, Taylor JM, et al: Rescue of fatal neonatal hemorrhage in factor V deficient mice by low level transgene expression. Thromb Haemost 83:70–77, 2000.
60. Miletich JP, Majerus DW, Majerus PW: Patients with congenital factor V deficiency have decreased factor Xa binding sites on their platelets. J Clin Invest 62:824–831, 1978.
61. Manotti C, Quintavalla R, Pini M, et al: Thromboembolic manifestations and congenital factor V deficiency: A family study. Haemostasis 19:331–334, 1989.
62. Fratantoni JC, Hilgartner M, Nachman RL: Nature of the defect in congenital factor V deficiency: Study in a patient with an acquired circulating anticoagulant. Blood 39:751–758, 1972.
63. Zehnder JL, Leung LL: Development of antibodies to thrombin and factor V with recurrent bleeding in a patient exposed to topical bovine thrombin. Blood 76:2011–2016, 1990.
64. Tracy PB, Giles AR, Mann KG, et al: Factor V (Quebec): A bleeding diathesis associated with a qualitative platelet factor V deficiency. J Clin Invest 74:1221–1228, 1984.
65. Hayward CP, Cramer EM, Kane WH, et al: Studies of a second family with the Quebec platelet disorder: Evidence that the degradation of the alpha-granule membrane and its soluble contents are not secondary to a defect in targeting proteins to alpha-granules. Blood 89:1243–1253, 1997.
66. Webster W, Roberts HR, Penick GD: Hemostasis in factor V deficiency. Am J Med Sci 248:194, 1964.
67. Sallah AS, Angchaisuksiri P, Roberts HR: Use of plasma exchange in hereditary deficiency of factor V and factor VIII. Am J Hematol 52:229–230, 1996.
68. Chediak J, Ashenhurst JB, Garlick I, Desser RK: Successful management of bleeding in a patient with factor V inhibitor by platelet transfusions. Blood 56:835–841, 1980.
69. Gonzalez-Boullosa R, Ocampo-Martinez R, Alarcon-Martinez MJ, et al: The use of activated recombinant factor VII during haemarthroses and synovectomy in a patient with congenital severe factor V deficiency. Haemophilia 11:167–170, 2005.
70. Alexander B, Goldstein R, Landwehr G, Cook CD: Congenital SPCA deficiency: A hitherto unrecognized coagulation defect with hemorrhage rectified by serum and serum fractions. J Clin Invest 30:596–606, 1951.
71. Giansily-Blaizot M, Schved JF: Potential predictors of bleeding risk in inherited factor VII deficiency. Thromb Haemost 94:901–906, 2005.
72. Mariani G, Mazzucconi MG: Factor VII congenital deficiency: Clinical picture and classification of the variants. Haemostasis 13:169–177, 1983.
73. Giansily-Blaizot M, Verdier R, Biron-Adreani C, et al: Analysis of biological phenotypes from 42 patients with inherited factor VII deficiency: Can biological tests predict the bleeding risk? Haematologica 89:704–709, 2004.
74. Ragni MV, Lewis JH, Spero JA, Hasiba U: Factor VII deficiency. Am J Hematol 10:79–88, 1981.
75. Mariani G, Herrmann FH, Schulman S, et al: Thrombosis in inherited factor VII deficiency. J Thromb Haemost 1:2153–2158, 2003.
76. Lusher J, Ingerslev J, Roberts H, Hedner U: Clinical experience with recombinant factor VIIa. Blood Coagul Fibrinolysis 9:119–128, 1998.
77. Morrissey JH, Macik BG, Neuenschwander PF, Comp PC: Quantification of activated factor VII levels in plasma using a tissue factor mutant selectively deficient in promoting factor VII activation. Blood 81:734–744, 1993.
78. Delmer A, Horellou MH, Andreu G, et al: Life-threatening intracranial bleeding associated with the presence of an antifactor VII antibody. Blood 74:229–232, 1989.
79. Dantzenberg MD, Saudubray JM, Girot R: Factor VII deficiency in homocysteinuria [abstract]. Thromb Haemost 50:409, 1983.
80. Weisdorf D, Hasegawa D, Fair DS: Acquired factor VII deficiency associated with aplastic anemia: Correction with bone marrow transplantation. Br J Haematol 71:409–413, 1989.

81. Seligsohn U, Shani M, Ramot B, et al: Hereditary deficiency of blood clotting factor VII and Dubin-Johnson syndrome in an Israeli family. Isr J Med Sci 5:1060–1065, 1959.

82. Seligsohn U, Shani M, Ramot B: Gilbert syndrome and factor VII deficiency. Lancet 1:1398, 1970.

83. Mariani G, Konkle BA, Ingerslev J: Congenital factor VII deficiency: Therapy with recombinant activated factor VII—A critical appraisal. Haemophilia 12:19–27, 2006.

84. Peyvandi F, Mannucci PM: Rare coagulation disorders. Thromb Haemost 82:1207–1214, 1999.

85. Hougie C, Barrow EM, Graham JB: Stuart clotting defect I. Segregation of an hereditary hemorrhagic state from the heterogeneous group heretofore called "stable factor" (SPCA, proconvertin, factor VII) deficiency. J Clin Invest 36:485–496, 1957.

86. Telfer TP, Denson KW, Wright DR: A "new" coagulation defect. Br J Haematol 2:308–316, 1956.

87. Cooper DN, Millar DS, Wacey A, et al: Inherited factor X deficiency: Molecular genetics and pathophysiology. Thromb Haemost 78:161–172, 1997.

88. Dewerchin M, Liang Z, Moons L, et al: Blood coagulation factor X deficiency causes partial embryonic lethality and fatal neonatal bleeding in mice. Thromb Haemost 83:185–190, 2000.

89. Peyvandi F, Mannucci PM, Lak M, et al: Congenital factor X deficiency: Spectrum of bleeding symptoms in 32 Iranian patients. Br J Haematol 102:626–628, 1998.

90. Currie MS, Stein AM, Rustagi PK, et al: Transient acquired factor X deficiency associated with pneumonia. N Y State J Med 84:572–573, 1984.

91. Smith SV, Liles DK, White DK 2nd, Brecher ME: Successful treatment of transient acquired factor X deficiency by plasmapheresis with concomitant intravenous immunoglobulin and steroid therapy. Am J Hematol 57:245–252, 1998.

92. Caimi MT, Redaelli R, Cattaneo D, et al: Acquired selective factor X deficiency in acute nonlymphocytic leukemia. Am J Hematol 36:65–66, 1991.

93. Nora RE, Bell WR, Noe DA, Sholar PW: Novel factor X deficiency: Normal partial thromboplastin time and associated spindle cell thymoma. Am J Med 79:122–126, 1985.

94. Ness PM, Hymas PG, Gesme D, Perkins HA: An unusual factor X inhibitor in leprosy. Am J Hematol 8:397–402, 1980.

95. Henson K, Files JC, Morrison FS: Transient acquired factor X deficiency: Report of the use of activated clotting concentrate to control a life-threatening hemorrhage. Am J Med 87:583–585, 1989.

96. Rao LV, Zivelin A, Iturbe I, Rapaport SI: Antibody-induced acute factor X deficiency: Clinical manifestations and properties of the antibody. Thromb Haemost 72:363–371, 1994.

97. Furie B, Greene E, Furie BC: Syndrome of acquired factor X deficiency and systemic amyloidosis in vivo studies of the metabolic fate of factor X. N Engl J Med 297:81–85, 1977.

98. Mumford AD, O'Donnell J, Gillmore JD, et al: Bleeding symptoms and coagulation abnormalities in 337 patients with AL-amyloidosis. Br J Haematol 110:454–460, 2000.

99. Greip PR, Kyle RA, Bowie EJ: Factor X deficiency in primary amyloidosis: Resolution after splenectomy. N Engl J Med 301:1050–1051, 1979.

100. Camoriano JK, Greipp PR, Bayer GK, Bowie EJ: Resolution of acquired factor X deficiency and amyloidosis with melphalan and prednisone therapy. N Engl J Med 316:1133–1135, 1987.

101. Breadell FV, Varma M, Martinez J: Normalization of plasma factor X levels in amyloidosis after plasma exchange. Am J Hematol 54:68–71, 1997.

102. Boggio L, Green D: Recombinant human factor VIIa in the management of amyloid-associated factor X deficiency. Br J Haematol 112:1074–1075, 2001.

103. Takabe K, Holman PR, Herbst KD, et al: Successful perioperative management of factor X deficiency associated with primary amyloidosis. J Gastrointest Surg 8:358–362, 2004.

104. Telgt DS, Macik BG, McCord DM, et al: Mechanism by which recombinant factor VIIa shortens the aPTT: Activation of factor X in the absence of tissue factor. Thromb Res 56:603–609, 1989.

105. Rosenthal RL, Dreskin OH, Rosenthal N: New hemophilia-like disease caused by deficiency of a third plasma thromboplastin factor. Proc Soc Exp Biol Med 82:171–174, 1953.

106. Seligsohn U: High gene frequency of factor XI (PTA) deficiency in Ashkenazi Jews. Blood 51:1223–1228, 1978.

107. Asakai R, Chung DW, Davie EW, Seligsohn U: Factor XI deficiency in Ashkenazi Jews in Israel. N Engl J Med 325:153–158, 1991.

108. Fujikawa K, Chung DW: Factor XI. In High KA, Roberts HR (eds): Molecular Basis of Thrombosis and Hemostasis. New York, Marcel Dekker, 1995, pp 257–268.

109. Lipscomb MS, Walsh PN: Human platelets and factor XI: Localization in platelet membranes of factor XI–like activity and its functional distinction from plasma factor XI. J Clin Invest 63:1006–1014, 1979.

110. Kitchens CS: Factor XI: A review of its biochemistry and deficiency. Semin Thromb Hemost 17:55–72, 1991.

111. Sidi A, Seligsohn U, Jonas P, Many M: Factor XI deficiency: Detection and management during urological surgery. J Urol 119:528–530, 1978.

112. Kitchens CS, Alexander J: Partial deficiency of coagulation factor XI as a newly recognized feature of Noonan syndrome. J Pediatr 102:224–227, 1983.

113. Lian EC, Deykin D, Harkness DR: Combined deficiencies of factor VIII (AHF) and factor XI (PTA). Am J Hematol 1:319–324, 1976.

114. Soff GA, Levin J, Bell WR: Familial multiple coagulation factor deficiencies II. Combined factor VIII, IX, and XI deficiency and combined factor IX and XI deficiency: Two previously uncharacterized familial multiple factor deficiency syndromes. Semin Thromb Hemost 7:149–169, 1981.

115. Tavori S, Brenner B, Tatarsky I: The effect of combined factor XI deficiency with von Willebrand factor abnormalities on haemorrhagic diathesis. Thromb Haemost 63:36–38, 1990.

116. Peter MK, Meili EO, von Felton A: Factor XI deficiency: Additional hemostatic defects are present in patients with bleeding tendency. Thromb Haemost 73:1442, 1995.

117. Vander Woude JC, Milam JD, Walker WE, et al: Cardiovascular surgery in patients with congenital plasma coagulopathies. Ann Thorac Surg 46:283–288, 1988.

118. Blatt PM, McFarland DH, Eifrig DE: Ophthalmic surgery and plasma prothrombin antecedent (factor XI) deficiency. Arch Ophthalmol 98:863–864, 1980.

119. Berliner S, Horowitz I, Martinowitz U, et al: Dental surgery in patients with severe factor XI deficiency without plasma replacement. Blood Coagul Fibrinolysis 3:465–468, 1992.

120. Rakocz M, Mazar A, Varon D, et al: Dental extractions in patients with bleeding disorders: The use of fibrin glue. Oral Surg Oral Med Oral Pathol 75:280–282, 1993.

121. Bern MM, Sahud M, Zhukov O, et al: Treatment of factor XI inhibitor using recombinant factor VIIa. Haemophilia 11:20–25, 2005.

122. Lawler P, White B, Pye S, et al: Successful use of recombinant factor VIIa in a patient with inhibitor secondary to severe factor XI deficiency. Haemophilia 8:145–148, 2002.

123. Bolton-Maggs PH, Colvin BT, Satchi BT, et al: Thrombogenic potential of factor XI concentrate. Lancet 344:748–749, 1994.

124. Stern DM, Nossel HL, Owen J: Acquired antibody to factor XI in a patient with congenital factor XI deficiency. J Clin Invest 69:1270–1276, 1982.

125. Ginsberg SS, Clyne LP, McPhedran P, et al: Successful childbirth by a patient with congenital factor XI deficiency and an acquired inhibitor. Br J Haematol 84:172–174, 1993.

126. Hedner U: NovoSeven as a universal haemostatic agent. Blood Coagul Fibrinolysis 11 (suppl 1): S107–S111, 2000.

127. Colman RW: Biologic activities of the contact favors in vivo: Potentiation of hypotension, inflammation, and fibrinolysis, and inhibition of cell adhesion, angiogenesis and thrombosis. Thromb Haemost 82:1568–1577, 1999.

128. Ratnoff OD, Colopy JE: A familial hemorrhagic trait associated with a deficiency of a clot-promoting fraction of plasma. J Clin Invest 34:602–613, 1954.

129. Bennett B, Ratnoff OD, Holt JB, Roberts HR: Hageman trait (factor XII deficiency): A probably second genotype inherited as an autosomal dominant characteristic. Blood 40:412–415, 1972.

129a. Halbmayer WM, Haushofer A, Schön R, et al: The prevalence of moderate and severe FXII (Hageman factor) deficiency among the normal population: Evaluation of the incidence of FXII deficiency among 300 healthy blood donors. Thromb Haemost 71:68–72, 1994.

130. Gordon EM, Donaldson VH, Saito H, et al: Reduced titers of Hageman factor (factor XII) in Orientals. Ann Intern Med 95:697–700, 1981.

130a. Kitchens CS: The contact system. Arch Pathol Lab Med 126: 1382–1386, 2002.

131. Criel A, Collen D, Masson PL: A case of IgM antibodies which inhibit the contact activation of blood coagulation. Thromb Res 12:883–892, 1978.

132. Clyne LP, Farber LR, Chopyk RL: Procainamide-induced circulating anticoagulants in a congenitally-defective factor XI patient. Folia Haematol Int Mag Klin Morphol Blutforsch 116:239–244, 1989.

133. Zucker S, Zarrabi MH, Romano GS, Miller F: IgM inhibitors of the contact activation phase of coagulation in chlorpromazine-treated patients. Br J Haematol 40:447–457, 1978.

134. Bux-Gewehr I, Morgenschweis K, Zotz RB, et al: Combined von Willebrand factor deficiency and factor XII deficiency. Thromb Haemost 83:514–516, 2000.

135. Mant MJ: Combined factor IX and XII deficiencies in both male and female members of a single family. Thromb Haemost 42:816–818, 1979.

136. Hathaway WE, Belhasen LP, Hathaway HS: Evidence for a new plasma thromboplastin factor. I. Case report, coagulation studies and physicochemical properties. Blood 26:521–532, 1965.

137. Saito H, Kojima T: Factor XII, prekallikrein, and high molecular weight kininogen. In High KA, Roberts HR (eds): Molecular Basis of Thrombosis and Hemostasis. New York, Marcel Dekker, 1995, pp 269–285.

138. Wong PY, Talamo RC, Williams GH: Kallikrein-kinin and renin-angiotensin systems in functional renal failure of cirrhosis of the liver. Gastroenterology 73:1114–1118, 1977.

139. Saito H, Ratnoff OD, Waldmann R, Abraham JP: Deficiency of a hitherto unrecognized agent, Fitzgerald factor, participating in surface-mediated reactions of clotting, fibrinolysis, generation of kinins, and the property of diluted plasma enhancing vascular permeability (PF/DIL). J Clin Invest 55:1082–1089, 1975.

140. Duckert F, Jung E, Shmerling DH: A hitherto undescribed congenital haemorrhagic diathesis probably due to fibrin stabilizing factor deficiency. Thromb Diath Haemorrh 5:179–186, 1960.

141. Lopaciuk S, Lovette KM, McDonagh J, et al: Subcellular distribution of fibrinogen and factor XIII in human blood platelets. Thromb Res 84:453–465, 1976.

142. Lai T, Greenberg CS: Factor XIII. In High KA, Roberts HR (eds): Molecular Basis of Thrombosis and Hemostasis. New York, Marcel Dekker, 1995, pp 287–308.

143. Bouhasin JD, Altay C: Factor 13 deficiency: Concentrations in relatives of patients and in normal infants. J Pediatr 72:336–341, 1968.

144. Fisher S, Rikover M, Naor S: Factor 13 deficiency with severe hemorrhagic diathesis. Blood 28:235–238, 1966.

145. Kobsydhi T, Terao T, Kojima T, et al: Congenital factor XIII deficiency with treatment of factor XIII concentrate and normal vaginal delivery. Gynecol Obstet Invest 29:235–238, 1990.

146. Kitchens CS, Newcomb TF: Factor XIII. Medicine 58:413–429, 1979.

147. Duckert F: Documentation of the plasma factor XIII deficiency in man. Ann N Y Acad Sci 202:190–199, 1972.

148. Anwar R, Miloszewski KJ: Factor XIII deficiency. Br J Haematol 107:468–484, 1999.

149. Otis PT, Feinstein DI, Rapaport SI, Patch MJ: An acquired inhibitor of fibrin stabilization associated with isoniazid therapy: Clinical and biochemical observations. Blood 44:771–781, 1974.

150. Lopaciuk S, Bykowska K, McDonagh JM, et al: Difference between type I autoimmune inhibitors of fibrin stabilization in two patients with severe hemorrhagic disorder. J Clin Invest 61:661–669, 1978.

151. Godal HC, Ly B: An inhibitor of activated factor XIII, inhibiting fibrin cross-linking but not incorporation of amino acid into casein. Scand J Haemotol 19:443–448, 1977.

152. Graham JE, Yount WJ, Roberts HR: Immunochemical characterization of a human antibody to factor XIII. Blood 41:661–669, 1973.

153. Lorand L, Velasco PT, Rinne JR, et al: Autoimmune antibody (IgG Kansas) against the fibrin stabilizing factor (factor XIII) system. Proc Natl Acad Sci U S A 85:232–236, 1988.

154. Tosetto A, Rodeghiero F, Gatto E, et al: An acquired hemorrhagic disorder of fibrin crosslinking due to IgG antibodies to FVIII, successfully treated with FXIII replacement and cyclophosphamide. Am J Hematol 48:34–39, 1995.

155. Kamitsuji H, Tani K, Yasui M, et al: Activity of blood coagulation factor XIII as a prognostic indicator in patients with Henoch-Schonlein purpura: Efficacy of factor XIII substitution. Eur J Pediatr 146:519–523, 1987.

156. Rasche H: Blood coagulation factor XIII and fibrin stabilization. Klin Wochenschr 53:1137–1145, 1977.

157. Fear JD, Miloszewski KJ, Losowsky MS: The half life of factor XIII in the management of inherited deficiency. Thromb Haemost 49:102–105, 1983.

158. Stenbjerg S: Prophylaxis in factor XIII deficiency [letter]. Lancet 2:257, 1980.

159. Godal HC: An inhibitor to fibrin stabilizing factor (FSF), factor XIII. Scand J Haematol 7:43–48, 1970.

160. Zhang B, McGee B, Yamaoka JS, et al: Combined deficiency of factor V and factor VIII is due to mutations in either LMANI or MCFD2. Blood 107:1903–1907, 2006.

161. McMillan CW, Roberts HR: Congenital deficiency of coagulation factors II, VII, IX and X: Report of a case. N Engl J Med 274:1313–1315, 1966.

162. Fregin A, Rost S, Wolz W, et al: Homozygosity mapping of a second gene locus for hereditary combined deficiency of vitamin K–dependent clotting factors to the centromeric region of chromosome 16. Blood 100:3229–3232, 2002.

163. Wu SM, Cheung WF, Frazier D, Stafford DW: Cloning and expression of the cDNA for human gamma-glutamyl carboxylase. Science 254:1634–1636, 1991.

164. Li T, Chang CY, Jin DY, et al: Identification of the gene for vitamin K epoxide reductase. Nature 427:493–494, 2004.

165. Rost S, Fregin A, Ivaskevicius V, et al: Mutations in VKORC1 cause warfarin resistance and multiple coagulation factor deficiency type 2. Nature 427:537–541, 2004.

166. Wu SM, Stanley TB, Mutucumarana VP, Stafford DW: Characterization of the gamma-glutamyl carboxylase. Thromb Haemost 78:599–604, 1997.

167. Brenner B, Tavori S, Zivelin A, et al: Hereditary deficiency of all vitamin K–dependent procoagulants and anticoagulants. Br J Haematol 75:537–542, 1990.

168. Goldsmith GH Jr, Pence RE, Ratnoff OD, et al: Studies on a family with combined functional deficiencies of vitamin K–dependent coagulation factors. J Clin Invest 69:1253–1260, 1982.

169. Sarin S, Mukhtar H, Mirza MA: Prolonged coagulopathy related to superwarfarin overdose. Ann Intern Med 142:156, 2005.

170. Chua JD, Friedenberg WR: Superwarfarin poisoning. Arch Intern Med 158:1929–1932, 1998.

170a. Laposata M, Van Cott EM, Lev MH: A 40-year-old woman with epistaxis, hematemesis, and altered mental status: Case records of the Massachusetts General Hospital. N Engl J Med 356:174–182, 2007.

171. Aoki N: Alpha-2-plasmin inhibitor. In High KA, Roberts HR (eds): Molecular Basis of Thrombosis and Hemostasis. New York, Marcel Dekker, 1995, pp 545–559.

172. Meyer K, Williams EC: Fibrinolysis and acquired alpha-2-plasmin inhibitor deficiency in amyloidosis. Am J Med 79:394–396, 1985.

173. Collen D, Bounameaux H, De Cock F, et al: Analysis of coagulation and fibrinolysis during intravenous infusion of recombinant human tissue–type plasminogen activator in patients with acute myocardial infarction. Circulation 76:511–517, 1986.

174. Owen MC, Brennan SO, Lewis JH, Carrell RW: Mutation of antitrypsin to antithrombin: Alpha 1-antitrypsin Pittsburgh (358 Met leads to Arg), a fatal bleeding disorder. N Engl J Med 309:694–698, 1983.

175. Vidaud D, Emmerich J, Alhenc-Gelas M, et al: Met 358 to Arg mutation of alpha 1-antitrypsin associated with protein C deficiency in a patient with mild bleeding tendency. J Clin Invest 89:1537–1543, 1992.

176. Prowse CV, Esnouf MP: The isolation of a new warfarin-sensitive protein from bovine plasma. Biochem Soc Trans 5:255–256, 1977.

177. Broze GJ Jr, Miletich JP: Human protein Z. J Clin Invest 73:933–938, 1984.

178. Miletich JP, Broze GK Jr: Human plasma protein Z antigen: Range in normal subjects and effect of warfarin therapy. Blood 69:1580–1586, 1987.

179. Kemkes-Matthes B, Matthes KJ: Protein Z deficiency: A new cause of bleeding tendency. Thromb Res 79:49–55, 1995.

180. Han X, Fiehler R, Broze GJ Jr: Isolation of a protein Z–dependent plasma protease inhibitor. Proc Natl Acad Sci U S A 95:9250–9255, 1998.

181. Han X, Huang ZF, Fiehler R, Broze GJ Jr: The protein Z–dependent protease inhibitor is a serpin. Biochemistry 38:10073–10078, 1999.

182. Yin ZF, Huang ZF, Cui J, et al: Prothrombotic phenotype of protein Z deficiency. Proc Natl Acad Sci U S A 97:6734–6738, 2000.

183. Kitchens CS: To bleed or not to bleed? Is that the question for the PTT? J Thromb Haemost 12:2607–2611, 2005.

Chapter 6

Nonhemophilic Inhibitors of Coagulation

Bruce M. Ewenstein, MD, PhD

INTRODUCTION

Although not often encountered in clinical practice, patients with acquired inhibitors of coagulation provide unique challenges to medical personnel and institutional resources. Acquired inhibitors of coagulation include circulating immunoglobulins, usually of the immunoglobulin G (IgG) class, that neutralize the activity of a specific coagulation protein or accelerate its clearance from the plasma. These inhibitors are defined as *allo*antibodies when they arise after blood product exposure in individuals with congenital factor deficiencies (discussed further in Chapter 4), and as *auto*antibodies when they occur among patients without a preexistent coagulation defect. Autoantibodies against coagulation factors are associated with a variety of clinical conditions characterized by disturbed immune function but are also encountered among patients whose only identifiable risk factor is advanced age. Nonhemophilic inhibitors are rare but are associated with significant morbidity and mortality and should be suspected in any patient who presents with signs and symptoms of bleeding in the absence of a personal or family history of a coagulation disorder.

Loss of tolerance to endogenously expressed coagulation proteins in affected patients is not fully understood, but it is likely to involve dysregulation of both B- and T-cell responses. The most frequently affected coagulation protein is factor VIII, which results in a condition that has been called *acquired hemophilia*. Factor VIII–specific CD4+ T cells and low levels of anti–factor VIII antibodies, including some with inhibitory activity, can be detected through immunologic methods in a significant number of apparently healthy subjects.[1–3] These findings suggest that perturbations of normal immune responses to factor VIII may play an important role in the development of clinically significant anti–factor VIII antibodies.[4] It remains possible that the pathogenic potential of autoantibodies that recognize factor VIII is also modulated through idiotypic determinants on these molecules.[5,6] The presence of anti-idiotypic antibodies may be responsible, in part, for the ability of pooled IgG to suppress anti–factor VIII activity in some patients.[7,8]

In general, the clinical and laboratory manifestations of nonhemophilic inhibitors resemble those of the corresponding inherited coagulation disorder, although often with important differences. This chapter focuses principally on the natural history, diagnosis, and clinical management of patients with acquired hemophilia; other inhibitors of coagulation are briefly reviewed. Lupus anticoagulants and antiphospholipid and antiphospholipid/protein antibodies that interfere with coagulation-based laboratory assays but are principally associated with venous and arterial thrombosis, pregnancy loss, and other clinical manifestations are discussed further in Chapter 19.

LABORATORY DIAGNOSIS

Screening Tests

In routine laboratory testing, simple factor deficiencies and specific inhibitors result in prolongation of partial prothrombin time (PTT), prothrombin time (PT), or both. These conditions can be distinguished through mixing studies. In the presence of a simple factor deficiency, mixtures of equal volumes of patient and normal plasmas in vitro will correct the abnormality. In contrast, the presence of an inhibitor in patient plasma will inactivate the target protein in normal plasma, and the PTT or PT will remain prolonged.[9] Inactivation is time and temperature dependent[10] and may require several hours to prolong the PTT, especially in cases of weak inhibitors. Typically, the PTT or PT is measured immediately after normal and patient test plasmas are mixed and after 1 and 2 hours of incubation at 37°C. Because certain coagulation proteins, including factor VIII, are heat labile, the PTT derived from mixtures of normal and patient plasmas must be compared with those of control mixtures of normal plasma and buffer incubated under the same conditions. Prolongation greater than 10 seconds over the control value is typically taken as a positive inhibitor screen. The sensitivity of the screening assay may be improved by increasing the proportion of patient plasma to normal plasma to 4:1.[9]

Inhibitor Specificity

The next step in evaluation of a patient with a prolonged screening test and a positive mixing study is to determine the specificity of the inhibitor. One goal is to distinguish inhibitors of specific coagulation pathway components from "lupus anticoagulants"—antibodies with specificity for phospholipid or phospholipid-binding proteins that may prolong the PTT but are not usually associated with clinical bleeding. This distinction is especially important in the evaluation of patients for whom no antecedent diagnosis of a factor deficiency was confirmed. A second goal is to properly identify the specific coagulation protein targeted by the inhibitor.

Table 6-1 Laboratory Tests to Distinguish Antibodies to Specific Coagulation Factors from Lupus Anticoagulants

Method	Result	
	Specific Inhibitor	Lupus Anticoagulant
Normalization of all factor assays with increasing dilution of patient plasma	Negative	Positive
Kinetics of prolongation	Slow	Immediate
Prolonged RVVT	Negative[a]	Positive
Phospholipid neutralization procedure	Negative	Positive

[a]Except in the presence of inhibitors to factors in the "common pathway."

Several methods are commonly employed for distinguishing lupus anticoagulants from inhibitors of factor VIII or other specific coagulation factors (Table 6-1).[11,12] The presence of a strong specific factor inhibitor may result in a modest reduction in the measurement of other factors when assays are performed at standard dilutions, leading to the false impression that the inhibitor is not specific. When assays are performed on a series of increasingly more dilute patient plasma samples, the apparent concentrations of all factors, except the one that is specifically inhibited, will rise into the normal range. In contrast, progressive normalization of all factor levels will be observed with increasing dilution of the test plasma that contains a lupus anticoagulant. Another commonly used technique, Russell's viper venom time (RVVT), makes use of an enzyme found in the venom of Russell's viper that promotes fibrin formation through the direct activation of factors V and X. The enzyme is dependent on the presence of phospholipid but independent of factor VIII or other intrinsic pathway factors. The RVVT is thus prolonged in the presence of antiphospholipid antibodies but not with inhibitors of intrinsic pathway proteins.[13] A third technique makes use of the observation that the addition of platelet membranes or hexagonal-phase phospholipid (phosphatidylethanolamine) will shorten the prolonged PTT caused by a lupus anticoagulant, but it will have little or no effect on prolongation of the PTT due to specific factor inhibitors.[14] Diagnosis of a lupus anticoagulant is supported by the detection of antibodies to cardiolipin, β_2-glycoprotein I (β_2GPI), or prothrombin (see later) through the use of quantitative immunoassays. However, it should be recognized that not all lupus anticoagulant sera yield positive results in these immunoassays.[15] Rarely, patients are encountered who have both lupus anticoagulant and specific factor VIII inhibitors, producing complex laboratory test results.[16,17] Such patients present primarily with bleeding.

Quantitative Assays of Coagulation Factor Inhibitors

Once the presence of a specific factor inhibitor has been established, it should be quantified because this result will influence treatment strategy. Methods are best characterized for anti–factor VIII inhibitors. The most widely used assay today is the Bethesda method, which measures residual factor VIII activity after dilutions of inhibitor patient plasma have been incubated with pooled normal plasma for 2 hours at 37°C.[18] Because factor VIII is labile, the residual factor must be compared (through mixture of control and patient plasmas) with factor VIII activity that remains after control plasma has been mixed with buffer under identical conditions.[19] The quantity (in Bethesda units [BU]) of inhibitor is defined as the reciprocal of the titer that produces 50% inhibition. The Bethesda assay may yield false-positive results because of nonspecific loss of factor VIII activity. The Nijmegen modification, which includes the addition of buffers in the assay to minimize shifts in pH, permits more accurate measurement of low-titer inhibitors.[20]

Inhibitor titers may be determined reliably only for antibodies that display second-order concentration dependence (type 1); the titer of antibodies with more complex kinetics (type 2) can only be approximated (Fig. 6-1). Particularly in

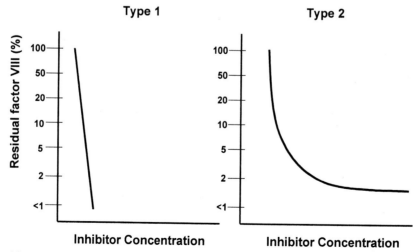

Figure 6-1 Inactivation of factor VIII by type 1 and type 2 inhibitors. Type 1 inhibitors, when present in excess, produce complete inactivation; a linear relationship exists between inhibitor concentration and the logarithm of residual factor VIII activity. Type 2 inhibitors, which are typical of non-hemophilic autoantibodies, do not produce complete inactivation of factor VIII. (Based on the work of Gawryl MS, Hoyer LW: Inactivation of factor VIII coagulant activity by two different types of human antibodies. Blood 60:1103–1109, 1982. Permission granted for the previous edition.)

the case of type 2 inhibitors, it is essential that dilutions of patient plasma that produce residual factor VIII activity as close to 50% as possible should be used when the inhibitor titer is calculated. This method has been extrapolated to the detection and quantification of other factor inhibitors as well.

Other assays of factor inhibitors that rely on immunologic rather than functional methods are extremely sensitive but are generally confined to research settings. These include immunodiffusion and enzyme-linked immunosorbent assay (ELISA).[21–23] Each of these methods is able to detect antibodies that accelerate clearance of the coagulation protein from the circulation without inhibiting its activity in vitro.[24] With the immunodiffusion assay, patient plasma is allowed to diffuse in an agarose gel that contains citrated plasma that is then incubated with a calcium-containing solution to initiate the coagulation cascade in situ. Inhibition of fibrin formation, evident as a clear ring in the gel, provides a sensitive measure of factor inhibitors. The distinct advantage of this system is that inhibitory activity is measurable even after factor replacement therapy has been provided. With the ELISA system, samples that contain the inhibitor are applied to wells in which factor VIII has been previously immobilized. Monospecific antisera are then added so that the immunoglobulin class and subclass and light-chain type of the inhibitor can be determined.

ACQUIRED INHIBITORS OF FACTOR VIII

Presentation and Natural History

The estimated incidence of acquired hemophilia is approximately 1.0 per million, although it is likely that not all affected patients are reported.[25,26] Bleeding manifestations are often severe and may occur spontaneously or after minor trauma. In contrast to patients with congenital factor VIII deficiency, in whom intra-articular bleeding is the archetypal manifestation, those with acquired hemophilia principally experience soft tissue bleeding. Clinical features include intramuscular hemorrhage (spontaneous or following minor stress such as an intramuscular injection) and bleeding in the gastrointestinal or urinary tract.[25–30] Retroperitoneal bleeding appears to be especially common and is sometimes fatal.[27,31] Hemorrhage limited to subcutaneous ecchymosis, although frequently dramatic (see Fig. 11-9), can be tolerated without specific therapy in the absence of more serious hemorrhage.

Overall mortality associated with acquired hemophilia has been reported at between 8% and 42%[25,28,32]; most hemorrhagic deaths occur within the first few weeks after presentation. Median age of patients at the time of diagnosis is 60 to 70 years (Fig. 6-2A)—a fact that may underscore, in part, the relatively high rates of morbidity and mortality that are associated with the disorder.[25–31] Acquired inhibitors occur with similar frequency in males and females (see Fig. 6-2B), although the age distribution for females is younger than that for males, likely because of the additional risk of postpartum inhibitors.

Concomitant Conditions

In approximately half of patients with inhibitors, no concomitant disease can be found. In the remainder of patients, the conditions most commonly associated with factor VIII inhibitors include connective tissue disease, inflammatory bowel disease, the puerperium, malignancy, and some dermatologic disorders (see Fig. 6-2C).[25,31]

The development of a postpartum inhibitor to factor VIII is a serious and potentially life-threatening complication of an otherwise normal pregnancy. Symptoms generally appear at term or within 3 months of delivery, and less commonly prior to parturition. If postpartum hemorrhage is the presentation and an acquired factor VIII inhibitor is possible, it is strongly advised that this matter be resolved prior to the performance of surgical or obstetric procedures. Severe vaginal bleeding is extremely common, as are soft tissue and intra-articular hemorrhages.[33] The vast majority of, if not all, postpartum inhibitors ultimately disappear, but this may take up to 2 years, with or without the use of immunosuppressive drugs.[34] Among patients whose inhibitors have abated, reemergence of the inhibitor in subsequent pregnancies appears to be rare. Indeed, some reports have described instances in which the inhibitor disappeared during a subsequent pregnancy.[35,36] Transplacental transfer of the inhibitor can be detected in the newborn and may lead to a severe, albeit transient, bleeding diathesis.[37,38]

Systemic lupus erythematosus (SLE) and rheumatoid arthritis are the most frequently encountered autoimmune disorders associated with factor VIII inhibitor development.[25,39–41] Moreover, several dermatologic conditions with a known autoimmune basis, such as psoriasis and pemphigus vulgaris, are also associated with acquired hemophilia.[25,39] Because these disorders are also associated with the development of antibodies to other coagulation factors and phospholipid-binding proteins (see later), special care must be taken to identify the specificity of the inhibitor in this group of patients.

Factor VIII inhibitors also arise among patients with a variety of solid tumors and hematologic malignancies. Perhaps the first reported case of acquired hemophilia, in 1940, was that of a 61-year-old man who died of hemorrhage after undergoing lymph node excision.[42] In view of the relationship between factor VIII inhibitor formation and altered immune status, it is not surprising that the most common association is with lymphoproliferative disorders.[25,43–47] Factor VIII inhibitors have been detected in association with numerous solid tumors, including neoplasms of the colon, pancreas, kidney, prostate, testes, brain, and lung.[25,29,31,44] As is often true in rare disease associations, it is uncertain whether these reports represent chance occurrences or potentially causative events.[44] For example, the use of radiation therapy or systemic chemotherapy may induce generalized immunologic alterations that predispose to autoantibody formation.

Severe drug reactions, most commonly to penicillin, sulfa antibiotics, chloramphenicol, and phenytoin, have been associated with factor VIII inhibitor formation.[48] It appears likely that alterations in the immunologic state induced by the hypersensitivity reaction, rather than the drug-specific antibody itself, are responsible for development of the inhibitor. Recent viral infections appear to be common among the rare nonhemophilic children who develop acquired inhibitors of coagulation.[49]

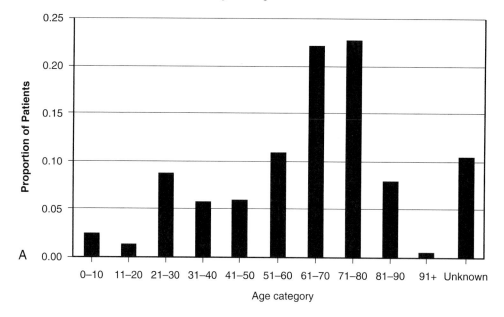

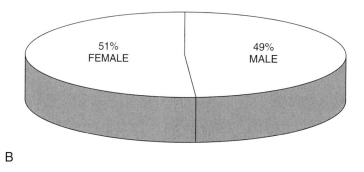

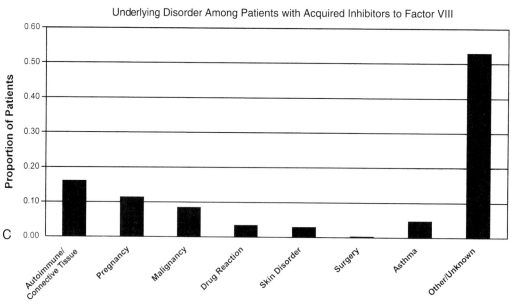

Figure 6-2 Demographics of patients with nonhemophilic inhibitors to factor VIII. **A.** Age distribution. **B.** Sex. **C.** Underlying disorder. In most patients, advanced age is the only identifiable risk factor. See text for references to primary data.

Immunochemistry of Factor VIII Inhibitors

Factor VIII circulates as cation-linked heterodimers in which heterogeneous 92- to 200-kD heavy chains (domains A1, A2, and B) are associated with 80-kD light chains (domains A3, C1, and C2).[50] In plasma, factor VIII is noncovalently bound to von Willebrand factor (VWF), which serves to localize factor VIII to sites of vascular injury and to protect it from inactivation by activated protein C (APC).[51] Activation of factor VIII by thrombin results in its release from VWF and promotion of binding to phospholipid surfaces on the platelet.[52] The VWF and phospholipid binding regions of factor VIII are found on the light chain. Detailed studies in which competitive binding and neutralization assays were used have shown that most factor VIII autoantibodies are directed against the C2 domain and other light-chain sequences.[53–55] Antibodies that recognize the A2 domain of the heavy chain have also been described. Unexpectedly, alloantibodies and autoantibodies bind to similar epitopes on factor VIII, although the pattern of reactivity tends to be simpler in nonhemophilic patients with factor VIII inhibitors.[53,54] Further elucidation of the immunochemical complexity of acquired factor VIII inhibitors ultimately may explain observed differences between laboratory assays and clinical manifestations.[56,57]

Anti–factor VIII antibodies exhibit a number of biochemical characteristics that are relevant to their detection and clinical manifestations. Almost all are high-affinity IgG immunoglobulins of restricted polyclonal origin.[58] A predominance of the IgG$_4$ subclass and of κ and λ light chains can be found with approximately equal frequency. IgG$_4$ antibodies do not fix complement; consequently, patients do not develop renal or vascular complications, even in the presence of endogenous factor VIII. Although the vast majority of inhibitors found in patients with acquired hemophilia are of the IgG class, isolated instances of IgM[47,59] and IgA[46] also have been reported. Progression from a predominantly IgM to an IgG profile was observed on at least one occasion.[60]

Factor VIII inhibitors promote the increased catabolism of factor VIII or interfere with coagulation function through a variety of mechanisms. These include inhibition of the interaction of factor VIII with phospholipid[61] or VWF[58,62] or factor IX,[63] and interference with thrombin-mediated factor VIII activation.[64,65] It is possible that some anti–factor VIII autoantibodies also interfere with VWF or platelet function, thus explaining their propensity to produce mucocutaneous bleeding.

Inactivation of factor VIII by acquired inhibitors is time and temperature dependent.[40] Two types of inactivation patterns are described (see Fig. 6-1).[66,67] Type 1 antibodies, when present in excess, produce complete inactivation of factor VIII, and a linear relationship exists between the concentration of inhibitor and the (logarithm of) residual factor VIII activity. This pattern of inactivation permits accurate measurement of inhibitor potency with the Bethesda assay. In contrast, type 2 antibodies do not produce complete inactivation unless the factor VIII is first dissociated from the VWF with which it is normally complexed.[68]

Patients with acquired hemophilia almost always develop inhibitors that exhibit type 2 inactivation kinetics, and often, residual factor VIII levels may be measured, even while patients are experiencing severe bleeding complications. Factor VIII inhibitors in individuals with congenital hemophilia characteristically exhibit type 1 kinetics. The reason for partial inhibition of factor VIII by type 2 antibodies is unclear but may be related to the target epitope(s) or to the formation of immune complexes.[68,69]

Treatment

When treatment strategies are considered, two objectives must be met: (1) immediate control of bleeding manifestations, if present, and (2) long-term suppression of the inhibitor, if possible. In both instances, one must take into consideration a variety of details, including the severity of the clinical symptoms, the patient's previous history of blood product exposure, the availability of therapeutic products, and the costs associated with treatment.

Management of Acute Bleeding

When possible, optimal management of bleeding is achieved through normalization of the plasma factor VIII level.[70] For patients with low-titer inhibitors (<5 BU), this goal can best be attained through the infusion of exogenous factor VIII in concentrations great enough to overwhelm the inhibitor, so that hemostatic levels of factor VIII are achieved and therapeutic efficacy assured. In the face of high-titer inhibitors (≥5 BU), this approach is not practical, and strategies to bypass the inhibitor are required (Fig. 6-3).

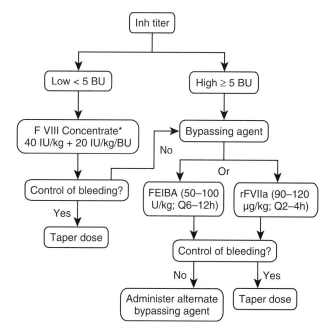

Figure 6-3 Suggested algorithm for the management of patients with nonhemophilic inhibitors to factor VIII who experience a serious bleeding event. Antifibrinolytics (e.g., ε-aminocaproic acid) should not be given concomitantly with FEIBA and should be used with caution in all patients with risk factors for thromboembolic disease. BU, Bethesda units; FEIBA, factor VIII inhibitor bypassing activity; inh, inhibitor; rFVIIa, recombinant activated factor VII.

Hemostatic Agents that "Bypass" the Inhibitor

When the inhibitor titer is high, as is generally the case, strategies to bypass the inhibitor must be used. These strategies consist of infusing activators of the extrinsic or common coagulation pathways, with the effect of generating thrombin in the absence of factor VIII.[71]

Historically, both prothombin complex concentrates (PCC) and activated prothrombin complex concentrates (APCC) have been used extensively to treat patients with factor VIII inhibitors, including those with acquired hemophilia.[72] In the only large, blinded study of the efficacy of PCC and APCC, patients with severe hemophilia, inhibitors, and acute hemarthroses received single doses of each of the two products infused at 50 to 75 U per kilogram; clinical improvement was noted in 52% and 64% of patients, respectively.[73] No comparable study has focused on patients with acquired hemophilia, although the use of APCC in the management of hemophilia A with inhibitors and acquired hemophilia is generally recommended.[74]

At this time, Factor Eight Inhibitor Bypassing Activity (FEIBA VH; Baxter Healthcare, Deerfield, Ill) remains the sole APCC available for general clinical use. The recommended dose of activated concentrate is 50 to 100 U per kilogram; maximum daily dose is 200 U per kilogram.[75] Sallah[76] reported an overall response rate of 86% for this APCC in the management of bleeding episodes in 34 patients with acquired hemophilia. Most received dosing regimens of 75 U per kilogram every 8 to 12 hours. A similar dosing regimen of 70 U per kilogram every 8 hours was successfully used[77] in the treatment of bleeding episodes and minor invasive procedures. FEIBA was similarly administered to 60 patients with factor VIII inhibitors, 6 of whom were given a diagnosis of acquired hemophilia, at an average dose of 70 U per kilogram every 8 to 12 hours.[78] In this series, the effective response rate was reported to be 81%.

The mechanisms by which APCC promotes hemostasis have recently become more fully elucidated. Reconstitution experiments with recombinant proteins showed that a complex of activated FX and prothrombin substantially reproduced the thrombin generating properties of FEIBA.[79] In the current model, other zymogens and activated factors in APCC may further enhance the hemostatic properties of the product.

Despite the proven usefulness of APCC in the treatment of patients with acute bleeding episodes who had inhibitors to factor VIII, these products have some limitations. APCC are derived from plasma, and the infectious risks associated with all plasma-derived products have been dramatically attenuated but cannot be fully eliminated.[80] Further, the absence of laboratory measurements that accurately reflect the pharmacodynamics of the product means that only clinical end points have been generally used to monitor treatment. Even with repeated infusions, a substantial proportion of patients appear to gain little clinical benefit. However, recent reports have suggested that the thrombin generation assay (TGA) may prove useful in assessment of the bioavailability of APCC, resulting in precise dosing adjustments.[81]

APCC has been associated with rare thrombotic events, including disseminated intravascular coagulation (DIC)[82] and myocardial infarction.[83] An incidence of 4 to 8 events per 10^5 infusions has been estimated from pharmacovigilance data.[84,85] Thromboembolic risk appears to be greatest among patients who exceed the recommended daily dose of 200 U per kilogram, and in those with significant other morbidities such as advanced liver or ischemic heart disease.[84] Finally, although the concentrates are often used to avoid exposure to factor VIII and anamnestic immune response, increases in factor VIII inhibitor titers have been reported in a small percentage of patients,[86] most likely resulting from the presence of small quantities of factor VIII in some products.[87] However, in patients with acquired hemophilia, in whom exposure to endogenous factor VIII is ongoing, this risk would appear to be negligible.

Recombinant Activated Factor VII

Recombinant activated human factor VII (rFVIIa; NovoSeven; Novo Nordisk, Denmark) is a procoagulant protein concentrate developed to "bypass" factor VIII or IX inhibitors.[88] Several plausible mechanisms of action have been defined. At physiologic concentrations, the activity of rFVIIa is absolutely dependent on tissue factor (TF), a membrane protein expressed on cellular components of the vascular wall that is exposed only at times of injury. The rFVIIa:TF complex activates factor X to Xa and thus promotes thrombin generation and fibrin formation. In the absence of the intrinsic pathway, tissue factor pathway inhibitor (TFPI) inhibits this activity, and only small amounts of thrombin are generated. Pharmacologic concentrations of rFVIIa may escape this inhibition by competing with zymogen factor VII for binding to TF,[89] or by directly generating Xa, and subsequently thrombin, on the surfaces of activated platelets.[90] The ability to activate factor X in the absence of a functional tenase complex provides a rationale for its use in the management of patients with factor VIII or factor IX inhibitors; its usefulness in treating patients with inhibitors to common pathway factors (V, X, and prothombin) would appear to be less well founded.[91]

Hay and colleagues[32] reported the use of rFVIIa to treat 74 bleeding episodes in 38 patients who participated in a compassionate use program. A median of 28 doses were infused over a median of 3.9 days. The response rate at 24 hours was good in 75% of the 60 bleeds in which rFVIIa was used as salvage therapy; a good response rate was seen in all 14 bleeds in which the drug was employed as first-line therapy. Smaller series have also shown rFVIIa to be effective in most patients with acquired hemophilia when used as salvage therapy.[92,93]

The recommended dose for rFVIIa is 90 µg per kilogram every 2 hours until hemostasis is achieved, or the drug is deemed ineffective. Typically, initial doses of 90 to 120 µg per kilogram every 2 hours have been used with a wide range of subsequent dosages, dosing intervals, and durations. Higher doses have been considered, especially in children with congenital hemophilia and inhibitors, with variable results.[94,95] rFVIIa appears to be more effective when treatment is initiated early, at least in the treatment of acute hemarthrosis.[96,97] Whether this is also true in acquired hemophilia has not been established. The feasibility of using rFVIIa by continuous infusion has also been considered.[98,99]

II

Many of the limitations previously described for the use of APCC also apply to rFVIIa. Laboratory markers that accurately predict clinical efficacy have yet to be developed. The PT shortens to approximately 7 seconds at FVII:C concentrations of approximately 5 U per milliliter, but this level of drug is not hemostatically effective in patients with inhibitors. FVII:C levels can be measured, but these values have been inconsistent with respect to clinical efficacy.

Variability among patients in ability to generate thrombin on activated platelet surfaces may influence the efficacy of rFVIIa, leading to the need for higher dosing and higher plasma levels in some patients.[100] More global tests of hemostasis, such as TGA and thromboelastography (TEG),[81,91] may eventually prove useful. Thromboembolic complications have been reported after the use of rFVIIa, some in patients with acquired hemophilia.[85,101,102] However, concomitant risk factors or the use of PCCs co-existed in most of these situations. It is important to note that antibodies to factor VII or rFVIIa have yet to be observed in infused patients, other than those with congenital factor VII deficiency, after repeated administration of these products.[103]

Factor VIII Replacement Therapy

When the inhibitor titer is low, human factor VIII concentrates may be used. The factor VIII present in intermediate-purity concentrates is complexed with VWF, and it has been proposed that these may be less susceptible to inactivation, especially by antibodies directed against the C2 domain.[104] Most autoantibodies, and some alloantibodies, neutralize porcine-derived factor VIII to a much lesser extent than factor VIII derived from human plasma[105]; however, porcine factor VIII concentrate (Hyate C; Ipsen, Maidenhead, UK) is no longer produced. A recombinant porcine factor VIII is currently undergoing clinical trials but is not yet commercially available.

In treating patients with hemophilia A, the initial dose of factor may be calculated roughly with the following formula: 40 IU factor VIII per kilogram + 20 IU factor VIII per kilogram per BU of inhibitor.[70] However, as was mentioned previously, inhibitor titers among patients with acquired hemophilia are notoriously inaccurate, and post-infusion factor VIII levels should be monitored closely as measured Bethesda titers may not be predictive of response. If the inhibitor titer has not yet been determined, one may consider the use of an empirically determined initial dose of 75 to 100 IU per kilogram.[106] A particularly useful strategy involves the administration of a bolus dose to neutralize the inhibitor, followed by a continuous infusion of factor to achieve hemostatic levels (30 to 50 IU/dL).[106–108] This approach takes advantage of the fact that the kinetics of factor VIII inhibition is time dependent, so that a steady state of uninhibited factor VIII can be achieved. The continuous, albeit low, availability of uncomplexed factor VIII may help to explain observed clinical improvement in response to factor VIII infusion, even among patients in whom increases in plasma factor VIII activity cannot be proved.

DDAVP

Intravenous administration of 1-deamino-8-D-arginine vasopressin (DDAVP [desmopressin]) at a dose of 0.3 μg

per kilogram results in rapid increases in VWF and factor VIII levels in normal individuals.[109] DDAVP may also increase circulating factor VIII sufficiently to treat minor non–life-threatening bleeding in patients with acquired hemophilia.[110–112] Treatment is generally effective in cases in which the inhibitor titer is low and the residual factor VIII level measurable. As might be predicted, DDAVP is associated with tachyphylaxis but does not produce anamnesis to factor VIII.

Transient Reduction in Inhibitor Titers

The treatment of a life-threatening hemorrhage in a patient with a high-titer inhibitor who has not responded to bypass strategies is particularly difficult. In such circumstances, a temporary reduction of the inhibitor titer may be attempted to improve the efficacy of exogenous factor VIII infusions. This can be accomplished through exchange plasmapheresis,[113] with or without extracorporeal immunoadsorption.[114] Because most factor VIII inhibitors are of the IgG class, the extent of reduction in titer is limited by the inability of plasmapheresis to directly access the extravascular space in which IgG is partly distributed. Nevertheless, it may be possible to achieve as much as a 90% reduction in inhibitor titer.[115] Volume replacement usually consists of normal plasma followed by factor VIII infusion, although factor concentrate has also been used in the initial replacement fluid in a preoperative setting. Plasmapheresis cannot be used in patients who are hemodynamically unstable, or in whom vascular access cannot be easily achieved (see Chapter 30).

Extracorporeal reduction in inhibitor titer can be improved dramatically by the addition of an immunoadsorption step.[116] Staphylococcal protein A, which binds with high affinity to the Fc portion of all IgG subclasses except IgG$_3$, provides an effective means of selectively depleting plasma of a variety of autoantibodies and alloantibodies. Because the predominant IgG subclass of factor VIII inhibitors is IgG$_4$, protein A appears to be ideally suited to the treatment of this disorder. For each plasma volume that is immunoadsorbed, plasma level is reduced by approximately 50%; thus, an 80% to 90% reduction in inhibitor titer is possible after three plasma volumes have been processed.[117] After adsorption exchange plasmapheresis has been completed, patients are infused with immune globulin and human or porcine factor VIII. An even more specific immunoadsorption method has been developed in which inhibitor plasma is passed through a column of agarose coupled to monoclonal antihuman IgG$_4$ antibodies.[118] Despite the inherent logic of these approaches and the favorable outcomes reported in small groups of patients, technical difficulties associated with the adsorption columns have prevented their widespread application.

Intravenous Immune Globulin

Intravenous administration of immune globulin (IVIg) (2 g/kg total dose administered in two or five daily fractions) results in at least partial suppression of factor VIII inhibitors in a subset of patients with acquired hemophilia.[6,119,120] In general, the best results are achieved in patients who have low initial antibody titers. The rapid decline in measurable titer that is observed in some patients[119,120] suggests that the success of intravenous IgG may be related to the presence of anti-idiotypic antibodies in plasma pools derived from normal donors.[7,121]

Immunosuppression of Factor VIII Inhibitors

The long-term goal in the treatment of patients with acquired inhibitors of factor VIII is eradication of the autoantibody. Although a small proportion of patients may never require hemostatic treatment, and spontaneous remissions are not uncommon,[27] most patients are likely to develop life- or limb-threatening hemorrhage, and the immediate initiation of immunosuppressive therapy as soon as the diagnosis of acquired hemophilia has been established is recommended.[74]

Once the decision for pharmacologic intervention has been made, the initial choice is most often between glucocorticoid alone[122] and glucocorticoids in combination with azathioprine or cyclophosphamide.[123] In a large, multicenter, retrospective study, clinical response was documented in 78 of 145 patients (54%) who received immunosuppression with one or more of these drugs, whereas only 11 of 39 (28%) patients improved without specific treatment.[25] In the only prospective, randomized study on the subject, patients were treated initially with prednisone alone at a dose of 1 mg per kilogram daily for 3 weeks.[124] If antibody continued to be detectable, patients were randomly assigned to receive additional prednisone, prednisone with oral cyclophosphamide (2 mg/kg/day), or cyclophosphamide alone. Approximately one third of patients responded to the initial prednisone course; approximately 50% of steroid-resistant patients responded to the cyclophosphamide-containing regimens. The combination of prednisone (50 to 80 mg/day) and oral cyclophosphamide (100 to 200 mg/day) was similarly effective in other small series of patients.[125,126] A prospective study reported a 91% response rate in 12 patients treated with repeated cycles of factor VIII concentrate, cyclophosphamide, vincristine, and prednisone, although none of the 11 good responders had initial antibody titers greater than 50 BU.[127] More favorable responses were also noted among patients with low-titer inhibitors in other studies.[122,124] It has been proposed that the addition of factor VIII to the regimen enhances responsiveness to immunosuppressive agents,[127] although this assertion has been disputed.[125] Cyclosporine may be useful for patients who are unresponsive to these agents.[98]

Recently, rituximab, a monoclonal antibody directed against CD20 antigen on B lymphocytes,[128] has been successfully used in the treatment of patients with acquired hemophilia. This drug is currently approved for use in non-Hodgkin's lymphoma (NHL), but it has proved effective in many autoimmune disorders.[129] Wiestner and colleagues[130–132] described eight patients with acquired hemophilia, including two with titers over 200 BU, who responded to rituximab with or without other immunosuppressive agents. Rapid and complete remission was achieved in 8 of 10 patients with rituximab alone. Patients who relapsed after cessation of the drug, could be successfully retreated with the previous regimen of rituximab. It is important to note that responses to rituximab have been observed after failure was observed with prednisone and/or other immunosuppressive regimens.[133] Typically, the dosing regimen was adopted from that used to treat patients with NHL—375 mg per meter squared intravenously given once weekly in 4-week cycles. Fever and rigors were observed in most patients. Serious infections and adverse immunologic reactions due to the development of anti-rituximab antibodies have each been reported in a small percentage of treated patients.

Immune tolerance induction (ITI) is a possibility for the eradication of alloantibodies that one may encounter as a complication in the management of patients with hemophilia A. This approach is discussed in Chapter 4.

INHIBITORS OF VITAMIN K–DEPENDENT PROTEINS

Inhibitors of Prothrombin and Thrombin

Antiprothrombin and antiphosphotidylserine/prothrombin antibodies are commonly detected as "lupus anticoagulants" in patients with SLE and have been described in a large proportion of patients in whom antiphospholipid syndrome has been diagnosed.[134–136] In this setting, their presence has been associated with increased thromboembolic risk.[136,137] Antiprothombin antibodies may also produce a reduction in the level of prothrombin sufficient to produce clinical bleeding.[138,139] Antithrombin antibodies are also commonly seen after exposure to bovine thrombin preparations in association with anti–factor V antibodies, in which they may be detected only as a laboratory abnormality or may contribute to the bleeding diathesis (see later).[140,141] Case reports, at least one with a fatal outcome, have described patients in whom antibodies against thrombin arose in the setting of autoimmune disease or liver cirrhosis.[142,143] In the laboratory, one observes prolonged PT, PTT, and thrombin time, which are not corrected in mixing studies.

The mechanisms by which antiprothrombin antibodies exert their influence are heterogeneous. Some hamper prothrombin activation by coagulation factors Xa and Va and thus behave in vitro as acquired phospholipid-dependent inhibitors.[134] In many instances, antibodies are directed against nonfunctional epitopes on prothrombin (e.g., fragment 1); they thus promote accelerated clearance of the coagulation factor from the circulation but are not detectable in mixing studies.[144] Nonneutralizing antiprothrombin antibodies have also been described in a patient without evidence of a lupus anticoagulant.[145] In one instance, an autoantibody was described that aberrantly activated prothrombin, thereby permitting subsequent neutralization by antithrombin III. The prothrombin molecule was not cleaved to thrombin and remained unable to convert fibrinogen to fibrin, resulting in a significant bleeding diathesis.[146]

Therapeutic benefit in patients with acquired antiprothrombin and antithrombin antibodies has been shown after therapy with prednisone,[145] danazol,[147] and high-dose immunoglobulin.[148,149] rFVIIa was successfully used to provide immediate hemostatic coverage in a patient with acquired hypothrombinemia who required a minor surgical procedure.[139]

Inhibitors of Factor IX

Inhibitors of factor IX arise in approximately 3% of patients with congenital factor IX deficiency after exposure to exogenous sources of the coagulation protein.[150] Factor IX inhibitors have also been reported in nonhemophilic patients in association with systemic autoimmune disorders.[151,152] In general, factor IX inhibitors are polyclonal immunoglobulins of the IgG class,[153] although at least one case of a factor IX inhibitor produced by monoclonal gammopathy has been reported.[154] In the laboratory, factor IX inhibitors are first detected by the failure of normal plasma to correct the PTT in mixing studies; these times may be quantified through modification of the Bethesda assay.[18] However, different from the behavior of most factor VIII antibodies in vitro, anti–factor IX antibodies induce an immediate loss of factor IX activity that does not require prolonged incubation.[151]

Inhibitors of Factor X

Acquired factor X deficiency occurs in approximately 5% of patients with systemic amyloid disease.[155] In contrast to other acquired factor deficiencies, the bleeding diathesis in this instance arises not from a circulating inhibitor, but from adsorption of factor X on the amyloid fibrils, particularly in the spleen.[156] Bleeding into soft tissues is often severe.[155] Replacement therapy with factor X, with the use of fresh frozen plasma or factor IX complex concentrates, is often only partially effective because of the shortened half-life of the infused factor. Splenectomy may produce a rapid improvement in factor X levels caused by the physical removal of amyloid binding sites.[157] Chemotherapy drugs, such as melphalan and prednisone, may further limit amyloid deposition.[158] rFVIIa was reported to be effective in achieving immediate hemostasis in a bleeding patient.[159]

INHIBITORS OF FACTOR XI

Factor XI is one of the contact phase coagulation factors; it displays both procoagulant (through direct action on factor IX) and antifibrinolytic (through activation of thrombin-activated fibrinolysis inhibitor [TAFI]) activities.[160] Factor XI inhibitors have been observed rarely among patients with congenital factor XI deficiency who have been exposed to exogenous factor XI.[161] Factor XI antibodies are also seen in association with a variety of autoimmune disorders, principally SLE.[162] Acquired factor XI deficiency has been observed rarely in association with a number of malignancies, particularly those of hematologic origin.[163,164] Many older reports of factor XI antibodies among patients with SLE and thrombosis are likely to be misdiagnosed lupus anticoagulants.[165] Bleeding manifestations in this setting appear to be decidedly uncommon.

The laboratory diagnosis of factor XI inhibitors is usually made on discovery of a prolonged PTT, normal PT, normal thrombin time, and lack of correction in mixing studies. Specific factor assays performed at progressive plasma dilutions yield a persistently low factor XI level, with normalization of remaining factors, although factor XII levels may remain falsely low unless sufficient dilutions of patient plasma are prepared.

Although patients with congenital factor XI deficiency who develop inhibitors usually do not develop spontaneous hemorrhage, perioperative bleeding has been reported to be severe.[161,166] Because titers of factor XI inhibitors

are generally low, adequate replacement therapy with fresh frozen plasma can sometimes be provided. Alternatively, factor IX complex concentrates, their active forms, or rFVIIa may be effective in achieving hemostasis.[88,167] High-dose prednisone, 60 to 80 mg per day, is often effective in suppressing the inhibitor.[162]

INHIBITORS OF FACTOR V

Numerous reports have described factor V inhibitors arising in individuals without a prior history of abnormal hemostasis. Approximately 20% of cases are idiopathic, but the most common associations involve recent surgery, drug exposure (aminoglycosides, β-lactam antibiotics), autoimmune disorders, and pregnancy.[168] Of these, the occurrence of factor V inhibitors after topical bovine thrombin preparations that contain bovine factor V have been administered is the best described and most important.[169,170] An immune response to bovine protein generates antibodies that cross-react with endogenous human factor V. Most of the inhibitors are composed of polyclonal IgG, although instances have been reported of IgG in association with IgM[171] or IgA.[172] Interference with the interaction between the C2 domains of factor Va and phospholipid was demonstrated in the analysis of one such inhibitor, and hemorrhagic manifestations appear to correlate well with the degree of inhibition of the prothrombinase complex.[173]

Factor V inhibitors initially are detected during routine laboratory evaluation by the prolongation of PT and PTT, both of which fail to correct on mixing with normal plasma. As in the case of lupus anticoagulants, the RVVT is prolonged, but factor V inhibitors can be distinguished from the latter by their failure to correct in the presence of excess phospholipid and by specific factor assays performed on progressive dilutions of patient plasma.

Clinical manifestations in the setting of factor V inhibitors are highly variable. Bleeding, which is seen in the great majority of cases, is typically severe and frequently fatal.[168,170,174,175] Mucocutaneous bleeding and bleeding at the surgical site are the most commonly observed events. In the postoperative setting, factor V inhibitors are first observed approximately 7 to 10 days after surgery and may intensify with repeated exposure to bovine preparations. In general, the titer of the inhibitor correlates with clinical severity. However, in some instances, little if any clinical bleeding is observed, even in postsurgical settings, despite overtly abnormal in vitro laboratory findings.[176]

Most factor V inhibitors that arise in association with bovine protein exposure appear to be of short duration, usually disappearing within 8 to 10 weeks; they can be managed expectantly in the absence of bleeding manifestations. Factor V inhibitors associated with other risk factors typically persist for significantly longer periods, and immunosuppressive therapy is usually warranted. Glucocorticoids, cyclophosphamide, and other regimens that contain these agents have been successful in the treatment of 65% to 74% of patients.[170,177] Immunomodulation with IVIg has also proved generally successful in some settings.[141] In many instances, exposure to bovine protein can be avoided by the use of a commercial fibrin sealant that contains virus-inactivated human fibrinogen, factor XIII, and thrombin.[178]

The management of acute bleeding with acquired factor V inhibitors can be especially challenging. Because these inhibitors interfere with prothrombinase complex formation, replacement therapy with fresh frozen plasma or the use of "bypassing agents" such as APCC or rFVIIa is likely to be of limited value.[168] Platelet transfusion, with response rates of 30% to 40%, appears to be an especially useful means of "bypassing" the inhibitor in that transfused factor V is stored in the intracellular α granules and becomes accessible to the inhibitor only after platelet activation has occurred.[177] Replacement therapy may become transiently feasible after rapid reduction in antibody titer achieved through the use of plasmapheresis or immunoadsorption.[179]

INHIBITORS OF FIBRINOGEN AND FACTOR XIII

Thrombin-mediated conversion of fibrinogen to fibrin, formation of a fibrin mesh, and crosslinking of the α and γ chains of fibrin by factor XIIIa make up the final steps in blood coagulation.[180] Rare inhibitors of factor XIII, some specifically characterized as immunoglobulins, have been reported in congenitally deficient patients who have received exogenous factor XIII, as well as in previously normal individuals. In the case of spontaneously acquired inhibitors, prior exposure to isoniazid[181] or procainamide[182] has also been implicated in the pathogenesis. It is known that isoniazid can be incorporated into protein by factor XIIIa, although the relationship of this action to inhibitor formation remains unclear.[183]

Inhibitors of factor XIII, principally immunoglobulins, act through a variety of molecular mechanisms to produce functional derangement. These include inhibition of thrombin activation, transamidase activity and fibrin crosslinking, and inhibition of factor XIIIa binding to fibrin.[182,184] In some cases, the antibody may exert the same effects by reacting with the crosslinking site on the fibrin substrate.[185] Other antibodies, both polyclonal and monoclonal, have been described that inhibit the conversion of fibrinogen to fibrin.[186,187] Generally, these antibodies can be detected in the laboratory by their effects on fibrin clot stability in dissociating agents such as 5M urea (urea clot solubility test).[182]

Clinically, patients with acquired defects in fibrin crosslinking often present with massive, and sometimes fatal, spontaneous hemorrhaging. These patients exhibit high-titer inhibitors and are not easily treated by factor XIII replacement therapy. In one reported case, resolution of an acute bleeding episode was achieved after plasma immunoadsorption was accomplished with staphylococcal protein A.[188] Fortunately, in many cases, the inhibitors regress spontaneously over time or in response to immunosuppressive agents such as cyclophosphamide.[189] Administration of a factor XIII concentrate can sometimes be sufficient to overwhelm the inhibitor and achieve transient hemostasis.[190]

INHIBITORS OF VON WILLEBRAND FACTOR

von Willebrand factor (VWF) is large, multimeric glycoprotein with two principal functions. It forms an essential bridge between platelets (via platelet glycoprotein-Ib-IX)

and subendothelial components (e.g., collagen) at sites of vascular injury, and it serves as a carrier protein for circulating factor VIII.[191] Acquired von Willebrand syndrome (AVWS), a collection of acquired disorders that resemble congenital forms of von Willebrand disease (VWD), is described in association with numerous other diseases.[192,193] Most common among these are lymphoproliferative disorders, monoclonal gammopathies, autoimmune diseases, and myeloproliferative disorders.[194-197] AVWS is also seen in association with acquired or congenital heart disease[198] and with Wilms tumor in the pediatric setting.[199] Several pathogenic mechanisms are described: adsorption of VWF, particularly high molecular weight forms, by tumor cells; loss of larger VWF multimers in the high–shear stress environment of an abnormal vasculature and specific or nonspecific binding of VWF to circulating immunoglobulins.[200,201] Most often, the latter represent true autoantibodies; less frequently, the paraprotein itself may be the offending agent. AVWS is also seen in some patients with hypothyroidism as a result of decreased synthesis and/or release of the VWF protein.[202]

In the laboratory, factor VIII, VWF antigen, and VWF ristocetin cofactor activity are reduced, although not always to the same extent (see Chapter 7). The absence of the largest multimeric forms of VWF and the decreased ratio of VWF activity to antigen, a pattern resembling congenital type 2A VWD, is frequently seen in cases caused by protein absorption. Among autoantibodies to VWF, approximately 15% inhibit function (e.g., VWF binding to platelet glycoprotein Ib) and therefore can be shown in mixing studies based on the VWF:RCo assay. Noninhibitory antibodies, which promote the accelerated clearance of factor VIII/VWF complexes, can be detected only with immunoassays that are available in research laboratories.[192]

The clinical manifestations of AVWS resemble those of congenital VWD (spontaneous mucocutaneous bleeding and postsurgical hemorrhage) and should be considered in all patients with recent onset of such symptoms in the absence of a personal or family history of VWD.[203] Bleeding from angiodysplastic lesions in the gastrointestinal tract is particularly common and often serious.[204] Overall, patients with autoantibodies to VWF are more severely affected than are those individuals with other forms of the disease.[205] Treatment of the underlying disease through surgical or medical means often leads to improvement in the bleeding diathesis associated with AVWS.[199,206] AVWS associated with SLE is typically responsive to glucocorticoids, and reduction in autoantibody titer and correction of laboratory parameters can often be accomplished with IVIg therapy in patients with monoclonal gammopathy.[192,193,204,207,208] Particularly in instances of non–immune-mediated AVWS, transient correction of factor VIII and VWF activity levels and favorable hemostatic responses may be achieved with DDAVP or VWF/factor VIII concentrates.[209-211] Patients with refractory AVWS have been successfully treated with rFVIIa.[212]

FINAL CONSIDERATIONS

The acquired disorders of coagulation described in this chapter are only infrequently encountered in general medical practice but are characteristically challenging to diagnose and costly to manage. Once considered, specialized laboratory evaluation is invariably required and consultation with a specialist with expertise in hemostasis is strongly advised. Often these conditions present as but one manifestation of other serious medical disorders and close and ongoing collaboration between the hematology consultant and referring physician is essential. A systematic approach to treatment, in the context of the frequently observed co-morbidities, is likely to lead to improvements in both the medical outcome and resource utilization.

REFERENCES

1. Algiman M, Dietrich G, Nydegger UE, et al: Natural antibodies to factor VIII (anti-hemophilic factor) in healthy individuals. Proc Natl Acad Sci U S A 89:3795–3799, 1992.
2. Gilles JG, Saint-Remy JM: Healthy subjects produce both anti-factor VIII and specific anti-idiotypic antibodies. J Clin Invest 94:1496–1505, 1994.
3. Reding MT, Wu H, Krampf M, et al: CD4+ T cell response to factor VIII in hemophilia A, acquired hemophilia, and healthy subjects. Thromb Haemost 82:509–515, 1999.
4. Reding MT, Wu H, Krampf M, et al: Sensitization of CD4+ T cells to coagulation factor VIII: Response in congenital and acquired hemophilia patients and in healthy subjects. Thromb Haemost 84:643–652, 2000.
5. Jerne NK: Towards a network theory of the immune system. Ann Immunol (Paris) 125C:373–389, 1994.
6. Sultan Y, Kazatchkine MD, Maisonneuve P, Nydegger UE: Anti-idiotypic suppression of autoantibodies to factor VIII (antihaemophilic factor) by high-dose intravenous gammaglobulin. Lancet 2:765–768, 1984.
7. Rossi F, Dietrich G, Kazatchkine MD: Anti-idiotypes against autoantibodies in normal immunoglobulins: Evidence for network regulation of human autoimmune responses. Immunol Rev 110:135–149, 1989.
8. Moffat EH, Furlong RA, Dannatt AHG, et al: Anti-idiotypes to factor VIII antibodies and their possible role in the pathogenesis and treatment of factor VIII inhibitors. Br J Haematol 71:85–90, 1989.
9. Lossing TS, Kasper CK, Feinstein DI: Detection of factor VIII inhibitors with the partial thromboplastin time. Blood 495:797, 1977.
10. Biggs R, Bidwell E: A method for the study of antihaemophilic globulin inhibitors with reference to six cases. Br J Haematol 5:379–395, 1959.
11. Goldsmith JC: Diagnosis of factor VIII versus nonspecific inhibitors. Semin Hematol 30:6, 1993.
12. Brandt JT, Barna LK, Triplett DA: On behalf of the Subcommittee on Lupus Anticoagulants/Antiphospholipid Antibodies of the ISTH: Laboratory identification of lupus anticoagulants: Results of the Second International Workshop for Identification of Lupus Anticoagulants. Thromb Haemost 74:1597–1603, 1995.
13. Thiagarajan P, Pengo V, Shapiro SS: The use of the dilute Russell viper venom time for the diagnosis of lupus anticoagulants. Blood 68:869–874, 1986.
14. Triplett DA, Barna LK, Unger GA: A hexagonal (II) phase phospholipid neutralization assay for lupus anticoagulant identification. Thromb Haemost 70:787–793, 1993.
15. Triplett DA, Brandt JT, Musgrave KA, Orr CA: The relationship between lupus anticoagulants and antibodies to phospholipid. JAMA 259:550–554, 1988.
16. Saxena R, Dhot PS, Saraya AK, et al: Simultaneous occurrence of factor VIIIC inhibitor and lupus anticoagulant. Am J Hematol 42:232–233, 1993.
17. Triplett DA: Simultaneous occurrence of lupus anticoagulant and factor VIII inhibitors. Am J Hematol 56:195–196, 1997.
18. Kasper CK: Blood—its derivatives and its problems—factor IX. Ann N Y Acad Sci 240:180, 1975.
19. Triplett DA: New methods in coagulation. Crit Rev Clin Lab Sci 15:25–84, 1981.
20. Verbruggen B, Novakova I, Wessels H, et al: The Nijmegen modification of the Bethesda assay for factor VIII:C inhibitors: Improved specificity and reliability. Thromb Haemost 73:247–251, 1995.
21. Ewing NP, Kasper CK: In vitro detection of mild inhibitors to factor VIII in hemophilia. Am J Clin Pathol 77:749–752, 1982.
22. Coots MC, Glueck HI, Miller MA: Agarose gel method: Its usefulness in assaying factor VIII inhibitors, evaluating treatment and suggesting a mechanism of action for factor IX concentrates. Br J Haematol 60:735–750, 1985.
23. Sanchez-Curenca JM, Carmona E, Villanueva MJ, Aznar JA: Immunological characterization of factor VIII inhibitors by a sensitive micro-ELISA method. Thromb Res 57:897–908, 1990.
24. Nilsson IM, Berntorp E, Zettervall O, Dahlback B: Noncoagulation inhibitory factor VIII antibodies after induction of tolerance to factor VIII in hemophilia A patients. Blood 75:378–383, 1990.
25. Green D, Lechner K: A survey of 215 non-hemophilic patients with inhibitors to factor VIII. Thromb Haemost 45:200–203, 1981.
26. Hoyer LW: Factor VIII inhibitors: A continuing problem [editorial]. J Lab Clin Med 121:385–387, 1993.
27. Lottenberg R, Kentro TB, Kitchens CS: Acquired hemophilia: A natural history study of 16 patients with factor VIII inhibitors receiving little or no therapy. Arch Intern Med 147:1077–1081, 1987.
28. Kessler CM, Ludlam CA, for the International Acquired Hemophilia Study Group: The treatment of acquired factor VIII inhibitors: Worldwide experience with porcine factor VIII concentrate. Semin Hematol 30:22–27, 1993.
29. Di Bona E, Schiavoni M, Castaman G, et al: Acquired haemophilia: Experience of two Italian centres with 17 new cases. Haemophilia 3:183–188, 1997.
30. Bossi P, Cabane J, Ninet J, et al: Acquired hemophilia due to factor VIII inhibitors in 34 patients. Am J Med 105:400–408, 1998.
31. Morrison AE, Ludlam CA, Kessler C: Use of porcine factor VIII in the treatment of patients with acquired hemophilia. Blood 81:1513–1520, 1993.
32. Hay CR, Negrier C, Ludlam CA: The treatment of bleeding in acquired haemophilia with recombinant factor VIIa: A multicentre study. Thromb Haemost 78:1463–1467, 1997.
33. Solymoss S: Postpartum acquired factor VIII inhibitors: Results of a survey. Am J Hematol 59:1–4, 1998.
34. Hauser I, Schneider B, Lechner K: Post-partum factor VIII inhibitors: A review of the literature with special reference to the value of steroid and immunosuppressive treatment. Thromb Haemost 73:1–5, 1995.
35. Voke J, Letsky E: Pregnancy and antibody to factor VIII. J Clin Pathol 30:928–932, 1977.
36. Coller BS, Hultin MB, Hoyer LW, et al: Normal pregnancy in a patient with a prior postpartum factor VIII inhibitor: With observations on pathogenesis and prognosis. Blood 58:619–624, 1981.
37. Vicente V, Alberca I, Gonzalez R, Alegre A: Normal pregnancy in a patient with a postpartum factor VIII inhibitor. Am J Hematol 24:107–109, 1987.
38. Ries M, Wolfel D, Maier-Brandt B: Severe intracranial hemorrhage in a newborn infant with transplacental transfer of an acquired factor VII:C inhibitor. J Pediatr 127:649–650, 1995.
39. Margolius A Jr, Jackson DP, Ratnoff OD: Circulating anticoagulants: A study of 40 cases and a review of the literature. Medicine (Baltimore) 40:145–202, 1961.
40. Shapiro SS, Hultin M: Acquired inhibitors to the blood coagulation factors. Semin Thromb Hemost 1:336–385, 1975.
41. Soriano RM, Matthews JM, Guerado-Parra E: Acquired haemophilia and rheumatoid arthritis. Br J Rheumatol 26:381–383, 1987.
42. Lozner EL, Joliffe LS, Taylor FHL: Haemorrhagic diathesis with prolonged coagulation time associated with a circulating anticoagulant. Am J Med Sci 199:318–383, 1940.
43. Kelsey PR, Leyland MJ: Acquired inhibitor to human factor VIII associated with paraproteinaemia and subsequent development of chronic lymphatic leukaemia. BMJ (Clin Res Ed) 285:174–175, 1982.
44. Hultin MB: Acquired inhibitors in malignant and nonmalignant disease states. Am J Med 91:9S–13S, 1991.
45. Sallah S, Nguyen NP, Abdallah JM, Hanrahan LR: Acquired hemophilia in patients with hematologic malignancies. Arch Pathol Lab Med 124:730–734, 2000.
46. Glueck HI, Hong R: A circulating anticoagulant in gamma-1A-multiple myeloma: Its modification by penicillin. J Clin Invest 44:1866–1881, 1965.
47. Castaldi PA, Penny R: A macroglobulin with inhibitory activity against coagulation factor VIII. Blood 35:370–376, 1970.
48. Green D: Cytotoxic suppression of acquired factor VIII:C inhibitors. Am J Med 91:14S–19S, 1991.
49. Brodeur GM, O'Neill PJ, Williams JA: Acquired inhibitors of coagulation in nonhemophiliac children. J Pediatr 96:439–441, 1980.

50. Kaufman RJ, Wasley LC, Dorner AJ: Synthesis, processing, and secretion of recombinant human factor VIII expressed in mammalian cells. J Biol Chem 263:6352–6362, 1988.

51. Koedam JA, Meijers JC, Sixma JJ, Bouma BN: Inactivation of human factor VIII by activated protein C: Cofactor activity of protein S and protective effect of von Willebrand factor. J Clin Invest 82:1236–1243, 1988.

52. Hill-Eubanks DC, Parker CG, Lollar P: Differential proteolytic activation of factor VIII–von Willebrand factor complex by thrombin. Proc Natl Acad Sci U S A 86:6508–6512, 1989.

53. Scandella D, Mattingly M, de Graaf S, Fulcher CA: Localization of epitopes for human factor VIII inhibitor antibodies by immunoblotting and antibody neutralization. Blood 74:1618–1626, 1989.

54. Prescott R, Nakai H, Saenko EL, et al: The inhibitor antibody response is more complex in hemophilia A patients than in most nonhemophiliacs with factor VIII autoantibodies. Recombinate and Kogenate Study Groups. Blood 89:3663–3671, 1997.

55. Nogami K, Shima M, Giddings JC, et al: Circulating factor VIII immune complexes in patients with type 2 acquired hemophilia A and protection from activated protein C–mediated proteolysis. Blood 97:669–677, 2001.

56. Collins P, Macartney N, Davies R, et al: A population based, unselected, consecutive cohort of patients with acquired haemophilia A. Br J Haematol 124:86–90, 2004.

57. Yee TT, Taher A, Pasi KJ, Lee CA: A survey of patients with acquired haemophilia in a haemophilia centre over a 28-year period. Clin Lab Haematol 22:275–278, 2000.

58. Hoyer LW, Gawryl MS, de la Fuente B: Immunochemical characterization of factor VIII inhibitors. Prog Clin Biol Res 150:73–85, 1984.

59. Tiarks C, Pechet L, Humphreys RE: Development of anti-idiotypic antibodies in a patient with a factor VIII autoantibody. Am J Hematol 32:217–221, 1989.

60. Marengo-Rowe AJ, Murff G, Leveson JE, Cook J: Hemophilia-like disease associated with pregnancy. Obstet Gynecol 40:56–64, 1972.

61. Arai M, Scandella D, Hoyer LW: Molecular basis of factor VIII inhibition by human antibodies: Antibodies that bind to the factor VIII light chain prevent the interaction of factor VIII with phospholipid. J Clin Invest 83:1978–1984, 1989.

62. Shima M, Nakai H, Scandella D, et al: Common inhibitory effects of human anti-C2 domain inhibitor alloantibodies on factor VIII binding to von Willebrand factor. Br J Haematol 91:714–721, 1995.

63. Fulcher CA: Immunochemistry of factor VIII:C inhibitor antibodies. Am J Med 91:6S–8S, 1991.

64. Lazarchick J, Ashby MA, Lazarchick JJ, Sens DA: Mechanism of factor VIII inactivation by human antibodies. IV. Antibody binding prevents factor VIII proteolysis by thrombin. Ann Clin Lab Sci 16:497–501, 1986.

65. Saenko EL, Shima M, Gilbert GE, Scandella D: Slowed release of thrombin-cleaved factor VIII from von Willebrand factor by a monoclonal and a human antibody is a novel mechanism for factor VIII inhibition. J Biol Chem 271:27424–27431, 1996.

66. Biggs R, Austen DE, Denson KW, et al: The mode of action of antibodies which destroy factor VIII. I. Antibodies which have second-order concentration graphs. Br J Haematol 23:125–135, 1972.

67. Biggs R, Austen DE, Denson KW, et al: The mode of action of antibodies which destroy factor VIII. II. Antibodies which give complex concentration graphs. Br J Haematol 23:137–155, 1972.

68. Gawryl MS, Hoyer LW: Inactivation of factor VIII coagulant activity by two different types of human antibodies. Blood 60:1103–1109, 1982.

69. Nogami K, Shima M, Hosokawa K, et al: Factor VIII C2 domain contains the thrombin-binding site responsible for thrombin-catalyzed cleavage at Arg1689. J Biol Chem 275:25774–25780, 2000.

70. Kasper CK: Treatment of factor VIII inhibitors. Prog Hemost Thromb 9:57–86, 1989.

71. Sultan Y, Loyer F: In vitro evaluation of factor VIII–bypassing activity of activated prothrombin complex concentrate, prothrombin complex concentrate, and factor VIIa in the plasma of patients with factor VIII inhibitors: Thrombin generation test in the presence of collagen-activated platelets. J Lab Clin Med 121:444–452, 1993.

72. Delgado J, Jimenez-Yuste V, Hernandez-Navarro F, Villar A: Acquired haemophilia: Review and meta-analysis focused on therapy and prognostic factors. Br J Haematol 121:21–35, 2003.

73. Lusher JM, Blatt PM, Penner JA, et al: Autoplex versus proplex: A controlled, double-blind study of effectiveness in acute hemarthroses in hemophiliacs with inhibitors to factor VIII. Blood 62:1135–1138, 1986.

74. Hay CR, Brown S, Collins PW, et al: The diagnosis and management of factor VIII and IX inhibitors: A guideline from the United Kingdom Haemophilia Centre Doctors Organisation. Br J Haematol 133:591–605, 2006.

75. Baxter Healthcare: FEIBA VH Anti-Inhibitor Coagulant Complex Vapor Heated [package insert]. Deerfield, Ill, Baxter Healthcare, 2004.

76. Sallah S: Treatment of acquired haemophilia with factor eight inhibitor bypassing activity. Haemophilia 10:169–173, 2004.

77. Holme PA, Brosstad F, Tjonnfjord GE: Acquired haemophilia: Management of bleeds and immune therapy to eradicate autoantibodies. Haemophilia 11:510–515, 2005.

78. Negrier C, Goudemand J, Sultan Y, et al: Multicenter retrospective study on the utilization of FEIBA in France in patients with factor VIII and factor IX inhibitors: Factor eight bypassing activity. French FEIBA Study Group. Thromb Haemost 77:1113–1119, 1997.

79. Turecek PL, Varadi K, Gritsch H, Schwarz HP: FEIBA: Mode of action. Haemophilia 10:3–9, 2004.

80. Luu H, Ewenstein B: FEIBA safety profile in multiple modes of clinical and home-therapy application. Haemophilia 10:10–16, 2004.

81. Varadi K, Turecek PL, Schwarz HP: Thrombin generation assay and other universal tests for monitoring haemophilia therapy. Haemophilia 10:17–21, 2004.

82. Rodeghiero F, Castronovo S, Dini E: Disseminated intravascular coagulation after infusion of FEIBA (factor VIII inhibitor bypassing activity) in a patient with acquired haemophilia. Thromb Haemost 48:339–340, 1982.

83. Sullivan DW, Purdy LJ, Billingham M, Glader BE: Fatal myocardial infarction following therapy with prothrombin complex concentrates in a young man with hemophilia A. Pediatrics 74:279–281, 1984.

84. Ehrlich HJ, Henzl MJ, Gomperts ED: Safety of factor VIII inhibitor bypass activity (FEIBA®): 10-Year compilation of thrombotic adverse events. Haemophilia 8:83–90, 2002.

85. Aledort LM: Comparative thrombotic event incidence after infusion of recombinant factor VIIa versus factor VIII inhibitor bypass activity. J Thromb Haemost 2:1700–1708, 2004.

86. Laurian Y, Girma JP, Lambert T, et al: Incidence of immune responses following 102 infusions of autoplex in 18 hemophilic patients with antibody to factor VIII. Blood 63:457–462, 1984.

87. Onder O, Hoyer LW: Factor VIII coagulant antigen in factor IX complex. Thromb Res 15:569–572, 1979.

88. Hedner U, Glazer S, Falch J: Recombinant activated factor VII in the treatment of bleeding episodes in patients with inherited and acquired bleeding disorders. Transfus Med Rev 7:78–83, 1993.

89. van't Veer C, Golden NJ, Mann KG: Inhibition of thrombin generation by the zymogen factor VII: Implications for the treatment of hemophilia A by factor VIIa. Blood 95:1330–1335, 2000.

90. Gabriel DA, Li X, Monroe DM III, Roberts HR: Recombinant human factor VIIa (rFVIIa) can activate factor FIX on activated platelets. J Thromb Haemost 2:1816–1822, 2004.

91. Sorensen B, Ingerslev J: Whole blood clot formation phenotype in hemophilia A and rare coagulation disorders: Patterns of response to recombinant factor VIIa. Thromb Haemost 2:102–110, 2003.

92. Scharrer I: Recombinant factor VIIa for patients with inhibitors to factor VIII or IX or factor VII deficiency. Haemophilia 5:253–259, 1999.

93. Arkin S, Blei F, Fetten J, et al: Human coagulation factor FVIIa (recombinant) in the management of limb-threatening bleeds unresponsive to alternative therapies: Results from the NovoSeven emergency-use programme in patients with severe haemophilia or with acquired inhibitors. Blood Coagul Fibrinolysis 11:255–259, 2000.

94. Kenet G, Lubetsky A, Luboshitz J, Martinowitz U: A new approach to treatment of bleeding episodes in young hemophilia patients: A single bolus megadose of recombinant activated factor VII (NovoSeven). J Thromb Haemost 1:450–455, 2003.

95. Santagostino E, Mancuso ME, Rocino A, et al: A prospective randomized trial of high and standard dosages of recombinant factor VIIa for treatment of hemarthroses in hemophiliacs with inhibitors. J Thromb Haemost 4:367–371, 2006.

96. Santagostino E, Gringeri A, Mannucci PM: Home treatment with recombinant activated factor VII in patients with factor VIII inhibitors: The advantages of early intervention. Br J Haematol 104:22–26, 1999.

97. Lusher JM: Acute hemarthroses: The benefits of early versus late treatment with recombinant activated factor VII. Blood Coagul Fibrinolysis 11 (suppl 1): S45–S49, 2000.

98. Schulman S, Bech Jensen M, Varon D, et al: Feasibility of using recombinant factor VIIa in continuous infusion. Thromb Haemost 75:432–436, 1996.

99. Mauser-Bunschoten E, de Goede-Bolder A, Wielenga J, et al: Continious infusion of recombinant factor VIIa in patients with haemophilia and inhibitors. N Engl J Med 53:249–255, 1998.

100. Hedner U: Dosing with recombinant factor VIIA based on current evidence. Semin Hematol 41:35–39, 2004.

101. Abshire T, Kenet G: Recombinant factor VIIa: Review of efficacy, dosing regimens, and safety in patients with congenital and acquired factor VIII or IX inhibitors. J Thromb Haemost 2:899–909, 2004.

102. O'Connell KA, Wood JJ, Wise RP, et al: Thromboembolic adverse events after use of recombinant human coagulation factor VIIa. JAMA 295:293–298, 2006.

103. Nicolaisen EM: Antigenicity of activated recombinant factor VII followed through nine years of clinical experience. Blood Coagul Fibrinolysis 9:S119–S123, 1998.

104. Suzuki T, Arai M, Amano K, et al: Factor VIII inhibitor antibodies with c2 domain specificity are less inhibitory to factor VIII complexed with von Willebrand factor. Thromb Haemost 76:749–754, 1996.

105. Shulman NR, Hirschman RJ: Acquired hemophilia. Trans Assoc Am Physicians 82:397, 1969.

106. Rubinger M, Rivard GE, Teitel J, Walker H: Inhibitor Subcommittee of the Association of Hemophilia Clinic Directors of Canada: Suggestions for the management of factor VIII inhibitors. Haemophilia 6 (suppl 1): 52–59, 2000.

107. Bona RD, Riberio M, Klatsky AU, et al: Continuous infusion of porcine factor VIII for the treatment of patients with factor inhibitors. Semin Hematol 30:32–35, 1993.

108. Rubinger M, Houston DS, Schwetz N, et al: Continuous infusion of porcine factor VIII in the management of patients with factor VIII inhibitors. Am J Hematol 56:112–118, 1997.

109. Mannucci PM: Desmopressin (DDAVP) in the treatment of bleeding disorders: The first 20 years. Blood 90:2515–2521, 1970.

110. de la Fuente B, Kasper CK, Rickles FR, Hoyer LW: Response of patients with mild and moderate hemophilia A and von Willebrand's disease to treatment with desmopressin. Ann Intern Med 103:6–14, 1985.

111. Chistolini A, Ghirardini A, Tirindelli MC, et al: Inhibitor to factor VIII in a non-haemophilic patient: Evaluation of the response to DDAVP and the in vitro kinetics of factor VIII. A case report. Nouv Rev Fr Hematol 29:221–224, 1987.

112. Mudad R, Kane WH: DDAVP in acquired hemophilia A: Case report and review of the literature. Am J Hematol 43:295–299, 1993.

113. Cobcroft R, Tamagnini G, Dormandy KM: Serial plasmapheresis in a haemophiliac with antibodies to FVIII. J Clin Pathol 30:763–765, 1977.

114. Gjorstrup P, Watt RM: Therapeutic protein A immunoadsorption: A review. Transfus Sci 11:281–302, 1990.

115. Slocombe GW, Newland AC, Colvin MP, Colvin BT: The role of intensive plasma exchange in the prevention and management of haemorrhage in patients with inhibitors to factor VIII. Br J Haematol 47:577–585, 1981.

116. Nilsson IM, Sundqvist SB, Freiburghaus C: Extracorporeal protein A–sepharose and specific affinity chromatography for removal of antibodies. Prog Clin Biol Res 150:225–241, 1984.

117. Gjorstrup P, Berntorp E, Larsson L, Nilsson IM: Kinetic aspects of the removal of IgG and inhibitors in hemophiliacs using protein A immunoadsorption. Vox Sang 61:244–250, 1991.

118. Regnault V, Rivat C, Vallet JP, et al: A potential new procedure for removing anti–factor VIII antibodies from hemophilic plasma. Thromb Res 45:51–57, 1984.

119. Sultan Y, Kazatchkine MD, Nydegger U, et al: Intravenous immunoglobulin in the treatment of spontaneously acquired factor VIII:C inhibitors. Am J Med 91:35S–39S, 1991.

120. Schwartz RS, Gabriel DA, Aledort LM, et al: A prospective study of treatment of acquired (autoimmune) factor VIII inhibitors with high-dose intravenous gammaglobulin. Blood 86:797–804, 1995.

121. Dietrich G, Algiman M, Sultan Y, et al: Origin of anti-idiotypic activity against anti–factor VIII autoantibodies in pools of normal human immunoglobulin G (IVIg). Blood 79:2946–2951, 1992.

122. Spero JA, Lewis JH, Hasiba U: Corticosteroids therapy for acquired F VIII:C inhibitors. Br J Haematol 48:635–642, 1981.

123. Green D: Suppression of an antibody to factor VIII by a combination of factor VIII and cyclophosphamide. Blood 37:381–387, 1971.

124. Green D: Immunosuppression of factor VIII inhibitors in nonhemophilic patients. Semin Hematol 30:28–31, 1993.

125. Shaffer LG, Phillips MD: Successful treatment of acquired hemophilia with oral immunosuppressive therapy. Ann Intern Med 127:206–209, 1997.

126. Bayer RL, Lichtman SM, Allen SL, et al: Acquired factor VIII inhibitors: Successful treatment with an oral outpatient regimen. Am J Hematol 60:70–71, 1990.

127. Lian EC, Larcada AF, Chiu AY: Combination immunosuppressive therapy after factor VIII infusion for acquired factor VIII inhibitor. Ann Intern Med 110:774–778, 1989.

128. Gopal AK, Press OW: Clinical applications of anti-CD20 antibodies. J Lab Clin Med 134:445–450, 1999.

129. George JN, Woodson RD, Kiss JE, et al: Rituximab therapy for thrombotic thrombocytopenic purpura: A proposed study of the Transfusion Medicine/Hemostasis Clinical Trials Network with a systematic review of rituximab therapy for immune-mediated disorders. J Clin Apher 21:49–56, 2006.

130. Wiestner A, Cho HJ, Asch AS, et al: Rituximab in the treatment of acquired factor VIII inhibitors. Blood 100:3426–3428, 2002.

131. Aggarwal A, Grewing R, Green RJ, et al: Rituximab for autoimmune haemophilia: A proposed treatment algorithm. Haemophilia 11:13–19, 2005.

132. Stasi R, Brunetto M, Stipa E, Amadori S: Selective B-cell depletion with rituximab for the treatment of patients with acquired hemophilia. Blood 103:4424–4428, 2004.

133. Abdallah A, Coghlan DW, Duncan EM, et al: Rituximab-induced long-term remission in patients with refractory acquired hemophilia. J Thromb Haemost 3:2589–2590, 2005.

134. Galli M, Barbui T: Antiprothrombin antibodies: Detection and clinical significance in the antiphospholipid syndrome. Blood 93: 2149–2157, 1999.

135. Horbach DA, van Oort E, Derksen RH, de Groot PG: The contribution of anti-prothrombin antibodies to lupus anticoagulant activity—discrimination between functional and non-functional anti-prothrombin antibodies. Thromb Haemost 79:790–795, 1998.

136. Bertolaccini ML, Atsumi T, Koike T, et al: Antiprothrombin antibodies detected in two different assay systems: Prevalence and clinical significance in systemic lupus erythematosus. Thromb Haemost 93:289–297, 2005.

137. Horbach DA, van Oort E, Donders RC, et al: Lupus anticoagulant is the strongest risk factor for both venous and arterial thrombosis in patients with systemic lupus erythematosus: Comparison between different assays for the detection of antiphospholipid antibodies. Thromb Haemost 78:967–968, 1996.

138. Fleck RA, Rapaport SI, Rao LVM: Anti-prothrombin antibodies and the lupus anticoagulant. Blood 2:512, 1988.

139. Holm M, Andreasen RB, Ingerslev J: Management of bleeding using recombinant factor VIIa in a patient suffering from bleeding tendency due to a lupus anticoagulant–hypoprothrombinemia syndrome. Thromb Haemost 82:1776–1778, 1999.

140. Sie P, Bezeaud A, Dupouy D, et al: An acquired antithrombin autoantibody directed toward the catalytic center of the enzyme. J Clin Invest 88:290–296, 1991.

141. Tarantino MD, Ross MP, Daniels TM, et al: Modulation of an acquired coagulation factor V inhibitor with intravenous immune globulin. J Pediatr Hematol Oncol 19:226–231, 1997.

142. La Spada AR, Skalhegg BS, Henderson R, et al: Brief report: Fatal hemorrhage in a patient with an acquired inhibitor of human thrombin. N Engl J Med 333:494–497, 1995.

143. Barthels M, Heimburger N: Acquired thrombin inhibitor in a patient with liver cirrhosis. Haemostasis 15:395–401, 1985.

144. Bajaj SP, Rapaport SI, Fierer J: A mechanism for the hypoprothrombinemia of the acquired hypoprothrombinemia–lupus anticoagulant syndrome. Blood 82:1776–1778, 1983.

145. Bajaj SP, Rapaport SI, Barclay S, Herbst KD: Acquired hypoprothrombinemia due to non-neutralizing antibodies to prothrombin: Mechanism and management. Blood 65:1538–1543, 1985.

146. Madoiwa S, Nakamura Y, Mimuro J, et al: Autoantibody against prothrombin aberrantly alters the proenzyme to facilitate formation of a complex with its physiological inhibitor antithrombin III without thrombin conversion. Blood 97:3783–3789, 2001.

147. Williams S, Linardic C, Wilson O, et al: Acquired hypoprothrombinemia: Effects of danazol treatment. Am J Hematol 53:272–276, 1996.

148. Pernod G, Arvieux J, Carpentier PH, et al: Successful treatment of lupus anticoagulant–hypoprothrombinemia syndrome using intravenous immunoglobulins. Thromb Haemost 78:969–970, 1997.

149. Barbui T, Finazzi G, Falanga A, Cortelazzo S: Intravenous gammaglobulin, antiphospholipid antibodies, and thrombocytopenia. Lancet 2:969, 1988.

150. Briet E, Reisner HM, Roberts HR: Inhibitors in Christmas disease. Prog Clin Biol Res 150:123–139, 1984.

151. Lechner K: Factor IX inhibitors: Report of two cases and a study of the biological, chemical and immunological properties of the inhibitors. Thromb Haemost 25:447–459, 1971.

152. Largo R, Sigg P, von Felton A, Straub PW: Acquired factor-IX inhibitor in a nonhaemophilic patient with autoimmune disease. Br J Haematol 26:129–140, 1974.

153. Reisner HM, Roberts HR, Krumholz S, Yount WJ: Immunochemical characterization of a polyclonal human antibody to factor IX. Blood 50:11–19, 1977.

154. Pike IM, Yount WJ, Puritz E, Roberts HR: Immunochemical characterization of a monoclonal G4 lambda human antibody to factor IX. Blood 40:1–10, 1972.

155. Gertz MA, Lacy MQ, Dispenzieri A: Amyloidosis: Recognition, confirmation, prognosis, and therapy. Proc Natl Acad Sci U S A 74:490–494, 1999.

156. Furie B, Voo L, McAdam KP, Furie BC: Mechanism of factor X deficiency in systemic amyloidosis. N Engl J Med 304:827–830, 1981.

157. Greipp PR, Kyle RA, Bowie EJ: Factor X deficiency in primary amyloidosis: Resolution after splenectomy. N Engl J Med 301:1050–1051, 1979.

158. Camoriano JK, Greipp PR, Bayer GK, Bowie EJ: Resolution of acquired factor X deficiency and amyloidosis with melphalan and prednisone therapy. N Engl J Med 316:1133–1135, 1987.

159. Boggio L, Green D: Recombinant human factor VIIa in the management of amyloid-associated factor X deficiency. Br J Haematol 12:1074–1075, 2001.

160. Minnema MC, Ten CH, Hack CE: The role of factor XI in coagulation: A matter of revision. Semin Thromb Hemost 25:419–428, 1999.

161. Schnall SF, Duffy TP, Clyne LP: Acquired factor XI inhibitors in congenitally deficient patients. Am J Hematol 26:323–328, 1987.

162. Reece EA, Clyne LP, Romero R, Hobbins JC: Spontaneous factor XI inhibitors: Seven additional cases and a review of the literature. Arch Intern Med 144:525–529, 1984.

163. Goodrick MJ, Prentice AG, Copplestone JA, et al: Acquired factor XI inhibitor in chronic lymphocytic leukaemia. J Clin Pathol 45:352–353, 1992.

164. Billon S, Blouch MT, Escoffre-Barbe M, et al: A case of chronic myelomonocytic leukaemia and factor XI deficiency with a circulating anticoagulant. Haemophilia 7:433–436, 2001.

165. Triplett DA, Brandt JT, Maas RL: The laboratory heterogeneity of lupus anticoagulants. Arch Pathol Lab Med 109:946–951, 1985.

166. Morgan K, Schiffman S, Feinstein D: Acquired factor XI inhibitors in two patients with hereditary factor XI deficiency. Thromb Haemost 51:371–375, 1984.

167. Rolovic Z, Elezovic I, Obrenovic B, Rizza C: Life-threatening bleeding due to an acquired inhibitor to factor XII-XI successfully treated with "activated" prothrombin complex concentrate (FEIBA). Br J Haematol 51:659, 1982.

168. Knobl P, Lechner K: Acquired factor V inhibitors. Baillieres Clin Haematol 11:305–318, 1998.

169. Zehnder JL, Leung LL: Development of antibodies to thrombin and factor V with recurrent bleeding in a patient exposed to topical bovine thrombin. Blood 76:2011–2016, 1990.

170. Streiff MB, Ness PM: Acquired FV inhibitors: A needless iatrogenic complication of bovine thrombin exposure. Transfusion 42:18–26, 2002.

171. Crowell EB Jr: Observations on a factor-V inhibitor. Br J Haematol 29:397–404, 1975.

172. Lane TA, Shapiro SS, Burka ER: Factor V antibody and disseminated intravascular coagulation. Ann Intern Med 89:182–185, 1978.

173. Ortel TL, Quinn-Allen MA, Charles LA, et al: Characterization of an acquired inhibitor to coagulation factor V: Antibody binding to the second C-type domain of factor V inhibits the binding of factor V to phosphatidylserine and neutralizes procoagulant activity. J Clin Invest 90:2340–2347, 1992.

174. Coots MC, Muhleman AF, Glueck HI: Hemorrhagic death associated with a high titer factor V inhibitor. Am J Hematol 4:193–206, 1978.

175. Ortel TL, Charles LA, Keller FG, et al: Topical thrombin and acquired coagulation factor inhibitors: Clinical spectrum and laboratory diagnosis. Am J Hematol 45:128–135, 1994.

176. Nesheim ME, Nichols WL, Cole TL, et al: Isolation and study of an acquired inhibitor of human coagulation factor V. J Clin Invest 77:406–415, 1986.

177. Chediak J, Ashenhurst JB, Garlick I, Desser RK: Successful management of bleeding in a patient with factor V inhibitor by platelet transfusions. Blood 56:835–841, 1980.

178. Alving BM, Weinstein JS, Finlayson JS, et al: Fibrin sealant: Summary of a conference on characteristics and clinical uses. Transfusion 35:783–790, 1995.

179. Tribl B, Knobl P, Derfler K, et al: Rapid elimination of a high-titer spontaneous factor V antibody by extracorporeal antibody-based immunoadsorption and immunosuppression. Ann Hematol 71:199–203, 1995.

180. McDonagh RP Jr, McDonagh J, Duckert F: The influence of fibrin cross-linking on the kinetics of urokinase-induced clot lysis. Br J Haematol 21:323–332, 1971.

181. Otis PT, Feinstein DI, Rapaport SI, Patch MJ: An acquired inhibitor of fibrin stabilization associated with isoniazid therapy: Clinical and biochemical observations. Blood 44:771–781, 1974.

182. Fukue H, Anderson K, McPhedran P, et al: A unique factor XIII inhibitor to a fibrin-binding site on factor XIIIA. Blood 79:65–74, 1992.

183. Lorand L, Campbell LK, Robertson BJ: Enzymatic coupling of isoniazid to proteins. Biochemistry 11:434–438, 1972.

184. Lopaciuk S, Bykowska K, McDonagh JM, et al: Difference between type I autoimmune inhibitors of fibrin stabilization in two patients with severe hemorrhagic disorder. J Clin Invest 61:1196–1203, 1978.

185. Rosenberg RD, Colman RW, Lorand L: A new haemorrhagic disorder with defective fibrin stabilization and cryofibrinogenaemia. Br J Haematol 26:269–284, 1974.

186. Coleman M, Vigliano EM, Weksler ME, Nachman RL: Inhibition of fibrin monomer polymerization by lambda myeloma globulins. Blood 39:210–223, 1972.

187. Marciniak E, Greenwood MF: Acquired coagulation inhibitor delaying fibrinopeptide release. Blood 53:81–92, 1979.

188. Gailani D: An IgG inhibitor against coagulation factor XIII: Resolution of bleeding after plasma immunoadsorption with staphylococcal protein A. Am J Med 92:110–112, 1992.

189. Nakamura S, Kato A, Sakata Y, Aoki N: Bleeding tendency caused by IgG inhibitor to factor XIII, treated successfully by cyclophosphamide. Br J Haematol 68:313–319, 1988.

190. Daly HM, Carson PJ, Smith JK: Intracerebral haemorrhage due to acquired factor XIII inhibitor—successful response to factor XIII concentrate. Blood Coagul Fibrinolysis 2:507–514, 1991.

191. Sadler JE: von Willebrand factor. J Biol Chem 266:22777–22780, 1991.

192. Veyradier A, Jenkins CS, Fressinaud E, Meyer D: Acquired von Willebrand syndrome: From pathophysiology to management. Thromb Haemost 84:175–182, 2000.

193. Tefferi A, Nichols WL: Acquired von Willebrand disease: Concise review of occurrence, diagnosis, pathogenesis, and treatment. Am J Med 103:536–540, 1997.

194. Mannucci PM, Lombardi R, Bader R, et al: Studies of the pathophysiology of acquired von Willebrand's disease in seven patients with lymphoproliferative disorders or benign monoclonal gammopathies. Blood 64:614–621, 1984.

195. Richard C, Cuadrado MA, Prieto M, et al: Acquired von Willebrand disease in multiple myeloma secondary to absorption of von Willebrand factor by plasma cells. Am J Hematol 35:114–117, 1990.

196. Simone JV, Cornet AJ, Abildgaard CF: Acquired von Willebrand's syndrome in systemic lupus erythematosus. Blood 6:806–812, 1968.

197. Carter C, Boughton BJ: Acquired von Willebrand's disease in myeloproliferative syndrome: Spontaneous remission during pregnancy. Thromb Haemost 67:387–388, 1992.

198. Warkentin TE, Moore JC, Morgan DG: Aortic stenosis and bleeding gastrointestinal angiodysplasia: Is acquired von Willebrand's disease the link? Lancet 340:35–37, 1992.

199. Scott JP, Montgomery RR, Tubergen DG, Hays T: Acquired von Willebrand's disease in association with Wilm's tumor: Regression following treatment. Blood 58:665–669, 1981.

200. Nitu-Whalley IC, Lee CA: Acquired von Willebrand syndrome: Report of 10 cases and review of the literature. Haemophilia 5:318–326, 1999.

201. Federici AB, Rand JH, Bucciarelli P, et al: Acquired von Willebrand syndrome: Data from an international registry. Subcommittee on von Willebrand Factor. Thromb Haemost 84:345–349, 2000.

202. Dalton RG, Dewar MS, Savidge GF, et al: Hypothyroidism as a cause of acquired von Willebrand's disease. Lancet 1:1007–1009, 1987.

II

203. Laffan M, Brown SA, Collins PW, et al: The diagnosis of von Willebrand disease: A guideline from the UK Haemophilia Centre Doctors' Organization. Haemophilia 10:199–217, 2004.

204. Fressinaud E, Meyer D: International survey of patients with von Willebrand disease and angiodysplasia. Thromb Haemost 70:527–528, 1993.

205. Mohri H, Motomura S, Kanamori H, et al: Clinical significance of inhibitors in acquired von Willebrand syndrome. Blood 91: 3623–3629, 1998.

206. Anderson RP, McGrath K, Street A: Reversal of aortic stenosis, bleeding gastrointestinal angiodysplasia, and von Willebrand syndrome by aortic valve replacement. Lancet 347:689–690, 1996.

207. Macik BG, Gabriel DA, White GC II, et al: The use of high-dose intravenous gamma-globulin in acquired von Willebrand syndrome. Arch Pathol Lab Med 112:143–146, 1988.

208. Michiels JJ, Berneman Z, Gadisseur A, et al: Immune-mediated etiology of acquired von Willebrand syndrome in systemic lupus erythematosus and in benign monoclonal gammopathy: Therapeutic implications. Semin Thromb Hemost 32:577–588, 2006.

209. Castaman G, Rodeghiero F, Di Bona E, Ruggeri M: Clinical effectiveness of desmopressin in a case of acquired von Willebrand's syndrome associated with benign monoclonal gammopathy. Blut 58:211–213, 1989.

210. Meyer D, Frommel D, Larrieu MJ, Zimmerman TS: Selective absence of large forms of factor VIII/von Willebrand factor in acquired von Willebrand's syndrome: Response to transfusion. Blood 54:600–606, 1979.

211. Morris ES, Hampton KK, Nesbitt IM, et al: The management of von Willebrand's disease–associated gastrointestinal angiodysplasia. Blood Coagul Fibrinolysis 12:143–148, 2001.

212. Meijer K, Peters FT, van der Meer J: Recurrent severe bleeding from gastrointestinal angiodysplasia in a patient with von Willebrand's disease, controlled with recombinant factor VIIa. Blood Coagul Fibrinolysis 12:211–213, 2001.

6

Chapter 7

von Willebrand Disease

Margaret E. Rick, MD

INTRODUCTION

von Willebrand disease (VWD), which is transmitted in an autosomal dominant fashion, is the most common of the inherited bleeding disorders. It is caused by a decrease in the quantity of circulating von Willebrand factor (VWF) or by a qualitatively abnormal VWF in the circulation. VWD also may rarely present as an acquired disorder. Patients come to medical attention because of skin and mucosal bleeding symptoms such as epistaxis, gum bleeding, or hemorrhage from other mucosal surfaces; symptoms may be so mild that they are not recognized by the patient and are discovered only during testing that occurs because another family member has VWD. Diagnosis depends on laboratory tests that measure the VWF antigen, VWF activity (ristocetin cofactor and/or collagen-binding activity), and factor VIII activity; classification of the type of VWD (types 1–3) depends on additional assays, including the VWF multimer assay and ristocetin-induced platelet aggregation (RIPA) studies. It is important to classify the type of VWD because VWD type influences choice of therapy. The treatment of choice in most cases is desmopressin, which releases synthesized VWF and factor VIII from body storage sites, transiently increasing their levels. Treatment of more severe VWD includes replacement therapy with plasma-derived concentrates of VWF. Other topical and antifibrinolytic therapy modalities are also used as adjuncts.

VWD is an inherited autosomal dominant bleeding disorder that is found in approximately 1% of the population when random laboratory screening is carried out.[1] Only a fraction of these individuals is symptomatic, however, and most have mild or moderate manifestations that do not significantly affect daily living activities. Estimates derived from patients attending hemostasis treatment centers indicate that the number of patients with symptomatic VWD is 23 to 110 per million; this estimate predicts that approximately 580,000 patients worldwide are at risk for bleeding from VWD.[2] Easy bruising, epistaxis, and oral bleeding with dental procedures are often the primary symptoms. In most cases, the bleeding results from decreased VWF-mediated binding of platelets to the vascular subendothelium and decreased VWF-mediated platelet–platelet interactions that occur in areas of high shear (arterial circulation).[3]

Biochemical and physiologic information about VWF has enhanced our understanding of the functions of this molecule and has allowed clarification of the terminology for its activities. VWF was originally believed to be a part of the same protein as coagulation factor VIII because these molecules circulate in plasma as a complex, the VWF acting as a carrier for factor VIII; VWF was called "factor VIII–related antigen" until the 1980s. (The current terminology and definitions are presented in Table 7-1.) Genetic information promoted the development of a new classification of VWD,[4,4a] and this is important not only for an understanding of the structure–function relationships of the protein, but also for the selection of optimal therapy for patients.

HISTORICAL OVERVIEW

Erik von Willebrand described the first patient with VWD in 1926, when he cared for a young patient and her extended family who lived on the Åland Islands in the Gulf of Bothnia. The proband was severely affected and died at the age of 13 years, when she had uncontrollable menstrual bleeding; 4 of her 11 siblings were also severely affected. After evaluating 66 other family members and identifying the disease in 24, von Willebrand recognized that the inheritance pattern of this disease was autosomal dominant, different from that seen in hemophilia A (which is sex-linked recessive), and he named the disorder "hereditary pseudohemophilia." He also recognized that patients' platelet counts were normal, and that this disease was different from the other inherited bleeding disorders known at that time.[5]

When the laboratory test for factor VIII was developed in the 1950s, it was shown that patients with VWD had decreased levels of factor VIII activity,[6] and that the bleeding could be corrected with transfusion of plasma or partially purified preparations of factor VIII.[7] Considerable debate focused on the nature of the von Willebrand protein until factor VIII and VWF were cloned in the 1980s[8–11]; before this, there was uncertainty about whether one bifunctional protein or two different proteins carried out the platelet-related functions (VWF) and the task of promoting fibrin formation (factor VIII). We now know that these are two entirely different molecules encoded by different genes, and that factor VIII is bound to VWF, forming a noncovalent complex in the circulation that prolongs factor VIII survival.[12,13]

PHYSIOLOGY AND STRUCTURE– FUNCTION RELATIONSHIPS

VWF has two primary functions (Table 7-2): It binds to both platelets and subendothelial structures, acting as a

Table 7-1 Nomenclature

Designation	Function	Assay
von Willebrand factor (VWF)	Multimeric glycoprotein that promotes platelet adhesion and aggregation and is a carrier for factor VIII in plasma	See below
von Willebrand factor activity (VWF:RCo)	Binding activity of VWF that causes binding of VWF to platelets in the presence of ristocetin with consequent agglutination	Ristocetin cofactor activity: Quantitate platelet agglutination after addition of ristocetin and VWF
	Ability of VWF to bind to collagen	Collagen-binding activity: Quantitate binding of VWF to collagen-coated plates (ELISA format)
von Willebrand factor antigen (VWF:Ag)	VWF protein as measured by protein assays; does not imply functional ability	Immunologic assays such as ELISA, RIA, Laurell electroimmunoassay
von Willebrand factor multimers	Size distribution and analysis of VWF multimers as assessed by agarose gel electrophoresis	VWF multimer assay: Electrophoresis in low-concentration agarose gel and visualization by monospecific antibody to VWF
Factor VIII (FVIII)	Circulating coagulation protein that is protected from clearance by VWF and is important in thrombin generation	Factor VIII activity: Plasma clotting test based on PTT assay using FVIII-deficient substrate; quantitates activity
Ristocetin-induced platelet aggregation (RIPA)	Test that measures the ability of patient VWF to bind to platelets in the presence of various concentrations of ristocetin	RIPA: Aggregation of patient PRP using various (low) concentrations of ristocetin

ELISA, enzyme-linked immunosorbent assay; RIA, radioimmunoassay; PTT, partial thromboplastin time; PRP, platelet-rich plasma.

Table 7-2 Functions of von Willebrand Factor

Platelet–Subendothelium Binding

von Willebrand factor (VWF) binds to platelet receptor glycoprotein Ib (GP-Ib) and to subendothelial collagen and other matrix molecules, binding platelets to damaged vessel.

Platelet–Platelet Binding

VWF binds to platelet receptor GP-Ib in areas with high shear (arterial circulation) and binds platelets together, causing platelet aggregation.

Carrier for Factor VIII in Plasma

VWF binds to factor VIII by a site in the aminoterminus of VWF, protecting factor VIII from proteolysis and prolonging its half-life.

bridging molecule for initial reactions during primary hemostasis,[3] and it binds factor VIII, averting proteolysis of factor VIII in the circulation.[14,15] VWF is a huge multimeric glycoprotein that is synthesized in endothelial cells and megakaryocytes.[16,17] The largest multimers are created by the polymerization of subunits that all contain the same binding sites (Fig. 7-1); these repeated binding sites make VWF particularly well suited to act as a bridge between cells and other structures of the vasculature. Synthesis of VWF includes the initial formation of a dimer between the basic subunits and subsequent multimerization of the dimers to form multimers of a magnitude greater than 20 million daltons. The newly synthesized VWF is secreted constitutively or is targeted to storage granules such as the Weibel-Palade bodies in endothelial cells or α granules in megakaryocytes.[18] These storage granules contain the larger, more hemostatic forms of VWF that are released upon stimulation with agonists such as thrombin, epinephrine, and fibrin.[19–21] The VWF within storage granules contains newly synthesized, even larger multimers than are usually found in the circulation. Limited proteolysis occurs in plasma and targets especially these very large prothrombotic multimers[18]; the protease, ADAMTS13 (a disintegrin and metalloproteinase with thrombospondin subunits), has been shown to be responsible for this cleavage.[22–24] Other evidence suggests that another protein, thrombospondin-1, may also reduce the size of these unusually large multimers by acting as a protein disulfide reductase.[25]

Also contained within the storage granules and released upon stimulation is a propolypeptide, von Willebrand antigen II, which contains a large sequence of the originally synthesized VWF that is cleaved near the time that multimerization takes place (see Fig. 7-1).[18]

The gene for VWF is located on chromosome 12, and a number of polymorphisms and mutations have been identified in the gene sequence, the latter most often in patients with qualitative defects of VWF (type 2 VWD) (reviewed in detail by Nichols and Ginsburg[26]). Many of the mutations responsible for type 2 VWD are located in areas of the gene that are responsible for the structure of important binding sites or cleavage sites in VWF (see Fig. 7-1). The genetic abnormalities responsible for many patients with VWD have not been identified. In type 1, approximately 50% to 65% of kindreds have recognized mutations accounting for their disease.[27,28,28a,28b]

A website that contains information on reported mutations and polymorphisms is administered by the University of Sheffield in the United Kingdom (http://www.shef.ac.uk/vwf/).

Platelet-Related Functions of von Willebrand Factor

VWF circulates in a tangled coil configuration,[29] enclosing some of the subunits and binding sites; the molecule likely

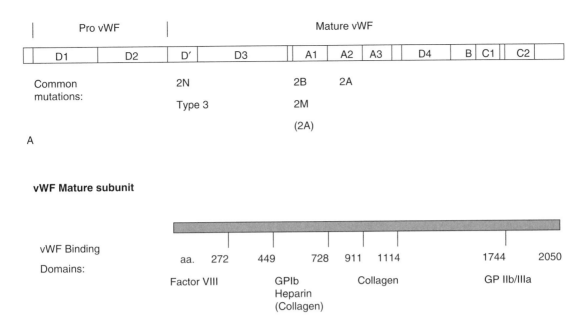

vWF mRNA

Figure 7-1 A, Von Willebrand factor (VWF) mRNA is shown, with domain designations noted inside the figure. Various types of VWD are shown in the areas where mutations that result in a particular type of VWD are most commonly found. **B,** The mature VWF subunit, aligned with the mRNA above, is depicted with amino acid numbering and binding sites shown below. (From Rose BD [ed]: UpToDate. Wellesley, MA, 2001. Copyright 2001 UpToDate, Inc.)

assumes a more linear configuration upon binding to a surface or when flowing through high-shear vessels in the arterial circulation.[30] The linear form allows the binding sites on many more of the subunits to become accessible for binding to receptors such as platelet glycoprotein Ib (GP-Ib)[31] and to subendothelial collagen, one of the important vascular cell molecules that binds VWF.[32] The binding of VWF to these ligands results in the tethering (adhesion) of platelets to the subendothelium in damaged blood vessels and in platelet–platelet interaction (aggregation) in high-shear vessels via a VWF bridge. The binding of VWF to platelet GP-Ib does not require prior activation of platelets and, in fact, such binding initiates intrinsic platelet activation.[33] VWF contains a second binding site for another platelet receptor, platelet glycoprotein IIb/IIIa (GP-IIb/IIIa), and this binding requires prior activation of platelets for exposure of the receptor. It is important in the later, irreversible binding of platelets to the subendothelium.[34] Other binding sites for heparin and sulfatides are also present in the VWF monomer.[35,36]

Factor VIII–Related Functions of von Willebrand Factor

VWF contains a binding site for factor VIII that protects factor VIII from proteolysis in the circulation.[14] This non-covalent interaction of VWF with factor VIII prolongs the half-life of factor VIII in the circulation by fivefold.[15] In addition to the platelet interactions described earlier, the binding and protection of factor VIII are other important functions of VWF. As one might anticipate, a defect in this part of the VWF molecule leads to a bleeding disorder in which one finds a decreased level of circulating factor VIII owing to its rapid clearance; the VWF-mediated platelet functions of VWD, however, are normal (see later, type 2 Normandy).

von Willebrand Factor Levels in Health and Disease

In addition to a broad normal range of VWF in plasma (≈30 IU/dL to 200 IU/dL), physiologic and pathologic conditions may alter the level of VWF in the circulation. Estrogen and thyroid hormone are important in regulating the synthesis of VWF,[37,38] and a low level of thyroid hormone can lead to clinically important decreases in VWF.[39] Levels of VWF are at their baseline in women during the follicular phase of their menstrual cycle, and despite considerable day-to-day variation, they are generally higher during the late luteal phase.[40] During the second and third trimesters of pregnancy, VWF increases by two- to threefold, often leading to "normal" levels of VWF in patients with mild VWD; VWF levels may fall within hours after delivery.[41] As an acute phase reactant, VWF (and factor VIII) levels are increased during the physiologic changes that occur with inflammation.[42] An important variation occurs in the level of VWF in subjects with different blood groups: Individuals with type O blood have circulating levels of VWF that are approximately 30 IU/dL lower than in those with type A, B, or AB.[43] The latter must be taken into account when one attempts to make a definitive diagnosis of VWD in a patient who presents with "slightly low" laboratory values for VWF (see Pitfalls in Making the Diagnosis of VWD, later).

The role of VWF in atherogenesis and coronary artery syndromes is still being defined. Although markedly decreased levels of VWF play a protective role in preventing the development of coronary atherosclerosis in an animal model with type 3 VWD, it has not yet been proved that extremely low VWF levels reduce atherosclerosis in humans.[44,45] However, studies of animals with more moderate (heterozygous) VWD and a few autopsy studies in humans with type 2 or type 3 VWD have shown that reduced VWF levels can prevent occlusive thrombi in atherosclerotic vessels.[46,47]

CLINICAL PRESENTATION

Patients with moderate and severe VWD present with bleeding symptoms in childhood or young adulthood; however, patients may present at any age because of the wide spectrum in the severity of bleeding symptoms. Males and females are equally affected, and most patients (with type 1 and some with type 2) have minimal, mild, or moderate disease. Because one of the primary functions of VWF is to support normal platelet function, the bleeding manifestations in patients with VWD are similar to those observed in platelet disorders—bruising and mucous membrane bleeding such as epistaxis, oral bleeding, menorrhagia, and gastrointestinal bleeding.[48] Patients may come to attention as a result of postsurgical bleeding, particularly that involving mucous membrane surfaces (e.g., tooth extractions, tonsillectomy) or the onset of menses. The most serious bleeding is generally gastrointestinal hemorrhage, and it can be life-threatening, particularly when it is associated with angiodysplasia.[49] The rare homozygous or doubly heterozygous (type 3) patients are severely affected and have low factor VIII levels (2 IU/dL to 10 IU/dL) associated with extremely low VWF levels; they have severe bleeding, which includes hemarthroses and soft tissue bleeding similar to the symptoms seen in hemophiliacs, in addition to platelet-related bleeding symptoms. Homozygotes most likely represent the cases originally described by von Willebrand.

The severity of bleeding can vary modestly among affected family members and, to a much lesser degree, within an individual patient. Recent evidence suggests that normal variation (polymorphisms) in the level of other "unrelated" components of hemostasis (e.g., the platelet collagen receptor) may affect the degree of bleeding in patients with mild VWD.[50] As mentioned earlier, levels of VWF (and hence bleeding tendency) also vary with inflammatory processes, adrenergic stimulation, and pregnancy, and during estrogen replacement therapy.

DIAGNOSIS

Laboratory Assays for von Willebrand Factor

Laboratory testing essential for the diagnosis of VWD includes the following (Table 7-3):

1. VWF antigen
2. VWF activity (measured as ristocetin cofactor activity and/or collagen-binding activity)

Table 7-3 Assays for Diagnosis of von Willebrand Disease

Diagnostic Assays
von Willebrand factor antigen
von Willebrand factor activity (measured as ristocetin cofactor and/or collagen-binding activity)
Factor VIII activity (abnormal only in moderate to severe von Willebrand disease [VWD])

Other Assays
Bleeding time (prolonged only in moderate to severe VWD)
Partial thromboplastin time (PTT) is not recommended as a "rule-out" test because it is too insensitive and results may be normal in VWD.

Assays for Classification
RIPA (ristocetin-induced platelet aggregation) or quantitative platelet-binding assay
von Willebrand factor multimers

3. Factor VIII activity (abnormal only in moderate or severe disease)
4. Tests that measure the ability of VWF to support platelet plug formation (platelet function analyzer [PFA-100] or bleeding time). These tests are also abnormal in intrinsic platelet disorders and are prolonged only in moderate and severe VWD (limited specificity and sensitivity), so although the PFA-100 may be helpful, its diagnostic value is debated.[51,52]

After the initial diagnosis of VWD, the following assays are used to classify the type of VWD:

1. Ristocetin-induced platelet aggregation (RIPA) or platelet-binding studies
2. VWF multimer studies

VWF antigen, activity, and multimer studies can also be performed on platelet VWF.[53] In rare cases of VWD, only the platelet VWF is decreased, and plasma levels are normal (designated "platelet-low" VWD).[54]

The VWF antigen (VWF:Ag) is generally assayed using an enzyme-linked immunosorbent assay (ELISA) method, although electroimmunoassays and radioimmunoassays may be used.[55] Automated turbidometric tests that use latex particles coated with antibodies to VWF have also been used; the addition of plasma dilutions containing VWF causes clumping of the particles, and the VWF can be thus quantified. False positives may be seen in patients with rheumatoid factors.[56]

VWF activity can be measured by a number of different functional tests, including the ristocetin cofactor (VWF:RCo) assay, which is the most commonly used assay and the "gold standard," despite the fact that standardization of it from laboratory to laboratory is difficult.[57] The test is performed by making dilutions of patient plasma (the source of VWF) and mixing the dilutions with normal platelets or platelet membrane fragments that have been washed to remove any adherent VWF; ristocetin, an antibiotic that promotes binding of VWF to platelets, is added at 1.0 to 1.2 mg/mL, and the time to platelet aggregation/agglutination is assessed visually or with a platelet aggregometer. The use of ristocetin for evaluation of VWF activity was first suggested by Howard and Firkin,[58] who discovered that this antibiotic caused thrombocytopenia in individuals who had normal VWF but not in VWF-deficient subjects. A number of automated ristocetin cofactor methods have been introduced, some using the same reagents noted above and others measuring direct VWF binding to a purified GP-Ib; these have varying diagnostic sensitivity.[59-61] A sensitive ELISA that measures binding of plasma VWF to GP-Ib looks promising as a more quantitative assay for VWF platelet binding; further experience with this assay will allow assessment of its usefulness in terms of the ristocetin cofactor assay.[62] It is important to inquire about the method used and its sensitivity if results are to be accurately interpreted for diagnostic purposes.

A second *VWF activity* can be measured by testing the collagen-binding activity (VWF:CB) of VWF. In this test, ELISA plates are coated with collagen, dilutions of normal or patient plasma are added, and bound VWF is measured with the use of an antibody. This assay is usually performed in conjunction with other tests such as the ristocetin cofactor and VWF:Ag.[63,64] In rare cases of VWD in which the mutation affects only the collagen-binding site, the diagnosis could be missed if VWF:CB is not performed.

Factor VIII activity is measured in a functional assay, generally with the use of a modified partial thromboplastin time (PTT) and clot end point. The PTT itself is also used as a screening test, although it is less sensitive than the factor VIII assay. Both of these tests are abnormal only when the patient has a sufficiently low level of VWF to cause a low factor VIII, or when the VWF has defective binding for factor VIII that leads to a low level of factor VIII. Normal values for these tests cannot be used as exclusionary criteria for VWD.

The *PFA-100* measures the ability of platelets in whole blood to form a plug that occludes an aperture in a membrane. It requires VWF and normal platelet function. Fresh citrated whole blood is aspirated at arterial shear rates through tubing to a collagen-coated membrane with a central aperture; epinephrine or ADP is added to the blood, in addition to the collagen, to activate the platelets. The end point is measured as the time necessary for the platelet plug to form, closing the aperture and reducing pressure in the system.[65] The sensitivity of the PFA-100 for the diagnosis of VWD is debated.[52]

Bleeding time is a global assessment of vascular integrity, platelet function, and plasma factors, including VWF. If it is prolonged, the bleeding time is helpful in the diagnosis of VWD, but a normal bleeding time may be found in mild and even moderate VWD.[66,67] Quick[68] reported a marked prolongation of bleeding time after aspirin ingestion in patients with mild type 1 VWD as compared with normal subjects. Although bleeding time often is more prolonged after aspirin ingestion in patients with VWD than in patients without VWD (a fact that emphasizes that patients should avoid aspirin), many patients do not want to undergo multiple bleeding times; this test is not widely used at the present time.

Ristocetin-induced platelet aggregation (RIPA) is different from the ristocetin cofactor test and is used to aid clinicians in classifying the type of VWD that a patient has. RIPA is used to detect a qualitative abnormality in VWF, a "gain of function" that occurs in type 2B VWD (see Classification below). In RIPA, the patient provides both platelets and VWF as platelet-rich plasma (PRP). Different

concentrations of ristocetin are added separately to the PRP (usually varying progressively in final concentration from 0.4 to 1.2 mg/mL), and the presence or absence of platelet aggregation is assessed on an aggregometer. If platelets aggregate with low concentrations of ristocetin (less than 0.7 mg/mL), the VWF may have a "gain of function" abnormality (see later, type 2B). The same information can be obtained by directly measuring the amount of VWF bound to normal platelets at different concentrations of ristocetin.[69]

VWF multimers are evaluated by electrophoresis of plasma in low-concentration (1% or lower) agarose gels, followed by detection with a specific antibody to VWF for visualization of multimers.[70] These gels are used to detect decreased or absent high molecular weight multimers of VWF, which occur in the more common subtypes within type 2 VWD (types 2A and 2B) (Fig. 7-2). The gels can also detect the unusually high molecular weight multimers of VWF that may be present in patients with thrombotic thrombocytopenic purpura and in the rare cases of an inherited defect in which larger than normal multimers are present in the circulation (see type 2M, later). Electrophoresis in agarose gels of slightly higher concentration (1.2% to 1.5%) is used to study the components making up each multimer.

The factor VIII–binding assay measures the ability of a patient's VWF to bind normal factor VIII. This assay is used to test for a qualitative abnormality in VWF that impairs binding of FVIII and results in loss of protection and low circulating FVIII levels (VWD type 2N, see Classification later). The test is performed by coating ELISA plates with the patient's VWF (usually by means of a capture antibody), removing any endogenous bound FVIII, and then adding a known quantity of purified FVIII. After washing, the bound purified FVIII is measured by a chromogenic assay for FVIII.

The ristocetin cofactor:VWF antigen ratio is used to detect VWF that has relatively less activity compared with antigen, including VWF with qualitative defects such as those seen in types 2A, 2B, and 2M VWD. Unfortunately, at this time, criteria for the "normal" ratio are not uniform among laboratories (normal ratio is usually set at >0.5 to 0.7), and very few laboratories have used their local reagents and methods to establish a "normal" reference range for normal individuals or those with type 1 VWD. This calculated value, however, when it is abnormally low, can be helpful in suggesting the need for a VWF multimer study.

Pitfalls in Making the Diagnosis of VWD

The diagnosis of mild type 1 von Willebrand disease (see Classification below) is difficult. There is neither a simple genetic screening test nor a qualitative defect that defines type 1 VWD, and because the lower range of normal VWF activity and antigen overlaps with the levels of patients with mild VWD, one cannot simply use a laboratory "cutoff" level with confidence. Levels below 20 IU/dL are more likely to be associated with a significant personal and family bleeding history and mutations in the VWF gene, but levels between 30 and 50 IU/dL may not be definitive for VWD.[28,71,72] The lower levels of VWF in normal individuals with blood type O add another level of complexity for the diagnosis. A further confounding fact is that

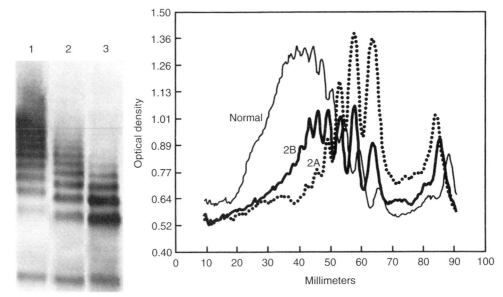

Figure 7-2 *Left*, Normal and variant von Willebrand factor (VWF) multimeric patterns. *Lane 1*, Normal VWF. *Lane 2*, Type 2B von Willebrand disease (VWD), showing decreased high molecular weight multimers. *Lane 3*, Type 2A VWD, showing a decrease in high and intermediate molecular weight multimers. *Right*, Densitometric tracing of lanes 1 to 3. (From Krizek DM, Rick ME: A rapid method to visualize von Willebrand factor multimers using agarose gel electrophoresis, immunolocalization and luminographic detection. Thromb Res 97:457–462, 2000, with permission from Elsevier Science.)

II

normal individuals report mild bleeding symptoms when asked in questionnaires, so a bleeding history cannot always be relied upon. For instance, up to 41% of normal subjects report bleeding after dental extractions, 28% report postoperative bleeding, 22% report epistaxis, and 68% report menorrhagia.[73–75] It may be helpful to repeat VWF testing 2 to 3 times at intervals in individuals and to test family members in some cases. However, continued testing may not clarify the dilemma and may lead to patient confusion. Additionally, it is important to avoid testing during the second and third trimesters of pregnancy when low VWF levels in patients may be elevated into the normal range; diagnosis should be delayed until several weeks after parturition.

It has been suggested that a category of "possible" VWD or "low" von Willebrand factor should be used, without the clinician actually making a diagnosis of von Willebrand disease in these individuals.[75a] Levels of VWF between 50 and 150 IU/dL might be viewed as optimal in terms of hemostasis and thrombosis, and slightly low levels, in the absence of a convincing bleeding history in the patient and family, may be better referred to as "low VWF" than VWD. No consensus has yet been reached among hemostasis experts about this, and vigorous discussion is ongoing. Regardless of the criteria used for the diagnosis of VWD, bleeding symptoms occur more frequently in subjects who have lower levels of VWF, and these individuals may benefit from prophylactic measures such as administration of desamino-D-arginine vasopressin (DDAVP) or antifibrinolytic medications in appropriate circumstances. These treatments do not require that a firm diagnosis for or against VWD be established, and they should be employed as appropriate in individuals with levels of VWF in the 30 to 50 IU/dL range, even in the absence of a definitive diagnosis.

Several papers concerning the diagnostic process for VWD have been published,[76,77] and a group has been assembled by the National Heart, Lung, and Blood Institute to evaluate the diagnosis and management of VWD; recommendations will be available in 2007.

CLASSIFICATION

VWD is classified into three types according to the results of laboratory and molecular genetic testing (Table 7-4):[4,4a] type 1, a partial quantitative deficiency of VWF, affecting approximately 70% to 75% of patients with VWD; type 2, a group of qualitative variants identified in approximately 20% to 25% of patients with VWD; and type 3, a rare homozygous or doubly heterozygous complete deficiency of VWF, which occurs in about 1 in every million persons.

Type 1

This dominantly inherited common type of VWD is usually associated with mild or moderate bleeding symptoms, although occasionally, bleeding can be severe, especially after administration of antiplatelet medications such as aspirin or other nonsteroidal anti-inflammatory medications. Bleeding may also be nonexistent, with "patients" discovered only through family studies. Childhood epistaxis is characteristic and may be outgrown after puberty. A number of mutations causing type 1 have been described, but many have not yet been identified. These mutations affect different areas of the gene and may reduce intracellular transport of the VWF dimer within the cell, or they may cause increased clearance of VWF from the circulation.[72,78]

VWF antigen and activity (ristocetin cofactor and collagen binding) are usually decreased concordantly, and factor VIII activity is decreased if the VWF deficiency is sufficiently severe (see Table 7-4). RIPA is decreased, and all VWF multimers are present (normal distribution). The bleeding time or PFA-100 will be prolonged if the deficiency is severe enough.

Table 7-4   Classification of von Willebrand Disease

Type	Inheritance	VWF Activity	RIPA	Multimer Pattern
Type 1 (Classic)	Autosomal dominant	↓	↓	Uniform ↓ but all multimers present
Type 2 (Variant)				
2A	Autosomal dominant (and recessive)	↓	↓	↓ Large and intermediate multimers
2B	Autosomal dominant	↓	↑	↓ Large multimers
2M	Autosomal dominant (and recessive)	↓	↓	Normal multimers
2N	Autosomal recessive	Normal	Normal	Normal multimers
Type 3 (Severe)	Autosomal recessive	↓↓	↓↓	Undetectable (usually cannot be visualized)

Type 2

Type 2 VWD is divided into four subtypes.

Type 2A

This subtype is usually inherited as an autosomal dominant trait and accounts for 10% to 15% of VWD cases. It usually is associated with moderate to severe bleeding symptoms. Mutations in type 2A cause a defect in the intracellular assembly and transport of VWF monomers (2A, type 1) or an increased susceptibility to proteolysis by ADAMTS13 (2A, type 2).[79,80] A number of mutations have been identified in the region that encodes the A2 domain of the VWF monomer, where a normal cleavage site is situated. Mutations are also described in the D2, D3, and A1 domains that result in a type 2A phenotype (see Fig. 7-1; see also Internet VWF database).

The VWF antigen is normal or decreased, and ristocetin cofactor activity is usually decreased out of proportion to the antigen, resulting in a decreased ratio of VWF activity to antigen. Factor VIII activity may be normal or decreased (see Table 7-4). RIPA is reduced, and the VWF multimers show an abnormal distribution, with an absence of high and intermediate molecular weight multimers (see Fig. 7-2). The bleeding time or PFA-100 is usually prolonged.

Type 2B

This subtype is transmitted as an autosomal dominant trait and usually manifests as moderate to severe disease; it accounts for approximately 5% of VWD cases. Mutations have been identified in an area of the gene that encodes the binding region for GP-Ib (see Fig. 7-1), and these give rise to a VWF molecule with a gain of function defect. These mutations cause the larger multimers of VWF to bind spontaneously to platelets in the circulation, resulting in removal of the multimers and, in some instances, thrombocytopenia[81,82]; the latter is likely due to the formation of small platelet aggregates and sequestration. The VWF antigen is normal or decreased, and the ristocetin cofactor is low because of the decrease or absence of the more functional high molecular weight multimers (leading to a reduced ratio of VWF activity to antigen, as in type 2A). On the other hand, the RIPA is increased, that is, there is aggregation of the patient's

PRP with concentrations of ristocetin lower than 0.6 mg/mL.[83] Factor VIII activity is normal or decreased, and VWF multimers usually show decreased or absent high molecular weight forms, usually less severe than those seen in type 2A.

A platelet defect that causes the same phenotype (fewer high molecular weight multimers of VWF and reduced ristocetin cofactor) is called platelet-type or pseudo–von Willebrand disease.[84,85] It is caused by an abnormal platelet GP-Ib receptor that binds normal VWF more avidly than usual, decreasing the number of high molecular weight multimers of VWF and often resulting in thrombocytopenia. Type 2B VWD and pseudo-VWD can be distinguished by a modification of the RIPA, with patient platelets mixed with normal plasma and, separately, patient plasma mixed with normal platelets. Type 2B VWD can also be distinguished from pseudo-VWD by genetic studies that indicate whether the mutation resides in the VWF gene or the platelet GP-Ib gene and by specific binding studies of VWF to platelets.

Type 2M

This subtype of VWD is an uncommon disorder that is usually inherited in an autosomal dominant manner. It presents as moderate or moderately severe disease and is characterized by reduced binding of the abnormal VWF to GP-Ib; however, all multimers are present, thus differentiating it from type 2A VWD.[4,4a] On gel electrophoresis, individual multimer bands may show abnormal patterns (formerly called types 1C and 1D)[86,87]; in other instances, larger than normal multimers are present in plasma (Vicenza variant),[88,89] or the variant VWF retains the propeptide within the multimers.[90] VWF antigen is variably decreased and ristocetin cofactor is more markedly decreased; factor VIII activity is reduced if the VWF is sufficiently low. Mutations that cause type 2M are clustered in the A1 domain in a separate area from the mutations that cause type 2B VWD.

Type 2N

One of the first two patients with type 2N VWD was described in France (in Normandy) and presented with a low factor VIII level that had been inherited in an autosomal pattern.[91,92] Patients with this subtype usually present with the constellation of autosomal inheritance and low factor VIII levels. Bleeding symptoms are moderate to moderately severe and include episodes of soft tissue bleeding and bleeding with invasive procedures that are more characteristic of factor VIII deficiency than the mucocutaneous bleeding usually seen in VWD. This variant is characterized by mutations in the aminoterminus of the VWF monomer within the binding site for factor VIII, which lead to decreased binding and diminished protection of factor VIII in the circulation.[93-96] The half-life of factor VIII is decreased from 8 to 12 hours to approximately 2 hours because of the lack of protection by VWF.[15] Platelet-related functions of VWF are usually intact, unless (uncommonly) a second mutation has been inherited in the other VWF allele that causes another VWF defect, such as those present in type 1 or a different type 2 VWD. Because the concentration of VWF in plasma is so much higher than the concentration of factor VIII, the binding defect must be inherited in a homozygous fashion, or a second defect must be present that limits synthesis of VWF by the other allele. Factor VIII levels are low (usually, 5 to 15 IU/dL), and the VWF antigen, ristocetin cofactor, RIPA, and VWF multimers are usually normal.

Because patients with type 2N VWD present with factor VIII deficiency, it is possible that they will be misdiagnosed with hemophilia A. The presence of an autosomal inheritance pattern and the presence or history of bleeding in women suggests that the patient and kindred should be tested for type 2N VWD. This is accomplished by testing the ability of the patient's VWF to bind factor VIII[91,92]; genetic studies are under way to establish this diagnosis.[93-96]

Type 3

Type 3 VWD is characterized by a severe deficiency of VWF and by a moderately severe deficiency of factor VIII. It is rare and is inherited in a homozygous or doubly heterozygous manner.[45] Patients present with mucocutaneous bleeding (from decreased VWF) and with soft tissue and joint bleeding (from decreased factor VIII). Deletions, compound heterozygous mutations, and nondeletion defects leading to decreased mRNA expression have been identified in these patients.[4,4a] Laboratory testing shows that VWF antigen is extremely low or unmeasurable, ristocetin cofactor is below the limits of detection, RIPA is absent, and VWF multimers usually cannot be visualized. Factor VIII activity is in the range of 2 to 10 IU/dL.

ACQUIRED VON WILLEBRAND DISEASE

Acquired VWD may appear spontaneously, or it may be associated with diseases that lead to decreased levels of VWF by one of several mechanisms: antibodies to VWF, increased proteolysis of VWF, abnormal binding to cells (usually tumor cells), or decreased synthesis. A number of recent reviews and an international survey have addressed this topic.[97-100]

The diagnosis of acquired VWD is made when decreased levels of VWF activity and antigen (and some-

times factor VIII activity) are detected in a patient who does not have a past history of bleeding and lacks a family history of bleeding. Antibodies to VWF most often occur in autoimmune or lymphoproliferative disease, and they may be difficult to identify in most patients with the use of functional studies[101-103]; other methods for antibody detection may be more sensitive.[104] Increased proteolysis occurs in patients with accelerated fibrinolysis, in those with noncyanotic congenital heart disease or high-grade aortic stenosis,[105,106] and possibly, in patients with myeloproliferative disease.[107,108] Tumor adsorption has been described in Wilms tumor,[109] and decreased synthesis has been described in hypothyroidism.[39,110] Some medications, such as valproic acid, dextrans, and hydroxyethyl starch, have also been associated with acquired VWD.[111-113]

TREATMENT

Inherited VWD

Selection of proper treatment depends on the type of VWD that a patient has, so a thorough laboratory evaluation should be completed before therapy is chosen, if time permits. In addition, the patient's general medical condition, associated illnesses, and medications (particularly aspirin-containing medications, nonsteroidal anti-inflammatory agents, or other antiplatelet agents) should be taken into account. These factors may influence decisions about the duration of treatment and whether to give additional medication or replacement therapy, including platelet concentrates, in cases of serious bleeding. The need for treatment in women with mild VWD may be minimized by scheduling elective minor surgical procedures during the latter half of the menstrual cycle, when slightly higher levels of VWF can be anticipated. In patients with type 1 VWD with atherosclerotic heart disease who need heart catheterization for evaluation or treatment, the choice of a short-acting nonsteroidal anti-inflammatory agent over aspirin is prudent for the procedure. No studies are available to assess the relative risk of long-term use of low-dose aspirin or other antiplatelet agents in patients with VWD who have atherosclerotic heart disease. If a patient with mild to moderate type 1 VWD is reliable and has a good understanding of VWD and how antiplatelet agents may aggravate bleeding, it is reasonable to give a trial of an antiplatelet agent to assess whether the patient has increased bruising or other bleeding. Depending on the response and the perceived relative risks presented by the heart disease compared with possible bleeding with VWD, a longer course of treatment may be given. Patients should be aware that they should discontinue the medication before undergoing invasive procedures (including dental work) and if any bleeding occurs.

Because no laboratory tests predict or correlate well with the severity of bleeding, it is necessary to monitor the patient clinically.[114] However, as a general and empirical goal, therapy is usually given in the amount predicted to increase the level of VWF activity and factor VIII to 50 to 100 IU/dL (Table 7-5).[115] In practice, it is often only the factor VIII level that may be available in a timely fashion for decision making, and this can be followed safely in many patients to evaluate therapy for adequate hemostasis,

Table 7-5   Treatment of Patients with von Willebrand Disease

Medication	Dose	Comments
DDAVP (desmopressin)	Intravenous (IV): 0.3 µg/kg in 50 mL saline over 20 min. Nasal spray: Weight >50 kg, 300 µg (1 spray in each nostril); <50 kg, 150 µg (1 spray in only one nostril)	Useful in most patients with type 1; variable in type 2.* Not useful in type 3. Patient should be given therapeutic trial before invasive procedure. May repeat dose after 12 hr and every 24 hr.† Tachyphylaxis and hyponatremia may occur; patients must be monitored.
VWF concentrates that contain all VWF multimers	Initial dose, 40–60 U/kg. Then, 20–30 U/kg q12h to keep VWF levels at 50%–100%, or to control clinical bleeding. Levels should be maintained for 3–10 days for major surgery.	Dose and duration based on clinical experience.

Antifibrinolytic agents:
  ε-Aminocaproic acid
  tranexamic acid
	50 mg/kg (maximum, 5 g dose) 4× daily
	25 mg/kg 3× daily
		Use alone or in conjunction with other therapy. Especially useful for mucosal bleeding (often for dental procedures).

IVIg (immune acquired inhibitors of VWF)	1 g/kg daily for 2 days; infusion over 8–12 hr	Use after trial of DDAVP or other measures in patients with acquired VWD, particularly when associated with autoimmune disease.

VWF, von Willebrand factor; IVIg, intravenous immune globulin; VWD, von Willebrand disease.
*Thrombocytopenia may worsen in some patients with type 2B disease.
†Total dose usually should not exceed 3 to 4 doses because of tachyphylaxis and possible hyponatremia.

as indicated by the clinical experience of experts who treat VWD.[116,117] Treatment modalities include DDAVP (desmopressin), replacement therapy with VWF-containing plasma products, antifibrinolytic and topical therapies, and estrogen (in women) (see Table 7-5).

DDAVP

DDAVP (desmopressin) is a synthetic analogue of antidiuretic hormone that causes release of VWF and factor VIII from body stores by an indirect mechanism that is not yet understood.[118] DDAVP is the treatment of choice in most patients with type 1 and in many with type 2 VWD.[119] It is administered in a much larger dose than the dose used for antidiuretic hormone replacement therapy.

Although most patients with type 1 VWD respond to DDAVP, it is recommended that patients undergo a trial before the first therapeutic use of the agent. DDAVP is given as an intravenous infusion at a dose of 0.3 µg/kg (not to exceed 20–25 µg) or as an intranasal spray at a dose of 300 µg (2 sprays) for patients who weigh more than 50 kg, or 150 µg (1 spray) for patients who weigh 50 kg or less. (It should be noted that this dose is 10-fold higher than the DDAVP dose used for replacement therapy in posterior pituitary gland disease.) For intravenous infusion, DDAVP is diluted in 50 mL saline and administered over 20 to 30 minutes. Levels of ristocetin cofactor, VWF antigen, and factor VIII should be determined before infusion and at 2 to 4 hours; the use of bleeding times to assess whether prolonged values decrease significantly 2 or 4 hours after infusion has declined because of patient concerns about multiple bleeding times, and because it is not necessary to normalize the bleeding time before a procedure is performed. An increase of two- to fivefold in VWF and factor VIII levels is expected 30 to 60 minutes after infusion; these values return to baseline in approximately 4 to 6 hours.[120]

Adverse effects include flushing, hypertension or hypotension, headache, and, rarely, tingling; these can usually be controlled by slowing the infusion of DDAVP. Although thrombosis has occurred after administration of DDAVP, it is uncertain whether this is causal.[121] Tachyphylaxis occurs after repeated administration, and serious hyponatremia has been observed, especially with concomitant intake of free water.[122] For these reasons, DDAVP administration is usually limited for any single procedure; it is usually given 0.5 to 2 hours before a procedure and may be repeated 8 to 12 hours later and daily on the following 2 to 3 days if necessary, while free water intake is limited and serum sodium concentrations are monitored.

DDAVP is useful in most patients with mild and moderate type 1 VWD, except those rare patients with type 1 who do not have normal levels of platelet VWF (platelet-low patients).[123] Patients with type 2A VWD respond variably to DDAVP,[124] and those with type 2B may experience a decrease in platelet counts following the increase in plasma levels of abnormal 2B VWF.[125] Despite this possible drawback, a number of patients with type 2B VWD have undergone procedures after administration of DDAVP, and any reduction in platelet count has usually normalized after 2 hours.[126] It is especially important to use a trial infusion to evaluate the effects of DDAVP in patients with type 2A and type 2B disease before they undergo surgery. DDAVP is not helpful in patients with type 3 VWD, who rarely have sufficient stores of VWF.

Intranasal DDAVP has proved extremely useful and convenient for patients because they are able to administer the medication "on the spot" when bleeding occurs without delaying treatment. A good example is its use in helping to control menstrual bleeding in women with VWD.[127] Oral bleeding and epistaxis have also been controlled by this method.

Replacement Therapy With VWF

Several preparations that contain VWF are available for use in patients with VWD. These include intermediate-purity factor VIII concentrates that contain VWF (not monoclonally purified or recombinant factor VIII concentrates, which lack VWF), more highly purified VWF concentrates, and cryoprecipitate. Most experts do not recommend cryoprecipitate unless no other VWF concentrate is available because of the potential for transmission of viruses.[128] The other concentrates mentioned here undergo a step such as pasteurization to decrease the risk of viral transmission.

The VWF concentrate available in the United States that is labeled with the concentration of ristocetin cofactor units per vial is Humate P (ZLB Behring). Others are available in Europe.[129,130] These concentrates are usually administered as a short (approximately 15 minute) intravenous infusion, although studies have shown that when therapy is needed for several days, the total dose used is reduced by 20 to 50 IU/dL when the concentrate is given by constant infusion.[131,132] The dose for major bleeding challenges is estimated at the amount that will raise the ristocetin cofactor to 50 to 100 IU/dL (loading dose, 40 to 60 U/kg; maintenance dose, 20 to 40 U/kg) (see Table 7-5). Repeat infusions may be necessary at 12-hour intervals for 3 to 10 days for major surgery or serious bleeding. If bleeding is not controlled by replacement therapy, patients may benefit from platelet transfusions, in addition to VWF.[133]

Replacement therapy is used for patients with type 3 VWD, for those with type 2 disease who do not respond to DDAVP, and for patients with the more severe type 1 disease who have not responded to DDAVP or have responded but need further long-range hemostatic support that cannot be provided with just 2 to 3 days of DDAVP therapy.

Antifibrinolytic Therapy

Both ε-aminocaproic acid (EACA) and tranexamic acid have been used alone and as adjuncts to other therapies for patients with VWD, particularly those with oral and other moderate mucous membrane bleeding. When given orally for this use, they are administered 3 or 4 times daily (see Table 7-5) for 3 to 7 days.[115] Doses must be adjusted in patients with renal failure. These medications may also be given by the intravenous route. Prolonged use of either medication may lead to thrombosis in susceptible patients.

Topical Agents

These agents are usually used for oral or nasal bleeding; they provide local therapy to the bleeding surface. Gelfoam or Surgicel (Johnson and Johnson and others) may be soaked in topical thrombin before application to the site. Micronized collagen (Avitene, C.R. Bard) and fibrin sealant have also been used topically[134] (see Chapter 29).

Estrogen

Estrogen can enhance the synthesis of VWF, and women with mild to moderate VWD may benefit from therapy with estrogen. Its use, however, has been tempered recently because of the potential adverse effects of estrogen. It is usually administered in doses equivalent to those used for hormone replacement therapy.[135]

von Willebrand Disease During Pregnancy

Because levels of VWF increase two- to threefold over baseline during the second and third trimesters of pregnancy, treatment typically is not needed during delivery in many patients with type 1 VWD. Qualitative defects present in type 2 VWF do not correct, however, and increases in VWF levels may be variable.[136] Additionally, VWF levels fall rapidly and excessive bleeding may occur in the weeks following delivery. DDAVP therapy is used after labor has been initiated in those patients who are responsive and have moderately severe disease with persistently lower levels of VWF during the third trimester; VWF replacement therapy is usually not required but should be used when patients are not responsive to DDAVP and bleeding occurs.[41,137] No standard recommendation can be made for the level of VWF that is safe for regional anesthesia; it is usually considered safe when VWF:RCo is 50 IU/dL or greater.[138]

Acquired von Willebrand Disease

Different mechanisms may lead to acquired VWD, and treatment may vary with the underlying pathophysiology. Treatment of an associated primary disease is usually undertaken in those cases where it can be identified; this is particularly important in unusual cases in which hypothyroidism is the underlying cause, because treatment with thyroid hormone normalizes VWF levels.[39,110] Many times, selection of a treatment regimen involves a process of empirical trials undertaken to determine which treatment is most useful; often, a trial of DDAVP is given initially, followed by replacement therapy (if DDAVP is unsuccessful in stopping bleeding). If neither is successful, a trial of high-dose intravenous immune globulin (IVIg) is recommended (1 g/kg daily for 2 days), particularly if the cause is believed to be an acquired inhibitor associated with autoimmune disease or a monoclonal gammopathy.[139] In all situations, response should be monitored by measurement of VWF and factor VIII levels over the first hours after treatment and by following clinical responses. Less commonly, plasmapheresis or extracorporeal immunoadsorption may be used to remove an antibody, at least temporarily, if clinical bleeding is occurring.[140] Immunosuppressive medications used for the treatment of underlying disease, such as rituximab, may decrease the antibody in some patients.

Practical Considerations for Therapy

Because of enhanced awareness and increased diagnosis of VWD, a number of patients who have an undocumented diagnosis of VWD may present emergently with bleeding that requires urgent treatment. A careful past bleeding history and family history can be particularly helpful to the clinician who is deciding whether the patient should receive treatment for VWD. If the patient does require treatment, it is likely that DDAVP may be used successfully and the patient can be spared exposure to blood products. For serious bleeding (brisk gastrointestinal or central nervous system bleeding), replacement therapy should be given, along with other therapy as indicated, to maintain VWF between 50 and 100 IU/dL, until a more definitive diagnosis can be established. Structural lesions may co-exist. After bleeding is controlled and baseline health returns for 3 to 4 weeks, the patient should be asked to return for a full evaluation and should be given information to carry that provides test results and recommendations for treatment in an emergency situation.

REFERENCES

1. Rodeghiero F, Castaman G, Dini E: Epidemiological investigation of the prevalence of von Willebrand's disease. Blood 69:454–459, 1987.
2. Sadler JE, Mannucci PM, Berntorp E, et al: Impact, diagnosis and treatment of von Willebrand disease. Thromb Haemost 84:160–174, 2000.
3. Ruggeri ZM, Ware J: von Willebrand factor. FASEB J 7:308–316, 1993.
4. Sadler JE: A revised classification of von Willebrand disease. For the Subcommittee on von Willebrand Factor of the Scientific and Standardization Committee of the International Society on Thrombosis and Haemostasis. Thromb Haemost 71:520–525, 1994.
4a. Sadler JE, Budde U, Eikenboom JC, et al: Working party on von Willebrand disease classification. Update on the pathophysiology and classification of von Willebrand disease: A report of the subcommittee on von Willebrand factor. J Thromb Haemost 4:2103–2114, 2006.
5. Nilsson IM: Von Willebrand's disease—Fifty years old. Acta Med Scand 201:497–508, 1977.
6. Alexander B, Goldstein R: Dual hemostatic defect in pseudohemophilia. J Clin Invest 32:551, 1953.
7. Nilsson IM, Blombäck M, Jorpes E, et al: V Willebrand's disease and its correction with human plasma fraction 1–0. Acta Med Scand 159:179–188, 1957.
8. Ginsburg D, Handin RI, Bonthron DT, et al: Human von Willebrand factor (VWF): Isolation of complementary DNA (cDNA) clones and chromosomal localization. Science 228:1401–1406, 1985.
9. Lynch DC, Zimmerman TS, Collins CJ, et al: Molecular cloning of cDNA for human von Willebrand factor: Authentication by a new method. Cell 41:49–56, 1985.
10. Sadler JE, Shelton-Inloes BB, Sorace JM, et al: Cloning and characterization of two cDNAs coding for human von Willebrand factor. Proc Natl Acad Sci U S A 82:6394–6398, 1985.
11. Verweij CL, de Vries CJ, Distel B, et al: Construction of cDNA coding for human von Willebrand factor using antibody probes for colony-screening and mapping of the chromosomal gene. Nucleic Acids Res 13:4699–4717, 1985.
12. Weiss HJ, Phillips LL, Rosner W: Separation of sub-units of antihemophilic factor (AHF) by agarose gel chromatography. Thromb Diath Haemorrh 27:212–219, 1972.
13. Rick ME, Hoyer LW: Immunologic studies of antihemophilic factor (AHF, Factor VIII). V. Immunologic properties of AHF subunits produced by salt dissociation. Blood 42:737–747, 1973.
14. Koedam JA, Meijers JC, Sixma JJ, Bouma BN: Inactivation of human factor VIII by activated protein C: Cofactor activity of protein S and protective effect of von Willebrand factor. J Clin Invest 82:1236–1243, 1988.
15. Brinkhous KM, Sandberg H, Garris JB, et al: Purified human factor VIII procoagulant protein: Comparative hemostatic response after infusion into hemophilic and von Willebrand disease dogs. Proc Natl Acad Sci U S A 82:8752–8756, 1985.
16. Jaffe E, Hoyer L, Nachman R: Synthesis of antihemophilic factor antigen by cultured endothelial cells. J Clin Invest 52:2757–2764, 1975.
17. Sporn L, Chavin S, Marder V: Biosynthesis of von Willebrand protein by human megakaryocytes. J Clin Invest 76:1102–1106, 1985.
18. Wagner DD: Cell biology of von Willebrand factor. Annu Rev Cell Biol 6:217–246, 1990.
19. Levine JD, Harlan JM, Harker LA, et al: Thrombin-mediated release of factor VIII–related antigen from human umbilical vein endothelial cells in culture. Blood 60:531–534, 1982.
20. Rickles FR, Hoyer LW, Rick ME, Ahr DJ: The effects of epinephrine infusion in patients with von Willebrand's disease. J Clin Invest 57:1618–1625, 1976.
21. Ribes JA, Francis CW, Wagner DD: Fibrin induces release of von Willebrand factor from endothelial cells. J Clin Invest 79:117–123, 1987.
22. Tsai HM: Physiologic cleavage of von Willebrand factor by a plasma protease is dependent on its conformation and requires calcium ion. Blood 87:4235–4244, 1996.
23. Furlan M, Robles R, Lamie B: Partial purification and characterization of a protease from human plasma cleaving von Willebrand factor to fragments produced by in vivo proteolysis. Blood 87:4223–4234, 1996.
24. Dong J, Moake JL, Nolasco L, et al: ADAMTS-13 rapidly cleaves newly secreted ultralarge von Willebrand factor multimers on the endothelial surface under flowing conditions. Blood 100:4033–4039, 2002.
25. Xie L, Chesterman CN, Hogg PJ: Control of von Willebrand factor multimer size by thrombospondin-1. J Exp Med 193:1341–1350, 2001.
26. Nichols WC, Ginsburg D: Reviews in molecular medicine: von Willebrand disease. Medicine 76:1–20, 1997.
27. O'Brien LA, James PD, Othman M, et al: For the Association of Hemophilia Clinic Directors of Canada: Founder von Willebrand factor haplotype associated with type 1 von Willebrand disease. Blood 102:549–557, 2003.
28. Bodó I, Katsumi A, Tuley EA, et al: Type 1 von Willebrand disease mutation Cys1149Arg causes intracellular retention and degradation of heterodimers: A possible general mechanism for dominant mutations of oligomeric proteins. Blood 98:2973–2979, 2001.
28a. James PD, Notley C, Hegadorn C, et al: The mutational spectrum of type 1 von Willebrand disease: Results from a Canadian cohort study. Blood 109:145–154, 2007.
28b. Goodeve A, Eikenboom J, Castaman G, et al: Phenotype and genotype of a cohort of families historically diagnosed with type 1 von Willebrand disease in the European study, Molecular and Clinical Markers for the Diagnosis and Management of Type 1 von Willebrand Disease (MCMDM-1VWD). Blood 109:112–121, 2007.
29. Fowler WE, Fretto LJ, Hamilton KK, et al: Substructure of human von Willebrand factor. J Clin Invest 76:1491–1500, 1985.
30. Siedlecki CA, Lestini BJ, Kottke-Marchant KK, et al: Shear dependent changes in the three-dimensional structure of human von Willebrand factor. Blood 88:2939–2950, 1996.
31. Mohri H, Fujimura Y, Shima M, et al: Structure of the von Willebrand factor domain interacting with glycoprotein Ib. J Biol Chem 263:17901–17904, 1988.
32. Santoro SA: Adsorption of von Willebrand factor/factor VIII by the genetically distinct interstitial collagens. Thromb Res 21:689–691, 1981.
33. De Marco L, Girolami A, Zimmerman TS, et al: Interaction of purified type IIB von Willebrand factor with the platelet membrane glycoprotein Ib induces fibrinogen binding to the glycoprotein IIb/IIIa complex and initiates aggregation. Proc Natl Acad Sci U S A 82:7424–7428, 1985.
34. Savage B, Shattil SJ, Ruggeri ZM: Modulation of platelet function through adhesion receptors: A dual role for glycoprotein IIb-IIIa (integrin alpha IIb beta 3) mediated by fibrinogen and glycoprotein Ib-von Willebrand factor. J Biol Chem 267:11300–11306, 1992.
35. Mohri H, Yoshioka A, Zimmerman TS, Ruggeri ZM: Isolation of the von Willebrand factor domain interacting with platelet glycoprotein Ib, heparin, and collagen, and characterization of its three distinct functional sites. J Biol Chem 264:17361–17367, 1989.
36. Roberts DD, Williams SB, Gralnick HR, Ginsburg V: von Willebrand factor binds specifically to sulfated glycolipids. J Biol Chem 26:3306–3309, 1986.
37. Harrison RL, McKee PA: Estrogen stimulates von Willebrand factor production by cultured endothelial cells. Blood 63:657–664, 1984.
38. Baumgartner-Parzer SM, Wagner L, Reining G, et al: Increase by tri-iodothyronine of endothelin-1, fibronectin and von Willebrand factor in cultured endothelial cells. J Endocrinol 154:231–239, 1997.
39. Dalton RG, Savidge GF, Matthews KB, et al: Hypothyroidism as a cause of acquired von Willebrand's disease. Lancet 1:1007–1009, 1987.
40. Kadir RA, Economides DL, Sabin CA, et al: Variations in coagulation factors in women: Effects of age, ethnicity, menstrual cycle, and combined oral contraceptive. Thromb Haemost 82:1456–1461, 1999.
41. Ito M, Yoshimura K, Toyoda N, Wada H: Pregnancy and delivery in patients with von Willebrand's disease. J Obstet Gynaecol Res 23:37–43, 1997.
42. Bennett B, Ratnoff OD: Changes in antihemophilic factor (AHF, factor 8) procoagulant activity and AHF-like antigen in normal pregnancy, and following exercise and pneumoencephalography. J Lab Clin Med 80:256–263, 1972.
43. Gill JC, Endres-Brooks J, Bauer PJ, et al: The effect of ABO blood group on the diagnosis of von Willebrand disease. Blood 69:1691–1695, 1987.
44. Fuster V, Bowie EJW, Lewis JC, et al: Resistance to arteriosclerosis in pigs with von Willebrand's disease: Spontaneous and high cholesterol diet–induced arteriosclerosis. J Clin Invest 61:722–730, 1978.

45. Mannucci PM, Bloom AL, Larrieu MJ, et al: Atherosclerosis and von Willebrand factor. I. Prevalence of severe von Willebrand's disease in western Europe and Israel. Br J Haematol 57:163–169, 1984.

46. Nichols TC, Bellinger DA, Tate DA, et al: von Willebrand factor and occlusive arterial thrombosis: A study in normal and von Willebrand's disease pigs with diet-induced hypercholesterolemia and atherosclerosis. Arteriosclerosis 10:449–461, 1990.

47. Federici AB, Mannucci PM, Fogato E, et al: Autopsy findings in three patients with von Willebrand disease type IIB and type III: Presence of atherosclerotic lesions without occlusive arterial thrombi. Thromb Haemost 70:758–761, 1993.

48. Miller CH, Graham JB, Goldin LR, Elston RC: Genetics of classic von Willebrand's disease. I. Phenotypic variation within families. Blood 54:117–136, 1979.

49. Ahr DJ, Rickles FR, Hoyer LW, et al: von Willebrand's disease and hemorrhagic telangiectasia: Association of two complex disorders of hemostasis resulting in life-threatening hemorrhage. Am J Med 62:452–458, 1977.

50. Di Paola J, Federici AB, Mannucci PM, et al: Low platelet alpha2beta1 levels in type I von Willebrand disease correlate with impaired platelet function in a high shear stress system. Blood 93:3578–3582, 1999.

51. Fressinaud E, Veyradier A, Truchaud F, et al: Screening for von Willebrand disease with a new analyzer using high shear stress: A study of 60 cases. Blood 91:1325–1331, 1998.

52. Quiroga T, Goycoolea M, Munoz B, et al: Template bleeding time and PFA-100 have low sensitivity to screen patients with hereditary mucocutaneous hemorrhages: Comparative study in 148 patients. J Thromb Haemost 2:892–898, 2004.

53. Gralnick HR, Williams SB, McKeown LP, et al: Platelet von Willebrand factor: Comparison with plasma von Willebrand factor. Thromb Res 38:623–633, 1985.

54. Weiss HJ, Pietu G, Rabinowitz R, et al: Heterogeneous abnormalities in the multimeric structure, antigenic properties, and plasma-platelet content of factor VIII/von Willebrand factor in subtypes of classic (type I) and variant (type IIA) von Willebrand's disease. J Lab Clin Med 101:411–425, 1983.

55. Ingerslev J: A sensitive ELISA for von Willebrand factor (VWF:Ag). Scand J Clin Lab Invest 47:143–149, 1987.

56. Veyradier A, Fressinaud E, Sigaud M, et al: A new automated method for von Willebrand factor antigen measurement using latex particles [letter]. Thromb Haemost 81:320–321, 1999.

57. Favaloro EJ, Smith J, Petinos P, et al: Laboratory testing for von Willebrand's disease: An assessment of current diagnostic practice and efficacy by means of a multi-laboratory survey. RCPA Quality Assurance Program (QAP) in Haematology Haemostasis Scientific Advisory Panel. Thromb Haemost 82:1276–1282, 1999.

58. Howard MA, Firkin BG: Ristocetin—A new tool in the investigation of platelet aggregation. Thromb Diath Haemorrh 26:362–369, 1971.

59. Miller CH, Platt SJ, Daniele C, Kaczor D: Evaluation of two automated methods for measurement of the ristocetin cofactor activity of von Willebrand factor. Thromb Haemost 88:56–59, 2002.

60. Redaelli R, Corno AR, Borroni L, et al: von Willebrand factor ristocetin cofactor (VWF:RCo) assay: Implementation on an automated coagulometer (ACL). J Thromb Haemost 3:2684–2688, 2005.

61. Fischer BE, Thomas KB, Dorner F: von Willebrand factor: Measuring its antigen or function? Correlation between the level of antigen, activity, and multimer size using various detection systems. Thromb Res 9:39–43, 1998.

62. Federici AB, Canciani MT, Forza I, et al: A sensitive ristocetin co-factor activity assay with recombinant glycoprotein Ibalpha for the diagnosis of patients with low von Willebrand factor levels. Haematologica 89:77–85, 2004.

63. Siekmann J, Turecek PL, Schwarz HP: The determination of von Willebrand factor activity by collagen binding assay. Haemophilia 4 (suppl 3):15–24, 1998.

64. Riddell AF, Jenkins PV, Nitu-Whalley IC, et al: Use of the collagen-binding assay for von Willebrand factor in the analysis of type 2M von Willebrand disease: A comparison with the ristocetin cofactor assay. Br J Haematol 116:187–192, 2002.

65. Mammen EF, Comp PC, Gosselin R, et al: PFA-100 system: A new method for assessment of platelet dysfunction. Semin Thromb Hemost 24:195–202, 1998.

66. Ratnoff OD, Bennett B: Clues to the pathogenesis of bleeding in von Willebrand's disease. N Engl J Med 289:1182–1183, 1983.

67. Abildgaard CF: Diagnosis of von Willebrand disease. Prog Clin Biol Res 324:263–268, 1990.

68. Quick AJ: Salicylates and bleeding: The aspirin tolerance test. Am J Med Sci 252:265–269, 1966.

69. Scott JP, Montgomery RR: The rapid differentiation of type IIb von Willebrand's disease from platelet-type (pseudo-) von Willebrand's disease by the "neutral" monoclonal antibody binding assay. Am J Clin Pathol 96:723–728, 1991.

70. Krizek DM, Rick ME: A rapid method to visualize von Willebrand factor multimers using agarose gel electrophoresis, immunolocalization and luminographic detection. Thrombosis Res 97:457–462, 2000.

71. Castaman G, Federici AB, Rodeghiero F, et al: Von Willebrand's disease in the year 2003: Towards the complete identification of gene defects for correct diagnosis and treatment. Haematologica 88:94–108, 2003.

72. Eikenboom JC, Matsushita T, Reitsma PH, et al: Dominant type 1 von Willebrand disease caused by mutated cysteine residues in the D3 domain of von Willebrand factor. Blood 88:2433–2441, 1996.

73. Drews CD, Dilley AB, Lally C, et al: Screening questions to identify women with von Willebrand disease. J Am Med Womens Assoc 57:217–218, 2002.

74. Sramek A, Eikenboom JC, Briet E, et al: Usefulness of patient interview in bleeding disorders. Arch Intern Med 155:1409–1415, 1995.

75. Silwer J: von Willebrand's disease in Sweden. Acta Paediatr Scand Suppl 238:1–159, 1973.

75a. Sadler JE: von Willebrand disease type 1: A diagnosis in search of a disease. Blood 101:2089–2093, 2003.

76. Laffan M, Brown SA, Collins PW, et al: The diagnosis of von Willebrand disease: A guideline from the UK Haemophilia Centre Doctors' Organization. Haemophilia 10:199–217, 2004.

77. Federici AB, Castaman G, Mannucci PM: for the Italian Association of Hemophilia Centers (AICE): Guidelines for the diagnosis and management of von Willebrand disease in Italy. Haemophilia 8:607–621, 2002.

78. Gavazova S, Gill JC, Scott JP, et al: A mutation in the D4 domain of von Willebrand factor (VWF) results in a variant of type 1 von Willebrand disease with accelerated in vivo VWF clearance. Blood 100(suppl 1):128a, 2002.

79. Lyons SE, Bruck ME, Bowie EJ, Ginsburg D: Impaired intracellular transport produced by a subset of type IIA von Willebrand disease mutations. J Biol Chem 267:4424–4430, 1992.

80. Gralnick HR, Williams SB, McKeown LP, et al: In vitro correction of the abnormal multimeric structure of von Willebrand factor in type IIa von Willebrand's disease. Proc Natl Acad Sci U S A 82:5968–5972, 1985.

81. Cooney KA, Ginsburg D: Comparative analysis of type 2b von Willebrand disease mutations: Implications for the mechanism of von Willebrand factor binding to platelets. Blood 87:2322–2328, 1996.

82. Gralnick HR, Williams SB, McKeown LP, et al: Von Willebrand's disease with spontaneous platelet aggregation induced by an abnormal plasma von Willebrand factor. J Clin Invest 76:1522–1529, 1985.

83. Ruggeri ZM, Pareti FI, Mannucci PM, et al: Heightened interaction between platelets and factor VIII/von Willebrand factor in a new subtype of von Willebrand's disease. N Engl J Med 302:1047–1051, 1980.

84. Weiss HJ, Meyer D, Rabinowitz R, et al: Pseudo–von Willebrand's disease: An intrinsic platelet defect with aggregation by unmodified human factor VIII/von Willebrand factor and enhanced adsorption of its high-molecular-weight multimers. N Engl J Med 306:326–333, 1982.

85. Miller JL, Kupinski JM, Castella A, Ruggeri ZM: von Willebrand factor binds to platelets and induces aggregation in platelet-type but not type IIB von Willebrand disease. J Clin Invest 72:1532–1542, 1983.

86. Ciavarella G, Ciavarella N, Antoncecchi S, et al: High-resolution analysis of von Willebrand factor multimeric composition defines a new variant of type I von Willebrand disease with aberrant structure but presence of all size multimers (type IC). Blood 66:1423–1429, 1985.

87. Lopez-Fernandez MF, Gonzalez-Boullosa R, Blanco-Lopez MJ, et al: Abnormal proteolytic degradation of von Willebrand factor after desmopressin infusion in a new subtype of von Willebrand disease (ID). Am J Hematol 36:163–170, 1991.

88. Mannucci PM, Lombardi R, Castaman G, et al: Von Willebrand disease "Vicenza" with larger-than-normal (supranormal) von Willebrand factor multimers. Blood 71:65–70, 1988.

89. Schneppenheim R, Federici AB, Budde U, et al: Von Willebrand disease type 2M "Vicenza" in Italian and German patients: Identification of the first candidate mutation (G3864A; R1205H) in 8 families. Thromb Haemost 83:136–140, 2000.

II

90. Montgomery RR, Dent J, Schmidt W, et al: Hereditary persistence of circulating pro von Willebrand factor (pro-VWF). Circulation 74 (suppl 2):406, 1986. Abstract.

91. Nishino M, Girma J-P, Rothschild C, et al: New variant of von Willebrand disease with defective binding to factor VIII. Blood 74:1591–1599, 1989.

92. Mazurier C, Dieval J, Jorieux S, et al: A new von Willebrand factor (VWF) defect in a patient with factor VIII (fVIII) deficiency but normal levels and multimeric patterns of both plasma and platelet VWF: Characterization of abnormal VWF/fVIII interaction. Blood 75:20–26, 1990.

93. Cacheris PM, Nichols WC, Ginsburg D: Molecular characterization of a unique von Willebrand disease variant: A novel mutation affecting von Willebrand factor/factor VIII interaction. J Biol Chem 266:13499–13502, 1991.

94. Gaucher C, Mazurier B, Jorieux S, et al: Identification of two point mutations in the von Willebrand factor gene of three families with the "Normandy" variant of von Willebrand disease. Br J Haematol 78:506–514, 1991.

95. Kroner PA, Friedman KD, Fahs SA, et al: Abnormal binding of factor VIII is linked with the substitution of glutamine for arginine 91 in von Willebrand factor in a variant form of von Willebrand disease. J Biol Chem 266:19146–19149, 1991.

96. Rick ME, Krizek DM: Identification of a His54Gln substitution in von Willebrand factor from a patient with defective binding of factor VIII. Am J Hematol 51:302–306, 1996.

97. Kumar S, Pruthi RK, Nichols WL: Acquired von Willebrand's syndrome: A single institution experience. Am J Hematol 72:243–247, 2003.

98. Veyradier A, Jenkins CS, Fressinaud E, Meyer D: Acquired von Willebrand syndrome: From pathophysiology to management. Thromb Haemost 84:175–182, 2000.

99. Michiels JJ, Budde U, van der Planken M, et al: Acquired von Willebrand syndromes: Clinical features, aetiology, pathophysiology, classification and management. Best Pract Res Clin Haematol 14:401–436, 2001.

100. Federici AB, Mannucci PM: Diagnosis and management of acquired von Willebrand syndrome. Clin Adv Hematol Oncol 1:169–175, 2003.

101. Handin RI, Martin V, Moloney WC: Antibody-induced von Willebrand's disease: A newly defined inhibitor syndrome. Blood 48:393–405, 1976.

102. Wautier JL, Levy-Toledano S, Caen JP: Acquired von Willebrand's syndrome and thrombopathy in a patient with chronic lymphocytic leukaemia. Scand J Haematol 16:128–134, 1976.

103. Mohri H, Motomura S, Kanamori H, et al: Clinical significance of inhibitors in acquired von Willebrand syndrome. Blood 91:3623–3629, 1998.

104. Siaka C, Rugeri L, Caron C, Goudemand J: A new ELISA assay for diagnosis of acquired von Willebrand syndrome. Haemophilia 9:303–308, 2003.

105. Gill JC, Wilson AD, Endres-Brooks J, Montgomery RR: Loss of the largest von Willebrand factor multimers from the plasma of patients with congenital cardiac defects. Blood 67:758–761, 1986.

106. Vincentelli A, Susen S, Le Tourneau T, et al: Acquired von Willebrand syndrome in aortic stenosis. N Engl J Med 349:343–349, 2003.

107. Eikenboom JCJ, van der Meer FJM, Briet E: Acquired von Willebrand's disease due to excessive fibrinolysis. Br J Haematol 81:618–620, 1992.

108. Budde U, Schaefer G, Mueller N, et al: Acquired von Willebrand's disease in the myeloproliferative syndrome. Blood 64:981–985, 1984.

109. Bracey AW, Wu AH, Aceves J, et al: Platelet dysfunction associated with Wilms tumor and hyaluronic acid. Am J Hematol 24:247–257, 1987.

110. Aylesworth CA, Smallridge RC, Rick ME, Alving BA: Acquired von Willebrand's disease: A rare manifestation of postpartum thyroiditis. Am J Hematol 50:217–219, 1995.

111. Kreuz W, Linde R, Funk M, et al: Valproate therapy induces von Willebrand disease type I. Epilepsia 33:178–184, 1992.

112. Aberg M, Hedner U, Bergentz SE: Effect of dextran on factor VIII (antihemophilic factor) and platelet function. Ann Surg 189:243–247, 1979.

113. Sanfelippo MJ, Suberviola PD, Geimer NF: Development of a von Willebrand-like syndrome after prolonged use of hydroxyethyl starch. Am J Clin Pathol 88:653–655, 1987.

114. Ratnoff OD, Saito H: Bleeding in von Willebrand's disease. N Engl J Med 290:1089, 1974.

115. Scott JP, Montgomery RR: Therapy of von Willebrand disease. Semin Thromb Hemost 19:37–47, 1993.

116. Lusher JM: Clinical guidelines for treating von Willebrand disease patients who are not candidates for DDAVP—A survey of European physicians. Haemophilia 4(suppl 3):11–14, 1998.

117. Mannucci PM: How I treat patients with von Willebrand disease. Blood 97:1915–1919, 2001.

118. Moffat EH, Giddings JC, Bloom AL: The effect of desamino-D-arginine vasopressin (DDAVP) and naloxone infusions on factor VIII and possible endothelial cell (EC) related activities. Br J Haematol 57:651–662, 1984.

119. Mannucci PM: Treatment of von Willebrand's disease. J Intern Med 740(suppl):129–132, 1997.

120. Aledort LM: Treatment of von Willebrand's disease. Mayo Clin Proc 66:841–846, 1991.

121. Mannucci PM, Lusher JM: Desmopressin and thrombosis. Lancet 2:675, 1989. Letter.

122. Mannucci PM, Bettega D, Cattaneo M: Patterns of development of tachyphylaxis in patients with haemophilia and von Willebrand disease after repeated doses of desmopressin (DDAVP). Br J Haematol 82:87–93, 1992.

123. Mannucci PM, Lombardi R, Bader R, et al: Heterogeneity of type I von Willebrand disease: Evidence for a subgroup with an abnormal von Willebrand factor. Blood 66:796–802, 1985.

124. Sutor AH: DDAVP is not a panacea for children with bleeding disorders. Br J Haematol 108:217–227, 2000.

125. Holmberg L, Nilsson EM, Borge L, et al: Platelet aggregation induced by 1-desamino-8-D-arginine vasopressin (DDAVP) in type 2 von Willebrand's disease. N Engl J Med 309:816–821, 1983.

126. Casonato A, Pontara E, Dannhaeuser D, et al: Re-evaluation of the therapeutic efficacy of DDAVP in type IIB von Willebrand's disease. Blood Coagul Fibrinolysis 5:959–964, 1994.

127. Lethagen S, Ragnarson Tennvall G: Self-treatment with desmopressin intranasal spray in patients with bleeding disorders: Effect on bleeding symptoms and socioeconomic factors. Ann Hematol 66:257–260, 1993.

128. Chang AC, Rick ME, Pierce LR, Weinstein MJ: Summary of a workshop on potency and dosage of von Willebrand factor concentrates. Haemophilia 4(suppl 3):1–6, 1998.

129. Pasi KJ, Williams MD, Enayat MS, Hill FG: Clinical and laboratory evaluation of the treatment of von Willebrand's disease patients with heat-treated factor VIII concentrate (BPL 8Y). Br J Haematol 75:228–233, 1990.

130. Goudemand J, Negrier C, Ounnoughene N, Sultan Y: Clinical management of patients with von Willebrand's disease with a VHP VWF concentrate: The French experience. Haemophilia 4(suppl 3):48–52, 1998.

131. Varon D, Martinowitz U: Continuous infusion therapy in haemophilia. Haemophilia 4:431–435, 1998.

132. Lubetsky A, Schulman S, Varon D, et al: Safety and efficacy of continuous infusion of a combined factor VIII–von Willebrand factor (VWF) concentrate (Haemate-P) in patients with von Willebrand disease. Thromb Haemost 81:229–233, 1999.

133. Castillo R, Escolar G, Monteagudo J, et al: Hemostasis in patients with severe von Willebrand disease improves after normal platelet transfusion and normalizes with further correction of the plasma defect. Transfusion 37:785–790, 1997.

134. Association of Hemophilia Clinic Directors of Canada: Hemophilia and von Willebrand's disease. 2. Management. CMAJ 153:147–157, 1995.

135. Alperin JB: Estrogens and surgery in women with von Willebrand's disease. Am J Med 73:367–371, 1982.

136. Conti M, Mari D, Conti E, et al: Pregnancy in women with different types of von Willebrand disease. Obstet Gynecol 68:282–285, 1986.

137. Walker ID, Walker JJ, Colvin BT, et al: Investigation and management of haemorrhagic disorders in pregnancy. Haemostasis and Thrombosis Task Force. J Clin Pathol 47:100–108, 1994.

138. Kadir RA, Lee CA, Sabin CA, et al: Pregnancy in women with von Willebrand's disease or factor XI deficiency. Br J Obstet Gynaecol 105:314–321, 1998.

139. Federici AB, Rand JH, Castaman G, et al: Treatment of acquired von Willebrand syndrome in patients with monoclonal gammopathy of uncertain significance: Comparison of three different therapeutic approaches. Blood 92:2707–2711, 1998.

140. Viallard JF, Pellegrin JL, Vergnes C, et al: Three cases of acquired von Willebrand disease associated with systemic lupus erythematosus. Br J Haematol 105:532–537, 1999.

Chapter 8

General Aspects of Thrombocytopenia, Platelet Transfusions, and Thrombopoietic Growth Factors

David J. Kuter, MD, DPhil

INTRODUCTION

Of the circulating blood cells, the platelet was the last to be fully described and its attributes determined. Although early studies by Osler, Hayam, and Bizzozero identified small particles in the blood, these were believed to be bacteria, fragments of red blood cells, or other hematopoietic elements.[1,2] It was not until the development of a novel blood staining method by James Homer Wright that the true identity of these circulating blood cells and their relationship to hemostasis became apparent.[3–5] After observing their common tinctorial properties, Wright showed that blood platelets (initially called "plates") arose from bone marrow megakaryocytes. He found that these megakaryocytes extended a portion of their cytoplasm into the bone marrow sinusoids and shed platelets into the circulation (Fig. 8-1).

These observations were carried one step further in 1910 by William Duke,[6] who described three patients at Massachusetts General Hospital who were bleeding and had low platelet counts, as determined by early cell counting procedures. He was able to show that "certain types of hemorrhagic disease may be attributed to an extreme reduction in the number of platelets." Indeed, Duke showed that on creating a venous shunt between a normal donor and a thrombocytopenic recipient, the platelet count would increase in the thrombocytopenic recipient, and bleeding would cease. Although platelet transfusions had unknowingly been given in the form of whole blood transfusions over many centuries, this was the first time it was shown that transfused platelets could ameliorate bleeding.

Since the time of these seminal observations, evaluation of disorders of blood platelets and of treatment of thrombocytopenia has become a common hematology consultation. Indeed, on a general inpatient hematology consultation service, approximately one third of all consultations are requested for assessment of thrombocytopenia (D. Kuter, personal observation, 2005). Some 5% to 10% of all hospitalized patients are thrombocytopenic, and for patients in medical and surgical intensive care units, this figure rises to as high as 30% to 35%. Indeed, some data suggest that thrombocytopenic patients suffer a twofold greater mortality rate than those who are not thrombocytopenic.[7–10]

The primary reason for evaluating any thrombocytopenic patient is to assess the risk of bleeding. In general, patients with platelet counts less than 20,000/μL are at increased risk of spontaneous bleeding and bleeding with procedures. These individuals are commonly the subjects of consultative hematology evaluations because they may need treatment with transfusions or more specific therapies to ameliorate the bleeding risk.

A more common source of hematology consultations are those patients with milder degrees of thrombocytopenia and platelet counts ranging from 20,000/μL to 50,000/μL. These individuals rarely have any risk of spontaneous bleeding but may have increased bleeding risk with procedures.

A final group of patients who are commonly the subject of hematology consultations are those with platelet counts ranging from 50,000/μL to 100,000/μL. Such patients do not have an increased risk of spontaneous bleeding and can probably undergo most procedures without an increased risk of major bleeding complications. Nonetheless, this patient population is oftentimes strikingly limited in its access to medical care. Surgeons are often reluctant to operate on patients whose platelet counts are in this range, albeit for poorly documented reasons. Epidural anesthesia for pregnant patients with platelet counts below 100,000/μL is often withheld; finally, procedures as routine as colonoscopy, dental extraction, dental prophylaxis, prostate biopsy, and breast biopsy are often not undertaken in patients whose platelet counts fall within this range. Effective antiviral treatment frequently is not administered to individuals with hepatitis C who have such mild thrombocytopenia.

Aside from the risk of bleeding, another reason for consultation on the thrombocytopenic patient is to determine whether some other underlying medical condition is involved. Thrombocytopenia is often associated with other diseases such as thrombotic thrombocytopenic purpura (TTP), hemolytic-uremic syndrome (HUS), systemic lupus erythematosus (SLE), heparin-induced thrombocytopenia, (HIT), and primary bone marrow disorders.

The goals of the hematology consultant in evaluating the thrombocytopenic patient consist of the following:

1. To assess the risk of bleeding
2. To diagnose the underlying cause of the thrombocytopenia
3. To treat the thrombocytopenia as indicated

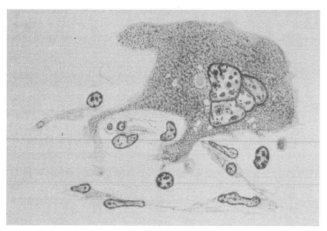

Figure 8-1 *(See also Color Plate 8-1.)* Megakaryocyte protruding into the bone marrow sinusoid and producing platelets. Camera lucida drawing by James Homer Wright.[5]

RELATION OF BLEEDING RISKS TO PLATELET COUNT

Except for situations in which the platelet count drop is indicative of other disorders, such as heparin-induced thrombocytopenia, antiphospholipid antibody syndrome, or collagen-vascular disorders, a platelet count above 100,000/μL is rarely associated with any significant bleeding risk or thrombotic difficulty. For the purposes of this discussion, clinically significant thrombocytopenia occurs when platelet counts are lower than 100,000/μL. As suggested earlier, such subjects can be roughly grouped into three categories. The first are those whose platelet counts are between 50,000/μL and 100,000/μL for whom spontaneous bleeding does not occur and for whom surgical bleeding risk is low. The second group includes those whose platelet counts are between 20,000/μL and 50,000/μL; for this group, spontaneous bleeding rarely occurs, but the risk of bleeding with surgical procedures may be increased. Finally, the group that is of greatest concern consists of those whose platelet counts are lower than 20,000/μL for whom the risk of spontaneous bleeding is increased and for whom surgical bleeding risks usually are increased.

Although seemingly intuitive, the relation of platelet count to bleeding risk is poorly defined. This is not only due to inadequate clinical studies but also to the inability of clinicians to measure accurately the second important platelet variable, platelet function. Indeed, in some situations of increased platelet destruction such as immune thrombocytopenic purpura (ITP), as the platelet count declines, mean platelet volume (MPV) rises, which tends to offset the decline in total platelet function. This increase in MPV has been attributed to "phylogenetic canalization," suggesting some feedback system wherein increased platelet volume (and hence increased function) tends to mitigate against decreased platelet numbers.[11] Alternatively, drugs or intrinsic platelet defects may reduce the function of platelets, thereby increasing the bleeding risk at any degree of thrombocytopenia. This is commonly seen in situations in which patients have taken antiplatelet agents such as aspirin, or when they are uremic. Fever and other medical conditions also affect hemostatic risk at any degree of thrombocytopenia.

Even though it is convenient to think of hemostatic risk solely as a function of platelet count, this is an oversimplification because of the many other variables that affect hemostatic risk. Rigid adherence to customary threshold values of 50,000/μL for surgical hemostasis and 5000/μL to 10,000/μL for prophylaxis is inappropriate. Nonetheless, these platelet numbers are generally helpful and are based on the following evidence.

One example of the increased risk of bleeding with thrombocytopenia is seen in studies that showed the relation of bleeding time to platelet count.[12] Below a platelet count of 100,000/μL, a linear relation is observed between the decline in platelet count and the increase in bleeding time. Although bleeding time is an unreliable predictor of bleeding risk,[13] this is perhaps the clearest visual demonstration of the relation between the decline in platelet count and the increase in bleeding risk.

Early studies in leukemic children showed a direct relation between platelet count and risk of spontaneous bleeding. As the logarithm of the platelet count fell below 100,000/μL, a linear increase was reported in the amount of hemorrhage that occurred. Most of this was accounted for by milder forms of hemorrhage such as petechiae, ecchymoses, and epistaxis, which tended to occur particularly when the count was below 50,000/μL. If only more major forms of hemorrhage were analyzed, an increase was evident as counts fell below 100,000/μL, but most bleeding events occurred at platelet counts lower than 10,000/μL; of this latter group, most bleeding events occurred at below 5000/μL. For both minor and major bleeding episodes, the authors emphasized that no threshold platelet count was used, but rather, a continuous increase in hemorrhagic risk was noted as platelet count fell. These often-quoted studies are confounded by the fact that many subjects were also treated with antipyretics that adversely affected platelet function, the use of capillary platelet counts, and the lack of adequate antibiotic treatment of these often febrile patients. Nonetheless, these studies confirm the relation between bleeding risk and platelet count and have been used (despite the authors' exhortations) to support the concept of the 50,000/μL threshold for surgical hemostasis and the 5000/μL to 10,000/μL threshold for prophylaxis.

More recent bleeding studies by Rebulla[14,15] and Wandt[16] have shown that in leukemic patients given chemotherapy, hemorrhage occurs to the same extent at 10,000/μL and at 20,000/μL.

A biologic estimate of the lowest effective platelet count comes from the work of Slichter,[17–19] who used 51Cr-labeled red blood cells (RBCs) to quantify fecal blood loss in stable aplastic thrombocytopenic patients who were treated only with anabolic steroids. At platelet counts above 10,000/μL, patients had a normal blood loss of less than 5 mL per day. At platelet counts of 5000/μL to 10,000/μL, this loss rose slightly to 9 ± 7 mL per day; however, at platelet counts below 5000/μL, this was markedly elevated to 50 ± 20 mL per day.

To assess further this apparent critical platelet threshold of 5000/μL to 10,000/μL, Hanson and Slichter[20] performed platelet kinetic studies in thrombocytopenic patients with platelet counts ranging from 12,000/μL to 70,000/μL. They found a fixed minimum requirement for 7100 platelets/μL per day to maintain vascular integrity; this was 18% of the normal daily turnover of 41,200 platelets/μL per day. These studies have provided the experimental explanation for current recommendations that prophylactic platelet transfusions should be given only to those patients whose platelet counts are lower than 5000/μL to 10,000/μL.[21,22]

One final pathophysiologic basis for the bleeding risk recommendations just described is supported by recent data on the precise role that platelet surface activation plays in the coagulation cascade. With the use of real-time measurements during clotting, thrombin generation appears to be maximal as long as the platelet count is above 10,000/μL; below this value, thrombin generation declines in direct proportion to the platelet count.[23,24]

THE BIOLOGY OF PLATELET PRODUCTION

As a pathophysiologic basis for clinical evaluation of the thrombocytopenic patient, a brief review of the biology of platelet production is helpful. This approach allows the hematology consultant to relate the various causes of thrombocytopenia to relevant aspects of platelet production.

The pluripotential stem cell gives rise through a stochastic differentiation process to precursor cells committed to megakaryocyte differentiation, called megakaryocyte colony-forming cells (Meg-CFCs).[25,26] The viability of the Meg-CFC depends on the presence of numerous hematopoietic cytokines, including thrombopoietin (TPO). Meg-CFCs are mitotically active until some triggering event, as yet unidentified, causes them to stop their mitotic divisions and enter a process called endomitosis, in which DNA replication ensues but neither the nucleus nor the cytoplasm undergoes division. This gives rise to polyploid megakaryocyte precursor cells that contain anywhere from 4 to 16 times the normal diploid complement of DNA—all contained within a single nuclear envelope. Initially, these cells are morphologically indistinct, but once they complete their endomitotic divisions, they grow into large, morphologically identifiable megakaryocytes.

Megakaryocytes occupy unique positions within the bone marrow. Early megakaryocyte precursor cells and stem cells occupy a niche close to the bone.[27-30] As megakaryocytes differentiate, they appear to follow a stromal cell–derived factor-1 (SDF-1) gradient and migrate close to the endothelial cells that line the bone marrow sinusoids. Cytoplasmic projections from the megakaryocytes then pass through the endothelial cell—not between its gap junctions—and appear in the bone marrow sinusoid, where they appear to undergo cleavage into platelets and long strands of megakaryocyte cytoplasm destined to become platelets (called "proplatelets").[27] Whether platelet production occurs entirely in the bone marrow sinusoids or in other tissues such as the lungs has been the subject of much speculation for decades.[31-34] What is clear is that platelets or proplatelets bud into the bone marrow sinusoid from megakaryocytes within the marrow. What is unclear is whether these proplatelets then undergo subsequent processing into platelets within the lung parenchyma. Mathematical models suggested that this occurs, although biochemical data have not supported this.[33-35]

Once in the circulation, the human platelet survives for 10 days; it then probably undergoes programmed cell death and is removed from the circulation. Data to support programmed cell death have come from several recent experiments but have not been conclusive.[36-38] An alternative hypothesis suggests that surface glycoprotein changes result in clearance of the older platelets by the reticuloendothelial cell system, such as that which occurs with senescent red cells. No evidence suggests that platelet activation plays a major role in platelet clearance; indeed, most platelets that enter the circulation do not undergo platelet activation before they undergo senescence and clearance. The tissue responsible for the clearance of senescent platelets has not been well defined. In animal models, splenectomy does not seem to alter the platelet life span; therefore, one can assume that clearance in humans also occurs through a nonsplenic mechanism.[39]

The key hematopoietic regulators of platelet production appear to be TPO and SDF-1. TPO is necessary for platelet production, and in its absence, platelet counts in animals and humans drop to about 10% of normal.[40] Nonetheless, platelets continue to be made, albeit from a reduced number of polyploid megakaryocytes. TPO appears to be made in a constitutive fashion by the liver, and its rate of synthesis is not affected by any known cytokine or disease.[26] The only exception appears to be the reduction in TPO production that occurs in patients with liver dysfunction such as chronic hepatitis and after partial hepatectomy[41,42]; in this setting, platelet count declines in direct proportion to the reduction that occurs in liver function. TPO is therefore made constitutively by the liver; it enters the circulation and is cleared by avid receptors on platelets and probably bone marrow megakaryocytes.[43-45] This results in a basal level of TPO that is necessary for normal megakaryocyte growth, polyploidization, and development.

The relationship of circulating TPO levels to platelet count depends on the nature of the thrombocytopenia.[46,47] In situations in which the marrow has been damaged and platelet production is decreased, TPO clearance is decreased and TPO levels rise. For example, in patients with aplastic anemia with platelet counts of 10,000/μL, TPO levels rise from normal values of about 100 pg per milliliter to 2000 to 3000 pg per milliliter. However, when thrombocytopenia is due to peripheral destruction of platelets, and when the megakaryocyte mass is normal or increased, net clearance of TPO may be nearly normal and TPO levels may not be elevated. An example is ITP in which the increased bone marrow megakaryocyte mass and the increased release of platelets into the blood result in almost normal TPO clearance and virtually normal TPO levels. Although TPO levels might be helpful in distinguishing between patients with decreased platelet production and those with increased platelet production, plasma TPO levels are not currently clinically available.

Less well appreciated is the role that SDF-1 plays in platelet production.[28] When SDF-1 was administered to thrombocytopenic animals that lacked TPO, platelet count rose to nearly normal levels. In normal healthy animals in which SDF-1 was transiently removed, platelet count fell. SDF-1 appears to guide megakaryocyte progenitors toward bone marrow sinusoids and to trigger their shedding of platelets. The main problem in platelet biology at the present time involves an understanding of the mechanism of platelet shedding from bone marrow megakaryocytes. This appears to be a very finely tuned mechanism that involves TPO, SDF-1, and endothelial cells.

As is discussed later, with this understanding of platelet biology, several general mechanisms for thrombocytopenia become apparent. Thrombocytopenia will occur if platelet destruction due to immune or nonimmune mechanisms overwhelms the compensatory ability of the bone marrow to increase platelet production. Thrombocytopenia will also arise from disorders that decrease platelet production. With reduced numbers of progenitor cells such as those seen after chemotherapy, the platelet count will certainly fall. If TPO production is reduced, such as after liver resection or in severe liver disease, a concomitant drop in platelet count occurs. Less well understood are the mechanisms by which other medications cause decreased platelet production. Recent data suggest that drugs such as gemcitabine and bortezomib may actually reduce platelet shedding from megakaryocytes with little effect on the number of megakaryocytes or their progenitors.[48] It has been suggested that this is due to alteration in the SDF-1 gradient.

CAUSES OF THROMBOCYTOPENIA

Table 8-1 lists a general classification of the causes of thrombocytopenia.

Laboratory artefact ("pseudothrombocytopenia") occurs in up to 0.2% of patients who have blood counts performed.[49–51] Although this may be due to the use of therapeutic antiplatelet antibodies such as abciximab,[52,53] most cases of pseudothrombocytopenia result from the clumping of platelets that occurs ex vivo in anticoagulated blood samples. Several mechanisms have been proposed for this.[54–57] Most involve conformational changes in the IIb-IIIa receptor that are due to the low divalent cation concentration and/or the lower temperature of anticoagulated blood; novel GPIIb/IIIa epitopes appear to be exposed that react with preexisting antibodies in the patient's blood, causing aggregation. In both of these situations, collecting the blood in an acid-citrate-dextrose (ACD; yellow-top) or heparinized (green-top) tube, as well as keeping samples at 37°C, usually prevents clumping and permits an accurate blood count. Although most modern cell counting devices "flag" samples that contain platelet clumps, review of the peripheral blood smear may be the only way to detect this phenomenon (Fig. 8-2). Certainly, patients reported to have a very low platelet count but who lack signs and symptoms of thrombocytopenia should be evaluated for pseudothrombocytopenia through review of the peripheral blood smear.

A second important but easily diagnosed cause of thrombocytopenia occurs primarily in intensive care unit and postsurgical patients who have received multiple RBC transfusions and developed dilutional thrombocytopenia. Given that fresh whole blood is rarely used anymore, transfusion with large amounts of packed RBCs, fresh frozen plasma (FFP), and fluids may result in dilution of platelets. In massive trauma, it is important that adequate platelet transfusions be provided, along with RBC and plasma transfusions.

A third cause of mild thrombocytopenia (with platelets usually in the 40,000/μL to 60,000/μL range) is the splenic sequestration commonly seen in patients with severe liver disease or other causes of splenomegaly. Because the body

Table 8-1 Causes of Thrombocytopenia

Artefact/cell counter malfunction
Dilution
Splenic sequestration
Decreased production
    Primary bone marrow disorders
        Aplastic anemia
        Myelodysplasia
        Acute leukemia
        Familial thrombocytopenia
        Thrombocytopenia with absent radius (TAR) syndrome
    Infection
        Human immunodeficiency virus
    Toxins/drugs
    Radiation
    Vitamin/nutritional deficiencies
        Vitamin B_{12}
        Iron deficiency, severe
    Metabolic disorders
        Hypothyroidism
        Adrenal insufficiency
        Gaucher disease
    Thrombopoietin deficiency
    Thrombopoietin receptor defect
Increased destruction
    Nonimmune
        Disseminated intravascular coagulation, acute and chronic
        Thrombotic thrombocytopenic purpura (TTP)/hemolytic-uremic syndrome (HUS)
        Giant cavernous hemangiomas
        Burns
        Sepsis
        Continuous venovenous hemofiltration
        Renal transplant rejection
        Intra-aortic balloon pump
        Cyclosporine A
        von Willebrand disease, type 2B
    Immune
        Fc mediated
            Heparin
            Immune complex
        Fab mediated
            Idiopathic thrombocytopenic purpura (ITP)
                Drug associated
                Idiopathic
        Posttransfusion purpura
        Neonatal isoimmune thrombocytopenia

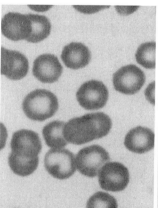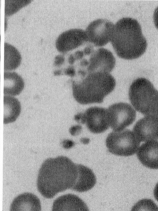

Figure 8-2 *(See also Color Plate 8-2.)* Platelet clumping (pseudo-thrombocytopenia). Peripheral blood smear of patient shows no platelets in one field *(left panel)* but large platelet clumps in another field *(right panel)*.

conserves the circulating platelet mass and not the platelet count, approximately one third of the total platelet mass is normally sequestered in the spleen.[58–62] With splenic enlargement, additional platelets become sequestered within the spleen.[60–62] In patients with liver disease and splenomegaly, the situation may be more complicated. Because the liver is the main source of TPO production, thrombocytopenia can be attributed to sequestration and diminished TPO levels.[63]

As with many other hematologic conditions, the two remaining major categories of thrombocytopenia can be attributed to decreased production of platelets or increased destruction of platelets, or some combination of the two.

Decreased platelet production occurs in many situations, ranging from bone marrow replaced by metastatic cancer to lack of bone marrow due to bone marrow failure syndromes. Toxins, ethanol ingestion, vitamin B_{12} deficiency, and some medications can decrease megakaryocyte endomitosis and inhibit megakaryocyte maturation.[64,65] Furthermore, some drugs such as gemcitabine and bortezomib may actually decrease the shedding of platelets from existing megakaryocytes. With these chemotherapies, the number of megakaryocytes may be normal or elevated, although effective platelet production (thrombopoiesis) may be reduced. Finally, it should not be forgotten that ITP is also a disease of decreased platelet production in that megakaryocytes may be undergoing programmed cell death from the antiplatelet antibody.[66,67] In human immunodeficiency virus (HIV) thrombocytopenia, megakaryocyte mass and megakaryocyte ploidy are markedly increased but effective thrombopoiesis from these megakaryocytes is markedly diminished, presumably because of early programmed cell death of these megakaryocytes.[68,69]

Disorders of increased platelet destruction are relatively common and include both nonimmune and immune disorders. Nonimmune thrombocytopenic disorders consist of disseminated intravascular coagulation (DIC), thrombotic thrombocytopenic purpura (TTP), and HUS, as well as pulmonary hypertension, veno-occlusive disease, and full-thickness burns. Immune causes of thrombocytopenia can be divided into those that are related to antigen/antibody complex deposition onto platelet Fc receptors and those in which the antibody Fab region directly binds to the platelet. An example of the former is heparin-induced thrombocytopenia (HIT), in which immune complexes cause platelet activation. An example of the latter is ITP, in which antibodies are directed against IIb/IIIa and Ib-IX glycoproteins on the platelet surface; this results in opsonization of platelets and their removal by FcγRIII receptors on macrophages in organs such as the spleen.

EVALUATION OF THE THROMBOCYTOPENIC PATIENT

For the hematology consultant, the urgency and pace of evaluation are determined by platelet count, extent of bleeding or thrombosis, the need for procedures, the presence of antiplatelet agents, the extent of nonhematologic symptoms, and concurrent anemia and/or leukopenia. The following general approach to evaluating the patient is useful

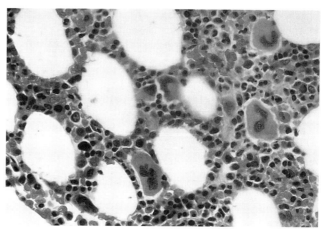

Figure 8-3 Bone marrow megakaryocytes in idiopathic thrombocytopenic purpura (ITP). Bone marrow biopsy of patient with chronic ITP shows increased megakaryocyte number and size, as well as increased megakaryocyte nucleus size (ploidy).

but should be individualized. Pseudothrombocytopenia should always first be excluded by a careful review of the blood smear. This examination also helps to assess for TTP and HUS because these usually preclude treatment with platelet transfusions. For patients on unfractionated or low molecular weight heparin, the drug should be stopped until HIT is excluded; the presence of HIT is another contraindication to platelet transfusion. Dilutional thrombocytopenia may be uncovered by a review of the transfusion record. The presence of splenic sequestration may be determined by physical examination or radiographic procedures such as ultrasound or computed tomography (CT). Finally, to determine whether platelet production is adequate, a bone marrow examination may be performed (Fig. 8-3).

As in the assessment of any other medical disorder, careful attention to the history and symptoms, physical examination findings, and appropriate laboratory investigations is essential. Although these suggestions are not meant to be exhaustive, the following approaches are often helpful in evaluating the thrombocytopenic patient.

Medical History

Given the potential myriad causes of thrombocytopenia, a careful history is in order. Prior platelet counts are important for documenting the chronicity of the thrombocytopenia and for excluding rare cases of familial thrombocytopenia and macrothrombocytopenia. Recent viral infections and vaccinations may cause transient thrombocytopenia. It is mandatory for the clinician to inquire about exposure to new medications such as antibiotics and antiplatelet drugs. The former (e.g., linezolide, vancomycin, nafcillin) commonly cause thrombocytopenia,[70,71] and the presence of the latter (e.g., aspirin, nonsteroidal anti-inflammatory drugs, ketorolac) may explain ongoing bleeding. Current or recent exposure to unfractionated or low molecular weight heparin must be documented. Excessive ethanol ingestion may directly cause thrombocytopenia, or it may occur indirectly through hepatic cirrhosis. In pregnant patients, platelet counts from prior pregnancies may suggest gestational thrombocytopenia or recurrence of ITP; a history of hypertension and proteinuria may indicate

HELLP (*H*emolysis, *E*levated *L*iver function tests, and *L*ow *P*latelets) syndrome. Recent headache, visual changes, confusion, or personality changes in patients with thrombocytopenia may suggest intracranial hemorrhage. A history of lymphoma or autoimmune disease (SLE, Hashimoto thyroiditis, anticardiolipin antibody syndrome) may suggest a diagnosis of ITP.

In hospitalized patients, a history of recent RBC or platelet transfusion may be associated with posttransfusion purpura (PTP). The response to prior platelet transfusions may also be helpful in assessing whether platelet destruction is ongoing; if such destruction is present, the corrected platelet count increment will be low and the rise in platelet count transient. The use of devices such as continuous venovenous hemofiltration[72] and intra-aortic balloon pump counterpulsation[73] is commonly associated with thrombocytopenia. The presence of renal failure may also predict an increased risk of hemorrhage due to uremic platelet dysfunction.

Symptoms and Signs of Thrombocytopenia

Patients will have symptoms or signs of thrombocytopenia in accordance with platelet count and platelet function.[10] Most thrombocytopenic patients have no symptoms and no signs. Such patients, as indicated earlier, usually have platelet counts above 50,000/µL and lack any significant platelet dysfunction. Such individuals are usually evaluated for assessment of the risk for future bleeding during procedures or for determination of the underlying cause of thrombocytopenia.

Patients who warrant the greatest amount of attention are those who have signs and symptoms of thrombocytopenia, usually with platelet counts less than 20,000/µL. Such individuals may have a wide range of bleeding complications, ranging from modest bruising to intracranial hemorrhage. Assessment of the patient for ongoing bleeding is of paramount importance for the consultant who is evaluating the patient at the bedside. Close examination of the patient for bruises and petechiae should be undertaken. In hospitalized bedridden patients, petechiae often occur on the back and dependent surfaces of the body rather than on the lower extremities, as is more common in ambulatory patients. Signs of "wet purpura" such as conjunctival hemorrhage, gum bleeding, and oral blood blisters are of great consequence and have been shown in some studies to herald more severe bleeding.[74,75] Patients should be assessed for evidence of gastrointestinal bleeding such as melena and a positive test for fecal occult blood. Thrombocytopenic women often have menorrhagia. Careful abdominal examination usually provides an adequate assessment of splenic size. Cutaneous signs of giant cavernous hemangioma may be found. Although they are uncommon, signs and symptoms of central nervous system (CNS) bleeding range from subtle events (e.g., headache, mild gait abnormalities, confusion) to catastrophic occurrences (e.g., paralysis, coma). CNS bleeding has been reported to occur in 0.2% to 1% of children with ITP.[74,75]

Signs of thrombosis should not be overlooked in thrombocytopenic patients. This is an important finding because it may indicate underlying disorders of platelet activation such as TTP, HUS, anticardiolipin antibody syndrome, DIC, and HIT.

Table 8-2 Comprehensive Laboratory Evaluation of Thrombocytopenia*

Review of peripheral blood smear
Mean platelet volume (MPV)
Platelet histogram
Complete blood count (CBC) drawn in heparinized or
   acid-citrate-dextrose (ACD) tube
CBC drawn and kept at 37°C
Prothrombin time (PT)
Partial thromboplastin time (PTT)
D-Dimer
Fibrin degradation products assay
PF4-heparin antibody test
Antiplatelet antibodies
Direct antiglobulin test
Reticulocyte count
Reticulated platelet assay
Antiphospholipid antibody assays
Antinuclear antibody (ANA)
Hepatitis C serology
Abdominal ultrasound
Abdominal computed tomography (CT)
Bone marrow examination
Blood urea nitrogen (BUN)
Creatinine

*In evaluation of the thrombocytopenic patient, some of these tests may be helpful; see text discussion.

Laboratory Investigations

A number of laboratory tests may be used to assess the thrombocytopenic patient (Table 8-2). The importance of reviewing the blood smear to exclude pseudothrombocytopenia has already been mentioned. The blood smear also reveals the relative size and granularity of platelets; large granular platelets (megathrombocytes) are characteristic of disorders of platelet destruction and may suggest a low bleeding risk[76,77]; hypogranular platelets may indicate myelodysplastic syndrome (MDS) and an increased bleeding risk. The mean platelet volume (MPV) and the platelet histogram help to confirm these visual findings. In addition, review of the smear reveals the presence of schistocytes that may be indicative of TTP, HUS, or DIC, or the presence of spherocytes, which might indicate Evans syndrome.

Measurement of the rate of platelet production may be assessed by flow cytometric measurement of reticulated platelets. However, this procedure has not been validated in most clinical settings and is not widely available.[63,78,79]

Repeating the complete blood count (CBC) without delay with a heparinized (green top) or citrate (yellow top) tube kept at 37°C will assist the clinician in evaluating for pseudothrombocytopenia. The presence of coagulopathies such as DIC may be detected with the use of prothrombin time (PT), partial thromboplastin time (PTT), D-dimer, and fibrin split product (FSP) assays. The PF4-heparin antibody test can be used to assess for HIT. Antibodies to human platelet antigen (HPA)-1a (PLA1) may be identified serologically to assess for PTP. ITP may be investigated with the use of antiplatelet antibodies, but this test has a poor predictive value[80]; rather, the direct antiglobulin test (DAT; Coombs test), antiphospholipid antibodies, antinuclear antibody (ANA), and hepatitis C serologies may be more helpful in revealing an autoimmune cause of thrombocytopenia.

Abdominal ultrasound or CT scan may be useful in assessing for splenomegaly or abdominal aortic dissection. A bone marrow examination may be useful but is often not required; thrombocytopenia rarely causes major hemorrhage with this procedure, and prophylactic platelet transfusions usually are not indicated.

Although platelet function tests cannot be reliably performed at platelet counts lower than 100,000/μL, most thrombocytopenic patients should have blood urea nitrogen (BUN) and creatinine checked for assessment of uremic platelet dysfunction.

TREATMENT OF PATIENTS WITH THROMBOCYTOPENIA

Although most patients with thrombocytopenia do not require immediate treatment, treatment of thrombocytopenia is often indicated when the patient has bleeding, reduced platelet function, platelets below 10,000/μL, or the need for procedures. As is discussed in the following sections, general treatment approaches include (1) specific treatment of the underlying cause; (2) platelet transfusions; (3) methods designed to enhance hemostatic function; and (4) the use of thrombopoietic growth factors.

Treatments for Specific Causes of Thrombocytopenia

If the condition is identified, treatment of the underlying cause of thrombocytopenia is indicated; treatment methods are discussed elsewhere. For TTP, treatment may include plasma exchange, as well as corticosteroids (see Chapter 24). For ITP, corticosteroids, intravenous immunoglobulin (IVIg) and splenectomy are commonly effective (see Chapter 9). For HIT, stopping the heparin and starting an alternative anticoagulant would be advised (see Chapter 25). Other drugs that are believed to cause thrombocytopenia should be discontinued.

Platelet Transfusions

Platelet transfusion is the mainstay for the treatment of thrombocytopenia. Each year, more than 2 million platelet transfusions are given at a cost of over $1 billion.[81–83] About 75% are apheresis platelets, and the rest are whole blood–derived platelet concentrates. About one third of all platelet transfusions are used to treat active bleeding; the rest are administered prophylactically.[84]

Although considerable consensus has been reached about the use of therapeutic platelet transfusions to treat bleeding in thrombocytopenic patients, much debate continues about the use of prophylactic platelet transfusions in the nonbleeding patient. Table 8-3 provides suggested guidelines for administration of platelet transfusions. In the following discussion, data are presented to support these recommendations.

What is the transfusion target for bleeding patients?

In bleeding patients, transfusion is indicated to increase platelet count to at least 40,000/μL until the bleeding stops, although some prefer a target of 100,000/μL.[82] These recommendations are not based on any clinical trial data.

Table 8-3 Platelet Transfusion Guidelines*

Platelet transfusions are contraindicated in the following situations:
Thrombotic thrombocytopenic purpura/hemolytic-uremic syndrome
Heparin-induced thrombocytopenia

Platelet transfusions may be of minimal effect in the following situations, and use should be limited to situations of life-threatening bleeding:
Idiopathic thrombocytopenic purpura (ITP)
Disseminated intravascular coagulation (DIC)
Platelet alloimmunization (with high panel-reactive antibody [PRA] titer and/or no demonstrable corrected count increment [CCI])
Patients with chronic thrombocytopenia due to aplastic anemia, myelodysplastic syndrome (MDS) in the absence of bleeding

Platelet transfusions can be administered in the following situations without restriction:
Active bleeding and platelet count <50,000/μL or demonstrable platelet function defect (uremia, known storage pool defect, after cardiac bypass)
Nonbleeding patients who have the following:
Temporary myelosuppression and platelets <10,000/μL (<20,000/μL if febrile or with minor bleeding)
Need for major surgery or central nervous system (CNS) procedures and platelet count <100,000/μL
Other surgery or procedures in which potential bleeding can be visualized or external pressure applied and platelet count <50,000/μL
Need for surgery or procedure in a patient with known platelet dysfunction (von Willebrand disease [VWD], uremia) for whom other measures (1-deamino-8-D-arginine vasopressin [DDAVP], dialysis) may be ineffective
Cardiac bypass patients who have the following:
Increased chest tube bleeding and no abnormal coagulation abnormalities with platelets <100,000/μL
Increased chest tube bleeding and known platelet function defect

*From Massachusetts General Hospital Transfusion Committee Guidelines based on AABB and other guidelines.[99]

What is an adequate platelet count for procedures?

In thrombocytopenic patients who are about to undergo procedures, the platelet target has not been established by clinical studies. The British Committee for Standards in Haematology has recommended the following:[85]

1. Routine dentistry—10,000/μL
2. Dental extractions—30,000/μL
3. Regional dental block—30,000/μL
4. Minor surgery—50,000/μL
5. Major surgery—80,000/μL

A recent study has suggested that a platelet count of 50,000/μL is safe in patients with ITP who are undergoing epidural anesthesia.[86]

When should prophylactic platelet transfusions be given?

Whether prophylactic platelet transfusions enhance survival and decrease bleeding has never been the subject of a placebo-controlled clinical trial. Certainly, clinical experience from William Duke to the present has convinced clinicians of their important effects in both areas.[87,88] A matter of concern involves the question of what platelet count "trigger" patients should be given. Although current data suggest that this trigger is probably 10,000/μL in most subjects (possibly 5000/μL in some), treatment of each patient should be individualized. Factors other than platelet count help the clinician to determine the overall bleeding risk of a thrombocytopenic patient. These include underlying disease, fever, infection, coagulopathy, and concurrent medications. For these reasons, the decision about prophylactic platelet transfusions must take into account the patient's condition and the clinical setting in which thrombocytopenia occurs.[14,15]

Several studies in leukemic patients have convincingly showed that a prophylactic platelet transfusion trigger of 10,000/μL (10,000/μL to 20,000/μL if febrile, bleeding, or undergoing procedures) results in the same rate of major bleeding as a transfusion trigger of 20,000/μL. In one study,[14] major bleeding (defined as any bleeding greater than petechial, mucosal, or retinal bleeding) occurred in 21.5% and 20% of patients, and on 3.1% and 2.0% of hospital days in the two groups, respectively. Red cell transfusions were the same in the two groups, but platelet transfusions were 21.5% fewer in the group transfused at 10,000/μL. In another study of leukemic patients,[16] bleeding complications (World Health Organization [WHO] grades 2 to 4) occurred in 18% of those transfused at 10,000/μL versus 17% of those transfused at 20,000/μL. Serious bleeding events (WHO grades 3 to 4) were unrelated to platelet count but were associated with local lesions, sepsis, or coagulation abnormalities. Those transfused at 10,000/μL required one third fewer platelet transfusions. Several other studies in patients with leukemia and stem cell transplants have also confirmed these findings.[89–91] It is possible that in patients without leukemia who are given chemotherapy, a trigger of 5000/μL may be adequate.[92]

What platelet product should be used?

At equivalent doses, pooled single-donor platelets have the same hemostatic benefit as apheresis platelets. Apheresis platelets are often preferred for presumed reasons of efficiency, testing, bacterial contamination, white blood cell (WBC) removal, reduced donor exposure, and possible future bacterial and viral inactivation. Platelets that have been leukoreduced by bedside filtration or apheresis are preferred in most situations to reduce alloimmunization, febrile nonhemolytic transfusion reactions, and cytomegalovirus (CMV) infection (something accomplished equally well by selection of CMV-negative donors). This is particularly important in patients who will be receiving repeated transfusions, in those who are immunocompromised, and in those receiving chemotherapy; it is probably not important in surgical patients or those who have experienced trauma. To eliminate the small risk of acquired graft-versus-host disease, platelets should be irradiated if obtained from a related donor, or if the recipient is highly immunocompromised.

What dose of platelets should be given?

The average whole blood–derived platelet concentrate is required to contain 5.5×10^{10} platelets, but it usually contains 8.0 to 9.0×10^{10} platelets.[93] Apheresis platelets are required to have on average 3.0×10^{11} platelets, but centers may collect 3 to 4 times that amount from any single donor. Administration of 1×10^{11} platelets for each meter

of body surface area should increase the platelet count by 8000/μL to 10,000/μL 1 hour after transfusion; this provides the basis for the corrected count increment (CCI). These anticipated increments are affected by multiple other variables ranging from fever to splenomegaly to alloimmunization.

In bleeding patients, the dose should be that which increases the platelet count to the target ranges described previously.

Unfortunately, the dose in prophylactic settings has not been well established. It has become customary to transfuse 4 to 6 U of whole blood–derived platelet concentrates or a single apheresis platelet unit. However, lower doses may be effective. In a recent trial, thrombocytopenic leukemic or transplant patients received a low dose (three random donor concentrates = 2×10^{11} platelets) or a standard dose (five random donor concentrates = 4×10^{11} platelets) of platelets. Minor bleeding events occurred in 20% of low-dose and 40% of standard-dose patients, and major bleeds occurred in 10.7% of low-dose and 7.3% of standard-dose patients; 25% fewer platelet units were used in the low-dose group.[94,95] A larger multicenter trial is currently under way to test the hemostatic benefits of various dose levels. Mathematical models suggest that small daily platelet doses are more economical and produce fewer donor exposures than do larger, less frequent transfusions.[96,97] In contrast, one study showed that larger doses of platelets markedly reduced the frequency of prophylactic platelet transfusions[98] and may have reduced bleeding.

What are the complications of platelet transfusions?

These are well described in other reviews and monographs.[99] In brief, these include bacterial infection, hepatitis, alloimmunization, febrile nonhemolytic transfusion reactions, urticarial reactions, and CMV infection .

Enhanced Hemostatic Function

In some thrombocytopenic patients, platelet transfusions may not be effective because of alloimmunization; in others, the platelet count may be moderately depressed (30,000/μL to 60,000/μL), but platelets are dysfunctional because of uremia. Others may refuse blood products. In such settings, efforts to enhance overall hemostatic function may be helpful.

In both situations, the use of antifibrinolytics such as ε-aminocaproic acid (EACA) (Amicar; Wyeth, Madison, NJ, USA) or tranexamic acid (Cyclokapron; Pharmacia, Mississauga, Canada) may be effective. (The latter agent is currently available only as an intravenous formulation.) Daily doses of 2 to 24 g of EACA have been found to decrease bleeding in immune and nonimmune thrombocytopenias.[100–102]

A more recent therapeutic option has been the use of recombinant factor VIIa (rFVIIa) (NovoSeven; Novo Nordisk, Princeton, NJ, USA). A recent report analyzed 24 cases of hemorrhage in patients with thrombocytopenia and hematologic malignancy.[103] All but one patient improved, and 46% experienced abrupt cessation of bleeding. This modality warrants further clinical study.

In addition to dialysis, a number of modalities improve platelet function in uremia. Whether these improve platelet function in nonuremic, thrombocytopenic patients has been the subject of anecdote only. By raising the hematocrit to greater than 30% through transfusion or erythroid growth factors, bleeding is reduced in uremic patients.[104–107] A proposed mechanism for this effect is that because red cells flow in the center of the blood vessel lumen, a higher hematocrit "pushes" the platelets to the periphery and increases interactions with the endothelium.[108] Other modalities that have proved effective involve the administration of DDAVP (1-deamino-8-D-arginine vasopressin), cryoprecipitate, and estrogens. Although DDAVP and cryoprecipitate work within 15 minutes and last for 4 to 6 hours, it may take weeks for the effects of estrogens to become apparent.

Thrombopoietic Growth Factors

Over the past decade, a number of hematopoietic growth factors have been shown to increase platelet production. These include interleukin (IL)-3, IL-6, and IL-11, as well as TPO and various TPO mimetics.[26] Of these, only IL-11 and the TPOs have been developed for clinical use. Although these therapies may ameliorate chronic thrombocytopenia, they will never replace platelet transfusions for the acute treatment of thrombocytopenia; with all of these treatment approaches, at least 5 days must pass before platelet count is increased, and usually 10 to 14 days are needed for maximal effect. Only one platelet growth factor, IL-11, has been approved by the U.S. Food and Drug Administration (FDA); TPOs and TPO mimetics are still in clinical development, but several should become available soon.[109]

IL-11

IL-11 is not required for platelet formation in normal physiology; animals that are deficient in it have normal platelet counts but are sterile.[110] Nonetheless, IL-11 increases megakaryocyte number and platelet count. In studies in patients undergoing standard chemotherapy, administration of a daily 50-μg per kilogram dose of recombinant IL-11 (oprelvekin) (Neumega; Wyeth Pharmaceuticals, Philadelphia, Pa, USA) reduced the need for platelet transfusions from 96% in the placebo group to 70% in the treated group.[111] Oprelvekin is currently FDA approved at that dose for the prevention of thrombocytopenia in patients undergoing nonmyeloablative chemotherapy who have experienced thrombocytopenia during a prior cycle, and for whom dose reduction is not appropriate. Oprelvekin is not widely used because of its significant adverse effects, which include dilutional anemia, fluid retention, congestive heart failure, arrhythmias, and anaphylaxis. At a daily dose of 10 μg per kilogram, some patients with bone marrow failure have had an increase in platelet count.[112]

Thrombopoietin and Thrombopoietin Mimetics

TPO, the primary regulator of platelet production in normal physiology, accounts for more than 90% of all platelet production.[113] The first generation of clinical thrombopoietins included recombinant human TPO (rHTPO, a glycosylated, full-length version of the native molecule) and pegylated recombinant human megakaryocyte growth and development factor (PEG-rHuMGDF, a nonglycosylated, truncated TPO coupled to polyethylene glycol). Both of these recombinant TPOs bound to the TPO receptor and were very potent stimulators of platelet production in healthy individuals. These platelet growth factors increased the nadir platelet count in patients undergoing nonmyeloablative chemotherapy and reduced the need for platelet transfusions.[114,115] In patients with ITP and MDS, they increased platelet counts,[116] and when given to platelet apheresis donors, they increased platelet yield.[98,117,118] However, in stem cell transplantation and acute leukemia treatments, they had no effect on time to platelet recovery or number of platelet transfusions.[119] These recombinant TPOs did increase the yield of CD34 cells when added to standard stem cell mobilization schemes, but the mobilized product was only marginally more effective during engraftment.[120] After antibodies developed against PEG-rHuMGDF and caused thrombocytopenia, development of both of these growth factors ceased.[121]

Recently, a second generation of platelet growth factors has been developed to avoid the problem of antibody formation. One of these, AMG-531, is a TPO mimetic that contains four peptides that bind and activate the TPO receptor and that are incorporated into the immunoglobulin Fc domain.[122,123] This molecule is not antigenic, has a half-life of longer than 120 hours, and is a potent stimulator of platelet production in healthy humans. It has been shown to normalize platelet count in more than 85% of patients with ITP, when given weekly by a subcutaneous route.[124]

A second family of platelet growth factors consists of the small nonpeptide molecules that bind the TPO receptor at a site distant from the binding site for TPO.[125–132] These dimerize and activate the TPO receptor and promote platelet production in healthy humans. One of these, eltrombopag, has been extensively developed and has been shown to normalize the platelet count in 85% of patients with ITP, when given orally on a daily basis. It also normalizes the platelet count in patients with thrombocytopenia due to liver disease.

Both AMG-531 and eltrombopag are in the late stages of clinical development and will probably initially receive FDA approval for the treatment of ITP. They should also be effective in treating thrombocytopenia related to liver disease, nonmyeloablative chemotherapy, and possibly MDS. Both should be effective in increasing platelet apheresis yields. So far, use of neither has shown any major toxicity.

Acknowledgments

This work was supported in part by NIH grants HL72299 and HL082889.

REFERENCES

1. Spaet T: Platelets: The blood dust. In Wintrobe M (ed): Blood, Pure and Eloquent, New York, McGraw-Hill, 1980, pp 549–571.
2. Kuter DJ: Cover art: The watercolor drawings of James Homer Wright. Stem Cells 16:ix–x, 1998.
3. Wright JH: A rapid method for the differential staining of blood films and malarial parasites. J Medical Res 7:138–144, 1902.
4. Wright JH: The origin and nature of blood plates. Boston Med Surg J 154:643–645, 1906.
5. Wright JH: The histogenesis of the blood platelets. J Morph 21:263–278, 1910.
6. Duke WW: The relationship of blood platelets to hemorrhagic disease: Description of a method for determining the bleeding time and coagulation time. JAMA 55:1185–1192, 1910.
7. Akca S, Haji-Michael P, de Mendonca A, et al: Time course of platelet counts in critically ill patients. Crit Care Med 30:753–756, 2002.

8. Vanderschueren S, De Weerdt A, Malbrain M, et al: Thrombocytopenia and prognosis in intensive care. Crit Care Med 28:1871–1876, 2000.

9. Stephan F, Hollande J, Richard O, et al: Thrombocytopenia in a surgical ICU. Chest 115:1363–1370, 1999.

10. Kuter DJ: Thrombocytopenia and thrombocytosis. In Furie B, Cassileth PA, Atkins MB, and Mayer RJ (eds): Clinical Hematology and Oncology: Presentation, Diagnosis, and Treatment, Philadelphia, Churchill Livingstone, 2003, pp 221–231.

11. von Behrens W: Evidence of phylogenic canalisation of the circulating platelet mass in man. Thromb Diath Haemorrh 27:159–172, 1972.

12. Harker LA, Slichter SJ: The bleeding time as a screening test for evaluation of platelet function. N Engl J Med 287:155–159, 1972.

13. Rodgers RP, Levin J: A critical reappraisal of the bleeding time. Semin Thromb Hemost 16:1–20, 1990.

14. Rebulla P, Finazzi G, Marangoni F, et al: The threshold for prophylactic platelet transfusions in adults with acute myeloid leukemia. N Engl J Med 337:1870–1875, 1997.

15. Rebulla P: Trigger for platelet transfusion. Vox Sang 78 (suppl 2): 179–182, 2000.

16. Wandt H, Frank M, Ehninger G, et al: Safety and cost effectiveness of a 10×10^9/L trigger for prophylactic platelet transfusions compared with the traditional 20×10^9/L trigger: A prospective comparative trial in 105 patients with acute myeloid leukemia. Blood 91:3601–3606, 1998.

17. Slichter SJ: Optimizing platelet transfusions in chronically thrombocytopenic patients. Semin Hematol 35:269–278, 1998.

18. Slichter SJ, LeBlanc R, Jones MK: Quantitative analysis of bleeding risk in cancer patients prophylactically transfused at platelet (PLT) counts (CTS) of, 5,000, 10,000, or 20,000. Blood 94:376a, 1999.

19. Slichter SJ, Harker LA: Thrombocytopenia: Mechanisms and management of defects in platelet production. Clin Haematol 7:523–539, 1978.

20. Hanson SR, Slichter SJ: Platelet kinetics in patients with bone marrow hypoplasia: Evidence for a fixed platelet requirement. Blood 66:1105–1109, 1985.

21. Slichter SJ: Relationship between platelet count and bleeding risk in thrombocytopenic patients. Transfus Med Rev 18:153–167, 2004.

22. Slichter SJ: Background, rationale, and design of a clinical trial to assess the effects of platelet dose on bleeding risk in thrombocytopenic patients. J Clin Apher 21:78–84, 2006.

23. Chantarangkul V, Clerici M, Bressi C, et al: Thrombin generation assessed as endogenous thrombin potential in patients with hyper- or hypocoagulability. Haematologica 88:547–554, 2003.

24. Chantarangkul V, Clerici M, Bressi C, Tripodi A: Standardization of the endogenous thrombin potential measurement: How to minimize the effect of residual platelets in stored plasma. Br J Haematol 124:355–357, 2004.

25. Kuter DJ: The Platelet. In Beck WS (ed): Hematology, 5th ed. Cambridge, Mass., MIT Press, pp 543–576, 1991.

26. Kuter DJ, Begley CG: Recombinant human thrombopoietin: Basic biology and evaluation of clinical studies. Blood 100:3457–3469, 2002.

27. Hamada T, Mohle R, Hesselgesser J, et al: Transendothelial migration of megakaryocytes in response to stromal cell–derived factor 1 (SDF-1) enhances platelet formation. J Exp Med 188:539–548, 1998.

28. Avecilla ST, Hattori K, Heissig B, et al: Chemokine-mediated interaction of hematopoietic progenitors with the bone marrow vascular niche is required for thrombopoiesis. Nat Med 10:64–71, 2004.

29. Heissig B, Ohki Y, Sato Y, et al: A role for niches in hematopoietic cell development. Hematology 10:247–253, 2005.

30. Kopp HG, Avecilla ST, Hooper AT, Rafii S: The bone marrow vascular niche: Home of HSC differentiation and mobilization. Physiology (Bethesda) 20:349–356, 2005.

31. Levine RF, Eldor A, Shoff PK, et al: Circulating megakaryocytes: Delivery of large numbers of intact, mature megakaryocytes to the lungs. Eur J Haematol 51:233–246, 1993.

32. Levine RF, Shoff P, Han ZC, Eldor A: Circulating megakaryocytes and platelet production in the lungs. Prog Clin Biol Res 356:41–52, 1990.

33. Trowbridge EA, Harley PJ: A stochastic model of pulmonary platelet production. J Math Appl Med Biol 5:45–63, 1988.

34. Trowbridge EA: Pulmonary platelet production: A physical analogue of mitosis? Blood Cells 13:451–465, 1988.

35. Trowbridge EA, Martin JF, Slater DN: Evidence for a theory of physical fragmentation of megakaryocytes, implying that all platelets are produced in the pulmonary circulation. Thromb Res 28:461–475, 1982.

36. Kuter DJ: Apoptosis in platelets during ex vivo storage. Vox Sang 83 (suppl 1): 311–313, 2002.

37. Bertino AM, Qi XQ, Li J, et al: Apoptotic markers are increased in platelets stored at 37 degrees C. Transfusion 43:857–866, 2003.

38. Xia Y, Li J, Bertino A, Kuter DJ: Thrombopoietin and the TPO receptor during platelet storage. Transfusion 40:976–987, 2000.

39. Berger G, Hartwell DW, Wagner DD: P-selectin and platelet clearance. Blood 92:4446–4452, 1998.

40. Gurney AL, Carver-Moore K, de Sauvage FJ, Moore MW: Thrombocytopenia in c-Mpl–deficient mice. Science 265:1445–1447, 1994.

41. Peck-Radosavljevic M, Zacherl J, Meng YG, et al: Is inadequate thrombopoietin production a major cause of thrombocytopenia in cirrhosis of the liver? J Hepatol 27:127–131, 1997.

42. Peck-Radosavljevic M, Wichlas M, Zacherl J, et al: Thrombopoietin induces rapid resolution of thrombocytopenia after orthotopic liver transplantation through increased platelet production. Blood 95:795–801, 2000.

43. Shivdasani RA, Fielder P, Keller GA, et al: Regulation of the serum concentration of thrombopoietin in thrombocytopenic NF-E2 knockout mice. Blood 90:1821–1827, 1997.

44. Yang C, Li YC, Kuter DJ: The physiological response of thrombopoietin (c-Mpl ligand) to thrombocytopenia in the rat. Br J Haematol 105:478–485, 1999.

45. Stoffel R, Wiestner A, Skoda RC: Thrombopoietin in thrombocytopenic mice: Evidence against regulation at the mRNA level and for a direct regulatory role of platelets. Blood 87:567–573, 1996.

46. Emmons RV, Reid DM, Cohen RL, et al: Human thrombopoietin levels are high when thrombocytopenia is due to megakaryocyte deficiency and low when due to increased platelet destruction. Blood 87:4068–4071, 1996.

47. Nichol JL: Thrombopoietin levels after chemotherapy and in naturally occurring human diseases. Curr Opin Hematol 5:203–208, 1998.

48. Lonial S, Waller EK, Richardson PG, et al: Risk factors and kinetics of thrombocytopenia associated with bortezomib for relapsed, refractory multiple myeloma. Blood 106:3777–3784, 2005.

49. Sweeney JD, Holme S, Heaton WA, et al: Pseudothrombocytopenia in plateletpheresis donors. Transfusion 35:46–49, 1995.

50. Cohen AM, Cycowitz Z, Mittelman M, et al: The incidence of pseudothrombocytopenia in automatic blood analyzers. Haematologia (Budap) 30:117–121, 2000.

51. Shalev O, Lotman A: Images in clinical medicine: Pseudothrombocytopenia. N Engl J Med 329:1467, 1993.

52. Sane DC, Damaraju LV, Topol EJ, et al: Occurrence and clinical significance of pseudothrombocytopenia during abciximab therapy. J Am Coll Cardiol 36:75–83, 2000.

53. Schell DA, Ganti AK, Levitt R, Potti A: Thrombocytopenia associated with c7E3 Fab (abciximab). Ann Hematol 81:76–79, 2002.

54. Veenhoven WA, van der Schans GS, Huiges W, et al: Pseudothrombocytopenia due to agglutinins. Am J Clin Pathol 72:1005–1008, 1979.

55. Onder O, Weinstein A, Hoyer LW: Pseudothrombocytopenia caused by platelet agglutinins that are reactive in blood anticoagulated with chelating agents. Blood 56:177–182, 1980.

56. Watkins SP, Shulman NR: Platelet cold agglutinins. Blood 36:153–158, 1970.

57. Kjeldsberg CP, Hershgold EJ: Spurious thrombocytopenia. JAMA 227:628–630, 1974.

58. Aster RH: Pooling of platelets in the spleen: Role in the pathogenesis of "hypersplenic" thrombocytopenia. J Clin Invest 45:645–657, 1966.

59. Aster RH: Studies of the mechanism of "hypersplenic" thrombocytopenia in rats. J Lab Clin Med 70:736–751, 1967.

60. De Gabriele G, Penington DG: Regulation of platelet production: "Thrombopoietin". Br J Haematol 13:210–215, 1967.

61. De Gabriele G, Penington DG: Physiology of the regulation of platelet production. Br J Haematol 13:202–209, 1967.

62. De Gabriele G, Penington DG: Regulation of platelet production: "Hypersplenism" in the experimental animal. Br J Haematol 13:384–393, 1967.

63. Koike Y, Yoneyama A, Shirai J, et al: Evaluation of thrombopoiesis in thrombocytopenic disorders by simultaneous measurement of reticulated platelets of whole blood and serum thrombopoietin concentrations. Thromb Haemost 79:1106–1110, 1998.

64. Harker LA: Kinetics of thrombopoiesis. J Clin Invest 47:458–465, 1968.

65. Harker LA, Finch CA: Thrombokinetics in man. J Clin Invest 48:963–974, 1969.

66. McMillan R, Wang L, Tomer A, et al: Suppression of in vitro megakaryocyte production by antiplatelet autoantibodies from adult patients with chronic ITP. Blood 103:1364–1369, 2004.

67. Ballem PJ, Segal GM, Stratton JR, et al: Mechanisms of thrombocytopenia in chronic autoimmune thrombocytopenic purpura: Evidence of both impaired platelet production and increased platelet clearance. J Clin Invest 80:33–40, 1987.

68. Ballem PJ, Belzberg A, Devine DV, et al: Kinetic studies of the mechanism of thrombocytopenia in patients with human immunodeficiency virus infection. N Engl J Med 327:1779–1784, 1992.

69. Harker LA, Carter RA, Marzec UM, et al: Correction of thrombocytopenia and ineffective platelet production in patients infected with human immunodeficiency virus (HIV) by PEG-rHu MGDF therapy. Blood 92:707a, 1998.

70. Kuter DJ, Tillotson GS: Hematologic effects of antimicrobials: Focus on the oxazolidinone, linezolid. Pharmacotherapy 21:1010–1013, 2001.

71. Gerson SL, Kaplan SL, Bruss JB, et al: Hematologic effects of linezolid: Summary of clinical experience. Antimicrob Agents Chemother 46:2723–2726, 2002.

72. Abel G, Kuter DJ: Association of thrombocytopenia with continuous venovenous hemofiltration. Blood 100:221a, 2002.

73. Vonderheide RH, Thadhani R, Kuter DJ: Association of thrombocytopenia with the use of intra-aortic balloon pumps. Am J Med 105:27–32, 1998.

74. Cohen YC, Djulbegovic B, Shamai-Lubovitz O, Mozes B: The bleeding risk and natural history of idiopathic thrombocytopenic purpura in patients with persistent low platelet counts. Arch Intern Med 160:1630–1638, 2000.

75. Butros LJ, Bussel JB: Intracranial hemorrhage in immune thrombocytopenic purpura: A retrospective analysis. J Pediatr Hematol Oncol 25:660–664, 2003.

76. Karpatkin S, Garg SK: The megathrombocyte as an index of platelet production. Br J Haematol 26:307–311, 1974.

77. Karpatkin S: Biochemical and clinical aspects of megathrombocytes. Ann N Y Acad Sci 201:262–279, 1972.

78. Ault KA, Rinder HM, Mitchell J, et al: The significance of platelets with increased RNA content (reticulated platelets): A measure of the rate of thrombopoiesis. Am J Clin Pathol 98:637–646, 1992.

79. Gyongyossy-Issa MI, Miranda J, Devine DV: Generation of reticulated platelets in response to whole blood donation or plateletpheresis. Transfusion 41:1234–1240, 2001.

80. Kelton JG, Powers PJ, Carter CJ: A prospective study of the usefulness of the measurement of platelet-associated IgG for the diagnosis of idiopathic thrombocytopenic purpura. Blood 60:1050–1053, 1982.

81. Heal JM, Blumberg N: Optimizing platelet transfusion therapy. Blood Rev 18:149–165, 2004.

82. Strauss RG: Low-dose prophylactic platelet transfusions: Time for further study, but too early for routine clinical practice. Transfusion 44:1680–1682, 2004.

83. Wallace EL, Churchill WH, Surgenor DM, et al: Collection and transfusion of blood and blood components in the United States, 1994. Transfusion 38:625–636, 1998.

84. McCullough J, Steeper TA, Connelly DP, et al: Platelet utilization in a university hospital. JAMA 259:2414–2418, 1988.

85. Guidelines for the use of platelet transfusions. Br J Haematol 122:10–23, 2003.

86. Webert KE, Mittal R, Sigouin C, et al: A retrospective 11-year analysis of obstetric patients with idiopathic thrombocytopenic purpura. Blood 102:4306–4311, 2003.

87. Roy AJ, Jaffe N, Djerassi I: Prophylactic platelet transfusions in children with acute leukemia: A dose response study. Transfusion 13:283–290, 1973.

88. Higby DJ, Cohen E, Holland JF, Sinks L: The prophylactic treatment of thrombocytopenic leukemic patients with platelets: A double blind study. Transfusion 14:440–446, 1974.

89. Heckman KD, Weiner GJ, Davis CS, et al: Randomized study of prophylactic platelet transfusion threshold during induction therapy for adult acute leukemia: 10,000/microL versus 20,000/microL. J Clin Oncol 15:1143–1149, 1997.

90. Zumberg MS, del Rosario ML, Nejame CF, et al: A prospective randomized trial of prophylactic platelet transfusion and bleeding incidence in hematopoietic stem cell transplant recipients: 10,000/L versus 20,000/microL trigger. Biol Blood Marrow Transplant 8:569–576, 2002.

91. Gmur J, Burger J, Schanz U, et al: Safety of stringent prophylactic platelet transfusion policy for patients with acute leukaemia. Lancet 338:1223–1226, 1991.

92. Fanning J, Hilgers RD, Murray KP, et al: Conservative management of chemotherapeutic-induced thrombocytopenia in women with gynecologic cancers. Gynecol Oncol 59:191–193, 1995.

93. Murphy S: Platelet transfusion. In Loscalzq J, Schafer A (eds): Platelet Transfusion Therapy in Thrombosis and Hemorrhage, Baltimore, Williams & Wilkins, 1998, pp 1119–1134.

94. Tinmouth A, Macdougall L, Fergusson D, et al: Reducing the amount of blood transfused: A systematic review of behavioral interventions to change physicians' transfusion practices. Arch Intern Med 165:845–852, 2005.

95. Tinmouth A, Tannock IF, Crump M, et al: Low-dose prophylactic platelet transfusions in recipients of an autologous peripheral blood progenitor cell transplant and patients with acute leukemia: A randomized controlled trial with a sequential Bayesian design. Transfusion 44:1711–1719, 2004.

96. Brecher ME, Hom EG, Hersh JK: Optimal platelet dosing. Transfusion 39:431–434, 1999.

97. Hersh JK, Hom EG, Brecher ME: Mathematical modeling of platelet survival with implications for optimal transfusion practice in the chronically platelet transfusion-dependent patient. Transfusion 38:637–644, 1998.

98. Goodnough LT, Kuter DJ, McCullough J, et al: Prophylactic platelet transfusions from healthy apheresis platelet donors undergoing treatment with thrombopoietin. Blood 98:1346–1351, 2001.

99. McFarland J: Platelet transfusion: Indications and adverse effects. In McCrae K (ed): Thrombocytopenia, New York, Taylor & Francis, 2006, pp 275–306.

100. Bartholomew JR, Salgia R, Bell WR: Control of bleeding in patients with immune and nonimmune thrombocytopenia with aminocaproic acid. Arch Intern Med 149:1959–1961, 1989.

101. Gardner FH, Helmer RE 3rd: Aminocaproic acid: Use in control of hemorrhage in patients with amegakaryocytic thrombocytopenia. JAMA 243:35–37, 1980.

102. Chakrabarti S, Varma S, Singh S, Kumari S: Low dose bolus aminocaproic acid: An alternative to platelet transfusion in thrombocytopenia? Eur J Haematol 60:313–314, 1998.

103. Brenner B, Hoffman R, Balashov D, et al: Control of bleeding caused by thrombocytopenia associated with hematologic malignancy: An audit of the clinical use of recombinant activated factor VII. Clin Appl Thromb Hemost 11:401–410, 2005.

104. Gordge MP, Leaker B, Patel A, et al: Recombinant human erythropoietin shortens the uraemic bleeding time without causing intravascular haemostatic activation. Thromb Res 57:171–182, 1990.

105. Vigano G, Benigni A, Mendogni D, et al: Recombinant human erythropoietin to correct uremic bleeding. Am J Kidney Dis 18:44–49, 1991.

106. el-Shahawy MA, Francis R, Akmal M, Massry SG: Recombinant human erythropoietin shortens the bleeding time and corrects the abnormal platelet aggregation in hemodialysis patients. Clin Nephrol 41:308–313, 1994.

107. Weigert AL, Schafer AI: Uremic bleeding: Pathogenesis and therapy. Am J Med Sci 316:94–104, 1998.

108. Anand A, Feffer SE: Hematocrit and bleeding time: An update. South Med J 87:299–301, 1994.

109. Kuter DJ: The promise of thrombopoietins in the treatment of ITP. Clin Adv Hematol Oncol 3:464–466, 2005.

110. Nandurkar HH, Robb L, Tarlinton D, et al: Adult mice with targeted mutation of the interleukin-11 receptor (IL11Ra) display normal hematopoiesis. Blood 90:2148–2159, 1997.

111. Tepler I, Elias L, Smith JW 2nd, et al: A randomized placebo-controlled trial of recombinant human interleukin-11 in cancer patients with severe thrombocytopenia due to chemotherapy. Blood 87:3607–3614, 1996.

112. Tsimberidou AM, Giles FJ, Khouri I, et al: Low-dose interleukin-11 in patients with bone marrow failure: Update of the M. D. Anderson Cancer Center experience. Ann Oncol 16:139–145, 2005.

113. de Sauvage FJ, Carver-Moore K, Luoh SM, et al: Physiological regulation of early and late stages of megakaryocytopoiesis by thrombopoietin. J Exp Med 183:651–656, 1996.

114. Fanucchi M, Glaspy J, Crawford J, et al: Effects of polyethylene glycol–conjugated recombinant human megakaryocyte growth and development factor on platelet counts after chemotherapy for lung cancer. N Engl J Med 336:404–409, 1997.

115. Vadhan-Raj S, Verschraegen CF, Bueso-Ramos C, et al: Recombinant human thrombopoietin attenuates carboplatin-induced severe thrombocytopenia and the need for platelet transfusions in patients with gynecologic cancer. Ann Intern Med 132:364–368, 2000.

116. Nomura S, Dan K, Hotta T, et al: Effects of pegylated recombinant human megakaryocyte growth and development factor in patients with idiopathic thrombocytopenic purpura. Blood 100:728–730, 2002.

8

117. Kuter DJ, Goodnough LT, Romo J, et al: Thrombopoietin therapy increases platelet yields in healthy platelet donors. Blood 98:1339–1345, 2001.

118. Vadhan-Raj S, Kavanagh JJ, Freedman RS, et al: Safety and efficacy of transfusions of autologous cryopreserved platelets derived from recombinant human thrombopoietin to support chemotherapy-associated severe thrombocytopenia: A randomised cross-over study. Lancet 359:2145–2152, 2002.

119. Schiffer CA, Miller K, Larson RA, et al: A double-blind, placebo-controlled trial of pegylated recombinant human megakaryocyte growth and development factor as an adjunct to induction and consolidation therapy for patients with acute myeloid leukemia. Blood 95:2530–2535, 2000.

120. Somlo G, Sniecinski I, ter Veer A, et al: Recombinant human thrombopoietin in combination with granulocyte colony-stimulating factor enhances mobilization of peripheral blood progenitor cells, increases peripheral blood platelet concentration, and accelerates hematopoietic recovery following high-dose chemotherapy. Blood 93:2798–2806, 1999.

121. Li J, Yang C, Xia Y, et al: Thrombocytopenia caused by the development of antibodies to thrombopoietin. Blood 98:3241–3248, 2001.

122. Broudy VC, Lin NL: AMG531 stimulates megakaryopoiesis in vitro by binding to Mpl. Cytokine 25:52–60, 2004.

123. Wang B, Nichol JL, Sullivan JT: Pharmacodynamics and pharmacokinetics of AMG 531, a novel thrombopoietin receptor ligand. Clin Pharmacol Ther 76:628–638, 2004.

124. Kuter DJ, Bussel J, Aledort L, et al: A phase 2 placebo controlled study evaluating the platelet response and safety of weekly dosing with a novel thrombopoietic protein (AMG 531) in thrombocytopenic adult patients with immune thrombocytopenic purpura. Blood 104:148a, 2004.

125. Duffy KJ, Darcy MG, Delorme E, et al: Hydrazinonaphthalene and azonaphthalene thrombopoietin mimics are nonpeptidyl promoters of megakaryocytopoiesis. J Med Chem 44:3730–3745, 2001.

126. Duffy KJ, Shaw AN, Delorme E, et al: Identification of a pharmacophore for thrombopoietic activity of small, non-peptidyl molecules. 1. Discovery and optimization of salicylaldehyde thiosemicarbazone thrombopoietin mimics. J Med Chem 45:3573–3575, 2002.

127. Duffy KJ, Price AT, Delorme E, et al: Identification of a pharmacophore for thrombopoietic activity of small, non-peptidyl molecules. 2. Rational design of naphtho(1,2-d)imidazole thrombopoietin mimics. J Med Chem 45:3576–3578, 2002.

128. Jenkins J, Nicholl R, Williams D, et al: An oral, non-peptide, small molecule thrombopoietin receptor agonist increases platelet counts in healthy subjects. Blood 104:797a, 2004.

129. Erickson-Miller C, Delorme E, Iskander M, et al: Species specificity and receptor domain interaction of a small molecule TPO receptor agonist. Blood 104:795a, 2004.

130. Erickson-Miller CL, Delorme E, Tian SS, et al: Discovery and characterization of a selective, non-peptidyl thrombopoietin receptor agonist. Blood 96:675a, 2000.

131. Erickson-Miller CL, Delorme E, Giampa L, et al: Biological activity and selectivity for Tpo receptor of the orally bioavailable, small molecule Tpo receptor agonist, SB-497115. Blood 104:796a, 2004.

132. Erickson-Miller CL, DeLorme E, Tian SS, et al: Discovery and characterization of a selective, nonpeptidyl thrombopoietin receptor agonist. Exp Hematol 33:85–93, 2005.

Chapter 9

Immune Thrombocytopenic Purpura

James N. George, MD • Kiarash Kojouri, MD, MPH

Immune thrombocytopenic purpura (ITP) is defined as isolated thrombocytopenia with no clinically apparent associated conditions or other causes of thrombocytopenia.[1-4] No specific criteria establish the diagnosis of ITP; the diagnosis requires the exclusion of other causes of thrombocytopenia.[1-4] ITP can be an acute disorder, with abrupt onset of bleeding symptoms and spontaneous resolution in several weeks or months. These clinical features may occur in adults,[5] but they are more common in children younger than 10 years old, in whom acute and spontaneously resolving ITP is the rule.[6-8] ITP can be a chronic disorder, with an insidious onset of minor bleeding symptoms and persistent, perhaps even permanent, thrombocytopenia. This thrombocytopenia may be unexpectedly discovered on routine blood studies in asymptomatic patients. This is the common clinical course in adults[9] and adolescents.[10] In some patients, long-term durable remission may be punctuated by an acute episode of symptomatic thrombocytopenia that may be caused by a viral illness and may not indicate recurrence of chronic, persistent thrombocytopenia. This chapter focuses on the issues of diagnosis and management of ITP in adults.

Because ITP is a persistent disorder, and because the mortality is negligible, the prevalence is great. The incidence of ITP in adults has been estimated in two recent prospective studies to be 16 to 27 patients newly given the diagnosis per million population per year.[11,12] Both of these studies[11,12] documented the following consistent and important observations: (1) The incidence of ITP has increased, principally because of heightened detection of asymptomatic patients with mild thrombocytopenia—an inevitable result of the wider use of routine platelet counts. Currently, as many as one third of patients with ITP may be discovered incidentally.[11-14] (2) A surprising observation was that incidence increases with age.[11,12] (3) The female predominance that was so characteristic present in previous case series and that was present in the study from Denmark[11] of patients younger than 60 years old was not evident in patients older than 60 years of age. Therefore, the common assumption that ITP in adults is primarily a disease of young women may be incorrect; ITP is now recognized with increasing frequency among older patients of either sex.

PATHOGENESIS

The principal cause of ITP is increased platelet destruction caused by antiplatelet autoantibodies. However, some studies have shown a concomitant lack of compensatory increase in marrow production of platelets, or even a decrease in platelet production, in patients with clinically typical ITP.[15] Dimished platelet production may be the result of suppression of marrow megakaryocytes by antiplatelet autoantibodies.[16-18] Interpretation of these observations is difficult because the methods required to document these abnormalities—increased destruction and relative marrow failure—are complex and are not easily reproducible. Measurement of antiplatelet antibodies is not a routine clinical laboratory test, and even in research laboratories, sensitivity and specificity are low and of limited clinical value.[19] Estimates of platelet kinetics to document platelet production rates are dependent on radioisotope labeling of autologous platelets, and these studies are technically difficult. For example, even though they may be preferred for avoidance of alloantibody sensitization,[15] the use of autologous platelets is associated with the risk that a patient's platelets that remain in the circulation may be younger and relatively less susceptible to destruction, and may therefore survive longer. This would be interpreted as indicating less platelet turnover and therefore less platelet production when compared with kinetic studies, in which isotope-labeled donor platelets from a normal subject who may have a shorter survival time are used.

In spite of these technical issues, the principal cause of increased platelet destruction is supported by in vivo studies in human volunteers that demonstrate the presence of antiplatelet antibodies in the plasma of patients with ITP. The initial classic report of Harrington, Hollingsworth, and others, in which they described infusing themselves with plasma from a woman with acute, severe ITP and the resulting prompt, profound thrombocytopenia,[20] has been retold in graphic detail.[21] Shulman and others subsequently extended these studies with quantitative assessment of infusions of ITP plasma into normal and asplenic subjects (Fig. 9-1).[22] Increasingly larger volumes of plasma from a patient with ITP that were transfused into a recipient who did not have ITP caused increasingly severe thrombocytopenia. Higher doses of ITP plasma were required to cause the same degree of thrombocytopenia in an asplenic subject, thus documenting the role of the spleen in removing antibody-sensitized platelets. Glucocorticoids administered to the recipient also blunted the ability of ITP plasma to cause thrombocytopenia when infused into a normal subject (see Fig. 9-1). In this series of investigations, an estimate of the titer of antiplatelet antibody could be deduced by infusion studies in normal subjects: Table 9-1 shows that patients with higher titers of antiplatelet antibodies were those with more severe ITP who were less responsive to treatment. The epitope specificity of antiplatelet antibodies may also contribute to the

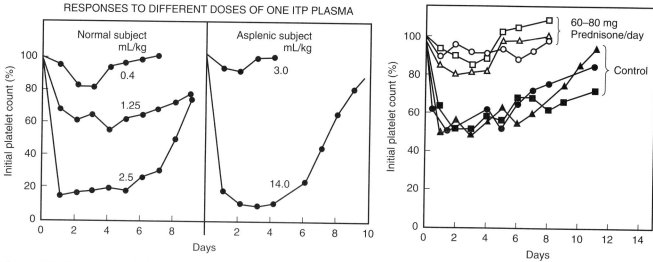

Figure 9-1 Responses to infusions of plasma from patients with ITP into normal subjects. The left two panels illustrate the occurrence of thrombocytopenia in a normal subject following different doses of plasma from a patient with ITP, as well as the results of infusion of the same ITP plasma into a splenectomized subject. Note that the ITP plasma dose that did not produce thrombocytopenia in the splenectomized subject was greater than the dose that produced marked thrombocytopenia in the normal subject. The right panel illustrates the effects of prednisone on response to ITP plasma. Plasma from a patient with ITP was infused into three normal subjects without and with treatment with prednisone, 60 to 80 mg/day. Prednisone was begun 3 hours, 1 day, or 3 days before the plasma was infused and was continued for a minimum of 7 days. Control infusions were given 1 and 2 months before, and 3 weeks after, treatment with prednisone was administered. (Adapted from Shulman NR, Weinrach RS, Libre EP, Andrews HL: The role of the reticuloendothelial system in the pathogenesis of idiopathic thrombocytopenic purpura. Trans Assoc Am Physicians 1965;78:374–390, with permission.)

Table 9-1   Correlation Between In Vivo Assessment of the Titer of Antiplatelet Antibody and Response to Treatment

Patient With ITP	Titer of Antiplatelet Antibody	Platelet Count (per μL)		
		Before Prednisone	*After Prednisone*	*After Splenectomy*
1	<1:3	12,000	70,000	200,000
2	<1:3	5000	200,000	400,000
3	<1:3	<1000	200,000	-
4	<1:3	2000	200,000	-
5	1:3	5000	100,000	-
6	1:20	5000	25,000	30,000
7	1:20	3000	10,000	10,000
8	1:20	9000	12,000	15,000
9	1:40	<1000	2000	2000
10	1:50	1500	2000	2000

Antiplatelet antibody titer was determined as the dilution of the plasma of each patient with immune thrombocytopenic purpura (ITP) that caused an approximately 50% decrease in platelet count in a normal recipient, similar to the dose of 1.25 mL/kg in Figure 9-1 *(left)*. If a plasma volume of 40 mL/kg is assumed, this plasma would have an estimated titer of 1:32. Plasma from patients with estimated titers of less than 1:3 did not cause a 50% decrease in a normal recipient's platelet count, even when 15 mL/kg (approximately 1 L) was infused. Patients 3, 4, and 5 did not undergo splenectomy. Adapted from Shulman NR, Weinrach RS, Libre EP, Andrews HL: The role of the reticuloendothelial system in the pathogenesis of idiopathic thrombocytopenic purpura. Trans Assoc Am Physicians 1965;78:374-390, with permission.

severity of bleeding symptoms. Antiplatelet antibodies that react with the fibrinogen-binding site of glycoprotein (GP)-IIb/IIIa may interfere with platelet function.[23]

EVALUATION OF A PATIENT WHO PRESENTS WITH ISOLATED THROMBOCYTOPENIA

An algorithm for a diagnostic approach to isolated thrombocytopenia is presented in Figure 9-2. Medical history, physical examination, and examination of peripheral blood smear are sufficient to exclude other possible causes of thrombocytopenia and to establish the diagnosis of ITP in most patients. Certainly, these time-honored activities are sufficient in patients with incidentally discovered asymptomatic thrombocytopenia; they may also be the only items that are essential for the evaluation of patients who present with severe, symptomatic thrombocytopenia. The response to treatment and the clinical course of symptomatic patients provide additional diagnostic confirmation.

Several features of peripheral blood morphology are critical in the diagnosis of ITP (Table 9-2). First, actual thrombocytopenia should be confirmed. No abnormalities of red

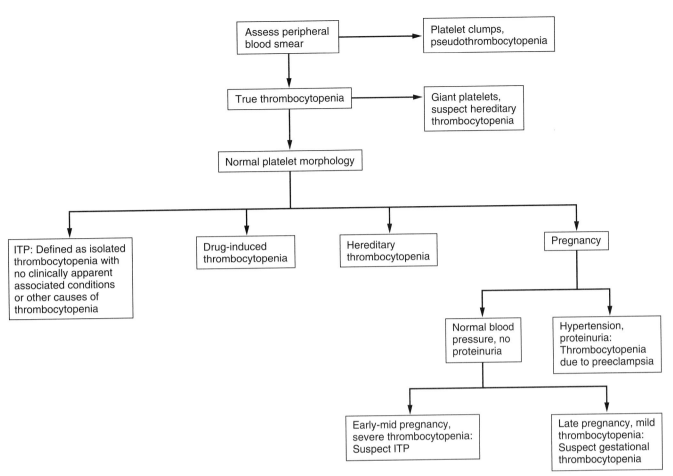

Figure 9-2 Algorithm for the evaluation of isolated thrombocytopenia in an otherwise healthy person. (From George NJ: Platelets. Lancet 2000;355:1531–1539, with permission from Elsevier Science.)

Table 9-2 The Peripheral Blood Smear in Immune Thrombocytopenic Purpura (ITP)

Features Consistent With the Diagnosis of ITP

Thrombocytopenia, with normal platelet size and morphology, or slightly larger than normal platelets

Normal red cell number and morphology. Exceptions may be abnormalities from expected associated conditions, such as iron deficiency from chronic bleeding, or incidental conditions, such as thalassemia minor

Normal white cell number and morphology

Features Not Consistent With the Diagnosis of ITP

Predominance of giant platelets with diameters similar to those of red cells

Red cell abnormalities, such as schistocytes, oval macrocytes, teardrop cells, and nucleated red cells

Leukocytosis or leukopenia with immature or abnormal cells

---

cell or white cell number or morphology should be present, other than expected associated conditions such as iron deficiency from chronic bleeding or incidental conditions such as thalassemia minor. Platelet morphology should be normal, although some reports describe a larger size of platelets in ITP, postulated to represent younger "stress" platelets produced in response to accelerated peripheral platelet destruction. However, the presence of truly giant platelets, approaching or exceeding the size of red blood cells, is

not consistent with the diagnosis of ITP but suggests the presence of congenital thrombocytopenia.[24]

Tests for antiplatelet antibodies are *not* recommended for the diagnostic evaluation of patients with suspected ITP.[1,3,4] Measurements of platelet-associated immunoglobulin (Ig)G merely reflect the plasma IgG concentration and platelet α granule content of plasma proteins.[25] In multiple studies, the sensitivity and specificity of commercial tests for antiplatelet antibody detection are poor,[19,26] and results with multiple assays for antiplatelet antibodies in which identical split samples were used in multiple research laboratories were inconsistent in one study.[27] Therefore, the possibility of misinformation is high.

Contrary to the opinion of some physicians, splenomegaly is rarely present in ITP. One large study reported palpable spleens in only 7 of 271 (2.6%) patients[28]—a frequency similar to the 2.9% incidence of palpable spleens noted in healthy college students.[29] Enlargement of the spleen should broaden the differential diagnosis to include thrombocytopenia that may be part of immune disorders characterized by an enlarged spleen, notably chronic lymphocytic leukemia. Additionally, the spleen may be enlarged when patients have concomitant Coombs-positive hemolytic anemia (so-called Evan syndrome) or when patients actually have hypersplenism rather than ITP.

The role of bone marrow aspirate examination is controversial. Some hematologists believe that it is necessary in all patients who present with a new observation of thrombocytopenia; other hematologists believe that a bone marrow aspirate examination in all patients with suspected ITP is inappropriate.[1] Guidelines for the evaluation of patients with suspected ITP have suggested that bone marrow aspirate examination conducted to exclude the possibility of myelodysplasia may be appropriate in patients older than 60 years of age.[1,3] Bone marrow aspirate examination may also be appropriate when a patient is unresponsive to initial treatment, or when splenectomy is considered.[1,3,4] However, in most patients, bone marrow aspirate examination is not helpful in the differential diagnosis. For example, other than in myelodysplasia and acquired pure megakaryocytic aplasia, bone marrow aspirate examination would not be helpful for the differential diagnostic possibilities listed in Table 9-3. Systematic studies in adults[30] and children[31] with suspected ITP have documented that bone marrow aspirate examination provided an alternative diagnosis only when abnormalities were identified during the initial evaluation by history, physical examination, and examination of the peripheral blood smear.

DIFFERENTIAL DIAGNOSIS OF ITP

The differential diagnosis of ITP includes all disorders that can manifest with unexpected observation of a low platelet count or purpura. Because the diagnosis of ITP requires

Table 9-3 Differential Diagnosis of Immune Thrombocytopenic Purpura (ITP)

Disorders	Clinical Features
Pseudothrombocytopenia	
EDTA-dependent clumping	Actual platelet count normal but falsely low on laboratory report because platelets are clumped in vitro and on blood smear
Platelet satellitism	Actual platelet count normal; in vitro platelets adhere to granulocytes or monocytes
Common Causes of Thrombocytopenia	
Drug-induced thrombocytopenia	Initially indistinguishable from ITP. Diagnosis established by prompt recovery on withdrawal of the drug and, in some circumstances, rechallenge. May also be caused by nutritional supplements, herbal remedies, foods
Pregnancy	Asymptomatic, mild thrombocytopenia common near term and may actually be an exacerbation of subclinical ITP. More severe thrombocytopenia may accompany preeclampsia/HELLP syndrome
Hypersplenism	Asymptomatic mild thrombocytopenia may be the initial clue to occult liver disease
Infection	Asymptomatic mild thrombocytopenia may occur with HIV infection, viral immunization, or EBV infection. More severe thrombocytopenia may be prominent with rickettsial infection, *Ehrlichia*, or leptospirosis
Less Common Causes of Thrombocytopenia	
Congenital thrombocytopenias	Typically mistaken for ITP and inappropriately treated
Bernard-Soulier syndrome	Giant platelets. Autosomal recessive, therefore consanguinity common. Bleeding symptoms greater than expected because of GP-Ib-IX abnormality and defective VWF binding
MYH9-related thrombocytopenia	Giant platelets, granulocyte inclusions. Autosomal dominant. Typically mild bleeding symptoms. Also, sensorineural deafness and nephritis may occur
Fanconi syndrome	Autosomal recessive, short stature. May manifest in adults with isolated thrombocytopenia but typically progresses to aplasia or myelodysplasia
Wiskott-Aldrich syndrome	X-linked. Small platelets. Typically associated with eczema and immunodeficiency but may manifest as isolated thrombocytopenia
Thrombocytopenia with absent radius	Autosomal recessive, associated with multiple skeletal anomalies. Typically manifests as severe thrombocytopenia in infancy but may cause mild thrombocytopenia in adults
Other uncharacterized congenital thrombocytopenias	May be autosomal dominant, recessive, or X-linked. Family history is the key to diagnosis
von Willebrand disease, type 2B	Autosomal dominant thrombocytopenia due to in vivo platelet clumping and clearance caused by abnormal VWF. Bleeding symptoms more serious than expected because of associated VWF deficiency
Myelodysplasia	May manifest as isolated thrombocytopenia in older patients
Chronic disseminated intravascular coagulation	May be detected initially because of thrombocytopenia
Thrombotic thrombocytopenic purpura-hemolytic-uremic syndrome	Typically acute onset with multiple organ dysfunction, but may have a prodrome of isolated thrombocytopenia
Acquired pure megakaryocytic aplasia	Indistinguishable from ITP until marrow aspirate is done because of poor response to treatment

EDTA, ethylenediaminetetraacetic acid; HELLP, syndrome of hemolytic anemia, elevated liver enzymes, and low platelet count; HIV, human immunodeficiency syndrome; EBV, Epstein-Barr virus; GP, glycoprotein; VWF, von Willebrand factor.

the exclusion of other causes of thrombocytopenia, the conditions listed in Table 9-3 must be considered.

Pseudothrombocytopenia

Pseudothrombocytopenia is consistently observed in 1 in 1000 subjects and is not related to the presence or absence of any disease (Figs. 9-3 and 9-4) (Table 9-4).[32–37] The most common cause of pseudothrombocytopenia is a "naturally occurring" autoantibody against a neo-epitope on GP-IIb/IIIa, exposed by the ethylenediaminetetraacetic acid (EDTA) anticoagulant used for routine blood counts.[38] In EDTA, these autoantibodies cause platelet clumping and falsely low platelet counts in vitro. Platelet counts in citrate-anticoagulated blood are usually, but not always, normal, as calcium chelation by citrate is not strong enough to alter the configuration of the GP-IIb/IIIa molecule. EDTA-dependent platelet agglutinins are of no clinical importance,[39] except that they may contribute to the acute thrombocytopenia that can occur with initial administration of GP-IIb/IIIa–blocking antithrombotic agents, which may cause structural alteration of GP-IIb/IIIa, similar to EDTA.[40] Pseudothrombocytopenia may result from in vitro platelet adherence ("satellitism") to leukocytes, typically granulocytes.[41] This phenomenon may occur only in EDTA-anticoagulated blood.[41] Either cause of pseudothrombocytopenia will be clearly seen during examination of the peripheral blood smear.

Drug-Induced Thrombocytopenia

Drug-induced thrombocytopenia cannot initially be distinguished from ITP. A careful history not only of drugs[42] but also of foods,[43] herbal remedies,[44,45] and nutritional products[46] must be obtained. Especially in patients with intermittent acute thrombocytopenia,[46] these agents must be excluded as the cause before a diagnosis of ITP can be confidently established. A critical purpose for the investigation of drug-induced thrombocytopenia is to emphasize to the patient that it is not only prescription drugs that may be involved. For example, quinine is probably the most commonly currently reported cause of drug-induced thrombocytopenia,[12,42] but patients may not recognize quinine as a "drug"; therefore, they may continue to use it, even after they have been advised to discontinue all medications.[46] Furthermore, quinine is present in tonic water,[47] as well as in over-the-counter nutritional supplements,[46] in sufficient concentrations to cause profound thrombocytopenia. Drug-dependent antibodies are not demonstrable in all patients with drug-induced thrombocytopenia.[48] Effective diagnostic strategies include observation of recovery from thrombocytopenia within 7 days after discontinuation of all drugs and other potentially causative compounds, and fortuitous observations after the offending agent is reintroduced.[42] Patients with symptomatic thrombocytopenia are typically treated with prednisone; therefore, even platelet

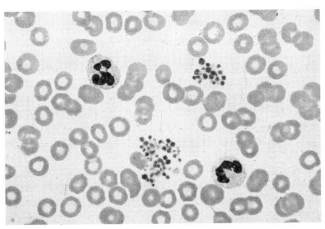

Figure 9-3 *(See also Color Plate 9-3.)* Platelet clumping. Note that several platelets clump to one another on the peripheral blood smear. This clumping is independent of the nearby neutrophils.

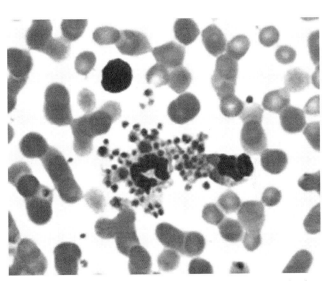

Figure 9-4 *(See also Color Plate 9-4.)* Platelet satellitism. Platelets adhere in a necklace-like pattern around two neutrophils yet do not clump together.

Table 9-4 Frequency of Pseudothrombocytopenia Caused by EDTA-Dependent Platelet Agglutinins	
Study	**Frequency**
Payne and Pierre:[32] All platelet counts for 1 yr at Mayo Clinic	124/143,000; 0.09%
Savage:[33] All platelet counts for 9 mo at Cleveland Clinic	154/135,806; 0.11%
Vicari et al:[34] All platelet counts for 1 yr at Istituto S. Raffaele, Milan	43/33,623; 0.13%
Garcia Suarez et al:[35] Ambulatory patients, Asturias Hospital, Madrid	23/20,760; 0.11%
Sweeney et al:[36] Healthy blood donors, Norfolk, Virginia	2/945; 0.21%
Bartels et al:[37] Hospital and clinic patients in The Netherlands	46/45,000; 0.10%

EDTA, ethylenediaminetetraacetic acid.

count recovery may not allow a distinction from ITP. Some "complete remissions" of ITP after prednisone is taken may actually be due to occult drug-induced thrombocytopenia. Continuing systematic reviews, updated through October 2006, have evaluated all published case reports with the use of standardized criteria for assessing the causal relationship of drugs to thrombocytopenia (http://moon.ouhsc.edu/jgeorge).

Pregnancy

Mild thrombocytopenia, typically with platelet counts above 70,000/μL, occurs in 5% of women as pregnancy approaches term, and it resolves spontaneously after delivery.[49] This abnormality has been called "gestational thrombocytopenia" or "incidental thrombocytopenia of pregnancy," and it has been deemed to be a pregnancy-related syndrome, distinct from ITP.[1] Diagnostic features include (1) asymptomatic, mild thrombocytopenia, (2) with no past history of thrombocytopenia (except possibly during a previous pregnancy), (3) occurring during late gestation, (4) that is not associated with fetal thrombocytopenia, and (5) that resolves spontaneously after delivery.[1] However, several observations suggest that gestational thrombocytopenia may be only a common, mild, and transient presentation of ITP, perhaps an exacerbation of platelet destruction for which compensation is normally provided by increased platelet production. First, multiple different methods for detecting antiplatelet antibodies could not distinguish patients with a clinical diagnosis of ITP from those with gestational thrombocytopenia who were diagnosed by the previous criteria.[50] Second, patients with ITP and mild or moderate thrombocytopenia may have lower platelet counts toward the end of pregnancy that return to previous levels after delivery.[51] This is consistent with clinical observations in other autoimmune disorders that can become exacerbated during pregnancy. For example, hemolysis increased in 18 of 19 patients with autoimmune hemolytic anemia during the third trimester of pregnancy and resolved during the first 3 months postpartum.[52] Third, the risk of neonatal thrombocytopenia may be related to the severity of maternal thrombocytopenia,[53] consistent with early observations on higher titers of antiplatelet antibodies in patients with severe ITP (see Table 9-1).[22] Therefore, it may be anticipated that women whose ITP becomes clinically apparent only during pregnancy, but who otherwise have normal platelet counts, would not be expected to have thrombocytopenic infants at birth.

Hypersplenism

Perhaps the most common cause of thrombocytopenia among hospitalized patients is the mild thrombocytopenia caused by splenic pooling due to portal hypertension and congestive splenomegaly. The most common cause of portal hypertension is intrinsic liver disease, but other causes include extrahepatic portal hypertension due to splanchnic venous thrombosis or systemic venous hypertension, such as from cardiopulmonary disease (see Chapter 39). In these patients, thrombocytopenia is typically mild, with platelet counts rarely below 40,000/μL and with most in the range of 50,000 to 90,000/μL. Total body platelet counts are actually normal, as is platelet survival; the only abnormality is passive pooling of most platelets in the congested, enlarged spleen.[54] Patients with severe thrombocytopenia associated with liver disease may also have decreased platelet production caused by decreased thrombopoietin synthesis in the liver.[55]

Infection

Human immunodeficiency virus (HIV) may cause thrombocytopenia that is indistinguishable from ITP due to infection of marrow stromal cells[56] (see Chapter 13). Other viral infections and even immunizations[57] commonly cause a decreased platelet count, although rarely to levels that are symptomatic. Thrombocytopenia mimicking ITP may be the initial manifestation of disseminated tuberculosis.[58] In some infections, such as Rocky Mountain spotted fever and ehrlichiosis,[59] severe and symptomatic thrombocytopenia may occur, but other systemic signs and symptoms distinguish these disorders from ITP (see Chapter 11).

Congenital Thrombocytopenias
(see Chapter 10)

Adults with newly recognized congenital thrombocytopenia are almost always mistakenly given the initial diagnosis of and treatment for ITP.[24] Many well-described syndromes of congenital thrombocytopenia have been described (see Table 9-3), but perhaps most common are disorders that fit no described syndrome.[24] Syndromes previously described as May-Hegglin anomaly, Epstein, Fechtner, and Sebastian syndromes, or Alport syndrome variants are now known to have the same genotypic origin: mutation of *MYH9*, the gene that encodes the nonmuscle myosin, heavy-chain IIA.[24,60] The key diagnostic feature is a family history of a low platelet count, which is often not initially recognized. Problematic with the misdiagnosis of ITP are unfortunate therapeutic interventions with glucocorticoids, rituximab, or even splenectomy that are not efficacious. Congenital thrombocytopenia should be considered in patients whose platelet counts are unresponsive to initial prednisone treatment, who have unusually large platelets or neutrophil inclusions (e.g., Döhle bodies) on their peripheral blood smear, who have other inherited anomalies such as skeletal deformities, or who have a family history of consanguinity, which increases the opportunity for expression of autosomal recessive traits.

The presence of truly giant platelets that are similar in diameter to red cells should suggest congenital thrombocytopenia (see Table 9-2). Inherited giant platelet disorders are heterogeneous, typically are associated with minimal bleeding symptoms, and often are initially misdiagnosed as ITP.[61-64] In some inherited syndromes, abnormalities such as skeletal deformities, nephritis, and sensorineural deafness may be associated (see Table 9-3). In some syndromes, a greater amount of bleeding may occur than would be expected for the degree of thrombocytopenia because of an associated platelet function defect, as in Bernard-Soulier syndrome, or an associated hemostatic disorder, as in von Willebrand disease, type 2B (see Table 9-3). However, most patients with congenital thrombocytopenia have no distinguishing clinical features other than moderate thrombocytopenia.[24,65,66]

Myelodysplasia

Myelodysplasia may manifest as isolated thrombocytopenia,[67,68] but this is uncommon. Patients with chronic ITP may have monoclonal hematopoiesis,[69] suggesting the possibility that in some patients, ITP and myelodysplasia may be overlapping syndromes.[70] Because myelodysplastic syndromes are much more frequent among older patients, bone marrow aspiration and biopsy are appropriate when patients present with apparent ITP at the age of 60 years or older.[1,3] This was, of course, a consideration in a recent epidemiologic study on the incidence of ITP[11] that documented a higher than expected occurrence among older men. However, in this study, most older patients had bone marrow examinations that were normal, and no patient with ITP from the study period subsequently developed a myelodysplastic syndrome.[11]

Disseminated Intravascular Coagulation

Although it is very rare for disseminated intravascular coagulation (DIC) to occur in the absence of an overt clinical cause, and even more rare for chronic, indolent DIC to present as isolated thrombocytopenia, this has been observed.[71] Patients with large hemangiomas may have localized intravascular coagulation, which may first be recognized in adulthood as asymptomatic thrombocytopenia. A comparable but more severe disorder that presents in infancy is the Kasabach-Merritt syndrome.[72] Recognition of this possibility is important for an awareness of the broad spectrum of abnormalities that can mimic ITP and lead to inappropriate treatment (see Chapter 12).

Thrombotic Thrombocytopenic Purpura–Hemolytic-Uremic Syndromes

The thrombotic thrombocytopenic purpura–hemolytic-uremic syndromes (TTP-HUS) typically present as acute severe illness with symptoms and signs of multiple organ dysfunction. However, patients may have a syndrome of isolated, asymptomatic thrombocytopenia that is indistinguishable from ITP. This is increasingly apparent with close follow-up of patients who have recovered from TTP-HUS. In these patients, incidentally discovered thrombocytopenia may or may not predict a relapse of acute TTP-HUS (see Chapter 24).

Acquired Pure Megakaryocytic Aplasia

Autoantibodies to thrombopoietin or megakaryocytes may cause severe thrombocytopenia associated with absent marrow megakaryocytes, which may be indistinguishable from ITP until a bone marrow aspiration is done. Patients may not respond to prednisone and intravenous immune globulin (IVIg) but can achieve durable remission with cyclosporine and antithymocyte globulin—the more intensive immunosuppressive regimen used for aplastic anemia.[73]

Thrombocytopenia Associated With Other Autoimmune Disorders

Patients in whom thrombocytopenia is part of a clinically overt autoimmune or lymphoproliferative[74] disorder are considered to be distinct from those with ITP because the clinical course is determined by the primary disease. For example, in patients with Graves disease and thrombocytopenia, thrombocytopenia often resolves with effective treatment of hyperthyroidism.[75] However, isolated abnormalities of serologic tests for antinuclear antibodies or antiphospholipid antibodies are frequently encountered in patients with typical ITP and do not influence its management or clinical course.[76–78]

MANAGEMENT OF ITP

The single goal in the management of ITP is to prevent major bleeding. Therefore, the practical goal is to maintain a safe platelet count. Cure is not a goal. Although simple in concept, this principle of management is essential for preventing the common occurrence of making adverse effects of treatment worse than symptoms of the disease.

What is a Safe Platelet Count?

The consistent clinical observation is that most patients with ITP never have clinically important bleeding, even when their platelet counts are very low. Easy bruising may be common and petechiae may be numerous, but truly extensive purpura with innumerable petechiae and extensive ecchymoses is very rare. These cutaneous bleeding symptoms are often referred to as "dry purpura,"[79] to distinguish them from overt mucous membrane bleeding, such as persistent epistaxis or gingival bleeding, referred to as "wet purpura." Wet purpura is less common but more alarming and may be associated with greater risk for major bleeding. The feared complication of ITP is intracranial hemorrhage, which is too rare to have a documented incidence among patients with ITP. Suggestions have been made that the incidence may be 0.1% to 1.0%,[1] but this high frequency, if true, would be relevant only to patients with severe and symptomatic thrombocytopenia.

Few platelets are required to provide adequate hemostasis. Clinical studies in other disorders, such as aplastic anemia[80] and thrombocytopenia after chemotherapy for acute leukemia,[81,82] suggest that spontaneous, clinically important bleeding does not occur with platelet counts above 5000 to 10,000/μL. Because younger platelets are assumed to have greater hemostatic capability than older platelets,[83] patients with ITP may have even less risk for bleeding at comparable platelet counts compared with patients with thrombocytopenia caused by marrow failure. Therefore, an analogy may be made to patients with hemophilia, in whom the presence of any measurable factor VIII or factor IX transforms a disease with severe bleeding risk to a clinically occult disorder.[84]

Initial Management of ITP in Children

Conservative management of ITP in children yields important lessons for its management in adults. Because spontaneous remission occurs in most children within several weeks to months, some pediatric hematologists believe that careful observation without specific treatment is sufficient, even when thrombocytopenia is severe.[6,85] Although platelet counts in children recover more quickly with glucocorticoid or IVIg treatment,[86] no studies have shown that more rapid recovery results in less bleeding. Although many pediatric hematologists treat children initially with IVIg or anti-D,[87] these agents are expensive, are not always promptly available, may require hospitalization, and produce frequent adverse side effects of headache with nausea and vomiting[88] that can mimic intracranial hemorrhage, causing severe alarm and thus requiring further diagnostic study.[88,89] Anti-D can cause severe intravascular hemolysis with frequently fatal DIC.[90]

For children whose ITP does not spontaneously resolve, conservative management without specific treatment remains a common practice. In a recent audit of 427 children with ITP in the United Kingdom, only 3 had undergone splenectomy.[91] Avoidance of splenectomy is in part related to the continuous occurrence of spontaneous remission in children, even after many years,[92,93] but this decision is made also because of concern for subsequent severe sepsis, particularly when splenectomy is performed before age 5.[94]

Although bleeding risks may be greater in older adults than in children because of comorbidities such as hypertension,[95,96] adults have the advantage of moderating their activity and avoiding trauma; these are difficult assignments for young children.

Initial Treatment of Adult Patients who have Incidentally Discovered Asymptomatic Thrombocytopenia

If the patient is asymptomatic, probably no specific therapy is indicated. However, in standard practice, the method of treatment of patients with ITP is linked to the level of thrombocytopenia. If it is assumed that a platelet count above 10,000/µL is safe,[80–82] then a reasonable belief would be that treatment is unnecessary for patients with platelet counts above 20,000/µL.[4] Although observation without specific treatment is a common standard of care for children who present with a new diagnosis of acute ITP, even when platelet counts are less than 10,000/µL,[6,85] in adults, because of uncertainty regarding the stability of persistent thrombocytopenia and because of the simplicity of initial oral prednisone therapy, initial treatment with prednisone is inevitably prescribed unless the platelet count is significantly higher than 10,000 to 20,000/µL.

Multiple case series have followed adult patients with newly diagnosed ITP and platelet counts above 20,000 to 50,000/µL[12–14,96,97] who were given no specific treatment. In these case series with median follow-up durations of 3 to 10 years, no adverse outcomes of major bleeding were reported. A few of these patients may develop more severe thrombocytopenia and may require treatment; also, in a few patients, the platelet count may spontaneously return to normal.[12,97] However, it appears that in most patients, incidentally detected mild thrombocytopenia is persistent for the duration of follow-up.[14] If no specific treatment is prescribed, then the interval for measuring the platelet count becomes an issue. If the interval between platelet counts seems too long, the patient becomes apprehensive and the physician may appear unconcerned. On the other hand, platelet counts measured too frequently may cause patient apprehension that results from an obsessive focus

on clinically unimportant variations. Resolution of this issue requires thorough patient education about the nature of ITP, its clinical course, its risks, and the goals of treatment. Resources for reliable patient education include the websites of the National Heart, Lung, and Blood Institute (http://dci.nhlbi.nih.gov/Disease/Itp/ITP_What Is.html), the ITP Support Association (http://itpsupport.uk), and the University of Oklahoma (http://ouhsc.edu/jgeorge). After several platelet counts have been taken to establish the consistency of thrombocytopenia, patients must be gradually weaned from dependence on knowing their current platelet count.

Initial Treatment of Adult Patients who Present with Severe Thrombocytopenia and Symptomatic Purpura

Adults with symptomatic purpura are treated initially with glucocorticoids.[4] Prednisone is a commonly used agent; the dosage is empirical, but 1 mg/kg/day given as a single dose is a common standard regimen, but lower doses may be as effective.[98] Most, but not all, patients respond with a decrease in formation of new petechiae and an increase in platelet count; then the dose is gradually tapered. A case can be made for more rapid tapering of prednisone to determine whether severe, symptomatic thrombocytopenia at presentation was perhaps a transient, reversible occurrence in the course of more mild ITP, or perhaps occult drug-induced thrombocytopenia.[12] If severe thrombocytopenia recurs on tapering of prednisone, this becomes an indication for splenectomy. Patients may urge withdrawal of prednisone because of the misery caused by symptoms of emotional lability, inability to concentrate, tremulousness, difficulty sleeping, and the inevitably depressing "moon facies." Of greater concern is that prednisone doses equivalent to or even less than physiologic cortisol secretion (2.5 to 5.0 mg prednisone/day) may cause bone loss within several months through impairment of normal diurnal cortisol secretion.[99,100] In spite of the rationale for quick tapering of the prednisone dose, some hematologists believe that a greater opportunity to achieve durable remission and to avoid splenectomy arises when a more prolonged course of prednisone therapy with gradual tapering is carried out.

An alternative initial glucocorticoid regimen is dexamethasone 40 mg/day given for 4 days.[101] In this report, 106 (85%) of 125 patients whose initial platelet counts were lower than 20,000/µL responded; 53 (50%) of those who responded maintained this safe platelet count without further treatment for the duration of follow-up (median, 2.5 yr).[101] If the success reported by this experience[101] is confirmed by outcomes described in subsequent reports, this regimen has the advantage of a brief course, although with a very high dose, of glucocorticoids. Short-term complications of mood disturbance and hyperglycemia may be important, but the destructive long-term complications of prolonged glucocorticoid treatment can be avoided.

IVIg and anti-D are treatments given to temporarily increase platelet count; they have occasionally been used in the initial treatment of patients with ITP. IVIg may cause systemic symptoms of myalgia, fever, nausea, and headache in one third of patients.[88] Actual aseptic meningitis may occur,[89] with signs mimicking intracranial hemorrhage. Acute renal failure has also been reported and appears related to osmotic injury to proximal renal tubules associated with the sucrose content of the IVIg product.[102,103] Therefore, older patients, those with preexisting renal insufficiency, and those who are receiving concomitant nephrotoxic drugs should be given IVIg only with caution.

An anti-Rh(D) product developed for the treatment of patients with ITP was based on the hypothesis that hemolysis caused by alloantibodies in IVIg may be the mechanism for blocking sequestration of autoantibody-coated platelets. This product is a preparation of anti-Rh(D) alloantibodies, often referred to simply as anti-D. Anti-D is easier to administer than IVIg (a 3- to 5-minute infusion compared with administration over several hours), but it is effective only in patients whose red cells are D positive and appears to be effective only in nonsplenectomized patients.[104] It causes fewer systemic symptoms, and the major and dose-limiting adverse effect is alloimmune hemolytic anemia; severe, life-threatening intravascular hemolysis with DIC has been reported.[90,105] Although the typical regimen of anti-D (50 to 75 μg/kg given once) costs less than a regimen of IVIg (the approximate cost for a course of IVIg in an adult is $10,000 to $15,000; for anti-D, $5000 to $8000), these are both expensive treatments. Much less expensive (approximately $100) is the use of intravenous methylprednisolone, which may have efficacy comparable with that of IVIg and anti-D.

A randomized clinical trial conducted to determine whether intermittent initial treatment of adults with anti-D may allow spontaneous remission to occur and splenectomy to be avoided, while avoiding complications of glucocorticoids has been performed.[106] Although splenectomy was deferred, it was not avoided,[106] consistent with other experiences in which spontaneous remissions of ITP were uncommon in adults.

Treatment of Patients with Acute Bleeding Due to Severe Thrombocytopenia

Patients must be alert for the symptoms and signs of acute bleeding, and physicians must be prepared for emergency care. For a bleeding emergency, in addition to conventional critical care measures, appropriate treatments include platelet transfusions, high-dose parenteral glucocorticoids, and IVIg.[1] Emergency splenectomy may also be important in providing more immediate and durable recovery from severe thrombocytopenia.[107] Despite a presumably short platelet survival time, platelet transfusions may provide substantial platelet count increments in some patients.[108,109] Continuous infusion of platelets to provide continual hemostatic support has been suggested.[110] High-dose glucocorticoids, such as 1 g/day of methylprednisolone given by intravenous infusion and repeated daily for 2 additional days, can rapidly increase the platelet count. IVIg, given as 1 g/kg/day for 2 days, increases the platelet count in most patients within 3 days. Furthermore, IVIg given before a platelet transfusion may increase the platelet count increment and prolong the duration of response.[111] In patients with critical bleeding who do not respond to these treatments, recombinant factor VIIa may be effective.[112,113]

Splenectomy

In adult patients who continue to have severe and symptomatic thrombocytopenia after initial glucocorticoid treatment, splenectomy is traditionally the next treatment consideration. Although splenectomy is not universally effective (or else it would be recommended sooner and more often), the relative efficacy of splenectomy is better than that of any other treatment given to patients with ITP.[114] The response to splenectomy may be prompt, supporting experimental observations (see Fig. 9-1) that the spleen is the principal source of removal of autoantibody-coated platelets. The response to splenectomy may also be durable, consistent with the spleen as the major source of autoantibody production. Most case series suggest that approximately two thirds of patients achieve and sustain a normal platelet count after splenectomy, thereby requiring no additional therapy.[114]

Historically, splenectomy was the first effective treatment for ITP; it was established long before glucocorticoid therapy was initiated in the 1950s. Numerous case series describe the results of splenectomy, but many of these reports describe patients who lived decades ago, when splenectomy was often performed as initial therapy at diagnosis and was routinely performed in children and adults. These earlier studies included patients who would now retrospectively be expected to have undergone spontaneous recovery; therefore, they consistently reported better than average outcomes. Even among adults, younger patients respond better to splenectomy than do older patients.[114] Although many other preoperative variables, such as previous response to prednisone or IVIg, or degree of splenic sequestration of radioisotope-labeled platelets, have been reported to correlate with patient response to splenectomy, none is sufficiently consistent to influence the decision to perform a splenectomy.[114]

Consistent with an apparent trend toward conservative management of adults with ITP attained by not treating patients with asymptomatic thrombocytopenia, the frequency of splenectomy appears to be decreasing. For example, in a case series of patients accrued from 1974 to 1994, 78 (51%) of 152 patients underwent splenectomy.[13] In a more recent case series, with patients accrued from 1993 to 1999, the rate of splenectomy was lower: 30 (12%) of 245 patients.[12] Also, a randomized controlled trial of anti-D given to prevent splenectomy noted a significantly decreased rate of splenectomy during the course of the study.[106]

The morbidity and mortality that result from splenectomy are often reported to be minimal, but mortality may be as high as 1%, and the rate of major complications may be as high as 10%.[114] These high rates are an important consideration when the decision regarding splenectomy is discussed; however, these rates of mortality and complications may not be greater than those associated with alternative treatment approaches for patients with severe and symptomatic thrombocytopenia. In preparation for splenectomy, the platelet count should be elevated by treatment with steroids and/or IVIg. If the patient is unresponsive to treatment and has severe, symptomatic thrombocytopenia, a platelet transfusion given when surgery begins may help hemostasis. The frequency of death and complications may be lessened by laparoscopic procedures.[114]

9

Because splenectomy will often be considered in adult patients who present with severe and symptomatic thrombocytopenia, it is appropriate for the clinician to immunize these patients on diagnosis, in anticipation of possible splenectomy. Earlier immunization provided before immunosuppression with prednisone becomes established may be more effective. Although the occurrence of overwhelming sepsis in adults after splenectomy is too rare for its incidence to be known, most reports of this lethal complication date from the era before pneumococcal immunization and modern antibiotic treatment were available; anecdotes of overwhelming sepsis continue to be reported.[115,116] Therefore, immunization at least 2 weeks before elective splenectomy is appropriate because the potential benefits of immunization outweigh its risks in all subjects. Current recommendations are that patients should be immunized with pneumococcal polysaccharide vaccine, *Haemophilus influenzae* b vaccine, and quadrivalent meningococcal polysaccharide vaccine.[1,3] Most cases of overwhelming sepsis in asplenic subjects are due to pneumococci.[115,116] Five years after undergoing splenectomy, patients should be revaccinated with pneumococcal vaccine. Children are routinely placed on daily oral prophylactic penicillin after splenectomy is performed, at least up until age 5 years but often into adolescence; this is not routine care for adults in the United States. In the United Kingdom, prophylaxis with daily oral penicillin is recommended for all subjects, both children and adults, after splenectomy,[117] although this practice is often not followed.[116] Splenectomized patients must be instructed to seek medical attention immediately when they have symptoms of fever and chills; this may be the single most important aspect of education for patients before splenectomy and in the management of patients after splenectomy. Possible long-term complications of splenectomy include myocardial infarction[118,119] and pulmonary hypertension[120] that may be related to protective immunity against atherosclerosis provided by splenic B cells.[121,122]

Treatment of Patients who have Failed to Respond to Prednisone and Splenectomy

The treatment of patients with chronic, refractory thrombocytopenia, defined as those who do not respond to initial treatment with prednisone followed by splenectomy,[123] is a dilemma. No clear priority of treatment strategies after splenectomy has been delineated. No evidence suggests that any treatment is more effective than another, or indicates which treatments result in more good than harm.[1,4,123,124] Although some patients with chronic, refractory ITP have significant morbidity, most patients do well, with or without additional treatment.[124–126]

But perhaps this dilemma is overstated in that many patients are safe and relatively asymptomatic with no specific treatment. Initial treatment of adults with newly diagnosed ITP is guided by platelet count; however, with initial prednisone prescribed for essentially all patients with platelet counts below 20,000 to 30,000/μL, the indications for treatment intervention in patients after failure of prednisone and splenectomy must be more stringent.[127] For these patients, the chance for success is less and the risk is great that the adverse effects of treatment will be worse than the symptoms of bleeding. For example, in one case series

of 134 patients, 4 deaths were caused by infection related to treatment compared with only 1 death that was caused by bleeding.[13] It may be appropriate to only carefully observe patients who have negligible bleeding symptoms, even if their platelet counts are very low, even less than 10,000/μL. However, in practice, patients with such low platelet counts are inevitably believed to be at risk for major bleeding and therefore are given some form of immunosuppressive treatment, often a sequence of several different treatments. Too often, sufficient motivation to merely observe the patient without treatment occurs only when the doctor and the patient become frustrated because the platelet count fails to increase despite intolerable adverse effects. For some patients, quality of life with no treatment is far better than that with any of the commonly prescribed treatments for chronic refractory ITP.

Treatment decisions are traditionally based solely on the severity of thrombocytopenia, but consideration of other factors is critical. The absence of overt bleeding should make physicians cautious about recommending aggressive immunosuppressive therapy. Treatment decisions must also consider assessment of lifestyle and other medical conditions that could influence the risks of bleeding and immunosuppressive treatment. Older patients, who have a greater frequency of hypertension and a greater risk of intracerebral hemorrhage,[95,96] may require higher platelet counts, but these patients are also more vulnerable to the adverse effects of treatment.[95] Younger patients with a more vigorous lifestyle may also require higher platelet counts. However, most patients, after experiencing limited efficacy and the major problems caused by immunosuppressive regimens, comfortably adapt to low platelet counts and minor bleeding symptoms. These issues illustrate the need for the physician and the patient to discuss and decide together future management approaches that are based on best estimates of the benefits and risks of treatment compared with the risks of no specific treatment.

A sequence of management options for patients with chronic refractory ITP is presented in Table 9-5. Even this sequence may overemphasize the need for treatment interventions. The most important consideration is to avoid basing treatment decisions solely on platelet count; instead, treatment intensity should be measured against actual bleeding symptoms. This rule was stated succinctly in Gilbert and Sullivan's *Mikado*: "Let the punishment fit the crime."[128]

Once a decision for intervention has been made, a choice is often made among the following regimens.

Glucocorticoids

In some patients, a safe platelet count can be maintained on very low doses, or even intermittent doses, of prednisone that do not cause disturbing adverse effects. However, even very low doses of prednisone may cause or contribute to osteoporosis.[99,100] One report describes success in 10 selected patients with a regimen adapted from the management of multiple myeloma: dexamethasone 40 mg/day for 4 days, repeated every 4 weeks.[129] Six of these patients had failed to respond to splenectomy, and all apparently responded with normal platelet counts sustained after treatment had been discontinued.[129] However, no subsequent reports have confirmed these results, and some reports have described serious adverse events with this regimen.[123]

Table 9-5　Sequence of Management Options for Patients with Chronic, Refractory Immune Thrombocytopenic Purpura (ITP)

Intervention	Indication	Outcome
Observation with supportive care	No bleeding symptoms; platelet count >20,000/μL	Stable asymptomatic thrombocytopenia may persist. Morbidity of any treatment may exceed risk of bleeding. Some patients with greater risk for bleeding may require treatment
Glucocorticoids	Bleeding symptoms; platelet count <20,000/μL	Goal is a safe platelet count with a minimal dose, such as (1) prednisone, 10 mg every other day, or (2) dexamethasone, 10-40 mg/day for 4 days, repeated every 4 weeks or as needed
Immunosuppressive agents/combinations	Bleeding symptoms unresponsive to glucocorticoids	Goal is a safe platelet count with control of bleeding symptoms
Investigational protocols	Severe bleeding symptoms unresponsive to conventional immunosuppressive combination regimens	Goal is a safe platelet count with control of bleeding symptoms
Observation with supportive care	Unresponsive to treatment	Some patients may have minimal or no bleeding in spite of persistent severe thrombocytopenia

This sequence is empirical and has not been validated by controlled clinical observations. The goal of management is to prevent major bleeding, which rarely occurs unless the platelet count is below 10,000/L, and to minimize risks associated with treatment. Aggressive immunosuppressive treatment is appropriate only for patients with severe symptomatic thrombocytopenia. For patients with major bleeding unresponsive to conventional regimens, investigational treatment is appropriate. Finally, some patients refractory to all treatments may actually have minimal or no bleeding symptoms in spite of prolonged, severe thrombocytopenia. Adapted from George JN, Kojouri K, Perdue JJ, Vesely SK: Management of patients with chronic refractory idiopathic thrombocytopenic purpura. Semin Hematol 2000;37:214-218, with permission.

Removal of Accessory Spleens

Accessory spleens are found and removed at the time of splenectomy in 15% to 20% of patients. Additional accessory spleens may be found at a later time in as many as 10% of patients who are refractory to splenectomy, or who relapse after splenectomy. In spite of suggestions of the efficacy of surgical removal of accessory spleens in patients with refractory or recurrent ITP, durable remissions have been very rarely reported in patients with severe thrombocytopenia.[123]

Helicobacter pylori eradication

Eradication of H. pylori from the gastric mucosa has been associated with improvement in patients with autoimmune disorders, including ITP.[130] However, data on the prevalence of H. pylori infection among patients with ITP and the effects of H. pylori eradication on platelet counts are not consistent; reports of success from Italy[131] and Japan[132,133] are more numerous than from the United States.[4,130,134] The appeal of this therapeutic approach, in spite of limited success rates, is the safety of antimicrobial therapy.[130]

Rituximab

Because of its selective immunosuppressive effects, the chimeric anti-CD20 monoclonal antibody, rituximab, has become a common therapy for patients who require treatment after failure of splenectomy.[4] Although it has been approved by the U.S. Food and Drug Administration (FDA) only for patients with refractory low-grade B-cell lymphoma, rituximab is now commonly used for many autoimmune disorders.[135] For ITP and most other autoimmune disorders, the regimen developed for lymphoma is used, that is, 375 mg/m^2 given intravenously weekly for 4 weeks. In contrast to other immunosuppressive regimens, infectious complications rarely occur with rituximab. The efficacy of rituximab is similar to that of other immunosuppressive agents; complete remission occurs in about 30% of patients.[123,127] A recent meta-analysis found a 63% response rate but a 3% fatality rate with rituximab use in chronic ITP.[127a]

Cyclophosphamide

Uncontrolled and selected case series have reported complete responses to cyclophosphamide in 20% to 40% of patients in whom previous treatment with prednisone and splenectomy was unsuccessful.[123,136-138] Complete responses have occurred after 1 to 6 months of treatment with daily oral cyclophosphamide, typically given in a dosage of 1 to 2 mg/kg/day, adjusted for leukopenia. Intermittent intravenous doses of 1000 mg/m^2, repeated at 4-week intervals for one to five doses, have also been recommended.[138] Risks associated with cyclophosphamide therapy include dose-related marrow suppression, which may exacerbate thrombocytopenia and may actually increase the risk for bleeding. Other potential risks include teratogenicity in pregnant women, infertility, alopecia, hemorrhagic cystitis, and potential leukemogenesis.

Vinca Alkaloids

Vinblastine and vincristine have been administered by intravenous bolus injection or by intravenous infusion; results are comparable with both agents regardless of method of administration.[123] A common approach is to give vincristine by intravenous bolus, 2 mg once weekly for up to 3 to 6 weeks, until the dose-related adverse effect of peripheral neuropathy inevitably occurs. A platelet count response may occur within several days, although in most responding patients, the platelet count returns to pretreatment levels within several weeks.[123]

Azathioprine

Uncontrolled and selected case series have reported approximately 20% complete responses with azathioprine given at a daily oral dose of 1 to 2 mg/kg.[123,137,139] The average time required for response is 4 months, and most patients require continued treatment to sustain a remission.[139] As with cyclophosphamide, marrow suppression may occur with worsening of thrombocytopenia, thereby increasing the risk for hemorrhage.

Danazol

Although danazol may cause sustained platelet count responses for as long as treatment is continued, durable responses after treatment is stopped probably do not occur.[123] Danazol may be more effective when given together with immunosuppressive agents.[4] The recommended dosages of danazol for ITP vary greatly, ranging from 50 mg/day[140] to 600 to 800 mg/day.[4,141] Adverse side effects include headache, nausea, breast tenderness, skin rash, and liver function abnormalities. Hirsutism and a deeper voice may occur in women. Particularly disturbing are reports of drug-induced thrombocytopenia in five patients given danazol for endometriosis or to stimulate erythropoiesis; in two of these patients, acute thrombocytopenia recurred with readministration of danazol.[142,143]

Combination Therapy

One report described the use of several different regimens, adapted from the treatment of patients with malignant lymphoma, in 10 patients with severe chronic refractory ITP; 5 had a complete response.[144] More recent reports have described patients treated with even more intensive chemotherapy, with[145] or without[146] peripheral blood stem cell support.

Other Treatments

Multiple other treatments have been used in patients with chronic refractory ITP. All are supported by anecdotal reports of success in a few patients, often in patients with only moderate thrombocytopenia who may have needed no treatment[123]; none can be recommended for routine use.

Investigational Treatment

A new approach to treatment, the use of thrombopoietic agents, is based on increasing platelet production rather than, as with all other therapies, decreasing platelet destruction. This concept is based on observations of inappropriately low platelet production rates[15] and relative endogenous thrombopoietin deficiency[147] in many patients with ITP. An initial trial reported increased platelet counts in three of four patients.[148] Current clinical trials with a thrombopoietin mimetic molecule have documented sustained platelet count responses in most patients with weekly subcutaneous injections.[149–151] Thrombopoietic agents may become effective maintenance therapy for patients with severe, symptomatic thrombocytopenia who do not achieve remission with standard treatment.

MANAGEMENT OF ITP IN PREGNANT WOMEN AND THEIR NEWBORN INFANTS

The diagnostic distinction between ITP and gestational thrombocytopenia, which was described earlier, is not relevant to management decisions. Mild thrombocytopenia, whatever the cause, requires no treatment; it can be expected to resolve after delivery, especially if thrombocytopenia first occurs late during the third trimester. Indications for treatment during pregnancy are not different from those for treatment of any other patient with ITP, except for the recommendation of greater caution with any intervention. Treatment with prednisone and intermittent IVIg is considered safe and appropriate when severe, symptomatic thrombocytopenia is present.[1] Splenectomy may also be appropriate for severe, symptomatic thrombocytopenia that is unresponsive to prednisone and IVIg, although the risk exists that miscarriage may be induced early during pregnancy and that premature labor may occur later during pregnancy; greater technical difficulty has also been noted because of the gravid uterus, with splenectomy that is performed late during pregnancy. Other than possibly exacerbating the severity of thrombocytopenia, pregnancy itself does not present risks for the patient with ITP. To decrease the risk of postpartum hemorrhage, some patients may require treatment with glucocorticoids or IVIg in anticipation of a scheduled delivery. Epidural anesthesia appears to be safe if the platelet count is greater than 50,000/μL.[152]

The major concern for a woman with ITP who is considering pregnancy is the risk to the newborn infant, who may be thrombocytopenic at birth from passive transfer of maternal antiplatelet antibodies and therefore may be at risk for bleeding. This risk occurs at delivery and during the first week of life; with the exception of a single report,[152] no thrombocytopenic bleeding in utero has been described, distinct from alloimmune thrombocytopenia, which can cause severe intrauterine fetal hemorrhage. Although two reports have documented a correlation between the severity of maternal ITP and an infant's platelet count at birth,[53,153] other data suggest no correlation.[152] Among all women with ITP, approximately 10% of their infants have platelet counts below 50,000/μL at birth, and 4% have platelet counts below 20,000/μL.[152,154]

In spite of the risk for neonatal thrombocytopenia, reports of intracranial hemorrhage among newborn infants are extremely rare. Most intracranial hemorrhages occur during the first several days after birth—not at birth.[154] This is so because platelet counts in infants born to mothers with ITP characteristically fall during the first few days after birth[155] because of the rapid development of splenic function after birth. Hyposplenism at birth is documented by the appearance of pitted red cells and Howell-Jolly bodies within the circulation[156]; these signs correlate with the degree of prematurity of the infant and disappear within the first 2 months of life. Decreasing platelet counts after birth in infants born to mothers with ITP are similar to observations in infants born with hereditary spherocytosis, in whom hemoglobin values are usually normal at birth but may decrease sharply during the first several weeks.[157] The important lesson to be learned from these observations is that most neonatal hemorrhage is preventable through careful observation of the infant's platelet count during the first weeks of life and effective treatment of patients with thrombocytopenia with glucocorticoids and IVIg as needed. These observations also support the current recommendation that caesarean section offers no advantage to the infant over routine vaginal delivery.[152]

REFERENCES

1. George JN, Woolf SH, Raskob GE, et al: Idiopathic thrombocytopenic purpura: A practice guideline developed by explicit methods for the American Society of Hematology. Blood 88:3–40, 1996.
2. Cines DB, Blanchette VS: Immune thrombocytopenic purpura. N Engl J Med 346:995–1008, 2002.
3. British Committee for Standards in Haematology: Guidelines for the investigation and management of idiopathic thrombocytopenic purpura in adults, children and in pregnancy. Br J Haematol 120:574–596, 2003.
4. Cines DB, Bussel JB: How I treat idiopathic thrombocytopenic purpura (ITP). Blood 106:2244–2251, 2005.
5. Dameshek W, Ebbe S, Greenberg L, Baldini M: Recurrent acute idiopathic thrombocytopenic purpura. N Engl J Med 269:647–653, 1963.
6. Dickerhoff R, von Ruecker A: The clinical course of immune thrombocytopenic purpura in children who did not receive intravenous immunoglobulins or sustained prednisone treatment. J Pediatr 137:629–632, 2000.
7. Zeller B, Helgestad J, Hellebostad M, et al: Immune thrombocytopenic purpura in childhood in Norway: A prospective, population-based registration. Pediatr Hematol Oncol 17:551–558, 2000.
8. Rosthoj S, Hedlund-Treutiger I, Rajantie J, et al: Duration and morbidity of newly diagnosed idiopathic thrombocytopenic purpura in children: A prospective Nordic study of an unselected cohort. J Pediatr 143:302–307, 2003.
9. George JN, El-Harake MA, Raskob GE: Chronic idiopathic thrombocytopenic purpura. N Engl J Med 331:1207–1211, 1994.
10. Lowe EJ, Buchanan GR: Idiopathic thrombocytopenic purpura diagnosed during the second decade of life. J Pediatr 141:253–258, 2002.
11. Frederiksen H, Schmidt K: The incidence of ITP in adults increases with age. Blood 94:909–913, 1999.
12. Neylon AJ, Saunders PWG, Howard MR, et al: Clinically significant newly presenting autoimmune thrombocytopenic purpura in adults: A prospective study of a population-based cohort of 245 patients. Br J Haematol 122:966–974, 2003.
13. Portielje JEA, Westendorp RGJ, Kluin-Nelemans HC, Brand A: Morbidity and mortality in adults with idiopathic thrombocytopenic purpura. Blood 97:2549–2554, 2001.
14. Vianelli N, Valdre L, Fiacchini M, et al: Long-term follow-up of idiopathic thrombocytopenic purpura in 310 patients. Haematologia 86:504–509, 2001.
15. Ballem PJ, Segal GM, Stratton JR, et al: Mechanisms of thrombocytopenia in chronic autoimmune thrombocytopenia purpura: Evidence for both impaired platelet production and increased platelet clearance. J Clin Invest 80:33–40, 1987.
16. Chang M, Nakagawa PA, Williams SA, et al: Immune thrombocytopenic purpura (ITP) plasma and purified ITP monoclonal autoantibodies inhibit megakaryocytopoiesis in vitro. Blood 102:887–895, 2003.
17. McMillan R, Wang L, Tomer A, et al: Suppression of in vitro megakaryocyte production by antiplatelet autoantibodies from adult patients with chronic ITP. Blood 103:1364–1369, 2004.
18. Houweerzijl EJ, Blom NR, van der Want JJL, et al: Ultrastructural study shows morphologic features of apoptosis and para-apoptosis in megakaryocytes from patients with idiopathic thrombocytopenic purpura. Blood 103:500–506, 2004.
19. Davoren A, Bussel J, Curtis BR, et al: Prospective evaluation of a new platelet glycoprotein (GP)-specific assay (PakAuto) in the diagnosis of autoimmune thrombocytopenia (AITP). Am J Hematol 78:193–197, 2005.
20. Harrington WJ, Minnich V, Hollingsworth JW, Moore CV: Demonstration of a thrombocytopenic factor in the blood of patients with thrombocytopenic purpura. J Lab Clin Med 38:1, 1951.
21. Altman LK: Black and Blue at the Flick of a Feather. Who Goes First? New York, Random House, 1987:273–282, 1987.
22. Shulman NR, Weinrach RS, Libre EP, Andrews HL: The role of the reticuloendothelial system in the pathogenesis of idiopathic thrombocytopenic purpura. Trans Assoc Am Phys 78:374–390, 1965.
23. Kosugi S, Tomiyama Y, Honda S, et al: Platelet-associated anti–GPIIb-IIIa autoantibodies in chronic immune thrombocytopenic purpura recognizing epitopes close to the ligand-binding site of glycoprotein (GP) IIb. Blood 98:1819–1827, 2001.
24. Drachman JG: Inherited thrombocytopenia: When a low platelet count does not mean ITP. Blood 103:390–398, 2004.
25. George JN: Platelet immunoglobulin G: Its significance for the evaluation of thrombocytopenia and for understanding the origin of alpha-granule proteins. Blood 76:859–870, 1990.
26. Raife TJ, Olson JD, Lentz SR: Platelet antibody testing in idiopathic thrombocytopenic purpura. Blood 89:1112–1113, 1997.
27. Berchtold P, Müller D, Beardsley D, et al: International study to compare antigen-specific methods used for the measurement of antiplatelet autoantibodies. Br J Haematol 96:477–483, 1997.
28. Doan CA, Bouroncle BA, Wiseman BK: Idiopathic and secondary thrombocytopenic purpura: Clinical study and evaluation of 381 cases over a period of 28 years. Ann Intern Med 53:861–876, 1960.
29. McIntyre OR, Ebaugh FGJr: Palpable spleens in college freshmen. Ann Intern Med 66:301–306, 1967.
30. Westerman DA, Grigg AP: The diagnosis of idiopathic thrombocytopenic purpura in adults: Does bone marrow biopsy have a place? Med J Aust 170:216–217, 1999.
31. Calpin C, Dick P, Poon A, Feldman W: Is bone marrow aspiration needed in acute childhood idiopathic thrombocytopenic purpura to rule out leukemia? Arch Pediatr Adolesc Med 152:345–347, 1998.
32. Payne BA, Pierre RV: Pseudothrombocytopenia: A laboratory artifact with potentially serious consequences. Mayo Clin Proc 59:123–125, 1984.
33. Savage RA: Pseudoleukocytosis due to EDTA-induced platelet clumping. Am J Clin Pathol 81:317–322, 1984.
34. Vicari A, Banfi G, Bonini PA: EDTA-dependent pseudothrombocytopaenia: A 12-month epidemiological study. Scand J Clin Lab Invest 48:537–542, 1988.
35. Garcia Suarez J, Calero MA, Ricard MP, et al: EDTA-dependent pseudothrombocytopenia in ambulatory patients: Clinical characteristics and role of new automated cell-counting in its detection. Am J Hematol 39:146–147, 1992.
36. Sweeney JD, Holme S, Heaton WAL, et al: Pseudothrombocytopenia in plateletpheresis donors. Transfusion 35:46–49, 1995.
37. Bartels PCM, Schoorl M, Lombarts AJPF: Screening for EDTA-dependent deviations in platelet counts and abnormalities in platelet distribution histograms in pseudothrombocytopenia. Scand J Clin Lab Invest 57:629–636, 1997.
38. Fiorin F, Steffan A, Pradella P, et al: IgG platelet antibodies in EDTA-dependent pseudothrombocytopenia bind to platelet membrane glycoprotein IIb. Am J Clin Pathol 110:178–183, 1998.
39. Bizzaro N: EDTA-dependent pseudothrombocytopenia: A clinical and epidemiological study of 112 cases, with 10-year follow-up. Am J Hematol 50:103–109, 1995.
40. George JN: Platelets. Lancet 355:1531–1539, 2000.
41. Kjeldsberg CR, Swanson J: Platelet satellitism. Blood 43:831–836, 1974.
42. George JN, Raskob GE, Shah SR, et al: Drug-induced thrombocytopenia: A systematic review of published case reports. Ann Intern Med 129:886–890, 1998.
43. Arnold J, Ouwehand WH, Smith G, Cohen H: A young woman with petechiae. Lancet 352:618, 1998.
44. Azuno Y, Yaga K, Sasayama T, Kimoto K: Thrombocytopenia induced by *Jui*, a traditional Chinese herbal medicine. Lancet 354:304–305, 1999.
45. Ohmori T, Nishii K, Hagihara A, et al: Acute thrombocytopenia induced by *Jui*, a traditional herbal medicine. J Thromb Haemost 2:1479–1480, 2004.
46. Kojouri K, Perdue JJ, Medina PJ, George JN: Occult quinine-induced thrombocytopenia. Oklahoma State Med J 93:519–521, 2000.
47. Siroty RR: Purpura on the rocks—with a twist. JAMA 235:2521, 1976.
48. Gentilini G, Curtis BR, Aster RH: An antibody from a patient with ranitidine-induced thrombocytopenia recognizes a site on glycoprotein IX that is a favored target for drug-induced antibodies. Blood 92:2359–2365, 1998.
49. Burrows RF, Kelton JG: Fetal thrombocytopenia and its relation to maternal thrombocytopenia. N Engl J Med 329:1463–1466, 1993.

50. Lescale KB, Eddleman KA, Cines DB, et al: Antiplatelet antibody testing in thrombocytopenic pregnant women. Am J Obstet Gynecol 174:1014–1018, 1996.

51. Moise KJ: Autoimmune thrombocytopenic purpura in pregnancy. Clin Obstet Gynecol 34:51–63, 1991.

52. Chaplin H, Cohen R, Bloomberg G, et al: Pregnancy and idiopathic autoimmune haemolytic anaemia: A prospective study during 6 months gestation and 3 months post-partum. Br J Haematol 24:219–229, 1973.

53. Valat AS, Caulier MT, Devos P, et al: Relationships between severe neonatal thrombocytopenia and maternal characteristics in pregnancies associated with autoimmune thrombocytopenia. Br J Haematol 103:397–401, 1998.

54. Aster RH: Pooling of platelets in the spleen: Role in the pathogenesis of "hypersplenic" thrombocytopenia. J Clin Invest 45:645–657, 1966.

55. Martin TG III, Somberg KA, Meng YG, et al: Thrombopoietin levels in patients with cirrhosis before and after orthotopic liver transplantation. Ann Intern Med 127:285–288, 1997.

56. Bahner I, Kearns K, Coutinho S, et al: Infection of human marrow stroma by human immunodeficiency virus-1 (HIV-1) is both required and sufficient for HIV-1–induced hematopoietic suppression in vitro: Demonstration by gene modification of primary human stroma. Blood 90:1787–1798, 1997.

57. Oski FA, Naiman JL: Effect of live measles vaccine on the platelet count. N Engl J Med 275:352–356, 1966.

58. Ghobrial MW, Albornoz MA: Immune thrombocytopenia: A rare presenting manifestation of tuberculosis. Am J Hematol 67:139–143, 2001.

59. Standaert SM, Dawson JE, Schaffner W, et al: Ehrlichiosis in a golf-oriented retirement community. N Engl J Med 333:420–425, 1995.

60. Seri M, Pecci A, Di Bari F, et al: MYH9-related disease: May-Hegglin anomaly, Sebastian syndrome, Fechtner syndrome, and Epstein syndrome are not distinct entities but represent a variable expression of a single illness. Medicine 82:203–215, 2003.

61. Mhawech P, Saleem A: Inherited giant platelet disorders: Classification and literature review. Am J Clin Pathol 113:176–190, 2000.

62. Noris P, Spedini P, Belletti S, et al: Thrombocytopenia, giant platelets, and leukocyte inclusion bodies (May-Hegglin anomaly): Clinical and laboratory findings. Am J Med 104:355–360, 1998.

63. Young G, Luban NL, White JG: Sebastian syndrome: Case report and review of the literature. Am J Hematol 61:62–65, 1999.

64. Rocca B, Ranelletti FO, Maggiano N, et al: Inherited macrothrombocytopenia with distinctive platelet ultrastructural and functional features. Thromb Haemost 83:35–41, 2000.

65. Iolascon A, Perrotta S, Amendola G, et al: Familial dominant thrombocytopenia: Clinical, biologic, and molecular studies. Pediatr Res 46:548–552, 1998.

66. Tonelli R, Strippoli P, Grossi A, et al: Hereditary thrombocytopenia due to reduced platelet production: Report on two families and mutational screening of the thrombopoietin receptor gene (c-mpl). Thromb Haemost 83:931–936, 2000.

67. Menke DM, Colon-Otero G, Cockerill KJ, et al: Refractory thrombocytopenia: A myelodysplastic syndrome that may mimic immune thrombocytopenic purpura. Am J Clin Pathol 98:502–510, 1992.

68. Qian J, Zue Y, Pan J, et al: Refractory thrombocytopenia, an unusual myelodysplastic syndrome with an initial presentation mimicking idiopathic thrombocytopenic purpura. Int J Haematol 81:142–147, 2005.

69. Sashida G, Ohyashiki JH, Ito Y, Ohyashiki K: Monoclonal constitution of neutrophils detected by PCR-based human androgen receptor gene assay in a subset of idiopathic thrombocytopenic purpura patients. Leuk Res 26:825–830, 2002.

70. George JN: Idiopathic thrombocytopenic purpura and myelodysplastic syndrome: Distinct entities or overlapping syndromes? Leuk Res 26:789–790, 2002.

71. Mosesson MW, Colman RW, Sherry S: Chronic intravascular coagulation syndrome: Report of a case with special studies of an associated plasma cryoprecipitate ("cryofibrinogen"). N Engl J Med 278:815–821, 1968.

72. Enjolras O, Wassef M, Mazoyer E, et al: Infants with Kasabach-Merritt syndrome do not have "true" hemangiomas. J Pediatr 130:631–640, 1997.

73. Leach JW, Hussein KK, George JN: Acquired pure megakaryocytic aplasia: Report of two cases with long-term responses to antithymocyte globulin and cyclosporine. Am J Hematol 62:115–117, 1999.

74. Garderet L, Aoudjhane M, Bonte H, et al: Immune thrombocytopenic purpura: First symptom of gamma/delta T-cell lymphoma. Am J Med 111:242–243, 2001.

75. Aggarwal A, Doolittle G: Autoimmune thrombocytopenic purpura associated with hyperthyroidism in a single individual. Southern Med J 90:933–936, 1997.

76. Kurata Y, Miyagawa S, Kosugi S, et al: High-titer antinuclear antibodies, anti-SSA/Ro antibodies and anti-nuclear RNP antibodies in patients with idiopathic thrombocytopenic purpura. Thromb Haemost 71:184–187, 1994.

77. Stasi R, Stipa E, Masi M, et al: Prevalence and clinical significance of elevated antiphospholipid antibodies in patients with idiopathic thrombocytopenic purpura. Blood 84:4203–4208, 1994.

78. Lipp E, Von Felten A, Sax H, et al: Antibodies against platelet glycoproteins and antiphospholipid antibodies in autoimmune thrombocytopenia. Eur J Haematol 60:283–288, 1998.

79. Crosby WH: Wet purpura, dry purpura. JAMA 232:744–745, 1975.

80. Slichter SJ, Harker LA: Thrombocytopenia: Mechanisms and management of defects of platelet production. Clin Haematol 7:523–539, 1978.

81. Wandt H, Frank M, Ehninger G, et al: Safety and cost effectiveness of a 10×10^9/L trigger for prophylactic platelet transfusions compared with the traditional 20×10^9/L trigger: A prospective comparative trial in 105 patients with acute myeloid leukemia. Blood 91:3601–3606, 1998.

82. Rebulla P, Finazzi G, Marangoni F, et al: The threshold for prophylactic platelet transfusions in adults with acute myeloid leukemia. N Engl J Med 337:1870–1875, 1997.

83. Alberio L, Safa O, Clemetson KJ, et al: Surface expression and functional characterization of alpha-granule factor V in human platelets: Effects of ionophore A23187, thrombin, collagen, and convulxin. Blood 95:1694–1702, 2000.

84. Kitchens CS: Occult hemophilia. Johns Hopkins Med J 146:255–259, 1980.

85. Bolton-Maggs PHB, Tarantino MD, Buchanan GR, et al: The child with immune thrombocytopenic purpura: Is pharmacotherapy or watchful waiting the best initial management? A panel discussion from the meeting of the American Society of Pediatric Hematology/Oncology. J Pediatr Hematol Oncol 26:146–151, 2004.

86. Blanchette VS, Luke B, Andrew M, et al: A prospective, randomized trial of high-dose intravenous immune globulin G therapy, oral prednisone therapy, and no therapy in childhood acute immune thrombocytopenic purpura. J Pediatr 123:989–995, 1993.

87. Vesely SK, Buchanan GR, Adix L, et al: Self-reported initial management for childhood idiopathic thrombocytopenic purpura: Results of a survey of members of the American Society of Pediatric Hematology/Oncology—2001. J Pediatr Hematol Oncol 25:130–133, 2003.

88. Kattamis AC, Shankar S, Cohen AR: Neurologic complications of treatment of childhood acute immune thrombocytopenic purpura with intravenously administered immunoglobulin G. J Pediatr 130:281–283, 1997.

89. Sekul EA, Cupler EJ, Dalakas MC: Aseptic meningitis associated with high-dose intravenous immunoglobulin therapy: Frequency and risk factors. Ann Intern Med 121:259–262, 1994.

90. Gaines AR: Disseminated intravascular coagulation associated with acute hemoglobinemia or hemoglobinuria following Rh immune globulin intravenous administration for immune thrombocytopenic purpura. Blood 106:1532–1537, 2005.

91. Bolton-Maggs PHB, Moon I: Assessment of UK practice for management of acute childhood idiopathic thrombocytopenic purpura against published guidelines. Lancet 350:620–623, 1997.

92. Reid MM: Chronic idiopathic thrombocytopenic purpura: Incidence, treatment, and outcome. Arch Dis Child 72:125–128, 1995.

93. Imbach P, Kuhne T, Muller D, et al: Childhood ITP: 12 months follow-up data from the prospective registry I of the intercontinental childhood ITP study group (ICIS). Pediatr Blood Cancer 1:6, 2005.

94. Gaston MH, Verter JI, Woods G, et al: Prophylaxis with oral penicillin in children with sickle cell anemia: A randomized trial. N Engl J Med 314:1593–1599, 1986.

95. Guthrie TH, Brannan DP, Prisant LM: Idiopathic thrombocytopenic purpura in the older adult patient. Am J Med Sci 296:17–21, 1988.

96. Cortelazzo S, Finazzi G, Buelli M, et al: High risk of severe bleeding in aged patients with chronic idiopathic thrombocytopenic purpura. Blood 77:31–33, 1991.

97. Stasi R, Stipa E, Masi M, et al: Long-term observation of 208 adults with chronic idiopathic thrombocytopenic purpura. Am J Med 98:436–442, 1995.

II

98. Bellucci S, Charpak Y, Chastang C, Tobelem G: Low doses of conventional doses of corticoids in immune thrombocytopenic purpura (ITP): Results of a randomized clinical trial in 160 children, 223 adults. Blood 71:1165–1169, 1988.

99. Lukert BP, Raisz LG: Glucocorticoid-induced osteoporosis: Pathogenesis and management. Ann Intern Med 112:352–364, 1990.

100. Reid IR: Glucocorticoid osteoporosis: Mechanisms and management. Eur J Endocrinol 137:209–217, 1997.

101. Cheng Y, Wong RSM, Soo YOY, et al: Initial treatment of immune thrombocytopenic purpura with high-dose dexamethasone. N Engl J Med 349:831–836, 2003.

102. Windrum P, Bharucha C, Desai ZR: Intravenous immunoglobulin therapy and renal dysfunction. Br J Haematol 101:592, 1998.

103. Epstein, JS, Zoon, KC: FDA important drug warning: Acute renal failure associated with the administration of immune globulin intravenous (human IGIV) products. FDA Warning Letter to Physicians 1998.

104. Scaradavou A, Woo B, Woloski BMR, et al: Intravenous anti-D treatment of immune thrombocytopenic purpura: Experience in 272 patients. Blood 89:2689–2700, 1997.

105. Gaines AR: Acute onset hemoglobinemia and/or hemoglobinuria and sequelae following RHo(D) immune globulin intravenous administration in immune thrombocytopenic purpura patients. Blood 95:2523–2529, 2000.

106. George JN, Raskob GE, Vesely SK, et al: Initial management of immune thrombocytopenic purpura in adults: A randomized controlled trial comparing intermittant anti-D with routine care. Am J Hematol 74:161–169, 2003.

107. Wanachiwanawin W, Piankijagum A, Sindhvananda K, et al: Emergency splenectomy in adult idiopathic thrombocytopenic purpura: A report of seven cases. Arch Intern Med 149:217–219, 1989.

108. Carr JM, Kruskall MS, Kaye JA, Robinson SH: Efficacy of platelet transfusions in immune thrombocytopenia. Am J Med 80:1051–1054, 1986.

109. Abrahm J, Ellman L: Platelet transfusion in immune thrombocytopenic purpura. JAMA 236:1847, 1976.

110. McMillan R: Therapy for adults with refractory chronic immune thrombocytopenic purpura. Ann Intern Med 126:307–314, 1997.

111. Baumann MA, Menitove JE, Aster RH, Anderson T: Urgent treatment of idiopathic thrombocytopenic purpura with single-dose gammaglobulin infusion followed by platelet transfusion. Ann Intern Med 104:808–809, 1986.

112. Gerotziafas GT, Zervas C, Gavrielidis G, et al: Effective hemostasis with rFVIIa treatment in two patients with severe thrombocytopenia and life-threatening hemorrhage. Am J Hematol 69:219–222, 2002.

113. Culic S: Recombinant factor VIIa for refractory haemorrhage in autoimmune idiopathic thrombocytopenic purpura. Br J Haematol 120:909–910, 2003.

114. Kojouri K, Vesely SK, Terrell DR, George JN: Splenectomy for adult patients with idiopathic thrombocytopenic purpura: A systematic literature review to assess long-term platelet count responses, prediction of response, and surgical complications. Blood 104:2623–2634, 2004.

115. Schilling RF: Estimating the risk for sepsis after splenectomy in hereditary spherocytosis. Ann Intern Med 122:187–188, 1995.

116. Waghorn DJ: Overwhelming infection in asplenic patients: Current best practice preventive measures are not being followed. J Clin Pathol 54:214–218, 2001.

117. Lortan JE: Management of asplenic patients. Br J Haematol 84:566–569, 1993.

118. Robinette CD, Fraumeni JF: Splenectomy and subsequent mortality in veterans of the 1939–1945 war. Lancet 2:127–129, 1977.

119. Schilling RF: Spherocytosis, splenectomy, strokes, and heart attacks. Lancet 350:1677–1678, 1997.

120. Hoeper MM, Niedermeyer J, Hoffmeyer F, et al: Pulmonary hypertension after splenectomy? Ann Intern Med 130:506–509, 1999.

121. Caligiuri G, Nicoletti A, Poirier B, Hansson GK: Protective immunity against atherosclerosis carried by B cells of hypercholesterolemic mice. J Clin Invest 109:745–753, 2002.

122. Witzum JL: Splenic immunity and atherosclerosis: A glimpse into a novel paradigm? J Clin Invest 109:721–724, 2002.

123. Vesely SK, Perdue JJ, Rizvi MA, et al: Management of adult patients with idiopathic thrombocytopenic purpura after failure of splenectomy: A systematic review. Ann Intern Med 140:112–120, 2004.

124. Provan D, Newland A: Fifty years of idiopathic thrombocytopenic purpura (ITP): Management of refractory ITP in adults. Br J Haematol 118:933–944, 2002.

125. McMillan R, Durette C: Long-term outcomes in adults with chronic ITP after splenectomy failure. Blood 104:956–960, 2004.

126. Bourgeois E, Caulier MT, Delarozee C, et al: Long-term follow-up of chronic autoimmune thrombocytopenic purpura refractory to splenectomy: A prospective analysis. Br J Haematol 120:1079–1088, 2003.

127. Kojouri K, George JN: Recent advances in the treatment of chronic refractory immune thrombocytopenic purpura. Int J Haematol 81:119–125, 2005.

127a. Arnold DM, Dentali F, Crowther MA, et al: Systemic review: Efficacy and safety of rituximab for adults with idiopathic thrombocytopenic purpura. Ann Intern Med 146:25–33, 2007.

128. George JN, Vesely SK: Immune thrombocytopenic purpura: Let the treatment fit the patient. N Engl J Med 349:903–905, 2003.

129. Andersen JC: Response of resistant idiopathic thrombocytopenic purpura to pulsed high-dose dexamethasone therapy. N Engl J Med 330:1560–1564, 1994.

130. Jackson S, Beck PL, Pineo GF, Poon M-C: Helicobacter pylori eradication: Novel therapy for immune thrombocytopenic purpura? A review of the literature. Am J Hematol 78:142–150, 2005.

131. Emilia G, Longo G, Luppi M, et al: Helicobacter pylori eradication can induce platelet recovery in idiopathic thrombocytopenic purpura. Blood 97:812–814, 2001.

132. Fujimura K, Kuwana M, Kurata Y, et al: Is eradication therapy useful as the first line of treatment in Helicobacter pylori–positive idiopathic thrombocytopenic purpura? Analysis of 207 eradicated chronic ITP cases in Japan. Int J Haematol 81:162–168, 2005.

133. Fujimura K: Helicobacter pylori infection and idiopathic thrombocytopenic purpura. Int J Haematol 81:113–118, 2005.

134. Michel M, Cooper N, Jean C, et al: Does Helicobacter pylori initiate or perpetuate immune thormbocytopenic purpura? Blood 103:890–896, 2003.

135. George JN, Woodson RD, Kiss JE, et al: Rituximab therapy for thrombotic thrombocytopenic purpura: A proposed study of the Transfusion Medicine/Hemostasis Clinical Trials Network with a systematic review of rituximab therapy for immune-mediated disorders. J Clin Apher 21:49–56, 2006.

136. Verlin M, Laros RK, Penner JA: Treatment of refractory thrombocytopenic purpura with cyclophosphamide. Am J Hematol 1:97–104, 1976.

137. Pizzuto J, Ambriz R: Therapeutic experience on 934 adults with idiopathic thrombocytopenic purpura: Multicentric trial of the cooperative Latin American group on hemostasis and thrombosis. Blood 64:1179–1183, 1984.

138. Reiner A, Gernsheimer T, Slichter SJ: Pulse cyclophosphamide therapy for refractory autoimmune thrombocytopenic purpura. Blood 85:351–358, 1995.

139. Quiquandon I, Fenaux P, Caulier MT, et al: Re-evaluation of the role of azathioprine in the treatment of adult chronic idiopathic thrombocytopenic purpura: A report on 53 cases. Br J Haematol 74:223–228, 1990.

140. Ahn YS, Mylvaganam R, Garcia RO, et al: Low-dose danazol therapy in idiopathic thrombocytopenic purpura. Ann Intern Med 107:177–181, 1987.

141. Ahn YS, Harrington WJ, Simon SR, et al: Danazol for the treatment of idiopathic thrombocytopenic purpura. N Engl J Med 308:1396–1399, 1983.

142. Arrowsmith JB, Dreis M: Thrombocytopenia after treatment with danazol. N Engl J Med 314:585, 1986.

143. Rabinowe SN, Miller KB: Danazol-induced thrombocytopenia. Br J Haematol 65:383–384, 1987.

144. Figueroa M, Gehlsen J, Hammond D, et al: Combination chemotherapy in refractory immune thrombocytopenic purpura. N Engl J Med 328:1226–1229, 1993.

145. Huhn RD, Fogarty PF, Nakamura R, et al: High-dose cyclophosphamide with autologous lymphocyte–depleted peripheral blood stem cell (PBSC) support for treatment of refractory chronic autoimmune thrombocytopenia. Blood 101:71–77, 2003.

146. Brodsky R, Petri M, Smith BD, et al: Immunoablative high-dose cyclophosphamide without stem cell rescue for refractory, severe autoimmune disease. Ann Intern Med 129:1031–1035, 1998.

147. Kosugi S, Kurata Y, Tomiyama Y, et al: Circulating thrombopoietin level in chronic immune thrombocytopenic purpura. Br J Haematol 93:704–706, 1996.

148. Nomura S, Dan K, Hotta T, et al: Effects of pegylated recombinant human megakaryocyte growth and development factor in patients with idiopathic thrombocytopenia purpura. Blood 100:728–730, 2002.

149. Bussel JB, George JN, Kuter DJ, et al: An open-label, dose-finding study evaluating the safety and platelet response of a novel thrombopoietic protein (AMG 531) in thrombocytopenic adult patients with immune thrombocytopenic purpura. Blood 102:86, 2003.

150. Kuter DJ, Bussel JB, Aledort L, et al: A phase 2 placebo controlled study evaluating the platelet count and safety of weekly dosing with a novel thrombopoietic protein (AMG531) in thrombocytopenic adult patients with immune thrombocytopenic purpura. Blood 104:148a–149a, 2004.

151. Bussel JB, Kuter DJ, George JN, et al: AMG 531, a thrombopoiesis-stimulating protein, for chronic ITP. N Engl J Med 355:1672–1681, 2006.

152. Webert KE, Mittal R, Sigourin C, et al: A retrospective 11-year analysis of obstetric patients with idiopathic thrombocytopenic purpura. Blood 102:4306–4311, 2003.

153. Payne SD, Resnik R, Moore TR, et al: Maternal characteristics and risk of severe neonatal thrombocytopenia and intracranial hemorrhage in pregnancies complicated by autoimmune thrombocytopenia. Am J Obstet Gynecol 177:149–155, 1997.

154. Burrows RF, Kelton JG: Pregnancy in patients with idiopathic thrombocytopenic purpura: Assessing the risks for the infant at delivery. Obstet Gynecol Surv 48:781–788, 1993.

155. Burrows RF, Kelton JG: Low fetal risks in pregnancies associated with idiopathic thrombocytopenic purpura. Am J Obstet Gynecol 163:1147–1150, 1990.

156. Holroyde CP, Oski FA, Gardner FH: The "pocked" erythrocyte: Red cell alterations in reticuloendothelial immaturity of the neonate. N Engl J Med 281:516–520, 1969.

157. Delhommeau F, Cynober T, Schischmanoff PO, et al: Natural history of hereditary spherocytosis during the first year of life. Blood 95:393–397, 2000.

Chapter 10

Congenital and Acquired Disorders of Platelet Function and Number

Shawn Jobe, MD, PhD • Jorge Di Paola, MD

INTRODUCTION

Platelet dysfunction and thrombocytopenia result from a variety of inherited and acquired disorders. When a patient with mucocutaneous bleeding is first evaluated, the list of differential diagnoses is usually extensive. Elements of the medical history, physical examination findings, and laboratory workup results are critically helpful to the clinician in determining whether the bleeding is due to a platelet disorder. The intent of this chapter is to provide the hematologist with a rational approach to common questions that arise during the evaluation of a patient with a suspected platelet defect. It is also intended to offer a brief discussion of the genetics, pathophysiology, and management of platelet-related bleeding disorders (Fig. 10-1).

HISTORICAL PERSPECTIVE

In 1918, Eduard Glanzmann, a Swiss pediatrician, described a group of individuals with a mucocutaneous bleeding disorder he then called *thrombasthenie* (weak platelets).[1] These patients exhibited grossly abnormal clot retraction yet normal platelet counts. Platelets appeared normal under the light microscope. About 50 years later, the identification of several nuclear families with thrombasthenia confirmed the inherited nature of the disorder, and in the late 1960s, platelet aggregation techniques showed the inability of thrombasthenic platelets to bind fibrinogen and aggregate after stimulation with physiologic agonists.[2,3]

In 1974, while using sodium dodecyl sulfate (SDS)–polyacrylamide gel electrophoresis, Nurden and Caen noted the absence of one of three major platelet membrane glycoproteins in platelets obtained from thrombasthenic patients.[4,5] Over the next few years, it was gradually recognized through the work of several laboratories that two glycoproteins, identified as IIb and IIIa, were absent in platelets from patients with Glanzmann thrombasthenia.[6,7]

In the early 1980s, platelets obtained from thrombasthenic patients were once again critical in the identification and characterization of the fibrinogen receptor glycoprotein (GP)-IIb/IIIa (also known as integrin $\alpha IIb\beta 3$) and in the subsequent development of monoclonal antibodies that recognize this molecule.[8–10] One of these monoclonal antibodies, 7E3, was evaluated further as an antiplatelet agent in different animal models.[11,12] These promising preclinical study results led to the development of the chimeric monoclonal antibody abciximab (Reopro), which, in subsequent clinical trials, showed its efficacy in the prevention of thrombosis and restenosis after percutaneous coronary interventions.[13,14]

Therefore, the study of individuals with Glanzmann thrombasthenia was essential in the development of the anti-IIb/IIIa antiplatelet agents abciximab, eptifibatide, and tirofiban. Translational research, in this case from bedside to bench and back to bedside, has represented a fundamental principle in platelet research over previous decades. Additional studies of rare, inherited platelet disorders will likely result in a better understanding of the platelet "machinery" and ultimately will lead to the development of new treatments that are beneficial to affected individuals and to patients with other bleeding and thrombotic illnesses.

CLINICAL MANIFESTATIONS OF PLATELET-RELATED BLEEDING AND TESTS OF PLATELET FUNCTION

Does the Patient Have a Platelet-Related Bleeding Disorder?

Although our understanding of the mechanisms of platelet dysfunction and thrombocytopenia has significantly improved since Glanzmann's initial case report was presented, tests and skills required for the identification of individuals with platelet-specific bleeding disorders have essentially remained unchanged. Typically, most individuals with a platelet-related bleeding disorder have their first encounter with a hematologist because of patient or physician concerns about excessive mucocutaneous bleeding, thrombocytopenia, or a family history of bleeding. Frequently, to exclude other causes of bleeding, a referring physician will have already performed several screening laboratory tests, including prothrombin time (PT), partial thromboplastin time (PTT), and fibrinogen level. Sometimes, other screening tests, such as bleeding time or the more recently developed Platelet Function Analyzer (PFA-100), may have been used. Therefore, on initial evaluation by the hematologist, including a history, physical examination, and careful evaluation of blood smear, most of the information that is critical for a correct diagnosis will have been obtained.

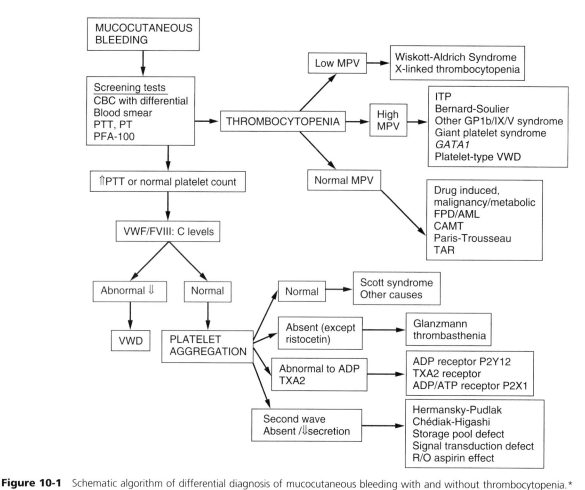

Figure 10-1 Schematic algorithm of differential diagnosis of mucocutaneous bleeding with and without thrombocytopenia.*
*For didactic reasons, not all described platelet disorders have been included.
CAMT, congenital amegakaryocytic thrombocytopenia; FPD/AML, familial platelet disorder/acute myeloid leukemia; MPV, mean platelet volume; TAR, thrombocytopenia with absent radii; TAX2, thromboxane A2; VWD, von Willebrand disease.

Bleeding associated with platelet disorders primarily involves the skin and mucous membranes. Spontaneous joint or deep muscle bleeds are relatively uncommon in patients with platelet disorders. Bleeding manifestations within the skin can be characterized by their size, elevation, and distribution. Petechiae, purpura, ecchymoses, and hematomas may be found (see Chapter 11). Close attention should also be given to the distribution and elevation of lesions because this information can be helpful to the clinician in distinguishing bleeding related to platelet disorders from that associated with other causes, such as vasculitic disease or nonaccidental injury. For example, the lesions associated with Henoch-Schönlein purpura, a leukocytoclastic vasculitic disease, are raised ("palpable purpura") and often appear in a classic distribution that involves dependent surfaces and the lower extremities. Unusual or regular patterns of skin lesions (e.g., handprint, linear pattern) may suggest the possibility of nonaccidental injury.

Platelet-related bleeding, including epistaxis, bleeding within the oral cavity, upper and lower gastrointestinal hemorrhage, hematuria, and menorrhagia, is also associated with mucosal surfaces. Menorrhagia is a common presenting symptom in young women, and it is estimated that up to 15% of women with menorrhagia will have platelet dysfunction or von Willebrand disease (VWD).[15,16] Platelet dysfunction should also be suspected

in the presence of increased bleeding after dental extraction, tonsillectomy, and other surgical procedures.

Screening methods have been used in an attempt to identify individuals with a high likelihood of developing a platelet-related bleeding disorder or VWD. A rapid assay with high sensitivity would be expected to lower the need for further, more costly, invasive testing. Bleeding time was the first of these methods to be widely used, but its clinical usefulness is questionable because of difficulties with standardization, reproducibility, and lack of sensitivity and specificity.[17] The recently introduced PFA-100 has also been proposed to have a role in the screening of individuals with suspected platelet dysfunction. The PFA-100 is a high-shear–stress-inducing device that simulates primary hemostasis by facilitating the flow of whole blood through an aperture cut into a membrane coated with collagen and adenosine diphosphate (ADP) (50 µg) or epinephrine (10 µg). Platelets adhere to the collagen-coated surface and aggregate at the rim of the aperture. The platelet plug enlarges until it occludes the aperture, causing cessation of blood flow. The time to cessation of flow is recorded as closure time (CT).

Initial studies focused on the efficacy of the PFA-100 in the evaluation of individuals with known VWD and severe platelet disorders, such as Glanzmann thrombasthenia and Bernard-Soulier syndrome (BSS). In these patient populations with VWD (von Willebrand factor [VWF] <25%) or severe platelet disorders, the sensitivity and specificity of the PFA-100 approach 90%. These results suggest that the PFA-100 could have usefulness as a diagnostic tool in the initial evaluation of individuals with a suspected platelet-related bleeding disorder.[18–20] Recently, however, the initial enthusiasm for the usefulness of the PFA-100 as a screening tool has diminished because of the low sensitivity (24% to 41%) of the device reported in individuals with mild platelet secretion defects or storage pool disorders.[21–23]

DIFFERENTIAL DIAGNOSIS OF PLATELET-RELATED BLEEDING

Is the Defect Acquired or Congenital?

After the decision has been made to pursue the investigation of platelet-related bleeding, a careful medical history, physical examination, and evaluation of platelet count and smear can rapidly narrow the diagnostic possibilities. Several elements of the history provide critical information and should be explored in detail. History should be obtained about medication usage, particularly the use of aspirin or nonsteroidal anti-inflammatory drugs (NSAIDs). Although aspirin and NSAIDs are the most highly recognized drugs or groups of drugs associated with platelet dysfunction, all medications should be evaluated because the list of possible interactions is long and will continue to grow.

Close evaluation of the family and past medical history may provide clues about whether the bleeding disorder is acquired or congenital. Platelet dysfunction may be related to other systemic disorders. Uremia from renal impairment may also cause platelet dysfunction. Cardiopulmonary bypass or extracorporeal membrane oxygenation (ECMO) may result in decreased effectiveness of circulating platelets. Careful evaluation of the peripheral blood smear and blood count, as well as assessment of hepatosplenomegaly and lymphadenopathy, may reveal the need for further workup for myeloproliferative disease, malignancy, or aplastic anemia.

Additional elements of the history, physical examination, and peripheral smear are especially useful in the differentiation of immune thrombocytopenic purpura (ITP) from a congenital platelet disorder. The persistence of neonatal thrombocytopenia or a low platelet count despite the use of several standard therapies (e.g., intravenous immune globulin [IVIg], steroids) for ITP also points toward a congenital cause of the thrombocytopenia. Bleeding symptoms out of proportion to the platelet count should prompt consideration of a congenital platelet disorder. Patients with ITP typically have minimal bleeding until their platelet count decreases to below 10,000/μL. Even at those low values, the presence of "fresh reticulated platelets" usually is enough to secure hemostasis. Bleeding observed at platelet counts greater than 30,000/μL suggests the presence of a coexisting underlying platelet dysfunction.

Many congenital platelet disorders are associated with other diseases, unique physical characteristics, or findings on the peripheral blood smear. For example, thrombocytopenia in the presence of auditory or renal dysfunction suggests an *MYH9*-related thrombocytopenia, and the presence of skeletal abnormalities may lead to the diagnosis of thrombocytopenia with absent radii (TAR) or amegakar-yocytic thrombocytopenia with radioulnar synostosis (see later in the chapter).

ACQUIRED PLATELET DISORDERS
(TABLE 10-1)

Medication-Related Disorders

Numerous medications have been associated with platelet dysfunction or thrombocytopenia. Inhibitors of platelet cyclooxygenase-1 (COX-1)—aspirin and NSAIDs—are the most commonly used drugs known to affect platelet function by decreasing the platelet production of the prostaglandin, thromboxane A2 (TXA2), which is a potent secondary mediator of platelet activation; its production within the platelet is mediated by the enzyme cyclooxygenase. Aspirin inhibits cyclooxygenase function through an irreversible covalent modification of the enzyme's active site; as little as 80 mg is required to completely inhibit TXA2.[24] Because of this irreversibility, the effectiveness of aspirin in inhibiting platelet function persists until platelets circulating at the time of administration are replaced (days).[25] NSAIDs, however, act as reversible competitive inhibitors of platelet cyclooxygenase, and the duration of platelet inhibition correlates with the half-life of the NSAID used (hours).

Both thienopyridines—ticlopidine and clopidogrel—inhibit platelet activation through covalent modification of the P2Y12 receptor, a platelet receptor for the secondary mediator ADP.[26,27] Both of these agents are prodrugs that require cytochrome P450–dependent pathways for their activation. Similar to aspirin, the effects of ticlopidine and clopidogrel persist during the entire life span of the platelet.

Inhibitors of the fibrinogen receptor, GP-IIb/IIIa, also block platelet function. The reversible competitive inhibitors tirofiban, eptifibatide, and abciximab are frequently administered in conjunction with vascular procedures, and all are rapidly cleared from the circulation after administration.

Several other drugs whose primary target is not the platelet may also cause platelet dysfunction. The β-lactam antibiotic penicillins and cephalosporins have been reported to affect platelet function. The mechanism of this inhibition is unclear, although it appears to be related to the effects of the drugs on agonist–platelet receptor interaction.[28] This effect typically occurs 2 to 3 days after initiation of treatment.[29] Drugs with primarily cardiovascular effects that may inhibit platelet function

---

Table 10-1 Acquired Disorders Associated With Platelet-Related Bleeding

Medication related
Renal failure/uremia
Cardiopulmonary bypass/extracorporeal membrane oxygenation (ECMO)
Hypersplenism (e.g., lysosomal storage diseases, portal hypertension)
Myeloproliferative disorders
Immune thrombocytopenia (neonatal, acute, chronic) (see Chapter 9)
Myelophthisic disorders (leukemia, metastasis, fibrosis)
Aplastic disorders (immune, congenital, infectious)

include nitrates, the calcium channel blockers,[30] and propranolol.[31] The nitrates act as nitric oxide (NO) donors. NO inhibits platelet function by decreasing platelet adhesion and recruitment to the forming thrombus.[32] Among the psychotropic agents, the selective serotonin reuptake inhibitors (SSRIs) and tricyclic antidepressants (TCAs) may inhibit platelet function by decreasing the serotonin content of platelet-dense granules. Retrospective clinical studies suggest an increased risk of bleeding in patients who receive SSRIs or TCAs.[33–35] Consumption of alcohol has long been associated with platelet function changes.[36] The impact of this effect appears to be sex dependent, and the effect is greater on men.[37] Both protective and detrimental effects on the cardiovascular system have been described, although moderate alcohol consumption seems to confer protection against cardiovascular disease.[38] Therefore, although it is clear that alcohol has definitive effects on platelet activation and other components of the hemostatic and vascular system, the extent of these effects and their clinical correlation with outcomes are unclear and require further investigation. Often, these agents with their mild antiplatelet effects combine with other mild hemostatic defects (such as VWD) to serve as a "second hit," resulting in a more apparent hemorrhagic condition.

Cardiopulmonary Bypass/Extracorporeal Membrane Oxygenation

Both cardiopulmonary bypass (CPB) and ECMO require circulation of blood over an artificial surface. Because the membrane lacks the antihemostatic properties of endothelium, platelets can become activated.[39,40] Platelet activation may result in platelet dysfunction and increased platelet clearance. With the use of flow cytometry for evaluation of platelet P-selectin expression and the formation of platelet–monocyte aggregates, increased platelet activation has been detected in patients after cardiopulmonary bypass.[41] Remaining circulating platelets also exhibit decreased expression of the VWF receptor GP-Ib and the fibrinogen receptor GP-IIb/IIIa, suggesting a possible explanation for platelet dysfunction. After CPB has ceased, normalization of the level of platelet receptors occurs gradually over 3 to 4 hours.[42,43] It is not clear which laboratory tests of platelet function are useful for identifying patients at excessive risk of post-bypass bleeding or thrombosis.[44,45] Because of this underlying platelet dysfunction, platelet transfusion is frequently employed in post–CPB hemorrhage despite the presence of an adequate platelet count (see Chapter 37).

Uremia

Patients with chronic renal failure and uremia have long been recognized to be at increased risk of bleeding. The cause of this tendency toward increased bleeding is multifactorial and has been related to vascular abnormalities, anemia, and defects of platelet function and adhesion.[46,47] Correction of the anemia of chronic renal failure with erythropoietin or red blood cell transfusion often results in normalization of abnormal bleeding times and improved platelet adhesion and aggregation.[48–50]

Additionally, multiple abnormalities of platelet function have been described. Among these are defects in platelet

adhesion noted in various in vitro flow models in which blood from uremic patients was used,[51,52] as well as decreased synthesis of the secondary mediator of platelet activation, TXA_2.[53] Many different circulating metabolites are increased in the uremic patient, and controversy continues regarding the identity of substances within uremic plasma that are responsible for observed hemostatic abnormalities. One of the metabolites that increases in uremic patients, guanidinosuccinic acid, can function as an NO donor and in some studies can recapitulate several observed defects. Phenolic acid has also been proposed as a candidate agent because it is present at concentrations within the plasma shown to affect platelet function in vitro.[54,55]

Management of bleeding in uremic patients can be challenging. 1-Deamino-8-D-arginine vasopressin (DDAVP) remains the agent of choice and has been shown to effectively shorten bleeding time in uremic patients.[56,57] However, 4 to 8 hours after its administration, bleeding time returns to baseline. Also, tachyphylaxis to repeated doses of DDAVP may occur.[58] Improvement of anemia through packed red cell transfusion may aid in hemostasis.[50] Because the bleeding is presumed to be due to the presence of circulating metabolites, dialysis has been recommended in some circumstances. The benefits of dialysis must, however, be weighed against the potential hazards of anticoagulation and exposure of platelets to an artificial membrane with the potential for undesired platelet activation. Platelet transfusion will be only transiently effective, in that the transfused platelets will be inhibited quickly within the uremic host. Recombinant factor VIIa (rFVIIa) has also been reported to effectively stop bleeding in uremic patients.[59,60] The use of rFVIIa should be carefully considered, however, because of the potential for thrombotic complications (e.g., catheter thrombosis).

Myeloproliferative Disorders

Both hemorrhagic and thrombotic complications have been reported in individuals with myeloproliferative disorders; however, reportedly, the most common manifestation is thrombosis (reviewed in Elliott and Tefferi[61]). Hemorrhage can be problematic, and several possible reasons have been cited for the observed platelet defect. Megakaryocytic clonal abnormalities have been proposed to result in the production of defective platelets.[62,63] Recently, the effect of JAK2 on the stability and localization of the thrombopoietin receptor c-MPL has been shown, indicating a possible mechanism for the platelet abnormalities seen in these syndromes.[64] Abnormal in vivo platelet activation may result in the premature release of platelet granules, causing an acquired platelet defect.[61,62] Loss of the highly hemostatic, large VWF multimers has been associated with essential thrombocythemia, resulting in an acquired form of VWD.[65] Concomitant use of antithrombotic agents increases the risk of bleeding in this patient population.

The use of platelet aggregation tests to define a set of patients with myeloproliferative disorders who are at risk for bleeding has limited clinical efficacy.[61]

Hypersplenism

Hypersplenism refers to the thrombocytopenia that (1) often occurs in individuals with splenic enlargement and (2) cannot be accounted for by other causes. Hypersplenism has been associated with a variety of diseases, including portal hypertension, lysosomal storage disorders, and myeloproliferative diseases.[66] Both increased pooling of the circulating platelet population within the enlarged spleen and immunologic mechanisms have been suggested as causes.[67,68] In general, platelet survival is normal but up to 50% to 90% of circulating platelets are sequestered in the large spleen. Thrombocytopenia associated with hypersplenism is usually mild (50,000 to 100,000/μL) and requires no specific treatment. Severe thrombocytopenia or thrombocytopenia that interferes with required therapy may require intervention, although this is rare. Different surgical approaches, including splenectomy, partial splenic embolization, and use of a distal splenorenal shunt, have been used and may result in long-term normalization of the platelet count.[69–71]

CONGENITAL PLATELET DISORDERS
(TABLE 10-2)

Congenital platelet disorders can be categorized according to several distinguishing characteristics. In many individuals, a family history of bleeding or thrombocytopenia allows identification of the inheritance pattern. Autosomal recessive, X-linked, and autosomal dominant inheritance patterns can be found in individuals with platelet-related bleeding. For example, in the evaluation of a patient with a suspected platelet defect, a history of a brother, maternal uncle, or grandfather with thrombocytopenia would suggest an X-linked disorder such as Wiskott-Aldrich syndrome (WAS) or *GATA1*-related thrombocytopenia as the cause. Also, a particular platelet aggregation pattern can often be diagnostic of a specific disorder, such as Bernard-Soulier syndrome or Glanzmann thrombasthenia. Finally, the presence of associated congenital malformations or abnormalities on the blood smear, within both platelets and leukocytes, may simplify the diagnostic workup.

As a first step in the evaluation, two values of the complete blood count—platelet count and mean platelet volume (MPV)—should be carefully reviewed because these can provide critical information in the differential diagnosis. Several platelet-related bleeding disorders are associated with thrombocytopenia; others have normal platelet count and morphology but clinical and laboratory evidence of platelet dysfunction.

Many of the congenital thrombocytopenias can also be characterized by their platelet size. The normal MPV is 7 to 11 fL, and platelets smaller or larger than this, as well as giant platelets, are unique to particular congenital thrombocytopenias.

Table 10-2 Reasons to Suspect a Congenital Platelet Disorder

Persistence of neonatal thrombocytopenia (onset at birth) or onset of bleeding symptoms in childhood

Family history of thrombocytopenia or mucocutaneous bleeding/bruising

Mucocutaneous bleeding/bruising out of proportion to the platelet count

Presence of associated clinical or laboratory features

Platelet count unresponsive to typical treatments for ITP

Typical causes of acquired platelet-related bleeding do not account for symptoms

---

These two features—platelet count and platelet size—then become excellent tools for classification of congenital platelet disorders. Although no clear definition can be provided for large versus giant platelets, on the basis of laboratory and clinical experience, we classify large platelets as those whose diameter is similar or larger to that of a lymphocyte; we reserve the definition of giant for those platelets that reach the diameter of a neutrophil.

Several other features of the blood smear should be also closely evaluated. Automated blood cell counters often base their assessment on cell size. Therefore, platelet counts are frequently underestimated in the large and giant platelet syndromes; thus, a manual count of the blood smear should also be performed. Additionally, several inherited disorders are associated with unique features observable in the neutrophil population; these cells should be scanned closely for the presence of unique features such as Döhle-like bodies (*MYH9*-related disorders) or giant cytoplasmic granules (Chédiak-Higashi syndrome).

CONGENITAL PLATELET DISORDERS WITH A NORMAL PLATELET COUNT

If a congenital platelet disorder is strongly suspected in an individual with a normal or near-normal platelet count, one of the first tests that should be considered is platelet aggregation. Platelet aggregation tests the ability of platelets to aggregate in stirred platelet-rich plasma (PRP) in response to a panel of platelet agonists. Typical agonists evaluated include collagen, ADP, arachidonic acid, ristocetin, and epinephrine. Upon stimulation, platelets within the suspension become activated, change shape, release their granular contents, and aggregate. All these events can be recorded by modern luminoaggregometry. When the turbid PRP is illuminated before addition of the agonist, transmitted light is scattered. Addition of the platelet agonist then results in an initial peak of increased transmission, corresponding to a rapid change in platelet shape. After this shape change, the amount of light transmitted increases because of platelet clumping or aggregation. Two phases of aggregation can then be evaluated—a primary reversible aggregation phase due to an immediate response of the platelets to exogenous agonists, and a secondary irreversible phase corresponding to the response of the platelets to secondary mediators endogenously released by the platelets (Fig. 10-2). Absence of, or a large decrease in, any of these components may be indicative of a particular congenital platelet disorder. Luminometry, used in combination with platelet aggregation, provides a sensitive evaluation of dense granular release of adenosine triphosphate (ATP). ATP released by platelets provides energy for the added light-producing enzyme luciferase, and a burst of light is recorded. In patients with a dense granular deficiency or platelet release defect, this burst will be impaired. Without the platelet's own "agonists" (e.g., ADP), often the secondary wave of platelet aggregation will be absent as well (Fig. 10-3). Electron microscopy can then be used to distinguish a dense granular deficiency from a platelet release defect. Closer evaluation of other platelet features by electron microscopy is often critically helpful as well.

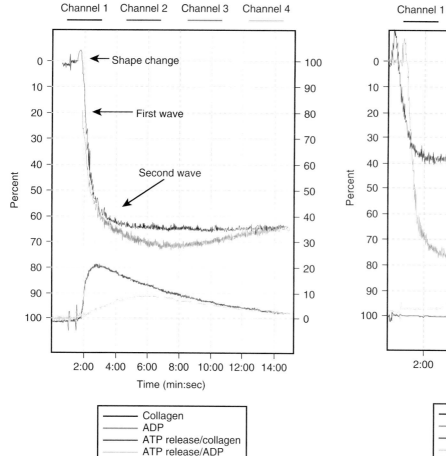

Figure 10-2 *(See also Color Plate 10-2.)* Normal aggregation pattern. Adenosine diphosphate (ADP) and collagen were used as agonists. The curve reflects percentage of aggregation as a function of time. The arrows indicate the different steps observed during platelet aggregation. The first wave of aggregation is caused by exogenous agonists, in this case, collagen and ADP; the second wave is due to endogenous release of dense granular content. Curves in green and black indicate adenosine triphosphate (ATP) release.

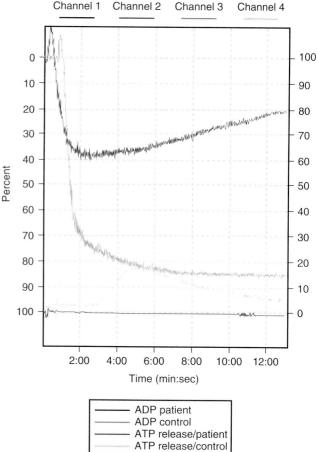

Figure 10-3 *(See also Color Plate 10-3.)* Abnormal aggregation pattern. Adenosine diphosphate (ADP) was used as an agonist. The first wave of aggregation (due to the exogenous agonist) is conserved in the patient and the normal control subject. However, the second wave of aggregation and adenosine triphosphate (ATP) release are absent in this patient, indicating an intrinsic defect in platelet activation. A similar pattern of aggregation and desaggregation is observed when platelets are inhibited by aspirin or nonsteroidal anti-inflammatory drugs (NSAIDs).

Although luminoaggregometry and electron microscopy provide useful information about many structural and functional components of platelets, it should be emphasized that not all aspects of platelet activation are evaluated by these tests. Platelet function defects have been described in patients with a normal platelet count and a normal pattern of platelet aggregation, such as occurs in Scott syndrome. Also, platelet aggregation presents some of the same issues that are encountered with other platelet tests. It is fairly accurate for diagnosing severe platelet disorders such as Glanzmann thrombasthenia and BSS, but it seems to lack sensitivity and specificity for milder platelet defects.

CONGENITAL PLATELET DISORDERS WITH NORMAL PLATELET COUNT AND ABNORMAL AGGREGATION (TABLE 10-3)

Glanzmann thrombasthenia

Glanzmann thrombasthenia (GT) represents the prototypical inherited platelet defect; it occurs as the result of mutations in the genes that encode for the two polypeptide chains that constitute the platelet fibrinogen receptor, integrin GP-IIb/IIIa. Its inheritance is autosomal recessive, and in most patients with GT, mutations within the gene *ITGA2B* (that encodes for IIb) or *ITGB3* (that encodes for IIIa) result in significantly low or absent surface levels of GP-IIb/IIIa, as measured by flow cytometry. The severe quantitative deficiency (<5%) is also known as type 1 GT, and the moderate decrease in surface expression (10% to 20%) is known as type 2 GT.[72,73]

Several different functional mutations have been identified in individuals with GT. Similar to other integrins, GP-IIb/IIIa requires an activation step before it can recognize its ligand. The series of intracellular events that facilitate exposure of the GP-IIb/IIIa fibrinogen binding site and allow fibrinogen to bind are known collectively as inside-out signaling. Mutations that affect the intracellular domain of GP-IIb/IIIa can consequently result in the impairment of inside-out signaling and GP-IIb/IIIa activation.[74,75] Mutations that prevent appropriate exposure of the fibrinogen binding site after activation but do not affect surface expression of GP-IIb/IIIa have also been reported to result in a very rare qualitative GT defect.[76,77] It is interesting to note that constitutive activation of GP-IIb/IIIa may also be

Table 10-3 Pattern of Inheritance of Hereditary Platelet Disorders and Gene Defects Responsible for Them

Pattern of Inheritance	Disease	Gene (Entrez Gene ID*)
X-linked	Wiskott-Aldrich syndrome	WAS (7454)
	X-linked thrombocytopenia	GATA1 (2623)
	X-linked dyserythropoiesis with or without anemia	
	X-linked thrombocytopenia/thalassemia	
	May-Hegglin anomaly	
	Fechtner syndrome	
	Sebastian syndrome	MYH9 (4627)
	Epstein syndrome	AML1 (861)
Autosomal dominant	Familiar platelet disorder/acute myeloid leukemia (FPD/AML)	Unknown
		HOXA11 (3207)
	Thrombocytopenia with absent radii (TAR)	GP1BA (2811)
	Amegakaryocytic thrombocytopenia with radioulnar synostosis	FLI1 (2313)
		Unknown
	Mediterranean macrothrombocytopenia	
	Velocardiofacial syndrome/DiGeorge	
	Platelet VWD/type 2B VWD	
	Paris-Trousseau syndrome/Jacobsen syndrome	
	White platelet syndrome	
	Glanzmann thrombasthenia	ITGA2B (3674) and ITGB3 (3690)
	Bernard-Soulier syndrome	
Autosomal recessive	Gray platelet syndrome	GP1BA (2811)
	Hermansky-Pudlak syndrome	Unknown
		HPS1 (3257)

*__Entrez Gene:__ http://www.ncbi.nlm.nih.gov/entrez/query.fcgi?db=gene

associated with GT. The *Cys560Arg* mutation results in the presence of GP-IIb/IIIa at decreased levels (20%) on the platelet surface. However, the remaining GP-IIb/IIIa has a constitutively high affinity for fibrinogen and exists in an activated conformation.[78]

Patients with GT typically present with moderate to severe mucocutaneous bleeding and often require multiple platelet transfusions from early infancy. However, the variability of bleeding phenotypes can be striking, even in patients with the same genetic mutation.[79] In all described subtypes of GT, platelet aggregation will be absent or greatly diminished in response to all agonists tested except for the agglutinating agent, ristocetin, which does not require interaction with the fibrinogen receptor. Flow cytometry in the experimental setting can then be used to distinguish the various subtypes; however, its clinical usefulness is uncertain.

Platelet transfusion is the treatment of choice for significant bleeding episodes in GT. However, in some cases, alloimmunization with platelet refractoriness has been described; this leaves the practicing hematologist with limited alternatives to treatment. Recently, the successful use of rFVIIa, alone or as a supplement to platelet transfusion, during bleeding episodes has been reported.[80] This concept is partially supported by experimental data that demonstrate enhanced GT platelet adhesion to collagen in the presence of rFVIIa through a tissue factor–independent pathway.[81] Before invasive procedures or surgeries are performed in severe cases of alloimmunization, the immunoadsorption protein A column has been successfully used to transitorily remove platelet antibodies.[82] Finally, a few patients with extremely severe bleeding due to alloimmunization have undergone bone marrow transplantation with full engraftment and resolution of the platelet defect.[83,84]

Other receptor defects

Several other receptor defects on the platelet surface have been implicated as causes of platelet dysfunction and bleeding. TXA2, collagen, and ADP receptor abnormalities have been described in several patients and families. Patients with these disorders are typically identified by the absence of an aggregation response to a particular agonist. A few examples are presented here. (For a more extensive review, see Rao.[85])

Individuals with a dominantly inherited mild bleeding diathesis and an impaired aggregation response to TXA2 have been found to have a mutation of the gene *TBAX2R* that encodes for the TXA2 receptor, resulting in defective signal transduction despite normal TXA2 binding activity.[86,87] Two platelet surface receptors—integrin $\alpha_2\beta_1$ and GP-VI—are critical for adhesion of platelets to collagen and collagen-induced signaling. Mutations in each of these receptors have been reported in patients with impaired aggregation to collagen and a bleeding diathesis.[88,89]

Mutations in the gene *P2RY12* that encodes for the P2Y12 receptor, the target of the antithrombotic compounds clopidogrel and ticlopidine, have been described; they result in a mild bleeding diathesis and a decreased aggregation response to ADP.[27,90] Also, a dominant negative mutation has been identified in the ADP/ATP receptor, *P2RX1*, which results in a moderate bleeding disorder with impaired ADP-induced aggregation.[91] In some families with a mild bleeding disorder, decreased density of $\alpha2$-adrenergic receptors and an abnormal aggregation response to epinephrine have been described.[92] However, it is noteworthy that up to 10% of "healthy controls" may exhibit an abnormal aggregation response to epinephrine.[93]

In summary, mutations in genes that encode for platelet receptors other than GPIIb/IIIa αIIbβ3 (fibrinogen receptor) and GP-Ibα (VWF receptor) have been described in isolated case reports or affected families. Bleeding manifestations appear to be mild, and the clinical impact is uncertain. Common polymorphisms in these genes may, however, act as modifiers of clinical bleeding when associated with an established underlying bleeding disorder such as VWD.[94,95]

Hermansky-Pudlak syndrome

Patients with the autosomal recessive disease, Hermansky-Pudlak syndrome (HPS), have dysfunctional platelets with absence of dense granules in association with oculocutaneous albinism. Mutations of the genes responsible for the packaging and formation of specialized lysosomes, such as melanosomes and platelet-dense granules, are responsible for the observed phenotypes. This disease exhibits considerable locus heterogeneity, and mutations in seven different genes can result in the HPS phenotype.[96] It is interesting to note that each of the seven genes affected in human disease has been identified in mouse models of HPS as well.[97,98] The most common of the seven HPS subtypes (HPS1-7), HPS-1, is caused by mutations in the HPS1 gene and is responsible for approximately 90% of cases. Most cases of HPS-1 occur in members of an extensive pedigree from the Caribbean island of Puerto Rico as the result of a founder effect.[96]

Although albinism and platelet dysfunction are predominant features in the early stages of this disease, several other organ systems appear to require appropriate trafficking of these specialized lysosomes.[96] Pulmonary fibrosis occurs in 60% of patients with HPS-1, and initiation of pulmonary symptoms typically occurs in the fourth decade of life.[99] Granulomatous colitis affects approximately 15% of HPS-1 patients, and ophthalmologic complications, including nystagmus and cataracts, occur frequently as well.

Patients with HPS typically have a mild bleeding diathesis. The platelet aggregation pattern demonstrates an absent second wave of aggregation, and luminometry shows no release. Electron micrographs show absence or extreme paucity of dense granules (Figs. 10-4 and 10-5). The treatment of choice for severe life-threatening hemorrhage in patients with HPS is platelet transfusion given to replace defective platelets. The antifibrinolytic agents, DDAVP, and rFVIIa have also been used with limited success.[100,101] Recently, it has been reported that administration of DDAVP to many Puerto Rican descendants did not significantly shorten bleeding time.[102]

Chédiak-Higashi syndrome

Although the characteristic deficiency of platelet-dense granules in Chédiak-Higashi syndrome (CHS) is similar to that seen in HPS, CHS is also characterized by neutropenia and pronounced immunodeficiency. CHS is frequently associated with the development of life-threatening lymphohistiocytic infiltration in the first decades of life, referred to as the accelerated phase.[103] Additionally, varying degrees of oculocutaneous albinism are noted. The blood

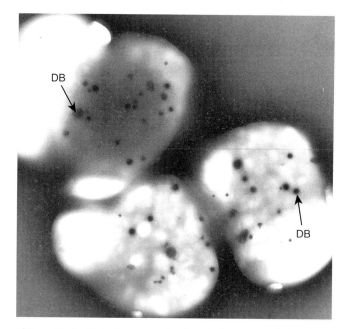

Figure 10-4 Platelets prepared by the whole mount technique from a normal individual. Electron opaque dense bodies (DB) are clearly present without fixation.

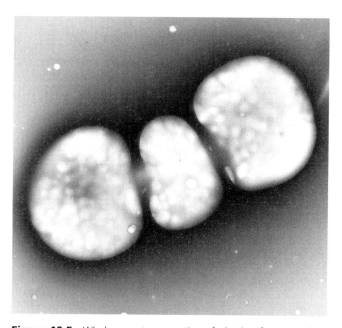

Figure 10-5 Whole mount preparation of platelets from a patient wth the Hermansky-Pudlak syndrome (HPS). Dense bodies are completely absent from the platelets. Together with albinism, this finding is diagnostic of HPS.

smear is remarkable for the presence of granulocytes with very large cytoplasmic granules.[103] Similar to HPS, the gene responsible for CHS, LYST, has a corresponding mutation in a mouse model and is presumed to play a role in vesicular trafficking.[103] Bone marrow transplant cures the hematologic manifestations of the illness, but neurologic aspects such as ataxia and decreased cognitive abilities continue to progress, manifesting later in life.[104] Management of bleeding complications is based on transfusion of platelets and antifibrinolytic agents.

Other Dense Granule Defects: Storage Pool Defect

In clinical practice, many patients identified as having dense granular deficiency or impaired dense granular release do not have the genetic syndromes described earlier. These patients are classified as having a storage pool defect, and diagnosis is usually based on the presence of a mild mucocutaneous bleeding disorder, along with lack or a diminished secondary wave of aggregation and absence or paucity of platelet-dense granules.

Defects of Intracellular Signaling Pathways

After agonist binding to a surface receptor (e.g., ADP to the receptor P2Y12), numerous downstream events occur through G-protein–coupled, tyrosine kinase, and prostaglandin-mediated signaling. Defects in these intracellular signaling pathways have been identified in several patients with a mild bleeding diathesis (for review, see Rao[85]) and varying patterns of platelet aggregation. Often, the aggregation response to multiple agonists will be affected.

GTP-binding proteins often function as a link between surface receptors and intracellular enzymes, and significantly decreased levels of the G-protein, $G\alpha_q$ have been found in a patient with a mild bleeding diathesis and decreased aggregation to multiple agonists.[105] In several patients, the production of TXA2 from arachidonic acid is impaired. Most of these individuals have been characterized as having a cyclooxygenase deficiency, but deficiencies in other enzymes within this pathway have been reported as well.[106–108] Various individuals with bleeding symptoms or decreased platelet activation have been shown to have other defective intracellular responses as well, such as altered calcium mobilization, decreased tyrosine kinase activity, and decreased phospholipase activity.[85]

Quebec Platelet Syndrome

The Quebec platelet syndrome is an autosomal dominant disorder described in two French-Canadian pedigrees. It is characterized by normal-appearing α granules seen under the electron microscope, with increased degradation of their content due to the accumulation of abnormally high amounts of urokinase-type plasminogen activator (u-PA).[109] This leads to increased spontaneous intracellular fibrinolytic activity with intraplatelet plasmin generation and normal to elevated u-PA plasma levels.[110] Affected individuals may exhibit low platelet counts and abnormal aggregation responses to collagen and ADP. The use of antifibrinolytic agents has been advocated; they have been shown to decrease bleeding risk during hemostatic challenge.[111]

Congenital Disorders With Normal Platelet Count and Normal Pattern of Aggregation

Scott Syndrome

The coagulation response requires the coordinated activities of both plasma-borne enzymes and platelets for optimal thrombus formation at the site of injury. Rapid exposure of negatively charged phospholipids, primarily phosphatidylserine, on the platelet surface follows platelet activation. Exposed phospholipids can then facilitate the activities of the plasma enzymes prothrombinase and tenase by providing a discrete surface for their localization at the injured site and by directly stimulating enzyme activity.[112]

In individuals with Scott syndrome, external exposure of negatively charged phospholipids is impaired in response to physiologic agonists or a calcium ionophore.[113–115] Patients heterozygous for the defect may exhibit intermediate responses. Recently, an individual with Scott syndrome has been identified who has a mutation in the membrane protein ABCA1.[116] However, the significance of this finding is uncertain in that patients with Tangier disease who have complete absence of ABCA1 have no impairment in platelet phosphatidlyserine exposure after platelet activation in response to varying concentrations of collagen and ionomycin.[117]

The few described patients with this rare syndrome have a mild bleeding diathesis. Platelet aggregation patterns are normal. Impairment of phosphatidlyserine exposure seen in these patients can be evaluated by flow cytometry with the use of labeled annexin V (a naturally occurring plasma protein with a high affinity for phosphatidlyserine). In individuals with Scott syndrome, annexin V binding is absent.[114] Bleeding episodes can be efficiently treated with platelet transfusion.

DISORDERS WITH THROMBOCYTOPENIA AND SMALL PLATELETS

Wiskott-Aldrich Syndrome/X-linked Thrombocytopenia

Wiskott-Aldrich syndrome/X-linked thrombocytopenia (WAS/XLT) is a moderate to severe X-linked thrombocytopenia that is often associated with eczema and immunodeficiency (reviewed in Ochs and colleagues[118,119]). The MPV in affected individuals ranges from 3.5 to 5.0 fL (Fig. 10-6). The phenotype of this disease is variable; some individuals exhibit only moderate thrombocytopenia (XLT), and others have severe disease that encompasses all components of WAS, including (1) eczema, ranging from mild to severe, (2) immunodeficiency with both cellular and humoral components, (3) autoimmune diseases, such as autoimmune

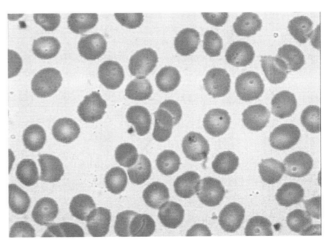

Figure 10-6 *(See also Color Plate 10-6.)* Wiskott-Aldrich syndrome. There are three platelets on this blood smear. Notice their small size. Department of Haematological Pathology, Tygerberg Hospital and University of Stellenbosch, South Africa, with permission.

hemolytic anemia,[120] and (4) increased risk of lymphoma, particularly in adulthood.

Patients with WAS/XLT have decreased or absent production of the Wiskott-Aldrich syndrome protein (WASp),[121] an intracellular protein critical for the regulation of actin polymerization and cellular signaling. The phenotype of patients with WAS mutations is most closely correlated with the degree of residual WASp expression in patients' lymphocytes.[122] Patients with a milder phenotype have been described to have intact WASp, although often in reduced amounts; in more severely affected individuals, WASp is absent or is present in a truncated form. Genotype–phenotype correlations have also been described; missense mutations are associated with milder disease, and nonsense mutations and larger gene deletions are associated with severe WAS.[122]

Although splenectomy has been reported to improve the platelet count in individuals with XLT, the consequences of asplenia could be catastrophic for individuals with severe underlying immunodeficiency.[118] Treatment of patients with WAS/XLT focuses on care for acute hemorrhage and prevention or treatment of infection and autoimmunity. Allogeneic bone marrow transplantation (BMT) may be curative and should be considered in severe cases, particularly when matched sibling donors are available.[118]

CONGENITAL DISORDERS WITH THROMBOCYTOPENIA AND NORMAL PLATELET SIZE

Familial Platelet Disorder/Acute Myeloid Leukemia

Familial platelet disorder/acute myeloid leukemia (FPD/AML) is an autosomal dominant disorder characterized by thrombocytopenia and platelet dysfunction associated with a strong predisposition to the development of hematologic malignancies. Up to 30% of affected individuals develop myelodysplasia or acute myeloid leukemia by the sixth decade of life.[123,124] Loss of function mutation within a single copy of the AML1 gene (also known as CBFA2 or RUNX1) has been shown to be responsible for FPD/AML.[124] AML1 is a transcription factor important in thrombopoiesis, and decreased expression of the AML1 protein resulting from the loss of a single AML1 allele has been proposed to be sufficient cause for the decrease in thrombopoiesis that is observed (gene dosage effect).[125,126]

Affected individuals are thrombocytopenic in the first decade of life and have an increased bleeding tendency. Abnormalities in platelet aggregation, particularly with arachidonic acid, have been noted. Myelodysplasia, acute myeloid leukemia, particularly of the M0 subtype, and lymphosarcoma have all been reported in affected individuals.[123,124]

Thrombocytopenia with Absent Radii

As the name of this autosomal recessive syndrome implies, TAR is characterized by neonatal thrombocytopenia and absent radii; various upper limb abnormalities, including phocomelia and abnormalities of the shoulder girdle, have also been reported. Other prominent features of this syndrome include renal and cardiac defects, skeletal abnormalities of the lower limbs, and a high incidence of

milk–protein allergy.[127,128] The gene responsible for TAR is unknown. Several candidate genes such as HOX (involved in skeletal development) and MPL (thrombopoietin receptor) have been excluded.[129,130] TAR combined with a chromosomal translocation involving 7p suggests that this region may be involved in the pathogenesis of TAR.[128] Other studies suggest that a blockade of megakaryocytic maturation and decreased responsiveness of megakaryocytic precursors to various cytokines underlie the observed thrombocytopenia.[131]

Although the thrombocytopenia observed in neonates with TAR may be severe and often requires multiple platelet transfusions for bleeding, it is notable for its gradual remission.[128] In older individuals, platelet counts within the lower limits of normal have been reported. Because of the reportedly high incidence of milk–protein allergy in individuals with TAR, removal of milk-containing products has been attempted and has been reported to improve thrombocytopenia.[128] It is significant that in the differential diagnosis of TAR, two other specific disorders also associated with limb abnormalities must be reported. These include Fanconi anemia (distinguished by the absence of thumbs and chromosomal breakage testing) and 22q11 microdeletion; this latter syndrome can also involve thrombocytopenia (see GP-Ib/IX/V receptor defects), which has been reported to cause limb abnormalities, including absent radii.[128]

Amegakaryocytic Thrombocytopenia with Radioulnar Synostosis

Although similar to TAR in its involvement of the hematopoietic and skeletal systems, amegakaryocytic thrombocytopenia with radioulnar synostosis represents a distinct syndrome caused by a mutation of the HOXA11,[132,133] a gene in the homeobox family that is involved in skeletal development. Individuals with this syndrome present with neonatal thrombocytopenia and proximal radioulnar synostosis combined with digital abnormalities such as syndactyly and clinodactyly.[132] Another common feature is hip dysplasia. Radioulnar synostosis may be identified on physical examination by limited pronation. Also in contrast to TAR, the natural history of this disorder often involves worsening thrombocytopenia and involvement of other blood cell lines, often requiring BMT.[132]

Congenital Amegakaryocytic Thrombocytopenia

Patients with congenital amegakaryocytic thrombocytopenia (CAMT) present with neonatal thrombocytopenia. Examination of the bone marrow reveals almost complete absence of megakaryocytes. Serum thrombopoietin (TPO) levels are markedly elevated, and when the few remaining megakaryocytes are evaluated following stimulation by TPO, no response is observed.[134,135] CAMT follows an autosomal recessive pattern. Mutations within both alleles of the MPL gene that encodes for the TPO receptor c-MPL have been identified in patients with CAMT, and the phenotype can be recapitulated in the mouse on disruption of the MPL gene.[134–136]

A gradual decline in other hematologic cell lines is frequently observed in patients with CAMT, and cases of aplasia have been reported. Allogeneic BMT, the only curative therapy, has been successfully used in the treatment of patients with CAMT.[134,135]

11q Terminal Deletion Disorder (Paris-Trousseau/Jacobsen Syndrome)

Patients with thrombocytopenia due to an 11q terminal deletion disorder (11q−) have platelets with abnormally large α granules and a distinct clinical syndrome. Abnormally large α granules, seen in a fraction of the platelet population, exhibit abnormal responses to thrombin. Numerous micromegakaryocytes may be identified on evaluation of the bone marrow.[137,138] Other clinical abnormalities associated with this syndrome include characteristic dysmorphic facies, abnormalities of the upper extremities, cardiovascular defects (>50% of cases), and mild to moderate mental retardation.[139]

The pathogenesis of thrombocytopenia associated with 11q− provides an example of a unique mechanism responsible for an autosomal dominant inherited disorder. The *FLI1* gene that encodes for a critically important transcription factor in platelet development known as FLI1 is located in the deleted region of chromosome 11.[138] Although this deficiency of FLI1 may account for the platelet disorder, one of the crucial remaining questions regarding the pathogenesis of 11q− thrombocytopenia is why the remaining copy of FLI1 is not sufficient for adequate platelet development. The answer may lie in the fact that only one of the two *FLI1* alleles is expressed (monoallelic expression) at a critical stage in megakaryocyte development. Heterozygous deficiency of *FLI1*, as occurs in patients with 11q−, would therefore result in the absence of FLI1 expression in a subset of megakaryocytes. Megakaryocytes expressing FLI1 from the unaffected allele develop normally, and those that attempt to express the deleted allele fail to do so and exhibit the affected phenotype (micromegakaryocyte). Therefore, monoallelic expression of FLI1 at a critical point in megakaryocyte development may account for the two distinct subpopulations of megakaryocytes/platelets observed in 11q− patients.[140]

Thrombocytopenia of 11q−, which can be severe at a young age, frequently resolves by adolescence.[139] However, despite resolution of thrombocytopenia, platelet structural abnormalities characteristic of 11q− can still be observed on evaluation of the peripheral blood smear. Bleeding manifestations of 11q− thrombocytopenia are variable, and some platelet abnormalities and clinical symptoms of bleeding may persist after the platelet count has been normalized.[139]

Other Familial Thrombocytopenias

Many hematologists are aware of individuals or families with congenital thrombocytopenia who do not fit any of the described categories. Investigation into the cause of the thrombocytopenia in these individuals may provide greater insight into platelet formation and function. For example, using linkage analysis, Drachman and colleagues[141] identified a gene located on the short arm of chromosome 10 as the cause of moderate thrombocytopenia in a pedigree with a mild bleeding diathesis. It is expected that the use of similar genetic techniques, along with a better understanding of platelet physiology, will allow the characterization of other families as well.

DISORDERS WITH THROMBOCYTOPENIA AND LARGE OR GIANT PLATELETS

GP-Ib/IX/V Receptor Defects (Bernard-Soulier Syndrome, Mediterranean Macrothrombocytopenia, and Velocardiofacial [DiGeorge] Syndrome)

The GP-Ib/IX/V complex, the primary platelet receptor for VWF, is composed of the products of four separate genes (*GP1BA*, *GP1BB*, *GP5*, and *GP9*). Mutations in the genes that encode for components of this receptor have been implicated in several thrombocytopenic syndromes, including Bernard-Soulier syndrome (BSS), Mediterranean macrothrombocytopenia, and thrombocytopenia observed in velocardiofacial (22q11 microdeletion) syndrome.

BSS is an autosomal recessive disorder characterized by the presence of giant platelets, with some platelets measuring up to 20 μM in diameter and thrombocytopenia ranging from 20,000/μL to nearly normal (Fig. 10-7).[72] The association of GP-Ibα, GP-Ibβ, and GP-IX is required for efficient transport of the complex to the platelet surface,[142] and homozygous or compound heterozygous mutations of each of these components have been identified in BSS.[72] Platelet aggregation studies exhibit a typical pattern of lack of response to ristocetin, even in the presence of added normal plasma.

Evaluation of BSS platelets reveals absence of the receptor on the platelet surface; however, variant forms of BSS, in which a nonfunctional GP-Ib/IX/V complex is expressed at low levels, have been identified.[72] Patients with BSS typically exhibit mucocutaneous bleeding manifestations, although the clinical presentation is variable. Platelet concentrates are the choice for life-threatening bleeds, but as in patients with Glanzmann thrombasthenia, alloimmunization may occur.[143] DDAVP and factor rVIIa have also been used with success.[144]

Autosomal dominant Mediterranean macrothrombocytopenia and velocardiofacial syndromes are disorders in which only a single allele of a component of the GP-Ib/IX/V complex is mutated. Different from BSS, these syndromes are characterized by large but not giant platelets and a mild bleeding diathesis. Linkage analysis of several families with the autosomal dominant Mediterranean

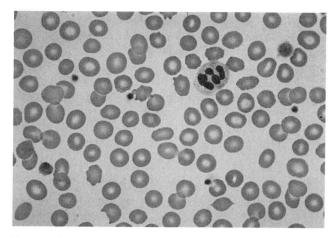

Figure 10-7 (See also Color Plate 10-7.) Bernard-Soulier syndrome. There are six platelets on this blood smear. Notice that two platelets are very large.

macrothrombocytopenia syndrome led to the identification of a heterozygous missense mutation (Ala156Val) of GP-Ibα as the cause of thrombocytopenia in 10 of 12 pedigrees analyzed.[145] Heterozygous absence of a component of the GP-Ib/IX/V complex also accounts for the thrombocytopenia observed in approximately 40% of patients with velocardiofacial syndrome (22q11), often referred to as DiGeorge syndrome.[146,147] The GP-Ib gene that encodes for GP-Ibβ is located within the commonly deleted region. It is interesting to note that only 60% of patients heterozygous for the absence of the GP-Ib/IX/V complex exhibit macrothrombocytopenia. Accordingly, manifestations of heterozygote carriers of mutations known to cause BSS are variable.

Platelet-type von Willebrand Disease (Gain of Function Mutation of GP-Ib/IX/V)

Platelet-type VWD, also known as pseudo-VWD, is an autosomal dominant disorder characterized by mild to moderate mucocutaneous bleeding, mild thrombocytopenia, and decreased plasma levels of the VWF high-molecular-weight multimers.[148] Mutations within the VWF binding domain of GP-Ibα and deletion of a portion of the macroglycopeptide region of GP-Ibα have been identified in patients with platelet-type VWD.[149,150] These gain of function mutations prompt GP-Ibα to exhibit an increased affinity for VWF, and spontaneous binding of VWF to platelets occurs. As a result, circulating plasma levels of VWF multimers are low, and thrombocytopenia is noted, presumably caused by the increased clearance of VWF/platelet complexes. Impaired platelet production may also contribute to thrombocytopenia, as evidenced by the presence of giant platelets on evaluation of several patients with platelet-type VWD. Mean platelet volume was elevated in three unrelated families who were tested, suggesting that macrothrombocytopenia may be a feature of this disorder as well.[151]

It is critical to differentiate this syndrome from type 2B VWD, a more common disorder that is caused by gain of function mutations within the VWF binding site for the platelet GP-1bα. This increased binding affinity also leads to rapid clearance of the platelet/VWF complex, mimicking the platelet-type phenotype. Increased platelet aggregation in response to low doses of ristocetin is noted in both syndromes; however, aggregation will occur in the platelet-type patient sample only if the patient's platelets instead of fixed control platelets are used.

Management of these two entities varies because VWF concentrates and DDAVP can worsen thrombocytopenia of platelet-type VWD because of the increased availability of VWF multimers and subsequent increased clearance of the patient's defective platelets.[152] Platelet replacement is the treatment of choice for bleeding episodes in platelet-type VWD.

MYH9-Related Thrombocytopenia (May-Hegglin, Sebastian, Fechtner, and Epstein Syndromes)

MYH9-related disease refers to a spectrum of autosomal dominant syndromes characterized by macrothrombocytopenia and varying degrees of nephritis, hearing loss, and cataracts. Previously, on the basis of their various clinical presentations, patients with *MYH9*-related disorders had been classified as having one of several different syndromes (May-Hegglin anomaly, Sebastian, Fechtner, and Epstein syndromes). The recent discovery of the causative gene for the May-Hegglin anomaly led to the recognition that these disorders are all the result of mutations within the same gene, *MYH9*.[153–155] All individuals from families with a mutation in the *MYH9* gene described to date exhibit some degree of macrothrombocytopenia (Figs. 10-8 and 10-9);

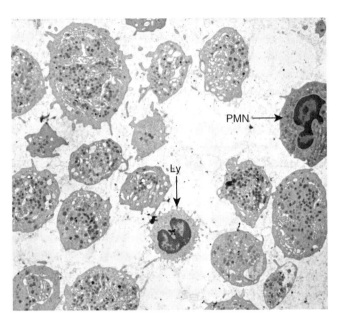

Figure 10-8 Low-magnification micrograph of platelets and leukocytes from a patient with May-Hegglin anomaly. Platelets appear normal, except for their large size. At least one platelet is larger than a polymorphonuclear leukocyte (PMN), and several are larger than a lymphocyte (Ly).

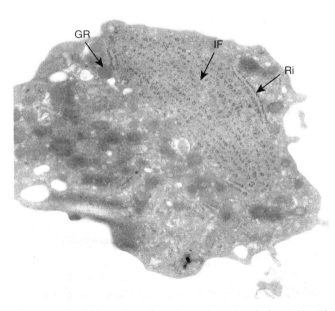

Figure 10-9 Thin section of a polymorphonuclear leukocyte (PMN) containing a spindle-shaped inclusion diagnostic of the May-Hegglin anomaly (MHA). Ribosomal (Ri) clusters are present on intermediate filaments (IF) in the long axis of the inclusion. The cell contains normal PMN organelles other than the MHA inclusion. Gr, granules.

however, the occurrence of other phenotypes is variable. In one study, families with 21 different causative mutations of *MYH9*-related disease were screened by audiology, urinalysis, and ophthalmologic evaluation. High-tone sensorineural hearing loss occurred in 83% of individuals with *MYH9* mutations. Of these individuals, 62% had some degree of nephritis, ranging from microscopic hematuria to renal failure, and ocular cataracts were observed in 23% of patients.[156] Other studies have reported a lower incidence of these manifestations. On close examination of the blood smear, polymorphonuclear inclusions called Döhle-like bodies can also be observed in almost all patients with *MYH9*-related disease (Fig. 10-10). Diagnosis of these disorders is dependent on the observation of macrothrombocytopenia in association with characteristic leukocyte inclusions.

The protein product of the *MYH9* gene is nonmuscle myosin heavy chain IIA, a component of nonmuscle myosin IIA. The precise biologic function of myosin IIA within the platelet is unknown, but it has been suggested that it serves as a molecular motor, facilitating changes in cell shape, phagocytosis, and organelle trafficking (for review, see Krendel and Mooseker[157]). The universal finding of thrombocytopenia in these syndromes is most likely related to the fact that human platelets exclusively express myosin IIA, whereas other tissues express multiple isoforms of myosin II (IIA, IIB, and IIC).[158] Consistent with the role of myosin IIA in platelet cytoskeletal organization, defective localization of myosin, tubulin, and multiple intracellular signaling molecules is seen before and after platelet activation in patients with May-Hegglin syndrome.[159,160]

Approximately 80% of identified myosin IIA mutations in patients with *MYH9*-related disorders are exclusively localized at five different amino acid residues of the 1961 amino acid protein.[161] Evaluation of patients with these common mutations has allowed investigators to make reliable genotype/phenotype associations. For example, mutation of the site for amino acid R702 is closely related to hearing loss and nephritis, and individuals with a mutation of the C-terminal residue E1841 have no kidney or hearing manifestations.[161]

Although bleeding symptoms are usually mild, platelets from these patients have been reported to lack the platelet shape change typically observed in platelet aggregation studies. Otherwise, the platelet aggregation pattern is normal, with the exception of an increased frequency of individuals with a defective response to epinephrine.[160]

GATA1-Related Thrombocytopenia

Mutations of the transcription factor *GATA1* have been described in several families who presented with X-linked macrothrombocytopenia and varying degrees of dyserythropoiesis or thalassemia.[162] *GATA1* is a transcription factor critical for normal megakaryocytopoiesis, and several different causative mutations have been identified within the region encoding its N-terminal zinc finger domain.[162,163] The N-terminal zinc finger functions as a DNA binding domain and in recruitment of the essential transcription cofactor *FOG1* to the promoter of platelet specific genes such as *ITGA2B* (which encodes for the IIb portion of the fibrinogen receptor GP-IIb/IIIa). Mutations within the N-terminal zinc finger domain that interfere with the DNA binding of *GATA1* or with its ability to interact with *FOG1* have been identified.[162]

Patients with thrombocytopenia due to a *GATA1* mutation typically have a moderate bleeding diathesis with a greater than expected amount of bleeding relative to the observed platelet count. On close inspection, the platelets of patients with *GATA1* mutations are large and have a paucity of α granules; cytoplasmic clusters of smooth endoplasmic reticulum are often noted.[164] Platelet function studies show abnormalities in platelet shape change after platelet activation, as well as impaired platelet activation, particularly with collagen.[165,166] The severity of the hematologic abnormalities associated with mutations in *GATA1* is highly variable; these abnormalities include thalassemia, mild marrow dyserythropoiesis, and transfusion dependent–anemia with marked anisocytosis and poikilocytosis.[162]

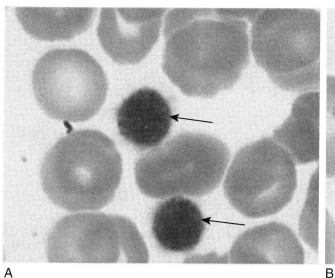
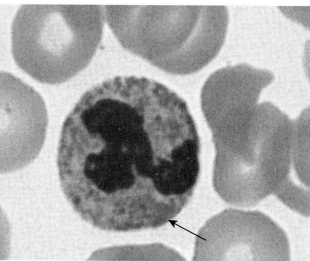

A   B

Figure 10-10 *(See also Color Plate 10-10.)* May-Hegglin syndrome. In panel **A,** notice the two large platelets. In panel **B,** the neutrophil contains a pale blue inclusion body.

Gray Platelet Syndrome

Gray platelet syndrome (GPS) is a mild to moderate bleeding diathesis characterized by the presence of macrothrombocytopenia and gray-appearing platelets on peripheral blood smear (Fig. 10-11).[167] Electron microscopy shows the presence of α-granules that are virtually empty (Figs. 10-12 and 10-13). Analysis of platelet content reveals severely decreased levels of several α-granule proteins, including fibrinogen, thrombospondin, and factor V.[167,168]

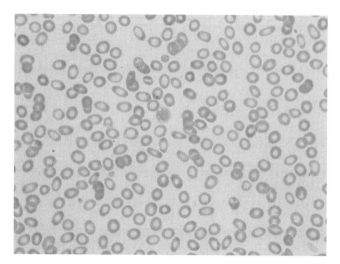

Figure 10-11 *(See also Color Plate 10-11.)* Gray platelet syndrome. There is a large ghost-like platelet near the middle. Its pale color is due to lack of stainable granules.

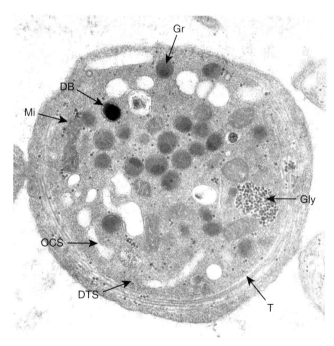

Figure 10-12 Thin section of a normal human platelet cut in the horizontal plane. A circumferential coil of microtubules (T) just under the cell membrane supports the discoid form. Numerous organelles, including α-granules (Gr), dense bodies (DB), and mitochondria (Mi), are randomly dispersed in the cytoplasm, which also contains single and masses of glycogen (Gly) particles. Two membrane systems are present, including the open canalicular system (OCS), continuous with the cell membrane, and the dense tubular system (DTS), derived from endoplasmic reticulum.

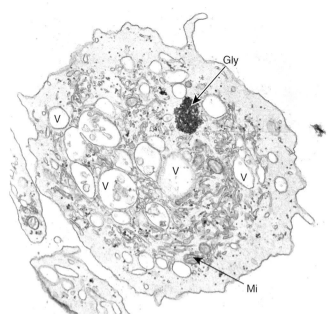

Figure 10-13 Single gray platelet syndrome (GPS) platelet. The absence of internal contents inside the α-granule vacuoles (V) is evident in this example. Glycogen (Gly), mitochondria (Mi), and other cytoplasmic contents are normal despite the large size of the GPS platelet.

Both autosomal recessive and dominant forms of GPS have been reported.[169,170] In some patients, GPS has been associated with a mild to severe myelofibrosis that on occasions is associated with extramedullary hematopoiesis.[170] In another described pedigree, gray-appearing neutrophils with absent granules are also observed.[171] These varying presentations and patterns of inheritance suggest locus heterogeneity, as seen in the Hermansky-Pudlak syndrome. To date, no gene has been assigned responsibility for GPS.

White Platelet Syndrome

This autosomal dominant macrothrombocytopenic syndrome was recently described in a large multigenerational pedigree from Minnesota.[172] The α-granule content of platelets was decreased, giving some platelets a gray appearance. Different from GPS, uniquely large, fully developed Golgi complexes were noted in a minority of circulating platelets. Mild to moderate bleeding symptoms were reported in affected patients, and platelet aggregation to all agonists tested was blunted (Table 10-4).

TREATMENT OF PATIENTS WITH PLATELET-RELATED BLEEDING (GENERAL GUIDELINES)

Transfusion of donor platelets is the optimal treatment for significant bleeds in most patients with congenital or acquired platelet disorders. DDAVP is the treatment of choice for individuals with bleeding and platelet dysfunction secondary to uremia and may provide some benefit in select individuals with other platelet disorders with mild to moderate bleeds. DDAVP facilitates clot formation by causing the release of VWF and FVIII from endothelial cells, thereby enhancing platelet adhesion. The potential

Table 10-4 Clinical and Laboratory Features Associated With Congenital Platelet Disorders

System	Clinical Manifestations	Disease
Skin	Eczema	Wiskott-Aldrich syndrome
	Albinism	Hermansky-Pudlak and Chédiak-Higashi syndromes
Skeletal	*Upper Extremities*	
	Absent radii, thumbs present, phocomelia	Thrombocytopenia, absent radii (TAR)
	Restricted pronation of the forearm	Amegakaryocytic thrombocytopenia with ulnar synostosis
	Hand abnormalities, syndactyly	Paris-Trousseau syndrome
		TAR
	Lower Extremities	
	Various anomalies	Amegakaryocytic thrombocytopenia with radioulnar synostosis
	Hip dysplasia	
Pulmonary	Fibrosis	Hermansky-Pudlak syndrome
Cardiac	Ventricular septal defects	DiGeorge sequence, velocardiofacial syndrome
	Tetralogy of Fallot	Paris-Trousseau syndrome
	Right aortic arch	TAR
Renal	Hematuria, proteinuria	*MYH9*
	Congenital malformations	TAR
Gastrointestinal	Milk–protein allergy	TAR
	Granulomatous colitis	Hermansky-Pudlak syndrome
Auditory	High-tone sensorineural hearing loss	*MYH9*-related thrombocytopenia
Ocular	Cataracts	*MYH9*-related thrombocytopenia
Neurologic	Mental retardation	11q terminal deletion
	Ataxia, cognitive defects	Chédiak-Higashi syndrome
Immunologic	Autoimmunity	*WAS/XLT*, Chédiak-Higashi syndrome
	Immunodeficiency	*WAS/XLT*, Chédiak-Higashi syndrome
Hematologic	Thalassemia/anemia	*GATA1* mutation
	AML (family/personal history)	Familial platelet disorder/acute myeloid leukemia
	Lymphoma	*WAS/XLT*
	Neutropenia	Chédiak-Higashi syndrome
	White blood cell giant cytoplasmic granules	Chédiak-Higashi syndrome
	Döhle-like bodies	*MYH9*-related thrombocytopenia

effectiveness of DDAVP in minor bleeds may be assessed in select patients with use of the PFA-100. In patients with congenital or acquired platelet disorders and a prolonged PFA-100 closure time, shortening of closure time may suggest that DDAVP will be of some benefit. However, the correlation with clinical outcomes has yet to be determined.

rFVIIa has been used with some success in individuals with congenital platelet disorders and is of particular benefit in those patients who are refractory to transfused platelets.[80,173] rFVIIa is believed to function by increasing thrombin generation at the site of vessel wall damage, thereby enhancing platelet recruitment and facilitating the use of alternate pathways for platelet aggregate formation.[81,174,175]

As expected, each treatment option is associated with specific adverse effects and complications that must be considered. Patients who receive multiple platelet transfusions may become refractory to the administration of donor platelet because of immunity to platelet-specific or human leukocyte antigen (HLA)-related antigens. In Glanzmann thrombasthenia, which is characterized by the absence of the fibrinogen receptor GP-IIb/IIIa on the platelet surface, both GP-IIb/IIIa and HLA antigens on the surface of donor platelets have been linked to the development of antibodies that result in increased platelet clearance and platelet transfusion refractoriness.[80]

Administration of DDAVP causes water retention, and appropriate precautions regarding fluid restriction must be taken to avoid possible serious electrolyte imbalance. Because of this complication, its use in children younger than 2 years of age should be approached with caution.[176] Tachyphylaxis to DDAVP will most likely develop if multiple successive doses of DDAVP are given.[58] It is important to mention that the use of aspirin and NSAIDs in patients with congenital platelet disorders should be avoided if possible because of the known effects of these drugs on platelet function.

The increasing off-label use of rFVIIa for acquired and congenital platelet conditions has triggered a large number of case reports and patient series.[60,80,173] However, only carefully designed clinical trials will prove the efficacy of this hemostatic agent in various platelet disorders related to bleeding. With any of the previously mentioned treatment options, the potential exacerbation of an underlying thrombotic condition should be carefully considered before treatment is initiated.[177]

CONCLUSIONS

Accurate diagnosis of congenital and acquired platelet disorders should have considerable impact on the care of patients with clinical bleeding. Appropriate treatments that avoid undesired adverse effects may be implemented, and safeguards for procedures and surgeries determined. Also, understanding the mode of transmission of hereditary disorders allows medical personnel to provide family counseling.

Once the diagnosis has been made, the real challenge for the practicing hematologist is to identify patients at risk for clinical bleeding. No global test of platelet function has been able to predict the population at risk, and treatment decisions are usually made on the basis of bleeding history or previous hemostatic challenge (e.g., surgeries).

It is hoped that newly discovered modifier genes in the hemostatic and vascular systems will provide new insights into the variability observed in clinical presentations. However understanding the impact of these modifiers requires time and carefully designed clinical trials. Meanwhile, the hematologist should judiciously use the tools that are currently available to provide the best care for patients with platelet-related bleeding.

ACKNOWLEDGMENT

The authors thank Dr. James White of the University of Minnesota for kindly providing all the electron micrographs for this chapter.

REFERENCES

1. Glanzmann E: Hereditäre Hämorrhagische thrombasthenic. Ein Beitrag zur Pathologie der Blutplättchen. Jahrbuch der Kinderheilkunde 1988:1–42, 1918.
2. Hardisty R, Dormandy K, Hutton R: Thrombasthenia: Studies on three cases. Br J Haematol 10:371–387, 1964.
3. Caen J, Castaldi P-A, Leclerc J-C, et al: Congenital bleeding disorders with long bleeding time and normal platelet count. Am J Med 41:4–26, 1966.
4. Nurden AT, Caen JP: An abnormal platelet glycoprotein pattern in three cases of Glanzmann's thrombasthenia. Br J Haematol 28:253–260, 1974.
5. Nurden AT, Caen JP: Specific roles for platelet surface glycoproteins in platelet function. Nature 255:720–722, 1975.
6. Hagen I, Nurden A, Bjerrum OJ, et al: Immunochemical evidence for protein abnormalities in platelets from patients with Glanzmann's thrombasthenia and Bernard-Soulier syndrome. J Clin Invest 65:722–731, 1980.
7. Phillips DR, Agin PP: Platelet membrane defects in Glanzmann's thrombasthenia: Evidence for decreased amounts of two major glycoproteins. J Clin Invest 60:535–545, 1977.
8. McEver RP, Baenziger NL, Majerus PW: Isolation and quantitation of the platelet membrane glycoprotein deficient in thrombasthenia using a monoclonal hybridoma antibody. J Clin Invest 66:1311–1318, 1980.
9. Coller BS, Peerschke EI, Scudder LE, et al: A murine monoclonal antibody that completely blocks the binding of fibrinogen to platelets produces a thrombasthenic-like state in normal platelets and binds to glycoproteins IIb and/or IIIa. J Clin Invest 72:325–338, 1983.
10. Coller BS: A new murine monoclonal antibody reports an activation-dependent change in the conformation and/or microenvironment of the platelet glycoprotein IIb/IIIa complex. J Clin Invest 76:101–108, 1985.
11. Coller BS, Folts JD, Scudder LE, Smith SR: Antithrombotic effect of a monoclonal antibody to the platelet glycoprotein IIb/IIIa receptor in an experimental animal model. Blood 68:783–786, 1986.
12. Coller BS, Folts JD, Smith SR, et al: Abolition of in vivo platelet thrombus formation in primates with monoclonal antibodies to the platelet GPIIb/IIIa receptor: Correlation with bleeding time, platelet aggregation, and blockade of GPIIb/IIIa receptors. Circulation 80:1766–1774, 1989.
13. Randomised placebo-controlled trial of abciximab before and during coronary intervention in refractory unstable angina: The CAPTURE study. The Lancet 349:1429–1435, 1997.
14. The EPIC Investigators: Use of a monoclonal antibody directed against the platelet glycoprotein IIb/IIIa receptor in high-risk coronary angioplasty. N Engl J Med 330:956–961, 1994.
15. Kadir RA, Economides DL, Sabin CA, et al: Frequency of inherited bleeding disorders in women with menorrhagia. Lancet 351: 485–489, 1998.
16. Bevan JA, Maloney KW, Hillery CA, et al: Bleeding disorders: A common cause of menorrhagia in adolescents. J Pediatr 138:856–861, 2001.
17. Peterson P, Hayes TE, Arkin CF, et al: The preoperative bleeding time test lacks clinical benefit: College of American Pathologists' and American Society of Clinical Pathologists' position article. Arch Surg 133:134–139, 1998.
18. Cattaneo M, Federici AB, Lecchi A, et al: Evaluation of the PFA-100 system in the diagnosis and therapeutic monitoring of patients with von Willebrand disease. Thromb Haemost 82:35–39, 1999.
19. Harrison P, Robinson MS, Mackie IJ, et al: Performance of the platelet function analyser PFA-100 in testing abnormalities of primary haemostasis. Blood Coagul Fibrinolysis 10:25–31, 1999.
20. Harrison P: The role of PFA-100 testing in the investigation and management of haemostatic defects in children and adults. Br J Haematol 130:3–10, 2005.
21. Quiroga T, Goycoolea M, Munoz B, et al: Template bleeding time and PFA-100 have low sensitivity to screen patients with hereditary mucocutaneous hemorrhages: Comparative study in 148 patients. J Thromb Haemost 2:892–898, 2004.
22. Harrison C, Khair K, Baxter B, et al: Hermansky-Pudlak syndrome: Infrequent bleeding and first report of Turkish and Pakistani kindreds. Arch Dis Child 86:297–301, 2002.
23. Cattaneo M, Lecchi A, Agati B, et al: Evaluation of platelet function with the PFA-100 system in patients with congenital defects of platelet secretion. Thromb Res 96:213–217, 1999.
24. Patrignani P, Filabozzi P, Patrono C: Selective cumulative inhibition of platelet thromboxane production by low-dose aspirin in healthy subjects. J Clin Invest 69:1366–1372, 1982.
25. Roth GJ, Majerus PW: The mechanism of the effect of aspirin on human platelets. I. Acetylation of a particulate fraction protein. J Clin Invest 56:624–632, 1975.
26. Savi P, Herbert JM: Clopidogrel and ticlopidine: P2Y12 adenosine diphosphate-receptor antagonists for the prevention of atherothrombosis. Semin Thromb Hemost 31:174–183, 2005.
27. Hollopeter G, Jantzen HM, Vincent D, et al: Identification of the platelet ADP receptor targeted by antithrombotic drugs. Nature 409:202–207, 2001.
28. Shattil SJ, Bennett JS, McDonough M, Turnbull J: Carbenicillin and penicillin G inhibit platelet function in vitro by impairing the interaction of agonists with the platelet surface. J Clin Invest 65:329–337, 1980.
29. Johnson GJ: Platelets, penicillins, and purpura: What does it all mean? J Lab Clin Med 121:531–533, 1993.
30. Glusa E, Bevan J, Heptinstall S: Verapamil is a potent inhibitor of 5-HT–induced platelet aggregation. Thromb Res 55:239–245, 1989.
31. Weksler BB, Gillick M, Pink J: Effect of propranolol on platelet function. Blood 49:185–196, 1977.
32. de Graaf JC, Banga JD, Moncada S, et al: Nitric oxide functions as an inhibitor of platelet adhesion under flow conditions. Circulation 85:2284–2290, 1992.
33. de Abajo FJ, Rodriguez LA, Montero D: Association between selective serotonin reuptake inhibitors and upper gastrointestinal bleeding: Population based case-control study. BMJ 319:1106–1109, 1999.
34. Movig KL, Janssen MW, de Waal Malefijt J, et al: Relationship of serotonergic antidepressants and need for blood transfusion in orthopedic surgical patients. Arch Intern Med 163:2354–2358, 2003.
35. van Walraven C, Mamdani MM, Wells PS, Williams JI: Inhibition of serotonin reuptake by antidepressants and upper gastrointestinal bleeding in elderly patients: Retrospective cohort study. BMJ 323:655–658, 2001.
36. Salem RO, Laposata M: Effects of alcohol on hemostasis. Am J Clin Pathol 123(suppl): S96–S105, 2005.
37. Mukamal KJ, Massaro JM, Ault KA, et al: Alcohol consumption and platelet activation and aggregation among women and men: The Framingham Offspring Study. Alcohol Clin Exp Res 29:1906–1912, 2005.

38. Serebruany VL, Lowry DR, Fuzailov SY, et al: Moderate alcohol consumption is associated with decreased platelet activity in patients presenting with acute myocardial infarction. J Thromb Thrombolysis 9:229–234, 2000.

39. Weerasinghe A, Taylor KM: The platelet in cardiopulmonary bypass. Ann Thorac Surg 66:2145–2152, 1998.

40. Plotz FB, van Oeveren W, Bartlett RH, Wildevuur CR: Blood activation during neonatal extracorporeal life support. J Thorac Cardiovasc Surg 105:823–832, 1993.

41. Rinder CS, Mathew JP, Rinder HM, et al: Modulation of platelet surface adhesion receptors during cardiopulmonary bypass. Anesthesiology 75:563–570, 1991.

42. Rinder CS, Bonan JL, Rinder HM, et al: Cardiopulmonary bypass induces leukocyte–platelet adhesion. Blood 79:1201–1205, 1992.

43. Kondo C, Tanaka K, Takagi K, et al: Platelet dysfunction during cardiopulmonary bypass surgery: With special reference to platelet membrane glycoproteins. Asaio J 39:M550–M553, 1993.

44. Mohnle P, Schwann NM, Vaughn WK, et al: Perturbations in laboratory values after coronary artery bypass graft surgery with cardiopulmonary bypass. J Cardiothorac Vasc Anesth 19:19–25, 2005.

45. Gelb AB, Roth RI, Levin J, et al: Changes in blood coagulation during and following cardiopulmonary bypass: Lack of correlation with clinical bleeding. Am J Clin Pathol 106:87–99, 1996.

46. Steiner RW, Coggins C, Carvalho AC: Bleeding time in uremia: A useful test to assess clinical bleeding. Am J Hematol 7:107–117, 1979.

47. Reverter JC, Escolar G, Sanz C, et al: Platelet activation during hemodialysis measured through exposure of p-selectin: Analysis by flow cytometric and ultrastructural techniques. J Lab Clin Med 124:79–85, 1994.

48. Zwaginga JJ, Ijsseldijk MJ, de Groot PG, et al: Treatment of uremic anemia with recombinant erythropoietin also reduces the defects in platelet adhesion and aggregation caused by uremic plasma. Thromb Haemost 66:638–647, 1991.

49. Moia M, Mannucci PM, Vizzotto L, et al: Improvement in the haemostatic defect of uraemia after treatment with recombinant human erythropoietin. Lancet 2:1227–1229, 1987.

50. Fernandez F, Goudable C, Sie P, et al: Low haematocrit and prolonged bleeding time in uraemic patients: Effect of red cell transfusions. Br J Haematol 59:139–148, 1985.

51. Castillo R, Lozano T, Escolar G, et al: Defective platelet adhesion on vessel subendothelium in uremic patients. Blood 68:337–342, 1986.

52. Zwaginga JJ, Ijsseldijk MJ, de Groot PG, et al: Defects in platelet adhesion and aggregate formation in uremic bleeding disorder can be attributed to factors in plasma. Arterioscler Thromb 11:733–744, 1991.

53. Remuzzi G, Benigni A, Dodesini P, et al: Reduced platelet thromboxane formation in uremia: Evidence for a functional cyclooxygenase defect. J Clin Invest 71:762–768, 1983.

54. Boccardo P, Remuzzi G, Galbusera M: Platelet dysfunction in renal failure. Semin Thromb Hemost 30:579–589, 2004.

55. Noris M, Remuzzi G: Uremic bleeding: Closing the circle after 30 years of controversies? Blood 94:2569–2574, 1999.

56. Gotti E, Mecca G, Valentino C, et al: Renal biopsy in patients with acute renal failure and prolonged bleeding time: A preliminary report. Am J Kidney Dis 6:397–399, 1985.

57. Watson AJ, Keogh JA: Effect of 1-deamino-8-D-arginine vasopressin on the prolonged bleeding time in chronic renal failure. Nephron 32:49–52, 1982.

58. Canavese C, Salomone M, Pacitti A, et al: Reduced response of uraemic bleeding time to repeated doses of desmopressin. Lancet 1:867–868, 1985.

59. Revesz T, Arets B, Bierings M, et al: Recombinant factor VIIa in severe uremic bleeding. Thromb Haemost 80:353, 1998.

60. Poon MC, d'Oiron R: Recombinant activated factor VII (Novo-Seven) treatment of platelet-related bleeding disorders. International Registry on Recombinant Factor VIIa and Congenital Platelet Disorders Group. Blood Coagul Fibrinolysis 11(suppl 1): S55–S68, 2000.

61. Elliott MA, Tefferi A: Thrombosis and haemorrhage in polycythaemia vera and essential thrombocythaemia. Br J Haematol 128:275–290, 2005.

62. Jensen MK, de Nully Brown P, Lund BV, et al: Increased platelet activation and abnormal membrane glycoprotein content and redistribution in myeloproliferative disorders. Br J Haematol 110:116–124, 2000.

63. Presseizen K, Friedman Z, Shapiro H, et al: Phosphatidylserine expression on the platelet membrane of patients with myeloproliferative disorders and its effect on platelet-dependent thrombin formation. Clin Appl Thromb Hemost 8:33–39, 2002.

64. Royer Y, Staerk J, Costuleanu M, et al: Janus kinases affect thrombopoietin receptor cell surface localization and stability. J Biol Chem 280:27251–27261, 2005.

65. Budde U, Scharf RE, Franke P, et al: Elevated platelet count as a cause of abnormal von Willebrand factor multimer distribution in plasma. Blood 82:1749–1757, 1993.

66. Gielchinsky Y, Elstein D, Hadas-Halpern I, et al: Is there a correlation between degree of splenomegaly, symptoms and hypersplenism?. A study of 218 patients with Gaucher disease. Br J Haematol 106:812–816, 1999.

67. Wadenvik H, Denfors I, Kutti J: Splenic blood flow and intrasplenic platelet kinetics in relation to spleen volume. Br J Haematol 67:181–185, 1987.

68. Noguchi H, Hirai K, Aoki Y, et al: Changes in platelet kinetics after a partial splenic arterial embolization in cirrhotic patients with hypersplenism. Hepatology 22:1682–1688, 1995.

69. Kercher KW, Carbonell AM, Heniford BT, et al: Laparoscopic splenectomy reverses thrombocytopenia in patients with hepatitis C cirrhosis and portal hypertension. J Gastrointest Surg 8:120–126, 2004.

70. Nio M, Hayashi Y, Sano N, et al: Long-term efficacy of partial splenic embolization in children. J Pediatr Surg 38:1760–1762, 2003.

71. Shilyansky J, Roberts EA, Superina RA: Distal splenorenal shunts for the treatment of severe thrombocytopenia from portal hypertension in children. J Gastrointest Surg 3:167–172, 1999.

72. Nurden AT, Nurden P: Inherited defects of platelet function. Rev Clin Exp Hematol 5:314–334, 2001.

73. Bellucci S, Caen J: Molecular basis of Glanzmann's thrombasthenia and current strategies in treatment. Blood Rev 16:193–202, 2002.

74. Chen YP, O'Toole TE, Ylanne J, et al: A point mutation in the integrin beta 3 cytoplasmic domain (S752→P) impairs bidirectional signaling through alpha IIb beta 3 (platelet glycoprotein IIb-IIIa). Blood 84:1857–1865, 1994.

75. Wang R, Shattil SJ, Ambruso DR, Newman PJ: Truncation of the cytoplasmic domain of beta3 in a variant form of Glanzmann thrombasthenia abrogates signaling through the integrin alpha(IIb)beta3 complex. J Clin Invest 100:2393–2403, 1997.

76. Loftus JC, O'Toole TE, Plow EF, et al: A beta 3 integrin mutation abolishes ligand binding and alters divalent cation-dependent conformation. Science 249:915–918, 1990.

77. French DL, Seligsohn U: Platelet glycoprotein IIb/IIIa receptors and Glanzmann's thrombasthenia. Arterioscler Thromb Vasc Biol 20:607–610, 2000.

78. Ruiz C, Liu CY, Sun QH, et al: A point mutation in the cysteine-rich domain of glycoprotein (GP) IIIa results in the expression of a GPIIb-IIIa (alphaIIbbeta3) integrin receptor locked in a high-affinity state and a Glanzmann thrombasthenia-like phenotype. Blood 98:2432–2441, 2001.

79. Peretz H, Seligsohn U, Zwang E, et al: Detection of the Glanzmann's thrombasthenia mutations in Arab and Iraqi-Jewish patients by polymerase chain reaction and restriction analysis of blood or urine samples. Thromb Haemost 66:500–504, 1991.

80. Poon MC, D'Oiron R, Von Depka M, et al: Prophylactic and therapeutic recombinant factor VIIa administration to patients with Glanzmann's thrombasthenia: Results of an international survey. J Thromb Haemost 2:1096–1103, 2004.

81. Lisman T, Moschatsis S, Adelmeijer J, et al: Recombinant factor VIIa enhances deposition of platelets with congenital or acquired alpha IIb beta 3 deficiency to endothelial cell matrix and collagen under conditions of flow via tissue factor–independent thrombin generation. Blood 101:1864–1870, 2003.

82. Vivier M, Treisser A, Naett M, et al: [Glanzmann's thrombasthenia and pregnancy: Contribution of plasma exchange before scheduled cesarean section]. J Gynecol Obstet Biol Reprod (Paris) 18:507–513, 1989.

83. Bellucci S, Devergie A, Gluckman E, et al: Complete correction of Glanzmann's thrombasthenia by allogeneic bone-marrow transplantation. Br J Haematol 59:635–641, 1985.

84. Bellucci S, Damaj G, Boval B, et al: Bone marrow transplantation in severe Glanzmann's thrombasthenia with antiplatelet alloimmunization. Bone Marrow Transplant 25:327–330, 2000.

85. Rao AK: Inherited defects in platelet signaling mechanisms. J Thromb Haemost 1:671–681, 2003.

86. Fuse I, Hattori A, Mito M, et al: Pathogenetic analysis of five cases with a platelet disorder characterized by the absence of thromboxane

A2 (TXA2)-induced platelet aggregation in spite of normal TXA2 binding activity. Thromb Haemost 76:1080–1085, 1996.

87. Hirata T, Kakizuka A, Ushikubi F, et al: Arg60 to Leu mutation of the human thromboxane A2 receptor in a dominantly inherited bleeding disorder. J Clin Invest 94:1662–1667, 1994.

88. Moroi M, Jung SM, Okuma M, Shinmyozu K: A patient with platelets deficient in glycoprotein VI that lack both collagen-induced aggregation and adhesion. J Clin Invest 84:1440–1445, 1989.

89. Nieuwenhuis HK, Akkerman JW, Houdijk WP, Sixma JJ: Human blood platelets showing no response to collagen fail to express surface glycoprotein Ia. Nature 318:470–472, 1985.

90. Cattaneo M, Zighetti ML, Lombardi R, et al: Molecular bases of defective signal transduction in the platelet P2Y12 receptor of a patient with congenital bleeding. Proc Natl Acad Sci U S A 100:1978–1983, 2003.

91. Oury C, Toth-Zsamboki E, Van Geet C, et al: A natural dominant negative P2X1 receptor due to deletion of a single amino acid residue. J Biol Chem 275:22611–22614, 2000.

92. Rao AK, Willis J, Kowalska MA, et al: Differential requirements for platelet aggregation and inhibition of adenylate cyclase by epinephrine: Studies of a familial platelet alpha 2-adrenergic receptor defect. Blood 71:494–501, 1988.

93. Scrutton MC, Clare KA, Hutton RA, Bruckdorfer KR: Depressed responsiveness to adrenaline in platelets from apparently normal human donors: A familial trait. Br J Haematol 49:303–314, 1981.

94. Di Paola J, Federici AB, Mannucci PM, et al: Low platelet alpha2-beta1 levels in type I von Willebrand disease correlate with impaired platelet function in a high shear stress system. Blood 93:3578–3582, 1999.

95. Kunicki TJ, Federici AB, Salomon DR, et al: An association of candidate gene haplotypes and bleeding severity in von Willebrand disease (VWD) type 1 pedigrees. Blood 104:2359–2367, 2004.

96. Gunay-Aygun M, Huizing M, Gahl WA: Molecular defects that affect platelet dense granules. Semin Thromb Hemost 30:537–547, 2004.

97. Huizing M, Boissy RE, Gahl WA: Hermansky-Pudlak syndrome: Vesicle formation from yeast to man. Pigment Cell Res 15:405–419, 2002.

98. Di Pietro SM, Dell'Angelica EC: The cell biology of Hermansky-Pudlak syndrome: Recent advances. Traffic 6:525–533, 2005.

99. Brantly M, Avila NA, Shotelersuk V, et al: Pulmonary function and high-resolution CT findings in patients with an inherited form of pulmonary fibrosis, Hermansky-Pudlak syndrome, due to mutations in HPS-1. Chest 117:129–136, 2000.

100. del Pozo AI, Jimenez-Yuste V, Villar A, et al: Successful thyroidectomy in a patient with Hermansky-Pudlak syndrome treated with recombinant activated factor VII and platelet concentrates. Blood Coagul Fibrinolysis 13:551–553, 2002.

101. Zatik J, Poka R, Borsos A, Pfliegler G: Variable response of Hermansky-Pudlak syndrome to prophylactic administration of 1-desamino 8D-arginine in subsequent pregnancies. Eur J Obstet Gynecol Reprod Biol 104:165–166, 2002.

102. Cordova A, Barrios NJ, Ortiz I, et al: Poor response to desmopressin acetate (DDAVP) in children with Hermansky-Pudlak syndrome. Pediatr Blood Cancer 44:51–54, 2005.

103. Introne W, Boissy RE, Gahl WA: Clinical, molecular, and cell biological aspects of Chediak-Higashi syndrome. Mol Genet Metab 68:283–303, 1999.

104. Tardieu M, Lacroix C, Neven B, et al: Progressive neurologic dysfunctions 20 years after allogeneic bone marrow transplantation for Chediak-Higashi syndrome. Blood 106:40–42, 2005.

105. Gabbeta J, Yang X, Kowalska MA, et al: Platelet signal transduction defect with Galpha subunit dysfunction and diminished Galphaq in a patient with abnormal platelet responses. Proc Natl Acad Sci U S A 94:8750–8755, 1997.

106. Defreyn G, Machin SJ, Carreras LO, et al: Familial bleeding tendency with partial platelet thromboxane synthetase deficiency: Reorientation of cyclic endoperoxide metabolism. Br J Haematol 49:29–41, 1981.

107. Lagarde M, Byron PA, Vargaftig BB, Dechavanne M: Impairment of platelet thromboxane A2 generation and of the platelet release reaction in two patients with congenital deficiency of platelet cyclooxygenase. Br J Haematol 38:251–266, 1978.

108. Matijevic-Aleksic N, McPhedran P, Wu KK: Bleeding disorder due to platelet prostaglandin H synthase-1 (PGHS-1) deficiency. Br J Haematol 92:212–217, 1996.

109. Kahr WH, Zheng S, Sheth PM, et al: Platelets from patients with the Quebec platelet disorder contain and secrete abnormal amounts of urokinase-type plasminogen activator. Blood 98:257–265, 2001.

110. Sheth PM, Kahr WH, Haq MA, et al: Intracellular activation of the fibrinolytic cascade in the Quebec platelet disorder. Thromb Haemost 90:293–298, 2003.

111. McKay H, Derome F, Haq MA, et al: Bleeding risks associated with inheritance of the Quebec platelet disorder. Blood 104:159–165, 2004.

112. Lentz BR: Exposure of platelet membrane phosphatidylserine regulates blood coagulation. Prog Lipid Res 42:423–438, 2003.

113. Weiss HJ, Lages B: Platelet prothrombinase activity and intracellular calcium responses in patients with storage pool deficiency, glycoprotein IIb-IIIa deficiency, or impaired platelet coagulant activity: A comparison with Scott syndrome. Blood 89:1599–1611, 1997.

114. Toti F, Satta N, Fressinaud E, et al: Scott syndrome, characterized by impaired transmembrane migration of procoagulant phosphatidylserine and hemorrhagic complications, is an inherited disorder. Blood 87:1409–1415, 1996.

115. Munnix IC, Harmsma M, Giddings JC, et al: Store-mediated calcium entry in the regulation of phosphatidylserine exposure in blood cells from Scott patients. Thromb Haemost 89:687–695, 2003.

116. Albrecht C, McVey JH, Elliott JI, et al: A novel missense mutation in ABCA1 results in altered protein trafficking and reduced phosphatidylserine translocation in a patient with Scott syndrome. Blood 106:542–549, 2005.

117. Nofer JR, Herminghaus G, Brodde M, et al: Impaired platelet activation in familial high density lipoprotein deficiency (Tangier disease). J Biol Chem 279:34032–34037, 2004.

118. Ochs HD: The Wiskott-Aldrich syndrome. Clin Rev Allergy Immunol 20:61–86, 2001.

119. Ochs HD, Notarangelo LD: Structure and function of the Wiskott-Aldrich syndrome protein. Curr Opin Hematol 12:284–291, 2005.

120. Dupuis-Girod S, Medioni J, Haddad E, et al: Autoimmunity in Wiskott-Aldrich syndrome: Risk factors, clinical features, and outcome in a single-center cohort of 55 patients. Pediatrics 111: e622–e627, 2003.

121. Derry JM, Ochs HD, Francke U: Isolation of a novel gene mutated in Wiskott-Aldrich syndrome. Cell 78:635–644, 1994.

122. Jin Y, Mazza C, Christie JR, et al: Mutations of the Wiskott-Aldrich syndrome protein (WASP): Hotspots, effect on transcription, and translation and phenotype/genotype correlation. Blood 104:4010–4019, 2004.

123. Dowton SB, Beardsley D, Jamison D, et al: Studies of a familial platelet disorder. Blood 65:557–563, 1985.

124. Song WJ, Sullivan MG, Legare RD, et al: Haploinsufficiency of CBFA2 causes familial thrombocytopenia with propensity to develop acute myelogenous leukaemia. Nat Genet 23:166–175, 1999.

125. Michaud J, Wu F, Osato M, et al: In vitro analyses of known and novel RUNX1/AML1 mutations in dominant familial platelet disorder with predisposition to acute myelogenous leukemia: Implications for mechanisms of pathogenesis. Blood 99:1364–1372, 2002.

126. Ichikawa M, Asai T, Saito T, et al: AML-1 is required for megakaryocytic maturation and lymphocytic differentiation, but not for maintenance of hematopoietic stem cells in adult hematopoiesis. Nat Med 10:299–304, 2004.

127. Hall JG, Levin J, Kuhn JP, et al: Thrombocytopenia with absent radius (TAR). Medicine (Baltimore) 48:411–439, 1969.

128. Greenhalgh KL, Howell RT, Bottani A, et al: Thrombocytopenia–absent radius syndrome: A clinical genetic study. J Med Genet 39:876–881, 2002.

129. Fleischman RA, Letestu R, Mi X, et al: Absence of mutations in the HoxA10, HoxA11 and HoxD11 nucleotide coding sequences in thrombocytopenia with absent radius syndrome. Br J Haematol 116:367–375, 2002.

130. Strippoli P, Savoia A, Iolascon A, et al: Mutational screening of thrombopoietin receptor gene (c-mpl) in patients with congenital thrombocytopenia and absent radii (TAR). Br J Haematol 103:311–314, 1998.

131. Letestu R, Vitrat N, Masse A, et al: Existence of a differentiation blockage at the stage of a megakaryocyte precursor in the thrombocytopenia and absent radii (TAR) syndrome. Blood 95:1633–1641, 2000.

132. Thompson AA, Woodruff K, Feig SA, et al: Congenital thrombocytopenia and radio-ulnar synostosis: A new familial syndrome. Br J Haematol 113:866–870, 2001.

133. Thompson AA, Nguyen LT: Amegakaryocytic thrombocytopenia and radio-ulnar synostosis are associated with HOXA11 mutation. Nat Genet 26:397–398, 2000.

134. van den Oudenrijn S, Bruin M, Folman CC, et al: Mutations in the thrombopoietin receptor, Mpl, in children with congenital

amegakaryocytic thrombocytopenia. Br J Haematol 110:441–448, 2000.

135. Ballmaier M, Germeshausen M, Schulze H, et al: *c-mpl* mutations are the cause of congenital amegakaryocytic thrombocytopenia. Blood 97:139–146, 2001.

136. Ihara K, Ishii E, Eguchi M, et al: Identification of mutations in the *c-mpl* gene in congenital amegakaryocytic thrombocytopenia. Proc Natl Acad Sci U S A 96:3132–3136, 1999.

137. Favier R, Jondeau K, Boutard P, et al: Paris-Trousseau syndrome: Clinical, hematological, molecular data of ten new cases. Thromb Haemost 90:893–897, 2003.

138. Breton-Gorius J, Favier R, Guichard J, et al: A new congenital dysmegakaryopoietic thrombocytopenia (Paris-Trousseau) associated with giant platelet alpha-granules and chromosome 11 deletion at 11q23. Blood 85:1805–1814, 1995.

139. Grossfeld PD, Mattina T, Lai Z, et al: The 11q terminal deletion disorder: A prospective study of 110 cases. Am J Med Genet A 129:51–61, 2004.

140. Raslova H, Komura E, Le Couedic JP, et al: FLI1 monoallelic expression combined with its hemizygous loss underlies Paris-Trousseau/Jacobsen thrombopenia. J Clin Invest 114:77–84, 2004.

141. Drachman JG, Jarvik GP, Mehaffey MG: Autosomal dominant thrombocytopenia: Incomplete megakaryocyte differentiation and linkage to human chromosome 10. Blood 96:118–125, 2000.

142. Sae-Tung G, Dong JF, Lopez JA: Biosynthetic defect in platelet glycoprotein IX mutants associated with Bernard-Soulier syndrome. Blood 87:1361–1367, 1996.

143. Peng TC, Kickler TS, Bell WR, Haller E: Obstetric complications in a patient with Bernard-Soulier syndrome. Am J Obstet Gynecol 165:425–426, 1991.

144. Nurden AT: Qualitative disorders of platelets and megakaryocytes. J Thromb Haemost 3:1773–1782, 2005.

145. Savoia A, Balduini CL, Savino M, et al: Autosomal dominant macrothrombocytopenia in Italy is most frequently a type of heterozygous Bernard-Soulier syndrome. Blood 97:1330–1335, 2001.

146. Van Geet C, Devriendt K, Eyskens B, et al: Velocardiofacial syndrome patients with a heterozygous chromosome 22q11 deletion have giant platelets. Pediatr Res 44:607–611, 1998.

147. Kato T, Kosaka K, Kimura M, et al: Thrombocytopenia in patients with 22q11.2 deletion syndrome and its association with glycoprotein Ib-beta. Genet Med 5:113–119, 2003.

148. Miller JL, Castella A: Platelet-type von Willebrand's disease: Characterization of a new bleeding disorder. Blood 60:790–794, 1982.

149. Othman M, Notley C, Lavender FL, et al: Identification and functional characterization of a novel 27-bp deletion in the macroglycopeptide-coding region of the *GPIBA* gene resulting in platelet-type von Willebrand disease. Blood 105:4330–4336, 2005.

150. Lopez JA, Andrews RK, Afshar-Kharghan V, Berndt MC: Bernard-Soulier syndrome. Blood 91:4397–4418, 1998.

151. Nurden P, Chretien F, Poujol C, et al: Platelet ultrastructural abnormalities in three patients with type 2B von Willebrand disease. Br J Haematol 110:704–714, 2000.

152. Miller JL, Kupinski JM, Castella A, Ruggeri ZM: von Willebrand factor binds to platelets and induces aggregation in platelet-type but not type IIB von Willebrand disease. J Clin Invest 72:1532–1542, 1983.

153. Heath KE, Campos-Barros A, Toren A, et al: Nonmuscle myosin heavy chain IIA mutations define a spectrum of autosomal dominant macrothrombocytopenias: May-Hegglin anomaly and Fechtner, Sebastian, Epstein, and Alport-like syndromes. Am J Hum Genet 69:1033–1045, 2001.

154. Kelley MJ, Jawien W, Ortel TL, Korczak JF: Mutation of *MYH9*, encoding non-muscle myosin heavy chain A, in May-Hegglin anomaly. Nat Genet 26:106–108, 2000.

155. Seri M, Cusano R, Gangarossa S, et al: Mutations in *MYH9* result in the May-Hegglin anomaly, and Fechtner and Sebastian syndromes: The May-Hegglin/Fechtner syndrome consortium. Nat Genet 26:103–105, 2000.

156. Seri M, Pecci A, Di Bari F, et al: *MYH9*-related disease: May-Hegglin anomaly, Sebastian syndrome, Fechtner syndrome, and Epstein syndrome are not distinct entities but represent a variable expression of a single illness. Medicine (Baltimore) 82:203–215, 2003.

157. Krendel M, Mooseker MS: Myosins: Tails (and heads) of functional diversity. Physiology (Bethesda) 20:239–251, 2005.

158. Maupin P, Phillips CL, Adelstein RS, Pollard TD: Differential localization of myosin-II isozymes in human cultured cells and blood cells. J Cell Sci 107:3077–3090, 1994.

159. Canobbio I, Noris P, Pecci A, et al: Altered cytoskeleton organization in platelets from patients with *MYH9*-related disease. J Thromb Haemost 3:1026–1035, 2005.

160. Noris P, Spedini P, Belletti S, et al: Thrombocytopenia, giant platelets, and leukocyte inclusion bodies (May-Hegglin anomaly): Clinical and laboratory findings. Am J Med 104:355–360, 1998.

161. Dong F, Li S, Pujol-Moix N, et al: Genotype–phenotype correlation in *MYH9*-related thrombocytopenia. Br J Haematol 130:620–627, 2005.

162. Crispino JD: *GATA1* in normal and malignant hematopoiesis. Semin Cell Dev Biol 16:137–147, 2005.

163. Nichols KE, Crispino JD, Poncz M, et al: Familial dyserythropoietic anaemia and thrombocytopenia due to an inherited mutation in GATA1. Nat Genet 24:266–270, 2000.

164. Freson K, Devriendt K, Matthijs G, et al: Platelet characteristics in patients with X-linked macrothrombocytopenia because of a novel GATA1 mutation. Blood 98:85–92, 2001.

165. Hughan SC, Senis Y, Best D, et al: Selective impairment of platelet activation to collagen in the absence of *GATA1*. Blood 105:4369–4376, 2005.

166. Balduini CL, Pecci A, Loffredo G, et al: Effects of the *R216Q* mutation of *GATA-1* on erythropoiesis and megakaryocytopoiesis. Thromb Haemost 91:129–140, 2004.

167. Gerrard JM, Phillips DR, Rao GH, et al: Biochemical studies of two patients with the gray platelet syndrome: Selective deficiency of platelet alpha granules. J Clin Invest 66:102–109, 1980.

168. Hayward CP, Weiss HJ, Lages B, et al: The storage defects in grey platelet syndrome and alphadelta-storage pool deficiency affect alpha-granule factor V and multimerin storage without altering their proteolytic processing. Br J Haematol 113:871–877, 2001.

169. Mori K, Suzuki S, Sugai K: Electron microscopic and functional studies on platelets in gray platelet syndrome. Tohoku J Exp Med 143:261–287, 1984.

170. Falik-Zaccai TC, Anikster Y, Rivera CE, et al: A new genetic isolate of gray platelet syndrome (GPS): Clinical, cellular, and hematologic characteristics. Mol Genet Metab 74:303–313, 2001.

171. Drouin A, Favier R, Masse JM, et al: Newly recognized cellular abnormalities in the gray platelet syndrome. Blood 98:1382–1391, 2001.

172. White JG, Key NS, King RA, Vercellotti GM: The White platelet syndrome: A new autosomal dominant platelet disorder. Platelets 15:173–184, 2004.

173. Poon MC, Demers C, Jobin F, Wu JW: Recombinant factor VIIa is effective for bleeding and surgery in patients with Glanzmann thrombasthenia. Blood 94:3951–3953, 1999.

174. Lisman T, Adelmeijer J, Heijnen HF, de Groot PG: Recombinant factor VIIa restores aggregation of alphaIIbbeta3-deficient platelets via tissue factor-independent fibrin generation. Blood 103:1720–1727, 2004.

175. Lisman T, Adelmeijer J, Cauwenberghs S, et al: Recombinant factor VIIa enhances platelet adhesion and activation under flow conditions at normal and reduced platelet count. J Thromb Haemost 3:742–751, 2005.

176. Das P, Carcao M, Hitzler J: DDAVP-induced hyponatremia in young children. J Pediatr Hematol Oncol 27:330–332, 2005.

177. O'Connell KA, Wood JJ, Wise RP, et al: Thromboembolic adverse events after use of recombinant human coagulation factor VIIa. JAMA 295:293–298, 2006.

Chapter 11

Purpura and Other Hematovascular Disorders

Marc Zumberg, MD • Craig S. Kitchens, MD

Confined to the vascular system, blood comes into contact only with endothelial cells, which line all macrovascular, microvascular, and sinusoidal systems. Disruption of this closed system leads to bleeding—either gross bleeding (characteristic of macrovascular hemorrhage) or extravasation into tissue or potential spaces (more typical of microvascular leakage). Table 11-1 depicts the nature, causes, consequences, and therapeutic approaches to bleeding, and even the types of physicians who address these issues. Bleeding occurs chiefly via at least one of two possible mechanisms: trauma and physical disruption or hemostatic failure; neither is necessarily exclusive. This chapter focuses on hemorrhagic processes that are due to nontraumatic weakening of the vascular wall at the microvascular or macrovascular level. The hematologist is called to consult on such events. The primary goal of this chapter is to present a systematic approach to and differential diagnosis of hemorrhage and purpura. Discussion of treatment provided to patients with each disease is not feasible, and the reader is referred to more in-depth reviews of each disease. Central to the theme of this chapter is the normality of the hemostatic system yet the failure of vessels through which normal blood flows.

Sudden hemorrhage (characteristic of macrovascular disruption) leads to alterations in blood volume; patients often present with shock and usually with pain. Purpura, ecchymoses, and especially petechiae are not characteristic. In microvascular disruption, leakage of red cells from extravasated blood displayed as petechiae and purpura is characteristic, but alterations in blood volume and blood pressure from blood loss are generally not. Uncommonly, shock due to infectious causes of purpura may occur.

Table 11-2 lists and defines multiple terms used in the discussion of various microvascular and macrovascular lesions.

Reports of purpura are common. During histories and physical examinations, up to 65% of healthy women and 25% of healthy men state that they bruise easily.[1] This is a common occurrence in general medical practice. Much of what is regarded by patients as excessive bleeding is actually mild day-to-day traumatic purpura. Defining characteristics of these benign "normal" lesions are that (1) they are never true (i.e., palpable) hematomas, (2) they number no more than four to six on the body at any one time, and (3) lesions are generally not larger than 3 cm in diameter.

Petechiae are pinpoint lesions that are brilliant "cayenne pepper red" when they first appear. Petechiae are usually smaller than 3 mm in diameter with sharply demarcated margins. They soon fade to a salmon color in a few days, becoming less demarcated, and then finally become brownish spots caused by retention of hemosiderin from extravasated blood. A new crop may occur, with the process repeating itself.

Ecchymosis refers to large extravasations that result from coalescence of separate petechial lesions or, more commonly, a bleed from a slightly larger vessel.

Purpura occurs as the initial presentation of a variety of illnesses that are further discussed in the section on microvascular disruption. Any leakage of blood may well be due to or exacerbated by hematologic causes; therefore, the hematologist may be consulted. Often, no true hemostatic defect is apparent; therefore, the hematologist must have broad medical knowledge and interest. Establishing the diagnosis from a broad differential diagnosis and opening various therapeutic and prognostic windows are keys.

A modicum of hemostatic tests can be ordered and initiated when the consultation occurs. Results of these tests, combined with findings of history and physical examination, usually help to differentiate hematologic causes from other causes (Table 11-3). A thorough list of prescribed, nonprescribed, borrowed, and over-the-counter medications, including herbal and alternative medicines (see Chapter 33), should be elicited. Systemic symptoms such as weight loss, chills, fevers, night sweats, and malaise are frequently described. A thorough examination should include auscultation of the heart and examination for lymphadenopathy and splenomegaly.

MACROVASCULAR DISRUPTION

Macrovascular disruption most often occurs suddenly as the result of trauma or severe atherosclerotic processes, such as a ruptured abdominal aortic aneurysm. Whereas management of macrovascular hemorrhage is beyond the scope of this text, reference is made here to disease processes for which the hematologist may be asked to consult and assist.

Causes of macrovascular hemorrhage can be grouped into six broad categories (Table 11-4). The first two, trauma and atherosclerotic processes, are not further discussed in this chapter. The four broad categories that may be called primary vascular disorders of the macrocirculation include disorders of connective tissue, infiltration of

Table 11-1 Characteristics of Macrovascular and Microvascular Vessel Bleeding

	Large Vessel	Small Vessel
Vessel	Typically named	Typically unnamed
Nature of bleeding	Sudden gush	Slow ooze
Primary promoter	Vessel wall	Hemostatic system
Pathophysiology	Trauma, disruption	Hemostatic failure
Physician	Surgeon	Hematologist
Therapeutic approach	Ligature, cautery	Diagnose and treat cause

macrovascular vessels with amyloid, inflammatory processes involving the macrocirculation, and certain arteriovenous malformations. Designation of a particular disorder as microvascular or macrovascular in origin is imperfect in that some processes may fit into either niche.

TRUE DISORDERS OF CONNECTIVE TISSUE

Ehlers-Danlos Syndrome

Ehlers-Danlos syndrome (EDS) encompasses clinical manifestations associated with a true collagen vascular disease.[2] (This section does not include discussion of rheumatic

Table 11-2 Terminology Used in This Chapter

Purpura	General term for nonblanching, bluish-purple lesions due to extravasated blood, fading over time to greenish-yellow lesions as those extravasated cells deteriorate.
Petechiae	Specific type of purpura with macular pinpoint lesions (3 mm) and well-demarcated borders.
Ecchymosis	Specific type of purpura that is a larger macular purpuric lesion due to confluence of petechiae or, more commonly, a larger hemorrhagic lesion. Borders are not sharply defined.
Palpable purpura	Purpuric lesions that appear to be raised (i.e., papular) and palpable because of infiltration of lesions with leukocytes.
Bruise	Lay term without specific meaning; a frequent chief complaint.
Hematoma	Palpable 1-cm or larger mass usually due to bleeding into or between tissue planes.
Vasculitis	Palpable purpura due to infectious, inflammatory, or immunologic mechanisms with white cell infiltration.
Necrotizing vasculitis	Infarctive necrosis of the skin due to vasculitis. Subsequent to necrosis, lesions may turn from purple to "gun-metal gray" or black.
Erythema	Reddened skin due to increased cutaneous blood flow from vasodilatation secondary to fever, exercise, or emotional factors. Ill-defined borders. Readily blanchable.
Telangiectases	Plural term for 1- to 4-mm dark-red masses of capillaries without extravasation that blanch to pressure. May be macular or somewhat papular.
Cherry angiomas	Very papular 1- to 4-mm cherry red "hard" hemangiomas that compress only with difficulty. A normal finding in middle-aged and older persons, particularly in the lower chest and upper abdominal area.
Spiders	Appropriately named lesions with a central 1- to 2-mm visible arteriole ("body") with "legs" branching centrifugally for 1 to 3 cm. Gentle pressure on the body occludes the arteriole, and the legs rapidly disappear.
Livedo reticularis	Purplish, faint, ill-defined reticular network of small vessels on the legs and occasionally arms.
Purple (or blue) toes	Ischemic toes and extremities from arteriolar infarction due to arteriolar emboli, especially from cholesterol embolization or thrombosis in the setting of heparin-induced thrombocytopenia.
Warfarin skin necrosis	Ischemic skin over fatty tissue resulting from capillary and venular infarction due to fibrin deposition.

Table 11-3 Evaluation of the Patient With Petechiae, Purpura, or Ecchymosis

Following a complete history and physical examination, the following laboratory examinations should be considered:

Always	Complete blood count and review of blood smear Partial thromboplastin time and prothrombin time
Additional tests to be considered if diagnosis not apparent	Thrombin time Fibrinogen level Analyses for fibrin degradation products and D-dimers
Additional tests to be considered in cases of cutaneous vasculitis	Skin biopsy Serologic tests for hepatitis B and C Antinuclear antibody (ANA) Antineutrophilic cytoplasmic antibody (ANCA) Rheumatoid factor (RF) Serum protein electrophoresis (SPEP) Complement Human immunodeficiency (HIV) antibodies
Additional tests to be considered in obscure cases	Blood cultures Viral studies Bone marrow aspirate/biopsy

Table 11-4 Macrovascular Disorders That May Lead to Hemorrhage

1. Trauma
2. Atherosclerosis
3. Disorders of connective tissue
   A. Ehlers-Danlos syndrome
   B. Osteogenesis imperfecta
   C. Pseudoxanthoma elasticum
   D. Marfan syndrome and cystic medial degeneration
4. Infiltration with amyloid
5. Inflammatory vasculitis
   A. Syphilis
   B. Tuberculosis
   C. Mycotic aneurysms
   D. Rheumatic disorders (RA, SLE, PAN, etc.)
   E. Kawasaki disease
6. Arteriovenous malformations
   A. Hemangiomas
   B. Kaposiform hemangioendothelioma
   C. Hereditary hemorrhagic telangiectasia

RA, rheumatoid arthritis; SLE, systemic lupus erythematosus; PAN, polyarteritis nodosa.

diseases such as lupus erythematosus, which previously were regarded as "collagen vascular diseases.") This clinically and genetically heterogeneous connective tissue disorder is characterized by abnormalities in genetic coding of various subtypes of collagen. Advances in our basic understanding of abnormalities of the various subtypes of EDS have been reviewed.[3,4] In brief, nine subtypes have been identified, and each subtype is characterized by specific genetic abnormalities; six subtypes are considered to be primary clinical variants and three are viewed as primary biochemical variants.[5]

Several groups have studied kindreds with EDS by seeking disorders of the hemostatic system, yet no thematic defects have been discovered.[6,7] Anstey and colleagues, in studying a group of 51 patients, found that only 8% exhibited any type of abnormal bleeding, and 82% of the group had normal findings on multiple plasma-based coagulation tests.[7] Hemostatic laboratory abnormalities observed in the remaining 18% of these patients were deemed to lack clinical significance. Therefore, the general consensus is that bleeding is due to alterations in the structure of collagen that result in weakened collagen or collagen that does not adequately enhance hemostasis. Most of the "bleeding" that these patients exhibit occurs because of the general tendency for their skin to be weak and thin and to heal poorly, leading to tears with subcutaneous bruising. These abnormalities cause so-called "cigarette paper skin," which is characteristic of patients with some EDS subtypes. Other problems noted in patients with this underlying connective tissue disorder include spontaneous dislocation of joints and the tendency to be "double jointed."

Among several subtypes of EDS, type IV appears to be one of the rarest, yet it has the worst hemorrhagic potential with respect to arterial hemorrhage.[8,9] The hematologist is most likely to encounter type IV EDS. Median survival appears to be 48 years for patients with this autosomal dominant subtype. The specific abnormality associated with type IV EDS is the production of abnormal type III collagen. This abnormality accounts for the structural compromise of these vessels, which, in turn, accounts for their tendency to rupture.

The primary cause of death in EDS is rupture of large intra-abdominal arteries. The secondary cause is colonic perforation. Freeman and colleagues[10] reviewed 90 surgical procedures encountered over a 20-year period; 41 were performed for colonic perforation, 17 for repair of arterial aneurysm, and 17 for spontaneous hemorrhage from ruptured arteries. In this study, 23% of patients died from a gastrointestinal problem, and 30% died of vascular complications. Their review showed that treatment with fresh frozen plasma, cryoprecipitate, or any other hemostatic agent did not aid the patient. It was also noted that attempts to repair these large, muscular arteries with the use of vascular clamps were fraught with complications. Maltz and associates[11] concluded that hemorrhaging vessels should be ligated, and that none should be clamped. Other conservative methods, such as a great reluctance to operate, use of bed rest, and the generous and continued use of external compression, were advocated.

Osteogenesis Imperfecta

Osteogenesis imperfecta (OI) is a true collagen-vascular disorder in which type I collagen is defective because of several flaws in the genes that encode for type I procollagen.[12] Type I collagen, which is found primarily in bone, ligaments, tendons, skin, sclerae, and dentin, is not a major component of blood vessels; therefore, disorders of type I collagen are not typically hemorrhagic in manifestation. Although OI is occasionally mentioned as a collagen-vascular disease characterized by hemorrhagic tendencies and purpuric lesions, bruising may be so minimal that it serves almost no diagnostic purpose in the management of OI. Indeed, modern reviews of this disorder fail to mention clinical hemostatic defects despite several surgical needs noted for patients with OI.[12,13]

Pseudoxanthoma Elasticum

Pseudoxanthoma elasticum (PXE) is another disease that results from derangement of tensile strength in connective tissues and occasionally may be associated with subcutaneous evulsion of tissue, resulting in minimal purpura. Purpura and bleeding, however, are not cardinal manifestations of this disease. PXE appears to be due to homozygous (or double heterozygous) inheritance of mutations involving the *ABCC6* gene, leading to degeneration of elastic fibers in the skin, retina, and cardiovascular system. The primary arteries that rupture are those of the gastric mucosa; thus, gastrointestinal bleeding may occur. This disease has recently been reviewed.[14,15]

Marfan Syndrome and Cystic Medial Degeneration

Marfan syndrome results from mutations in genes that encode for production of fibrillin-1, a component of normal connective tissue.[16] This autosomal dominant syndrome has several defining features that include a marked tendency toward dissection of the aorta with aneurysmal formation, the chief cause of death in this syndrome. Bleeding or bruising of the skin is rare and hemostatic defects are not encountered, despite the frequent need for corrective cardiothoracic surgery in this disorder.[17]

11

The histologic lesion that is uniformly seen in the aortic wall of Marfan syndrome is called cystic medial degeneration. Many patients have the identical histologic lesion but do not share any of the other features of Marfan syndrome. Most often, these patients are older than those with Marfan syndrome and appear to have no familial pattern of inheritance. The cause of cystic medial degeneration of the aorta is unknown, but the effects on the aorta and resultant aneurysmal formation and treatment are the same as those for Marfan syndrome.

LARGE VESSEL INFILTRATION

Amyloidosis and its hemorrhagic manifestations are generally microvascular in nature but may involve the great vessels of the brain; thus, they are discussed here. Amyloidosis is not a single disorder, but a series of disorders, all which have in common the misfolding of any number of proteins, giving rise to beta-pleated sheets that reside beneath the basement membrane of multiple structures, including blood vessels. All of these proteins have in common the characteristic birefringent apple green color seen on staining of affected tissue with Congo red in polarized light, as well as a typical pattern of microfibrils on electron microscopy.[18] Over 20 types of amyloid have been described, and each abnormality has subtle variations in its clinical manifestation.[19] Vessel wall strength may be reduced; thus, simple mechanical stress or sheer force may result in bleeding, which is seen in 28% of patients with amyloidosis.[20] Purpura about the face (Fig. 11-1) seems especially common in amyloidosis and is discussed in greater detail in the Microvascular Purpura section of this chapter. Of interest, spontaneous rupture of the spleen has been described in amyloidosis and in fact may be the presenting symptom.[21]

A unique subtype of amyloidosis that clearly has hemorrhagic macrovascular ramifications is cerebral amyloid angiopathy (CAA), which has in the past been referred to as congophilic angiopathy. Subtypes of CAA may be sporadic or familial; all have as yet undetermined causes.[22,23] In CAA, amyloid deposition of the cerebral arteries is characteristic. CAA is extremely common and may be present in nearly one half of all elderly individuals at autopsy. CAA is one of the leading causes of spontaneous cerebral hemorrhage, accounting for about 10% to 15% of all such bleeds.[23] CAA has medical-legal implications, in that many older patients are given long-term anticoagulation therapy, which is often blamed for the hemorrhagic event, even though the true underlying cause is frequently CAA.[24] A peculiar and uncertain relationship has been noted between CAA and Alzheimer disease, in that cerebral vessels that contain amyloid are seen in 80% of patients with Alzheimer disease.[25]

INFLAMMATORY PROCESSES

Any one of several inflammatory processes may involve large vessels and subsequently may lead to their rupture and hemorrhage.

Infectious causes have historically included syphilitic aortitis. Although this disorder is rarely seen now, in previous eras, it was the prevalent cause of aortic aneurysm. Tuberculous arteritis can conceivably affect any artery.[26] Mycotic aneurysms[27] may accompany almost any infection but are classically seen in subacute bacterial endocarditis[28]; unfortunately, they may lead to hemorrhage, particularly in the central nervous system. Human immunodeficiency virus (HIV) infection has been implicated as a cause of inflammatory vasculitis resulting from large vessel damage.[29]

Any of the classic inflammatory rheumatic diseases, such as rheumatoid arthritis, polyarteritis nodosa, relapsing polychondritis, Behçet syndrome,[30] giant cell arteritis,[31] and systemic lupus erythematosus,[32] occasionally involve large vessels characterized by inflammation, weakening, and eventual rupture and sudden hemorrhage. Probably, the best understood relation is with rheumatoid vasculitis,[33] which, paradoxically, may occur in older patients with quiescent "burned-out" arthritic manifestations, yet may perforate large arteries. Kawasaki disease involves an inflammatory process of the arteries that occurs in childhood; in a small number of patients, panvasculitis occurs, with particular reference to coronary vessels, which may lead to aneurysmal dilatation of these vessels.[34]

ARTERIOVENOUS MALFORMATIONS/ HEMANGIOMAS

Recent discoveries have changed our knowledge and understanding of the pathogenesis of this anatomic disorder. Whereas in the past, most terms used to define these entities as separate diseases were based on epidemiology, clinical presentations, or even treatment, an explosion in our understanding of the basic science of vascular endothelial growth has already begun to change not only our understanding but even our classification of these disorders. Ultimately, no doubt, new treatments will be found as our level of knowledge increases. Accordingly, processes as diverse as Kaposi sarcoma, hereditary hemorrhagic telangiectasia, and diabetic retinopathy may have more in common than we would otherwise ever have imagined.[35]

Many of these processes have at their core abnormal and sustained proliferation of endothelial cells caused by upregulation of growth-promoting factors or inhibition of growth-promoting apoptosis.[36] Indeed, in hereditary hemorrhagic telangiectasia (HHT), circulating levels of vascular

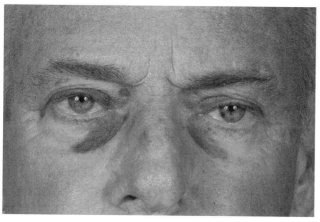

Figure 11-1 (See also Color Plate 11-1.) Spontaneous periorbital purpura in a patient with systemic amyloidosis.

endothelial cell growth factor (VEGF) are consistently higher than normal, and a tendency toward even higher levels has been noted among those patients with HHT who bleed more than other patients with HHT.[37] It is hypothesized that most features of HHT are due to persistence of the activation phase of angiogenesis caused by perturbations in VEGF.

Our understanding of these processes has realigned our thinking regarding hemangiomas, particularly those occurring in children.[38] The International Society for the Study of Vascular Anomalies has produced a new classification scheme that is based on whether the lesion is a tumor (i.e., due to vascular proliferation) or a malformation (i.e., due to structural abnormalities associated with slow endothelial cell turnover).[39] This group carefully dissected what were previously (and probably erroneously) considered to be two manifestations of the same process, namely, localized disseminated intravascular coagulation (DIC) and "cavernous hemangioma" (previously known as the Kasabach-Merritt syndrome). Students of this disease now argue that what up to this point has been called Kasabach-Merritt syndrome is actually a localized form of coagulation activation that produces thrombocytopenia and arguably DIC; however, most often, it is confined to a unique vascular anomaly, namely, kaposiform hemangioendothelioma (KHE).[40] Most vascular lesions, particularly the common hemangiomas of infancy, do not exhibit the Kasabach-Merritt phenomena, namely, localized DIC and DIC-like changes.

Mulliken and associates defined differences between KHE and otherwise benign infantile hemangioma.[41] Vascular lesions, whether KHE or not, that exhibit the Kasabach-Merritt phenomenon, have recently been reviewed by Hall.[42] These lesions were initially described by Kasabach and Merritt in 1940[43] and were believed to be seen in only about 1% of cases of hemangioma. Neither the site nor the size of the vascular lesion predicts the syndrome. The Kasabach-Merritt phenomenon is very serious, with a mortality rate of about 40%. Patients can "bleed into" these highly vascular tumors. Not many specimens undergo biopsy, but the vast majority of patients who have true Kasabach-Merritt phenomena actually have KHE—not benign hemangioma. Therapy includes arterial embolization and general support of the patient with fresh frozen plasma (FFP) or platelet infusion. Some have advocated the use of glucocorticosteroids, 2 to 3 mg/kg/day. It is hoped that breakthroughs in antiangiogenic sciences may result in therapies based on antiangiogenic strategies.

Hereditary Hemorrhagic Telangiectasia

Whereas most of the hemangiomas that appear in infancy spontaneously involute over the years, the lesions of HHT (Osler-Weber-Rendu syndrome [OWR]) slowly progress over decades. As has been mentioned, perturbations of VEGF are most certainly associated with the slow, continued hyperproliferation of microcirculatory endothelial cells, giving rise to characteristic telangiectasia. Because blood remains intravascular in HHT, the lesions are easily blanched by external pressure, a key feature distinguishing telangiectasia from purpura.

HHT remains arguably the most understood and most common of this group of vascular proliferative lesions.

Understanding of the molecular basis of this disease has resulted in division into two types of HHT, namely, HHT-1 and HHT-2. Disorders of endoglin, located on chromosome 9q33-34, are those which determine that a kindred has HHT-1, whereas genes encoding for the activin A receptor, which are encoded on chromosomes 12q13, account for those kindred that have HHT-2. Both of these genes are heavily expressed in endothelial cells, and most lesions have in common loss of function mutations.[44] Rapid growth in this field, as in other areas of human genetics, is documented by the cataloguing of at least 57 genetic defects that lead to HHT-1 and 50 that lead to HHT-2.[45] A mouse model for HHT-2 exists.[46] It appears that homozygosity for HHT is lethal in mice and man.[47]

As experience with HHT has progressed, the poorly appreciated but long known interrelations between bothersome cutaneous otolaryngologic (ENT) lesions of HHT and systemic arterial venous malformations (AVMs) have been solidified. Jacobson[48] estimates that 70% of all patients with AVMs have as their root cause HHT, type 1 or type 2, as do 10% of all patients with central nervous system (CNS) AVMs.

Pulmonary AVMs in HHT can cause considerable morbidity and mortality, ranging from high cardiac output heart failure to massive intrathoracic hemorrhage.[49] These as well as other AVMs may worsen with pregnancy, especially given increased blood volume and cardiac output during pregnancy.[50] Diagnosis and management of this situation in pregnancy have been addressed, and it has been concluded that embolotherapy is effective and safe in pregnancy.[51]

Primary symptoms that lead to the diagnosis and treatment of HHT involve persistent ENT bleeding (Table 11-5). In a study of recalcitrant epistaxis, Shah and colleagues[52] noted that among 76 patients, 66% had mild epistaxis (correlating with one or two short episodes of epistaxis per week), 21% had moderate epistaxis (meaning one or two brief episodes per day), and 13% had severe (daily bleeds longer than 30 minutes) epistaxis. Their perceived requirement for red cell transfusion among 76 patients with HHT mirrored the degree of bleeding; of those patients labeled as having mild epistaxis, none required transfusions; those labeled with moderate epistaxis required 1 to 10 transfusions per year, and those labeled severe required more than 10 units of blood per year.

Pathophysiology of HHT is explained by increased elaboration of VEGF, leading to enhanced microcirculatory

Table 11-5 Characteristics of Patients With HHT

Positive family history	70%–95%
Epistaxis	90%–95%
Cutaneous telangiectasia	70%–75%
Visceral involvement	20%–25%
Gastrointestinal involvement	12%–15%
Hepatic AVMs	8%–30%
Pulmonary AVMs	5%–20%
Central nervous system AVMs	4%–10%

HHT, hereditary hemorrhagic telangiectasia; AVM, arteriovenous malformation.
From Larson.[59]

growth, which slowly increases over the decades, leading to AVMs that slowly grow into frank telangiectases characteristic of the disorder. The architecture of these AVMs is that of abnormally large capillaries, meaning that there is no smooth muscle investiture of these very large, even visible vessels that yet have the architectural makeup of capillaries. Hence, vasoconstriction to minimize bleeding is not anatomically possible.

Multiple methods for arresting epistaxis have been advocated[53]; these include packing, electrocautery, cryosurgery, arterial embolization, arterial ligation, and hormonal manipulation. Various types of laser apparatus also may be used. Whereas each of these methods has its advocate, the fact that none of them has clearly been established as having precedence over the others is problematic. None of these treatments has been studied in an evidence-based format, and the preferences and resources of one's local otolaryngologists may well determine the approach taken until the best treatment for epistaxis of HHT is determined. Daily use of nasal lubricants and avoidance of low-humidity environments seem effective. Websites exist for North American (www.hht.org) and European (www.telangiectasia.co.uk) patients.

One group has developed diagnostic criteria for HHT. Each finding is given a score of 1. Findings include epistaxis, the presence of telangiectases, visceral AVMs, and a positive history of a first-degree relative with similar findings. A score of 2 leads to possible diagnosis of HHT, and a score of 3 or 4 is definitive.[54]

Although ENT manifestations of this disease are most problematic, it is now becoming clear that systemic AVMs are equally serious. Primary causes of death in HHT consist of hemorrhage due to pulmonary and CNS AVMs. CNS AVMs in particular may become sites of abscess; therefore, prophylactic administration of antibiotics in a manner similar to that used in the prevention of endocarditis has been advocated by many for dental work and for gastrointestinal/genitourologic (GI/GU) procedures.[55,56]

AVMs of HHT are cumulative and progressive. Abdalla and colleagues[57] noted that 26% of a cohort with HHT-1 developed visceral lesions upon screening for such, and 30% of kindred with HHT-2 had similar lesions.[57] Lesions of the liver can be sought by ultrasound. One group[58] found that if the diameter of the hepatic artery is greater than 7 mm, the probability of hepatic hypervascularity was high, whereas if the hepatic artery is smaller than 7 mm, such is not the case. The average size of the hepatic artery among patients with hepatic AVMs due to HHT was 11.3 mm, whereas lesions in controls measured 4.6 mm and in patients with cirrhosis, only 4.8 mm. Larson[59] found that 30% of patients with liver disease due to AVMs of HHT developed signs of high cardiac output congestive heart failure, portal hypertension, biliary ischemia, liver failure, and, in some cases, hepatic encephalopathy. Debate continues about whether embolization of large hepatic AVMs is less dangerous than liver transplantation in affected patients. Embolization of hepatic AVMs is associated with complications in up to 40% of patients who undergo the procedure.[59]

Elsewhere in the gastrointestinal (GI) tract, telangiectases are common along the large and small intestines and are a frequent cause of persistent GI hemorrhage and iron deficiency. Longacre and colleagues[60] found a correlation between the number of lesions seen in the GI tract on endoscopy and the number of transfusions needed per year. Those patients with fewer than 7 visible lesions required 9 units of blood per year, those with 7 to 19 lesions needed on average 13 units of blood per year, and patients with more than 20 lesions used an average of 28 units of blood per year. Neither estrogen therapy, danazol, ε-aminocaproic acid (EACA), nor any combination thereof yielded reproducible or dependable success; 50% of patients appeared to respond to any therapeutic maneuver. Standard of care remains elusive. Video capsule endoscopy has been successful in finding the cause (including HHT) of obscure chronic GI hemorrhage.[61]

Central nervous system lesions occur less frequently (5% to 10% of patients with HHT) and tend to occur later in life. Obviously, the seriousness of hemorrhage is great. It is estimated that mortality associated with a CNS bleed from an AVM is between 53% and 81%.[62] It appears that males have approximately a four-times higher risk than females of developing a spontaneous CNS bleed, and the entire group has a 1.8% chance per year of developing this complication. HHT with large AVMs may involve the spinal cord.[63]

These data have caused considerable debate in the literature regarding screening for CNS lesions. Students of this disorder from the United Kingdom[64] strongly suggest that magnetic resonance imaging (MRI) should be used to screen even asymptomatic patients with HHT, whereas Maher and colleagues[65] in the United States, in their review of patients from the Mayo Clinic, found a low incidence (4%) of CNS AVMs in patients with HHT who had no symptoms. They argue that this figure is low and that outcomes after a CNS bleed may be not as bleak as was originally believed; therefore, they do not favor screening of asymptomatic patients. However, among a cadre of patients with HHT known to have pulmonary AVMs, 30% had experienced symptoms such as transient ischemic attacks (TIAs) or infarction of the brain; therefore, CNS screening of patients known to have pulmonary AVMs is rational.

Despite several excellent reviews on the management of HHT[55,60,66] very little mention is made of aggressive replacement of iron through intravenous administration. Anemia of HHT is due to profound iron deficiency. Iron replacement in its least efficient form, namely, transfusion of blood is the prevalent method of treating patients with severe anemia. Given that the rate of maximal absorption from the GI tract of medicinal and/or food iron is sufficient only to make 8 to 12 ml. of blood each day, even in the most compliant of patients, it is understandable that oral replenishment of iron is sufficient only in the mildest cases of HHT. Because hemorrhagic loss from ENT and GI bleeding is lifelong and progressive, the routine administration of parenteral iron is rational yet grossly underused. At this institution, we follow patients' serum ferritin levels, and as soon as they begin to drop, yet before the development of microcytic anemia, we routinely infuse total replacement doses of iron in the form of 2 g of iron dextran, which is enough iron to generate the equivalent of 8 units of blood. Our average patient with HHT requires 1 to 2 such administrations per year, whereas some exceptional patients require 4 to 6 administrations per year.

When aggressive periodic iron infusion is used, it is the exception that patients with HHT require transfusions.[67] The rare patient who is intolerant of iron infusion may have to be given oral iron replacement, supplemented occasionally by transfusion. Given that patients will need such treatment over their lifetime, once one can establish that a patient is tolerant of intravenous iron, outpatient maintenance therapy becomes much more rational and acceptable to all parties involved. Additionally, blood-borne infections and multiple alloantibody formation are minimized.

MICROVASCULAR HEMORRHAGE

Purpura is a general term that describes either small punctate lesions called petechiae or larger lesions called ecchymoses (see Table 11-2 for terminology). *Purpura* is derived from the Latin term for purple—the color generated by the extravasation of red cells into the skin. Extravasation may result from coagulation disorders, physical trauma, or systemic conditions that lead to alterations in the microvasculature. Purpura, which is due to extravasation of blood from the microcirculation, consisting of the smallest arterioles, capillaries, and postcapillary venules, is thus a disorder of the microcirculation.

The hematologist may be consulted to evaluate patients with purpura because the differential diagnosis of disorders that may result in purpura includes many hematologic processes. Because purpuric disorders require careful consideration of hematologic and dermatologic causes, the hematologist should be familiar with hematologic purpura, as well as its imitators. One may wish to coconsult with a dermatologist for many patients. The differential diagnosis of disorders that lead to purpuric lesions encompasses a considerable range of processes, from mild chronic dermatologic disorders to rapidly progressive, life-threatening illnesses such as meningococcemia with DIC.

Although HHT (also known as Osler-Weber-Rendu syndrome) is not truly a purpuric disorder because blood is not extravasated, discussion of HHT syndrome traditionally is placed among discussions of nonthrombocytopenic purpura. HHT also was discussed in the previous section because of its multiple macrovascular manifestations. Later in the chapter, we will address other hematovascular perturbations of skin that are included in the differential diagnosis of purpura.

HISTORICAL PERSPECTIVE

Because of their ready visibility, purpuric lesions have been described throughout history. Victims of the bubonic plague, which circled the globe in the Middle Ages, killing untold millions of people, often were purpuric (hence "Black Death"), which led to the rapid recognition of the affliction and banishment by others. Typhus is claimed to have killed more soldiers throughout history than all battles combined.[68] Scurvy, particularly the prevention of scurvy, which was appreciated and practiced by the British Navy, was highly instrumental in England's defeat of Napoleon's navy at Trafalgar because the French did not practice scurvy prevention. Before the adoption of antiscorbutic measures by the British Navy, 1500 patients with scurvy

were admitted to the main naval hospital in England each year. After antiscorbutic policies were initiated, scurvy was essentially eliminated from the British Navy, and extant records reveal only two cases in the 5-year period following Alfred Lord Nelson's destruction of the French Navy in 1805. This story has been engagingly recounted in the medical literature.[69]

Although purpura had been known for centuries, scientific interest in these lesions was established in the 18th century, when Werlhof, then serving as court physician to King George II of England, accurately described what is now called acute idiopathic thrombocytopenic purpura (ITP).[70] At the very beginning of the 19th century, Willan[71] reviewed purpura and proposed five categories in the first rudimentary attempt to explain purpura as a rightfully circumscribed area of clinical science. The five subtypes of purpura that he described consisted of the following: (1) purpura simplex, (2) purpura hemorrhagica, (3) purpura urticans, (4) purpura senilis, and (5) purpura contagiosa. More likely than not, the five subtypes of purpura that he explained 200 years ago would now be regarded as, respectively, purpura simplex, acute ITP, Henoch-Schönlein purpura, senile purpura, and meningococcemia, as well as other acute bacterial infections related to purpura. Approximately 100 years later, at the turn of the 19th century, purpura was reviewed by Austin Flint in his textbook.[72] Scientists' understanding of purpura had not substantially advanced since the time of Willan's review. Flint clearly separated clinical purpura from hemophilia and traumatic hemorrhage. He preferred the term *purpura rheumatica* to *purpura urticans* and clearly described what we now refer to as Henoch-Schönlein purpura (HSP). He did not like Willan's term, *purpura hemorrhagica*, because he recognized that all purpura was indeed hemorrhagic. He preferred to revert to the older European name for ITP, namely, *morbus maculosus Werlhofii*, or Werlhof disease. Although he did not use a separate descriptive category for scurvy, he correctly described the two primary differences between ITP and scurvy—gum swelling and bleeding characteristic of advanced scurvy but not of ITP—and that ITP did not respond to dietetic manipulation, as did scurvy. William Osler in a major textbook of medicine in that era (competing with that of Flint) gave a similar account of purpura.[73] He again clearly separated hemophilia from the purpuric disorders. Revealing his strength in observational medicine, he was the first to accurately describe petechiae, differentiating them from ecchymoses. He described cases of purpura following iodine administration, which were probably the result of iodine-induced cutaneous vasculitis. He preferred the term *cachectic purpura* to *senile purpura*. Osler also clearly distinguished HHT (now one of the several diseases bearing his name, OWR syndrome) from hemophilia, while recognizing that both were hereditary hemorrhagic diatheses.[74]

That thrombocytopenia was causally related to the petechiae of ITP was recognized by the end of the 19th century. The existence of nonthrombocytopenic purpura received a large boost in credibility when Wolbach[75] in 1919 described that purpura in Rocky Mountain spotted fever was associated with the infestation of rickettsiae in the walls of microcirculatory vessels. In 1942, Wintrobe opined that although thrombocytopenia was characteristic in ITP, in many purpuric diseases, platelet counts were normal;

he therefore concluded that "some obscure change in the capillary endothelium" must account for at least some cases of nonthrombocytopenic purpura.[76] In 1948, Haden and colleagues[77] showed that cutaneous hemorrhage could occur with a normal platelet count and a normal clotting system. They promulgated the concept of "increased capillary fragility," a term that by virtue of its accuracy, has continued to be used up to now. In 1952, Spaet,[78] and in 1953, Ackroyd[79] clearly, convincingly, and permanently established vascular damage as the primary cause of nonthrombocytopenic purpura. Study of the microcirculation and endothelial biology in particular became possible with electron microscopy, endothelial cell culture, and other modern biomedical techniques.

MICROVASCULAR STRUCTURE–FUNCTION INTERRELATIONS

Study of the fine structure of the microcirculation was pioneered by Majno.[80] The microcirculation is defined as terminal arterioles, capillaries, and postcapillary venules. Figure 11-2 depicts a normal capillary, which will be used as the model of the basic microvascular structural unit. The primary anatomic difference between capillaries and arterioles, as well as postcapillary venules, is that both of the latter have an investiture of smooth muscle cells that control blood flow. The capillary, by anatomic definition, lacks smooth muscle investiture because its function is not to regulate traffic; rather, as the "business end" of the circulation, it is the site of unimpeded gas, fluid, and nutrient exchange. Accordingly, its structure is simple. The primary structural unit is a series of two to five endothelial cells that are joined by tight junctions. Endothelial cells are now known to be extremely influential, providing a great deal of secretory activity on both luminal and

abluminal surfaces and assuming, under appropriate stimulation, a neutral, antithrombotic, or prothrombotic stance (see Chapter 3). The subendothelial basement membrane is immediately beneath the closed circle of endothelial cells. This ill-defined material probably affords some degree of structural integrity but chiefly is highly procoagulant in the event that blood makes contact with it by virtue of a breach in the endothelial membrane. Liberally scattered both longitudinally and circumferentially around capillaries are collagen bundles, which offer resilience against mechanical stresses. Around capillaries are pericytes, whose function is probably largely one of support. Accordingly, the four chief functioning members of the structure of the capillary circulation that keep the circulatory system closed are (1) the endothelium; (2) the subendothelial basement membrane; (3) collagen; and (4) pericytes.

The histologic hallmark of purpura is extravasation of red blood cells from the microcirculation. Figure 11-3 shows light microscopic examination of a biopsy specimen of a single petechia in which red cells have extravasated from a nearby capillary. In Figure 11-4, extravasated red cells abound, with at least one phagocytized by a tissue macrophage. Iron from the heme of red blood cells remains in the skin, causing hemosiderin deposition characteristic of the extremities of patients who have had long-standing purpura.

PATHOPHYSIOLOGIC CATEGORIES OF PURPURA

Table 11-6 presents a classification of purpura and hematovascular lesions.

Purpura Not Associated with Known Microvascular Pathology

Frequently, purpura is identified in which no known anatomic aberration of the microcirculation occurs. These conditions are truly purpuric in that if one chooses to biopsy such lesions, extravasated red cells are seen.

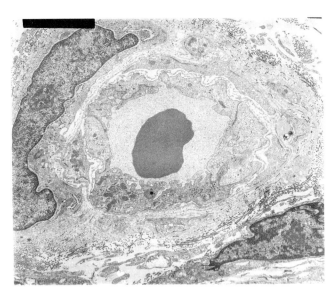

Figure 11-2 Electron micrograph of a normal capillary. This capillary consists of parts of five endothelial cells. A red cell is in the lumen. The thickness of the endothelium is approximately 2500 μm. Supporting tissue includes the basement membrane immediately on the abluminal side of the endothelium. Darker bands of collagen are seen longitudinally and circumferentially around the capillary. The two large nuclei are those of pericytes.

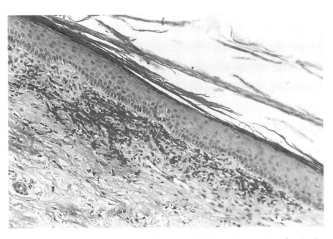

Figure 11-3 (*See also Color Plate 11-3.*) Light micrograph of a single petechia. Beneath the skin, one sees the longitudinal cut of a capillary from which innumerable red cells have extravasated and are trapped in the interstitial connective tissue. The diameter of the entire field is roughly that of a petechia, namely on the order of 1 mm.

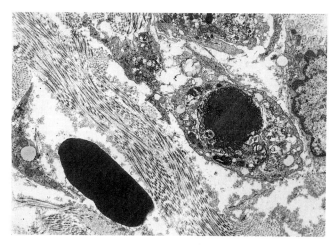

Figure 11-4 Electron micrograph of a petechia. Two extravasated red cells are apparent. The one on the bottom left is in the interstitial space surrounded by bundles of collagen. The one on the right has been phagocytized by a macrophage and is being degraded. The cytoplasm of the macrophage contains residual material from previous red cell ingestion.

Table 11-6 Microvascular Disorders That May Lead to Hemorrhage

1. Purpura not associated with known microvascular pathology
   A. Mechanical causes of purpura
   B. Factitious and psychogenic purpura
   C. Purpura simplex
   D. Bruises and hematomas
   E. Progressive pigmented purpuras (PPPs)
2. Purpura associated with abnormalities of platelets
   A. Immune thrombocytopenic purpura (ITP)
   B. Disorders of platelet function
3. Cutaneous vasculitis and leukocytoclastic vasculitis
4. Microbial endothelial damage
   A. Rickettsial diseases
   B. Leptospiral diseases
   C. Parvovirus B19 infection
   D. Viral hemorrhagic fevers
5. Decreased microvascular mechanical strength
   A. Scurvy
   B. Hypercortisolism
   C. "Senile," "Atrophic," or "Actinic" purpura
   D. Heritable disorders of connective tissue
   E. Amyloidosis
   F. Hereditary hemorrhagic telangiectasia
6. Purpura due to microthrombi
   A. Disseminated intravascular coagulation (DIC)
   B. Warfarin skin nercrosis
   C. Fat embolism
   D. Myeloblastemia
   E. Thrombotic thrombocytopenic purpura (TTP)
   F. Heparin-induced thrombocytopenia (HIT)
   G. Cholesterol emboli
7. Purpura associated with endothelial malignancies

Mechanical Purpura

The mechanical strength of the capillary unit is finite; thus, any pressure that exceeds that limit could well lead to extravasation of red cells. A vacuum of 200 mm Hg over normal skin will extravasate red cells.[81,82] That the human mouth can generate this much suction is exemplified by lesions about the neck known as "hickeys." Petechiae on the face and neck may result from increased venous pressure after vomiting or seizures, or even from prolonged hanging upside down by one's feet to alleviate back pain.[83] Purpura on the palms and soles of the feet may result from leisure activities such as weight-lifting or from traumatic blows from one's avocation or occupation.[84] Formation of petechiae may be seen following choking,[85] asphyxiation,[86] seizure,[87] barotrauma,[88] and electrocution,[89] and even a few may be seen on normal infants.[90] The chief diagnostic criterion is the history of activities prior to the appearance of purpura.

Factitious Purpura

When patients with purpura provide a history that is vague or not credible, one should suspect factitious purpura. A variety of suction devices have been applied to every imaginable part of the body to produce purpura for whatever gain the patient may seek. Figure 11-5 shows a pattern of purpura that clearly suggests that the patient raked reachable parts of his body with a gardening implement. Factitious purpura is more common than one may at first appreciate but can be suspected when the patient has been seen repeatedly by multiple physicians with no hemostatic or underlying medical conditions found. This purpura tends to be well circumscribed and is found chiefly in areas that can be readily reached by the patient.

Psychogenic Purpura

This is an unusual form of purpura that is increasingly regarded as factitious in origin.[91–93] It is indisputable that patients with this type of purpura harbor major deep emotional disturbances and a great deal of unresolved emotional conflict. Lesions of this type of purpura usually begin with bruises that are heralded after a variable lead time by a feeling of warmth, stinging, or swelling. Later, an ecchymotic lesion might appear. These bruises can vary from small to rather large. They have many of the features of factitious purpura in that they are often linear, have well-demarcated edges, and chiefly occur in areas that can

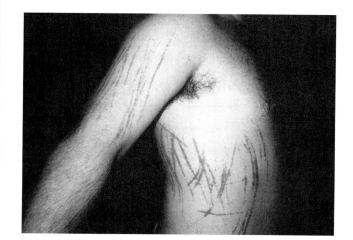

Figure 11-5 (*See also Color Plate 11-5.*) Factitious purpura. These long linear lesions with very sharply demarcated borders appear only in places that the patient can reach. All hemostatic tests were normal, and no evidence suggested an underlying medical disorder. These lesions were probably produced when the patient traumatized his skin with a gardening implement.

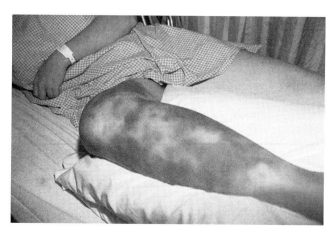

Figure 11-6 (*See also Color Plate 11-6.*) Factitious purpura. This patient has diffuse purpura on one leg without true hematoma formation; the other leg has no lesions at all. All hemostatic studies were normal. She had underlying psychological problems and later admitted to causing these lesions by beating her leg with a hairbrush.

be reached by the patient (Fig. 11-6). The relationship of this disorder to autoerythrocyte sensitization as described by Gardner and Diamond[94] is uncertain.

Purpura Simplex

This vascular phenomenon is a nonpathologic normal process. Many people have small bruises that are associated with trauma of daily living. Women bruise or report bruising more frequently than men.[95] Figure 11-7 shows an ecchymotic area on the lateral surface of the thigh. It is striking how frequently these bruises appear about 30 inches above the floor—the height of most furniture, cabinets, and tables about the house or at work. Purpura simplex may result from being pinched; such lesions are also referred to as "devil's pinches" if an individual has no recall of being pinched. Because this purpura is not of pathologic origin, further evaluation is not necessary. Such patients may safely undergo surgery or invasive procedures.

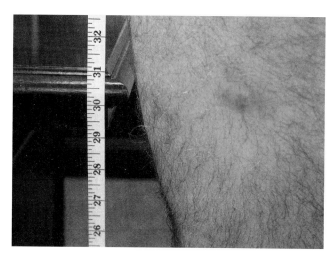

Figure 11-7 (*See also Color Plate 11-7.*) Simple bruise due to day-to-day trauma. Such bruises are caused by encounters with objects on a daily basis. As shown, these lesions occur on the external surface of the thigh and are typically 30 inches above the ground, as this is the height of most American furniture, desks, and countertops.

Bruises and Hematomas

Bruises (including purpura simplex) are not palpable (i.e., not true hematomas) but are flat within the surface of the skin. Bruises result from trauma but of course can be exacerbated by platelet or coagulation defects to become larger bruises or even hematomas. Simple bruises have been somewhat arbitrarily defined as smaller than 3 cm in diameter and not palpable; they usually number no more than four to six over the body. "Normal bruising" has been quantified in healthy infants, of whom 13% may have up to four bruises up to 10-mm maximum diameter. Such bruises tend to occur over bony prominences and increase in frequency as the child's mobility increases.[96] Bruises not confined to bony prominences or in unusual places (soles or palms) may raise questions of abuse. If bruises are larger and more numerous, consideration may be given to a hemostatic defect, especially if the masses are palpable (i.e., true hematomas). Figure 11-8 shows a large hematoma of the shin after an athletic incident that served as the diagnostic event for a teenager with heretofore undiagnosed mild hemophilia A with 7% of normal factor VIII activity. Large ecchymotic areas with hematoma formation (Fig. 11-9) provide the typical presentation of factor VIII inhibitors, as discussed in Chapter 6.

Progressive Pigmented Purpura

A variety of dermatologic diseases have no known underlying cause but are characterized by long periods of progressive crops of purpuric lesions about the legs. Dermatologists have subdivided these progressive pigmented purpuras (PPPs) into a variety of categories, such as progressive pigmented purpura

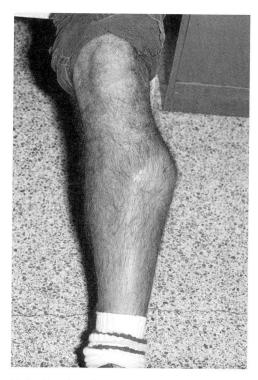

Figure 11-8 (*See also Color Plate 11-8.*) True hematoma in a previously undiagnosed hemophiliac. This 22-year-old college athlete developed a large hematoma over the external surface of his leg after a baseball game in which his leg was stepped on by another player. The patient was found to have 7% of normal factor VIII activity.

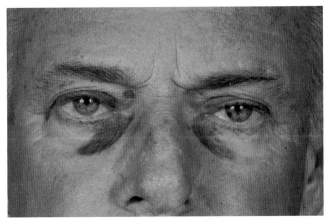

Color Plate 11-1 Spontaneous periorbital purpura in a patient with systemic amyloidosis.

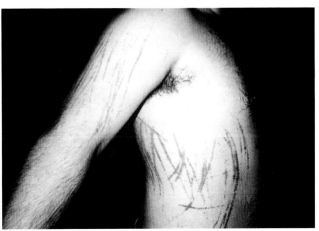

Color Plate 11-5 Factitious purpura. These long linear lesions with very sharply demarcated borders appear only in places that the patient can reach. All hemostatic tests were normal, and no evidence suggested an underlying medical disorder. These lesions were probably produced when the patient traumatized his skin with a gardening implement.

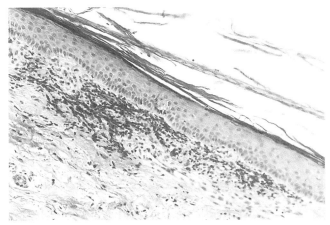

Color Plate 11-3 Light micrograph of a single petechia. Beneath the skin, one sees the longitudinal cut of a capillary from which innumerable red cells have extravasated and are trapped in the interstitial connective tissue. The diameter of the entire field is roughly that of a petechia, namely on the order of 1 mm.

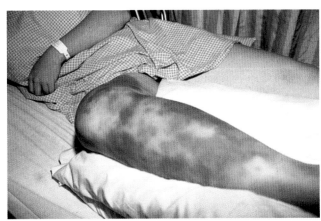

Color Plate 11-6 Factitious purpura. This patient has diffuse purpura on one leg without true hematoma formation; the other leg has no lesions at all. All hemostatic studies were normal. She had underlying psychological problems and later admitted to causing these lesions by beating her leg with a hairbrush.

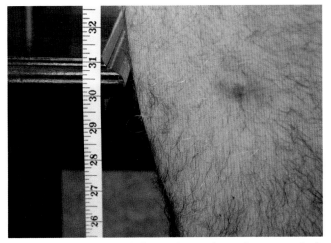

Color Plate 11-7 Simple bruise due to day-to-day trauma. Such bruises are caused by encounters with objects on a daily basis. As shown, these lesions occur on the external surface of the thigh and are typically 30 inches above the ground, as this is the height of most American furniture, desks, and countertops.

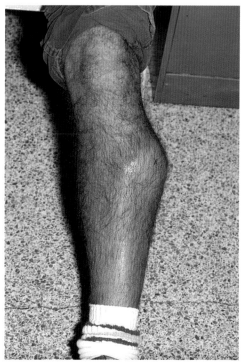

Color Plate 11-8 True hematoma in a previously undiagnosed hemophiliac. This 22-year-old college athlete developed a large hematoma over the external surface of his leg after a baseball game in which his leg was stepped on by another player. The patient was found to have 7% of normal factor VIII activity.

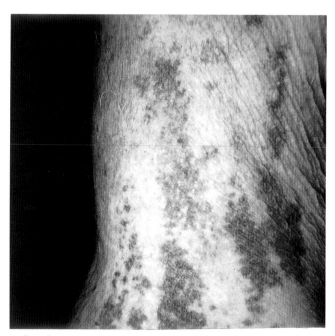

Color Plate 11-10 Capillary fragility. This man developed petechiae on his upper arm in the area underneath a blood pressure cuff following determination of his blood pressure. His platelet count was found to be 5000/L, and he was diagnosed as having idiopathic thrombocytopenic purpura (ITP).

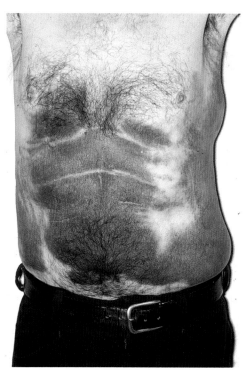

Color Plate 11-9 Extensive subcutaneous hemorrhage in a patient with acquired hemophilia. This patient's extrathoracic hematoma occurred following mild trauma to the skin over his left scapula. Over the next several days, he bled several units of blood and was found to have a high titer antibody against factor VIII.

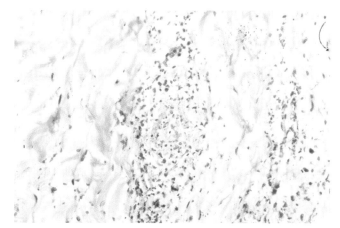

Color Plate 11-12 Leukocytoclastic vasculitis. This photomicrograph shows a central capillary surrounded by extravasated red cells and neutrophils in varying grades of disintegration ("nuclear dust"). This infiltrative process gives rise to the notion of "palpable purpura."

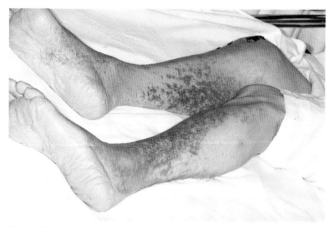

Color Plate 11-13 Palpable purpura. This man had an upper respiratory tract infection, received antibiotics, and several days later developed cutaneous vasculitis typical of palpable purpura.

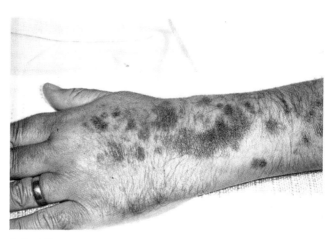

Color Plate 11-16 Hypercortisolism. Subcutaneous purpura is seen in this man's arm, as is slight edema consistent with his hypercortisolism due to long-term, high-dose glucocorticosteroid therapy.

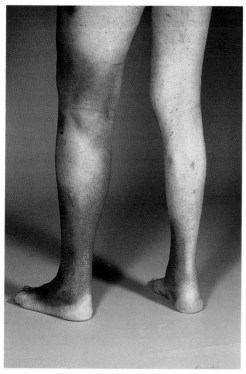

Color Plate 11-15 Scurvy. These large, platelike ecchymotic areas are characteristic of scurvy. They promptly resolved following resumption of a normal diet.

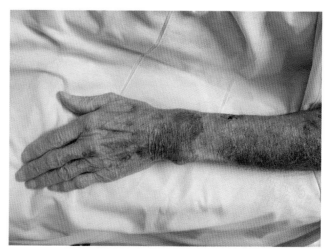

Color Plate 11-17 Actinic or solar purpura. The skin of this man's forearm is very thin; the tendons of the hand are visible. The skin can easily be torn away. The purpura consists of sheets of extravasated red cells. It is not palpable.

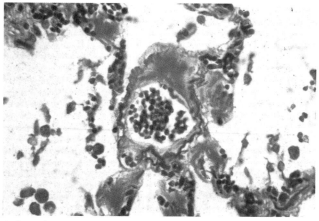

Color Plate 11-18 Amyloidosis. This small vessel is encased in amorphous material between the endothelial wall and the basement membrane, resulting in increased capillary fragility.

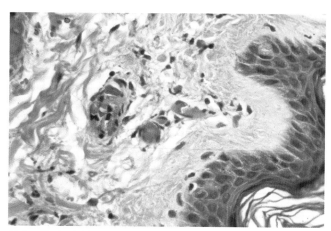

Color Plate 11-21 Meningococcal purpura. Skin biopsy shows several capillaries tensely engorged with fibrin deposition (disseminated intravascular coagulation [DIC]), which can lead to rupture of the microcirculation, as well as ischemic infarction of the skin.

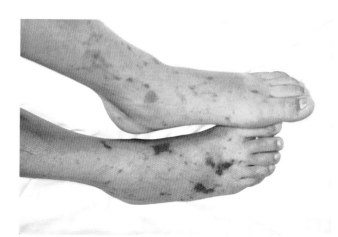

Color Plate 11-20 Meningococcal purpura. This young woman presented with fever and headache. Her early, bright red petechiae rapidly became darker; the characteristic "gun-metal gray" necrosis was apparent.

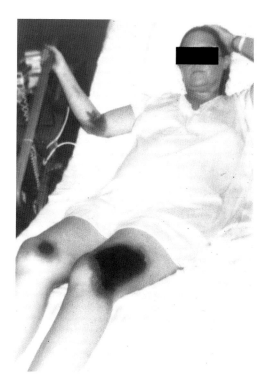

Color Plate 11-22 Warfarin skin necrosis. This woman was administered warfarin and developed painful infarctive lesions a few days later; lesions are shown here as necrotic eschars.

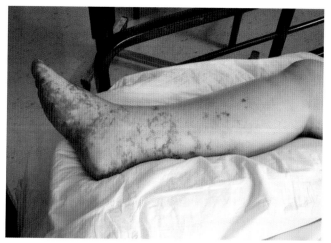

Color Plate 11-23 Cholesterol embolization. This man had severe peripheral vascular disease and had recently undergone cardiac catheterization. The lesions resemble livido reticularis but are painful and darker, and the margins are more easily delineated. Additionally, ischemic blisters are seen in this case, near the Achilles tendon.

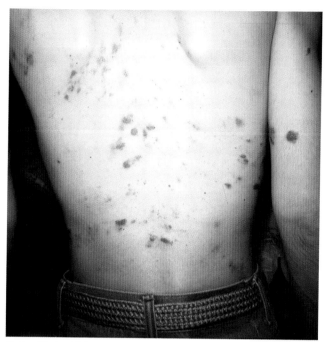

Color Plate 11-24 Kaposi sarcoma. These fleshy tumors are purpuric as a result of extravasated blood cells, yet they are most purpuric in their early stages.

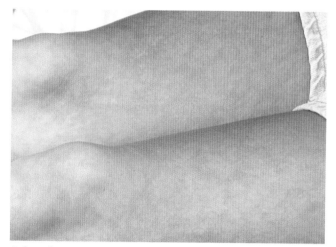

Color Plate 11-25 Livido reticularis. This young woman with antiphospholipid syndrome exhibits the lacy, evanescent-appearing, weblike pattern characteristic of this skin disorder. A more advanced (but less typical) case is shown as "Images in Clinical Medicine," N Engl J Med 356:284, 2007.

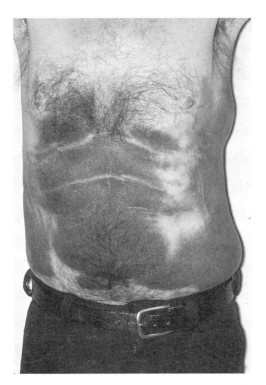

Figure 11-9 (*See also Color Plate 11-9*.) Extensive subcutaneous hemorrhage in a patient with acquired hemophilia. This patient's extrathoracic hematoma occurred following mild trauma to the skin over his left scapula. Over the next several days, he bled several units of blood and was found to have a high titer antibody against factor VIII.

of Schamberg, telangiectodes of Majocchi, lichen aureus, and Gougerot-Blum purpura.[97] These disorders are similar on skin biopsy, with specific absence of leukocytoclastic vasculitis, but many display mononuclear pericapillaritis. Results of laboratory examinations such as complete blood count (CBC) and immunologic tests are normal. Electron microscopic studies in these disorders have failed to show any abnormalities in the capillaries. These disorders have no major sequelae, and therapy is primarily cosmetic.

Purpura Associated With Abnormalities of Platelets

Thrombocytopenic purpura results most commonly from mild trauma with profound thrombocytopenia (20,000/μL or less) but may also be found in patients with qualitative platelet defects.

Thrombocytopenic Purpura

Spontaneous purpura and epistaxis are most frequently seen in severe thrombocytopenia (less than 10,000/dL) and, as such, sudden, spontaneous petechial hemorrhage is the clinical hallmark of acute ITP (see Chapter 9). Purpura probably results from two closely related but separate pathophysiologic events. Clearly, platelets serve a reparative function in the microcirculation, in that they are called on to bridge breaches in the endothelium through adhesion to disrupted endothelium and subendothelial tissues with subsequent aggregation. However, lack of this reparative process does not readily explain the concept of increased

capillary fragility. Petechiae, ecchymosis, and epistaxis occur during severe thrombocytopenia, even without trauma. Examples of capillary fragility include the ring of petechiae around the arm under a blood pressure cuff following blood pressure determination (Fig. 11-10) and petechiae that appear after one simply scratches oneself. This is likely due to intense capillary fragility resulting from severe thrombocytopenia. In experimental animals and humans with severe thrombocytopenia, the microvascular endothelium undergoes morphologic changes, including extreme thinning of the endothelium from its normal 2000 to 3000 μm to 20 to 50 μm, or even, in some places, to narrow fenestrations composed only of endothelial cell membranes (Fig. 11-11). Clearly, such endothelial lesions afford virtually no strength against mechanical stresses or pressure and, in fact, may spontaneously leak red cells. Of interest, capillary membrane thickness reverts toward normal even without quantitative improvement in platelets after administration of glucocorticosteroids.[98,99]

Purpura Associated With Abnormal Platelet Function

Occasionally, platelets are sufficient in number but their quality is such that hemostatic failure manifested as purpura or epistaxis may occur. Theoretically, this can be seen with antiplatelet agents such as aspirin or any of the newer agents that are being increasingly used in the treatment of patients with ischemic heart disease.[100] Whether an accompanying endothelial morphologic disturbance occurs by virtue of qualitative platelet defects, as in quantitative defects, is not known. Congenital defects of platelet function that cause purpura, such as Bernard-Soulier syndrome or Glanzmann thrombasthenia, are discussed in Chapter 10. Chapter 33 discusses various over-the-counter and

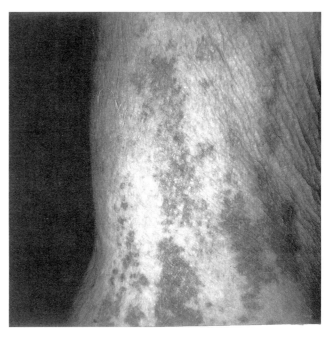

Figure 11-10 (*See also Color Plate 11-10*.) Capillary fragility. This man developed petechiae on his upper arm in the area underneath a blood pressure cuff following determination of his blood pressure. His platelet count was found to be 5000/μL, and he was diagnosed as having idiopathic thrombocytopenic purpura (ITP).

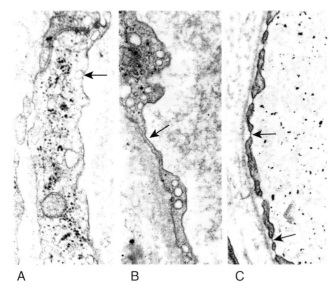

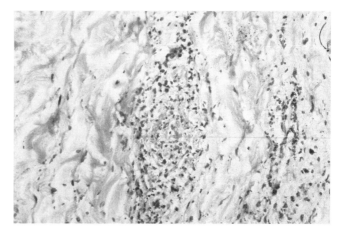

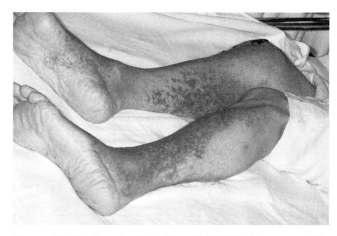

Figure 11-11 Electron micrograph of capillaries in experimental thrombocytopenia. (**A**) A capillary from a nonthrombocytopenic control animal. The endothelial membrane has a thickness of approximately 2000 to 2500 μm. The arrow points to a normal vesicle. (**B**) The endothelium has been thinned *(arrow)* nearly to the same size as the normal vesicle. (**C**) Even further thinning is shown *(arrows)*, to the point where the endothelium has become fenestrated, an anatomic finding not characteristic of cutaneous capillaries. The lumen of the capillary is oriented to the right in all three panels. (From Kitchens CS: Amelioration of endothelial abnormalities by prednisone in experimental thrombocytopenia in the rabbit. J Clin Invest 60:1129–1134, 1977, with permission.)

Figure 11-12 *(See also Color Plate 11-12.)* Leukocytoclastic vasculitis. This photomicrograph shows a central capillary surrounded by extravasated red cells and neutrophils in varying grades of disintegration ("nuclear dust"). This infiltrative process gives rise to the notion of "palpable purpura."

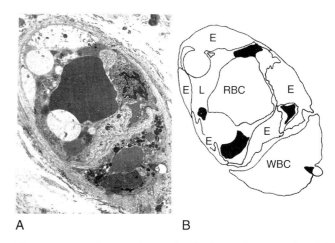

Figure 11-13 *(See also Color Plate 11-13.)* Palpable purpura. This man had an upper respiratory tract infection, received antibiotics, and several days later developed cutaneous vasculitis typical of palpable purpura.

complementary medicines that decrease platelet function and may result in purpuric lesions, especially when an underlying platelet defect coexists.

Cutaneous Vasculitis

Cutaneous vasculitis (CV) is one of the most common causes of nonthrombocytopenic purpura and, because of its frequent association with significant underlying medical disease, is of interest to the hematologist and the internist. That CV is often associated with diseases of rheumatic origin led early investigators such as William Osler and Austin Flint to refer to this as *purpura rheumatica*. We now frequently refer to CV also by its chief clinical attribute (*palpable purpura*) or its histologic hallmark (*leukocytoclastic vasculitis*). In leukocytoclastic vasculitis (LCV), the smallest vessels in the skin are encased by sheets of neutrophils in various stages of disintegration, often referred to as "nuclear dust" (Fig. 11-12). Heavy infiltration by leukocytes is what actually gives rise to the perception of palpability in palpable purpura (Fig. 11-13). It is hypothesized that this pathologic event results from leakage of immune complexes through the vessel wall into the subendothelial area. These complexes then induce the egress of leukocytes. Subsequently, the neutrophils disintegrate, releasing their proteolytic enzymes into the area around the adjacent vessel, causing digestion and disruption of the endothelial membrane, with subsequent egress of red cells (Fig. 11-14). When LCV is acutely severe, it is called *necrotizing vasculitis.*

Figure 11-14 Electron micrograph of leukocytoclastic vasculitis. (**A**) A capillary with an extravasated granulocyte (white blood cell [WBC]) at the lower pole. The endothelial cell (E) on the top has become ballooned and is nonviable. (**B**) A key, with RBC representing a red blood cell, L, the lumen, and the blackened areas representing electron-dense immune complexes.

The list of disorders associated with CV is long and varied (Table 11-7). These are best categorized as rheumatic in origin and are associated with requisite immune complexes. The predominance of CV in children is called *primary CV* because no obvious chronic underlying cause can be found. Most (89%) pediatric primary CV is associated with some combination of palpable purpura, arthralgia, colicky abdominal pain, and evidence of nephritis and is commonly referred to as Henoch-Schönlein purpura (HSP). In a large series,[101] these findings occurred in 100%, 70%, 70%, and 50%, respectively, of patients who were deemed to have HSP. No chronic underlying disease occurs. The other 11% of pediatric cases represent acute hypersensitivity reactions. Only about 1% of CV in children and young adults is determined to result from some underlying and more serious chronic disease.

In adults, again, most cases (63%) are deemed primary CV, but two thirds are labeled acute hypersensitivity vasculitis, with only one third meeting the criteria for HSP. Hypersensitivity to drugs is a common cause of CV. Roughly one third of all adult CV is found to be secondary; in Table 11-7, the most common causes are lupus erythematosus, cryoglobulinemia,[102,103] chronic hepatitis C,[104] Sjögren syndrome, polyarteritis nodosa, Churg-Strauss syndrome,[105] rheumatoid arthritis, and subacute bacterial endocarditis.[106]

As was mentioned previously, CV is often referred to by its historical name of Henoch-Schönlein purpura when it is associated with any two or three of the following four cardinal features: symmetrical petechial process, abdominal pain, large joint arthralgia or swelling, and evidence of nephritis. Others have found that the diagnosis of HSP is facilitated by ultrasound of the abdomen, which can frequently show edematous bowel walls with visible blood flow.[107] Indeed, the line between the disease classically referred to as HSP, especially when adult and childhood variations are taken into account, and the increasingly used

term CV has blurred,[108] and in fact, some[109] have questioned why the term HSP continues to be used, as the distinction occasionally is arbitrary, especially if one uses preemptory criteria such as an age cutoff and whether or not microvascular deposition of immunoglobulin (Ig)A is found. If a specific chronic underlying disease is not encountered and the patient has arthralgia, nephritis, or abdominal pain, perhaps the more narrow term *HSP* is best. If no cause can be found and criteria for HSP are not met, *primary hypersensitivity vasculitis* is the term that is used, denoting a hypersensitivity reaction to some commonly occurring viral infection, medications used to treat such upper respiratory tract infections, or the use of other drugs.

Primary CV is indicated not only by the lack of an obvious underlying disease but also by normal results of almost all routine laboratory studies, with the exception of the sedimentation rate, which is greatly elevated in 69% of cases. Studies that return with normal results include CBC, coagulation profile, serum studies for cryoglobulins, serologic studies for antinuclear antibodies (ANAs), serum complement levels, and antineutrophil cytoplasmic antibodies (ANCAs).[110] A proposed guideline for the evaluation of palpable purpura[108] includes studies shown in Table 11-3. More specific studies are guided by one's clinical index of suspicion for a specific underlying disorder.

The diagnosis of secondary CV is not difficult to make when one notices palpable purpura in a patient known to have a disorder such as lupus erythematosus, subacute bacterial endocarditis, or other immune complex illness. On the other hand, evaluation of CV may lead to the discovery of an important underlying disease first manifested by palpable purpura.

The prognosis for primary CV is excellent; complete recovery occurs in 90% of cases in adults and children with primary CV. Frequently, especially in childhood, the process spontaneously resolves over weeks. Prognosis in the secondary types depends on the prognosis of the underlying disease, particularly the presence or absence of nephropathy, which determines the outcome in many adults.[111]

One unusual and fairly rare cause of CV is benign hypergammaglobulinemic purpura of Waldenström.[112] This process is seen chiefly in women with episodic bursts of palpable purpura that are clearly dependent in distribution and exacerbated by prolonged standing or the wearing of tight clothes. As its name implies, the hallmark is a broad-based polyclonal increase in immunoglobulins that does not appear to be associated with any other known disease, and therefore, by definition, is negative for evidence of chronic viral hepatitis. ANA and other serologic tests for lupus may be positive, as may analysis for rheumatoid factor and ANCA. Treatment is rarely indicated, and the process is not known to progress to any other disease.

Golfer's vasculitis[113] has been recently described in healthy men who play golf in hot environments. The lesions are those of CV on usual and histologic examination. Tests as outlined in Table 11-3 are negative, and vasculitis tends to spontaneously disappear within a week. This represents most likely the same process as that described by Ramelet[114]—exercise-induced purpura; the only exception is that Ramelet ascribed the purpuric disorder to "major muscular activity," a term hardly descriptive of golf.

Table 11-7 Disorders Associated With Cutaneous Vasculitis

Primary	Secondary
Idiopathic	Systemic lupus erythematosus
Hypersensitivity reaction*	Chronic hepatitis B
Upper respiratory tract	Chronic hepatitis C
infection, viral or bacterial	Cryoglobulinemia
Drugs	Sjögren syndrome
Penicillin	Polyarteritis nodosa
Iodine	Rheumatoid arthritis
Aspirin	Mixed connective tissue
Antibiotics	syndrome
Analgesics	Subacute bacterial endocarditis
NSAIDs	Wegener granulomatosis
Thiazides	Churg-Strauss syndrome
Colchicine	Hypergammaglobulinemic
	purpura of Waldenström
	Myelodysplastic syndromes
	Malignancies

*Hypersensitivity reactions frequently are called Henoch-Schönlein purpura (HSP) if the patient has colicky gastrointestinal symptoms, gastrointestinal bleeding, hematuria or other evidence of nephritis, and large joint arthralgias or swelling and is not on medication known to be associated with hypersensitivity vasculitis.
NSAIDs, nonsteroidal anti-inflammatory drugs.

Purpura Associated With Microbial Endothelial Damage

The endothelium may be the site of residence and proliferation of microorganisms, or it can be directly attacked by microorganisms. Either situation may lead to destruction of the endothelial membrane with resultant extravasation of red cells.

Rickettsial Disease

The best-studied rickettsial disease involving purpura is Rocky Mountain spotted fever (RMSF), due to *Rickettsia rickettsii*. This agent is an obligate endothelial cell organism, and its endothelial presence was shown as early as 1919 by Wolbach.[75] The petechial rash may be first detectable on the first day of illness but generally is not clearly manifest until the third or fourth day. These spots become larger than most petechiae, growing to 5 to 6 mm in diameter, and may have vague borders that blend into erythema. One unusual feature is that the spots also may appear on the palms and soles. The seriousness of the disease is enhanced by the invasion of the vasculature of all organs by the organism and an intense increase in vascular permeability brought about by destruction of endothelial cell integrity. This results in simultaneous edema and intravascular hypovolemia with characteristic increases in serum concentrations of blood urea nitrogen and creatinine. Although mild thrombocytopenia occurs, it is not believed to be the genesis of hemorrhage. True disseminated intravascular coagulation (DIC) is rare. The hematologist may be asked to consult for evaluation of mild thrombocytopenia in a febrile patient with multiorgan failure who is not improving despite antibiotics. The hematologist may be the first practitioner to suspect RMSF. Other rickettsial diseases may be associated with petechial rashes, but none as extensively as RMSF.

Leptospiral Disease

Leptospirosis is due to systemic invasion by the spirochete genus *Leptospira*. In its severe form, often known as Weil disease, nearly all tissues are invaded by this microbe. Endothelial damage gives rise to the vasculitis, capillary leak syndrome, and petechial rash that are characteristic of the disorder. Other hemorrhagic phenomena can be abetted by the modest thrombocytopenia and DIC that may occur. Penicillins are usually the antibiotic group of choice for therapy.

Parvovirus B19 Infection

This virus may cause a variety of hematologic disorders, such as pure red cell aplasia or hypoplastic pancytopenia. It is also the agent of "fifth disease." Recently, it has been reported to cause a peculiar "socks and gloves" petechial rash that is self limited.[115–117] On skin biopsy, no evidence for vasculitis is found, so endothelial damage is speculated to be the cause of blood extravasation.

Viral Hemorrhagic Fevers

Several viruses have been incriminated as destroying endothelial cells, resulting in various hemorrhagic fevers. Owing in part to the global distribution of these illnesses, typically in remote areas, detailed investigation into these diseases has been severely limited. Whereas bleeding may also be due in part to accompanying thrombocytopenia or even DIC, petechial manifestations of these hemorrhagic fevers are believed to represent endothelial damage caused by direct invasion and destruction. These hemorrhagic fevers include Lassa fever, Rift Valley fever, dengue, yellow fever, and Marburg fever.[117a] The mortality rate of these diseases varies from rather low to extremely high.[118,119] A periodically discovered and rediscovered hemorrhagic fever with a mortality rate as high as 90% is Ebola hemorrhagic fever, which directly causes endothelial cell damage.[120] Hemorrhage in all these disorders not only is cutaneous in the way of purpura but also involves multiple organs, the dysfunction of which results from hemorrhage and ultimately causes death. Unfortunately, treatment is nonexistent. If any of these viral hemorrhagic diseases is seriously considered in the differential diagnosis, especially in persons who have recently been abroad, rapid consultation with infectious disease experts and the Centers for Disease Control and Prevention in Atlanta is mandatory.[121]

Purpura Associated With Decreased Microvascular Mechanical Strength

The following disorders have in common that the structural integrity of the microvascular unit, shown in Figure 11-2, has been compromised. Many investigators have tried to ascribe platelet defects and mild coagulation disorders as causative or additive in this classification of purpura, but none of these theories has stood the test of time.

Scurvy

We have alluded to scurvy previously in the Historical Perspective section of this chapter. Scurvy was the first hemorrhagic disease to have a specific cure following Lind's study of this disabling bleeding disorder.[69] Scorbutic bleeding is characterized by perifollicular hemorrhage, large if not even huge, flat, platelike ecchymoses (Fig. 11-15), and hypertrophic spongy, bleeding gums. The disease is only rarely seen now because of improved dietary habits; severe chronic inveterate alcoholics with poor nutrition represent most current patients with scurvy. Scurvy, however, has been reported in pediatric populations[122] and those on exceptionally low-carbohydrate diets.[123]

The disease is diagnosed clinically by its appearance. One may send blood samples for vitamin C level determination in equivocal cases. The response to vitamin C administration either pharmacologically or dietarily is gratifying and rapid. The disorder is due to the inability to crosslink fibers of collagen at proline sites, as vitamin C is necessary to convert proline into hydroxyproline for participation in crosslinking of the helical structure of collagen. Microvascular strength and structure are enormously compromised by virtue of weakened collagen synthesis.

Hypercortisolism

Hypercortisolism, whether exogenous or endogenous, also results in decreased collagen strength. Cortisol is known to decrease collagen synthesis, and because collagen catabolism is not affected, collagen becomes scarce, resulting in capillary fragility. Purpura is seen primarily on the extensor surfaces of the forearms (Fig. 11-16). Purpura is a presenting sign in about 25% of cases.[124] The skin is thin, which accounts for the superficial appearance of extravasated

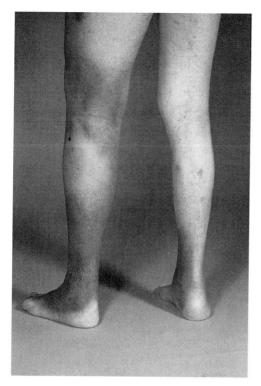

Figure 11-15 (*See also Color Plate 11-15.*) Scurvy. These large, platelike ecchymotic areas are characteristic of scurvy. They promptly resolved following resumption of a normal diet.

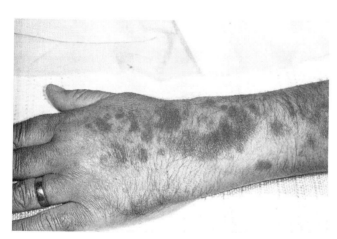

Figure 11-16 (*See also Color Plate 11-16.*) Hypercortisolism. Subcutaneous purpura is seen in this man's arm, as is slight edema consistent with his hypercortisolism due to long-term, high-dose glucocorticosteroid therapy.

blood. Treatment involves cessation of cortisone administration in exogenous hypercortisolism or correction, if possible, of endogenous sources, resulting in the increased production of cortisol. Vitamin C administration has not been shown to help in the management of these patients.

"Senile," "Atrophic," or "Actinic" Purpura

This type of purpura is common in older and debilitated patients, but it is hardly limited to the elderly, as any extremely ill patient who exhibits weight loss and negative nitrogen balance is subject to this process. It is also seen in fairly healthy patients who have excessive solar exposure,

which increases breakdown of collagen. Accordingly, the extensor surfaces of the forearms are characteristic locations of this purpura, particularly in those who work outdoors with short or no sleeves. The skin has the appearance on close examination of being extremely thin across the extensor surfaces of the arms and the backs of the hands (Fig. 11-17). Should the skin undergo biopsy, the dermal–epidermal junction is found to be thin, with characteristically flattened rete pegs. Patients often report that just the slightest trauma or stretching of the skin can cause the skin to physically rupture, with subcutaneous bleeding. No specific treatment is available. Vitamin C is not efficacious in this disorder. Hemostasis is normal.

Heritable Disorders of Connective Tissue

Rare inherited metabolic disorders of connective tissue may result in large vessel hemorrhage, as was discussed in the first section of this chapter. Subcutaneous hemorrhage may be encountered yet essentially is never of diagnostic importance in that these heritable disorders are usually quite obvious to all. Bleeding in these disorders usually is more likely to occur as the result of tearing of fragile subcutaneous tissues and skin than as the result of spontaneous purpuric lesions. No persistent coagulation or platelet abnormality has been elucidated. No specific treatment is available. Surgical hemostasis is normal, but healing is impaired.

Amyloidosis

Macrovascular hemorrhage due to amyloidosis was discussed in the first section of this chapter. Purpuric bleeding may very well be one of the initial findings that leads to the correct diagnosis. Purpuric bleeding was detected in 15% of all cases of amyloidosis in one large review.[125] Amyloid material is deposited between the endothelium and the basement membrane (Fig. 11-18) and therefore can be found in the vasculature of any organ. Amyloid not only leads to probable increased capillary fragility but also, for arterioles, impedes the ability of those vessels to constrict, thereby failing to limit regional flow and bleeding from injured vessels. Coagulation abnormalities are frequent,

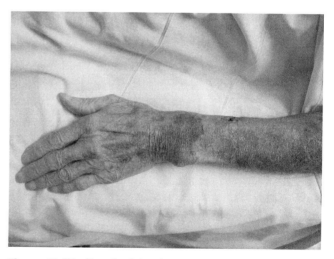

Figure 11-17 (*See also Color Plate 11-17.*) Actinic or solar purpura. The skin of this man's forearm is very thin; the tendons of the hand are visible. The skin can easily be torn away. The purpura consists of sheets of extravasated red cells. It is not palpable.

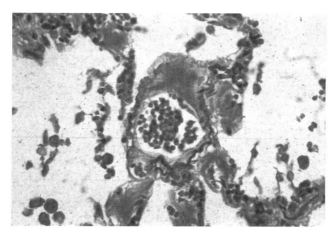

Figure 11-18 (*See also Color Plate 11-18.*) Amyloidosis. This small vessel is encased in amorphous material between the endothelial wall and the basement membrane, resulting in increased capillary fragility.

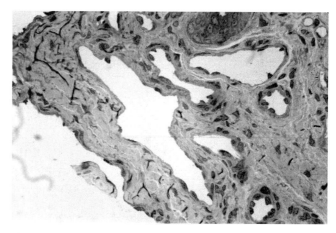

Figure 11-19 Light microphotograph of Osler-Weber-Rendu syndrome. This section has been made through a telangiectasis. No extravasated red cells are observed. Red blood cells have been washed out of the lumina of these vessels during preparation. Toward the top and also on the right-hand edge are several normal capillaries. Toward the center are several larger vessels, and in the extreme lower left-hand corner, is the lumen of an even larger vessel. The walls of all these vessels are anatomically those of a capillary, that is, thin-walled consisting only of an endothelial cell. These anatomic characteristics give insufficient strength to vessels larger than capillaries, which leads to increased hemorrhage.

multiple, and of varying patterns in amyloidosis[126–128] which may confuse the diagnostician about the true cause of the purpura, which is the deposition of amyloid. The distribution of purpura is somewhat unusual in that it is not nearly as dependent as most purpuric lesions are but seems more likely to occur along pressure points, with a peculiar periorbital predilection (see Fig. 11-1).

Hereditary Hemorrhagic Telangiectasia

This disorder is also referred to as Osler-Weber-Rendu syndrome (OWR). HHT is an accurate term in that it describes key elements of the disease. HHT is not truly a purpuric disorder because no extravasation of red cells occurs; rather, they remain in the intravascular space until the lesions rupture. Because of this, telangiectases blanch easily on external pressure. Additionally, a telangiectatic lesion is typically 2 to 3 mm in diameter, slightly larger than a nonblanchable petechia. This disorder is discussed under Purpuric Diseases, as it is traditionally classified in reviews. The hemorrhagic component of the disorder is due to decreased mechanical strength of the microvasculature (Fig. 11-19). HHT was discussed in depth in the section on Macrovascular Hemorrhage.

Numerous attempts to identify coagulation defects have usually not borne out any consistent defect. Individual cases of concomitant von Willebrand disease and HHT syndrome have been reported.

A surgical approach to any problem should not be discounted for fear of bleeding, as HHT is not a primary hemostatic defect. Patients may undergo surgery for these AVMs or other procedures not related to their HHT without risk of excessive bleeding.

Telangiectases are not limited to HHT. Many otherwise normal persons have a few telangiectases while having no family history of characteristic hemorrhage. Lesions may become even more prominent during pregnancy. Telangiectases are seen in some other disorders, particularly as part of the CREST syndrome (calcinosis, Raynaud phenomenon, esophageal dysmotility, sclerodactyly, and telangiectasia) of scleroderma. They may also result from actinic damage or from therapeutic radiation.

Purpura Associated With Microthrombi

The microcirculation may become obstructed by emboli, which may cause microinfarction and disruption of the endothelial membrane with subsequent extravasation of red cells. These dermal emboli cause purpuric lesions. In its most expressive form, the process is called *purpura fulminans*. Because microthrombi often simultaneously occur in other organs, end organ damage may occur, leading to multiorgan dysfunction syndrome (MODS).

Disseminated Intravascular Coagulation

Multiple causes give rise to the syndrome called *disseminated intravascular coagulation (DIC)*. Tissue samples or autopsy specimens frequently show occlusive deposition of fibrin, particularly in the microcirculation. These emboli lead to purpuric skin lesions and frank purpura fulminans. One of the foremost causes of the latter is meningococcemia, which results in characteristic rapidly progressive necrotizing purpura fulminans (Figs. 11-20 and 11-21). Fibrin deposition is not limited to the skin; MODS is the most frequent cause of death in DIC. Recognition and treatment of disorders associated with DIC are more thoroughly discussed in Chapters 12 and 13. Morbidity and mortality in purpura fulminans are high, averaging about 50%.[129,130] An underlying thrombophilic disorder such as factor V Leiden mutation may coexist in patients whose illness progresses to purpura fulminans.[131]

Warfarin Skin Necrosis

This is a special cause of fibrin deposition that appears limited to the dermal microcirculation.[132,133] This process was previously believed to be due to an idiosyncratic toxic reaction to warfarin. It is now believed to be due to the precipitous drop in levels of protein C following initiation of warfarin administration. The half-life of protein C is only 4 to 5 hours; therefore, a rapid decrease in this

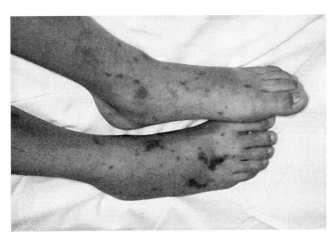

Figure 11-20 (*See also Color Plate 11-20.*) Meningococcal purpura. This young woman presented with fever and headache. Her early, bright red petechiae rapidly became darker; the characteristic "gun-metal gray" necrosis was apparent.

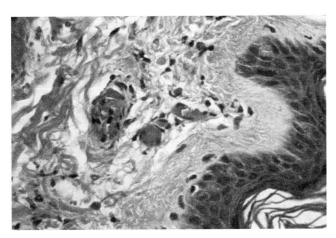

Figure 11-21 (*See also Color Plate 11-21.*) Meningococcal purpura. Skin biopsy shows several capillaries tensely engorged with fibrin deposition (disseminated intravascular coagulation [DIC]), which can lead to rupture of the microcirculation, as well as ischemic infarction of the skin.

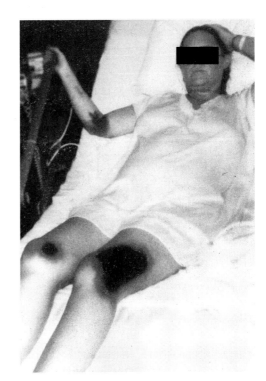

Figure 11-22 (*See also Color Plate 11-22.*) Warfarin skin necrosis. This woman was administered warfarin and developed painful infarctive lesions a few days later; lesions are shown here as necrotic eschars.

anticoagulant occurs before a decrease is noted in procoagulant factors II, VII, IX, and X. This is believed to induce an early hypercoagulable state. Levels of protein C may already be low for genetic reasons or because of further consumption during the thrombotic process. A further decrease in protein C levels allows for relative localized hypercoagulability in the microcirculation, the site of the primary action of protein C. Because protein S is the cofactor of protein C, congenital or acquired protein S deficiency is also a risk factor for warfarin skin necrosis.

This process is normally heralded first by a stinging or burning sensation about 2 to 4 days after the initiation of warfarin therapy. The site becomes hemorrhagic a day or two later. For some reason, warfarin skin necrosis occurs more frequently in women than men (9:1 ratio) and usually develops in areas in where generous adipose tissue is found, such as the thighs, buttocks, or breasts. If the condition is not recognized and treated promptly, the site becomes necrotic and assumes the appearance of a large burn eschar, usually requiring subsequent skin grafting (Fig. 11-22). On biopsy, fibrin deposition is prominent in the microcirculation. This process is not as common as it used to be when large doses of warfarin (up to 1 mg/kg) were used as a "loading dose." It is best prevented by not loading patients with warfarin but starting with a dose that approximates the estimated maintenance dose. It may also be rarer now because patients with active thromboses are first aggressively administered heparin. If the diagnosis of warfarin skin necrosis is entertained, prompt initiation of heparin therapy and cessation of warfarin is considered the best treatment. Vitamin K should be administered intravenously. A similar pattern of unopposed decrease in protein C levels may be seen with intermittent stopping and restarting of warfarin and nearly certainly explains warfarin skin necrosis that occurs in patients reported to develop this syndrome during long-term warfarin therapy. Initiation of warfarin therapy should follow heparin therapy, and these should overlap for 4 to 5 days in patients known to have protein C or S deficiency or those with a personal or family history of warfarin skin necrosis. Warfarin skin necrosis is extremely unlikely following initiation of warfarin for treatment of patients with stroke or for prophylaxis in atrial fibrillation, because a large, fresh clot is not present, and this population is not believed to harbor patients with congenital deficiency of protein C or S. Accordingly, heparin therapy is not routinely given first to such patients unless the history suggests an underlying thrombophilia. Warfarin skin necrosis may also complicate warfarin therapy in patients with heparin-induced thrombocytopenia (see Chapter 25).

Fat Embolism Syndrome

Petechiae are characteristic of fat embolism syndrome. These petechiae have a fairly unusual distribution in that they are scattered most often about the neck, shoulders, and especially the axillary folds in the upper chest area. They are occasionally seen on the conjunctivae. It is believed that this distribution may be due to the fact that these are counterdependent areas of the body. Thus, circulating fat particles may rise and embolize in this pattern. These petechiae rarely represent a problem in and of themselves, but their presence may serve to suggest or diagnose fat embolism syndrome.[134–136]

Fat embolism is apparently much more common than fat embolism syndrome. If one looks for fat embolism particularly with the use of bronchoalveolar lavage (BAL) and staining of pulmonary macrophages for neutral fat, fat may be seen in as many as 60% of patients who undergo instrumentation of long bone fractures. Fat can also be seen traversing the cardiac circulation through transesophageal echocardiography performed at the time of long bone manipulation. Fat embolism may also be seen after liposuction.

Among trauma cases, fat embolism syndrome is diagnosed in approximately 0.5%, if it is not actively sought; however, it is diagnosed in 10% to 20% of all trauma cases when evidence is prospectively sought, specifically, through close examination of patients with trauma and hypoxemia. Fat embolism syndrome is seen in up to 60% of autopsies involving blunt trauma.

This syndrome is characterized by petechiae in the characteristic distribution in 60% of cases, and by shortness of breath and hypoxia in 50%. Thirty percent of patients experience confusion or coma. Retinal changes may occur, and platelet count may drop slightly in 50% of cases. Fever is characteristic, and diagnosis hinges on recognition of the probability of this syndrome. Its peak incidence is between 24 and 72 hours after the traumatic event.

Treatment is believed to be nonspecific and supportive. Because of the apparent association (if it is not a precipitating factor) with hypovolemic shock, low blood pressure should be aggressively treated. Hypoxemia needs to be addressed. Putative treatments include steroids, heparin, or aspirin. Although all of these may have some efficacy, no evidence-based study has proved their efficacy.[137]

Myeloblastemia

Leukostasis syndromes typically manifest through central nervous system dysfunction and hypoxia when cerebral and pulmonary capillary beds are involved.[138] Leukostasis is most typically seen with a large number of circulating myeloblasts and promyelocytes such as in blast crisis of chronic myelogenous leukemia. These large malignant myeloid cells may also embolize within the dermal microcirculation and cause infarctive lesions that are far in excess of the degree of thrombocytopenia that may accompany leukemia and its treatment. The most appropriate therapy is cytoreduction of malignant cells.

Thrombotic Thrombocytopenic Purpura (TTP)

This interesting disease is discussed thoroughly in Chapter 24. Although platelet aggregates induce thrombosis in many tissues, a paucity of cutaneous purpura is noted, despite its name. Nonetheless, petechial, purpuric, and infarctive lesions are occasionally present but are often overshadowed by other manifestations of this disorder.

Heparin-Induced Thrombocytopenia With Thrombosis (HIT)

Purpura and embolic ischemia but rarely petechiae are characteristic of this disorder. Ischemia of the extremities in patients who have received or are receiving heparin and in those who have become thrombocytopenic should alert the practitioner to this possibility. HIT is discussed in Chapter 25.

Blue Toe Syndrome, Purple Toe Syndrome, and Cholesterol Emboli Syndrome

These are different terms for what most likely are variations of the same process.[133,139–141] Whether they occur during heparin administration, during warfarin administration, following abdominal trauma, following cardiac catheterization, or even spontaneously, the unifying points are (1) that all these patients have significant underlying atherosclerosis, and (2) that the histologic picture is one of cholesterol crystals in the arterioles of biopsied lesions.

In the past, the purple (or blue) discoloration of the toes that occurred when patients were administered an oral or a parenteral anticoagulant was believed to be a reaction to the anticoagulants. It is far more likely that these lesions are due to the underlying process for which the anticoagulants were indicated. Use of anticoagulants results in remodeling of the clots that commingle among large atherosclerotic plaques, allowing bleeding into the atherosclerotic plaques or freeing up of cholesterol crystals, which then embolize distally.

This process resembles livedo reticularis but differs in that it is usually significantly bluer and is quite painful because of the ischemia. This appears to be strictly an arteriolar embolization syndrome in that deposition of fibrin that one sees in the venules in warfarin skin necrosis is not encountered. The process may progress to involve not only purple or blue toes but through-and-through necrosis of the toes and feet, as well as significant parts of the soft tissue, usually of the legs and sometimes into the lower flank and back (Fig. 11-23).

Occasionally, the differential diagnosis is not straightforward and includes HIT, antiphospholipid syndrome (APLS), warfarin skin necrosis, and cholesterol emboli, which may be clarified if there is a recent history of manipulation or trauma of the arterial system. When it occurs spontaneously, one can often be led astray by many findings that suggest a vasculitis, including weight loss, anorexia, fever, anemia, eosinophilia, and a very high erythrocyte sedimentation rate. Calf muscle tenderness may coexist with elevations in serum creatine kinase level, both of which can broaden the differential diagnosis; however, this is believed to be due to an ischemic myositis from infarcts that are simultaneously taking place within the calf muscles.

Assessment should be focused on the arterial system. Echocardiography that includes the aortic arch is indicated, as is imaging of the entire aorta. Ankle-to–brachial pressure index may be helpful, but sometimes arterial pulses are palpable and half the time are even described as bounding. There is usually a very high probability that cholesterol crystal deposition will be found on skin biopsy of appropriate material.

These conditions are serious, not only because of the ischemia and the risk of amputation but because of the underlying atherosclerosis itself. Treatment probably is best

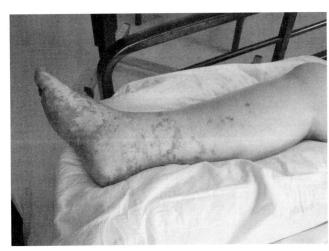

Figure 11-23 *(See also Color Plate 11-23.)* Cholesterol emboliza-tion. This man had severe peripheral vascular disease and had recently undergone cardiac catheterization. The lesions resemble livido reticu-laris but are painful and darker, and the margins are more easily deli-neated. Additionally, ischemic blisters are seen in this case, near the Achilles tendon.

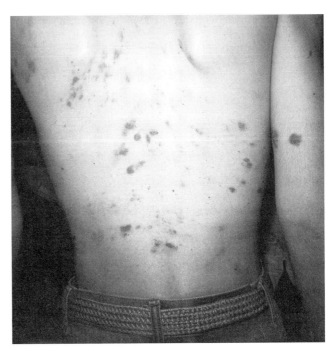

Figure 11-24 *(See also Color Plate 11-24.)* Kaposi sarcoma. These fleshy tumors are purpuric as a result of extravasated blood cells, yet they are most purpuric in their early stages.

provided by minimizing or totally avoiding additional in-vasive procedures of the arterial system; if catheterization studies are necessary, consideration should be given to use of the upper extremity.

Purpura Associated With Vascular Malignancy

Endothelial cells, similar to other cells, may become malig-nant. Although multiple rare endothelial malignancies exist, the prototypic and most common form is Kaposi sarcoma (KS).[142] This disease in the past was very rare; however, it became more common in the 1980s because of its associa-tion with acquired immunodeficiency syndrome (AIDS).

The hematologist from time to time will be asked to see a patient with a purpuric lesion that proves to be KS (Fig. 11-24). KS typically starts as an ecchymotic-appearing macular lesion that progresses to a plaque or nodular le-sion. KS has become more common in the AIDS pandemic and is believed to be due to the opportunistic coinfection of human immunodeficiency virus (HIV)-positive patients with Kaposi sarcoma herpes virus (KSHV), which is also known as human herpes virus type 8 (HHV8). Although KS is seen chiefly in homosexual men and at one time was the AIDS-defining illness in approximately one half of such patients, a dramatic decrease has occurred over the past decade, with KS being found in only about 15% of patients with AIDS and in 1% of newly diagnosed HIV-positive patients.[143] A variety of dermal processes are included in the differential diagnosis, but a very important clue, typical of all purpuric lesions, is that the early KS lesion does not blanch on external pressure. As lesions be-come larger, more plaquelike, and nodular, they are clearly distinguished from purpura. The diagnosis may ultimately depend on biopsy, which can be undertaken without exces-sive risk of hemorrhage despite the vascular nature of the tumor.

Research into this tumor has generated a wealth of information on angiogenesis.[144] The sarcomatous tissue produces vascular endothelial growth factor (VEGF), which greatly stimulates further proliferation of endothelial cells. This accounts for the massing of endothelial cells in an at-tempt to make channels, referred to as "vascular slits," the histologic hallmark of this lesion. Also found is a swirling arrangement of spindle-shaped cells admixed with the an-giogenic component. These spindle cells stain for smooth muscle actin, which suggests their relation to vascular cells. These cells also produce matrix metalloproteinase 2 (MMP-2), as well as a collagenase and other enzymes that tend to degrade the hemostatic membrane and may very well facilitate migration of endothelial cells among the growing lesion and extravasation of red cells.

The lesions rarely cause severe morbidity and mortality but often do cause cosmetic and other less life-threatening burdens. As KS progresses, an increased number of life-threatening lesions may occur, particularly in the respiratory tract, mouth, and gastrointestinal tract.[145]

Other Hematovascular Findings of Hematologic Interest

For completeness, several disorders of interest that are germane to this topic and the differential diagnosis are presented here.

Livedo Reticularis

Livedo reticularis is commonly seen and, in the correct clinical setting, is indicative of APLS. Livedo reticularis has a dusky, ill-defined violaceous reticular pattern that is seen primarily on the legs and occasionally on the arms (Fig. 11-25). It vaguely resembles a pair of blue or purple fishnet stockings. It may be seen transiently in normal people, especially if they are in a cool environment. Anti-cardiolipin antibodies were found in roughly one half of

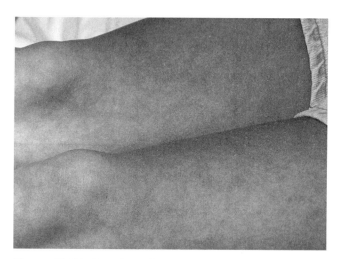

Figure 11-25 *(See also Color Plate 11-25.)* Livido reticularis. This young woman with antiphospholipid syndrome exhibits the lacy, evanescent-appearing, weblike pattern characteristic of this skin disorder. A more advanced (but less typical) case is shown as "Images in Clinical Medicine," N Engl J Med 356:284, 2007.

65 patients with livedo reticularis studied by Asherson and colleagues.[146] Livedo reticularis may also be seen in lupus without APLS and in other rheumatic disorders. Sneddon recognized the association of livedo reticularis with cerebrovascular accidents; this disorder was referred to as Sneddon syndrome although it now appears he was recording two manifestations of APLS.[147]

Histopathologic samples of livedo reticularis show a slight endotheliitis, usually without necrotizing features. Should necrotic lesions be encountered, the process may be called *livedoid vasculitis*. Following necrotization, small cutaneous porcelain-white ulcerations, called *atrophie blanche*, result.[148]

Livedo reticularis serves as one of the minor diagnostic criteria for APLS (see Chapter 19). Therapy other than the treatment of underlying disease is not indicated. Other dermal manifestations of APLS have been recently reviewed by Gibson and colleagues.[149]

Urticarial Vasculitis

Whereas typical urticaria is commonplace and self limited, a subtype has been called *urticarial vasculitis*. These edematous lesions look like typical urticaria, except that their appearance includes a considerable vasculitic component. On biopsy, some degree of neutrophilic perivascular infiltrate is usually apparent. Clinically, this type of urticaria differs from common urticaria in that it usually lasts longer than 24 hours, is actually painful, and is sometimes described as burning; also, sometimes, when the lesions clear, a slight amount of residual purpura is seen. It is associated with hypocomplementemia. Some patients also have arthritis and abdominal pain.[150]

Purpuric Contact Dermatitis

Contact dermatitis is a common skin disorder known to all practitioners. It is a small subtype of dermatitis, and lesions, particularly those that appear to be elicited by contact with various textile dyes in clothing, are purpuric. Extravasated red cells are seen on biopsy, but no vasculitis is apparent.[151]

Acute Hemorrhagic Edema of Infants

Dermatologists have described this as the alarmingly sudden onset of hemorrhagic edema in children that involves particularly the face. Onset is very rapid, but fortunately, the condition proves to be benign and usually goes away in about a week. On biopsy, intense leukocytoclastic vasculitis is seen. This appears to be different from Henoch-Schönlein purpura, in that the disease is more benign and sudden in its coming and going.[152–154]

Hemangiomas

These soft bluish tumors are common in infancy and usually spontaneously regress.[38] Persistent huge cavernous hemangiomas have a worse prognosis and may require aggressive treatment. The Kasabach-Merritt syndrome is thrombocytopenic hemorrhage that results from DIC or hyperfibrinolysis, or both when it occurs in patients with a subtype of giant hemangioma that was recently renamed kaposiform hemangioendothelioma (KHE).[40–42] The hemostatic defect is believed to result from activation of the coagulation and fibrinolytic systems through stagnation of blood creeping through the maze of entangled vessels in these large lesions.

Cherry Angiomas

These appear as cherry red, small, 1- to 3-mm domed papules over the upper abdomen and lower chest that occur in the second half of life. They consist of proliferated capillaries with vessels that are not as large as those in HHT syndrome; cherry angiomas do not blanch nearly as easily or completely as the telangiectases of HHT syndrome. At one time, they were also known as de Morgan spots and were believed to herald internal malignancy, but this is no longer held as true.

Spiders

These vascular lesions are noted by their 1- to 3-cm "legs" that radiate out from a 1- to 2-mm central body. The body of the spider angioma is a dermal arteriole with anastomoses to the legs. Gentle pressure on the head causes collapse of the spider and disappearance of the legs. Spiders are seen in aging, cirrhosis, and pregnancy and require no specific therapy. Vascular spiders are occasionally of cosmetic concern.

Erythema

A simple increased supply of blood to the skin dilates normal dermal vessels with resultant reddening of the skin, especially the skin of the face. Erythema has no clear-cut borders but blanches with pressure or application of cold to decrease cutaneous blood flow. Erythema may result from a hot environment, hyperthermia, fever, mild viral infection ("slapped cheeks" of fifth disease), or emotional phenomena.

CONSULTATION CONSIDERATIONS

In hospitalized patients with purpura, high probabilities exist for CV, DIC, amyloidosis, and livedo reticularis, as well as for the above-mentioned classic hemostatic diatheses. Essentially all patients in the category of purpura due to microthrombi will be hospitalized because of their underlying illness. In healthy ambulatory patients, the most commonly encountered processes are senile purpura, purpura simplex, PPPs, OWR syndrome, CV, and factitious purpura.

Clues exist in the distribution of purpura. Postictal petechiae, petechiae secondary to fat embolization, telangiectases of OWR syndrome, and the purpura associated with amyloidosis occur about the head and face. Mouth bleeding from boggy gums should signal the possibility of scurvy. Body and trunk ecchymoses and purpura are seen with hemophilia, factor VIII inhibitors, concomitant anticoagulant use, amyloidosis, and even purpura simplex, especially when the patient's activities involve leaning over and bearing weight on the lower rib cage.

Dependent purpura is seen in acute and chronic ITP, PPPs, CV, and scurvy. Livedo reticularis is seen most commonly on the legs. Painful acral purpuric lesions are indicative of ischemia from emboli such as those seen in subacute bacterial endocarditis, cholesterol embolization, or cardioembolization from atrial myxoma or nonbacterial thrombotic emboli (marantic endocarditis).[155] The nearly mirror image, symmetrical involvement of the legs and trunk in the palpable purpura of CV is noteworthy. A high degree of asymmetry should increase the index of suspicion for a factitious process.

Acute-onset purpura generally has a worse prognosis than chronic purpura, and haste must be used to evaluate for and rule out infectious causes, DIC, cholesterol embolism, and other catastrophic processes such as TTP and DIC in the microthrombotic category. Long-standing purpuric lesions may well be HHT, PPPs, purpura simplex, purpura secondary to heritable connective tissue disorders, or chronic ITP. Hemosiderin deposits in the dependent portions of the legs connote chronicity due to accumulation of heme iron retained in the cutaneous macrophages. Both senile (atrophic or actinic) purpura and purpura secondary to hypercortisolism are essentially limited to the extensor surfaces of the forearms, a pattern that essentially is diagnostic for either of these disorders.

LABORATORY EVALUATION

The hematologist will nearly always order a CBC with a platelet count and differential white cell count, as well as a prothrombin time and a partial thromboplastin time for screening purposes. Such practice is both understandable and defensible. Otherwise, the laboratory should be used primarily to rule out or rule in other specific disorders in a manner not unlike those listed in Table 11-3, which are used to specifically evaluate for secondary causes of CV.

The bleeding time or platelet function assay (PFA) is normal, except in qualitative and quantitative platelet disorders. Normal bleeding time is consistent with the fact that other purpuric disorders do not primarily interfere with platelet–endothelial interaction, as is tested by bleeding time.

Skin biopsy is frequently helpful and is usually ordered in collaboration with a dermatologist. It is particularly useful in establishing CV, PPPs, amyloidosis, KS, and senile purpura if these diagnostic considerations are not otherwise straightforward, thus justifying further testing.

COST CONTAINMENT

The modest laboratory evaluation just described will considerably curtail costs. A reasonable knowledge base of purpura and a good history and physical examination are typically all that are needed to establish the diagnosis in most patients with purpura. This approach leads to the accurate diagnosis of mechanical purpura, factitious purpura, purpura simplex, PPPs, many causes of CV, RMSF, scurvy, hypercortisolism, senile purpura, heritable disorders of connective tissue, OWR syndrome, DIC, warfarin skin necrosis, fat embolism syndrome, cholesterol emboli, and associated nonpurpuric hematovascular disorders such as livedo reticularis, angiomas, and spiders.

TREATMENT ISSUES

Clearly, treatment begins with a correct diagnosis. No hematologic treatment is necessary for many patients (e.g., purpura simplex, PPPs, primary CV), but hematologic treatment is indicated for others (e.g., ITP, TTP, DIC, HHT). Nonhematologic treatment is indicated for a third group (e.g., psychiatric evaluation in factitious purpura; rheumatologic evaluation in many cases of secondary CV; antibiotics for RMSF, subacute bacterial endocarditis, or meningococcemia; dietary management for scurvy). This review does not cover all treatment aspects for all causes of purpura.

With the obvious exceptions of patients with a qualitative or quantitative platelet defect, hemophilia, or an acquired coagulation factor inhibitor, and those on anticoagulants, purpuric patients do not harbor a systemic hemorrhagic diathesis. Accordingly, those patients with HHT, senile purpura, purpura simplex, PPPs, CV, scurvy, heritable disorders of connective tissue, and KS may undergo invasive and operative procedures without fear of hemostatic failure. Patients with amyloidosis fall between these two groups and may require special consideration before undergoing an elective invasive procedure.

MEDICAL-LEGAL CONSIDERATIONS

In patients with bruising and hematoma, consideration must always be given to the possibility of trauma due to abuse. Although abused patients may present with bruising as their sole problem, nonabused patients may be falsely accused of having been abused simply because of the presence of purpuric lesions. Parents who do not know that a child has von Willebrand disease or mild hemophilia may be accused of abuse.

REFERENCES

1. Lackner H, Karpatkin S: On the "easy bruising" syndrome with normal platelet count. Ann Intern Med 83:190–196, 1975.
2. Myllyharju J, Kivirikko KI: Collagens and collagen-related diseases. Ann Med 33:4–6, 2001.
3. Mao JR, Bristow J: The Ehlers-Danlos syndrome: On beyond collagens. J Clin Invest 107:1063–1069, 2001.
4. de Paepe A: The Ehlers-Danlos syndrome: A heritable collagen disorder as cause of bleeding. Thromb Haemost 75:379–386, 1996.

5. Solomon JA, Abrams L, Lichtenstein GR: GI manifestations of Ehlers-Danlos syndrome. Am J Gastroenterol 91:2282–2288, 1996.

6. Nuss R, Manco-Johnson M: Hemostasis in Ehlers-Danlos syndrome: Patient report and literature review. Clin Pediatr 34:552–555, 1995.

7. Anstey A, Mayne K, Winter M, et al: Platelet and coagulation studies in Ehlers-Danlos syndrome. Br J Dermatol 125:155–163, 1991.

8. Germain DP: Clinical and genetic features of vascular Ehlers-Danlos syndrome. Ann Vasc Surg 16:391–397, 2002.

9. Dowton SB, Pincott S, Demmer L: Respiratory complications of Ehlers-Danlos syndrome type IV. Clin Genet 50:510–514, 1996.

10. Freeman RK, Swegle J, Sise MJ: The surgical complications of Ehlers-Danlos syndrome. Am Surg 62:869–873, 1996.

11. Maltz SB, Fantus RJ, Mellett MM, et al: Surgical complications of Ehlers-Danlos syndrome type IV: Case report and review of the literature. J Trauma 51:387–390, 2001.

12. Byers PH: Osteogenesis imperfecta: Perspectives and opportunities. Curr Opin Pediatr 12:603–609, 2000.

13. Cole WG: Advances in osteogenesis imperfecta. Clin Orthop 401:6–16, 2002.

14. Ohtani T, Furukawa F: Pseudoxanthoma elasticum. J Dermatol 29:615–620, 2002.

15. Ringpfeil F, Pulkkinen L, Uitto J: Molecular genetics of pseudoxanthoma elasticum. Exp Dermatol 10:221–228, 2001.

16. Aburawi EH, O'Sullivan J, Hasan A: Marfan's syndrome: A review. Hosp Med 62:153–157, 2001.

17. Hopkins RA: Aortic valve leaflet sparing and salvage surgery: Evolution of techniques for aortic root reconstruction. Eur J Cardiothorac Surg 24:886–897, 2003.

18. Skinner M, Falk RH: The systemic amyloidoses: An overview. Adv Intern Med 45:107–137, 2000.

19. Merlini G, Bellotti V: Molecular mechanisms of amyloidosis. N Engl J Med 349:583–596, 2003.

20. Mumford AD, O'Donnell J, Gillmore JD, et al: Bleeding symptoms and coagulation abnormalities in 337 patients with AL-amyloidosis. Br J Haematol 110:454–460, 2000.

21. Oran B, Wright DG, Seldin DC, et al: Spontaneous rupture of the spleen in AL amyloidosis. Am J Hematol 74:131–135, 2003.

22. Rensink AAM, deWaal RM, Kremer B, et al: Pathogenesis of cerebral amyloid angiopathy. Brain Res Rev 43:207–223, 2003.

23. Revesz T, Ghiso J, Lashley T, et al: Cerebral amyloid angiopathies: A pathologic, biochemical and genetic view. J Neuropathol Exp Neurol 62:885–898, 2003.

24. Fewel ME, Thompson BG Jr, Hoff JT: Spontaneous intracerebral hemorrhage: A review. Neurosurg Focus 15:e1, 2003.

25. Rosano J, Hyler EM, O'Donnell HC, et al: Warfarin-associated hemorrhage and cerebral amyloid angiopathy: A genetic and pathologic study. Neurology 55:947–951, 2000.

26. Long R, Guzman R, Greenberg H, et al: Tuberculous mycotic aneurysm of the aorta: Review of published medical and surgical experience. Chest 115:522–531, 1999.

27. Cina CS, Arena GO, Fiture AO, et al: Ruptured mycotic thoracoabdominal aortic aneurysms: A report of three cases and a systematic review. J Vasc Surg 33:861–867, 2001.

28. Chukwudelunzu F, Brown RD Jr, Wijdicks EF, et al: Subarachnoid haemorrhage associated with endocarditis: Case report and literature review. Eur J Neurol 9:423–427, 2002.

29. Chetty R, Batitang S, Nair R: Large artery vasculopathy in HIV-positive patients: Another vasculitic enigma. Hum Pathol 31:374–379, 2000.

30. Cakir O, Eren N, Ulku R, et al: Bilateral subclavian arterial aneurysm and ruptured aorta pseudoaneurysm in Behçet's disease. Ann Vasc Surg 16:516–520, 2002.

31. Neunninghoff DM, Hunder GG, Christianson JH, et al: Incidence and predictors of large-artery complications (aortic aneurysm, aortic dissection, and/or large-artery stenosis) in patients with giant cell arteritis: A population-based study over 50 years. Arthritis Rheum 48:3522–3531, 2003.

32. Ohara N, Miyata T, Kurata A, et al: Ten years' experience of aortic aneurysm associated with systemic lupus erythematosus. Eur J Vasc Endovasc Surg 19:288–293, 2000.

33. Turesson C, O'Fallon WM, Crowson CS, et al: Extra-articular disease manifestations in rheumatoid arthritis: Incidence, trends and risk factors over 46 years. Ann Rheum Dis 62:722–727, 2003.

34. Burns JC, Kushner HI, Bastian JF, et al: Kawasaki disease: A brief history. Pediatrics 106:E27, 2000.

35. Timar J, Dome B, Fazekas K, et al: Angiogenesis-dependent diseases and angiogenesis therapy. Pathol Oncol Res 7:85–94, 2001.

36. Bell CD: Endothelial cell tumors. Microsc Res Tech 60:165–170, 2003.

37. Cirulli A, Liso A, D'Ovidio F, et al: Vascular endothelial growth factor serum levels are elevated in patients with hereditary hemorrhagic telangiectasia. Acta Haematol 110:29–32, 2003.

38. Drolet BA, Esterly NB, Frieden IJ: Hemangiomas in children. N Engl J Med 341:173–181, 1999.

39. Enjolras O, Mulliken JB: Vascular tumors and vascular malformations (new issues). Adv Dermatol 13:375–423, 1997.

40. Tsung WYW, Chan JKC: Kaposi-like infantile hemangioendothelioma: A distinctive vacular neoplasm of the retroperitoneum. Am J Surg Pathol 15:982–989, 1991.

41. Mulliken JB, Anupindi S, Ezekowitz RAB, et al: Case records of the Massachusetts General Hospital: A newborn girl with a large cutaneous lesion, thrombocytopenia and anemia. N Engl J Med 350:1764–1775, 2004.

42. Hall GW: Kasabach-Merritt syndrome: Pathogenesis and management. Br J Haematol 112:851–862, 2001.

43. Kasabach HH, Merritt KK: Capillary hemangioma with extensive purpura: Report of a case. Am J Dis Child 59:1063–1070, 1940.

44. Marchuk DA, Srinivasan S, Squire TL, et al: Vascular morphogenesis: Tales of two syndromes. Hum Mol Genet 12:R97–R112, 2003.

45. van den Driesche S, Mummery CL, Westermann CJ: Hereditary hemorrhagic telangiectasia: An update on transforming growth factor beta signaling in vasculogenesis and angiogenesis. Cardiovasc Res 58:20–31, 2003.

46. Srinivasan S, Hanes MA, Dickens T, et al: A mouse model for hereditary hemorrhagic telangiectasia (HHT) type 2. Hum Mol Genet 12:473–482, 2003.

47. Karabegovic A, Shinawi M, Cymerman U, et al: No live individual homozygous for a novel endoglin mutation was found in a consanguineous Arab family with hereditary haemorrhagic telangiectasis. J Med Genet 41:e119, 2004.

48. Jacobson BS: Hereditary hemorrhagic telangiectasia: A model for blood vessel growth and enlargement. Am J Pathol 156:737–742, 2000.

49. Gammon RB, Miksa AK, Keller FS: Osler-Weber-Rendu disease and pulmonary arteriovenous fistulas. Chest 98:1522–1524, 1990.

50. Shovlin CL, Winstock AR, Peters AM, et al: Medical complications of pregnancy in hereditary hemorrhagic telangiectasia. Q J Med 88:879–887, 1995.

51. Gershon AS, Faughnan ME, Chon KS, et al: Transcatheter embolotherapy of maternal pulmonary arteriovenous malformations during pregnancy. Chest 119:470–477, 2001.

52. Shah RK, Dhingra JK, Shapshay SM: Hereditary hemorrhagic telangiectasia: A review of 76 cases. Laryngoscope 112:767–773, 2002.

53. Sabba C: A rare and misdiagnosed bleeding disorder: Hereditary hemorrhagic telangiectasia. J Thromb Haemost 3:2201–2210, 2005.

54. Shovlin CL, Guttmacher AE, Buscarini E, et al: Diagnostic criteria for hereditary hemorrhagic telangiectasia (Rendu-Osler-Weber syndrome). Am J Med Genet 91:66–67, 2000.

55. Begbie ME, Wallace GM, Shovlin CL: Hereditary haemorrhagic telangiectasia (Osler-Weber-Rendu syndrome): A view from the 21st century. Postgrad Med J 79:18–24, 2003.

56. Dong SL, Reynolds SF, Steiner IP: Brain abscess in patients with hereditary hemorrhagic telangiectasia: Case report and review of the literature. J Emerg Med 20:247–251, 2001.

57. Abdalla SA, Geisthoff UW, Bonneau D, et al: Visceral manifestations in hereditary haemorrhagic telangiectasia type 2. J Med Genet 40:494–502, 2003.

58. Caselitz M, Bahr MJ, Bleck JS, et al: Sonographic criteria for the diagnosis of hepatic involvement in hereditary hemorrhagic telangiectasia (HHT). Hepatology 37:1139–1146, 2003.

59. Larson AM: Liver disease in hereditary hemorrhagic telangiectasia. J Clin Gastroenterol 36:149–158, 2003.

60. Longacre AV, Gross CP, Gallitelli M, et al: Diagnosis and management of gastrointestinal bleeding in patients with hereditary hemorrhagic telangiectasia. Am J Gastroenterol 98:59–65, 2003.

61. Ali A, Santisi JM, Vargo J: Video capsule endoscopy: A voyage beyond the end of the scope. Cleve Clin J Med 71:415–425, 2004.

62. Easey AJ, Wallace GM, Hughes JM, et al: Should asymptomatic patients with hereditary haemorrhagic telangiectasia (HHT) be screened for cerebral vascular malformations? Data from 22,061 years of HHT patient life. J Neurol Neurosurg Psychiatry 74:743–748, 2003.

63. Rodesch G, Hurth M, Alvarez H, et al: Spinal cord intradural arteriovenous fistulae: Anatomic, clinical, and therapeutic considerations in a series of 32 consecutive patients seen between 1981 and 2000 with emphasis on endovascular therapy. Neurosurgery 57:973–983, 2004.

64. Mandzia J, Henderson K, Faughnan M, et al: Compelling reasons to screen brain in HHT. Stroke 32:2957–2958, 2001.

65. Maher CO, Piepgras DG, Brown RD Jr, et al: Cerebrovascular manifestations in 321 cases of hereditary hemorrhagic telangiectasia. Stroke 32:877–882, 2001.

66. Sabba C, Pasculli G, Cirulli A, et al: Rendu-Osler-Weber disease: Experience with 56 patients. Ann Ital Med Int 17:173–179, 2002.

67. Silverstein SB, Rodgers GM: Parental iron therapy options. Am J Hematol 76:74–78, 2004.

68. Jones HW, Tocantins LM: The history of purpura hemorrhagica. Ann Med Hist 5:349–359, 1933.

69. Bullet AJ: How Lind, as much as Nelson, broke the power of Napoleon. Resident Staff Physician 39:85–88, 1993.

70. Werlhof PG, Wichmann JE: Opera Medica: Hamnoverae, imp fractorem, 1775–1776, p 748.

71. Willan R: On cutaneous diseases. (London, Johnson, 1808, as referenced by Jones and Tocantins, ref 92.) Ann Med Hist 5:349, 1933.

72. Flint A: A Treatise in the Principles and Practice of Medicine, 6th ed. Philadelphia, Lea Brothers, 1886, pp 1130–1134.

73. Osler W: The Principles and Practice of Medicine, 2nd ed. New York, Appleton, 1896, pp 343–350.

74. Osler W: On a family form of recurring epistaxis, associated with multiple telangiectases of skin and mucous membranes. Bull Johns Hopkins Hosp 12:333–337, 1901.

75. Wolbach SB: Studies on Rocky Mountain spotted fever. J Med Res 41:1–197, 1919.

76. Wintrobe MM: Clinical Hematology, 1st ed. Philadelphia, Lea & Febiger, 1942, p 154.

77. Haden RL, Schneider RH, Underwood LC: Abnormal hemorrhage with normal platelet count and normal clotting. Ann NY Acad Sci 49:641–646, 1948.

78. Spaet TH: Vascular factors in the pathogenesis of hemorrhagic syndromes. Blood 7:641–652, 1952.

79. Ackroyd JF: Allergic purpura, including purpura due to foods, drugs, and infections. Am J Med 14:605–632, 1953.

80. Majno G: Ultrastructure of the vascular membrane. In Hamilton WF (ed): Handbook of Physiology, sec 2, vol III: Washington, DC, Am Physiol Soc, 1965, p 2293.

81. Elliott RHE: The suction test for capillary resistance in thrombocytopenic purpura. JAMA 110:1177–1179, 1938.

82. Urkin J, Katz M: Suction purpura. Isr Med Assoc J 2:711, 2000.

83. Friberg TR, Weinreb RN: Ocular manifestations of gravity inversion. JAMA 253:1755–1757, 1985.

84. Rashkovsky I, Safadi R, Zlotogorski A: Black palmar macules: Palmar petechiae ("black palm"). Arch Dermatol 134:1020, 1023–1024, 1998.

85. Ely SF, Hirsch CS: Asphyxial deaths and petechiae: A review. J Forensic Sci 45:1274–1277, 2000.

86. Maxeiner H: Congestion bleedings of the face and cardiopulmonary resuscitation: An attempt to evaluate their relationship. Forensic Sci Int 117:191–198, 2001.

87. Grunfeld J, Klein C: Seizure-induced purpura: A rare but useful clue. Isr Med Assoc J 3:779, 2001.

88. Mader C: Barotrauma in diving. Wien Med Wochenschr 151:126–130, 1999.

89. Karger B, Suggeler O, Brinkmann B: Electrocution: Autopsy study with emphasis on "electrical petechiae." Forensic Sci Int 23:126, 210–213, 2002.

90. Downes AJ, Crossland DS, Mellon AF: Prevalence and distribution of petechiae in well babies. Arch Dis Child 86:291–292, 2002.

91. Ratnoff OD: Psychogenic bleeding. In Ratnoff OD and Forbes CD (eds): Disorders of Hemostasis, 3rd ed. Philadelphia, WB Saunders, 1996.

92. Uthman IW, Moukarbel GV, Salman SM, et al: Autoerythrocyte sensitization (Gardner-Diamond) syndrome. Eur J Haematol 65:144–147, 2000.

93. Yucel B, Kiziltan E, Aktan M: Dissociative identity disorder presenting with psychogenic purpura. Psychosomatics 41:279–281, 2000.

94. Gardner FH, Diamond LK: Autoerythrocyte sensitization: A form of purpura producing painful bruising following autosensitization to red blood cells in certain women. Blood 10:675–690, 1955.

95. Lackner H, Karpatkin S: On the "easy bruising" syndrome with normal platelet count. Ann Intern Med 83:190–196, 1975.

96. Carpenter RF: The prevalence and distribution of bruising in babies. Arch Dis Child 80:363–366, 1999.

97. Kim HJ, Skidmore RA, Woosley JT: Pigmented purpura over the lower extremities: Purpura annularis telangiectodes of Majocchi. Arch Dermatol 134:1477, 1480, 1998.

98. Kitchens CS: Amelioration of endothelial abnormalities by prednisone in experimental thrombocytopenia in the rabbit. J Clin Invest 60:1129–1134, 1977.

99. Kitchens CS, Pendergast JF: Human thrombocytopenia is associated with structural abnormalities of the endothelium which are ameliorated by glucocorticosteroid administration. Blood 67:203–206, 1986.

100. Tsuda T, Okamoto Y, Sakaguchi R, et al: Purpura due to aspirin-induced platelet dysfunction aggravated by drinking alcohol. J Int Med Res 29:374–380, 2001.

101. Kraft DM, McKee D, Scott C: Henoch-Schönlein purpura: A review. Am Fam Physician 58:405–411, 1998.

102. Dammacco F, Sansonno D, Piccoli C, et al: The cryoglobulins: An overview. Eur J Clin Invest 31:628–638, 2001.

103. Morra E: Cryoglobulinemia. Washington, DC, American Society of Hematology Education Program, 2005, pp 368–372.

104. Della Rossa A, Tavoni A, Baldini C, Bombardieri S: Mixed cryoglobulinemia and hepatitis C virus association: Ten years later. Isr Med Assoc J 3:430–434, 2001.

105. Sable-Fourtassou R, Cohyen P, Mahr A, et al: Antineutrophil cytoplasmic antibodies and the Churg-Strauss syndrome. Ann Intern Med 143:632–638, 2004.

106. Crowson AN, Mihm MC Jr, Magro CM: Cutaneous vasculitis: A review. J Cutan Pathol 30:161–173, 2003.

107. Shirahama M, Umeno Y, Tomimasu R, et al: The value of colour Doppler ultrasonography for small bowel involvement of adult Henoch-Schönlein purpura. Br J Radiol 71:788–791, 1998.

108. Blanco R, Martinez-Taboada VM, Rodriguez-Valverde V, et al: Cutaneous vasculitis in children and adults: Associated diseases and etiologic factors in 303 patients. Medicine 77:403–418, 1998.

109. Piette WW: What is Schönlein-Henoch purpura, and why should we care? Arch Dermatol 133:515–518, 1997.

110. Martinez-Taboada VM, Blanco R, Garcia-Fuentes M, et al: Clinical features and outcome of 95 patients with hypersensitivity vasculitis. Am J Med 102:186–191, 1997.

111. Blanco R, Martinez-Taboada VM, Rodriguez-Valverde V, et al: Henoch-Schönlein purpura in adulthood and childhood: Two different expressions of the same syndrome. Arthritis Rheum 40: 859–864, 1997.

112. Malaviya AN, Kaushik P, Budhiraja S, et al: Hypergammaglobulinemic purpura of Waldenstrom: Report of 3 cases with a short review. Clin Exp Rheumatol 18:518–522, 2000.

113. Kelly RI, Opie J, Nixon R: Golfer's vasculitis. Australasian J Dermatol 46:11–14, 2005.

114. Ramelet AA: Exercise-induced purpura. Dermatology 208:293–296, 2004.

115. Halasz CLG, Cormier D, Den M: Petechial glove and sock syndrome caused by parvovirus B19. J Am Acad Dermatol 27:835–838, 1992.

116. Veraldi S, Rizzitelli G, Scarabelli G, et al: Papular-purpuric "gloves and socks" syndrome. Arch Dermatol 132:975–977, 1996.

117. Grilli R, Izquierdu MJ, Farina MC, et al: Papular-purpuric "gloves and socks" syndrome: Polymerase chain reaction demonstration of parvovirus B19 DNA in cutaneous lesions and sera. J Am Acad Dermatol 41:793–796, 1999.

117a. Bausch DG, Nichol ST, Muyembe-Tamfum JJ, et al: Marburg hemorrhagic fever associated with multiple genetic lineages of virus. N Engl J Med 355:909–919, 2006.

118. Schnittler H-J, Feldmann H: Viral hemorrhagic fever: A vascular disease? Thromb Haemost 89:967–972, 2003.

119. Ndayimirije N, Kindhauser MK: Marburg hemorrhagic fever in Angola: Fighting fear and a lethal pathogen. N Engl J Med 352: 2155–2157, 2005.

120. Connolly BM, Steele KE, Davis KJ, et al: Pathogenesis of experimental Ebola virus infection in guinea pigs. J Infect Dis 179 (suppl 1): S203–S217, 1999.

121. Borio L, Inglesby T, Peters W, et al: Hemorrhagic fever viruses as biological weapons: Medical and public health management. JAMA 287:2391–2405, 2002.

122. Weinstein M, Babyn P, Zlotkin S: An orange a day keeps the doctor away: Scurvy in the year 2000. Pediatrics 108:e55, 2001.

123. Levin NA, Greer KE: Scurvy in an unrepentant carnivore. Cutis 66:39–44, 2000.

124. Giraldi FP, Moro M, Cavagnini F: Gender-related differences in the presentation and course of Cushing's disease. J Clin Endocrinol Metab 88:1554–1558, 2003.

125. Gertz MA, Lacy MQ, Dispenzieri A: Amyloidosis. Hematol Oncol Clin North Am 13:1211–1233, 1999.

126. Mumford AD, O'Donell J, Gillmore JD, et al: Bleeding symptoms and coagulation abnormalities in 337 patients with AL-amyloidosis. Br J Haematol 110:454–460, 2000.

127. Boggio L, Gren D: Recombinant human factor VIIa in the management of amyloid-associated factor X deficiency. Br J Haematol 112:1074–1075, 2001.

128. Emori Y, Sakugawa M, Niiya K, et al: Life-threatening bleeding and acquired factor V deficiency associated with primary systemic amyloidosis. Blood Coagul Fibrinolysis 13:555–559, 2002.

129. Faust SN, Heyderman RS, Levin M: Disseminated intravascular coagulation and purpura fulminans secondary to infection. Bailliere's Clin Haematol 13:179–197, 2000.

130. Gamper G, Oschatz E, Herkner H, et al: Sepsis-associated purpura fulminans in adults. Wien Klin Wochenschr 113:107–112, 2001.

131. Gürgey A, Aytac S, Kanra G, et al: Outcome in children with purpura fulminans: Report on 16 patients. Am J Hematol 80:20–25, 2005.

132. McKnight JT, Maxwell AJ, Anderson RL: Warfarin necrosis. Arch Fam Med 1:105–108, 1992.

133. Sallah S, Thomas DP, Roberts HR: Warfarin and heparin-induced skin necrosis and the purple toe syndrome: Infrequent complications of anticoagulant treatment. Thromb Haemost 78:785–790, 1997.

134. Muller C, Rahn BA, Pfister U, et al: The incidence, pathogenesis, diagnosis and treatment of fat embolism. Orthopaedic Rev 23:107–117, 1994.

135. Pell ACH, Hughes D, Keating J, et al: Fulminating fat embolism syndrome caused by paradoxical embolism through a patent foramen ovale. N Engl J Med 329:926–929, 1993.

136. Fabian TC: Unraveling the fat embolism syndrome. N Engl J Med 329:961–963, 1993.

137. Mellor A, Soni N: Fat embolism. Anaesthesia 56:145–154, 2001.

138. McKee LC Jr., Collins RD: Intravascular leukocyte thrombi and aggregates as a cause of morbidity and mortality in leukemia. Medicine 53:463–478, 1974.

139. Donohue KG, Saap L, Falanga V: Cholesterol crystal embolization: An atherosclerotic disease with frequent and varied cutaneous manifestations. J Eur Acad Dermatol Venereol 17:504–511, 2003.

140. Bashore TM, Gehrig T: Cholesterol emboli after invasive cardiac procedures. J Am Coll Cardiol 42:217–218, 2003.

141. O'Leary KJ, Horn K: Blue-tinged toes. Am J Med 118:1105–1107, 2005.

142. Antman K, Chang Y: Kaposi's sarcoma. N Engl J Med 342:1027–1038, 2000.

143. Samet JH, Muz P, Cabral P, et al: Dermatologic manifestations in HIV-infected patients: A primary care perspective. Mayo Clin Proc 74:658–660, 1999.

144. Kroll MH, Shandera WX: AIDS-associated Kaposi's sarcoma. Hosp Pract April: 85–102, 1998.

145. Dezube BJ: Clinical presentation and natural history of AIDS-related Kaposi's sarcoma. Hematol Oncol Clin North Am 10:1023–1029, 1996.

146. Asherson RA, Mayou SC, Merry P, et al: The spectrum of livedo reticularis and anticardiolipin antibodies. Br J Dermatol 120:215–221, 1989.

147. Sneddon JB: Cerebrovascular lesions and livedo reticularis. Br J Dermatol 77:180–185, 1965.

148. Maessen-Visch MG, Koedam MI, Hamulyak K, et al: Atrophie blanche. Int J Dermatol 38:161–172, 1999.

149. Gibson GE, Su WPD, Pittelkow MR: Antiphospholipid syndrome and the skin. J Am Acad Dermatol 36:971–982, 1997.

150. Mehregan DR, Hall MG, Gibson LE: Urticarial vasculitis: A histopathologic and clinical review of 72 cases. J Am Acad Dermatol 26:441–448, 1992.

151. Lazarov A, Cordoba M: Purpuric contact dermatitis in patients with allergic reaction to textile dyes and resins. J Eur Acad Dermatol Venereol 14:101–105, 2000.

152. Garty BZ, Ofer I, Finkelstein Y: Acute hemorrhagic edema of infancy. Isr Med Assoc J 4:228–229, 2002.

153. Poyrazoglu HM, Per H, Gunduz Z, et al: Acute hemorrhagic edema of infancy. Pediatr Int 45:697–700, 2003.

154. da Silva Manzoni AP, Viecili JB, de Andrade CB, et al: Acute hemorrhagic edema of infancy: A case report. Int J Dermatol 4:48–51, 2004.

155. McAllister SM, Bornstein AM, Callen JP: Painful acral purpura. Arch Dermatol 134:789–791, 1998.

Chapter 12

Disseminated Intravascular Coagulation

Carrie LaBelle, MD • Craig S. Kitchens, MD

An enormous amount has been written about disseminated intravascular coagulation (DIC). During the 1970s and 1980s, it was rather fashionable to report on yet another "cause" of DIC. Over the past three decades, however, it has become increasingly clear that DIC, rather than being a specific disease, really represents a pathophysiologic final common pathway of the coagulation system gone awry. That single understanding brings into focus that DIC is an "intermediary mechanism of disease"[1] and collapses the nearly infinite list of causes into an understandable and functional process. Less time is now spent on indexing new and unique causes of DIC, with the thrust toward recognizing the underlying and initiating process of DIC and directing therapy toward that cause. The central role of tissue factor and various cytokines in the initiation and continuation of coagulation up to and including DIC has been elucidated and will be the focus of Chapter 13.

Even the terminology has been controversial. DIC has been called *defibrination syndrome, acquired afibrinogenemia, consumptive coagulopathy,* and *consumptive thrombohemorrhagic disorder.* Although each term certainly has its advocates and rationale for use, the term *disseminated intravascular coagulation,* and "DIC" in particular, seems to be rooted in our medical vocabulary, and so DIC will be used in this chapter. Additionally, microvascular thrombosis appears to be a major pathologic mechanism, resulting in multiorgan dysfunction syndrome (MODS). MODS is the chief cause of death among patients experiencing processes that initiate DIC. Hence, an association between DIC and MODS has been identified.

HISTORICAL OVERVIEW

The end result of DIC has been long known. The "Black Death" refers to the intense peripheral gangrene and bleeding resulting from thrombosis and defibrination of the plague that scourged the earth over the second millennium. That fatal bleeding could occur with various obstetric emergencies has been known also for centuries.[2] In 1834, de Blainville[3] was able to induce fatal massive intravascular thrombosis in animals through the rapid infusion of brain tissue. Nauyn,[4] 40 years later, observed similar manifestations when animals were infused with hemolyzed red cells. In 1884, Foa and Pellacani[5] elaborated on de Blainville's experiment by showing that extracts of several organs when infused could cause both thrombosis and hemorrhage. In further studying de Blainville's model, Wooldridge[6] in 1893 infused brain tissue slowly rather than rapidly, as did de Blainville, and showed that the animals did not die of massive intravascular thrombosis but rather, their blood became unclottable and, further, that after this state had been achieved, rapid infusions of more brain tissue did not cause any outward harm to the animal. It was Mills[7] in 1921 who observed that the latter findings were in fact due to selective defibrination that occurred with slow infusion of brain tissue and that the secondary rapid infusion failed to cause thrombosis because the animal had been defibrinated. In 1957, Krevans and colleagues[8] studied defibrination after hemolytic transfusion reactions in humans and made seminal observations regarding what we would now call DIC. At about that same time, Schneider[9] infused placental tissue into rabbits and was able to induce hemorrhage in these animals, thus offering a peek into the mechanism of DIC characteristic of obstetric catastrophes. In the late 1960s, Merskey's[10] laboratory developed a test to detect serum fibrin degradation products (FDPs) and thus opened the door to laboratory investigation of DIC. Additional studies into the fate of fibrinogen and the mechanism of FDP production in DIC were conducted by Marder's group.[11] Corrigan and colleagues[12] made rapid advances in the elucidation of DIC associated with septicemia, focusing on meningococcemia. McKay[1] catalogued the knowledge base regarding DIC in 1965, making it a distinct clinical entity. In 1968, microangiopathic hemolysis to include that seen in DIC was described.[13] The rapid growth in experience and knowledge was again thoroughly reviewed by Colman in 1972.[14] The notion of a pristine laboratory approach to diagnosing DIC was dismantled when Merskey[15] pointed out that not everything that appears to be DIC by laboratory criteria may be DIC, whereas sometimes true DIC may not "fit" if the primary criteria are laboratory findings rather than the underlying illness and the overall clinical picture. Mant and King[16] appropriately argued that DIC may be severe and acute, and Sack and colleagues[17] clearly and accurately described chronic DIC associated with neoplasia. Causes of DIC are heterogeneous and signs and symptoms are varying.[18]

During the next 30 years and up to the present, innumerable papers have been written on the initiation and control of normal hemostasis and the pathologic end result, DIC. These discoveries are discussed in greater detail in the following pages.

PHYSIOLOGY AND PATHOPHYSIOLOGY

Coagulation is initiated by interruption of the endothelial lining of the vascular system or by entry of tissue factor (TF) into the blood. With the former mechanism, the intrinsic clotting system may be activated by interaction of blood with subendothelial tissue and collagen; with the latter, TF, which is within all or most cells with the exception of unperturbed endothelial and peripheral blood cells and is released with cellular disruption,[19] causes activation of the tissue factor (extrinsic) clotting system. It appears that the extrinsic TF-driven system is the predominant force in hemostasis. Provided that the impetus is durable or protracted enough to sustain a procoagulant force, thrombin will be generated. During this cascade of activation, each step must pass through physiologic hurdles, be they potential inactivation of activated serine proteases (factors XIa, Xa, IXa, VIIa, and IIa) by antithrombin III (ATIII) or degradation of activated cofactors (factors Va and VIIIa) by the protein C system. Should thrombin be eventually generated, it must continue to evade ATIII as well as endothelial-bound thrombomodulin (TM) to finally convert fibrinogen to fibrin. All of this is quite physiologic following a surgical incision or other event for which hemostasis is regarded as desirable. When a breach in the circulatory system has been corrected, it is then appropriate for any remaining procoagulants, but especially thrombin, to be neutralized by these physiologic inhibitors. By virtue of the fact that a clot begets its own dissolution by incorporation of plasminogen, which is then activated by the fibrinolytic system, the clot remains in place for a while until it eventually is cleared by the action of plasmin. Any excess plasmin is neutralized by its inhibitor, α_2-plasmin inhibitor (α_2-PI). This all physiologically happens continually. One could arguably claim that events that could lead to DIC occur every day, but DIC does not routinely happen because these are tightly regulated events.

What separates the pathophysiologic process of DIC from physiologic clotting is the combination of nonphysiologic, sustained, and excessive initiation of coagulation (obstetric catastrophes, sepsis, cancer, trauma) and the eventual inability to neutralize circulating activated products of coagulation because of deficiencies in the inhibitory system (congenital deficiencies, hepatic insufficiency, or impaired circulation), such that the initiating stimulus for coagulation is not neutralized. If the stimulus is massive, sustained, and/or not neutralized, the resultant procoagulant wave soon inundates physiologic inhibitors, resulting in free, circulating, unopposed thrombin and plasmin, the two key agents responsible for DIC. Table 12-1 lists the inhibitors that are overcome in the genesis of DIC. Each inhibitor system is in place to neutralize a key hemostatic force listed on the left, each of which is key in the initiation and sustainment of DIC. Any attempt by their individual inhibitors to hold these in check will be overwhelmed by the continued amassing of procoagulants. The pathologic consequence of overwhelming the inhibitors is listed to the right. In fact, the clinical and laboratory manifestations of DIC can be explained by pathologic circulation of thrombin and plasmin. Thrombin will result in the pathologic intravascular clotting of fibrinogen, especially in the microcirculation, and deposition of platelets in nonphysiologic areas and consumption of coagulation factors; plasmin degrades fibrinogen, fibrin, and multiple coagulation factors, thus generating FDPs and D-dimer characteristic of DIC (Fig. 12-1). Of interest in profound DIC is that circulating levels of plasminogen activator inhibitor-1 (PAI-1) paradoxically increase by virtue of being an acute phase reactant greatly intensified by cytokines.[20] This increase in PAI-1 efficiently downregulates the fibrinolytic system, which correlates with more massive thrombosis, MODS, and death.[21] During infusion of *Escherichia coli* endotoxin into normal human subjects, circulating levels of tissue plasminogen activator (tPA) initially increase and fibrinolysis is promoted; however, with continual infusion, levels of PAI-1 greatly increase, resulting in a total loss of tPA functional activity.[22] D-dimer is the specific FDP generated by plasmin lysis of two γ-chain fragments of fibrin that have been crosslinked by the action of activated factor XIII. Because factor XIII activation requires the presence of thrombin and the only initiator of fibrinolysis is plasmin, this D-dimer complex serves as a "footprint," proving

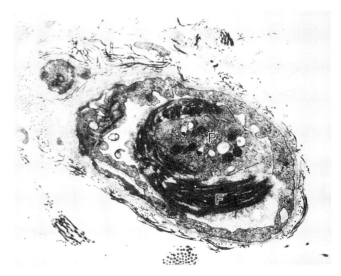

Figure 12-1 Electron micrograph of a capillary in experimental disseminated intravascular coagulation (DIC). The intact capillary contains a network of fibrin (F) and an occluded platelet (P) ($\times$13,000).

Table 12-1 Hemostatic Consequences of Loss of Inhibitors in Disseminated Intravascular Coagulation

Key Hemostatic Forces	Inhibitor	Consequence of Loss of Inhibitor
Tissue factor (TF)	Tissue factor pathway inhibitor (TFPI)	Enhanced thrombin generation
Activated factors V and VIII	Protein C and protein S	Enhanced thrombin generation
Activated coagulation factors, especially thrombin	Antithrombin III (ATIII)	Enhanced fibrin formation and platelet activation
Tissue plasminogen activator (tPA)	Plasminogen activator inhibitor, type 1 (PAI-1)	Enhanced fibrinolytic activation with decrease in PAI-1 and enhanced thrombosis with increase in PAI-1 (see text)
Plasmin	α_2-plasmin inhibitor (α_2-PI)	Unopposed fibrinolysis

the prior dual existence of thrombin and plasmin in the circulation.[23,24]

CAUSES OF DISSEMINATED INTRAVASCULAR COAGULATION

Whereas DIC was previously regarded as a specific disorder, it is now held that DIC, much as fever, hyponatremia, or abdominal pain, is a manifestation of a pathologic process. These are all abnormalities but are not recognized diseases. Rather, they are always due to some underlying cause. Accordingly, recognizing DIC in a patient implies that an underlying process is becoming such a burden on the patient's hemostatic system that the patient's situation is becoming increasingly unstable. DIC should be regarded as an indicator of a severe disease process or injury that is blatantly obvious (e.g., burns, trauma, cardiopulmonary collapse, carcinomatosis, sepsis), yet occasionally DIC serves as part of the original diagnosis, which may help to establish the presence of an underlying process. Common examples include recognition of DIC as distinguishing meningococcemia from viral headache and fever in a young healthy patient, establishing acute promyelocytic leukemia (APL) in a previously uncertain type of leukemia, and differentiating an obstetric catastrophe such as abruptio placentae or placenta previa from an otherwise mildly complicated labor and delivery. Table 12-2 lists several processes that may induce DIC.

INITIATION OF DISSEMINATED INTRAVASCULAR COAGULATION

Following is a brief outline of the physiologic activation of coagulation that may help to explain how continued and unchecked activation results in the clinical syndrome known as DIC.

Figure 12-2 is a crude attempt to illustrate key events in DIC. Any graphic attempting to exhaustively demonstrate all the on-going reactions, interactions, and counteractions would be functionally unfathomable; accordingly, this chart admittedly greatly simplifies the seminal points of DIC. For instance, the direct infusion of substances (snake venoms) that activate directly either prothrombin or factor X[25] is not portrayed by this simplification. The key role of the liver in holding in check DIC by the clearance of activated factors is also not satisfactorily addressed. The importance of the liver was revealed by the pioneering works of Deykin.[26] Key inhibitors of coagulation are represented by letters at proposed control points, although they too are greatly simplified. For example, Sandset and colleagues[27] showed that elimination of the TF pathway inhibitor (TFPI) from experimental animals proved that TFPI was an important governor of experimental DIC.

Nonetheless, Figure 12-2 does depict the general flow of events. Effects of vascular injuries that occur are not as neatly divided into activation of the extrinsic (TF-driven) clotting system or the intrinsic (contact system–driven) system as was previously held. Accordingly, in the box on the left, initiation by tissue damage, endothelial injury, and exposure of blood to bacterial products, necrotic cells, and subendothelial tissue is probably correctly depicted as activating both the intrinsic and extrinsic systems. However, the role of the intrinsic system appears to actually be less important than that of the TF-driven extrinsic system in initiating DIC.[28,29] Endotoxin and other bacterial products can activate the contact system.[30] Those systems result in the generation of thrombin, which is absolutely essential to normal or perturbed hemostasis. Thrombin then activates platelets, clots fibrinogen, and activates factors V, VIII, and XIII. All of these create a profound prothrombotic force. When their inhibitors as depicted by A (TFPI) and B (ATIII) are overwhelmed, thrombin generation becomes pathologic and DIC starts.

Circulating thrombin binds to TM. When thrombin binds to TM to make a thrombin:TM complex, thrombin metamorphoses from a powerful procoagulant to a powerful anticoagulant by virtue of it activating proteins C and S, which, in turn, enhance the fibrinolytic system by neutralizing PAI-1. The product of the fibrinolytic system is the conversion of plasminogen to circulating plasmin. Other enhancers of fibrinolysis include endotoxin, interleukin-1 (IL-1), IL-6, factor XIIa, and fibrin, as well as tumor necrosis factor (TNF), which releases endothelial tPA and u-PA (urokinase-type plasminogen activator). Just as important as the keystone role of thrombin in DIC is the role of plasmin, as it causes degradation not only of fibrin but also of fibrinogen and factors V, VIII, and XIII. Degradation of fibrinogen and fibrin results in the characteristic "footprints" of circulating FDPs and D-dimer. Attempting to check plasminogen activation is PAI-1, whose concentration is greatly increased in the inflammatory reaction. If levels of PAI-1 greatly increase, the fibrinolytic system totally shuts down, potentiating catastrophic thrombosis. The inhibitor of plasmin, α_2-PI, also attempts to keep plasmin activity under control but is overwhelmed in DIC.

DIC may be characterized along three different axes, representing tempo, extent, and clinical manifestation

Table 12-2 Processes that May Induce Disseminated Intravascular Coagulation

Tissue Damage
Trauma
Crush injuries
Central nervous system
  injuries
Heatstroke
Burns
Hemolytic transfusion reaction
Acute transplant rejection

Neoplasia
Cancers
Leukemias
Cancer chemotherapy
Tumor lysis syndrome

Miscellaneous
Shock
Cardiac arrest
Near drowning, especially in
  fresh water
Fat embolism
Aortic aneurysm
Giant hemangiomas
Bites by certain snakes

Infection
Gram-positive bacteria
Gram-negative bacteria
Spirochetes
Rickettsiae
Protozoa
Fungi
Viruses

Obstetric Conditions
Abruptio placentae
Placenta previa, accreta,
  and percreta
Retained dead fetus
  syndrome
Amniotic fluid embolism
Uterine atony
Therapeutic abortion
Toxemia of pregnancy

12

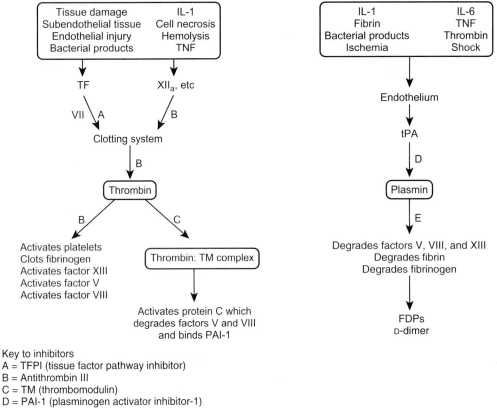

Figure 12-2 A brief overview outlining forces initiating coagulation that could lead to disseminated intravascular coagulation (DIC). Key to the generation of DIC is circulating thrombin and plasmin free of physiologic inhibition.

(Table 12-3). It is acknowledged that this simplistic approach may represent some degree of overlap; however, it offers a glimpse into the multiple and varied ways that DIC can manifest. The tempo axis distinguishes DIC as acute or chronic. The classic diseases representing acute DIC include most of the sepsis syndromes, DIC secondary to trauma, and cardiopulmonary collapse. Chronic DIC is represented by the retained dead fetus syndrome, large intra-abdominal aortic aneurysms, and Trousseau syndrome.

Regarding extent, localized causes of DIC include abdominal aortic aneurysm (AAA), an empyema or necrotic gallbladder, or an obstetric catastrophe such as placenta previa or abruptio placentae. Systemic causes include most leukemias and lymphomas, carcinomatosis, sepsis, heatstroke, and burns.

The third axis for consideration is clinical manifestation, which can be thrombotic, hemorrhagic, or, occasionally, both. An example of the thrombotic arm is Trousseau syndrome, whereas examples of almost pure hemorrhagic DIC would include abruptio placentae or hemolytic transfusion reaction.

FIVE ILLUSTRATIVE CAUSES OF DISSEMINATED INTRAVASCULAR COAGULATION

Closed Head Injury

Closed head injury is a model for acute, severe DIC.[31] In experimental head injury in rats, fixed amounts of head trauma result in reproducible amounts of fibrin deposition in the microcirculation.[32] The same investigators[33] found that among patients with head injury, a correlation could be made between extent of head injury, hemostatic defects, and worsening clinical outcome. Olson and associates[34] confirmed these findings in a large series of patients with head injuries. Head injuries not only lead to neurologic damage, paralysis, and venous stasis, they also cause coagulation activation because damaged brain tissue serves as the source of tissue thromboplastin released into the circulation. Selladurai and colleagues[35] prospectively studied

Table 12-3 The Three Axes of Disseminated Intravascular Coagulation, with Clinical Examples

Axis	Example
Tempo	
Acute	Meningococcemia
Chronic	Retained dead fetus syndrome
Extent	
Localized	Abdominal aortic aneurysm
Systemic	Acute promyelocytic leukemia
Manifestation	
Hemorrhagic	Abruptio placentae
Thrombotic	Trousseau syndrome

204 patients with acute closed head injury using readily available coagulation tests and found that 38% had moderate or severe alterations of such global tests, thus supporting the diagnosis of DIC. They noticed an increasing incidence of DIC with decreasing Glasgow coma scores ($P < .0001$). Patients whose laboratory data suggested DIC had worse overall outcomes than those without such findings. Fujii and associates[36] pointed out that for these hemostatic manifestations to occur, the damaged neural tissue had to transverse from the parenchyma into the circulation via the subarachnoid space. DIC associated with closed head injury is usually rather brisk and self limited because the spillage of brain tissue into the circulation usually ceases. On the other hand, closed head injury often has such a high mortality rate that the patient may expire from the primary injury.

Abdominal Aortic Aneurysm

Abdominal aortic aneurysm (AAA) serves as a model for chronic compensated DIC in that the platelet count can be low, high, or normal, as can the fibrinogen concentration. Most frequently, DIC in AAA is recognized when the platelet count is somewhat low, in the 40,000 to 80,000/µL range, and analysis for serum FDP is positive. It is believed that the rough saccular nature of the aneurysm allows pockets of clotting to take place, and therefore, some degree of localized DIC occurs. Of interest, microangiopathic hemolytic anemia changes in red cells may be seen, as well as laboratory evidence of intravascular hemolysis, including decreased levels of serum haptoglobin and the presence of urine hemosiderin. Low-dose heparin, such as 5000 units administered subcutaneously twice daily, or low molecular weight heparin (LMWH) has been advocated to attenuate chronic DIC and allow the platelet count to increase, so the patient may be a better surgical candidate.[37] The platelet count may increase yet fluctuate on its own. Oba and colleagues[38] opine that because the cause of the DIC is the aneurysm itself, rather than spending days to weeks administering heparin to such patients and waiting for improvement, the clinician should surgically approach the aneurysm as soon as possible. Aboulafia and Aboulafia[39] reportedly found evidence of such chronic DIC in 2 of 67 consecutive cases of AAA. They reviewed reports of 34 cases of DIC associated with AAA and concluded that DIC was a variable process and that often the platelet count improved whether heparin was administered or not. They also suggested that the best approach was surgical correction of the AAA. It is not clear whether the presence of DIC added to the overall surgical morbidity of AAA.

Acute Bilateral Renal Cortical Necrosis

Acute bilateral renal cortical necrosis (BRCN) is a rare cause of acute renal failure (ARF) and may represent acute DIC with preponderance of impact on the renal microvasculature. Two lines of evidence suggest that this process may well be a limited form of DIC.[40,41] The first is that the list of precipitating illnesses is the same as the list for DIC with special reference to all manner of obstetric emergencies,[42,43] sepsis,[44] and shock.[40] Second, extreme deposition of fibrin is frequently seen in the renal microcirculation,

particularly if renal biopsy is done early in the process, although this event does not happen frequently, given the laboratory perturbations of DIC. This finding sets BRCN apart from the more common acute tubular necrosis (ATN), also seen in many similarly ill patients. Because hypotension and hypoperfusion are common in both BRCN and ATN, differentiation by clinical means is frequently difficult.

The histologic pattern is extremely reminiscent of those found in the generalized Shwartzman reaction seen in laboratory animals that have been administered repeated doses of endotoxin.[45] Whereas in DIC of unknown cause, fibrin deposition can be seen in any organ, in BRCN, the renal vasculature is disproportionately involved. Whether local "second hits" (renal endothelial damage, or unknown host effects) destine this vascular bed is a matter of conjecture. The initial clinical picture of nearly all cases of BRNC is characterized by hypotension, suggesting that hypoperfusion to the point of overcoming renal autoregulatory defense mechanisms may well be a major contributing factor. Additionally, experimental models show that the high levels of PAI-1 seen in BRCN play an important antifibrinolytic role,[46] and that PAI-1 can be blocked by anti–PAI-1 antibodies, which results in marked histologic reduction of renal fibrin deposition.[47]

The pattern of ischemic necrosis is unusual in that sparing of a thin rim of perfused viable tissue immediately under the renal capsule and at the corticomedullary junction can be seen, thus causing the brunt of the thwarted circulation to be directed at the interlobular and afferent arterioles. Clinically, this is important in that magnetic resonance imaging (MRI) showing such a pattern might be the prime or even sole early suggestion of BRNC.[48]

BRNC has become less common with improved obstetric intensive care and the use of high-risk teams providing prepartum care for those patients who might otherwise be at risk for this disorder. Similar arguments can be made regarding nonobstetric causes because of improved interventional and intensive care.

Treatment hinges on prompt diagnosis, correction of hypoperfusion, and measures taken to address other contributory factors. Renal failure is extremely common, and usually, renal replacement therapy is required. Whether anticoagulant therapy is efficacious is unclear but, on the basis of the histologic deposition of fibrin, one is tempted to use it.

Placental Abnormalities

Placental abnormalities are a rare yet significant cause of obstetric DIC morbidity and mortality. Placenta previa (the implantation of the placenta in such a position as to occlude the cervical canal) is most common, occurring in 10% of women who had a previous caesarean section. This abnormality is not discussed further here. A subtype of placenta previa is placenta accreta, which may occur in about 1% of women who have undergone caesarean section; rarer yet is placenta percreta, which occurs in about 1 in 10,000 pregnancies.[49–51] The term *placenta accreta* implies the pathologic implantation of the placenta deep into the myometrium. *Placenta percreta* implies dissection of the placenta with the use of its proteolytic and coagulation proteins through the uterine wall along the line of a previous injury such as a caesarean section.[52] Once in the peritoneal cavity, the placenta may implant itself ectopically onto the bladder or any other available tissues. Although all these placental abnormalities are fairly rare, without question they are becoming more common as the rate of caesarean section increases. When the pregnancy is otherwise normal, whether the fetus survives is a function of its success in establishing an adequate vascular supply. If inadequate, the fetus may not survive; if adequate, gestation may progress normally, yet at parturition, the placenta fails to be delivered because it is extrauterine.

Diagnosis can be made prepartum by imaging,[50,53,54] especially in women with a high index of suspicion, such as those with multiple prior caesarean sections. The density of abnormal vasculature with vascular spaces represents the diagnostic criteria (sometimes called "Swiss cheese appearance") and the source of characteristic hemorrhage, which may occur prematurely or at parturition because these vessels are large and multiple. Management of this event is largely handled surgically with liberal use of fluid and blood products, as well as internal uterine artery ligation or coil embolization.[50,51,54]

The failed third stage of labor presents the question of whether one should leave the placenta in situ or pursue the retained ectopic placenta; both of these approaches have been advocated. In situations in which it is left in, the placenta sometimes undergoes spontaneous involution.[55,56] Leaving the placenta in place can be associated with a delayed DIC–hyperfibrinolysis situation, probably caused by the necrosing retained products of conception. Methotrexate has been administered to hasten involution or to otherwise curtail the hemorrhagic picture, with both good[57] and poor results reported.[58]

In the diagnosis and management of such cases, the hematologist should be aware of these rare conditions, particularly in the rare patient with retained implanted placenta of placenta percreta.

Acute Promyelocytic Leukemia

Acute promyelocytic leukemia (APL) represents a particular leukemic subtype that is highly associated with DIC and hyperfibrinolysis. It is mentioned here because advances in its treatment have resulted in substantial improvement in survival. Prior to the availability of all-transretinoic acid (ATRA) induction therapy, patients with APL had rates of extreme and frequently lethal hemorrhage as high as 50%.[59] Now, with the routine availability of ATRA therapy, the hemorrhagic rate is much lower, although still about 3% of patients die of hemorrhage before therapy is started, and another 3% die of hemorrhage during the first week of induction with ATRA. Another 2% to 3% die after the first week.[60] Because it appears that early therapy is associated with a less intense and/or an abbreviated coagulopathy, experts in APL therapy recommend that ATRA be administered as early as possible to control hemorrhage, even if this means not awaiting results of sophisticated genetic confirmation of the diagnosis. The malignant cells of APL cause increased generation of thrombin associated with brisk fibrinolysis, which may be part of the DIC; others have believed that it may be an event that is primarily induced by APL malignant cells.[61] With early and aggressive ATRA therapy

combined with aggressive supportive therapy, up to 90% of patients may achieve remission, and an estimated 70% are curable.[62] Supportive therapy is aimed primarily at anticipation and early diagnosis of hemorrhagic complications, which may very well be the acute presentation of APL. Fibrinogen sources are often suggested in quantities sufficient to keep the fibrinogen level at approximately 150 mg/dL and platelet counts higher than 30,000/μL during induction with ATRA.[60] The role of heparin therapy with or without antifibrinolytic therapy, given to prevent the development of the coagulopathy or to ameliorate it once it has started, has never been established in a controlled study.

DIAGNOSIS OF DISSEMINATED INTRAVASCULAR COAGULATION

The most common clinical manifestations of DIC are bleeding, thrombosis, and concomitant bleeding and thrombosis, often with resultant dysfunction of one or many organs. This is what the clinician sees. Bleeding occurs from all incisions, mildly traumatized mucosal membranes, and intravenous (IV) sites, and in the urine. Occasionally, thrombosis is the first clinical observation. This can occur in the form of ecchymoses, which may rapidly progress to purpura fulminans (the manifestation of subdermal microthrombosis with skin necrosis), a cold pulseless limb, or sudden loss of vision or some other neurologic catastrophe resulting from thrombosis.

The diagnosis of DIC is, indeed, a clinical diagnosis (Table 12-4).[16] Because such patients are already at such high clinical suspicion for DIC, only a few simple and readily available laboratory tests are necessary to confirm the diagnosis. These include prothrombin time (PT), partial thromboplastin time (PTT), thrombin time (TT), platelet count, FDP level, and blood smear. PT and PTT, in clinically severe and life-threatening DIC, are prolonged in approximately 50% to 75% of cases by virtue of consumption of many coagulation factors. TT is significantly prolonged in approximately 70% to 80% of cases because levels of fibrinogen may be low whereas FDPs may be high, both of which serve to prolong the TT. The platelet count is moderately reduced, or at least lower than seen on previous pre-DIC observations, about 80% to 90% of the time. Usually, the initial platelet count is not lower than 30,000 to 40,000/μL. Analysis for FDPs yields abnormal findings 95% of the time (i.e., high sensitivity); when FDPs are

---

Table 12-4 Clinical Diagnostic Criteria for Disseminated Intravascular Coagulation

- Patient bleeding, thrombosing, or both, typically with progressive organ dysfunction
- An underlying illness or process that may cause tissue damage, cell death, or production/release of tissue factor
- Usually some perturbation exists of simple, readily available tests such as thrombin time (TT), prothrombin time (PT), partial thromboplastin time (PTT), fibrin degradation products (FDP)/D-dimer, and platelet count. These values may markedly change as the clinical situation changes.

increased and D-dimers (i.e., high specificity) are concomitantly present in patients for whom the clinical suspicion for DIC is high, virtually 100% will indeed have DIC.[23] Examination of the blood smear confirms the thrombocytopenia and reveals schistocytic hemolysis in about one half of cases.

Some have written extensively on more detailed laboratory evaluations of DIC. Because various factors are consumed, measurement of any of the classic coagulation factors may reveal reduced levels, as well as reduced levels of ATIII, plasminogen, and α_2-PI. The difficulties associated with a pure laboratory approach are several (Table 12-5). First, this approach implies that consideration of a diagnosis of DIC should begin in the laboratory, whereas, in fact, this occurs at the bedside. Second, DIC presents an extremely dynamic situation in which its initiation may be extremely brisk, yet brief, such as occurs with intermittent sepsis from a necrotic gallbladder, empyema, or abscess. This initiating force for DIC may be so rapid that by the time the clinical manifestations of DIC are observed, laboratory parameters may already have been righted by reparative mechanisms before the tests are ordered, samples collected, tests performed, and results reported and interpreted. These more sophisticated tests require a considerable amount of time, laboratory expertise, and expense and, in the authors' opinion, are unlikely to yield more clinically useful information than is provided by the simple tests described.

Others[21,63,64] have advocated more aggressive incorporation of laboratory data to support a diagnosis of DIC. Bick[63] has evaluated and ranked more than 20 tests that may be used in formulating such a diagnosis. These tests arguably are frequently but not always altered in DIC. One might object that availability of many of these tests is much more restricted compared with tests that we have favored, which are readily available in almost any clinical setting. Using elaborate laboratory data, Reister and colleagues[64] formulated four different levels of DIC (DIC I to DIC IV), claiming that progression of DIC through these phases is supported by progressive perturbations of 11 laboratory tests. Gando and colleagues[21] established a score using four laboratory tests and three clinical situations. They also stated that by following this score, they were able to separate patients into survivors (those whose scores decreased over the next 5 days) and nonsurvivors (those whose scores remained high for the 5-day period). They noted that higher scores correlated not only with clinical deterioration of the patient but with progressive organ failure until MODS developed. Gando's report[21]

Table 12-5 Reasons Why Laboratory Findings are of Secondary Importance in the Diagnosis of Disseminated Intravascular Coagulation

- There is always an underlying problem that presents its own varied perturbations of many tests.
- Tests represent static "snapshots" of a highly dynamic situation.
- Special tests frequently are esoteric, and results arrive long after the dynamic situation has changed.
- Diagnostic test results rarely direct or redirect therapy and may confuse the clinical picture.

---

parenthetically noted that an increase in PAI-1 level was the best predictor for lethality of DIC, whereas Wada and colleagues[65] found no such correlation between PAI-1 levels and the prediction of patient outcomes. Not only are laboratory data in DIC potentially confusing, but results may show trends in opposing directions when acute DIC is compared with chronic DIC or when compensated and decompensated DIC are compared.[66] Accordingly, unless and until such interesting laboratory findings prove more predictive and cost effective, the conservative use of inexpensive and rapidly available tests seems most prudent. The International Society of Thrombosis and Haemostasis (ISTH) Subcommittee on DIC published a scoring grid in 2001 in order to facilitate laboratory diagnosis of DIC and validated the utility of this simplified approach in 2007.[67,67a]

DIFFERENTIAL DIAGNOSIS OF DISSEMINATED INTRAVASCULAR COAGULATION

Several situations should be considered in the differential diagnosis of DIC because clinical manifestations or laboratory abnormalities of other disorders may mimic DIC. Most common among these is severe hepatic cirrhosis, whose laboratory coagulation abnormalities mimic DIC (see Chapter 39). In patients with hepatic cirrhosis, decreased levels of hemostatic factors, including fibrinogen, ATIII, protein C, protein S, and plasminogen, are due to impaired production and not usually to enhanced activation, as would be found in DIC.[68] Because the liver clears the small quantity of FDPs as the result of physiologic production, decreased clearance with hepatic disease results in an accumulation of FDPs in the blood. Portal hypertension with hypersplenism is also characteristic of advanced cirrhosis, hence thrombocytopenia is frequently encountered. Bleeding varices and gastritis in these patients are due not to DIC but to hepatic failure and portal hypertension.

Dilutional coagulopathy may cause diagnostic confusion with DIC or may coexist with DIC, but it does not cause DIC in the sense of a pathologic overproduction of thrombin. One working definition for dilutional coagulopathy is the result of infusion of blood, blood products, or crystalloid fluids infused at a volume to compensate for the loss of blood equal to the total blood volume of a patient within a 24-hour period. Because packed red cells, platelet concentrates, plasma, and crystalloid fluids, separately or together, are not equal to native blood in any respect, one must appreciate that any test, such as platelet count, PT, or PTT, cannot emulate the results of a stable patient. Troubles arise when one tries to make clinical decisions that are based on the results of static tests in the midst of a most dynamic emergency, using tests that were neither designed nor able to do this.[69]

As are depicted in Table 12-6, the results of such basic coagulation tests cannot help the clinician to discriminate between DIC, dilutional coagulopathy, and severe hepatic failure. Regarding Table 12-6, assume that Case 1 represents a 55-year-old patient with severe alcoholic cirrhosis who is presently stable but has splenomegaly, ascites, jaundice, and severely deranged hepatic synthetic function. Case 2 could be considered a 40-year-old healthy woman

Table 12-6 Laboratory Testing is Limited in Discriminating Among Three Clinical Situations

	Case #1* Chronic, Stable, Severe Hepatic Insufficiency		Case #2* Dilutional Coagulopathy		Case #3* Disseminated Intravascular Coagulation	
	Level	*Score*	*Level*	*Score*	*Level*	*Score*
ISTH DIC TESTS						
Platelet count/μL	80,000	1	70,000	1	60,000	1
D-dimer, μg/mL	2	2	2	2	3	2
PT, seconds prolonged	6	2	7	2	6	2
Fibrinogen, mg/dL	85	1	70	1	90	1
Total ISTH score		6		6		6
Other Coagulation Tests[†]						
ATIII level, % normal (nL)	30–50		30–50		30–50	
Plasminogen level, % nL	30–50		30–50		30–50	
Most coagulation factors, % nL	30–50		30–50		30–50	
Factor VIII activity, % nL	80–200		30–50		50–80	
PTT 1:1 mix with plasma	Usually corrects		Always corrects		Rarely corrects	
Other Features						
Pathophysiology	Decreased protein synthesis		Effects of dilution		Increased consumption	
Thrombin generation	Intact but sluggish		Maintained		Excessive	
Systemic hemorrhage	Few		None		Characteristic	
Systemic thrombosis	Rare		None		Characteristic	
Hematologic treatment	Nonspecific		Platelets, fresh frozen plasma, cryoprecipitate		Aimed at instigating circumstance	

ISTH, International Society of Thrombosis and Haemostasis; DIC, disseminated intravascular coagulation; PT, prothrombin time; ATIII, antithrombin III; PTT, partial thromboplastin time.
*See text for case details.
†These levels represent ranges typically encountered within such patient scenarios.

undergoing an elective hysterectomy during which ligation of an artery was incomplete and, because of postoperative hemorrhage, she became hypotensive, during which time she was resuscitated with 6 liters of saline, 6 units of FFP, and 6 units of blood. Consider the third case to be an example of classic DIC involving a healthy 47-year-old man with gallstones, who suddenly became febrile, septic, and hypotensive, and whose blood cultures subsequently grew out Gram-negative rods. Changes in the patient's clinical condition, whether or not blood or volume replacement was administered, were more important than changes in hemostatic test results.[70] Improvement seen on tests of a deteriorating patient is not as desirable as those noted in an improving patient with distorted laboratory tests. Dilutional coagulopathy is thoroughly discussed in Chapter 46, but it is mentioned here because of its association and confusion with DIC. They may coexist. In simple terms, two primary clinical situations may eventuate dilutional coagulopathy. The first is elective surgery in which unexpected massive hemorrhage (such as from a ruptured major artery or a ligature failure) results in massive blood and fluid infusion to the extent that it represents a rather pure form of dilutional coagulopathy. The second is the trauma patient who not only is experiencing severe hemorrhage, but also has multiple fractures or punctures of various organs with concomitant sepsis, hypovolemia, and shock with acidosis, which would represent dilutional coagulopathy coexisting with DIC. Indeed, it is the massive production of tissue factor and other cytokines within the trauma patient that initiates DIC, distinguishing that situation from the relatively controlled situation of events in an elective surgery patient. Both hypothermia and acidosis are appreciated as limiting physiologic coagulation (i.e.,

thrombin generation) and enhancing the fibrinolytic system, both of which may exacerbate clinical bleeding.[71] Following therapeutic phereses in which volume is replaced with albumin administration, fibrinogen level, PT, and PTT, and platelet count due to this dilutional coagulopathy may be considerably altered, but microvascular hemorrhage is rarely encountered. Considerable surgical and critical care debate is ongoing regarding whether, when, and with what the massively injured trauma patient should be infused.[72] As is discussed in Chapter 46, prompt exploration to minimize hemorrhage, thereby minimizing dilutional coagulopathy in the first place, is becoming the accepted trauma surgery standard.

Measurable decreases in plasma fibrinogen (typically elevated in pregnancy) and increases in serum FDP are found during the immediate postpartum period, even in uncomplicated deliveries. These measurable changes should be viewed not as pathologic but as physiologic. However, in an appropriate clinical setting such as massive hemorrhage, these changes may support a diagnosis of DIC.

The differential diagnosis of DIC may include the HELLP (Hemolysis, Elevated Liver function tests, and Low Platelets) syndrome, which is discussed thoroughly in Chapter 35.[73] Indeed, distinguishing among DIC, acute fatty liver of pregnancy, preeclampsia, eclampsia, massive thrombosis, thrombotic thrombocytopenic purpura (TTP), and the HELLP syndrome[74,75] can present a challenge. Table 12-7 lists some differences among these presentations. Treatment for patients with the HELLP syndrome centers around delivery of the child and placenta as soon as is feasible. Delivery is timed closely with the obstetrician. If possible, waiting a few extra days will enhance

Table 12-7 Differential Diagnosis of Disseminated Intravascular Coagulation

Feature	Acute DIC (e.g., sepsis)	Chronic DIC (e.g., Trousseau syndrome)	Thrombotic Storm	HELLP	TTP	Primary Hyperfibrinolysis
Patient population	Patients with severe obstetric, medical, or surgical illness	Patients with cancer	Patients with hypercoagulability	Pregnant patients	Usually otherwise healthy	Prostate cancer, post CAB
Mechanism	Tissue damage and release of thromboplastins and cytokines	Tumor cell release of procoagulants or cell death	Uncontrolled hypercoagulability	Placental factors?	Platelet microthrombi	Direct plasminogen activation
Course	Usually acute	Subacute/chronic	Subacute	Subacute	Acute	Acute
Thrombosis*	Usually microcirculation	Arteries, veins, and microcirculation	Multiple veins and arteries	Nil	Microvascular	Nil
Hemorrhage	Frequent	Nil	Nil	Nil	Microvascular	Massive
Coagulation parameters	Usually abnormal	Usually normal	Normal	Normal	Normal	Abnormal
Platelet count	Low	Variable	Normal	Low	Low	Normal
Response to heparin	Nil	Fair	Good	NA	NA	NA
Response to warfarin after heparin	Nil	Nil	Good	NA	NA	NA
Prognosis with aggressive therapy	Good if underlying cause corrected	Poor	Good	Improved after delivery	Improved with plasma therapy	May be self limited; consider EACA
Hemolysis	Microangiopathic	Microangiopathic	None	Microangiopathic	Microangiopathic	None

DIC, disseminated intravascular coagulation; HELLP, *H*emolysis, *E*levated *L*iver function tests, and *L*ow *P*latelets) syndrome; TTP, thrombotic thrombocytopenic purpura; CAB, coronary artery bypass; NA, not applicable; EACA, ε-aminocaproic acid.
*Without anticoagulant therapy.

12

the viability of the fetus, as this syndrome often comes to light at the beginning of the third trimester.[76] Paradoxically, the HELLP syndrome frequently deteriorates 2 to 4 days before or after delivery. One must be on guard at that time for the possibility of overt thrombosis. In fact, one can justify prophylactic administration of heparin immediately postpartum if the platelet count is not less than 20,000/μL. Distinguishing between the HELLP syndrome and DIC can be difficult or impossible, as it is clear that the HELLP syndrome can degenerate to DIC. Van Dam and colleagues[76] and De Boer and associates[77] studied this transition and found that laboratory manifestations heralding a worsening of the HELLP syndrome into probable DIC included progression of the PT and PTT from normal to abnormal, the progressive appearance of serum FDPs, and a decrease in the plasma ATIII level.

Although TTP (discussed in Chapter 24) is clearly a thrombotic process with major organ damage resulting from pathologic intravascular deposition of large aggregates of platelets, it is not regarded as representative of DIC. The PT, PTT, TT, and FDP level are nearly always normal. Microangiopathic hemolysis is a hallmark.

A thrombin-like enzyme, crotalase, found in the venom of the Eastern diamondback rattlesnake (*Crotalus adamantus*), partially clots fibrinogen.[25] However, it does not activate platelets or bind to ATIII, which distinguishes its actions from those of thrombin. Although laboratory findings after envenomation by the Eastern diamondback rattlesnake are highly reminiscent of DIC, neither thrombotic nor hemorrhagic complications usually occur.

It has been long known that there is an association between thromboembolic disease and carcinoma. If thromboembolism occurs as described by Trousseau over 100 years ago,[78] the process is appropriately known as Trousseau syndrome. The approximate two- to threefold incidence of bland deep venous thrombosis (DVT) found in patients with cancer is not usually regarded as Trousseau syndrome. Rather, Trousseau syndrome is a subset of the hypercoagulability associated with carcinoma and is recognized by specific characteristics (Table 12-8). Trousseau syndrome is now regarded as chronic DIC, as elaborated by Sack and colleagues.[17] The syndrome is particularly associated with

adenocarcinoma, and frequently, the tumor is occult.[79] It is believed to be due to the release of procoagulant products from tumors, one of which is TF.[79,80] Indeed, these authors showed an association between malignant tissue TF concentrations and hypercoagulability. The metastatic potential of a tumor may be related to TF expression in or on the malignant cells.[79,81]

Many studies have been undertaken to find laboratory abnormalities that would be sensitive and specific enough to establish the diagnosis of Trousseau syndrome, but these variables have not gained much popularity because of their inherent variability. Situations such as Trousseau syndrome have been referred to as *chronic compensated DIC* by Mammen,[66] who observed that the simplest tests such as platelet count, PT, partial thromboplastin time (PTT), and fibrinogen level can yield results that are low, normal, or high. Typically, but not always, the ATIII level is decreased and the concentration of FDP increased in Trousseau syndrome.

Trousseau syndrome is recognized by its features, as listed in Table 12-8. A particularly useful diagnostic criterion is the recurrent nature of DVT, which is usually controlled by heparin but then recurs almost as soon as heparin therapy is withdrawn after initiation of warfarin therapy, regardless of the international normalized ratio (INR) achieved.[79] The vessels involved may be veins, particularly those in unusual places such as superficial veins in the thorax and abdomen, subclavian veins, and especially cerebral veins.[82,83] Arterial thromboses also occur and may be sudden, catastrophic, life-threatening, or fatal.[17,84] Therapy is challenging. Warfarin therapy fails.[79,85] Heparin, often given in very large doses, is required to keep the PTT at target levels, or at least to maintain the heparin concentration at therapeutic levels, such as 0.3 to 0.8 U/mL, which can be achieved with large doses of standard unfractionated heparin, even on an outpatient basis. Some have resorted to continuous infusion of heparin to avoid peaks and troughs of heparin levels.[85] Whether LMWH is more efficacious than standard heparin in this situation is not certain.[86] However, if one does use LMWH, measurement of LMWH levels by anti-Xa activity to validate sufficient concentrations for long-term ambulatory therapy appears rational. At least one patient who developed heparin-induced thrombocytopenia was treated on a long-term basis with lepirudin.[87] The patient may succumb to uncontrolled venous and arterial thrombosis of Trousseau syndrome or to therapy, as metastases may hemorrhage. The thrombohemorrhagic syndrome is as lethal as the primary tumor.[88,89] The prognosis is poor owing to the nature of the malignancy and its thrombohemorrhagic manifestations.[84,86]

The fibrinolytic system may be activated independent of the coagulation system. Activation of the fibrinolytic system in the overwhelming majority of cases of DIC is the secondary physiologic result of thrombosis. In some circumstances, the fibrinolytic system may be activated in a primary fashion. The existence of primary hyperfibrinolysis has been debated for some time, and it probably does exist in select instances. In this situation, bleeding may be significant, but thrombosis is not a feature. Primary hyperfibrinolysis may result in some cases of carcinoma[90] or acute promyelocytic leukemia, as such cells may elaborate plasminogen activators.[91] Late phases of cardiopulmonary bypass (rewarming) and orthotopic liver transplant

---

Table 12-8 Features of Trousseau Syndrome

Clinical

Recurrent migratory thrombophlebitis

Unusual sites of thrombosis: axillary/subclavian veins; superficial veins of the neck, thorax, or abdomen; visceral or cerebral veins

Failure to respond clinically to warfarin

Usually respond clinically to heparin but may relapse immediately after discontinuation

May simultaneously experience arterial thrombosis and hemorrhage

Associated with nonbacterial thrombotic endocarditis

Tumor typically small or occult adenocarcinoma

Laboratory

No laboratory test sensitive or specific

Platelets and antithrombin III (ATIII) levels are usually decreased

Red blood cells may show changes consistent with microangiopathic hemolysis (washout of the donor liver) also are associated with a brisk release of endogenous tPA, resulting in probably the most common cause of bleeding after cardiopulmonary bypass and liver transplantation.[92,93] In keeping with this hypothesis, the use of antifibrinolytic agents is associated with decreased hemorrhage during such procedures. Obviously, infusion of pharmacologic plasminogen activators, such as streptokinase or tPA, causes a primary hyperfibrinolytic state. Hemorrhage may be brisk but often is self limited, especially after cardiovascular surgery or liver transplantation. Coagulation tests, which reflect the very low fibrinogen level and high level of FDP, include prolonged TT, PT, and PTT. Platelet count and ATIII level are normal or near normal, and microangiopathic hemolytic anemia is conspicuously absent. If the condition is not self limited and DIC (thrombosis) can be excluded, treatment with antifibrinolytic agents such as ε-aminocaproic acid (EACA) or tranexamic acid may be carefully attempted.

CONSEQUENCES OF DISSEMINATED INTRAVASCULAR COAGULATION

The consequences, often life-threatening or fatal, of DIC involve multiorgan failure, resulting in what is now called *multiorgan dysfunction syndrome* (MODS) (Table 12-9). At autopsy, target organs are found to be damaged and rendered ineffective by hemorrhage into the organ and thromboses. Both events tend to occur more often at the microcirculatory level than at the macrocirculatory level. Liver function test results may deteriorate at an alarming rate. This may be due not only to hemorrhage and infarction of the organ, but also to circulatory collapse with so-called shock liver. Clearly, preexisting liver disease makes this syndrome worse.[26] Because of the liver's key role in clearance of activated factors and its role in synthesis of hemostatic factors, sustained liver function is key to survival. Additionally, the liver has been shown to be central to the host's survival in sepsis.

Cardiac abnormalities are revealed by the appearance of elevated levels of serum cardiac enzymes, such as creatine kinase (CK), or cardiac rhythm disturbances due to destruction of the cardiac conduction system. Central nervous system abnormalities include seizures, mental status alterations, and behavioral abnormalities that may appear to be psychiatric in origin. Decreased renal function often occurs because of microinfarction of the filtering and collecting tubular apparatus. Usually, oliguria is the harbinger

---

Table 12-9 Multiorgan Dysfunction Syndrome as a Consequence of Disseminated Intravascular Coagulation

Pertubation of liver function tests
Leakage of cardiac enzymes, indicating ischemia
Cardiac rhythm disturbances
Central nervous system abnormalities
Oliguria
Decreased renal function
Acute respiratory distress syndrome (ARDS)
Gastrointestinal tract mucosal ulceration with bleeding
Adrenal insufficiency
Purpura fulminans

---

of renal insufficiency and is quickly followed by elevation of serum creatinine and/or blood urea nitrogen (BUN). Adult respiratory distress syndrome (ARDS) is a very common and frequently lethal manifestation of sepsis with shock; it occurs most often in situations severe enough to result in DIC. Gastrointestinal manifestations appear chiefly as mucosal ulcerations with subsequent bleeding. Adrenal glands may infarct and then necrose, leaving the patient adrenally insufficient. Skin manifestations include petechiae from bleeding and infarctive necrosis, with the prime example being purpura fulminans (see Chapter 11). The onset of MODS, especially with progressive and sequential organ failure despite therapeutic efforts, accurately forecasts lethality.

A probable role of the von Willebrand factor cleaving protease (ADAMTS13) in DIC has recently been suggested. Low levels of plasma ADAMTS13 have been detected in patients with DIC. Crawley and colleagues[96a] have demonstrated that plasmin and thrombin can proteolytically inactivate ADAMTS13. As both thrombin and plasmin circulate in DIC, it is plausible that ADAMTS13 reductions encountered in DIC are explained, at least in part, by these discoveries. Ono and colleagues[96b] demonstrated that patients with DIC with plasma ADAMTS13 levels lower than 20% of normal were three times more likely to experience renal failure than patients with DIC with levels higher than 20% of normal. The finding of increased levels of unusually large von Willebrand factor multimers in patients with ADAMTS13 levels lower than 20% suggested a causal relationship with renal failure.

It is impossible to accurately predict lethality of DIC for two reasons. The first is that by its very definition, DIC may include a range of patients, from those who will have no immediate mortality (those with liver disease presenting with laboratory data mimicking DIC) to those who have long-range mortality (those with AAA or chronic DIC from neoplasia), to those with a relatively high acute mortality (those with acute leukemias, crush injuries, and shock), and finally, to those with exceedingly high mortality (those with septic shock or meningococcemia). Second, each initiating process is recognized and treated in a different fashion, and the overall approach to the patient and his or her morbidity hinges on those processes. The process of DIC is less important regarding lethality than are the host, the disease, and its treatment. Mant and King[16] showed that 85% of patients with acute, severe DIC expired. Most expired, in their opinion, from the underlying disease and not from DIC itself. Wada and colleagues[65] showed that of 395 patients with DIC, a total of 25% died. Study patients comprised 154 with leukemia (of whom 21% died) and 241 who did not have leukemia but had cancer, sepsis, or other infectious diseases (of whom 28% died).

Predictors of death based on laboratory criteria are even more difficult to establish. Some have claimed that specific laboratory data did[21] or did not[65] predict death. Of interest and seemingly paradoxically, higher plasma fibrinogen levels predicted a higher rate of MODS and eventual death. Higher fibrinogen levels connote higher levels of fibrinolytic inhibition (presumably from higher levels of PAI-1), resulting in more microinfarction-enhancing MODS.[94] The more often laboratory abnormalities manifest and the greater the degree of alteration that occurs, the more likely the patient is to expire. Additionally, hepatic insufficiency is as an effective predictor of mortality as is shock. At autopsy, many patients who die of DIC have ARDS and MODS. Multiple interrelationships exist between DIC, ARDS, MODS, and systemic inflammatory response syndrome (SIRS).[95] These may be separate factors that reveal a very ill patient with processes that are progressively killing the patient or, more likely, they may all be different manifestations of an evolving fatal process.[21,27,66,95,96] From a clinical point of view, one may predict at least a 25% to 50% mortality rate if the presenting syndrome of a very ill patient is DIC, MODS, ARDS, or SIRS, and the patient fails to rapidly improve. The mortality rate is even higher if the presenting syndrome is conjoined by or progresses to include another of the DIC, MODS, SIRS, or ARDS consortium.

TREATMENT OF PATIENTS WITH DISSEMINATED INTRAVASCULAR COAGULATION

Because DIC is a grave consequence of a serious underlying disease, it would seem reasonable that primary treatment should be directed at control of that disease. Such has become increasingly accepted, although stating this fact is easier than accomplishing it. This approach is so successful that, when it can be accomplished, identification of DIC in a patient sanctions the use of aggressive therapy directed toward the primary process. The author knows of no clinical setting in which this is more successful than in a case of DIC that results from an obstetric emergency. Women may present in labor with massive bleeding and all the laboratory and clinical manifestations of DIC. The appropriate treatment is now recognized by obstetricians to be evacuation of the uterus. Time should not be spent in studying or trying to analyze in great depth the individual parameters of DIC; rather, the patient should be taken to the delivery suite, with resuscitation of blood pressure and volume by appropriate fluids, and the uterus evacuated. It is remarkable that a patient who is severely hemorrhaging can become hemostatically normal within a few hours of evacuation of the uterus. The success of this situation additionally underscores the marked restorative ability of an otherwise healthy person with normal hepatic function and a normal circulatory system to rectify these hemostatic abnormalities.

DIC may result from bacterial sepsis that occurs as a complication of an empyema, necrotic gallbladder, or other abscess. Again, time should not be spent analyzing various patterns and parameters of laboratory data in attempts to stratify, stage, or correct the DIC; rather, this situation is a medical and surgical emergency, neither of which will get better until the abscess is drained. Too frequently, surgical colleagues request "correction of the coagulopathy" before the abscess is drained, when it is precisely drainage of the abscess that will lead to correction of the coagulopathy. It is far more likely that the patient will die from bleeding and/or thrombosis from the DIC while one vainly attempts to correct the DIC, rather than from the minimal amount of bleeding that may occur with prompt drainage of the abscess to which the DIC will respond.

Table 12-10 presents a treatment schema for DIC. First, treating the underlying cause is the mainstay of treatment for patients with DIC. Second, and almost equally important, is resuscitation of the patient's circulatory system. It would be difficult to overestimate the value of the liver in neutralizing activated coagulation products and reconstituting normal procoagulant and inhibitory proteins.[97] Hepatic circulation will not be maximal and hence correction of blood abnormalities will not be maximal until hepatic perfusion is normalized by correction of volume, electrolyte, pH, temperature, and blood pressure abnormalities. Failure to correct the initiating process and preexisting hepatic hypoperfusion are harbingers of a bad outcome.

The role of fresh frozen plasma (FFP) and/or platelet transfusion appears to be simultaneously uncertain yet necessary. For thrombocytopenia to be a key potentiator of hemorrhage in patients, the platelet count is usually substantially below $50,000/\mu L$. Similarly, if depletion of fibrinogen and other coagulation factors is to be clinically significant, levels must be below approximately 50 to 60 mg/dL and below 25% of normal levels, respectively. Otherwise, administration of fibrinogen, FFP, or platelet transfusions is not indicated because these pertubations are the result of DIC and not the cause of bleeding. However, if the patient is hemorrhaging and the platelet count is less than $50,000/\mu L$, transfusing platelets to keep the platelet count in the range of 50,000 to $75,000/\mu L$ seems reasonable. Equally, in a patient who is bleeding with a fibrinogen concentration of less than 50 to 60 mg/dL, fibrinogen may be infused in the form of FFP or, preferably, cryoprecipitate in amounts needed to raise the fibrinogen level to that minimal level. Usually 10 "units" of

Table 12-10	Treatment of Disseminated Intravascular Coagulation	
Treatment	**Example**	**Rationale**
Treat underlying cause	Abruptio placentae	Interrupt cause of DIC
Resuscitation	Maintain blood pressure, correct acid/base balance	Maximize blood flow from areas of activation to clearance by liver
Replacement	Fresh frozen plasma and platelet transfusions	Provide enough procoagulant materials to control hemostasis
Antithrombin III	Severe liver disease with concomitant DIC	Replace severely decreased levels of ATIII
Heparin therapy	Trousseau syndrome, purpura fulminans, abdominal aortic aneurysm	May decrease ongoing thrombosis
Antifibrinolytic therapy	Kasabach-Merritt syndrome, prostate cancer	Occasionally used to control fibrinolysis, but only after administration of heparin

DIC, disseminated intravascular coagulation; ATIII, antithrombin III.

cryoprecipitate (each containing about 200 mg of fibrinogen) will suffice. Rarely are other blood coagulation factor levels lower than 25% of normal; accordingly, FFP is rarely recommended for the replacement of other coagulation factors.

If ATIII is considered to be the primary inhibitor of circulating thrombin, it would seem that ATIII infusion would be efficacious in treating DIC. ATIII is available in FFP but has more recently become available as a purified concentrate. Infusion in DIC has not been rigorously established, but its use certainly is rational. In experimental models, ATIII infusions blunt lethality, DIC, and SIRS in response to infusion of lethal amounts of *E. coli*.[98] Preliminary studies[99,100] have proved the safety and efficacy of ATIII concentrates, particularly in septic shock syndromes and in patients whose liver insufficiency is such that an acquired ATIII deficiency state exists. ATIII may be administered in amounts sufficient to support the ATIII level in the range of 100% of normal. This may be approximated by the infusion of 100 units of ATIII per kilogram of body weight. This formula is complicated by the variable and often brief half-life of ATIII in DIC. For clinical purposes, ATIII in otherwise normal patients has an overall half-life of approximately 24 hours; in DIC, it may be as brief as 3 or 4 hours. Should ATIII concentrates be employed, frequent measurement of ATIII levels is indicated to help regulate the infusion. At this time, infusion of ATIII concentrates generally is not recommended.[101]

Activated protein C infusion has shown some initial success in decreasing mortality in patients with severe sepsis[102] and is discussed further in Chapter 13.

Direct thrombin inhibitors such as hirudin have the theoretical advantage of neutralizing thrombin, a key participant in DIC, while not acting as a direct anticoagulant. In preliminary human DIC studies, several laboratory markers improved, but overall survival was uncertain when this evolving treatment modality was used.[103]

Heparin therapy remains extremely controversial. In some studies, the infusion of heparin has seemed to increase not only death, but particularly, hemorrhagic death.[16] It is intellectually attractive to administer heparin to decrease thrombotic events; its use may be even more reasonable when the clinical axis of thrombosis versus hemorrhage is more toward the thrombotic end. Accordingly, its use in Trousseau syndrome has been established as not only rational but lifesaving.[88] It may also be useful in purpura fulminans, APL, and AAA, each of which represents a subacute thrombotic form of DIC. When heparin is used in situations in which coagulation test results are abnormal, one cannot monitor it with the usual coagulation tests, so it must be given empirically. One commonly recommended method is to administer approximately 8 to 10 U/kg of standard heparin per hour by constant intravenous infusion. In more chronic DIC such as Trousseau syndrome, one may monitor heparin administration by PTT or plasma heparin levels.

Antifibrinolytic inhibitors such as EACA are occasionally advocated in patients who are on the extreme hemorrhagic end of the thrombotic-hemorrhagic axis. Such agents are very effective in blocking fibrinolysis and therefore must be used with caution. Patients with massive fibrinolysis may be considered candidates for EACA therapy; however, EACA should not be administered unless heparin has previously been infused to block the prothrombotic arm of DIC before the antifibrinolytic arm is blocked. A 4-g intravenous loading dose followed by 1 g every 2 hours intravenously for 24 hours may be tried. If bleeding does not decrease within 24 hours, it is unlikely to do so later.

Recombinant factor VIIa (discussed extensively in Chapter 27) has been used in select cases of DIC associated with obstetric emergencies,[104] malignancies,[105] and cerebral injuries.[106] Whereas thus far in these few cases, factor VIIa was administered after all other methods failed, the efficacy of factor VIIa seemed impressive, and the feared complication of thrombosis was not frequently reported. Further work is anticipated.

CONSULTATION CONSIDERATIONS

Patients who are consulted on usually fall into the following two groups: (1) those with rather typical severe acute DIC in which bleeding, hypotension, and organ failure generate the consultation; or (2) stable patients whose laboratory data make the referring practitioner consider the possibility of DIC.

Promptness in consultation is in order. Because of the great usefulness of readily available and inexpensive global tests such as PT, PTT, TT, FDP level, and complete blood count (CBC), it is strongly advisable that these tests should be repeated immediately in one's preparation to see the patient. One should insist that blood samples be drawn through a fresh venipuncture and not through intraarterial or intravenous lines that may contain blood, saline, or heparin. Very frequently, one finds that a new, fresh, reliable set of data is of more use than a set that may have been obtained 1 or 2 days in the past, let alone any disinformation generated from an incorrectly obtained sample. The consultant should have an open dialogue with the coagulation laboratory technicians because discussion heightens the hematology technician's involvement in the patient's problem. The technician's expertise frequently generates data or observations not immediately available to the consultant that may be helpful. The laboratory technician may be the first to observe schistocytes on the blood smear, signifying microangiopathic hemolysis; vacuolization of white cells, signifying sepsis; or spontaneous lysis of a test tube clot, signifying high levels of plasmin activity.

During the consultation, one must think extremely broadly as an internist rather than just as a subspecialist—a comment justified by the extraordinarily broad range of differential diagnoses and initiating processes involved in DIC. The consultant may be the first to recognize petechiae on a febrile patient, thus securing a working diagnosis of meningococcemia and justifying rapid, aggressive antibiotic treatment, or the peripheral stigmata of chronic liver disease, which, heretofore not appreciated, would indicate that the patient's laboratory data are more consistent with chronic liver insufficiency than with acute DIC.

Should it be determined that an invasive procedure such as drainage of an abscess or evacuation of the uterus may be needed, the surgeon, obstetrician, or invasive radiologist must appreciate that the necessity of the procedure overrides concern regarding "coagulopathy," because the cure for the coagulopathy is the procedure itself.

COST CONTAINMENT ISSUES

Patients with DIC are typically so ill that they are usually cared for in an intensive care unit, so hospital costs are truly considerable. Blood replacement costs can escalate if one does elect to use large quantities of FFP or platelet transfusions. Blood products should be used in moderation, perhaps, as indicated earlier in this chapter, with the aim of keeping the platelet count higher than 25,000 to 50,000/μL and/or the fibrinogen level higher than 50 mg/dL with active bleeding. Most practitioners would not transfuse platelets or FFP unless such critical levels are reached; transfusion at levels above these cutoffs has not been shown to improve clinical outcomes.

Perhaps the most important area for cost containment in DIC is the use of the laboratory. The routine laboratory tests advocated in this chapter such as CBC, TT, PT, PTT, and FDP level are generally available and are useful to the clinician in making a diagnosis in the current clinical setting.[67a] Their rapid turnaround and low cost justify their use. Select tests such as ATIII, D-dimer, and fibrinogen levels may be of intermittent use. Not only are most of the other tests that some have advocated extremely expensive, but also, because of their relative nonavailability, more often than not, test results are returned to the practitioner too late to be of clear use in daily bedside decision making.

MEDICAL-LEGAL CONSIDERATIONS

One might expect medical-legal concerns to arise periodically because DIC may be difficult to diagnose, it is typically associated with a wide variety of dire clinical circumstances, and it is known to have a high rate of mortality. On the other hand, no clear standards of care or practice guidelines have been established for the recognition or treatment of DIC. Physicians are held to practice in a manner consistent with good medical care and are required to approach the patient as any reasonable and prudent physician would do. As in any dire clinical situation, frank and open discussion with the patient and family is in order.

Potential areas of controversy include failure to obtain a sufficiently detailed history or physical examination, documentation of facts, and interpretation of the myriad of laboratory data. This may be another reason to limit laboratory data and focus on those tests that one is accustomed to ordering, reviewing, and interpreting. Treatment is sharply focused on the initiating cause of DIC; therefore, treatment for DIC itself would hardly be expected to be a standard of care issue, as it is anecdotal and controversial. It has not even been established whether one should use heparin, or how much FFP or platelet transfusion support patients require. Use of antifibrinolytics is extremely controversial, and one should probably not employ those agents unless heparin or some other antithrombotic agent is first administered.

REFERENCES

1. McKay DG:DIC: An Intermediary Mechanism of Disease. New York, Harper-Hoeber, 1965, p 493.
2. Hunter J: A Treatise on the Blood, Inflammation, and Gun-Shot Wounds. Philadelphia, Webster, 1817.
3. DeBlainville HMD: Injection de matiere cerebrale dans les veins. Gaz Med Paris (ser 2) 2:524–567, 1834.
4. Nauyn B: Unterschungen Ober Blutgirinnung Im Lebenden Tiere und Ihre Folgen. Arch Exp Pathol Pharmak 1:1, 1873.
5. Foa P, Pellacani P: Sul Fermento Fibrinogeno: Sulle Azioni Tossiche, Escercitate da Alcuni Organi Fresch. Arch Sci Med (Torino) 7:113, 1884.
6. Wooldridge LD: In Horsley V and Starling E (eds): On the Chemistry of the Blood and Other Scientific Papers. London, Kegan, Paul, Trench, Trubner, and Co, 1893.
7. Mills CA: The action of tissue extracts in the coagulation of blood. J Biol Chem 46:167–192, 1921.
8. Krevans JR, Jackson DP, Conley CL, et al: The nature of the hemorrhagic disorders accompanied by hemolytic transfusions in man. Blood 12:834–843, 1957.
9. Schneider C: Etiology of fibrinopenia: Fibrination defibrination. Ann NY Acad Sci 75:634–675, 1959.
10. Merskey C, Kleiner GJ, Johnson AJ: Quantitative estimation of split products of fibrinogen in human serum, relation to diagnosis and treatment. Blood 28:1–18, 1966.
11. Marder VJ, Shulman HR, Carroll WR: High molecular weight derivatives of human fibrinogen produced by plasmin. I. Physicochemical and immunological characterization. J Biol Chem 244:211–219, 1969.
12. Corrigan JJ: Changes in the blood coagulation system associated with septicemia. N Engl J Med 279:851–856, 1968.
13. Bull B, Rubenberg M, Dacie J, et al: Microangiopathic haemolytic anemia: Mechanisms of red-cell fragmentation. Br J Haematol 14:643–652, 1968.
14. Colman RW, Robboy SJ, Minna JD: DIC: An approach. Am J Med 52:679–689, 1972.
15. Merskey C: Defibrination syndrome or. . .? Blood 41:599–603, 1973.
16. Mant MJ, King EG: Severe acute DIC. Am J Med 67:557–563, 1979.
17. Sack GH, Levin J, Bell WR: Trousseau's syndrome and other manifestations of chronic disseminated coagulopathy in patients with neoplasms: Clinical, pathologic and therapeutic features. Medicine (Baltimore) 56:1–37, 1977.
18. Okajima K, Sakamoto Y, Uchiba M: Heterogenity in the incidence and clinical manifestations of disseminated intravascular coagulation. Am J Hematol 65:215–222, 2000.
19. Semeraro N, Colucci M: Tissue factor in health and disease. Thromb Haemost 78:759–764, 1997.
20. Gabay C, Kushner J: Acute-phase proteins and other systemic responses to inflammation. N Engl J Med 340:448–454, 1999.
21. Gando S, Kameve T, Nanzaki S, et al: Disseminated intravascular coagulation is a frequent complication of systemic inflammatory response syndrome. Thromb Haemost 75:224–228, 1996.
22. Suffredini AF, Harpel PC, Parrillo JE: Promotion and subsequent inhibition of plasminogen activation after administration of intravenous endotoxin to normal subjects. N Engl J Med 320:1165–1172, 1989.
23. Carr JM, McKinney M, McDonagh J: Diagnosis of disseminated intravascular coagulation: Role of D-dimer. Am J Clin Pathol 91:280–287, 1989.
24. Mombelli G, Fiori G, Monotto R, et al: Fibrinopeptide A in liver cirrhosis: Evidence against a major contribution of disseminated intravascular coagulation to coagulopathy of chronic liver disease. J Lab Clin Med 121:83–90, 1993.
25. Kitchens CS: Hemostatic aspects of envenomation by North American snakes. Hematol Oncol Clin North Am 6:1189–1195, 1992.
26. Deykin D: The role of the liver in serum-induced hypercoagulability. J Clin Invest 45:256–263, 1966.
27. Sandset PM, Warn-Cramer BJ, Maki SL, et al: Immunodepletion of extrinsic pathway inhibitor sensitizes rabbits to endotoxin-induced intravascular coagulation and the generalized Shwartzman reaction. Blood 78:1496–1502, 1991.
28. Pixley RA, De La Cadena R, Page JD, et al: The contact system contributes to hypotension but not disseminated intravascular coagulation in lethal bacteremia: In vivo use of a monoclonal anti–factor XII antibody to block contact activation in baboons. J Clin Invest 92:61–68, 1993.
29. Levi M, ten Cate H: Disseminated intravascular coagulation. N Engl J Med 341:586–592, 1999.
30. Tapper H, Herwald H: Modulation of hemostatic mechanisms in bacterial infectious diseases. Blood 96:2329–2337, 2000.
31. Goodnight SH: Defibrination after brain-tissue destruction: A serious complication of head injury. N Engl J Med 290:1043–1047, 1974.

32. Van der Sande JJ, Emiss JJ, Lindeman J: Intravascular coagulation: A common phenomenon in minor experimental head injury. J Neurosurg 54:21–25, 1981.

33. Van der Sande JJ, Veltkamp JJ, Boekhout-Mussert RJ, et al: Hemostasis and computerized tomography in head injury: Their relationship to clinical features. J Neurosurg 55:718–724, 1981.

34. Olson JD, Kaufman HH, Moake J, et al: The incidence and significance of hemostatic abnormalities in patients with head injuries. Neurosurgery 24:825–832, 1989.

35. Selladurai BM, Vickneswaran M, Duraisamy S, et al: Coagulopathy in acute head injury: A study of its role as a prognostic indicator. Br J Neurosurg 11:398–404, 1997.

36. Fujii Y, Takeuchi S, Harada A, et al: Hemostatic activation in spontaneous intracranial hemorrhage. Stroke 32:883–890, 2001.

37. Jelenska MM, Szmidt J, Bojakowski K, et al: Compensated activation of coagulation in patients with abdominal aortic aneurysm: Effects of heparin treatment prior to elective surgery. Thromb Haemost 92:997–1002, 2004.

38. Oba J, Shiiya N, Matsui Y, et al: Preoperative disseminated intravascular coagulation (DIC) associated with aortic aneurysm: Does it need to be corrected before surgery? Surg Today 25:1011–1014, 1995.

39. Aboulafia DM, Aboulafia ED: Aortic aneurysm–induced disseminated intravascular coagulation. Ann Vasc Surg 10:396–405, 1996.

40. Brady HR, Singer GG: Acute renal failure. Lancet 346:1533–1540, 1995.

41. Thadhani R, Pascual M, Bonventre JV: Acute renal failure. N Engl J Med 334:1448–1460, 1996.

42. Pertuiset N, Grunfeld JP: Acute renal failure in pregnancy. Baillieres Clin Obstet Gynaecol 8:333–351, 1994.

43. Kleinknecht D, Grunfeld JP, Gomez PC, et al: Diagnostic procedures and long-term prognosis in bilateral renal cortical necrosis. Kidney Int 4:390–400, 1973.

44. Marotto MS, Marotto PC, Sztajnbok J, Seguro AC: Outcome of acute renal failure in meningococcemia. Ren Fail 19:807–810, 1997.

45. Brozna JP: Shwartzman reaction. Semin Thromb Hemost 16:326–332, 1990.

46. Kitching AR, Kong YZ, Huang XR, et al: Plasminogen activator inhibitor-1 is a significant determinant of renal injury in experimental crescentic glomerulonephritis. J Am Soc Nephrol 14:1487–1495, 2003.

47. Montes R, Declerck PH, Calvo A, et al: Prevention of renal fibrin deposition in endotoxin-induced DIC through inhibition of PAI-1. Thromb Haemost 84:65–70, 2000.

48. Francois M, Tostivint I, Mercadal L, et al: MR imaging features of acute bilateral renal cortical necrosis. Am J Kidney Dis 35:745–748, 2000.

49. Gielchinsky Y, Rojansky N, Fasouliotis SJ, Ezra Y: Placenta accreta—Summary of 10 years: A survey of 310 cases. Placenta 23:210–214, 2002.

50. Hudon L, Belfort MA, Broome DR: Diagnosis and management of placenta percreta: A review. Obstet Gynecol Surv 53:509–517, 1998.

51. Abbas F, Talati J, Wasti S, et al: Placenta percreta with bladder invasion as a cause of life threatening hemorrhage. J Urol 164:1270–1274, 2000.

52. Merviel P, Evain-Brion D, Challier JC, et al: The molecular basis of embryo implantation in humans. Zentralbl Gynakol 123:328–339, 2001.

53. Taipale P, Orden MR, Berg M, et al: Prenatal diagnosis of placenta accrete and percreta with ultrasonography, color Doppler, and magnetic resonance imaging. Obstet Gynecol 104:537–540, 2004.

54. Dinkel HP, Durig P, Schnatterbeck P, Triller J: Percutaneous treatment of placenta percreta using coil embolization. J Endovasc Ther 10:158–162, 2003.

55. Alkazaleh F, Geary M, Kingdom J, et al: Elective non-removal of the placenta and prophylactic uterine artery embolization postpartum as a diagnostic imaging approach for the management of placenta percreta: A case report. J Obstet Gynaecol Can 26:743–746, 2004.

56. Clement D, Kayem G, Cabrol D: Conservative treatment of placenta percreta: A safe alternative. Eur J Obstet Gynecol Reprod Biol 114:108–109, 2004.

57. Henrich W, Fuchs I, Ehrenstein T, et al: Antenatal diagnosis of placenta percreta with planned in situ retention and methotrexate therapy in a woman infected with HIV. Ultrasound Obstet Gynecol 20:90–93, 2002.

58. Butt K, Gagnon A, Delisle MF: Failure of methotrexate and internal iliac balloon catheterization to manage placenta percreta. Obstet Gynecol 99:981–982, 2002.

59. Barbui T, Finazzi G, Falanga A: The impact of all-trans-retinoic acid on the coagulopathy of acute promyelocytic leukemia. Blood 91:3093–3102, 1998.

60. Sanz MA, Tallman MS, Lo-Coco F: Tricks of the trade for the appropriate management of newly diagnosed acute promyelocytic leukemia. Blood 105:3019–3025, 2005.

61. Kwann HC, Wang J, Boggio LN: Abnormalities in hemostasis in acute promyelocytic leukemia. Hematol Oncol 20:33–41, 2002.

62. Ohno R, Asou N, Ohnishi K: Treatment of acute promyelocytic leukemia: Strategy toward further increase of cure rate. Leukemia 17:1454–1463, 2003.

63. Bick RL: Disseminated intravascular coagulation: Pathophysiological mechanisms and manifestations. Semin Thromb Hemost 24:3–18, 1998.

64. Reister F, Heyl W, Rath W: Coagulation disorders in pregnancy. Biomed Prog 10:62–67, 1997.

65. Wada H, Wakita Y, Nakase T, et al: Outcome of disseminated intravascular coagulation in relation to the score when treatment was begun. Thromb Haemost 74:848–852, 1995.

66. Mammen EF: The haematological manifestations of sepsis. J Antimicrob Chemother 41:17–24, 1998.

67. Taylor FB Jr, Toh C-H, Hoots WK, et al: Towards definition, clinical and laboratory criteria, and a scoring system for disseminated intravascular coagulation. Thromb Haemost 86:1327–1330, 2001.

67a. Toh CH, Hoots WK, on behalf of the SSC on Disseminated Intravascular Coagulation of the ISTH: The scoring system of the scientific and standardisation committee on disseminated intravascular coagulation of the international society on thrombosis and haemostasis: A 5-year overview. J Thromb Haemost 5:604–606, 2007.

68. Ben-Ari Z, Osman E, Hutton RA, et al: Disseminated intravascular coagulation in liver cirrhosis: Fact or fiction? Am J Gastroenterol 94:2977–2982, 1999.

69. Kitchens CS: To bleed or not to bleed? Is that the question for the PTT? J Thromb Haemost 3:2605–2611, 2005.

70. Hardy JF, De Moerloose P, Samama M, et al: Massive transfusion and coagulopathy: Pathophysiology and implications for clinical management. Can J Anaesth 51:293–310, 2004.

71. Cosgriff N, Moore EE, Sauaia A, et al: Predicting life-threatening coagulopathy in the massively transfused trauma patient: Hypothermia and acidosis revisited. J Trauma 42:857–861, 1997.

72. MacIntyre L, Hebert PC: To transfuse or not in trauma patients: A presentation of the evidence and rationale. Curr Opin Anesthesiol 15:179–185, 2002.

73. Stone JH: HELLP syndrome: Hemolysis, elevated liver enzymes, and low platelets. JAMA 280:559–562, 1998.

74. Kitchens CS: Thrombotic storm: When thrombosis begets thrombosis. Am J Med 104:381–385, 1998.

75. Egerman RS, Sibai RM: Imitators of preeclampsia and eclampsia. Clin Obstet Gynecol 42:551–562, 1999.

76. Van Dam PA, Renier M, Baekelandt M, et al: Disseminated intravascular coaglation and the syndrome of hemolysis, elevated liver enzymes, and low platelets in severe preeclampsia. Obstet Gynecol 73:97–102, 1989.

77. De Boer K, Buller HR, ten Cate JW, et al: Coagulation studies in the syndrome of haemolysis, elevated liver enzymes and low platelets. Br J Obstet Gynaecol 98:42–47, 1991.

78. Trousseau A: Phlegmasia alba dolens: Clinique Medicale de l'Hotel-Dieu de Paris. The New Sydenham Society 3:94, 1865.

79. Callander N, Rapaport SI: Trousseau's syndrome. West J Med 158:364–371, 1993.

80. Callander NS, Varki N, Mohan LV: Immunohistochemical identification of tissue factor in solid tumors. Cancer 70:1194–1201, 1992.

81. Shigemori C, Wada H, Matsumoto K, et al: Tissue factor expression and metastatic potential of colorectal cancer. Thromb Haemost 80:894–898, 1998.

82. Hickey WF, Garnick MB, Henderson IC, et al: Primary cerebral venous thrombosis in patients with cancer: A rarely diagnosed paraneoplastic syndrome. Am J Med 73:740–750, 1982.

83. Tasi SH, Juan CH, Dai MS, Kao WY: Trousseau's syndrome related to adenocarcinoma of the colon and cholangiocarcinoma. Eur J Neurol 11:493–496, 2004.

84. Ridgon EE: Trousseau's syndrome and acute arterial thrombosis. Cardiovasc Surg 8:214–218, 2000.

85. Alderman CP, McClure AF, Jersmann HP, Scott SD: Continuous subcutaneous heparin infusion for treatment of Trousseau's syndrome. Ann Pharmacother 29:710–713, 1995.

86. Walsh-McMonagle D, Green D: Low-molecular-weight heparin in the management of Trousseau's syndrome. Cancer 80:649–655, 1997.

87. Andreescu AC, Cushman M, Hammond JM, Wood ME: Trousseau's syndrome treated with long-term subcutaneous lepirudin (case report and review of the literature). J Thromb Thrombolysis 11: 33–37, 2001.

88. Bell WR, Starksen NF, Tong S, et al: Trousseau's syndrome: Devastating coagulopathy in the absence of heparin. Am J Med 79:423–430, 1985.

89. Woerner EM, Rowe RL: Trousseau's syndrome. Am Fam Physician 38:195–201, 1988.

90. Meijer K, Smid WM, Geerards S, et al: Hyperfibrinogenolysis in disseminated adenocarcinoma. Blood Coagul Fibrinolysis 9:279–283, 1998.

91. Menell JS, Cesarman GM, Jacovina AT, et al: Annexin II and bleeding in acute promyelocytic leukemia. N Engl J Med 340:994–1004, 1999.

92. Kallis P, Tooze JA, Talbot S, et al: Aprotinin inhibits fibrinolysis, improves platelet adhesion and reduces blood loss. Eur J Cardiothorac Surg 8:315–323, 1994.

93. Boylan JF, Klinck JR, Sandler AN, et al: Tranexamic acid reduces blood loss, transfusion requirements, and coagulation factor use in primary orthotopic liver transplantation. Anesthesiology 85:1043–1048, 1996.

94. Wada H, Mori Y, Okabayashi K, et al: High plasma fibrinogen level is associated with poor clinical outcome in DIC patients. Am J Hematol 72:1–7, 2003.

95. Rangel-Frausto MS, Pittet D, Costigan M, et al: The natural history of the systemic inflammatory response syndrome (SIRS). JAMA 273:117–123, 1995.

96. Gando S, Nakanishi Y, Tedo I: Cytokines and plasminogen activator inhibitor-1 in posttrauma disseminated intravascular coagulation: Relationship to multiple organ dysfunction syndrome. Crit Care Med 23:1835–1842, 1995.

96a. Crawley JT, Lam JK, Rance JB, et al: Proteolytic inactivation of ADAMTS13 by thrombin and plasmin. Blood 105:1085–1093, 2005.

96b. Ono T, Mimuro J, Madoiwa S, et al: Severe secondary deficiency of von Willebrand factor-cleaving protease (ADAMTS13) in patients with sepsis-induced disseminated intravascular coagulation: Its correlation with development of renal failure. Blood 107:528–534, 2006.

97. Wells MJ, Sheffield WP, Blajchman MA: The clearance of thrombin–antithrombin and related serpin–enzyme complexes from the circulation: Role of various hepatocyte receptors. Thromb Haemost 81:325–327, 1999.

98. Minnema MC, Chang CK, Jansen PM, et al: Recombinant human antithrombin III improves survival and attenuates inflammatory responses in baboons lethally challenged with Escherichia coli. Blood 95:1117–1123, 2000.

99. Baudo F, Caimi TK, de Cataldo F, et al: Antithrombin III (ATIII) replacement therapy in patients with sepsis and/or postsurgical complications: A controlled double-blind, randomized, multicenter study. Intensive Care Med 24:336–342, 1998.

100. Inthorn D, Hoffmann JN, Hartl WH, et al: Antithrombin III supplementation in severe sepsis: Beneficial effects on organ dysfunction. Shock 8:328–334, 1997.

101. Wheeler AP, Bernard GR: Treating patients with severe sepsis. N Engl J Med 340:207–214, 1999.

102. Bernard GR, Vincent J-L, Laterre P-F, et al: Efficacy and safety of recombinant human activated protein C for severe sepsis. N Engl J Med 344:699–709, 2001.

103. Saito M, Asakura H, Jokaji H, et al: Recombinant hirudin for the treatment of disseminated intravascular coagulation in patients with haematological malignancy. Blood Coagul Fibrinolysis 6:60–64, 1995.

104. Segal S, Shemesh IY, Blumenthal R, et al: Treatment of obstetric hemorrhage with recombinant activated factor VII (rFVIIa). Arch Gynecol Obstet 268:266–267, 2003.

105. Sallah S, Husain A, Nguyen NP: Recombinant activated factor VII in patients with cancer and hemorrhagic disseminated intravascular coagulation. Blood Coagul Fibrinolysis 15:577–582, 2004.

106. Morenski JD, Tobias JD, Jimenez DF: Recombinant activated factor VII for cerebral injury–induced coagulopathy in pediatric patients: Report of three cases and review of the literature. J Neurosurg 98:611–616, 2003.

Chapter 13

The Cross-Talk of Inflammation and Coagulation in Infectious Disease and Their Roles in Disseminated Intravascular Coagulation

Eefje Jong, MD • Eric C.M. van Gorp, MD • Marcel Levi, MD • Hugo ten Cate, MD

Viral, bacterial, fungal, and parasitic infections may all cause disturbances in hemostasis, which can eventually lead to thrombohemorrhagic complications such as disseminated intravascular coagulation (DIC), hemolytic-uremic syndrome (HUS), thrombotic thrombocytopenic purpura (TTP), or even vasculitis. Symptoms and signs may be absent in cases of subclinical activation of the coagulation cascade, or they may be overt in cases of bleeding, thrombosis, or both.[1] None of the clinical signs and symptoms is pathogen specific, and in general, signs and symptoms depend on the severity of the infection and the response of the host. In this chapter, we discuss general aspects and pathogen-specific aspects of the cross-talk between coagulation and inflammation. We focus on the pathophysiology of Gram-negative sepsis as a prototypic model of an inflammation-coagulation–regulated syndrome. In addition, we discuss recently developed and clinically tested anticoagulants designed to intervene in DIC and sepsis.

DIC is associated with a high rate of mortality in both bacterial and nonbacterial disease; for this reason, the acronym has been referred to as "Death Is Coming."[2,3] According to criteria developed by the International Society for Thrombosis and Haemostasis (ISTH), DIC (see Chapter 12) is "an acquired syndrome characterised by the intravascular activation of coagulation with loss of localisation arising from different causes. It can originate from and cause damage to the microvasculature, which if sufficiently severe, can produce organ dysfunction."[4] One consequence of DIC may indeed be fibrinous occlusion of small and midsize vessels, contributing to multiorgan failure (MOF). Because of consumption of coagulation factors and activation of the fibrinolytic system, life-threatening hemorrhage may occur. The severity of bleeding ranges from localized oozing from arterial or venous puncture sites to more systemic complications, such as petechiae, purpura, ecchymosis, intestinal bleeding such as hemoptysis, or frank hematuria. Purpura fulminans is observed in the course of bacterial infection with meningococci and pneumococci, as well as in other bacterial and viral infections.[5] The typical thrombohemorrhagic syndrome described by Waterhouse and Friderichsen in 1911 includes fever, cyanosis, a purpuric rash, and circulatory collapse. Internal bleeding within organs may be confined and asymptomatic but can also cause systemic circulatory failure when localized in critical organs such as the adrenals.

Often, a patient with DIC has microvascular fibrin formation and bleeding at the same time, which hampers the clinician's choice of appropriate treatment.[2,6] Local thromboembolic disease, that is, deep venous thrombosis and pulmonary embolism, may theoretically occur in viral and bacterial infections, particularly in bedridden patients with comorbidity. In a thromboembolism prevention study of low-dose subcutaneous standard heparin for hospitalized patients with infectious diseases, morbidity due to thromboembolic disease was significantly reduced in the heparin group compared with the group that was given no prophylaxis. However, no beneficial effect of prophylaxis was noted on mortality due to thromboembolic complications.[7]

HUS and TTP are regarded as variants of a single syndrome characterized by thrombocytopenia, hemolytic anemia, fever, renal abnormalities, and neurologic disturbances. For a discussion of TTP and HUS, the reader is referred to Chapter 24. Vasculitis is characterized by local or more generalized vascular changes, resulting from ischemia caused by luminal occluding of thrombi of small blood vessels in the upper part of the dermis or bleeding due to local tissue damage (see Chapters 11 and 16).[6,8]

GENERAL ASPECTS OF PRIMARY HEMOSTASIS, COAGULATION, AND FIBRINOLYSIS

The hemostatic mechanism consists of primary hemostasis and coagulation on the one hand, and natural anticoagulant mechanisms and fibrinolysis on the other hand. Under physiologic conditions, these mechanisms are balanced. The tissue factor (TF) pathway is considered to be the main route for activation of the coagulation cascade in sepsis. Initiating factors comprise the membrane-bound glycoprotein TF and plasma protein factor VIIa.[9,10] TF is induced by proinflammatory mediators, including cytokines, C-reactive protein, and advanced glycated end products in circulating blood cells and on microparticle fragments.[11–13] On expression at the cell surface, TF interacts with factor VII in its zymogen or activated form, and the catalytic complex activates factors IX and X, resulting in the generation of thrombin and subsequently fibrin (Fig. 13-1).[14] In contrast to current hypotheses, a recent study indicates that factor XII is not irrelevant for procoagulant activity because platelet-dependent thrombosis is reduced in factor XII–deficient mice.[15] However, in patients with sepsis and other infections, a significant contribution of factor XII in generating fibrin has not yet been proved. A more prominent role of the kinin–kallikrein system relates to regulation of vascular tone and permeability, also through interactions with the complement system.[16] In addition, factor XII is an activator of fibrinolysis, which also may be relevant in infectious disease, but not much is known yet about its particular functions.[17]

Coagulation is balanced by different inhibitory mechanisms. The first mechanism is made up of circulating inhibitors of blood coagulation (e.g., antithrombin III [ATIII], proteins C [PC] and S, and the TF pathway inhibitor [TFPI]). A second inhibitory mechanism consists of the glycocalyx-associated glycosaminoglycans such as heparan sulfate, endothelial protein C receptor (EPCR), and thrombomodulin (TM), all of which facilitate the inhibitory activity of ATIII and activated protein C (APC).[18] The third mechanism, fibrinolysis, may be activated primarily and thus independently of activation of the coagulation cascade, or secondarily in response to fibrin formation. It is activated by tissue plasminogen activator (tPA) and urokinase-type plaminogen activator (uPA) after their synthesis and release from the endothelial cell. These activators initiate the conversion of plasminogen to plasmin, which hydrolyzes polymerized fibrin strands into soluble fibrin degradation products. An important inhibitor of this

system is plasminogen activator inhibitor-1 (PAI-1). Severe infections result in an imbalance between primary hemostasis and coagulation with anticoagulant mechanisms and fibrinolysis, as is explained later.[19] During these events, endothelial cells at the tissue–blood interface become of crucial importance.

ENDOTHELIAL ACTIVATION AND ITS EFFECTS ON COAGULATION DURING INFLAMMATION

Vascular endothelial cells play a central role in all mechanisms that contribute to inflammation-induced activation of coagulation. During acute infection, the endothelium is activated by pathogens or indirectly via inflammatory mediators, and the major regulatory antithrombotic properties become inactivated (Fig. 13-2).[18,20,21] Proinflammatory cytokines, including interleukin (IL)-1,[22,23] tumor necrosis factor (TNF)-α and IL-6,[24] induce TF within endothelial cells, which may be shed in part as soluble TF.[25] Shedding of soluble TF may perhaps explain why it has been difficult to detect endothelial TF by immunohistochemistry in animal studies.[26] The same proinflammatory cytokines appear to downregulate the anticoagulant receptors TM and EPCR, as well as cellular glycosaminoglycans.[27] Proteolytic cleavage of the receptors TM and EPCR may also occur owing to enzymes such as elastase, which are secreted by activated neutrophils. Soluble TF probably does not activate clotting,[28] and soluble TM may continue to function as a cofactor for activation of thrombin activatable fibrinolytic inhibitor (TAFI), which would slow down fibrinolysis and worsen DIC.[29] Given interactions with inflammation (see later), it is also most likely that loss of TM and EPCR from the cell surface, such as has been demonstrated in the microvasculature of patients with sepsis,[30] leads to enhanced inflammatory

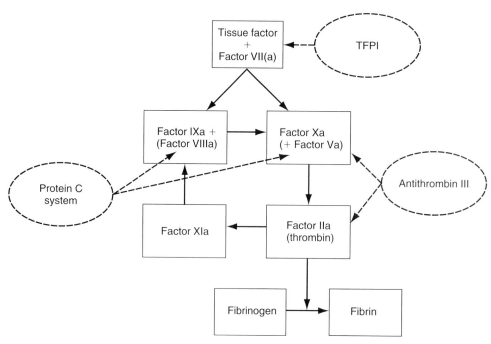

Figure 13–1 The core of the coagulation cascade related to fibrin formation and the three major natural anticoagulant pathways (*dotted ovals*).

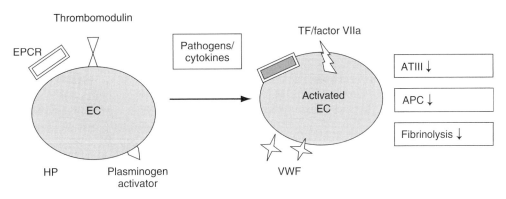

Figure 13–2 Endothelial cell and infection. Under normal conditions, endothelial cells (EC) contain anticoagulant agents, such as thrombomodulin, heparan sulfate (HP), and plasminogen activator. Stimulation by pathogens and/or cytokines activates endothelial cells (EPCR, endothelial protein C receptor). Tissue factor (TF) and von Willebrand factor (VWF) are expressed. Subsequently, the coagulation cascade is activated through the TF pathway, as described in Figure 13-1. Furthermore, normal antithrombotic properties are lost, such as antithrombin III (ATIII), activated protein C (APC), and fibrinolysis. Activation of endothelial cells produces a procoagulant state.[29]

responses in vivo. The net effect of these changes in endothelial cell function likely is of a procoagulant and proinflammatory nature.

TFPI is synthesized and stored in endothelial cells. However, no evidence suggests that depletion or dysfunction of TFPI occurs as part of an infectious disease such as sepsis, and its clinical role in inflammation and infection must be further substantiated.[31–33]

Studies have shown that the PC system is critically important in inflammation and infection.[34,35] On binding, thrombin TM catalyzes PC activation, and APC appears to be a modifier of inflammation, apoptosis, and wound healing,[36–41] although its precise anti-inflammatory actions in vivo remain unclear.[42]

The TM molecule has two properties that differentiate it from PC. First, the lectin-like domain of TM has direct anti-inflammatory properties in mice,[43] not only as an integral part of TM but also as a soluble molecule. Second, TM sequesters high-mobility group B-1 (HMGB-1), providing another anti-inflammatory defense mechanism.[44] EPCR, by it sequence homology with major histocompatibility complex class I (MHC I) CD1, may also play a role in inflammation, but details of this remain unknown.[34] Overexpression of EPCR enhances the level of APC in vivo; such mice are also protected against lipopolysaccharide (LPS).[45]

ATIII directly mediates cellular responses through anti-inflammatory effects that are partly antagonized by heparin (which may explain why patients with sepsis given ATIII did worse in cases of heparin comedication).[34] In septic baboons, high doses of ATIII markedly attenuated proinflammatory activity.[46]

Another important endothelial cell mechanism is provided by cellular protease activated receptors (PARs). These receptors are widely distributed among different cell types, but PAR-1 and PAR-2 are present on endothelial cells.[47,48] Here, these receptors are linked to cell signaling functions that modulate endothelium-dependent relaxation and contraction, angiogenesis, vascular permeability, and expression of P-selectin, intercellular adhesion molecule (ICAM), and vascular cell adhesion molecule (VCAM) on stimulation. Phosphorylation of cellular proteins turns down the expression of the receptor, thus maintaining a regulated level of activity. Thrombin, trypsin, and

APC are agonists of PAR-1,[47,48] and PAR-2 is activated mainly by factors Xa and VIIa (in competition with binding to TF, which also drives cell signaling functions).[49] A recent study comparing the kinetics of PAR-1 cleavage on endothelial cells by APC or thrombin indicates that APC can indeed cleave and activate PAR-1, but it is ≈104-fold less potent than thrombin, and the concentrations required are substantially higher than endogenous APC concentrations in vivo.[50] From this perspective, thrombin seems the preferred agonist of PAR-1 on endothelial cells, potentially regulating a range of cellular functions.[51] Specifically, the activated coagulation system, especially thrombin, can stimulate endothelial cells to express proinflammatory cytokines, such as IL-6, IL-8, and monocyte chemotactic protein-1 (MCP-1).[19,20] Endothelial cells are also able to express adhesion molecules and growth factors that may not only promote the inflammatory response but also increase the coagulation response. Interactions between platelets and endothelial cells, as well as between platelets and neutrophils, are important links in the onset of inflammation. In endothelial cells, the Weibel-Palade body secretes von Willebrand factor and P-selectin, which support platelet rolling. Inflamed endothelium supports leukocyte rolling, and activated platelets in contact with leukocytes and endothelial cells release a number of mediators of the inflammatory response.[52] Such mediators include CD40-ligand, lipoxygenases, prostaglandins, and so forth.

Of potential procoagulant importance are microparticles that are released on activation and apoptosis of cells and that originate from virtually any blood cell.[53] These microparticles have shown procoagulant activity by carrying TF or other enzymes in a number of disease states, including meningococcal sepsis.[13]

COAGULATION AND INFLAMMATORY DISORDERS ASSOCIATED WITH VARIOUS PATHOGENS

Inflammatory Networks in Gram-Negative Sepsis

By definition, sepsis is a systemic inflammatory response syndrome that occurs in a patient with a documented or

13

highly suspected infection (based on culture or Gram stain and/or focus of infection).[54] Although nowadays, most cases of bacterial sepsis are due to Gram-positive microorganisms, most studies of the pathophysiology of infection in relation to coagulation have focused on Gram-negative bacteria. Gram-negative bacteria make and shed an endotoxin, an LPS component of the membrane, which is in large part responsible for the sepsis syndrome. Experimental models of live bacteria or purified LPS have been extensively applied in the study of the mechanisms of sepsis and of the patterns of release of cytokines, coagulation, and fibrinolytic proteins and peptides. Before addressing the relevant outcomes of such model studies, we briefly discuss here the mechanisms involved in Gram-negative sepsis in humans. More extensive reviews on this subject have been recently published.[54–57]

Common Gram-negative bacteria that cause septic shock include opportunistic normal flora of the intestines or genitourinary system such as *Escherichia coli*, *Klebsiella* species, *Enterobacter* species, and *Proteus* species. Other opportunistic Gram-negative pathogens are *Neisseria* species and *Pseudomonas aeruginosa*.[58,59]

Endotoxin plays a pivotal role in development of the sepsis syndrome.[60,61] It can be detected in the blood of patients with Gram-negative sepsis, although this remains technically challenging. In some cases, such as meningococcemia, but also in more "common" infections, a reasonable correlation between plasma levels of endotoxin and outcomes has been described.[62,63]

The introduction of Gram-negative bacteria and LPS into the bloodstream induces a host response through binding of LPS to LPS-binding protein (LBP) that is interacting with the opsonic receptor CD14, which exists in membrane-bound and soluble forms. Cells that do not express CD14 may respond to LPS through the soluble CD14 molecule.[55] The LPS–CD14 complex triggers one of the family of Toll-like receptors (TLRs), of which TLR-4 is most relevant for inducing an array of host response effects. The innate immune response includes the release of inflammation-modulating cytokines (e.g., IL-1, IL-6, IL-8, TNF-α, interferon-β, and IL-10) from activated monocytes and macrophages.

In general, the host response serves to counteract infection; thus, an adequate initial proinflammatory response is critical in combating all infections. Indeed, attempts to counteract specific proinflammatory cytokines such as IL-1 or TNF-α (pneumonia, peritonitis) have been generally disappointing in clinical trials.[57,64] During the recovery phase, anti-inflammatory cytokines are important in limiting inflammatory damage to the host. Hence, the balance between proinflammatory and anti-inflammatory response signals (including cytokine release) is critical to the clinical outcomes of patients with infection.

In sepsis, the early cytokine storm appears within 30 to 90 minutes after LPS exposure. The next phase consists of activation of neutrophils and nitrous oxide, further cytokine release, and the formation of kinins, complement products, and lipid mediators,[55,57] and the tissue response to infection is initiated by the expression of cellular adhesion molecules. An increase in HMGB-1 appears about 24 hours after LPS stimulation and is considered an important "late" mediator of severe sepsis but not of septic shock.[65] This notion raises another important issue, that is, the

difference in immunology between sepsis and septic shock.[54] Sepsis follows a protracted course over several days, and HMGB-1 may have a profound impact on its pathogenesis, contributing to epithelial cell barrier dysfunction and acute cardiac arrest, but without overt pathologic sequelae. In contrast, septic shock is the typical picture dominated by TNF-α, with features of hemorrhagic necrosis in the bowel, inflammation in the kidneys and lungs, and adrenal necrosis. Serum concentrations of TNF-α and HMGB-1 may help to distinguish these features.

Early Events in Sepsis in Relation to Blood Coagulation: LPS Studies

The above scenario of inflammatory response to sepsis is important in appreciating the effects on blood coagulation, which is an evolutionary conserved element of the innate immune system.[34] This means that in cases of invading organisms, whether these are bacteria or viruses, an immediate coagulation response occurs that should assist in limiting morbidity.

Early events after infection are probably mimicked well by the infusion of LPS in volunteers or animals, particularly primates. A single dose of 2 to 4 ng/kg LPS elicits a symptomatic inflammatory and an asymptomatic procoagulant response, the latter characterized by immediate generation of TF mRNA in blood leukocytes (likely mononuclear cells)[66] and exposure of TF to trigger factor (F) X conversion to Xa.[67] Early rises in TNF-α and IL-6 occur at between 30 and 90 minutes, and the early procoagulant response, including generation of FXa, follows the same time course. This phase is followed by a slower, more sustained generation of thrombin, indicated by a rise in prothrombin fragments 1 and 2 (F1+2) and thrombin: ATIII (TAT) complexes in plasma, with a peak at 4 to 6 hours after LPS. A fibrinolytic response also follows a biphasic course, with an early rise in tPA and a subsequent rise in PAI-1, which shuts off fibrinolytic activity in blood. The net result of these reactions contributes to DIC in patients with sepsis.[68] Studies by Taylor and colleagues[69] have further indicated that after a single LPS injection, a sustained response reflecting neutrophil activation (elastase release) and damage of other cell types follows, indicated by increases in soluble fibrin, soluble TM, and soluble TF, and even a rise in lactate that reflects microvascular perturbation during a 48-hour period.[69]

Early and Late Effects Merge in Models of Sepsis and DIC

Animal models have been used to study the kinetics of early hyperinflammatory responses in humans and primates challenged with LPS. To mimic sepsis in a disease-like way, other models are required that more thoroughly reflect the condition wherein bacteria remain present in the circulation for a longer time, or a disease process remains active (such as in models of cecal ligation and puncture, peritonitis, local infection, etc.). Here, we focus on the sepsis model in baboons because this model has been fundamental in the development of the inhibitors APC, TFPI, and ATIII for testing in clinical trials.

In the model originally developed by Hinshaw,[70] live *E. coli* are injected intravenously, targeting reversible (sublethal) or irreversible (lethal) sepsis in a dose-dependent way. In sublethal concentrations, four stages can be distinguished: an inflammatory stage (0–2 hours), a coagulopathic stage (2–6 hours), a cell injury stage (6–10 hours), and a cell degeneration stage (>10 hours).[71] In a lethal (LD100) inoculation of E. coli, the four phases tend to merge in an overwhelming sepsis.

In the baboon model, inhibitors of the TF system (TFPI, anti-TF, FVIIai), PC, and APC, as well as ATIII, each successfully prevented death from sepsis associated with a marked attenuation of systemic inflammation and coagulopathy.[72–74] These studies were fundamental in elucidating the concept that coagulation and its inhibitors are of major importance in coagulation-inflammation cross-talk, as well as in survival from sepsis. Although the limited clinical efficacy of APC appears to support the animal data, other major phase 3 trials with TFPI and ATIII have been disappointing (see later). These negative clinical data also cast doubt on the value of primate models in the study of human sepsis; however, these doubts should not diminish the importance of the fundamental pathways and interactions that have emerged from these animal studies. As outlined by Esmon,[75] a variety of factors differentiate sepsis models in primates from patients with sepsis; the absence of underlying morbidity or comorbidity may be one of the most relevant differences. Although healthy baboons behave similarly to healthy volunteers in showing a hyperimmune response to bacterial challenge, patients often are older with a number of significant comorbid conditions like diabetes, heart failure, and atherosclerosis that may alter the inflammatory response. Another major difference concerns the timing of the intervention in the disease process. Anticoagulant agents with potential anti-inflammatory effects (like APC, ATIII, and TFPI) may benefit patients only during a particular phase of the disease and may even harm those whose inflammatory system should not be impaired.

In this regard, it is also fundamentally important to recognize the fact that many, if not all, coagulation enzymes and inhibitors have a number of often counteracting properties, for instance, thrombin is a potent anticoagulant under normal conditions but also is the most powerful procoagulant in thrombosis. These considerations are vital in a determination of the appropriate timing of interventions in the individual patient; however, at this time, proper laboratory predictors for guiding individual treatment are not available.

GRAM-POSITIVE BACTERIA

The role of Gram-positive bacterial pathogens in the pathogenesis of sepsis has received little attention because these organisms were believed to be quantitatively less important than Gram-negative bacteria. However, recent data indicate that Gram-positive pathogens are increasing in prevalence in septic patients.[54,76–78] Common Gram-positive bacteria that may cause septic shock include Staphylococcus aureus, Streptococcus pneumoniae, Enterococcus species that make up the normal flora of the intestines, and Streptococcus pyogenes. These organisms arise from skin, wounds, or soft tissue structures and catheter sites rather than from enteric or genitourinary sites.

One of the fundamental differences between Gram-positive and Gram-negative bacteria is the way in which they initiate disease. Endotoxin, the sine qua non of Gram-negative bacteria, is not present in Gram-positive bacteria, although the cell wall contains specific components that are able to mimic some of the properties of endotoxin-inducing proinflammatory cytokines from mononuclear cells.[79] It is important to note that Gram-positive bacteria produce exotoxins. Some toxins act locally to help bacteria survive by killing nearby white blood cells. Other toxins help organisms to disseminate in host tissues by degrading the proteins of the connective tissue matrix. Still other toxins diffuse far from the site where they are synthesized.[80]

The mode of action of exotoxin from the clostridial species (gas gangrene, antibiotic-associated colitis), diphtheria (Corynebacterium diphtheriae), food poisoning (Bacillus cereus, S. aureus), and anthrax (Bacillus anthracis) is highly specific and well understood. For Gram-positive bacteria associated with septic shock, however, toxins of a different type seem to be involved. Cases of menstruation-associated staphylococcal infection in healthy women (the staphylococcal toxic shock syndrome) were associated with the production of toxic shock syndrome toxin-1, a so-called superantigen.[81,82] Superantigens do not require previous processing and highly specific presentation by antigen-presenting cells. They are able to activate more lymphocytes than conventionally processed antigens. The peak response to these cytokines occurs 50 to 75 hours after the challenge, in contrast to the 1- to 5-hour response to endotoxin.[83]

Staphylococcal infections usually are localized infections like an abscess, as occurs in furuncles. If the staphylococci spread to the subcutaneous and submucosal tissue, cellulitis may develop. If bacteria sustain the host immune response, they may cause metastatic abscesses in highly vascularized organs like bones, lungs, and kidneys. More severe staphylococcal infections are associated with the production of superantigens. These superantigens may cause purpura fulminans and DIC[84]; a possible mechanism involves the induction of spontaneous platelet aggregation by staphylococcal peptidoglycan.[85] Only rare cases of HUS or TTP associated with staphylococcal infection have been described.[86]

In infection with S. pneumoniae, the main virulence factor and principal antigen is a capsular polysaccharide rather than an exotoxin. The classic manifestation is pneumococcal pneumonia in which bacteremia can be shown in 25% of patients and is indicative of more severe illness. DIC and purpura fulminans have been described in a few case reports.[87] Certain other respiratory pathogens, especially Haemophilus influenzae type b and Klebsiella pneumoniae, also have similar polysaccharide capsular antigens and do not produce exotoxins. Activation of inflammation and coagulation by these organisms also appears to occur through the CD14 mechanism, but less is known about the signal transduction pathways.[83] The tempo of cytokine response is much slower than in Gram-negative infection.[88]

Leptospirosis, especially in those with Weil syndrome, may present with hemoptysis, epistaxis, intestinal bleeding, adrenal hemorrhage, hematuria, and even subarachnoid hemorrhage.[89] The pathogenesis may be primary activation of coagulation or diffuse vasculitis, resulting in bleeding or ischemia of the vascularized tissue.[90,91] TTP, with bleeding as the presenting symptom, may also occur in the course of Weil syndrome.[92]

VIRAL INFECTIONS

Viruses may influence the coagulation system in various ways; one general route of entry for a number of viruses may be provided by invasion of endothelial cells. This has been shown to occur for herpes simplex virus (HSV),[24,93] adenovirus, (para-)influenzavirus, poliovirus, echovirus, measles virus, mumps virus, cytomegalovirus (CMV),[94–98] and human immunodeficiency virus (HIV). Infection of endothelial cells has also been shown for hemorrhagic fever (HF) caused by dengue, Marburg, Ebola, Hantaan, and Lassa HF viruses, which increases the possibility that hemorrhage occurs as the result of endothelial cell activation and enhanced permeation to blood cells, particularly in combination with thrombocytopenia. A procoagulant response may be caused by increased expression of TF and secretion of PAI-1.

Severe coagulation disorders occur in HF.[1] Among the viral HFs, dengue,[90–92] Marburg,[99,100] and Ebola[101–103] are the most prominent, and dengue is the most prevalent. Dengue fever (DF) is a self-limited, non-specific illness characterized by fever, headache, myalgia, and constitutional symptoms caused by the dengue virus (serotypes 1–4). The cardinal feature that differentiates dengue hemorrhagic fever (DHF) from DF is not hemorrhage but increased vascular permeability that results from capillary leakage.[104–106] The underlying mechanisms responsible for bleeding in dengue infection remain poorly understood. Thrombocytopenia is universal in DHF. Platelet function is abnormal with impaired platelet aggregation. Through the capillary leak, plasma levels of coagulation proteins are decreased. Some evidence suggests specific activation of the endothelial cells by dengue virus, which liberates TF, PAI-1, and TM.[107,108] Dengue virus isolates can bind to and activate plasminogen directly and activate fibrinolysis.[109] The plasmin generated can specifically degrade both fibrin and fibrinogen. A possible scenario for the coagulation disorders associated with dengue infection may be that dengue virus primarily activates fibrinolysis in the absence of a thrombotic stimulus, degrading fibrinogen directly and prompting secondary activation of various procoagulant mechanisms. Bleeding in patients with dengue infection may result from a combination of thrombocytopenia, dysfunctional platelets, and increased fibrinolysis.[108] DIC is not frequently encountered in other viral infections but has been found in cases of rotavirus,[110,111] varicella,[112,113] rubella, rubeola, and influenza infections.[113–118]

HIV is associated with both venous and arterial disease.[119] In epidemiologic studies on the occurrence of venous thrombotic disease in HIV-infected patients, the overall risk of venous thrombotic disease may be roughly 2- to 10-fold higher in comparison with a healthy population of similar age. Important risk factors for the development of venous thrombosis in these patients could be severity of HIV infection and the therapeutic introduction of protease inhibitors. Changes in procoagulant and anticoagulant factors, including acquired defects in ATIII and the protein C and S systems, may contribute to a

hypercoagulable state in blood and may explain the apparently increased risk of venous thrombotic disease. Infection with HIV leads to activation of endothelial cells and subsequent expression of TF. Another triggering factor of the coagulation cascade in patients with HIV could be stimulation of microvesicles, small cellular remnants originating from platelets, endothelial cells, and CD4 lymphocytes.[120–129] DIC is only sporadically associated with HIV. HIV infection may also be accompanied by vasculitis syndromes such as polyarteritis nodosa, Henoch-Schönlein purpura, and leukocytoclastic vasculitis.[130–136] Thrombotic microangiopathy, for example, TTP and HUS, has been described in HIV infection.[137–139] Bleeding disorders may occur as the result of thrombocytopenia, a common hematologic complication of HIV infection. The most common cause is now known to be immune thrombocytopenic purpura (ITP).[140] Decreased production owing to megakaryocyte infection is also suggested, as is marrow infiltration by infectious organisms or neoplasms.[141] Adverse drug effects may cause impaired platelet function and thrombocytopenia.[142] The hemophagocytic syndrome is an uncommon complication of HIV infection.[143–145]

Vasculitis is well documented in CMV infection,[146,147] occurring predominantly in the vasculature of the gastrointestinal tract where it causes colitis,[148,149] the central nervous system where it causes cerebral infarction,[150,151] and the skin where it results in petechiae, papular purpura, localized ulcers, or a diffuse maculopapular eruption.[1,152] Hepatitis B and C infections may cause polyarteritis-like vasculitis.[153–155] Parvovirus B19 has been suggested to be associated with vasculitis-like syndromes, including Kawasaki disease, polyarteritis nodosa, and Wegener granulomatosis.[156–158] These associations are also discussed in Chapter 11.

FUNGAL AND PARASITIC INFECTIONS

Data on fungal and parasitic infections are scarce and are limited to smaller studies and case reports. Fungal infections such as systemic candidiasis or aspergillosis are a common major clinical complication in immunocompromised patients and may lead to DIC and the development of MOF.[159,160] The mechanism of activation of the coagulation cascade works through a complex network of proinflammatory and anti-inflammatory cytokines, resulting in deficiencies of ATIII, PC and protein S (PS), and TFPI. Additional inhibition of the fibrinolytic system by elevated plasma concentrations of PAI-1 ultimately may lead to DIC and the development of MOF. Subsequent depletion of clotting factors and platelets also can result in severe hemorrhage.[161–165] *Candida albicans*–derived substances lead to arteritis in an animal model of coronary arteritis.[166]

DIC is seen in less than 5% of patients with severe falciparum malaria.[167] It tends to occur more commonly in patients with cerebral malaria, pregnancy, and secondary bacterial infection. DIC may aggravate the other complications of malaria, including cerebral malaria, renal failure, pulmonary edema, and hemorrhage, and predicts a worse outcome.[168–170]

The presence of low-grade DIC has been described in patients with advanced hepatosplenic schistosomiasis and trypanosomiasis.[171,172]

TREATMENT OF PATIENTS WITH DISSEMINATED INTRAVASCULAR COAGULATION AND INFECTION

The cornerstone in the treatment of patients with hemostatic abnormalities and severe infection, such as sepsis, is the specific use of appropriate antibiotics and control of the infectious source. However, in many cases, additional supportive treatment, aimed at circulatory and respiratory support and replacement of organ function, is required. Coagulation abnormalities may proceed, even after proper treatment has been initiated. In those cases, supportive measures taken to manage the coagulation disorder may be considered and may positively affect morbidity and mortality.[173] Increased insight into the various mechanisms that play roles in the coagulation abnormalities associated with infection has indeed been helpful in the development of such supportive management strategies.

Plasma and Platelet Substitution Therapy

Low levels of platelets and coagulation factors may increase the risk of bleeding. However, plasma or platelet substitution therapy should not be instituted on the basis of laboratory results alone; it is indicated only in patients with active bleeding and in those requiring an invasive procedure or otherwise at risk for bleeding complications.[174] The suggestion that administration of blood components might "add fuel to the fire" has in fact never been proved in clinical or experimental studies. The presumed efficacy of treatment with plasma, fibrinogen, cryoprecipitate, or platelets is not based on randomized controlled trials but appears to represent rational therapy in bleeding patients or in those at risk for bleeding with a significant depletion of these hemostatic factors.[175] It may be necessary to use large volumes of plasma to improve the coagulation defect. Coagulation factor concentrates, such as prothrombin complex concentrate, may overcome this obstacle, but these compounds may lack essential factors, such as factor V. Moreover, in the older literature, caution is advocated with the use of prothrombin complex concentrates in DIC because these may worsen coagulopathy through traces of activated factors in the concentrate. It is, however, not clear whether this is relevant for the concentrates that are currently in use. Specific deficiencies in coagulation factors may be corrected by administration of purified coagulation factor concentrates or, in the case of fibrinogen, cryoprecipitate.

Anticoagulants

Experimental studies have shown that heparin can at least partially inhibit the activation of coagulation in sepsis.[176] Uncontrolled case series in patients with sepsis and DIC have claimed to be successful. However, a beneficial effect of heparin on clinically important outcome events in patients with DIC has never been demonstrated in controlled clinical trials.[177] Also, the safety of heparin treatment is debatable in patients with DIC, who are prone to bleeding. Therapeutic doses of heparin are rational in patients with clinically overt thromboembolism or extensive fibrin deposition, as occurs in purpura fulminans or acral ischemia. Patients with sepsis may benefit from prophylaxis to prevent venous thromboembolism, which may not be achieved with standard low-dose subcutaneous heparin.[178] Theoretically, the most logical anticoagulant agent for use in DIC is directed against TF activity. Potential agents include recombinant TFPI, active site–inhibited factor VIIa, and recombinant NAPc2, a potent and specific inhibitor of the ternary complex between tissue factor/factor VIIa and factor Xa.[179] Phase 2 trials of recombinant TFPI in patients with sepsis showed promising results,[180] but a recently completed phase 3 trial did not show an overall survival benefit in patients who were treated with TFPI.[181] It is interesting to note that in an a priori defined subgroup of patients with an international normalized ratio (INR) <1.2, TFPI treatment was associated with more favorable outcomes.

Restoration of Anticoagulant Pathways

In view of the deficient state of physiologic anticoagulant pathways in patients with sepsis, restoration of these inhibitors may offer a rational approach.[182] Because ATIII is one of the most important physiologic inhibitors of coagulation, and because preclinical results have been successful, the use of ATIII concentrates in patients with DIC has been studied relatively intensively. Most randomized, controlled trials consisted of patients with sepsis, septic shock, or both. All trials showed some beneficial effect in terms of improved laboratory parameters, shortening of the duration of DIC, or even improvement in organ function.[183] In more recent clinical trials, very high doses of ATIII concentrate were used to attain supraphysiologic plasma levels. A series of relatively small trials showed a modest reduction in mortality in ATIII-treated patients[184–186]; however, this effect did not reach statistical significance in any of the trials. A large-scale, multicenter, randomized controlled trial conducted to directly address this issue showed no significant reduction in the mortality of patients with sepsis who were treated with ATIII concentrate.[187] It is interesting to note that post hoc subgroup analyses revealed some benefit in patients who did not receive concomitant heparin, but this observation needs prospective validation.

On the basis of the notion that depression of the protein C system may significantly contribute to the pathophysiology of DIC, supplementation of APC might be beneficial.[188] A beneficial effect of recombinant human APC was shown in two randomized controlled trials. First, in a dose-ranging clinical trial, 131 patients with sepsis were enrolled.[189] Included patients received APC by continuous infusion at doses ranging from 12 μg/kg/hr to 30 μg/kg/hr, or they were given placebo. In accordance with D-dimer plasma levels, the optimal dose of recombinant human APC was determined to be 24 μg/kg/hr. A clear trend toward lower mortality was noted in patients who received higher doses of APC. In these patients, a 40% reduction in relative risk of mortality was shown, although this was not statistically significant (because of the size of the trial). The potential benefit of APC was shown for duration of mechanical ventilation, shock, and length of intensive care unit (ICU) stay, as well as for days free of systemic inflammatory response. A subsequent phase 3 trial of APC concentrate in patients with sepsis was prematurely stopped because of its efficacy in reducing mortality in these patients.[190] All-cause mortality at 28 days after inclusion was 24.7% in the APC group versus 30.8% in the control group (19.4% relative risk reduction). Administration of APC was shown to cause amelioration of coagulation abnormalities; APC-treated patients also had less organ failure.[191] In view of the previously described effects that APC has on inflammation, part of the success may have been caused by a beneficial effect on inflammatory pathways.[192]

A recent analysis of this trial showed that patients who met criteria for DIC, according to the DIC scoring system of the ISTH, received a relatively greater benefit with APC treatment than did patients who did not have overt DIC.[193] Relative risk reduction in mortality of patients with sepsis and DIC who received APC was 38%, in comparison with a relative risk reduction of 18% in patients with sepsis who did not have DIC. This seems to underscore the importance of the coagulation derangement in the pathogenesis of sepsis and the point of impact that restoration of microvascular anticoagulant pathways may provide in the treatment of sepsis. Recombinant human APC has been licensed in most countries for the treatment of patients with severe sepsis and two or more failing organs. The most frequently encountered adverse effect of APC is bleeding. In a phase 3 study conducted in patients with severe sepsis, the incidence of major bleeding (i.e., bleeding reported as a serious adverse event) during the infusion period was 2.4% in the APC group as compared with 1.0% in the control group ($P = .02$).[190] During the 28-day study period, the incidence of major bleeding was 3.5% in the APC group and 2.0% in the placebo group ($P = .06$). Gastrointestinal bleeding was the most frequent bleeding complication in both groups. Most bleeding episodes were procedure related or occurred in patients with a severely deranged coagulation system (partial thromboplastin time [PTT] > 120 sec or INR > 3.0), whereas spontaneous bleeding was rare. Of note, severe thrombocytopenia (i.e., platelet count <50,000/μL) was an exclusion criterion for the trial, but patients with lower platelet counts appeared to benefit more from the administration of APC compared with patients with higher platelet counts. Ongoing studies focus on the concomitant use of heparin in patients given APC and the efficacy of APC in patients with less severe sepsis. Recent data indicate that recombinant APC in patients with severe sepsis but with a low risk of dying (APACHE [Acute Physiology And Chronic Health Evaluation] score <25 or single organ failure) provides no survival benefit over placebo but increases the risk of serious bleeding.[194] Therefore, APC should be considered only in patients with severe sepsis who are also at increased risk of death.

REFERENCES

1. van Gorp EC, Suharti C, ten Cate H, et al: Review: Infectious diseases and coagulation disorders. J Infect Dis 180:176–186, 1999.
2. Levi M, ten Cate H: Disseminated intravascular coagulation. N Engl J Med 341:586–592, 1999.
3. Toh CH, Dennis M: Disseminated intravascular coagulation. Br Med J 327:974–977, 2003.
4. Taylor FBJ, Toh CH, Hoots WK, et al: Towards definition, clinical and laboratory criteria, and a scoring system for disseminated intravascular coagulation. Thromb Haemost 86:1327–1330, 2001.
5. Dempfle CE: Coagulopathy of sepsis. Thromb Haemost 91:213–224, 2004.
6. Ackerman AB, Chongchitnant N, Sanchez J, et al: Inflammatory diseases. In Histologic Diagnosis of Inflammatory Skin Diseases, 2nd ed. Baltimore, Williams & Wilkins, 1997, pp 170–186.
7. Gardlund B: Randomised controlled trial of low dose heparin for prevention of fatal pulmonary embolism in patients with infectious diseases: The heparin prophylaxis study group. Lancet 347:1357–1361, 1996.
8. Lie JT: Vasculitis associated with infectious agents. Curr Opin Rheumatol 8:26–29, 1996.
9. Ruf W, Edgington TS: Structural biology of tissue factor, the initiator of thrombogenesis in vivo. FASEB J 8:385–390, 1994.
10. Mann KG, van't Veer C, Cawthern K, et al: The role of tissue factor pathway in initiation of coagulation. Blood Coagul Fibrinolysis 9 (suppl 1): S3–S7, 1998.
11. Camerer E, Kolsto AB, Prydz H: Cell biology of tissue factor, the principal initiator of blood coagulation. Thromb Res 81:1–41, 1996.
12. Edgington TS, Mackman N, Fan ST, et al: Cellular immune and cytokine pathways resulting in tissue factor expression and relevance to septic shock. Nouv Rev Franc d Hematol 34 (suppl): S15–S27, 1992.
13. Nieuwland R, Berckmans RJ, McGregor S, et al: Cellular origin and procoagulant properties of microparticles in meningococcal sepsis. Blood 95:930–935, 2000.
14. Levi M, ten Cate H, Van der Poll T, et al: Pathogenesis of disseminated intravascular coagulation in sepsis. JAMA 270:975–979, 1993.
15. Renne T, Pozgajova M, Gruner S, et al: Defective thrombus formation in mice lacking coagulation factor XII. J Exp Med 202:271–281, 2005.
16. Shariat-Madar Z, Schmaier AH: The plasma kallikrein/kinin and renin angiotensin systems in blood pressure regulation in sepsis. J Endotoxin Res 10:3–13, 2004.
17. Braat EA, Dooijewaard G, Rijken DC: Fibrinolytic properties of activated FXII. Eur J Biochem 263:904–911, 1999.
18. Wiel E, Vallet B, ten Cate H: The endothelium in intensive care. Crit Care Clin 21:403–416, 2005.
19. Levi M, Keller TT, van Gorp ECM, et al: Infection and inflammation and the coagulation system. Cardiovasc Res 60:26–39, 2003.
20. Aird WC: Vascular bed–specific hemostasis: Role of endothelium in sepsis pathogenesis. Crit Care Med 29:S28–S34, 2001.
21. Keller TT, Mairuhu ATA, de Kruif MD, et al: Infections and endothelial cells. Cardiovasc Res 60:40–48, 2003.
22. Bevilacqua M, Pober J, Wheeler M, et al: Interleukin-1 activation of vascular endothelium: Effects on procoagulant activity and leucocyte adhesion. Am J Pathol 121:394–403, 1985.
23. Schorer A, Kaplan M, Rao G, et al: Interleukin-1 stimulates endothelial cells tissue factor production and expression by a prostaglandin-independent mechanism. Thromb Haemost 56:256–259, 1986.
24. Etingin OR, Silverstein RL, Hajjar DP: Identification of a monocyte receptor on herpes virus-infected cells. Proc Natl Acad Sci USA 88:7200–7203, 1991.
25. Szotowski B, Antoniak S, Poller W, et al: Procoagulant soluble tissue factor is released from endothelial cells in response to inflammatory cytokines. Circ Res 96:1233–1239, 2005.
26. Osterud B, Bjorklid E: The tissue factor pathway in disseminated intravascular coagulation. Semin Thromb Hemost 27:605–617, 2001.
27. Esmon CT: Introduction: Are natural anticoagulants candidates for modulating the inflammatory response to endotoxin? Blood 95:113–116, 2000.
28. Butenas S, Bouchard BA, Brummel-Ziedins KE, et al: Tissue factor activity in whole blood. Blood 105:2764–2770, 2005.
29. Bajzar L, Nesheim M, Morser J, et al: Both cellular and soluble forms of thrombomodulin inhibit fibrinolysis by potentiating the activation of thrombin-activable fibrinolysis inhibitor. J Biol Chem 273:2792–2798, 1998.
30. Faust SN, Levin M, Harrison OB, et al: Dysfunction of endothelial protein C activation in severe meningococcal sepsis. N Engl J Med 345:408–416, 2001.
31. Iversen N, Brandtzaeg P, Sandset PM, et al: TFPI fractions in plasma from patients with systemic meningococcal disease. Thromb Res 108:347–353, 2002.
32. Gando S, Kameue T, Morimoto Y, et al: Tissue factor production not balanced by tissue factor pathway inhibitor in sepsis promotes poor prognosis. Crit Care Med 30:1729–1734, 2002.
33. Creasey AA, Reinhart K: Tissue factor pathway inhibitor activity in severe sepsis. Crit Care Med 29 (7 suppl): S126–S129, 2001.

34. Esmon CT: Interactions between the innate immune and blood coagulation systems. Trends Immunol 25:536–542, 2004.

35. Esmon CT: The protein C pathway. Chest 124 (3 suppl): 26S–32S, 2003.

36. Taylor FB, Kinasewitz G: Activated protein C in sepsis. J Thromb Haemost 2:708–717, 2004.

37. Brueckmann M, Hoffmann U, de Rossi L, et al: Activated protein C inhibits the release of macrophage inflammatory protein-1-alpha from THP cells and from monocytes. Cytokine 26:106–113, 2004.

38. Schoots IG, Levi M, van Vliet AK, et al: Inhibition of coagulation and inflammation by activated protein C or antithrombin reduces intestinal ischemia/reperfusion injury in rats. Crit Care Med 32:1375–1383, 2004.

39. Nick JA, Coldren CD, Geraci MW, et al: Recombinant human activated protein C reduces human endotoxin–induced pulmonary inflammation via inhibition of neutrophil chemotaxis. Blood 104:3878–3885, 2004.

40. Franscini N, Bachli EB, Blau N, et al: Gene expression profiling of inflamed human endothelial cells and influence of activated protein C. Circulation 110:2903–2909, 2004.

41. Jackson CJ, Xue M, Thompson P, et al: Activated protein C prevents inflammation yet stimulates angiogenesis to promote wound healing. Wound Repair Regen 13:284–294, 2005.

42. Dhainaut JF, Yan SB, Margolis BD, et al: Drotrecogin alfa (activated) (recombinant human activated protein C) reduces host coagulopathy response in patients with severe sepsis. Thromb Haemost 90: 642–653, 2003.

43. Conway EM, Van de Wouwer M, Pollefeyt S, et al: The lectin-like domain of thrombomodulin confers protection from neutrophil-mediated tissue damage by suppressing adhesion molecule expression via nuclear factor kappaB and mitogen-activated protein kinase pathways. J Exp Med 196:565–577, 2002.

44. Abeyama K, Stern DM, Ito Y, et al: The N-terminal domain of thrombomodulin sequesters high-mobility group-B1 protein, a novel antiinflammatory mechanism. J Clin Invest 115:1267–1274, 2005.

45. Li W, Zheng X, Gu J, et al: Overexpressing endothelial cell protein C receptor alters the hemostatic balance and protects mice from endotoxin. J Thromb Haemost 3:1351–1359, 2005.

46. Minnema MC, Chang AC, Jansen PM, et al: Recombinant human antithrombin III improves survival and attenuates inflammatory responses in baboons lethally challenged with Escherichia coli. Blood 95:1117–1123, 2000.

47. Hirano K, Kanaide H: Role of protease-activated receptors in the vascular system. J Atheroscler Thromb 10:211–225, 2003.

48. Riewald M, Ruf W: Science review: Role of coagulation protease cascades in sepsis. Crit Care 7:123–129, 2003.

49. Versteeg HH: Tissue factor as an evolutionary conserved cytokine receptor: Implications for inflammation and signal transduction. Semin Hematol 41 (suppl 1): 168–172, 2004.

50. Ludeman MJ, Kataoka H, Srinivasan Y, et al: PAR1 cleavage and signaling in response to activated protein C and thrombin. J Biol Chem 280:13122–13128, 2005.

51. Minami T, Sugiyama A, Wu SQ, et al: Thrombin and phenotypic modulation of the endothelium. Arterioscler Thromb Vasc Biol 24:41–53, 2004.

52. Wagner DD: New links between inflammation and thrombosis. Arterioscler Thromb Vasc Biol 25:1321–1324, 2005.

53. Diamant M, Tushuizen ME, Sturk A, et al: Cellular microparticles: New players in the field of vascular disease? Eur J Clin Invest 34:392–401, 2004.

54. Annane D, Bellisant E, Cavaillon JM: Septic shock. Lancet 365:63–78, 2005.

55. Cohen J: The immunopathogenesis of sepsis. Nature 420:885–891, 2002.

56. Hotchkiss RS, Karl IE: The pathophysiology and treatment of sepsis. N Engl J Med 348:138–150, 2003.

57. Cross AS, Opal SM: A new paradigm for the treatment of sepsis: Is it time to consider combination therapy? Arch Intern Med 138:502–505, 2003.

58. Young LS: Gram-negative sepsis. In Mandell GL, Douglas RG Jr, and Bennett JE (eds): Principles and Practice of Infectious Diseases, 3rd ed. New York, Churchill Livingstone, 1990, pp 611–636.

59. Bone RG: Gram-negative sepsis: A dilemma of modern medicine. Clin Microbiol Rev 6:57–68, 1993.

60. Chaby R: Lipopolysaccharide-binding molecules: Transporters, blockers and sensors. Cell Mol Life Sci 61:1697–1713, 2004.

61. Braude AI: Bacterial endotoxins. In Braude AI (ed): Infectious Diseases and Medical Microbiology, 2nd ed. Philadelphia, WB Saunders, 1986, pp 51–60.

62. Brandtzaeg P, Kerrulf P, Gaustad P, et al: Plasma endotoxin as a predictor of multiple organ failure and death in systemic meningococcal disease. J Infect Dis 159:195–204, 1989.

63. Danner RL, Elin RJ, Hosseini JM, et al: Endotoxemia in human septic shock. Chest 99:169–175, 1991.

64. Polderman KH, Girbes ARJ: Drug intervention trials in sepsis: Divergent results. Lancet 363:1721–1723, 2004.

65. Lotze MT, Tracey KJ: High-mobility group box 1 protein (HMGB1): Nuclear weapon in the immune arsenal. Nature Rev 5:331–342, 2005.

66. Franco RF, de Jonge E, Dekkers PE, et al: The in vivo kinetics of tissue factor messenger RNA expression during human endotoxemia: Relationship with activation of coagulation. Blood 96:554–559, 2000.

67. van der Poll T, Buller HR, ten Cate H, et al: Activation of coagulation after administration of tumor necrosis factor to normal subjects. N Engl J Med 322:1622–1627, 1990.

68. Biemond BJ, Levi M, ten Cate H, et al: Plasminogen activator and plasminogen activator inhibitor I release during experimental endotoxaemia in chimpanzees: Effects of interventions in cytokine and coagulation cascades. Clin Sci (Colch) 88:587–594, 1995.

69. Taylor FB Jr, Wada H, Kinasewitz G: Description of compensated and uncompensated disseminated intravascular coagulation (DIC) responses (non-overt and overt DIC) in baboon models of intravenous and intraperitoneal Escherichia coli sepsis and in the human model of endotoxemia: Toward a better definition of DIC. Crit Care Med 28:S12–S19, 2000.

70. Hinshaw LB: Development of animal models for application to clinical trials in septic shock. Prog Clin Biol Res 308:835–846, 1989.

71. Taylor FB Jr: Staging of the pathophysiologic responses of the primate microvasculature to Escherichia coli and endotoxin: Examination of the elements of the compensated response and their links to the corresponding uncompensated lethal variants. Crit Care Med 29:S78–S89, 2001.

72. Randolph MM, White GL, Kosanke SD, et al: Attenuation of tissue thrombosis and hemorrhage by ala-TFPI does not account for its protection against E. coli: A comparative study of treated and untreated non-surviving baboons challenged with LD100 E. coli. Thromb Haemost 79:1048–1053, 1998.

73. Taylor FB Jr, Emerson TE Jr, Jordan R, et al: Antithrombin-III prevents the lethal effects of Escherichia coli infusion in baboons. Circ Shock 26:227–235, 1988.

74. Taylor FB Jr, Chang A, Esmon CT, et al: Protein C prevents the coagulopathic and lethal effects of Escherichia coli infusion in the baboon. J Clin Invest 79:918–925, 1987.

75. Esmon CT: Why do animal models (sometimes) fail to mimic human sepsis? Crit Care Med 32:S219–S222, 2004.

76. Geerdes HF, Ziegler D, Lode H, et al: Septicemia in 980 patients at a university hospital in Berlin: Prospective studies during four selected years between 1979 and 1989. Clin Infect Dis 15:991–1002, 1992.

77. Bochud PY, Calandra T, Francioli P: Bacteremia due to viridans streptococci in neutropenic patients: A review. N Engl J Med 97:256–264, 1994.

78. Bone RC: Gram-positive organisms and sepsis. Arch Intern Med 154:26–34, 1994.

79. Timmerman CP, Mattsson E, Martinez-Martinez L, et al: Induction of release of tumor necrosis factor from human monocytes by staphylococci and staphylococcal peptidoglycans. Infect Immun 61:4167–4172, 1993.

80. Schaechter M, Medoff G, Eisenstein BI: Mechanisms of Microbial Disease, 3rd ed. Baltimore, Williams & Wilkins, 1993, pp 162–175.

81. Rago JV, Schlievert PM: Mechanisms of pathogenesis of staphylococcal and streptococcal superantigens. Curr Top Microbiol Immunol 225:81–97, 1998.

82. Kotb M: Bacterial pyrogenic exotoxins as superantigens. Clin Microbiol Rev 8:411–426, 1995.

83. Opal SM, Cohen J: Clinical gram-positive sepsis: Does it fundamentally differ from gram-negative bacterial sepsis? Crit Care Med 27:1608–1616, 1999.

84. Kravitz GR, Dries DJ, Peterson ML, et al: Purpura fulminans due to Staphylococcus aureus. Clin Infect Dis 40:941–947, 2005.

85. Kessler CM, Nussbaum E, Tuazon CU: Disseminated intravascular coagulation associated with Staphylococcus aureus septicaemia is mediated by peptidoglycan-induced platelet aggregation. J Infect Dis 164:101–107, 1991.

86. Niv E, Segev A, Ellis MH: *Staphylococcus aureus* bacteremia as a cause of early relapse of thrombotic thrombocytopenic purpura. Transfusion 40:1067–1070, 2000.

87. Carpenter CT, Kaiser AB: Purpura fulminans in pneumococcal sepsis: Case report and review. Scand J Infect Dis 29:479–483, 1997.

88. Andersson J, Nagy S, Bjork L, et al: Bacterial toxin–induced cytokine production studied at the single-cell level. Immunol Rev 127:69–96, 1992.

89. Lecour H, Mirande M, Mavgro C, et al: Human leptospirosis: A review of 50 cases. Infection 17:8–12, 1989.

90. Mairuhu ATA, MacGillavry MR, Setiati TE, et al: Is clinical outcome of dengue-virus infections influenced by coagulation and fibrinolysis? A critical review of evidence. Lancet Infect Dis 3:33–41, 2003.

91. Guzman MG, Kouri G: Dengue: An update. Lancet Infect Dis 2:33–42, 2002.

92. Laing RW, Teh C, Toh CH: Thrombotic thrombocytopenic purpura (TTP) complicating leptospirosis: A previously underscribed association. J Clin Pathol 43:961–962, 1990.

93. Visser MR, Tracy PB, Vercelotti GM, et al: Enhanced thrombin generation and platelet binding on herpes simplex virus–infected endothelium. Proc Natl Acad Sci USA 85:8227–8230, 1988.

94. van Dam-Mieras MCE, Muller AD, van Hinsbergh VWM, et al: The procoagulant response of cytomegalovirus infected endothelial cells. Thromb Haemost 68:364–370, 1992.

95. van Dam-Mieras MCE, Bruggeman CA, Muller AD, et al: Induction of endothelial cells procoagulant activity by cytomegalovirus infection. Thromb Res 47:69–75, 1987.

96. Dudding L, Haskel S, Clark BD, et al: Cytomegalovirus infection stimulates expression of monocyte associated mediator genes. J Immunol 143:3343–3352, 1989.

97. Smith PD, Saini SS, Raffeld M, et al: Cytomegalovirus induction of tumor necrosis factor-α by human monocytes and mucosal macrophages. J Clin Invest 90:1642–1648, 1992.

98. Almeida GD, Porada CD, St. Jeor S, et al: Human cytomegalovirus alters interleukin-6 production by endothelial cells. Blood 83:370–376, 1994.

99. Hayes EB, Gubler DJ: Dengue and dengue hemorrhagic fever. Pediatr Infect Dis J 11:311–317, 1992.

100. Sumarmo DJ, Wultur H, Jahja E, et al: Clinical observations on virologically confirmed fatal dengue infections in Jakarta, Indonesia. Bull World Health Organ 61:693–701, 1983.

101. Kuberski T, Rosen L, Reed D, et al: Clinical and laboratory observations on patients with primary and secondary dengue type I infections with hemorrhagic manifestations in Fiji. Am J Trop Med 26:775–783, 1977.

102. Egbring R, Slenczka W, Baltzer G: Clinical manifestations and mechanism of the hemorrhagic diathesis in Marburg viral disease. In Martini GA Siegert R (eds): Marburg Virus Disease, New York, Springer-Verlag, 1971, pp 41–48.

103. Gear JSS, Cassel GA, Gear AJ, et al: Outbreak of Marburg virus disease in Johannesburg. Br Med J 4:489–493, 1975.

104. Report of the WHO international study team: Ebola hemorrhagic fever in Sudan, 1976. Bull World Health Organ 56:247–270, 1978.

105. Report of the WHO international study team: Ebola hemorrhagic fever in Zaire, 1976. Bull World Health Organ 56:271–293, 1978.

106. Geisbert TW, Young HA, Jahrling PB: Mechanisms underlying coagulation abnormalities in Ebola hemorrhagic fever: Overexpression of tissue factor in primate monocytes/macrophages is a key event. J Infect Dis 188:1618–1629, 2003.

107. Rigau-Perez JG, Clark GC, Gubler DJ, et al: Dengue and dengue haemorrhagic fever. Lancet 352:971–977, 1998.

108. Halstead SB: Antibody, macrophages, dengue virus infection, shock and hemorrhage: A pathogenetic cascade. Rev Infect Dis 11 (suppl 4): S830–S839, 1989.

109. Wills BA, Oragui EE, Stephens AC, et al: Coagulation abnormalities in dengue hemorrhagic fever: Serial investigations in 167 Vietnamese children with dengue shock syndrome. Clin Infect Dis 35:277–285, 2002.

110. Monroy V, Ruiz BH: Participation of dengue virus in the fibrinolytic process. Virus Genes 21:197–208, 2000.

111. Marder VJ, Feinstein DI, Francis CW, et al: Consumptive thrombohemorrhagic disorders. In Colman RW, Hirsh J, Marder VJ, et al (eds): Hemostasis and Thrombosis: Basic Principles and Clinical Practice, 3rd ed. Philadelphia, JB Lippincott, 1994, pp 1023–1063.

112. Limbos MA, Lieberman JM: Disseminated intravascular coagulation associated with rotavirus gastroenteritis: Report of two cases. Clin Infect Dis 22:834–836, 1996.

113. WHO Scientific Working Group: Rotavirus and other viral diarrheas. Bull World Health Organ 58:183–198, 1980.

114. Lee S, Ito N, Inagaki T, et al: Fulminant varicella infection complicated with acute respiratory distress syndrome, and disseminated intravascular coagulation in an immunocompetent young adult. Intern Med 12:1205–1209, 2004.

115. Anderson DR, Schwartz J, Hunter NJ, et al: Varicella hepatitis: A fatal case in a previously healthy, immunocompetent adult. Arch Intern Med 154:2101–2105, 1994.

116. McKay DG, Margaretten W: Disseminated intravascular coagulation in virus diseases. Arch Intern Med 120:129–152, 1967.

117. Linder M, Müller-Berghaus G, Lasch HG, et al: Virus infection and blood coagulation. Thromb Diath Haemorrh 23:1–11, 1970.

118. Talley NA, Assumpcae CAR: Disseminated intravascular clotting complicating viral pneumonia due to influenza. Med J Aust 2:763–766, 1971.

119. Davison AM, Thomson D, Robson JS: Intravascular coagulation complicating influenza A virus infection. Br Med J 1:654–655, 1973.

120. Whitaker AN, Bunce I, Graeme ER: Disseminated intravascular coagulation and acute renal failure in influenza A2 infection. Med J Aust 2:196–201, 1974.

121. Settle H, Glueck HI: Disseminated intravascular coagulation associated with influenza. Ohio State Med J 71:541–543, 1975.

122. Klein SK, Slim EJ, de Kruif MD, et al: Is chronic HIV infection associated with venous thrombotic disease? A systemic review. Neth J Med 63:129–136, 2005.

123. Jenkins RE, Peters BS, Pinching AJ: Thromboembolic disease in AIDS is associated with cytomegalovirus. AIDS 5:1540–1543, 1991.

124. Hassell KL, Kressin DC, Neumann A, et al: Correlation of antiphospholipid antibodies and protein S deficiency with thrombosis in HIV-infected men. Blood Coag Fibrinol 5:455–462, 1994.

125. Howling SJ, Shaw PJ, Miller RF: Acute pulmonary embolism in patients with HIV disease. Sex Transm Infect 75:25–29, 1999.

126. Laing RBS, Brettle RP, Leen CLS: Venous thrombosis in HIV infection. Int J STD AIDS 7:82–85, 1996.

127. George SL, Swindells S, Knudson R, et al: Unexplained thrombosis in HIV-infected patients receiving protease inhibitors: Report of seven cases. Am J Med 107:624–626, 1999.

128. Sullivan PS, Dworkin MS, Jones JL, et al: Epidemiology of thrombosis in HIV-infected individuals. AIDS 14:321–324, 2000.

129. Saif MW, Bona R, Greenberg B: AIDS and thrombosis: Retrospective study of 131 HIV-infected patients. AIDS Patient Care STDS 15:311–320, 2001.

130. Saber AA, Aboolian A, LaRaja RD, et al: HIV/AIDS and the risk of deep vein thrombosis: A study of 45 patients with lower extremity involvement. Am Surg 67:645–647, 2001.

131. Copur AS, Smith PR, Gomez V, et al: HIV infection is a risk factor for venous thromboembolism. AIDS Patient Care STDS 16:205–209, 2002.

132. Fultz SL, McGinnis KA, Skanderson M, et al: Association of venous thromboembolism with human immunodeficiency virus and mortality in veterans. Am J Med 116:420–423, 2004.

133. Libman BS, Quinsmorio FP, Stimmler MM: Polyarteritis nodosa–like vasculitis in human immunodeficiency virus infection. J Rheumatol 22:351–355, 1995.

134. Calabrese LH: Vasculitis and infection with human immunodeficiency virus infection. Rheum Dis Clin North Am 17:131–147, 1991.

135. Gherardi R, Belec I, Mhiri C, et al: The spectrum of vasculitis in human immunodeficiency virus infected patients. Arthritis Rheum 36:1164–1174, 1993.

136. Oehler R: Vaskulitis bei HIV infizierten patienten. Med Klin 15: 327–329, 1993.

137. Gervasoni C, Ridolfo AL, Vaccarezza M, et al: Thrombotic microangiopathy in patients with acquired immunodeficiency syndrome before and during the era of introduction of highly active antiretroviral therapy. Clin Infect Dis 35:1534–1540, 2002.

138. Sahud MA, Claster S, Liu L, et al: Von Willebrand factor–cleaving protease inhibitor in a patient with human immunodeficiency syndrome–associated thrombotic thrombocytopenic purpura. Br J Hematol 116:909–911, 2002.

139. Gruszecki AC, Wehrli G, Ragland BD, et al: Management of a patient with HIV infection–induced anemia and thrombocytopenia who presented with thrombotic thrombocytopenic purpura. Am J Hematol 69:228–231, 2002.

140. Paterson DL, Swindells S, Mohr J, et al: Adherence to protease inhibitor therapy and oucomes in patients with HIV infection. Ann Intern Med 133:21–30, 2000.

141. Zauli G, Catani L, Gibellini D, et al: Impaired survival of bone marrow GPIIb/IIIa+ megakaryocytic cells as an additional pathogenetic mechanism of HIV-1 related thrombocytopenia. Br J Hematol 45:82–85, 1996.

142. Volberding PA, Baker KR, Levine AM: Human immunodeficiency virus hematology. Hematology 294–313, 2003.

143. Fardet L, Blum L, Kerob D, et al: Human herpesvirus 8–associated hemophagocytic lymphohistiocytosis in human immunodeficiency virus–infected patients. Clin Infect Dis 37:285–291, 2003.

144. Castiletti C, Preziosi R, Bernardini G, et al: Hemophagocytic syndrome in a patient with acute human immunodeficiency virus infection. Clin Infect Dis 38:1792–1793, 2004.

145. Chen TL, Wong WW, Chiou TJ: Hemophagocytic syndrome: An unusual manifestation of acute human immunodeficiency virus infection. Int J Hematol 78:450–452, 2003.

146. Golden MP, Hammer SM, Wanke CA, et al: Cytomegalovirus vasculitis: Case reports and review of literature. Medicine 73:246–255, 1994.

147. Ho DD, Rota TR, Andrews CA, et al: Replication of human cytomegalovirus in endothelial cells. J Infect Dis 150:956–957, 1984.

148. Goodman MD, Porter DD: Cytomegalovirus vasculitis with fatal colonic hemorrhage. Arch Pathol 96:281–284, 1973.

149. Foucar E, Mukai K, Foucar K, et al: Colon ulceration in lethal cytomegalovirus infection. Am J Clin Pathol 76:788–801, 1981.

150. Booss J, Dann PR, Winkler SR, et al: Mechanisms of injury to the central nervous system following experimental cytomegalovirus infection. Am J Otolaryngol 11:313–317, 1990.

151. Koeppen AH, Lansing LS, Peng SK, et al: Central nervous system vasculitis in cytomegalovirus infection. J Neurol Sci 51:395–410, 1981.

152. Lin CS, Penha PD, Krishman MN, et al: Cytomeglic inclusion disease of the skin. Arch Dermatol 117:282–284, 1981.

153. Sergent JS, Lockshin MD, Christian CL, et al: Vasculitis with hepatitis B antigenemia. Medicine 55:1–18, 1976.

154. Carson CW, Conn DL, Czaja AJ, et al: Frequency and significance of antibodies to hepatitis C virus in polyarteritis nodosa. J Rheumatol 20:304–309, 1993.

155. Quint L, Deny P, Guillevin L, et al: Hepatitis C virus in patients with polyarteritis nodosa: Prevalence in 38 patients. Clin Exp Rheumatol 9:253–257, 1991.

156. Leruez-Ville M, Laugé A, Morinet F, et al: Polyarteritis nodosa and parvovirus B19. Lancet 344:263–264, 1994.

157. Nikkari S, Mertsola J, Korvenranta H, et al: Wegener's granulomatosis and parvovirus B19 infection. Arthritis Rheum 37:1707–1708, 1994.

158. Yoto Y, Kudoh T, Haseyama K, et al: Human parvovirus B19 infection in Kawasaki disease. Lancet 344:58–59, 1994.

159. Kambayashi J, Ogawa Y, Kosaki G: Fungal sepsis and DIC in surgical patients. Nippon Geka Gakkai Zasshi 84:882–885, 1983.

160. Philippidis P, Naiman JM, Sibinga MS, et al: Disseminated intravascular coagulation in *Candida albicans* septicaemia. J Pediatr 78:683–688, 1971.

161. Pizzo PA: Management of fever in patients with cancer and treatment-induced neutropenia. N Engl J Med 54:6–15, 1993.

162. Rinaldi MG: Invasive aspergillosis. Rev Infect Dis 5:1061–1077, 1983.

163. Young RC, Bennett JE, Vogel CI, et al: Aspergillosis: The spectrum of disease in 98 patients. Medicine 49:147–173, 1970.

164. Vervloet MG, Thijs LG, Hack CE, et al: Derangements of coagulation and fibrinolysis in critically ill patients with sepsis and septic shock. Semin Thromb Hemost 24:33–44, 1998.

165. Grothues F, Welte T, Grote HJ, et al: Floating aortic thrombus in systemic aspergillosis and detection by transoesophageal echocardiography. Crit Care Med 30:2355–2358, 2002.

166. Oharaseki T, Kameoka Y, Kura F, et al: Susceptibility loci to coronary arteritis in animal model of Kawasaki disease induced with *Candida albicans*–derived substances. Microbiol Immunol 49:181–189, 2005.

167. Banzal S, Ayoola EA, El Sammani EE, et al: The clinical pattern and complications of severe malaria in the Gizan region of Saudi Arabia. Ann Saudi Med 19:378–379, 1999.

168. Tanabe K, Shimada K: Incidences of DIC complication in Japanese patients with malaria. Kansenshogaku Zasshi 64:1019–1023, 1990.

169. Takaki K, Aoki T, Akeda H, et al: A case of *Plasmodium vivax* malaria with findings of DIC. Kansenshogaku Zasshi 65:488–492, 1991.

170. Mehta KS, Halankar AR, Makwana PD, et al: Severe acute renal failure in malaria. J Postgrad Med 47:24–26, 2001.

171. Tanabe K: Haemostatic abnormalities in hepatosplenic schistosomiasis mansoni. Parasitol Int 52:351–359, 2003.

172. Robins-Browne RM, Schneider J, Metz J: Thrombocytopenia in trypanosomiasis. Am J Trop Med Hyg 24:226–231, 1975.

173. Levi M: Current understanding of disseminated intravascular coagulation. Br J Haematol 124:567–576, 2004.

174. Alving BM, Spivak JL, DeLoughery TG: Consultative hematology: Hemostasis and transfusion issues in surgery and critical care medicine. In McArthur JR, Schechter GP, Schrier SL (eds): Hematology, 320–341, 1998 (The American Society of Hematology Education Program Book).

175. de Jonge E, Levi M, Stoutenbeek CP, et al: Current drug treatment strategies for disseminated intravascular coagulation. Drugs 55:767–777, 1998.

176. du Toit H, Coetzee AR, Chalton DO: Heparin treatment in thrombin-induced disseminated intravascular coagulation in the baboon. Crit Care Med 19:1195–1200, 1991.

177. Feinstein DI: Diagnosis and management of disseminated intravascular coagulation: The role of heparin therapy. Blood 60:284–287, 1982.

178. Dorffler-Melly J, de Jonge E, Pont AC, et al: Bioavailability of subcutaneous low-molecular-weight heparin to patients on vasopressors. Lancet 359:849–850, 2002.

179. Vlasuk GP, Bergum PW, Bradbury AE, et al: Clinical evaluation of rNAPc2, an inhibitor of the fVIIa/tissue factor coagulation complex. Am J Cardiol 80:66S, 1997.

180. Abraham E, Reinhart K, Svoboda P, et al: Assessment of the safety of recombinant tissue factor pathway inhibitor in patients with severe sepsis: A multicenter, randomized, placebo-controlled, single-blind, dose escalation study. Crit Care Med 29:2081–2089, 2001.

181. Abraham E, Reinhart K, Opal S, et al: Efficacy and safety of tifacogin (recombinant tissue factor pathway inhibitor) in severe sepsis: A randomized controlled trial. JAMA 290:238–247, 2003.

182. de Jonge E, van der Poll T, Kesecioglu J, et al: Anticoagulant factor concentrates in disseminated intravascular coagulation: Rationale for use and clinical experience. Semin Thromb Hemost 27:667–674, 2001.

183. Levi M, ten Cate H, van der Poll T: Disseminated intravascular coagulation: State of the art. Thromb Haemost 82:695–705, 1999.

184. Fourrier F, Chopin C, Huart JJ, et al: Double-blind, placebo-controlled trial of antithrombin III concentrates in septic shock with disseminated intravascular coagulation. Chest 104:882–888, 1993.

185. Eisele B, Lamy M, Thijs LG, et al: Antithrombin III in patients with severe sepsis: A randomized, placebo-controlled, double-blind multicenter trial plus a meta-analysis on all randomized, placebo-controlled, double-blind trials with antithrombin III in severe sepsis. Intensive Care Med 24:663–672, 1998.

186. Baudo F, Caimi TM, de Cataldo F, et al: Antithrombin III (ATIII) replacement therapy in patients with sepsis and/or postsurgical complications: A controlled double-blind, randomized, multicenter study. Intensive Care Med 24:336–342, 1998.

187. Warren BL, Eid A, Singer P, et al: Caring for the critically ill patient: High-dose antithrombin III in severe sepsis: A randomized controlled trial. JAMA 286:1869–1878, 2001.

188. Levi M, de Jonge E, van der Poll T: Rationale for restoration of physiological anticoagulant pathways in patients with sepsis and disseminated intravascular coagulation. Crit Care Med 29 (7 suppl): S90–S94, 2001.

189. Bernard GR, Ely EW, Wright TJ, et al: Safety and dose relationship of recombinant human activated protein C for coagulopathy in severe sepsis. Crit Care Med 29:2051–2059, 2001.

190. Bernard GR, Vincent JL, Laterre PF, et al: Efficacy and safety of recombinant human activated protein C for severe sepsis. N Engl J Med 344:699–709, 2001.

191. Vincent JL, Angus DC, Artigas A, et al: Effects of drotrecogin alfa (activated) on organ dysfunction in the PROWESS trial. Crit Care Med 31:834–840, 2003.

192. Levi M, van der Poll T, Buller HR: Bidirectional relation between inflammation and coagulation. Circulation 109:2698–2704, 2004.

193. Dhainaut JF, Yan SB, Joyce DE, et al: Treatment effects of drotrecogin alfa (activated) in patients with severe sepsis with or without overt disseminated intravascular coagulation. J Thromb Haemost 2:1924–1933, 2004.

194. Abraham E, Laterre PF, Garg R, et al: Drotrecogin alfa (activated) for adults with severe sepsis and a low risk of death. N Engl J Med 353:1332–1341, 2005.

Part III

Thrombotic Processes

Chapter 14

Thrombophilia: Clinical and Laboratory Assessment and Management

John A. Heit, MD

INTRODUCTION

Symptomatic thrombosis is due to dysregulation of the normal hemostatic response to vessel wall "injury" that occurs with exposure to a clinical risk factor (e.g., surgery, trauma, inflammation, hospitalization for acute medical illness). Vessel wall injury may be anatomic (e.g., venous endothelial microtears within vein valve cusps due to stasis, rupture of a lipid-rich atherosclerotic plaque)[1-3] or "nonanatomic" (e.g., cytokine-mediated endothelial expression of adhesion molecules, downregulation of thrombomodulin expression, related to the "acute inflammatory response").[4,5] However, the vast majority of individuals who are exposed to a clinical risk factor do not develop symptomatic thrombosis. We now recognize that clinical thrombosis is a multifactorial (complex) disease that becomes manifest when a person with an underlying predisposition to thrombosis (e.g., a thrombophilia) is exposed to additional risk factors. Emerging evidence suggests that individual variation in the regulation of the procoagulant, anticoagulant, fibrinolytic, and acute inflammation/innate immunity pathways likely accounts for those exposed individuals who actually develop clinical thrombosis.

Thrombophilia is defined as a predisposition or susceptibility to thrombosis. Thrombophilia is not a disease per se, but it may be associated with a disease (e.g., cancer), drug exposure (e.g., oral contraceptives), or a medical condition (e.g., pregnancy, postpartum; "acquired thrombophilia"; Table 14-1); thrombophilia may also be inherited (Table 14-2). This concept is important because disease susceptibility does not imply an absolute requirement for primary or secondary prevention, or for treatment. Most persons with a thrombophilia do not develop thrombosis. Thus, a thrombophilia must be considered in the context of other risk factors for incident thrombosis or predictors of recurrent thrombosis when the need for primary or secondary prophylaxis, respectively, is estimated. With rare exceptions, therapy for acute thrombosis is no different for those with versus those without a recognized thrombophilia.

Thrombophilia may manifest clinically as one or more of several thrombotic disorders ("phenotypes"; Table 14-3). The predominant clinical manifestation of thrombophilia is venous thromboembolism (VTE), the chief components of which are deep vein thrombosis (DVT) and pulmonary embolism (PE).[6,7] Consequently, this chapter focuses on the role of thrombophilia in VTE. In particular, this chapter describes recent comprehensive studies of the epidemiology of VTE that reported racial demography and included the full spectrum of disease that occurred within a well-defined geographic area over time, separated by event type, incident versus recurrent event, and level of diagnostic certainty, as well as studies of VTE recurrence that included a relevant duration of follow-up.

Thrombophilia may also rarely present as purpura fulminans (i.e., neonatalis or adult)[8] or as warfarin-induced skin necrosis.[9-12] Although it is biologically plausible to hypothesize that patients with atherosclerotic arterial occlusive disease and an underlying thrombophilia who experience an atherosclerotic plaque rupture are more likely to develop a symptomatic thrombosis,[13] most clinical studies have failed to show a consistent association between thrombophilia and myocardial infarction or stroke.[14-19] Thrombophilia may also manifest as (recurrent) fetal loss,[20-23] and possibly as stillbirth and complications of pregnancy[24,25] (e.g., intrauterine growth restriction,[26,27] severe preeclampsia,[28] abruptio placentae) (see Chapter 36).

Unfortunately, no single laboratory assay or simple set of assays will identify all thrombophilias. Consequently, a battery of complex and potentially expensive assays is usually required. Many of these laboratory analytes are affected by other conditions (e.g., warfarin reduces protein C and S levels) such that the correct interpretation of results may be complicated and always requires clinical correlation. This chapter addresses several fundamental questions that all clinicians must answer when faced with the task of assessing a person or a patient for a possible thrombophilia. In addition, this chapter addresses how the results of such testing should be interpreted, and how results might alter primary prophylaxis, acute therapy, or secondary prevention of thrombosis. Detailed descriptions of the known thrombophilias are appended, including information on special coagulation laboratory interpretation. Most likely, several thrombophilic disorders have yet to be discovered.

INDICATIONS FOR THROMBOPHILIA TESTING: WHY SHOULD I TEST FOR THROMBOPHILIA?

No absolute indications for clinical diagnostic thrombophilia testing have been determined. Potential relative indications may include general population screening, selected screening of populations that are potentially "enriched" for a thrombophilia(s) (e.g., asymptomatic or symptomatic

Table 14-1 Acquired or Secondary Thrombophilia

Strongly supportive data

Active malignant neoplasm
Chemotherapy (L-asparaginase, thalidomide, antiangiogenesis therapy)
Myeloproliferative disorders
Heparin-induced thrombocytopenia and thrombosis (HIT)
Nephrotic syndrome
Intravascular coagulation and fibrinolysis/disseminated intravascular coagulation (ICF/DIC)
Thrombotic thrombocytopenic purpura (TTP)
Oral contraceptives
Estrogen therapy
Pregnancy/postpartum state
Tamoxifen and raloxifene therapy (selective estrogen receptor modulator [SERM])
Antiphospholipid antibodies (lupus anticoagulant, anticardiolipin antibody, anti–β_2-glycoprotein I antibody)
Paroxysmal nocturnal hemoglobinuria (PNH)
Wegener granulomatosis

Supportive data

Inflammatory bowel disease
Thromboangiitis obliterans (Buerger disease)
Behçet syndrome
Varicose veins
Systemic lupus erythematosus
Venous vascular anomalies (e.g., Klippel-Trénaunay syndrome)
Progesterone therapy
Infertility "therapy"
Hyperhomocysteinemia
Human immunodeficiency virus (HIV) infection
Dehydration
Inappropriate use of erythropoietin

Table 14-2 Hereditary (Familial or Primary) Thrombophilia

Strongly supportive data

Antithrombin III deficiency
Protein C deficiency
Protein S deficiency
Activated protein C (APC) resistance
Factor V Leiden
Prothrombin 20210
Homocystinuria

Supportive data

Increased plasma factors I (fibrinogen), II (prothrombin), VIII, IX, and XI
Hyperhomocysteinemia
Dysfibrinogenemia
Hypoplasminogenemia and dysplasminogenemia
Hypofibrinolysis
Reduced protein Z and Z-dependent protease inhibitor (ZPI)
Reduced tissue factor pathway inhibitor (TFPI)
Sickle cell disease

Weakly supportive data

Tissue plasminogen activator (tPA) deficiency
Increased plasminogen activator inhibitor (PAI-1) levels
Methylene tetrahydrofolate reductase (MTHFR) polymorphisms
Factor XIII polymorphisms
Increased thrombin-activatable fibrinolysis inhibitor (TAFI)

Table 14-3 Thrombophilia: Clinical Manifestations

Purpura fulminans (neonatalis or adult)
Superficial or deep vein thrombosis, pulmonary embolism
Thrombosis of "unusual" venous circulations (e.g., cerebral, hepatic, mesenteric, and renal veins; possibly arm, portal, and ovarian veins)
Warfarin-induced skin necrosis
Possibly arterial thrombosis (e.g., stroke, acute myocardial infarction)
(Recurrent) fetal loss
Possibly intrauterine growth restriction
Possibly stillbirth
Possibly severe gestational hypertension (preeclampsia)
Possibly abruptio placentae

family members of patients with a known familial thrombophilia, especially first-degree relatives) or populations at increased risk for thrombosis (e.g., prior to pregnancy, oral contraception or estrogen therapy, high-risk surgery, chemotherapy with angiogenesis inhibitors), testing of symptomatic patients with an incident thrombotic event (e.g., incident VTE, stillbirth or another complication of pregnancy, incident arterial thrombosis in a young person without other arterial disease), or testing of symptomatic patients with recurrent thrombosis, "idiopathic" thrombosis, thrombosis at a young age (e.g., ≤45 years for venous thrombosis, ≤55 years for arterial thrombosis), or thrombosis in unusual vascular territories (e.g., cerebral vein, portal vein, hepatic vein, mesenteric vein or artery, renal vein) (see Chapter 16). With the exception of general population screening (which is not recommended), all of these potential indications are controversial and must be considered in the context of the clinical presentation.

Counseling and Screening Asymptomatic Family Members

Thrombophilia testing, and especially genetic testing, of asymptomatic family members should be done with caution. Family members (and patients) should first receive genetic counseling and are most appropriately tested only after consent is obtained. Counseling should include the reasons for testing, such as the potential for avoiding clinical thrombosis by risk factor modification or prophylaxis (for the family member and for his or her children), and the reasons for not testing, such as stigmatization and mental anguish,[29] the potential effect on obtaining personal health insurance or employment, and the possibility of nonpaternity.

Thrombophilia testing should be done if the results are likely to change medical management. The risk of idiopathic ("unprovoked") thrombosis associated with thrombophilia, although increased, is still insufficient to warrant chronic primary prophylaxis (e.g., warfarin anticoagulation), even for thrombophilias with high penetrance (e.g., antithrombin III deficiency, homozygous factor V Leiden carriers), with the possible exception of paroxysmal nocturnal hemoglobinuria.[30] Thus, primary "prophylaxis" typically involves avoidance or modification of risk exposure, or prophylaxis when such exposures are unavoidable.

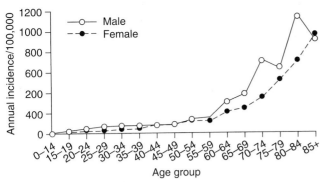

Figure 14-1 Annual incidence of venous thromboembolism by age and sex. Silverstein M, Heit J, Mohr D, et al: Trends in the incidence of deep vein thrombosis and pulmonary embolism: A 25-year population-based, cohort study. Arch Intern Med 158:585–593, 1998.

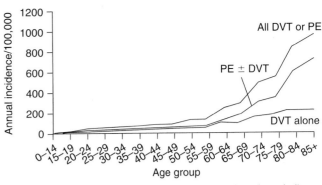

Figure 14-2 Annual incidence of all venous thromboembolism, deep vein thrombosis (DVT) alone, and pulmonary embolism with or without DVT (PE ± DVT) by age. Silverstein M, Heit J, Mohr D, et al: Trends in the incidence of deep vein thrombosis and pulmonary embolism: A 25-year population-based, cohort study. Arch Intern Med 158:585–593, 1998.

When counseling a family member (or patient) regarding the risk of thrombosis associated with a thrombophilia, it is most useful to provide the "absolute" risk (e.g., incidence) of thrombosis among persons with that particular thrombophilia. For example, the relative risk of VTE among heterozygous factor V Leiden carriers who receive oral contraceptives is increased about 30-fold; however, the incidence is only about 300 per 100,000 woman-years, or about 0.3% per woman-year.[31,32] Thus, the absolute risk provides information on both the baseline risk of VTE (e.g., about 10 to 46 per 100,000 woman-years for women of reproductive age[31,33]) and the relative risk (e.g., relative risk [RR] of 30 for women who are factor V Leiden carriers and are taking oral contraceptives).

When the absolute risk of thrombosis is estimated, it is especially important to factor in the effects of age on the baseline incidence of VTE. For example, among women of potentially perimenopausal age (i.e., ages 50 to 54 years), the incidence of VTE is 123 per 100,000 woman-years,[34] and this incidence increases exponentially thereafter (Fig. 14-1). Among women who are factor V Leiden carriers of perimenopausal age, the relative risk of VTE associated with hormone therapy may be increased 7- to 15-fold.[32,35–38] However, although the relative risk for VTE is less with hormone therapy than with oral contraceptives, the absolute risk is substantially higher (e.g., ≈900 to 1800 per 100,000 woman-years, or ≈1% to 2% per woman-year) because of the increased baseline incidence associated with age. Given recent studies questioning the benefit of postmenopausal hormone therapy,[39] most women likely would choose to avoid such therapy if they were known to be carriers of thrombophilia. Thus, it may be relatively cost-effective to perform thrombophilia screening for an asymptomatic perimenopausal or postmenopausal woman with a known history of familial thrombophilia who is considering hormone therapy.[40]

Primary Prevention of Incident Venous Thromboembolism

VTE is a major health problem, with at least 300,000 first-lifetime cases per year reported in the United States.[34,41] Observed survival after VTE is significantly less than expected, especially after PE.[42] For about one quarter of patients with acute PE, the initial clinical presentation is sudden death.

After controlling for other comorbid diseases, survival is significantly reduced for up to 3 months after PE. PE accounts for an increasing proportion of VTE, with increasing age for each sex (Fig. 14-2).[34] Hence, as the average U.S. population age increases, the total number of incident VTE events per year will increase, and an increasing number of these events will be PE. Because of markedly reduced survival after PE, the number of U.S. deaths due to VTE per year also will increase. In addition to reduced survival, VTE and its common complication, namely, venous stasis syndrome, significantly reduce quality of life.[43] VTE patients have a 17-fold increased risk of U.S. venous stasis syndrome.[44] The 20-year cumulative incidence rates of venous stasis syndrome after venous VTE and after proximal deep vein thrombosis are about 25% and 40%, respectively (see Chapter 17).[45,46] Primary prevention of VTE, by risk factor modification or by appropriate prophylaxis of U.S. patients at risk, is essential for improving survival and preventing complications. However, despite improved prophylaxis regimens and more widespread use of prophylaxis, the overall incidence of VTE has been relatively constant at about 1 per 1000 since 1979.[34,41,44,47]

To avoid or modify risk, or appropriately target prophylaxis, patients at risk for VTE must first be identified. In the absence of a central venous catheter or active cancer, the incidence of VTE among children and adolescents is very low (<1 per 100,000 for ages 15 years and younger), and the incidence increases exponentially after age 50 to 55 years to about 1000 per 100,000 for persons who are 85 years of age or older.[34,48–50] The incidence of VTE increases significantly with age for both idiopathic and secondary VTE, suggesting that the risk associated with advancing age may be due to the biology of aging rather than simply to an increased exposure to risk factors due to advancing age.[34,47,51–54] The incidence is slightly higher for women during childbearing years and higher for men after age 50 to 55 years. The incidence of VTE also varies by race. Compared with white Americans, African Americans have a 30% higher incidence, and Asian and Native Americans have up to a 70% lower incidence; Hispanics have an incidence that is intermediate between that of whites and Asian Americans.[51,55–59]

Additional independent risk factors for VTE, as well as the magnitude of risk associated with each, are shown in Table 14-4.[60–65] Compared with residents in the community, hospitalized residents have a greater than 150-fold increased incidence of acute VTE.[44] Hospitalized and nursing home residents together account for almost 60% of all incident VTE events that occur in the community.[61] Thus, hospital confinement provides an important opportunity to significantly reduce VTE incidence. Of note, hospitalization for medical illness and for surgery accounts for almost equal proportions of VTE (22% and 24%, respectively), emphasizing the need to provide prophylaxis to both of these risk groups.

The risk among surgery patients can be further stratified on the basis of patient age, type of surgery, and presence of active cancer.[66,67] The incidence of postoperative VTE is increased for surgical patients who are 65 years of age or older. High-risk surgical procedures include neurosurgery; major orthopaedic surgery of the leg; thoracic, abdominal, or pelvic surgery for malignancy; renal transplantation; and cardiovascular surgery.[67] After controlling for age, type of surgery and type of cancer, additional independent risk factors for incident VTE after major surgery include increasing body mass index, intensive care unit confinement for longer than 6 days, immobility, infection, and varicose veins.[41,68] The risk from surgery may be reduced with neuraxial (spinal or epidural) anesthesia compared with general anesthesia.[69]

Independent risk factors for incident VTE among patients hospitalized for acute medical illness include increasing age and body mass index, active cancer, neurologic disease with extremity paresis, immobility, fracture, and prior superficial vein thrombosis.[41,70,71] Active cancer accounts for almost 20% of incident VTE events that occur in the community.[61] VTE risk among patients with active cancer can be further stratified by tumor site, presence of distant metastases, and whether active chemotherapy is being provided. Although all patients with active cancer are at risk, this risk appears to be greater with pancreatic cancer, lymphoma, malignant brain tumor, cancer of the liver, leukemia, and colorectal and other digestive cancers,[72–74] and in patients with distant metastases.[75] Patients with cancer who are given immunosuppressive or cytotoxic chemotherapy are at even higher risk for VTE,[60,75] including therapy with L-asparaginase,[76] thalidomide[77] and other angiogenesis inhibitors,[78] tamoxifen,[79,80] and erythropoietin.[81]

A central venous catheter or transvenous pacemaker now accounts for about 9% of incident VTE.[61] Unfortunately, neither warfarin nor low molecular weight heparin (LMWH) prophylaxis is effective in preventing catheter-induced thrombosis, and therefore are not recommended.[66] Prior superficial vein thrombosis is an independent risk factor for subsequent DVT or PE remote from the episode of superficial thrombophlebitis (Table 14-4).[60] The risk of DVT imparted by varicose veins is uncertain and appears to be higher among persons younger than 40 years of age.[60] Long haul (>6 hours) air travel is associated with a slightly increased risk for VTE that is preventable with elastic stockings.[82,83] Studies regarding the protective effects of coenzyme A reductase inhibitor (statin) therapy against VTE have provided conflicting results.[84,85] In addition, the risk associated with atherosclerosis or other risk factors for atherosclerosis (e.g., diabetes mellitus) remains uncertain.[86–89] Body mass index, current or past tobacco smoking, chronic obstructive pulmonary disease, and renal failure are not independent risk factors for VTE.[60] The risk associated with congestive heart failure, independent of hospitalization, is low.[60,64]

Among women, additional risk factors for VTE include oral contraceptive use and hormone therapy,[90,91] pregnancy, and the postpartum period.[33,63] The greatest risk may occur during early use of oral contraceptives[92] and hormone therapy.[91] This risk may be less with second-generation oral contraceptives or progesterone alone compared with first- or third-generation oral contraceptives (see Chapter 34).[93,90] For women with disabling perimenopausal symptoms that cannot be controlled with nonestrogen therapy,[35,39,94] esterified oral estrogen or transdermal estrogen therapy may confer less risk than oral conjugated equine estrogen therapy.[95–97] Although VTE can occur at any time during pregnancy,[98] the highest incidence has been noted during the first two postpartum weeks, especially for older mothers.[99] Independent risk factors for pregnancy-associated VTE include tobacco smoking and prior superficial vein thrombosis.[100] Women who are given therapy with the selective estrogen receptor modulators, tamoxifen[80,101–104] and raloxifene,[105,106] also are at increased risk for VTE.

Other conditions associated with VTE include heparin-induced thrombocytopenia, myeloproliferative disorders (especially uncontrolled polycythemia rubra vera and essential thrombocythemia),[80,107,108] intravascular coagulation and fibrinolysis/disseminated intravascular coagulation (ICF/DIC), nephrotic syndrome,[109] paroxysmal nocturnal hemoglobinuria,[30] thromboangiitis obliterans (Buerger disease), plasma exchange for thrombotic thrombocytopenic purpura,[110] Behçet syndrome, systemic lupus erythematosus,[111] Wegener granulomatosis,[112] inflammatory bowel disease,[113] homocystinuria,[114] and possibly, hyperhomocysteinemia.[115–117]

Table 14-4 Independent Risk Factors for Deep Vein Thrombosis or Pulmonary Embolism[60]

Baseline Characteristic	Odds Ratio	95% CI
Hospitalization		
Hospitalization for acute medical illness	7.98	4.49, 14.18
Hospitalization for major surgery	21.72	9.44, 49.93
Trauma	12.69	4.06, 39.66
Malignancy without chemotherapy	4.05	1.93, 8.52
Malignancy with chemotherapy	6.53	2.11, 20.23
Prior central venous catheter or transvenous pacemaker	5.55	1.57, 19.58
Prior superficial vein thrombosis	4.32	1.76, 10.61
Neurologic disease with extremity paresis	3.04	1.25, 7.38
Serious liver disease	0.10	0.01, 0.71

CI, confidence interval.

Heit J, Silverstein M, Mohr D, et al: Risk factors for deep vein thrombosis and pulmonary embolism: A population-based case-control study. Arch Intern Med 160:809–815, 2000.

Recent family-based studies indicate that VTE is highly heritable and follows a complex mode of inheritance involving environmental interaction.[118–120] Inherited reductions in plasma natural anticoagulants (e.g., antithrombin III, protein C, protein S) have long been recognized as uncommon but potent risk factors for VTE.[121–124] More recent discoveries of additional reduced natural anticoagulants[125–130] or anticoagulant cofactors,[131] impaired downregulation of the procoagulant system (e.g., activated protein C resistance, factor V Leiden),[19,99,132,133] increased plasma concentrations of procoagulant factors (e.g., factors I [fibrinogen], II [prothrombin], VIII, IX, and XI)[134–144] and increased basal procoagulant activity,[145–147] impaired fibrinolysis,[148] and increased basal innate immunity activity and reactivity[149,150] have added new paradigms to the list of inherited or acquired disorders that predispose to thrombosis (thrombophilia). These plasma hemostasis-related factors or markers of coagulation activation correlate with increased thrombotic risk and are highly heritable.[118,151–154] Inherited thrombophilias interact with such clinical risk factors (e.g., environmental exposures) as oral contraceptives,[31,92,155] pregnancy,[156] hormone therapy,[36–38] surgery,[157,158] and cancer[159] to compound the risks associated with incident VTE. Similarly, genetic interaction increases the risk of incident venous thromboembolism.[160] Thus, it may be reasonable to consider thrombophilia testing of asymptomatic male and female family members with a known family history of familial thrombophilia.

Secondary Prevention of Recurrent VTE

VTE recurs frequently; about 30% of patients develop recurrence within the next 10 years (Table 14-5).[161] A recent modeling study suggested that more than 900,000 incident or recurrent VTE events occurred in the United States in 2002.[162] The hazard ratio varies with time since the incident event and is highest within the first 6 to 12 months (Fig. 14-3).[161,163] Additional independent predictors of recurrence and the hazard ratio associated with each are shown in Table 14-6; these include male sex,[161,163–165] increasing patient age and body mass index, neurologic disease with extremity paresis, and active malignancy.[45,47,161,166,167] Other predictors of recurrence include "idiopathic" (as opposed to provoked) VTE,[163,168–170] a persistent lupus anticoagulant and/or high-titer antiphospholipid antibody,[168,171] antithrombin III, protein C or protein S deficiency,[124,172] compound heterozygous carriers for more than one familial thrombophilia (e.g., heterozygous for the factor V Leiden and prothrombin 20210 mutations) or homozygous carriers,[173–181] possibly increased procoagulant factor VIII[182] and factor IX[176] levels, decreased tissue factor pathway inhibitor (TFPI) levels,[179] and persistent residual DVT.[183]

Data regarding the risk of recurrent VTE among isolated heterozygous carriers for the factor V Leiden or the prothrombin 20210 mutation are conflicting.[19] In a recent meta-analysis, pooled results from 10 studies involving 3104 patients with incident VTE revealed that the factor V Leiden mutation was present in 21.4% of patients and was associated with a 1.41-fold increased risk for recurrent

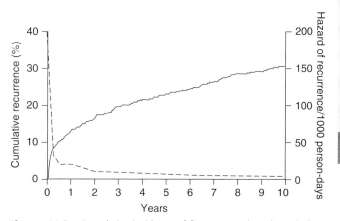

Figure 14-3 Cumulative incidence of first venous thromboembolism recurrence (—) and the hazard of first recurrence per 1000 person-days (- - -). Heit J, Mohr D, Silverstein M, et al: Predictors of recurrence after deep vein thrombosis and pulmonary embolism: A population-based cohort study. Arch Intern Med 160:761–768, 2000.

Table 14-5 Cumulative Incidence and Hazard of Venous Thromboembolism Recurrence[161]

Time to Recurrence	Venous Thromboembolism Recurrence	
	Cumulative Recurrence %	Hazard of Recurrence Per 1000 Person-days (±SD)
0 days	0.0	0
7 days	1.6	170 (30)
30 days	5.2	130 (20)
90 days	8.3	30 (5)
180 days	10.1	20 (4)
1 year	12.9	20 (2)
2 years	16.6	10 (1)
5 years	22.8	6 (1)
10 years	30.4	5 (1)

Heit J, Mohr D, Silverstein M, et al: Predictors of recurrence after deep vein thrombosis and pulmonary embolism: A population-based cohort study. Arch Intern Med 160:761–768, 2000.

Table 14-6 Independent Predictors of Venous Thromboembolism Recurrence[60]

Characteristic	Hazard Ratio	95% CI
Age*	1.17	1.11, 1.24
Body mass index†	1.24	1.04, 1.47
Neurologic disease with extremity paresis	1.87	1.28, 2.73
Active malignancy		
Malignancy with chemotherapy	4.24	2.58, 6.95
Malignancy without chemotherapy	2.21	1.60, 3.06

*Per decade increase in age.
†Per 10-kg/m² increase in body mass index. Heit J, Mohr D, Silverstein M, et al: Predictors of recurrence after deep vein thrombosis and pulmonary embolism: A population-based cohort study. Arch Intern Med 160:761–768, 2000.

VTE (95% confidence interval [CI], 1.14 to 1.75).[184] Similarly, pooled results from nine studies involving 2903 patients revealed that the prothrombin 20210 mutation was present in 9.7% and was associated with a 1.72-fold increased risk of recurrence (95% CI, 1.27 to 2.31). The estimated population-attributable risks for recurrence were 9.0% and 6.7% for the factor V Leiden and prothrombin 20210 mutations, respectively.

An increased D-dimer measured at least one month after warfarin therapy was stopped may be a predictor of DVT recurrence independent of residual venous obstruction.[185,186] Secondary prophylaxis with anticoagulation therapy should be considered for patients with these characteristics. Although the incident event type (DVT vs PE) is not a predictor of recurrence, patients with recurrence are significantly more likely to recur with the same event type as the incident event type.[187,188] Because the 7-day case fatality rate is significantly higher for recurrent PE (34%) than for recurrent DVT alone (4%),[188,189] secondary prophylaxis should be considered for incident PE, especially for patients with chronically reduced cardiopulmonary functional reserve.

DIAGNOSTIC THROMBOPHILIA TESTING: WHO SHOULD BE TESTED?

Current Recommendations

Currently recommended indications for thrombophilia testing include idiopathic or recurrent venous thromboembolism; a first episode of venous thromboembolism at a "young" age (e.g., ≤45 years); a family history of venous thromboembolism (in particular, a first-degree relative with thrombosis at a young age); venous thrombosis in an unusual vascular territory (e.g., cerebral, hepatic, mesenteric, or renal vein thrombosis) (see Chapter 16); and neonatal purpura fulminans or warfarin-induced skin necrosis (see Chapter 11).[17,190–192] When two or more of these thrombosis characteristics are present, the prevalence of at least one of antithrombin III, protein C, or protein S deficiency, as well as the factor V Leiden and prothrombin 20210 mutations, is increased.[193–196] Consequently, a "complete" laboratory investigation (*vide infra*) is recommended for patients who meet these criteria, and more selective testing (e.g., activated protein C resistance/factor V Leiden, prothrombin 20210 mutation) is recommended for other patients (Table 14-7).[191]

However, the prevalence of hereditary thrombophilia (e.g., activated protein C [APC] resistance, factor V Leiden) is substantial among patients with a first-lifetime VTE (Table 14-8). Because knowledge of a hereditary thrombophilia may be important for estimating the risk of VTE recurrence,[184,197] testing for a hereditary thrombophilia should be considered for patients with a first-lifetime thrombosis and should not be limited to patients with recurrent VTE. Moreover, although patients with idiopathic or recurrent VTE may have a higher prevalence of a recognized thrombophilia, these patients should be considered for secondary prophylaxis regardless of the results of thrombophilia testing. In addition, the prevalence of hereditary thrombophilia (e.g., APC resistance) is substantial among patients with a first-lifetime episode of VTE at an older age (see Table 14-8). Therefore, testing for a hereditary thrombophilia should not be limited to patients with a first-lifetime episode of VTE prior to age 40 to 50 years. Although persons with a deficiency of antithrombin III, protein C, or protein S are more likely to experience thrombosis at a younger age,[20] genetic interaction (e.g., factor V Leiden or prothrombin 20210 mutations combined with antithrombin III, protein C, or protein S deficiency) compounds the risk of thrombosis[160,198–201] such that testing among patients with a first thrombosis after age 45 years should not be limited to APC resistance (factor V Leiden) or the prothrombin 20210 mutation.[202]

Recent evidence suggests that a family history of VTE does not increase the likelihood that a recognized familial thrombophilia will be identified.[203] The cumulative lifetime incidence (penetrance) of thrombosis among carriers of the most common familial thrombophilia (factor V Leiden) is only about 10%.[99] Therefore, many patients with VTE with an inherited thrombophilia do not have a family history of thrombosis. Consequently, thrombophilia testing should not be limited to symptomatic patients with a family history of VTE.

The most common manifestation of familial thrombophilia consists of DVT of the leg veins and PE.[7] Except for catheter-induced thrombosis, all VTE is likely associated with an underlying thrombophilia. Therefore, limiting testing to patients with thrombosis in unusual vascular territories will cause most patients with an identifiable familial (or acquired) thrombophilia to be missed.

Several additional issues should be considered when one is addressing the question of whether to perform testing for a possible thrombophilia. For example, the prevalence of hereditary thrombophilia (e.g., factor V Leiden, prothrombin 20210) among patients with VTE differs substantially by race.[204–208] However, the question of whether testing should be modified on the basis of race has not been directly addressed. Factor V Leiden and prothrombin 20210 mutation carrier frequency among asymptomatic African Americans, Asian Americans, and Native Americans, as well as among African Americans with VTE, is extremely low,[207] such that test selection for hereditary thrombophilia likely should be tailored to patient race. The risk of VTE during pregnancy or the postpartum period and the risk of recurrent fetal loss are increased among patients with acquired or hereditary thrombophilia. Women with these obstetric disorders should be tested. Recent evidence suggests that patients who develop acute VTE in the presence of active malignancy are also more likely to have an underlying thrombophilia.[159] Nevertheless, thrombophilia testing for patients with thrombosis associated with active cancer or another risk exposure (e.g., surgery, hospitalization for acute medical illness, trauma, neurologic disease with extremity paresis, upper extremity thrombosis in the presence of a central venous catheter or transvenous pacemaker) is controversial.

Suggested Revised Recommendations

All patients with VTE, regardless of age, sex, race, location of venous thrombosis, initial or recurrent event, or family history of VTE, should be considered for testing for an acquired or hereditary thrombophilia. Women with recurrent fetal loss or complications of pregnancy and patients

Table 14-7   Laboratory Evaluation for Suspected Familial or Acquired Thrombophilia

(Suggested tests to be performed selectively on the basis of clinical judgment)

General

   Blood: CBC, peripheral smear, ESR, chemistries, PSA, β-HCG, CA-125, ANA (dsDNA, RF, ENA)
   PA/lateral CXR, UA, mammogram
   Colon imaging, especially if no prior screening (proctosigmoidoscopy, colonoscopy)
   Chest imaging for smokers (CT, MRI)
   ENT consultation, especially for smokers
   UGI/upper endoscopy
   Abdominal imaging (CT, MRI, ultrasound)
   Angiography

Special Coagulation Laboratory Testing

   Platelets

      HIT testing: plasma anti-PF4/glycosaminoglycan (heparin) antibodies ELISA; platelet ^{14}C-serotonin release assay; heparin-
         dependent platelet aggregation

   Plasma Coagulation

      Prothrombin time, PTT (with phospholipid "mixing" procedure if inhibited)
      Thrombin time/reptilase time
      Dilute Russell's viper venom time (with confirmatory procedures)
      Mixing studies (inhibitors)
      Specific factor assays (as indicated)

   Fibrinolytic System

      Fibrinogen
      Plasma fibrin D-dimer
      Soluble fibrin monomer complex (SFMC)

   Natural Anticoagulant System

      Antithrombin III (activity, antigen)
      Protein C (activity, antigen)
      Protein S (activity, total and free antigen)
      Activated protein C (APC) resistance ratio (second generation; factor V-deficient plasma mixing study)

   Direct Genomic DNA Mutation Testing

      Factor V Leiden gene (depending on the result of the APC resistance ratio)
      Prothrombin 20210

   Additional General Testing

      Anticardiolipin (antiphospholipid) antibodies (immunoglobulin [Ig]G and IgM isotypes); anti-β$_2$-glycoprotein I antibodies
      Plasma homocysteine (basal, postmethionine load)

   Additional Selective Testing

      Flow cytometry for PNH
      Plasma ADAMTS13 activity
      Plasminogen (activity)

CBC, complete blood count; ESR, erythrocyte sedimentation rate; PSA, prostate-specific antigen; β-HCG, β-human chorionic gonadotropin; CA-125, cancer antigen 125; ANA, antinuclear antibody; dsDNA, double-stranded DNA; RF, rheumatoid factor; ENA, extractable nuclear antigen; PA, posteroanterior; CXR, chest x-ray; UA, urinalysis; CT, computed tomography; MRI, magnetic resonance imaging; ENT, ear, nose, and throat; UGI, upper gastrointestinal; HIT, heparin-induced thrombocytopenia; ELISA, enzyme-linked immunosorbent assay; PTT, partial thromboplastin time; PNH, paroxysmal nocturnal hemoglobinuria; ADAMTS13, a *d*isintegrin and *m*etalloproteinase with *t*hrombospondin. subunits.

with unexplained arterial thrombosis also most likely should be tested. These recommendations are controversial and are not universally accepted.

DIAGNOSTIC THROMBOPHILIA TESTING: FOR WHAT SHOULD I TEST?

A complete history and physical examination is mandatory in the evaluation of individuals with a recent or remote history of thrombosis, with special attention given to age at onset, location of prior thromboses, and results of objective diagnostic studies undertaken to document thrombotic episodes. An inquiry regarding interval imaging to establish a new baseline is particularly important when recurrent thrombosis is diagnosed in the same vascular territory as a previous thrombosis. For patients with an uncorroborated history of DVT, noninvasive venous vascular laboratory or venous duplex ultrasound evidence of venous outflow obstruction (e.g., residual vein thrombosis) or (possibly) venous valvular incompetence may be helpful in corroborating the clinical history.

Patients should be questioned carefully about diseases, exposures, conditions, or drugs that are associated with thrombosis (see Tables 14-1 and 14-4). A family history of thrombosis may provide insight for a potential familial thrombophilia, especially in first-degree relatives. Thrombosis may be the initial manifestation of a malignancy, so a complete review of systems directed at symptoms of (occult) malignancy is important, including whether indicated screening tests for normal health maintenance (e.g., mammography, colon imaging) are current. Ethnic background should be considered, given the extremely low prevalence of factor V Leiden and prothrombin 20210 mutations in

Table 14-8 Familial or Acquired Thrombophilia: Estimated Prevalence by Population, and Incidence and Relative Risk of Incident or Recurrent Venous Thromboembolism by Thrombophilia

| Thrombophilia | Prevalence (Whites, %) | | | Incident VTE | | Recurrent VTE | |
	Normal	Incident VTE	Recurrent VTE	Incidence* (95% CI)	Relative Risk (95% CI)	Incidence* (95% CI)	Relative Risk (95% CI)
Antithrombin III deficiency	0.02–0.04	1–2	2–5	500 (320, 730)	17.5 (9.1, 33.8)	10,500 (3800, 23,000)	2.5
Protein C deficiency	0.02–0.05	2–5	5–10	310 (530, 930)	11.3 (5.7, 22.3)	5100 (2500, 9400)	2.5
Protein S deficiency	0.01–1	1–3	5–10	710 (530, 930)	32.4 (16.7, 62.9)	6500 (2800, 11,800)	2.5
Factor V Leiden[†‡]	3–7	12–20	50–50	150 (80, 260)	4.3[‡] (1.9, 9.7)	3500 (1900, 6100)	1.3 (1.0, 3.3)
Prothrombin 20210[†]	1–3	3–8	15–20	350	1.9 (0.9, 4.1)		1.4 (0.9, 2.0)
Combined[§]	-	-	-	840 (560, 1220)	32.4 (16.7, 62.9)	5000 (2000, 10,300)	-
Hyperhomocysteinemia	-	-	-	-	-	-	2.5
Antiphospholipid Ab	-	-	-	-	-	-	2.5
Factor VIII (>200 IU/dL)	-	-	-	-	-	-	1.8 (1.0, 3.3)

*Per 100,000 person–years.
[†]Heterozygous carriers.
[‡]Homozygous carriers relative risk, 80.
[§]Combined factor V Leiden and prothrombin 20210.
VTE, venous thromboembolism; CI, confidence interval; Ab, antibody.

individuals of African American, Asian American, and Native American ancestries.[204-207,209]

The physical examination should include a careful peripheral pulse examination and examination of the extremities for signs of superficial thrombosis or DVT and vascular anomalies, as well as a skin examination for venous stasis syndrome (e.g., leg swelling, stasis pigmentation and/or dermatitis, stasis ulcer), varicose veins, livedo reticularis, skin infarction, or other evidence of microcirculatory occlusive disease. Given the strong association of thrombosis with active cancer, a careful examination for lymphadenopathy, hepatosplenomegaly, and abdominal or rectal mass should be performed, along with breast and pelvic examinations for women and testicular and prostate examinations for men (see Chapter 23).

Laboratory evaluation for individuals with thrombosis should be selective and based on the history and physical examination (see Table 14-7); assessment may include a complete blood count with peripheral smear, serum protein electrophoresis, serum chemistries for electrolytes and liver and renal function, prostate-specific antigen, carcinoembryonic antigen, α-fetoprotein, β-human chorionic gonadotropin (HCG), cancer antigen ([CA]-125), antinuclear antibody (ANA) (double-stranded DNA [dsDNA], rheumatoid factor [RF], extractable nuclear antigen [AUA]), and urinalysis. Elevations in hematocrit or platelet count may indicate the presence of a myeloproliferative disorder, which can be associated with venous or arterial thrombosis. Secondary polycythemia may also provide evidence of an underlying occult malignancy. Leukopenia and thrombocytopenia can be found in paroxysmal nocturnal hemoglobinuria, which is characterized by intravascular hemolysis and thrombotic sequelae. The development of thrombosis and thrombocytopenia concurrent with heparin administration should always prompt consideration of heparin-induced thrombocytopenia (see Chapter 25). The peripheral smear should be reviewed for evidence of red cell fragmentation that would indicate microangiopathic hemolytic anemia, such as occurs with ICF/DIC (see Chapter 12). In individuals with malignancy, chronic ICF/DIC may result in venous or arterial thrombosis. A leukoerythroblastic picture with nucleated red cells or immature white cells suggests the possibility of marrow infiltration by tumor.

A chest x-ray should be performed. More detailed imaging (e.g., chest, abdominal, or pelvic computed tomography [CT] or magnetic resonance imaging [MRI]; angiography) should be performed only if there are other independent reasons to suspect an occult malignancy or other arterial disease (in the case of arterial thrombosis). Routine screening for occult cancer in patients who present with idiopathic VTE has not been shown to improve cancer-related survival and is not warranted in the absence of clinical features and abnormal basic laboratory findings suggestive of underlying malignancy.[210,211] Sputum cytology, an ear, nose, and throat (ENT) examination, and upper gastrointestinal (GI) endoscopy should be considered for tobacco smokers or others at risk for esophageal or gastric cancer. In addition to a Papanicolaou (Pap) smear, endometrial sampling should be considered for women at risk for endometrial cancer.

Recommended assays for initial and reflex special coagulation testing for a familial or acquired condition are provided in Table 14-7. Detailed discussions regarding the interpretation and nuances of specific assays are provided at the end of this chapter, along with a description of the biochemistry, molecular biology, and epidemiology of each thrombophilia.

Arterial Thrombosis

Aside from antiphospholipid antibodies (e.g., lupus anticoagulant, anticardiolipin antibody, anti–β_2-glycoprotein I antibodies), heparin-induced thrombocytopenia, myeloproliferative disorders, homocystinuria, and possibly, hyperhomocysteinemia, a familial or acquired thrombophilia appears to be an unusual cause of stroke, myocardial infarction, or other organ or skin infarction.[17,192] A young patient with organ or skin infarction in the absence of one of the previously mentioned disorders, or with no risk factors for atherosclerosis (e.g., diabetes mellitus, hypertension, hyperlipidemia, cocaine or tobacco exposure) or cardioembolism (e.g., cardiac arrhythmia, patent foramen ovale), should be carefully evaluated for "esoteric" or occult arterial disease (Table 14-9). One should not conclude that organ infarction must be due to a "hypercoagulable disorder" simply because the patient is young or lacks common risk factors for atherosclerosis or arterial thromboembolism. A detailed inquiry into constitutional or specific symptoms of vasculitis (primary or secondary), infection (systemic [e.g., endocarditis] or local [e.g., infected aneurysm with artery-to-artery embolism), atheroembolism, trauma (accidental, thermal, or occupational), dissection, vasospasm, or vascular anomaly is required. In addition to a careful pulse examination (including examination for aneurysmal disease), evidence of microcirculatory

Table 14-9 "Esoteric" Causes of Arterial Thrombosis

Cardioembolism (e.g., atrial fibrillation, left ventricular or atrial septal aneurysm, endocarditis [infectious or noninfectious], atrial septal defect [ASD] or patent foramen ovale [PFO] with "paradoxical" embolism, cardiac tumors)
Artery-to-artery embolism (thromboembolism, cholesterol, tumor, infection)
Arterial dissection (large and small vessels)
Fibromuscular dysplasia (cervical and renal arteries)
Cystic adventitial disease
Arterial aneurysmal disease with thrombosis in situ
Trauma
Arterial entrapment (e.g., thoracic outlet syndrome, popliteal entrapment, common femoral entrapment at the inguinal ligament)
Vasculitis (primary or secondary)
Thromboangiitis obliterans
Arterial wall infection
Vasospasm
Vascular tumors
Vascular anomalies
Thermal injury (erythromelalgia, pernio [chilblains], frostbite)
Occupational trauma (e.g., hypothenar hammer hand syndrome)
Hyperviscosity syndromes
Cold agglutinins
Cryoglobulinemia
Cocaine abuse

occlusive disease of the hand (e.g., livedo, skin or nail bed infarction, ulcer) should prompt a search for endocarditis (infectious and noninfectious), thoracic outlet syndrome, or other causes of repetitive arterial trauma (e.g., hypothenar hammer hand syndrome, "jackhammer" or "volleyball" hand), atheroembolism, and thermal injury. Such physical findings in the foot should involve a similar search plus an evaluation for abdominal aortic or popliteal artery aneurysmal disease with atherothromboembolism or thromboembolism. Fibromuscular disease typically affects the carotid and renal arteries and may manifest as stroke or renal infarct due to carotid and renal artery dissection or embolism, respectively. Because the vascular supply to the organs cannot be directly palpated or observed, arteriography is required to evaluate organ infarction.

In general, duplex ultrasonography and CT or MRI angiography do not provide sufficient resolution to exclude these arteriopathies, with the exception of carotid artery disease. Contrast arteriography should be performed by a vascular physician (i.e., vascular radiologist, vascular surgeon, vascular medicine/cardiologist) who is experienced in diagnosing occult vascular disease, including careful and detailed selective arteriography of the involved and upstream vascular territory with selective vasodilator injection and magnified views, where appropriate.

TIMING OF DIAGNOSTIC THROMBOPHILIA TESTING: WHEN SHOULD I TEST?

Many of the natural anticoagulant and procoagulant plasma proteins are acute phase reactants. Acute thrombosis can transiently reduce levels of antithrombin III and occasionally proteins C and S. Consequently, testing should not be performed during the acute phase of thrombosis or during pregnancy. A delay of at least 6 weeks after the acute thrombosis, or after delivery, usually allows sufficient time for acute phase reactant proteins to return to baseline. Heparin therapy can lower antithrombin III activity and antigen levels and may impair interpretation of clot-based assays for a lupus anticoagulant. A delay of at least 5 days after heparin is stopped prior to testing[212] is usually feasible. Warfarin therapy reduces the activity and antigen levels of vitamin K–dependent factors, including proteins C and S. Rarely, warfarin has also been shown to elevate antithrombin III levels into the lower normal range in individuals with a hereditary deficiency.[213] Many authorities recommend delaying testing until the effects of warfarin therapy also have resolved. In those in whom temporary discontinuation of anticoagulation is not practical, heparin can be substituted for warfarin. However, the effects of warfarin on protein S levels may not resolve for up to 6 weeks. Moreover, the clinical decision regarding secondary prophylaxis may depend on the results of special coagulation testing. For these patients, testing for protein C or S deficiency may be done during stable warfarin anticoagulation, with adjustment of protein C and S levels for the warfarin effect by comparison with the levels of other vitamin K–dependent proteins with similar plasma half-lives (e.g., factors VII and II [prothrombin], respectively). If levels of protein C or S are within the normal range, then

the diagnosis of deficiency may be reliably excluded. However, any abnormal result should be confirmed after the patient has been taken off warfarin therapy for a sufficient amount of time to allow warfarin effects to resolve (if possible), or through testing of a first-degree family member. Direct leukocyte genomic DNA testing for factor V Leiden and prothrombin 20210 mutations is unaffected by anticoagulation therapy; such testing can be performed at any time.

DIAGNOSTIC THROMBOPHILIA TESTING: HOW DO I MANAGE PATIENTS WITH THROMBOPHILIA?

Primary Prophylaxis

All patients should receive appropriate antithrombotic prophylaxis when exposed to thrombotic risk factors (e.g., surgery, trauma, hospitalization for acute medical illness; see Table 14-4).[66] Despite accumulating evidence that an underlying thrombophilia increases the risk of clinical thrombosis among individuals exposed to a clinical risk factor, thrombophilia screening for such persons in the absence of a known family history of familial thrombophilia is not recommended at this time.[32] Current recommendations regarding VTE prophylaxis for surgery or hospitalization for medical illness are based solely on clinical characteristics[66]; in general, prophylactic regimens are not altered on the basis of a known inherited or acquired thrombophilia. However, given emerging evidence that a thrombophilia does increase the risk of symptomatic VTE after high-risk surgery,[157,158] in the absence of contraindications, such patients should be considered for a longer duration (e.g., "out-of-hospital") of prophylaxis.[214]

At present, general screening of asymptomatic women for a thrombophilia prior to initiation of oral contraceptive therapy or prior to conception is not recommended. However, it may be appropriate to screen asymptomatic women family members of a proband with a known familial thrombophilia. Anticoagulant prophylaxis is recommended for asymptomatic women with antithrombin III deficiency or homozygosity/double heterozygosity for factor V Leiden and/or prothrombin 20210 mutations during pregnancy and the puerperium (see Chapter 36).

Acute Therapy

In general, patients with a familial or acquired thrombophilia and a first-lifetime VTE should be managed in standard fashion with intravenous unfractionated heparin at doses sufficient to prolong the partial thromboplastin time (PTT) into the laboratory-specific therapeutic range, as referenced to plasma heparin levels (0.2 to 0.4 U/mL using protamine sulfate titration, or 0.3 to 0.7 anti-Xa IU/mL) or with LMWH or fondaparinux (see Chapter 15).[215,216] Among patients with impaired renal function (e.g., creatinine clearance of ≤30 mL/minute), peak LMWH levels (obtained 3 hours after subcutaneous injection) should be monitored and the dose adjusted to maintain a LMWH (anti-Xa activity) level of 0.5 to 1.0 anti-Xa IU/mL. Fondaparinux is not approved for use among patients with renal insufficiency.

Patients with a prolonged baseline PTT due to a lupus anticoagulant likely should be treated with LMWH rather than unfractionated heparin (UFH) because of difficulties associated with use of the PTT for monitoring and adjusting the UFH dose. Patients with acute DVT may be managed as outpatients. However, a brief hospitalization may be appropriate for edema reduction, along with fitting of a 30- to 40-mm Hg calf-high graduated compression stocking for patients with severe edema. Compared with patients with DVT alone, those with PE have significantly worse survival rates. Such patients may need to be hospitalized at least briefly to ensure that they are hemodynamically stable. Hemodynamically stable patients with PE who have normal cardiopulmonary functional reserve may be managed as outpatients with the use of LMWH therapy. Subsequent oral anticoagulation should be adjusted to prolong the international normalized ratio (INR) to a target of 2.5, with a therapeutic range of 2.0 to 3.0. Heparin and oral anticoagulation therapy should be overlapped by at least 5 days (regardless of the INR) and until the INR has been within the therapeutic range for at least two consecutive days. Warfarin therapy for lupus anticoagulant patients should not be monitored with INR point-of-care devices.

Special attention may be required for patients with deficiencies of antithrombin III or protein C. Some patients with antithrombin III deficiency are heparin resistant and may require larger doses of unfractionated heparin to obtain an adequate anticoagulant effect, as measured by the PTT. Antithrombin III concentrate can be used in special circumstances, such as with recurrent thrombosis despite adequate anticoagulation, unusually severe thrombosis, or difficulty achieving adequate anticoagulation.[217] It is also reasonable to treat antithrombin III–deficient patients with concentrate before major surgeries or in unusual obstetric situations when the risks of bleeding from anticoagulation are unacceptable.[218] Antithrombin III concentrate appears to have a low risk of transmitting blood-borne infection and is supplied as 500 IU per 10 mL or 1000 IU per 20 mL. An initial loading dose should be calculated to increase the antithrombin III level to 120%, assuming an expected rise of 1.4%/IU/per kilogram transfused over the baseline antithrombin III level. For example, for a patient with a baseline antithrombin III level of 57%, the calculated dose is $(120 - 57) 1.4 = 45$ IU per kilogram. The dose should be administered over 10 to 20 minutes, and a 20-minute postinfusion antithrombin III level should be measured. In general, plasma antithrombin levels of 80% to 120% can be maintained by administration of 60% of the initial loading dose every 24 hours.

Hereditary protein C deficiency may be associated with warfarin-induced skin necrosis due to a transient hypercoagulable state. Initiation of warfarin at standard doses leads to a decrease in protein C anticoagulant activity to approximately 50% of baseline within the first day. Consequently, treatment with warfarin should be started only after the individual is receiving full therapeutic doses of heparin, and the dose of warfarin should be increased gradually, after starting from a relatively low dose (e.g., 2 mg). Individuals with a history of warfarin-induced skin necrosis may be anticoagulated after receiving a source of exogenous protein C via fresh frozen plasma or an investigational protein C concentrate. This offers a bridge until a stable level of anticoagulation can be achieved.

The total duration of anticoagulation for acute therapy should be individualized in accordance with the circumstances of the thrombotic event. In general, a duration of 3 months appears to be adequate for thrombosis related to transient risk factors,[168,219] and patients with persistent risk factors require at least 3 to 6 months.[168,215,216,219,220]

Secondary Prophylaxis

It is important to make a distinction between acute therapy and secondary prophylaxis. Acute therapy aims to prevent extension or embolism of an acute thrombosis, and it must continue for a sufficient duration of time and intensity to ensure that the acute thrombus has lysed or become organized and the "activated" acute inflammatory/innate immunity system has returned to baseline.[221] As discussed earlier, the most appropriate duration of acute therapy varies among individual patients but probably is between 3 and 6 months.

Beyond about 6 months, the aim of continued anticoagulation is not to prevent acute thrombus extension or embolism but instead to prevent recurrent thrombosis (e.g., secondary prophylaxis). VTE is now viewed as a chronic disease (likely because all such patients have an underlying, if not recognized, thrombophilia) with episodic recurrences.[41,222] All randomized clinical trials that tested different durations of anticoagulation showed that as soon as anticoagulation is stopped, VTE begins to recur.[168,169,219,220,223–227] Thus, anticoagulation therapy does not "cure" VTE.[228] When the full spectrum of venous thromboembolic disease is considered, the rate of recurrence after acute therapy is stopped differs according to the duration of anticoagulation, but this is so because the rate of recurrence varies (decreases, yet the risk curve never becomes "flat") according to (increasing) time since the incident event—not the duration of anticoagulation.[161,166,226]

The decision regarding a recommendation for secondary prophylaxis is complex and depends on estimates of the risk of unprovoked VTE recurrence while the patient is not receiving secondary prophylaxis, the risk of anticoagulant-related bleeding, and the consequences of both, as well as the patient's individual preference.[229] Clinical predictors of VTE recurrence and the hazard ratios associated with each are presented above and in Table 14-6.[161] In addition, a meta-analysis of the relative risks of recurrence associated with a familial or acquired thrombophilia is presented in Table 14-8.[230]

Secondary prophylaxis after a first episode of VTE is controversial and should be recommended only after careful consideration of the risks and benefits. In general, secondary prophylaxis is not recommended after a first-lifetime episode, especially if the event was provoked by a transient (e.g., surgery, hospitalization for acute medical illness, trauma, oral contraceptive use, pregnancy, the puerperium) clinical risk factor.

Secondary prophylaxis may be recommended for idiopathic, recurrent, or life-threatening VTE (e.g., PE, especially in association with persistently reduced cardiopulmonary functional reserve due to chronic cardiopulmonary disease; phlegmasia with threatened venous gangrene; purpura fulminans); persistent clinical risk factors (e.g., active cancer, chronic neurologic disease with extremity paresis, other persistent secondary causes of thrombophilia

14

223

[see Table 14-1])[161,163]; a persistent lupus anticoagulant and/or high-titer anticardiolipin or anti–β_2-glycoprotein I antibody[168,171,231]; antithrombin III, protein C, or protein S deficiency[7,124,172,232]; increased basal factor VIII activity[182] or substantial hyperhomocysteinemia[233]; compound heterozygous carriers for more than one familial thrombophilia (e.g., heterozygous for factor V Leiden and prothrombin 20210 mutations) or homozygous carriers[173–179,181]; and possibly, a persistently increased plasma fibrin D-dimer[186] or residual posttreatment venous obstruction.[183,234] The risk of recurrence among isolated heterozygous carriers for the factor V Leiden or prothrombin 20210 mutations is relatively low and is likely insufficient to warrant secondary prophylaxis after a first-lifetime thrombotic event in the absence of other independent predictors of recurrence.[184] A family history of VTE is not a predictor of an increased risk for VTE recurrence[235] and should not influence the decision regarding secondary prophylaxis. However, the quality of anticoagulation (i.e., time within the therapeutic INR range) during acute therapy is a predictor of the long-term risk of recurrence.[236,237] Because of the high risk of recurrent VTE due to warfarin failure among patients with active cancer, the most recent American College of Chest Physicians (ACCP) Consensus Conference on Antithrombotic and Thrombolytic Therapy recommended LMWH as secondary prophylaxis as long as the cancer remains active.[238,239]

The risks of recurrent VTE must be weighed against the risks of bleeding from anticoagulant (warfarin)-based secondary prophylaxis. The relative risk of major bleeding is increased about 1.5-fold for every 10-year increase in age,[226,230,240–242] and about twofold for patients with active cancer.[167,226,230,238–240] Additional risk factors for bleeding include a history of prior gastrointestinal bleeding or stroke, or one or more comorbid conditions, including recent myocardial infarction, anemia (hematocrit <30%), impaired renal function (serum creatinine >1.5 mg per deciliter),[243,244] impaired liver function, and thrombocytopenia. Moreover, the ability to perform activities of daily living should be considered because of the increased risk of bleeding associated with falls. The patient's prior anticoagulation experience during acute therapy should also be considered; patients with unexplained wide variations in the INR and noncompliant patients likely should not receive secondary prophylaxis. Finally, the method by which the anticoagulation effect of secondary prophylaxis with warfarin will be monitored and the warfarin dose adjusted should be considered; the efficacy and safety of such care, when rendered through an "anticoagulation clinic" or when "self-managed" at home, are superior to those associated with usual medical care.[245–247] With appropriate patient selection and management, the risk of major bleeding can be reduced to 1% per year, or less.[248–250]

Because the risk of VTE recurrence decreases over time since the incident event,[161] because the risk of anticoagulant-related bleeding also may vary over time,[242] and because our knowledge base changes, the indications for secondary prophylaxis must be continually reevaluated; it is inappropriate to simply recommend "lifelong" or "indefinite" anticoagulation therapy.

Common myths and misunderstandings regarding thrombophilia are presented in Table 14-10.

Table 14-10 Thrombophilia Myths and Misunderstandings

In clinical decision making, the presence of an acquired or familial thrombophilia "outweighs" clinical risk factors.

"Negative thrombophilia testing" excludes the presence of an acquired or familial thrombophilia.

Oral contraceptives are contraindicated for women with thrombophilia.

Acute therapy for thrombosis is always different for patients with thrombophilia.

Heparin or warfarin "resistance" must indicate a "hypercoagulable disorder."

Symptomatic patients with thrombophilia require lifelong anticoagulation.

Cerebral, retinal, myocardial, hepatic, splenic, bowel, or renal arterial infarction at a young age must represent a hypercoagulable disorder.

SPECIFIC THROMBOPHILIAS: PRIMARY OR FAMILIAL

Impaired "Natural" Anticoagulant Pathway

Antithrombin III Deficiency

Antithrombin III is a single-chain plasma glycoprotein (432 amino acids; molecular weight [M_r], 58 kDa; plasma concentration, 2.5 μM) that is synthesized in the liver.[251] Antithrombin III is a serine protease inhibitor (SERPIN) that acts as a pseudosubstrate to inhibit factors IIa (thrombin), IXa, Xa, XIa, and XIIa, and kallikrein and plasmin, through covalent binding of Arg393 within the antithrombin III reactive site loop to the serine protease active site. Antithrombin III inhibitory activity is increased approximately 1000-fold by the catalyst, glycosaminoglycan (e.g., heparin). The antithrombin III plasma half-life is 60 to 70 hours, and the thrombin:antithrombin (TAT) complex is cleared by the liver.[252]

The antithrombin III gene is located on the long arm of chromosome 1 (1q23-q25); it contains seven exons (1, 2, 3A, 3B, 4, 5, and 6) that span 13.5 kilobases (kb). Congential antithrombin III deficiency is inherited as an autosomal dominant disorder, with an estimated prevalence of 70 to 160 per 100,000. Antithrombin III has two major active functional sites: the reactive site and the heparin-binding site located at the amino terminus of the molecule. Congenital antithrombin III deficiency can be classified into two general categories. Type I deficiency is characterized by a concordant reduction in antithrombin III function (activity) and protein (antigen) levels to about 50% of normal plasma. Over 80 point mutations, and 9 whole or partial gene deletions (>30 bp) have been described in individuals with type I deficiency.[253] Type II deficiency is characterized by a normal antithrombin III antigen level with reduced activity due to a dysfunctional protein. This category has been further subdivided into three subtypes, depending on the genetic defect: type IIa mutations affect the antithrombin III active site; type IIb mutations involve the heparin-binding site; and type IIc includes a pleiotropic group of 11 distinct mutations near the antithrombin III "reactive loop." Homozygous types I and IIa mutations are embryonically lethal and heterozygous types I and IIa mutations have a higher prevalence of thrombosis compared with heterozygous type IIb mutations. However, homozygous type IIb mutations are not embryonically lethal and may be associated with venous and arterial thromboses.[254] Type IIc mutations also have reduced plasma antigen levels, possibly caused by reduced synthesis and secretion, and increased catabolism.

Functional antithrombin III activity assays use a synthetic peptide that mimics the natural substrate of thrombin, to which is attached a "reporter" group (e.g., para-nitroaniline) that forms a "chromogenic substrate." Cleavage of the specific synthetic peptide by thrombin releases the reporter group, which emits a color (yellow) at a specific light wavelength (405 nm). In this assay, patient plasma (the source of antithrombin III) is incubated with an excess of thrombin and heparin. During the first phase of the reaction, heparin catalyzes the patient antithrombin III to bind and inhibit thrombin in a 1:1 stoichiometry. The remaining "free" thrombin, which is inversely proportional to the patient plasma antithrombin III, is then quantitated through cleavage of the chromogenic substrate. Some assays use inhibition of factor Xa rather than thrombin to decrease potential confounding by heparin cofactor II (which inhibits thrombin but not factor Xa).[255] More recent commercial assays minimize the effects of nonspecific substrate cleavage by other proteases (e.g., plasmin) or the effects of heparin cofactor II by the addition of protease inhibitors (e.g., aprotinin) and the use of bovine thrombin (which is not inhibited by heparin cofactor II), respectively. Antithrombin III antigen levels are typically tested by enzyme-linked immunosorbent assay (ELISA) or latex immunoassay (LIA). The antithrombin III activity and antigen level reference range is about 80% to 130%,[256] although each laboratory should determine its own laboratory-specific reference range according to the methods and equipment used in the laboratory. The typical interassay coefficient of variation (CV) ranges from 3% to 5%, and possibly up to 10%.

Both assays may be affected by such preanalytic variables as hemolysis, lipemia, high hematocrit (>55%), or a clotted sample (as are all "clot-based" coagulation assays). LIAs may be spuriously increased in the presence of high levels of rheumatoid factor or dysproteinemia. Normal antithrombin III activity and antigen levels are unaffected by sex or tobacco use. However, antithrombin III levels are lower in neonates and approach adult levels by about age 1 year; after 1 year of age, levels may be slightly higher than those of adults until about age 16 years.[257] Modest reductions are also found in women on oral contraceptives or estrogen therapy,[258,259] and warfarin therapy may tend to normalize reduced antithrombin III levels.[213] Acquired causes of decreased antithrombin III levels include impaired synthesis (liver disease, malnutrition, premature infancy, inflammatory bowel disease, and burns) and increased consumption (acute thrombosis, heparin therapy, intravascular coagulation and fibrinolysis [ICF/DIC], sepsis, hemolytic transfusion reaction, malignancy, L-asparaginase therapy, and urinary protein loss [nephrotic syndrome]).[260,261] Patients with low antithrombin III levels should have this finding confirmed on a subsequent sample after acquired causes have been excluded. Family studies may also be useful in confirming a diagnosis of congenital antithrombin III deficiency.

Heterozygosity for antithrombin III deficiency can be found in approximately 4% of families with inherited thrombophilia and in 1% of consecutive patients with an initial episode of deep VTE.[6,262] The incidence and relative risk of a first-lifetime (incident) and recurrent venous thromboembolism are presented in Table 14-8.

Protein C Deficiency

Protein C is a vitamin K–dependent plasma glycoprotein that is synthesized in the liver as a single-chain molecule (M_r, 62 kDa).[251] However, most plasma protein C consists of a two-chain molecule (light- and heavy-chain) that results from cleavage at Arg157-Thr158 prior to secretion. The protein C plasma concentration (65 nM) is about 100-fold lower than the antithrombin III plasma concentration (2.5 μM). The protein C plasma half-life is 6 to 7 hours.

Protein C is the zymogen precursor to the serine protease—activated protein C. Protein C is cleaved at Arg169-Leu170 by the thrombin:thrombomodulin complex on the endothelial cell surface (facilitated by endothelial protein C receptor) to form activated protein C. Activated protein C (along with phospholipid, calcium, and its cofactor, protein S) acts as a potent anticoagulant through cleavage/inactivation of factors VIIIa and Va; it thus downregulates the rate of thrombin generation by a huge factor. The protein C aminoterminal light chain (155 amino acids; M_r, 21 kDa) functions in calcium and phospholipid binding, protein C activation, and interaction with protein S; it contains the γ-carboxyglutamic acid (Gla)-rich domain and two epidermal growth factor (EGF)-like domains. The carboxyterminal heavy chain (250 amino acids; M_r, 41 kDa) contains the serine protease catalytic domain. Activated protein C is inhibited by an α_1-proteinase inhibitor (protein C inhibitor-1) and α_2-macroglobulin.

The protein C (PROC) gene is located on the long arm of chromosome 2 (2q13-q14) and contains 9 exons that span 11 kb. Congenital protein C deficiency is inherited as an autosomal dominant disorder but with variable penetrance; more than 160 unique mutations spread throughout the PROC gene have been identified. The estimated prevalence of protein C deficiency ranges from 200 to 400 per 100,000 (see Table 14-8).[263,264] Congenital protein C deficiency is classified as two types. Type I deficiency consists of concordant reduction in protein C activity and antigen level; it accounts for about 75% of all congenital protein C deficiencies. Approximately 60% of type I deficiency mutations are missense mutations that likely cause decreased protein synthesis or intracellular protein degradation. However, type I deficiency also is caused by promoter and 5′-untranslated region mutations that disrupt binding of transcription factors, as well as splice junction and small insertion/deletion mutations that cause premature stop codons. Type II deficiencies are due to missense mutations that cause synthesis of dysfunctional protein C; functional plasma protein C activity is reduced, yet protein C antigen levels are normal. Examples include mutation within the catalytic active site, the Gla domain, and the propeptide cleavage site.

Functional protein C assays may be clot-based or amidolytic; both use the protein C activator, Protac, from the venom of the Southern Copperhead snake (*Agkistrodon contortrix contortrix*) to activate patient protein C. Clot-based assays may be modified PTT- or prothrombin time

(PT)-based, and they determine the patient's (activated) protein C level by measuring prolongation of the clotting time. In contrast, amidolytic assays determine the patient's (activated) protein C level by measuring color from a reporter group (para-nitroaniline) released by cleavage of a synthetic ("chromogenic") peptide substrate. Clot-based protein C activity assays have the potential to detect abnormalities due to mutation within several different protein C domains, as well as factors VIII and V; amidolytic assays detect only mutations within the catalytic active site.[265] However, interfering substances that prolong the baseline clotting time (e.g., heparin, direct thrombin inhibitors, lupus anticoagulant, uremia[266]) may preclude interpretation of clot-based assays, and high factor VIII levels (as occurs with an acute phase reaction) may cause underestimation of protein C activity when measured by PTT-based assays. Finally, most clot-based assays require predilution of the patient's plasma in protein C–deficient plasma to correct for possible protein S deficiency. Neither clot-based nor amidolytic assays measure all functional aspects of protein C, such as the ability of protein C to interact with thrombin, thrombomodulin, phospholipids, or endothelial cell protein C receptor. Consequently, although clot-based assays may have the highest sensitivity in screening patients for hereditary protein C deficiency,[262] most laboratories use an amidolytic assay because it is more reproducible and less susceptible to interfering substances.[267] Rarely, however, some type II protein C deficiencies may have normal amidolytic functional activity and antigen levels but abnormal clot-based functional activity and may be missed.[268] Protein C antigen levels are determined by ELISA, which typically is performed only when protein C activity is reduced.

The normal adult protein C plasma level ranges from about 70% to 140%, but each laboratory must determine its own laboratory-specific reference range. Levels of protein C antigen in the heterozygous deficiency state overlap with those in the normal population, thus making it difficult to define the diagnosis in some patients. In general, antigen levels of 60% to 70% represent borderline values and warrant repeat testing. Protein C antigen levels may also vary according to age. Protein C levels in newborns are 20% to 40% of normal adult levels,[269] and preterm infants have even lower levels.[270] Neonates with significant perinatal thrombosis may have levels suggestive of homozygous deficiency.[271] In adults, protein C levels typically increase by 4% per decade.[264] Adult levels are independent of age and sex but may be higher in postmenopausal women. Acquired reduction in protein C occurs because of decreased synthesis/posttranslational modification (e.g., liver disease, vitamin K deficiency, warfarin therapy) or increased turnover (e.g., acute thrombosis, ICF/DIC, sepsis, impaired renal function, postoperative state, adult respiratory distress syndrome [ARDS], plasma exchange, breast cancer, massive hemorrhage).[212] A particularly severe form of acquired protein C deficiency has been reported in association with purpura fulminans and ICF/DIC in individuals with acute meningococcal infection.[8,272] In contrast to antithrombin III, antigenic concentrations of vitamin K–dependent plasma proteins, including protein C, are often increased in individuals with nephrotic syndrome.[273] Patients with low protein C levels should have this finding confirmed on a subsequent sample after acquired causes have been excluded. Family studies may also be useful in

confirming a diagnosis of congenital protein C deficiency. Warfarin therapy reduces functional and, to a lesser extent, antigenic measurements of protein C, thus complicating diagnosis of the deficiency state.[268] For patients who are stably anticoagulated on warfarin, a suspicion of congenital protein C deficiency may be raised when protein C activity is discordantly reduced compared with factor VII activity, a vitamin K–dependent zymogen with a similar plasma half-life.[274] However, definitive diagnosis requires repeated measurements after the patient has been off warfarin therapy for at least 1 week, preferably longer. If it is not possible to discontinue warfarin therapy because of the severity of the thrombotic diathesis, such individuals may be studied while receiving heparin therapy, which does not alter plasma protein C levels. In addition, family studies may be helpful. The incidence and relative risk of first-lifetime (incident) and recurrent VTE are presented in Table 14-8.

Protein S Deficiency

Protein S is a vitamin K–dependent plasma glycoprotein (635 amino acids; M_r, 70 kDa) that is predominantly synthesized in the liver but also in the endothelial cells, megakaryocytes, and Leydig cells of the testis.[275] Protein S is a nonenzymatic cofactor for APC-mediated inactivation of factors VIIIa and Va. In addition, protein S may exhibit APC-independent anticoagulant activity by directly binding and inhibiting factor VIIIa in the tenase complex, as well as factors Va and Xa in the prothrombinase complex. The aminoterminal end of the molecule consists of a Gla domain, an aromatic ring amino acid domain, a thrombin-sensitive region, and four EGF-like domains; the carboxyterminal end includes a sex hormone–binding globulin-like domain rather than a serine protease domain. Approximately 60% to 70% of total plasma protein S circulates noncovalently bound in 1:1 stoichiometry to a complement regulatory protein, C4b-binding protein (C4BPβ+), and is inactive. The remainder circulates as "free" protein S (plasma concentration, 150 nM) with a plasma half-life of 96 hours.

The protein S (PROS, PSa) gene is located on the short arm of chromosome 3 (3p11.1–3p11.2) and consists of 15 exons that span 80 kb. In addition, a protein S pseudogene (PSβ) with 96.5% homology to PSa is located within 4 centimorgans (cM) of the PROS gene. Congenital protein S deficiency is inherited as an autosomal dominant disorder with variable penetrance. The prevalence of protein S deficiency in the normal population is about 200 per 100,000 (see Table 14-8).

Of the known congenital deficiencies that may lead to thrombophilia, testing and interpretation are most difficult for protein S deficiency. On the basis of total and free plasma protein S antigen levels, protein S deficiency was initially categorized into three phenotypes; all three have reduced protein S activity. Type I protein S deficiency consists of reduced total and free protein S antigen levels,[276,277] type II is made up of normal total and free protein S antigen levels, and type III comprises normal total protein S antigen levels but reduced free protein S antigen. However, mutations have been identified in only 44% of individuals with a type III phenotype, raising the possibility that some of these cases represent acquired abnormalities.[278] More recent studies show that many patients with type III deficiency have the same molecular defect as those with type I deficiency, and that the age-related increase in C4BPβ+ but not protein S leads to the type III phenotype.[200,275] About two thirds of protein S–deficient patients have a type I phenotype, and one third have a type III phenotype; the type II phenotype is rare. However, because most laboratories previously screened for protein S deficiency with a free protein S antigen assay, and because of our inability to measure all protein S anticoagulant activities, the true prevalence of type II protein S deficiency is unknown.

Plasma protein S (e.g., APC cofactor) activity assays are modified PTT- or PT-based assays in which patient protein S levels are directly proportionate to protein S cofactor activity in APC-mediated prolongation of the clotting time. In the PTT-based functional protein S assay, patient plasma is diluted in protein S–deficient plasma; fixed amounts of APC and factor Va are added, and the clotting time is measured. PT-based assays are performed similarly, or the patient's native protein C may be activated to APC by the addition of Protac. Early-generation assays yielded falsely low protein S activity in the presence of APC resistance, the factor V Leiden mutation, or increased factor II (prothrombin), VII, or VIII activities. In addition, prolongation of baseline PTT due to heparin or a lupus anticoagulant rendered the assay uninterpretable. More recent generation assays are less susceptible to such interference because of greater dilution of patient plasma in protein S–deficient plasma, addition of an increased amount of factor Va, and inclusion of polybrene to neutralize any heparin effect. However, increased factor VIII activity (as occurs with acute thrombosis or any other cause of an acute phase reaction) still may cause falsely low protein S activity with PTT-based assays.

Early assays of plasma protein S protein levels typically measured total protein S antigen by ELISA. Free protein S antigen levels were measured in the plasma supernatant after precipitation of protein S:C4b-binding protein complexes with 3.75% polyethylene glycol (PEG) 6000. More recent assays measure free protein S antigen directly and without the need for PEG precipitation with the use of a monoclonal antibody ELISA that is specific for free protein S antigen.

Assays for protein S activity or free protein S antigen level may be used for initial testing for protein S deficiency.[275] A screening assay for protein S activity may identify type II protein S deficiency that would be missed with a free protein S antigen assay. However, protein S activity assays are subject to potential interference and should be used with caution as initial testing. A low protein S activity should be confirmed with an assay for free protein S antigen. If the initial protein S test result is low with either method, the result should be confirmed on a different sample collected after it has been ensured that all potentially acquired causes of protein S deficiency have been excluded or corrected. Routine testing of total protein S antigen levels is unnecessary but may be useful if the free protein S antigen level and/or protein S activity is low.

Neonatal protein S levels are approximately 35% and approach adult levels by about 1 year of age.[275] Protein S levels are generally lower among premenopausal than among postmenopausal women, and levels increase with age for both men and women. Levels are reduced by vitamin K deficiency, oral (vitamin K antagonist) anticoagulants, liver disease, acute thrombosis,[279] sepsis, ICF/DIC, human immunodeficiency virus (HIV) infection,[280] and

L-asparaginase therapy, and among women, by oral contraceptives, pregnancy, and estrogen therapy. Although total protein S antigen measurements are generally increased in individuals with nephrotic syndrome, free protein S antigen levels and protein S activity may be reduced because of the loss of free protein S in the urine and elevations in C4b-binding protein levels.[273] For patients who are stably anticoagulated on warfarin, a suspicion of congenital protein S deficiency may be raised when protein S activity is discordantly reduced compared with factor II (prothrombin) activity, a vitamin K–dependent zymogen with a similar plasma half-life. However, definitive diagnosis requires repeated measurements after the patient has been off warfarin therapy for at least 4 to 6 weeks, preferably longer. If it is not possible to discontinue warfarin because of the severity of the thrombotic diathesis, such individuals can be studied while receiving heparin therapy, which does not alter free protein S antigen levels. Family studies may also be useful in confirming a diagnosis of congenital protein S deficiency. The incidence and relative risk of first-lifetime (incident) and recurrent VTE are presented in Table 14-8.

Deficiencies of Other Natural Anticoagulants (TFPI, Protein Z, Z-Dependent Protease Inhibitor, and Heparin Cofactor II)

Tissue factor pathway inhibitor (TFPI) is a 32 kDa (276 amino acid) plasma protein and a Kunitz-type protease inhibitor of factor Xa and tissue factor:factor VIIa catalytic activity.[281,282] The TFPI gene is located on the short arm of chromosome 2 (q32) and consists of 9 exons that span 70 kb. TFPI has a complex intravascular distribution. A major proportion (60% to 80%) of intravascular TFPI is normally bound to the vascular endothelium; this pool is mobilized to circulating blood after the injection of heparins.[283] Plasma contains only a minor fraction (20% to 30%) of intravascular TFPI, which is largely associated with lipoproteins.[284] Consequently, measurement of TFPI is difficult. Moreover, international standards for calibration of TFPI assays are not yet available. Several studies have reported that TFPI increases somewhat with age, possibly in relation to hormonal state.[285,286] Plasma TFPI levels are lowest in women on oral contraceptives, and premenopausal women have lower levels compared with postmenopausal women and men.[286–288] Postmenopausal women who receive hormone therapy also have lower TFPI levels.[289]

TFPI knockout mice die in utero from thrombosis.[290] Immunodepletion of TFPI in rabbits lowers the threshold for tissue factor–induced thrombosis,[291,292] and exogenous recombinant TFPI protects against DIC[293] and VTE.[294,295] Hormone therapy reduces plasma TFPI levels by 30% to 50% and may contribute to the risk of thrombosis associated with exogenous estrogen therapy.[289] Plasma TFPI levels below the 10th percentile are a weak risk factor for DVT (odds ratio [OR], 1.1 to 1.7),[286] and patients with DVT may have slightly lower mean TFPI levels compared with controls.[125,296–298]

Protein Z is a 62-kDa vitamin K–dependent plasma protein that circulates in blood almost entirely as a noncovalent complex with a protein Z–dependent protease inhibitor (ZPI) with a plasma concentration of 2.6 ± 1 μg per milliliter.[128,129,299,300] The ZPI plasma concentration is 3.8 μg per milliliter (53 nM). Protein Z catalyzes the inhibition of factor Xa by ZPI by 1000-fold. Protein Z increases rapidly during the first months of life, and adult levels are reached during puberty.[264,301] Protein Z deficiency compounds the risk of thrombosis among carriers of the factor V Leiden mutation.[302] Reduced protein Z levels may increase the risk of an adverse pregnancy outcome.[303] Low plasma protein Z levels have also been reported in patients with antiphospholipid antibodies.[304] Studies undertaken to test for an association between ischemic stroke and protein Z deficiency have reached contradictory conclusions.[305,306]

Heparin cofactor II is a serine protease inhibitor (SERPIN) synthesized in the liver that circulates in blood at a plasma concentration of ≈ 1 μM.[307] Heparin cofactor II solely inhibits thrombin, and the rate of thrombin inhibition is increased more than 1000-fold by heparin, heparan sulfate, or dermatan sulfate. The physiologic function of heparin cofactor II is unknown. Heparin cofactor II knockout mice undergo normal fetal development, are born at the expected mendelian frequency, and have subsequent normal growth and survival with no increased rate of spontaneous thrombosis. However, such mice have a shorter time to thrombosis in an arterial injury model. At least 15 families with heparin cofactor II deficiency have been reported. Data from these families suggest that heparin cofactor II deficiency is a weak risk factor for VTE; usually, the risk for thrombosis is compounded when it is combined with other thrombophilias.[307]

These data suggest that deficiency of TFPI, protein Z and/or ZPI, and heparin cofactor II may be important risk factors for thrombosis, but current data are insufficient to support routine assay of these analytes as part of a diagnostic thrombophilia evaluation.

Enhanced Procoagulant Pathway: Increased Plasma Procoagulant Levels

Increased Fibrinogen (Factor I) Level

Fibrinogen (factor I) is a 340-kDa soluble glycoprotein that is synthesized in the liver.[308] Thrombin cleaves fibrinogen, yielding fibrinopeptides A and B and fibrin monomers. Fibrin monomers self-assemble to form soluble fibrin polymers that are crosslinked by factor XIIIa to form insoluble (crosslinked) fibrin. Increased fibrinogen levels may enhance thrombus formation by altering the kinetics of coagulation, augmenting platelet interaction due to increased binding to the platelet glycoprotein-IIb/IIIa ($\alpha_{IIb}\beta_3$) receptor, and increasing plasma viscosity, and through formation of less porous fibrin networks, leading to impaired fibrinolysis.[309]

An increased fibrinogen level is epidemiologically strongly associated with myocardial infarction, stroke, and peripheral vascular disease.[310–317] A plasma fibrinogen level >500 mg/dL combined with thrombosis has been associated with incident DVT in two studies.[318,319] However, an increased fibrinogen level was not significantly associated with VTE in other studies and did not compound the risk for thrombosis among factor V Leiden carriers.[320,321] Fibrinogen levels increase with age, which may, in part, explain the increased risk of VTE that is associated with increasing age.[135]

Routine measurement of fibrinogen to assess individual thrombotic risk is controversial.[308] No threshold measurement for defining hyperfibrinogenemia has been determined,

and no universal standardization system has been developed for the fibrinogen assay. Moreover, significant intra-individual variation in fibrinogen levels has been noted over time, suggesting the need for serial determinations before diagnosing hyperfibrinogenemia.

Increased Prothrombin (Factor II) Level/Prothrombin 20210 Mutation

Prothrombin (factor II) is a vitamin K–dependent plasma protein that is synthesized in the liver. In the final common coagulation pathway, factor Xa within the prothrombinase complex (factors Va and phospholipid) cleaves an activation peptide (prothrombin fragment 1.2) from prothrombin, yielding thrombin that cleaves fibrinogen to yield fibrin, and activates platelets and factors V, VIII, XI, and XIII to form an insoluble hemostatic plug. Plasma prothrombin activity ranges from about 70% to 130%, and the amount of thrombin formed is directly proportionate to the plasma prothrombin concentration.[322]

In a population-based, candidate gene, case-controlled study from the Netherlands, a common variation within the 3'-untranslated region (UTR) of the prothrombin gene (prothrombin 20210) was associated with a threefold increased risk of VTE.[137,196] The prothrombin 20210 carrier frequency among VTE cases was 6.2% compared with 2.3% (1.2% allele frequency) among healthy controls. These findings have been confirmed in populations from Brazil, Italy, Sweden, and the United Kingdom, with VTE relative risks ranging from 2.8 to 11.5.[137,323]

The prothrombin gene is located on chromosome 11 and consists of 14 exons and 13 introns that span 21 kb. The prothrombin 20210 mutation is located at the 3'-UTR polyadenylation cleavage site and is a gain of function mutation leading to increased plasma prothrombin levels.[324–326] The incidence and relative risk of first-lifetime (incident) and recurrent VTEs are presented in Table 14-8. In the initial study, 87% of prothrombin 20210 carriers were in the highest quartile of plasma prothrombin levels.[196] Prothrombin 20210 carriers have indirect evidence of increased thrombin generation.[327] The prothrombin 20210 polymorphism is a founder mutation that arose 20,000 to 30,000 years ago.[388] The carrier frequency is highest among persons of Southern European ancestry (3%), and the carrier frequency in Northern Europeans is lower (1.7%).[137] The prothrombin 20210 allele is uncommon among Asians and African Americans (carrier frequency, 0.4%), and it accounts for <0.5% of VTE cases in the latter population.[206,207]

Depending on the population, about 3% to 8% of patients with incident VTE and 15% to 20% of those with recurrent VTE will be prothrombin 20210 carriers (see Table 14-8). VTE risk among prothrombin 20210 carriers is compounded by concomitant deficiency of antithrombin III, protein C or protein S, or factor V Leiden, as well as other exposures, such as oral contraceptives, pregnancy, or hormone therapy.[137,328] The prothrombin 20210 mutation has also been associated with recurrent fetal loss and complications of pregnancy.[21] The prothrombin 20210 mutation generally is not associated with myocardial infarction or stroke in older populations, but it may interact with other exposures (e.g., tobacco smoking, hormone therapy) to increase the risk of arterial thrombosis in younger populations.[137,329]

Identification of prothrombin 20210 mutation carriers requires direct DNA-based genotyping assays; the plasma prothrombin activity is not sufficiently sensitive for carrier testing.[137]

Increased Factors VII, VIII, IX, X, and XI, and von Willebrand Factor

Factor VII is a 50-kDa, vitamin K–dependent zymogen synthesized by the liver that is critical for initiation of tissue factor–induced coagulation (extrinsic pathway).[308] The tissue factor–factor VIIa pathway is believed to be the major mechanism for initiating thrombin generation. Increased factor VII levels are seen in patients who use certain types of oral contraceptives[330] and in those who are pregnant[331] or have hyperlipidemia,[332] as well as during obesity and aging.[308] In the Northwick Park Heart Study, increased basal factor VII levels were significantly associated with subsequent death from ischemic heart disease.[333] However, in more recent studies, an increased factor VII level was not an independent risk factor for arterial[311,315,334–336] or venous thrombosis.[318]

Factor VIII is a 330-kDa glycoprotein that is synthesized in nonhepatocyte liver cells and endothelium, and that circulates in blood bound to von Willebrand factor (VWF) at a mean plasma concentration of 0.1 ng per milliliter (0.6 nM).[308] Thrombin (or factor Xa) activates factor VIII to factor VIIIa. Factor VIIIa is the cofactor for intrinsic system activation of factor X by factor IXa in the presence of phospholipids and calcium. Factor VIII activity is an acute phase reactant that increases with acute stress, chronic inflammation, and exogenous estrogen administration. Factor VIII levels also vary with ABO blood type; factor VIII activity is about 15% lower for those with type O blood group compared with type A or B. In addition, factor VIII activity is labile and may be decreased by 10% to 20% with improper sample collection and processing, including freeze-thaw. Increased basal factor VIII activity is, in part, heritable.[141,337–339] The level of plasma VWF and ABO blood type account for about one third of the population variability of factor VIII.[340]

Increased factor VIII activity was first associated with thrombosis more than 40 years ago.[341] Subsequent studies have shown that basal factor VIII activity >150% confers about a five- to sevenfold increased risk for incident[139,141,319,342,343] and recurrent VTE.[141,182] Combined increased factor IX and factor VIII antigen levels are associated with an eightfold relative risk of VTE.[143] In addition, increased factor VIII activity interacts with the factor V Leiden mutation to compound the risk for thrombosis.[342,344] Increased factor VIII activity also confers a 1.5- to twofold increased risk for arterial thrombosis (see Table 14-8).[345–348] In a recent case-controlled study, the risk of VTE associated with increased factor VIII activity (>270%) was increased almost ninefold, but risk varied by patient age.[136] Factor VIII cutoffs for a 95% specificity by age were 238% for subjects <40 years of age, 248% for ages 40 to 55 years, 261% for ages 56 to 70 years, and 313% for ages >70 years. The upper limit of normal (150%) for factor VIII was not of clinical use, and a much higher cutoff (>270%) was proposed. In addition, age-specific cutoffs were recommended for clinical use.

Factor VIII activity typically is measured with a PTT-based one-stage clotting assay. Although a factor VIII activity assay is available in many laboratories, the reported reference range may vary by more than threefold (e.g., 55% to 205%).[349] Immunoassays (e.g., ELISA) are commercially available for use in measuring factor VIII antigen levels.[339] In general, ELISAs show narrower coefficients of variation than clotting assays and are not influenced by spurious factors, such as partial clotting activation during blood drawing. Most other commercially available immunoassays are limited in their ability to bind to factor VIII in plasma.[308]

Factor IX is a 57-kDa vitamin K–dependent zymogen that is synthesized in the liver. Factor IX is activated by factor VIIa or factor XIa.[308] In turn, factor IXa together with factor VIIIa activates factor X. Factor IX levels increase with age and with the use of oral contraceptives.[350] After correction for age, sex, oral contraceptive use, factor VIII, factor XI, and other vitamin K–dependent clotting factors, increased plasma factor IX (antigen level >129%, or activity level >150%) is associated with a two- to 2.3-fold (95% CI, 1.3 to 3.2) increased risk for incident VTE.[143,351]

Factor X is a 59-kDa vitamin K–dependent zymogen that is synthesized by the liver. Factor X is activated to factor Xa by the tissue factor–factor VIIa (extrinsic) pathway or by the factor IXa–factor VIIIa (intrinsic) pathway.[308] In conjunction with the cofactor, factor Va, factor Xa catalyzes the conversion of prothrombin to thrombin. Increased factor X levels have been reported in users of oral contraceptives and during pregnancy.[331] In univariate analyses, increased factor X antigen levels were associated with a 1.6-fold increased risk of VTE.[352] However, after adjusting for other vitamin K–dependent coagulation factor levels, factor X was not an independent risk factor for VTE. Similarly, increased factor X activity is not an independent risk factor for myocardial infarction.[334]

Factor XI is a 143-kDa zymogen that is synthesized in the liver and megakaryocytes, and that circulates in blood at a plasma concentration of 4 to 6 μg per milliliter (≈30 nM).[308] Factor XI is activated to the serine protease, factor XIa, by factor XIIa (as part of the contact activation or intrinsic coagulation pathway) or by thrombin (as part of "feedback" activation).[353] After adjusting for inherited risk factors, age, sex, and oral contraceptives, factor XI antigen levels above the 90th percentile (>121%) are associated with a 2.2-fold (95% CI, 1.5 to 3.2) increased risk of VTE.[144] Factor XIa formed by thrombin creates positive feedback, leading to even higher levels of thrombin that can activate thrombin-activatable fibrinolysis inhibitor.[354] Inhibition of fibrinolysis may account for an association of factor XI levels with VTE.

VWF is a large multimeric protein that is synthesized in endothelial cells and megakaryocytes. VWF functions as a ligand to tether platelets to the site of a blood vessel injury and as a carrier protein for plasma factor VIII.[308] VWF is stored within endothelial cell Weibel-Palade bodies and platelet α granules. VWF levels vary with blood type. Individuals with type O blood have the lowest levels, those with type AB have the highest levels, and those with types A and B have intermediate levels. VWF levels increase with age and may be higher in women than in men.[355,356] VWF is an acute phase reactant that is rapidly released from endothelial cells in response to a variety of agonists, including epinephrine, bradykinin, and vasopressin and its analogues (1-deamino-8-D-arginine vasopressin [DDAVP]).

14

The concentration in blood can increase chronically in response to inflammation, infection, cancer, trauma, female hormones, sepsis, and other stimuli.

Univariate analyses from prospective studies have shown that an increased basal VWF antigen level is associated with a 1.2-fold increased risk of coronary heart disease and stroke.[311,317] However, VWF was not an independent risk factor after adjustments were made for smoking, hypertension, diabetes, and lipid profile. In contrast, in the ECAT (European Concerted Action on Thrombosis) Angina Pectoris study, an increased VWF antigen level was significantly associated with an increased risk of myocardial infarction or sudden cardiac death in patients with a history of angina pectoris after adjusting for age, field center, and other risk factors (RR > 1.24).[356] Other studies have shown a significant association between VWF antigen level and ischemic heart disease after adjusting for age, sex, and other risk factors[357]; a significant association with acute myocardial infarction,[358] recurrent myocardial infarction,[359] stroke,[360] and peripheral arterial disease[316] after adjusting for age and sex, but not after adjustment for other risk factors; an association with fatal ischemic heart disease but not all ischemic heart disease after adjusting for blood group[347]; and no association between VWF levels and stroke.[315] An increased VWF level was not an independent risk factor for VTE after adjusting for factor VIII activity.[139] Therefore, an increased VWF level does not appear to be an independent predictor of thrombotic risk but is part of a larger complex of hemostatic alterations associated with inflammation, atherosclerosis, and arterial thrombosis.

Current procoagulant factor activity assays were developed to identify factor deficiencies among patients with clinical bleeding disorders; however, extant tests have not been established to precisely measure excesses among patients with thrombotic presentations. In general, factor activities of 35% to 40% or higher are associated with normal or near normal hemostasis. In contrast, an increase in factor activity as small as 15% may be associated with a significant risk for thrombosis. International standards for procoagulant factors are neither widely available nor routinely used to calibrate most assays.[308] In a recent College of American Pathologists survey, plasma laboratories were asked to assay several procoagulant factor activities. The between-laboratory coefficient of variation for a sample with an approximately normal level of factor ranged from 11.6% for factor X activity to 20.4% for factor IX activity. Because of the lack of widely used calibrators and the imprecision of individual assay methods, a single cutoff value for risk that will apply to all methods has not yet been defined. Consequently, routine assays of procoagulant factor activities to assess individual thrombosis risk are not recommended at this time.[308]

Increased Homocysteine (Homocystinuria; Hyperhomocysteinemia)/Methylene-Tetrahydrofolate Reductase (MTHFR)

Homocysteine is a sulfhydryl amino acid that is an intermediary between methionine and cysteine. Homocysteine cycles to methionine in an intracellular demethylation/remethylation pathway, where dietary methionine is demethylated to form homocysteine, and homocysteine is subsequently remethylated to form methionine (Fig. 14-4).[115] The remethylation pathway requires inclusion of the enzyme, methionine synthase, and the essential cofactor, cobalamin (vitamin B_{12}). In this reaction, methyltetrahydrofolate "donates" a methyl group to "remethylate" homocysteine to form methionine. Methyltetrahydrofolate is derived through reduction of 5,10-methylenetetrahydrofolate in a reaction catalyzed by the enzyme, methylenetetrahydrofolate reductase (MTHFR). When methionine is present in excess or cysteine synthesis is required, homocysteine cycles to cysteine in a transsulfuration pathway. In the transsulfuration pathway, homocysteine is condensed with serine to form cystathionine in a reaction that requires the enzyme, cystathionine β-synthase (CBS), and the essential cofactor, pyridoxal 5′-phosphate (vitamin B_6; see Fig. 14-4). Cystathionine is subsequently hydrolyzed to cysteine and α-ketobutyrate. The remethylation pathway is primarily responsible for regulating fasting plasma homocysteine levels (e.g., dependent on folate, vitamin B_{12}, MTHFR); the resulfuration pathway mainly regulates higher plasma homocysteine levels, as occurs in the postprandial state or after a methionine load (e.g., dependent on vitamin B_6, CBS).[115]

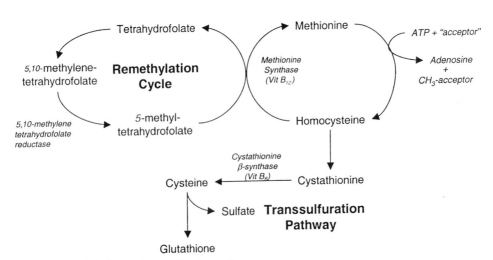

Figure 14-4 Homocysteine remethylation and transsulfuration pathways.

The initial association of one or more childhood features of mental retardation, ectopia lentis, marfanoid habitus, premature atherosclerosis, and VTE with homocystinuria was noted longer than 40 years ago.[361,362] As opposed to "normal" fasting plasma homocysteine levels of 5 to 15 μmol per liter, homocystinuric individuals have levels in the range of 100 to 400 μmol per liter. Plasma homocysteine reference ranges may vary according to population characteristics, including dietary intake of methionine and vitamins B_6 and B_{12} or folic acid. In about 90% to 95% of cases, homocystinuria is due to an inherited deficiency of CBS; the remainder of cases are due to a deficiency in the remethylation pathway (e.g., severe deficiency of methionine synthase or MTHFR). The CBS gene is located on the long arm of chromosome 21 (q22). The most frequent CBS mutations leading to homocystinuria include homozygosity for T833C, G919A, and A1224C; the population carrier frequency for these mutations is 0.3% to 1.0%.[115] Heterozygotes may have normal fasting homocysteine levels but increased levels within 4 to 8 hours after methionine loading. However, abnormal results from loading tests are not specific for heterozygous CBS deficiencies.[363]

The observation of arterial and venous thrombosis due to severe hyperhomocysteinemia suggested the hypothesis that mild (15 to 30 μmol per liter) or moderate (31 to 100 μmol per liter) hyperhomocysteinemia might be associated with incident or recurrent thrombosis at an older age.[114] This hypothesis has been tested in case-controlled and prospective cohort study designs with conflicting conclusions. A meta-analysis of 27 case-controlled studies determined that the risk for coronary, cerebrovascular, and peripheral arterial disease was increased 1.6-, 1.5- and 6.8-fold, respectively, per 5 μmol per liter increase in total plasma homocysteine.[364] Compared with the lowest four quintiles, a large case-controlled study found that patients in the top plasma homocysteine quintile had a 2.2-fold (95% CI, 1.6 to 2.9) increased risk for vascular disease.[365] Single case-controlled studies and meta-analyses of these studies have detected a similar risk for incident and recurrent VTE, with about a 2.5- to threefold increased risk.[115,117,233,366–368]

Case-controlled studies, however, cannot establish causality. Previous studies have shown that homocysteine levels may increase for an unknown duration after an acute thrombotic event, suggesting that hyperhomocysteinemia may be an effect of thrombosis rather than a cause.[115,368] In support of this hypothesis, prospective cohort studies found no increase in relative risk, or only a weakly increased risk, of arterial vascular disease or incident VTE with hyperhomocysteinemia.[115,116,368–372] One study found an increased risk for idiopathic but not secondary VTE,[205] and several studies found an increased risk for recurrent VTE.[116,233,373] Hyperhomocysteinemia may interact with other risk factors (e.g., factor V Leiden) to compound the risk for VTE.[205,374] However, prospective clinical trials of homocysteine-lowering (vitamin) therapy have failed to show a benefit in reducing recurrent stroke, myocardial infarction, or VTE.[373,375–377] Taken together, these findings question the benefit of measuring basal or post–methionine load plasma homocysteine levels. Nevertheless, hyperhomocysteinemia, whether causal or a marker for some other

cause, appears to be a consistent predictor of increased risk for recurrent VTE. Consequently, homocysteine levels may be useful in assessing the need for secondary prophylaxis with oral vitamin K inhibitors (e.g., warfarin).

Hyperhomocysteinemia may be due to inherited or acquired disorders. Deficiencies of vitamins B_6, B_{12}, or folic acid are common acquired causes. Two common polymorphisms within the MTHFR gene (C677T and A1298C) increase the risk of hyperhomocysteinemia among homozygous carriers who become deficient in folic acid or vitamin B_{12}.[115] The MTHFR C677T polymorphism encodes for substitution of valine for alanine, and the A1298C polymorphism encodes for a glutamic acid-to-alanine substitution. Both polymorphisms are associated with reduced in vitro MTHFR enzymatic activity, and both are quite common, with a minor allele carrier frequency approaching 40%; about 10% of the U.S. white population are homozygous carriers. These MTHFR polymorphisms are uncommon among African Americans.[378] Combined heterozygotes may have a mildly increased risk for hyperhomocysteinemia with a deficiency of vitamin B_{12} or folic acid. However, in the absence of hyperhomocysteinemia, homozygous or combined heterozygous carriers are not at increased risk for arterial or venous thrombosis.[115,363,368] In a recent meta-analysis of 40 case-controlled studies, individuals with the MTHFR C677T genotype had a 16% increased risk for coronary heart disease, but significant heterogeneity was seen between studies of European and American populations, suggesting an interaction with folate status.[379] Consequently, routine genotyping for these polymorphisms is neither useful nor recommended.[115]

Other common acquired causes for hyperhomocysteinemia include impaired renal or liver function, hypothyroidism, psoriasis, inflammatory bowel disease, rheumatoid arthritis, organ transplantation, and drugs (e.g., anticonvulsants, levodopa, niacin, bile acid sequestrants, methotrexate, thiazides, cyclosporin A).[115] Social (e.g., physical inactivity, tobacco smoking, coffee consumption) and demographic (increasing age, postmenopausal status, male sex) characteristics also may cause mild hyperhomocysteinemia. Exogenous estrogens (e.g., oral contraceptives, hormone therapy) may decrease plasma homocysteine levels.

About 70% of homocysteine in plasma circulates while bound to albumin; about 30% is oxidized to disulfides and 2% or less as free homocysteine.[115] Total plasma homocysteine is usually assayed with high-pressure liquid chromatography or immunoassay after reduction of all homocystine moieties to homocysteine. Basal plasma homocysteine levels are usually measured on a fasting blood sample. A post–methionine load sample is usually collected 3 to 6 hours after oral ingestion of 0.1 g of L-methionine per kilogram of body weight. About 25% to 45% of patients with a normal basal homocysteine level will exhibit hyperhomocysteinemia after methionine loading. Blood samples collected in ethylenediaminetetraacetic acid (EDTA) must remain on ice until the plasma can be separated as homocysteine is produced and exported by blood cells. Laboratories should develop local population- and sex-specific reference ranges. As noted previously, homocysteine levels may remain elevated for several months after an acute thrombotic event, such that measurement of plasma homocysteine levels should be delayed accordingly.

Enhanced Procoagulant Pathway: Impaired Downregulation of Procoagulant Activity

Activated Protein C Resistance/Factor V Leiden

Protein C is a plasma protein zymogen (pre-enzyme) that is activated by the thrombin:thrombomodulin complex on the endothelial cell membrane luminal surface to activated protein C (APC), a serine protease that cleaves and inactivates procoagulant factors VIIIa and Va, thus downregulating further thrombin generation. When added to plasma ex vivo, APC causes progressive prolongation of the clotting time (e.g., PTT, PT) in a dose-dependent manner. In 1993, Dahlbäck and coworkers[380] reported three apparently unrelated patients with idiopathic recurrent VTE whose plasma was resistant to the anticoagulant effect of exogenous addition of activated protein C, called APC resistance. With the use of a simple assay for APC resistance that consisted of the ratio of PTT after the addition of a fixed amount of APC (sufficient to prolong the PTT about twofold) divided by the baseline PTT (e.g., normal APC ratio, 2), APC resistance (defined as APC ratio <2) was noted to segregate in families with a mendelian autosomal dominant inheritance pattern, and it was found to be associated with VTE.[194,381]

Procoagulant factors V and VIII are large (300+ kDa) template proteins that catalyze assembly of the prothrombinase and "tenase" complexes, respectively, on negatively charged phospholipid (e.g., activated platelet surface membrane). Factors V and VIII are "activated" (FVa, FVIIIa) by proteolytic cleavage of an activation peptide (B domain) by thrombin. FVa and FVIIIa markedly accelerate the rate of activation of prothrombin to thrombin and thus are key regulatory points for downregulation of procoagulant activity. Activated protein C inactivates FVa and FVIIIa via cleavage of FVa at three different amino acid positions (R[arginine]306, R506, and R679), and at two FVIIIa positions (R336 and R562), within the heavy chains of each. Initial APC cleavage at the R506 position is required for optimal exposure and subsequent rapid inactivation of FVa by APC cleavage at positions R306 and R679.[382]

The factor V gene is located on the long arm of chromosome 1 (1q21–1q25) and is closely linked to the antithrombin gene. FVa isolated from APC-R patient plasma was noted to be resistant to inactivation by APC.[383] Subsequent work identified a single point mutation (guanine to adenine) at the 1691 position of the heavy chain of factor V that encodes for substitution of a glutamine (Q) for arginine (R) at amino acid position 506, now called factor V Leiden.[384] Carriers of the factor V Leiden mutation have normal factor V procoagulant activity but impaired downregulation of this activity, as shown by increased basal prothrombin fragment 1.2 (an activation fragment generated when prothrombin is converted to thrombin), consistent with increased basal thrombin production.[385] Factor V Leiden carriers also have reduced rates of thrombolysis, possibly caused by increased activity of thrombin-activated fibrinolysis inhibitor (TAFI).[386,387]

The first-generation PTT-based APC resistance (ratio) assay could not be interpreted in the presence of an abnormal baseline PTT (i.e., as may occur with a lupus anticoagulant, or heparin or oral anticoagulation) and was only

85% to 95% sensitive for the factor V Leiden mutation. Assay results were sensitive to the choice of reagents (PTT reagent and APC and calcium chloride concentration), instrument (mechanical, photo-optical), preanalytic conditions (centrifugation, storage, fresh or frozen samples), and several patient-related factors (e.g., pregnancy, oral contraceptive therapy, factor VIII and prothrombin activities). Residual platelets in frozen/thawed samples could falsely lower the APC resistance ratio. Prolonged centrifugation, double centrifugation, or postcentrifugation plasma filtration was required prior to sample freezing.

Alternative (non–PTT-based) assays, including assays based on PT, factor Xa–clotting time, Russell's viper venom time, and Textarin time, have been developed. The major advantage of all these assays is insensitivity to FVIII activity. "Second–generation" PT- or PTT-based assays with predilution (1:10) in factor V–deficient plasma (immunodepleted) have been developed to normalize all other factors that might affect the APC resistance ratio (e.g., FVIII, prothrombin, protein S, other vitamin K dependent factors reduced in oral anticoagulation therapy) and possibly prevent interference by heparin or the presence of a lupus-like anticoagulant. These assays are 100% sensitive for the factor V Leiden mutation but are insensitive to other causes of APC resistance (e.g., oral contraceptives, pregnancy). Nevertheless, a second-generation APC resistance assay is recommended for screening for APC resistance.

APC resistance is associated with VTE. Depending on the assay used, 95% to 100% of patients with APC resistance are factor V Leiden carriers. Factor V Leiden is common among white populations of Northern European ancestry.[19] Factor V Leiden is a founder mutation that occurred 30,000 years ago.[388] No survival disadvantage is evident among factor V Leiden carriers.[99] About 10% of factor V Leiden carriers develop VTE over their lifetime.[99] The risk of VTE among factor V Leiden carriers increases with age; most events occur in carriers older than 50 to 55 years of age (Table 14-11).[99,133] Homozygous factor V Leiden carriers have an 80-fold increased risk of thrombosis, and environmental exposures or other genetic risk factors may compound that risk.[389,390] Penetrance of the thrombosis phenotype is increased among patients with multiple genetic defects (e.g., concomitant antithrombin III, protein C, or protein S deficiency).[19] Thrombosis phenotype penetrance is dependent on clinical risk factor exposure (genetic/environmental interaction), such as oral contraceptives, pregnancy, or surgery. The reported risk of recurrent VTE among factor V Leiden carriers varies.[19] The risk of recurrence is increased among homozygous factor V Leiden carriers, and among combined heterozygous factor V Leiden and prothrombin 20210 carriers. In a recent meta-analysis, pooled results from 10 studies involving 3104 patients with incident VTE revealed that the factor V Leiden mutation was present in 21.4% of patients and was associated with a 1.41-fold increased risk for recurrent VTE (95% CI, 1.14 to 1.75).[184] Factor V Leiden (along with other hereditary thrombophilias) is associated with increased fetal loss. Factor V Leiden does not appear to be associated with arterial events such as acute myocardial infarction, coronary artery disease, or stroke.[19]

Table 14-11   Age-Specific Annual Incidence (95% Confidence Interval [CI]) and Relative Risk of First-Lifetime Venous Thromboembolism Among Factor V Leiden Carriers

Age group (years)		15–30	40–59	50–59	>60	>70
Author						
Ridker, 1997	Incidence*	—	0	197 (72–428)	258 (95–561)	783 (358–1486)
	Relative risk[†]	—	—	2.7	2.7	4.2
Middeldorp, 1998	Incidence*	250 (120–490)	470 (230–860)	820 (350–1610)	110 (240–3330)	—
	Relative risk[†]	~15	4.3	2.4	2.8	—
Simioni, 1999	Incidence*	182 (59–424)	264 (86–616)	380 (104–973)	730 (150–2128)	—
	Relative risk[†]	3.6	3.7	1.4	~700	—
Heit, 2005	Incidence*	0 (0–112)	61 (7–219)	244 (98–502)	764 (428–1260)	—
	Relative risk[†]	~1 (0–1.22)	1.96 (0.24–7.04)	1.73 (0.70–3.56)	3.61 (2.02–5.95)	—

*Per 100,000 person-years.
[†]Compared to patients without factor V Leiden.

Impaired Fibrinolysis Pathway

With the use of an assay for global clot lysis, hypofibrinolysis (as reflected by a prolonged clot lysis time) was associated with a 1.6-fold increased risk of VTE.[148] In this assay, the clot lysis time is at least partially dependent on plasma levels of the proteins involved in fibrinolysis, including plasminogen, α_2-plasmin inhibitor, and plasminogen activator inhibitor-1 (PAI-1).

Plasminogen Deficiency

Plasminogen is a 92-kDa protein that is present in blood as the inactive precursor of the serine protease, plasmin.[391,392] Plasminogen is converted to plasmin by cleavage at the Arg561-Val562 peptide bond by tissue-type or urokinase-type plasminogen activator (tPA and uPA, respectively). Activation of plasminogen by tPA is the major physiologic pathway that leads to lysis of fibrin clots. The interaction between tPA and plasminogen is relatively slow. Annexin II is a cofactor on endothelial cells that binds plasminogen and tPA and catalyzes activation of plasminogen by tPA. The other major protein cofactor for the activation of plasminogen by tPA is fibrin. Both plasminogen and tPA have a relatively high affinity for fibrin (but not fibrinogen) and are incorporated into the fibrin clot that is forming. Coordinated binding of plasminogen and tPA to fibrin localizes activation of plasmin to the matrix of the clot, where tPA and plasmin are relatively protected from inhibition by PAI-1 and α_2-plasmin inhibitor, respectively. Plasmin progressively lyses the fibrin clot, releasing multiple varying degradation products, including a specific degradation product, D-dimer. The rate and extent of fibrinolysis are affected by the activity of factor XIIIa; the more the fibrin clot is crosslinked, the more resistant it is to lysis.

Homozygous plasminogen deficiency is associated with ligneous conjunctivitis, characterized by the formation of proliferative pseudomembranes on the conjunctiva and other mucous membranes.[393,394] However, the clinical importance of plasminogen deficiency as a risk factor for thrombosis is uncertain.

In family studies, thrombosis does not segregate with plasminogen deficiency.[392] Moreover, no consistent clinical evidence of an association between homozygous plasminogen deficiency or decreased tPA and risk of thrombosis is apparent. Consequently, determination of plasminogen or tPA concentration (activity or antigen) should not be part of the routine evaluation of patients with thrombophilia. In addition, no indication for routine assessment of genetic abnormalities or polymorphisms of plasminogen or tPA has been identified in the evaluation of risk for VTE or arterial thrombosis.[392]

Increased PAI-1/Reduced Plasminogen Activator

PAI-1 is a 52-kDa single-chain plasma glycoprotein that is synthesized in the liver and endothelial cells; its synthesis is regulated by several physiologic mediators, including endotoxin, interleukin-1, fibroblast growth factor-2, and lipids.[395] Plasma levels increase after surgery is performed. PAI-1 is a member of the SERPIN family and the primary inhibitor of tPA. Plasma PAI-1 is stabilized in its active form through interaction with vitronectin in plasma. Although increased plasma PAI-1 activity theoretically may become prothrombotic through downregulation of intravascular thrombolysis clearance, the results of studies that tested for an association of venous or arterial thrombosis with increased PAI-1 level or PAI-1 polymorphisms are conflicting.[395] The predictive value of PAI-1 plasma concentrations is uncertain, and several important physiologic covariates are involved in the regulation of plasma levels. Common polymorphisms in the PAI-1 gene may affect plasma concentrations. However, currently available data do not support the routine measurement of PAI-1 plasma levels or genotype in the evaluation of thrombophilia.

Increased Factor XIII Activity/Factor XIII Polymorphisms

Plasma factor XIII is zymogen that circulates as a tetramer of two pairs of nonidentical A and B subunits.[396] Factor XIII is activated to factor XIIIa by thrombin cleavage of an activation peptide from the two A subunits, which then dissociate from the B chains in the presence of calcium ions to form the active enzyme. Factor XIII is also found in the soluble fraction of platelets, but platelet factor XIII is composed only of α-chain dimers.

14

Factor XIIIa is a transamidase that catalyzes the formation of intermolecular (γ-glutamyl)-lysine covalent crosslinks in fibrin. One set of crosslinks forms rapidly between two fibrin α chains of adjacent fibrin monomers with reciprocal antiparallel bonding between Lys and Gln residues near the carboxylterminus of the chain. Factor XIIIa also crosslinks the fibrin α chain in a more complex pattern, ultimately resulting in large crosslinked fibrin polymers. α-Chain crosslinking proceeds more slowly than γ-chain crosslinking, and other plasma proteins, including α_2-plasmin inhibitor, fibronectin, and VWF, are also crosslinked to the α chain.

Crosslinking increases fibrin strength and imparts resistance to lysis by plasmin, contributing to the stability of fibrin clots. Factor XIIIa also participates in other physiologic processes, including clot retraction, cell migration, and wound healing.

Factor XIII deficiency (see Chapter 5) results in a bleeding disorder that is inherited as an autosomal recessive trait with variable severity. Mutations of the A and B subunits have been associated with a bleeding tendency, and a large number of different mutations have been identified.

Four common polymorphisms are found within the factor XIII gene; these may produce amino acid changes at Val34Leu, Pro564Leu, Val650Ile, and Glu651Gln. The common Val34Leu mutation in the factor XIII A subunit is located only three amino acids away from the thrombin cleavage site (Arg37-Gly38). Thrombin activates factor XIII 34Leu more rapidly and at lower concentration than 34Val.[397-399] Early activation of factor XIII leads to early crosslinking of fibrin, which inhibits lateral aggregation of the fibrin fibers such that the fibers are thinner and the fibrin clot is less porous. Thin fibrin fibers are relatively resistant to plasmin degradation,[400] suggesting that factor XIII 34Val could be a risk factor for symptomatic thrombosis by producing a thrombus that is less susceptible to clearance by fibrinolysis.

However, contradictory to what would be predicted from fibrin structure, studies that determined the risk of VTE among factor XIII 34Leu carriers relative to noncarriers have reported a protective effect or no effect on risk.[401-406] Recent studies suggest a complex interaction between the factor XIII 34Leu mutation and plasma fibrinogen levels. Similar to the factor XIII 34Leu variant, high fibrinogen levels lead to a less porous and therefore less permeable fibrin clot with thin fibers, which would predict less susceptibility to fibrinolysis and an increased risk for thrombosis. Indeed, high fibrinogen levels are associated with an increased risk of myocardial infarction and premature coronary artery disease[407,408] and VTE.[135,318] However, at high fibrinogen concentrations, clot permeability is increased among factor XIII 34Leu homozygotes.[409] This interaction would predict a protective effect of 34Leu at high fibrinogen levels. A recent study did report a reduced risk of VTE among factor XIII 34Leu carriers with high fibrinogen levels,[123] although the protective effect was limited to men. Similarly, case-controlled studies have reported that factor XIII 34Leu is protective from coronary artery disease and stroke,[17,410] although the 34Leu polymorphism has also been associated with resistance to fibrinolytic therapy for acute myocardial infarction.[411]

Clearly, additional studies are needed to resolve the complex interaction between factor XIII activity and genotype, fibrinogen concentration and fibrin structure, and risk of thrombosis. The data are insufficient at this time to warrant routine assay of factor XIII activity or genotyping for common factor XIII polymorphisms as part of a diagnostic evaluation of thrombophilia.[396]

Dysfibrinogenemia

The dysfibrinogemias are a heterogeneous group of disorders that may cause alterations in the conversion of fibrinogen to fibrin. Approximately 300 abnormal fibrinogens have been reported with a wide variation in phenotypic expression, ranging from asymptomatic to a bleeding diathesis to recurrent VTE.[412] Fewer than 20 cases of variant fibrinogens have been reported to be associated with thrombotic complications.

Increased Thrombin-Activatable Fibrinolytic Inhibitor

Thrombin-activatable fibrinolytic inhibitor (TAFI) is a 55-kDa carboxypeptidase B–like proenzyme that is synthesized in the liver and circulates in blood at a plasma concentration of 4 to 15 µg per milliliter (70 to 275 nM).[412-418] TAFI is activated by thrombin cleavage at Arg93 to form the active enzyme, carboxypeptidase U (also called TAFIa); thrombomodulin accelerates thrombin-mediated activation of TAFI by 1250-fold.[413] Thrombin-mediated activation of factor XI generates large amounts of additional thrombin via the intrinsic pathway, which results in TAFI-dependent downregulation of fibrinolysis.[417,419,420] TAFIa inhibits fibrinolysis by removing carboxyterminal lysine residues from partially degraded fibrin polymers and preventing the binding of the fibrinolytic components, plasminogen and tPA, thereby limiting plasmin formation.[414] Plasma TAFI antigen levels appear to be lower among premenopausal women but otherwise do not appear to vary by age or sex.[421-423] An assay for functional TAFI has been developed that is based on (1) activation of TAFI with thrombin:thrombomodulin and (2) the amount of TAFIa activity generated.[415]

Increased plasma TAFI levels and/or increased generation of TAFIa theoretically may be prothrombotic, and single studies have shown that increased plasma TAFI levels are weak risk factors for incident[424] and recurrent[189] VTE. High TAFI levels have also been associated with incident stroke,[425] although the association with coronary artery disease is less certain.[426] However, the data are insufficient at this time to warrant routine assay of TAFI activity as part of a diagnostic evaluation of thrombophilia.

PAROXYSMAL NOCTURNAL HEMOGLOBINURIA

Paroxysmal nocturnal hemoglobinuria (PNH) manifests as hemolytic anemia, bone marrow failure, and thrombophilia, and is due to nonmalignant clonal expansion of one or more hematopoietic stem cells that have acquired a somatic mutation in the X-linked PIG-A gene, resulting in deficiency of glycosyl phosphatidylinositol (GPI)-anchored proteins such as the complement regulatory proteins, CD55 and CD59.[427] Despite its rarity, PNH has served as a diagnostic dilemma, as an unusual but highly virulent form of thrombophilia, and as an example of a unique clinical profile because of its thrombotic manifestations. Whereas DVT and PE are reported in PNH, an unusual overrepresentation of hepatic vein thrombosis (HVT), mesenteric vein thrombosis (MVT), cerebral vein thrombosis (CVT), and excess morbidity and mortality has been observed during pregnancy.[427a] In their review of 125 patients with PNH, Ray and colleagues[428] reported that DVTs and PEs together accounted for only 34% of all thromboses, and HVT alone constituted 29% and CVT 20% of all thrombotic events.

The disorder is rare and usually affects adults. It seems to have a common but not totally understood relationship with prior bone marrow problems, aplastic anemia in particular. It occurs in about 1 to 10 individuals per million and appears to be worldwide in its distribution. Its three primary manifestations consist of (1) thrombotic events (discussed here), (2) paroxysmal episodes of hemolysis with hemoglobinemia, and (3) hematopoietic marrow failure that manifests as any mixture of pancytopenia, myelodysplastic syndrome, and, within this population, a tendency toward evolution into acute leukemia.[429] Hemolysis and hematopoietic failure are not further addressed in this chapter.

The median age of patients at the time of diagnosis was 42 years, and median survival was reported to be 10 years in a 1995 review.[430] A leading, if not *the* leading, cause of death was venous thrombosis. In this review, 40% of patients experienced various thrombotic episodes during their illness. Of interest, spontaneous and lasting remissions of PNH may recur. Long-term anticoagulant therapy enhanced overall survival.[427,430] A 2004 review[431] reported a longer survival, which may mean additional diagnoses of subtle, less virulent PNH categories and/or improvement in therapy. Investigators reported that patients of European ancestry experience more thrombotic events than Asians, and those Western patients' current survival appears to be on the order of 20 years, whereas in those of Asian extraction with fewer thrombotic events, survival is as long as 30 years. Asian patients appear to have more difficulty than Western patients with bone marrow aplasia. An additional risk for thrombosis is evident in African American and Latin American patients with PNH.[432]

Laboratory diagnosis historically involved the sucrose hemolysis test and the Ham acidified hemolysis test, but recently, these tests have been supplanted by flow cytometric detection of CD59-negative cells.[433] As tests become more sensitive, one can expect that more patients with CD59-negative cells will be identified. Of interest, the finding of CD59-negative cells is not specific for PNH as patients with myeloproliferative disorders (especially essential thrombocythemia) and aplastic anemia may harbor small clones of CD59-deficient cells.[434,435]

The red cell defect can be quantified through determination of the number of polymorphonuclear white cells that are negative for the CD59 antigen.[431] Patients who have a larger CD59-negative clone seem to have the worst symptoms, particularly thrombotic symptoms. Those with smaller PNH clones seem to express fewer thromboses but are more prone to bone marrow failure. Patients with shrinkage of their PNH clone may be especially subject to marrow failure. No patients with a PNH clone <60% in one series were found to have experienced thrombosis, whereas at least half of all patients with PNH clones ≥60% manifested

thrombosis. It was estimated that for each 10% increase in PNH clone, the odds ratio for risk of thrombosis increased by 1.64.[436] These facts must be used in calculating the risks of anticoagulant therapy in patients who have not yet had a thrombotic manifestation.

One group that studied 56 patients with PNH sought evidence for additional thrombophilic risk factors to determine whether risks were additive. It was surprising that among 56 patients, no increase in the frequency of factor V Leiden mutation was noted.[437] It remains to be seen whether these data can be duplicated for other thrombophilic disorders among patients with PNH.

Despite the relative rarity of PNH, all investigators have been intrigued by the strong proclivity among these patients to present with HVT or CVT. Among reviews of patients with HVT, the density of those who have PNH is noteworthy. PNH also seems to be overrepresented in CVT.

Louwes and colleagues[438] detected shortened platelet survival, as well as decreased platelet production, among patients with PNH. Using kinetic studies, investigators identified enhanced uptake of platelets within abdominal vessels and hypothesized increased adherence of platelets to the endothelium within abdominal vessels in patients with PNH. This may explain, in part, the tendency of patients with PNH to experience intra-abdominal thromboses.

An increase in circulating procoagulant microparticles (MPs) has been detected in the plasma of patients with PNH.[439,440,441] Hugel[439] found increased circulating MPs seemingly of platelet origin in the plasma of patients with PNH, and they argued that these could serve as procoagulant phospholipid platforms in the plasma of such patients. Others[440] detected increased platelet activation and platelet MP formation, as well as laboratory evidence for increased hypercoagulability (positive plasma thrombin:antithrombin III complexes as well as D-dimers) and markedly elevated levels of tissue factor (TF).

Given the frequency of thrombotic manifestations of PNH, all reviews suggest that anticoagulation is indicated and is usually effective.[427,430,433,442,443] Antithrombotic therapy, probably provided for an indefinite period, appears to be indicated for nearly all patients who have had prior thrombosis. The use of anticoagulants for primary prevention of thromboembolic phenomena is controversial but certainly seems rational in patients with PNH clones greater than 50% to 60%[436] and perhaps is less indicated in patients of Asian ancestry.[431]

PNH is particularly virulent among pregnant patients. Ray and colleagues[428] reviewed the literature regarding pregnancy in patients with PNH. They studied 20 reports involving 33 pregnancies and found a thrombosis rate of 12%. It also appears that some patients progress to thrombosis despite seemingly aggressive and adequate prophylaxis.[440,444] The all-cause mortality rate was 21%. Half of patients were delivered before they reached term. A 9% perinatal mortality rate was reported.

In their review of PNH and pregnancy, Ray and associates[428] recommended heparin (7500 to 10,000 units twice daily) or enoxaparin (75 to 100 anti-Xa units per kilogram once daily) for thromboprophylaxis, beginning early in the first trimester and continuing for at least 4 to 6 weeks postpartum. In patients with PNH who have concomitant thrombocytopenia with a platelet count of less than

50,000/µL, such therapy may be trying. Because of the extreme degree of hypercoagulability at term, one should be cautious regarding the usual lowering or cessation of thromboprophylaxis at the time of delivery, as this action seems to be frequently associated with a thrombotic event. Careful discussion with the obstetrician is warranted.

REFERENCES

1. Samuels P, Webster D: The role of venous endothelium in the inception of thrombosis. Ann Surg 136:422–438, 1952.
2. Stewart G, Ritchie W, Lynch P: Venous endothelial damage produced by massive sticking and emigration of leukocytes. Am J Pathol 74:507–521, 1974.
3. Fuster V, Moreno P, Fayad Z, et al: Atherothrombosis and high-risk plaque: Part I: Evolving concepts. J Am Coll Cardiol 46:937–954, 2005.
4. Esmon C: Protein-C: Biochemistry, physiology, and clinical implications. Blood 62:1155, 1983.
5. Cines D, Pollak E, Buck C, et al: Endothelial cells in physiology and in the pathophysiology of vascular disorders. Blood 91:3527–3561, 1999.
6. Heijboer H, Brandjes D, Büller H, et al: Deficiencies of coagulation-inhibiting and fibrinolytic proteins in outpatients with deep vein thrombosis. N Engl J Med 323:1512–1516, 1990.
7. Vossen C, Conard J, Fontcuberta J, et al: Familial thrombophilia and lifetime risk of venous thrombosis. J Thromb Haemost 2:1526–1532, 2004.
8. Auletta M, Headington J: Purpura fulminans: A cutaneous manifestation of severe protein C deficiency. Arch Dermatol 124:1387–1391, 1988.
9. Branson H, Katz J, Marble R, Griffin J: Inherited protein C deficiency and coumarin-responsive chronic relapsing purpura fulminans in a newborn infant. Lancet 2:1165–1168, 1983.
10. Comp P, Elrod J, Karzenski S: Warfarin-induced skin necrosis. Semin Thromb Haemost 16:293–298, 1990.
11. Friedman K, Marlar R, Houson J, et al: Warfarin-induced skin necrosis in a patient with protein S deficiency. Blood 68:333a, 1986.
12. Makris M, Bardhan G, Preston F: Warfarin induced skin necrosis associated with activated protein C resistance. Thromb Haemost 75:523–524, 1996.
13. Inbal A, Freimark D, Modan B, et al: Synergistic effects of prothrombotic polymorphisms and atherogenic factors on the risk of myocardial infarction in young males. Blood 93:2189–2190, 1999.
14. Coller B: Deficiency of plasma protein S, protein C, or antithrombin III and arterial thrombosis. Arterioscler Thromb 7:456, 1987.
15. Johnson E: Premature arterial disease associated with familial antithrombin III deficiency. Thromb Haemost 63:13, 1990.
16. Douay X, Lucas C, Caron C, et al: Antithrombin, protein C and protein S levels in 127 consecutive young adults with ischemic stroke. Acta Neurol Scand 98:124–127, 1998.
17. Lane D, Grant P: Role of hemostatic gene polymorphisms in venous and arterial thrombotic disease. Blood 95:1517–1532, 2000.
18. Price D, Ridker P: Factor V Leiden mutation and the risks for thromboembolic disease: A clinical perspective. Ann Intern Med 127:895–903, 1997.
19. Press R, Bauer K, Kujovich J, Heit J: Clinical utility of Factor V Leiden (R506Q) testing for the diagnosis and management of thromboembolic disorders. Arch Pathol Lab Med 126:1304–1318, 2002.
20. Vossen C, Preston F, Conard J, et al: Hereditary thrombophilia and fetal loss: A prospective follow-up study. J Thromb Haemost 2:529–596, 2004.
21. Lissalde-Lavigne G, Fabbro-Peray P, Cochery-Nouvellon E, et al: Factor V Leiden and prothrombin G20210A polymorphisms as risk factors for miscarriage during a first intended pregnancy: The matched case-control 'NOHA first' study. J Thromb Haemost 3:2178–2184, 2005.
22. Brenner B, Nowak-Gottl U, Kosch A, et al: Diagnostic studies for thrombophilia in women on hormonal therapy and during pregnancy, and in children. Arch Pathol Lab Med 126:1296–1303, 2002.
23. Dilley A, Benito C, Hooper W, et al: Mutations in the factor V, prothrombin and MTHFR genes are not risk factors for recurrent fetal loss. J Maternal-Fetal Neonat Med 11:176–182, 2002.
24. Dizon-Townson D, Miller C, Sibai B, et al: National Institute of Child Health and Human Development Maternal-Fetal Medicine Units Network: The relationship of the factor V Leiden mutation and pregnancy outcomes for mother and fetus. Obstet Gynecol 106:517–524, 2005.
25. Robertson L, Wu O, Langhorne P, et al: The Thrombosis: Risk and Economic Assessment of Thrombophilia Screening (TREATS) Study: Thrombophilia in pregnancy: A systematic review. Br J Haematol 132:171–196, 2006.
26. Franchi F, Cetin I, Todros T, et al: Intrauterine growth restriction and genetic predisposition to thrombophilia. Haematologica 89:444–449, 2004.
27. Infante-Rivard C, Rivard G, Yotov W, et al: Absence of association of thrombophilia polymorphisms with intrauterine growth restriction. N Engl J Med 347:19–25, 2002.
28. Mello G, Parretti E, Marozio L, et al: Thrombophilia is significantly associated with severe preeclampsia: Results of a large-scale, case-controlled study. Hypertension 46:1270–1274, 2005.
29. Bank I, Scavenius M, Buller H, Middeldorp S: Social aspects of genetic testing for factor V leiden mutation in healthy individuals and their importance for daily practice. Thromb Res 113:7–12, 2004.
30. Parker C, Omine M, Richards S, et al: Diagnosis and management of paroxysmal nocturnal hemoglobinuria. Blood 106:3699–3706, 2005.
31. Vandenbroucke J, Koster T, Briet E, et al: Increased risk of venous thrombosis in oral-contraceptive users who are carriers of factor V Leiden mutation. Lancet 344:1453–1457, 1994.
32. Wu O, Robertson L, Langhorne P, et al: Oral contraceptives, hormone replacement therapy, thrombophilias and risk of venous thromboembolism: A systematic review. The Thrombosis: Risk and Economic Assessment of Thrombophilia Screening. Thromb Haemost 94:17–25, 2005.
33. Heit J, Kobbervig C, James A, et al: Trends in the incidence of deep vein thrombosis and pulmonary embolism during pregnancy or the puerperium: A 30-year population-based study. Ann Intern Med 143:697–706, 2005.
34. Silverstein M, Heit J, Mohr D, et al: Trends in the incidence of deep vein thrombosis and pulmonary embolism: A 25-year population-based, cohort study. Arch Intern Med 158:585–593, 1998.
35. Shanafelt T, Barton D, Adjei A, Loprinzi C: Pathophysiology and treatment of hot flashes. Mayo Clin Proc 77:1207–1218, 2002.
36. Herrington D, Vittinghoff E, Howard T, et al: Factor V Leiden, hormone replacement therapy, and risk of venous thromboembolic events in women with coronary disease. Arterioscler Thromb Vasc Biol 22:1012–1017, 2002.
37. Rosendaal F, Vessey M, Rumley A: Hormonal replacement therapy, prothrombotic mutations and the risk of venous thrombosis. Br J Haematol 116:851–854, 2002.
38. Cushman M, Kuller L, Prentice R, et al: Estrogen plus progestin and risk of venous thrombosis. JAMA 292:1573–1580, 2004.
39. Hulley S, Grady D, Bush T, et al: Randomized trial of estrogen plus progestin for secondary prevention of coronary heart disease in postmenopausal women. JAMA 180:605–613, 1998.
40. Wu O, Robertson L, Twaddle S, et al: The Thrombosis: Risk and Economic Assessment of Thrombophilia Screening (TREATS) Study. Screening for thrombophilia in high-risk situations: A meta-analysis and cost-effectiveness analysis. Br J Haematol 131:80–90, 2005.
41. Heit J: Venous thromboembolism: Disease burden, outcomes and risk factors: State of the art. J Thromb Haemost 3:1611–1617, 2005.
42. Heit J, Silverstein M, Mohr D, et al: Predictors of survival after deep vein thrombosis and pulmonary embolism: A population-based, cohort study. Arch Intern Med 159:445–453, 1999.
43. Kahn S, M'Lan C, Lamping D, et al: The Veines Study Group: The influence of venous thromboembolism on quality of life and severity of chronic venous disease. J Thromb Haemost 2:2152–2155, 2004.
44. Heit J, Melton L, Lohse C, et al: Incidence of venous thromboembolism in hospitalized patients versus community residents. Mayo Clin Proc 76:1102–1110, 2001.
45. Prandoni P, Lensing A, Cogo A, et al: The long-term clinical course of acute deep vein thrombosis. Ann Intern Med 125:1–7, 1996.
46. Mohr D, Silverstein M, Heit J, et al: The venous stasis syndrome after deep venous thrombosis or pulmonary embolism: A population-based study. Mayo Clin Proc 75:1249–1256, 2000.
47. Cushman M, Albert W, Tsai RH, et al: Deep vein thrombosis and pulmonary embolism in two cohorts: The longitudinal investigation of thromboembolism etiology. Am J Med 117:19–25, 2004.
48. Massicote M, Dix D, Monagle P, et al: Central venous catheter related thrombosis in children: Analysis of the Canadian Registry of Venous Thromboembolic Complications. J Pediatr 133:770–776, 1998.
49. van Ommen C, Heijboer H, Büller H, et al: Venous thromboembolism in childhood: A prospective two-year registry in The Netherlands. J Pediatr 139:676–681, 2001.

50. Tormene D, Simioni P, Prandoni P, et al: The incidence of venous thromboembolism in thrombophilic children: A prospective cohort study. Blood 100:2403–2405, 2002.

51. White R, Zhou H, Romano P: Incidence of idiopathic deep venous thrombosis and secondary thromboembolism among ethnic groups in California. Ann Intern Med 128:737–740, 1998.

52. Oger E: Incidence of venous thromboembolism: A community-based study in western France. Thromb Haemost 83:657–660, 2000.

53. Stein P, Hull R, Kayali F, et al: Venous thromboembolism according to age: Impact of an aging population. Arch Intern Med 164: 2260–2265, 2004.

54. Kobbervig C, Heit J, Petterson T, et al: The effect of patient age on the incidence of idiopathic vs. secondary venous thromboembolism: A population-based cohort study. Blood 104:957a, 2004.

55. Klatsky A, Armstrong M, Poggi J: Risk of pulmonary embolism and/or deep venous thrombosis in Asian-Americans. Am J Cardiol 85:1334–1337, 2000.

56. Stein P, Kayali F, Olson R, Milford C: Pulmonary thromboembolism in American Indians and Alaskan Natives. Arch Intern Med 164:1804–1806, 2004.

57. Hooper W, Holman R, Heit J, Cobb N: Venous thromboembolism hospitalizations among American Indians and Alaska Natives. Thromb Res 108:273–278, 2002.

58. Stein P, Kayali F, Olson R, Milford C: Pulmonary thromboembolism in Asians/Pacific Islanders in the United States: Analysis of data from the National Hospital Discharge Survey and the United States Bureau of the Census. Am J Med 116:435–442, 2004.

59. White R, Zhou H, Murin S, Harvey D: Effect of ethnicity and gender on the incidence of venous thromboembolism in a diverse population in California in 1996. Thromb Haemost 93:298–305, 2005.

60. Heit J, Silverstein M, Mohr D, et al: Risk factors for deep vein thrombosis and pulmonary embolism: A population-based case-control study. Arch Intern Med 160:809–815, 2000.

61. Heit J, O'Fallon W, Petterson T, et al: Relative impact of risk factors for deep vein thrombosis and pulmonary embolism: A population-based study. Arch Intern Med 162:1245–1248, 2002.

62. Cogo A, Bernardi E, Prandoni P, et al: Acquired risk factors for deep-vein thrombosis in symptomatic outpatients. Arch Intern Med 154:164–168, 1994.

63. Rosendaal F: Risk factors for venous thrombotic disease. Thromb Haemost 82:610–619, 1999.

64. Samama M: An epidemiologic study of risk factors for deep vein thrombosis in medical outpatients. Arch Intern Med 160: 3415–3420, 2000.

65. Jones T, Ugalde V, Franks P, et al: Venous thromboembolism after spinal cord injury: Incidence, time course, and associated risk factors in 16,240 adults and children. Arch Phys Med Rehabil 86:2240–2247, 2005.

66. Geerts W, Pineo G, Heit J, et al: Prevention of venous thromboembolism: The Seventh ACCP Conference on Antithrombotic and Thrombolytic Therapy. Chest 126 (suppl 3): 338S–400S, 2004.

67. White R, Zhou H, Romano P: Incidence of symptomatic venous thromboembolism after different elective or urgent surgical procedures. Thromb Haemost 90:446–455, 2003.

68. White R, Gettner S, Newman J, Romano P: Predictors of rehospitalization for symptomatic venous thromboembolism after total hip arthroplasty. N Engl J Med 343:1758–1764, 2000.

69. Sharrock N, Haas S, Hargett M, et al: Effects of epidural anesthesia on the incidence of deep vein thrombosis after total knee replacement. J Bone Joint Surg Am 73:502–506, 1991.

70. Alikhan R, Cohen A, Combe S, et al: Risk factors for venous thromboembolism in hospitalized patients with acute medical illness. Arch Intern Med 164:963–968, 2004.

71. Zakai N, Wright J, Cushman M: Risk factors for venous thrombosis in medical inpatients: Validation of a thrombosis risk score. Thromb Haemost 2:2156–2161, 2004.

72. Heit J, Petterson T, Bailey K, Melton LI: The influence of tumor site on venous thromboembolism risk among cancer patients: A population-based study. Congress of the American Society of Hematology. Blood 104:711a, 2004.

73. Chew H, Wun T, Harvey D, et al: Incidence of venous thromboembolism and its effect on survival among patients with common cancers. Arch Intern Med 166:458–464, 2006.

74. Stein P, Beemath A, Meyers F, et al: Incidence of venous thromboembolism in patients hospitalized with cancer. Am J Med 119:60–68, 2006.

75. Blom J, Vanderschoot J, Ostindier M, et al: Incidence of venous thrombosis in a large cohort of 66,329 cancer patients: Results of a record linkage study. J Thromb Haemost 4:529, 2006.

76. Kucek O, Kwaan H, Gunnak W, et al: Thromboembolic complications associated with L-asparaginase therapy. Cancer 55:702, 1985.

77. Zangari M, Anaissie E, Barlogie B, et al: Increased risk of deep-vein thrombosis in patients with multiple myeloma receiving thalidomide and chemotherapy. Blood 98:1614–1615, 2001.

78. Kuenen B, Rosen L, Smit E, et al: Dose-finding and pharmacokinetic study of cisplatin, gemcitabine, and SU5416 in patients with solid tumors. J Clin Oncol 20:1657–1667, 2002.

79. Pritchard K, Paterson A, Paul N, et al: Increased thromboembolic complications with concurrent tamoxifen and chemotherapy in a randomized trial of adjuvant therapy for women with breast cancer. National Cancer Institute of Canada Clinical Trials Group Breast Cancer Site Group. J Clin Oncol 14:2731–2737, 1996.

80. Heit J, Farmer S, Petterson T, et al: Novel risk factors for venous thromboembolism: A population-based, case-control study. Blood 106:463A, 2005.

81. Wun T, Law L, Harvey D, et al: Increased incidence of symptomatic venous thrombosis in patients with cervical carcinoma treated with concurrent chemotherapy, radiation, and erythropoietin. Cancer 98:1514–1520, 2003.

82. Dalen J: Economy class syndrome: Too much flying or too much sitting? Arch Intern Med 163:2674, 2003.

83. Chee Y-L, Watson J: Air travel and thrombosis. Br J Haematol 130:671–680, 2005.

84. Ray J, Mamdani M, Tsuyuki R, et al: Use of statins and the subsequent development of deep vein thrombosis. Arch Intern Med 161:1405–1410, 2001.

85. Doggen C, Lemaitre R, Smith N, et al: HMGCoA reductase inhibitors and the risk of venous thrombosis among postmenopausal women. J Thromb Haemost 2:700–701, 2004.

86. Prandoni P, Bilora F, Marchiori A, et al: An association between atherosclerosis and venous thrombosis. N Engl J Med 348:1435–1441, 2003.

87. Tsai A, Cushman M, Rosamond W, et al: Cardiovascular risk factors and venous thromboembolism incidence. Arch Intern Med 162:1182–1189, 2002.

88. Petterson T, Agmon Y, Meissner I, et al: Atherosclerosis as a risk factor for venous thromboembolism: A population-based cohort study. Blood 104:708a, 2004.

89. Glynn R, Rosner B: Comparison of risk factors for the competing risks of coronary heart disease, stroke, and venous thromboembolism. J Epidemiol 162:975–982, 2005.

90. Gomez E, van der Poel S, Jansen J: Rapid simultaneous screening of factor V Leiden and G20210A prothrombin variant by multiplex polymerase chain reaction on whole blood. Blood 91:2208–2209, 1995.

91. Curb D, Prentice R, Bray P, et al: Venous thrombosis and conjugated equine estrogen in women without a uterus. Arch Intern Med 166:729–736, 2006.

92. Bloemenkamp K, Rosendaal F, Helmerhorst F, Vandenbroucke J: Higher risk of venous thrombosis during early use of oral contraceptives in women with inherited clotting defects. Arch Intern Med 160:49–52, 2000.

93. World Health Organization Collaborative Study of Cardiovascular Disease and Steroid Hormone, C: Cardiovascular disease and use of oral and injectable progesterone-only contraceptives and combined injectable contraceptives: Results of an international, multicenter, case-control study. Contraception 57:315–324, 1998.

94. Pandya K, Morrow G, Roscoe J, et al: Gabapentin for hot flashes in 420 women with breast cancer: A randomized double-blind placebo-controlled trial. Lancet 366:818–824, 2005.

95. Smith N, Heckbert S, Lemaitre R, et al: Esterified estrogens and conjugated equine estrogens and the risk for venous thrombosis. JAMA 292:1581–1587, 2004.

96. Scarabin P, Oger E, Plu-Bureau G: Differential association of oral and transdermal oestrogen replacement therapy with venous thromboembolism risk. Lancet 362:428–432, 2003.

97. Straczek C, Oger E, Yon de Jonage-Canonico M, et al: Estrogen and Thromboembolism Risk (ESTHER) Study Group: Prothrombotic mutations, hormone therapy, and venous thromboembolism among postmenopausal women: Impact of the route of estrogen administration. Circulation 112:3495–3500, 2005.

98. James A, Tapson V, Goldhaber S: Thrombosis during pregnancy and the postpartum period. Am J Obstet Gynecol 193:216–219, 2005.

99. Heit J, Sobell J, Li H, Sommer S: The incidence of venous thromboembolism among Factor V Leiden carriers: A community-based cohort study. J Thromb Haemost 3:305–311, 2005.

100. Danilenko-Dixon D, Heit J, Watkins T, et al: Risk factors for deep vein thrombosis and pulmonary embolism during pregnancy or the

postpartum period: A population-based case-control study. Am J Obstet Gynecol 184:104–110, 2001.

101. Fisher B, Costantino J, Wickerham D, et al: Tamoxifen for prevention of breast cancer: Report of the National Surgical Adjuvant Breast and Bowel Project P-1 Study. J Natl Cancer Inst 90:1371–1388, 1998.

102. Meier C, Jick H: Tamoxifen and risk of idiopathic venous thromboembolism. Br J Pharmacol 45:608–612, 1998.

103. McCaskill-Stevens W, Bryant J, Costantino J, et al: Incidence of contralateral breast cancer (CBC), endometrial cancer (EC), and thromboembolic events (TE) in African American (AA) women receiving tamoxifen for treatment of primary breast cancer. Proc Am Soc Clin Oncol 19:70a, 2000.

104. Weitz I, Israel V, Liebman H: Tamoxifen-associated venous thrombosis and activated protein C resistance due to factor V Leiden. Cancer 79:2024–2027, 1997.

105. Cummings S, Eckert S, Krueger K, et al: The effect of raloxifene on risk of breast cancer in postmenopausal women: Results from the MORE randomized trial. Multiple Outcomes of Taloxifene Evaluation. JAMA 281:2189–2197, 1998.

106. Grady D, Ettinger B, Moscarelli E, et al: Safety and adverse effects associated with raloxifene: Multiple outcomes of raloxifene evaluation. Obstet Gynecol 104:837–844, 2004.

107. Schafer A: Bleeding and thrombosis in the myeloproliferative disorders. Blood 64:1–12, 1984.

108. Cortelazzo S, Viero P, Finazzi G, et al: Incidence and risk factors for thrombotic complications in a historical cohort of 100 patients with essential thrombocythemia. J Clin Oncol 8:556–562, 1990.

109. Llach F: Hypercoagulability, renal vein thrombosis, and other thrombotic complications of nephrotic syndrome. Kidney Int 28:429–439, 1985.

110. Yarranton H, Machin S: An update on the pathogenesis and management of acquired thrombotic thrombocytopenic purpura. Curr Opin Neurol 16:367–373, 2003.

111. Calvo-Alen J, Toloza S, Fernandez M, et al: Systemic lupus erythematosus in a multiethnic U.S. cohort (LUMINA). XXV. Smoking, older age, disease activity, lupus anticoagulant, and glucocorticoid dose as risk factors for the occurrence of venous thrombosis in lupus patients. Arthritis Rheum 52:2060–2068, 2005.

112. Merkel P, Lo G, Holbrook J, et al: High incidence of venous thrombotic events among patients with Wegener Granulomatosis: The Wegener's Granulomatosis Occurrence of Thrombosis (WeCLOT) Study. Ann Intern Med 142:620–626, 2005.

113. Srirajaskanthan R, Winter M, Muller A: Venous thrombosis in inflammatory bowel disease. Eur J Gastroenterol Hepatol 17:697–700, 2005.

114. McCully K: Vascular pathology of homocysteinemia: Implications for the pathogenesis of arteriosclerosis. Am J Pathol 56:111–128, 1969.

115. Key N, McGlennen R: Hyperhomocyst(e)inemia and thrombophilia. Arch Pathol Lab Med 126:1367–1375, 2002.

116. Tsai A, Cushman M, Tsai M, et al: Serum homocysteine, thermolabile variant of methylene tetrahydrofolate reductase (MTHFR), and venous thromboembolism: Longitudinal Investigation of Thromboembolism Etiology (LITE). Am J Hematol 72:192–200, 2003.

117. den Heijer M, Lewington S, Clarke R: Homocysteine, MTHFR and risk of venous thrombosis: A meta-analysis of published epidemiological studies. J Thromb Haemost 3:292–299, 2005.

118. Souto J, Almasy L, Borrell M, et al: Genetic susceptibility to thrombosis and its relationship to physiological risk factors: The GAIT study. Genetic Analysis of Idiopathic Thrombophilia. Am J Human Genet 67:1452–1459, 2000.

119. Larsen T, Sorensen H, Skytthe A, et al: Major genetic susceptibility for venous thromboembolism in men: A study of Danish twins. Epidemiology 14:328–332, 2003.

120. Heit J, Phelps M, Ward S, et al: Familial segregation of venous thromboembolism. J Thromb Haemost 2:731–736, 2004.

121. Sanson B, Simioni P, Tormene D, et al: The incidence of venous thromboembolism in asymptomatic carriers of a deficiency of antithrombin, protein C, or protein S: A prospective cohort study. Blood 94:3702–3706, 1999.

122. Folsom A, Aleksic N, Wang N, et al: Protein C, antithrombin, and venous thromboembolism incidence: A prospective population-based study. Arterioscler Thromb Vasc Biol 22:1018–1022, 2002.

123. Vossen C, Rosendaal F: The protective effect of the factor XIII Val34-Leu mutation on the risk of deep venous thrombosis is dependent on the fibrinogen level. Thromb Haemost 3:1102–1103, 2005.

124. Vossen C, Walker I, Svensson P, et al: Recurrence rate after a first venous thrombosis in patients with familial thrombophilia. Arterioscler Thromb Vasc Biol 25:1992–1997, 2005.

125. Bombeli T, Piccapietra B, Boersma J, Fehr J: Decreased anticoagulant response to tissue factor pathway inhibitor in patients with venous thromboembolism and otherwise no evidence of hereditary or acquired thrombophilia. Thromb Haemost 91:80–86, 2004.

126. Broze G Jr: Human protein Z. J Clin Invest 73:933–938, 1984.

127. Yin Z, Huang Z, Cui J, et al: Prothrombotic phenotype of protein Z deficiency. Proc Natl Acad Sci U S A 97:6734–6738, 2000.

128. Han X, Fiehler R, Broze G Jr: Isolation of a protein Z–dependent plasma protease inhibitor. Proc Natl Acad Sci U S A 95:9250–9255, 1998.

129. Han X, Huang Z, Fiehler R, Broze G Jr: The protein Z–dependent protease inhibitor is a serpin. Biochemistry 38:11073–11078, 1999.

130. Souri M, Koseki-Kuno S, Iwata H, et al: A naturally occurring E30Q mutation in the Gla domain of protein Z causes its impaired secretion and subsequent deficiency. Blood 105:3149–3154, 2005.

131. Uitte de Willige S, de Visser M, Houwing-Duistermaat J, et al: Genetic variation in the fibrinogen gamma gene increases the risk for deep venous thrombosis by reducing fibrinogen gamma levels. Blood 106:4176–4183, 2005.

132. Folsom A, Cushman M, Tsai M, et al: A prospective study of venous thromboembolism in relation to factor V Leiden and related factors. Blood 88:2720–2725, 2002.

133. Juul K, Tybjærg-Hansen A, Schnohr P, Nordestgaard B: Factor V Leiden and the risk for venous thromboembolism in the adult Danish population. Ann Intern Med 140:330–337, 2004.

134. Chandler W, Rodgers G, Sprouse J, Thompson A: Elevated hemostatic factors as potential risk factors for thrombosis. Arch Pathol Lab Med 126:1405–1414, 2002.

135. van Hylckama Vlieg A, Rosendaal F: High levels of fibrinogen are associated with the risk of deep venous thrombosis mainly in the elderly. J Thromb Haemost 1:2677–2678, 2003.

136. Wells P, Langlois N, Webster M, et al: Elevated factor VIII is a risk factor for idiopathic venous thromboembolism in Canada—Is it necessary to define a new upper reference range for factor VIII? Thromb Haemost 93:842–846, 2005.

137. McGlennen R, Key N: Clinical and laboratory management of the prothrombin G20210A mutation. Arch Pathol Lab Med 126:1319–1325, 2002.

138. Folsom A, Cushman M, Tsai M, et al: Prospective study of the G20210A polymorphism in the prothrombin gene, plasma prothrombin concentration, and incidence of venous thromboembolism. Am J Hematol 71:285–290, 2002.

139. Koster T, Blann A, Briët E, et al: Role of clotting factor VIII in effect of von Willebrand factor on occurrence of deep vein thrombosis. Lancet 345:152–155, 1995.

140. MacCallum P, Meade T, Cooper J, et al: Clotting factor VIII and risk of deep-vein thrombosis. Lancet 345:804, 1995.

141. Kraaigenhagen R, Anker P, Koopman M, et al: High plasma concentration of Factor VIIIc is a major risk factor for venous thromboembolism. Thromb Haemost 83:5–9, 2000.

142. Bank I, Libourel E, Middeldorp S, et al: Elevated levels of FVIII:C within families are associated with an increased risk for venous and arterial thrombosis. J Thromb Haemost 3:79–84, 2005.

143. van Hylckama Vlieg A, van der Linden I, Bertina R, Rosendaal F: High levels of factor IX increase the risk of venous thrombosis. Blood 95:3678–3682, 2000.

144. Meijers J, Tekelenburg W, Bouma B, et al: High levels of coagulation factor XI as a risk factor for venous thrombosis. N Engl J Med 342:696–701, 2000.

145. Tripodi A, Chantarangkul V, Martinelli I, et al: A shortened activated partial thromboplastin time is associated with the risk of venous thromboembolism. Blood 104:3631–3634, 2004.

146. Folsom A, Cushman M, Heckbert S, et al: Prospective study of fibrinolytic markers and venous thromboembolism. J Clin Epidemiol 56:598–603, 2003.

147. Cushman M, Folsom A, Wang L, et al: Fibrin fragment D-dimer and the risk of future venous thrombosis. Blood 101:1243–1248, 2003.

148. Lisman T, de Groot P, Meijers J: Reduced plasma fibrinolytic potential is a risk factor for venous thrombosis. Blood 105:1102–1105, 2005.

149. Andre P, Hartwell D, Hrachovinova I, et al: Pro-coagulant state resulting from high levels of soluble P-selectin in blood. Proc Natl Acad Sci U S A 97:13835–13840, 2000.

150. Reitsma P, Rosendaal F: Activation of innate immunity in patients with venous thrombosis: The Leiden Thrombophilia Study. J Thromb Haemost 2:619–622, 2004.

151. de Lange M, Snieder H, Ariens R, et al: The genetics of haemostasis: A twin study. Lancet 357:101–105, 2001.

152. Ariëns R, de Lange M, Snieder H, et al: Activation markers of coagulation and fibrinolysis in twins: Heritability of the prethrombotic state. Lancet 359:667–671, 2002.

153. Vossen C, Hasstedt S, Rosendaal F, et al: Heritability of plasma concentrations of clotting factors and measures of a prethrombotic state in a protein C–deficient family. J Thromb Haemost 2: 242–247, 2004.

154. Morange P, Tregouet D, Frere C, et al: Biological and genetic factors influencing plasma factor VIII levels in a healthy family population: Results from the Stanislas cohort. Br J Haematol 128:91–99, 2004.

155. van Hylckama Vlieg A, Rosendaal F: Interaction between oral contraceptive use and coagulation factor levels in deep venous thrombosis. J Thromb Haemost 1:2189–2190, 2003.

156. Martinelli I, De Stefano V, Taioli E, et al: Inherited thrombophilia and first venous thromboembolism during pregnancy and puerperium. Thromb Haemost 87:791–795, 2002.

157. Lindahl T, Lundahl T, Nilsson L, Andersson C: APC-resistance is a risk factor for postoperative thromboembolism in elective replacement of the hip or knee: A prospective study. Thromb Haemost 81:18–21, 1999.

158. Salvati E, Della Valle A, Westrich G, et al: The John Charnley Award: Heritable thrombophilia and development of thromboembolic disease after total hip arthroplasty. Clin Orthop Rel Res 441, 2005.

159. Blom J, Doggen C, Osanto S, Rosendaal F: Malignancies, prothrombotic mutations, and the risk of venous thrombosis. JAMA 293:715–722, 2005.

160. Libourel EIB, Meinardi J, Balje-Volkers C, et al: Co-segregation of thrombophilic disorders in factor V Leiden carriers: The contributions of factor VIII, factor XI, thrombin activatable fibrinolysis inhibitor and lipoprotein(a) to the absolute risk of venous thromboembolism. Haematologica 87:1068–1073, 2002.

161. Heit J, Mohr D, Silverstein M, et al: Predictors of recurrence after deep vein thrombosis and pulmonary embolism: A population-based cohort study. Arch Intern Med 160:761–768, 2000.

162. Heit J, Cohen A, Anderson FJ: Estimated annual number of incident and recurrent, non-fatal and fatal venous thromboembolism (VTE) events in the U.S. Blood 106:267A, 2005.

163. Christiansen S, Cannegieter S, Koster T, et al: Thrombophilia, clinical factors, and recurrent venous thrombotic events. JAMA 293:2351–2361, 2005.

164. Kyrle P, Minar E, Bialonczyk C, et al: The risk of recurrent venous thromboembolism in men and women. N Engl J Med 350:2558–2563, 2004.

165. Baglin T, Luddington R, Brown K, Baglin C: High risk of recurrent venous thromboembolism in men. J Thromb Haemost 2:2152–2155, 2004.

166. Hansson P, Sorbo J, Eriksson H: Recurrent venous thromboembolism after deep vein thrombosis: Incidence and risk factors. Arch Intern Med 160:769–774, 2000.

167. Prandoni P, Lensing A, Piccioli A, et al: Recurrent venous thromboembolism and bleeding complications during anticoagulant treatment in patients with cancer and venous thrombosis. Blood 100:3484–3488, 2002.

168. Kearon C, Gent M, Hirsh J, et al: A comparison of three months of anticoagulation with extended anticoagulation for a first episode of idiopathic venous thromboembolism. N Engl J Med 340:901–907, 1999.

169. Agnelli G, Prandoni P, Santamaria M, et al: Three months versus one year of oral anticoagulant therapy for idiopathic deep venous thrombosis. N Engl J Med 345:165–169, 2001.

170. Baglin T, Luddington R, Brown K, Baglin C: Incidence of recurrent venous thromboembolism in relation to clinical and thrombophilic risk factors: Prospective cohort study. Lancet 362:523–526, 2003.

171. Schulman S, Svenungsson E, Granqvist S: Anticardiolipin antibodies predict early recurrence of thromboembolism and death among patients with venous thromboembolism following anticoagulant therapy. Duration of Anticoagulation Study Group. Am J Med 104:332–338, 1998.

172. van den Belt A, Sanson B-J, Simioni P, et al: Recurrence of venous thromboembolism in patients with familial thrombophilia. Arch Intern Med 157:227–232, 1997.

173. De Stefano V, Marinelli I, Mannucci P, et al: The risk of recurrent deep vein thrombosis among heterozygous carriers of both factor V Leiden and the G20210A prothrombin mutation. N Engl J Med 341:801–806, 1999.

174. Lindmarker P, Schulman S, Sten-Linder M, et al: The risk of recurrent venous thromboembolism in carriers and non-carriers of the G1691A allele in the coagulation factor V gene and the G20210a allele in the prothrombin gene. Thromb Haemost 81:684–689, 1999.

175. Meinardi J, Middeldorp S, de Kam P, et al: The incidence of recurrent venous thromboembolism in carriers of factor V Leiden is related to concomitant thrombophilic disorders. Br J Haematol 116:625–631, 2002.

176. Weltermann A, Eichinger S, Bialonczyk C, et al: The risk of recurrent venous thromboembolism among patients with high factor IX levels. J Thromb Haemost 1:28–32, 2003.

177. Santamaria M, Agnelli G, Taliani M, et al: Thrombophilic abnormalities and recurrence of venous thromboembolism in patients treated with standardized anticoagulant treatment. Thromb Res 116:301–306, 2005.

178. Garcia-Fuster M, Forner M, Fernandez C, et al: Long-term prospective study of recurrent venous thromboembolism in patients younger than 50 years. Pathophysiol Haemost 34:6–12, 2005.

179. Hoke M, Kyrle P, Minar E, et al: Tissue factor pathway inhibitor and the risk of recurrent venous thromboembolism. Thromb Haemost 94:787–790, 2005.

180. De Stefano V, Chiusolo P, Paciaroni K, et al: Prothrombin G20210A mutant genotype is a risk factor for cerebrovascular ischemic disease in young patients. Blood 91:3562–3565, 1998.

181. Margaglione M, D'Andrea G, Colaizzo D, et al: Coexistence of factor V Leiden and Factor II A20210 mutations and recurrent venous thromboembolism. Thromb Haemost 82:1583–1587, 1999.

182. Kyrle P, Minar E, Mirschl M, et al: High plasma levels of factor VIII and the risk of recurrent venous thromboembolism. N Engl J Med 343:457–462, 2000.

183. Prandoni P, Lensing A, Prins M, et al: Residual venous thrombosis as a predictive factor of recurrent venous thromboembolism. Ann Intern Med 137:955–960, 2002.

184. Ho W, Hankey G, Quinlan D: Risk of recurrent venous thromboembolism in patients with common thrombophilia: A systematic review. Arch Intern Med 166:729–736, 2006.

185. Eichinger S, Minar E, Bialonczyk C, et al: D-dimer levels and risk of recurrent venous thromboembolism. JAMA 290:1071–1074, 2003.

186. Cosmi B, Legnani C, Cini M, et al: D-dimer levels in combination with residual venous obstruction and the risk of recurrence after anticoagulation withdrawal for a first idiopathic deep vein thrombosis. Thromb Haemost 94:969–974, 2005.

187. Murin S, Romano P, White R: Comparison of outcomes after hospitalization for deep venous thrombosis or pulmonary embolism. Thromb Haemost 88:407–414, 2002.

188. Heit J, Farmer S, Petterson T, et al: Venous thromboembolism event type (PE±DVT vs. DVT alone) predicts recurrence type and survival. Blood 100:149a, 2002.

189. Eichinger S, Weltermann A, Minar E, et al: Symptomatic pulmonary embolism and the risk of recurrent venous thromboembolism. Arch Intern Med 164:92–96, 2004.

190. DeStefano V, Finazzi G, Mannucci P: Inherited thrombophilia: Pathogenesis, clinical syndromes and management. Blood 87:3531–3544, 1996.

191. Bauer K: Management of thrombophilia. J Thromb Haemost 1:1429–1434, 2003.

192. Van Cott E, Laposata M, Prins M: Laboratory evaluation of hypercoagulability with venous or arterial thrombosis. Arch Pathol Lab Med 126:1281–1295, 2002.

193. Mateo J, Oliver A, Borrell M: Laboratory evaluation and clinical characteristics of 2,132 consecutive unselected patients with venous thromboembolism—Results of the Spanish multicentric study on thrombophilia (EMET Study). Thromb Haemost 77:444–451, 1997.

194. Svensson P, Dahlbäck B: Resistance to activated protein C as a basis of venous thrombosis. N Engl J Med 330:517–522, 1994.

195. Griffin J, Evatt B, Wideman C: Anticoagulant protein C pathway defective in majority of thrombophilia patients. Blood 82:1989–1993, 1993.

196. Poort S, Rosendaal F, Reitsma P, et al: A common genetic variation in the 3′-untranslated region of the prothrombin gene is associated with elevated plasma prothrombin levels and an increase in venous thrombosis. Blood 88:398–3703, 1996.

197. Kyrle P: The optimal duration of secondary thromboprophylaxis in patients with venous thromboembolism: The importance of thrombophilia screening. Wien Med Wochenschr 155:17–21, 2005.

198. van Boven H, Reitsma P, Rosendaal F, et al: Factor V Leiden (FV R506Q) in families with inherited antithrombin deficiency. Thromb Haemost 75:417–421, 1996.

199. Koeleman B, Reitsma P, Allaart C, Bertina R: Activated protein C as an additional risk factor for thrombosis in protein C–deficient families. Blood 84:1031–1035, 1994.

200. Zöller B, Berntsdotter A, Carcia de Frutos P, Dahlbäck B: Resistance to activated protein C as an additional genetic risk factor in hereditary deficiency of protein S. Blood 85:3518–3523, 1995.

201. van Boven H, Vandenbroucke J, Briet E, Rosendaal F: Gene-gene and gene-environment interactions determine the risk of thrombosis in families with inherited antithrombin deficiency. Blood 94:2590–2594, 1999.

202. De Stefano V, Rossi E, Paciaroni K, et al: Different circumstances of the first venous thromboembolism among younger or older heterozygous carriers of the G20210A polymorphism in the prothrombin gene. Haematologica 88:61–66, 2003.

203. Ruud E, Holmstrom H, Brosstad F, Wesenberg F: Diagnostic value of family histories of thrombosis to identify children with thrombophilia. Pediatr Hematol Oncol 22:453–462, 2005.

204. Rees D, Cox M, Clegg J: World distribution of factor V Leiden. Lancet 346:1133–1134, 1995.

205. Ridker P, Hennekens C, Selhub J: Interrelation of hyperhomocyst(e)inemia, factor V Leiden, and risk of future venous thromboembolism. Circulation 95:1777–1782, 1997.

206. Rosendaal F, Doggen C, Zvelin A: Geographic distribution of the 20210 G to A prothrombin variant. Thromb Haemost 79:706–708, 1998.

207. Dilley A, Austin H, Hooper W, et al: Prevalence of the prothrombin 20210 G-to-A variant in blacks: Infants, patients with venous thrombosis, patients with myocardial infarction, and control subjects. J Lab Clin Med 132:452–455, 1998.

208. Downing LJ, Wakefield TW, Strieter RM, et al: Anti–P-selectin antibody decreases inflammation and thrombus formation in venous thrombosis. J Vasc Surg 25:816–827, 1997.

209. Dowling N, Austin H, Dilley A, et al: The epidemiology of venous thromboembolism in Caucasians and African-Americans: The GATE study. J Thromb Haemost 1:80–87, 2003.

210. Piccioli A, Lensing A, Prins M, et al: Prandoni Investigators Group: Extensive screening for occult malignant disease in idiopathic venous thromboembolism: A prospective randomized clinical trial. J Thromb Haemost 2:884–889, 2004.

211. Lee A: Screening for occult cancer in patients with idiopathic venous thromboembolism. J Thromb Haemost 1:2273–2274, 2003.

212. Kottke-Marchant K, Duncan A: Antithrombin deficiency: Issues in laboratory diagnosis. Arch Pathol Lab Med 126:1326–1336, 2002.

213. Kitchens CS: Amelioration of antithrombin III defidiency by coumarin administration. Am J Med Sci 293:403–406, 1987.

214. O'Donnell M, Linkins L, Kearon C, et al: Reduction of out-of-hospital symptomatic venous thromboembolism by extended thromboprophylaxis with low-molecular-weight heparin following elective hip arthroplasty: A systematic review. Arch Intern Med 163:1362–1366, 2003.

215. Buller H, Agnelli G, Hull R, et al: Antithrombotic therapy for venous thromboembolic disease: The Seventh ACCP Conference on Antithrombotic and Thrombolytic Therapy. Chest 126:401S–428S, 2004.

216. Buller H, Sohne M, Middeldorp S: Treatment of venous thromboembolism. J Thromb Haemost 3:1554–1560, 2005.

217. Bucur S, Levy J, Despotis G, et al: Uses of antithrombin III concentrate in congenital and acquired deficiency states. Transfusion 38:481–498, 1998.

218. Menache D: Replacement therapy in patients with hereditary antithrombin III deficiency. Semin Thromb Haemost 28:31–38, 1991.

219. Pinede L, Ninet J, Duhaut P, et al: Investigators of the "Duree Optimale du Traitement AntiVitamines K" (DOTAVK), S: Comparison of 3 and 6 months of oral anticoagulant therapy after a first episode of proximal deep vein thrombosis or pulmonary embolism and comparison of 6 and 12 weeks of therapy after isolated calf deep vein thrombosis. Circulation 103:2453–2460, 2001.

220. Schulman S, Rhedin A, Lindmarker P, et al: A comparison of six weeks with six months of oral anticoagulant therapy after a first episode of venous thromboembolism. Duration of Anticoagulation Trial Study Group. N Engl J Med 332:1661–1665, 1995.

221. van Aken B, den Heijer M, Bos G, et al: Recurrent venous thrombosis and markers of inflammation. Thromb Haemost 83:536–539, 2000.

222. Heit J, Alfred C, Lokken T, et al: Thrombomodulin mutations as potential risk factors for venous thromboembolism: A populationbased case-control study. Blood 98:90b, 2001.

223. Schulman S, Granqvist S, Holmström M, et al: The duration of oral anticoagulation therapy after a second episode of venous thromboembolism. N Engl J Med 336:393–398, 1997.

224. Agnelli G, Prandoni P, Becattini C, et al: Warfarin Optimal Duration Italian Trial Investigators: Extended oral anticoagulant therapy after a first episode of pulmonary embolism. Ann Intern Med 139:19–25, 2003.

225. Kearon C, Ginsberg J, Anderson D, et al: Comparison of 1 month with 3 months of anticoagulation for a first episode of venous thromboembolism associated with a transient risk factor. J Thromb Haemost 2:743–749, 2004.

226. van Dongen C, Vink R, Hutten B, et al: The incidence of recurrent venous thromboembolism after treatment with vitamin K antagonists in relation to time since first event: A meta-analysis. Arch Intern Med 163:1285–1293, 2003.

227. Kyrle P, Eichinger S: The risk of recurrent venous thromboembolism: The Austrian Study on Recurrent Venous Thromboembolism. Wien Medizin Wochenschr 115:471–474, 2003.

228. Schulman S, Lindmarker P, Holmstrom M, et al: Post-thrombotic syndrome, recurrence, and death 10 years after the first episode of venous thromboembolism treated with warfarin for 6 weeks or 6 months. J Thromb Haemost 4:732–742, 2006.

229. Locadia M, Bossuyt P, Stalmeier P, et al: Treatment of venous thromboembolism with vitamin K antagonists: Patients' health state valuations and treatment preferences. Thromb Haemost 92:1336–1341, 2004.

230. Vink R, Kraaijenhagen R, Levi M, Buller H: Individualized duration of oral anticoagulant therapy for deep vein thrombosis based on a decision model. J Thromb Haemost 1:2523–2530, 2003.

231. Forastiero R, Martinuzzo M, Pombo G, et al: A prospective study of antibodies to beta2-glycoprotein I and prothrombin, and risk of thrombosis. J Thromb Haemost 3:1231–1238, 2005.

232. Comp P, Esmon C: Recurrent venous thromboembolism in patients with a partial deficiency of protein S. N Engl J Med 311:1525–1528, 1984.

233. Eichinger S, Stumpflen A, Hirschl M, et al: Hyperhomocysteinemia is a risk factor of recurrent venous thromboembolism. Thromb Haemost 80:566–569, 1998.

234. Hull R, Marder V, Mah A, et al: Quantitive assessment of thrombus burder predicts the outcome of treatment for venous thrombosis: A systematic review. Am J Med 118:456–464, 2005.

235. Hron G, Eichinger S, Weltermann A, et al: Family history for venous thromboembolism and the risk for recurrence. Am J Med 119:50–53, 2006.

236. Hull R, Raskob G, Hirsh J: Continuous intravenous heparin compared with intermittent subcutaneous heparin in the initial treatment of proximal-vein thrombosis. N Engl J Med 315:1109–1114, 1986.

237. Palareti G, Legnani C, Cosmi B, et al: Poor anticoagulation quality in the first 3 months after unprovoked venous thromboembolism is a risk factor for long-term recurrence. J Thromb Haemost 3:955–961, 2005.

238. Lee A, Levine M, Baker R, et al: Low-molecular-weight heparin versus coumarin for the prevention of recurrent venous thromboembolism in patients with cancer. N Engl J Med 349:146–153, 2003.

239. Hutten B, Prins M, Gent M, et al: Incidence of recurrent thromboembolic and bleeding complications among patients with venous thromboembolism in relation to both malignancy and achieved international normalized ratio: A retrospective analysis. J Clin Oncol 18:3078–3083, 2000.

240. van der Meer F, Rosendaal F, Vandenbroucke J, Briet E: Assessment of a bleeding risk index in two cohorts of patients treated with oral anticoagulants. Thromb Haemost 76:12–16, 1996.

241. Landefeld CS, Goldman L: Major bleeding in outpatients treated with warfarin: Incidence and prediction by factors known at the start of outpatient therapy. Am J Med 87:144–152, 1989.

242. Torn M, Bollen W, van der Meer F, et al: Risks of oral anticoagulant therapy with increasing age. Arch Intern Med 165:1527–1532, 2005.

243. Wells P, Anderson D, Rodger M, et al: Evaluation of D-dimer in the diagnosis of suspected deep-vein thrombosis. N Engl J Med 349:1227–1235, 2003.

244. Beyth RJ, Quinn LM, Landefeld CS: Prospective evaluation of an index for predicting the risk of major bleeding in outpatients treated with warfarin. Am J Med 105:91–99, 1998.

245. Gitter M, Jaeger T, Petterson T, et al: Bleeding and thromboembolism during anticoagulant therapy: A population-based study in Rochester, Minn. Mayo Clin Proc 70:725–733, 1995.

III

246. Chiquette E, Amato M, Bussey H: Comparison of an anticoagulation clinic with usual medical care: Anticoagulation control, patient outcomes, and health care costs. Arch Intern Med 158:1641–1647, 1998.

247. Cromheecke M, Levi M, Colly L, et al: Oral anticoagulation self-management and management by a specialist anticoagulation clinic: A randomised cross-over comparison. Lancet 356:97–102, 2000.

248. Ridker P, Goldhaber S, Danielson E, et al: PREVENT Investigators: Long-term, low-intensity warfarin therapy for the prevention of recurrent venous thromboembolism[comment]. N Engl J Med 348:1425–1434, 2003.

249. Kearon C, Ginsberg J, Kovacs M, et al: Comparison of low-intensity warfarin therapy with conventional-intensity warfarin therapy for long-term prevention of recurrent venous thromboembolism. N Engl J Med 349:631–639, 2003.

250. Fanikos J, Grasso-Correnti N, Shah R, et al: Major bleeding complications in a specialized anticoagulation service. J Cardiol 96:595–598, 2005.

251. Kottke-Marchant K, Comp P: Laboratory issues in diagnosing abnormalities of protein C, thrombomodulin, and endothelial cell protein C receptor. Arch Pathol Lab Med 126:1337–1348, 2002.

252. Perry D: Antithrombin and its inherited deficiencies. Blood Rev 8:37–55, 1994.

253. Lane D, Bayston T, Olds R, et al: Antithrombin mutation database: 2nd 1997 update. For the Plasma Coagulation Inhibitors Subcommittee of the Scientific and Standardization Committee of the International Society on Thrombosis and Haemostasis. Thromb Haemost 77:197–211, 1997.

254. Finazzi G, Caccia R, Barbui T: Different prevalance of thromboembolism in the subtypes of congenital antithrombin deficiency. Thromb Haemost 58:1094, 1987.

255. Demers C, Henderson P, Blajchman M, et al: An antithrombin III assay based on factor Xa inhibition provides a more reliable test to identify congenital antithrombin III deficiency than an assay based on thrombin inhibition. Thromb Haemost 69:231–235, 1993.

256. Tait R, Walker I, Islam S, et al: Influence of demographic factors on antithrombin III activity in a healthy population. J Haematol 84:476–480, 1993.

257. Andrew M, Vegh P, Johnston M, et al: Maturation of the hemostatic system during childhood. Blood 80:1998–2005, 1992.

258. Weenink G, Kahle L, Lamping R, et al: Antithrombin III in oral contraceptive users and during normotensive pregnancy. Acta Obstet Gynecol Scand 63:57–61, 1984.

259. Caine Y, Bauer K, Barzegar S, et al: Coagulation activation following estrogen administration to postmenopausal women. Thromb Haemost 6:392–395, 1992.

260. Von Kaulla E, Von Kaulla K: Antithrombin 3 and diseases. Am J Clin Pathol 48:69–80, 1967.

261. Kauffmann R, Veltkamp J, Van Tilburg N, Van Es L: Acquired antithrombin III deficiency and thrombosis in the nephrotic syndrome. Am J Med 65:607–613, 1978.

262. Lane D, Mannucci P, Bauer K, et al: Inherited thrombophilia: Part 1. Thromb Haemost 76:651–662, 1996.

263. Tait R, Walker I, Reitsma P, et al: Prevalence of protein C deficiency in the healthy population. Thromb Haemost 73:87–93, 1995.

264. Miletich J, Sherman L, Broze GJ: Absence of thrombosis in subjects with heterozygous protein C deficiency. N Engl J Med 317:991–996, 1987.

265. Francis RJ, Seyfert U: Rapid amidolytic assay of protein C in whole plasma using an activator from the venom of Agkistrodon contortrix. 87:619–625, 1987.

266. Faioni E, Franchi F, Krachmalnicoff A, et al: Low levels of the anticoagulant activity of protein C in patients with chronic renal insufficiency: An inhibitor of protein C is present in uremic plasma. Thromb Haemost 66:420–425, 1991.

267. Sorensen P, Knudsen F, Nielsen A, Dyerberg J: Protein C activity in renal disease. Thromb Res 38:243–249, 1985.

268. Vigano D'Angelo S, Comp P, Esmon C, D'Angelo A: Relationship between protein C antigen and anticoagulant activity during oral anticoagulation and in selected disease states. J Clin Invest 77:416–425, 1986.

269. Manco-Johnson M, Marlar R, Jacobson L: Severe protein C deficiency in newborn infants. J Pediatr 113:359–363, 1988.

270. Karpatkin M, Mannuccio MP, Bhogal M, et al: Low protein C in the neonatal period. Br J Haematol 62:137–142, 1986.

271. Polack B, Pouzol P, Amiral J, Kolodie L: Protein C level at birth. Thromb Haemost 52:188–191, 1984.

272. Gerson W, Dickerman J, Bovill E, Golden E: Severe acquired protein C deficiency in purpura fulminans associated with disseminated intravascular coagulation: Treatment with protein C concentrate. Pediatrics 91:418–422, 1993.

273. Vigano-D'Angelo S, D'Angelo A, Kaufman CJ, et al: Protein S deficiency occurs in the nephrotic syndrome. Ann Intern Med 107:42–47, 1987.

274. Jones D, Mackie I, Winter M, et al: Detection of protein C deficiency during oral anticoagulant therapy—Use of the protein C:factor VII ratio. Blood Coagul Fibrinolysis 2:407–411, 1991.

275. Goodwin A, Rosendaal F, Kottke-Marchant K, Bovill E: A review of the technical, diagnostic, and epidemiologic considerations for protein S assays. Arch Pathol Lab Med 126:1349–1366, 2002.

276. Schwarz H, Fischer M, Hopmeier P, et al: Plasma protein S deficiency in familial thrombotic disease. Blood 64:1297–1300, 1984.

277. Comp P, Doray D, Patton D, Esmon C: An abnormal plasma distribution of protein S occurs in functional protein S deficiency. Blood 67:504–508, 1986.

278. Borgel D, Gandrille S, Aiach M: Protein S deficiency. Thromb Haemost 78:351–356, 1997.

279. D'Angelo A, Vigano-D'Angelo S, Esmon C, Comp P: Acquired deficiencies of protein S: Protein S activity during oral anticoagulation, in liver disease, and in disseminated intravascular coagulation. J Clin Invest 81:1445–1454, 1988.

280. Stahl C, Wideman C, Spira T, et al: Protein S deficiency in men with long-term human immunodeficiency virus infection. Blood 81:1801–1807, 1993.

281. Broze GJ: Tissue factor pathway inhibitor. Thromb Haemost 74:90–93, 1995.

282. Sandset P: Tissue factor pathway inhibitor (TFPI): An update. Haemostasis 23:154–165, 1996.

283. Sandset P, Abildgaard U, Larsen M: Heparin induces release of extrinsic coagulation pathway inhibitor (EPI). Thromb Res 50:803–813, 1988.

284. Novotny W, Girard T, Miletich J, Broze GJ: Purification and characterization of the lipoprotein-associated coagulation inhibitor from human plasma. J Biol Chem 264:18832–18837, 1989.

285. Sandset P, Larsen M, Abildgaard U, et al: Chromogenic substrate assay of extrinsic pathway inhibitor (EPI): Levels in the normal population and relation to cholesterol. Blood Coagul Fibrinolysis 2:425–433, 1991.

286. Dahm A, Van Hylckama Vlieg A, Bendz B, et al: Low levels of tissue factor pathway inhibitor (TFPI) increase the risk of venous thrombosis. Blood 101:4387–4392, 2003.

287. Harris G, Stendt C, Vollenhoven B, et al: Decreased plasma tissue factor pathway inhibitor in women taking combined oral contraceptives. Am J Hematol 60:175–180, 1999.

288. Kluft C: Effects on haemostasis variables by second and third generation combined oral contraceptives: A review of directly comparative studies. Curr Med Chem 7:585–591, 2000.

289. Hoibraaten E, Qvigstad E, Andersen T, et al: The effects of hormone replacement therapy (HRT) on hemostatic variables in women with previous venous thromboembolism: Results from a randomized, double-blind, clinical trial. Thromb Haemost 85:775–781, 2001.

290. Huang Z, Higuchi D, Lasky N, Broze GJ: Tissue factor pathway inhibitor gene disruption produces intrauterine lethality in mice. Blood 90:944–951, 1997.

291. Sandset P, Warn-Cramer B, Maki S, Rapaport S: Immunodepletion of extrinsic pathway inhibitor sensitizes rabbits to endotoxin-induced intravascular coagulation and the generalized Shwartzman reaction. Blood 78:1496–1502, 1991.

292. Sandset P, Warn-Cramer B, Rao L, et al: Depletion of extrinsic pathway inhibitor (EPI) sensitizes rabbits to disseminated intravascular coagulation induced with tissue factor: Evidence supporting a physiologic role for EPI as a natural anticoagulant. Natl Acad Sci U S A 88:708–712, 1991.

293. Bajaj M, Bajaj S: Tissue factor pathway inhibitor: Potential therapeutic applications. Thromb Haemost 78:471–477, 1997.

294. Holst J, Lindblad B, Bergqvist D, et al: Antithrombotic properties of a truncated recombinant tissue factor pathway inhibitor in an experimental venous thrombosis model. Haemostasis 23:112–117, 1993.

295. Kaiser B, Fareed J: Recombinant full-length tissue factor pathway inhibitor (TFPI) prevents thrombus formation and rethrombosis after lysis in a rabbit model of jugular vein thrombosis. Thromb Haemost 76:615–620, 1996.

296. Van Dreden P, Grosley M, Cost H: Total and free levels of tissue factor pathway inhibitor: A risk factor in patients with factor V Leiden? Blood Coagul Fibrinolysis 10:115–116, 1999.

297. Ariens R, Alberio G, Moia M, Mannucci P: Low levels of heparin-releasable tissue factor pathway inhibitor in young patients with thrombosis. Thromb Haemost 81:203–207, 1999.

298. Amini-Nekoo A, Futers T, Moia M, et al: Analysis of the tissue factor pathway inhibitor gene and antigen levels in relation to venous thrombosis. Br J Haematol 113:537–543, 2001.

299. Han X, Fiehler R, Broze G Jr: Characterization of the protein Z–dependent protease inhibitor. Blood 96:3049–3055, 2000.

300. Broze GJ: Protein Z–dependent regulation of coagulation. Thromb Haemost 86:8–13, 2001.

301. Yurdakok M, Gurakan B, Ozbag E, et al: Plasma protein Z levels in healthy newborn infants. Am J Hematol 48:206–207, 1995.

302. Kemkes-Matthes B, Nees M, Kuhnel G, et al: Protein Z influences the prothrombotic phenotype in Factor V Leiden patients. Thromb Res 106:183–185, 2002.

303. Paidas M, Ku D, Lee M, et al: Protein Z, protein S levels are lower in patients with thrombophilia and subsequent pregnancy complications. J Thromb Haemost 3:497–501, 2005.

304. McColl M, Deans A, Maclean P, et al: Plasma protein Z deficiency is common in women with antiphospholipid antibodies. Br J Haematol 120:913–914, 2003.

305. Vasse M, Guegan-Massardier E, Borg J, et al: Frequency of protein Z deficiency in patients with ischaemic stroke. Lancet 357:933–934, 2001.

306. Wuillemin W, Demarmels BF, Mattle H, Lammle B: Frequency of protein Z deficiency in patients with ischaemic stroke. Lancet 358:840–841, 2001.

307. Tollefsen D: Heparin cofactor II deficiency. Arch Pathol Lab Med 126:1394–1400, 2002.

308. Chandler W, Rodgers G, Sprouse J, Thompson A: Elevated hemostatic factor levels as potential risk factors for thrombosis. Arch Pathol Lab Med 126:1405–1414, 2002.

309. Koenig W: Fibrin(ogen) in cardiovascular disease: An update. Thromb Haemost 89:601–609, 2003.

310. Thompson S, Kienast J, Pyke S, et al: Hemostatic factors and the risk of myocardial infarction and death. N Engl J Med 332:635–641, 1995.

311. Folsom A, Wu K, Rosamond W, et al: Prospective study of hemostatic factors and incidence of coronary heart disease: The atherosclerosis risk in communities. Circulation 96:1102–1108, 1997.

312. Zito F, Di Castelnuovo A, Amore C, et al: Bcl I polymorphism in the fibrinogen beta-chain gene is associated with the risk of familial myocardial infarction by increasing plasma fibrinogen levels: A case-control study in a sample of GISSI-2 patients. Arterioscler Thromb Vasc Biol 17:3489–3494, 1997.

313. de Maat M, Kastelein J, Jukema J, et al: -455G/A polymorphism of the beta-fibrinogen gene is associated with the progression of coronary atherosclerosis in symptomatic men: Proposed role for an acute-phase reaction pattern of fibrinogen. REGRESS Group. Arterioscler Thromb Vasc Biol 18:265–271, 1998.

314. Stec J, Silbershatz H, Tofler G, et al: Association of fibrinogen with cardiovascular risk factors and cardiovascular disease in the Framingham Offspring Population. Circulation 102:1634–1638, 2000.

315. Smith F, Lee A, Fowkes F, et al: Hemostatic factors as predictors of ischemic heart disease and stroke in the Edinburgh Artery Study. Arterioscler Thromb Vasc Biol 17:3321–3328, 1997.

316. Smith F, Lee A, Hau C, et al: Plasma fibrinogen, haemostatic factors and prediction of peripheral arterial disease in the Edinburgh Artery Study. Blood Coagul Fibrinolysis 11:43–50, 2000.

317. Folsom A, Rosamond W, Shahar E, et al: Prospective study of markers of hemostatic function with risk of ischemic stroke. The Atherosclerosis Risk in Communities (ARIC) Study Investigators. Circulation 100:736–742, 1999.

318. Koster T, Rosendaal F, Reitsma P, et al: Factor VII and fibrinogen levels as risk factors for venous thrombosis. Thromb Haemost 71:719–722, 1994.

319. Kamphuisen P, Eikenboom J, Vos H, et al: Increased levels of factor VIII and fibrinogen in patients with venous thrombosis are not caused by acute phase reactions. Thromb Haemost 81:680–683, 1999.

320. Austin H, Hooper W, Lally C, et al: Venous thrombosis in relation to fibrinogen and factor VII genes among African-Americans. J Epidemiol 53:997–1001, 2000.

321. Billon S, Escoffre-Barbe M, Mercier B, et al: Fibrinogen is not an additional risk factor of thromboembolic disease in factor V Leiden patients. Thromb Haemost 81:659–660, 1999.

322. Butenas S, van't Veer C, Mann K: "Normal" thrombin generation. Blood 94:2169–2178, 1999.

323. Hillarp A, Zoller B, Svensson P, Dahlback B: The 20210 A allele of the prothrombin gene is a common risk factor among Swedish outpatients with verified deep venous thrombosis. Thromb Haemost 78:990–992, 1997.

324. Gehring N, Frede U, Neu-Yilik G, et al: Increased efficiency of mRNA 3′ end formation: A new genetic mechanism contributory to hereditary thrombophilia. Nat Genet 28:389–392, 2001.

325. Soria J, Almasy L, Souto J, et al: Linkage analysis demonstrates that the prothrombin G20210A mutation jointly influences plasma prothrombin levels and risk of thrombosis. Blood 95:2780–2875, 2000.

326. Danckwardt S, Gehring N, Neu-Yilik G, et al: The prothrombin 3′ end formation signal reveals a unique architecture that is sensitive to thrombophilic gain-of-function mutations. Blood 10:428–435, 2004.

327. Kyrle P, Mannhalter C, Beguin S, et al: Clinical studies and thrombin generation in patients homozygous or heterozygous for the G20210A mutation in the prothrombin gene. Arterioscler Thromb Vasc Biol 18:1287–1291, 1998.

328. Martinelli I, Mannucci P, De Stefano V, et al: Different risks of thrombosis in four coagulation defects associated with inherited thrombophilia: A study of 150 families. Blood 92:2353–2358, 1998.

329. Bank I, Libourel E, Middeldorp S, et al: Prothrombin 20210A mutation: A mild risk factor for venous thromboembolism but not for arterial thrombotic disease and pregnancy-related complications in a family study. Arch Intern Med 164:1932–1937, 2004.

330. Poller L, Tabiowo A, Thomson J: Effects of low-dose oral contraceptives on blood coagulation. Br Med J 3:218–221, 1968.

331. Schafer A: The primary and secondary hypercoagulable states. In Schafer AI, (ed): Molecular Mechanisma of Hypercoagulable States., Landes Bioscience and Chapman & Hall, London, 1997, pp 1–48.

332. Constantino M, Merskey C, Kudzma D, Zucker M: Increased activity of vitamin K–dependent clotting factors in human hyperlipoproteinaemia: Association with cholesterol and triglyceride levels. Thromb Haemost 38:465–474, 1977.

333. Meade T, Mellows S, Brozovic M, et al: Haemostatic function and ischaemic heart disease: Principal results of the Northwick Park Heart Study. Lancet 2:533–537, 1986.

334. Redondo M, Watzke H, Stucki B, et al: Coagulation factors II, V, VII, and X, prothrombin gene 20210G A transition, and factor V Leiden in coronary artery disease: High factor V clotting activity is an independent risk factor for myocardial infarction. Thromb Vasc Biol 19:1020–1025, 1999.

335. Iacoviello L, Di Castelnuovo A, De Knijff P, et al: Polymorphisms in the coagulation factor VII gene and the risk of myocardial infarction. N Engl J Med 338:79–85, 1998.

336. Doggen C, Manger Cats V, Bertina R, et al: A genetic propensity to high factor VII is not associated with the risk of myocardial infarction in men. Thromb Haemost 80:281–285, 1998.

337. Kamphuisen P, Lensen R, Houwing-Duistermaat J, et al: Heritability of elevated factor VIII antigen levels in factor V Leiden families with thrombophilia. Br J Haematol 109:519–522, 2000.

338. Schambeck C, Hinney K, Haubitz I, et al: Familial clustering of high factor VIII levels in patients with venous thromboembolism. Arterioscler Thromb Vasc Biol 21:289–292, 2001.

339. Kamphuisen P, Rosendaal F, Eikenboom J, et al: Factor V antigen levels and venous thrombosis: Risk profile, interaction with factor V leiden, and relation with factor VIII antigen levels. Arterioscler Thromb Vasc Biol 20:1382–1386, 2000.

340. Kamphuisen P, Eikenboom J, Bertina R: Elevated factor VIII levels and the risk of thrombosis. Arterioscler Thromb Vasc Biol 21:731–738, 2001.

341. Penick G, Dejanov I, Roberts H, Webster W: Elevation of factor 8 in hypercoagulable states. Thromb Diath Haemorrhag 20:39–48, 1966.

342. De Mitrio V, Marino R, Scaraggi F, et al: Influence of factor VIII/von Willebrand complex on the activated protein C–resistance phenotype and on the risk for venous thromboembolism in heterozygous carriers of the factor V Leiden mutation. Blood Coagul Fibrinolysis 10:409–416, 1999.

343. O'Donnell J, Mumford A, Manning R, Laffan M: Elevation of FVIII: C in venous thromboembolism is persistent and independent of the acute phase response. Thromb Haemost 83:10–13, 2000.

344. Lensen R, Bertina R, Vandenbroucke J, Rosendaal F: High factor VIII levels contribute to the thrombotic risk in families with factor V Leiden. Br J Haematol 114:380–386, 2001.

345. Rosendaal F: Factor VIII and coronary heart disease. Eur J Epidemiol 8 (suppl), 71–75, 1992.

346. Reiner A, Siscovick D, Rosendaal F: Hemostatic risk factors and arterial thrombotic disease. Thromb Haemost 85:584–595, 2001.

347. Meade T, Cooper J, Stirling Y, et al: Factor VIII, ABO blood group and the incidence of ischaemic heart disease. J Haematol 88:601–607, 1994.

III

348. Tracy R, Arnold A, Ettinger W, et al: The relationship of fibrinogen and factors VII and VIII to incident cardiovascular disease and death in the elderly: Results from the cardiovascular health study. Arterioscler Thromb Vasc Biol 19:1776–1783, 1999.

349. Mansvelt E, Laffan M, McVey J, Tuddenham E: Analysis of the F8 gene in individuals with high plasma factor VIII:C levels and associated venous thrombosis. Thromb Haemost 80:561–565, 1998.

350. Lowe G, Rumley A, Woodward M, et al: Epidemiology of coagulation factors, inhibitors and activation markers: The Third Glasgow MONICA Survey. I. Illustrative reference ranges by age, sex and hormone use. Br J Haematol 97:775–784, 1997.

351. Lowe G, Woodward M, Vessey M, et al: Thrombotic variables and risk of idiopathic venous thromboembolism in women aged 45–64 years: Relationships to hormone replacement therapy. Thromb Haemost 83:530–535, 2000.

352. de Visser M, Poort S, Vos H, et al: Factor X levels, polymorphisms in the promoter region of factor X, and the risk of venous thrombosis. Thromb Haemost 85:1011–1017, 2001.

353. Walsh P: Factor XI. In Colman RW, Hirsh J, and Marder VJ, et al, (eds): Hemostasis and Thrombosis, 4th ed. Philadelphia, Lippincott Williams & Wilkins, 2001, pp 191–201.

354. Bouma B, Mosnier L, Meijers J, Griffin J: Factor XI dependent and independent activation of thrombin activatable fibrinolysis inhibitor (TAFI) in plasma associated with clot formation. Thromb Haemost 82:1703–1708, 1999.

355. Conlan M, Folsom A, Finch A, et al: Associations of factor VIII and von Willebrand factor with age, race, sex, and risk factors for atherosclerosis. The Atherosclerosis Risk in Communities (ARIC) Study. Thromb Haemost 70:380–385, 1993.

356. Haverkate F, Thompson S, Duckert F: Haemostasis factors in angina pectoris: Relation to gender, age and acute-phase reaction. Results of the ECAT Angina Pectoris Study Group. Thromb Haemost 73:561–567, 1995.

357. Rumley A, Lowe G, Sweetnam P, et al: Factor VIII, von Willebrand factor and the risk of major ischaemic heart disease in the Caerphilly Heart Study. Br J Haematol 105:110–116, 1999.

358. Thogersen A, Jansson J, Boman K, et al: High plasminogen activator inhibitor and tissue plasminogen activator levels in plasma precede a first acute myocardial infarction in both men and women: Evidence for the fibrinolytic system as an independent primary risk factor. Circulation 98:2241–2247, 1998.

359. Wiman B, Andersson T, Hallqvist J, et al: Plasma levels of tissue plasminogen activator/plasminogen activator inhibitor-1 complex and von Willebrand factor are significant risk markers for recurrent myocardial infarction in the Stockholm Heart Epidemiology Program (SHEEP) study. Arterioscler Thromb Vasc Biol 20:2019–2023, 2000.

360. Qizilbash N, Duffy S, Prentice C, et al: Von Willebrand factor and risk of ischemic stroke. Neurology 49:1552–1556, 1997.

361. Carson N, Neill D: Metabolic abnormalities detected in a survey of mentally backward individuals in Northern Ireland. Arch Dis Child 37:505–513, 1962.

362. Mudd S, Skovby F, Levy H, et al: The natural history of homocystinuria due to cystathionine beta-synthase deficiency. Am J Human Genet 37:1–31, 1985.

363. Kluijtmans L, den Heijer M, Reitsma P, et al: Thermolabile methylenetetrahydrofolate reductase and factor V Leiden in the risk of deep-vein thrombosis. Thromb Haemost 79:254–258, 1998.

364. Boushey C, Beresford S, Omenn G, Motulsky A: A quantitative assessment of plasma homocysteine as a risk factor for vascular disease: Probable benefits of increasing folic acid intakes. JAMA 274:1049–1057, 1995.

365. Graham I, Daly L, Refsum H, et al: Plasma homocysteine as a risk factor for vascular disease. The European Concerted Action Project. JAMA 277:1775–1781, 1997.

366. den Heijer M, Koster T, Blom H, et al: Hyperhomocysteinemia as a risk factor for deep vein thrombosis. N Engl J Med 334:759–762, 1996.

367. den Heijer M, Rosendaal F, Blom H, et al: Hyperhomocysteinemia and venous thrombosis: A meta-analysis. Thromb Haemost 80:874–877, 1998.

368. Frederiksen J, Juul K, Grande P, et al: Methylenetetrahydrofolate reductase polymorphism (C677T), hyperhomocysteinemia, and risk of ischemic cardiovascular disease and venous thromboembolism: Prospective and case-control studies from the Copenhagen City Heart Study. Blood 104:3046–3051, 2004.

369. Danesh J, Lewington S: Plasma homocysteine and coronary heart disease: Systematic review of published epidemiological studies. J Cardiovasc Risk 5:229–232, 1998.

370. Folsom A, Nieto F, McGovern P, et al: Prospective study of coronary heart disease incidence in relation to fasting total homocysteine, related genetic polymorphisms, and B vitamins: The Atherosclerosis Risk in Communities (ARIC) study. Circulation 98:204–210, 1998.

371. Ridker P, Manson J, Buring J, et al: Homocysteine and risk of cardiovascular disease among postmenopausal women. JAMA 281:1817–1821, 1999.

372. Collaboration HS: Homocysteine and risk of ischemic heart disease and stroke: A meta-analysis. JAMA 288:2015–2055, 2002.

373. den Heijer M, Willems H, Blom H, et al Homocysteine lowering by B vitamins and the secondary prevention of deep-vein thrombosis and pulmonary embolism: A randomized, placebo-controlled double blind trial. Blood 109:139–144, 2007.

374. Cattaneo M, My T, Bucciarelli P, et al: A common mutation in the methylenetetrahydrofolate reductase gene (C677T) increases the risk for deep-vein thrombosis in patients with mutant factor V (factor V: Q506). Thromb Vasc Biol 17:1662–1666, 1997.

375. Toole J, Malinow M, Chambless L, et al: Lowering homocysteine in patients with ischemic stroke to prevent recurrent stroke, myocardial infarction, and death: The Vitamin Intervention for Stroke Prevention (VISP) randomized controlled trial. JAMA 291:565–575, 2004.

376. Bonaa K, Njolstad I, Ueland P, et al: Homocysteine lowering and cardiovascular events after acute myocardial infarction. N Engl J Med 354:1578–1588, 2006.

377. Lonn E, Yusuf S, Arnold MJ, et al: HOPE 2 Investigators: Homocysteine lowering with folic acid and B vitamins in vascular disease. N Engl J Med 354:1557–1567, 2006.

378. Botto L, Yang Q: Methylenetetrahydrofolate reductase gene variants and congenital anomalies. Am J Epidemiol 151:862–877, 2000.

379. Klerk M, Verhoef P, Clarke R, et al: MTHFR Studies Collaboration Group: T polymorphism and risk of coronary heart disease: A meta-analysis. JAMA 288:2023–2031, 2002.

380. Dahlbäck B, Carlsson M, Svensson P: Familial thrombophilia due to a previously unrecognized mechanism characterized by poor anticoagulant response to activated protein C: Prediction of a cofactor to activated protein C. Proc Natl Acad Sci U S A 90:1004–1008, 1993.

381. Koster T, Rosendaal F, de Ronde H, et al: Venous thrombosis due to poor anticoagulant response to activated protein C: Leiden Thrombophilia Study. Lancet 342:1503–1506, 1993.

382. Kalafatis M, Bertina R, Rand M, Mann K: Characterization of the molecular defect in FV R506Q. J Biol Chem 270:4053–4057, 1995.

383. Sun X, Evatt B, Griffin J: Blood coagulation factor Va abnormality associated with resistance to activated protein C in venous thrombophilia. Blood 83:3120–3125, 1994.

384. Bertina R, Koeleman B, Koster T, et al: Mutation in blood coagulation factor V associated with resistance to activated protein C. Nature 369:64–67, 1994.

385. Martinelli I, Bottasso B, Duca F, et al: Heightened thrombin generation in individuals with resistance to activated protein C. Thromb Haemost 75:270–274, 1996.

386. Bajzar L, Nesheim M, Tracy P: The profibrinolytic effect of activated protein C in clots formed from plasma is TAFI-dependent. Blood 88:2093–2100, 1996.

387. Bajzar L, Kalafatis M, Simioni P, Tracy P: An antifibrinolytic mechanism describing the prothrombotic effect associated with factor V Leiden. J Biol Chem 271:22949–22952, 1996.

388. Zivelin A, Griffin J, Xu X, et al: A single genetic origin for a common Caucasian risk factor for venous thrombosis. Blood 89:397–402, 1997.

389. Rosendaal F, Koster T, Vandenbroucke J, Reitsma P: High risk of thrombosis in patients homozygous for factor V Leiden (activated protein C resistance). Blood 85:1504–1508, 1995.

390. Ehrenforth S, Nemes L, Mannhalter C, et al: Impact of environmental and hereditary risk factors on the clinical manifestation of thrombophilia in homozygous carriers of factor V:G1691A. J Thromb Haemost 2:430–436, 2004.

391. Bachman F: Plasminogen-plasmin enzyme system. In Colman RW, Hirsh J, Marder VJ, et al: Hemostasis and Thrombosis, 4th ed. Philadelphia, Lippincott Williams & Wilkins, 2001, pp 275–320.

392. Brandt J: Plasminogen and tissue-type plasminogen activator deficiency as risk factors for thromboembolic disease. Arch Pathol Lab Med 126:1379–1381, 2002.

393. Schuster V, Mingers A, Seidenspinner S, et al: Homozygous mutations in the plasminogen gene of two unrelated girls with ligneous conjunctivitis. Blood 90:958–966, 1997.

394. Schott D, Dempfle C, Beck P, et al: Therapy with a purified plasminogen concentrate in an infant with ligneous conjunctivitis and homozygous plasminogen deficiency. N Engl J Med 339:1679–1686, 1998.

395. Francis C: Plasminogen activator inhibitor-1 levels and polymorphisms. Arch Pathol Lab Med 126:1401–1404, 2002.

396. Francis C: Factor XIII polymorphisms and venous thromboembolism. Arch Pathol Lab Med 126:1391–1393, 2002.

397. Ariens R, Philippou H, Nagaswami C, et al: The factor XIII V34L polymorphism accelerates thrombin activation of factor XIII and affects cross-linked fibrin structure. Blood 96:988–995, 2000.

398. Trumbo T, Maurer M: Examining thrombin hydrolysis of the factor XIII activation peptide segment leads to a proposal for explaining the cardioprotective effects observed with the factor XIII V34L mutation. J Biol Chem 275:20627–20631, 2000.

399. Undas A, Brzezinska-Kolarz B, Brummel-Ziedins K, et al: Factor XIII Val34Leu polymorphism and gamma-chain cross-linking at the site of microvascular injury in healthy and coumadin-treated subjects. J Thromb Haemost 3:2015–2021, 2005.

400. Carr MJ, Alving B: Effect of fibrin structure on plasmin-mediated dissolution of plasma clots. Blood Coagul Fibrinolysis 6:567–573, 1995.

401. Catto A, Kohler H, Coore J, et al: Association of a common polymorphism in the factor XIII gene with venous thrombosis. Blood 93:906–908, 1999.

402. Corral J, Gonzalez-Conejero R, Iniesta J, et al: The FXIII Val34Leu polymorphism in venous and arterial thromboembolism. Haematologica 85:293–297, 2000.

403. Franco R, Reitsma P, Lourenco D, et al: Factor XIII Val34Leu is a genetic factor involved in the etiology of venous thrombosis. Thromb Haemost 81:676–679, 1999.

404. Renner W, Koppel H, Hoffmann C, et al: Prothrombin G20210A, factor V Leiden, and factor XIII Val34Leu: Common mutations of blood coagulation factors and deep vein thrombosis in Austria. Thromb Res 99:35–39, 2000.

405. Van Hylckama Vlieg A, Komanasin N, Ariens R, et al: Factor XIII Val34Leu polymorphism, factor XIII antigen levels and activity and the risk of deep venous thrombosis. Br J Haematol 119:169–175, 2002.

406. Margaglione M, Bossone A, Brancaccio V, et al: Factor XIII Val34Leu polymorphism and risk of deep vein thrombosis. Thromb Haemost 84:1118–1119, 2000.

407. Fatah K, Silveira A, Tornvall P, et al: Proneness to formation of tight and rigid fibrin gel structures in men with myocardial infarction at a young age. Thromb Haemost 76:535–540, 1996.

408. Fatah K, Hamsten A, Blomback B, Blomback M: Fibrin gel network characteristics and coronary heart disease: Relations to plasma fibrinogen concentration, acute phase protein, serum lipoproteins and coronary atherosclerosis. Thromb Haemost 68:130–135, 1992.

409. Lim B, Ariens R, Carter A, et al: Genetic regulation of fibrin structure and function: Complex gene-environment interactions may modulate vascular risk. Lancet 361:1424–1431, 2003.

410. Elbaz A, Poirier O, Canaple S, et al: The association between the Val34Leu polymorphism in the factor XIII gene and brain infarction. Blood 95:586–591, 2000.

411. Marin F, Gonzalez-Conejero R, Lee K, et al: A pharmacogenetic effect of factor XIII valine 34 leucine polymorphism on fibrinolytic therapy for acute myocardial infarction. J Am Coll Cardiol 45:25–29, 2005.

412. McDonagh J: Dysfibrinogenemia and other disorders of fibrinogen structure or function. In Colman RW, Hirsh J, and Marder VJ, et al, (eds): Hemostasis and Thrombosis, 4th ed. Philadelphia, Lippincott Williams & Wilkins, 2001, pp 856–892.

413. Bajzar L, Morser J, Nesheim M: TAFI, or plasma procarboxypeptidase B, couples the coagulation and fibrinolytic cascades through the thrombin-thrombomodulin complex. J Biol Chem 271:16603–16608, 1996.

414. Bouma B, Marx P, Mosnier L, Meijers J: Thrombin-activatable fibrinolysis inhibitor (TAFI, plasma procarboxypeptidase B, procarboxypeptidase R, procarboxypeptidase U). Thromb Res 101:329–354, 2001.

415. Mosnier L, von dem Borne P, Meijers J, Bouma B: Plasma TAFI levels influence the clot lysis time in healthy individuals in the presence of an intact intrinsic pathway of coagulation. Thromb Haemost 80:829–835, 1998.

416. Bouma B, Meijers J: Thrombin-activatable fibrinolysis inhibitor (TAFI, plasma procarboxypeptidase B, procarboxypeptidase R, procarboxypeptidase U). J Thromb Haemost 1:1566–1574, 2003.

417. Bajzar L: Thrombin activatable fibrinolysis inhibitor and an antifibrinolytic pathway. Arterioscler Thromb Vasc Biol 20:2511–2518, 2000.

418. Nesheim M: TAFI. Fibrinolysis Proteol 13:72–77, 1999.

419. von dem Borne P, Meijers J, Bouma B: Feedback activation of factor XI by thrombin in plasma results in additional formation of thrombin that protects fibrin clots from fibrinolysis. Blood 86:3035–3042, 1995.

420. Von dem Borne P, Bajzar L, Meijers J, et al: Thrombin-mediated activation of factor XI results in a thrombin-activatable fibrinolysis

inhibitor–dependent inhibition of fibrinolysis. J Clin Invest 90:2323–2327, 1997.

421. Chetaille P, Alessi M, Kouassi D, et al: Plasma TAFI antigen variations in healthy subjects. Thromb Haemost 83:902–905, 2000.

422. Juhan-Vague I, Renucci J, Grimaux M, et al: Thrombin-activatable fibrinolysis inhibitor antigen levels and cardiovascular risk factors. Arterioscler Thromb Vasc Biol 20:2156–2161, 2000.

423. Santamaria A, Borrell M, Oliver A, et al: Association of functional thrombin-activatable fibrinolysis inhibitor (TAFI) with conventional cardiovascular risk factors and its correlation with other hemostatic factors in a Spanish population. Am J Hematol 76:348–352, 2004.

424. van Tilberg N, Rosendaal F, Bertina R: Thrombin activatable fibrinolysis inhibitor and the risk for deep vein thrombosis. Blood 95:2855–2859, 2000.

425. Leebeek F, Goor M, Guimaraes A, et al: High functional levels of thrombin-activatable fibrinolysis inhibitor are associated with an increased risk of first ischemic stroke. J Thromb Haemost 3:2211–2218, 2005.

426. Morange P, Tregouet D, Frere C, et al: The Prime Study Group: TAFI gene haplotypes, TAFI plasma levels and future risk of coronary heart disease: The PRIME study. J Thromb Haemost 3:1503–1510, 2005.

427. Young NS: Paroxysmal nocturnal hemoglobinuria: Current issues in pathophysiology and treatment. Curr Hematol Rep 4:103–109, 2005.

427a. Ziakas PD, Poulou LS, Rokas GI, et al: Thrombosis in paroxysmal nocturnal hemoglobinuria: Sites, risks, outcome: An overview. J Thromb Haemost 5:642–645, 2007.

428. Ray JG, Burows RF, Ginsberg JS, Burrows EA: Paroxysmal nocturnal hemoglobinuria and the risk of venous thrombosis: Review and recommendations for management of the pregnant and nonpregnant patient. Haemostasis 30:103–117, 2000.

429. Rosse WF, Nishimura J: Clinical manifestations of paroxysmal nocturnal hemoglobinuria: Present state and future problems. Int J Hematol 77:113–120, 2003.

430. Hillmen P, Lewis SM, Bessler M, et al: Natural histort of paroxysmal nocturnal hemoglobinuria. N Engl J Med 333:1253–1258, 1995.

431. Nishimura J, Kanakura Y, Ware RE, et al: Clinical course and flow cytometric analysis of paroxysmal noctural hemoglobinuria in the United States and Japan. Medicine 83:193–207, 2004.

432. Araten DJ, Thaler HT, Luzzatto L: High incidence of thrombosis in African-American and Latin-American patients with paroxysmal nocturnal haemoglobinuria. Thromb Haemost 93:8–91, 2005.

433. Smith LJ: Paroxysmal nocturnal hemoglobinuria. Clin Lab Sci 17:172–177, 2004.

434. Melitis J, Terpos E, Samarkos M, et al: Detection of CD55 and/or CD59 deficient red cell populations in patients with aplastic anaemia, myelodysplastic syndromes and myeloproliferative disorders. Haematologia 31:7–16, 2001.

435. Krauss JS: Laboratory diagnosis of paroxysmal nocturnal hemoglobinuria. Ann Clin Lab Sci 33:401–406, 2003.

436. Moyo VM, Mukhina GL, Garrett ES, Brodsky RA: Natural history of paroxysmal nocturnal haemoglobinuria using modern diagnostic assays. Br J Haematol 126:133–138, 2004.

437. Nafa K, Bessler M, Mason P, et al: Factor V Leiden mutation investigated by amplification created restriction enzyme site (ACRES) in PNH patients with and without thrombosis. Haematologica 81:540–542, 1996.

438. Louwes H, Vellenga E, de Wolf JT: Abnormal platelet adhesion on abdominal vessels in asymptomatic patients with paroxysmal nocturnal hemoglobinuria. Ann Hematol 80:573–576, 2001.

439. Hugel B, Socie G, Vu T, et al: Elevated levels of circulating procoagulant microparticles in patients with paroxysmal nocturnal haemoglobinuria and aplastic anemia. Blood 93:3451–3456, 1999.

440. Liebman HA, Feinstein DI: Thrombosis in patients with paroxysmal nocturnal hemoglobinuria is associated with markedly elevated plasma levels of leukocyte-derived tissue factor. Thromb Res 111:235–238, 2003.

441. Simak J, Holada K, Risitano AM, et al: Elevated circulating endothelial membrane microparticles in paroxysmal nocturnal haemoglobinuria. Br J Haematol 125:804–813, 2004.

442. Hall C, Richards S, Hillmen P: Primary prophylaxis with warfarin prevents thrombosis in paroxysmal nocturnal hemoglobinuria (PNH). Blood 102:3587–3591, 2003.

443. Meyers G, Parker CJ: Management issues in paroxysmal nocturnal hemoglobinuria. Int J Hematol 77:125–132, 2003.

444. Bjorge L, Ernst P, Haram KO: Paroxysmal noctural hemoglobinuria in pregnancy. Acta Obstet Gynecol Scand 82:1067–1071, 2003.

III

Chapter 15

Deep Vein Thrombosis and Pulmonary Embolism

Samuel Z. Goldhaber, MD

Venous thromboembolism (VTE) comprises deep vein thrombosis (DVT) and pulmonary embolism (PE). VTE constitutes the third most common cardiovascular disease, after acute coronary syndrome and stroke.[1] DVT and PE afflict individuals over a wide age range, from teenagers to the elderly. This illness strikes all socioeconomic groups in developed Western countries. Because the morbidity and mortality of VTE are favorably affected by modern therapy, accurate and prompt diagnosis is very important.

The diagnosis of VTE is often elusive. The greatest challenge for the clinician is to have sufficient clinical suspicion to consider the diagnosis. DVT and PE often manifest without classic symptoms or signs. DVT often mimics a harmless muscle cramp. In a multicentered VTE registry at 70 North American medical centers, 170 of 808 patients (21%) were given diagnoses more than 1 week after symptom onset, and 40 of 808 (5%) received diagnoses more than 3 weeks after symptom onset. On average, 80% of the delay in diagnosis occurred between symptom onset and medical evaluation.[2]

PE is notoriously difficult to diagnose and has earned the description of "the Great Masquerader." However, attention to the clinical setting, risk factors, and differential diagnosis, coupled with ordering the appropriate imaging tests, often result in an accurate and timely diagnosis.

DIAGNOSIS

Deep Vein Thrombosis

Clinical Considerations

Figure 15-1 is an algorithm for DVT diagnosis. The most commonly reported symptom is a cramp or "charley horse" in the lower calf that gets worse with walking, that does not abate, and that gradually worsens after several days. The discomfort begins as a transient, nagging sensation, but it may eventually become persistent.

Edema may develop. Swelling is usually most prominent in the calf but can be limited to the ankle or even the foot. When thigh edema occurs because of DVT, one should consider the possibility of pelvic vein thrombosis. If the leg is diffusely edematous, DVT is less unlikely. Much more common is an acute exacerbation of venous insufficiency due to postphlebitic syndrome. Occasionally, erythema accompanies leg edema. Erythema may signify concomitant superficial phlebitis with saphenous vein involvement or coexisting cellulitis.

The differential diagnosis (Table 15-1) includes ruptured Baker cyst, often manifested by sudden, excruciating calf discomfort. Fever and chills usually suggest cellulitis rather than DVT, although DVT may occur concomitantly. The clinical probability of DVT can be estimated with the use of the formal Wells DVT Scoring System,[3] yet this approach is rarely used. I have never witnessed its use first-hand. Likelihood is usually estimated by *gestalt*.

Some favor stopping the DVT workup and not ordering a venous ultrasound if the clinical probability is low and a D-dimer enzyme–linked immunosorbent assay (ELISA) is normal. However, the prevailing approach is to image virtually all patients suspected of having DVT. The terminology of the ultrasound report may cause miscommunication. The distal portion of the deep femoral vein is called the *superficial femoral vein*. Despite the use of the term *superficial*, this is a large deep vein, and patients with superficial femoral vein thrombosis should be treated for DVT. Patients should not be discharged with the mistaken diagnosis of superficial thrombophlebitis.[4]

With upper extremity venous thrombosis, asymmetry may be noted in the supraclavicular fossae or in the girth of the upper arms.[5,6] Also, a prominent superficial venous pattern may be seen over the anterior chest wall. This condition occurs most commonly (1) as a complication of a chronic indwelling central venous catheter, or (2) in otherwise healthy individuals who have been overexerting themselves with activities such as weightlifting (see Chapter 16).

Venous Ultrasonography

Usually, the venous ultrasound examination definitively detects or excludes symptomatic DVT. It is safe to withhold anticoagulation after negative results have been obtained on comprehensive duplex ultrasonography.[7] However, new or progressive symptoms should prompt further testing. Occasionally, imaging test results are equivocal because of the patient's body habitus, recent leg trauma or surgery, or profound edema that limits compression of vascular structures. Under these circumstances, one should consider using other imaging modalities such as computed tomography (CT) venography, magnetic resonance venography, or invasive contrast venography.[8]

Venous ultrasound is less reliable for screening asymptomatic patients. In a meta-analysis of asymptomatic

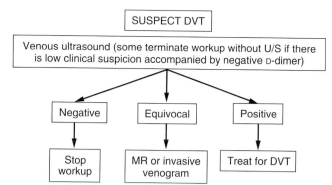

Figure 15-1 Diagnosis of deep vein thrombosis (DVT).

Table 15-1 Differential Diagnosis of Deep Vein Thrombosis

1. Superficial thrombophlebitis
2. Ruptured Baker cyst
3. Cellulitis
4. Venous insufficiency/postphlebitic syndrome
5. Varicose veins
6. Erythema nodosum

---

patients after orthopaedic surgery, when venous ultrasound was compared with invasive contrast venography as the gold standard, ultrasonography had a sensitivity of 62%, a specificity of 97%, and a positive predictive value of 66% in detecting proximal DVT.[9] Of 100 consecutive patients who had undergone craniotomy, 13 had proximal DVT with contrast venography, and only 38% of these had concomitant abnormalities on ultrasound evaluation. Overall, ultrasound identified only 13 of 26 patients with proximal or isolated calf DVT.[10] Should one leg be found to harbor a DVT, it is advisable for the clinician to study the other leg, even if it is presently asymptomatic.

Magnetic Resonance Venography

Magnetic resonance venography is especially useful for assessing pelvic vein and upper extremity thrombosis and for defining the extent of upper extremity vein thrombosis. Magnetic resonance imaging (MRI) can also be used to estimate the age of thrombus on the basis of "spin" characteristics of the image. Among patients with normal venous ultrasound examination findings, a substantial proportion of the DVTs that are responsible for PE originate in the pelvic veins.[11] For leg DVT diagnosis, MRI agrees closely with contrast venography.[12]

Catheter-Based Venography

Invasive contrast venography[13] is rarely performed as a diagnostic test. However, for catheter-based intervention, contrast venography is the first step when one is considering thrombolysis, suction embolectomy, angioplasty, or stenting.

Pulmonary Embolism

Clinical Evaluation

The most important step involved in successfully diagnosing PE is simply to include PE in the differential diagnosis when the symptoms, signs, and clinical setting suggest this condition. If PE is considered, one should pay careful attention to the chest x-ray (Table 15-2) and electrocardiogram (Table 15-3) to determine whether they are consistent with PE, or if they point toward another diagnosis, such as pneumonia or acute myocardial infarction. Too often, PE is overlooked because it mimics so many other illnesses (Table 15-4).

After the diagnosis is considered as a possibility, the next step for the clinician is to consider the likelihood of PE. This can be done in a formal model or by *gestalt*. With clinical *gestalt*, accurate determination of pretest probability appears to increase with clinical experience. In a study at the Brigham and Women's Hospital's emergency department, a trend was observed toward increasing accuracy with increasing experience, with respect to true-positive assessments, true-negative assessments, and likelihood ratios.[14]

When the clinician assesses for possible PE, the clinical context and the patient's symptoms are the two most helpful findings. The clinician should ask whether the patient was predisposed to PE. Regarding symptoms, the most important clue is the presence of otherwise unexplained shortness of breath. Pleuritic chest pain usually occurs with small peripheral PE near the pleural lining, where nerve innervation is plentiful. Ironically, PE associated with dyspnea but no chest pain tends to be anatomically large and at times massive, whereas painful pleuritic PE tends to be anatomically small.

Table 15-2 Chest X-Ray Findings

Dilated pulmonary arteries, especially the right descending pulmonary artery
Pulmonary infarction (Hampton hump)
Lack of pulmonary vascularity (Westermark sign)
Dilated azygous vein (indicating tricuspid regurgitation due to right ventricular dysfunction)

Table 15-3 Electrocardiographic Findings

Tachycardia (often absent in previously healthy younger patients)
S in lead I; Q in lead III; inverted T in lead III
Right bundle branch block (sometimes incomplete right bundle branch block)
New atrial fibrillation or atrial flutter
Rightward QRS axis

Table 15-4 Illnesses That Mimic Pulmonary Embolism

Anxiety/hyperventilation
Pleurisy/acute viral illness
Pneumonia
Myocardial infarction
Dissection of the aorta
Pericardial tamponade

Small PE in the distal pulmonary vasculature may cause pulmonary infarction. This infarction is usually small but painful. It can cause so much pain that splinting of the chest and resulting atelectasis lead to secondary pneumonia. Pulmonary infarction is characterized by low-grade fever, tachypnea, and pain with inspiration or changing position. Hemoptysis is frequent in infarction and less common in PE without infarction. The pain may not respond to high-dose narcotics but usually abates with the use of nonsteroidal anti-inflammatory agents.

Use of a formal clinical scoring model is becoming more widely accepted as an accurate, efficient, and inexpensive way to triage patients according to the clinical probability of PE. The best known model is the Wells DVT Scoring System, which continues to be revised and modified.[15] In 1998, Wells[15] tested a clinical model in a prospective cohort study of 1239 inpatients and outpatients with suspected PE. These investigators showed that by using a clinical scoring system, they could stratify patients into 3 groups: low probability in 734 patients (3.4% with PE), moderate in 403 patients (28% with PE), and high in 102 patients (78% with PE).

The Wells criteria have been modified into a decision rule that dichotomizes patients according to PE unlikely with 4 or fewer score points versus PE likely with more than 4 score points (Table 15-5). This modified simple clinical decision rule can be used by the clinician as the first step in deciding whether to pursue blood test screening with D-dimer, or to go directly to imaging with chest CT scanning.[16]

Regardless of whether *gestalt* or Wells criteria are used to assess PE likelihood, it is important for the consultant to perform a directed history (Table 15-6) and physical examination (Table 15-7). Pertinent positive and negative findings are useful when one is predicting the clinical likelihood of PE, and they rapidly assist the consultant in understanding specific circumstances relevant to the patient who is being evaluated.

Screening With Blood Tests

Room air arterial blood gas analysis was the classic screening blood test used to triage patients with suspected PE. However, in the Prospective Investigation of PE Diagnosis (PIOPED) study, hypoxemia did not discriminate well between patients suspected of PE who actually had PE at pulmonary angiography and those whose pulmonary

Table 15-6 A "Directed" History for Suspected Pulmonary Embolism

"What did you notice that made you think you needed medical attention?"
"Did you have breathlessness?"
"Did you have chest pain? If so, did it occur with taking a deep breath or changing position?"
"Have you had a prior DVT or PE?"
"Is there a family history of DVT or PE?"
"What do you think might predispose you to DVT or PE? Surgery? Trauma? Cancer? Birth control pills or hormone replacement? Immobility? Stress?"
"Do you smoke cigarettes?"
"What is your exercise routine?"

DVT, deep vein thrombosis; PE, pulmonary embolism.

Table 15-7 A "Directed" Physical Examination for Suspected Pulmonary Embolism

General appearance: Ill or healthy-looking? Anxious or calm?
Respiratory rate and whether respirations are shallow, deep, or labored
Neck vein distention
Lung auscultation: Is there dullness at the base? Is there a pleural rub?
Cardiac examination: Is there a right ventricular heave (manifested by a left parasternal lift)? Is S2 accentuated? Is there a distinct P2? Is there a murmur of tricuspid regurgitation (often a II/VI systolic murmur best heard at the left lower sternal border that increases to III/VI with inspiration)?
Abdomen: Is there hepatojugular reflux?
Legs: Is there leg or calf swelling or tenderness? Unilateral? Bilateral?

angiograms were normal.[17] Normal values for the alveolar-arterial oxygen gradient also failed to exclude the diagnosis of PE in this study.[18]

Plasma D-dimer is the most useful screening test for patients with suspected PE. Even in the presence of PE, endogenous albeit ineffective fibrinolysis causes plasmin to digest some of the fibrin clot from the PE. The digested portion circulates as D-dimers that can be recognized by commercially available high-sensitivity monoclonal antibody kits. An elevated D-dimer is sensitive but not specific for PE.[19] Other causes of D-dimer elevation include conditions that mimic PE and even those conditions predisposing to PE (Table 15-8).

Not all D-dimer testing is the same. Quantitative rapid ELISA D-dimer testing appears to provide the most reliable results for exclusion of DVT and PE.[20] In the emergency department of Brigham and Women's Hospital, investigators mandated during a single calendar year that physicians order D-dimer ELISA tests on all patients suspected of acute PE. Of 1106 D-dimer assays, 559 were elevated, and 547 were normal. Only 2 of 547 had PE despite a normal D-dimer. The sensitivity of the D-dimer ELISA for acute PE was 96%. A high negative predictive value is the most important feature of an excellent screening test. In this study, the negative predictive value was 99.6%. Thus, with ruling out of PE by D-dimer testing, fewer chest CT scans

Table 15-5 Pulmonary Embolism Clinical Decision Rule

PE is unlikely with ≤4 score points.
PE is likely with >4 score points.

Variable	Points
Signs, symptoms of DVT	3.0
Alternative diagnosis less likely than PE	3.0
Heart rate > 100/minute	1.5
Immobilization or surgery within 4 weeks	1.5
Prior PE or DVT	1.5
Hemoptysis	1.0
Cancer	1.0

DVT, deep vein thrombosis; PE, pulmonary embolism.

Table 15-8 Common Causes of D-Dimer Elevation Other Than Pulmonary Embolism

Myocardial infarction
Congestive heart failure
Pneumonia
Sepsis
Advanced cancer
Surgery
Second or third trimester of pregnancy

III

and lung scans were required.[21] The safety of D-dimer testing in ruling out PE and halting evaluation for PE in those patients with a high clinical probability of PE has not been firmly established.[22]

Lung Scans

If clinical probability and D-dimer testing do not exclude suspected PE, the next major step is to order an imaging test. Lung scanning is rarely diagnostic[23] and has therefore fallen out of favor. By 2001, in the United States, a higher proportion of PE imaging tests were performed with chest CT than with lung scans.[24] Nowadays, lung scans are done only for patients with renal insufficiency, those with severe intravenous contrast reactions, and pregnant women (to minimize radiation).

Chest CT Scans

The introduction of the chest CT scan changed my professional life as a PE consulting doctor.[25] Before CT scanning became available, the most frequently posed question was: "Does this patient have a PE?" Most consult questions focused on interpretations of lung scans, which were usually reported as nondiagnostic. However, some consultant cases involved queries about patients with low-probability lung scans but high clinical suspicion. As a practical matter, PE consultants could not from a practical standpoint recommend diagnostic pulmonary angiography on every patient who had been evaluated with an equivocal lung scan. One has to practice the art and the science of medicine. After the patient had been exhaustively examined, with review of every detail of history and attempts to elicit every possible physical sign that would clarify the likelihood of PE, one had only three options: (1) Treat empirically for PE, (2) declare "no PE," or (3) recommend invasive pulmonary angiography. Nowadays, with the advent of chest CT scans, the consultant is less haunted by the possibility of excessive diagnosis or underdiagnosis of PE.

Multislice CT for PE diagnosis is a technological marvel. Multiple generations of CT scanners are used, but even first-generation machines deliver images that are dramatic in clarity, rapidly acquired, and accurate in delineating the proximal pulmonary arterial tree.[26] A 16-slice scanner can image the entire chest with submillimeter resolution and a breath-hold of less than 10 seconds.[27] The latest generation of scanners can image sixth-order vessels and visualize thrombi so small that their clinical importance is uncertain.[28]

The chest CT scan can first make the "yes" or "no" diagnosis of PE. If PE is present, the CT will provide information on size and location that is crucial to planning the management strategy. A central, saddle PE is readily seen and is amenable to surgical or catheter embolectomy. Multiple small peripheral PEs exclude a mechanical approach.

The chest CT scan can provide "one stop" access to diagnostic and prognostic information (Table 15-9). CT scan of the chest includes the central upper extremity veins and can be extended to the pelvic and deep leg veins, often pinpointing the location of the DVT that served as the source of the PE. In addition, careful review of the right ventricular size in relation to the left ventricular size can provide clues regarding the presence of pulmonary hypertension and the likelihood of right heart failure. These observations are important because they signify that the CT scan can be used as a prognostic tool and as a diagnostic tool.

If no PE is present, CT can often provide another plausible explanation for symptoms such as dyspnea that led to the PE workup. Most common is a pneumonia that is not well visualized on chest x-ray. At times, important incidental findings are noted that can be lifesaving, such as an early lung carcinoma causing no symptoms whatsoever.

A single-center study[29] and two overviews[30,31] recently analyzed the reliability of CT scanning as the primary diagnostic test performed to exclude PE. All three studies required a minimum of 3 months of patient follow-up. Chest CT scanning was found to be at least as reliable as traditional invasive contrast pulmonary angiography. With normal CT scans that excluded PE, it was safe to withhold anticoagulation. CT scanning certainly avoids the myriad of complications that can occur with invasive pulmonary angiography,[32] including cardiac perforation, pericardial tamponade, precipitation of ventricular tachycardia or fibrillation, and development of pseudoaneurysm or infection at the vascular access site.

Echocardiography

Transthoracic echocardiography is usually normal in patients with PE. The thrombus itself is difficult to visualize. Interpretation of the echocardiogram depends on indirect clues, such as right ventricular dilatation and hypokinesis, septal flattening and paradoxical septal

Table 15-9 Information to be Gleaned from the Chest Computed Tomography Scan

Is PE present or excluded? If PE is excluded, is there CT evidence for dissection of the aorta or pericardial effusion or tamponade?
If PE is present, what are the locations of the emboli? Are they central and accessible to surgical or catheter therapy?
Are there concomitant pulmonary parenchymal problems, such as pulmonary infarction, atelectasis, or pneumonia?
What is the diameter of the right ventricle compared with the left ventricle? Is the interventricular septum displaced toward the left ventricle?
Is thrombus visualized in the pelvic, leg, or arm veins?
Is thrombus visualized in any arterial vessel (thereby suggesting paradoxical embolism in the presence of PE)?

PE, pulmonary embolism; CT, computed tomography.

motion, and diastolic left ventricular impairment. These findings are often absent in patients with PE of small to moderate size. If present, they are especially useful in patients with PE that has been confirmed directly by chest CT. Right ventricular dysfunction on echocardiogram is far more useful for prognosis than for diagnosis.[33] Transesophageal echocardiography facilitates direct visualization of PE in the right or left main pulmonary artery. It provides a tool for prompt decision making in patients with hemodynamic compromise, in whom confirmation of the diagnosis is essential before thrombolysis or embolectomy is performed.[34]

Magnetic Resonance Angiography

This modality is especially useful for patients with renal insufficiency or contrast allergy. In addition to direct thrombus imaging, lung perfusion-ventilation MRI is under development.[35] Beware that the FDA issued an alert in December 2006 that gadolinium, the contrast agent for MRI, is associated with development of a rare form of kidney disease.

Integrated Diagnostic Approach

Disparate clinical assessment tools and imaging modalities may overwhelm both the clinician who seeks consultation and the consultant. It is important to choose carefully from the array of diagnostic options and to select those tests that will be most helpful in a particular circumstance.

The most fundamental question is whether the patient has a PE. A systematic approach to assessment with an accepted and validated diagnostic protocol maximizes efficiency and success (Fig. 15-2). If the workup is negative, the consultant should try to find an alternative explanation for the symptoms and signs that suggested the diagnosis. If the workup reveals PE, the consultant should determine whether the PE is acute, subacute, or chronic. The consultant should then proceed with risk stratification and recommendations for therapy, as discussed in the remainder of this chapter.

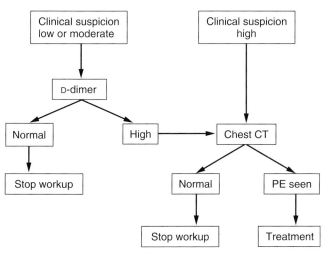

Figure 15-2 Diagnosis of pulmonary embolism (PE).

RISK STRATIFICATION

Risk stratification is the key to successful treatment of patients with DVT and PE (Table 15-10). Low-risk patients have excellent outcomes with anticoagulation alone. Higher risk PE patients may benefit from consideration for more aggressive therapy with thrombolysis or embolectomy.

Clinical evaluation and fundamental parameters such as general appearance, respiratory rate, oxygen saturation level, heart rate, and blood pressure constitute the foundation for PE risk assessment. However, patients who have been previously healthy will often maintain normal vital signs despite anatomically large PE. Thus, contemporary risk assessment moves beyond the classic clinical evaluation and adds key elements, including measurement of cardiac biomarkers and determination of right ventricular size and function.

Cardiac Biomarkers

Cardiac troponins and NT-pro brain natriuretic peptide (NT-proBNP) and brain natriuretic peptide (BNP) have emerged as promising tools for risk stratification.[36] Elevated troponin levels in patients with PE are transient and small, compared with those in patients with acute coronary syndrome. In acute PE, troponin levels correlate with extent of right ventricular dysfunction.[37–41] Myocardial ischemia due to alterations in oxygen supply and demand of the failing right ventricle play major roles in the pathogenesis of troponin level elevation.[42]

The stimulus for natriuretic synthesis and secretion is cardiomyocyte stretch. Elevations in BNP and NT-proBNP are associated with right ventricular dysfunction in acute PE.[43–48] Normal levels of natriuretic peptides imply low risk for patients with PE.

Elevated cardiac biomarker levels indicate that further risk stratification is warranted owing to limited specificity of the assays for predicting right ventricular dysfunction. In patients with PE who have normal biomarker levels, echocardiography is unlikely to provide additional prognostic information.[49]

Echocardiography

Right ventricular dysfunction on echocardiography (Table 15-11) is an independent predictor of mortality in patients with PE.[50,51] Among 1035 patients in the International Cooperative PE Registry (ICOPER) who presented

Table 15-10 Risk Stratification
Clinical assessment (Hemodynamically stable? Ill or healthy appearing?)
Anatomic size of clot
Oxygen saturation?
Elevation of cardiac biomarkers (e.g., troponin or BNP)?
Right ventricular enlargement (on chest CT or echo)
Right ventricular dysfunction (on echo)
Pulmonary hypertension (estimated on echo)

BNP, brain natriuretic peptide; CT, computed tomography; echo, echocardiography.

Table 15-11 Echocardiographic Abnormalities in Pulmonary Embolism

Abnormality	Comments
Right ventricular dilatation	Right-to-left ventricular diameter ratio >0.9 in the apical four-chamber view
Reduced (<50%) respiratory variability of dilated (>2 cm) inferior vena cava	Suggests increased central venous pressure
Flattening or paradoxical motion of the interventricular septum	Suggests pulmonary hypertension
Tricuspid regurgitation jet velocity >2.6 mL/sec	Indicates pulmonary arterial systolic hypertension
Right ventricular systolic hypokinesis	Indicates right ventricular dysfunction
McConnell sign: Hypokinesis of the free wall but preserved apical motion	Specific for pulmonary embolism
Pulmonary artery thrombi	Rarely seen with transthoracic echo; more commonly observed with transesophageal echo
Right atrial or ventricular thrombi	Usually free floating
Patent foramen ovale; atrial septal defect	Seen with color duplex interrogation or echo "bubble" study

echo, echocardiography.

with systolic blood pressure ≥90 mm Hg and who underwent echocardiography within 24 hours of diagnosis, 405 had right ventricular hypokinesis, and 630 had preserved right ventricular function.[52] The 30-day survival rates were 83.7% and 90.6%, respectively (P < .001).

Detection on echocardiography of a patent foramen ovale or an atrial septal defect is an ominous prognostic sign.[53] Another adverse prognostic finding is free floating right heart thrombus. In ICOPER, patients with right heart thrombus had increased mortality, primarily within the subgroup that was treated conservatively with only heparin (24% vs 8%).[54]

Combined Troponin Elevation Plus Right Ventricular Enlargement

In a series of 141 patients with PE for whom both echocardiographic and troponin data were reported, those with both elevated troponin levels and right ventricular enlargement were at significantly greater risk of death after PE than those with only one or no adverse prognostic marker. The 30-day mortality rates were 5% for normal troponin and normal echocardiography, 9% for right ventricular dilatation alone, 23% for elevated troponin alone, and 38% for the lethal combination of right ventricular enlargement and elevated troponin. The adjusted hazard ratio for death within 30 days associated with right ventricular enlargement on echocardiogram and normal troponin was 2.2. For elevated troponin and no right ventricular enlargement on echocardiogram, the hazard ratio was 4.9. With the combination of troponin and right ventricular enlargement, the hazard ratio was 7.2.[55]

Chest CT

Chest CT can be used to risk stratify and diagnose PE. With multislice CT scanners, standardized cardiac views provide valuable information about the size of the right ventricle compared with the left ventricle. In 63 patients with acute PE, the presence of right ventricular enlargement on the reconstructed CT four-chamber view correlated with the presence of right ventricular dysfunction on echocardiogram.[56]

Right ventricular enlargement on chest CT helps the clinician to identify patients with PE who are at especially high risk of death. In 431 consecutive patients with acute PE, right ventricular enlargement on the reconstructed CT four-chamber view was an independent predictor of 30-day mortality (hazard ratio, 5.2).[57]

PARENTERAL ANTICOAGULATION

Rapidly initiated, adequately dosed parenteral anticoagulation provides the foundation of treatment for DVT and PE. Initial treatment with oral anticoagulation alone leads to paradoxical thrombosis and triples the rate of recurrent VTE compared with the standard approach.[58] The mechanism is probably acute depletion of protein C, which causes rebound thrombosis.

Unfractionated Heparin

Bolus followed by continuous intravenous infusion of unfractionated heparin remains the most widely employed strategy for the initial management of acute PE. The heparin dose is titrated to the partial thromboplastin time (PTT), usually with the use of a target of 60 to 80 seconds. Many nomograms are available for heparin dosing.[59] In the United States, the most popular nomogram is the Raschke nomogram, which boluses initially with 80 U/kg, immediately followed by an infusion of 18 U/kg/hr.[60]

Although continuous intravenous unfractionated heparin has been used for about 40 years, it is the most frequent cause of medication errors associated with anticoagulant therapy in the hospital. The root of these errors is most often related to the infusion device and to parenteral delivery problems. More advanced infusion devices with drug libraries, dosing guardrails, bar code readers, and dose calculators are being introduced.[61]

Subcutaneously administered anticoagulation has become increasingly popular in avoiding intravenous parenteral anticoagulation. Adjusted-dose subcutaneous heparin can be given safely and effectively to treat patients with DVT.[62,63] However, this approach requires that PTTs be obtained and is cumbersome when used to maintain the target therapeutic range.

Low Molecular Weight Heparin

Subcutaneously administered low molecular weight heparin (LMWH) has become the first-line anticoagulant in the treatment of patients with DVT. A meta-analysis suggests that LMWH reduces the mortality rate compared with unfractionated heparin, with no increase in major bleeding complications.[64] LMWH also appears to be highly cost effective, even for inpatient management of DVT.[65] However, proponents of unfractionated heparin argue that previous studies with unfractionated heparin used subtherapeutic ranges for the PTT target and dispute that LMWH is superior to unfractionated heparin.[66] Nevertheless, the ability to provide fixed, weight-based dosing without laboratory coagulation monitoring and the ability to avoid intravenous therapy have influenced most practitioners to favor LMWH.

For treatment of patients with DVT with LMWH, the most widely used regimen is enoxaparin 1.0 mg/kg twice daily.[67] An alternative dosing regimen is enoxaparin 1.5 mg/kg once daily.[68] A head-to-head comparison of tinzaparin versus dalteparin showed no differences with respect to efficacy and safety in a randomized trial for outpatient treatment of VTE.[69] The LMWH reviparin, appears more effective than unfractionated heparin in reducing the size of DVT. It is also more effective than unfractionated heparin for preventing recurrent DVT.[70]

Because of success in managing DVT with LMWH, interest in the use of LMWH to treat patients with acute PE has been increasing. A study in which subcutaneous tinzaparin was compared with intravenous unfractionated heparin found that tinzaparin appeared to be as effective and safe in patients with acute PE.[71] An individual patient data meta-analysis showed that the efficacy and safety of enoxaparin versus unfractionated heparin for DVT treatment are not modified by the presence of symptomatic PE.[72] Another meta-analysis found that fixed-dose LMWH appears to be as effective and safe as dose-adjusted intravenous unfractionated heparin for the initial treatment of nonmassive PE.[73]

In patients with cancer and VTE, a randomized trial of 672 patients compared dalteparin as a bridge to oral anticoagulation with dalteparin as monotherapy without oral anticoagulation. During the 6-month study period, a 52% reduction in recurrent VTE occurred in the dalteparin monotherapy group, without any difference in the bleeding complication rate.[74] It also appears that enoxaparin can be given as monotherapy to patients with acute PE with no differences in efficacy or safety compared with a strategy that "bridges" to warfarin.[75,76]

Fondaparinux

Fondaparinux is a synthetic and selective inhibitor of factor Xa. It is FDA approved as a "bridge" to warfarin therapy in patients with acute DVT or PE. Its pharmacokinetic properties allow a simple, fixed-dose, once-daily subcutaneous injection that is weight based and that does not require laboratory coagulation monitoring. In a trial of 2205 patients with symptomatic acute DVT, fixed-dose fondaparinux (5.0 mg for <50 kg, 7.5 mg for 50–100 kg, and 10.0 mg for >100 kg) was at least as effective and safe as twice-daily weight-adjusted enoxaparin.[77] In a separate trial of 2213 patients with symptomatic acute PE, fondaparinux given in the same once-daily subcutaneous dosing regimen was at least as effective and safe as adjusted-dose continuous infusion intravenous unfractionated heparin.[78]

THROMBOLYSIS

Thrombolytic therapy as an adjunct to parenteral anticoagulation should be considered for patients with painful iliofemoral DVT or for those with PE with adverse prognostic factors such as elevated cardiac biomarkers, moderate or severe right ventricular enlargement, or moderate or severe right ventricular hypokinesis.

The Management Strategies and Prognosis in Pulmonary Embolism Trial-3 (MAPPET-3) is the largest single randomized, controlled PE trial of thrombolysis plus heparin versus heparin alone. Alteplase, the thrombolytic agent, was administered as a peripheral intravenous infusion of 100 mg over 2 hours. The primary end point was in-hospital death or clinical deterioration requiring escalation of treatment, defined as catecholamine infusion, repeat thrombolysis, mechanical ventilation, cardiopulmonary resuscitation, or embolectomy. The end point of escalation of therapy was higher in the heparin alone group (25% vs 10% in the heparin plus alteplase group). However, the difference was driven primarily by the administration of thrombolysis, which was considered a "soft" and controversial part of the composite end point.[79] A meta-analysis of randomized trials found that a benefit was suggested in those with hemodynamically unstable PE who were at highest risk of recurrence or death.[80]

The indications for PE thrombolysis continue to generate controversy. A recent analysis from ICOPER found no benefit for thrombolysis among patients with massive PE, defined as those presenting with a systolic arterial pressure lower than 90 mm Hg.[81]

Lytic therapy administered systemically or ("catheter-directed") regionally may have a role in the treatment of patients with acute DVT. The rationale for lytic therapy is that if clot lysis was rapidly successful, then decompression of the extremity would occur faster and perhaps would be limb saving in cases of impending venous gangrene, resulting in less venous valvular destruction and, over the long term, less chronic venous insufficiency.[82–85] Despite years of use, none of these hypotheses has been adequately addressed, let alone answered, by appropriate randomized control trials (RCTs). Registries of catheter-directed lytic therapy documenting prompt efficacy do not prove superiority over systemically administered thrombolytic therapy or adequate heparin-based anticoagulant therapy. Evidence favoring catheter-directed thrombolytic therapy is strongest in cases of acute impending venous gangrene.[86,87] Thrombolysis is frequently used to treat large, fresh thromboses of the veins of the arm and iliofemoral veins, especially in younger, otherwise healthy patients who are expected to have a low hemorrhagic risk and a long lifetime of less troublesome postphlebitic syndrome.

EMBOLECTOMY

Pulmonary embolectomy should be considered for patients with PE who are at high risk of death or major nonfatal complications and who cannot safely receive treatment with thrombolysis because of a prohibitively high bleeding risk. At Brigham and Women's Hospital, we perform about one pulmonary embolectomy per month and 30-day survival exceeds 90%. Our success is based in part on an integrated medical-surgical thrombosis service that rapidly consults on high-risk PE patients. The objectives are (1) to refer patients to surgery on the basis of risk stratification, and (2) to make a disposition prior to the onset of irreversible cardiogenic shock and multisystem organ failure.[88] At certain centers, surgical pulmonary embolectomy, which had been virtually abandoned, is making a successful renaissance.[89,90]

Catheter embolectomy promises to be a less invasive approach for patients with PE who have a poor prognosis and contraindications to thrombolysis.[91] Integration of catheter thrombectomy into the therapeutic armamentarium has been hampered by technical problems, including poor steerability, mechanical hemolysis, and distal embolization of the thrombus. A novel catheter is under development that aspirates, macerates, and removes the thrombus through an aspiration port.[92]

INFERIOR VENA CAVAL FILTERS

Two major indications for inferior vena caval (IVC) filters are as follows: (1) inability of the patient to tolerate anticoagulation because of major bleeding, and (2) recurrent PE despite adequate anticoagulation. However, filter insertion has increased for "softer" indications such as prophylaxis in high-risk or trauma patients, anatomically large DVT, or "free-floating" DVTs.[93]

Over a 20-year period in the United States, the frequency of IVC filter insertion has increased by more than 20-fold.[94] The most recent trend has been to insert retrievable IVC filters.[95] In a prospective DVT registry of 5451 patients with ultrasound-confirmed DVT from 183 U.S. study sites, 781 (14%) received IVC filters.[96] IVC filters, used in both short-term[97] and long-term follow-up,[98] appear to reduce the risk of PE but increase the risk of DVT, with no effect on overall survival. Patients with IVC filters have a higher rate of rehospitalization for VTE than do those with DVT who are not given IVC filters[99] (see Chapter 31).

INTEGRATED APPROACH TO INITIAL MANAGEMENT

Acute DVT

Most patients with small or moderate leg DVT are at low risk of complications and receive LMWH as a "bridge" to oral anticoagulation with warfarin (Fig. 15-3). An alternative and equally effective strategy is to prescribe fondaparinux as a "bridge" to warfarin. Symptomatic patients with isolated calf DVT should receive anticoagulation and should not be subjected to a strategy of "observe and rescan for proximal propagation."

A pivotal management issue is whether patients should be treated at home or in the hospital. Although home treatment is becoming more popular, certain caveats should be kept in mind. Table 15-12 lists contraindications to home treatment of DVT.

For patients with large or massive DVT, a decision must be made as to whether catheter-directed thrombolysis is appropriate.[100] Massive DVT with purplish skin discoloration is called phlegmasia cerulea dolens. This term refers to a spectrum of large DVT, ranging from iliofemoral thrombosis to venous gangrene and necrosis. Venous engorgement with increased pressure in the capillaries leads to massive leg edema and potential arterial inflow compromise. Patients should be followed for possible progression to a compartment syndrome, for which urgent fasciotomy may be required if arterial flow becomes impaired.

For those patients with DVT who have active bleeding or a tendency to bleed, insertion of an IVC filter should be considered. When the duration of bleeding is believed to be short, placement of a retrievable filter is preferable to use of a permanent filter.

Patients with septic thrombophlebitis should receive broad coverage antibiotics plus full anticoagulation, usually with continuous intravenous unfractionated heparin. They should remain hospitalized until the fever subsides and the pain and erythema caused by the phlebitis have abated.

Patients with only an initial superficial thrombophlebitis may respond to conservative measures such as nonsteroidal anti-inflammatory agents. If superficial phlebitis persists, a 1-month course of half-dose anticoagulation, such as with enoxaparin 1 mg/kg once daily as monotherapy without warfarin, is often highly effective.

Acute PE

The key to successful management is rapid and accurate risk stratification (Fig. 15-4). Low-risk patients have excellent outcomes with anticoagulation alone. However, thrombolysis or embolectomy should be considered, in addition to anticoagulation, for high-risk patients.[101] Rapid institution of definitive therapy usually improves the acutely decompensated right ventricle.[102]

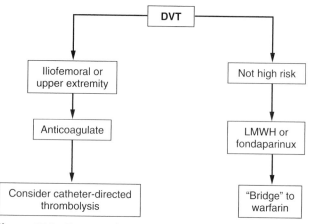

Figure 15-3 Treatment for deep vein thrombosis (DVT).

Table 15-12 **Contraindications to Home Treatment of Patients With Deep Vein Thrombosis**
The patient has leg pain or is unable to walk comfortably.
Massive thigh or calf swelling has been noted.
Pelvic vein thrombosis occurs, in addition to leg DVT.
The upper arm is markedly swollen.
Thrombolysis, catheter embolectomy, or IVC filter placement has been planned.
Low likelihood of compliance with prescribed treatment.
Homeless.
Phoneless.

DVT, deep vein thrombosis; IVC, inferior vena caval.

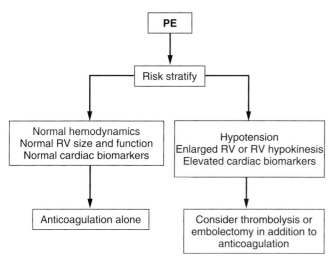

Figure 15-4 Risk stratification for pulmonary embolism (PE).

Massive PE with hemodynamic compromise warrants special consideration. The clinician may use high-dose unfractionated heparin in larger than usual doses. A minimum bolus of 10,000 units followed by a continuous infusion of at least 1250 units per hour serves as a cornerstone of therapy. Empirical observation reveals that standard doses of heparin often fail to achieve therapeutic levels of anticoagulation. Although rapid administration of 500 mL of normal saline is acceptable for restoring adequate blood pressure, fluids should be used with extreme caution. In right ventricular failure, fluid administration exacerbates right ventricular wall stress, intensifies right ventricular ischemia, and causes further interventricular septal shift toward the left ventricle, thereby worsening left ventricular compliance and filling. Therefore, the clinician should have a low threshold for initiating pressors, such as dopamine or dobutamine.[103] A temporary improvement in hemodynamics facilitates more definitive therapy with thrombolysis or embolectomy.

Acute PE can lead to chronic thromboembolic pulmonary hypertension[104] (see Chapter 45). Previously considered a rare event, the incidence is high and seems progressive: 1.0% at 6 months, 3.1% at 1 year, and 3.8% at 2 years.[104] The best therapy for established chronic thromboembolic pulmonary hypertension is pulmonary thromboendarterectomy, a complex operation that can restore normal cardiopulmonary function.[105] For nonsurgical candidates, balloon pulmonary angioplasty may be considered.[106]

LONG-TERM ANTICOAGULATION

Warfarin anticoagulation provides the foundation for long-term prevention of recurrent DVT and PE. Warfarin, patented in 1948 and introduced commercially in 1954, is the 20th most frequently prescribed drug in the United States, with more than 24,000,000 prescriptions written annually in the United States alone.

For the initial treatment of patients with DVT or PE, the target international normalized ratio (INR) is usually between 2.0 and 3.0. An overview of bleeding complications revealed that the rate of intracranial bleeding was 1.15 per 100 patient-years, and the case fatality rate of major bleeding was 13%.[107] Centralized telephone-based anticoagulation services can improve safety.[108] Self-monitoring of INR and learning how to self-dose warfarin, analogous to the common practice among patients with insulin-dependent diabetes of blood sugar testing and self-dosing, can lower the complication rate even further[109] (see Chapter 40). Rapid turnaround genetic testing may personalize warfarin dosing and eliminate much of the "guess work" in prescribing the initial dose.

Risk of Recurrence After Warfarin is Discontinued

Clinical and thrombophilic risk factors for recurrent DVT and PE are present after warfarin is discontinued. In general, clinical risk factors are more predictive than is laboratory thrombophilia evaluation. Patients with provoked DVT or PE after surgery, trauma, pregnancy, or hormone replacement therapy are ordinarily at low risk of recurrence, as long as these specific risk factors are negated and further avoided.

Patients with a first symptomatic PE have a higher risk of recurrent VTE than do those who originally present with DVT without symptoms of PE. In a study from Vienna, Austria, the relative risk of recurrence was more than twice as high in patients who initially presented with PE.[110] The risk that patients may have a PE rather than a DVT as the recurrent event was 4 times higher compared with the risk in patients who presented originally with DVT and no symptoms of PE.[110] For unknown reasons, men have a higher risk of recurrence than women.[111,112]

Impact of Thrombophilia

The Leiden Thrombophilia Study enrolled and followed 474 patients with VTE for a mean of 7 years; complete follow-up was provided in 94%. The incidence rate of recurrence was highest during the first 2 years after the event. The risk of thrombotic event recurrence was twice as high among patients whose initial event was idiopathic. Prothrombotic laboratory abnormalities did not appear to play an important role in the risk of recurrent VTE.[113] However, other studies found that prothrombin gene mutation,[114] hyperhomocysteinemia,[115] and antiphospholipid antibody syndrome[116] increased the risk of recurrent events. Whether factor V Leiden increases the risk of recurrence remains controversial[117,118] (see Chapter 14).

Optimal Duration of Anticoagulation

It is clear that 6 months of anticoagulation halves the recurrent VTE rate compared with 6 weeks of therapy.[119] It is also evident that indefinite anticoagulation should be instituted after a second episode of VTE has occurred.[120] A meta-analysis indicates that with lifelong therapy, one needs to treat about nine patients to prevent a single episode of VTE. The long-term bleeding risk in the population that has successfully received anticoagulation for 6 months is very low.[121]

For patients with idiopathic VTE, indefinite duration anticoagulation was shown to be superior to 3 to 6 months of anticoagulation in three separate randomized, controlled trials of the extended treatment strategy. A Canadian study[122] investigated warfarin given in the standard therapeutic INR range of 2.0 to 3.0. An American study[123] examined warfarin in the low-intensity INR range of 1.5 to 2.0. A European study[124] examined ximelagatran, an oral direct thrombin inhibitor, as the therapeutic anticoagulant agent. All three extended treatment strategies were successful.

Another approach to determining duration of therapy in patients with DVT used residual venous thrombosis visualized on venous ultrasound examination. Patients with residual disease at 3 months underwent serial ultrasound examinations until their studies normalized, or until they had undergone 36 months of follow-up. At 3 months, only 39% of patients had normal ultrasound examinations. By 36 months, 74% of patients had normal studies. The likelihood of recurrent DVT was 2.4 times higher among patients whose ultrasound results showed residual venous thrombosis.[125]

Another alternative strategy involves measuring D-dimer levels 1 month after anticoagulation is discontinued. In an Italian study, VTE recurrence was 2.4 times greater among patients whose D-dimer levels failed to normalize.[126] A study from Vienna found that the recurrence rate was 40% lower with D-dimer levels between 250 and 500 ng/mL (the upper portion of the normal range) and 70% lower for levels below 250 ng/mL.[127]

REFERENCES

1. Goldhaber SZ, Elliott CG: Acute pulmonary embolism: Part I—Epidemiology, pathophysiology, and diagnosis. Circulation 108:2726–2729, 2003.
2. Elliott CG, Goldhaber SZ, Jensen RL: Delays in diagnosis of deep vein thrombosis and pulmonary embolism. Chest 128:3372–3376, 2005.
3. Wells PS, Anderson DR, Bormanis J, et al: Value of assessment of pretest probability of deep-vein thrombosis in clinical management. Lancet 350:1795–1798, 1997.
4. Bundens WP, Bergan JJ, Halasz NA, et al: The superficial femoral vein: A potentially lethal misnomer. JAMA 274:1296–1298, 1995.
5. Joffe HV, Goldhaber SZ: Upper extremity deep vein thrombosis. Circulation 106:1874–1880, 2002.
6. Joffe HV, Kucher N, Tapson VF, et al: Upper-extremity deep vein thrombosis: A prospective registry of 592 patients. Circulation 110:1605–1611, 2004.
7. Stevens SM, Elliott CG, Chan KJ, et al: Withholding anticoagulation after a negative result on duplex ultrasonography for suspected symptomatic deep venous thrombosis. Ann Intern Med 140:985–991, 2004.
8. Loud PA, Katz DS, Belfi L, et al: Imaging of deep venous thrombosis in suspected pulmonary embolism. Semin Roentgenol 40:33–40, 2005.
9. Wells PS, Lensing AW, Davidson BL, et al: Accuracy of ultrasound for the diagnosis of deep venous thrombosis in asymptomatic patients after orthopedic surgery: A meta-analysis. Ann Intern Med 122:47–53, 1995.
10. Jongbloets LM, Lensing AW, Koopman MM, et al: Limitations of compression ultrasound for the detection of symptomless postoperative deep vein thrombosis. Lancet 343:1142–1144, 1994.
11. Stern JB, Abehsera M, Grenet D, et al: Detection of pelvic vein thrombosis by magnetic resonance angiography in patients with acute pulmonary embolism and normal lower limb compression ultrasonography. Chest 122:115–121, 2002.
12. Fraser DG, Moody AR, Morgan PS, et al: Diagnosis of lower-limb deep venous thrombosis: A prospective blinded study of magnetic resonance direct thrombus imaging. Ann Intern Med 136:89–98, 2002.
13. Hull R, Hirsh J, Sackett DL, et al: Clinical validity of a negative venogram in patients with clinically suspected venous thrombosis. Circulation 64:622–625, 1981.
14. Kabrhel C, Camargo CA Jr, Goldhaber SZ: Clinical gestalt and the diagnosis of pulmonary embolism: Does experience matter? Chest 127:1627–1630, 2005.
15. Wells PS, Ginsberg JS, Anderson DR, et al: Use of a clinical model for safe management of patients with suspected pulmonary embolism. Ann Intern Med 129:997–1005, 1998.
16. van Belle A, Buller HR, Huisman MV, et al: Effectiveness of managing suspected pulmonary embolism using an algorithm combining clinical probability, D-dimer testing, and computed tomography. JAMA 295:172–179, 2006.
17. Stein PD, Goldhaber SZ, Henry JW, Miller AC: Arterial blood gas analysis in the assessment of suspected acute pulmonary embolism. Chest 109:78–81, 1996.
18. Stein PD, Goldhaber SZ, Henry JW: Alveolar-arterial oxygen gradient in the assessment of acute pulmonary embolism. Chest 107:139–143, 1995.
19. Brown MD, Rowe BH, Reeves MJ, et al: The accuracy of the enzyme-linked immunosorbent assay D-dimer test in the diagnosis of pulmonary embolism: A meta-analysis. Ann Emerg Med 40:133–144, 2002.
20. Stein PD, Hull RD, Patel KC, et al: D-dimer for the exclusion of acute venous thrombosis and pulmonary embolism: A systematic review. Ann Intern Med 140:589–602, 2004.
21. Dunn KL, Wolf JP, Dorfman DM, et al: Normal D-dimer levels in emergency department patients suspected of acute pulmonary embolism. J Am Coll Cardiol 40:1475–1478, 2002.
22. Righini M, Aujesky D, Roy PM, et al: Clinical usefulness of D-dimer depending on clinical probability and cutoff value in outpatients with suspected pulmonary embolism. Arch Intern Med 164:2483–2487, 2004.
23. Gottschalk A, Sostman HD, Coleman RE, et al: Ventilation-perfusion scintigraphy in the PIOPED study. Part II. Evaluation of the scintigraphic criteria and interpretations. J Nucl Med 34:1119–1126, 1993.
24. Stein PD, Kayali F, Olson RE: Trends in the use of diagnostic imaging in patients hospitalized with acute pulmonary embolism. Am J Cardiol 93:1316–1317, 2004.
25. Goldhaber SZ: How chest CT for the diagnosis of pulmonary embolism (PE) has changed my professional life: Reflections from a PE doctor. Semin Roentgenol 40:8–10, 2005.
26. Goldhaber SZ: Multislice computed tomography for pulmonary embolism: A technological marvel. N Engl J Med 352:1812–1814, 2005.
27. Schoepf UJ, Goldhaber SZ, Costello P: Spiral computed tomography for acute pulmonary embolism. Circulation 109:2160–2167, 2004.
28. Ravenel JG, Kipfmueller F, Schoepf UJ: CT angiography with multidetector-row CT for detection of acute pulmonary embolus. Semin Roentgenol 40:11–19, 2005.
29. van Strijen MJ, de Monye W, Schiereck J, et al: Single-detector helical computed tomography as the primary diagnostic test in suspected pulmonary embolism: A multicenter clinical management study of 510 patients. Ann Intern Med 138:307–314, 2003.
30. Moores LK, Jackson WL Jr, Shorr AF, Jackson JL: Meta-analysis: Outcomes in patients with suspected pulmonary embolism managed with computed tomographic pulmonary angiography. Ann Intern Med 141:866–874, 2004.
31. Quiroz R, Kucher N, Zou KH, et al: Clinical validity of a negative computed tomography scan in patients with suspected pulmonary embolism: A systematic review. JAMA 293:2012–2017, 2005.
32. Stein PD, Athanasoulis C, Alavi A, et al: Complications and validity of pulmonary angiography in acute pulmonary embolism. Circulation 85:462–468, 1992.
33. Goldhaber SZ: Echocardiography in the management of pulmonary embolism. Ann Intern Med 136:691–700, 2002.
34. Pruszczyk P, Torbicki A, Kuch-Wocial A, et al: Diagnostic value of transoesophageal echocardiography in suspected haemodynamically significant pulmonary embolism. Heart 85:628–634, 2001.
35. van Beek EJR, Wild JM, Fink C, et al: MRI for the diagnosis of pulmonary embolism. J Magn Reson Imaging 18:627–640, 2003.
36. Kucher N, Goldhaber SZ: Cardiac biomarkers for risk stratification of patients with acute pulmonary embolism. Circulation 108:2191–2194, 2003.
37. Konstantinides S, Geibel A, Olschewski M, et al: Importance of cardiac troponins I and T in risk stratification of patients with acute pulmonary embolism. Circulation 106:1263–1268, 2002.
38. Kucher N, Wallmann D, Carone A, et al: Incremental prognostic value of troponin I and echocardiography in patients with acute pulmonary embolism. Eur Heart J 24:1651–1656, 2003.

39. Janata K, Holzer M, Laggner AN, Mullner M: Cardiac troponin T in the severity assessment of patients with pulmonary embolism: Cohort study. BMJ 326:312–313, 2003.

40. Pruszczyk P, Bochowicz A, Torbicki A, et al: Cardiac troponin T monitoring identifies high-risk group of normotensive patients with acute pulmonary embolism. Chest 123:1947–1952, 2003.

41. Giannitsis E, Muller-Bardorff M, Kurowski V, et al: Independent prognostic value of cardiac troponin T in patients with confirmed pulmonary embolism. Circulation 102:211–217, 2000.

42. Meyer T, Binder L, Hruska N, et al: Cardiac troponin I elevation in acute pulmonary embolism is associated with right ventricular dysfunction. J Am Coll Cardiol 36:1632–1636, 2000.

43. Kucher N, Printzen G, Doernhoefer T, et al: Low pro-brain natriuretic peptide levels predict benign clinical outcome in acute pulmonary embolism. Circulation 107:1576–1578, 2003.

44. Kucher N, Printzen G, Goldhaber SZ: Prognostic role of brain natriuretic peptide in acute pulmonary embolism. Circulation 107:2545–2547, 2003.

45. Nagaya N, Nishikimi T, Okano Y, et al: Plasma brain natriuretic peptide levels increase in proportion to the extent of right ventricular dysfunction in pulmonary hypertension. J Am Coll Cardiol 31:202–208, 1998.

46. Pruszczyk P, Kostrubiec M, Bochowicz A, et al: N-terminal pro-brain natriuretic peptide in patients with acute pulmonary embolism. Eur Respir J 22:649–653, 2003.

47. ten Wolde M, Tulevski II, Mulder JW, et al: Brain natriuretic peptide as a predictor of adverse outcome in patients with pulmonary embolism. Circulation 107:2082–2084, 2003.

48. Tulevski II, Hirsch A, Sanson BJ, et al: Increased brain natriuretic peptide as a marker for right ventricular dysfunction in acute pulmonary embolism. Thromb Haemost 86:1193–1196, 2001.

49. Binder L, Pieske B, Olschewski M, et al: N-terminal pro-brain natriuretic peptide or troponin testing followed by echocardiography for risk stratification of acute pulmonary embolism. Circulation 112:1573–1579, 2005.

50. Ribeiro A, Lindmarker P, Juhlin-Dannfelt A, et al: Echocardiography Doppler in pulmonary embolism: Right ventricular dysfunction as a predictor of mortality rate. Am Heart J 134:479–487, 1997.

51. Torbicki A, Galie N, Covezzoli A, et al: Right heart thrombi in pulmonary embolism: Results from the International Cooperative Pulmonary Embolism Registry. J Am Coll Cardiol 41:2245–2251, 2003.

52. Kucher N, Rossi E, De Rosa M, Goldhaber SZ: Prognostic role of echocardiography among patients with acute pulmonary embolism and a systolic arterial pressure of 90 mm Hg or higher. Arch Intern Med 165:1777–1781, 2005.

53. Konstantinides S, Geibel A, Kasper W, et al: Patent foramen ovale is an important predictor of adverse outcome in patients with major pulmonary embolism. Circulation 97:1946–1951, 1998.

54. Torbicki A, Galie N, Covezzoli A, et al: Right heart thrombi in pulmonary embolism: Results from the International Cooperative Pulmonary Embolism Registry. J Am Coll Cardiol 41:2245–2251, 2003.

55. Scridon T, Scridon C, Skali H, et al: Prognostic significance of troponin elevation and right ventricular enlargement in acute pulmonary embolism. Am J Cardiol 96:303–305, 2005.

56. Quiroz R, Kucher N, Schoepf UJ, et al: Right ventricular enlargement on chest computed tomography: Prognostic role in acute pulmonary embolism. Circulation 109:2401–2404, 2004.

57. Schoepf UJ, Kucher N, Kipfmueller F, et al: Right ventricular enlargement on chest computed tomography: A predictor of early death in acute pulmonary embolism. Circulation 110:3276–3280, 2004.

58. Brandjes DP, Heijboer H, Buller HR, et al: Acenocoumarol and heparin compared with acenocoumarol alone in the initial treatment of proximal-vein thrombosis. N Engl J Med 327:1485–1489, 1992.

59. Bernardi E, Piccioli A, Oliboni G, et al: Nomograms for the administration of unfractionated heparin in the initial treatment of acute thromboembolism—An overview. Thromb Haemost 84:22–26, 2000.

60. Raschke RA, Reilly BM, Guidry JR, et al: The weight-based heparin dosing nomogram compared with a "standard care" nomogram: A randomized controlled trial. Ann Intern Med 119:874–881, 1993.

61. Fanikos J, Stapinski C, Koo S, et al: Medication errors associated with anticoagulant therapy in the hospital. Am J Cardiol 94:532–535, 2004.

62. Hirsch DR, Lee TH, Morrison RB, et al: Shortened hospitalization by means of adjusted-dose subcutaneous heparin for deep venous thrombosis. Am Heart J 131:276–280, 1996.

63. Prandoni P, Carnovali M, Marchiori A: Subcutaneous adjusted-dose unfractionated heparin vs fixed-dose low-molecular-weight heparin in the initial treatment of venous thromboembolism. Arch Intern Med 164:1077–1083, 2004.

64. Gould MK, Dembitzer AD, Doyle RL, et al: Low-molecular-weight heparins compared with unfractionated heparin for treatment of acute deep venous thrombosis: A meta-analysis of randomized, controlled trials. Ann Intern Med 130:800–809, 1999.

65. Gould MK, Dembitzer AD, Sanders GD, Garber AM: Low-molecular-weight heparins compared with unfractionated heparin for treatment of acute deep venous thrombosis: A cost-effectiveness analysis. Ann Intern Med 130:789–799, 1999.

66. Raschke R, Hirsh J, Guidry JR: Suboptimal monitoring and dosing of unfractionated heparin in comparative studies with low-molecular-weight heparin. Ann Intern Med 138:720–723, 2003.

67. Levine M, Gent M, Hirsh J, et al: A comparison of low-molecular-weight heparin administered primarily at home with unfractionated heparin administered in the hospital for proximal deep-vein thrombosis. N Engl J Med 334:677–681, 1996.

68. Merli G, Spiro TE, Olsson CG, et al: Subcutaneous enoxaparin once or twice daily compared with intravenous unfractionated heparin for treatment of venous thromboembolic disease. Ann Intern Med 134:191–202, 2001.

69. Wells PS, Anderson DR, Rodger MA, et al: A randomized trial comparing 2 low-molecular-weight heparins for the outpatient treatment of deep vein thrombosis and pulmonary embolism. Arch Intern Med 165:733–738, 2005.

70. Breddin HK, Hach-Wunderle V, Nakov R, Kakkar VV: Effects of a low-molecular-weight heparin on thrombus regression and recurrent thromboembolism in patients with deep-vein thrombosis. N Engl J Med 344:626–631, 2001.

71. Simonneau G, Sors H, Charbonnier B, et al: A comparison of low-molecular-weight heparin with unfractionated heparin for acute pulmonary embolism. The THESEE Study Group. Tinzaparine ou Heparine Standard: Evaluations dans l'Embolie Pulmonaire. N Engl J Med 337:663–669, 1997.

72. Mismetti P, Quenet S, Levine M, et al: Enoxaparin in the treatment of deep vein thrombosis with or without pulmonary embolism: An individual patient data meta-analysis. Chest 128:2203–2210, 2005.

73. Quinlan DJ, McQuillan A, Eikelboom JW: Low-molecular-weight heparin compared with intravenous unfractionated heparin for treatment of pulmonary embolism: A meta-analysis of randomized, controlled trials. Ann Intern Med 140:175–183, 2004.

74. Lee AY, Levine MN, Baker RI, et al: Low-molecular-weight heparin versus a coumarin for the prevention of recurrent venous thromboembolism in patients with cancer. N Engl J Med 349:146–153, 2003.

75. Kucher N, Quiroz R, McKean S, et al: Extended enoxaparin monotherapy for acute symptomatic pulmonary embolism. Vasc Med 10:251–256, 2005.

76. Kucher N, Quiroz R, McKean S, et al: Extended enoxaparin monotherapy for acute symptomatic pulmonary embolism. Vasc Med 10:251–256, 2005.

77. Buller HR, Davidson BL, Decousus H, et al: Fondaparinux or enoxaparin for the initial treatment of symptomatic deep venous thrombosis: A randomized trial. Ann Intern Med 140:867–873, 2004.

78. Buller HR, Davidson BL, Decousus H, et al: Subcutaneous fondaparinux versus intravenous unfractionated heparin in the initial treatment of pulmonary embolism. N Engl J Med 349:1695–1702, 2003.

79. Konstantinides S, Geibel A, Heusel G, et al: Heparin plus alteplase compared with heparin alone in patients with submassive pulmonary embolism. N Engl J Med 347:1143–1150, 2002.

80. Wan S, Quinlan DJ, Agnelli G, Eikelboom JW: Thrombolysis compared with heparin for the initial treatment of pulmonary embolism: A meta-analysis of the randomized controlled trials. Circulation 110:744–749, 2004.

81. Kucher N, Rossi E, De Rosa M, Goldhaber SZ: Massive pulmonary embolism. Circulation 113:577–582, 2006.

82. Janssen MC, Wollersheim H, Schultze-Kool LJ, Thein T: Local and systemic thrombolytic therapy for acute deep vein thrombosis. Neth J Med 63:81–90, 2005.

83. Acharya G, Singh K, Hansen JB, et al: Catheter-directed thrombolysis for the management of postpartum deep vein thrombosis. Acta Obstet Gynecol Scand 84:155–158, 2005.

84. Laiho MK, Oinonen A, Sugano N, et al: Preservation of venous valve function after catheter-directed and systemic thrombolysis for deep vein thrombosis. Eur J Vasc Endovasc Surg 28:391–396, 2004.

85. Couturaud F, Kearon C: Treatment of deep vein thrombosis. Semin Vasc Med 1:43–54, 2001.

86. Arcasoy SM, Vachani A: Local and systemic thrombolytic therapy for acute venous thromboembolism. Clin Chest Med 24:73–91, 2003.

87. Wells PS, Forster AJ: Thrombolysis in deep vein thrombosis: Is there still an indication? Thromb Haemost 86:499–508, 2001.

88. Leacche M, Unic D, Goldhaber SZ, et al: Modern surgical treatment of massive pulmonary embolism: Results in 47 consecutive patients after rapid diagnosis and aggressive surgical approach. J Thorac Cardiovasc Surg 129:1018–1023, 2005.

89. Sukhija R, Aronow WS, Lee J, et al: Association of right ventricular dysfunction with in-hospital mortality in patients with acute pulmonary embolism and reduction in mortality in patients with right ventricular dysfunction by pulmonary embolectomy. Am J Cardiol 95:695–696, 2005.

90. Meneveau N, Seronde MF, Blonde MC, et al: Management of unsuccessful thrombolysis in acute massive pulmonary embolism. Chest 129:1043–1050, 2006.

91. Goldhaber SZ: Integration of catheter thrombectomy into our armamentarium to treat acute pulmonary embolism. Chest 114: 1237–1238, 1998.

92. Kucher N, Windecker S, Banz Y, et al: Percutaneous catheter thrombectomy device for acute pulmonary embolism: In vitro and in vivo testing. Radiology 236:852–858, 2005.

93. Pacouret G, Alison D, Pottier J-M, et al: Free-floating thrombus and embolic risk in patients with angiographically confirmed proximal deep venous thrombosis. Arch Intern Med 157:305–308, 1997.

94. Stein PD, Kayali F, Olson RE: Twenty-one-year trends in the use of inferior vena cava filters. Arch Intern Med 164:1541–1545, 2004.

95. Stein PD, Alnas M, Skaf E, et al: Outcome and complications of retrievable inferior vena cava filters. Am J Cardiol 94:1090–1093, 2004.

96. Jaff MR, Goldhaber SZ, Tapson VF: High utilization rate of vena cava filters in deep vein thrombosis. Thromb Haemost 93:1117–1119, 2005.

97. Decousus H, Leizorovicz A, Parent F, et al: A clinical trial of vena caval filters in the prevention of pulmonary embolism in patients with proximal deep-vein thrombosis. Prevention du Risque d'Embolie Pulmonaire par Interruption Cave Study Group. N Engl J Med 338:409–415, 1998.

98. Eight-year follow-up of patients with permanent vena cava filters in the prevention of pulmonary embolism: The PREPIC (Prevention du Risque d'Embolie Pulmonaire par Interruption Cave) randomized study. Circulation 112:416–422, 2005.

99. White RH, Zhou H, Kim J, Romano PS: A population-based study of the effectiveness of inferior vena cava filter use among patients with venous thromboembolism. Arch Intern Med 160:2033–2041, 2000.

100. Wood KE: Major pulmonary embolism: Review of a pathophysiologic approach to the golden hour of hemodynamically significant pulmonary embolism. Chest 121:877–905, 2002.

101. Piazza G, Goldhaber SZ: The acutely decompensated right ventricle: Pathways for diagnosis and management. Chest 128:1836–1852, 2005.

102. Kucher N, Goldhaber SZ: Management of massive pulmonary embolism. Circulation 112:e28–e32, 2005.

103. Hoeper MM, Mayer E, Simonneau G, Rubin LJ: Chronic thromboembolic pulmonary hypertension. Circulation 113:2011–2020, 2006.

104. Pengo V, Lensing AW, Prins MH, et al: Incidence of chronic thromboembolic pulmonary hypertension after pulmonary embolism. N Engl J Med 350:2257–2264, 2004.

105. Jamieson SW, Kapelanski DP, Sakakibara N, et al: Pulmonary endarterectomy: Experience and lessons learned in 1,500 cases. Ann Thorac Surg 76:1457–1462, 2003;discussion 1462–1464..

106. Feinstein JA, Goldhaber SZ, Lock JE, et al: Balloon pulmonary angioplasty for treatment of chronic thromboembolic pulmonary hypertension. Circulation 103:10–13, 2001.

107. Linkins LA, Choi PT, Douketis JD: Clinical impact of bleeding in patients taking oral anticoagulant therapy for venous thromboembolism: A meta-analysis. Ann Intern Med 139:893–900, 2003.

108. Witt DM, Sadler MA, Shanahan RL, et al: Effect of a centralized clinical pharmacy anticoagulation service on the outcomes of anticoagulation therapy. Chest 127:1515–1522, 2005.

109. Heneghan C, Alonso-Coello P, Garcia-Alamino JM, et al: Self-monitoring of oral anticoagulation: A systematic review and meta-analysis. Lancet 367:404–411, 2006.

110. Eichinger S, Weltermann A, Minar E, et al: Symptomatic pulmonary embolism and the risk of recurrent venous thromboembolism. Arch Intern Med 164:92–96, 2004.

111. Kyrle PA, Minar E, Bialonczyk C, et al: The risk of recurrent venous thromboembolism in men and women. N Engl J Med 350: 2558–2563, 2004.

112. Baglin T, Luddington R, Brown K, Baglin C: High risk of recurrent venous thromboembolism in men. J Thromb Haemost 2:2152–2155, 2004.

113. Christiansen SC, Cannegieter SC, Koster T, et al: Thrombophilia, clinical factors, and recurrent venous thrombotic events. JAMA 293:2352–2361, 2005.

114. Miles JS, Miletich JP, Goldhaber SZ, et al: G20210A mutation in the prothrombin gene and the risk of recurrent venous thromboembolism. J Am Coll Cardiol 37:215–218, 2001.

115. Eichinger S, Stumpflen A, Hirschl M, et al: Hyperhomocysteinemia is a risk factor of recurrent venous thromboembolism. Thromb Haemost 80:566–569, 1998.

116. Crowther MA, Ginsberg JS, Julian J, et al: A comparison of two intensities of warfarin for the prevention of recurrent thrombosis in patients with the antiphospholipid antibody syndrome. N Engl J Med 349:1133–1138, 2003.

117. Simioni P, Prandoni P, Lensing AW, et al: The risk of recurrent venous thromboembolism in patients with an Arg506→Gln mutation in the gene for factor V (factor V Leiden). N Engl J Med 336:399–403, 1997.

118. Eichinger S, Weltermann A, Mannhalter C, et al: The risk of recurrent venous thromboembolism in heterozygous carriers of factor V Leiden and a first spontaneous venous thromboembolism. Arch Intern Med 162:2357–2360, 2002.

119. Schulman S, Rhedin AS, Lindmarker P, et al: A comparison of six weeks with six months of oral anticoagulant therapy after a first episode of venous thromboembolism. Duration of Anticoagulation Trial Study Group. N Engl J Med 332:1661–1665, 1995.

120. Schulman S, Granqvist S, Holmstrom M, et al: The duration of oral anticoagulant therapy after a second episode of venous thromboembolism. The Duration of Anticoagulation Trial Study Group. N Engl J Med 336:393–398, 1997.

121. Ost D, Tepper J, Mihara H, et al: Duration of anticoagulation following venous thromboembolism: A meta-analysis. JAMA 294:706–715, 2005.

122. Kearon C, Ginsberg JS, Kovacs MJ, et al: Comparison of low-intensity warfarin therapy with conventional-intensity warfarin therapy for long-term prevention of recurrent venous thromboembolism. N Engl J Med 349:631–639, 2003.

123. Ridker PM, Goldhaber SZ, Danielson E, et al: Long-term, low-intensity warfarin therapy for the prevention of recurrent venous thromboembolism. N Engl J Med 348:1425–1434, 2003.

124. Schulman S, Wahlander K, Lundstrom T, et al: Secondary prevention of venous thromboembolism with the oral direct thrombin inhibitor ximelagatran. N Engl J Med 349:1713–1721, 2003.

125. Prandoni P, Lensing AW, Prins MH, et al: Residual venous thrombosis as a predictive factor of recurrent venous thromboembolism. Ann Intern Med 137:955–960, 2002.

126. Palareti G, Legnani C, Cosmi B, et al: Predictive value of D-dimer test for recurrent venous thromboembolism after anticoagulation withdrawal in subjects with a previous idiopathic event and in carriers of congenital thrombophilia. Circulation 108:313–318, 2003.

127. Eichinger S, Minar E, Bialonczyk C, et al: D-dimer levels and risk of recurrent venous thromboembolism. JAMA 290:1071–1074, 2003.

Chapter 16

Venous Thromboses at Unusual Sites

Marc Zumberg, MD • Craig S. Kitchens, MD

Deep venous thrombosis (DVT) and its associated condition, pulmonary embolism (PE), represent the most commonly encountered examples of venous thromboembolism (VTE). DVT and PE were discussed thoroughly in Chapter 15. VTE that occurs at unusual locations, for example, in the intracerebral or intra-abdominal venous circulation, is being diagnosed with increasing frequency. In this chapter, we discuss VTEs at unusual sites. These events are associated with acquired and congenital hypercoagulable disorders and, although less frequently encountered than DVT, they account for a disproportionate amount of morbidity and mortality. Modern radiographic imaging and improved clinical understanding have resulted in more timely diagnosis and institution of effective treatment. In fact, owing to the sensitivity of modern radiographic imaging, these VTEs may be detected in asymptomatic individuals as incidental findings on studies done for other purposes, thus leading to difficult management decisions. Whereas in the past these unusual VTEs were autopsy suite curiosities, we now have the opportunity to deal with them in life, thus minimizing morbidity and mortality.

HISTORICAL ASPECTS

Many founders of what we now call internal medicine complemented their vast clinical practice through precise observations made at the autopsy table. Both William Osler[1] and Austin Flint,[2] in their textbooks written a century ago, discussed unusual sites of VTE. They both recognized that these conditions were characterized by vague and often subacute symptoms, and that diagnosis was only rarely made in life and was more often noted at autopsy. These observations pertained to thromboses of the hepatic veins, cerebral veins and sinuses, portal vein, and renal veins. Although Virchow[3] speculated 30 years before the Osler and Flint textbooks were written that abnormalities would be found in blood, in addition to inflammation and impaired circulation (thus creating Virchow's triad), neither Osler nor Flint referenced his theory. Rather, they resorted to pathophysiologic theories that we now regard as somewhat unusual. For instance, the known association of cerebral venous and sinus thrombosis with the puerperium was explained by propagation of clots from pelvic veins up through venous complexes along the spinal column and into the brain. They also speculated that renal vein thrombosis was caused by DVTs of the legs that embolized to a renal vein. Those pathogenic mechanisms are no longer embraced. We now hold that these clots are formed in situ, yet they may also coexist with VTE at other locations—an association that early investigators did not appreciate. These great observational

clinicians believed that most of these events were idiopathic, although an association was made with marantic conditions and chronic infections.

Progress in our knowledge of this area of medicine has been exciting and intellectually satisfying as we have witnessed the replacement of theory, dogma, and the unknown by scientific discovery. Idiopathic causes are dwindling and have been replaced by more specific diagnoses (Table 16-1).[4] The tempo of knowledge acquisition has been rapid if one recalls that antithrombin III (ATIII) deficiency, the first thrombophilic disease discovered (which vindicated Virchow), was described in 1965, followed by protein C deficiency in 1981 and protein S deficiency in 1984. The factor V Leiden mutation and the prothrombin 20210 mutation were described in 1994 and 1996, respectively. Other acquired hematologic conditions such as the antiphospholipid antibody syndrome (APLS), paroxysmal nocturnal hemoglobinuria (PNH), and heparin-induced thrombocytopenia (HIT) have also been associated with thrombosis at unusual sites.[5–8] Undiscovered disorders will no doubt be found in ensuing years. Not only has the idiopathic category been eroded, but pathogenic mechanisms have given way to more reasonable concepts. Most thrombotic events are still best explained by a "double hit," in which an underlying hypercoagulable condition exists, yet an additional provocation such as pregnancy, surgery, infection, travel, or some other condition tips the hemostatic scales in favor of thrombosis. Contributing provocations may be revealed in approximately 50% of cases of thrombosis through a thorough history, with the remaining one half of cases remaining seemingly spontaneous and idiopthic.[9]

The role of diagnostic imaging in the 21st century is nowhere better exemplified than in the use of modern radiology to elucidate thromboses at unusual sites. Computed tomography (CT) is limited in some aspects, particularly in detecting cerebral vein and sinus thromboses, but it is excellent for imaging visceral thromboses. Ultrasonography with Doppler flow has also been extremely useful in the diagnosis of visceral thromboses. In many cases, magnetic resonance imaging/angiography (MRI/MRA) is the most sensitive and specific tool used by clinicians to diagnose thromboses at unusual sites.[10,11]

IMPORTANCE TO THE PATIENT AND THE CLINICIAN

DVT and PE remain the *sine qua non* of hypercoagulability. With the use of ATIII deficiency as the prototypic hypercoagulable disease, data are available to show that 25% of all

Table 16-1   Inherited and Acquired Hypercoagulable Conditions Associated with Thromboses at Unusual Sites

Congenital
Antithrombin III deficiency
Protein C deficiency
Protein S deficiency
Factor V Leiden mutation/activated protein C resistance
Prothrombin 20210 gene mutation
Hyperhomocysteinemia

Acquired
Cancer
Myeloproliferative disease
   Polycythemia vera rubra
   Essential thrombocytosis
Antiphospholipid antibody syndrome
Heparin-induced thrombocytopenia
Paroxysmal nocturnal hemoglobinuria (PNH)

Table 16-3   Facts Regarding Patients with Thromboses at Unusual Sites

- Thrombophilia will account for 75% of these unusual and rare conditions.
- Twenty-five percent of thrombophilic patients will experience at least one of these conditions in their lifetime.
- These conditions cause considerable degrees of morbidity and mortality if not diagnosed and treated aggressively.
- Familiarity with hypercoagulable patients allows the hematologist to maintain a high index of suspicion for these rare conditions.
- Anticoagulation or antifibrinolytic therapy is the mainstay of treatment in most thrombophilic conditions.

patients with ATIII deficiency will at some time manifest their thrombophilia as thrombosis at an unusual site (Table 16-2).[12–15] Thromboses may occur as the initial presentation of thrombophilia, may coexist with DVT/PE, or may arise later in the course, once the diagnosis of hypercoagulability has been established in patients or their kindred. A clue to the correct diagnosis of a thrombosis at an unusual site often is found in a past personal or family history of thromboembolism. Data presented by DeStefano and associates[9] substantiate the role of a heightened index of suspicion in the thrombophilic patient when the differential diagnosis of vague subacute symptoms is considered. Whereas such symptoms may signify uncertain meaning in patients without hypercoagulability, these same symptoms in a thrombophilic patient may very well prompt a diagnosis of cerebral or visceral thrombosis.

One could charge that the hematology community has been somewhat passive in the diagnosis, management, and follow-up of these patients, instead yielding to organ-specific physicians such as the hepatologist to treat a patient with hepatic vein thrombosis, the nephrologist for the patient with renal thrombosis, and the neurologist for the patient with cerebral vein thrombosis. It is obvious

that the pathophysiologic link among these three examples is hypercoagulability, and that the affected organ is primarily an "innocent bystander." A single organ that manifests a thrombosis in no way protects other organs or sites from thrombosis in patients with hypercoagulability. By virtue of their experience with a cohort of hypercoagulable patients, hematologists are in a unique position to make a prompt and preemptive diagnosis, guide initial treatment, and make long-term management decisions (Table 16-3).

INTRA-ABDOMINAL THROMBOSIS

The hepatic, portal, and mesenteric venous systems are sites of unusual thrombosis that can manifest with dramatic clinical and radiologic findings. Recognition of the anatomy of this region is imperative for the consultant hematologist who wishes to make effective treatment recommendations.

Mesenteric Venous Thrombosis

Overview

Mesenteric venous thrombosis (Table 16-4) is distinct and is much less common than mesenteric arterial thrombosis.[16] Although rare, it ranks as the third most common site of venous thrombosis behind the lungs and the limbs.[17] Mesenteric arterial thrombosis is usually seen in older, hypertensive, and often diabetic patients who present with an acute abdominal catastrophic event that rapidly leads to ischemia and death of the abdominal organs supplied

Table 16-2   Thromboses at Unusual Sites and the Role of Hypercoagulability

Established
Cerebral venous thrombosis
Mesenteric vein thrombosis
Hepatic venous thrombosis
Purpura fulminans
Splenic vein thrombosis
Portal vein thrombosis
Renal vein thrombosis
Axillary vein thrombosis
Placental infarction
Adrenal hemorrhage

Probable
Retinal vein thrombosis
Pituitary hemorrhage
Pelvic vein thrombosis

Table 16-4   Mesenteric Venous Thrombosis: Clinical Vignettes

Vague abdominal pain is insidious in onset.
Pain is out of proportion to physical findings.
Kidney, ureter, and bladder (KUB) findings are nondiagnostic.
Computed tomographic scanning with contrast or magnetic resonance imaging with gadolinium is necessary for proper diagnosis.
Frank gastrointestinal bleeding is rare.
If left untreated, it will evolve into a surgical abdomen.
Primary preinfarctive treatment consists of anticoagulant or thrombolytic therapy.

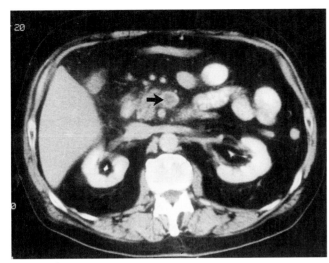

Figure 16-1 Mesenteric vein thrombosis. This computed tomographic scan with contrast shows an engorged superior mesenteric vein (*arrow*) that is distended with clot and outlined by a thin rim of dye.

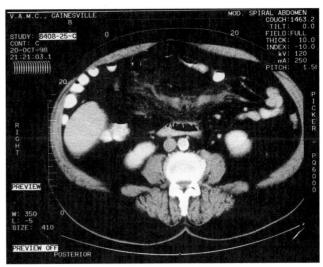

Figure 16-2 "Misty mesentery." This computed tomographic scan with contrast shows the mesentery as strands in a weblike configuration caused by edema and inflammation. This situation may have several causes, but in this case, mesenteric vein thrombosis is most likely due to leakage of bacteria and bacterial products from the compromised ischemic small bowel. After successful treatment was provided, follow-up images were normal.

by the superior mesenteric artery. A detailed description of mesenteric artery thrombosis is outside the scope of this chapter but is provided in other sources.[18] As compared with mesenteric artery occlusion, thrombosis of the superior and inferior mesenteric veins is less common and less precipitous; it is often subacute in nature. Superior mesenteric vein thrombosis has historically been difficult to diagnose because less sophisticated radiographic images, such as flat plates and upright views of the abdomen, as well as various barium studies, are nonspecific and often do not lead to the diagnosis. Diagnosis of mesenteric vein thrombosis is now more readily made, even if accidentally, by CT with vascular contrast. The thrombosed superior mesenteric vein is seen as a large, distended vessel that does not fill appropriately with contrast (Fig. 16-1). The bowel wall may be thick and edematous. We have observed several cases of a "misty mesentery"[19] on abdominal CT, caused by inflammation and edema from mesenteric vein thrombosis (Fig. 16-2). This finding totally resolves with successful treatment of the thrombosis.

Two adjacent articles in *Annals of Surgery* in 1895 provided seminal insight into mesenteric vein thrombosis. Delatour[20] described a fatal case of mesenteric infarction that occurred after an enlarged spleen had been electively removed to treat a patient with what was most likely a myeloproliferative disorder. He opined that the hematologic condition "so changed her blood that coagulation was easily induced." Elliot[21] was able to remove infarcted bowel in a living patient yet noted that the patient concomitantly had bilateral femoral vein and portal vein thrombosis, thus suggesting an underlying hypercoagulable condition.

Causes

Causes of mesenteric vein thrombosis are multiple. One must cautiously read older reviews of mesenteric vein thrombosis that garnered patients before the modern era of hypercoagulability because, by definition, causes could not include the thrombophilic diseases that had yet to be described. In one study, mesenteric vein thrombosis accounted for 0.01% of all surgical admissions and surgical autopsies,[22] and in another study, 0.06% of all surgical admissions.[23] Clearly, this is a rare disease. On the other hand, in a cross-sectional study, mesenteric vein thrombosis was found to have occurred in 3% of patients who were known to have a deficiency of ATIII, protein C, or protein S[9]; in another cross-sectional study, mesenteric vein thrombosis was found in 10% of patients with ATIII deficiency, in 6% of those with protein C deficiency, and in 4% of patients with protein S deficiency. One can estimate that the incidence of mesenteric vein thrombosis is increased at least 100-fold in patients who have an identified deficiency of one of these anticoagulant proteins. Pabinger and Schneider reported that 80% of patients who had thrombophilia and mesenteric vein thrombosis had a prior history of a previous DVT or PE.[15] Recent studies of patients with mesenteric vein thrombosis have discovered prothombotic disorders in 45% to 82% of cases.[17,24,25] In these studies, factor V Leiden was found in 18% to 25% of cases, and the prothrombin 20210 mutation in 25% to 45% of cases.[17,24] Combined defects were seen in more than one third of cases.[17,24] Recently, the *JAK*2 mutation has been detected in 17% of patients with splanchnic venous thrombosis; most had no evidence of myeloproliferation at the time of the thrombosis.[25a]

Whereas mesenteric vein thrombosis may appear to occur spontaneously in patients with thrombophilia, an additional provocation may be detected in about one half of cases. This fact more likely than not accounts for older reviews that include such "causes" of mesenteric vein thrombosis as cirrhosis, heart failure, intra-abdominal malignancy, peritonitis, intra-abdominal abscess, abdominal trauma, and abdominal surgery.[26] Although these provocations may well induce thrombosis in hypercoagulable patients, they prove to be the sole cause in only a minority of cases.[27] Synergy between an underlying hypercoagulable disorder and a provocation is frequent. For example, we have seen several patients with APLS whose long-term oral anticoagulant therapy had unwisely been held in preparation for colonoscopy with polypectomy; they developed abdominal pain several days later and were subsequently given a diagnosis of mesenteric vein thrombosis. The unopposed hypercoagulable disorder coupled with inflammation and bacterial showering from the biopsy site may have provoked thrombosis in these high-risk patients.

Signs and Symptoms

Symptoms of mesenteric vein thrombosis are vague and nonspecific.[4,28] Abdominal pain is usually of insidious onset. The patient cannot find a position or maneuver that makes the pain disappear. In contrast to most abdominal catastrophes, bowel movements continue, and frequently, the patient continues to eat. Nausea is seen in less than one half of cases. Typically, the pain continues for days to weeks, and several evaluations may yield no diagnosis. When transmural ischemia occurs, gastrointestinal bleeding, perforation, and peritonitis may ensue. Hematochezia, hemetemesis, or melena occurs in only 15% of patients, although occult blood may be detected in one half of cases.[27] When intra-abdominal disease is the main underlying cause, thrombosis usually occurs in proximal large vessels and then extends distally; however, the reverse is often true when underlying thombophilia is the main cause.[27]

Abdominal pain appears to be far worse than one can account for on the basis of physical examination findings. Rebound tenderness is not present unless the bowel is infarcted. Laboratory data show hemoconcentration and white cell count usually in the 15,000 to 30,000/μL range. Routine abdominal radiographs are nearly always normal. The natural history of the process is such that if a diagnosis is not made after 10 to 20 days, the intestines undergo ischemic infarction. At that time, the symptoms evolve into those of a classic surgical abdomen, with rebound tenderness, rigidity, and increased morbidity and mortality due to venous infarction of the intestine.

Diagnosis

Diagnosis is best made by helical CT scan or CT angiography, which confirms the diagnosis in 90% of cases.[11,27] Doppler ultrasonography is also accurate but is operator dependent and may be limited by bowel gas.[11] MRI with gadolinium and MRA are also highly accurate but may be less readily available.[25] Helical CT has remained our diagnostic test of choice.

If the patient undergoes surgery before the correct diagnosis has been made, the surgeon usually finds a dusky but not frankly gangrenous intestinal wall (unless through-and-through infarction has taken place) and bounding mesenteric arterial pulses. When ischemia or infarction is present, viability is not as clearly demarcated as in cases of acute arterial infarction. Second-look laparotomy has been advocated as an approach that is useful for minimizing the amount of resected bowel during the initial operation.[29,30] When the bowel wall is transected, tiny wormlike clots extrude from engorged veins at the edge of the resected bowel in a peculiar but pathognomonic way. Histologic examination shows extensive hyperemia and hemorrhage, and the degree of infarction is determined by the duration of ischemia.

Treatment

Surgery is to be avoided as the primary diagnostic method unless an acute surgical abdomen and obvious bowel infarction are detected. A thickened or edematous bowel wall on imaging itself does not imply infarction. Surgical exploration has been replaced by radiologic exploration. Once the thrombotic cause of the disorder has been discovered, it should be approached vigorously with aggressive anticoagulant therapy, even in the face of hemodynamically stable active gastrointestinal bleeding. Thrombolytic therapy has also been used with success.[31] We have employed systemic thrombolysis with excellent results without excessive hemorrhage. Some clinicians have advocated catheter-directed thrombolytic therapy, but this is not a universally accepted approach.[25,32] Early surgical series that were reported before anticoagulant therapy or modern radiologic imaging became available described a mortality rate of about 65%, which was an improvement over the initial natural history of the disease treated with only supportive care, for which mortality was estimated to be 95%. If the diagnosis is made at surgery and is followed promptly by anticoagulant therapy, observed mortality drops to approximately 35%. If the diagnosis is made radiographically and patients are treated promptly with anticoagulants with no surgical intervention, mortality averages about 10%.[4]

Because the pathogenesis of this abdominal catastrophe is thrombosis, it is appropriate that therapy should be directed toward minimizing thrombotic potential. Such an approach is appropriate and additionally targets, even if inadvertently, thromboses at other sites that the patient may harbor and of which the practitioner may be unaware. Modern reviews advocate early diagnosis and prompt aggressive anticoagulant or thrombolytic therapy.[25–27] Mesenteric vein thrombosis has a high rate of recurrence, which usually occurs within 30 days of presentation and typically at the anastomotic site in patients who have undergone surgery, further supporting the need for early and adequate anticoagulation.[27]

Because of the seriousness of this event and the fact that most patients have already sustained a previous DVT or PE, unless a definitive precipitant event (e.g., use of oral contraceptives) is found and reversed, we favor indefinite anticoagulant therapy with warfarin, even in the face of esophageal varices, to maintain an international normalized ratio (INR) in the range of 2.0 to 3.0.[27a]

Splenic Vein Thrombosis

Overview

Splenic vein thrombosis (Table 16-5) is often subtle and is rarely recognized at the time of initial thrombosis. However, vague acute abdominal pain and new-onset splenomegaly may lead to imaging studies that show acute splenic vein

---

Table 16-5   Splenic Vein Thrombosis: Clinical Vignettes

Vague abdominal pain, new-onset splenomegaly, or variceal bleeding may be noted.

Significant cytopenias are rare.

Liver function test results remain normal, and hepatomegaly is not typically seen.

The condition is often associated with intra-abdominal disease or surgery.

Splenectomy is recommended for recurrent variceal bleeding.

thrombosis. More often, splenic vein thrombosis is discovered during the evaluation of a patient with vague chronic abdominal pain or chronic splenomegaly or thrombocytopenia, or it may be detected serendipitously during the evaluation of pancreatitis or pancreatic carcinoma. Splenic vein thrombosis may complicate sclerotherapy for esophageal varices.[33]

Causes

Splenic vein thrombosis has been described in all types of hypercoagulable disorders, whether congenital or acquired. In this disorder, however, local intra-abdominal events, whether or not they are accompanied by hypercoagulable disorders, directly lead to a significant percentage of splenic vein thromboses. The chief offenders are pancreatitis and pancreatic carcinoma because of the intimate contact of the splenic vein with the pancreas. Pancreatitis is found to be the initiating event that leads to discovery of isolated splenic vein thrombosis in up to 65% of cases.[34] Splenic vein thrombosis has also been described in abdominal trauma and after abdominal surgery. It complicates 11% of all splenectomies but occurs at a much higher rate among patients who have had their spleens removed for hematologic indications.[35] Thus, the condition that warrants splenectomy (such as a myeloproliferative disorder) probably is more "hypercoagulable" than the operation per se. Splenic vein thrombosis has been related historically to splenectomy for immune thrombocytopenic purpura (ITP). That connection now is most likely due to the association of ITP with APLS, which explains both the ITP and the splenic vein thrombosis.[36]

Signs and Symptoms

A common presentation for chronic splenic vein thrombosis is variceal bleeding, especially from the stomach and lower esophagus. Varices develop in 17% to 55% of patients with isolated splenic vein thrombosis.[34] When varices occur in the setting of normal serum liver function test results and no hepatomegaly but isolated splenomegaly, the diagnosis of splenic vein thrombosis should be strongly considered.[37] This syndrome has been referred to as "left-sided portal hypertension." Up to 71% of patients with splenic vein thrombosis develop splenomegaly, although few develop significant cytopenias.[34,38] Because removal of the spleen relieves venous collateral outflow, splenectomy cures the portal hypertensive gastropathy, and esophageal hemorrhage usually ceases at this time as well.[34,37,39] Splenectomy remains a treatment choice when variceal bleeding is frequent, but it is controversial as a means of prophylaxis in the face of nonbleeding varices.[34]

Diagnosis

The signs and symptoms of splenic vein thrombosis are nonspecific. The diagnosis is most commonly made through ultrasonography, CT, or MRI.[35]

Treatment

Should the diagnosis of acute splenic vein thrombosis be made, anticoagulation is indicated not only to stop the process but also to limit potential propagation of thrombosis into the mesenteric and portal veins.[35] Long-term anticoagulant therapy is indicated, particularly if the patient has an

Table 16-6 Portal Vein Thrombosis: Clinical Vignettes
Painless splenomegaly with ascites is a common presentation.
Normal hepatic function is noted in extrahepatic thrombosis.
Thrombosis related to hepatic cirrhosis usually results in abnormal test findings.
Anticoagulation is recommended if underlying thrombophilia is suspected.
Anticoagulation is controversial if cirrhosis is the underlying cause.

underlying hypercoagulable condition. Most practitioners would maintain an INR at 2.0 to 3.0 with continued use of warfarin. Continued follow-up by the hematologist is also appropriate because a significant number of patients with idiopathic splenic vein thrombosis who do not currently have manifestations of a myeloproliferative disorder do develop them over time.[40]

Portal Vein Thrombosis

Overview

Similar to splenic vein thrombosis, portal vein thrombosis (Table 16-6) usually is not recognized in its acute phase. It is characterized by relatively painless increasing splenomegaly and ascites without concomitant worsening of hepatic function. Portal vein thrombosis appears to have been described first by Belfour and Stewart in 1869.[41] Portal vein thrombosis has been described in the recent literature in association with most of the acquired or congenital hypercoagulable disorders.[42] However, it also continues to be seen in patients with common variety portal hypertension, especially when due to hepatic cirrhosis. A recent review by Amitrano and colleagues[43] revealed an 11% incidence of portal vein thrombosis in 701 cirrhotic patients examined on Doppler ultrasound.

Causes/Signs and Symptoms

Almost one half of patients in whom portal vein thrombosis was detected remained asymptomatic.[43] It remains to be seen whether these two risk factors, namely, hypercoagulability and portal hypertension, are synergistic in the genesis of portal vein thrombosis.[44] Because proteins C and S and ATIII levels are low in patients with liver disease, it is likely that deficiencies in these clotting factors, especially if all are depressed, represent a secondary phenomenon.[45,46] A congenital or acquired thrombophilic condition was detected in 37% of patients with portal vein thrombosis in a recent case-controlled multicenter trial.[47] In other series, approximately 70% of patients with portal vein thrombosis were noted to have thrombophilic mutations.[43–45] In a recent study of cirrhotic patients, 13% and 35% of patients with portal vein thrombosis harbored the factor V Leiden or prothrombin 20210 gene mutation, respectively, compared with 8% and 2.5% of cirrhotic patients without portal vein thrombosis (PVT).[44] On the contrary, in a recent review by Pinto and coworkers,[48] hereditary thrombophilia did not seem to play a significant role in children and adolescents with PVT. However, in an Egyptian study, El-Karaksy[49] identified hereditary thrombophilia in 62% of 40 children investigated at a single center. Factor V Leiden (30%),

16

protein C deficiency (28%), and the prothrombin 20210 gene mutation (15%) were the most common conditions diagnosed. Other clinicians argue that even in cirrhotic patients, thrombophilia likely plays a contributing role and should be investigated.[45]

Other causes of portal vein thrombosis include intra-abdominal neoplasia, especially carcinoma of the pancreas; infection, with particular reference to spontaneous bacterial peritonitis; and abdominal trauma, including surgery. Additionally, sclerotherapy for esophageal varices has been implicated in several cases. Portal vein thrombosis may complicate neonatal umbilical vein catheterization but is not further discussed here. Hypercoagulability should be considered strongly in patients who have no history of hepatic disease, intra-abdominal infection, or an inflammatory or neoplastic process. As with splenic vein thromboses, the myeloproliferative disorders (acquired causes of hypercoagulability) are notoriously common, particularly when patients are followed long enough to manifest a previously occult myeloproliferative disorder.[50] When splenectomy is performed in patients with myeloproliferative disorders, the incidence of portal vein and mesenteric vein thromboses is approximately 30% for patients not given prophylactic anticoagulation.[51,52] Accordingly, when splenectomy is performed in patients with a known hypercoagulable or myeloproliferative disease, antithrombotic prophylaxis is strongly indicated.

Diagnosis

The diagnosis of portal vein thrombosis is usually made through noninvasive radiologic methods.[50] With color Doppler techniques, the direction of portal vein blood flow can be determined reliably. Contrast CT and MRI/MRA are equally powerful but somewhat more expensive (Fig. 16-3).

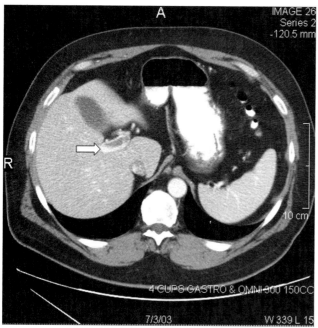

Figure 16-3 Portal vein thrombosis. This computed tomographic scan with contrast shows a distended portal vein that is partially occluded; the thrombus (arrow) is outlined by a rim of contrast material.

Treatment

Management of portal vein thrombosis depends on the manifestations of the process. If the process produces acute variceal hemorrhage, attention should be paid to that disorder. Discussion of the treatment of patients with variceal esophageal hemorrhage is not within the scope of this chapter; however, patients with pure portal vein thrombosis who do not have liver disease (so-called extrahepatic thrombosis) generally survive acute upper gastrointestinal hemorrhage far better than those who have liver disease. If portal vein thrombosis is believed to be secondary to an intra-abdominal process such as infection, neoplasia, or other inflammation, therapy should be directed toward those problems. Chronic portal hypertension due to chronic portal vein thrombosis is occasionally treated surgically through various decompressive mechanisms, but long-term anticoagulant therapy is increasingly considered.[27a,45,50]

The role of anticoagulant therapy has been somewhat controversial, but as more patients have presented and more proof has accrued that this disorder is frequently a manifestation of hypercoagulability, anticoagulant therapy has become more attractive.[45,53,54] This therapeutic option is particularly appealing for those patients who do not have prior portal hypertension on the basis of intrinsic liver disease but who have experienced spontaneous thrombosis due to a hypercoagulable disorder. In these conditions, it is rational to initiate acute anticoagulant therapy so as not only to reverse the thrombotic process but to minimize further progression of the thrombosis into the splenic or mesenteric veins.[45,54] In fact, in a small study by Sheen and associates,[55] resolution of thrombosis was noted in 5 of 9 patients who were treated with heparin followed by oral anticoagulant therapy.[55] Anticoagulant therapy is also strongly indicated in patients who have undergone a shunt procedure for decompression of chronic portal hypertension due to chronic portal vein thrombosis. In this situation, the patient's well-being is dependent on the shunt remaining patent; therefore, anticoagulant therapy, particularly for an identified underlying hypercoagulable disorder, is the treatment of choice. Concern about increased bleeding in patients with esophageal varices treated with concomitant anticoagulant therapy is always raised but may be more theoretical than based on actual experience; ironically, because anticoagulant therapy addresses the underlying pathophysiology, bleeding over time seems better controlled.[27a,45,54] In fact, recent reviews have suggested that anticoagulant therapy in the treatment of patients with portal vein thrombosis increased neither the risk nor the severity of gastrointestinal bleeding, and no deaths occurred on anticoagulant therapy.[45] We treat those patients with esophageal varices from portal hypertension due solely to hypercoagulable disorders with long-term warfarin therapy, while maintaining an INR of 2.0 to 3.0. Patients treated with long-term oral anticoagulant therapy have been described who have recanalized their portal veins, thereby reversing portal hypertension.[50] Thrombolytic therapy has been tried in a small number of cases with encouraging results; use of thrombolytic therapy is most attractive when thrombosis is fairly acute.[56] Data are limited on whether and how treatment should be provided for asymptomatic cirrhotic patients who were incidentally found to have portal vein thrombosis on imaging done

Table 16-7   Renal Vein Thrombosis: Clinical Vignettes

The classic triad of acute flank pain, hematuria, and sudden deterioration of renal function is seen in only a minority of cases.

Worsening renal insufficiency with peripheral edema is an increasingly common presentation.

Nephrotic syndrome, especially when due to glomerulonephritis, is a major risk factor.

Anticoagulant and thrombolytic therapies are the treatments of choice.

Often associated with thromboses at other sites.

for unrelated reasons. Patients with grade 2 to 4 portal vein thrombosis who require liver transplantation have a worse prognosis, a greater number of in-hospital complications, and greater mortality than those given transplants without portal vein thrombosis.[57]

Renal Vein Thrombosis

Overview

The association of renal vein thrombosis (Table 16-7) with renal disease, with particular reference to the nephrotic syndrome, has been known since 1840.[58] Previous debate focused on whether renal vein thrombosis caused the nephrotic syndrome or vice versa; it is now appreciated that the nephrotic syndrome is the preexistent problem, and the hypercoagulability of the nephrotic syndrome gives rise to thrombosis not only of renal veins but also of veins throughout the body, and frequently to pulmonary embolism.[59,60] One putative mechanism for this hypercoagulability is that of decreased plasma levels of ATIII resulting from urinary loss of this small plasma protein, paralleling the degree of albuminuria. Others have described a decrease in free protein S explained by urinary loss or by excessive binding to increased levels of C4b-binding protein characteristic of nephrotic syndrome.[61,62] The latter mechanism is especially attractive for APLS, which is increasingly recognized as one of the most common conditions associated with the nephrotic syndrome.[63–65]

Renal vein thrombosis may also occur in neonates during periods of acute dehydration. Whether these sporadic cases of renal vein thrombosis are associated with an underlying hypercoagulable disorder is currently unknown. Recent articles have reported on the association of hereditary thrombophilia with neonatal renal vein thrombosis. Mitchell noted a 50% incidence of prothombotic abnormalities in patients screened, but these usually occurred in association with other known risk factors such as prematurity, central venous catheterization, or a diabetic mother.[66] A separate multicenter case-controlled study showed an odds ratio of 10.9 for thrombophilia in neonates and infants with renal vein thrombosis.[67] A 10-year follow-up study noted a risk for in utero renal vein thrombosis in patients with the factor V Leiden mutation.[68]

The classic syndrome of acute renal vein thrombosis, namely, acute flank pain, hematuria, and sudden deterioration of renal function, is seen in only about 10% to 20% of all adults with renal vein thrombosis. Remaining patients have a more chronic variety that is usually detected by subtle worsening of renal insufficiency, progressive

proteinuria, and edema, usually without pain or hematuria. Nephrotic syndrome in adults appears to be more thrombogenic than in children, and nephrotic syndrome due to membranous nephropathy appears to be more thrombogenic than nephrotic syndrome related to diabetes.[69]

Causes

The chronic form of renal vein thrombosis occurs much more commonly than is appreciated and, accordingly, if one waits for symptoms, the disorder will be underdiagnosed. Cross-sectional studies have shown that as many as 30% to 50% of all patients with chronic nephrotic syndrome have evidence of renal vein thrombosis.[69,70] Renal vein thrombosis has also been noted to be an important cause of graft loss following transplantation, and the potential role of thrombophilia has been explored.[71] Functional renal vein thrombosis with acute worsening of renal function may be seen in patients in whom a suprarenal inferior vena cava (IVC) filter has been deployed, which subsequently fills with clots.

Thrombosis resulting from hypercoagulability with renal vein thrombosis may be self-perpetuating.[72] Concurrent PE is seen in 20% to 30% of patients in whom renal vein thrombosis has been diagnosed. Among these patients with PE, only 5% are symptomatic.[69,73] Renal vein thrombosis is bilateral in half of cases. Clots protrude from the renal vein into the IVC in 40% of cases. Anticoagulant therapy is the hallmark of successful treatment, although increasingly, systemic thrombolytic therapy is advocated; the few available case reports in which the use of thrombolytic therapy is reported describe gratifying results in acute situations.[73,74] Etoh and colleagues[75] have described several patients with the nephrotic syndrome who experienced multiple concomitant thromboses of the renal, portal, and splenic veins. The general systemic nature of such hypercoagulability and the potential involvement of multiple sites warrant systemic rather than catheter-directed therapy. Systemic thrombolytic therapy should be considered, especially in those patients with acute renal failure, bilateral renal vein thrombosis, or concomitant thromboses at other sites.[65]

Diagnosis

The diagnosis is aided by a high index of suspicion in the occasional patient with preexisting acute or chronic renal insufficiency who then develops flank pain, hematuria, and sudden worsening of renal failure or, more commonly, unexplained worsening renal insufficiency, as well as in the azotemic patient who has an increase in proteinuria and peripheral edema. Renal vein thrombosis is also known to occur in patients without renal disease who have other hypercoagulable disorders. Regardless of presentation, the diagnosis is best confirmed by imaging on ultrasonography with Doppler flow or on MRI/MRA after discussion with the radiologist of one's suspicion of renal vein thrombosis (Fig. 16-4).[76]

Treatment

The role of long-term anticoagulation with warfarin is debatable, but such therapy appears to be efficacious in the prevention of recurrent thrombosis of the renal vein or elsewhere. It is not known whether long-term oral anticoagulant therapy will help preserve renal function, given the

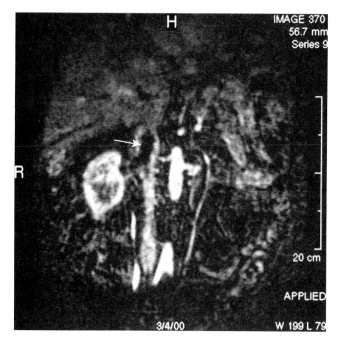

Figure 16-4 Renal vein thrombosis. This magnetic resonance angiography scan shows a large clot in the right renal vein that is extending (*arrow*) as a large mass into the suprarenal inferior vena cava.

natural slow deterioration of renal function in patients with ongoing renal disease. However, rapid return of renal function to the patient's long-term baseline level is expected with successful treatment in the acute syndrome.[73]

Hepatic Venous Thrombosis

Overview

Hepatic venous thrombosis (Table 16-8), previously known as Budd-Chiari syndrome, has been an area of semantic confusion since it was first described.[77] The history of this disorder has been detailed by Wang and Jones.[78] The English internist Budd described a case of thrombotic occlusion of the hepatic veins in 1845, and the Austrian pathologist Chiari reported on autopsies of 10 patients who had intrahepatic venous thrombosis. Osler[79] described a case of obliteration of the IVC by fibrotic stenosis at the orifices of the hepatic veins. It has become increasingly

clear that two entities that initially appeared to be similar are now regarded as two distinct disorders. These two entities differ in locality, tempo, lethality, and other manifestations. It is interesting that most scholars believe that obliterative hepatocavopathy (which is seen in Africa, India, and Asia) is the end result of thrombosis, resulting in formation of webs and intravascular diaphragms or scarring and obliteration of the vessels, as described by Osler. Whether both the Eastern and Western types of this syndrome are due to thrombosis, and, if so, why it would manifest as an acute veno-occlusive disease in the Western world and a chronic fibrosing disease in Africa, India, and Asia, are not known.

Many clinicians advocate use of the term *hepatic venous thrombosis* for the Western disease and the cumbersome term *obliterative hepatocavopathy* for the Eastern type.[80–83] The remainder of this discussion centers around the more acute thrombotic disease, for which we will use the term *hepatic venous thrombosis*, which includes hepatic outflow obstruction at the level of the main hepatic veins to the distal venules. *Veno-occlusive disease* refers to a nonthrombotic obstruction of sinusoids or central hepatic veins due to injury of the sinusoidal wall and seen most commonly as a complication of bone marrow transplantation; this condition is not discussed further here.[77]

Our understanding of hepatic vein thrombosis has been changed by rapid diagnosis, which is possible because of advances in radiographic imaging and in therapeutic options (Figs. 16-5 and 16-6). It is believed that this disease has an excellent prognosis when it is detected early and is limited to only the peripheral smaller hepatic veins. If larger veins are partially occluded, morbidity is about 30%, and in cases with total obstruction of the major hepatic vessels and suprahepatic IVC, mortality is 67%.[84,85] The current overall 10-year survival is estimated at 75%.[5]

Causes

Hepatic venous thrombosis is due principally to hypercoagulable disorders yet is exacerbated frequently by provocations such as pregnancy, use of estrogen-containing birth control pills, and infection. The syndrome is acute and is

---

Table 16-8 Hepatic Venous Thrombosis: Clinical Vignettes

Acute abdominal pain with hepatomegaly, rapid-onset ascites, and grossly elevated transaminases is a common presentation.

It is commonly associated with an underlying hereditary or acquired thrombophilia, such as polycythemia vera, essential thrombocytosis, antiphospholipid antibody syndrome, and paroxysmal nocturnal hemoglobinuria.

Prognosis is much improved through early anticoagulation or thrombolytic therapy, as compared with surgery and transplantation, as provided in historic controls.

Vascular decompression/shunting procedures are treatment options that should be considered if evidence of portal hypertension is found. Timing of these procedures remains controversial.

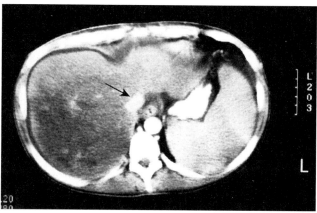

Figure 16-5 Hepatic venous thrombosis. This computed tomographic scan with contrast shows an enlarged, tense liver with a heterogenous perfusion pattern. At this level, the hepatic veins should be clearly outlined by contrast media as they enter the contrast-filled inferior vena cava (*arrow*). They are not visualized because of total thrombosis of the hepatic veins.

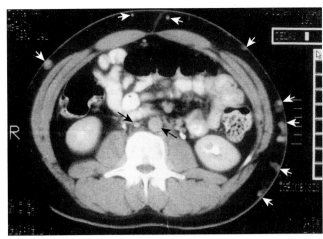

Figure 16-6 Obliteration of the inferior vena cava (IVC) with extensive collateral flow. In this case of chronic hepatic vein thrombosis, the IVC is obliterated. The aorta (*right black arrow*) and the azygos vein (*left black arrow*) are seen. Multiple large subcutaneous collaterals are apparent in the abdominal wall (*white arrows*).

recognized clinically by the triad of acute painful abdomen, sudden enlargement of the liver, and ascites, with these symptoms noted in 82%, 86%, and 100% of cases, respectively.[83] In acute cases of hepatic venous thrombosis, a lag of 1 or 2 days in elevation of standard liver function tests results may initially obscure the diagnosis.[86]

Diagnosis

Diagnosis can also be made through liver biopsy,[87] which may reveal the early phase of the disease when thrombosis is limited to the smaller hepatic veins. Sinusoidal congestion, loss of hepatocytes, centrilobular fibrosis, hepatic outflow obstruction, and venous engorgement are often seen. Lack of visualization of thombosis does not rule out the syndrome, and thrombosis may not always be apparent in biopsy specimens.[5] Constrictive pericarditis and congestive heart failure remain in the differential, and similar findings may be revealed on liver biopsy. The disease may also have a more insidious course, with more extensive microscopic changes observed on liver biopsy (i.e., fibrosis) than might be predicted from the apparently short clinical course.[77]

Before recent descriptions of the factor V Leiden mutation and the prothrombin 20210 mutation, Valla and Benhamou[82] opined that approximately 30% of cases were due to myeloproliferative disorders (notoriously polycythemia vera), and about 10% of all cases were due to PNH alone. Given the rarity of PNH, the penetrance of hepatic venous thrombosis in that rare disease is exceptional.[87a] It has been estimated that hepatic vein thrombosis is observed in 1% of patients with myeloproliferative disorders and 12% of patients with PNH.[5] As Valla and Benhamou[82] have shown, acute hepatic venous thrombosis may be the initial presentation of myeloproliferative disorder, and occasionally, these hematologic disorders may not become clinically apparent until after years of follow-up. The newly described somatic mutation *JAK2* is believed to be rather sensitive and specific in detecting myeloproliferative disorder even years prior to usual laboratory manifestations. Patel and colleagues[87b] report positive assays for *JAK2* in 59% of patients with hepatic venous thrombosis, thus representing the largest single group of disorders associated with hepatic venous thrombosis.

JAK2 should be tested for in patients with hepatic and other splanchnic venous thrombosis.[25a,87c] More recent reviews indicate that APLS is the second most common cause of the disease,[6,88] accounting for approximately 30% of cases, and congenital thrombophilic disorders account for up to another 30% of cases.[42,89] Acquired and congenital thrombophilic conditions and other risk factors can now be detected in at least 75% of patients.[90] In a recent review, factor V Leiden accounted for 25% to 30% of cases, and protein C deficiency 20% of cases; a combined thrombophilic defect was seen in 25% of cases of hepatic vein thrombosis. Fifty-five percent of those afflicted by hepatic vein thrombosis were oral contraceptive users compared with the expected prevalence of 25% in the general female population.[5] Other recent reviews have shown similar results, and the odds ratio for hepatic venous thrombosis has been estimated to be 11 for the factor V Leiden mutation, 7 for protein C deficiency, and 2 for the prothrombin gene mutation.[91,92] Interpretation of low protein C, protein S, and antithrombin III levels must be made with caution in the face of liver disease; therefore, their contribution to hepatic vein thrombosis remains uncertain.

With the advent of modern radiographic imaging, the diagnosis of hepatic vein thrombosis is made increasingly early. Imaging now is very effective; ultrasonography combined with Doppler flow yields the diagnosis very rapidly in 85% of cases. Using the combination of ultrasonography, MRI/MRA, and occasional angiography, Valla and Benhamou[82] confirmed the diagnosis rapidly in more than 90% of cases. The initial goal in the management of hepatic vein occlusion is to relieve hepatic outflow obstruction.[93] The natural history of this disease has therefore improved since the introduction of anticoagulation, although no randomized trials exist.[5] Many experts favor early initiation of heparin,[5,77,82,83,94] and others advocate an early, aggressive role of thrombolytic therapy, whether it is given systematically or by local infusion.[78,95,95a] If short segment thrombosis is noted or ascites cannot be controlled, some reports favor angioplasty and wall stenting.[77] Patency rates of 80% to 90% have been noted with this approach.[5] The success of the early use of thrombolytic therapy coupled with anticoagulants has resulted in the use of orthotopic liver transplantation as the therapy of last resort for those patients who have not benefited from thrombolytic therapy, or for those who present late with fulminant hepatic failure and coma.[83,85,89] Long-term management should include long-term anticoagulant therapy provided to prevent local recurrence of thrombus and systemic manifestations of any underlying hypercoagulable disorder.[78,83,88,96]

Treatment

If symptomatic portal hypertension persists and if vascular decompressive procedures are indicated, various types of decompressive surgery are available; these have been reviewed elsewhere.[78,81] Some argue for earlier surgical decompression.[97] The goal of these shunting procedures is to convert the portal vein into a venous outflow tract of the liver. Transjugular intrahepatic portosystemic shunts (TIPS) are minimally invasive and have been found to be beneficial in controlling ascites in chronic hepatic vein thrombosis, but stenosis requiring revision has been noted in up to 50% of cases in some series.[93,98–100] Other types of surgical portosystemic shunts have been described that have proved to be beneficial in controlling refractory ascites.[5,90,101]

Others argue that surgical decompression should be the initial treatment of choice, and, if thrombophilic conditions are found, anticoagulation should follow the surgical procedure.[97] If patients develop end-stage liver disease or if shunts fail, liver transplantation remains a viable option for many, with 5-year survival reported as high as 95%.[90,100]

CEREBRAL VENOUS THROMBOSIS

Overview

Cerebral venous thrombosis (Table 16-9) refers to thrombosis of the superficial or deep cerebral veins and of the dural venous sinuses. Blood from the brain drains through small cerebral veins into larger veins, which empty into the dural sinuses; these are themselves drained by the internal jugular veins.[102] The main cerebral venous sinuses affected by thrombosis are the superior sagittal sinus (72%) and the lateral sinuses (70%).[10] This condition, similar to most conditions discussed in this chapter, is diagnosed more frequently because of increased knowledge of its existence and increased ease of diagnosis through modern imaging techniques. Cerebral vein thrombosis remains rare, with an estimated annual incidence of 3 to 7 cases per million.[103]

Gates and Barnett have reviewed the history of cerebral venous thrombosis,[104] noting that Ribes first described cerebral venous thrombosis in 1825 in a man with disseminated carcinoma. Three years later, Abercrombie described cerebral venous thrombosis in a woman in her puerperium. In 1873, Parrot described neonatal cerebral venous thrombosis. Gowers in 1888 associated cerebral venous thrombosis with both congestive heart failure and cachexia. In 1904, Nonne first used the term *pseudotumor cerebri*. In an important neurosurgical review in 1966,[105] Krayenbuhl clearly separated infectious from noninfectious causes of cerebral venous thrombosis. He was prescient in stating that neurosurgery had a limited and decreasing role in the treatment of this disease, and that anticoagulant therapy was the treatment of choice. He further correctly pointed out that as opposed to other ischemic brain syndromes, central nervous system dysfunction due to cerebral venous thrombosis has an outstanding recovery rate, often with no permanent sequelae if treated aggressively and appropriately.[106,107]

Table 16-9 Cerebral Venous/Sinus Thrombosis: Clinical Vignettes

Headaches (75%), papilledema (49%), fevers (45%), seizures (37%), and altered mental status (30%) are frequent, yet subacute, presentations.

It is important to differentiate infectious from idiopathic risk factors.

High-estrogen states are significant risk factors.

Hereditary thrombophilias are significant risk factors, especially in combination with high-estrogen states.

Magnetic resonance imaging/venography is the imaging study of choice; computed tomographic scans may be falsely negative.

Anticoagulation is recommended with noninfectious causes.

Most patients have good clinical recovery.

---

*Data from Ameri A, Bousser MG: Cerebral venous thrombosis. Neurol Clin 10:87–111, 1992.

A recent international study of 624 patients with cerebral vein thrombosis revealed that 79% of patients had a full recovery or minimal residual symptoms.[106] In the Venous Thrombosis Portuguese Collaborative Study Group (VENOPORT) study, 82% of patients followed prospectively recovered completely.[107] The prognosis may be worse in the elderly, however.[108]

Causes

In the preantibiotic era, the most common causes of thrombophlebitis in the skull and its contents were chronic suppurative infection due to inner ear infection, skull osteomyelitis, and erysipelas. Infectious causes have been thoroughly reviewed.[109]

The puerperium represents a strong provocation for hypercoagulability and particularly thrombosis at unusual sites; however, this association is nowhere more apparent than in cerebral venous thrombosis. The reason for these repeated observations is unknown. Cerebral venous thrombosis appears to be the only thrombosis at an unusual site that has a strong sex predilection, with a 3:1 ratio favoring women; the difference is explained by the puerperium and/or the use of oral contraceptive agents.[110–113] Although cerebral vein thrombosis is often related to pregnancy, the recurrence rate appears to be low, and subsequent pregnancy is not thought to be contraindicated.[114] Cerebral venous thrombosis has been associated with all known hypercoagulable disorders, both congenital and acquired. A prothrombotic risk factor or direct cause for cerebral vein thrombosis is identified in up to 85% of affected patients.[103] Hereditary thrombophilia can be found in 20% to 30% of these cases.[114,115] Recent series have also documented a relative risk for cerebral venous thrombosis of 6 to 10 among patients having factor V Leiden mutation and a relative risk of 10 to 21 caused by the prothrombin 20210 mutation.[110–112,116,117,117a] Data document that risk factors are not simply additive: A relative risk for cerebral venous thrombosis of 8 to 22 exists in patients who use birth control pills, and a relative risk of 10 has been noted in women who have the prothrombin 20210 mutation; the relative risk factor escalates to 150 among women with the prothrombin 20210 mutation who also use oral contraceptives.[110] A fourfold increase in cerebral vein thrombosis was recently noted in patients with hyperhomocysteinemia in one study, and a sevenfold increase in another.[117,118] A recent pediatric study found at least 1 prothrombotic risk factor in 55% of patients with cerebral vein thrombosis as compared with 21% of controls.[119]

Diagnosis

As dangerous as the disease is, the diagnosis is often delayed because of its nonspecific and nonsensitive subacute presentation and fairly broad differential diagnosis. It is believed that symptoms are caused by increased intracranial pressure due to venous congestion and by local inflammation due to phlebitis.[117] Headaches are experienced in the vast majority of cases. Papilledema occurs in approximately half of cases. When headache and papilledema occur without focal neurologic signs, the term *pseudotumor cerebri* may be used.[120] Although pseudotumor cerebri has several sources of origin besides cerebral venous thrombosis, this condition remains one of its more important causes. Typically, the headache progresses over several days and is followed by confusion, stupor, and finally,

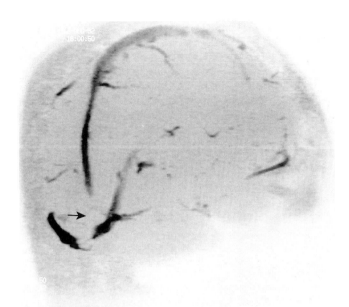

Figure 16-7 Cerebral venous thrombosis. This oblique magnetic resonance image shows a contrast-outlined superior sagittal sinus and both transverse sinuses. A large clot occupies the torcular Herophili, which is not visualized because contrast medium was not used (arrow).

Table 16-10 Outcomes of Cerebral Venous Thrombosis With and Without Heparin Therapy

	Historical Study*		Level 1 Study†	
	Heparin	No Heparin	Heparin	No Heparin
Complete recovery	85%	53%	80%	10%
Some sequelae	15%	20%	20%	60%
Died	0%	27%	0%	30%

*Data from Bousser M-G, Chiras J, Bories J, et al: Cerebral venous thrombosis: A review of 38 cases. Stroke 16:199–210, 1985.
†Data from Einhaupl KM, Villringer A, Meister W: Heparin treatment in sinus venous thrombosis. Lancet 338:597–600, 1991.

Table 16-11 Outcomes of Cerebral Venous Thrombosis With and Without Nadroparin

	Nadroparin	Placebo
Poor Outcome or Barthel Index of Activity of Daily Living Score <13		
3 weeks	20%	24%
12 weeks	13%	21%

Data from DeBruijn STFM, Stam J, for the Cerebral Venous Thrombosis Study Group: Randomized placebo-controlled trial of anticoagulant treatment with low molecular-weight heparin for cerebral sinus thrombosis. Stroke 30:484–488, 1999.

coma, if the process is not interrupted. Seizures occur much more commonly than in arterial stroke.[114] A recent review has suggested that patients older than 65 years of age may present differently with fewer symptoms, suggestive of isolated intracranial hypertension, but with an increased frequency of depressed levels of consciousness and mental status changes.[108] Conspicuously absent are sensory loss and motor weakness. Examination of the cerebrospinal fluid and electroencephalogram shows nonspecific findings that do not support other entries within the differential diagnosis. CT has usually been performed by this time in the evaluation but is notoriously nonspecific, if not even misleading. The classic "empty delta sign" is seen in only 21% of cases.[10,102,114] A normal CT scan is found in 25% to 30% of cases and should never be used to exclude this important diagnosis.[114] The diagnosis is best established by MRI/MRV (Fig. 16-7),[103,121–123] which has essentially replaced standard four-vessel angiography and is sensitive for diagnosing the subtype known as deep cerebral venous thrombosis; this includes thrombosis of the internal cerebral veins and/or the great vein of Galen.[122–124] Once the diagnosis has been made, prompt and aggressive therapy is indicated to avoid or reverse cerebral herniation. The lingering fear of hemorrhage with anticoagulant therapy is probably based on older reports of the natural history of cerebral venous thrombosis that terminates in intracerebral hemorrhage because of infarctive ischemia. Both historical[125] and level 1[126] studies have shown that patients who are treated with heparin achieve approximately 80% full recovery, with only 15% to 20% having any sequelae. A very small number or no patients die when administered heparin. Conversely, as shown in Table 16-10, of patients who do not receive heparin, approximately 25% die and 50% survive but with sequelae, with only 25% experiencing complete recovery. A recently published study in which low molecular weight heparin was used showed a nonstatistically significant trend toward benefit in the treatment group (Table 16-11).[127,128]

A meta-analysis of these data revealed an absolute risk reduction for mortality by 14% and death or dependency by 15%, although these findings were not statistically significant because of the small sample size (79 patients in the two studies combined). An increased rate of intracranial hemorrhage was not seen in these trials. Although these findings are not statistically significant, because of the trend in favor of anticoagulation, we and other physicians have adopted the use of early anticoagulation in the treatment plans of patients with cerebral vein thrombosis.[10,102,103,106,114,127,129,130,130a]

Treatment

Improvement with heparin therapy has been noted as early as the second or third day of therapy,[126] even in patients who have evidence of some "petechial" hemorrhage on imaging. Evidence for hemorrhage should no longer be viewed as an absolute contraindication to heparin therapy.[124,126] In a study involving small numbers of patients with the rarer subtype of deep cerebral venous thrombosis, none of 7 patients receiving heparin therapy died, and all 10 patients who did not receive heparin therapy died.[122] Most reviews of the subject agree that vigorous heparin therapy followed by warfarin is the treatment of choice.[10,102,103,112–114,120–122] However, in cases of cerebral vein thrombosis due to obvious underlying intracranial infection, the role of anticoagulation remains uncertain.

A growing number of patients have been treated successfully with thrombolytic agents without experiencing undue bleeding. Thrombolytic therapy cannot be routinely recommended at this time but should be given consideration because of its uniformly high efficacy. The safety of thrombolytic therapy compared with standard heparin therapy has not been evaluated rigorously, and a recent Cochrane Database review showed that no randomized trials have been performed.[131] A recent literature review of thrombolytic therapy reported a 17% incidence of intracranial hemorrhage, a 21% incidence of extracranial hemorrhage, and a 12% incidence of death or dependency.[132] It has been suggested that thrombolytic therapy may be reserved for use as initial therapy in those with significant CNS compromise, especially in those who are comatose.[106,114,132] Patients should be maintained on long-term warfarin in doses sufficient to keep the INR at 2.0 to 3.0 for at least 3 to 6 months, with consideration for indefinite therapy if a reversible cause is not corrected.[10]

RETINAL VEIN/ARTERY THROMBOSIS

Overview

The history of our knowledge of retinal vein occlusion (Table 16-12), which is often divided into branch retinal vein occlusion (BRVO) and central retinal vein occlusion (CRVO), has been reviewed by Williamson.[133]

Previous reviews and indeed some recent reviews in the ophthalmology literature continue to focus on the time-honored observation of an apparent correlation between retinal artery occlusion, BRVO, and CRVO and increased plasma fibrinogen level, age, dyslipidemia, diabetes mellitus, hypertension, hyperviscosity, and decreased exercise.[133–138] It is curious that none of these reviews addresses the possibility of an association with hypercoagulable disorders, and one[133] minimizes the role of anticoagulant therapy in afflicted patients.

A renaissance of investigation into retinal vein thrombosis began in the 1990s and continues to this day.[134] Although reported results of several studies are seemingly mutually incompatible, several groups have noted an association between the presence of antiphospholipid antibodies and retinal vein occlusion, as well as other retinal disorders.[135–137] In a recent review of 40 patients with retinal thrombosis, 22.5% had evidence of antiphospholipid antibodies compared with 5% in a reference population.[138] Case reports include an association with APLS in a young woman who had depressed levels of free protein S.[139] Glueck and associates[140] noted that 43% of their patients had laboratory evidence consistent with APLS, but only 3% in a control group had such laboratory evidence. In one study in Saudi Arabia,[141] 50% of patients with retinal venous occlusion had laboratory evidence of APLS. In a recent review of

thrombophilia in retinal vein occlusion, the odds ratio for retinal vein occlusion was estimated to be 3.9 for those with anticardiolipin antibodies as compared with those without detected antibodies.[137] A sixfold increase was noted in patients who harbored the factor V Leiden mutation in a single study[140]; another study group reported a twofold increase in factor V Leiden,[142] a third group[143] described an eightfold increase, and in a fourth group, a threefold increase was seen.[144] In a single report, 8.3% of patients with retinal vein occlusion tested positive for the prothrombin 20210 mutation compared with 0% in a control group.[145] Multiple other studies[137,146–152] failed to find an increased incidence of factor V Leiden mutation, but some have found evidence of resistance to activated protein C at a rate 5 times higher than that of controls.

One group reported that resistance to activated protein C was the most common cause of retinal vein occlusion in the young,[154] and another[153] found that it was the most common (25%) laboratory-identified risk factor among patients with CRVO. Of interest, the same investigator[154] a year later was unable to duplicate those findings when he reported that among 55 patients with retinal vein occlusion, the incidence of resistance to activated protein C was precisely the same as in his control group. A recent review comparing patients with CRVO with a normal cohort found that in only 2 of 9 studies was the incidence of resistance to activated protein C and/or factor V Leiden mutation significantly increased.[155] Gottlieb and colleagues[156] were unable to find any evidence of increased resistance to activated protein C or factor V Leiden mutation in 21 of their patients, and Delahousse[157] determined that the incidence of prothrombin 20210 mutation was precisely the same (3.6%) in his patients with retinal vein occlusion as in a control group.

Greiner and coworkers[158] reported an incidence of factor V Leiden of 27% among patients with CRVO. In a pooled analysis of 232 patients with CRVO, only 7 patients with the prothrombin 20210 mutation were identified—a number similar to that expected in the Caucasian population at large.[155] The incidence of factor V Leiden or prothrombin 20210 mutation was not increased in a recent study of 136 patients with retinal artery occlusion.[159] Compelling evidence appears to link elevated homocysteine levels to retinal vascular events,[137,160] although not all study findings have been positive.[161,162] One study found a 60% incidence of hyperhomocysteinemia in patients with ocular venous occlusion.[163] Several recent studies have shown higher risks of retinal artery and vein occlusion in patients with elevated homocysteine levels,[164–168] although others have not confirmed this association.[150,169] In one recent study, hyperhomocysteinemia was found to have an odds ratio of 8.9 for retinal vein occlusion—the highest ratio among all thrombophilic risk factors that were investigated.[137]

Causes

A causative role of abnormalities in the fibrinolytic system has been suggested by some clinicians, as summarized by Fegan, but this remains controversial.[155,165] It is difficult to resolve these differing data, but recent evidence published over the past several years suggests the possibility of an underlying disorder such as factor V Leiden mutation, prothrombin 20210 mutation, resistance to activated protein C, hyperhomocysteinemia, and particularly, APLS in patients with retinal vein thrombosis.[137,170–172,172a] Some

---

Table 16-12 Retinal Vein Thrombosis: Clinical Vignettes

Painless loss of vision is a typical presentation.
Risk factors for retinal artery thrombosis also apply to retinal vein thrombosis.
The role of inherited thrombophilia is controversial.
Data on antiphospholipid antibody syndrome are the most convincing.
The role of anticoagulant or thrombolytic therapy is controversial.

---

editorialists[141,155,170,171,173] urge an open mind and indicate that larger studies need to be done; others argue against an association of thrombophilia with retinal vascular occlusion.[174,175] They also note that much as with hypercoagulability and thrombosis in other sites, it may take a combination of a hypercoagulable disorder and a second provocation, such as age, diabetes, hypertension, and hyperfibrinogenemia in cases of CRVO, for the process to become manifest.

Diagnosis

Other matters to consider include the unique anatomy of the optic sheath, through which both the retinal vein and the retinal artery travel. Accordingly, perturbations of the retinal artery due to hypertension, diabetes, or aging may encroach upon the adjacent retinal vein. Thus, in contrast to other venous thrombotic disorders, typical risk factors for arterial thrombosis are significant and likely are more important than or, at a minimum, synergistic with the aforementioned hereditary thrombophilic states. Giorgi and colleagues[176] recommended long-term warfarin therapy in patients with retinal vein occlusion believed to be due to a thrombotic process.[176] Although oral anticoagulant therapy has been successfully used by others,[177,178] studies have yet to be done to establish the best therapy. One author strongly recommends against anticoagulation and states that it is contraindicated in patients with an increased bleeding risk.[175]

Treatment

Given our referral pattern of patients who are likely to have hereditary thrombophilia, along with the variable and poor prognosis with recent and recurrent retinal vessel thrombosis, we tend to anticoagulate patients with retinal vein occlusion, especially the young.[179] In older patients with retinal artery occlusion and other obvious risk factors, decisions are made on a case-by-case basis, but recommendations often include therapy aimed at improving atherosclerotic risk factors and the use of antiplatelet agents.

Some centers[180,181] have administered systemic intravenous thrombolytic therapy in both acute and subacute retinal vein occlusion and have reported very good results. In fact, vision in half of patients significantly improved, even though therapy was provided weeks after the occlusion occurred. Recent reports of local catheter-directed lytic therapy and of intravitreal infusion of tissue plasminogen activator (tPA) have shown variable success.[182–184]

Patients with this disorder should be monitored, and consideration should be given to thrombolytic therapy in an acute or subacute phase, depending on the level of visual impairment and the expertise of local interventional radiologists. Long-term oral anticoagulant therapy in doses designed to maintain an INR of 2.0 to 3.0 seems reasonable, especially if no obvious underlying disorder is found.

UPPER EXTREMITY THROMBOSIS

Overview

The prevalence of thrombosis of the vessels of the upper extremity (UE) (Table 16-13) is reported to be 2 per

Table 16-13 Upper Extremity Thrombosis: Clinical Vignettes

Swelling of a unilateral extremity, chest wall, or the face is a common presentation that is dependent on which specific vein is thrombosed.

It is less commonly associated with clinically significant pulmonary embolism as compared with lower extremity thrombosis.

Intravenous catheters or devices are a significant risk factor.

Anatomic abnormalities need to be evaluated and ruled out.

Recent data do not support routine primary prophylactic anticoagulation for central venous access devices.

Initial treatment includes anticoagulation and consideration of removal of intravenous devices, if present.

Surgical decompression is warranted in the presence of thoracic outlet syndrome.

100,000 patient-years but appears to be increasing, probably because of the combination of increased ease of diagnosis through modern imaging and increased use of intravascular devices such as indwelling catheters that are placed into those vessels.[185] The superficial veins of the upper extremities include the cephalic, basilic, and cubital veins, which drain into the deep system. The axillary vein is the first named deep vessel. It is joined by the brachial and cephalic veins, which continue into the chest as the subclavian vein. The subclavian and internal jugular veins form the brachiocephalic vein, which drains into the superior vena cava (SVC).

Causes

Although the incidence and causes of thrombosis of these vessels vary according to the perspective of the physician and the clinic reporting them, roughly one third are found to be due to so-called primary or effort thrombosis, often associated with an anatomic abnormality (Paget-Schroetter syndrome), at least one third are due to the presence of indwelling catheters, and the remaining one third appear to be more or less idiopathic, including those due to hypercoagulable situations. Concomitant use of oral birth control pills may increase the risk because of other factors. Of course, any of these causes may be additive, as Virchow would have predicted. A recent single institution study showed that in 60% of cases of upper extremity DVT, a catheter had been inserted into the thrombosed vessel, and in 46%, cancer was the underlying diagnosis.[186] Only 29% had no apparent cause. Thrombophilic situations, including ATIII deficiency, have been associated with axillary and subclavian vein thromboses. However, the inherited hypercoagulable disorders may play a lesser role in arm venous thrombosis than in deep[187] or superficial[188] vein thrombosis of the leg, in that a large quantity of the data is observational, with varying results.[189] APLS and Trousseau syndrome are common among the acquired causes of hypercoagulability.[190–192] In one study, 25% of patients who presented with idiopathic UE DVT were found to have a malignancy within the subsequent year.[189] The occurrence of thrombophilic defects in patients with UE DVT ranges from 8% to 61% in the literature, much of which is retrospective and descriptive of few patients.[185,193] A recent review documented at least one thrombophilic defect in 61% of patients examined; factor V Leiden (12.9%), prothrombin 20210 gene mutation (20%), and elevated homocysteine levels (16%) were the most prevalent.[185] In another study, the odds ratio for UE DVT was 6.2 for factor V Leiden, 5.0 for the prothrombin 20210 gene mutation, and 4.9 for anticoagulant protein deficiencies.[194] However, the prevalence of factor V Leiden and of the prothrombin 20210 gene mutation was not increased in a separate study by Leebeek and colleagues.[195] Catheter-related UE DVT may be present in as many as 72% of cases of catheter placement, if they are prospectively radiographically investigated.[196] In an epidemiologic study, the presence of a catheter was the strongest risk factor for thrombosis, with an odds ratio greater than 7.[197] In patients with idiopathic UE DVT, the odds ratio for a hypercoagulable condition was 4.1 as compared with those with effort-related thrombosis.[198]

UE DVT accounts for only about 1% to 4% of all DVTs.[193] The subclavian vein, the internal jugular vein, and the axillary veins seem to be the most commonly thrombosed deep veins of the UE, possibly because of the frequency of catheterization of these vessels.[199] A male/female predilection of about 2:1 has been reported, largely due to effort thrombosis, which is seen most often among younger males. UE DVT occurs bilaterally about 10% of the time, especially with effort thrombosis.

Signs and Symptoms

Signs and symptoms of the disorder include swelling (100%), venous engorgement (82%), pain (73%), mild cyanosis of the involved arm (55%), and a palpable cord (26%).[200] The palpable cord often is appreciated only in the very dome of the axilla, where the enlarged, tender, inflamed subclavian vein may be palpated. Fortunately, UE venous gangrene occurs in only about 1% of all cases.[200] Death from embolism-related pulmonary hypertension has been rarely reported. Debate is ongoing about the frequency of PE that originates from axillary or subclavian vein thrombosis; rates of 7% to 9% are frequently quoted.[186] More recent reviews quote rates as high as 33%.[201] Such emboli, however, are often asymptomatic and are only infrequently of sufficient size to cause circulatory compromise, which is characteristic of the large emboli originating from the legs.[186,191]

Effort thrombosis (Paget-Schroetter syndrome) may result from prolonged heavy use of the arms, particularly when the arms are maintained in somewhat less than usual positions. Examples include prolonged weightlifting, pole vaulting, painting ceilings, playing racquet sports, and taking rifle practice. A subset of patients with effort vein thrombosis is found to have some type of thoracic outlet obstruction, including anatomic abnormalities of the veins coursing under the first rib or the scalene muscle (Fig. 16-8). This fact is often discovered on follow-up venography of a previously thrombosed vessel. The degree of venous obstruction is best appreciated when the arm is raised above the head during venography. The rate of postphlebitic syndrome is uncertain but has been approximated as high as 90% in some series.[201]

The use of various indwelling catheters into veins of the arm, the subclavian vein, and the internal jugular vein is a frequent trigger for UE vein thrombosis (see Chapter 32). In a prospective study of patients admitted to intensive care units, Timsit and colleagues[202] found that 33% of internal jugular vein catheter placements and 10% of subclavian vein catheter placements were associated with thromboses of

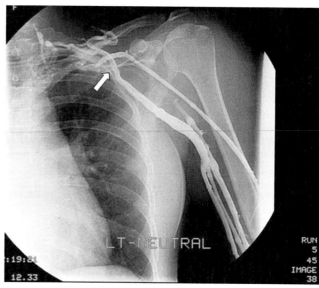

Figure 16-8 Thoracic outlet syndrome. Left upper extremity venogram shows large, contorted collateral veins arising from the axillary vein, rather than diving through the thoracic cage as the left subclavian vein. Removal of the first rib may relieve the pathologic obstruction. Narrowing of the subclavian vein is apparent, along with obliteration of normal flow (arrow).

those contiguous vessels when in place for 9 ± 5 days. A positive correlation was noted between older patients and those who were not receiving thromboprophylaxis with heparin. Catheter-related thrombosis also resulted in a 2.6-fold increase in risk for catheter-related sepsis. It is unknown whether catheter-related thrombosis is associated with underlying thrombophilic conditions.

Diagnosis

The subclavian and axillary veins may be associated with tumors that are caused (1) by resultant hypercoagulability associated with the tumor (including Trousseau syndrome), or (2) by direct pressure from a tumor mass, most commonly lung cancer and lymphoma.

Thrombosis of these vessels is best documented through the use of imaging techniques, typically starting with ultrasonography. These thromboses may be found serendipitously on imaging of the thorax for other reasons. The index of suspicion should be heightened in anyone with a newly swollen, tender arm with increased, engorged surface veins. A concern is cephalad propagation of thromboses up into the internal jugular and even into the cerebral venous drainage system; this is manifested by signs and symptoms of cerebral venous thrombosis, notably headache and papilledema.[203]

Treatment

Once the diagnosis has been made, most experts recommend anticoagulant therapy, although it is often underused.[189,197] Withholding anticoagulant therapy has not led to good outcomes; the result has often been a chronically swollen, heavy, and disfigured arm. Accordingly, treatment with anticoagulants and thrombolytic therapy have been proposed, whether they are given systemically or, in the case of thrombolytics, are site directed.[185,189,199,204–209] Anticoagulation has supplanted the indication for acute thrombectomy.[209,209a] Thrombolytic therapy was shown by one group[199] to result in a 50% reduction in residual signs and symptoms of UE postphlebitic syndrome. Thrombolytic therapy should be considered seriously for the rare person who presents with UE venous gangrene.[207] If anticoagulation is absolutely contraindicated in a patient with severe underlying lung disease, such that even a small pulmonary embolism may be considered life threatening, then an SVC filter could be considered. The efficacy and safety of SVC filters remain unproved, however.[189]

If a patient is subsequently found to have thoracic outlet obstruction, surgery is indicated, with selected use of first rib resection with or without scalenectomy, and appears to improve long-term results. Otherwise, an approximately 50% relapse rate is reported in these patients who do not undergo anatomic relief of their obstruction.[208,209] Others have recently recorded a more favorable long-term prognosis with conservative therapy alone.[210]

Previous studies have suggested that unmonitored prophylactic use of low-dose (1 mg daily) warfarin[211] or low-dose low molecular weight heparin[212] decreases the risk of UE DVT in patients with long-term catheter or central venous line placement. A study comparing these two treatment modalities in a prospective fashion showed no difference in efficacy.[213] However, more recent trials do not support these data, and recent recommendations from the American College of Chest Physicians (ACCP) recommend against routine prophylaxis in patients with cancer with central venous catheters.[214,215]

LEMIERRE SYNDROME

Overview

In 1936, Lemierre[216] described a rather rare syndrome that still bears his name. This consists of the triad of pharyngitis, thrombosis of the internal jugular vein (IJV), and severe metastatic infection, particularly to the lungs and large joints. Because this description was provided during the preantibiotic era, his observations were essentially those of the natural history of this aggressive course caused by the Gram-negative anaerobe *Fusobacterium necrophorum*, a normal oral cavity inhabitant. Indeed, 18 of his 20 patients died from this unique type and location of septic thrombophlebitis.

Now, with the broad use of antibiotics, the defining criteria employed by Lemierre have become blurred and modified, so one might expect the disorder to not unfold as originally defined.[217] Indeed, to some purists, if the triad is not as described, a patient does not have the true syndrome as described by Lemierre. Therefore, the characteristics and even the use of the eponym have been modified, and it is often now referred to as postanginal sepsis. Unfortunately, the disease is recognized and diagnosed less often than it should be; it is a dangerous condition if it remains unidentified and untreated.[218]

Diagnosis

Realizing the alteration of the natural history, Chirinos and coworkers[218] more recently described the evolution of the manifestations of Lemierre syndrome. Their diagnostic criteria consisted of pharyngitis plus thrombosis of the IJV

and/or culture positive for *Fusobacterium necrophorum*. Now that aggressive antibiotic therapy is available, the mortality rate in this review has dropped to only 5%, and, although pulmonary infiltrates are common, pulmonary cavitation is now rare.[218] Investigators described that the chief clinical clue leading to correct diagnosis in 70% of cases was a culture (usually of blood) that was positive for *Fusobacterium necrophorum*.[218] Additionally, detection of an IJV thrombosis was the deciding factor in 16% of cases, most of which did not involve positive blood culture findings. Most often, the IJV thrombosis was stumbled upon through imaging, typically by ultrasound, during evaluation of a tender swollen neck, particularly when it occurred parallel to the sternocleidomastoid muscle.

The reason to include this diagnosis in this chapter is that the hematologist may well be asked to consult on what otherwise may appear to be an isolated IJV thrombosis. This is especially true now that cases are typically diagnosed earlier and without an advanced inflammatory presentation, as had been initially described.

Treatment

The role of anticoagulant therapy in septic thrombophlebitis is uncertain. Most patients with Lemierre syndrome respond to antibiotic therapy, especially when the extent of the IJV thrombosis is limited. However, use of anticoagulant therapy seems justified, should the thrombotic process extend farther down into the great vessels of the chest and arm or, especially, cephalad into the vessels draining the head.[219]

Cutaneous Microvascular Thrombosis (Purpura Fulminans)

Overview

Thrombosis of the dermal microvasculature results in discoloration and infarction of the skin and subcutaneous tissues. In its most dramatic and florid state, this process is referred to as *purpura fulminans* (Table 16-14).[220,221] Although it is not limited to disseminated intravascular coagulation (DIC), purpura fulminans is characteristically seen in this condition; the reader is referred to Chapters 11 (purpura) and 12 (DIC) for additional details.

Causes

The leading category of causes of purpura fulminans is infectious disease,[222] which can be viral, bacterial, rickettsial, or protozoan. Key to the pathophysiology of infectious purpura fulminans are unchecked thrombin production

---

Table 16-14 Cutaneous Microvascular Thrombosis: Clinical Vignettes

Causes are often infectious.
In the neonate it is associated with homozygous protein C or protein S deficiency.
The roles of other inherited thrombophilic conditions are uncertain.
Treatment should include activated protein C concentrates used in inherited deficiency states.

---

and collapse of the fibrinolytic system, primarily through gross reductions in protein C and protein S and a concomitant increase in plasminogen activator inhibitor-1 (PAI-1).[223] In at least one case, transient severe depression of protein S was due to transient autoantibodies directed against protein S.[223]

Symptoms

Dermal necrosis related to capillary infarction is the hallmark of warfarin skin necrosis, which is discussed in Chapter 11. Warfarin skin necrosis may occur in patients who have congenital or acquired deficiency of protein C or protein S,[224–228] and occasionally, in patients with PNH.[229,230]

Skin necrosis occurs spontaneously in newborns who are homozygous for protein S or protein C deficiency.[231,232] In these situations, consanguinity may be encountered. Neonatal purpura fulminans has also been described in patients doubly heterozygous for protein C deficiency[233] or protein S deficiency.[234]

Diagnosis

Some investigators have questioned why only some patients with diseases such as meningococcemia develop purpura fulminans, but other patients with the same illness do not.[221] They speculate that these patients also might harbor an underlying thrombophilia that may aid and abet microcirculatory thrombosis or that large increases in PAI-1 levels seen in patients with purpura fulminans may be restricted to unique hyperreactors. An increasing number of reports[235–241] have involved patients ranging in age from infancy through adolescence to full adulthood who have had infectious disease associated with excessive purpura fulminans, all of whom were found to be heterozygous for the factor V Leiden mutation. In another report,[242] seven children with purpura fulminans from varicella infection were all found to have strong lupus anticoagulants and transient severe deficiency of protein S. These findings have led some[239,243] to recommend routine screening for congenital thrombophilic disorders in patients who exhibit purpura fulminans. On the other hand, Westendorp and colleagues[244] analyzed blood from patients who survived meningococcemia and from the parents of those patients who died. Although they found evidence for congenital thrombophilia in 7 of 50 consecutive patients, they determined that this incidence was the same as that in the general population. This question is an interesting point that has not yet been resolved.

Treatment

Therapy depends on prompt diagnosis and, in cases associated with DIC, therapy should be directed toward any treatable underlying cause. Treatment of patients with warfarin skin necrosis is discussed in Chapter 11. Owing to the central role of depletion of protein C, many have advocated infusion with activated protein C concentrates,[221] and limited case reports have shown a hint of efficacy (see Chapter 13). A therapeutic trial has been advocated by some,[245,246] and others[247] have proposed the use of tPA therapy. Because of extensive skin loss, these patients are best treated in a burn unit.[248]

Long-term replacement therapy with protein C has been advocated for the rare unfortunate children with homozygous deficiency of protein C. This has been administered intravenously[249] or, more recently, subcutaneously.[250]

OVARIAN VEIN THROMBOSIS

Overview

Thrombosis of the ovarian veins (Table 16-15) occurs almost exclusively during the postpartum period.[251] It occurs rarely ($\approx$1 in every 2000 deliveries), although in an extensive prospective study, Witlin and colleagues[252] found only 11 cases out of 77,000 deliveries over a 10-year period, representing an incidence of less than 0.01%. It is interesting to note that all these cases were associated with vaginal delivery, but in other series, the incidence was much higher after cesarean section, accounting for 87% of cases.[253] In Witlin's review,[252] investigators were unable to find features peculiar to or unusual about the nature of the pregnancy or the delivery predisposing to thrombosis. The typical patient was admitted 7 to 13 days postpartum, usually for the combination of fever, right pelvic pain, and leukocytosis. The admitting diagnosis was endometritis in three quarters of cases, and in the other one quarter, pyelonephritis; no patient was suspected to have postpartum ovarian vein thrombosis. Patients are regarded as clinically infected and are typically treated with antibiotics.

Symptoms

Two different forms of pelvic thrombophlebitis have been described. Ovarian vein thrombosis, as discussed in this chapter, typically manifests with fever and abdominal pain and is amenable to diagnosis on CT. The second form, deep septic thrombophlebitis, more commonly begins with high spiking fevers despite antibiotic therapy, but the patient feels well and comfortable between fevers. The condition is difficult to diagnosis on imaging. These two conditions are often discussed separately in the literature.

Diagnosis

Because of the overwhelming predominance of ovarian vein thrombosis occurring in the right pelvic vein as opposed to the left pelvic vein by virtue of the unique drainage of the right ovary, appendicitis is often included in the differential diagnosis. When patients' symptoms fail

---

Table 16-15 Ovarian Vein Thrombosis: Clinical Vignettes

Fever, right-sided abdominal pain, or leukocytosis unresponsive to antibiotic therapy is the most common presentation.
This is likely a complication of septic thrombophlebitis.
This is seen almost exclusively postpartum; less commonly, it occurs following gynecologic surgery.
Ultrasound, computed tomographic scanning, and magnetic resonance imaging are imaging studies of choice.
Heparin is recommended for initial treatment until symptoms resolve, but the role for extended anticoagulation is uncertain.
Few adverse long-term sequelae have been reported.

to respond to antibiotic therapy, deeper diagnostic consideration is required. The correct diagnosis is almost always made on the basis of the combination of failure to respond to antibiotics and visualization of abdominal and pelvic contents on modern imaging. One group found that MRI, CT, and ultrasonography had sensitivities and specificities as follows: 92% and 100%, 100% and 99%, and 50% and 99%, respectively. Imaging led to correct diagnosis in 76 consecutive cases of postpartum fever refractory to antibiotic therapy.[254] The thrombosed postpartum ovarian vein may be surprisingly large.

Treatment

Therapeutic efforts initially consist of antibiotics and are directed toward anticoagulation once the diagnosis has been made. Most experts recommend the initial use of heparin in the treatment of patients with ovarian vein thrombosis on the basis of rapid resolution of clinical symptoms in treated patients.[255] Whereas it is often cited in the obstetric literature that defervescence of fever in response to heparin therapy occurs characteristically within 24 to 48 hours, Witlin and colleagues[252] found in their study that the response usually requires 3 to 4 days. A recent series has questioned the need for anticoagulation. These authors randomly assigned 15 patients to antimicrobials, plus or minus heparin, and found no difference in the number of days of fever and hospitalization.[256] Our group favors initial anticoagulant therapy but does not necessarily prescribe anticoagulation with warfarin for longer than 3 to 6 months unless an underlying thrombophilic mutation is identified, because this unique DVT is always associated with the provocation of pregnancy or gynecologic surgery.

Ovarian vein thrombosis is believed to be due to septic thrombophlebitis.[257,258] Because modern imaging yields the correct diagnosis, surgical exploration is no longer required. Taking advantage of cases found at surgery in premodern imaging days, however, Munsick and Gillanders[258] cultured the clots excised from thrombosed ovarian veins and found that in six of seven cases, they were able to culture bacteria, thereby solidifying the theory that this is in fact septic thrombophlebitis. The postpartum state is already one of increased thrombotic risk, given hypercoagulability, but the dilated ovarian vein with slow flow further increases the risk. Minimal evidence suggests that this condition is associated with congenital thrombophilia. One case of protein C[259] deficiency, one case of protein S deficiency, and two cases of antiphospholipid antibody syndrome have been implicated.[260,261] A recent review, however, found that 11 of 22 patients with ovarian vein thrombosis had a thrombophilic condition with negative personal and family histories of prior VTE.[262] These experts suggested that warfarin may be administered for several months after the diagnosis has been established and initial heparin therapy provided. They were not certain about the role of antibiotics but noted that almost all patients had already completed a course of antibiotics prior to discharge. Although it is known that thrombi from the ovarian vein may protrude into the IVC or veins of the legs, clinically significant PE is very rare, and no cases of death due to PE have been reported in patients with ovarian vein thrombosis. The absence of adverse long-term sequelae has been noted with ovarian vein thrombosis, and the relapse rate with subsequent pregnancy is low.[252,253] Excellent

imaging studies of postpartum ovarian vein thrombosis have been published.[261] A smaller version of ovarian vein thrombosis has also been found in nonpregnant women, usually incidentally when clinicians are staging an oncologic disorder. Those having ovarian vein thromboses associated with malignancy have a worse prognosis, accounting for all the deaths in one series.[261a] Patients with these asymptomatic thromboses of the ovarian veins probably do not need to be treated with heparin, but the argument could be made for serial monitoring of the process.[262]

OTHER SITES OF THROMBOSES

Adrenal Gland

It is now believed that adrenal gland hemorrhage is (Table 16-16) initiated by thrombosis of the adrenal veins. The unique anatomy of the adrenal vein, with its rich arterial supply but only a single draining vein, may predispose this site to thrombosis.[7] Thrombosis is followed by infarction and subsequent hemorrhage[263] into this highly vascular organ. Adrenal vein hemorrhage occurs in stressful situations and is increasingly recognized in association with lupus anticoagulant syndrome, APLS, heparin-induced thrombocytopenia with thrombosis,[264] and purpura fulminans. In fact, in recent reviews, it has been noted that 10% to 26% of patients with catastrophic antiphospholipid antibody syndrome (CAPS) have adrenal failure, which may be the first clinical sign of CAPS in more than one third of cases.[8] Whereas, traditionally, adrenal gland hemorrhage had been detected at autopsy, it is now often recognized in life in patients who are in stressful situations and develop fever, hypotension, and abdominal or back pain of uncertain cause. Routine laboratory evaluation is not helpful in the acute situation, and therapy should hinge on clinical suspicion—not on laboratory results. Enlargement and hemorrhage of the gland subsequently are observed when abdominal exploration is performed by CT scanning (Fig. 16-9).[265] Despite secondary hemorrhage, initial management of the condition often involves anticoagulation, given the underlying thrombosis, especially in known hypercoagulable conditions.[7,8] Treatment of patients with adrenal insufficiency with mineralocorticosteroids is of paramount importance.

Table 16-16 Adrenal Infarction with Secondary Hemorrhage: Clinical Vignettes

Typical clinical presentation includes vague abdominal or back pain with hypotension requiring pressor support, especially in stressful situations.
It is commonly associated with antiphospholipid antibody syndrome.
Computed tomographic imaging is the diagnostic modality of choice.
Adrenal hormone studies are of little diagnostic value in the acute setting.
Anticoagulation is recommended despite overt hemorrhage.
Empirical replacement therapy of patients with adrenal insufficiency should be strongly considered.

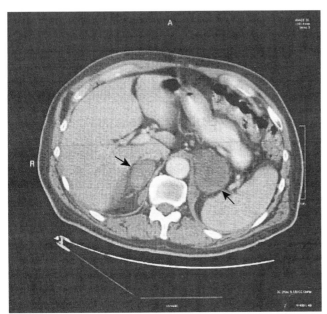

Figure 16-9 Adrenal gland hemorrhage. This computed tomographic scan with contrast shows bilateral adrenal hemorrhage (*arrows*) that is more advanced on the left.

Pituitary Gland

Hemorrhagic infarction related to thrombosis of the pituitary gland has been described as a cause of hypopituitarism in patients with APLS.[266] This diagnosis may be entertained in the appropriate clinical setting in patients who exhibit evidence of hypopituitarism.

Placenta

Antiphospholipid antibody syndrome[267–269] has long been regarded as a major cause of infarctive placental dysfunction (Table 16-17), but other hypercoagulable disorders are now also implicated through the systematic evaluation of women who have experienced late fetal loss and stillbirth.[267,270] The role of inherited thrombophilia as a cause of intrauterine growth retardation (IUGR), preeclampsia, and placental abruption remain controversial.[267,269] Pathologic evaluation of the placenta in cases of recurrent fetal loss also supports the causative role of thrombophilia.[267,269] Thrombotic changes and infarcts of the placental circulation are seen in a significant proportion of cases. Placental thrombotic infarcts may be maternal or fetal.[269] However, the frequent finding of thrombosis on the maternal side, in conjunction with the fact that heparin can prevent fetal loss but does not cross the placental circulation, argues that thrombosis on the maternal side of the placental circulation is of primary

Table 16-17 Infarctive Placental Dysfunction: Clinical Vignettes

Inherited and acquired thrombophilia may play a role in diverse fetal complications, especially with recurrent or second or third trimester miscarriage.
Recent data have shown the safety and efficacy of low molecular weight heparin in preventing fetal loss.
This topic is covered in greater detail in Chapter 36.

importance.[269] Kuperminc and colleagues[271] found that among 110 women with complications of pregnancy associated with abnormal placenta vasculature, 71 (65%) had laboratory evidence of thrombophilia compared with 18% among controls ($P < .001$).[271]

A complete review of the role of thrombophilia in pregnancy-related complications is beyond the scope of this chapter (see Chapter 36), but an increasing number of studies and reviews on this topic have been published.[267–270,272–274] A meta-analysis has recently shown that factor V Leiden and the prothrombin 20210 mutation were associated with early and late fetal loss (odds ratio, 2 to 8).[272] A recent review of the European Prospective Cohort on Thrombophilia (EPCOT) showed only a small increase in fetal loss among carriers of thrombophilic mutations (odds ratio, 1.4 to 1.6, depending on the mutation).[273] Brenner and colleagues[275] found factor V Leiden mutation in 32% of patients with fetal loss compared with only 10% in controls ($P<.001$). Gris and coworkers[276] identified similar defects in 21% of women with late fetal loss or stillbirth compared with 4% in controls. These last two reports additionally confirmed that those harboring more than one hypercoagulable defect had a higher rate of fetal wastage (increasing from 7% with one abnormality to 23% with more than one), consistent with the synergism of risk factors described for thromboses at other sites.[277] Martinelli and colleagues[278] calculated a relative risk of late fetal loss of 3.0 for women heterozygous for the factor V Leiden or prothrombin 20210 mutation. Among women known to have a deficiency of protein S, protein C, or ATIII, fetal loss was experienced in 22% of pregnancies when the women were not prophylactically treated with anticoagulants; among control women without these deficiencies, 11% experienced fetal loss.[279] Although positive and negative data exist for most of the mutations studied, recent reviews suggest roles of factor V Leiden, antiphospholipid antibody syndrome, hyperhomocysteinemia, and the prothrombin gene mutation in recurrent pregnancy loss.[271,272,274] Although deficiencies of ATIII, protein C, and protein S are much less common and their significance is therefore more difficult to prove, data suggest that these mutations also increase the risk of fetal loss.[274] Although less information is available on congenital hypercoagulable disorders compared with APLS (see Chapter 36), recent data suggest that it may be prudent to administer anticoagulant therapy to such women throughout pregnancy and the puerperium, to increase the chances for a live birth.[270,280,281] Newer data have supported the efficacy of low molecular weight heparin in increasing the chances of a viable pregnancy in women with recurrent fetal loss.[270] In a study by Brenner and associates,[282] doses of enoxaparin ranging from 40 to 80 mg per day (determined by the number of underlying thrombophilic risk factors) resulted in a live birth in 75% of gestations compared with 20% in previous pregnancies.[282]

CONSULTATION CONSIDERATIONS

The consultant hematologist will be asked to see patients with thromboses at unusual sites through differing pathways. First, the patient with an established hypercoagulable history may develop nonspecific yet serious signs and symptoms that defy diagnosis. However, the knowledgeable physician is justified in elevating to very high on the list thrombosis at an unusual site from a rarity buried in the differential diagnosis, when the patient is known to be thrombophilic. Second, the consulting hematologist could (and should) be asked to make anticoagulation recommendations in thrombophilic patients before the time of a planned or urgent surgical procedure, or after it has been performed. In a third instance, the hematologist will be asked to evaluate a patient who develops an unusual thrombosis for an underlying hypercoagulable disorder.

As in all internal medicine, the history and physical examination are fundamental. One should search aggressively for clues in the past history for signs or symptoms of a previous thrombosis. Subtle signs include varicose veins, hemosiderin deposition in the skin of the legs, and chronic edema. Family history should be combed for evidence of members with unexplained sudden death or a thrombophilic history, or who are on long-term warfarin therapy.

It is important to work closely with other specialists to plan for long-term management. Thrombosis is the unifying pathologic event in the genesis of syndromes with expressions as varied as abnormal liver function test results from hepatic vein thrombosis to altered mental status from cerebral venous thrombosis. Physicians who may not have received training or whose interest may not be attuned to thromboembolism may need special guidance and assistance in therapeutic maneuvers, especially ophthalmologists and obstetricians/gynecologists. Radiologists are essential in the diagnostic pursuit, in that special techniques, special contrasts, and special timing are all needed when modern expensive imaging studies are performed.

LABORATORY EVALUATION

It is ironic that laboratory evaluation is best *not* carried out during the acute part of a VTE because thrombosis itself and treatment thereof may affect levels of protein C, protein S, and ATIII, and possibly, detection of anticardiolipin antibodies. DNA-based testing through polymerase chain reaction (PCR) analyses, such as detection of the factor V Leiden mutation or the prothrombin 20210 mutation, will not be affected by these events, but results will usually be delayed by several days. It is important to query family members who visit the patient because frequently, a family member will have a history of a previous thrombosis. It should be noted that the presence or absence of thrombophilia will not change immediate management decisions; therefore, evaluation is likely best delayed until after the acute event, when a hematologist can guide, monitor, and interpret the results of ordered tests.

COST CONTAINMENT ISSUES

Frequently, the consulting physician will have already ordered an expensive battery of tests for hypercoagulability in a patient who has had an acute VTE and is under therapy. These will be difficult to interpret and, if abnormal, the results may have been altered by the acute condition or by therapy. Although these funds will have already been spent,

it is important to clarify in the medical record for future reference the clinical condition and medications the patient was receiving at the time the test samples were drawn. An incorrect diagnosis on a discharge summary is extremely difficult to undo. Frequently, a significant delay or even discharge may occur before results are returned, and many parties will have long forgotten these details. Cost containment is also favorably affected by rapid diagnosis of the thrombosis and rapid therapy, even if it includes expensive thrombolytic agents, because these may significantly decrease hospital stay, morbidity and mortality, and, frequently, the occurrence of extremely expensive procedures such as orthotopic liver transplantation in cases of hepatic vein thrombosis.

REFERENCES

1. Osler W: The Principles and Practice of Medicine 2nd ed. New York, Appleton, 1896.
2. Flint A: Treatise in the Principles and Practice of Medicine, 6th ed. Philadelphia, Lea Brothers, 1886.
3. Virchow R: Gesammette Abhandlungen zur Wissenschaftlichen Medicin.Frankfort, Meidinger Sohn, 1856, p 477.
4. Kitchens CS: Evolution of our understanding of the pathophysiology of primary mesenteric venous thrombosis. Am J Surg 163:346–348, 1992.
5. Valla DC: Hepatic vein thrombosis (Budd-Chiari syndrome). Semin Liver Dis 22:5–14, 2002.
6. Espinosa G, Font J, Garcia-Pagan JC, et al: Budd-Chiari syndrome secondary to antiphospholipid syndrome: Clinical and immunologic characteristics of 43 patients. Medicine (Baltimore) 80:345–354, 2001.
7. Espinosa G, Cervera R, Font J, et al: Adrenal involvement in the antiphospholipid syndrome. Lupus 12:569–572, 2003.
8. Espinosa G, Santos E, Cervera R, et al: Adrenal involvement in the antiphospholipid syndrome: Clinical and immunologic characteristics of 86 patients. Medicine (Baltimore) 82:106–118, 2003.
9. DeStefano V, Leone G, Mastrangelo S, et al: Clinical manifestations and management of inherited thrombophilia: Retrospective analysis and follow-up after diagnosis of 238 patients with congenital deficiency of antithrombin III, protein C, protein S. Thromb Haemost 72:352–358, 1994.
10. Allroggen H, Abbott RJ: Cerebral venous sinus thrombosis. Postgrad Med J 76:12–15, 2000.
11. Bradbury MS, Kavanagh PV, Bechtold RE, et al: Mesenteric venous thrombosis: Diagnosis and noninvasive imaging. Radiographics 22:527–541, 2002.
12. Thaler E, Lechner K: Antithrombin III deficiency and thromboembolism. Clin Haematol 10:369–390, 1981.
13. Cosgriff TM, Bishop DT, Hershgold EJ, et al: Familial antithrombin III deficiency: Its natural history, genetics, diagnosis and treatment. Medicine (Baltimore) 62:209–220, 1983.
14. Winter JH, Fenech A, Ridley W, et al: Familial antithrombin III deficiency. Q J Med 51:373–395, 1982.
15. Pabinger I, Schneider B: Thrombotic risk in hereditary antithrombin III, protein C, or protein S deficiency: A cooperative, retrospective study. Gesellschaft fur Thrombose und Hamostaseforschung (GTH) Study Group on Natural Inhibitors. Arterioscler Thromb Vasc Biol 16:742–748, 1996.
16. Clavien PA, Durig M, Harder F: Venous mesenteric infarction: A particular entity. Br J Surg 75:252–255, 1988.
17. Amitrano L, Brancaccio V, Guardascione MA, et al: High prevalence of thrombophilic genotypes in patients with acute mesenteric vein thrombosis. Am J Gastroenterol 96:146–149, 2001.
18. Sreenarasimhaiah J: Diagnosis and management of intestinal ischaemic disorders. BMJ 326:1372–1376, 2003.
19. Mindelzun RE, Jeffrey RE Jr, Lane MJ, et al: The misty mesentery on CT: Differential diagnosis. AJR Am J Roentgenol 167:61–65, 1996.
20. Delatour H: Thrombosis of mesenteric vein as a cause of death after splenectomy. Ann Surg 21:24–28, 1895.
21. Elliot J: The operative relief of gangrene of the intestine due to occlusion of the mesenteric vessels. Ann Surg 21:9–23, 1895.
22. Hansen H, Christofferson JK: Occlusive mesenteric infarction: A retrospective study of 83 cases. Acta Chir Scand 472:103–108, 1976.

16

23. Ottinger LAW: A study of 136 patients with mesenteric infarction. Surg Gynecol Obstet 124:251–261, 1967.

24. Agaoglu N, Mustafa NA, Turkyilmaz S: Prothrombotic disorders in patients with mesenteric vein thrombosis. J Invest Surg 16:299–304, 2003.

25. Morasch MD, Ebaugh JL, Chiou AC, et al: Mesenteric venous thrombosis: A changing clinical entity. J Vasc Surg 34:680–684, 2001.

25a. Colaizzo D, Amitrano L, Tiscia GL, et al: The JAK2 V617F mutation frequently occurs in patients with portal and mesenteric venous thrombosis. J Thromb Haemost 5:55–61, 2007.

26. Chen MC, Brown MC, Willson RA, et al: Mesenteric vein thrombosis: Four cases and review of the literature. Dig Dis 14:382–389, 1996.

27. Kumar S, Sarr MG, Kamath PS: Mesenteric venous thrombosis. N Engl J Med 345:1683–1688, 2001.

27a. Kitchens CS, Weidner MH, Lottenberg R:: Chronic oral anticoagulant therapy for extrahepatic visceral thrombosis is safe. J Thromb Thrombolysis 23:223–228, 2007.

28. Abdu RA, Zakhour BJ, Dallis DJ: Mesenteric venous thrombosis—1911 to 1984. Surgery 101:383–388, 1987.

29. Khodadadi J, Rozencwajg J, Nacasch N, et al: Mesenteric vein thrombosis: The importance of a second-look operation. Arch Surg 115:315–317, 1980.

30. Levy PJ, Krausz MM, Manny J: The role of second-look procedure in improving survival time for patients with mesenteric venous thrombosis. Surg Gynecol Obstet 170:287–291, 1990.

31. Robin P, Gruel Y, Lang Y, et al: Complete thrombolysis of mesenteric vein occlusion with recombinant tissue-type plasminogen activator. Lancet 1:1391, 1988.

32. Haskal ZJ, Edmond J, Brown R: Mesenteric venous thrombosis. N Engl J Med 346:1252–1253, 2002.

33. Leach SD, Meier GH, Gusberg RJ: Endoscopic sclerotherapy: A risk factor for splanchnic venous thrombosis. J Vasc Surg 10:9–12, 1989.

34. Weber SM, Rikkers LF: Splenic vein thrombosis and gastrointestinal bleeding in chronic pancreatitis. World J Surg 27:1271–1274, 2003.

35. Petit P, Bret PM, Atri M, et al: Splenic vein thrombosis after splenectomy: Frequency and role of imaging. Radiology 190:65–68, 1994.

36. Diz-Kucukkaya R, Hacihanefioglu A, Yenerel M, et al: Antiphospholipid antibodies and antiphospholipid syndrome in patients presenting with immune thrombocytopenic purpura: A prospective cohort study. Blood 98:1760–1764, 2001.

37. Han DC, Feliciano DV: The clinical complexity of splenic vein thrombosis. Am Surg 64:558–561, 1998.

38. Madsen MS, Petersen TH, Sommer H: Segmental portal hypertension. Ann Surg 204:72–77, 1986.

39. Elizalde JI, Castells A, Panes J, et al: Portal hypertensive gastropathy in splenic vein thrombosis. J Clin Gastroenterol 19:310–312, 1994.

40. Teofili L, DeStefano V, Leone G, et al: Hematological causes of venous thrombosis in young people: High incidence of myeloproliferative disorder as underlying disease in patients with splanchnic venous thrombosis. Thromb Haemost 67:297–301, 1992.

41. Belfour G, Stewart T: Case of enlarged spleen complicated by ascites, both depending upon varicose dilation and thrombosis. Edinburgh Med J 14:589–598, 1869.

42. Janssen HL, Meinardi JR, Vleggaar FP, et al: Factor V Leiden mutation, prothrombin gene mutation, and deficiencies in coagulation inhibitors associated with Budd-Chiari syndrome and portal vein thrombosis: Results of a case-control study. Blood 96:2364–2368, 2000.

43. Amitrano L, Guardascione MA, Brancaccio V, et al: Risk factors and clinical presentation of portal vein thrombosis in patients with liver cirrhosis. J Hepatol 40:736–741, 2004.

44. Amitrano L, Brancaccio V, Guardascione MA, et al: Inherited coagulation disorders in cirrhotic patients with portal vein thrombosis. Hepatology 31:345–348, 2000.

45. Valla DC, Condat B: Portal vein thrombosis in adults: Pathophysiology, pathogenesis and management. J Hepatol 32:865–871, 2000.

46. Fisher NC, Wilde JT, Roper JT, et al: Deficiency of natural anticoagulant proteins C, S, and antithrombin in portal vein thrombosis: A secondary phenomenon? Gut 46:534–539, 2000.

47. Janssen HL, Meinardi JR, Vleggaar FP, et al: Factor 5 Leiden mutation, prothrombin gene mutation, and deficiencies in coagulation inhibitors associated with Budd-Chiari syndrome and portal vein thrombosis: Results of a case-control study. Blood 96:3314–3315, 2001.

48. Pinto RB, Silveira TR, Bandinelli E, et al: Portal vein thrombosis in children and adolescents: The low prevalence of hereditary thrombophilic disorders. J Pediatr Surg 39:1356–1361, 2004.

49. El-Karaksy H, El Koofy N, El Hawary M, et al: Prevalence of factor V Leiden mutation and other hereditary thrombophilic factors in Egyptian children with portal vein thrombosis: Results of a single-center case-control study. Ann Hematol 83:712–715, 2004.

50. Cohen J, Edelman RR, Chopra S: Portal vein thrombosis: A review. Am J Med 92:173–182, 1992.

51. Broe PJ, Conley CL, Cameron JL: Thrombosis of the portal vein following splenectomy for myeloid metaplasia. Surg Gynecol Obstet 152:488–492, 1981.

52. Valla D, Casadevall N, Huisse MG, et al: Etiology of portal vein thrombosis in adults: A prospective evaluation of primary myeloproliferative disorders. Gastroenterology 94:1063–1069, 1988.

53. Amitrano L, Guardascione MA, Brancaccio V, et al: Portal and mesenteric venous thrombosis in cirrhotic patients. Gastroenterology 123:1409–1410, 2002.

54. Condat B, Pessione F, Hillaire S, et al: Current outcome of portal vein thrombosis in adults: Risk and benefit of anticoagulant therapy. Gastroenterology 120:490–497, 2001.

55. Sheen CL, Lamparelli H, Milne A, et al: Clinical features, diagnosis and outcome of acute portal vein thrombosis. QJM 93:531–534, 2000.

56. Schafer C, Zundler J, Bode JC: Thrombolytic therapy in patients with portal vein thrombosis: Case report and review of the literature. Eur J Gastroenterol Hepatol 12:1141–1145, 2000.

57. Yerdel MA, Gunson B, Mirza D, et al: Portal vein thrombosis in adults undergoing liver transplantation: Risk factors, screening, management, and outcome. Transplantation 69:1873–1881, 2000.

58. Rayer P: Traite des maladies des reins et des alteret lens de la secretions urinaire. Baillieve 2:550–559, 1840.

59. Llach F: Hypercoagulability, renal vein thrombosis, and other thrombotic complications of nephrotic syndrome. Kidney Int 28:429–439, 1985.

60. Laville M, Aguilera D, Maillet PJ: The prognosis of renal vein thrombosis: A re-evaluation of 27 cases. Nephrol Dial Transplant 3:247–256, 1988.

61. Vigano- D'Angelo S, D'Angelo A, Kaufman CE Jr, et al: Protein S deficiency occurs in the nephrotic syndrome. Ann Intern Med 107:42–47, 1987.

62. Gouault-Heilmann M, Gadelha-Parente T, Levent M, et al: Total and free protein S in nephrotic syndrome. Thromb Res 49:37–42, 1988.

63. Ko WS, Lim PS, Sung YP: Renal vein thrombosis as first clinical manifestation of the primary antiphospholipid syndrome. Nephrol Dial Transplant 10:1929–1931, 1995.

64. Morgan RJ, Feneley RC: Renal vein thrombosis caused by primary antiphospholipid syndrome. Br J Urol 74:807–808, 1994.

65. Asherson RA, Buchanan N, Baguley E, et al: Postpartum bilateral renal vein thrombosis in the primary antiphospholipid syndrome. J Rheumatol 20:874–876, 1993.

66. Kuhle S, Massicotte P, Chan A, et al: A case series of 72 neonates with renal vein thrombosis: Data from the 1–800-NO-CLOTS Registry. Thromb Haemost 92:729–733, 2004.

67. Heller C, Schobess R, Kurnik K, et al, for the Childhood Thrombophilia Study Group: Abdominal venous thrombosis in neonates and infants: Role of prothrombotic risk factors—A multicentre case-control study. Br J Haematol 111:534–539, 2000.

68. Zigman A, Yazbeck S, Emil S, et al: Renal vein thrombosis: A 10-year review. J Pediatr Surg 35:1540–1542, 2000.

69. Harris RC, Ismail N: Extrarenal complications of the nephrotic syndrome. Am J Kidney Dis 23:477–497, 1994.

70. Valasquez F, Garcia P, Ruiz M: Idiopathic nephrotic syndrome of the adult with asymptomatic thrombosis of the renal vein. Am J Nephrol 8:457–462, 1988.

71. Giustacchini P, Pisanti F, Citterio F, et al: Renal vein thrombosis after renal transplantation: An important cause of graft loss. Transplant Proc 34:2126–2127, 2002.

72. Kitchens CS: Thrombotic storm: When thrombosis begets thrombosis. Am J Med 104:381–385, 1998.

73. Markowitz GS, Brignol F, Burns ER, et al: Renal vein thrombosis treated with thrombolytic therapy: Case report and brief review. Am J Kidney Dis 25:801–806, 1995.

74. Lam KK, Lui CC: Successful treatment of acute inferior vena cava and unilateral renal vein thrombosis by local infusion of recombinant tissue plasminogen activator. Am J Kidney Dis 32:1075–1079, 1998.

75. Etoh Y, Ohsawa I, Fujita T, et al: Nephrotic syndrome with portal, splenic and renal vein thrombosis: A case report. Nephron 92:680–684, 2002.

76. Kanagasundaram NS, Bandyopadhyay D, Brownjohn AM, et al: The diagnosis of renal vein thrombosis by magnetic resonance angiography. Nephrol Dial Transplant 13:200–202, 1998.

77. Janssen HL, Garcia-Pagan JC, Elias E, et al: Budd-Chiari syndrome: A review by an expert panel. J Hepatol 38:364–371, 2003.

78. Wang Z, Jones R: Budd-Chiari syndrome. Curr Probl Surg 33:83–211, 1996.

79. Osler W: Case of obliteration of vena cava inferior, with great stenosis of orifices of hepatic veins. J Anat Physiol 13:291–294, 1878.

80. Dilawari JB, Bambery P, Chawla Y, et al: Hepatic outflow obstruction (Budd-Chiari syndrome): Experience with 177 patients and a review of the literature. Medicine (Baltimore) 73:21–36, 1994.

81. Okuda K, Kage M, Shrestha SM: Proposal of a new nomenclature for Budd-Chiari syndrome: Hepatic vein thrombosis versus thrombosis of the inferior vena cava at its hepatic portion. Hepatology 28:1191–1198, 1998.

82. Valla D, Benhamou JP: Obstruction of the hepatic veins or suprahepatic inferior vena cava. Dig Dis 14:99–118, 1996.

83. Min AD, Atillasoy EO, Schwartz ME, et al: Reassessing the role of medical therapy in the management of hepatic vein thrombosis. Liver Transpl Surg 3:423–429, 1997.

84. Maddrey WC: Hepatic vein thrombosis (Budd-Chiari syndrome). Hepatology 4 (suppl 1): 44S–46S, 1984.

85. Valla D, Dhumeaux D, Babany G, et al: Hepatic vein thrombosis in paroxysmal nocturnal hemoglobinuria: A spectrum from asymptomatic occlusion of hepatic venules to fatal Budd-Chiari syndrome. Gastroenterology 93:569–575, 1987.

86. Gentil-Kocher S, Bernard O, Brunelle F, et al: Budd-Chiari syndrome in children: Report of 22 cases. J Pediatr 113:30–38, 1988.

87. Nakamura H, Uehara H, Okada T, et al: Occlusion of small hepatic veins associated with systemic lupus erythematosus with the lupus anticoagulant and anti-cardiolipin antibody. Hepatogastroenterology 36:393–397, 1989.

87a. Ziakas PD, Poulou LS, Rokas GI, et al: Thrombosis in paroxysmal nocturnal hemoglobinuria: Sites, risks, outcome: An overview. J Thromb Haemost 5:642–645, 2007.

87b. Patel RK, Lea NC, Heneghan MA, et al: Prevalence of the activating JAK2 tyrosine kinase mutation V617F in the Budd-Chiari syndrome. Gastroenterology 130:2031–2038, 2006.

87c. De Stefano V, Fiorini A, Rossi E, et al: Incidence of the JAK2 V617F mutation among patients with splanchnic or cerebral venous thrombosis and without overt chronic myeloproliferative disorders. J Thromb Haemost 5:708–714, 2007.

88. Pelletier S, Landi B, Piette JC, et al: Antiphospholipid syndrome as the second cause of non-tumorous Budd-Chiari syndrome. J Hepatol 21:76–80, 1994.

89. Mahmoud A, Elias E: New approaches to the Budd-Chiari syndrome. J Gastroenterol Hepatol 11:1121–1123, 1996.

90. Menon KV, Shah V, Kamath PS: The Budd-Chiari syndrome. N Engl J Med 350:578–585, 2004.

91. Mohanty D, Shetty S, Ghosh K, et al: Hereditary thrombophilia as a cause of Budd-Chiari syndrome: A study from Western India. Hepatology 34:666–670, 2001.

92. Janssen HL, Meinardi JR, Vleggaar FP, et al: Factor V Leiden mutation, prothrombin gene mutation, and deficiencies in coagulation inhibitors associated with Budd-Chiari syndrome and portal vein thrombosis: Results of a case-control study. Blood 96:2364–2368, 2000.

93. Olzinski AT, Sanyal AJ: Treating Budd-Chiari Syndrome: Making rational choices from a myriad of options. J Clin Gastroenterol 30:155–161, 2000.

94. Langnas AN: Budd-Chiari syndrome: Decisions, decisions. Liver Transpl Surg 3:443–445, 1997.

95. Raju GS, Felver M, Olin JW, et al: Thrombolysis for acute Budd-Chiari syndrome: Case report and literature review. Am J Gastroenterol 91:1262–1263, 1996.

95a. Kuo GP, Brodsky RA, Kim HS: Catheter-directed thrombolysis and thrombectomy for the Budd-Chiari syndrome in paroxysmal nocturnal hemoglobinuria in three patients. J Vasc Interv Radiol 17: 383–387, 2006.

96. Campbell DA Jr, Rolles K, Jamieson N, et al: Hepatic transplantation with perioperative and long term anticoagulation as treatment for Budd-Chiari syndrome. Surg Gynecol Obstet 166:511–518, 1988.

97. Orloff MJ, Daily PO, Orloff SL, et al: A 27-year experience with surgical treatment of Budd-Chiari syndrome. Ann Surg 232:340–352, 2000.

98. Kavanagh PM, Roberts J, Gibney R, et al: Acute Budd-Chiari syndrome with liver failure: The experience of a policy of initial interventional radiological treatment using transjugular intrahepatic portosystemic shunt. J Gastroenterol Hepatol 19:1135–1139, 2004.

99. Rossle M, Olschewski M, Siegerstetter V, et al: The Budd-Chiari syndrome: Outcome after treatment with the transjugular intrahepatic portosystemic shunt. Surgery 135:394–403, 2004.

100. Mancuso A, Fung K, Mela M, et al: TIPS for acute and chronic Budd-Chiari syndrome: A single-centre experience. J Hepatol 38:751–754, 2003.

101. Xu PQ, Ma XX, Ye XX, et al: Surgical treatment of 1360 cases of Budd-Chiari syndrome: 20-year experience. Hepatobiliary Pancreat Dis Int 3:391–394, 2004.

102. Allroggen H, Abbott RJ: Cerebral venous sinus thrombosis. Postgrad Med J 76:12–15, 2000.

103. Stam J: Thrombosis of the cerebral veins and sinuses. N Engl J Med 352:1791–1798, 2005.

104. Gates P, Barnett H: Venous disease: Cortical veins and sinuses. In Barnett H, Stein B, and Mohr J, (eds): Stroke: Pathophysiology, Diagnosis, and Management. New York, Churchill Livingstone, 1986.

105. Krayenbuhl HA: Cerebral venous and sinus thrombosis. Clin Neurosurg 14:1–24, 1966.

106. Ferro JM, Canhao P, Stam J, et al: Prognosis of cerebral vein and dural sinus thrombosis: Results of the International Study on Cerebral Vein and Dural Sinus Thrombosis (ISCVT). Stroke 35:664–670, 2004.

107. Ferro JM, Lopes MG, Rosas MJ, et al: Long-term prognosis of cerebral vein and dural sinus thrombosis: Results of the VENOPORT study. Cerebrovasc Dis 13:272–278, 2002.

108. Ferro JM, Canhao P, Bousser MG, et al: Cerebral vein and dural sinus thrombosis in elderly patients. Stroke 36:1927–1932, 2005.

109. Southwick FS: Septic thrombophlebitis of major dural venous sinuses. Curr Clin Top Infect Dis 15:179–203, 1995.

110. Martinelli I, Sacchi E, Landi G, et al: High risk of cerebral-vein thrombosis in carriers of a prothrombin-gene mutation and in users of oral contraceptives. N Engl J Med 338:1793–1797, 1998.

111. Martinelli I, Landi G, Merati G, et al: Factor V gene mutation is a risk factor for cerebral venous thrombosis. Thromb Haemost 75:393–394, 1996.

112. Zuber M, Toulon P, Marnet L, et al: Factor V Leiden mutation in cerebral venous thrombosis. Stroke 27:1721–1723, 1996.

113. Reschiens M: Coagulation studies, factor V Leiden, and anticardiolipin antibodies in 40 cases of cerebral venous thrombosis. Stroke 27:1724–1730, 1996.

114. Masuhr F, Mehraein S, Einhaupl K: Cerebral venous and sinus thrombosis. J Neurol 251:11–23, 2004.

115. Weih M, Junge-Hulsing J, Mehraein S, et al: Hereditary thrombophilia with ischemic stroke and sinus thrombosis: Diagnosis, therapy and meta-analysis. Nervenarzt 71:936–945, 2000.

116. Gadelha T, Andre C, Juca AA, et al: Prothrombin 20210A and oral contraceptive use as risk factor for cerebral venous thrombosis. Cerebrovasc Dis 19:49–52, 2004.

117. Ventura P, Cobelli M, Marietta M, et al: Hyperhomocysteinemia and other newly recognized inherited coagulation disorders (factor V Leiden and prothrombin gene mutation) in patients with idiopathic cerebral vein thrombosis. Cerebrovasc Dis 17:153–159, 2004.

117a. Dentali F, Crowther M, Ageno W: Thrombophilic abnormalities, oral contraceptives, and risk of cerebral vein thrombosis: A meta-analysis. Blood 107:2766–2773, 2006.

118. Martinelli I, Battaglioli T, Pedotti P, et al: Hyperhomocysteinemia in cerebral vein thrombosis. Blood 102:1363–1366, 2003.

119. Heller C, Heinecke A, Junker R, et al: Cerebral venous thrombosis in children. Circulation 108:1362–1367, 2003.

120. Parnass SM, Goodwin JA, Patel DV, et al: Dural sinus thrombosis: A mechanism for pseudotumor cerebri in systemic lupus erythematosus. J Rheumatol 14:152–155, 1987.

121. Uziel Y, Laxer RM, Blaser S, et al: Cerebral vein thrombosis in childhood systemic lupus erythematosus. J Pediatr 126:722–727, 1995.

122. Crawford SC, Digre KB, Palmer CA, et al: Thrombosis of the deep venous drainage of the brain in adults: Analysis of seven cases with review of the literature. Arch Neurol 52:1101–1108, 1995.

123. Madan A, Sluzewski M, van Rooij WJ, et al: Thrombosis of the deep cerebral veins: CT and MRI findings with pathologic correlation. Neuroradiology 39:777–780, 1997.

124. Erbguth F, Brenner P, Schuierer G, et al: Diagnosis and treatment of deep cerebral vein thrombosis. Neurosurg Rev 14:145–148, 1991.

125. Bousser MG, Chiras J, Bories J, et al: Cerebral venous thrombosis: A review of 38 cases. Stroke 16:199–213, 1985.

126. Einhaupl KM, Villringer A, Meister W, et al: Heparin treatment in sinus venous thrombosis. Lancet 338:597–600, 1991.

127. Benamer HT, Bone I: Cerebral venous thrombosis: Anticoagulants or thrombolytic therapy? J Neurol Neurosurg Psychiatry 69:427–430, 2000

128. DeBruijn SF, Stam J: Randomized, placebo-controlled trial of anticoagulant treatment with low-molecular-weight heparin for cerebral sinus thrombosis. Stroke 30:484–488, 1999.

129. Stam J, DeBruijn SF, DeVeber G: Anticoagulation for cerebral sinus thrombosis. Cochrane Database Syst Rev 4:CD002005, 2002.

130. Stam J, DeBruijn S, deVeber G: Anticoagulation for cerebral sinus thrombosis. Stroke 34:1054–1055, 2003.

130a. Dentali F, Gianni M, Crowther MA, et al: Natural history of cerebral vein thrombosis: A systematic review. Blood 108:1129–1134, 2006.

131. Ciccone A, Canhao P, Falcao F, et al: Thrombolysis for cerebral vein and dural sinus thrombosis. Cochrane Database Syst Rev 1: CD003693, 2004.

132. Canhao P, Falcao F, Ferro JM: Thrombolytics for cerebral sinus thrombosis: A systematic review. Cerebrovasc Dis 15:159–166, 2003.

133. Williamson TH: Central retinal vein occlusion: What's the story? Br J Ophthalmol 81:698–704, 1997

134. Hunt BJ: Activated protein C and retinal vein occlusion. Br J Ophthalmol 80:194, 1996.

135. Dunn JP, Noorily SW, Petri M, et al: Antiphospholipid antibodies and retinal vascular disease. Lupus 5:313–322, 1996.

136. Williams GA, Sarrafizadeh R: Antiphospholipid antibodies and retinal thrombosis in patients without risk factors: A prospective case-control study. Am J Ophthalmol 130:538–539, 2000.

137. Janssen MC, den Heijer M, Cruysberg JR, et al: Retinal vein occlusion: A form of venous thrombosis or a complication of atherosclerosis? A meta-analysis of thrombophilic factors. Thromb Haemost 93:1021–1026, 2005.

138. DeMoerloose P, Bounameaux HR, Mannucci PM: Screening test for thrombophilic patients: Which tests, for which patient, by whom, when, and why? Semin Thromb Hemost 24:321–327, 1998

139. Prince HM, Thurlow PJ, Buchanan RC, et al: Acquired protein S deficiency in a patient with systemic lupus erythematosus causing central retinal vein thrombosis. J Clin Pathol 48:387–389, 1995.

140. Glueck CJ, Bell H, Vadlamani L, et al: Heritable thrombophilia and hypofibrinolysis: Possible causes of retinal vein occlusion. Arch Ophthalmol 117:43–49, 1999.

141. Abu El-Asrar AM, Al Momen AK, Amro S, et al: Prothrombotic states associated with retinal venous occlusion in young adults. Int Ophthalmol 20:197–204, 1996.

142. Linna T, Ylikorkala A, Kontula K, et al: Prevalence of factor V Leiden in young adults with retinal vein occlusion. Thromb Haemost 77:214–216, 1997.

143. Albisinni R, Coppola A, Loffredo M, et al: Retinal vein occlusion and inherited conditions predisposing to thrombophilia. Thromb Haemost 80:702–703, 1998.

144. Greiner K, Hafner G, Dick B, et al: Retinal vascular occlusion and deficiencies in the protein C pathway. Am J Ophthalmol 128:69–74, 1999.

145. Albisinni R, Coppola A, Loffredo M, et al: Retinal vein occlusion and inherited conditions predisposing to thrombophilia. Thromb Haemost 80:702–703, 1998.

146. Williamson TH, Rumley A, Lowe GD: Blood viscosity, coagulation, and activated protein C resistance in central retinal vein occlusion: A population controlled study. Br J Ophthalmol 80:203–208, 1996.

147. Larsson J, Olafsdottir E, Bauer B: Activated protein C resistance in young adults with central retinal vein occlusion. Br J Ophthalmol 80:200–202, 1996.

148. Ciardella AP, Yannuzzi LA, Freund KB, et al: Factor V Leiden, activated protein C resistance, and retinal vein occlusion. Retina 18:308–315, 1998.

149. Yesim F, Demirci K, Guney D, et al: Prevalence of factor V Leiden in patients with retinal vein occlusion. Acta Ophthalmol Scand 77:631–633, 1999.

150. Cruciani F, Moramarco A, Curto T, et al: MTHFR C677T mutation, factor II G20210A mutation and factor V Leiden as risks factor for youth retinal vein occlusion. Clin Ter 154:299–303, 2003.

151. Kalayci D, Gurgey A, Guven D, et al: Factor V Leiden and prothrombin 20210 A mutations in patients with central and branch retinal vein occlusion. Acta Ophthalmol Scand 77:622–624, 1999.

152. Scott JA, Arnold JJ, Currie JM, et al: No excess of factor V:Q506 genotype but high prevalence of anticardiolipin antibodies without antiendothelial cell antibodies in retinal vein occlusion in young patients. Ophthalmologica 215:217–221, 2001.

153. Guven D, Sayinalp N, Kalayci D, et al: Risk factors in central retinal vein occlusion and activated protein C resistance. Eur J Ophthalmol 9:43–48, 1999.

154. Larsson J, Sellman A, Bauer B: Activated protein C resistance in patients with central retinal vein occlusion. Br J Ophthalmol 81:832–834, 1997.

155. Fegan CD: Central retinal vein occlusion and thrombophilia. Eye 16:98–106, 2002.

156. Gottlieb JL, Blice JP, Mestichelli B, et al: Activated protein C resistance, factor V Leiden, and central retinal vein occlusion in young adults. Arch Ophthalmol 116:577–579, 1998.

157. Delahousse B, Arsene S, Piquemal R, et al: The 20210A allele of the prothrombin gene is not a risk factor for retinal vein occlusion. Blood Coagul Fibrinolysis 9:447–448, 1998.

158. Greiner K, Peetz D, Winken A, et al: Genetic thrombophilia in patients with retinal vascular occlusion. Intern Ophthalmol 23:155–160, 2001.

159. Weger M, Renner W, Pinter O, et al: Role of factor V Leiden and prothrombin 20210A in patients with retinal artery occlusion. Eye 17:731–734, 2003.

160. Yildirim C, Yaylali V, Tatlipinar S, et al: Hyperhomocysteinemia: A risk factor for retinal vein occlusion. Ophthalmologica 218:102–106, 2004.

161. Larsson J, Hultberg B, Hillarp A: Hyperhomocysteinemia and the MTHFR C677T mutation in central retinal vein occlusion. Acta Ophthalmol Scand 78:340–343, 2000.

162. Boyd S, Owens D, Gin T, et al: Plasma homocysteine, methylene tetrahydrofolate reductase C677T and factor II G20210A polymorphisms, factor VIII, and VWF in central retinal vein occlusion. Br J Ophthalmol 85:1313–1315, 2001.

163. DeBruijne EL, Keulen-de Vos GH, Ouwendijk RJ: Ocular venous occlusion and hyperhomocysteinemia. Ann Intern Med 130:78, 1999.

164. Weger M, Stanger O, Deutschmann H, et al: The role of hyperhomocysteinemia and methylenetetrahydrofolate reductase (MTHFR) C677T mutation in patients with retinal artery occlusion. Am J Ophthalmol 134:57–61, 2002.

165. Marcucci R, Bertini L, Giusti B, et al: Thrombophilic risk factors in patients with central retinal vein occlusion. Thromb Haemost 86:772–776, 2001.

166. Vine AK: Hyperhomocysteinemia: A risk factor for central retinal vein occlusion. Am J Ophthalmol 129:640–644, 2000.

167. Brown BA, Marx JL, Ward TP, et al: Homocysteine: A risk factor for retinal venous occlusive disease. Ophthalmology 109:287–290, 2002.

168. Weger M, Stanger O, Deutschmann H, et al: Hyperhomocyst(e)inemia, but not methylenetetrahydrofolate reductase C677T mutation, as a risk factor in branch retinal vein occlusion. Ophthalmology 109:1105–1109, 2002.

169. Parodi MB, Di Crecchio L: Hyperhomocysteinemia in central retinal vein occlusion in young adults. Semin Ophthalmol 18:154–159, 2003.

170. Salomon O, Huna-Baron R, Moisseiev J, et al: Thrombophilia as a cause for central and branch retinal artery occlusion in patients without an apparent embolic source. Eye 15:511–514, 2001.

171. Ingerslev J: Thrombophilia: A feature of importance in retinal vein thrombosis. Acta Ophthalmol Scand 77:619–621, 1999.

172. Adamczuk YP, Iglesias Varela ML, Martinuzzo ME, et al: Central retinal vein occlusion and thrombophilia risk factors. Blood Coagul Fibrinolysis 13:623–626, 2002.

172a. Palmowski-Wolfe AM, Denninger E, Geisel J, et al: Antiphospholipid antibodies in ocular arterial and venous occlusive disease. Ophthalmologica 221:41–46, 2007.

173. Greaves M: Aging and the pathogenesis of retinal vein thrombosis. Br J Ophthalmol 81:810–811, 1997.

174. Chak M, Wallace GR, Graham EM, et al: Thrombophilia: Genetic polymorphisms and their association with retinal vascular occlusive disease. Br J Ophthalmol 85:883–886, 2001.

175. Hayreh SS: Management of central retinal vein occlusion. Ophthalmologica 217:167–188, 2003.

176. Giorgi D, Gabrieli CB, Bonomo L: The clinico-ophthalmological spectrum of antiphospholipid syndrome. Ocul Immunol Inflamm 6:269–273, 1998.

177. Wiechens B, Schroder JO, Potzsch B, et al: Primary antiphospholipid antibody syndrome and retinal occlusive vasculopathy. Am J Ophthalmol 123:848–850, 1997.

178. Prisco D, Marcucci R: Retinal vein thrombosis: Risk factors, pathogenesis and therapeutic approach. Pathophysiol Haemost Thromb 32:308–311, 2002.

179. Recchia FM, Carvalho-Recchia CA, Hassan TS: Clinical course of younger patients with central retinal vein occlusion. Arch Ophthalmol 122:317–321, 2004.

III

180. Hattenbach LO, Steinkamp G, Scharrer I, et al: Fibrinolytic therapy with low-dose recombinant tissue plasminogen activator in retinal vein occlusion. Ophthalmologica 212:394–398, 1998.

181. Elman MJ: Thrombolytic therapy for central retinal vein occlusion: Results of a pilot study. Trans Am Ophthalmol Soc 94:471–504, 1996.

182. Schmidt DP, Schulte-Monting J, Schumacher M: Prognosis of central retinal artery occlusion: Local intraarterial fibrinolysis versus conservative treatment. Am J Neuroradiol 23:1301–1307, 2002.

183. Lahey JM, Kearney JJ, Cheung MC: Sequential treatment of central retinal vein occlusion with intravitreal tissue plasminogen activator and intravitreal triamcinolone. Br J Ophthalmol 88:1100–1101, 2004.

184. Weiss JN, Bynoe LA: Injection of tissue plasminogen activator into a branch retinal vein in eyes with central retinal vein occlusion. Ophthalmology 108:2249–2257, 2001.

185. Hendler MF, Meschengieser SS, Blanco AN, et al: Primary upper-extremity deep vein thrombosis: High prevalence of thrombophilic defects. Am J Hematol 76:330–337, 2004.

186. Mustafa S, Stein PD, Patel KC, et al: Upper extremity deep venous thrombosis. Chest 123:1953–1956, 2003.

187. Martinelli I, Cattaneo M, Panzeri D, et al: Risk factors for deep venous thrombosis of the upper extremities. Ann Intern Med 126:707–711, 1997.

188. Martinelli I, Cattaneo M, Taioli E, et al: Genetic risk factors for superficial vein thrombosis. Thromb Haemost 82:1215–1217, 1999.

189. Joffe HV, Goldhaber SZ: Upper-extremity deep vein thrombosis. Circulation 106:1874–1880, 2002.

190. Painter TD, Karpf M: Deep venous thrombosis of the upper extremity: Five years experience at a university hospital. Angiology 35:743–749, 1984.

191. Becker DM, Philbrick JT, Walker FB: Axillary and subclavian venous thrombosis: Prognosis and treatment. Arch Intern Med 151:1934–1943, 1991.

192. Lindblad B, Tengborn L, Bergqvist D: Deep vein thrombosis of the axillary-subclavian veins: Epidemiologic data, effects of different types of treatment and late sequelae. Eur J Vasc Surg 2:161–165, 1988.

193. Kommareddy A, Zaroukian MH, Hassouna HI: Upper extremity deep venous thrombosis. Semin Thromb Hemost 28:89–99, 2002.

194. Martinelli I, Battaglioli T, Bucciarelli P, et al: Risk factors and recurrence rate of primary deep vein thrombosis of the upper extremities. Circulation 110:566–570, 2004.

195. Leebeek FW, Stadhouders NA, van Stein D, et al: Hypercoagulability states in upper-extremity deep venous thrombosis. Am J Hematol 67:15–19, 2001.

196. Marinella MA, Kathula SK, Markert RJ: Spectrum of upper-extremity deep venous thrombosis in a community teaching hospital. Heart Lung 29:113–117, 2000.

197. Joffe HV, Kucher N, Tapson VF, et al: Upper-extremity deep vein thrombosis: A prospective registry of 592 patients. Circulation 110:1605–1611, 2004.

198. Heron E, Lozinguez O, Alhenc-Gelas M, et al: Hypercoagulable states in primary upper-extremity deep vein thrombosis. Arch Intern Med 160:382–386, 2000.

199. Schmittling ZC, McLafferty RB, Bohannon WT, et al: Characterization and probability of upper extremity deep venous thrombosis. Ann Vasc Surg 18:552–557, 2004.

200. Hurlbert SN, Rutherford RB: Primary subclavian-axillary vein thrombosis. Ann Vasc Surg 9:217–223, 1995.

201. Shah MK, Burke DT, Shah SH: Upper-extremity deep vein thrombosis. South Med J 96:669–672, 2003.

202. Timsit JF, Farkas JC, Boyer JM, et al: Central vein catheter-related thrombosis in intensive care patients: Incidence, risks factors, and relationship with catheter-related sepsis. Chest 114:207–213, 1998.

203. Birdwell BG, Yeager R, Whitsett TL: Pseudotumor cerebri: A complication of catheter-induced subclavian vein thrombosis. Arch Intern Med 154:808–811, 1994.

204. Ameli FM, Minas T, Weiss M, et al: Consequences of "conservative" conventional management of axillary vein thrombosis. Can J Surg 30:167–169, 1987.

205. Druy EM, Trout HH III, Giordano JM, et al: Lytic therapy in the treatment of axillary and subclavian vein thrombosis. J Vasc Surg 2:821–827, 1985.

206. Wilson JJ, Zahn CA, Newman H: Fibrinolytic therapy for idiopathic subclavian-axillary vein thrombosis. Am J Surg 159:208–210, 1990.

207. Hicken GJ, Ameli FM: Management of subclavian-axillary vein thrombosis: A review. Can J Surg 41:13–25, 1998.

208. Malcynski J, O'Donnell TF Jr, Mackey WC, et al: Long-term results of treatment for axillary subclavian vein thrombosis. Can J Surg 36:365–371, 1993.

209. Azakie A, McElhinney DB, Thompson RW, et al: Surgical management of subclavian-vein effort thrombosis as a result of thoracic outlet compression. J Vasc Surg 28:777–786, 1998.

209a. Bernardi E, Pesavento R, Prandoni P: Upper extremity deep venous thrombosis. Semin Thromb Hemost 32:729–736, 2006.

210. Heron E, Lozinguez O, Emmerich J, et al: Long-term sequelae of spontaneous axillary-subclavian venous thrombosis. Ann Intern Med 131:510–513, 1999.

211. Bern MM, Lokich JJ, Wallach SR, et al: Very low doses of warfarin can prevent thrombosis in central venous catheters: A randomized prospective trial. Ann Intern Med 112:423–428, 1990.

212. Monreal M, Alastrue A, Rull M, et al: Upper extremity deep venous thrombosis in cancer patients with venous access devices: Prophylaxis with a low molecular weight heparin (Fragmin). Thromb Haemost 75:251–253, 1996.

213. Mismetti P, Mille D, Laporte S, et al: Low-molecular-weight heparin (nadroparin) and very low doses of warfarin in the prevention of upper extremity thrombosis in cancer patients with indwelling long-term central venous catheters: A pilot randomized trial. Haematologica 88:67–73, 2003.

214. Geerts WH, Pineo GF, Heit JA, et al: Prevention of venous thromboembolism: The Seventh ACCP Conference on Antithrombotic and Thrombolytic Therapy. Chest 126:338S–400S, 2004.

215. Karthaus M, Kretzschmar A, Kroning H, et al: Dalteparin for prevention of catheter-related complications in cancer patients with central venous catheters: Final results of a double-blind, placebo-controlled phase III trial. Ann Oncol 17:289–296, 2006.

216. Lemierre A: Septicaemias and anaerobic organisms. Lancet 1:701–703, 1936.

217. Riordan T, Wilson M: Lemierre's syndrome: More than a historical curiosa. Postgrad Med J 80:328–334, 2004.

218. Chirinos JA, Lichtstein DM, Garcia J, et al: The evolution of Lemierre syndrome: Report of 2 cases and review of the literature. Medicine (Baltimore) 81:458–465, 2002.

219. Lustig LR, Cusick BC, Cheung SW, et al: Lemierre's syndrome: Two cases of postanginal sepsis. Otolaryngol Head Neck Surg 112:767–772, 1995.

220. Seagle MB, Bingham HG: Purpura fulminans. Ann Plast Surg 20:576–581, 1988.

221. Smith OP, White B: Infectious purpura fulminans: Diagnosis and treatment. Br J Haematol 104:202–207, 1999.

222. Darmstadt GL: Acute infectious purpura fulminans: Pathogenesis and medical management. Pediatr Dermatol 15:169–183, 1998.

223. Bergmann F, Hoyer PF, D'Angelo SV, et al: Severe autoimmune protein S deficiency in a boy with idiopathic purpura fulminans. Br J Haematol 89:610–614, 1995.

224. Moreb J, Kitchens CS: Acquired functional protein S deficiency, cerebral venous thrombosis, and coumarin skin necrosis in association with antiphospholipid syndrome: Report of two cases. Am J Med 87:207–210, 1989.

225. DeFranzo AJ, Marasco P, Argenta LC: Warfarin-induced necrosis of the skin. Ann Plast Surg 34:203–208, 1995.

226. Goldberg SL, Orthner CL, Yalisove BL, et al: Skin necrosis following prolonged administration of coumarin in a patient with inherited protein S deficiency. Am J Hematol 38:64–66, 1991.

227. Dominey A, Kettler A, Yiannias J, et al: Purpura fulminans and transient protein C and S deficiency. Arch Dermatol 124:1442–1443, 1988.

228. Madden RM, Gill JC, Marlar RA: Protein C and protein S levels in two patients with acquired purpura fulminans. Br J Haematol 75:112–117, 1990.

229. Draelos ZK, Hansen RC: Hemorrhagic bullae in an anemic woman: Paroxysmal nocturnal hemoglobinuria (PNH). Arch Dermatol 122:1326–1330, 1986.

230. Rietschel RL, Lewis CW, Simmons RA, et al: Skin lesions in paroxysmal nocturnal hemoglobinuria. Arch Dermatol 114:560–563, 1978.

231. Marlar RA, Montgomery RR, Broekmans AW: Diagnosis and treatment of homozygous protein C deficiency: Report of the Working Party on Homozygous Protein C Deficiency of the Subcommittee on Protein C and Protein S, International Committee on Thrombosis and Haemostasis. J Pediatr 114:528–534, 1989.

232. Alessi MC, Aillaud MF, Paut O, et al: Purpura fulminans in a patient homozygous for a mutation in the protein C gene: Prenatal diagnosis in a subsequent pregnancy. Thromb Haemost 75:525–526, 1996.

16

233. Soria JM, Morell M, Jimenez-Astorga C, et al: Severe type I protein C deficiency in a compound heterozygote for Y124C and Q132X mutations in exon 6 of the PROC gene. Thromb Haemost 74:1215–1220, 1995.

234. Pung-Amritt P, Poort SR, Vos HL, et al: Compound heterozygosity for one novel and one recurrent mutation in a Thai patient with severe protein S deficiency. Thromb Haemost 81:189–192, 1999.

235. Jackson RT, Luplow RE III: Adult purpura fulminans and digital necrosis associated with sepsis and the factor V mutation. JAMA 280:1829–1830, 1998.

236. Woods CR, Johnson CA: Varicella purpura fulminans associated with heterozygosity for factor V leiden and transient protein S deficiency. Pediatrics 102:1208–1210, 1998.

237. Gurgey A: Clinical manifestations in thrombotic children with factor V Leiden mutation. Pediatr Hematol Oncol 16:233–237, 1999.

238. Pipe SW, Schmaier AH, Nichols WC, et al: Neonatal purpura fulminans in association with factor V R506Q mutation. J Pediatr 128:706–709, 1996.

239. Inbal A, Kenet G, Zivelin A, et al: Purpura fulminans induced by disseminated intravascular coagulation following infection in 2 unrelated children with double heterozygosity for factor V Leiden and protein S deficiency. Thromb Haemost 77:1086–1089, 1997.

240. Dogan Y, Aygun D, Yilmaz Y, et al: Severe protein S deficiency associated with heterozygous factor V Leiden mutation in a child with purpura fulminans. Pediatr Hematol Oncol 20:1–5, 2003.

241. Ozbek N, Atac FB, Verdi H, et al: Purpura fulminans in a child with combined heterozygous prothrombin G20210A and factor V Leiden mutations. Ann Hematol 82:118–120, 2003.

242. Manco-Johnson MJ, Nuss R, Key N, et al: Lupus anticoagulant and protein S deficiency in children with postvaricella purpura fulminans or thrombosis. J Pediatr 128:319–323, 1996.

243. Sackesen C, Secmeer G, Gurgey A, et al: Homozygous factor V Leiden mutation in a child with meningococcal purpura fulminans. Pediatr Infect Dis J 17:87, 1998.

244. Westendorp RG, Reitsma PH, Bertina RM: Inherited prethrombotic disorders and infectious purpura. Thromb Haemost 75:899–901, 1996.

245. Rintala E, Seppala OP, Kotilainen P, et al: Protein C in the treatment of coagulopathy in meningococcal disease. Crit Care Med 26:965–968, 1998.

246. Smith OP, White B, Vaughan D, et al: Use of protein-C concentrate, heparin, and haemodiafiltration in meningococcus-induced purpura fulminans. Lancet 350:1590–1593, 1997.

247. Aiuto LT, Barone SR, Cohen PS, et al: Recombinant tissue plasminogen activator restores perfusion in meningococcal purpura fulminans. Crit Care Med 25:1079–1082, 1997.

248. Brown DL, Greenhalgh DG, Warden GD: Purpura fulminans: A disease best managed in a burn center. J Burn Care Rehabil 19:119–123, 1998.

249. Muller FM, Ehrenthal W, Hafner G, et al: Purpura fulminans in severe congenital protein C deficiency: Monitoring of treatment with protein C concentrate. Eur J Pediatr 155:20–25, 1996.

250. Sanz-Rodriguez C, Gil-Fernandez JJ, Zapater P, et al: Long-term management of homozygous protein C deficiency: Replacement therapy with subcutaneous purified protein C concentrate. Thromb Haemost 81:887–890, 1999.

251. Ballem P: Acquired thrombophilia in pregnancy. Semin Thromb Hemost 24 (suppl 1): 41–47 1998.

252. Witlin AG, Sibai BM: Postpartum ovarian vein thrombosis after vaginal delivery: A report of 11 cases. Obstet Gynecol 85:775–780, 1995.

253. Witlin AG, Mercer BM, Sibai BM: Septic pelvic thrombophlebitis or refractory postpartum fever of undetermined etiology. J Matern Fetal Med 5:355–358, 1996.

254. Twickler DM, Setiawan AT, Evans RS, et al: Imaging of puerperal septic thrombophlebitis: Prospective comparison of MR imaging, CT, and sonography. Am J Roentgenol 169:1039–1043, 1997.

255. Josey WE, Staggers SR Jr: Heparin therapy in septic pelvic thrombophlebitis: A study of 46 cases. Am J Obstet Gynecol 120:228–233, 1974.

256. Brown CE, Stettler RW, Twickler D, et al: Puerperal septic pelvic thrombophlebitis: Incidence and response to heparin therapy. Am J Obstet Gynecol 181:143–148, 1999.

257. Isada NB, Landy HJ, Larsen JW Jr: Postabortal septic pelvic thrombophlebitis diagnosed with computed tomography: A case report. J Reprod Med 32:866–868, 1987.

258. Munsick RA, Gillanders LA: A review of the syndrome of puerperal ovarian vein thrombophlebitis. Obstet Gynecol Surv 36:57–66, 1981.

259. Melissari E, Kakkar VV: Congenital severe protein C deficiency in adults. Br J Haematol 72:222–228, 1989.

260. Giraud JR, Poulain P, Renaud-Giono A, et al: Diagnosis of postpartum ovarian vein thrombophlebitis by color Doppler ultrasonography: About 10 cases. Acta Obstet Gynecol Scand 76:773–778, 1997.

261. Salomon O, Apter S, Shaham D, et al: Risk factors associated with postpartum ovarian vein thrombosis. Thromb Haemost 82:1015–1019, 1999.

261a. Wysokinska EM, Hodge D, McBane RD 2nd: Ovarian vein thrombosis: Incidence of recurrent venous thromboembolism and survival. Thromb Haemost 96:126–131, 2006.

262. Simons GR, Piwnica-Worms DR, Goldhaber SZ: Ovarian vein thrombosis. Am Heart J 126:641–647, 1993.

263. Asherson RA, Hughes GR: Hypoadrenalism, Addison's disease and antiphospholipid antibodies. J Rheumatol 18:1–3, 1991.

264. Warkentin TE: Clinical presentation of heparin-induced thrombocytopenia. Semin Hematol 35:9–16, 1998.

265. Caron P, Chabannier MH, Cambus JP, et al: Definitive adrenal insufficiency due to bilateral adrenal hemorrhage and primary antiphospholipid syndrome. J Clin Endocrinol Metab 83:1437–1439, 1998.

266. Pandolfi C, Gianini A, Fregoni V, et al: Hypopituitarism and antiphospholipid syndrome. Minerva Endocrinol 22:103–105, 1997.

267. Kupferminc MJ: Thrombophilia and pregnancy. Reprod Biol Endocrinol 1:111, 2003.

268. Abbate R, Sofi F, Gensini F, et al: Thrombophilias as risk factors for disorders of pregnancy and fetal damage. Pathophysiol Haemost Thromb 32:318–321, 2002.

269. Brenner B: Thrombophilia and fetal loss. Semin Thromb Hemost 29:165–170, 2003.

270. Adelberg AM, Kuller JA: Thrombophilias and recurrent miscarriage. Obstet Gynecol Surv 57:703–709, 2002.

271. Kupferminc MJ, Eldor A, Steinman N, et al: Increased frequency of genetic thrombophilia in women with complications of pregnancy. N Engl J Med 340:9–13, 1999.

272. Rey E, Kahn SR, David M, Shrier I: Thrombophilic disorders and fetal loss: A meta-analysis. Lancet 361:901–908, 2003.

273. Vossen CY, Preston FE, Conard J, et al: Hereditary thrombophilia and fetal loss: A prospective follow-up study. J Thromb Haemost 2:592–596, 2004.

274. Kujovich JL: Thrombophilia and pregnancy complications. Am J Obstet Gynecol 191:412–424, 2004.

275. Brenner B, Sarig G, Weiner Z, et al: Thrombophilic polymorphisms are common in women with fetal loss without apparent cause. Thromb Haemost 82:6–9, 1999.

276. Gris JC, Quere I, Monpeyroux F, et al: Case-control study of the frequency of thrombophilic disorders in couples with late foetal loss and no thrombotic antecedent—The Nimes Obstetricians and Haematologists Study 5 (NOHA5). Thromb Haemost 81:891–899, 1999.

277. Rosendaal FR: Thrombosis in the young: Epidemiology and risk factors: A focus on venous thrombosis. Thromb Haemost 78:1–6, 1997.

278. Martinelli I, Taioli E, Cetin I, et al: Mutations in coagulation factors in women with unexplained late fetal loss. N Engl J Med 343:1015–1018, 2000.

279. Sanson BJ, Friederich PW, Simioni P, et al: The risk of abortion and stillbirth in antithrombin-, protein C-, and protein S-deficient women. Thromb Haemost 75:387–388, 1996.

280. Empson M, Lassere M, Craig JC, et al: Recurrent pregnancy loss with antiphospholipid antibody: A systematic review of therapeutic trials. Obstet Gynecol 99:135–144, 2002.

281. Rosone M, Tabsh K, Waserstrum N: Heparin therapy for pregnant women with lupus anticoagulant or anticardiolipin antibodies. Obstet Gynecol 75:630–634, 1990.

282. Brenner B, Hoffman R, Blumenfeld Z, et al: Gestational outcome in thrombophilic women with recurrent pregnancy loss treated by enoxaparin. Thromb Haemost 83:693–697, 2000.

Chapter 17

Prevention, Diagnosis, and Treatment of the Postphlebitic Syndrome

Reagan W. Quan, MD • David L. Gillespie, MD

INTRODUCTION/EPIDEMIOLOGY

The incidence of deep venous thrombosis (DVT) of the lower extremity is 250,000 cases per year, or 1 of 1000 persons in the United States annually.[1] The postphlebitic syndrome, consisting of persistent pain, edema, hyperpigmentation, induration of the skin, and stasis ulceration,[2] is a well-recognized complication of acute DVT, estimated to affect up to 4% of the general population.[3] The most likely cause of the postphlebitic syndrome is venous hypertension that results from outflow obstruction and venous reflux, causing damage to venous valves. This venous hypertension is then transmitted to the skin microcirculation, leading to tissue hypoxia and lymphatic obstruction.[4] Two thirds of patients with postphlebitic symptoms have evidence of a clinically or phlebographically proven DVT.[5] Five to ten years may be required for the postphlebitic syndrome to become evident, although in some studies, most cases were recognized within the first 2 years of the acute thrombotic event.[4] In one study of patients with acute DVT, 17% showed symptoms the first week after the acute episode; this increased to 37% after the first month and 69% after the first year.[5] Approximately 25% to 33% of individuals with a history of DVT remain asymptomatic over the long term.[3,6] Studies have reported that 67% to 80% of patients have symptoms and abnormal venous hemodynamics[7,8] after DVT.

The presence of abnormal venous hemodynamics, with incompetent valves and reflux on a chronic basis, constitutes chronic venous insufficiency (CVI). Over time, CVI may lead to the symptom complex that we know as postphlebitic syndrome. The terms *chronic venous insufficiency* and *postphlebitic syndrome* are often used interchangeably. However, the former term represents the pathophysiologic situation, and the latter is a complex of resultant symptoms.

The postphlebitic syndrome varies from mild edema with minimal discomfort to incapacitating limb swelling with pain and ulceration. Mild postphlebitic skin changes and hyperpigmentation are observed in 15% to 30%,[3,9] and severe signs of postphlebitic syndrome and marked trophic skin changes progressing to ulceration are observed in 2% to 10% of patients from 5 to 10 years after their DVT,[3,6,8,9] regardless of the initial site of thrombosis. Severe CVI can be highly debilitating and frustrating to patient and physician. Successful treatment is fraught with difficulty, patient noncompliance, and recurrence, despite the initial success of the treatment.[10] The incidence of severe CVI appears to increase with age.[11]

Retrospective studies report that in more than 80% of affected limbs, cutaneous ulceration resulted 10 years after a DVT. Recent studies suggest a lower incidence of severe changes after an episode of DVT.[3] Some studies suggest that the aggressive use of heparin may have reduced the incidence of serious long-term changes in the postphlebitic syndrome,[12] but other studies have reported that even with adequate laboratory control of anticoagulation, up to 30% of patients will show extension of their DVT.[3]

Most studies have shown that patients who develop venous reflux after DVT have incompetence of the deep venous system, whereas about 15% have reflux of the superficial venous system alone.[5] Venous thrombosis results in destruction of the delicate bicuspid venous valves that promote antegrade flow of blood from the leg. During the process of walking, with each step, the gastrocsoleus muscle complex compresses lower extremity veins and propels the column of blood toward the heart. With the destruction of the venous valves, however, blood is free to reflux into the distal extremity. This results in a persistently elevated ambulatory venous pressure (AVP). The combination of a persistently elevated AVP and other factors yet to be fully elucidated results in the chronic skin changes of the lower extremity that we recognize as evidence of CVI, or the postphlebitic syndrome. Although some data suggest that this is most closely associated with the development of incompetent venous valves, the mechanism by which incompetence occurs, as well as its time course, is not completely understood.[2] For example, 15% of normal people have some degree of venous reflux, most often in the superficial veins.[5]

PATHOPHYSIOLOGY

The venous system of the lower extremity comprises three anatomic components: the superficial, perforator, and deep venous systems. The postphlebitic syndrome may be the result of abnormalities in one or more of these systems. CVI may be primary or secondary. Primary CVI, or idiopathic CVI, is usually due to primary valvular insufficiency. Secondary CVI is acquired and is typically a postphlebitic event.[11,13] In primary valvular insufficiency, all symptoms of typical CVI are identified, yet patients have no prior history or imaging evidence of previous thrombosis. Patients with secondary CVI experience the consequences of the two major sequelae of DVT: obstruction to outflow due to the presence of residual thrombus, and reflux due to valvular damage.[3,5,14] Obstructive symptoms are most commonly associated with acute thrombosis, which usually improves with recanalization of the vessel[11] and collateral formation around an area of occlusion.[2,15] Residual obstruction to outflow results from failure to recanalize the major deep veins of the leg. It is believed that reflux results from irreversible valve destruction. This results in valvular insufficiency that prevents efficient function of the calf muscle pump. Distal venous hypertension develops equal to the hydraulic pressure of the vertical column of blood extending without impedence from the heart to the ankle in the standing position.[3,16] A common dilemma is whether valvular incompetence or venous outflow obstruction is the more important factor in the development of symptoms.[15] Although it is likely a combination of both, reflux is usually believed to be the primary pathologic problem. As such, symptoms are more closely associated with valvular incompetence than with residual obstruction.[2,7,11,13] Many patients with severe reflux have only mild symptoms; additional factors must therefore contribute to the development of severe postphlebitic syndrome.[17] Chronic venous obstruction plays at least a secondary role in the sequelae of postphlebitic syndrome.[7] It has been proposed that primary deep venous insufficiency in the thigh may play a role in the development of distal DVT by allowing reflux, which induces stasis. Valve destruction by DVT then appears to increase reflux, although this has not been proved in any prospective studies.[12,18]

After DVT occurs, recanalization commences. In one study of patients treated with heparin, lysis of thrombi with recanalization was present in 44% of cases at 7 days, 94% at 30 days, and 100% at 90 days. This is not, however, a simple straightforward sequence, because many patients showed extension of thrombus despite therapeutic doses of anticoagulants. Some patients showed extension of thrombus as early as 7 days into their course, and some as late as between 30 and 180 days.[2] Incomplete recanalization or inadequate formation of collaterals may leave residual obstruction, resulting in venous hypertension. In the process of recanalization, however, some damage occurs to the venous valves, which ultimately results in valvular incompetence, reflux, and venous hypertension. Several mechanisms play a role in the recanalization of the thrombus; these include retraction of the thrombus, peripheral fragmentation, central softening of the thrombus, and spontaneous fibrinolysis.[2,7] Lytic clefts form around the valve cusps; this has been attributed to local fibrinolytic activity that may be greater on the valve cusps than in the surrounding endothelium. This fibrinolytic activity appears to be more efficient in small veins, suggesting a higher concentration of fibrinolytic activity at these sites. Such increased efficiency may contribute to valve preservation. It also appears that very large and very small thrombi are more likely to recanalize rapidly and that certain veins, such as the posterior tibial vein, which has a large number of valves, may have a decreased incidence of reflux. Analysis of lysis times of the thrombi in vivo suggests that early recanalization is important in preserving valve integrity.[2,7] It has been postulated that rapid resolution of the thrombus may preserve valvular function and decrease the incidence of postphlebitic syndrome. In one study, early lysis

with the use of fibrinolytic agents resulted in a better clinical outcome after DVT than did stabilization of the thrombus with heparin.[2] The theory that early and complete lysis reduces the incidence of the postphlebitic syndrome has been the basis for the use of early, aggressive thrombolysis in selected patients with acute DVT.

Factors that contribute to the development of valvular incompetence are not completely understood. After thrombosis has resolved, changes in the vein walls and valve degeneration occur within a few months, leading to postphlebitic reflux.[19] A strong association has long been established between severe postphlebitic syndrome and venous reflux, which is probably the major pathophysiologic component of ulceration.[17,18] The valve cusps rarely are involved through fibrocellular organization.[7] However, because of the surrounding inflammatory processes, loss of elasticity results in impairment of venous wall compliance.[18] The development of reflux, which coincides with or is preceded by complete clot lysis within a venous segment, has been reported as early as 7 days after onset of the DVT.[2] Some patients have transient reflux associated with recanalization. Because of incomplete clot lysis, valves are prevented from closing completely. With complete lysis, these valves eventually become functional again.[7] In other cases, venous valvular incompetence develops much later than recanalization. Doppler data suggest that incompetence occurs between 2 and 5 months after a DVT.[2] Van Bemmelen and coworkers[20] proposed that the development of venous incompetence is a two-stage process. Initially, the vein dilates in response to proximal venous obstruction. Valvular incompetence occurs because the cusps of the valves are not large enough to coapt with the increased venous diameter.[20] At this stage, which occurs between the first and second months, the incompetence is reversible. By approximately the sixth month, the valves are completely destroyed and thus permanently incompetent.[7] Therefore, the presence of thrombus may not be the primary factor responsible for the development of valvular incompetence. These studies suggest that long-term permanent destruction may be related to the development of venous hypertension.[2] Investigators have attempted to document the chronologic changes of venous physiology that occur after major thromboses. Akesson and coworkers[21] studied 20 patients for longer than 5 years after an acute iliofemoral thrombosis was treated with conventional anticoagulation. Radionuclide angiography showed that 70% of patients had obstructive lesions of the iliac vein, with only minor changes occurring from 6 months to 5 years. Despite this, plethysmographic evaluation showed that venous outflow improved over time. Venous reflux, however, worsened with time. The authors concluded that, although venous outflow continually improves after iliofemoral thromboses, valvular competence and muscle pump function continually deteriorate.[21]

Obstruction to outflow, although not the primary cause of the postphlebitic syndrome, may be more common than has been realized, and may in fact be present in as many as one third of patients with severe symptoms.[3,15] It seems that collaterals may be sufficient sometimes to accommodate resting but not ambulatory flow.[2,15] Duplex abnormalities consistent with previous DVT often suggest the coexistence of reflux and chronic obstruction.[11] Venous obstruction, particularly of the proximal veins, is more often implicated as the cause of the uncommon symptom of venous claudication, defined as pain in the limb while walking. This symptom is due to venous hypertension that results from occlusion of the proximal veins.[5]

Increasing severity of the postphlebitic syndrome seems to be related to the site and extent of the DVT.[5,11,22] Residual venous abnormalities in the popliteal and tibial veins are associated with an increased likelihood that an individual will develop the postphlebitic syndrome.[14,22] Isolated disease of the superficial system is most frequently responsible for the development of CVI, which occurs in 18% to 30% of patients. Isolated perforator vein incompetence is uncommon and occurs in less than 5% of individuals. Most individuals with severe CVI have combined abnormalities that involve all three venous systems.[11] In another study, in which the incidence of symptoms was correlated with the site of disease, swelling was increased by distal reflux or a combination of proximal and distal reflux, regardless of which system was involved. Absence of superficial reflux was associated with a low incidence of ulceration, even in the presence of deep venous insufficiency.[5]

It has been suggested that vena caval filters have an association with the postphlebitic syndrome by virtue of the associated incidence of inferior vena caval thrombosis. In a recent comprehensive review of all the literature related to vena caval filters, however, the incidence of postphlebitic syndrome after vena caval interruption ranged from 14% to 41%, according to the type of filter used,[23] whereas the incidence of postphlebitic syndrome after DVT is recognized to be as high as 80%.[7,8] Further study would be required, therefore, before we can say that vena caval filters are associated with an increased incidence of postphlebitic syndrome. The relatively low incidence of postphlebitic syndrome associated with the filters is likely to be a reflection of relatively short follow-up.

At the microscopic level, cutaneous blood flow regulation is disturbed in severe CVI. The feedback system between the transmural pressure in the postcapillary venules and the precapillary resistance that regulates arterioles is altered. Postural feedback remains disturbed and upregulated even after a venous ulcer has healed.[24] Skin biopsy specimens from patients affected by CVI show marked structural derangements. These include collapsed, thickened, and reduplicated basement membranes of the blood vessels, numerous and complex interdigitations between contiguous endothelial cells, and a lack of open junctions, as well as extensive fibrosis in the connective tissue matrix. As a consequence, the capacity for fluid exchange is reduced in CVI.[25]

Four major areas of basic science in the development of lipodermatosclerosis (defined as thickening and induration of the skin) and ulceration associated with the postphlebitic syndrome have been investigated: (1) the role of cellular apoptosis, (2) the regulation of tissue fibrosis by transforming growth factor (TGF)-β, (3) leukocyte activation in the microcirculation of the skin, and (4) the role of matrix metalloproteinases in tissue remodeling.

Mendez and coworkers[26] have shown that wound fibroblasts grown from biopsy specimens of venous ulcers show an abnormally high rate of apoptosis as compared with fibroblasts from normal tissue. They also found that growth rates of wound fibroblasts were significantly lower in all patients than were those of normal fibroblasts.

Pappas and coworkers[27] have shown increased levels of TGF-β in dermal biopsy specimens of patients with advanced CVI as compared with normal tissue biopsy specimens. They showed that pathologic dermal degeneration in patients with CVI seems to be associated with increased production of TGF-β in patients with skin induration, hyperpigmentation, and lipodermatosclerosis. In addition, they found significantly increased production of TGF-β in the skin of patients with lipodermatosclerosis and active ulcers as compared with healthy skin. Finally, they were also able to show significantly increased production of TGF-β in lower calf skin biopsy specimens as compared with lower thigh skin biopsy specimens from the same patient.

Saharay and coworkers[28] have shown that venous hypertension results in sequestration of activated neutrophils and monocytes in the microcirculation of the leg in patients with venous disease. They postulate that these cells bind to the endothelium and release L-selectin.[28] Shoab and coworkers[29] reported on the efficacy of treating patients with CVI with oral micronized flavonoid fraction. In this study, they demonstrated decreased surface expression of L-selectin by neutrophils and monocytes, as well as reduction of endothelial activity of intercellular adhesion molecule (ICAM)-1 and vascular cell adhesion molecule (VCAM) with the administration of oral flavonoid 500 mg twice daily for 60 days.[29] The clinical significance of their findings is yet to be determined.[30]

Increased proteolytic activity by proteases, particularly matrix metalloproteinases (MMPs), is a key feature in venous leg ulcer formation. It is believed that the proteolytic effect of MMPs initiates an elevated turnover of the extracellular matrix, with breakdown of the matrix resulting in venous ulceration.[31,32] Further research is needed before we will understand the role of MMPs in venous stasis ulcer formation.

SYMPTOMS

Clinical features of the postphlebitic syndrome include pain, edema, pigment deposition resulting in hyperpigmentation, and, ultimately, ulceration.[5,16,33] In one fifth of patients, however, no evidence of antecedent deep venous occlusion is apparent.[34] Typically, unilateral lower leg swelling occurs. In milder cases, symptoms consist of pain and edema. The early edema that follows a DVT is secondary to residual obstruction, and the late edema that forms part of the postphlebitic syndrome is related to valvular insufficiency.[2] The pain is more often described as an ache, throb, or heaviness that worsens with prolonged standing and as the day progresses. Earlier in the course, the edema is pitting and may resolve with appropriate compression. It also worsens with prolonged standing and as the day progresses. As the disease progresses, the skin becomes chronically thickened and permanently indurated (lipodermatosclerosis) (Fig. 17-1), and subdermal scarring occurs.[11] It is not uncommon to see evidence of previously healed ulcers. Areas of hyperpigmentation are usually located in the anteromedial lower leg and appear as clusters of multiple brownish spots. Over time, these may coalesce and appear as a single large area of hyperpigmentation that involves the entire anteromedial mid to distal leg, or gaiter zone. Ulceration, when present, classically appears in the medial aspect of the mid to distal leg.

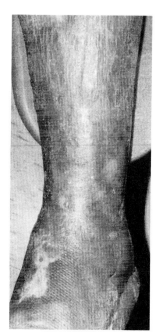

Figure 17-1 Postphlebitic syndrome. Note areas of hyperpigmentation and healed and healing ulcers.

Ulcers are usually painless. Any significant pain or tenderness should raise the suspicion of infection. Ulcers are often moist and covered by exudate.

The CEAP (Clinical, Etiologic, Anatomic, and Pathophysiologic) classification is used to categorize the severity of CVI.[35] CEAP is therefore a clinical classification. A numeric value can be assigned to each of the four categories; in practice, the clinical, or "C," category is most frequently used. The higher the number, the worse is the process. A "C" value of 0 indicates symptoms only with no identified venous disease. C1 indicates telangiectasias, reticular veins, or malleolar flares; C2 indicates the presence of varicose veins; C3 indicates edema without skin changes; C4 indicates the presence of skin changes, including brawny edema, venous eczema, thickening, pigmentation, and lipodermatosclerosis; C5 indicates a history of a previously healed ulcer; and C6 indicates the presence of an active ulceration[10,11] (Table 17-1). This classification is useful in providing a guide on how likely it is that a more complex form of therapy will be required in a particular patient. It also facilitates interinstitutional studies.[36]

DIFFERENTIAL DIAGNOSIS

In considering the diagnosis of postphlebitic syndrome, as in any other condition, a differential diagnosis should be entertained. The conditions to be considered will vary, depending on the stage and severity of the disease. In patients who have leg edema only, conditions that cause peripheral edema should be considered. Most prominent in the differential are lymphedema (primary or secondary, or hereditary in cases of Milroy disease), congestive heart failure, cirrhosis, nephrotic syndrome and other conditions associated with hypoproteinemia, and possibly hypothyroidism and hyperthyroidism.

In patients who present with an ulcer, the differential diagnosis includes arterial insufficiency, vasculitis, hypertensive (or Martorell) ulcer, pyoderma gangrenosum, squamous cell carcinoma, calciphylaxis, and other less common conditions.

A history of DVT and the presence of findings associated with venous insufficiency, such as hyperpigmentation and lipodermatosclerosis, assist in the diagnosis. Venous stasis ulcers are often located in the medial malleolar area and, unless infected, are not painful. Most often, the correct diagnosis can be established on the basis of history and physical examination alone.

RISK FACTORS

Multiple risk factors for the development of postphlebitic syndrome have been identified. Trauma to the venous wall, venous stasis, and hypercoagulability are the most common risk factors. Generally, we associate the development of postphlebitic syndrome with the previous occurrence of DVT, which is true in about 80% of patients.[34] The remaining 20% of patients, with no antecedent history of DVT, experience primary venous insufficiency, or, equally possible, a subclinical DVT. Some reports suggest that this number may be even higher. In a study in which ascending venography was performed on 51 limbs with postphlebitic syndrome, 32 had no radiologic evidence of recent or old thrombophlebitis. Instead, they had normal-appearing veins, which suggested primary incompetence of the deep and/or perforating venous valves rather than thrombophlebitis as the cause.[36] Older age, male sex, and obesity are also strongly associated with the development of CVI.[37] Somewhat less common associations consist of malignancy, superficial varicosities, family history of DVT, recent travel involving sitting for longer than 6 hours, cardiac failure, and pregnancy.[2] Some patients also essentially

Table 17-1 Clinical, Etiologic, Anatomic, and Pathophysiologic (CEAP) Classification of Venous Insufficiency

	CEAP Classification	
Class	**Clinical Characteristics**	**Clinical Significance**
C0	No identified venous disease	Minimally symptomatic disease; not generally
C1	Telangiectasia	considered candidates for perforating vein surgery,
C2	Varicose veins	although superficial ablation is appropriate for C2
C3	Edema	or greater
C4	Skin changes: Brawny edema, venous eczema, thickening, pigmentation, and lipodermatosclerosis	C4-6 are considered candidates for perforating vein surgery
C5	Previously healed ulcer	
C6	Active ulceration	

III

exist in a sitting position while eating, watching television, and even sleeping while sitting in a chair or recliner with their legs dependent all night. This activity can and should be avoided.

Deficiencies of the fibrinolytic system have been well documented in patients with the postphlebitic syndrome.[7] Those with inherited or acquired hypercoagulable states are also at risk for postphlebitic syndrome.[38] For example, the prevalence of antithrombin III (ATIII)-deficient patients among those with the postphlebitic syndrome is reported at between 2% and 3%. Conversely, postphlebitic syndrome may be an initial presentation of ATIII deficiency.[39] Diagnosis and treatment of the disorder with long-term warfarin therapy are indicated to reduce the incidence of recurrent venous thrombosis and the risk of pulmonary embolism.[40] Patients with DVT also may have lower levels of tissue plasminogen activator (tPA) or higher levels of plasminogen activator inhibitor (PAI-1).[2]

Other miscellaneous causes of lower extremity DVT include compression of the iliac vein, which was described by Thurner and May[41] and is now known as May-Thurner syndrome. In these patients, the left common iliac vein is compressed against the vertebral column by the overlying right common iliac artery. This results in constant pulsation, which causes reactive changes in the vein and luminal narrowing with subsequent stasis and DVT.[42]

DIAGNOSIS

The postphlebitic syndrome is most often a clinical diagnosis that is based on the typical signs and symptoms of pain, edema, hyperpigmentation and induration of the skin, and ulceration. More specific information is sometimes needed to differentiate the syndrome from DVT, or when surgical intervention is under consideration. As many as two thirds of patients who present with new symptoms after documented DVT actually have postphlebitic syndrome, which can often mimic or coexist with acute DVT. A skin biopsy, however, is neither necessary nor indicated to make the diagnosis of postphlebitic syndrome.

Duplex Scanning

Duplex scanning is the most common modality used to diagnose a DVT. Venous obstruction is indicated by the absence of spontaneous, augmentable, and phasic flow on pulsed-wave Doppler. Additional observations include the presence of thrombus visualized on B-mode ultrasonography and incompressibility of the vein in transverse section under probe pressure.[43] Absence of flow is considered the best method by which total occlusion of a venous segment can be determined.[2,3,44] To assist in the diagnosis of postphlebitic syndrome, duplex scanning can be used to diagnose chronic venous changes, indicated by the presence of incompetent valves and reflux, or to differentiate old from fresh clot on the basis of sonographic appearance of the thrombus.[43] Color flow Duplex scanning is the diagnostic test of choice for identifying the presence of reflux in the superficial, deep, and perforator systems. Competency of the saphenofemoral and saphenopopliteal junctions, the common femoral vein, and the origins of the deep and superficial femoral veins should be documented. Reflux should be evaluated with the patient in the standing position. Reflux of the lower leg is elicited by manual compression of the calf with sudden release or with the use of a rapid cuff deflator.[20]

Incompetency of the tibioperoneal veins is best evaluated with the patient sitting with the foot at rest supported off the floor. Duplex criteria for reflux within the deep system consist of retrograde flow that persists for longer than 0.5 second. Visualization of a venous lumen that directly connects a superficial and a deep vein is diagnostic of perforator vein incompetence.[2,5,11,33] Most surgically significant incompetent perforating veins are located on the medial calf. Medial calf–perforating veins generally link the posterior tibial vein with tributaries of the saphenous system, most commonly the posterior arch vein. The two clusters corresponding to Cockett II and III are the most commonly involved and are located between 7 and 9 cm and 10 and 12 cm proximal to the inferior border of the medial malleolus.

Air Plethysmography

Air plethysmography (APG) is a noninvasive test that provides reproducible information about degree of venous outflow obstruction, and reflux and efficiency of the calf pump.[45,46] An air-filled plastic bladder placed around the proximal calf is used to measure changes in the volume of the leg. These changes and the rates of these changes after certain maneuvers designed to fill or empty the venous system reflect the degree of venous obstruction. These maneuvers are done when the patient is supine, upright, or exercising. A series of measurements is obtained during the APG to assess the patient (Table 17-2). Immediately after a DVT appears, the venous outflow fraction (OF) is reduced because of obstruction. However, as recanalization and collateralization progress, OF gradually returns to normal and can become completely normal in a patient with evident postphlebitic syndrome. As the degree of reflux worsens, an increase in venous filling index and residual volume fraction (RVF) is observed. These changes are characteristic of valvular incompetence.[5,11]

Ambulatory Venous Pressure

An elevated AVP is the hallmark of chronic venous insufficiency and the postphlebitic syndrome. To measure the AVP, a catheter is inserted into a vein in the dorsum of the foot of the affected extremity, and the venous pressure is transduced while the patient is ambulating on a treadmill. This is cumbersome and invasive, and for these reasons, it is not frequently done. Investigations have shown that the RVF measurement during APG correlates directly with increased AVP.[47] However, because various operations have recently been proposed to correct or bypass malfunctioning valves, precise demonstration of pathologic change is required for selection of the appropriate procedure and evaluation of results.[36] Other tests, such as magnetic resonance imaging and radionuclide scintigraphy, may be useful in selected patients.[48]

Intravascular Ultrasound

A newer but more invasive form of ultrasound imaging is intravascular ultrasound (IVUS). With the use of percutaneous venous access, a guidewire-based catheter ultrasound

Table 17-2 Measurements Used to Assess Severity of Venous Obstruction and Insufficiency

Air Plethysmography (APG)			
Ejection fraction	EF	Fraction of the blood volume expelled by the calf pump after a single tiptoe maneuver	Evaluates calf pump function
Maximal venous volume	MVV	Maximum volume reached by the extremity, compared with baseline, when dependent and not weight bearing	Evaluates obstruction
Residual volume fraction	RVF	Fraction of blood volume remaining after 10 tiptoe maneuvers, which are designed to completely empty the extremity	Evaluates calf pump function
Venous filling index	VFI	Rate of filling of the venous system when going from supine with the leg elevated to an upright position	Evaluates reflux
Venous outflow	VO	Volume of blood passively expelled from the elevated extremity by the action of gravity	Evaluates obstruction

device is inserted into the vein lumen. Intraluminal imaging allows for visualization of the thrombus or stricture and measuring of the luminal diameter or vessel wall. This also enables users to verify that wire access is intraluminal versus subluminal or extraluminal. In areas where traditional color flow Duplex is limited, such as in the pelvic or truncal central veins, with obesity, and with significant scarring or fibrosis from a reoperative field, IVUS offers distinct advantages. In cases where exact sizing of the vein diameter is needed for angioplasty or stenting, measuring with IVUS may aid in prevention of vessel fracture.

Computed Tomography Venography

For arterial imaging, many studies have shown that computed tomography (CT) angiography is equivalent to digital subtraction angiography. Although conventional digital subtraction venography remains the gold standard, CT venography (CTV) offers contrast and spatial resolution, along with extraluminal information and multiplanar differentiation of venous and arterial structures.

In body cavities where the venous system is tortuous, such as in the thorax and the pelvis, venous imaging does not conform well to any single 2-dimensional (2D) plane.[49] Luminal diameters and stenotic vein segments are distorted by 2D venography. Similar to CT angiography for use in preoperative planning for aortic stent grafting, CT venography may be helpful for venous stenting.

Magnetic Resonance Venography

Magnetic resonance venography (MRV) is another modality that may be used to diagnose and stage central venous obstruction. It can reliably predict sites for central venous access. As an alternative to carbon dioxide venography or contrast venography for patients with contraindications to intravenous contrast, MRV can define patent and occluded veins, especially in the chest.

With the use of 2D time-of-flight MRV, slow or partial occlusion of the vessels may be detected. This modality is helpful in the evaluation of axillary-subclavian venous obstruction or thrombophlebitis. In a study by Muller and Triller,[50] 19 patients with malignant central vein obstruction were evaluated by digital subtraction venography and MRV for stent placement planning. MRV was found to be superior.

Venography

Venography may be used to show level of reflux and degree of venous obstruction. In ascending venography, a vein of the foot is cannulated and contrast is administered in an antegrade fashion. As contrast fills the veins from below, venous anatomy and any obstruction to venous outflow become evident (Fig. 17-2). Ascending venography may, however, fail to reveal the most proximal anatomy. Ascending venography may also be used to show perforator incompetence. With the use of tourniquets placed to obstruct the greater saphenous vein, contrast injected into a dorsal foot vein should reveal only the deep system. If perforator vein flow from the deep to the superficial system is shown, those perforator veins are seen to be incompetent.

In descending venography, a more proximal vein, such as the contralateral common femoral vein, is accessed, and contrast is injected in a retrograde fashion into the desired system. As contrast fills and distends the veins from above, the venous valves and their ability or inability to prevent reflux become evident. Descending venography cannot reveal distal disease in the presence of a competent

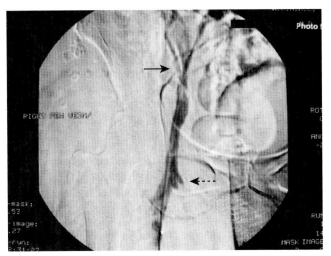

Figure 17-2 Ascending venography. **Solid arrow** shows obstruction. **Broken arrow** indicates valvular anatomy.

proximal femoral valve because the valve prevents contrast from filling the most distal vein.[3]

PREVENTION

Prevention of the postphlebitic syndrome centers on prevention of venous valvular damage and reduction of AVP. For the vast majority of patients, this means preventing DVT, or, once a DVT has occurred, minimizing damage to the venous valves with aggressive, adequate therapy. Healthcare professionals are responsible not only for recognizing and treating thromboembolic disorders, but also for taking all possible measures needed to prevent recurrences. Individuals who have developed a venous thromboembolism remain at an elevated risk of recurrence; this rate is about 3% to 6% during the first 3 months, and although it is lower from then on, it remains elevated for years (see Chapter 14). This possibility is greater in patients with permanent risk factors such as inherited abnormalities of hemostasis than in those with posttraumatic or postoperative venous thrombosis.[6,51] Hospitalized individuals are at increased risk of DVT because of immobility, trauma, and underlying conditions that promote a hypercoagulable state. These patients should be assessed for the need for a prophylactic regimen such as compression devices that prevent stasis of blood in the extremities and/or the use of anticoagulants. Once a DVT has occurred, prompt resolution is probably the best measure that could be taken to minimize long-term impact. Clinically suspected DVT should be confirmed by objective tests because further evaluation often reveals a different diagnosis.[43]

Although anticoagulation is critical for stabilizing the thrombus and reducing the incidence of pulmonary embolism after a DVT, anticoagulants may not prevent the sequelae of postphlebitic syndrome.[52] Unfortunately, no validated method is capable of predicting its occurrence.[53] The failure of anticoagulants to prevent postphlebitic syndrome probably stems from their failure to clear the thrombus.[53]

The long-term clinical implications regarding the development of postphlebitic syndrome after isolated calf DVT, which has been estimated to occur in 5% to 33% of all patients with DVT, are not clear. If not treated with anticoagulation, at least 8% of patients will have propagation of the thrombus proximally. The incidence of postphlebitic syndrome in this population has been reported to range between 3% and 37%. The incidence of ulceration, however, is extremely low.[54] On the basis of this information, a patient with DVT localized to the calf should be treated for 3 to 6 months with anticoagulation. Prior to discontinuation of anticoagulation, a follow-up Duplex ultrasound study should be performed to monitor for clot propagation; if the clot has propagated, then continued anticoagulation therapy is required. The use of compression stockings, although perhaps not as critical, given the low incidence of ulceration, is probably still advisable to reduce the incidence of some of the less severe sequelae of postphlebitic syndrome.

The use of thrombolytic agents to treat patients with acute DVT is believed to reduce the sequelae of postphlebitic syndrome by affecting valve preservation. Although this has not been proved definitively, several studies suggest that this is true. Because of large differences in the reported incidence of late postphlebitic syndrome after DVT, it has been suggested, however, that a minimal reopening rate is required to be of clinical value to the individual patient.[53] Thrombolytic therapy is most effective when initiated within 14 days of the onset of DVT. Thrombolytic therapy, however, has a higher incidence of hemorrhagic complications ($\approx$5% to 15%) (see Chapter 28). Until conclusive evidence proves its benefits, it should probably be reserved for those patients with massive DVT or DVT associated with relevant clinical signs, most often, for those with iliofemoral thrombosis.[1,55] The rationale of venous valve preservation is more attractive in young, healthy patients (e.g., postpartum patients) than in patients with short survival (e.g., patients with cancer). It should also be considered in patients who have failed to respond to standard therapy, and in those with a renal allograft on the same side as the DVT, in whom extension to the renal vein could result in loss of the transplant. The use of an inferior vena caval filter to prevent embolization during thrombolytic treatment is not necessary.[1] The use of catheter-directed thrombolysis may reduce the incidence of systemic complications and provide more complete lysis,[56] although this approach ignores the fact that 30% to 40% of such patients also have a coexisting pulmonary embolus or undetected DVT elsewhere. Although a large portion of the literature on thrombolysis has been based on urokinase therapy, because of its variable availability on the market, the more frequent choice has been tPA. Anticoagulation therapy, instead of thrombolysis, will probably continue to be the mainstay of therapy because of aspects such as limited extent of thrombosis, absence of tissue loss, complications associated with thrombolysis, and, unfortunately, delay in referral for treatment beyond the 7 days or so when thrombolysis is most effective.[57]

Open venous thrombectomy is rarely indicated and is not frequently used in modern medicine. It should be considered only in instances of DVT involving the iliofemoral venous segment, and when the age of the clot is believed to be less than 72 hours.[58,59] It is particularly indicated in the patient with phlegmasia cerulea dolens (see Chapter 14), in whom the inherent delay associated with thrombolytic therapy would be unacceptable because rapid results are necessary to save the limb and possibly the patient's life. Even if vascular patency is restored in a good percentage of cases, it is not particularly effective in preventing postphlebitic syndrome.[52] Open thrombectomy for venous thrombosis below the inguinal ligament has not been consistently beneficial. In the setting of widespread metastatic disease, rethrombosis rates are too high to justify thrombectomy in some patients.[58] Alternatively, aggressive anticoagulant therapy is indicated.

Following management of acute DVT, compression is probably the most important form of management for preventing the more debilitating form of CVI, which is ulceration. It has been suggested that early application of external compression in patients with acute DVT may prevent the sequelae of postphlebitic syndrome. A randomized trial that compared the use of stockings with the use of no stockings after a first episode of DVT showed reduced development of postphlebitic syndrome by 50% at 2 years in patients who wore the stockings when compared with those who did not wear the stockings.[4] Patients who have no symptoms often will not wear the stockings, even though they have been prescribed.[3] Although the precise mechanism is unknown, it is believed that they stimulate the development of collaterals, reduce transcapillary filtration, increase fibrinolytic activity, and reduce overdistention of the venous system.[4,7] It is recommended that the use of appropriately sized, graded compression stockings should be initiated within 2 to 3 weeks from the time of initial diagnosis, and they should be used for at least two[4] and perhaps up to five years.[9]

TREATMENT

Pharmacologic Treatment

The role of pharmacology in the treatment of patients with postphlebitic syndrome has been very limited. Although several products have been suggested to provide benefit, none has been established as routine clinical practice. Pentoxifylline is reported to improve the healing rate of venous leg ulcers. The mechanism of action of pentoxifylline is believed to be a downregulating effect in leukocyte activation. This in turn reduces leukocyte-derived free radicals, proteolytic enzymes, cytokines, and a number of other noxious mediators.[60] Another product is venostat, an herbal medicine commercially available as Venastat (Boehringer Ingelheim Corporation, Ingelheim, Germany). It is marketed for the treatment of patients with varicose veins and venous stasis among other conditions. As is the case with many herbal medicines, minimal or no scientific literature is available regarding its effectiveness.

Medical Therapy

The mainstay of treatment for patients with postphlebitic syndrome is compression. Graded compression stockings are used to mechanically reduce ambulatory venous pressure. Stockings are typically available in three degrees of compression: moderate compression provides 15 to 20 mmHg, firm compression, 20 to 30 mmHg, and extra firm compression, 30 to 40 mmHg. No firm data favor the use of knee-high stockings rather than thigh-high stockings, but compliance seems better with the knee-high devices. For the patient with minimal symptoms, moderate compression and even leg elevation at the end of the day are reasonable alternatives. For the patient with mild to moderate symptoms of heaviness, achiness, and edema, firm compression is a reasonable starting point. To prevent recurrence, compression stockings should be used continually in the patient who has experienced previous ulcer formation; in the compliant patient, most limbs are adequately controlled with graded compression stockings.[3] It is recommended that the patient put the stocking on in the morning when edema is at its least, before ambulating, and wear it all day. Stockings can be removed at night when the patient sleeps in the supine position and venous pressure is reduced to 0 mm Hg. Because of loss of their elasticity, stockings should be replaced approximately every 6 months. For patients who have previously had an ulcer, conservative treatment has initial treatment failure and recurrence rates at 1 to 3 years that range from 54% to 69%. In a study in which compliance with the use of

stockings was compared with noncompliance, the compliant group had a recurrence rate of 29%, but the noncompliant group had a 100% recurrence rate, at 3 years. If the data were recalculated, the recurrence rate would be closer to 30% in the first year.[10]

Patients with advanced CVI (CEAP 6) require daily care of their venous ulcer, in addition to compression therapy. The ulcer should be cleaned properly with saline, and a gentle detergent solution should be followed by adequate debridement. Various wound dressing alternatives are commercially available. The Unna boot is probably the best known. The dressing contains zinc oxide as the active ingredient, combined with a semirigid compression dressing. The goal is to apply the dressing with the use of the model of graded compression, in which the highest degree of compression is present at the foot, beginning just proximal to the toes, and the least compression is noted proximally, immediately below the knee. After application, "boots" are kept in place for 3 to 7 days, depending on the amount of wound drainage and dressing soilage that are present. A sponge dressing may be added to the Unna boot to absorb wound exudate.

Duoderm (ConvaTec, Princeton, NJ) is an example of this type of dressing. The use of a sponge dressing by itself does not improve healing rate, but in combination with compression, it has been shown to result in faster healing rates than the Unna boot alone.[61] A second type of nonelastic stocking is the CircAid (Metro Medical, Nashville, Tenn) legging. It consists of multiple pliable yet unyielding adjustable layers that are attached with the use of Velcro. This device is considered by some providers to be easier to apply than stockings.[62] This inelastic device has been shown to maintain limb size and reduce venous volume better than stockings.[63] A trial of sequential compression pump therapy is worthwhile for patients with severe postphlebitic syndrome. A sustained beneficial response can be expected in 80% of patients; this is slightly decreased to 75% with long-term continued use.[64] Pump therapy increases the transcutaneous pressure of oxygen; this is associated with a rise in skin temperature and a decrease in edema.[65]

Surgical Treatment

Various surgical alternatives have been developed over the years in an attempt to deal with the late sequelae of postphlebitic syndrome. Some procedures attempt to eliminate venous hypertension in the superficial system by eliminating diseased portions of the superficial system and by ligating incompetent perforating veins. Other procedures are aimed at reducing reflux and venous hypertension by restoring or reconstructing the valvular system. In any particular patient, surgery should be directed at the affected component, as identified by the proper preoperative studies.

Ligation and Stripping and Flush Ligation

Surgical treatment of patients with postphlebitic syndrome should be guided by preoperative venous testing.[66] In an effort to preserve the great saphenous vein (GSV) for potential later use for coronary artery bypass graft or lower extremity bypass, surgical ablation of varicose veins should be selective and guided by preoperative color flow Duplex and/or APG or continuous-wave Doppler.

III

Radiofrequency Ablation

As an alternative to conventional vein stripping, radiofrequency ablation (RFA) of the GSV has emerged as one of the earliest forms of minimally invasive endovenous treatments for saphenous vein incompetence. This approach uses a percutaneous technique, whereby radiofrequency energy is delivered through a catheter to achieve heat-induced venous endothelial injury that results in venous spasm and luminal shrinkage. Through the Seldinger technique, the distal GSV is entered with a vascular sheath. Under ultrasound guidance, a tumescent solution (50 mL of 1% lidocaine and 1 mL of epinephrine [1:1000] diluted in 1 L of 0.9% saline solution) is injected around the vein from the knee to the groin. The Closure System (VNUS Medical Technologies Inc., San Jose, Calif) treats 3-mm-diameter to 12-mm-diameter incompetent saphenous varicose veins. The RFA catheter tip is inserted into the vascular sheath and is advanced in an ascending fashion toward the saphenofemoral venous junction. The temperature of the RFA catheter tip is maintained between 82°C and 90°C. The advancement of the catheter, at a rate of 2 to 3 cm per second, is guided by ultrasound to prevent entry into and subsequent ablation of the femoral vein, snagging against valve leaflets, and accidental entry into venous side branches. After vein ablation has been completed, the leg is wrapped with a Kerlex (Kendall Co., Mansfield, Mass) inner layer and an ACE bandage (Becton Dickinson, Franklin, NJ) outer layer. RFA endovenous ablation has been shown to be comparable with vein ligation and stripping. The venous occlusion rate has been reported between 83% and 100%.[67,68] The complication rate ranges between 4% and 23%.[69,70] Complications include leg edema, cellulitis, thrombophlebitis, skin color changes, thermal injury, nerve injury, and femoral vein thrombosis or injury.

Endovenous Laser Treatment

Instead of using radiofrequency energy to obliterate the vein lumen, endovenous laser treatment (EVLT) uses laser-derived thermal energy to cause localized endothelial venous damage. Similar to RFA ablation, the vein is injected with tumescent solution under ultrasound guidance. The distal GSV is cannulated with a 5 Fr vascular sheath. Through an over-the-wire technique, a 810-nm laser diode catheter is advanced toward the saphenofemoral junction; this is verified by ultrasound. With the laser delivering continuous energy of 12 to 15 W, the catheter tip is withdrawn toward the knee at a rate of 1 cm per 2 sec until the catheter tip is located 2 cm proximal to the medial femoral condyle. Again, after the procedure has been completed, the leg is wrapped in a two-layered compressive dressing, as described for RFA ablation. Both RFA and EVLT have high rates of venous obliteration, with slightly higher rates for EVLT ranging from 98% to 100%.[71,72] Complications for EVLT range up to 10%[72] and are similar to those for RFA. In a direct comparison of early efficacy and complications, both techniques yielded >90% GSV occlusion at 1 month (94.4% for EVLT vs 90.9% for RFA). In three of 54 patients (6%) treated with EVLT, a common femoral vein (CFV) thrombus developed, with one patient requiring an inferior vena cava (IVC) filter for a free-floating thrombus.[83]

Subfascial Endoscopic Perforator Surgery

The first report from the NASEPS (North American Subfascial Endoscopic Perforator Surgery) registry emphasized the importance of superficial reflux as a cause of venous ulceration.[74] Perforator interruption, however, has remained a controversial issue.[10] The superficial system is managed by removal of the incompetent branches after these have been identified and marked. The perforator system has recently been the object of renewed interest with the advent of subfacial endoscopic perforator surgery (SEPS). Patients are not generally considered candidates for this type of procedure unless their CVI is rated CEAP 4 or higher. This procedure recreates in a minimally invasive fashion what previous procedures such as the Linton operation did, namely, ligature and interruption of communication between the superficial and deep venous systems of the lower extremity—the perforating veins. The recurrence rate of ulceration after a Linton flap operation of the lower extremities is 14.5% at 6 months to 10 years follow-up.[75] However, the Linton operation was associated with a high wound complication rate and required an extensive incision in the leg. The success rate of the SEPS procedure is very similar to that of the Linton operation, with about 84% of ulcers healed in one study at a median time of 54 days. The recurrence rate, in the same study, was 28% at 2 years. The wound complication rate, however, was 6%, which is lower than for open procedures. A very high failure rate was noted in patients with residual venous occlusion. In four of nine patients, the ulcer failed to heal, and the other five had recurrence. A clear association has also been found to exist between missed or recurrent perforators and ulcer recurrence.[10]

Valve Reconstruction

Various operations have been designed with the purpose of recreating a normal valvular system. Options include valve transposition, reconstruction, and transplantation.[76–78] In valve transposition, a normal segment of vein is swung into position to replace the diseased segment. In valve reconstruction, the wall of the vein may be folded and sutured in place to recreate valve function. In valve transplantation, a normal segment of vein from a distant position is removed and interposed in the area of disease.

Surgical repair of an incompetent femoral vein as an adjunct to conventional stripping of varices and subfascial interruption of perforating veins is associated with a 90% success rate.[79] Isolated disease of the more proximal (iliofemoral) valves does not seem to correlate with disease severity, yet distal incompetence, or combined distal and proximal incompetence, does appear to correlate with disease severity. Thus, the value of proximal vein reconstruction is uncertain.[40] Furthermore, venous pressure measurements do not always return to normal after surgery.[77] Failure of venous pressure to normalize in the presence of an otherwise successful operation may sometimes be explained by the presence of residual obstruction in association with reflux.[3]

Surgical Treatment for Patients with Venous Obstruction

Surgical alternatives are available for the rare patient who presents with symptoms associated with the presence of clinically significant chronic venous obstruction. The principal goal of these alternatives is to bypass the obstructed area. Various options have been described; these include the use of autologous or prosthetic material. Described configurations include saphenofemoral venous crossover,[80] femorofemoral crossover with expanded polytetrafluoroethylene (ePTFE),[81] cross-pubic bypass, and saphenopopliteal bypass.[82] Recently, percutaneous angioplasty and stenting have been used for the treatment of May-Thurner syndrome and more extensive iliocaval thrombosis.[83]

Catheter-Directed Thrombolysis, Thrombectomy, and Stenting

Systemic anticoagulation is the standard of care for the treatment of patients with acute DVT or pulmonary embolism (PE). This mode of treatment prevents propagation of the thrombus but does not protect against valvular incompetence and venous outflow obstruction, which may lead to the development of postthrombotic syndrome.[84] Catheter-directed thrombolysis and/or thrombectomy with selective endovascular stenting has been shown to be an effective alternative to systemic anticoagulation for the treatment of patients with acute DVT.[85]

Indications for thrombolysis treatment include acute symptoms lasting ≤14 days, thrombosis of two or more major deep venous segments, ambulatory capacity, and no contraindications to thrombolysis, such as allergy to thrombolytic agents, coagulopathy, recent surgery, previous stroke, brain lesions, recent gastrointestinal bleeding, severe hypertension, pregnancy, bacterial endocarditis, severe hypertension, and recent severe trauma. Catheter-directed thrombolysis has also been used in chronic DVT (symptoms >14 days), acute-on-chronic DVT, and recurrent DVT. However, the response rate and patency rates are significantly lower.

After DVT has been diagnosed by Duplex ultrasound, venographic examination is performed from the popliteal vein to the IVC. In our practice, an ascending venogram is performed from the ipsilateral ankle or foot to access the distal extent of the thrombus. This is followed by a descending venogram with sheath access from the contralateral common femoral vein, crossing over the IVC bifurcation into the ipsilateral iliac vein. From the contralateral side, a hydrophilic, pliable wire (under catheter guidance) is passed through the entire length of the thrombosed vein segments.

If the thrombus is soft, as evidenced by easy passage of the pliable wire, a pulsed mechanical thrombectomy is performed prior to thrombolysis. Through debulking of the thrombus, the surface area of the residual thrombus is increased for improved thrombolysis. We use an Angiojet Thrombectomy System (Possis Medical Inc., Minneapolis, Minn), which is a catheter-based impeller at the distal tip that produces a pulsed jet vortex. Another mechanical thrombectomy device is the Amplatx device (Microvena Corp., White Bear Lake, Minn). The clot is mascerated into subcapillary-sized particles, which are then aspirated into the suction catheter.

Thrombolysis is performed through a Cragg-McNamara infusion catheter, with tissue tPA provided at 1 to 2 mg per hour after a 2-mg bolus. Additionally, through the side port of the sheath, unfractionated heparin is infused at 500 U per hour to prevent thrombosis at the access site. After 12 to 24 hours, the patient returns for repeat venography. If residual thrombus remains, tPA is continued for another

24 hours. If the thrombus has resolved but flow-limiting stenosis is observed in a vein segment, then selective endovascular stenting is performed with a balloon expandable stent. After the intervention has been completed, patients are treated with oral anticoagulation with or without clopidogrel.

The efficacy of catheter-directed thrombolysis for lower extremity deep venous thrombosis has been reported by Mewissen and associates in a review of a national multicenter registry.[86] In this study, 221 patients with iliofemoral DVT and 79 patients with femoropopliteal DVT were treated with catheter-directed urokinase infusion. After thrombolysis was performed, endovascular stenting was completed in 99 iliac veins and five femoral veins. The 1-year primary patency rate was 60%. In another study by Jackson and colleagues,[85] mechanical thrombectomy was added to catheter-directed thrombolysis and stenting. In this series of 28 patients, 15.5-month follow-up revealed 80% long-term patency.

Percutaneous Angioplasty and Stenting

Endovascular surgery has emerged as a new modality for the treatment of patients with CVI and central venous stricture or obstruction from complications of lower extremity deep vein thrombosis. For some patients, IVC and/or iliac vein stenosis may be the cause of lower extremity edema or stasis dermatitis with or without skin ulceration, despite prior GSV stripping and stab avulsion. In a series by Raju and coworkers,[87] balloon angioplasty and stent placement were performed in 304 limbs with symptomatic CVI.[87] At 24 months, primary and secondary stent patency rates were 71% and 90%, respectively. Limb swelling decreased from 88% before stenting to 53% after stenting. The incidence of a pain-free limb increased from 51% to 71%. Cumulative recurrence for ulcer healing was 62% at 2 years after stenting.

The left common iliac vein is sometimes compressed by the overlying right common iliac artery. In May-Thurner syndrome, flow through the left common iliac vein is severely impeded because of external compression between the artery and the pelvic brim, as well as intraluminal web formation (venous spur) from within the vein. The acquired venous stenosis may result in left leg pain, edema, and ileofemoral DVT. When a DVT is found in this syndrome, the patient should be treated with catheter-directed thrombolysis, as was described previously. Otherwise, endoluminal stenting with self-expanding stents and balloon angioplasty, or balloon expandable stents have yielded high patency rates with low morbidity in multiple, small case series with up to 1 year of follow-up.

Retroperitoneal fibrosis is an uncommon condition. Its origin is uncertain but has been correlated with the ingestion of methysergide and now is believed to be associated with ergotamine, hydralazine, methyldopa, and β blockers. Classically, the disease involves encasement of the ureters. In more uncommon circumstances, iliocaval stenosis or occlusion may occur. Surgical exploration and iliocaval lysis have been disappointing. Endovenous stenting has been used with success.[88]

Venous Bypass Procedures

Currently, most cases of iliocaval stenosis or occlusion can be effectively treated with percutaneous stenting with or without angioplasty. In patients with unilateral iliac vein or inferior vena cava occlusion who have failed endovenous treatment, surgical therapy may be indicated.

In patients who have failed endovenous stenting of a unilateral iliac venous occlusion, a Palma-Dale operation or an interposition spiral vein graft may be performed. The contralateral GSV is harvested, and a crossover saphenous vein transposition is performed to create a femorofemoral venous bypass. In addition, a distal arteriovenous fistula is created on the side of the venous obstruction, to improve graft patency. The 4-year primary and secondary patency rates of 18 saphenous vein crossover grafts were 77% and 83%, respectively.[89] However, cross-femoral venous ePTFE grafts, even with an arteriovenous fistula, are associated with early graft thrombosis. Alternatively, an occluded iliac vein segment may be resected and reconstructed with a spiral vein graft. The 10-month patency for spiral grafts is 67%.

In the case of concomitant iliac and vena caval occlusion, iliocaval or femorocaval bypass with ePTFE may be used. Primary and secondary patency rates at 2 years for five iliocaval and eight femorocaval prosthetic bypass grafts were 38% and 54%, respectively.[89]

CONSULTATION CONSIDERATIONS

Prevention of the postphlebitic syndrome should be the goal of every practitioner who manages DVT. Prevention should begin with the prescription of compression stockings; these can be ordered by physicians of any practice specialty. In cases of iliofemoral thrombosis, preventive measures might involve thrombolysis, and consultation with a vascular surgeon should be considered.

Patients with evidence of established postphlebitic syndrome with active ulcers, new or recurrent, who continue to show evidence of progression despite compression therapy or who have associated varicose veins should be evaluated by a vascular surgeon.

Surgeons and hematologists can work best together if they communicate with each other within their particular institutions to gain an understanding of each other's practices in the management of postphlebitic syndrome.

CONCLUSIONS

Postphlebitic syndrome occurs as dermatologic destruction of the microscopic lymphatics, caused by persistent lower extremity venous hypertension. It is usually caused by valvular destruction after DVT. The mainstay of therapy is prevention through DVT prevention. Early venous thrombolysis decreases the incidence of the disorder. The goal of treatment of patients with the postphlebitic syndrome is to reduce venous hypertension associated with ambulation. Reduction in venous hypertension helps to prevent advanced CVI with ulceration (CEAP 6). Most patients with CVI may be treated with skin emollients and compression stockings. Surgical therapy for the postphlebitic syndrome is aimed at eliminating venous reflux through ligation or stripping of varicose veins, or valve reconstruction.

Unfortunately, reduction in ambulatory venous hypertension does not restore skin affected by lipodermatosclerosis to its healthy state. Patients require lifelong compression therapy and skin care. Ultimately, understanding and prevention of the postphlebitic syndrome will occur when investigators gain a better understanding of its cause.

REFERENCES

1. Silverstein MD, Heit JA, Mohr DN, et al: Trends in the incidence of deep venous thrombosis and pulmonary embolism: A 25-year population-based study. Arch Intern Med 158:585–593, 1998.
2. Killewich LA, Bedford GR, Beach KW, et al: Spontaneous lysis of deep venous thrombi: Rate and outcome. J Vasc Surg 9:89–97, 1989.
3. Johnson BF, Manzo RA, Bergelin RO, et al: Relationship between changes in the deep venous system and the development of the post-thrombotic syndrome after an acute episode of lower limb deep vein thrombosis: A one to six year follow-up. J Vasc Surg 21:307–313, 1995.
4. Brandjes DPM, Buller HR, Heijboer H, et al: Randomized trial of effect of compression stockings in patients with symptomatic proximal-vein thrombosis. Lancet 349:759–762, 1997.
5. Labropoulos N, Leon M, Nicolaides AN, et al: Venous reflux in patients with previous deep venous thrombosis: Correlation with ulceration and other symptoms. J Vasc Surg 20:20–26, 1994.
6. Leizorovicz A: Long-term consequences of deep vein thrombosis. Haemostasis 28 (suppl 3): 1–7, 1998.
7. Meissner MH, Manzo RA, Bergelin RO, et al: Deep venous insufficiency: The relationship between lysis and subsequent reflux. J Vasc Surg 18:596–608, 1993.
8. Lindner DJ, Edwards JM, Phinney ES, et al: Long-term hemodynamic and clinical sequelae of lower extremity deep vein thrombosis. J Vasc Surg 4:436–442, 1986.
9. Franzeck UK, Schalch I, Bollinger A: On the relationship between changes in the deep veins evaluated by duplex sonography and the postthrombotic syndrome 12 years after deep vein thrombosis. Thromb Haemost 77:1109–1112, 1997.
10. Gloviczki P, Bergan JJ, Rhodes JM, et al: Mid-term results of endoscopic perforator vein interruption for chronic venous insufficiency: Lessons learned from the North American Subfascial Endoscopic Perforator Surgery registry. J Vasc Surg 29:489–502, 1999.
11. Padberg FT: Endoscopic subfascial perforating vein ligation: Its complementary role in the surgical management of chronic venous insufficiency. Ann Vasc Surg 13:343–354, 1999.
12. Van Dongen CJ, Prandoni P, Frulla M, et al: Relation between quality of anticoagulation treatment and the development of the postthrombotic syndrome. J Thromb Haemost 3:939–942, 2005.
13. Masuda EM, Kistner RL: Long-term results of venous valve reconstruction: A four- to twenty-one-year follow-up. J Vasc Surg 19:391–403, 1994.
14. Johnson BF, Manzo RA, Bergelin RO, et al: The site of residual abnormalities in the leg veins in long-term follow-up after deep vein thrombosis and their relationship to the development of the post-thrombotic syndrome. Int Angiol 15:14–19, 1996.
15. Illig KA, Ouriel K, DeWeese JA, et al: Increasing the sensitivity of the diagnosis of chronic venous obstruction. J Vasc Surg 24:176–178, 1996.
16. Cardon JM, Cardon A, Joyeux A, et al: Use of ipsilateral greater saphenous vein as a valved transplant in management of post-thrombotic deep venous insufficiency: Long-term results. Ann Vasc Surg 13:284–289, 1999.
17. Milne AA, Stonebridge PA, Bradbury AW, et al: Venous function and clinical outcome following deep vein thrombosis. Br J Surg 81:847–849, 1994.
18. Perrin M, Hiltbrand B, Bayon JM: Results of valvuloplasty in patients presenting with deep venous insufficiency and recurring ulceration. Ann Vasc Surg 13:524–532, 1999.
19. Plagnol P, Ciostek P, Grimaud JP, et al: Autogenous valve reconstruction technique for post-thrombotic reflux. Ann Vasc Surg 13:339–342, 1999.
20. van Bemmelen PS, Bedford G, Beach K, et al: Quantitative segmental evaluation of venous valvular reflux with duplex ultrasound scanning. J Vasc Surg 10:425–431, 1989.
21. Akesson H, Brudin L, Dahlstrom JA, et al: Venous function assessed during a 5 year period after acute ilio-femoral venous thrombosis treated with anticoagulation. Eur J Vasc Surg 4:43–48, 1990.
22. Monreal M, Martorell A, Callejas JM, et al: Venographic assessment of deep vein thrombosis and risk of developing post-thrombotic syndrome: A prospective study. J Intern Med 233:233–238, 1993.

17

23. Streiff MB: Vena caval filters: A comprehensive review. Blood 95:3669–3677, 2000.

24. Junger M, Hahn M, Klyscz T, et al: Influence of healing on the disturbed blood flow regulation in venous ulcers. Vasa 25:341–348, 1996.

25. Scelsi R, Scelsi L, Cortinovis R, et al: Morphological changes of dermal blood and lymphatic vessels in chronic venous insufficiency of the leg. Int Angiol 13:308–311, 1994.

26. Mendez MV, Stanley A, Park HY, et al: Fibroblasts cultured from venous ulcers display cellular characteristics of senescence. J Vasc Surg 28:876–883, 1998.

27. Pappas PJ, You R, Rameshwar P, et al: Dermal tissue fibrosis in patients with chronic venous insufficiency is associated with increased transforming growth factor–beta₁ gene expression and protein production. J Vasc Surg 30:1129–1145, 1999.

28. Saharay M, Shields DA, Porter JB, et al: Leukocyte activity in the microcirculation of the leg in patients with chronic venous disease. J Vasc Surg 26:265–273, 1997.

29. Shoab SS, Porter J, Scurr JH, et al: Endothelial activation response to oral micronised flavonoid therapy in patients with chronic venous disease: A prospective study. Eur J Vasc Endovasc Surg 17:313–318, 1999.

30. Shoab SS, Porter JB, Scurr JH, et al: Effect of oral micronized purified flavonoid fraction treatment on leukocyte adhesion molecule expression in patients with chronic venous disease: A pilot study. J Vasc Surg 31:456–461, 2000.

31. Herouy Y, Nockowski P, Schopf E, et al: Lipodermatosclerosis and the significance of proteolytic remodeling in the pathogenesis of venous ulceration. Int J Mol Med 3:511–515, 1999.

32. Herouy Y, May AE, Pornschlegel G, et al: Lipodermatosclerosis is characterized by elevated expression and activation of matrix metalloproteinases: Implications for venous ulcer formation. J Invest Dermatol 111:822–827, 1998.

33. Halliday P: Development of the postthrombotic syndrome: Its management at different stages. World J Surg 14:703–710, 1990.

34. Jacobs P: Pathogenesis of the postphlebitic syndrome. Annu Rev Med 34:91–105, 1983.

35. Kistner RL, Eklof B, Masuda EM: Diagnosis of chronic venous disease of the lower extremities: The "CEAP" classification. Mayo Clin Proc 71:338–345, 1996.

36. Train JS, Schanzer H, Peirce ED, et al: Radiological evaluation of the chronic venous stasis syndrome. JAMA 258:941–944, 1987.

37. Scott TE, LaMorte WW, Gorin DR, et al: Risk factors for chronic venous insufficiency: A dual case-control study. J Vasc Surg 22:622–628, 1995.

38. Gillespie DL, Carrington L, Griffen J, et al: Resistance to activated protein C: A common, inherited cause of venous thrombosis. Ann Vasc Surg 10:174–177, 1996.

39. Jackson MR, Olsen SB, Gomez ER, et al: Use of antithrombin III concentrates to correct antithrombin III deficiency during vascular surgery. J Vasc Surg 22:804–807, 1995.

40. Phifer TJ, Mills GM: Occult antithrombin III deficiency: A potentially lethal complication of the postphlebitic limb. J Vasc Surg 11:586–590, 1990.

41. Thurner J, May R: [Problems of phlebopathology with special reference to phlebosclerosis]. Zentralbl Phlebol 6:404–482, 1967.

42. Blattler W, Blattler IK: Relief of obstructive pelvic venous symptoms with endoluminal stenting. J Vasc Surg 29:484–488, 1999.

43. Salcuni M, Fiorentino P, Pedicelli A, et al: Diagnostic imaging in deep vein thrombosis of the limbs. Rays 21:328–339, 1996.

44. Barloon TJ, Bergus GR, Seabold JE: Diagnostic imaging of lower limb deep venous thrombosis. Am Fam Phys 56:791–801, 1997.

45. Christopoulos DG, Nicolaides AN, Szendro G, et al: Air-plethysmography and the effect of elastic compression on venous hemodynamics of the leg. J Vasc Surg 5:148–159, 1987.

46. Gillespie DL, Cordts P, Hartono C, et al: The role of air plethysmography in monitoring the results of venous surgery. J Vasc Surg 16:647–678, 1992.

47. Christopoulos D, Nicolaides AN, Cook A, et al: Pathogenesis of venous ulceration in relation to the calf muscle pump function. Surgery 106:829–835, 1989.

48. Cronnan JJ: Venous thromboembolic disease: The role of US. Radiology 186:619–630, 1993.

49. Lawler LP, Fishman EK: Thoracic venous anatomy Multidetector row CT evaluation. Radiol Clin N Am 41:545–560, 2003.

50. Muller MF, Triller J: [The significance of magnetic resonance venography in the pre-interventional clarification of a malignant superior venous obstruction. Rofo 169:253–259, 1998.

51. Prandoni P, Lensing AW, Prins MR: Long-term outcomes after deep venous thrombosis of the lower extremities. Vasc Med 3:57–60, 1998.

52. Halstuk K, Mahler D, Baker WH: Late sequelae of deep venous thrombosis: Diagnostic and therapeutic considerations. Am J Surg 147:216–220, 1984.

53. Breddin HK: Treatment of deep vein thrombosis: Is thrombosis regression a desirable endpoint? Semin Thromb Hemost 23:179–183, 1997.

54. Masuda EM, Kessler DM, Kistner RL, et al: The natural history of calf vein thrombosis: Lysis of thrombi and development of reflux. J Vasc Surg 28:67–74, 1998.

55. Cina G, Marra R, Cotroneo AR, et al: Treatment of deep vein thrombosis. Rays 21:397–416, 1996.

56. Semba CP, Dake MD: Catheter-directed thrombolysis for iliofemoral venous thrombosis. Semin Vasc Surg 9:26–33, 1996.

57. Rutherford RB: Pathogenesis and pathophysiology of the postthrombotic syndrome: Clinical implications. Semin Vasc Surg 9:21–25, 1996.

58. Solis MM, Ranval TJ, Thompson BW, et al: Results of venous thrombectomy in the treatment of deep vein thrombosis. Surg Gynecol Obstet 177:633–639, 1993.

59. Ganger KH, Nachbur BH, Ris HB, et al: Surgical thrombectomy versus conservative treatment for deep venous thrombosis: Functional comparison of long-term results. Eur J Vasc Surg 3:438–439, 1989.

60. Dormandy JA: Pharmacologic treatment of venous leg ulcers. J Cardiovasc Pharmacol 25 (suppl 2): S61–S65, 1995.

61. Cordts PR, Hanrahan LM, Rodriguez AA, et al: A prospective, randomized trial of Unna's boot versus Duoderm CGF hydroactive dressing plus compression in the management of venous leg ulcers. J Vasc Surg 15:480–486, 1992.

62. Vernick SH, Shapiro D, Shaw FD: Legging orthosis for venous and lymphatic insufficiency. Arch Phys Med Rehabil 68:459–461, 1987.

63. Bergan JJ, Sparks SR: Non-elastic compression: An alternative in management of chronic venous insufficiency. J Wound Ostomy Continence Nurs 27:83–89, 2000.

64. Ginsberg JS, Magier D, Mackinnon B, et al: Intermittent compression units for severe post-phlebitic syndrome: A randomized cross-over study. CMAJ 160:1303–1306, 1999.

65. Kolari PJ, Pekanmaki K, Pohjola RT: Transcutaneous oxygen tension in patients with post-thrombotic leg ulcers: Treatment with intermittent pneumatic compression. Cardiovasc Res 22:138–141, 1988.

66. Villavicencio JL, Gillespie DL, Pikoulis E, et al: Superficial varicose veins. In Raju S, Villavicencio JL (eds): Therapeutic Options in Venous Surgery. Baltimore, Williams & Wilkins, 1997, pp 373–390.

67. Wagner WH, Levin PM, Cossman DV, et al: Early experience with radiofrequency ablation of the greater saphenous vein. Ann Vasc Surg 18:42–47, 2004.

68. Rautio T, Ohinmaa A, Perala J, et al: Endovenous obliteration versus conventional stripping operation in the treatment of primary varicose veins: A randomized controlled trial with comparison of the cost. J Vasc Surg 35:958–965, 2002.

69. Weiss RA, Weiss MA: Controlled radiofrequency endovenous occlusion using a unique radiofrequency catheter under duplex guidance to eliminate saphenous varicose vein reflux: A 2 year follow-up. Dermatol Surg 28:38–42, 2002.

70. Lurie F, Creton D, Eklof B, et al: Prospective randomized study of endovenous radiofrequency obliteration (Closure procedure) versus ligation and stripping in a selected patient poplutation (EVOLVeS study). J Vasc Surg 38:207–214, 2003.

71. Min RJ, Khilnani N, Zimmet SE: Endovenous laser treatment of saphenous vein reflux: Long-term results. J Vasc Intervent Radiol 14:991–996, 2003.

72. Proebstle TM, Gul D, Lehr HA, Kargl A, Knop J: Infrequent early recanalization of greater saphenous vein after endovenous laser treatment. J Vasc Surg 38:511–516, 2003.

73. Puggioni A, Kalra M, Carmo M, Mozes G, Gloviczki P: Endovenous laser therapy and radiofrequency ablation of the great saphenous vein: Analysis of early efficacy and complications. J Vasc Surg 43:488–493, 2005.

74. Gloviczki P, Bergan JJ, Menawat SS, et al: Safety, feasibility, and early efficacy of subfascial endoscopic perforator surgery: A preliminary report from the North American registry. J Vasc Surg 25:94–105, 1997.

75. Szostek M, Skorski M, Zajac S, et al: Recurrences after surgical treatment of patients with post-thrombotic syndrome of the lower extremities. Eur J Vasc Surg 2:191–192, 1988.

76. Nash T: Long-term results of vein valve transplants placed in the popliteal vein for intractable post-phlebitic venous ulcers and preulcer skin changes. J Cardiovasc Surg 29:712–716, 1988.

77. Taheri SA, Lazar L, Elias S, et al: Surgical treatment of postphlebitic syndrome with vein valve transplant. Am J Surg 144:221–224, 1982.

78. Goff JM, Gillespie DL, Rich NM: Long-term follow-up of a superficial femoral vein injury: A case report from the Vietnam Vascular Registry. J Trauma 44:209–211, 1997.

79. Kistner RL: Surgical repair of the incompetent femoral vein valve. Arch Surg 110:1336–1342, 1975.

80. Haas GE: Saphenofemoral veins crossover bypass grafting in iliofemoral vein obstruction. J Am Osteopath Assoc 89:511–518, 1989.

81. Yamamoto N, Takaba T, Hori G, et al: Reconstruction with insertion of expanded polytetrafluoroethylene (ePTFE) for iliac obstruction. J Cardiovasc Surg 27:697–702, 1986.

82. Bergan JJ, Yao JS, Flinn WR, et al: Surgical treatment of venous obstruction and insufficiency. J Vasc Surg 3:174–181, 1986.

83. Telian SH, Tretter JF, Watabe JT, et al: May-Thurner syndrome: Report of five cases treated with catheter-directed thrombolysis and stent placement. Curr Surg 56:428–436, 1999.

84. Johnson BF, Manzo RA, Bergelin RO, Srandness DE Jr: Relationship between changes in the deep venous system and the development of the post-thrombotic syndrome after an acute episode of lower limb deep venous thrombosis: One-to-six year follow-up. J Vasc Surg 21:307–312, 1995.

85. Jackson LM, Wang XJ, Dudrick SJ, Gersten GD: Catheter-directed thrombolysis and/or thrombectomy with selective endovascular stenting as alternatives to systemic anticoagulation for treatment of acute deep vein thrombosis. Am J Surg 190:864–868, 2005.

86. Mewissen MW, Seabrook GR, Meissner MH, Cynamon J, Labropoulos N, Haughton SH: Catheter-directed thrombolysis for lower extremity deep venous thrombosis: Report of a national multicenter registry. Radiology 211:39–49, 1999.

87. Raju S, Owen S, Neglen P: The clinical impact of iliac venous stent in the management of chronic venous insufficiency. J Vasc Surg 35:8–15, 2002.

88. Hartung O: Endovascular treatment of iliocaval occlusion caused by retroperitoneal fibrosis: Later results of two cases. J Vasc Surg 36:849–852, 2002.

89. Jost CJ, Gloviczki P, Cherry KJ, et al: Surgical reconstruction of iliofemoral veins and the inferior vena cava for non-malignant occlusive disease. J Vasc Surg 33:320–327, 2001.

Chapter 18

Thrombocytosis: Essential Thrombocythemia and Reactive Causes

Craig M. Kessler, MD • Jan Jacques Michiels, MD, PhD

INTRODUCTION

Thrombocytosis is defined as a platelet count above 350,000 to 400,000/μL, which is the upper limit of the normal reference range. Thrombocytosis may be categorized as familial, reactive, or secondary nonclonal processes (reactive thrombocytosis [RT]), or as the manifestation of a primary myeloproliferative disorder (MPD)—usually an autonomous and clonal process. This differentiation between RT- and MPD-associated thrombocytosis is critical because the clinical and laboratory features, as well as recommendations for management, are altogether different for each entity.[1] Thrombocytosis, when it is autonomous and clonal in origin, is designated as essential thrombocythemia (ET), a myeloproliferative disorder characterized by predominant megakaryocytic hyperplasia. However, thrombocytosis can also complicate any of the chronic MPDs, including polycythemia vera (PV), chronic myeloid leukemia (CML), myeloid metaplasia with myelofibrosis (MMM) (representing the transformation of these other MPDs), and de novo primary myelofibrosis.

REACTIVE THROMBOCYTOSIS

RT is caused by increased megakaryocyte production of platelets mediated by a physiologically normal megakaryocyte response to elevated circulating levels of cytokines. Megakaryocyte development is stimulated by various growth factors and cytokines, including thrombopoietin (TPO), interleukin (IL)-1, IL-3, IL-6, IL-11, granulocyte colony-stimulating factor, granulocyte-macrophage colony-stimulating factor, and stem cell factor. Elevated levels of IL-1, IL-6, IL-4, and C-reactive protein are found in patients with RT, whereas normal levels are observed in individuals with primary thrombocythemia.[2–4] Controversy is ongoing as to whether the degree of elevation of endogenous plasma levels of TPO can be used to distinguish a clonal process from RT. In those studies in which TPO levels were found to be significantly higher in patients with primary thrombocytosis versus those with RT (whose levels were essentially equal to those of normal healthy individuals), the difference was attributed to defective platelet- and megakaryocyte-dependent TPO clearance due to a reduced number of TPO receptors on ET platelets.

In general, RT is a much more common cause of elevated platelet counts than ET or thrombocythemia due to various MPDs (Fig. 18-1). RT is a common epiphenomenon of inflammatory (e.g., rheumatoid arthritis, inflammatory bowel disease) and neoplastic disease states, iron deficiency, and acute blood loss (Table 18-1). Secondary thrombocytosis is much more commonly encountered in clinical practice than is the primary process.[5,6] In one study of 280 patients with extreme thrombocytosis (platelet count, ≥1,000,000/μL), 82% were found to have secondary causes of thrombocytosis, and only 14% had MPDs that produced elevated platelet counts.[5] In another study, the causes of thrombocytosis in 732 patients included ET and the thrombocythemia associated with various MPDs in 12.3% and RT in 87.7%. RT was the result of tissue damage, infection, malignancy, and other rare or miscellaneous diseases (see Fig. 18-1). Therefore, a careful history and physical examination should be done and relevant laboratory data obtained to exclude causes of RT. Elevated levels of C-reactive protein, IL-6, erythrocyte sedimentation rate, and plasma fibrinogen suggest the presence of RT.[3] ET is considered a distinct entity, and its diagnosis is based on exclusion of reactive causes of elevated platelet count or on demonstration on bone marrow biopsy of increased numbers of large megakaryocytes.[7,8] Detection of the JAK2-V617F tyrosine kinase mutation is consistent with the diagnosis of ET but not with the presence of RT. Table 18-2 lists important clinical and laboratory features that may help the clinician to differentiate between diagnoses of ET and RT. RT is typically asymptomatic and is not associated with the thrombohemorrhagic complications seen in many patients with ET. Management of any secondary thrombocytosis basically involves treatment for the underlying condition that is responsible for the elevated platelet count.

FAMILIAL OR HEREDITARY THROMBOCYTOSIS

Familial thrombocytosis is a very rare condition in which extremely high platelet counts have been observed in multiple individuals in successive generations; it affects both sexes and is usually transmitted through an autosomal dominant inheritance mode.[9–13] This disorder appears to be mediated by heterogeneous gene mutations, which, in several well-defined families, have resulted in gain of function for the TPO gene[14–16] and the c-MPL receptor gene.[17] Each gain of function mutation in the TPO gene is associated

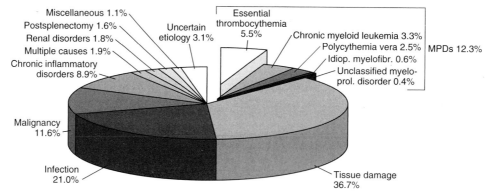

Figure 18-1 Causes of thrombocytosis in 732 patients. (From Griesshammer M, Bangerter M, Sauer T, et al: Aetiology and clinical significance of thrombocytosis: Analysis of 732 patients with an elevated platelet count. J Intern Med 245:295–300, 1999.)

Table 18-1   Causes of Thrombocytosis

- Pseudothrombocytosis
- Primary thrombocytosis
  Chronic myeloproliferative disorders: essential thrombocythemia, polycythemia vera, chronic myelogenous leukemia, agnogenic myeloid metaplasia/myelofibrosis
  Myelodysplastic syndromes: 5q- syndrome, idiopathic acquired sideroblastic anemia
  Hereditary or familial thrombocytosis
- Reactive or secondary thrombocytosis
  Bacterial infections and tuberculosis
  Inflammatory diseases
  Advanced malignancies
  Acute blood loss and hemolytic anemias
  Postsplenectomy or asplenia (congenital or functional)
  Rebound after chemotherapy-induced thrombocytopenia
  Iron deficiency

---

with overexpression of mRNA, causing TPO overproduction with increased plasma levels of TPO and increased platelet counts. Nevertheless, other mechanisms must be responsible for the development of hereditary thrombocythemia because in many other families, no mutations have been detected in the genes that code for TPO or its receptor, c-MPL.[18,19] Familial thrombocytosis due to a gain of function mutation in the TPO gene or in c-MPL is polyclonal and lacks the JAK2-V617F mutation. Clinical and laboratory features of familial thrombocythemia are similar to those of acquired ET, in which no TPO gene or c-MPL receptor gene mutation has yet been recognized. A TPO-independent mechanism has also been invoked for the extreme thrombocytosis observed in some African Americans, who are homozygous positive for the K39N missense mutation in the c-MPL gene.[20]

ESSENTIAL THROMBOCYTHEMIA

Although the ability of clinicians to establish disease clonality, to detect JAK2-V617F gene polymorphism, and to monitor elevated levels of TPO may suggest that ET can be distinguished easily from other phenotypically similar conditions associated with thrombocytosis, diagnosis of ET continues to rely heavily on exclusion of the secondary causes of elevated platelet counts (see Table 18-1 and Fig. 18-1).[1,5,6] For instance, through careful examination of the peripheral blood smear, the clinician can confirm or exclude the presence of "pseudothrombocytosis," an artefactual epiphenomenon generated by automated complete blood cell count analyzers, which frequently misidentify as platelets basophilic amorphous deposits of cryoglobulins, erythrocyte or white cell fragments, or cellular inclusions. This is most likely to occur in patients with chronic lymphocytic

---

Table 18-2   Laboratory and Clinical Characteristics of Essential Thrombocythemia and Reactive Thrombocytosis

Feature	Essential Thrombocythemia	Reactive Thrombocytosis
Thrombosis or hemorrhage	Present	Absent
Splenomegaly	Occasionally present	Typically absent
Abnormal platelet morphology and platelet aggregates on peripheral blood smear	Present	Absent
Bone marrow reticulum/fibrosis	Present	Absent
Clusters of dysplastic megakaryocytes in bone marrow	Present	Absent
Increased acute phase reactants (IL-6, C-reactive protein)	Absent	Present
Spontaneous colony formation in in-vitro cell cultures	Present	Absent
Abnormal cytogenetics	Occasionally present	Absent
Suboptimal platelet aggregation responses in in-vitro/spontaneous platelet aggregation	Present	Absent
JAK2 mutation	Frequently present	Absent

leukemia and extreme leukocytosis, in those with thrombotic thrombocytopenic purpura or massive burn injury with brisk intravascular hemolysis, and in postsplenectomy individuals with microspherocytosis in whom the presence of Howell-Jolly bodies is detected. Large numbers of giant platelets or so-called megakaryocytic fragments on the peripheral blood smear are very consistent with thrombocytosis due to an MPD rather than to a reactive process. Thus, the diagnostic workup of ET should also include cytogenetic screening for the Philadelphia chromosome (or the bcr/abl gene rearrangement) and other chromosome abnormalities because thrombocytosis and megakaryocytic hyperplasia, particularly the del(5q) syndrome, may be prominent presenting features of chronic myelogenous leukemia and myelodyplastic syndrome (MDS). Coexistence of thrombocytosis and ringed sideroblasts within the bone marrow aspirate should suggest the possibility of MDS (refractory anemia with ringed sideroblasts), but the presence of grade 3 to 4 myelofibrosis in the marrow would be more consistent with MPD.

MPD-associated thrombocythemia (polycythemia rubra vera, agnogenic myeloid metaplasia, idiopathic myeloid metaplasia, or ET) is characterized by the autonomous proliferation of platelets by megakaryocytes that reside in an abnormal marrow microenvironment and/or perhaps by megakaryocytes that are intrinsically hypersensitive to TPO stimulation.[1,21] Spontaneous megakaryocyte and/or erythroid colony formation in in vitro cell cultures is seen in 80% of patients with ET.[1] This type of abnormal growth is not observed in reactive or secondary thrombocytosis; therefore, this test, if available, may provide a useful means of distinguishing between benign and myeloproliferative causes of thrombocytosis.[1]

Although ET is the most common of the MPDs, it is a relatively uncommon disease state with an undetermined true incidence. For ET, reported annual incidence rates have ranged from 0.59 to 2.53 per 100,000 inhabitants (Table 18-3).[21–27] Prevalence is approximately 30 per 100,000 inhabitants. The Olmstead County study estimated that the annual incidence of ET is approximately 2.38 patients per 100,000 population[24]; however, the increasing use of automated blood counters has led to the detection of a significant number of incidental asymptomatic cases of ET. This is reflected in a 3.2-fold increase in the annual incidence of ET diagnosis in Denmark; diagnosis of this condition increased from 0.31 per 100,000 population in 1977 to 1.00 per 100,000 by 1998.[25] Two additional published studies have confirmed this recent phenomenon.[22,23]

Also, the incidence of ET is approximately twofold higher in females than in males.[23–25]

Pathogenesis of Essential Thrombocythemia

In 1981, ET was first recognized as a disease that arises from clonal platelet expansion by pluripotent stem cells. With the use of X-chromosome–linked gene probes, such as those used for glucose-6-phosphate dehydrogenase (G6PD), phosphoglycerate kinase, hypoxanthine phosphoribosyl transferase, and later, human androgen receptor (HUMARA) and reverse transcriptase polymerase chain reaction (RT-PCR) analysis of RNA transcripts from genes for iduronate-2-sulphatase (IDS), palmitoylated membrane protein p55, and G6PD, the study of larger populations of patients with ET became possible.[28–31]

TPO, as the primary regulator of platelet production, stimulates the growth and differentiation of megakaryocyte progenitor cells in vitro and in vivo. TPO binds to c-MPL receptors (the product of the c-MPL proto-oncogene) on the platelet membrane surface and is subsequently internalized and degraded.[32] Plasma TPO levels are regulated normally by total platelet and megakaryocyte mass, and are highly elevated in patients with aplastic anemia. It is interesting to note that TPO levels are normal or slightly elevated in ET despite an expanded megakaryocyte and platelet mass.[33] Dysregulation of the TPO–c-MPL system in ET is suggested. In fact, patients with ET have markedly decreased expression of c-MPL protein on their platelet membranes (and decreased mRNA expression), resulting in reduced TPO-binding capacity, impaired uptake and catabolism of TPO, and decreased clearance of TPO from the circulation. These findings explain the normal or slightly increased plasma TPO levels that occur in ET[34–36] and suggest that megakaryocytes in ET may be hypersensitive to the stimulatory effects of TPO on production of platelets in vivo.[6] It has not yet been determined how reliable the detection of reduced expression of c-MPL would be as a diagnostic marker for ET and primary thrombocytosis versus secondary causes for elevated platelet counts. Because TPO levels may be elevated in reactive and clonal thrombocytosis, TPO assays available to date cannot reliably be used to differentiate between these two conditions.[37–39]

Since the time that the JAK2-V617F mutation was discovered to be the cause of trilinear MPD, including ET, PV, and myelofibrosis, clinicians have come to appreciate that ET is pathogenetically heterogeneous, and that

---

Table 18-3 Incidences of Essential Thrombocythemia from Five Different Population-Based Studies, Adjusted to a Standard Population[27]

Author	Years	Location	Adjusted to	Number of Included Patients	Annual Incidence per 100,000 Inhabitants
Mesa et al, 1999[24]	1976–1995	Minnesota, USA	USnccp	39	2.53
Ridell et al, 2000[22]	1983–1992	Göteborg, Sweden	ESP	72	1.28
Jensen et al, 2000[25]	1977–1998	Copenhagen, Denmark	ESP	96	0.59
Johansson et al, 2004[23,27]	1983–1999	Göteborg, Sweden	ESP	153	1.55
Girodon et al, 2005[26]	1980–1999	Côte d'Ór, France	ESP	156	1.43

ESP, European Standard Population; USnccp, United States north central Caucasian population in 1990.[27] (From Johansson P: Epidemiology of the myeloproliferative disorders polycythemia vera and essential thrombocythemia. Sem Thromb Hemost 32:171–173, 2006.)

clonal thrombopoiesis is frequent.[40–44] Combined results of clonality assays and a PCR test for the JAK2-V617F mutation have shown that clonal proliferation occurs in up to 90% of patients with ET.[45,46] Half of these and most patients with PV have the JAK2-V617F mutation.[47–49] No consistent gene or chromosomal defect or causal gene association for ET has been identified to date.

Criteria for the Diagnosis of Essential Thrombocythemia

In 1923, Minot and Buckman[50] recognized the occurrence of multiple hemorrhagic episodes, along with very high platelet counts, in a patient with MPD. In 1934, Epstein and Goedel,[51] two Austrian hematologists, introduced the term *hemorrhagic thrombocythemia* for the association of recurrent hemorrhages with extreme thrombocytosis (vasculärer Schrumpfmilz) that had persisted for longer than 10 years. In 1960, Gunz[52] refined the definition of hemorrhagic thrombocythemia to a clinical syndrome of recurrent spontaneous hemorrhage, often preceded by thromboses, and extremely high platelet counts, usually in excess of 1,000,000/μL, that is frequently accompanied by splenomegaly and hypochromic anemia and a tendency to develop erythrocytosis (PV) between hemorrhagic episodes. In 1975, this entity was designated ET by the Polycythemia Vera Study Group (PVSG),[53] which at that time established the diagnostic criteria for ET as (1) platelet counts in excess of 1,000,000/μL, (2) bone marrow characterized by marked megakaryocytic hyperplasia, and (3) absence of PV, the Ph1 chromosome, and significant myelofibrosis.[54] These parameters were intended to exclude RT and other clonal causes of thrombocytosis (CML, PV, and the hypercellular stage of idiopathic myelofibrosis), which currently are more specifically excluded through PCR assays that detect the *bcr/abl* gene rearrangement when the Ph1 chromosome is absent and cytogenetic studies undertaken to detect del (5q), which is associated with a type of MDS that often manifests as thrombocytosis.[64–66]

In the late 1970s and early 1980s, several reports[55–61] showed that symptomatic patients with ET usually presented with microvascular peripheral or cerebral circulation disturbances when platelet counts ranged between 400,000 and 1,000,000/μL. This prompted the PVSG to lower the platelet count criterion for the diagnosis of ET to an arbitrary minimum of 600,000/μL[62] (Table 18-4). In addition, the PVSG endorsed the presence of a normal serum ferritin level concurrent with normal red blood cell MCV as sufficient evidence to exclude both reactive thrombocytosis caused by iron deficiency and PV masked by iron deficiency as the causes of thrombocytosis (see Table 18-4).[63]

The most prominent and consistent laboratory abnormality seen in ET, as defined by PVSG criteria, is a platelet count elevated to more than 600,000/μL.[61,62] In most studies, average platelet count at diagnosis is around 1,000,000/μL.[67,68] Hematocrit is usually normal unless the clinical course is complicated by bleeding or iron deficiency. Mild leukocytosis (range, 10,000 to 20,000/μL) is commonly seen and may be associated with myeloid immaturity and left shift in the differential count. Basophilia and/or eosinophilia may be present, as it is in other MPDs. Serum potassium levels may be spuriously elevated because of the very high platelet count observed in the presence of normal renal function (pseudohyperkalemia, i.e., increased serum yet normal plasma potassium levels).[61,69–71] This pseudohyperkalemia is explained by the release of potassium from platelets during in vitro coagulation and clot retraction.[70,71] Measurement of plasma potassium provides a more accurate assessment. One fourth of patients may have elevated serum lactate dehydrogenase and uric acid levels. Leukocyte alkaline phosphatase is normal in most patients, although abnormally increased or reduced levels are not uncommon.[67,72]

Assays for formation of spontaneous endogenous erythroid colonies (EECs) and spontaneous megakaryocytic colonies (EMCs) may be useful in distinguishing between ET and RT.[73] In one study, EEC had a diagnostic sensitivity of 65% for ET, and only one of 88 RT cases was EEC positive.[73] EEC-positive ET actually represents latent PV or PV masked by bleeding or chemotherapy.[74,75] In two representative studies of patients with ET[76,77] (n = 204) and RT (n = 59), the frequency of EMC in ET was modest (sensitivity, 63% and 69%; specificity, 100%), and diagnostic sensitivities rose to 77% and 92% when EMC results were combined with EEC data.[73] Although such in vitro assays are meaningful from a pathophysiologic perspective, they are difficult and expensive to perform and are reserved primarily for use in clinical research efforts.

A retrospective analysis of 143 patients with ET revealed that early ET can exist with platelet counts ranging from slightly above normal to 600,000/μL, despite the fact that PVSG diagnostic criteria for ET are not met. Bone marrow biopsies showed an increased number of loosely clustered large and giant megakaryocytes with mature cytoplasm and hyperploid multilobulated nuclei, consistent with ET.[61,65,78–86] In the overall population of patients with ET in this study,[78] bone marrow morphology in biopsy material showed normal cellularity in 52%, consistent with ET, and increased cellularity in 48%, which was attributed to erythroid hyperplasia in 17% (consistent with early PV that mimics ET) and myeloid hyperplasia in 45% (consistent with early or overt PV or prefibrotic chronic idiopathic myelofibrosis [CIMF-0]) (Table 18-5).[79]

In 2001, World Health Organization (WHO) bone marrow criteria attempted to differentiate between true ET, early PV mimicking ET, and extreme thrombocytosis, the latter of which is the presenting prominent feature in more than 90%

Table 18-4 Polycythemia Vera Study Group Criteria for Diagnosis of Essential Thrombocytosis

- Platelet count >600,000/μL
- Hematocrit <40%, or normal red cell mass (males <36mL/kg, females <32mL/kg)
- No cause for reactive thrombocytosis
- Absence of iron deficiency documented by stainable iron in marrow or normal serum ferritin or normal RBC mean corpuscular volume
- Absence of Philadelphia chromosome and *bcr/abl* gene rearrangement
- Absence of collagen fibrosis of marrow or, if present, it should be less than one third biopsy area without marked splenomegaly and without leukoerythroblastic reaction
- No cytogenetic or morphologic evidence of myelodysplastic syndrome

Table 18-5 Grading of Bone Marrow Fibrosis in Chronic Idiopathic Myelofibrosis (CIMF)

CIMF Classification	Characteristics
CIMF-0	Scattered linear reticulin with no intersections corresponding to normal bone marrow
CIMF-1	Loose network of reticulin with many intersections, particularly in perivascular areas
CIMF-2	Diffuse and dense increase in reticulin with extensive intersections, occasionally with focal bundles of collagen and/or osteosclerosis
CIMF-3	Diffuse and dense increase in reticulin with extensive intersections and coarse bundles of collagen, often associated with osteosclerosis.

Barosi G, Bordessoule D, Briere J, et al: Response criteria for myelofibrosis with myeloid metaplasia: Results of an initiative of the European Myelofibrosis Network (EUMNET). Blood 106:2849–2853, 2005.

of cases of prefibrotic CIMF (Table 18-6).[79–83] CIMF-0 is characterized by hypercellular bone marrow caused by a dual proliferation of megakaryocytes and myeloid precursors, along with relatively decreased erythropoiesis. Dense clusters of atypical immature megakaryocytes contain irregular "cloudlike nuclei," which are almost never seen in ET and PV (see Table 18-6).[79–83]

When WHO bone marrow criteria were applied retrospectively to 539 patients who had previously been diagnosed with ET according to PVSG criteria (platelet counts >600,000/μL),[79,91–93] true ET was corroborated in 21%, CIMF-0 in 27%, CIMF-1 in 40%, and CIMF-2 in 13%.[92]

According to PVSG criteria, approximately 50% of patients with ET present with spontaneous EEC[73–75] and increased polycythemia rubra vera (PRV)-1 expression,[74,87,88] together with low serum erythropoietin (EPO) levels.[87,89] EEC+/PRV-1+ ET is associated with higher risks for microvascular and major thrombotic complications as compared with EEC−/PRV-1− ET.[87,88] PRV-1–positive ET may represent a pathobiologically distinct subgroup of ET in which patients are at increased risk for the development of thrombotic complications and for eventual emergence of PV (Table 18-7).[88] The JAK2-V617F mutation has been strongly correlated with PRV-1 overexpression and the ability to form spontaneous EEC in all three subtypes of MPD.[90] Comparison of the laboratory features of JAK2-V617F positivity with those of JAK2 wild-type ET clearly shows that JAK2-V617F–positive ET is

Table 18-6 Clinical Peripheral Blood Criteria and World Health Organization (WHO) Bone Marrow Criteria for the Diagnosis of Essential Thrombocythemia (ET), Early-Stage Polycythemia Vera (PV) Mimicking ET, and Thrombocythemia as the Presenting Features of Prefibrotic Chronic Idiopathic Myelofibrosis (CIMF-0) Mimicking ET

Clinical Peripheral Blood Criteria of ET	Pathologic Criteria for ET, PV, and CIMF; WHO Bone Marrow Criteria
A1 Persistent increase in platelet count: in excess of 400,000/μL; grade I, 400,000–1,000,000/μL, and grade II, >1,000,000/μL A2 Normal spleen or only minor splenomegaly on ultrasound A3 Normal or increased leukocyte alkaline phosphatase (LAP) score, normal erythrocyte sedimentation rate (ESR) and increased mean platelet volume (MPV; some large platelets) A4 Spontaneous megakaryocyte colony formation (CFU-Meg) or spontaneous endogenous erythroid colony formation (EEC) A5 Normal or slightly increased hemoglobin (male <18.5 g/dL, female <16.5 g/dL) and hematocrit (male <51%, female <48%) A6 Low serum erythropoietin (EPO) level (early PV mimicking ET) A7 JAK2-V617F mutation (polymerase chain reaction [PCR] test) A8 No signs or causes of reactive thrombocytosis (RT) A9 No leukoerythroblastosis and no teardrop erythrocytes A10 No preceding or other allied subtypes of chronic myeloid leukemia (CML), CIMF, or myelodysplastic syndrome (MDS) and absence of the Philadelphia chromosome (*bcr/abl* gene)	**True ET** Predominant proliferation of enlarged megakaryocytes with hyperlobulated nuclei and mature cytoplasm, lacking conspicuous cytologic abnormalities. No proliferation or immaturity of granulopoiesis or erythropoiesis; no or only borderline increase in reticulin **Early PV mimicking ET** Increased cellularity with trilineage myeloproliferation (i.e., panmyelosis). Proliferation and clustering of small to giant (pleomorphic) megakaryocytes; no pronounced inflammatory reaction (plasmacytosis, cellular debris). Absence of bone marrow features consistent with congenital polycythemia and secondary erythrocytosis; no or only borderline increase in reticulin **Prefibrotic CIMF mimicking (false) ET** Megakaryocytic and granulocytic myeloproliferation and relative reduction of erythroid precursors; abnormal clustering and increase in atypical giant to medium-sized megakaryocytes containing clumpy (cloudlike) lobulated nuclei and definitive maturation defects; no or only borderline increase in reticulin

(From WHO classification of the chronic myeloproliferative diseases (CMPD) polycythemia vera, chronic idiopathic myelofibrosis, essential thrombocythemia, and CMPD unclassifiable. WHO Classification of Tumours. Tumours of Haematopoiesis and Lymphoid Tissues. Lyon, France, IARC 2001 pp 31–42; Michiels JJ, Thiele J: Clinical and pathological criteria for the diagnosis of essential thrombocythemia, polycythemia vera and idiopathic myelofibrosis (agnogenic myeloid metaplasia). Int J Hematol 76:133–145, 2002; Michiels JJ: Bone marrow histopathology and biological markers as specific clues to the differential diagnosis of essential thrombocythemia, polycythemia vera and prefibrotic or fibrotic myeloid metaplasia. Hematol J 5:93–102, 2004; Thiele J, Kvasnicka HM, Orazi A: Bone marrow histopathology in myeloproliferative disorders: Current diagnostic approach. Sem Hematol 42:184–195, 2005; and Thiele J, Kvasnicka HM: Clinicopathological criteria for the differential diagnosis of thrombocythemia in various myeloproliferative disorders. Sem Thromb Hemost 32:219–230, 2006.)

18

Table 18-7 ET According to New Clinical and WHO Bone Marrow Criteria

ET	Hereditary ET	True ET	Early PV Mimicking ET	Prefibrotic CIMF False ET
Incidence	< 0.001	20–30	20–30	40–60
Serum EPO	Normal	Normal	Decreased ↓	Normal
Platelets ×10^3/µL	>400	>400	>400	>400
Erythrocytes	N	N	N/↑	N/↓
Hematocrit	N	N	N/↑	N/↓
Bone marrow:	ET picture	ET picture	PV picture	CIMF picture
Megakaryocytes	(————————Large, giant, and mature————————)			Abnormal
Splenomegaly	–	– / +	– / +	+ / –
JAK2-V617F	Neg (–)	– / +	++	+ / –
EEC	Neg (–)	– / +	++	+ / –
PVR-1	Not applicable	– / +	++	+ / –
Clonality	Polyclonal	Polyclonal/Monoclonal	Monoclonal	Monoclonal

EEC, endogenous erythroid colony formation.

characterized by increased levels of hemoglobin and hematocrit, elevated neutrophil counts, and higher leukocyte alkaline phosphatase (LAP) scores, but by lower values for serum EPO, serum ferritin, and mean corpuscular volume (MCV); increased cellularity of the bone marrow is seen in biopsy material. These properties indicate that JAK2-V617F–positive ET probably represents a "forme fruste of PV" that is consistent with early PV that mimics ET (see Table 18-7).[37] In contrast, patients with JAK2 wild-type ET have significantly higher platelet counts and usually show a clinical picture of true ET with normal serum EPO levels, normal PRV-1 expression, and normal LAP scores.[37]

Life expectancy in true ET is normal when transformation or progression to myelofibrosis does not occur but is compromised in those with prefibrotic CIMF-0 or early fibrotic CIMF-1 mimicking ET (false ET). This is due to an increased tendency of patients to develop worsening myelofibrosis and splenomegaly during long-term follow-up.[91,93] In one large study, 10-year relative (age-adjusted) survival rates were 99.1% ± 7.8% for true ET, 80.8% ± 11.7% for CIMF-0, and 67.3% ± 17.8% for CIMF-1.[93]

Coagulation Laboratory Features of Essential Thrombocythemia: The Paradox of In Vivo Platelet Activation and Impaired Platelet Function

Elevated levels of plasma β-thromboglobulin, increased generation of thromboxane B$_2$, and enhanced expression of P-selectin (CD62P) and thrombospondin on platelet surface membranes have been observed in patients with ET.[94–98] These findings suggest that enhanced in vivo platelet activation occurs in patients with ET and may predispose them to hypercoagulable complications.[94–98] These laboratory changes are not detected in patients with RT.[94,95] A recent study of patients with ET and thrombocythemia associated with PV revealed that markers of in vivo platelet activation (CD62P [P-selectin] and CD63 antigens measured by flow cytometry) were significantly more elevated in those who experienced arterial thromboses or erythromelalgia[99] than in healthy controls and those thrombocythemic patients without thrombotic events. Individuals with arterial thromboses and/or erythromelalgia also exhibited evidence of endothelial cell activation (increased levels of plasma soluble vascular cell adhesion molecule-1 [sVCAM-1]).[99] Cause/effect relationships were not obvious in this cohort because laboratory markers for platelet and endothelial cell activation remained elevated after cytoreductive therapy was provided. A possible pathophysiologic link was suggested by the observation that patients with ET had higher percentages of circulating platelet/neutrophil and platelet/monocyte complexes in conjunction with higher monocyte tissue factor (mTF) expression as compared with healthy controls.[100] Enhanced platelet–leukocyte interaction is known to facilitate leukocyte adhesion and activation, as well as tissue factor (TF) transfer between monocytes and platelets. These events may modulate activation of coagulation by release of TF and formation of circulating microparticles rich in TF and may mediate damage to the endothelium. Consistent with this hypothesis is that monocyte activation (CD11b expression) and mTF expression were significantly higher in patients with ET who had a history of thrombosis than in patients without thrombosis.[100] Aspirin inhibits platelet–granulocyte interactions[101–103]; this inhibition provides a rationale for aspirin use to reduce the intrinsic hypercoagulability associated with ET and PV.[104,105] In toto, these data support the concept that spontaneous platelet activation and subsequent platelet–neutrophil and platelet–monocyte aggregation precipitate or exacerbate inflammatory responses and thrombogenesis in the end-arterial circulation of patients with ET (Fig. 18-2).[61,106,107] Thus, patients with ET and PV along with microvascular ischemic or thrombotic complications have shortened platelet survival; increased plasma levels of β-thromboglobulin (β-TG), platelet factor 4 (PF4), and thrombomodulin (TM); and increased urinary excretion of thromboxane B$_2$ (TxB$_2$).[108–110] Subsequent inhibition of platelet cyclo-oxygenase (COX-1) by aspirin is followed by symptomatic relief of microvascular ischemic and throm-

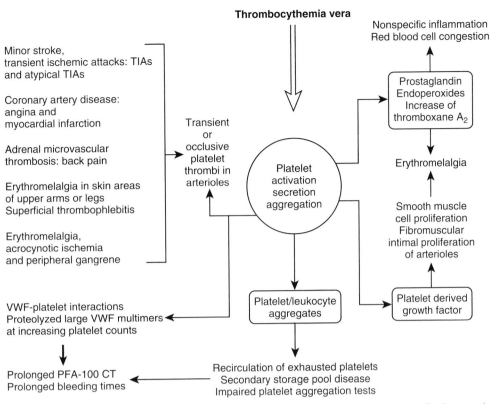

Figure 18-2 The clinical spectrum of microvascular circulation disturbances, including erythromelalgic ischemic complications, atypical transient ischemic cerebral attacks (TIAs), ocular manifestations, and coronary artery disease, is caused by platelet-mediated thrombotic processes in the peripheral, cerebral, and coronary microvascular circulation. The paradox of in vivo platelet activation and impaired platelet aggregation tests can readily be explained by recirculation of exhausted platelets with secondary storage pool disease. At increasing platelet counts, large von Willebrand factor (VWF) multimers are proteolyzed, leading to prolonged platelet function analyzer (PFA)-100 closure times (CTs) and bleeding times.

botic complications; reversal of shortened platelet survival; reduction of increased β-TG, PF4, and TM plasma levels; and normalization of increased TxB$_2$ excretion.[106–110]

Contrary to evidence of in vivo platelet activation, in vitro platelet aggregation responses in patients with ET are usually suboptimal after agonists are added.[111,112] Spontaneous platelet aggregation or hyperaggregability is variably observed.[56,67,68] Platelet function tests that characteristically differentiate ET from RT include (1) absent second wave of platelet aggregation after addition of epinephrine to platelet-rich plasma from patients with ET, (2) increased adenosine diphosphate (ADP) aggregation threshold in ET, and (3) reduced secretion of dense body products from ET platelets (e.g., serotonin during arachidonic acid or collagen-induced aggregation).[111,112] Bleeding time is usually normal at platelet counts between 400,000 and 1,000,000/μL.[111] Platelets in ET are characterized by acquired storage pool disease; by defects in the structure and function of surface membrane glycoproteins (GPs) and receptors, very likely due to downregulated adrenergic GP-Ib-IX and GP-IIb/IIIa receptors on activated platelets; and by their ability to form aggregates with activated leukocytes.[111,112]

Findings of ex vivo traditional platelet aggregation studies in which platelet-rich plasma from 55 patients with ET was used have been compared with simultaneous results obtained with platelet function analyzer (PFA)-100 closure times.[113] Aggregation results were abnormal in 75% of patients with ET; impaired responses to epinephrine were

noted in 58%, to collagen in 38%, and to ADP in 11%. Analysis of the whole group revealed a statistically significantly decreased response to epinephrine and collagen as compared with 26 normal controls. PFA-100 closure times were prolonged in 74% (41 of 55) of patients with ET: 38 with the collagen/epinephrine cartridge and 23 with the collagen/ADP cartridge (some with defects using both cartridges).[113] This study did not attempt to correlate abnormal PFA-100 closure times with occurrence of clinical bleeding.

The paradox that in vivo platelet activation and impaired platelet function may coexist in ET can be explained by the fact that ET platelets are "hypersensitive" and can be activated spontaneously by high shear stress in the arterial microvasculature. This causes platelets to secrete their granular contents to promote the formation of von Willebrand factor (VWF) protein–mediated platelet aggregates. These aggregates transiently plug the microcirculation; eventually, the platelets disaggregate and recirculate as "exhausted" or "spent" platelets, which are functionally deficient by virtue of their acquired "secondary" storage pool disease. This pattern is apparent on in vitro platelet function assays (see Fig. 18-2).[94–113]

From the clinical perspective, when VWF-mediated platelet aggregates plug the microcirculation, they release into the local milieu potent vasoactive and inflammatory secretion products, which, in turn, may precipitate vasomotor symptoms, such as erythromelalgia, acroparesthesia, migraine-like headaches, and atypical transient ischemic attacks (TIAs) (see Fig. 18-2). Paresis, visual disturbances, and epileptic seizures have also been reported.[114–118] VWF-rich platelet thrombi have been observed in skin punch biopsy specimens of erythromelalgic lesions in untreated patients with ET[108]; they probably also occur in the cerebral, ocular, coronary, and abdominal microcirculation, if left untreated (see Fig. 18-2).[94–113] Erythromelalgia and atypical and typical cerebral or ocular migraine-like TIAs in ET rapidly and dramatically resolve after administration of aspirin, which reveals an additional compelling indication of the critical role of platelet activation in vivo and the contribution of prostaglandin endoperoxides to induced thrombotic complications in ET.[56–61,106–110,115–117]

Clinical Features and Thrombohemorrhagic Complications

ET was originally classified as a hemorrhagic disease associated with thrombocytosis.[51–54] More recent observations indicate that thrombotic episodes, particularly microvascular episodes, occur far more frequently in ET than do hemorrhagic complications. This may reflect increased awareness and the earlier age of ET diagnosis when thrombocytosis is detected on routine complete blood count (CBC). When extreme thrombocytosis complicates other MPDs, differences are noted in patterns of clinical hemostatic manifestations as compared with ET.[111] For instance, bleeding and thrombosis occur very infrequently in individuals with CML, despite the presence of extreme thrombocytosis. Idiopathic myelofibrosis associated with extreme thrombocytosis is rarely complicated by hypercoagulable thrombotic events. Patients with PV and thrombocytosis are more prone to thrombotic episodes, particularly when their hematocrit levels are elevated (see later), although bleeding complications may occur concurrently. Despite these generalized observations, the literature has failed to show a clear correlation between platelet count and incidences of hemorrhage or thrombosis in patients with MPD with uncontrolled thrombocytosis.[119]

Patients with ET with platelet counts above 1,000,000/μL present with high incidences of bleeding and thrombotic complications.[54] Symptomatic manifestations related to the arterial microcirculation, especially in peripheral and cerebral regions, constitute the most frequent clinical complications in ET.[55,60,111] Patients may present with paresthesias and erythromelalgia, characterized by warm, markedly erythematous, and congested extremities and an intensely painful burning sensation over the fingers, soles, and toes. If left untreated, erythromelalgia can lead to acrocyanosis or gangrene of the fingers and toes. Other associated complications may include migraine-like headaches, atypical and typical TIAs, ocular ischemic manifestations, and peripheral arterial occlusive disease of the lower extremities.[56–61,65,72,114–117] These symptoms are most likely due to platelet activation in the microcirculation and microthrombi formation, which are so promptly relieved by low doses of aspirin (81 mg) that the response serves as a diagnostic criterion (see Fig. 18-2).

The published incidence of major thrombosis has ranged from about 25% to 30% in unselected individuals with ET.[67,68,120–127] An analysis of 11 retrospective clinical studies comprising 809 patients with ET[128] reported the overall incidence of thromboembolic complications

as 58% and of overall bleeding events as 17%; thromboembolic events without concurrent bleeding occurred in 42%, bleeding without thrombosis was reported in 1.4%, and absence of bleeding or thrombotic symptoms was noted in 36%.[128] The incidence of deep venous thrombosis, including portal and splenic vein thrombosis, was reportedly 4%, but the incidence of Budd-Chiari syndrome was not recorded.[128] Arterial thrombotic problems in this cohort of 809 patients with ET were described as microcirculatory in 41%, with 24% involving upper and lower extremities and 17% involving the cerebral circulation.

The literature is imprecise as to the frequency of thrombohemorrhagic complications at time of presentation of ET. Of 809 patients with ET in 11 retrospective studies analyzed, between 31% and 83% presented with minor and/or major arterial complications. Significantly, 27% to 70% of these patients had end-arterial microvascular signs and symptoms, reported as acroparesthesias, burning red or blue toes or fingers (erythromelalgia), peripheral ischemia, poorly localized neurologic symptoms, and blurred vision or headache.[128] Four percent to 38% of patients with ET presented with bleeding complications.[128] This variability in manifestations and longitudinal symptoms probably reflects the heterogeneity of the patient population studied and differences in the definition of thrombohemorrhagic complications; however, age at diagnosis of ET also is very important in this regard because major thrombohemorrhagic manifestations are less frequent before the age of 60 years. Analysis of the overall patient population with ET indicates that the median age at presentation is approximately 60 years, with only 10% to 25% of patients presenting when younger than 40 years old. In addition, one third of ET diagnoses are established in asymptomatic individuals.[67,68,120,121,124,128] At ages younger than 60 years, ET is more common among females, but thereafter, no sex predilection is known. The annual incidence of major thrombotic complications in ET is significantly greater in those older than 60 years of age (15%) compared with those younger than 40 years of age (2%).[125] Thrombosis-free survival (TFS) was noted to be normal in those diagnosed when younger than 60 years and without a prior history of venous or arterial thromboembolic episodes.[122,125] Most major thrombotic events in ET occur in those with prior hypercoagulable histories and cardiovascular risk factors. The potential contribution of the hereditary hypercoagulable state (factor V Leiden, prothrombin gene mutation, deficiency of antithrombin III, protein S, or protein C) to the incidence of thrombotic complications in patients with ET has not yet been established.[131]

A thrombocythemic patient with ET or PV may "shift" from being primarily thrombosis prone to becoming a "bleeder," as the disease progresses and platelet counts increase during long-term follow-up.[51,52,118] Major hemorrhagic complications usually affect the gastrointestinal tract and are frequently associated with, precipitated by, and exacerbated by concurrent use of antiplatelet-aggregating medications.[118,134–138] Large hematomas, hemarthroses, and intraocular, posttraumatic, or postsurgical bleeding rarely occur. Uncontrolled thrombocytosis is also a definite risk factor for these major bleeding events.[118,119] Minor bleeding is characteristic among those with qualitative or quantitative platelet disorders or VWD (Fig. 18-3)[111];

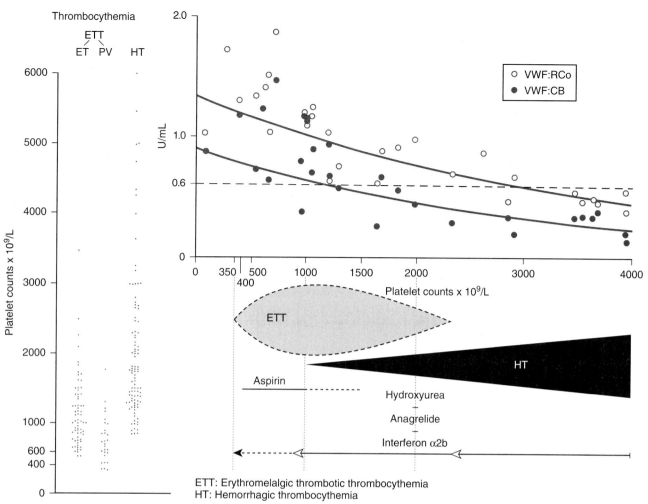

Figure 18-3 Correlation between clinical signs and symptoms and platelet counts in essential thrombocythemia (ET) and polycythemia vera (PV). The concept of platelet-mediated microvascular thrombosis and bleeding in thrombocythemia and the relationship between platelet counts and functional von Willebrand factor (VWF) levels (VWF ristocetin cofactor activity [VWF:RCo] and VWF collagen binding activity [VWF:CB]) in patients with erythromelalgic thrombotic thrombocythemia (ETT) and hemorrhagic thrombocythemia (HT) are shown here. Note the progressive decrease in VWF:RCo and VWF:CB that occurs at increasing platelet counts. As the platelet count rises, risks of bleeding increase because of reduced VWF protein activities. Erythromelalgic symptoms are an indication for aspirin, but loss of VWF protein activity is a relative contraindication for the use of aspirin in thrombocythemic patients (ET and PV). (From Schafer AI: Bleeding and thrombosis in the myeloproliferative disorders. Blood 64:1–12, 1984.)

mucosal hemorrhagic manifestations, such as epistaxis, ecchymoses, and gingival bleeding, predominate.

In a study of 100 consecutive case histories of MPD-associated hemorrhagic thrombocythemia, 50 had gastrointestinal blood loss (melena and/or hematemesis or chronic occult blood loss), 34 had manifestations of cutaneous bleeding (subcutaneous hematomas and ecchymoses), 33 had episodes of epistaxis, 15 experienced gingival bleeding, and 29 had bleeds related to trauma or surgery.[118] Petechiae were never seen. Bleeding symptoms occurred at a mean platelet count of greater than 2,000,000/μL (compared with thrombotic complications, which occurred at a mean platelet count of approximately 1,100,000/μL)[118] and often were associated with the development of acquired VWD (Figs. 18-3 and 18-4).

Decreases in VWF protein function (ristocetin cofactor activity; VWF:RCo) and in ability to bind to collagen (VWF:CB) and the loss of large VWF multimers are significantly correlated in ET and other MPDs with extremely increased platelet counts (see Fig. 18-4).[134–138] At platelet counts in excess of 1,000,000/μL, the absolute

values of VWF antigen (VWF:Ag) and factor VIII:C usually remain normal as VWF:RCo and VWF:CB decrease. This results in decreased ratios of VWF:RCo/VWF:Ag and VWF:CB/VWF:Ag, consistent with acquired variant type 2A von Willebrand disease. Also, plasma concentration of the large VWF multimers is decreased (confirmed on sodium dodecyl sulfate [SDS] chromatography of VWF protein) through their increased adsorption to platelet surfaces as platelet counts rise (see Fig. 18-4).[134–138] Reduction of the platelet count to <1,000,000/μL usually restores the multimeric integrity of the VWF protein with reversal of bleeding tendencies.[134–136] Deficient VWF:RCo and VWF:CB may also be corrected to low normal levels.[133–138] Altered VWF structure and function and qualitative platelet defects are not features of RT; thus, clinical bleeding is typically not observed in that condition.[137]

Physical examination is usually unremarkable in early ET. Some patients may have moderate or progressive splenomegaly and/or hepatomegaly indicative of CIMF,[61,67,68] particularly as the disease progresses to MMM.[61,67,68,129]

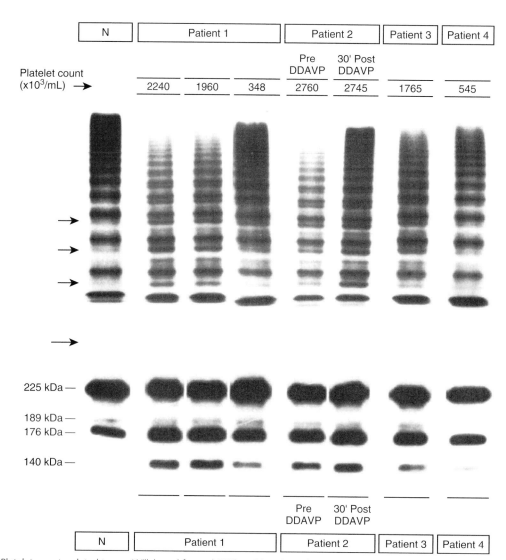

Figure 18-4 Platelet counts related to von Willebrand factor (VWF) multimeric analysis with medium-resolution agarose gel in four patients with essential thrombocythemia. Medium-resolution agarose gel separates each oligomer into at least three bands—one main and two satellite bands—the so-called triplet structure, which is typically pronounced because of proteolysis of large VWF in von Willebrand disease types 2A and 2B and is also seen in the three patients with ET and high platelet counts. Absence of large VWF at platelet counts of approximately 2,000,000/μL is associated with increased VWF degradation bands (176 and 140 kDa), reappearance of large VWF multimers after 1-deamino-8-D-arginine vasopressin (DDAVP), and correction of the VWF multimeric pattern to nearly normal at platelet counts of 348,000/μL and 545,000/μL. (Modified from Budde U, Scharf RE, Franke P, et al: Elevated platelet count as a cause of abnormal von-Willebrand factor multimer distribution in plasma. Blood 82:1749–1757, 1993.)

However, the prevalence of splenomegaly in ET is much less than the 70% incidence observed in PV.[130]

The natural history and life expectancy of individuals with ET have been difficult to ascertain in an accurate manner. Most clinical studies of ET have been retrospective in nature with limited follow-up times, small sample sizes, and a predominance of young women. A large longitudinal study of 187 consecutive patients with ET reported that those diagnosed before 55 years of age had a significantly shorter life expectancy than did healthy age-matched controls.[124] In this study, arterial thromboses occurred more frequently in ET than did venous thrombotic events (ratio, 3.1:1).[124] About 60% of venous thromboses were noted to involve splanchnic veins and cerebral venous sinuses.[60,124] RT is not associated with significant risks for thromboembolism. Life expectancy for patients with ET has recently been redefined through a retrospective analysis of a substantial cohort of 322 individuals followed for a median of longer than 13

years.[132] In this cohort, with a median age of 54 years (82.9% treated with cytoreductive therapy, 62.4% treated with aspirin), median survival time was 18.9 years, and survival during the first decade of disease was similar to that in a normal, healthy control group. On the other hand, as disease progressed over time, survival statistics worsened for patients with ET. At 20 years after diagnosis of ET, median survival was approximately 50% compared with 70% for controls.[132] Age at diagnosis of ET (> 60 years), leukocytosis, smoking, and diabetes mellitus were independent predictors of decreased survival and adverse thrombotic complications.[132] Short-term life expectancy has not been affected substantially by the rare progression of ET into acute leukemia or transformation of ET into MMM. In older studies, overall progression of ET to acute leukemia or development of MMM has been observed in 3% to 5% of cases, with acute leukemia occurring predominantly in older patients and in those who previously received treatment with radiophosphorus or alkylating agents.[67,68,129] The Mayo Clinic cohort recorded a relatively low incidence of leukemic or myeloid disease transformation over the first 10 years of the disease (1.4% and 9.1%, respectively) with substantially increased incidences of acute leukemia to 24% and 58.8%, respectively, with myeloid disease transformation during the third decade of ET.[132]

Similar trends in the natural history and life expectancy of ET were reported in a recent retrospective study of 231 consecutive Chinese patients with ET,[133] all of whom received hydroxyurea at diagnosis or during follow-up. Age over 60 years was the sole prognostic factor for overall survival and was a predominant risk factor for nonfatal major thrombosis with a TFS of 60% after 10 years as compared with a TFS of 90% at age younger than 60 years.[133] However, thrombosis was not a risk factor for survival, in that only 2 of 231 patients with ET (0.9%) died from thrombosis. Of 20 deaths in this cohort, 5 patients died between 62 and 90 years of age from acute myelogenous leukemia (AML)/MDS/MF, 2 died as a result of major thrombosis, 2 died because of severe bleeding, 3 died from carcinoma, and 8 died from pneumonia or chronic obstructive respiratory disease unrelated to ET.[133]

Prognostic Indicators for Thrombosis and Hemorrhage in ET

Numerous risk factors that predispose patients with ET to thrombotic and hemorrhagic complications have been identified and used to develop risk stratification paradigms for treatment planning. Age and prior history of cardiovascular disease and/or thromboembolic events have emerged as primary prognostic factors for future or recurrent thrombotic complications in ET. Age older than 60 years is associated with an annual incidence of thrombosis of almost 15%, compared with 6.7% at age 40 to 60 years, and less than 2% in those younger than 40 years of age.[122] The likelihood of thrombosis during follow-up was tenfold greater in those not on aspirin with a prior history of major thrombosis, irrespective of age (3.4% incidence per patient-year for those without and 31.4% per patient-year for those with a history of major thrombosis).[122] When aspirin is administered to patients with ET, TFS approaches normal and age is eliminated as a risk factor for such complications.[139]

Other risk factors besides age and history of prior thrombotic events may contribute to thrombotic tendencies. In a series of young women with ET, Tefferi[140] reported recurrent thrombosis in 45% of those with and 13% of those without a history of prior thrombosis. The contributions of obesity, oral estrogen contraceptive use, and smoking must be clarified in this population. The role of hypercholesterolemia in the development of thrombosis in ET is also unclear. Although one study reported a 59.5% incidence of thrombosis among patients with ET with hypercholesterolemia,[123] no increased risk has been noted by others.[122,124] Furthermore, no increased risks for thrombosis in ET were observed with other vascular risk factors, such as diabetes, essential hypertension,[78,122–124] and sex.[121,124] Cigarette smoking was linked to an increased incidence of ischemic complications in one study[61] but not in others.[78,122–124] Leukocytosis (>15,000/μL) also has recently been recognized as an independent predictor of major thrombotic events.[132]

In general, platelet count is *not* a reliable predictor for development of thromboses in individual patients with ET.[68,120–123,126] Although most thrombotic events are associated with platelet counts higher than 500,000 to 600,000/μL,[120,124] even while patients are on aspirin, it is not uncommon for thrombotic, neurologic, or peripheral vascular symptoms to be diagnosed at lower platelet counts.[127] Extreme thrombocytosis (1,000,000 to 1,500,000/μL) appears to increase the risk of spontaneous bleeding events, particularly from the gastrointestinal tract, with concomitant use of aspirin or other antiplatelet aggregation agents.[68,118,120,135,139]

Analysis of risk factors is important in determining which patients need cytoreductive therapy and when treatment should begin. Stratification of patients into low-, intermediate-, and high-risk categories for thrombohemorrhagic complications is recommended to establish the risk:benefit ratio for treatment because some cytoreductive medications have significant adverse effects and potentially are leukemogenic.[122,141–143] Patients of any age with a prior history of thrombosis, extreme thrombocytosis, and/or thrombotic or hemorrhagic symptoms should be classified as high risk. Those older than 60 years of age with platelet counts above 450,000/μL are also classified as high risk by most physicians, but in the absence of previous thrombosis and vascular risk factors, they are better labeled as intermediate risk.[139] Healthy patients with ET who are older than 60 to 65 years and have no vascular risk factors, no symptoms while on low-dose aspirin, and platelet counts lower than 1,000,000/μL are not at high risk for major thrombosis and therefore should not be treated with anagrelide or hydroxyurea.[139,142,143] Individuals of any age with extreme thrombocytosis (>1,500,000/μL) but without active thrombohemorrhagic symptoms are considered to be at intermediate risk.[122,140] It is unclear whether cardiovascular risk factors (e.g., diabetes mellitus, hypertension, hyperlipidemia) contribute to mortality or morbidity in ET, but clearly, these risk factors should be addressed. Patients with ET who are younger than 60 years of age, asymptomatic, and without a previous history of thrombosis and cardiovascular risks but who have an elevated platelet count (in excess of 1,000,000/μL and less than 1,500,000/μL) have been designated as at low risk for major thromboembolic or hemorrhagic events.[122,140] However, it remains unclear whether low-risk individuals with ET should be treated. Most clinicians advocate a "wait and watch" policy. Careful monitoring of bleeding time, PFA-100 closure times, and VWF parameters seems warranted for symptomatic patients with ET with platelet counts between 1,000,000/μL and 1,500,000/μL while on low-dose aspirin, because they are at increased risk of bleeding complications.[142,143] These considerations suggest that more aggressive cytoreductive therapy with newer nonleukemogenic agents, like anagrelide or interferon (IFN)-α, should be considered in patients with ET with platelet counts in excess of 1.000,000/μL, irrespective of age, to maintain platelet counts lower than 600,000 to 400,000/μL.

Treatment of Patients with Essential Thrombocythemia

In patients with ET, the occurrence of thrombotic complications is related to increased platelet count and enhanced function but is not exclusively dependent on degree of platelet elevation.[144]

Reducing the platelet count to normal (<400,000/µL) in *symptomatic* patients with ET through the use of cytoreductive medications is clearly associated with a significant reduction in the frequency of minor and major venous and cerebral arterial thrombotic events. In fact, recurrent thromboses are unusual, even without aspirin use, as long as platelet counts are maintained within the normal range.[115–117,139,142–146] In patients with ET with a platelet count greater than 600,000/µL (uncontrolled thrombocytosis), the incidence of cerebral arterial thrombosis was 180 times higher than the epidemiologic expected rate in a normal population.[147] In this controlled, prospective study of 100 consecutive patients with ET, 63% of arterial cerebral ischemic attacks were associated with platelet counts higher than 1,000,000/µL. After busulfan therapy had been administered to reduce platelet counts, the subsequent incidence of cerebral ischemic events was reduced to 37% when platelet count ranged from 650,000 to 990,000/µL, and no events occurred at counts lower than 650,000/µL.[147] In another prospective trial, 114 high-risk patients with ET were randomly assigned to receive no myelosuppressive therapy or hydroxyurea to maintain platelet counts lower than 600,000/µL.[148] After a median follow-up of 27 months, 2 (3.6%) patients in the hydroxyurea arm (one with stroke and one with deep vein thrombosis) versus 14 (24%) in the untreated group (one with cerebrovascular accident [CVA]; 12 with minor microvascular thrombotic events, including TIAs in five and peripheral digital ischemia in five; one with deep vein thrombosis [DVT]; and two with superficial thrombophlebitis) experienced thrombotic complications of ET.[148] Although this striking difference (P < .003) suggests at first glance that cytoreduction of platelet counts is the primary means of preventing thrombosis in high-risk patients with ET, another possible explanation for these observations may be the fact that 10 of 14 symptomatic patients in the control group were not receiving treatment with platelet-inhibiting medications (aspirin or ticlopidine) at the time of their thrombotic events.[148] This could also account for the unusually high incidence of microvascular arterial events reported in the control arm as compared with the hydroxyurea arm.[139,146]

Important hints for the optimal treatment of patients with ET have been provided by the British Medical Research Council's primary thrombocythemia (PT-1) study, in which 809 high-risk patients with ET were randomly assigned to receive hydroxyurea (an antineoplastic agent with nonspecific myelosuppressive properties acquired through inhibition of DNA synthesis) combined with aspirin (75 mg per day) or anagrelide (a specific inhibitor of megakaryocytopoiesis and thrombopoiesis) combined with aspirin.[149] No statistically significant differences in the incidence of specific major arterial thrombotic events (CVA, angina, or myocardial infarction), pulmonary embolism, or death due to thrombosis or hemorrhage were reported between the two arms of the study.[149] However, when composite end points were considered, anagrelide plus aspirin was associated with increased risk for the development of all types of arterial thromboses (P = .004), primarily those attributable to a greater than fivefold enhanced incidence of TIAs (P < .001), compared with hydroxyurea combined with low-dose aspirin. This is difficult to explain because the extent of reduction in platelet counts was equivalent between the two treatment arms,

and because aspirin has been shown to effectively prevent atypical and typical TIAs in ET.[115–117] Thus, control of platelet count alone should not be regarded as the exclusive surrogate end point by which the efficacy of a treatment strategy for ET should be judged. A more likely explanation for the apparent superiority of hydroxyurea over anagrelide in the PT-1 study lies in the observation that hydroxyurea, in contrast to the specific effects of anagrelide on platelet counts, conveys broader myelosuppressive activity that also affects platelets, leukocytes, and erythrocytes. Growing evidence suggests that leukocytes may play an important role in the pathogenesis of thrombosis in ET.[132] Perhaps counterintuitive to this discussion is the fact that a significantly decreased rate of venous thromboembolism (VTE) (pulmonary embolism and DVT) was seen in the anagrelide cohort compared with the hydroxyurea group (P = .006). Evidence suggests that the JAK2-V617F gene mutation is associated with predisposition to VTE as opposed to arterial events in patients with ET.[47]

Traditionally, the decision to initiate treatment for ET has been based on clinical symptoms and signs and risk factor analysis, and not merely on diagnosis, platelet number, or function (Table 18-8). It remains unclear whether young (younger than 60 years old), asymptomatic (low-risk) patients should receive treatment. In a prospective study of 65 untreated patients with ET who were younger than 65 years of age, had no history of thrombosis or hemorrhage, and had platelet counts lower than 1,500,000/µL, the incidence of thrombosis was 1.91 cases per 100 patient-years versus 1.5 cases of thrombosis in a normal, age- and sex-matched control population after a median follow-up of 4.1 years.[140] This was not statistically significant, but 25 of these patients (38%) needed low-dose aspirin to control ET-related microvascular symptoms.[140] Pregnancy and surgery were not associated with an increased incidence of thrombosis in these patients with ET. In contrast, cytoreductive therapy is clearly indicated for those patients with ET who have symptoms or who have risk factors for thrombosis or hemorrhage, including age older than 60 years, prior history of major thrombosis, or extreme thrombocytosis (platelet count >1,000,000/µL).[122,142,143,148] Hydroxyurea administration is the preferred treatment modality for patients with ET who are older than 60 to 65 years of age; anagrelide or IFN-α should be considered for the treatment of patients with ET who are younger than 60 to 65 years of age.[131] Patients should be advised to cease smoking, to avoid taking estrogen-containing medications, and to seek proper management of hypertension and diabetes, each of which is an independent risk factor for hypercoagulability and major thrombosis. Treatment options designed to reduce platelet counts in ET are listed in Table 18-8.

Hydroxyurea Therapy

Hydroxyurea is a nonalkylating S-phase–specific myelosuppressive agent with a mechanism of action that is not platelet specific. It inhibits ribonucleotide diphosphate reductase, the enzyme that catalyzes the conversion of ribonucleotide diphosphates to corresponding deoxyribose forms. Clinical experiments indicate that hydroxyurea treatment reduces hematopoietic progenitor growth and CD34-positive cells in PV and ET.[151] It is administered

Table 18-8   Risk Stratification and Management Guidelines for Essential Thrombocythemia

Age, years	Platelet count, ×10³/μL	Microvascular Symptoms	Prior History of Major Thrombosis or Bleeding	Vascular Risk	Risk of ET	Guideline
18–90	>1500	–	–	–	High	Platelet reduction to below 1000, and add aspirin
18–90	>400	–	Yes	–	High	Platelet reduction plus aspirin
18–90	<1000	Yes	No	No	Low	Low-dose aspirin
<60	<1500	No	No	No	Low	Wait and see, aspirin uncertain
<60	>1000 but <1500	Yes	No	No	Moderate	Platelet reduction to below 1000 plus aspirin
>60–65	<1000	Yes/no	No	No	Moderate	Low-dose aspirin
>60–65	<1000	Yes/no	No	Yes	High	Platelet reduction plus low-dose aspirin
>60–65	>1000	–	–	–	High	Platelet reduction plus low-dose aspirin

For all patients, manage cardiovascular risk factors; advise against smoking.
May consider low-dose aspirin in asymptomatic patients if no other contraindications are present and platelet counts are <1500 × 10³/μL.
Consider continuation of aspirin after platelet reduction is attained in patients with high-risk ET, if no contraindications are present.
Consider anagrelide as first-line therapy in patients younger than 65 years of age with no cardiac disease.[150]
Consider pegylated interferon-α as an alternative first-line nonleukemogenic agent in patients younger than 65 years of age.
Consider hydroxyurea as first-line therapy for patients 60 to 65 years of age or older.
Consider low-dose aspirin and pegylated interferon-α, if indicated, in pregnancy.

orally and appears to have good bioavailability. Hydroxyurea is predominantly used to treat patients with MPDs, in CML to control leukocytosis, in ET to reduce platelet counts, and in PV to reduce red cell mass and elevated platelet counts. The starting dose is 15 to 20 mg/kg/day orally, taken as a single dose. Subsequent dosing traditionally has been titrated to maintain platelet counts lower than 600,000 per microliter without excessive lowering of neutrophil counts. Recent data suggest that patients with ET may benefit further from platelet counts reduced to lower than 400,000/μL and maintained at that level. Dose modifications should be considered for patients with renal insufficiency. Continuous treatment with hydroxyurea has been shown to reduce platelet counts to lower than 500,000/μL within the first 8 weeks in 80% of patients.[152–154] Advantages of hydroxyurea include its convenience, efficacy, and low level of toxicity. Major short-term adverse effects include reversible myelosuppression manifested as neutropenia and macrocytic anemia. Other adverse effects include nausea, vomiting, diarrhea, skin changes and ulceration (including severe painful ankle ulceration), and, rarely, drug fever. Sudden withdrawal is associated with rebound elevations in platelet count.[155–157]

In the 1970s and 1980s, hydroxyurea was considered the drug of choice for reducing platelet counts in ET because of the significant risk that secondary acute leukemias may be associated with the administration of alkylating agents or radioactive phosphorus (^{32}P). Hydroxyurea is definitely effective in reducing the incidence of thrombotic complications in high-risk patients with ET.[148,149] A recent update of the data generated by the original prospective, randomized, controlled study continues to show a significantly better TFS in the hydroxyurea-treated ET cohort after a median follow-up of 73 months. Thrombotic complications occurred in 45% of patients in the untreated high-risk group with ET versus 9% of patients in the hydroxyurea treatment cohort.[158] In the PT-1 study, TFS was sig-

nificantly superior in the hydroxyurea/aspirin arm in JAK2-V617F–positive ET compared with the anagrelide/aspirin arm. TFS was equal in both treatment arms in JAK2-V617F–negative ET.[47] This suggests that hydroxyurea combined with low-dose aspirin should become the first-line treatment option in patients with JAK2-V617F–positive ET. Prospective, randomized studies are needed to confirm this premise.

Considerable concern that administration of hydroxyurea in ET accelerates the transformation of ET into AML has been prompted by the observation that leukemia-free survival appears significantly reduced in patients with ET who were given treatment with hydroxyurea plus busulfan (some patients had received busulphan prior to randomization) versus an untreated ET control group; however, cancer-free survival was equivalent between the hydroxyurea alone group and the untreated control group.[74]

Numerous other studies have challenged the relative leukemogenic safety of hydroxyurea.[152–154,159–162] All incidence data must be interpreted carefully because a natural, albeit low, progression of untreated ET to AML is apparent. The rate of background transformation to AML has been difficult to quantitate because most data were collected before PCR assays were available to exclude the presence of the *bcr/abl* gene. Furthermore, 17p chromosome deletions in patients with ET[159] have been associated with a higher risk of AML and suggest that some cohorts of patients with ET may be particularly susceptible and heretofore were not stratified in clinical studies. The incidence of transformation to AML is estimated to be approximately 3.5% at a median follow-up of 8.2 years when hydroxyurea is used alone.[159] This risk increases to 14% when hydroxyurea is combined with other agents, in this study, pipobroman. A high proportion of leukemia cases (41%) possessed deletions of the 17p chromosome, which were accompanied by morphologic evidence of dysgranulopoiesis and the presence of p53 mutations.[159] Thus, it appears that hydroxyurea administered as single-agent therapy carries an intrinsically small but definite genotoxic and mutagenic risk of inducing secondary malignancy. This risk increases significantly when hydroxyurea is administered in combination with other chemotherapy agents. Nevertheless, it is reasonable to continue to consider hydroxyurea the drug of choice for elderly patients (over 60 to 65 years of age) who have not received prior chemotherapy because its cost:benefit ratio, tolerability, and safety profile are superior to those of anagrelide, IFN-α, and the alkylating agents (Table 18-9).[148,149,163] In younger patients at high risk of thrombosis or hemorrhage, or in those given prior chemotherapy, anagrelide or IFN-α should be considered as the initial treatment choice.[131] Administration of hydroxyurea may be a particularly effective and rapid means of shrinking spleen size over 2 to 3 months in those patients with ET who have massive splenomegaly.

Anagrelide Therapy

Anagrelide is an imidazo (2-1-b) quinazolin-2-1 compound that was originally developed as an antithrombotic agent because of its powerful antiaggregating effect on platelets. It inhibits cyclic nucleotide phosphodiesterase and the release of arachidonic acid from phospholipase, possibly by inhibiting phospholipase A2. When anagrelide was first administered to humans, it had a potent thrombocytopenic effect, which had not been observed previously in any animal model system. Because anagrelide produces thrombocytopenia at doses significantly lower than those required to inhibit platelet aggregation, the potential risk that clinically important hemorrhagic complications may be precipitated is miniscule. Anagrelide has little or no immediate effect on myelopoiesis or erythropoiesis, but its long-term use has been associated with a 5% to 10% reduction in hemoglobin concentration in approximately one third of patients with ET.[164,165] This latter effect of anagrelide is probably mediated by an effect on EPO levels because it can be readily reversed in vivo by the administration of therapeutic doses of recombinant EPO.

The specific mechanism by which anagrelide induces thrombocytopenia remains unclear. The seminal clinical study, published by Silverstein and coworkers,[164] showed that anagrelide does not alter the cellularity of bone marrow, the number of megakaryocytes in the bone marrow, or the survival of circulating platelets.[164] Anagrelide does not inhibit the proliferation of megakaryoctyic-committed progenitor cells (colony forming units-megakaryocyte [CFU-M]) in vivo, although suprapharmacologic concentrations may inhibit megakaryocyte colony expansion in cell culture systems. Therefore, anagrelide-induced thrombocytopenia does not arise as the result of direct stem cell toxicity or from direct inhibition of megakaryocytopoiesis.[166] Anagrelide alters the maturation of megakaryocytes and thereby decreases their size and affects their morphology.[167] A left shift is observed in the distribution of morphologic stages and decreased ploidy. The intracellular processes influenced by anagrelide have not been elucidated. In addition, it is not known whether anagrelide or a metabolite of the drug possesses the primary platelet-lowering property (see Table 18-9). Anagrelide in large concentrations can inhibit platelet aggregation in vitro; however, this mechanism is independent of its effects on thrombopoiesis and is rarely a significant issue from the clinical perspective.

The elimination half-life of anagrelide from the circulation is 76 hours. Seventy-five percent of the administered dose is excreted in the urine over 6 days, and 10% is excreted in feces. The recommended initial dose of anagrelide is 0.5 mg two or four times daily. This dose should be increased by a maximum of 0.5 mg/d/wk until the desired reduction in platelet count is achieved. The ideal maximum dose of anagrelide should not exceed 10 mg per day or 3 mg per dose.[168] Dose adjustments may be necessary if renal failure occurs.

Anagrelide is licensed for use in the United States and Europe for the treatment of patients with thrombocythemia associated with all MPDs. The broadest experience with anagrelide has been generated by the multicenter phase 2 clinical trial conducted by the Anagrelide Study Group.[165] Of 577 patients with primary thrombocythemia (median platelet count, 990,000/μL), a 94% response rate (defined as reduction in platelet count by 50%, or maintenance at levels lower than 600,000/μL for at least 4 weeks) was reported in individuals with ET who were treated with anagrelide. Patients initially received 1 mg anagrelide orally every 6 hours, which was later reduced to 0.5 mg four times a day, with increases of 0.5 mg per day every 5 to 7 days, depending on platelet count response. The median time to maximal response was 11 days and the dose needed to achieve a response ranged from 0.5 to 9.0 mg/day. However, 95% of patients responded to a dose of 4 mg per day or less.[165]

Table 18-9 Comparisons of HU, IFN-α and Anagrelide[131]

	HU	IFN-α	Anagrelide
Route of administration	PO	SC	PO
Selectivity of platelet reduction	No	No	Yes
Leukemogenicity	Yes	No	No
Hematologic side effects	++	++	+
Tolerability	Very good	Fair/poor	Good/fair
Possibility to induce remission	No	Yes	No
Use in pregnancy	No	Yes	No
Regression of splenomegaly	Yes	Yes	No
Price	Low (1500 mg/d)	Moderate (3 MIU/d)	High (2.0 mg/d)

HU = hydroxyurea; IFN-α = interferon alpha. (Modified from Schwarz J, Pytlik R, Doubek M, et al: Analysis of risk factors: The rationale of the guidelines of the Czech Hematological Society for the diagnosis and treatment of Philadelphia-chromosome negative myeloproliferative disorders with thrombocythemia. Sem Thromb Hemostas; 32:231–245, 2006.)

The rapid and effective control of thrombocythemia by anagrelide would be expected to substantially reduce the incidence and severity of thrombotic and hemorrhagic complications in ET. In fact, the number of adverse events appears to be reduced proportionately to the decrease in platelet counts, but as indicated in the original nonrandomized studies that examined anagrelide use, the relationship was not linear. This suggests that other variables, such as total leukocyte counts, leukocyte properties, or intrinsic biochemical or physiologic characteristics of affected individuals with ET, may influence its clinical course (e.g., inherited hypercoagulability). Similar findings have been observed when hydroxyurea was used to control thrombocythemia. It is possible that markedly decreasing the elevated platelet counts in ET, no matter by what means or medications, is more critical than how they are reduced. One possible advantage that anagrelide has over hydroxyurea is that the "picket fence" or "peak-valley" pattern of platelet count reduction and rebound can be avoided. Fluctuating doses of hydroxyurea, necessitated by its effects on white blood cells, lead to a peak-valley effect on platelet counts compared with the stable plateau of platelet count reduction produced by anagrelide. Consistent control of platelet counts may reduce the risk of thrombosis; only randomized, controlled, appropriately prolonged studies with both of these medications will reveal whether this is a real or theoretical advantage for anagrelide therapy in ET.

Major adverse effects noted with anagrelide administration are neurologic, gastrointestinal, and cardiac in nature (Table 18-10). These may be severe enough to cause patients to discontinue the medication. Petit and coworkers[169] reported a 13% dropout rate in studies of anagrelide. Most neurologic and gastrointestinal adverse effects develop during the first 2 weeks of therapy and resolve on average within 2 weeks. Postural hypotension may be produced at higher dosing levels. In most cases, diuretics can control the fluid retention and peripheral edema induced by anagrelide use over time. Substantial normocytic and normochromic anemia is seen in about 25% of patients. Birgegard[170] recently reviewed the use of anagrelide in thrombocythemic (ET and PV) patients (Table 18-11). Platelet-lowering efficacy in seven studies was 70% to 80% in thrombocythemia, and response was rapid, with most patients reaching treatment goals within a few weeks.[169,171–176] Some studies do not give separate response results for ET and PV, and response criteria vary between studies. Adverse effects, which are common and are caused primarily by the vascular effects, include palpitations, headache, loose stools/diarrhea, and edema. Some adverse effects are time limited, but late dropout from therapy is not uncommon; the total dropout rate in prospective studies is 30% to 50%. Cardiac insufficiency may be worsened in patients with previous heart failure, and special caution is warranted in such patients.

In Europe, anagrelide was registered as a second-line therapy for thrombocythemia due to any MPD after a randomized, controlled, prospective study undertaken to compare the safety and efficacy of anagrelide with hydroxyurea revealed considerably more selective platelet-lowering effects compared with hydroxyurea.[149] In ET, anagrelide is often used as first-line therapy, especially in younger patients, because of concern about increased risk of leukemia with cytotoxic, potentially leukemogenic agents, such as hydroxyurea.[131] Given that dose escalation of anagrelide or hydroxyurea may be problematic in some patients because of adverse effects associated with either agent, combination of the two medications in lower doses is a

Table 18-10 Major Adverse Effects and Their Relative Frequencies Associated with Anagrelide Use

Cardiovascular
Fluid retention or edema (24%)
Congestive heart failure (2.5%)
Palpitations and tachycardia (36%)
Irregular pulse (2.5%)
New or worsening angina (0.9%)

Neurologic
Headache (30%)
Dizziness (8%)

Gastrointestinal
Nausea (19%)
Diarrhea (15%)
Gas, eructation, and bloating (8%)

Others (rare)
Rash and hyperpigmentation
Pulmonary fibrosis
Liver function abnormalities

Table 18-11 Response Rates for Patients with Thrombocythemia (ET and PV) and Dropout Frequency in Treatment Studies in Which More than 30 Patients were Receiving Anagrelide[170]

Study	Total, N	ET, n	PV, n	CR%, Total	CR%, ET	CR%, PV	Stopped Therapy, %
Anagrelide Study Group, 1992[165]	577	335	68	93	93	85	16
Petitt et al, 1997[169]	942	546	113	?	81	74	–
Petrides et al, 1998[171]	48	48	–	–	87	–	–
Storen and Tefferi, 2001[172]	35	35	–	74	74	–	18
Birgegard et al, 2004[173]	60	42	17	67	76	41	50
Steurer et al, 2004[174]	97	79	16	51(77)*	–	?	10
Penninga et al, 2004[175]	52	36	16	75	?	?	40
Fruchtman et al, 2005[176]	1618	934	208	–	67	61	45

*CR criterion: Platelets <450,000/µL. If <600,000/µL is used to define CR, the response rate is 77%.
ET, essential thrombocythemia; PV, polycythemia vera; CR, complete remission.
(From Birgegard G: Anagrelide treatment in myeloproliferative disorders. Sem Thromb Hemostas 32:260–266, 2006.)

practical option that is already used by many clinicians yet without basis in any published study.

Cardiac adverse effects are observed in more than one third of patients during anagrelide use, and it may be contraindicated in those with uncontrolled arrhythmia.[165,169,170] Many individuals report frequent anxiety-provoking palpitations that are dose related and temporally related to caffeine ingestion. Restriction of caffeine intake and/or dose reduction often relieves or eliminates symptomatic palpitations; occasionally, β-blocker medication may be necessary. Vasodilatory effects on the peripheral vasculature and potent inotropic properties of anagrelide may induce cardiac symptoms. Rarely, a cardiomyopathy may occur. This may be particularly problematic in elderly individuals but may respond to, or be reversed by, the use of diuretics.[165,169,170] Severe headaches are reported in approximately one third of patients and are often described as "vascular" or "migraine-like." These are probably the result of the peripheral vasodilatory effects of anagrelide and may lead to intolerance of the medication in a substantial number of patients. Those with a history of migraine may be particularly susceptible to this effect. Reduction of caffeine intake may be helpful. Finally, anagrelide is contraindicated in pregnancy because it crosses the placental barrier and may lead to fetal thrombocytopenia.[169,170]

Observations from this randomized clinical trial in which hydroxyurea was compared with anagrelide (patients in both arms also received low-dose aspirin [75 mg]) confirmed the expected high incidence of anagrelide-induced adverse effects (37%).[149] This implies that about 60% of high-risk patients with ET do very well without adverse effects and with no leukemic risk during long-term use of anagrelide. In contrast, 18% of the hydroxyurea cohort also withdrew because of adverse effects and for other reasons over short-term follow-up (2.5 years); this is a higher proportion than clinicians would have expected. Of concern was the higher incidence of transformation to myelofibrosis ($P = .01$) in the anagrelide plus aspirin group, which suggested some fibrogenic predisposition of this regimen.[149] However, on follow-up examination of bone marrow (BM) specimens from another group of patients administered anagrelide, the platelet-lowering medication failed to show stimulation of myelofibrosis in ET.[177] Long-term follow-up study of hydroxyurea compared with anagrelide in patients with ET to assess survival, major thrombosis, serious skin toxicity, transformation to acute leukemia and myelodysplasia, and potential fibrogenic potential is warranted.

Recombinant Interferon-α

Recombinant IFN-α was first studied as alternative therapy for the treatment of patients with PV; it was noted to reduce thrombocytosis and erythrocytosis in approximately two thirds of patients.[178] Occasionally, massive splenomegaly disappeared and intense pruritus was ameliorated. Recombinant IFN-α administration significantly reduced the platelet count in approximately 85% of patients with ET and had beneficial effects on spleen size in about one third of recipients.[178] Numerous clinical trials have assessed the efficacy of IFN-α in reducing platelet count in MPDs.[179–188] IFN-α was found to suppress the proliferation of pluripotent and lineage-committed hematopoietic progenitors and to

inhibit the growth of megakaryocyte progenitors in vivo and in vitro.[189–192] IFN-α also reduces thrombopoiesis and causes modest shortening of platelet mean life span.[193] IFN-α does not cross the placenta[194] and is not known to be teratogenic; it has been used safely in pregnant women with CML and is the drug of choice for the treatment of pregnant patients with ET. IFN-α administration circumvents theoretical concerns about the potential risks of teratogenicity with hydroxyurea and anagrelide. IFN-α is nonleukemogenic and nongonadotoxic, yet it controls thrombocythemia very efficiently.

Recombinant IFN-α is administered usually at doses of 3 million U given subcutaneously three times weekly. The response rate with regard to thrombocythemia approaches 90%, and after initial cytoreduction is achieved, the interferon dose usually can be reduced. Discontinuation results in rapid relapse of thrombocythemia, which usually responds to the resumption of interferon therapy.[178–180,184,185] Sustained remissions have been documented in some patients after IFN-α therapy, suggesting that IFN-α has an antiproliferative effect on the neoplastic clone.[179,181,182,195] One clinical study demonstrated decelerated proliferation of the neoplastic clone in five of seven patients who were given IFN-α for ET.[195] IFN-α also antagonizes the action of platelet-derived growth factor (PDGF), a product of megakaryopoiesis, which initiates fibroblast proliferation. IFN-α may reduce inherent risks of progressive myelofibrosis and leukemogenesis in ET and other MPDs through its antiproliferative and immunomodulatory effects. No randomized studies have yet compared the safety, efficacy, leukemia-free survival, and thrombohemorrhagic event-free survival of recombinant IFN-α with hydroxyurea or anagrelide in ET.

Major disadvantages of recombinant IFN-α in ET include its associated adverse effects and its high cost.[196] Almost all patients experience an influenza-like syndrome during induction with fever, chills, myalgias, headache, and arthralgias. These symptoms are frequently controlled with acetaminophen. Long-term treatment may result in fatigue, anorexia, weight loss, alopecia, and autoimmune disease, including autoimmune thyroiditis, autoimmune hemolytic anemia, autoimmune thrombocytopenia, and symmetrical polyarthropathy. Patients may also develop clinically significant neuropsychiatric symptoms, including altered mentation, confusion, and deep depression.[178,184,196] The treating physician must be aware of suicidal ideation in those with prior personal and/or family history of depression. Neutralizing antibodies to recombinant IFN-α therapy may develop, leading to a rise in platelet count. Therapy with leukocyte IFN-α has been tried in such situations with excellent response.[197] In a review of 273 cases, IFN-α therapy was terminated in 25% of patients. The most common reasons for withdrawal were interferon-related adverse effects in 55% and patient refusal in 10%.[196] Many adverse effects dissipate over time with continued administration of the drug. Recombinant IFN-α is a very attractive therapeutic option for ET because it can (1) suppress the neoplastic clone, (2) efficiently lower platelet counts, (3) reduce and reverse massive splenomegaly and progression of myelofibrosis, and (4) circumvent potential teratogenicity of anagrelide, hydroxyurea, and alkylating agents, as well as leukemogenicity of hydroxyurea and alkylating agents. Nevertheless, IFN-α remains underutilized in this disease, perhaps because of its price and its spectrum of adverse effects. It has been reserved primarily for use in patients with ET who are pregnant or who have massive splenomegaly.

Pegylated (PEG)-IFN-α is a chemically modified IFN-α that is produced by covalently attaching polymers of ethylene glycol (PEG) of varying average molecular weights, endowing PEG-IFN-α with a superior pharmacokinetic and pharmacodynamic profile, thus yielding a drug that can be given weekly. For this reason, PEG-IFN-α has proved to be a potential therapeutic agent in clinical trials of patients with bcr/abl-negative thrombocythemia, including ET and PV. PEG-IFN-α is probably more effective and better tolerated than other treatments and can be considered as a nonleukemogenic alternative cytoreductive therapy in younger patients with ET. Two large phase 3 trials in which the activity and toxicity profiles of two slightly different recombinant PEG-IFN-α molecules were compared with those of two standard recombinant IFN-α molecules in patients with chronic phase CML showed a clear superiority of PEG-IFN-α over standard IFN-α in terms of both efficacy and tolerability.[198,199] In a phase 2 study of 36 high-risk patients with ET, sustained treatment with PEG-IFN-α-2b was effective and safe in reducing platelet counts and had a toxicity comparable with that of conventional interferon.[200] The complete remission rate at 1 year was 67%, and 23 of 36 patients with ET (64%) remained on long-term PEG-IFN-α-2b.[201] In a phase 2 study conducted by the Nordic MPD Study Group, PEG-IFN-α-2b given at an initial dose of 0.5 μg per kilogram once weekly was administered to patients with PV (n = 22) and ET (n = 20).[201] Fifteen patients had previously received cytoreductive therapy. Four (10%) patients discontinued therapy initially because of toxicity, and 9 more were taken off study at 6 months because of adverse effects or insufficient response. At 12 months, 20 (48%) patients remained in complete remission, but 22 (52%) had discontinued therapy, primarily because of side effects—a higher rate than in previous trials.[201] The Italian GIMEMA Cooperative Group similarly reported on a large multicenter phase 2 study designed to evaluate the safety and tolerability of 2 years of treatment with PEG-IFN-α-2b.[202,203] Ninety patients with high-risk ET (30 men, 60 women) were included, of whom 60% had been previously treated with cytoreductive agents. During the first year of therapy, PEG-IFN-α-2b was given at 25 μg weekly with escalation up to 100 μg weekly until a platelet count of <500,000/μL was reached. After 12 months of therapy, 79% of patients were still receiving PEG-IFN-α-2b (at a mean value of 50 ± 22 μg weekly), and 64 (71%) had achieved the target platelet count. At 24 months, reduced platelet count had been sustained in 75%, and the prevalence of splenomegaly had decreased from 22% to 6%.[202] According to the bone marrow criteria proposed by WHO (see Table 18-6), two thirds of ET cases at baseline were categorized as having true ET (23%), CIMF-0 (pre-MF, 17%), CIMF-1 (early MF, 40%), CIMF-2/3 (classic MF, 3%), and MPD-Unclassified (17%).[203] No patient with true ET showed bone marrow evolution while on PEG-IFN-α-2b treatment, whereas those with CIMF-1/2/3 experienced an increase in marrow fibrosis. More important, the rate of complete hematologic remission at the end of the first year was higher with true ET (93%) than

in CIMF-0 (60%) and CIMF-1/2 (71%) patients.[203] Overall, these data suggest that evolution (natural history) to myelofibrosis is very rare among patients with true ET, and that these patients achieve significantly higher response rates with PEG-IFN-α-2b therapy than are attained by those with thrombocythemia associated with prefibrotic CIMF-0 or early fibrotic CIMF-1 (false ET).

Alkylating Agents and Radiophosphorus

The use of alkylating chemotherapeutic agents, such as busulfan, melphalan, and chlorambucil, was considered for the treatment of patients with ET after these agents had been successful in reducing and controlling the thrombocythemia associated with PV in PVSG protocols. Similar good to excellent platelet responses also have been observed in ET; however, 11.3% and 3.5% incidences of secondary acute leukemia associated with administration of chlorambucil and busulfan, respectively, have led to abandonment of their widespread use in both ET and PV. The risk that acute leukemias may develop in patients given chlorambucil was 2.3 times that in patients given radioactive phosphorus and 13 times that in patients who were treated by phlebotomy alone.[204]

Radiophosphorus (^{32}P) was equally successful in controlling thrombocythemic states; however, this agent also has been generally avoided, except in exceptional clinical situations, because of its inherent oncogenesis. The incidence of acute leukemia was 9.6% at 10 years post administration in the PVSG protocol, and the expected number of gastrointestinal tract and skin cancers had doubled, beginning 2 to 3 years after ^{32}P administration.[205]

At this time, the availability of relatively safer cytoreductive drugs, such as hydroxyurea, anagrelide, and IFN-α, has resulted in the use of busulfan and ^{32}P only in high-risk patients with ET who cannot tolerate other medications, and whose life expectancy is considered to be less than 10 years. Busulfan 2 to 4 mg may be given orally daily with careful monitoring of platelet and whole blood counts. After initial control of platelet count is achieved, only intermittent courses of the drug are required. This limits the adverse effects experienced with use of the drug; these include bone marrow aplasia, skin pigmentation, amenorrhea, and pulmonary fibrosis.[152,206]

^{32}P is a pure β emitter isotope with a half-life of 14.3 days and a maximum tissue range of 8 mm. Both oral and intravenous forms have been used to control thrombocythemia associated with ET or PV.[207-209] In one study, normalization of full blood count was achieved in 50% of patients after a single administration of ^{32}P and in 73% after two treatments. Because oral ^{32}P may be more leukemogenic than the intravenous form, ^{32}P is usually administered intravenously at 2.3 mCi per meter squared (capped at 5 mCi per meter squared). Repeat dosing (possibly escalated by 25% with a cap of 7 mCi per meter squared) should be delayed for at least 3 months and should be administered only if adequate platelet control has not been achieved.

Pipobroman is a piperazine derivative that is structurally similar to alkylating agents but appears to act as a metabolic competitor of pyrimidine bases.[108,112] Most experience with this medication has been derived from its wide use in France and Italy for the treatment of patients with ET and PV.[210–214] It is not licensed for use in the United States. A randomized prospective study of hydroxyurea and pipobroman in 292 patients with PV revealed equal efficacy for both in disease control and an equal risk of leukemogenesis of approximately 10% at 13 years.[221] Gastrointestinal toxicity, the predominant adverse effect, was sufficiently severe to cause discontinuation of pipobroman in 5.6%. In contrast, hydroxyurea toxicity was essentially limited to mucocutaneous adverse effects that included acne, oral aphthous ulcers (20%), and especially leg ulcers (9%). These mucocutaneous adverse effects generally appear late, 5 years or longer after initial treatment. Leg ulcers healed only when hydroxyurea was stopped and was replaced by pipobroman.[221]

The incidence of AML/MDS has ranged between 0% and 16% in clinical studies that compared pipobroman with hydroxyurea in PV.[159,215,216,222] In patients with PV who were younger than 65 years, rates of AML/MDS were 12% and 19% in the hydroxyurea and pipobroman groups, respectively, with median time to transformation of 10.5 years.[215,216] In both groups, 40% of observed cases of AML/MDS occurred after the twelfth year of follow-up. Half of patients who developed AML/MDS in the hydroxyurea group had received more than one cytoreductive drug, whereas in the pipobroman group, 85% of patients with AML/MDS had been given only pipobroman.[216]

Pipobroman has not been used widely in ET. In two uncontrolled studies involving 21 and 24 patients, hematologic remission and platelet control were attained in 86% and 92% of cases, respectively, with no observed secondary leukemia; however, the follow-up duration was relatively short in these studies.[223,224]

A registry of consecutive patients in whom high-risk ET was newly diagnosed and patients were treated with hydroxurea as first-line therapy and were prospectively followed has revealed a 9.3% incidence of AML after a median duration of 8 years of hydroxyurea administration.[216] Transformation to AML was the major cause of death (22%). Cytogenetics at diagnosis was the only parameter associated with evolution to AML: 28% of patients who developed AML had an abnormal karyotype, compared with 8% in the overall population.

Aspirin

The rationale for administration of aspirin in low doses (81 mg per day) in patients with ET is based on its irreversible inhibition of platelet cyclo-oxygenase (COX) activity and its excellent therapeutic and prophylactic profile in the control of platelet-mediated microcirculatory thrombotic disturbances.[56,60,61,72,106–111,115–117,139,143] Similar benefits, although of briefer duration, may be observed with the use of nonsteroidal anti-inflammatory drugs (NSAIDs), which may be used as an alternative in cases of aspirin allergy. Aspirin is particularly useful in the treatment of patients with erythromelalgia and acral cyanosis[56,60,61,106–110] (see Figs. 18-2 and 18-3) and in the prevention of thrombotic complications (i.e., TIAs, amaurosis fugax, and unstable angina).[115–117,139] These benefits are observed even when platelet counts remain elevated. Low-dose aspirin (75 to 100 mg per day) is very effective in preventing or reversing potential platelet microthromboembolic complications associated with the

in vitro phenomenon of spontaneous platelet aggregation in patients with thrombocythemia (ET or PV).[217] High doses of aspirin (more than 325 mg/day) or aspirin used in combination with other medications with antiplatelet aggregation properties (such as dipyridamole or NSAIDs) should be avoided in ET because of the significantly increased incidence of gastrointestinal bleeding that has been reported. Fortunately, the incidence of serious bleeding, generally, and specifically associated with the use of aspirin, is much lower in ET than in PV. Care should be taken when aspirin is administered in the presence of qualitative platelet defects (as determined by platelet aggregation studies). Aspirin exacerbates bleeding episodes in patients with ET at platelet counts in excess of $1,000,000 \pm 100,000/\mu L$ because of acquired VWD, which results from loss of the highest-molecular-weight multimers of circulating VWF protein.[72,134–138,143] Other medications with anticoagulant or antiplatelet activities, such as warfarin, sulfinpyrazone, dipyridamole, and ticlopidine, do not convey the same salutary effects in ET as are conferred by aspirin.[111,130,142,218]

Plateletpheresis in Essential Thrombocythemia

Rapid reduction in extremely elevated platelet counts (usually $>1,000,000/\mu L$) in ET is necessitated when emergent symptomatic or life-threatening thromboembolic and hemorrhagic complications occur. Cytoreductive agents may be initiated concurrently for long-term control; however, in certain clinical situations, such as pregnancy, the use of anagrelide and myelosuppressive medications may be contraindicated. Therefore, plateletpheresis, accomplished via the physical removal of platelets with an automated apheresis apparatus, can provide immediate and efficient benefits (see Chapter 30). Plateletpheresis is only a temporary measure, however, and other cytoreductive strategies will be needed.[219–221] RT is not symptomatic and does not require plateletpheresis.

PREGNANCY AND ESSENTIAL THROMBOCYTHEMIA

Pregnancy may be complicated by spontaneous abortion, premature delivery, or abruptio placentae caused by placental infarcts. Pregnancy is a special clinical circumstance in ET because approximately 50% of such pregnancies are complicated by spontaneous miscarriage, intrauterine fetal death, abruptio placentae, intrauterine growth retardation, premature delivery, and preeclampsia. This rate is considerably higher than that observed in the general population and may be due to placental vessel thrombosis and subsequent infarction. Spontaneous miscarriage occurs most commonly during the first trimester and is unrelated to the degree of thrombocytosis or the type of treatment (including no treatment) given to the patient with ET.[222,223] According to the observations of Beressi and coworkers,[224] pregnancies that persist until term are not usually complicated by thrombohemorrhagic events or catastrophes at delivery. Smoking should be avoided particularly during pregnancy because it may precipitate potential hypercoagulability or platelet hyperaggregability. Hemorrhagic complications are uncommon in pregnancy. In some cases, decreased platelet count and even spontaneous remission of thrombocytosis have been noted to occur during pregnancy, perhaps as the result of hemodilution effects. Pregnancy is usually successful in such individuals.[225]

In a recent review of the literature, it was discerned that about 300 cases of pregnancy have been reported in patients with ET, and fewer than 50 pregnancies have been reported in patients with PV.[226] Live birth rates are approximately 60% in ET and 58% in PV. Spontaneous abortion during the first trimester is the most frequent fetal complication, occurring in 31% of ET pregnancies and in 22% of PV pregnancies, respectively.[226] Major maternal complications are more frequent in PV than in ET (44.4% vs 7.7%).[226] Treatment of patients with ET with low-dose aspirin during pregnancy seems to reduce complications; this approach also seems beneficial during pregnancy in patients with PV. In high-risk pregnancies, the additional use of low molecular weight heparin and/or IFN-α should be considered.[226]

Management options during pregnancy should be tailored according to the perceived risk of thrombohemorrhagic complications. Low-risk (platelet count lower than 1,000,000/μL, asymptomatic, and no prior history of thrombosis) and intermediate-risk (platelet count higher than 1,000,000/μL, asymptomatic, and no history of thrombosis) pregnant women with ET or PV can usually be treated through careful observation alone with administration of low-dose aspirin. A successful pregnancy retention and delivery rate of 75% has been reported in association with aspirin administration compared with 43% in untreated women.[121] Moderate-dose aspirin (325 mg or less per day) is preferred to minimize bleeding risks and to minimize blood loss during delivery. Some have advocated that aspirin be stopped at least 1 week prior to delivery and then resumed postpartum.[226,227]

For women with ET (i.e., not RT) with high-risk pregnancy or those anticipated to be at high risk when pregnant (any high platelet count associated with prior miscarriage, neurovascular symptoms, prior thrombosis, hypertension, smoking, obesity, etc.), low-dose aspirin use should be combined with aggressive reduction of platelet counts. Cytoreduction can be achieved effectively with IFN-α, which does not cross the placenta and is unlikely to be teratogenic. No birth defects have been associated with the use of IFN-α during pregnancies complicated by ET or CML.[222,227–230] Nevertheless, package inserts list pregnancy as a contraindication for use. The adverse effects of IFN-α may be difficult to tolerate during pregnancy, and the cost is considerable.

Hydroxyurea has been used successfully and safely in pregnant patients with ET, CML, and sickle cell disease, despite its theoretical teratogenicity. Its initiation is often delayed until the second trimester. Currently, anagrelide is avoided during pregnancy because of its potential to cause fetal hemorrhage and teratogenicity.[169,170,226] Additional experience is needed before the safety of anagrelide use during pregnancy can be established. This may occur with monitoring of administration of anagrelide in pregnant women who are intolerant of IFN-α or hydroxyurea. Alkylating chemotherapeutic drugs like busulfan should not be prescribed because of their increased risks of teratogenicity, although they have been used safely during pregnancies

that occurred in association with Hodgkin disease and non-Hodgkin lymphomas. With the availability of these other options, there is no reason for clinicians to administer ^{32}P for platelet reduction in pregnant patients with ET. Plateletpheresis decreases platelet counts rapidly and safely, but its benefits are only temporizing until a more permanent solution to thrombocythemia can be implemented.

SUMMARY: TREATMENT STRATEGIES FOR PATIENTS WITH ESSENTIAL THROMBOCYTHEMIA

Treatment of patients with ET should be individualized, based on stratification of risk, and modified according to extenuating clinical circumstances (e.g., pregnancy). The treatment of high-risk individuals is very straightforward. Treatment decisions regarding low- and intermediate-risk patients with ET are considerably more difficult because of a dearth of properly performed, adequately sized, randomized, controlled, prospective studies. In the United States, treatment of these individuals generally has been more aggressive than the available literature would support; however, this has occurred in response to numerous medical-legal claims that arise when one of these individuals develops a life-threatening or fatal thrombohemorrhagic event. Complications are very infrequent in low- and intermediate-risk patients, and the risk:benefit ratio of cytoreductive therapies remains to be established.

REFERENCES

1. Pearson TC: Diagnosis and classification of erythrocytosis and thrombocytosis. Baillieres Clin Haematol 11:695–720, 1998.
2. Hsu H-C, Tsai W-H, Jiang M-L, et al: Circulating levels of thrombopoietin and inflammatory cytokines in patients with clonal and reactive thrombocytosis. J Lab Clin Med 134:392–397, 1999.
3. Tefferi A, Ho TC, Ahmann CJ, et al: Plasma interleukin-6 and C-reactive protein levels in reactive versus clonal thrombocytosis. Am J Med 97:374–378, 1994.
4. Haznedaroglu IC, Ertenli I, Ozcebe OI, et al: Megakaryocyte-related interleukins in reactive thrombocytosis versus autonomous thrombocythemia. Acta Haematol 95:107–111, 1996.
5. Buss DH, Cashell AW, O'Connor ML, et al: Occurrence, etiology and clinical significance of extreme thrombocytosis: A study of 280 cases. Am J Med 96:247–253, 1994.
6. Griesshammer M, Bangerter M, Sauer T, et al: Aetiology and clinical significance of thrombocytosis: Analysis of 732 patients with an elevated platelet count. J Intern Med 245:295–300, 1999.
7. Axelrad AA, Eskinazi D, Amato D: Hypersensitivity of circulating progenitor cells to megakaryocyte growth and development of factor (PEG-rHu MGDF) in essential thrombocythemia. Blood 96:3310–3321, 2000.
8. Michiels JJ: Diagnostic criteria of the myeloproliferative disorders (MPD): Essential thrombocythemia, polycythemia vera and chronic megakaryocytic granulocytic metaplasia. Neth J Med 51:57–64, 1997.
9. Fickers M, Speck B: Thrombocythemia, familial occurrence and transition into blastic crisis. Acta Haemat 51:257–265, 1974.
10. Eyster ME, Saletan SL, Rabellino EM, et al: Familial essential thrombocythemia. Am J Med 80:497–502, 1986.
11. Kikuchi M, Tayama T, Hayakawa H, et al: Familial thrombocytosis. Br J Haematol 89:900–902, 1995.
12. Schlemper RJ, van der Mass APC, Eikenboom JCJ, et al: Familial essential thrombocythemia: Clinical characteristics of 11 cases in one family. Ann Hematol 68:153–158, 1994.
13. Janssen JWG, Anger BR, Drexler HG, et al: Essential thrombocythemia in two sisters originating from different stem cell levels. Blood 75:1633–1636, 1990.

14. Wiestner A, Schlemper RJ, Mass APC, et al: An activating splice donor mutation in the thrombopoietin gene causes hereditary thrombocythaemia. Nat Gene 18:49–52, 1998.

15. Kondo T, Okabe M, Sanada M, et al: Familial essential thrombocythemia associated with one-base deletion in the 5'-untranslated region of the thrombopoietin gene. Blood 92:1091–1096, 1998.

16. Ghilardi N, Wiestner A, Kikuchi M, et al: Hereditary thrombocythaemia in a Japanese family is caused by a novel mutation in the thrombopoietin gene. Br J Haematol 107:310–316, 1999.

17. Ding J, Komatsu H, Wakita A, et al: Familial essential thrombocythemia associated with a dominant-positive activating mutation of the c-MPL gene, which encodes for the receptor for thrombopoietin. Blood 103:4198–4200, 2004.

18. Kunishima S, Mizuno S, Naoe T, et al: Genes for thrombopoietin and c-MPL are not responsible for familial thrombocythemia: A case study. Br J Haematol 100:383–386, 1998.

19. Wiester A, Padosch SA, Ghilardi N: Hereditary thrombocythaemia is a genetically heterogeneous disorder: Exclusion of TPO and mpl in two families with hereditary thrombocythaemia. Br J Haematol 110:104–109, 2000.

20. Moliterno AR, Williams DM, Gutierrez-Alamillo, et al: Mpl Baltimore: A thrombopoietin receptor polymorphism associated with thrombocytosis. Proc Natl Acad Sci U S A 101:11444–11447, 2004.

21. Michiels JJ, Juvonen E: Proposal for revised diagnostic criteria of essential thrombocythemia and polycythemia vera by the Thrombocythemia Vera Study Group. Semin Thromb Hemost 23:339–347, 1997.

22. Ridell B, Carneskog J, Wedel H, et al: Incidence of chronic myeloproliferative disorders in the city of Göteborg, Sweden 1983–1992. Eur J Haematol 65:267–271, 2000.

23. Johansson P, Kutti J, Andreasson B, et al: Trends in the incidence of chronic Philadelphia chromosome negative (Ph-) myeloproliferative disorders in the city of Göteborg, Sweden, during 1983–99. J Intern Med 256:161–165, 2004.

24. Mesa RA, Silverstein MN, Jacobsen SJ, et al: Population-based incidence and survival figures in essential thrombocythemia and agnogenic myeloid metaplasia: An Olmsted County Study, 1976–1995. Am J Hematol 61:10–15, 1999.

25. Jensen MK, de Nully Brown P, Nielsen OJ, et al: Incidence, clinical features and outcome of essential thrombocythaemia in a well defined geographical area. Eur J Haematol 65:132–139, 2000.

26. Girodon F, Jooste V, Maynadié M, et al: Incidence of chronic Philadelphia chromosome negative (Ph-) myeloproliferative disorders in the Côte d'Or area, France, during 1980–99. J Intern Med 258:90–91, 2005.

27. Johansson P: Epidemiology of the myeloproliferative disorders polycythemia vera and essential thrombocythemia. Semin Thromb Hemost 32:171–173, 2006.

28. Fialkow PJ, Faguet GB, Jacobson RJ, et al: Evidence that essential thrombocythemia is a clonal disorder with origin in a multipotent stem cell. Blood 58:916–919, 1981.

29. Briere J, el-Kassar N: Clonality markers in polycythaemia and primary thrombocythaemia. Bailliere Clin Haematol 11:787–801, 1998.

30. El-Kassar N, Hetet G, Briere J, et al: Clonality analysis of hematopoiesis in essential thrombocythaemia, advantages of studying T-lymphocytes and platelets. Blood 89:129–134, 1997.

31. Harrison CN, Gale RE, Machin SJ, et al: A large proportion of patients with a diagnosis of essential thrombocythemia do not have a clonal disorder and may be at lower risk of thrombotic complications. Blood 93:417–424, 1999.

32. Kaushansky K: Thrombopoietin. N Engl J Med 339:746–753, 1998.

33. Wang JC, Chen C, Novetsky AD, et al: Blood thrombopoietin levels in clonal thrombocytosis and reactive thrombocytosis. Am J Med 104:451–455, 1998.

34. Horikawa Y, Matsuma I, Hashimoto K, et al: Markedly reduced expression of platelet c-mpl receptor in essential thrombocythemia. Blood 90:4031–4038, 1997.

35. Kiladjian J, el-Kassar N, Hetet G, et al: Study of the thrombopoietin receptor in essential thrombocythemia. Leukemia 11:1821–1826, 1997.

36. Matsumura I, Horikawa Y, Kanakura Y: Functional roles of thrombopoietin C-mpl–system in essential thrombocythemia. Leukemia Lymphoma 32:351–358, 1999.

37. Harrison CN, Gale RE, Pezella F, et al: Platelet c-mpl expression is dysregulated in patients with essential thrombocythaemia but this is not of diagnostic value. Br J Haematol 107:139–147, 1999.

38. Espanol I, Hernandez A, Cortes M, et al: Patients with thrombocytosis have normal or slightly elevated thrombopoietin levels. Haematologica 84:312–316, 1999.

39. Verbeek W, Faulhaber M, Griesinger F, et al: Measurement of thrombopoietin levels: Clinical and biologic relationships. Curr Opin Haematol 7:143–149, 2000.

40. James C, Ugo V, Le Couedic PF, et al: A unique clonal JAK2 mutation leading to constitutive signalling causes polycythemia vera. Nature 434:1144–1148, 2005.

41. Levine RL, Wadleigh M, Cools J, et al: Activating mutation in the tyrosine kinase JAK2 in polycythemia vera, essential thrombocythemia and myeloid metaplasia with myelofibrosis. Cancer Cells 7:387–397, 2005.

42. Kralovics R, Passamonti F, Buser AS, et al: A gain-of-function mutation of JAK2 in myeloproliferative disorders. N Engl J Med 352:1779–1790, 2005.

43. Baxter EJ, Scott LM, Campbell PJ, et al: Acquired mutation of the tyrosine kinase in human myeloproliferative disorders. Lancet 365:1054–1061, 2005.

44. Jones AV, Kreil S, Xoi K, et al: Widespread occurrence of the JAK2 V617F mutation in chronic myeloproliferative disorders. Blood 106:2162–2168, 2005.

45. Levine RL, Belisle C, Wadleigh M, et al: X-inactivation based clonality analysis and quantitative JAK2 V617F assessment reveals a strong association between clonality and JAK2 V617F in PV but not in ET/MMM, and identifies a subset of JAK2 V617F negative ET and MMM patients with clonal hematopoiesis. Blood 107:4139–4141, 2006.

46. Kiladjian JJ, Elkassar N, Cassinat B, et al: Essential thrombocythemias without V617F JAK2 mutation are clonal hematopoietic stem cell disorders. Leukemia 20:1181–1183, 2006.

47. Campbell P, Scott LM, Buck G, et al: Definition of essential thrombocythemia and relation of essential thrombocythemia to polycythaemia vera based on JAK2 V617F mutation status: A prospective study. Lancet 366:1945–1953, 2005.

48. Wolansky AP, Lasho TL, Schwager SM, et al: JAK2 V617 mutation in essential thrombocythaemia: Clinical associations and long-term relevance. Br J Haematol 131:208–213, 2005.

49. Antonioli E, Guglielmelli P, Pancrazzi A, et al: Clinical implications of the JAK2 V617F mutation in essential thrombocythemia. Leukemia 19:1847–1849, 2005.

50. Minot GR, Buckman TE: Erythremia (polycythemia rubra vera). Am J Med Sci 166:469–489, 1923.

51. Epstein E, Goedel A: Hamorrhagische thrombozythamie bei vascularer schrumpfmilz. Virchows Archiv A [Pathol Anat Histopathol] 292:233–248, 1934.

52. Gunz FW: Hemorrhagic thrombocythemia: A critical review. Blood 15:706–723, 1960.

53. Laszlo J: Myeloproliferative disorders (MPD): Myelofibrosis, myelosclerosis, extramedullary hematopoiesis, undifferentiated MPD and hemorrhagic thrombocythemia. Semin Hematol 12:409–432, 1975.

54. Iland HJ, Laszlo J, Peterson P, et al: Essential thrombocythemia: Clinical and laboratory characteristics at presentation. Trans Assoc Am Phys XCVI:165–174, 1983.

55. Annetts DL, Tracy GD: Idiopathic thrombocythemia presenting with ischemia of the toes. Med J Austr 2:180–182, 1966.

56. Vreeken J, Van Aken WS: Spontaneous aggregation of blood platelets as a cause of idiopathic and recurrent painful toes and fingers. Lancet II:1394–1397, 1971.

57. Preston FE, Emmanuel IG, Winfield DA, et al: Essential thrombocythemia and peripheral gangrene. Br Med J 3:548–552, 1974.

58. Singh AK, Weitherley-Mein G: Microvascular occlusive lesions in primary thrombocythemia. Br J Haematol 36:553–564, 1977.

59. Redding KG: Thrombocythemia as a cause of erythromelalgia. Arch Dermatol 113:468–471, 1977.

60. Vera JC: Antiplatelet agents in the treatment of thrombotic complications of primary thrombocythemia. CMAJ 120:60–61, 1979.

61. Michiels JJ, Abels J, Steketee J, et al: Erythromelalgia caused by platelet-mediated arteriolar inflammation and thrombosis in thrombocythemia. Ann Intern Med 102:466–471, 1985.

62. Murphy S, Iland H, Rosenthal D, et al: Essential thrombocythemia: An interim report from the Polycythemia Vera Study Group. Semin Hematol 23:177–182, 1986.

63. Murphy S, Peterson P, Iland H, et al: Experience of the Polycythemia Vera Study Group with essential thrombocythemia: A final report on diagnostic criteria, survival, and leukemic transition by treatment. Semin Hematol 34:29–39, 1997.

64. Swolin B, Weinfeld A, Ridell B, et al: On the 5q-deletion: Clinical and cytogenetic observation in ten patients and review of literature. Blood 58:986–993, 1981.

65. Michiels JJ, ten Kate FJ: Erythromelalgia in thrombocythemia of various myeloproliferative disorders. Am J Hematol 39:131–136, 1992.

66. Schmitt-Graeff A, Thiele J, Zuk I, et al: Essential thrombocythemia with ringed sideroblasts: A heterogenous spectrum of diseases, but not a distinct entity. Haematologica 87:392–399, 2002.

67. Hehlmann R, Jahn M, Baumann B, et al: Essential thrombocythemia: Clinical characteristics and course of 61 cases. Cancer 61:2487–2496, 1988.

68. Bellucci S, Janvier M, Tobelem G, et al: Essential thrombocythaemia: Clinical evolutionary and biological data. Cancer 56:2440–2447, 1986.

69. Howard MR, Ashwell S, Bond LR, et al: Artefactual serum hyperkalemia and hypercalcemia in essential thrombocythemia. J Clin Pathol 53:105–109, 2000.

70. Wulkan RW, Michiels JJ: Pseudohyperkalemia in thrombocythemia. J Clin Chem Clin Biochem 28:489–491, 1990.

71. Michiels JJ: Pseudohyperkalemia and platelet count in thrombocythemia. Am J Hematol 42:42–43, 1990.

72. Michiels JJ, van Genderen PJJ, Lindemans J, et al: Erythromelalgic, thrombotic and hemorrhagic manifestations of 50 cases of thrombocythaemia. Leukemia Lymphoma 22(suppl): 147–156, 1996.

73. Westwood NB, Pearson TC: Diagnostic applications of haematopoietic progenitor culture techniques in polycythaemias and thrombocythaemias. Leukemia Lymphoma 22(suppl 1): 95–103, 1996.

74. Shih LY, Lee CT: Identification of masked polycythemia vera from patients with idiopathic thrombocytosis by endogenous erythroid colony assay. Blood 83:744–748, 1994.

75. Liu E, Jelinek J, Pastore YD, et al: Discrimination of polycythemias and thrombocytoses by novel simple, accurate clonality assays and comparison with PRV-1expression and BFU-e responses to erythropoietin. Blood 101:3294–3301, 2003.

76. Juvonen E, Ikkala E, Oksanen K, et al: Megakaryocyte and erythroid colony formation in essential thrombocythaemia and reactive thrombocytosis: Diagnostic value and correlation to complication. Br J Haematol 83:192–197, 1993.

77. Florensa L, Besses C, Woessner S, et al: Endogenous megakaryocyte and erythroid colony formation from blood in essential thrombocythemia. Leukemia 9:271–273, 1995.

78. Lengfelder E, Hochhaus A, Kronawitter U, et al: Should a platelet count of 600 × 10⁹/l be used as a diagnostic criterion in essential thrombocythemia? An analysis of the natural course including early stages. Br J Haematol 100:15–23, 1998.

79. WHO classification of the chronic myeloproliferative diseases (CMPD) polycythemia vera, chronic idiopathic myelofibrosis, essential thrombocythemia and CMPD unclassifiable In: WHO Classification of Tumours: Tumours of Haematopoiesis and Lymphoid Tissues. Lyon, France, IARC, 2001, pp 31–42.

80. Michiels JJ, Thiele J: Clinical and pathological criteria for the diagnosis of essential thrombocythemia, polycythemia vera and idiopathic myelofibrosis (agnogenic myeloid metaplasia). Int J Hematol 76:133–145, 2002.

81. Michiels JJ: Bone marrow histopathology and biological markers as specific clues to the differential diagnosis of essential thrombocythemia, polycythemia vera and prefibrotic or fibrotic myeloid metaplasia. Hematol J 5:93–102, 2004.

82. Thiele J, Kvasnicka HM, Orazi A: Bone marrow histopathology in myeloproliferative disorders: Current diagnostic approach. Semin Hematol 42:184–195, 2005.

83. Thiele J, Kvasnicka HM: Clinicopathological criteria for the differential diagnosis of thrombocythemia in various myeloproliferative disorders. Semin Thromb Hemost 32:219–230, 2006.

84. Thiele J, Kvasnicka HM, Zankovich R, et al: The value of bone marrow histopathology for the differentiation between early stage polycythemia vera and secondary (reactive) polycythemias. Haematologica 86:368–374, 2001.

85. Thiele J, Kvasnicka HM, Muehlhausen K, et al: Polycythemia rubra vera versus secondary polycythemias: A clinicopathological evaluation of distinctive features in 199 patients. Pathology Res Pract 197:77–84, 2001.

86. Thiele J, Kvasnicka HM, Diehl V: Initial (latent) polycythemia vera with thrombocytosis mimicking essential thrombocythemia. Acta Haematol 113:213–219, 2005.

87. Johansson P, Andreason B, Safai-Kutti S, et al: The presence of a significant association between elevated PRV-1 mRNA expression and low plasma erythropoietin concentration in essential thrombocythemia. Eur J Haematol 70:358–362, 2003.

88. Griesshammer M, Klippel S, Strunk E, et al: PRV-1 mRNA expression discriminates two types of essential thrombocythemia. Ann Hematol 83:364–370, 2004.

89. Messinezy M, Westwood NB, El-Hemaida I, et al: Serum erythropoietin values in erythrocytosis and in primary thrombocythaemia. Br J Haematol 117:47–53, 2002.

90. Goerttler PS, Steimle C, Maerz E, et al: The JAK2 V617F mutation, PRV-1 overexpression and EEC formation define a similar cohort of MPD patients. Blood 106:2862–2864, 2005.

91. Thiele J, Kvasnicka HM: Chronic myeloproliferative disorders with thrombocythemia: A comparative study of two classifications systems (PVSG-WHO) on 839 patients. Ann Hematol 82:148–152, 2003.

92. Thiele J, Kvasnicka HM: A critical reappraisal of the WHO classification of the chronic myeloproliferative disorders. Leukemia Lymphoma 47:381–396, 2006.

93. Kvasnicka HM, Thiele J: The impact of clinicopathological studies on staging and survival in essential thrombocythemia, chronic idiopathic myelofibrosis, and polycythemia rubra vera. Semin Thromb Hemost 32(4 Pt 2):362–371, 2006.

94. Zahavi J, Zahavi M, Firsteter E, et al: An abnormal pattern of multiple platelet function abnormalities and increased thromboxane generation in patients with primary thrombocytosis and thrombotic complications. Eur J Haematol 47:326–332, 1991.

95. Griesshammer M, Beneke H, Nussbaumer B, et al: Increased platelet surface expression of P-selectin and thrombospondin as markers of platelet activation in essential thrombocythaemia. Thromb Res 96:191–196, 1999.

96. Landolfi R, Ciabattoni G, Patrinani P, et al: Increased thromboxane biosynthesis in patients with polycythemia vera: Evidence for aspirin-suppressible platelet activation in vivo. Blood 80:1965–1971, 1992.

97. Rocca B, Ciabattoni G, Tartaglione R, et al: Increased thromboxane biosynthesis in essential thrombocythemia. Thromb Haemost 74:1225–1230, 1995.

98. Bellucci S, Ignatova E, Jaillet N, et al: Platelet activation in patients with essential thrombocythemia is not associated with vascular endothelial cell damage as judged by the level of plasma thrombomodulin, protein S, PAI-1, t-PA and vWF. Thromb Haemost 70:736–742, 1993.

99. Karakantza M, Giannakoulas NC, Zikos P, et al: Markers of endothelial and in vivo platelet activation in patients with essential thrombocythemia vera. Int J Hematol 79:253–259, 2004.

100. Arellano-Rodrigo E, Alvarez-Larran A, Reverter JC, et al: Increased platelet and leukocyte activation as contributing mechanisms for thrombosis in essential thrombocythemia and correlation with the JAK2 mutational status. Haematologica 91:169–175, 2006.

101. Evangelista V, Celardo A, Dell'Elba G, et al: Platelet contribution to leukotriene production in inflammation: In vivo evidence in the rabbit. Thromb Haemost 81:442–448, 1999.

102. Maugeri N, Evangelista V, Piccardoni P, et al: Transcellular metabolism of arachidonic acid: Increased platelet thromboxane generation in the presence of activated polymorphonuclear leukocytes. Blood 80:447–451, 1992.

103. Chlopicki S, Lomnicka M, Gryglewski RJ: Obligatory role of lipid mediators in platelet-neutrophil adhesion. Thromb Res 110:287–292, 2003.

104. Falanga A, Marchetti M, Evangelista V, et al: Polymorphonuclear leukocyte activation and hemostasis in patients with essential thrombocythemia and polycythemia vera. Blood 96:4261–4266, 2000.

105. Falanga A, Marchetti M, Barbui T, et al: Pathogenesis of thrombosis in essential thrombocythemia and polycythemia vera: The role of neutrophils. Semin Hematol 42:239–247, 2005.

106. Michiels JJ, ten Kate FJ, Vuzevski VD, et al: Histopathology of erythromelalgia in thrombocythemia. Histopathology 8:669–678, 1984.

107. Van Genderen PJJ, Michiels JJ: Erythromelalgia: A pathognomonic microvascular thrombotic complication in essential thrombocythemia and polycythemia vera. Semin Thromb Hemost 23:357–363, 1997.

108. Van Genderen PJJ, Lucas IS, van Strik R, et al: Erythromelalgia in essential thrombocythemia is characterized by platelet activation and endothelial cell damage but not by thrombin generation. Thromb Haemost 76:333–338, 1996.

109. Van Genderen PJJ, Michiels JJ, van Strik R, et al: Platelet consumption in thrombocythemia complicated by erythromelalgia: Reversal by aspirin. Thromb Haemost 73:210–214, 1995.

110. Van Genderen PJJ, Prins F, Michiels JJ, et al: Thromboxane-dependent platelet activation in vivo precedes arterial thrombosis in thrombocythaemia: A rationale for the use of low-dose aspirin as an antithrombotic agent. Br J Haematol 104:438–441, 1999.

111. Schafer AI: Bleeding and thrombosis in the myeloproliferative disorders. Blood 64:1–12, 1984.

112. Finazzi G, Budde U, Michiels JJ: Bleeding time and platelet function in essential thrombocythemia and other myeloproliferative disorders. Leukemia Lymphoma 22(suppl 1): 71–78, 1996.

113. Cesar JM, de Miguel D, Garcia Avello A, et al: Platelet dysfunction in primary thrombocythemia using the platelet function analyzer, PFA-100. Am J Clin Pathol 123:772–777, 2005.

114. Jabaily J, Iland HJ, Laszlo J, et al: Neurologic manifestations of essential thrombocythemia. Ann Intern Med 99:513–518, 1983.

115. Michiels JJ, Koudstaal PJ, Mulder AH: Transient neurologic and ocular manifestations in primary thrombocythemia. Neurology 43:1107–1110, 1993.

116. Michiels JJ, Van Genderen PJJ, Janssen PHP, et al: Atypical transient ischemic attacks in thrombocythemia of various myeloproliferative disorders. Leukemia Lymphoma 22(suppl 1): 65–70, 1996.

117. Koudstaal P, Koudstaal A: Neurologic and visual symptoms in essential thrombocythemia: Efficacy of low-dose aspirin. Semin Thromb Hemost 23:365–370, 1997.

118. Van Genderen PJ, Michiels JJ: Erythromelalgic, thrombotic and hemorrhagic manifestations of thrombocythaemia. Presse Med 23:73–77, 1994.

119. Kessler CM, Klein HG, Havlik RJ: Uncontrolled thrombocytosis in chronic myeloproliferative disorders. Br J Haematol 50:157–163, 1982.

120. Fenaux P, Simon M, Caulier T, et al: Clinical course of essential thrombocythaemia in 147 cases. Cancer 66:549–556, 1990.

121. Colombi M, Radaelli F, Zocchi L, et al: Thrombotic and hemorrhagic complications in essential thrombocythemia: A retrospective study of 103 patients. Cancer 67:2926–2930, 1991.

122. Cortelazzo S, Viero P, Finazzi G: Incidence and risk factors for thrombotic complications in a historical cohort of 100 patients with essential thrombocythemia. J Clin Oncol 8:556–562, 1990.

123. Besses C, Cervantes F, Pereira A, et al: Major vascular complications in essential thrombocythemia: A study of the predictive factors in a series of 148 patients. Leukemia 13:150–154, 1999.

124. Bazzan M, Tamponi G, Schinco P, et al: Thrombosis free survival and life expectancy in 187 consecutive patients with essential thrombocythemia. Ann Hematol 78:539–543, 1999.

125. Gugliotta L, Marchioli R, Fiacchini M, et al: Epidemiological, diagnostic, therapeutic and prognostic aspects of essential thrombocythemia in a retrospective study of the GIMMC group in two thousand patients. Blood 90(suppl 1): 348a, 1997.

126. Watson KV, Key N: Vascular complications of essential thrombocythaemia. Br J Haematol 83:198–203, 1993.

127. Regev A, Stark P, Blickstein D, et al: Thrombotic complications in essential thrombocythemia with relatively low platelet counts. Am J Hematol 56:168–172, 1997.

128. Griesshammer M, Bangerter M, Van Vliet HHDM, et al: Aspirin in essential thrombocythemia: Status quo and quo vadis. Semin Thromb Hemost 23:371–377, 1997.

129. Cervantes F, Alvarez-Larran A, Talarn C, et al: Myelofibrosis with myeloid metaplasia following essential thrombocythemia: Actuarial probability, presenting characteristics and evolution in a series of 195 patients. Br J Haematol 118:786–790, 2002.

130. Murphy S: Diagnostic criteria and prognosis in polycythemia vera and essential thrombocythemia. Semin Hematol 36(suppl 2): 9–13, 1999.

131. Schwarz J, Pytlik R, Doubek M, et al: Analysis of risk factors: The rationale of the guidelines of the Czech Hematological Society for the diagnosis and treatment of Philadelphia-chromosome negative myeloproliferative disorders with thrombocytosis. Semin Thromb Hemost 32:231–245, 2006.

132. Wolansky AP, Schwager SM, McClure RF, et al: Essential thrombocythemia beyond the first decade: Life expectancy, long-term complication rates, and prognostic factors. Mayo Clin Proc 81:159–166, 2006.

133. Chim C-S, Kwong Y-L, Lie K-W, et al: Long-term outcome of 231 patients with essential thrombocythemia. Arch Intern Med 165:2651–2658, 2005.

134. Budde U, Scharf RE, Franke P, et al: Elevated platelet count as a cause of abnormal von-Willebrand factor multimer distribution in plasma. Blood 82:1749–1757, 1993.

135. Fabris F, Casonato A, Del Ben MG, et al: Abnormalities of von Willebrand factor in myeloproliferative disease: A relationship with bleeding diathesis. Br J Haematol 63:75–83, 1986.

136. Van Genderen PJ, van Vliet H, Prins FJ, et al: The excessive prolongation of the bleeding time by aspirin in essential thrombocythemia is related to a decrease of large von Willebrand factor multimers in plasma. Ann Hematol 75:215–220, 1997.

137. van Genderen PJ, Budde V, Michiels JJ, et al: The reduction of large von-Willebrand factor multimers in plasma in essential thrombocythemia is related to the platelet count. Br J Haematol 93:962–965, 1996.

138. Michiels JJ: Acquired von-Willebrand disease due to increasing platelet count can readily explain the paradox of thrombosis and bleeding in thrombocythemia. Clin Appl Thromb Hemost 59:147–151, 1999.

139. Van Genderen PJ, Mulder PG, Waleboer M, et al: Prevention and treatment of thrombotic complications in essential thrombocythaemia: Efficacy and safety of aspirin. Br J Haematol 97:179–184, 1997.

140. Tefferi A: Risk Based Management in Essential Thrombocythemia. In: American Society of Hematology Educational Program Book. Washington, DC, American Society of Hematology, 1999, p 172.

141. Tefferi A, Solberg LA, Silverstein MN: A clinical update in polycythemia vera and essential thrombocythemia. Am J Med 109:141–149, 2000.

142. Michiels JJ: Aspirin and platelet-lowering agents for the prevention of vascular complications in essential thrombocythemia. Clin Appl Thromb Hemost 5:247–251, 1999.

143. Michiels JJ, Berneman Z, Van Bockstaele D, et al: Clinical and laboratory features, pathobiology of platelet-mediated thrombosis and bleeding complications and the molecular etiology of essential thrombocythemia and polycythemia vera: Therapeutic implications. Semin Thromb Hemost 32:174–207, 2006.

144. Pearson TC: The risk of thrombosis in essential thrombocythemia and polycythemia vera. Semin Oncol 29(3 suppl 10): 16–21, 2002.

145. Michiels JJ: Normal life expectancy and thrombosis-free survival in aspirin treated essential thrombocythemia. Clin Appl Thromb Hemost 5:30–36, 1999.

146. Van Genderen PJ, Michiels JJ: Hydroxyurea in essential thrombocytosis. N Engl J Med 333:802–803, 1985.

147. Lahuerta-Palacios JJ, Bornstein R, Fernandez-Debora FJ, et al: Controlled and uncontrolled thrombocytosis: Its clinical role in essential thrombocytosis. Cancer 61:1207–1212, 1988.

148. Cortelazzo S, Finazzi G, Ruggeri M, et al: Hydroxyurea for patients with essential thrombocythemia and a high risk of thrombosis. N Engl J Med 332:1132–1136, 1995.

149. Harrison C, Campbell PJ, Buck G, et al: Hydroxyurea compared with anagrelide in high-risk essential thrombocythaemia. N Engl J Med 353:33–45, 2005.

150. Petrides PE: Anagrelide: A decade of clinical experience with its use for the treatment of primary thrombocythemia. Expert Opin Pharmacother 5:1781–1798, 2004.

151. Andreasson B, Swolin B, Kutti J: Hydroxyurea treatment reduces haematopoietic progenitor growth and CD34 positive cells in polycythemia vera and essential thrombocythaemia. Eur J Haematol 64:188–193, 2000.

152. Barbui T, Finazzi G: Management of essential thrombocythemia. Crit Rev Oncol Hematol 29:257–266, 1999.

153. Finazzi G, Barbui T: Treatment of essential thrombocythemia with special emphasis on leukemogenic risk. Ann Hematol 78:389–392, 1999.

154. Löfvenberg E, Wahlin A: Management of polycythemia vera, essential thrombocythaemia and myelofibrosis with hydroxyurea. Eur J Haematol 41:375–381, 1988.

155. Daoud MS, Gibson LE, Pittelkow MR: Hydroxyurea dermopathy: A unique lichenoid eruption complicating long term therapy with hydroxyurea. J Am Acad Dermatol 36:178–182, 1997.

156. Best P, Daoud MS, Pittelkow MR, et al: Hydroxyurea induced leg ulceration in 14 patients. Ann Intern Med 128:29–32, 1998.

157. Starmans-Kool MJ, Fickers MM, Pannebakker MA: An unwanted side-effect of hydroxyurea in a patient with idiopathic myelofibrosis. Ann Hematol 70:279–280, 1995.

158. Finazzi G, Ruggeri M, Rodeghiero F, et al: Second malignancies in patients with essential thrombocythaemia treated with busulfan and hydroxyurea: Long term follow up of a randomized clinical trial. Br J Haematol 110:577–583, 2000.

159. Sterkers Y, Preudhomme C, Laï J-L, et al: Acute myeloid leukemia and myelodysplastic syndromes following essential thrombocythemia treated with hydroxyurea: High proportion of cases with 17p deletion. Blood 91:616–622, 1998.

160. Randi ML, Fabris F, Girolami A: Leukemia and myelodysplasia effect of multiple cytotoxic therapy in essential thrombocythemia. Leukemia Lymphoma 37:379–385, 2000.

161. Nand S, Stock W, Godwin J, et al: Leukemogenic risk of hydroxyurea therapy in polycythemia vera, essential thrombocythemia and myeloid metaplasia with myelofibrosis. Am J Hematol 52:42–46, 1996.

162. Liozon E, Brigaudeau C, Trimoreau F, et al: Is treatment with hydroxyurea leukemogenic in patients with essential thrombocythemia? An analysis of three new cases of leukaemia transformation and review of the literature. Hematol Cell Ther 39:11–18, 1997.

163. Barbui T, Finazzi G: When and how to treat essential thrombocythemia. N Engl J Med 353:85–86, 2005.

164. Silverstein MN, Petitt RM, Solberg LA, et al: Anagrelide: A new drug for treating thrombocytosis. N Engl J Med 318:1292–1294, 1988.

165. Anagrelide Study Group: Anagrelide, a therapy for thrombocythemic states: Experience in 577 patients. Am J Med 92:69–76, 1992.

166. Mazur EM, Rosmarin AG, Sohl PA, et al: Analysis of the mechanism of anagrelide induced thrombocytopenia in humans. Blood 79:1931–1937, 1992.

167. Solberg LA, Tefferi A, Oles KJ, et al: The effects of anagrelide on human megakaryocytopoiesis. Br J Haematol 99:174–180, 1997.

168. Spencer CM, Brogden RN: Anagrelide: A review of its pharmacodynamic and pharmacokinetic properties and therapeutic potential in the treatment of thrombocythaemia. Drugs 47:809–822, 1994.

169. Petitt RM, Silverstein MN, Petrone ME: Anagrelide for control of thrombocythemia in polycythemia and other myeloproliferative disorders. Semin Hematol 34:51–54, 1997.

170. Birgegard G: Anagrelide treatment in myeloproliferative disorders. Semin Thromb Hemost 32:260–266, 2006.

171. Petrides PE, Beykirch MK, Trapp OM: Anagrelide, a novel platelet lowering option in essential thrombocythaemia: Treatment experience in 48 patients in Germany. Eur J Haematol 61:71–76, 1998.

172. Storen EC, Tefferi A: Long-term use of anagrelide in young patients with essential thrombocythemia. Blood 97:863–866, 2001.

173. Birgegard G, Bjorkholm M, Kutti J, et al: Adverse effects and benefits of two years of anagrelide treatment for thrombocythemia in chronic myeloproliferative disorders. Haematologica 89:520–527, 2004.

174. Steurer M, Gastl G, Jedrzejczak WW, et al: Anagrelide for thrombocytosis in myeloproliferative disorders: A prospective study to assess efficacy and adverse event profile. Cancer 101:2239–2246, 2004.

175. Penninga E, Jensen BA, Hansen PB, et al: Anagrelide treatment in 52 patients with chronic myeloproliferative diseases. Clin Lab Haematol 26:335–340, 2004.

176. Fruchtman SM, Petitt RM, Gilbert HS, et al: Anagrelide: Analysis of long-term efficacy, safety and leukemogenic potential in myeloproliferative disorders. Leuk Res 29:481–491, 2005.

177. Thiele J, Kvasnicka HM, Schmitt-Graeff A: Effects of anagrelide on megakaryopoiesis and platelet production. Semin Thromb Hemost 32:352–361, 2006.

178. Elliott MA, Tefferi A: Interferon alpha therapy in polycythemia vera and essential thrombocythemia. Semin Thromb Hemost 23:464–472, 1997.

179. Sacchi S: The role of α-interferon in essential thrombocythaemia, polycythaemia vera and myelofibrosis with myeloid metaplasia (MMM): A concise update. Leukemia Lymphoma 19:13–20, 1995.

180. Giles FJ: Maintenance therapy in the myeloproliferative disorders: The current options. Br J Haematol 79(suppl 1): 92–95, 1991.

181. Sacchi S, Tabilio A, Leoni P, et al: Sustained complete hematological remission in essential thrombocythemia after discontinuation of long-term α-IFN treatment. Ann Hematol 66:245–246, 1993.

182. Kasparu H, Bernhart M, Krieger O, et al: Remission may continue after termination of rIFNα-2b treatment for essential thrombocythemia. Eur J Haematol 48:33–36, 1992.

183. Bentley M, Taylor K, Grigg A, et al: Long-term interferon-alpha 2A does not induce sustained hematologic remission in younger patients with essential thrombocythemia. Leukemia Lymphoma 36:123–128, 1999.

184. Gisslinger H, Linkesch W, Fritz E, et al: Long-term interferon therapy for thrombocytosis in myeloproliferative diseases. Lancet 1:634–637, 1989.

185. Middelhoff G, Boll I: A long-term clinical trial of interferon alpha therapy in essential thrombocythemia. Ann Hematol 64:207–209, 1992.

186. Pogliani EM, Rossini F, Miccolis I, et al: Alpha interferon as initial treatment of essential thrombocythemia: An analysis after two years of follow up. Tumori 81:245–248, 1995.

187. Rametta V, Ferrara F, Marottoli V, et al: Recombinant interferon alpha-2b as treatment of essential thrombocythemia. Acta Haematol 91:126–129, 1994.

188. Gisslinger H, Chott A, Scheithauer W, et al: Interferon in essential thrombocythaemia. Br J Haematol 79(suppl 1): 199142–47, 1991.

189. Gauser A, Carlo-Stella C, Greher J, et al: Effect of recombinant interferons alpha and gamma on human bone marrow derived megakaryocytic progenitor cells. Blood 70:1173–1179, 1987.

190. Broxmeyer HE, Lu L, Platzer E, et al: Comparative analysis of the influences of human gamma, alpha and beta interferons on human multipotential (CFU-GEMM), erythroid (BFU-E) and granulocyte-macrophage (CFU-GM) progenitor cells. J Immunol 131:1300–1305, 1983.

191. Carlo-Stella C, Cazzola M, Gasner A, et al: Effects of recombinant alpha and gamma interferons on the in-vitro growth of circulating hematopoietic progenitor cells (CFU-GEMM, CFU-MK, BFU-E and CFU-GM) from patients with myelofibrosis with myeloid metaplasia. Blood 70:1014–1019, 1987.

192. Gugliotta L, Bagnara GP, Catani L, et al: In vivo and in vitro inhibitory effect of α-interferon on megakaryocyte colony growth in essential thrombocythemia. Br J Haematol 71:177–181, 1989.

193. Wadenvik H, Kutti J, Ridell B, et al: The effect of α-interferon on bone marrow megakaryocytes and platelet production rate in essential thrombocythemia. Blood 77:2103–2108, 1991.

194. Waysbort A, Giroux M, Mansat V, et al: Experimental study of transplacental passage of alpha interferon by two assay techniques. J Antimicrob Chemother 37:1232–1237, 1993.

195. Sacchi S, Gugliotta L, Papineschi F, et al: Alfa-interferon in the treatment of essential thrombocythemia: Clinical results and evaluation of its biological effects on the hematopoietic neoplastic clone. Leukemia 12:289–294, 1998.

196. Lengfelder E, Griesshammer M, Hehlmann R, et al: Interferon-alpha in the treatment of essential thrombocythemia. Leukemia Lymphoma 22(suppl 1): 135–142, 1996.

197. Törnebohm-Roche E, Merup M, Lockner D, et al: α-2a Interferon therapy and antibody formation in patients with essential thrombocythemia and polycythemia vera with thrombocytosis. Am J Hematol 48:163–167, 1994.

198. Lipton JH, Khoroshko ND, Golenkov AN, et al: Pegasys CML Study Group. Two-year survival data from a randomized study of peginterferon ALFA-2a (40 kD) versus interferon α-2a in patients with chronic myelogenous leukemia. [abstract 3363]. American Society of Hematology Annual Meeting, San Diego, CA, 2003.

199. Michallet M, Maloisel F, Delain M, et al: Pegylated recombinant interferon alpha-2b vs recombinant interferon alpha-2b for the initial treatment of chronic-phase chronic myelogenous leukemia: A phase III study. Leukemia 18:309–315, 2004.

200. Langer C, Lengfelder E, Thiele J, et al: Pegylated interferon for the treatment of high risk essential thrombocythemia: Results of a phase II study. Haematologica 90:1333–1338, 2005.

201. Samuelsson J, Hasselbalch H, Bruserud O, et al A phase II trial of pegylated interferon alpha-2b therapy for polycythemia vera and essential thrombocythemia: Feasibility, clinical and biologic effects, and impact on quality of life. Cancer 106:2397–2405, 2006.

202. Gugliotta L, Bulgarelli S, Vianelli N, et al: PEG intron treatment in 90 patients with essential thrombocythemia (ET): Final report of a phase II study. Blood 106;2005. Abstract 2600.

203. Gugliotta L, Bulgarelli S, Asioli S, et al: Bone marrow evaluation according to the PVSG and WHO criteria in 90 essential thrombocythemia (ET) patients treated with PEG interferon alpha-2b: Preliminary results. Blood 106;2005. Abstract 4962.

204. Berk PD, Goldberg JD, Silverstein MN: Increased incidence of acute leukemia in polycythemia vera associated with chlorambucil therapy. N Engl J Med 304:441–447, 1981.

205. Najean Y, Rain J: The very long-term evolution of polycythemia vera: An analysis of 318 patients initially treated by phlebotomy or ^{32}P between 1969 and 1981. Semin Hematol 34:6–16, 1997.

206. Van De Pette JE, Prochazka AV, Pearson TC, et al: Primary thrombocythaemia treated with busulphan. Br J Haematol 62:229–237, 1986.

207. Leukemia and Hematosarcoma Cooperative Group; European Organization for Research on Treatment of Cancer (E.O.R.T.C): Treatment of polycythemia vera by radiophosphorus or busulphan: A randomized trial. Br J Cancer 44:75–80, 1981.

208. Brandt L, Anderson H: Survival and risk of leukaemia in polycythaemia vera and essential thrombocythaemia treated with oral radiophosphorus: Are safer drugs available? Eur J Haematol 54:21–26, 1995.

209. Balan KK, Critchley M: Outcome of 259 patients with primary proliferative polycythaemia (PPP) and idiopathic thrombocythaemia (IT) treated in a regional nuclear medicine department with phosphorus-32: A 15 year review. Br J Radiol 70:1169–1173, 1997.

210. Council on Drugs: Evaluation of two antineoplastic agents: Pipobroman (Vercyte) and thioguanine. JAMA 200:139–140, 1967.

211. Najean Y, Rain J-D: Treatment of polycythemia vera: The use of hydroxyurea and pipobroman in 292 patients under the age of 65 years. Blood 90:3370–3377, 1997.

212. Messora C, Bensi L, Vanzanelli P, et al: Myelodysplastic transformation in a case of essential thrombocythemia treated with pipobroman. Haematologica 81:51–53, 1996.

213. Mazzucconi MG, Francesconi M, Chistolini A, et al: Pipobroman therapy of essential thrombocythemia. Scand J Haematol 37:306–309, 1986.

214. Brusamolino E, Canevari A, Salvaneschi L: Efficacy trial of pipobroman in essential thrombocythemia: A study of 24 patients. Cancer Treat Rep 68:1339–1342, 1984.

215. Kiladjian JJ, Gardin C, Renoux M, et al: Long-term outcomes of polycythemia vera patients treated with pipobroman as initial therapy. Hematol J 4:198–207, 2003.

216. Chomienne C, Rain JD, Briere J, et al: Risk of leukemic transformation in PV and ET patients. Pathol Biol (Paris) 52:289–293, 2004.

217. Landolfi R, Marchioli R, Kutti J, et al: Efficacy and safety of low-dose aspirin in polycythemia vera: Results of the ECLAP trial. N Engl J Med 350:114–124, 2004.

218. Michiels JJ, Berneman Z, Schroyens W, et al: Platelet-mediated thrombotic complications in patients with ET: Reversal by aspirin, platelet reduction, and not by coumadin. Blood Cells Mol Dis 36:199–205, 2006.

219. Taft EG, Babcock RB, Scharfman WB, et al: Plateletpheresis in the management of thrombocytosis. Blood 50:927–933, 1977.

220. Goldfinger D, Thompson R, Lowe C, et al: Long-term plateletpheresis in the management of primary thrombocytosis. Transfusion 19:336–338, 1979.

221. Baron BW, Mick R, Baron JM: Combined plateletpheresis and cytotoxic chemotherapy for symptomatic thrombocytosis in myeloproliferative disorders. Cancer 72:1209–1218, 1993.

222. Griesshammer M, Heimpel H, Pearson TC: Essential thrombocythemia and pregnancy. Leukemia Lymphoma 22(suppl 1): 157–163,1996.

223. Griesshammer M, Grunewald M, Michiels JJ: Acquired thrombophilia in pregnancy: Essential thrombocythemia. Semin Thromb Hemost 29:205–212, 2003.

224. Beressi AH, Tefferi A, Silverstein MN, et al: Outcome analysis of 34 pregnancies in women with essential thrombocythemia. Arch Intern Med 155:1217–1222, 1995.

225. Samuelsson J, Swolin B: Spontaneous remission during two pregnancies in a patient with essential thrombocythaemia. Leukemia Lymphoma 25:597–600, 1997.

226. Griesshammer M, Struve S, Harrison C: Essential thrombocythemia/polycythemia vera and pregnancy: The need of an observational study. Semin Thromb Hemost 32(4 Pt 2):422–429, 2006.

227. Eliyahn S, Shalev E: Essential thrombocythemia during pregnancy. Obstet Gynecol Surv 52:243–247, 1997.

228. Milano V, Gabrielli S, Rizzo N, et al: Successful treatment of essential thrombocythaemia in a pregnancy with recombinant interferon-α2a. J Maternal-Fetal Med 5:74–78, 1996.

229. Pardini S, Careddu MF, Dore F, et al: Essential thrombocythemia and pregnancy. Haematologica 80:392–393, 1995.

230. Delage R, Demers C, Cantine G: Treatment of essential thrombocythemia during pregnancy with interferon-α. Obstet Gynecol 87:814–817, 1996.

Chapter 19

The Antiphospholipid Syndrome: Clinical Presentation, Diagnosis, and Patient Management

Jacob H. Rand, MD • Miles B. Levin, MD • Barbara M. Alving, MD

INTRODUCTION AND HISTORICAL COMMENTS

Although the antiphospholipid *syndrome* (APLS) was first described as a distinct entity about 20 years ago, antibodies to phospholipid-binding proteins—(antiphospholipid–protein *antibodies* [APLA])—were observed more than 30 years earlier. They were initially recognized as "circulating anticoagulants" because of their interference in phospholipid-dependent coagulation reactions and by their causing a biologic false-positive syphilis test due to antibody-mediated recognition of cardiolipins.[1,2] These in vitro anticoagulants became known as lupus anticoagulants (LAs)—a misnomer that persists to the present—because they were often detected in patients with underlying systemic lupus erythematosus (SLE). Forty years ago, Bowie and colleagues[3] recognized their association with thrombotic events in patients with SLE. Recognition of APLS[4] followed the development of quantitative immunoassays for APLA and the awareness that elevated levels of these antibodies were, in some patients, associated with thrombosis, fetal loss, and thrombocytopenia. During the past 20 years, sensitive quantitative tests for antibody detection have become available,[5] and over the past 15 years, plasma proteins that serve as antigens for these antibodies have been identified.[6–8]

The progressive elucidation of APLS has resulted in several different terms for the tests, target antigens, and related proteins; these are summarized in the glossary (Table 19-1). Individuals may have immunoglobulin (Ig)G, IgM, or IgA APLA. Approximately 90% of patients who test positive for LA also test positive for anticardiolipin antibodies (ACAs), which are actually antibodies against phospholipid-binding proteins.[9] However, no direct correlation has been made between the potency of LA activity and the titers of ACA as determined through enzyme-linked immunosorbent assays (ELISA); this may reflect the heterogeneity of the APLA.[4,9,10] Despite difficulties inherent in comparisons of studies in which only a single test for LA or only an ELISA has been used, associations between well-defined clinical conditions and the presence of APLA have emerged. This chapter describes the immunology, clinical presentations, and approaches to the diagnosis and management of treatment as they relate to patients who will generally be referred for consultation.

IMMUNOLOGY AND PATHOPHYSIOLOGY OF ANTIPHOSPHOLIPID ANTIBODIES

In the context of APLS, the term "antiphospholipid antibodies" is a misnomer that refers to a heterogeneous family of autoimmune immunoglobulins that are directed not against phospholipids, but against plasma proteins (also referred to as "cofactors") that bind to anionic phospholipids. Although β_2-glycoprotein I (β_2GPI) is believed to be the major target of the antibodies, several other phospholipid-binding cofactors have been identified; among these are prothrombin, protein C, protein S, and annexin A5. APLA detected in ELISA are directed against these proteins, which are bound to anionic phospholipids that coat the plastic microtiter plates.[7,11–14] The anionic phospholipid that is involved in this reaction in vivo is believed to be phosphatidylserine; however, the most widely used assays contain cardiolipin as the anionic phospholipid, with β_2GPI and prothrombin as cofactors.[13,15]

β_2-Glycoprotein I (β_2GPI)

β_2GPI, or apoprotein H, is a 50-kDa proline-rich glycoprotein that is present in plasma at a concentration of approximately 150 to 200 μg/mL. The protein is composed of five repeating stretches of $\approx$60 amino acid domains that bear homology to other members of the complement control protein superfamily (Fig. 19-1).[14,16,17] The fifth short chain consensus repeat (SCR) domain deviates structurally from domains I through IV in that its carboxyterminus bears hydrophobic and cationic amino acids. The affinity of this protein for anionic phospholipid membrane arises through the attraction of the cationic domain for the polar heads of the phospholipids and the insertion of the flexible hydrophobic loop into the hydrophobic portion of the bilayer.[16,18]

Recent evidence has defined an epitope that is recognized by thrombogenic APLA to domain I of β_2GPI and has localized it to Gly40-Arg43.[19,20] In a study of 198 patients with SLE, APLS, and "lupus-like" disease, investigators found that plasmas with detectable anti-β_2GPI antibodies that had Gly40-Arg43 specificity correlated highly with LA activity and with a history of thrombosis (odds ratio, 18.9 vs 1.1). In contrast, plasmas with anti-β_2GPI

Table 19-1 Glossary of Terms Used in Discussion of Antiphospholipid Antibodies

Antiphospholipid syndrome (APLS): Characterized by venous and/or arterial thrombosis, thrombocytopenia, or recurrent fetal loss in association with demonstrable antiphospholipid–protein antibodies.

Antiphospholipid–protein antibodies (APLA) or antiphospholipid antibodies: Immunoglobulin (Ig)G, IgM, or IgA antibodies directed against proteins such as prothrombin or β_2-glycoprotein I (β_2GPI) that bind to phospholipids. APLA may be described as lupus anticoagulant (LA) activity or by the particular immunoassay procedure used for their detection.

Lupus anticoagulant (LA): Antibody against a phospholipid-binding protein such as prothrombin or β_2GPI that induces prolongation of an in vitro phospholipid-dependent clotting assay. These may be detected by several different methods, including but not limited to dilute Russell's viper venom time, partial thromboplastin time (PTT), tissue thromboplastin inhibition time, kaolin clotting time, and textarin/ecarin time. Results of these various LA tests do not correlate well with each other.

Anticardiolipin antibodies (ACA): Antibodies against β_2GPI that have been detected in an enzyme-linked immunosorbent assay (ELISA) containing cardiolipin as the phospholipid-binding β_2GPI (which is present in the assay).

Antiphosphatidylserine antibodies: Antibodies against β_2GPI that have been detected in an ELISA that contains phosphatidylserine as the phospholipid-binding β_2GPI.

Anti-β_2GPI antibodies: Antibodies against β_2GPI that are detected in an ELISA that contains this phospholipid-binding protein adsorbed to the surfaces of microtiter plate wells.

---

risk in patients who tested positive for LA and ACA compared with those who tested positive in only one of the two tests.[22-24] Accumulating evidence for the role of a specific epitope in the APLA disease process may explain the suboptimal specificity of current clinical APLA tests (see "Laboratory Diagnosis of APLA"). Conversely, some anti-β_2GPI antibodies as currently detected are nonpathogenic, and some APLS-related thrombotic episodes may be due to different populations of autoantibodies (e.g., antiprothrombin).

Investigation into disease mechanism(s) in APLS has been especially challenging. A major problem is that APLA exhibit diverse effects in vitro because of the many biologic processes that involve phospholipids and phospholipid membranes. The heterogeneity of APLA, even in individual patients, as shown on clonal analysis,[25] adds to the difficulty of defining the pathogenesis of APLS. Some of the main hypotheses that have been proposed to account for the pathogenic mechanisms in APLS are listed in Table 19-2.[26-51]

The physiologic function of β_2GPI has not yet been established; the protein may play a scavenging role for anionic phospholipids after apoptosis.[52,53] Deficiencies of β_2GPI in humans have not been associated with any disorders, including thrombosis,[54] and do not appear to affect coagulation reactions.[55] β_2GPI-null mice do not manifest any obvious significant abnormalities.[56] Transgenic mice have impaired thrombin generation, and the offspring of heterozygous mice contained fewer than the expected percentage of homozygotes for β_2GPI-null disrupted alleles.[56] The latter observation suggests that β_2GPI may play an undefined role in the reproductive process.

Data from animal studies indicate that APLA may play a causal role in the development of thrombosis and that they are not simply an epiphenomenon. Mice immunized against β_2GPI develop APLA and pregnancy wastage.[37,57] Furthermore, mice that have been passively immunized with β_2GPI or that have received human antibodies to β_2GPI develop fetal wastage and susceptibility to thrombosis.[58-61]

Several possible causes of thrombosis have been postulated; however, none has gained exclusive acceptance. Anti–endothelial cell antibodies, which are a common aspect of APLS, may cause endothelial injury, thereby inducing tissue factor

---

antibodies that did not recognize the Gly40-Arg43 domain did not correlate with a history of thrombosis or with LA activity.[20] These findings of two different types of β_2GPI antibodies were followed by a retrospective study that showed an odds ratio for thrombosis of 42.3 for patients with β_2GPI–dependent lupus anticoagulant activity compared with 1.6 for those with LA activity independent of β_2GPI antibodies.[21] These findings contrast with those from prior studies that showed only modest increases in thrombogenic

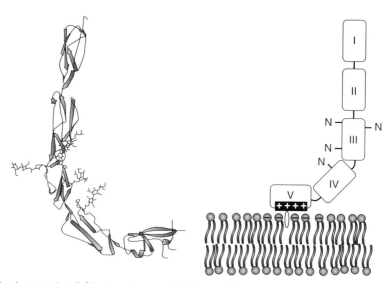

Figure 19-1 Structure of β_2-glycoprotein I *(left)* and mechanism of binding of β_2-glycoprotein I to the phospholipid surface. (From de Groot PG, Bouma B, Lutters BC, et al: J Autoimmunity 15:87–89, 2000; reprinted with permission from Elsevier.)

Table 19-2 Proposed Mechanisms for the Antiphospholipid Syndrome

Injury to endothelium[26]
Induction of receptors for cell adhesion molecules on endothelium[27,28]
Induction of tissue factor expression on monocytes and on endothelial cells[29,30]
Inhibition of heparin:antithrombin III complexes[31–33]
Interference with protein C pathway[34–36]
Complement activation[37,38]
Platelet activation[39–42]
Disruption of annexin A5 shield[43]
Induction of apoptosis[44,45]
Altered eicosanoid synthesis[46]
Increase in plasminogen activator inhibitor-1[47]
Cross-reactivity to oxidized low-density lipoprotein[48,49]
Impairment in autoactivation of factor XII and reduced fibrinolysis[50,51]

Table 19-3 Phospholipid-Dependent Coagulation Reactions

1. Tissue factor–factor VII/VIIa–mediated activation of factors X and IX
2. Factor IXa and factor VIIIa activation of factor X to factor Xa
3. Factor Xa and factor Va activation of prothrombin to thrombin

(TF) production and exposure of membrane phospholipid.[62] Circulating β_2GPI could then bind to the phospholipids, and the APLA could in turn bind to the complex, thus inducing further damage.[62] Other investigators have shown that APLA can recognize heparin or heparin bound to β_2GPI, thereby inhibiting the interaction of heparin with antithrombin III.[31–33] Several in vitro studies have suggested that APLA promote thromboses by inhibiting the ability of protein C to inactivate factors Va and VIIIa.[34–36] Complement activation also appears to play a role in the thrombotic process in APLS.[37,63]

Conflicting evidence has been gathered on the effects of APLA on platelets. APLA may activate platelets,[42,64] but at least two groups have reported that APLA can bind directly to circulating platelets without inducing platelet activation or aggregation.[40,65] Others have shown that APLA can bind to activated platelets, although this binding does not affect the release reaction or aggregation.[66] Most human hybridoma LAs do not bind to resting platelets in vitro.[67] Galli and coworkers[68] reported that 40% of patients with APLS and thrombocytopenia had antibodies against glycoprotein (GP)-IIb/IIIa and/or GP-Ib/IX, and that APLA did not bind to resting platelets.

Increasing evidence supports the concept that APLA and, in particular, β_2GPI:anti-β_2GPI complexes, may displace the potent anticoagulant, annexin A5 (previously known as annexin V) from anionic procoagulant phospholipid surfaces. Annexin A5 is derived from a family of proteins with a canonical structure consisting of repetitive homologous domains of about 70 amino acids. This protein clusters on exposed phospholipid membrane surfaces, forming a two-dimensional crystalline array[43,69–71] that shields the phospholipids for availability from phospholipid-dependent coagulation reactions.[70] It has recently been shown with atomic force microscopy that APLA can displace annexin A5 from procoagulant surfaces, thereby accelerating coagulation reactions.[71] Furthermore, annexin displacement is dependent on anti-β_2GPI antibodies. These antibodies have been reported to correlate with clinical manifestations of thrombosis in patients with APLA.[72]

Annexin A5 may play an antithrombotic role in physiologic conditions such as those present in the placental circulation, where it is expressed by trophoblasts whose apical surfaces are covered by a layer of annexin A5.[73] When mice were infused with anti–annexin A5 antibodies, varying degrees of fetal wastage occurred, including thrombosis and necrosis.[74] In one study, infusion of pregnant mice with APLA from patients with APLS reduced annexin A5 levels and accelerated the coagulation of plasma on cultured trophoblasts, endothelial cells,[75] and platelets.[76,77] Thus, annexin A5 may have an antithrombotic effect on the surfaces of cells lining the placenta and in the systemic vasculature, which can be disrupted by APLA.

LA Effects Explained

For most APLA, immune recognition requires antigen binding to a suitable anionic phospholipid surface.[11,12,78,79] Engagement of the F(ab) portions of an IgG APLA with two adjacent antigen molecules such as β_2GPI or prothrombin at the anionic surface enhances the binding of the complex to the surface.[11,12,78,79] Because most reactions that control the process of blood coagulation occur at the phospholipid surface, (Table 19-3) these stable trimolecular complexes of IgG and two phospholipid-binding protein molecules block the proper assembly of the phospholipid-dependent coagulation system, thereby producing the LA effect. Thus, in the confirmatory LA tests described later, this sequestering effect is overcome by the addition of excess phospholipids, which allow the coagulation reaction to proceed unhindered.

The paradox of why lupus anticoagulants promote thrombosis may be explained by the fact that APLA/β_2GPI complexes disrupt the ordered crystallization of the two-dimensional annexin A5 shield over phospholipid bilayers (Fig. 19-2). Consequently, the antibody/β_2GPI complexes expose a substantially greater quantity of phospholipids by disrupting the annexin A5 shield than they block by direct binding.[76,80,81]

Triggers for Hematologic Consultation

The diverse clinical presentation of APLS results in a variety of avenues through which patients are referred for consultation. Common subjects for consultation are young patients, without other known risk factors, who have sustained a stroke or who have had unexplained venous thromboembolism (VTE) (Table 19-4). Other patients are referred with a previous diagnosis of APLS and the need to confirm the diagnosis. Obstetricians send women with multiple pregnancy losses. Patients with lupus are referred for evaluation because of known association with APLS.

However, other conduits for consultation exist for which little is known about appropriate treatment. Patients with a prior diagnosis of APLS who have been without symptoms for several years may wish to discuss potential changes in therapy. Surgeons send patients for an elevated partial thromboplastin time (PTT) found incidentally on preoperative testing. Some obstetricians test for APLA

19

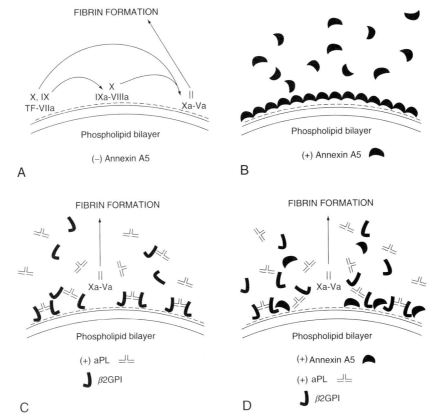

Figure 19-2 Proposed model for the "lupus anticoagulant effect" paradox and for a "lupus procoagulant effect:" **A,** Anionic phospholipids (negative charges), when exposed on the apical surface of the cell membrane bilayer, serve as potent cofactors for the assembly of three different coagulation complexes—the tissue factor (TF):VIIa complex, the IXa:VIIIa complex, and the Xa:Va complex—and thereby accelerate blood coagulation. TF complexes yield factor IXa or factor Xa, the IXa complex yields factor Xa, and the Xa formed from both of these reactions is the active enzyme in the prothrombinase complex that yields factor IIa (thrombin), which, in turn, cleaves fibrinogen to form fibrin. **B,** Annexin A5, in the absence of antiphospholipid antibodies (APLA), serves as a potent anticoagulant by forming a crystal lattice over the anionic phospholipid surface, shielding it from availability for assembly of the phospholipid-dependent coagulation complexes. **C,** In the absence of annexin A5, APLA:β_2GPI complexes prolong coagulation times, compared with control antibodies. This occurs via antibody recognition of domain I on the β_2GPI, which results in dimers and pentamers of antibody:β_2GPI complexes that have high affinity for phospholipid via domain V. These high-affinity complexes reduce the quantity of anionic phospholipids available for binding of coagulation factors. This results in a "lupus anticoagulant" effect in conditions with limited quantities of anionic phospholipids. **D,** In the presence of annexin A5, antiphospholipid antibodies, via interaction with β_2GPI, disrupt the ability of annexin A5 to form ordered crystals on the phospholipid surface. This results in a net increase in the amount of anionic phospholipid available for promoting coagulation reactions. APLA:β_2GPI complexes expose significantly more phospholipids by disrupting the annexin A5 shield than they block by direct binding. This manifests in the net acceleration of coagulation in vitro (i.e., a "lupus procoagulant effect") and in vivo (i.e., in thrombophilia). (Reprinted with permission from Rand JH: Molecular pathogenesis of the antiphospholipid syndrome. Circ Res 90:29–37, 2002.)

Table 19-4 Common Indications for Testing for Antiphospholipid Syndrome

Clinical

Venous thromboembolism (deep venous thrombosis, pulmonary embolism, and thrombosis in less common sites)
Peripheral arterial thrombosis
Myocardial infarction
Stroke or transient ischemic attack (<55 years old without other risk factors)
Pregnancy complications, including recurrent fetal loss, intrauterine growth retardation, preeclampsia, and HELLP (*h*emolytic anemia, *e*levated *l*iver enzymes, *l*ow *p*latelets) syndrome
SLE (systemic lupus erythematosus)

in women who have not had recurrent miscarriages. Patients with neurologic deficits or ophthalmic manifestations with serologic evidence for APLA must be differentiated from patients with multiple sclerosis and other neurologic conditions.

This is only a sampling of the reasons for which patients are referred for consultation. This chapter focuses on the patient population in the former paragraph and, where appropriate, suggests guidelines that may be helpful to the consultant.

ANTIPHOSPHOLIPID SYNDROME: CLINICAL DIAGNOSIS

APLS should be considered in patients who present with one or more of the following clinical conditions: VTE, arterial thrombosis (stroke, myocardial infarction), or recurrent pregnancy loss,[82–84] particularly in the absence of other thrombophilic risk factors. Associated conditions, particularly in patients with SLE or other autoimmune disorders, include thrombocytopenia, vasculitic rash, transient ischemic attack, arthralgia, dermal necrosis of digits, livedo reticularis, valvular heart disease, and pulmonary hypertension (Table 19-5).[85] The diagnosis is confirmed if the patient tests

Table 19-5 Clinical Manifestations of the Antiphospholipid Syndrome

Venous or arterial thromboembolism in typical or atypical locations
Multiple pregnancy losses
Thrombocytopenia
Stroke
Livedo reticularis, necrotizing skin vasculitis, skin ulcers
Cardiac valvular lesions
Coronary artery disease
Arthralgia, arthritis
Hemolytic anemia
Pulmonary hypertension, acute respiratory distress syndrome
Atherosclerosis, peripheral artery disease
Retinal disease
Adrenal failure, hemorrhagic adrenal infarction
Gastrointestinal manifestations: Budd-Chiari syndrome, mesenteric and portal vein obstructions, hepatic infarction, esophageal necrosis, gastric and colonic ulceration, gallbladder necrosis
Catastrophic antiphospholipid syndrome (CAPS) with microangiopathy

positive for autoantibodies that are detected in phospholipid-dependent clotting assays as LA, or as ACA in ELISA that contain cardiolipin, along with β_2-glycoprotein I (β_2GPI). Patients should be tested with both types of assay (immunologic and coagulation), and more than one negative test for LA is needed to rule out the diagnosis of APLS in a patient with a clinical presentation consistent with this disorder. Research criteria for diagnosing APLS, which have recently been updated in Sydney, Australia, require that tests should be positive for LA or for moderate to high levels of ACA (IgG, IgM, or anti-β_2GPI) on two occasions at least 12 weeks apart (Table 19-6).[84-89] The requirement for sustained positivity for APLA is given because results may be positive only transiently and may be unrelated to clinical symptoms.[90]

The syndrome is known as secondary APLS if it occurs in patients who have another identifiable autoimmune connective tissue disorder, usually SLE. In this patient group, the female/male ratio for development of APLS is 7:1, similar to the sex ratio for SLE (9:1 to 10:1).[91,92] The prevalence of ACA in patients with SLE is variable; frequencies range from 16% to 39%,[93-103] although incidences as high as 86% have been reported.[104] LA is also commonly detected in patients with SLE; frequencies range from 11% to 30%,[96,99,105] and significant overlap is seen in ACA detected in LA-positive plasma.

In the absence of SLE or other autoimmune connective tissue disorders, APLS is considered a primary APLS.[91] The multicentered Euro-Phospholipid Project gathered clinical and immunologic data from 1000 unselected patients who met proposed preliminary criteria for the classification of definite APLS[83]; investigators found that 53% of the cohort had primary APLS and 41% had APLS with SLE or lupus-like conditions.[91] They also calculated a female/male ratio of 3.5:1 for primary APLS ($P < .005$) compared with a 5:1 ratio overall.[91] The age of onset was between 15 and 50 years in 85% of patients. Patients who developed APLS after the age of 50 (n = 127; 12.7%) were most often male (34% vs 16%). In a retrospective analysis, it was noted that most patients with APLS did not progress to SLE.[106] Regardless, management of primary and secondary APLS is the same and the prognosis does not appear to

be different; some advocate eliminating the primary/secondary designation altogether.[84,107]

An accelerated subentity of APLS that consists of disseminated macrovascular and microvascular occlusions resulting in multiorgan failure is known as the catastrophic antiphospholipid syndrome (CAPS). This disorder, which is reported in less than 1% of all patients with APLS, is defined by thrombotic occlusions in at least three organs/tissues that occur within a week ("thrombotic storm"), along with laboratory confirmation of APLA. Histologically, small vessel occlusion predominates, in contrast to the large vessel thromboses that are common in standard APLS.[108] The differential diagnosis in some circumstances may include other microangiopathic syndromes such as thrombotic thrombocytopenic purpura, hemolytic-uremic syndrome, and heparin-induced thrombocytopenia. In addition, many critically ill patients have false-positive results on LA assays[109] (e.g., from coagulation factor deficiencies, caused by heparin administration) that further complicate the diagnosis. Although the cause of CAPS is unknown, infection is associated as a triggering factor in up to 20% of patients.[108] Because of tissue necrosis and the resultant "cytokine storm," many patients go on to develop acute respiratory distress syndrome and require mechanical ventilation. Even with optimal treatment, the mortality rate is approximately 48%.[108,110]

Neurologic Manifestations of Antiphospholipid Syndrome

Neurologic manifestations of APLS include single or recurrent cerebral infarct, severe vascular headache, transient ischemic attack, and visual disturbance (Table 19-7).[111] Recurrent strokes are more likely in patients with APLS who also have hypertension or other risk factors for cerebrovascular disease, such as cigarette smoking and hyperlipidemia.[111] As many as 80% of patients with primary APLS have at least one of these additional risk factors. Cerebral angiography performed on such patients shows large vessel occlusion with "cutoffs" or stenosis, without evidence of vasculitis and generally without systemic atherosclerosis.

Although arterial events are less frequent than venous events in APLS, ischemic stroke and transient ischemic attacks account for 50% of all arterial manifestations.[91,112] Such an event, particularly in a young adult, warrants an APLA investigation. In one prospective study, 18% of adults (aged 15 to 44 years) who had sustained ischemic stroke or a transient ischemic attack tested positive for ACA. Patients with ACA had a higher probability of recurrent events than those who did not have the antibody.[113]

Among older populations, one large study showed no association between stroke and the presence of ACA. In the nested, case-controlled Physicians' Health Study, which was composed of men aged 40 to 84 years, IgG ACA levels in 61 participants with ischemic stroke were not significantly different from those of controls ($P > .2$), and there was no evidence to suggest increased risk for stroke in those with higher APLA levels.[114] The Antiphospholipid Antibodies and Stroke Study (APASS) group recently completed the first prospective study of the role of APLA in recurrent ischemic stroke in collaboration with the Warfarin versus Aspirin Recurrent Stroke Study (WARSS) group.[23] The WARSS group was a controlled and blinded study that

Table 19-6 Sydney Consensus Statement on Classification Criteria for the Antiphospholipid Syndrome[84]

Antiphospholipid antibody syndrome (APLS) is present if at least one of the clinical criteria and one of the laboratory criteria that follow are met.*

Clinical criteria:

1. Vascular thromboses:[†]

    One or more clinical episodes[‡] of arterial, venous, or small vessel thrombosis[§] in any tissue or organ. Thrombosis must be confirmed by objective validated criteria (i.e., unequivocal findings of appropriate imaging studies or histopathology). For histopathologic confirmation, thrombosis should be present without significant evidence of inflammation in the vessel wall.

2. Pregnancy morbidity:

    (a) One or more unexplained deaths of a morphologically normal fetus at or beyond the 10th week of gestation, with normal fetal morphology documented by ultrasound or by direct examination of the fetus, or

    (b) One or more premature births of a morphologically normal neonate before the 34th week of gestation because of (i) eclampsia or severe preeclampsia defined according to standard definitions, or (ii) recognized features of placental insufficiency,[¶] or

    (c) Three or more unexplained consecutive spontaneous abortions before the 10th week of gestation, with maternal anatomic or hormonal abnormalities and paternal and maternal chromosomal causes excluded.

    In studies of populations of patients who have more than one type of pregnancy morbidity, investigators are strongly encouraged to stratify groups of subjects according to a, b, or c above.

Laboratory criteria:*

1. Lupus anticoagulant (LA) present in plasma on two or more occasions at least 12 weeks apart, detected according to the guidelines of the International Society on Thrombosis and Haemostasis (Scientific Subcommittee on LAs/Phospholipid-Dependent Antibodies).[86]

2. Anticardiolipin antibody (ACA) of immunoglobulin (Ig)G and/or IgM isotype in serum or plasma, present in medium or high titer (i.e., >40 GPL [1 µg of IgG antiphospholipid antibody {APLA}] or MPL [1 µg of IgM APLA], or >the 99th percentile), on two or more occasions, at least 12 weeks apart, measured by a standardized enzyme-linked immunosorbent assay (ELISA).[87,88]

3. Anti-β_2-glycoprotein I antibody of IgG and/or IgM isotype in serum or plasma (in titer >the 99th percentile), present on two or more occasions, at least 12 weeks apart, measured by a standardized ELISA, according to recommended procedures.[89]

*Classification of APLS should be avoided if less than 12 weeks or more than 5 years separate the positive APLA test from the clinical manifestation.
[†]Coexisting inherited or acquired factors for thrombosis are not reasons for excluding patients from APLS trials. However, two subgroups of APS patients should be recognized, according to (a) the presence, or (b) the absence of additional risk factors for thrombosis. Indicative (but not exhaustive) causes include age (>55 in men, and >65 in women) and the presence of any established risk factors for cardiovascular disease (hypertension, diabetes mellitus, elevated low-density lipoprotein [LDL] or low high-density lipoprotein [HDL] cholesterol, cigarette smoking, family history of premature cardiovascular disease, body mass index $\geq$30 kg/m^{-2}, microalbuminuria, estimated glomerular filtration rate [GFR] <60 mL min^{-1}), inherited thrombophilias, oral contraceptive, use nephrotic syndrome, malignancy, immobilization, and surgery. Thus, patients who fulfill criteria should be stratified according to contributing causes of thrombosis.
[‡]A thrombotic episode in the past could be regarded as a clinical criterion, provided that thrombosis is proved by appropriate diagnostic means and that no alternative diagnosis or cause of thrombosis is found.
[§]Superficial venous thrombosis is not included in the clinical criteria.
[¶]Generally accepted features of placental insufficiency include (1) abnormal or nonreassuring fetal surveillance test(s) (e.g., a nonreactive nonstress test, suggestive of fetal hypoxemia), (2) abnormal Doppler flow velocimetry waveform analysis suggestive of fetal hypoxemia (e.g., absent end-diastolic flow in the umbilical artery), (3) oligohydramnios (e.g., an amniotic fluid index $\leq$5 cm), or (4) a postnatal birth weight lower than the 10th percentile for gestational age.
**Investigators are strongly advised to classify patients with APLS into one of the following categories: I, more than one laboratory criterion present (any combination); IIa, LA alone present; IIb, ACA alone present; IIc, anti-β_2GPI antibody alone present.
(Reprinted with permission from Miyakis S, Lockshin MD, Atsumi T, et al: International consensus statement on an update of the classification criteria for definite antiphospholipid syndrome [APS]. J Thromb Haemost 4:295–306, 2006.)

sought to compare the risk of recurrent ischemic stroke in patients randomly assigned to aspirin (325 mg/day) or warfarin (target International Normalized Ratio [INR], 2.2; range, 1.4 to 2.8). The APASS trial included 890 patients on warfarin and 882 patients on aspirin; no increase was found in the rates of recurrent thrombotic events associated with baseline APLA status as measured at the time of initial stroke. Since this study began, before the Sydney and Sapporo[83] clinical criteria were formalized for APLS diagnosis, APLA-positive patients were not formally retested, which may account for the surprisingly high percentage of participants with APLA positivity (41%). It is interesting to note that the 7% of patients with baseline positivity for both LA and ACA tended to have a higher rate of recurrence than did those who were negative on both antibodies (32% vs 24%; RR, 1.36; 95% CI, 0.97–1.92; P = .07).

In a prospective case-controlled study that included whites, African Americans, and Hispanic patients, APLA

was found to be an independent stroke risk factor in all groups, causing a fourfold increase in risk for ischemic stroke.[115] Although this point has not yet been clarified, data suggest that for patients who have transient ischemic attacks at a young age, or for those who have these events in association with other features of APLS, testing for ACA and LA appears to be warranted. However, indiscriminate testing of an otherwise general patient population with cerebrovascular events is not indicated.[116]

Antiphospholipid Antibodies and Cardiac Dysfunction

An increased incidence of cardiac valvular lesions and myocardial dysfunction occurs in patients with both primary and secondary APLS, as well as in patients with SLE alone.[117–121] Prospective studies that used two-dimensional echocardiography to detect cardiac abnormalities in

Table 19-7 Neurologic Manifestations Associated with Antiphospholipid Antibodies

One or more episodes of the following occurring in
individuals at a relatively young age (<55 years):
   Vascular dementia
   Antiphospholipid antibody (APLA) multi-infarct dementia
   Transient ischemic attack
   Epilepsy
   Migraine
   Chorea
   Amaurosis fugax
   Retinal infarction
   Myelopathy
   Acute ischemic encephalopathy
   Sneddon syndrome

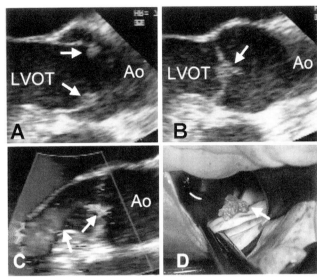

Figure 19-3 Transesophageal echocardiogram from a 35-year-old woman with antiphospholipid syndrome (APLS) showing the aortic valve in the long axis in systole (**A**) and diastole (**B**). *Arrows* show focal, nodular, symmetrical thickening of the aortic valve tips. **C,** Color flow imaging (shown here in black and white) shows aortic regurgitation *(arrow)*. **D,** Aortic valve with a platelet–fibrin thrombus *(arrows)* seen before resection. LVOT, left ventricular outflow tract; Ao, Aorta. (From Qaddoura F, Connolly H, Grogan M, et al: Valve morphology in antiphospholipid antibody syndrome: Echocardiographic features. Echocardiography 22:255–259, 2005; reprinted with permission from Blackwell Publishing.)

patients with primary and secondary APLS have found significant associations with valvular lesions. A study from Mexico found valvular lesions in 17 of 29 (71%) consecutive patients with APLS.[122] A prospective study in London identified valvular lesions in 38% of 55 patients with recently diagnosed APLS, and only in 4% in a control group of 55 healthy volunteers.[123] Studies have shown that at least one half of patients with cardiac lesions have other features of APLS.[91,117,122] Serial studies in these patients have indicated that hemodynamically significant cardiac valvular disease can develop over time,[119,122,123] and that these patients may be at increased risk for cerebroembolic events.[122,124–126] Intramural cardiac thrombosis occurs rarely.[127] These studies emphasize the value of echocardiographic screening for all patients with APLS.[123,128]

Sterile valvular lesions, known as Libman-Sacks endocarditis, are similar to those that occur in patients with SLE; they consist mainly of superficial or intravalvular fibrin deposits at various stages of fibroblastic organization and neovascularization, sometimes accompanied by mononuclear cell infiltration.[129,130] Echocardiographic findings include generally diffuse and symmetrical valve thickening; when localized thickening is noted, it involves the leaflet midportion or base (Fig. 19-3). In contrast to rheumatic heart disease, chordal thickening, fusion, and calcification are rarely seen and, when present, are not prominent.[129,131] The lesions, which appear as small clusters, most frequently affect the mitral valve, then the aortic valve; they may produce no symptoms, or they may cause valvular insufficiency or stenosis if significant thickening occurs.[117–121,129–135]

Evidence suggests an immunologic origin, with APLA deposition initiating the valvular damage. This leads to superficial thrombosis, subendocardial mononuclear cell infiltration, and eventually, fibrosis or calcification.[122,129] Histologically, most studies suggest that fibrin deposits are the major findings with minimum inflammation.[130,131] A role for corticosteroid therapy remains unclear in the absence of significant underlying inflammation. Although administration of steroids may dramatically reduce an inflammatory condition and may facilitate healing of valvular vegetations, this treatment may result in marked scarring and deformity of the valve, thereby leading to valve dysfunction.[135]

Nevertheless, clinical and hemodynamic responses have been reported in some cases, suggesting that a moderate inflammatory process is present.[136] Therefore, it is recommended that a short course of high-dose corticosteroids

be given, with echocardiographic follow-up[128] and appropriate anticoagulation treatment. Although case reports have described valvular improvement with anticoagulation, most studies cited earlier found that no benefit was derived from the use of anticoagulation.[122,130,135]

APLA have been associated with myocardial microvasculopathy that is sufficiently severe to induce myocardial infarction, even in patients with normal coronary arteries.[133] In the multicentered Euro-Phospholipid Project of 1000 patients with APLS (described previously), 2.8% of patients initially presented with a myocardial infarction (MI), and 5.5% had an MI in the course of their disease.[91] This suggests a possible role for screening for APLA in patients at low risk for coronary artery disease. However, in a different cohort study of the survivors of MI divided into those younger or older than 51 years of age, ACA (measured as both IgG and IgM isotypes) was not an independent risk factor for overall mortality, reinfarction, or thrombotic stroke.[124] The multivariate analysis was adjusted for age and high-density lipoprotein (HDL) cholesterol. The more recent Hopkins Lupus Cohort[137] study, which prospectively followed 380 patients with SLE (92% female; mean age, 46±12 years), evaluated whether APLA were predictive of atherosclerosis and/or coronary artery disease. Patients with LA were more likely to have an MI than those who tested negative for LA (22% vs 9%); however, elevated ACA levels also were not associated with an increased risk for MI. These findings are consistent with other studies that show the LA to be a stronger risk factor for thrombosis than ACA in the APLS.[13,79,138] Many studies have reported mixed results when investigating APLA as an independent risk factor for mortality, reinfarction, or nonhemorrhagic stroke.[130] In general, screening of all patients who develop an MI for the presence of APLA is not cost effective.

Table 19-8 Dermatologic Manifestations of Antiphospholipid Syndrome

Livedo reticularis
Sneddon syndrome
Skin ulceration
Necrotizing vasculitis
Cutaneous gangrene
Superficial thrombophlebitis
Pseudovasculitic lesions
Subungual hemorrhage
Anetoderma

Dermatologic Manifestations

Dermatologic manifestations are common; they occur in up to 40% to 50% of patients with APLS and as the presenting symptoms in 29% to 40% of patients.[91,139–141] Cutaneous manifestations are diverse, ranging from minor signs to life-threatening conditions such as widespread cutaneous necrosis (Table 19-8). The most frequently encountered skin lesions are livedo reticularis and skin ulcers.

Livedo reticularis is observed in 25% of patients with APLS[91,139]; it is characterized by a mottled purple reticular pattern that involves the upper and lower limbs and often the trunk and buttocks (see Fig. 11-25 in Chapter 11). The pattern is generally disseminated, with incomplete circular segments of irregular fine or wide ramifications. Microscopically, skin biopsy specimens do not usually reveal histopathologic changes, and they rarely contain thrombi, unless the patient has catastrophic APLS.[139,142,143] The arterial subset of APLS[139,144] may be related to Sneddon syndrome. First described in 1965, Sneddon syndrome is characterized by widespread livedo reticularis and recurrent ischemic cerebrovascular events with variable APLA positivity (0% to 85%).[145] Livedo may be observed in otherwise healthy patients, especially women after cold exposure; livedo may also be noted in patients with vasculitic and infectious conditions (e.g., syphilis, tuberculosis).[143]

Other APLS-related cutaneous manifestations include subungual hemorrhage, necrotizing vasculitis, thrombophlebitis, anetoderma, pseudovasculitic lesions, skin ulcerations, and digital gangrene. In the latter conditions, noninflammatory thromboses in small arteries and veins throughout the dermis and subcutaneous fat tissue are the primary histologic findings.[142] The presence of IgA ACA has been independently associated with skin ulcers, chilblain lupus, and vasculitis.[146] Treatments have included anticoagulation, immunosuppression,[147] and local measures such as autologous skin transplantation.[148]

Fetal Loss and Antiphospholipid Syndrome

Please see Chapter 36, "Management of Thrombophilia and APLS During Pregnancy."

Bleeding Complications and Antiphospholipid Syndrome

Although APLS is generally associated with thrombotic manifestations, bleeding complications may occasionally be encountered. Consultants should consider the following differential diagnosis in appropriate patients who have laboratory or clinical evidence of a bleeding disorder: prothrombin deficiency, presence of antibody inhibitor to coagulation factors, acquired von Willebrand disease, acquired platelet function abnormalities, and thrombocytopenia. The recognition that prothrombin time (PT) prolongation may, in some patients, be partially due to the LA effect should prompt the use of prothrombin assays insensitive to the LA. As always, when patients with APLS and concurrent bleeding diatheses are treated, the clinician cannot rely solely on laboratory results as a prognosticator for bleeding risk. A recent study found significantly prolonged bleeding times in 21 of 27 consecutive patients with consistent LA, normal von Willebrand factor (VWF), and normal platelet function, who were not exposed to aspirin or nonsteroidal anti-inflammatory drugs (NSAIDs).[149]

Thrombocytopenia is frequently present in APLS and is usually mild. Two studies, including the Euro-Phospholipid Project group study of 1000 patients with APLS, found that 30% of patients had episodes of thrombocytopenia (<100,000 platelets/μL).[91,150] When patients with idiopathic autoimmune thrombocytopenia (ITP) were examined in the absence of other autoimmune disease, elevated levels of ACA were noted in 15% to 66% of patients.[151–153] One recent study[153] showed elevated ACA in the acute exacerbation or relapse of ITP, with subsequent decline to undetectable levels on remission. More specifically, this study found ACA IgG to be more prevalent in the acute stage, and IgM more prevalent in stable disease. However, LA was negative in all patients, and β_2GPI was the least common target antigen. Although another study correlated thrombocytopenia in patients with APLS with higher rates of epilepsy, arthritis, livedo reticularis, skin ulceration, and cardiac valve thickening and dysfunction,[150] overall, the presence of APLA does not appear to affect outcome.

Patients who have LA may have slight prolongation of PT, depending on the sensitivity of the thromboplastin reagent used. However, patients who have significant prolongation of the PT (>2 to 3 seconds above the upper limit of normal) should be evaluated for a true acquired deficiency of factor II (prothrombin). In a study of patients with LA, SLE, and/or other autoimmune connective tissue disorders, most had IgG antibodies to prothrombin; only 30% of patients with antibodies had a detectable prothrombin deficiency.[154] Prothrombin deficiency, when it does occur in patients with LA, appears to be due to the binding of the antibody to prothrombin in vivo, which results in increased clearance.

An acquired deficiency of prothrombin with clinical symptoms of bleeding may be the initial presenting feature in a patient who will later develop other manifestations of APLS (and possibly SLE as well). Autoimmune-based prothrombin deficiency may also be suspected in a patient who is receiving warfarin as treatment for thrombotic complications of APLS, and who develops a gradually increasing INR for no apparent reason. Evaluation includes measurement of coagulation factor levels (II, V, VII, and X) in the extrinsic system and possible alterations in warfarin dose.

Multiple case reports of other factor deficiencies and antibody inhibitors have been found among patients with APLS, particularly those with inhibitors to factor VIII.[155] Caution is warranted in that the LA effect may be potent enough to cause apparent factor deficiencies in the assay system. When this is suspected, PTT reagents that are insensitive to the LA effect may be used for more accurate results.

Antibody production can be suppressed by administration of corticosteroids and azathioprine, as was demonstrated in one patient in whom PT was normal 7 days after treatment had been initiated.[156] In another study, the use of corticosteroid therapy alone increased the prothrombin level, even when prothrombin/antibody complexes were still detectable.[157]

More recently, several reports have indicated efficacy for rituximab, a chimeric anti-CD20 monoclonal antibody, in the treatment of patients with autoimmune disorders such as ITP, autoimmune hemolytic anemia (AIHA), SLE, and vasculitides.[109,158–160] B-cell depletion in autoimmune disease may lower the pathogenic autoantibody levels associated with these syndromes, including APLS. One report described a marked response in a patient with ITP with LA and ACA who was refractory to steroids and azathioprine. Soon after initiation of rituximab, platelet counts returned to normal; within 14 months, ACA IgG levels became negative and anti-β2GPI was markedly lowered.[160]

Laboratory Diagnosis of APLA

It is currently accepted that the detection of ACA for the diagnosis of APLS should be dependent on β2GPI. Also, prolongation of clotting assays for the LA effect should be confirmed by neutralization with excess phospholipids. Despite these generally accepted principles, the sensitivities and specificities of these methods vary widely, and no single test is sufficient for diagnosis. Therefore, when the disorder is suspected, a battery of available tests (Table 19-9) is required. Conversely, no array of negative results can conclusively exclude the diagnosis.

Lupus Anticoagulant

Currently, the detection of LA appears to be more specific for APLS than the ACA assay. In two recent studies in which antibody profiles for the diagnosis of APLS were analyzed, a positive LA test was independently associated

Table 19-9 Diagnostic Tests for the Antiphospholipid Syndrome

Immunoassays
Serologic test for syphilis
Anticardiolipin antibodies
Anti–β2-glycoprotein I (β2GPI) antibodies
Antiprothrombin antibodies
Antiphosphatidylserine antibodies

Coagulation Tests
Partial thromboplastin time (PTT)
—With mixing incubation studies
—With antiphospholipid antibody (APLA)-sensitive and -insensitive PTT reagents
—Platelet neutralization procedure (PNP)
Dilute Russell's viper venom time (dRVVT)
Kaolin clotting time
Tissue thromboplastin inhibition test
Hexagonal phase array test
Textarin/ecarin test

with VTE and arterial thrombosis with odds ratios of 4.4 and 3.6, respectively. When LA was also associated with ELISA-based tests, the odds ratios increased to 10.1 and 33, respectively.[24,54] This is consistent with previous studies; in a meta-analysis of the risk of VTE in patients with APLA, with exclusion of patients with SLE, the mean odds ratio for LA was 11.0.[161] More recently, in a systemic literature review, five of five studies reported a significant association of LA with thrombosis, with odds ratios ranging from 5.7 to 9.4 (Fig. 19-4).[13] A positive LA is consistently associated with increased risks for arterial and venous events and is more predictive than ELISA-based assays.

In general, a lupus anticoagulant is suspected when one of several screening assays, such as PTT, is prolonged. A suspected LA is further evaluated by means of an inhibitor screen, such as a mixing study, to rule out factor-specific inhibitors. LA usually prolongs the coagulation time of test plasma and normal plasma, immediately after mixing. Conversely, demonstration of a factor VIII inhibitor usually requires incubation after mixing, before the PTT becomes

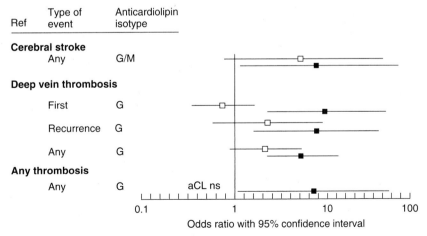

Figure 19-4 Comparison of lupus anticoagulants (■) and anticardiolipin antibodies (□) for their association with thrombosis: Compilation of 5 studies on 753 patients and 234 controls. aCL, anticardiolipin antibodies. (Modified from Galli M, Luciani D, Bertolini G, et al: Lupus anticoagulants are stronger risk factors of thrombosis than anticardiolipin antibodies in the antiphospholipid syndrome: A systematic review of the literature. Blood 101:1827–1832, 2003. Reprinted with permission from the publisher).

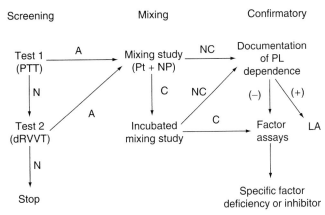

Figure 19-5 Approach to the diagnosis of lupus anticoagulant. Repeating the partial thromboplastin time (PTT) with a reagent known to be insensitive to lupus anticoagulant (LA) can facilitate documentation of whether an LA is present.[86] A, abnormal; C, corrected; N, normal; NC, no correction; NP, normal plasma; PL, phospholipid; pt, patient; LA, lupus anticoagulant. Modified from Brandt JT, Triplett DA, Alving B, et al, on behalf of the Subcommitte on Lupus Anticoagulant/Antiphospholipid Antibody of the Scientific and Standardisation Committee of the ISTH: Criteria for the diagnosis of lupus anticoagulants: An update. Thromb Haemost 74:1185–1190, 1995).

prolonged. The phospholipid-dependent nature of LA is then confirmed by correction of the LA effect through the addition of excess phospholipid. Also, the clinician should check to see whether PTT becomes normalized when an LA-insensitive PTT reagent is used (Fig. 19-5).[86]

Coagulation factor levels are measured for the purpose of excluding a true factor deficiency or the presence of another inhibitor. If patient plasma has a prolonged PTT and a normal PT, factors VIII, IX, XI, and XII, as well as high molecular weight kininogen and prekallikrein, are measured. Frequently, LA is sufficiently potent to effect an apparent decrease in these coagulation factors. These apparent decreases in activity of the "contact factors" (factors XI and XII, as well as prekallikrein and high molecular weight kininogen) due to LA may provide the foundation for anecdotal reports in which contact factor deficiencies are associated with hypercoagulability.[162]

Factor activity should increase toward the true value when measured in serial dilutions of patient plasma (i.e., because results among various dilutions are inconsistent, often referred to in the laboratory literature as inhibitory kinetics, or the "crossing lines" artifact). Progressive dilution of plasma also dilutes the inhibitory activity of LA and allows for more accurate determination of factor activity. Another option is to use PTT reagents that are relatively insensitive to LA. If the patient has a true factor inhibitor, determination of the factor level will not be influenced by the dilution at which the plasma is tested. If PT is also prolonged, then measurement of factors VII, X, V, and II should be included. Occasionally, in plasma with LA, the PT may also be slightly prolonged in the absence of a true factor deficiency.[163,164] The most common true factor deficiency associated with the LA is prothrombin deficiency, as described earlier.

A major limitation of the clinical usefulness of LA results is the often considerable variation among laboratories, assays, and reagents used. Of available assays, none is 100% sensitive or specific. A recent compilation of quality assurance surveys

from several international agencies over the past decade found an overall intermediate interlaboratory coefficient of variation (generally <20%).[165] However, multiple studies have shown that LA activity is predictive and specific for the occurrence of thrombosis and pregnancy loss, even more so than the ACA and the anti-β_2GPI ELISA assays.[54,79,166] Furthermore, despite interlaboratory variations among individual assays, the surveys discussed earlier found that the use of LA test panels yields an overall error rate < 5%.[165]

Other considerations regarding laboratory diagnosis of LA include the heterogeneous nature of the target protein antigens that produce the LA effect and the frequent interlaboratory disagreements encountered when plasmas known to have weak LA activity are analyzed. Also, the effect of LA on phospholipid-dependent coagulation assays depends on the depletion of platelets and platelet fragments from plasma. A normal PTT alone is insufficient to exclude LA, and additional screening assays such as dilute Russell's viper venom time or kaolin clotting time should be used before the diagnosis is ruled out. Alternatively, a patient with an equivocal LA result should be evaluated for concurrent deficiencies of specific coagulation factors, especially if symptoms of a bleeding diathesis are present.

Immunoassays

The other arm for APLS diagnosis is the identification of ACA, antiphosphatidylserine, anti-β_2GPI, and antiprothrombin antibodies. The first of these to be developed, the anticardiolipin test, was initially encountered as a biologic false-positive Venereal Disease Research Laboratory (VDRL) test for syphilis. Cardiolipin is an intracellular membrane phospholipid that is recognized by antibodies produced in response to syphilitic infection. In contrast to APLA, syphilitic anticardiolipins are not phospholipid dependent and can recognize cardiolipin epitopes directly.[167] Also, the conventional ACA assay is nonspecific in that it can detect a range of antibodies, including anti–human β_2GPI, antibodies to bovine β_2GPI, and direct ACA, to name a few.

These assays are designed to measure the level of APLA in patient sera in a quantitative fashion, with the use of microtiter plates coated with cardiolipin or another negatively charged phospholipid and containing β_2GPI.[5,168,169] After an incubation period has passed, plates are washed and antibodies are detected with the use of labeled antihuman IgG or IgM. Test results are expressed in units of MPL or GPL (1 MPL is equal to 1 µg of IgM APLA, and 1 GPL is equal to 1 µg of IgG APLA). Antibody concentrations are described qualitatively as high positive, moderately positive, low positive, or negative.[170–172] Appropriate reference ranges must be validated for each laboratory and patient population. Elevated levels of IgA ACA alone are rare, and the clinical relevance of this test has been debated. However, occasionally, IgA ACA positivity is found and is shown to be associated with the major clinical manifestations of APLS, thus making it clinically useful.[173,174]

ACA as risk factors for thrombosis are not as strong as LA, and studies have shown that only 50% of their associations with thrombosis reached statistical significance.[13] In a systemic literature review, only 15 of 28 studies showed significant associations between ACA and thrombosis. Statistical significance improved depending on the type of thrombosis; ACA were associated more with cerebral stroke and myocardial infarction than with VTE (Fig. 19-6). In all

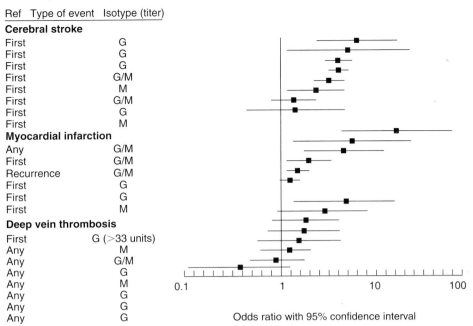

Ref	Type of event	Isotype (titer)
Cerebral stroke		
	First	G
	First	G
	First	G
	First	G/M
	First	M
	First	G/M
	First	G
	First	M
Myocardial infarction		
	Any	G/M
	First	G/M
	Recurrence	G/M
	First	G
	First	G
	First	M
Deep vein thrombosis		
	First	G (>33 units)
	Any	M
	Any	G/M
	Any	G
	Any	M
	Any	G
	Any	G
	Any	G

Odds ratio with 95% confidence interval

Figure 19-6 Anticardiolipin antibodies and thrombosis: Analysis of 11 cross-sectional, case-control, and ambispective studies on 1883 cases and 2469 controls. Odds ratios with 95% confidence intervals (CIs) are grouped according to site and type of thrombosis and antibody isotype. (Modified from Galli M, Luciani D, Bertolini G, et al: Lupus anticoagulants are stronger risk factors of thrombosis than anticardiolipin antibodies in the antiphospholipid syndrome: A systematic review of the literature. Blood 101:1827–1832, 2003. Reprinted with permission from the publisher).

studies, a correlation was noted between higher antibody titers and increased odds ratios for thrombosis. This is consistent with the Sydney consensus classification criteria,[83] which use only medium to high ACA and/or anti-β_2GPI antibody titers in evaluation of APLS.

Although β_2GPI is believed to be the major protein cofactor for APLA, most studies find that ACA is more predictive of thrombosis, both arterial and venous. In a systemic literature review, 34 of 60 studies (none prospective) showed significant associations between anti-β_2GPI and thrombosis, but with greater odds ratios for ACA associations.[79] In two subsequent studies, the odds ratios for β_2GPI-associated thrombosis were 2.4 and 2.7 when tests were performed independently of other APLA assays.[24,54] In a recent prospective study in which 194 consecutive patients who tested positive for LA and/or ACA were followed, the rate of thrombosis was 7.3% per patient-year among patients with APLA with anti-β_2GPI and/or antiprothrombin antibodies, as compared with 2.2% among those who tested negative.[22] This study further supports the association of greater relative risk for thrombosis in patients with antibodies against more than one phospholipid-binding protein.

Prothrombin is considered to be the second major cofactor for APLA. However, in a systemic literature review, only 17 of 46 studies were noted to have found a significant statistical association with thrombosis, irrespective of antibody type.[79] Thus, the clinical usefulness of detection in practice has yet to be established.

ACA and anti-β_2GPI immunoassays appear to be less well controlled and reliable compared with LA testing. In a recent multilaboratory quality assurance program, high interlaboratory variation in numeric results was found in 12 serum samples tested for ACA IgG, ACA IgM, and IgG β_2GPI. In semiquantitative reporting, a 100% consensus was reached on only 4 of 36 occasions (11%). General consensus (i.e., >90% of participating laboratories agreed that a given serum sample gave a result of either positive or negative) was attained on only 13 of 36 occasions.[175]

Attempts have been made to standardize ACA testing.[87,176] The first international workshop defined GPL and MPL units as 1 μg of affinity-purified immunoglobulin (Ig)G and IgM antibody; this information was distributed to participating laboratories. However, secondary standards, calibrated against initial sera, from individual laboratories and companies are composed of a heterogeneous mix of polyclonal IgG and IgM antibodies. Consequently, these antibodies have differing ranges of binding avidity from batch to batch, and they behave differently when standard curves are constructed. This explains the development of semiquantitative reporting (i.e., low, medium, high) of ACA results.[88]

Of the wide selection of APLA tests currently available for clinical use, only LA is consistently associated with thrombosis. Results of studies on ACA and anti-β_2GPI antibodies are less convincing and partially controversial. An explanation may be that phospholipid-dependent clotting assays measure a functional capability of APLA, rather than providing a quantitative measurement of a heterogeneous population of antibodies with uncertain thrombogenic properties.[13,79,165] With the recent identification of a subpopulation of β_2GPI antibodies that have a high correlation for thrombosis and LA positivity, newer assays targeted to detect antibodies against the specific Gly40-Arg43 portion of β_2GPI may prove to be the most specific and sensitive method of APLA testing.

APLA Presenting as a Laboratory Abnormality

The prevalence of LA and ACA in normal populations has been reported in several studies. ACA and LA in normal control populations are found at rates from 1.0% to 5.6% and from 1.0% to 3.6%, respectively[24,103,177]; they show seasonal variability with increased prevalence during the winter months.[178] These frequencies are similar in normal pregnant women.[179] In the "frail" elderly group, ACA have been reported to be significantly more prevalent, particularly after cerebrovascular events, than in normal controls, including older individuals (>63 years) without chronic illness.[180] Contradicting the latter finding of no relative increase in ACA among the healthy elderly compared with the general population was a study of 89 healthy women, with a mean age of 86 years (range, 75 to 102 years).[181] ACA and β₂GPI antibodies were elevated in 64% and 32%, respectively, of participants, suggesting that the prevalence of elevated ACA increases with age. The latter study is particularly important given the overall higher occurrence of thrombotic events in elderly patients. A prospective, nested, case-control study of 317 patients with elevated ACA and 655 control patients from the Longitudinal Investigation of Thromboembolism Etiology (LITE) cohort of 20,000 disease-free participants, found no association between elevated titers of ACA and VTE.[182] Odds ratios comparing IgG and IgM ACA above the 95th percentile and within quintiles were not statistically significant. The conclusion of investigators was that this population does not require anticoagulation on the basis of an elevated ACA alone.

LA is frequently found in patients hospitalized for a wide variety of disorders; it is a common cause of unexplained prolongation of the PTT in patients referred for consultation.[183] In a prospective study of 177 patients with elevated PTT admitted to an acute care general hospital, 53% of cases were attributed to an LA.[184]

Specific conditions other than APLS that are associated with APLA include carcinoma, infection, end-stage renal disease, and autoimmune disorders such as rheumatoid arthritis and Sjögren syndrome.[185-190] The use of drugs such as procainamide, hydralazine, chlorpromazine, quinidine, isoniazid, and methyldopa, which are also associated with the development of SLE, has been implicated as well.[191-196] LA activity associated with the IgG or IgM isotype may be detected months after drugs such as procainamide have been discontinued.[195,197] Although thromboembolic events have been described in several patients who developed LA in association with procainamide, reports of such events appear to be uncommon.[194,195,198-200] One study reported moderate to high APLA in 21% (14 of 66) of cardiac patients taking procainamide compared with no APLA elevations in 30 control cardiac patients. Overall, a frequent history of noncardiac thrombi was reported in the procainamide group (25.7%); however, no association with APLA positivity was found.[201]

Among patients given chlorpromazine, APLA (detected as LA or in ELISA) developed in approximately 40%; this may occur as early as 3 months after initiation of treatment.[192,193] One group reported that phenothiazines other than chlorpromazine did not induce LA; however, LA that occurred in patients on chlorpromazine persisted when patients were switched to other phenothiazines.[192] Other investigators have found APLA in 27% of patients given phenothiazines other than chlorpromazine.[193] Patients with detected APLA may express it as LA only or as ACA, which is usually of the IgM isotype.[191,193] Additional frequent immunologic abnormalities include positive tests for antinuclear antibodies (ANA)[192,202] and antibodies to native DNA.[202] It is unlikely that LA positiv-

ity is a risk factor for thrombosis in these patients. Only 3 of 96 patients given phenothiazines who had LA or ACA developed thrombosis over a median 5-year follow-up period.[191]

Another significant drawback to many anticardiolipin immunoassays is that they cannot distinguish "autoimmune" from "infectious" antibodies. Because the latter are not typically associated with thrombotic complications, these immunoassays as a group may underrate the true value of anticardiolipin antibodies for diagnosing APLS.

In a study of patients with hepatitis C, 37.3% of infected patients were positive for ACA (IgG and/or IgM); however, mean titers of each isotype were significantly lower than those found in the APLS group. Furthermore, no thrombotic events occurred among ACA-positive patients with hepatitis C.[203] In a study of patients with APLS with and without HCV, the HCV-positive group had a lower frequency of the more typical features of APLS, such as peripheral thrombosis and neurologic features, and a higher prevalence of atypical features of APLS, such as myocardial infarction and intra-abdominal thrombotic events.[204]

In the autoimmune variety of hepatitis (AIH), elevated levels of ACA were reported in 51% of patients with AIH. ACA were associated with more severe hepatic disease, including cirrhosis, with no APLS symptoms.[205] Patients with end-stage renal disease are also known to have elevated ACA (up to 1 in 5 patients tested).[186,190,206] Although no thrombotic risks are associated with these patients post transplantation, high titers of ACA may represent a risk factor for thrombosis.[206]

Elevated levels of ACA have been measured in patients with human immunodeficiency virus (HIV),[207-211] Lyme disease,[212] ornithosis, adenovirus, rubella, and chickenpox, as well as in those who have undergone vaccination against smallpox,[213] or who have syphilis. The presence of LA does not appear to increase the risk for thrombosis in these patients. In a study by McNally and colleagues,[214] sera from 114 patients with infection (syphilis, tuberculosis, and *Klebsiella* infection) were tested for IgG antibodies against β₂GPI and cardiolipin. All patients tested negative for antibodies to β₂GPI; the incidence of ACA in these patients according to their underlying infection was as follows: tuberculosis, 6%: *Klebsiella* infection, 5%; and syphilis, 64%. Similar results were found in HIV-positive patients who had low titers of β₂GPI antibodies after findings of elevated ACA.[208,215] In a retrospective analysis of 28 men with AIDS, 90% of whom were receiving highly active antiretroviral therapy (HAART), only two tested positive for LA, although 34 thrombotic events occurred during a 42-month period.[216] Although thrombotic complications may occur in patients with HIV,[217] specifically in patients with CD4 counts <200/mm³, APLS with its manifestations is infrequent in patients with HIV, and APLA screening is not warranted.[210,215,218,219]

Treatment of Patients Who Have the Antiphospholipid Syndrome

Major issues in the management of patients with APLS and thrombosis are the intensity of anticoagulation that should be given, the duration of anticoagulation, and the appropriate method of monitoring. One goal is to reduce other risk factors for thrombosis, such as uncontrolled hypertension, smoking, and use of oral contraceptives.[220] Treatment of asymptomatic patients with LA or with moderate or high titers of ACA in the absence of SLE is controversial (see later). Some studies recommend protection with low-dose aspirin (80 mg/day) and/or hydroxychloroquine supplemented by anticoagulation with warfarin or heparin at times of increased risk for thrombosis.[220] It is anticipated that clinical trials currently in progress will address this issue.[221,222] At the present time, screening for APLA in asymptomatic patients should be discouraged.

Patients with SLE who have persistent elevation of ACA have a significantly increased odds ratio (5.4) for a peripheral thromboembolic event compared with those patients with SLE who test positive for APLA on only one occasion.[92] The Hopkins Lupus Cohort study, which prospectively followed 380 patients, found that 20 years after SLE had been diagnosed, patients with LA had a 50% chance of having had a VTE.[137] These patients should be considered on an individual basis for prophylactic anticoagulation.

Patients with APLS may present with an initial thrombotic event followed by additional thrombotic episodes, leading to severe morbidity or death if adequate anticoagulation is not promptly achieved.[223] Thus, before any other interventions such as placement of vena caval filters or plasmapheresis are considered, consultants should be convinced that anticoagulation has been maximized. This may also require consideration of thrombolytic therapy for select patients.

Oral Anticoagulation Intensity

The optimum intensity of oral anticoagulation therapy has been a matter of debate since it became clear that anticoagulation was effective in the prevention of recurrent thrombosis in patients with APLS.[224–228] This subject has recently been systematically reviewed.[229] Two of these studies retrospectively studied 70[226] and 147[227] patients with APLS and found a lower rate of recurrent thrombosis when the INR was maintained at higher than 3.0. Obvious concerns are that the high-intensity regimen (INR >3.0) has been shown to be associated with a high risk (20%) of clinically important bleeding in a series of 3 randomized trials[230–232] and in more recent studies.[233] A more recent retrospective study,[224] which included 66 patients with APLS treated to a target INR of 3.5, concluded that risks of intracranial and fatal bleeding were similar to those in groups of patients treated to standard anticoagulation target INR (2.0 to 3.0).

To help resolve this debate, the Warfarin in the Anti-Phospholipid Syndrome (WAPS) trial from Europe[234] and a similar Canadian study[235] conducted independent prospective trials of 114 and 109 patients with APLS, respectively. Patients were randomly assigned to receive warfarin with a target INR of 2.0 to 3.0 (moderate intensity) or 3.0 to 4.0 (high intensity), to determine whether high-intensity anticoagulation was superior in preventing recurrent thrombosis without significantly increasing bleeding risks. In the Canadian study, recurrent thrombosis occurred in 2 of 58 patients (3.4%) given conventional therapy and in 6 of 56 patients (10.7%) who received high-intensity therapy (hazard ratio, 3.1; 95% confidence interval [CI], 0.6 to 15). The WAPS trial reported similar results, with recurrent thrombosis in 3 of 55 patients (5.5%) given conventional therapy and in 6 of 54 patients (11.1%) receiving high-intensity warfarin treatment (hazard ratio, 1.97; 95% CI, 0.49 to 7.89). Although investigators in both studies recognized the limited statistical power, both concluded that high-intensity warfarin therapy was not superior to standard treatment for thromboprophylaxis. The WAPS study reported an increased rate of minor hemorrhagic complications in the high-intensity treatment cohort. On the basis of these results, the 2004 edition of the *ACCP Conference on Antithrombotic and Thrombolytic Therapy: Evidence-Based Guidelines*[211] recommends a target INR of 2.0 to 3.0 in the treatment of patients with DVT and APLS; however, some patients may warrant higher INR targets or treatment with low molecular weight heparin to prevent recurrent thromboses.

In considering treatment recommendations based on these trials, the consultant should be aware of limitations that were noted.[236,237] Most of the patients included in these two studies had VTE. Furthermore, neither trial reached the expected sample size, and both excluded large numbers of patients because they had already experienced recurrent events while receiving oral anticoagulation treatment. The Canadian study also excluded patients with recent strokes, so that 76% of participants in this study had previous VTE only. Additionally, patients in the high-intensity group from this study had subtherapeutic levels of anticoagulation 43% of the time, which contributed to 6 of 8 recurrent thrombotic events in which INR was between 2.0 and 3.0.

Although this debate focuses on the intensity of warfarin treatment in the prevention of venous and arterial thrombosis, the situation may be different for patients with APLA and stroke. Recent results of the prospective, randomized, double-blinded APASS and WARSS trials indicate that aspirin is as efficacious as warfarin given at standard intensity in the prevention of recurrent thrombo-occlusive events, regardless of APLA status.[23] The Sydney criteria for the diagnosis of APLS[84] include retesting after 12 weeks for an APLS diagnosis; the APASS study recommended APLA testing only at the time of stroke. The high rate of APLA in this cohort (41%) likely indicated transient APLA—not definitive APLS. If the outcome had remained unchanged (i.e., with use of the Sydney criteria), these results would have been more conclusive.

This discussion focuses on the desire of clinicians to minimize levels of anticoagulation and associated risks of bleeding. However, published data have not shown increased frequency or severity of bleeding complications in patients with APLS treated with oral anticoagulation, even with high-intensity therapy (INR >3.0), when compared with cohorts of patients treated to a lower target INR.[224,234,235] Perhaps this may be partially attributed to the lower average age of this population compared with patients with atrial fibrillation.[237]

Case reports have been published describing patients with cerebral APLS who develop symptoms such as headache, dysarthria, confusion, and so forth, when their target INR of high-intensity treatment drops to below 3.0.[238,239] Given that cerebrovascular disease in APLS has greater morbidity and mortality with a greater number of disabling sequelae, many would argue that the risks of bleeding are outweighed by the potential benefits in patients with APLS.

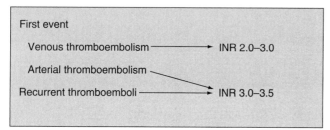

Figure 19-7 Recommended oral anticoagulation intensity for first antiphospholipid syndrome (APLS) thromboembolic events and recurrent thromboemboli that are refractory to conventional anticoagulant therapy.

Patients with APLS and VTE are at high risk for recurrence if anticoagulation is discontinued after a first episode of VTE.[226,227,240] In a retrospective study of patients with primary and secondary APLS, discontinuation of warfarin resulted in recurrent thrombotic events in nearly 70% over a median follow-up of 82 months (range, 12 to 258 months); rate of recurrence was highest during the first 6 months. In contrast, continuation of warfarin (INR, 2.5 to 4.0) resulted in a 90% rate of freedom from thrombosis over a 5-year period.[227]

In summary, it is recommended that patients with APLS should be treated with standard-intensity anticoagulation after the first VTE, and with high-intensity anticoagulation after a recurrence of VTE while on standard therapy. High-intensity anticoagulation is recommended after the first arterial event, provided that no contraindications are noted (Fig. 19-7). Furthermore, anticoagulation should be continued on an indefinite basis as long as the risks and consequences of bleeding are lower than the risk of thrombosis.[224] Low-dose aspirin may be added, depending on whether or not thrombotic manifestations such as superficial thrombophlebitis persist.

Monitoring of the International Normalized Ratio

One report has described variability in INR results for patients with LA who also had an increased baseline PT; this may result in underusage of warfarin.[241] However, two other studies have shown that the INR is not artificially prolonged in such patients.[242,243] In one study, variability in INR measurements was greatly increased when a recombinant tissue factor was used as the PT reagent.[242]

Secondary Therapies

Several studies have indicated that the antimalarial drug hydroxychloroquine (HCQ) might reduce platelet aggregation and blood viscosity.[244,245] In the 1980s and early 1990s, retrospective studies reported that patients with SLE who were treated with HCQ had fewer thrombotic events.[246,247] In a mouse model, APLA-induced thrombus formation was reduced in animals given HCQ.[59,248] These findings and proposed thrombotic mechanisms were supported by an in vitro study that showed that HCQ suppressed the activation of platelets by APLA primed with low doses of thrombin agonist receptor peptide (TRAP).[249] A longitudinal cohort study was performed in 272 Chinese patients with APLS who were administered the following treatments: hydroxychloroquine (152), warfarin (17), prednisolone (203), azathioprine (112), and aspirin (38). Investigators reported fewer thrombotic complications among patients taking HCQ compared with those not receiving the drug (odds ratio, 0.17; 95% CI, 0.07 to 0.44; $P<.0001$).[250]

Unresolved issues of HCQ administration involve adverse effects and safety during pregnancy. For the latter, HCQ is recommended only for malaria, but recent studies support its continued use in patients with SLE because no increase in the rate of birth defects has been reported.[251] In other populations, the primary serious adverse effect involves retinal pigment epithelium from HCQ, which can lead to retinal toxicity. Debate has focused on the optimum ophthalmologic screening, the reversibility of early effects, and whether a risk even exists at low HCQ doses.[252,253] Overall, it is conceivable that HCQ may be of benefit in patients who cannot tolerate high-intensity oral anticoagulation.

The role of corticosteroids or plasmapheresis has not been well documented for patients with APLS without CAPS or pregnancy. Case reports from transplant recipients have suggested that immunosuppressive regimens are inadequate for providing protection against thrombotic events, including graft rejection, in patients with APLS.[190,254] Even at the risk of bleeding, many prefer continued anticoagulation perioperatively rather than risking allograft thrombosis.[190] Immunosuppressive treatments are generally reserved for patients with CAPS. Asherson and colleagues[108–110,255] have documented more than 230 cases since 1992 and recommends intravenous (IV) heparin and corticosteroids as first-line treatments. Intravenous immunoglobulin (IVIg)[108,255] and plasmapheresis[108–110] are appropriate second-line therapies for removal of pathogenic antibodies. Fresh frozen plasma may also be added to help replenish diminished clotting factors. Third-line therapies such as cyclophosphamide have not been very effective. However, because trigger factors such as infection have been identified in 20% of Asherson's cases, any infection must be rigorously treated with appropriate antibiotics. As mentioned previously, rituximab (anti-CD20), which is used to treat B-cell non-Hodgkin lymphoma, has been used with some success in the treatment of patients with autoimmune disorders; subsequent declines in APLA titers have been noted.[158,160,256]

Despite seemingly adequate therapy, the mortality rate for CAPS is approximately 50%.[108] Once recovery ensues, patients usually have a stable course but require continued anticoagulant therapy. One paper reported that 66% of patients with CAPS who survived the initial catastrophic event remained symptom free over an average follow-up of 63 months. However, 26% of survivors experienced additional APLS-related events—not of the CAPS variety.[257]

COST CONTAINMENT AND MEDICAL-LEGAL ASPECTS OF TESTING FOR LUPUS ANTICOAGULANT AND ANTIPHOSPHOLIPID SYNDROME

LA testing is ordered primarily (1) to evaluate an unexplained (and unexpected) prolongation of the PTT, and (2) to assess an individual who presents with clinical features suggestive of APLS. In the first case, in which testing is done for prolonged PTT, at the present time, if the patient does not have a history of thrombosis, embolism, pregnancy loss, or SLE, the finding of LA does not mean that additional tests for ACA or cofactors must be performed. It is recommended that patients who have prolonged PTT and LA should also be tested for appropriate coagulation factor activities, especially if they are about to undergo a major invasive procedure.

Plasma from patients may show artefactually low levels of factor VIII activity if a potent LA is present. However, in this case, the factor VIII activity will increase as the plasma sample is diluted, thus reducing the potency of the LA effect and allowing more adequate assessment of factor activity. For patients with a specific factor VIII–inhibiting antibody, factor VIII activity is truly decreased, and the same level of activity is achieved at all plasma dilutions in the test system. Testing factor activities provide a safeguard against missing a possible factor deficiency. For example, a factor VIII deficiency due to an inhibitor antibody might be present in combination with LA, or an antibody against factor VIII might be mistakenly described as an LA. At a clinical level, patients with true factor VIII deficiency will have bleeds, especially ecchymoses, whereas those patients with artefactual factor VIII deficiency will not.

Laboratory confirmation of APLS is expensive and should be performed thoroughly once initiated. If testing commences for the evaluation of possible APLS, at least two different tests for LA should be performed, as well as the ELISA for ACA, to establish or exclude the diagnosis. If a test is positive, then the evaluation should be repeated in 12 weeks to confirm the persistence of the abnormality. Once the diagnosis has been established, no evidence currently suggests that subsequent changes in APLA positivity would modify treatment. Patients with a history of thrombosis who are given a diagnosis of APLS are at high risk for recurrent thrombotic events. These patients may be candidates for the use of home monitoring devices to measure INR, given that continued and adequate anticoagulation is essential (see Chapter 40).

The consultant should be wary of ordering tests in the absence of clinical manifestations or without a history of SLE because of the uncertainty of treatment based exclusively on a positive APLA assay. Administration of warfarin places patients at risk for bleeding; withholding treatment makes patients at pre-APLS stage more susceptible to thrombosis.

CONCLUSION

Although the pathophysiology of APLS has not been established, it is clear that APLS is a major cause of human morbidity and mortality, both of which are ameliorated by anticoagulant therapy. The specificity of autoantibodies is now becoming better defined, and diagnostic testing and criteria for establishing the diagnosis have been greatly refined. A major issue is that of treatment[228]; the optimum type, duration, and intensity of anticoagulation still have not been completely specified, but with the development of cooperative international clinical trials, some of these issues may soon be resolved. APLS is a disorder that encompasses many specialties: hematology, neurology, obstetrics, and rheumatology. Thus, the approach to patients with this disorder must be truly interdisciplinary.

REFERENCES

1. Mueller JF, Ratnoff O, Heinle RW: Observations on the characteristics of an unusual circulating anticoagulant. J Lab Clin Med 38:254–261, 1951.

2. Margolius A Jr, Jackson DP, Ratnoff OD: Circulating anticoagulants: A study of 40 cases and a review of the literature. Medicine (Baltimore) 40:145–202, 1961.

3. Bowie WEJ, Thompson JH, Pascuzzi CA, et al: Thrombosis in systemic erythematosus despite circulating anticoagulants. J Clin Invest 62:416–430, 1963.

4. Hughes GR: The antiphospholipid syndrome. Lupus 5:345–346, 1996.

5. Harris EN, Gharavi AE, Boey ML, et al: Anticardiolipin antibodies: Detection by radioimmunoassay and association with thrombosis in systemic lupus erythematosus. Lancet 2:1211–1214, 1983.

6. McNeil HP, Simpson RJ, Chesterman CN, et al: Anti-phospholipid antibodies are directed against a complex antigen that includes a lipid-binding inhibitor of coagulation: Beta 2-glycoprotein I (apolipoprotein H). Proc Natl Acad Sci U S A 87:4120–4124, 1990.

7. Galli M, Comfurius P, Maassen C, et al: Anticardiolipin antibodies (ACA) directed not to cardiolipin but to a plasma protein cofactor. Lancet 335:1544–1547, 1990.

8. Matsuura E, Igarashi Y, Fujimoto M, et al: Anticardiolipin cofactor(s) and differential diagnosis of autoimmune disease. Lancet 336:177–178, 1990.

9. Alving BM, Barr CF, Tang DB: Correlation between lupus anticoagulants and anticardiolipin antibodies in patients with prolonged activated partial thromboplastin times. Am J Med. 88:112–116, 1990.

10. McNeil HP, Chesterman CN, Krilis SA: Immunology and clinical importance of antiphospholipid antibodies. Adv Immunol 49:193–280, 1991.

11. Willems GM, Janssen MP, Comfurius P, et al: Kinetics of prothrombin-mediated binding of lupus anticoagulant antibodies to phosphatidylserine-containing phospholipid membranes: An ellipsometric study. Biochemistry 41:14357–14363, 2002.

12. Arnout J, Wittevrongel C, Vanrusselt M, et al: Beta-2-glycoprotein I dependent lupus anticoagulants form stable bivalent antibody beta-2-glycoprotein I complexes on phospholipid surfaces. Thromb Haemost 79:79–86, 1998.

13. Galli M, Luciani D, Bertolini G, et al: Lupus anticoagulants are stronger risk factors for thrombosis than anticardiolipin antibodies in the antiphospholipid syndrome: A systematic review of the literature. Blood 101:1827–1832, 2003.

14. Roubey RA: Immunology of the antiphospholipid syndrome: Antibodies, antigens, and autoimmune response. Thromb Haemost 82:656–661, 1999.

15. Galli M, Comfurius P, Barbui T, et al: Anticoagulant activity of beta 2-glycoprotein I is potentiated by a distinct subgroup of anticardiolipin antibodies. Thromb Haemost 68:297–300, 1992.

16. Bouma B, de Groot PG, van den Elsen JM, et al: Adhesion mechanism of human beta(2)-glycoprotein I to phospholipids based on its crystal structure. EMBO J 18:5166–5174, 1999.

17. de Groot G, Bouma B, Lutters BC, et al: Structure–function studies on beta 2-glycoprotein I. J Autoimmun 15:87–89, 2000.

18. Hunt J, Krilis S: The fifth domain of beta 2-glycoprotein I contains a phospholipid binding site (Cys281-Cys288) and a region recognized by anticardiolipin antibodies. J Immunol 152:653–659, 1994.

19. Iverson GM, Reddel S, Victoria EJ, et al: Use of single point mutations in domain I of beta 2-glycoprotein I to determine fine antigenic specificity of antiphospholipid autoantibodies. J Immunol 169:7097–7103, 2002.

20. de Laat B, Derksen RH, Urbanus RT, et al: IgG antibodies that recognize epitope Gly40-Arg43 in domain I of beta 2-glycoprotein I cause LAC, and their presence correlates strongly with thrombosis. Blood 105:1540–1545, 2005.

21. de Laat HB, Derksen RH, Urbanus RT, et al: Beta2-glycoprotein I–dependent lupus anticoagulant highly correlates with thrombosis in the antiphospholipid syndrome. Blood 104:3598–3602, 2004.

22. Forastiero R, Martinuzzo M, Pombo G, et al: A prospective study of antibodies to beta2-glycoprotein I and prothrombin, and risk of thrombosis. J Thromb Haemost 3:1231–1238, 2005.

23. Levine SR, Brey RL, Tilley BC, et al: Antiphospholipid antibodies and subsequent thrombo-occlusive events in patients with ischemic stroke. JAMA 291:576–584, 2004.

24. de Groot PG, Lutters B, Derksen RH, et al: Lupus anticoagulants and the risk of a first episode of deep venous thrombosis. J Thromb Haemost 3:1993–1997, 2005.

25. Lieby P, Soley A, Levallois H, et al: The clonal analysis of anticardiolipin antibodies in a single patient with primary antiphospholipid

syndrome reveals an extreme antibody heterogeneity. Blood 97:3820–3828, 2001.

26. Simantov R, LaSala JM, Lo SK, et al: Activation of cultured vascular endothelial cells by antiphospholipid antibodies. J Clin Invest 96:2211–2219, 1995.

27. Pierangeli SS, Espinola RG, Liu X, et al: Thrombogenic effects of antiphospholipid antibodies are mediated by intercellular cell adhesion molecule-1, vascular cell adhesion molecule-1, and P-selectin. Circ Res 88:245–250, 2001.

28. Meroni PL, Raschi E, Camera M, et al: Endothelial activation by aPL: A potential pathogenic mechanism for the clinical manifestations of the syndrome. J Autoimmun 15:237–240, 2000.

29. Visvanathan S, Geczy CL, Harmer JA, et al: Monocyte tissue factor induction by activation of beta 2-glycoprotein-I-specific T lymphocytes is associated with thrombosis and fetal loss in patients with antiphospholipid antibodies. J Immunol 165:2258–2262, 2000.

30. Roubey RA: Tissue factor pathway and the antiphospholipid syndrome. J Autoimmun 15:217–220, 2000.

31. Santoro SA: Antiphospholipid antibodies and thrombotic predisposition: Underlying pathogenetic mechanisms. Blood 83:2389–2391, 1994.

32. Pengo V, Biasiolo A, Fior MG: Binding of autoimmune cardiolipin–reactive antibodies to heparin: A mechanism of thrombosis? Thromb Res 78:371–378, 1995.

33. Shibata S, Harpel PC, Gharavi A, et al: Autoantibodies to heparin from patients with antiphospholipid antibody syndrome inhibit formation of antithrombin III–thrombin complexes. Blood 83:2532–2540, 1994.

34. Freyssinet JM, Wiesel ML, Gauchy J, et al: An IgM lupus anticoagulant that neutralizes the enhancing effect of phospholipid on purified endothelial thrombomodulin activity: A mechanism for thrombosis. Thromb Haemost 55:309–313, 1986.

35. Tsakiris DA, Settas L, Makris PE, et al: Lupus anticoagulant—Antiphospholipid antibodies and thrombophilia: Relation to protein C–protein S–thrombomodulin. J Rheumatol 17:785–789, 2000.

36. Cariou R, Tobelem G, Bellucci S, et al: Effect of lupus anticoagulant on antithrombogenic properties of endothelial cells: Inhibition of thrombomodulin-dependent protein C activation. Thromb Haemost 60:54–58, 1988.

37. Salmon JE, Girardi G, Holers VM: Complement activation as a mediator of antiphospholipid antibody induced pregnancy loss and thrombosis. Ann Rheum Dis 61 (suppl 2): ii46–ii50, 2002.

38. Holers VM, Girardi G, Mo L, et al: Complement C3 activation is required for antiphospholipid antibody–induced fetal loss. J Exp Med 195:211–220, 2002.

39. Arnout J: The pathogenesis of the antiphospholipid syndrome: A hypothesis based on parallelisms with heparin-induced thrombocytopenia. Thromb Haemost 75:536–541, 1996.

40. Out HJ, de Groot PG, van Vliet M, et al: Antibodies to platelets in patients with anti-phospholipid antibodies. Blood 77:2655–2659, 1991.

41. Arnout J, Vermylen J: Current status and implications of autoimmune antiphospholipid antibodies in relation to thrombotic disease. J Thromb Haemost 1:931–942, 2003.

42. Joseph JE, Harrison P, Mackie IJ, et al: Increased circulating platelet–leucocyte complexes and platelet activation in patients with antiphospholipid syndrome, systemic lupus erythematosus and rheumatoid arthritis. Br J Haematol 115:451–459, 2001.

43. Voges D, Berendes R, Burger A, et al: Three-dimensional structure of membrane-bound annexin V: A correlative electron microscopy–X-ray crystallography study. J Mol Biol 238:199–213, 1994.

44. Nakamura N, Ban T, Yamaji K, et al: Localization of the apoptosis-inducing activity of lupus anticoagulant in an annexin V-binding antibody subset. J Clin Invest 101:1951–1959, 1998.

45. Bordron A, Dueymes M, Levy Y, et al: The binding of some human antiendothelial cell antibodies induces endothelial cell apoptosis. J Clin Invest 101:2029–2035, 1998.

46. Schorer AE: Discordant effects on eicosanoids and fibrin degradation products in two murine models of antiphospholipid antibody. Thromb Res 85:295–304, 1997.

47. Ames PR, Tommasino C, Iannaccone L, et al: Coagulation activation and fibrinolytic imbalance in subjects with idiopathic antiphospholipid antibodies: A crucial role for acquired free protein S deficiency. Thromb Haemost 76:190–194, 1996.

48. Ames PR: Antiphospholipid antibodies, thrombosis and atherosclerosis in systemic lupus erythematosus: A unifying 'membrane stress syndrome' hypothesis. Lupus 3:371–377, 1994.

49. Vaarala O: Antibodies to oxidised LDL. Lupus 9:202–205, 2000.

50. Schousboe I, Rasmussen MS: Synchronized inhibition of the phospholipid mediated autoactivation of factor XII in plasma by beta 2–glycoprotein I and anti-beta 2–glycoprotein I. Thromb Haemost 73:798–804, 1995.

51. Cugno M, Cabibbe M, Galli M, et al: Antibodies to tissue-type plasminogen activator (tPA) in patients with antiphospholipid syndrome: Evidence of interaction between the antibodies and the catalytic domain of tPA in 2 patients. Blood 103:2121–2126, 2004.

52. Manfredi AA, Rovere P, Heltai S, et al: Apoptotic cell clearance in systemic lupus erythematosus. II. Role of beta2-glycoprotein I. Arthritis Rheum 41:215–223, 1998.

53. Manfredi AA, Rovere P, Galati G, et al: Apoptotic cell clearance in systemic lupus erythematosus. I. Opsonization by antiphospholipid antibodies. Arthritis Rheum 41:205–214, 1998.

54. Bancsi LF, van der Linden I, Bertina RM: Beta 2-glycoprotein I deficiency and the risk of thrombosis. Thromb Haemost 67:649–653, 1992.

55. Oosting JD, Derksen RH, Entjes HT, et al: Lupus anticoagulant activity is frequently dependent on the presence of beta 2-glycoprotein I. Thromb Haemost 67:499–502, 1992.

56. Sheng Y, Reddel SW, Herzog H, et al: Impaired thrombin generation in beta 2-glycoprotein I null mice. J Biol Chem 276:13817–13821, 2001.

57. Garcia CO, Kanbour-Shakir A, Tang H, et al: Induction of experimental antiphospholipid antibody syndrome in PL/J mice following immunization with beta 2 GPI. Am J Reprod Immunol 37:118–124, 1997.

58. Blank M, Faden D, Tincani A, et al: Immunization with anticardiolipin cofactor (beta-2-glycoprotein I) induces experimental antiphospholipid syndrome in naive mice. J Autoimmun 7:441–455, 1994.

59. Pierangeli SS, Harris EN: In vivo models of thrombosis for the antiphospholipid syndrome. Lupus 5:451–455, 1996.

60. Pierangeli SS, Barker JH, Stikovac D, et al: Effect of human IgG antiphospholipid antibodies on an in vivo thrombosis model in mice. Thromb Haemost 71:670–674, 1994.

61. Olee T, Pierangeli SS, Handley HH, et al: A monoclonal IgG anticardiolipin antibody from a patient with the antiphospholipid syndrome is thrombogenic in mice. Proc Natl Acad Sci U S A 93:8606–8611, 1996.

62. Greaves M, Hill MB, Phipps J, et al: The pathogenesis of the antiphospholipid syndrome. Thromb Haemost 76:817–818, 1996.

63. Pierangeli SS, Harris EN: Probing antiphospholipid-mediated thrombosis: The interplay between anticardiolipin antibodies and endothelial cells. Lupus 12:539–545, 2003.

64. Vega-Ostertag M, Harris EN, Pierangeli SS: Intracellular events in platelet activation induced by antiphospholipid antibodies in the presence of low doses of thrombin. Arthritis Rheum 50:2911–2919, 2004.

65. Lin YL, Wang CT: Activation of human platelets by the rabbit anticardiolipin antibodies. Blood 80:3135–3143, 1992.

66. Shi W, Chong BH, Chesterman CN: Beta 2-glycoprotein I is a requirement for anticardiolipin antibodies binding to activated platelets: Differences with lupus anticoagulants. Blood 81:1255–1262, 1993.

67. Rauch J, Meng QH, Tannenbaum H: Lupus anticoagulant and antiplatelet properties of human hybridoma autoantibodies. J Immunol 139:2598–2604, 1987.

68. Galli M, Beretta G, Daldossi M, et al: Different anticoagulant and immunological properties of anti-prothrombin antibodies in patients with antiphospholipid antibodies. Thromb Haemost 77:486–491, 1997.

69. Mosser G, Ravanat C, Freyssinet JM, et al: Sub-domain structure of lipid-bound annexin-V resolved by electron image analysis. J Mol Biol 217:241–245, 1991.

70. Andree HAM, Hermens WT, Hemker HC, et al: Displacement of factor Va by annexin V. In Andree HAM (ed): Phospholipid Binding and Anticoagulant Action of Annexin V. Maastricht, The Netherlands, Universitaire Pers Maastricht, 1992.

71. Rand JH, Wu XX, Quinn AS, et al: Human monoclonal antiphospholipid antibodies disrupt the annexin A5 anticoagulant crystal shield on phospholipid bilayers: Evidence from atomic force microscopy and functional assay. Am J Pathol 163:1193–1200, 2003.

72. Hanly JG, Smith SA: Anti-beta2-glycoprotein I (GPI) autoantibodies, annexin V binding and the anti-phospholipid syndrome. Clin Exp Immunol 120:537–543, 2000.

73. Krikun G, Lockwood CJ, Wu XX, et al: The expression of the placental anticoagulant protein, annexin V, by villous trophoblasts: Immunolocalization and in vitro regulation. Placenta 15:601–612, 1994.

74. Wang X, Campos B, Kaetzel MA, et al: Annexin V is critical in the maintenance of murine placental integrity. Am J Obstet Gynecol 180:1008–1016, 1999.

75. Rand JH, Wu XX, Andree HA, et al: Pregnancy loss in the antiphospholipid-antibody syndrome: A possible thrombogenic mechanism. N Engl J Med 337:154–160, 1997.

76. Rand JH, Wu XX, Andree HAM, et al: Antiphospholipid antibodies accelerate plasma coagulation by inhibiting annexin-V binding to phospholipids: A "lupus procoagulant" phenomenon. Blood 92:1652–1660, 1998.

77. Tomer A: Antiphospholipid antibody syndrome: Rapid, sensitive, and specific flow cytometric assay for determination of anti-platelet phospholipid autoantibodies. J Lab Clin Med 139:147–154, 2002.

78. Field SL, Chesterman CN, Dai YP, et al: Lupus antibody bivalency is required to enhance prothrombin binding to phospholipid. J Immunol 166:6118–6125, 2001.

79. Galli M, Barbui T: Antiphospholipid syndrome: Clinical and diagnostic utility of laboratory tests. Semin Thromb Hemost 31:17–24, 2005.

80. Simmelink MJ, Horbach DA, Derksen RH, et al: Complexes of anti-prothrombin antibodies and prothrombin cause lupus anticoagulant activity by competing with the binding of clotting factors for catalytic phospholipid surfaces. Br J Haematol 113:621–629, 2001.

81. Rand JH: Molecular pathogenesis of the antiphospholipid syndrome. Circ Res 90:29–37, 2002.

82. Greaves M: Antiphospholipid antibodies and thrombosis. Lancet 353:1348–1353, 1999.

83. Wilson WA, Gharavi AE, Koike T, et al: International consensus statement on preliminary classification criteria for definite antiphospholipid syndrome: Report of an international workshop. Arthritis Rheum 42:1309–1311, 1999.

84. Miyakis S, Lockshin MD, Atsumi T, et al: International consensus statement on an update of the classification criteria for definite antiphospholipid syndrome (APS). J Thromb Haemost 4:295–306, 2006.

85. Asherson RA: Phospholipid-Binding Antibodies. Boston, CRC Press Inc, 1991.

86. Brandt JT, Triplett DA, Alving B, et al: On behalf of the Subcommittee on Lupus Anticoagulant/Antiphospholipid Antibody of the Scientific and Standardisation Committee of the ISTH: Criteria for the diagnosis of lupus anticoagulants: An update. Thromb Haemost 74:1185–1190, 1995.

87. Harris EN, Pierangeli SS: Revisiting the anticardiolipin test and its standardization. Lupus 11:269–275, 2002.

88. Wong RC, Adelstein S, Gillis D, et al: Development of consensus guidelines for anticardiolipin and lupus anticoagulant testing. Semin Thromb Hemost 31:39–48, 2005.

89. Reber G, Tincani A, Sanmarco M, et al: For the Standardization Group of the European Forum on Antiphospholipid Antibodies: Proposals for the measurement of anti-beta2-glycoprotein I antibodies. J Thromb Haemost 2:1860–1862, 2004.

90. Vila P, Hernandez MC, Lopez Fernandez MF, et al: Prevalence, follow-up and clinical significance of the anticardiolipin antibodies in normal subjects. Thromb Haemost 72:209–213, 1994.

91. Cervera R, Piette JC, Font J, et al: Antiphospholipid syndrome: Clinical and immunologic manifestations and patterns of disease expression in a cohort of 1,000 patients. Arthritis Rheum 46:1019–1027, 2002.

92. Long AA, Ginsberg JS, Brill-Edwards P, et al: The relationship of antiphospholipid antibodies to thromboembolic disease in systemic lupus erythematosus: A cross-sectional study. Thromb Haemost 66:520–524, 1991.

93. Merkel PA, Chang Y, Pierangeli SS, et al: The prevalence and clinical associations of anticardiolipin antibodies in a large inception cohort of patients with connective tissue diseases. Am J Med 101:576–583, 1996.

94. Alarcon-Segovia D, Deleze M, Oria CV, et al: Antiphospholipid antibodies and the antiphospholipid syndrome in systemic lupus erythematosus: A prospective analysis of 500 consecutive patients. Medicine 68:353–365, 1989.

95. Buchanan RR, Wardlaw JR, Riglar AG, et al: Antiphospholipid antibodies in the connective tissue diseases: Their relation to the antiphospholipid syndrome and forme fruste disease. J Rheumatol 16:757–761, 1989.

96. Cervera R, Font J, Lopez-Soto A, et al: Isotype distribution of anticardiolipin antibodies in systemic lupus erythematosus: Prospective analysis of a series of 100 patients. Ann Rheum Dis 49:109–113, 1990.

97. Worrall JG, Snaith ML, Batchelor JR, et al: SLE: A rheumatological view. Analysis of the clinical features, serology and immunogenetics of 100 SLE patients during long-term follow-up. Q J Med 74:319–330, 1990.

98. Jones HW, Ireland R, Senaldi G, et al: Anticardiolipin antibodies in patients from Malaysia with systemic lupus erythematosus. Ann Rheum Dis 50:173–175, 1991.

99. Cervera R, Khamashta MA, Font J, et al: For the European Working Party on Systemic Lupus Erythematosus: Systemic lupus erythematosus: Clinical and immunologic patterns of disease expression in a cohort of 1,000 patients. Medicine (Baltimore) 72:113–124, 1993.

100. Kutteh WH, Lyda EC, Abraham SM, et al: Association of anticardiolipin antibodies and pregnancy loss in women with systemic lupus erythematosus. Fertil Steril 60:449–455, 1993.

101. Axtens RS, Miller MH, Littlejohn GO, et al: Single anticardiolipin measurement in the routine management of patients with systemic lupus erythematosus. J Rheumatol 21:91–93, 1994.

102. Cucurull E, Gharavi AE, Diri E, et al: IgA anticardiolipin and anti–beta2-glycoprotein I are the most prevalent isotypes in African American patients with systemic lupus erythematosus. Am J Med Sci 318:55–60, 1999.

103. Petri M: Classification and epidemiology of the antiphospholipid syndrome. In Asherson RA, Cervera R, and Piette, J-C et al (eds): The Antiphospholipid Syndrome II. Philadelphia, Elsevier, 2002.

104. Picillo U, Migliaresi S, Marcialis MR, et al: Longitudinal survey of anticardiolipin antibodies in systemic lupus erythematosus: Relationships with clinical manifestations and disease activity in an Italian series. Scand J Rheumatol 21:271–276, 1992.

105. Mayumi T, Nagasawa K, Inoguchi T, et al: Haemostatic factors associated with vascular thrombosis in patients with systemic lupus erythematosus and the lupus anticoagulant. Ann Rheum Dis 50:543–547, 1991.

106. Gomez-Puerta JA, Martin H, Amigo MC, et al: Long-term follow-up in 128 patients with primary antiphospholipid syndrome: Do they develop lupus? Medicine (Baltimore) 84:225–230, 2005.

107. Harris EN, Pierangeli SS: Primary, secondary, catastrophic antiphospholipid syndrome: Is there a difference? Thromb Res 114:357–361, 2004.

108. Asherson RA: The catastrophic antiphospholipid (Asherson's) syndrome in 2004: A review. Autoimmun Rev 4:48–54, 2005.

109. Uthman I, Shamseddine A, Taher A: The role of therapeutic plasma exchange in the catastrophic antiphospholipid syndrome. Transfus Apheresis Sci 33:11–17, 2005.

110. Asherson RA, Cervera R, Piette JC, et al: Catastrophic antiphospholipid syndrome: Clues to the pathogenesis from a series of 80 patients. Medicine (Baltimore) 80:355–377, 2001.

111. Levine SR, Deegan MJ, Futrell N, et al: Cerebrovascular and neurologic disease associated with antiphospholipid antibodies: 48 cases. Neurology 40:1181–1189, 1990.

112. Levine JS, Branch DW, Rauch J: The antiphospholipid syndrome. N Engl J Med 346:752–763, 2002.

113. Nencini P, Baruffi MC, Abbate R, et al: Lupus anticoagulant and anticardiolipin antibodies in young adults with cerebral ischemia. Stroke 23:189–193, 1992.

114. Ginsburg KS, Liang MH, Newcomer L, et al: Anticardiolipin antibodies and the risk for ischemic stroke and venous thrombosis. Ann Intern Med 117:997–1002, 1992.

115. Tuhrim S, Rand JH, Wu XX, et al: Elevated anticardiolipin antibody titer is a stroke risk factor in a multiethnic population independent of isotype or degree of positivity. Stroke 30:1561–1565, 1990.

116. Brey RL: Management of the neurological manifestations of APS: What do the trials tell us? Thromb Res 114:489–499, 2004.

117. Leung WH, Wong KL, Lau CP, et al: Association between antiphospholipid antibodies and cardiac abnormalities in patients with systemic lupus erythematosus. Am J Med 89:411–419, 1990.

118. Nihoyannopoulos P, Gomez PM, Joshi J, et al: Cardiac abnormalities in systemic lupus erythematosus: Association with raised anticardiolipin antibodies. Circulation 82:369–375, 1990.

119. Khamashta MA, Cervera R, Asherson RA, et al: Association of antibodies against phospholipids with heart valve disease in systemic lupus erythematosus. Lancet 335:1541–1544, 1990.

120. Galve E, Ordi J, Barquinero J, et al: Valvular heart disease in the primary antiphospholipid syndrome. Ann Intern Med 116:293–298, 1992.

121. Gleason CB, Stoddard MF, Wagner SG, et al: A comparison of cardiac valvular involvement in the primary antiphospholipid syndrome

versus anticardiolipin-negative systemic lupus erythematosus. Am Heart J 125:1123–1129, 1993.

122. Zavaleta NE, Montes RM, Soto ME, et al: Primary antiphospholipid syndrome: A 5-year transesophageal echocardiographic followup study. J Rheumatol 31:2402–2407, 2004.

123. Cervera R, Khamashta MA, Font J, et al: High prevalence of significant heart valve lesions in patients with the 'primary' antiphospholipid syndrome. Lupus 1:43–47, 1991.

124. Sletnes KE, Smith P, Abdelnoor M, et al: Antiphospholipid antibodies after myocardial infarction and their relation to mortality, reinfarction, and non-haemorrhagic stroke. Lancet 339:451–453, 1992.

125. Pope JM, Canny CL, Bell DA: Cerebral ischemic events associated with endocarditis, retinal vascular disease, and lupus anticoagulant. Am J Med 90:299–309, 1991.

126. Perez-Villa F, Font J, Azqueta M, et al: Severe valvular regurgitation and antiphospholipid antibodies in systemic lupus erythematosus: A prospective, long-term, followup study. Arthritis Rheum 53: 460–467, 2005.

127. Leventhal LJ, Borofsky MA, Bergey PD, et al: Antiphospholipid antibody syndrome with right atrial thrombosis mimicking an atrial myxoma. Am J Med 87:111–113, 1989.

128. Petri MA: Classification criteria for antiphospholipid syndrome: The case for cardiac valvular disease. J Rheumatol 31:2329–2330, 2004.

129. Lev S, Shoenfeld Y: Cardiac valvulopathy in the antiphospholipid syndrome. Clin Rev Allergy Immunol 23:341–348, 2002.

130. Cervera R: Coronary and valvular syndromes and antiphospholipid antibodies. Thromb Res 114:501–507, 2004.

131. Qaddoura F, Connolly H, Grogan M, et al: Valve morphology in antiphospholipid antibody syndrome: Echocardiographic features. Echocardiography 22:255–259, 2005.

132. Ford PM, Ford SE, Lillicrap DP: Association of lupus anticoagulant with severe valvular heart disease in systemic lupus erythematosus. J Rheumatol 15:597–600, 1988.

133. Kattwinkel N, Villanueva AG, Labib SB, et al: Myocardial infarction caused by cardiac microvasculopathy in a patient with the primary antiphospholipid syndrome. Ann Intern Med 116:974–976, 1992.

134. Chartash EK, Lans DM, Paget SA, et al: Aortic insufficiency and mitral regurgitation in patients with systemic lupus erythematosus and the antiphospholipid syndrome. Am J Med 86:407–412, 1989.

135. Hojnik M, George J, Ziporen L, et al: Heart valve involvement (Libman-Sacks endocarditis) in the antiphospholipid syndrome. Circulation 93:1579–1587, 1996.

136. Nesher G, Ilany J, Rosenmann D, et al: Valvular dysfunction in antiphospholipid syndrome: Prevalence, clinical features, and treatment. Semin Arthritis Rheum 27:27–35, 1997.

137. Petri M: The lupus anticoagulant is a risk factor for myocardial infarction (but not atherosclerosis): Hopkins Lupus Cohort. Thromb Res 114:593–595, 2004.

138. Pengo V, Biasiolo A, Pegoraro C, et al: Antibody profiles for the diagnosis of antiphospholipid syndrome. Thromb Haemost 93:1147–1152, 2005.

139. Frances C, Niang S, Laffitte E, et al: Dermatologic manifestations of the antiphospholipid syndrome: Two hundred consecutive cases. Arthritis Rheum 52:1785–1793, 2005.

140. Asherson RA, Khamashta MA, Ordi Ros J, et al: The "primary" antiphospholipid syndrome: Major clinical and serological features. Medicine 68:366–374, 1989.

141. Vianna JL, Khamashta MA, Ordi Ros J, et al: Comparison of the primary and secondary antiphospholipid syndrome: A European multicenter study of 114 patients. Am J Med 96:3–9, 1994.

142. Asherson RA, Frances C, Iaccarino L, et al: The antiphospholipid antibody syndrome: Diagnosis, skin. Clin Exp Rheumatol 24: S46–S51, 2006.

143. Battagliotti CA: Skin manifestations of antiphospholipid syndrome. In Khamashta MA (ed): Hughes Syndrome. Singapore, Springer, 2006.

144. Toubi E, Krause I, Fraser A, et al: Livedo reticularis is a marker for predicting multi-system thrombosis in antiphospholipid syndrome. Clin Exp Rheumatol 23:499–504, 2005.

145. Frances C, Papo T, Wechsler B, et al: Sneddon syndrome with or without antiphospholipid antibodies: A comparative study in 46 patients. Medicine (Baltimore) 78:209–219, 1999.

146. Tajima C, Suzuki Y, Mizushima Y, et al: Clinical significance of immunoglobulin A antiphospholipid antibodies: Possible association with skin manifestations and small vessel vasculitis. J Rheumatol 25:1730–1736, 1998.

147. Dessein PH, Lamparelli RD, Phillips SA, et al: Severe immune thrombocytopenia and the development of skin infarctions in a patient with an overlap syndrome. J Rheumatol 16:1494–1496, 1989.

148. Fiehn C, Breitbart A, Germann G: Autologous skin transplantation for widespread cutaneous necrosis in secondary antiphospholipid syndrome. Ann Rheum Dis 60:908–910, 2001.

149. Urbanus RT, de Laat HB, de Groot PG, et al: Prolonged bleeding time and lupus anticoagulant: A second paradox in the antiphospholipid syndrome. Arthritis Rheum 50:3605–3609, 2004.

150. Krause I, Blank M, Fraser A, et al: The association of thrombocytopenia with systemic manifestations in the antiphospholipid syndrome. Immunobiology 210:749–754, 2005.

151. Harris EN, Gharavi AE, Hegde U, et al: Anticardiolipin antibodies in autoimmune thrombocytopenic purpura. Br J Haematol 59:231–234, 1985.

152. Stasi R, Stipa E, Masi M, et al: Prevalence and clinical significance of elevated antiphospholipid antibodies in patients with idiopathic thrombocytopenic purpura. Blood 84:4203–4208, 1994.

153. Bidot CJ, Jy W, Horstman LL, et al: Antiphospholipid antibodies in immune thrombocytopenic purpura tend to emerge in exacerbation and decline in remission. Br J Haematol 128:366–372, 2005.

154. Edson JR, Vogt JM, Hasegawa DK: Abnormal prothrombin crossed-immunoelectrophoresis in patients with lupus inhibitors. Blood 64:807–816, 1984.

155. Rodriguez V, Reed AM, Kuntz NL, et al: Antiphospholipid syndrome with catastrophic bleeding and recurrent ischemic strokes as initial presentation of systemic lupus erythematosus. J Pediatr Hematol Oncol 27:403–407, 2005.

156. Bajaj SP, Rapaport SI, Fierer DS, et al: A mechanism for the hypoprothrombinemia of the acquired hypoprothrombinemia-lupus anticoagulant syndrome. Blood 61:684–692, 1983.

157. Fleck RA, Rapaport SI, Rao LV: Anti-prothrombin antibodies and the lupus anticoagulant. Blood 72:512–519, 1988.

158. Erdozain JG, Ruiz-Irastorza G, Egurbide MV, et al: Sustained response to rituximab of autoimmune hemolytic anemia associated with antiphospholipid syndrome. Haematologica 89:ECR34, 2004.

159. Bosly A, Keating MJ, Stasi R, et al: Rituximab in B-cell disorders other than non-Hodgkin's lymphoma. Anticancer Drugs 13 (suppl 2): S25–S33, 2002.

160. Tomietto P, Gremese E, Tolusso B, et al: B cell depletion may lead to normalization of anti-platelet, anti-erythrocyte and antiphospholipid antibodies in systemic lupus erythematosus. Thromb Haemost 92:1150–1153, 2004.

161. Wahl DG, Guillemin F, De-Maistre E, et al: Meta-analysis of the risk of venous thrombosis in individuals with antiphospholipid antibodies without underlying autoimmune disease or previous thrombosis. Lupus 7:15–22, 1998.

162. Kitchens CS: The contact system. Arch Pathol Lab Med 126: 1382–1386, 2002.

163. Lazarchick J, Kizer J: The laboratory diagnosis of lupus anticoagulants. Arch Pathol Lab Med 113:177–180, 1989.

164. Triplett DA, Brandt JT, Maas RL: The laboratory heterogeneity of lupus anticoagulants. Arch Pathol Lab Med 109:946–951, 1985.

165. Favaloro EJ: Learning from peer assessment: The role of the external quality assurance multilaboratory thrombophilia test process. Semin Thromb Hemost 31:85–89, 2005.

166. Somers E, Magder LS, Petri M: Antiphospholipid antibodies and incidence of venous thrombosis in a cohort of patients with systemic lupus erythematosus. J Rheumatol 29:2531–2536, 2002.

167. Roubey RA, Pratt CW, Buyon JP, et al: Lupus anticoagulant activity of autoimmune antiphospholipid antibodies is dependent upon beta 2-glycoprotein I. J Clin Invest 90:1100–1104, 1992.

168. Loizou S, McCrea JD, Rudge AC, et al: Measurement of anti-cardiolipin antibodies by an enzyme-linked immunosorbent assay (ELISA): Standardization and quantitation of results. Clin Exp Immunol 62:738–745, 1985.

169. Smolarsky M: A simple radioimmunoassay to determine binding of antibodies to lipid antigens. J Immunol Methods 38:85–93, 1980.

170. Harris EN: The Second International Anti-cardiolipin Standardization Workshop/The Kingston Anti-Phospholipid Antibody Study (KAPS) Group. Am J Clin Pathol 94:476–484, 1990.

171. Lockshin MD: Antiphospholipid antibody and antiphospholipid antibody syndrome. Curr Opin Rheumatol 3:797–802, 1991.

172. Stewart MW, Etches WS, Russell AS, et al: Detection of antiphospholipid antibodies by flow cytometry: Rapid detection of antibody isotype and phospholipid specificity. Thromb Haemost 70:603–607, 1993.

173. Samarkos M, Davies KA, Gordon C, et al: Clinical significance of IgA anticardiolipin and anti-beta(2)-GP1 antibodies in patients with sys-

temic lupus erythematosus and primary antiphospholipid syndrome. Clin Rheumatol 25:199–204, 2005.

174. Pierangeli SS, Harris EN: Clinical laboratory testing for the antiphospholipid syndrome. Clin Chim Acta 357:17–33, 2005.

175. Favaloro EJ, Wong RC, Silvestrini R, et al: A multilaboratory peer assessment quality assurance program–based evaluation of anticardiolipin antibody, and beta2-glycoprotein I antibody testing. Semin Thromb Hemost 31:73–84, 2005.

176. Harris EN, Pierangeli S, Birch D: Anticardiolipin wet workshop report: Fifth International Symposium on Antiphospholipid Antibodies. Am J Clin Pathol 101:616–624, 1994.

177. Shi W, Krilis SA, Chong BH, et al: Prevalence of lupus anticoagulant and anticardiolipin antibodies in a healthy population. Aust N Z J Med 20:231–236, 1990.

178. Luong TH, Rand JH, Wu XX, et al: Seasonal distribution of antiphospholipid antibodies. Stroke 32:1707–1711, 2001.

179. Petri M: Epidemiology of the antiphospholipid antibody syndrome. J Autoimmun 15:145–151, 2000.

180. Juby AG, Davis P: Prevalence and disease associations of certain autoantibodies in elderly patients. Clin Invest Med 21:4–11, 1998.

181. Richaud-Patin Y, Cabiedes J, Jakez-Ocampo J, et al: High prevalence of protein-dependent and protein-independent antiphospholipid and other autoantibodies in healthy elders. Thromb Res 99:129–133, 2000.

182. Runchey SS, Folsom AR, Tsai MY, et al: Anticardiolipin antibodies as a risk factor for venous thromboembolism in a population-based prospective study. Br J Haematol 119:1005–1010, 2002.

183. Kitchens CS: Prolonged activated partial thromboplastin time of unknown etiology: A prospective study of 100 consecutive cases referred for consultation. Am J Hematol 27:38–45, 1988.

184. Chang WJ, Sum C, Kuperan P: Causes of isolated prolonged activated partial thromboplastin time in an acute care general hospital. Singapore Med J 46:450–456, 2005.

185. Keane A, Woods R, Dowding V, et al: Anticardiolipin antibodies in rheumatoid arthritis. Br J Rheumatol 26:346–350, 1987.

186. Vaidya S, Sellers R, Kimball P, et al: Frequency, potential risk and therapeutic intervention in end-stage renal disease patients with antiphospholipid antibody syndrome: A multicenter study. Transplantation 69:1348–1352, 2000.

187. Boxer M, Ellman L, Carvalho A: The lupus anticoagulant. Arthritis Rheum 19:1244–1248, 1976.

188. Schleider MA, Nachman RL, Jaffe EA, et al: A clinical study of the lupus anticoagulant. Blood 48:499–509, 1976.

189. Elias M, Eldor A: Thromboembolism in patients with the 'lupus'-type circulating anticoagulant. Arch Intern Med 144:510–515, 1984.

190. Knight RJ, Schanzer H, Rand JH, et al: Renal allograft thrombosis associated with the antiphospholipid antibody syndrome. Transplantation 60:614–615, 1995.

191. Canoso RT, de Oliveira RM: Chlorpromazine-induced anticardiolipin antibodies and lupus anticoagulant: Absence of thrombosis. Am J Hematol 27:272–275, 1988.

192. Canoso RT, Sise HS: Chlorpromazine-induced lupus anticoagulant and associated immunologic abnormalities. Am J Hematol 13:121–129, 1982.

193. Lillicrap DP, Pinto M, Benford K, et al: Heterogeneity of laboratory test results for antiphospholipid antibodies in patients treated with chlorpromazine and other phenothiazines. Am J Clin Pathol 93:771–775, 1990.

194. Bell WR, Boss GR, Wolfson JS: Circulating anticoagulant in the procainamide-induced lupus syndrome. Arch Intern Med 137:1471–1473, 1977.

195. Edwards RL, Rick ME, Wakem CJ: Studies on a circulating anticoagulant in procainamide-induced lupus erythematosus. Arch Intern Med 141:1688–1690, 1981.

196. Hess E: Drug-related lupus. N Engl J Med 318:1460–1462, 1988.

197. Heyman MR, Flores RH, Edelman BB, et al: Procainamide-induced lupus anticoagulant. South Med J 81:934–936, 1988.

198. List AF, Doll DC: Thrombosis associated with procainamide-induced lupus anticoagulant. Acta Haematol 82:50–52, 1989.

199. Li GC, Greenberg CS, Currie MS: Procainamide-induced lupus anticoagulants and thrombosis. South Med J 81:262–264, 1988.

200. Asherson RA, Zulman J, Hughes GR: Pulmonary thromboembolism associated with procainamide induced lupus syndrome and anticardiolipin antibodies. Ann Rheum Dis 48:232–235, 1989.

201. Merrill JT, Shen C, Gugnani M, et al: High prevalence of antiphospholipid antibodies in patients taking procainamide. J Rheumatol 24:1083–1088, 1997.

202. Zarrabi MH, Zucker S, Miller F, et al: Immunologic and coagulation disorders in chlorpromazine-treated patients. Ann Intern Med 91:194–199, 1979.

203. Dalekos GN, Kistis KG, Boumba DS, et al: Increased incidence of anti-cardiolipin antibodies in patients with hepatitis C is not associated with aetiopathogenetic link to anti-phospholipid syndrome. Eur J Gastroenterol Hepatol 12:67–74, 2000.

204. Ramos-Casals M, Cervera R, Lagrutta M, et al: Clinical features related to antiphospholipid syndrome in patients with chronic viral infections (hepatitis C virus/HIV infection): Description of 82 cases. Clin Infect Dis 38:1009–1016, 2004.

205. Liaskos C, Rigopoulou E, Zachou K, et al: Prevalence and clinical significance of anticardiolipin antibodies in patients with type 1 autoimmune hepatitis. J Autoimmun 24:251–260, 2005.

206. Forman JP, Lin J, Pascual M, et al: Significance of anticardiolipin antibodies on short and long term allograft survival and function following kidney transplantation. Am J Transplant 4:1786–1791, 2004.

207. Cohen AJ, Philips TM, Kessler CM: Circulating coagulation inhibitors in the acquired immunodeficiency syndrome. Ann Intern Med 104:175–180, 1986.

208. Guglielmone H, Vitozzi S, Elbarcha O, et al: Cofactor dependence and isotype distribution of anticardiolipin antibodies in viral infections. Ann Rheum Dis 60:500–504, 2001.

209. Petrovas C, Vlachoyiannopoulos PG, Kordossis T, et al: Anti-phospholipid antibodies in HIV infection and SLE with or without anti-phospholipid syndrome: Comparisons of phospholipid specificity, avidity and reactivity with beta2-GPI. J Autoimmun 13:347–355, 1999.

210. Ankri A, Bonmarchand M, Coutellier A, et al: Antiphospholipid antibodies are an epiphenomenon in HIV-infected patients. AIDS 13:1282–1283, 1999.

211. Buller HR, Agnelli G, Hull RD, et al: Antithrombotic therapy for venous thromboembolic disease: The Seventh ACCP Conference on Antithrombotic and Thrombolytic Therapy. Chest 126:401S–428S, 2004.

212. Mackworth-Young CG, Harris EN, Steere AC, et al: Anticardiolipin antibodies in Lyme disease. Arthritis Rheum 31:1052–1056, 1988.

213. Vaarala O, Palosuo T, Kleemola M, et al: Anticardiolipin response in acute infections. Clin Immunol Immunopathol 41:8–15, 1986.

214. McNally T, Purdy G, Mackie IJ, et al: The use of an anti–beta 2-glycoprotein-I assay for discrimination between anticardiolipin antibodies associated with infection and increased risk of thrombosis. Br J Haematol 91:471–473, 1995.

215. Asherson RA, Shoenfeld Y: Human immunodeficiency virus infection, antiphospholipid antibodies, and the antiphospholipid syndrome. J Rheumatol 30:214–219, 2003.

216. Majluf-Cruz A, Silva-Estrada M, Sanchez-Barboza R, et al: Venous thrombosis among patients with AIDS. Clin Appl Thromb Hemost 10:19–25, 2004.

217. Turhal NS, Peters V, Rand J: Antiphospholipid syndrome in HIV infection: Report on four cases and review of literature. Allergy Clin Immunol Int J World Allergy Org 13:268–271, 2001.

218. Saif MW, Bona R, Greenberg B: AIDS and thrombosis: Retrospective study of 131 HIV-infected patients. AIDS Patient Care STDS 15:311–320, 2001.

219. Hassoun A, Al Kadhimi Z, Cervia J: HIV infection and antiphospholipid antibody: Literature review and link to the antiphospholipid syndrome. AIDS Patient Care STDS 18:333–340, 2004.

220. Khamashta MA: Management of thrombosis in the antiphospholipid syndrome. Lupus 5:463–466, 1996.

221. Erkan D, Yazici Y, Peterson MG, et al: A cross-sectional study of clinical thrombotic risk factors and preventive treatments in antiphospholipid syndrome. Rheumatology (Oxford) 41:924–929, 2002.

222. Finazzi G, Brancaccio V, Moia M, et al: Natural history and risk factors for thrombosis in 360 patients with antiphospholipid antibodies: A four-year prospective study from the Italian Registry. Am J Med 100:530–536, 1996.

223. Kitchens CS: Thrombotic storm: When thrombosis begets thrombosis. Am J Med 104:381–385, 1998.

224. Ruiz-Irastorza G, Khamashta MA, Hunt BJ, et al: Bleeding and recurrent thrombosis in definite antiphospholipid syndrome: Analysis of a series of 66 patients treated with oral anticoagulation to a target international normalized ratio of 3.5. Arch Intern Med 162:1164–1169, 2002.

225. Krnic BS, O'Connor CR, Looney SW, et al: A retrospective review of 61 patients with antiphospholipid syndrome: Analysis of factors influencing recurrent thrombosis. Arch Intern Med 157:2101–2108, 1997.

226. Rosove MH, Brewer PM: Antiphospholipid thrombosis: Clinical course after the first thrombotic event in 70 patients. Ann Intern Med 117:303–308, 1992.

227. Khamashta MA, Cuadrado MJ, Mujic F, et al: The management of thrombosis in the antiphospholipid-antibody syndrome. N Engl J Med 332:993–997, 1995.

228. Schulman S, Svenungsson E, Granqvist S, Duration of Anticoagulation Study Group: Anticardiolipin antibodies predict early recurrence of thromboembolism and death among patients with venous thromboembolism following anticoagulant therapy. Am J Med 104:332–338, 1998.

229. Lim W, Crowther MA, Eikelboom JW: Management of antiphospholipid antibody syndrome: A systematic review. JAMA 295:1050–1057, 2006.

230. Hull R, Delmore T, Carter C, et al: Adjusted subcutaneous heparin versus warfarin sodium in the long-term treatment of venous thrombosis. N Engl J Med 306:189–194, 1982.

231. Hull R, Delmore T, Genton E, et al: Warfarin sodium versus low-dose heparin in the long-term treatment of venous thrombosis. N Engl J Med 301:855–858, 1979.

232. Hull R, Hirsh J, Jay R, et al: Different intensities of oral anticoagulant therapy in the treatment of proximal-vein thrombosis. N Engl J Med 307:1676–1681, 1982.

233. Oden A, Fahlen M: Oral anticoagulation and risk of death: A medical record linkage study. BMJ 325:1073–1075, 2002.

234. Crowther MA, Ginsberg JS, Julian J, et al: A comparison of two intensities of warfarin for the prevention of recurrent thrombosis in patients with the antiphospholipid antibody syndrome. N Engl J Med 349:1133–1138, 2003.

235. Finazzi G, Marchioli R, Brancaccio V, et al: A randomized clinical trial of high-intensity warfarin vs. conventional antithrombotic therapy for the prevention of recurrent thrombosis in patients with the antiphospholipid syndrome (WAPS). J Thromb Haemost 3:848–853, 2005.

236. Rickles FR, Marder VJ: Moderate dose oral anticoagulant therapy in patients with the antiphospholipid syndrome? No. J Thromb Haemost 3:842–843, 2005.

237. Khamashta MA, Hunt BJ: Moderate dose oral anticoagulant therapy in patients with the antiphospholipid syndrome? No. J Thromb Haemost 3:844–845, 2005.

238. Letellier E, Hughes GR: "Listen to the patient": Anticoagulation is critical in the antiphospholipid (Hughes) syndrome. J Rheumatol 30:897, 2003.

239. Al-Matar M, Jaimes J, Malleson P: Chorea as the presenting clinical feature of primary antiphospholipid syndrome in childhood. Neuropediatrics 31:107–108, 2000.

240. Kearon C, Gent M, Hirsh J, et al: A comparison of three months of anticoagulation with extended anticoagulation for a first episode of idiopathic venous thromboembolism. N Engl J Med 340:901–907, 1999.

241. Moll S, Ortel TL: Monitoring warfarin therapy in patients with lupus anticoagulants. Ann Intern Med 127:177–185, 1997.

242. Robert A, Le Querrec A, Delahousse B, et al: Control of oral anticoagulation in patients with the antiphospholipid syndrome: Influence of the lupus anticoagulant on International Normalized Ratio. Groupe Methodologie en Hemostase du Groupe d'Etudes sur l'Hemostases et la Thrombose. Thromb Haemost 80:99–103, 1998.

243. Lawrie AS, Purdy G, Mackie IJ, et al: Monitoring of oral anticoagulant therapy in lupus anticoagulant positive patients with the antiphospholipid syndrome. Br J Haematol 98:887–892, 1997.

244. Bertrand E, Cloitre B, Ticolat R, et al: [Antiaggregation action of chloroquine]. Med Trop (Mars) 50:143–146, 1990.

245. Jancinova V, Nosal R, Petrikova M: On the inhibitory effect of chloroquine on blood platelet aggregation. Thromb Res 74:495–504, 1994.

246. Petri M, Hochberg M, Hellmann D, et al: Incidence of and predictors of thrombotic events in SLE: Protective role of hydroxychloroquine. Arthritis Rheum 35:S54, 1992.

247. Wallace DJ: Does hydroxychloroquine sulfate prevent clot formation in systemic lupus erythematosus? Arthritis Rheum 30:1435–1436, 1987.

248. Edwards MH, Pierangeli S, Liu X, et al: Hydroxychloroquine reverses thrombogenic properties of antiphospholipid antibodies in mice. Circulation 96:4380–4384, 1997.

249. Espinola RG, Pierangeli SS, Gharavi AE, et al: Hydroxychloroquine reverses platelet activation induced by human IgG antiphospholipid antibodies. Thromb Haemost 87:518–522, 2002.

250. Mok MY, Chan EY, Fong DY, et al: Antiphospholipid antibody profiles and their clinical associations in Chinese patients with systemic lupus erythematosus. J Rheumatol 32:622–628, 2005.

251. Costedoat-Chalumeau N, Amoura Z, Huong du LT, et al: Safety of hydroxychloroquine in pregnant patients with connective tissue diseases: Review of the literature. Autoimmun Rev 4:111–115, 2005.

252. Lai TY, Chan WM, Li H, et al: Multifocal electroretinographic changes in patients receiving hydroxychloroquine therapy. Am J Ophthalmol 140:794–807, 2005.

253. Marmor MF: Hydroxychloroquine at the recommended dose (< or = 6.5 mg/kg/day) is safe for the retina in patients with rheumatoid arthritis and systemic lupus erythematosus. Clin Exp Rheumatol 22:143–144, 2004.

254. Bronster DJ, Gousse R, Fassas A, et al: Anticardiolipin antibody–associated stroke after liver transplantation. Transplantation 63:908–909, 1997.

255. Asherson RA: The catastrophic antiphospholipid syndrome, 1998: A review of the clinical features, possible pathogenesis and treatment. Lupus 7 (suppl 2): S55–S62, 1998.

256. Harner KC, Jackson LW, Drabick JJ: Normalization of anticardiolipin antibodies following rituximab therapy for marginal zone lymphoma in a patient with Sjogren's syndrome. Rheumatology (Oxford) 43:1309–1310, 2004.

257. Erkan D, Asherson RA, Espinosa G, et al: Long term outcome of catastrophic antiphospholipid syndrome survivors. Ann Rheum Dis 62:530–533, 2003.

Chapter 20

Hemostatic Aspects of Cardiovascular Medicine

Richard C. Becker, MD

INTRODUCTION

The evolution of cardiovascular medicine is based soundly on a progressively advanced understanding of vascular biology, hemostasis, and thrombosis. Indeed, pharmacotherapies for the prevention and treatment of coronary atherothrombosis are the end results of several productive decades of investigation, highlighted by strong collaborative efforts between the cardiology, pathology, and hematology communities in response to several fundamental observations and clinically relevant questions that include the following: (1) What are the anatomic and physiologic effects of atherosclerotic vascular disease? (2) How does atherosclerosis influence the complex and delicate balance between thrombosis and thromboresistance? (3) Can intrinsic thrombotic potential in atherosclerotic vascular disease be selectively modulated pharmacologically without compromising protective hemostasis (and patient safety)? and (4) Are untapped opportunities available for translating an existing knowledge of congenital hemostatic disorders into the development of new and widely affordable treatments?

This chapter is designed to summarize the rapid evolution of cardiovascular medicine with particular emphasis on antithrombotic therapy, its evidence-based use in routine clinical practice, and the practical management of drug-induced hemostatic impairment.

SCOPE OF THE PROBLEM

According to recent studies conducted by the American Heart Association,[1] an estimated 1.2 million Americans will develop angina pectoris or experience an acute myocardial infarction in 2007. The cost of cardiovascular disease and stroke, projected to exceed $403 billion, includes the direct costs of health care expenditures (e.g., physicians and other health care professionals, hospitals, rehabilitation programs and nursing home services, medications, and home health care) and indirect costs (loss of productivity as a result of morbidity and mortality).

HISTORICAL PERSPECTIVES IN CARDIOVASCULAR MEDICINE

The rapid transformation of fluid blood to a gel-like substance (clot) has been a topic of great interest since the days of Plato and Aristotle.[2,3] However, it was not until the early 18th century that blood clotting was recognized as a complex mechanism that could be used to stem blood loss after vascular injury.[4]

The microscope played a pivotal role in enhancing understanding of coagulation. In the mid-17th century, Marcello Malpighi separated the individual components of a blood clot into fibers, cells, and serum.[5] Fibers were later found to be derived from a plasma precursor (fibrinogen) and were given the name fibrin.[6] Further advances in the mid-19th century included the recognition of an enzyme (later called thrombin) that was capable of coagulating fibrinogen.[7]

In the latter half of the 19th century, the scientific community began to appreciate that thrombin could not be a constituent of normal plasma (otherwise, clotting would occur continuously and at random).[8] This fundamental construct was vital to an understanding of coagulation, and it remains in situations in which inactive precursors are activated precisely where and when they are needed only to be quickly neutralized where and when they are not needed. It also introduced the possibility that blood contained many, if not all, of the necessary elements for intravascular coagulation and served as the template for the theory of intrinsic coagulation.

Coagulation Cascade: Past and Present

Scientists have long known that blood coagulates soon after it comes into contact with a foreign surface, and that some surfaces are more likely to precipitate clotting than others. This provided an early foundation for the study of hereditary disorders of coagulation.[9,10] Our understanding of extrinsic coagulation followed the pioneering work of several preeminent scientists,[11–14] all of whom described blood coagulation after infusion of tissue suspensions (tissue factor, thromboplastin). A revised theory of extrinsic coagulation suggested that exposed tissue surfaces (from damaged blood vessels) were capable of stimulating blood clot formation. Later discoveries included information on the direct contributions of calcium, phospholipid, and other essential components of the prothrombinase complex (factors Va, Xa) to blood coagulation.

Platelets

The contribution of platelets to blood coagulation can be traced back to Alfred Donné, who in 1842, described circulating globules seen under the newly developed microscope lens.[15] Despite his astute observations, the clinical importance of platelets in hemostasis was not appreciated until the end of the 19th century, when William Osler at age 25 first reported platelet aggregation,[16] and Hayem proposed platelet plugs as a critical means of stemming blood loss after tissue injury.[17]

Electron microscopy subsequently provided direct evidence that platelets adhered to damaged blood vessels and could subsequently become "activated" by one or more biochemical (e.g., adenosine diphosphate, epinephrine, thrombin) or mechanical (e.g., shear stress) stimuli.

Fibrinolysis

The inability of blood to remain clotted after death was observed as early as the days of Hippocrates.[18] Pioneering work near the end of the 18th century described the process of fibrinolysis and a mechanism whereby a circulating precursor (plasminogen) generated an active enzyme (plasmin) capable of degrading clotted blood.[19,20]

The era of fibrinolysis began with the work of Gratia, who observed in 1921 that clots could be dissolved by staphylococcal extracts.[21] Tillett and Garner[22] later found that bacteria-free filtrates of β-hemolytic streptococci contained a substance (streptokinase) capable of dissolving blood clots. Soon thereafter, the groundbreaking work of Sol Sherry and coworkers[23] highlighted the potential use of fibrinolytics in treating humans with thrombotic disorders.

Early Developments in Cardiovascular Medicine

Aspirin

The potential role of aspirin in the prevention and treatment of cardiovascular disease had been recognized by clinicians for decades; however, landmark observations made during the Second International Study of Infarct Survival (ISIS-2)[24] placed antithrombotic therapy with aspirin at the forefront of current management strategies for acute myocardial infarction (MI).

Myocardial Reperfusion

The recognition that sudden, complete coronary arterial occlusion was the proximate cause of acute ST segment elevation MI, coupled with the work of Reimer and Jennings highlighting the "wavefront phenomenon" of myocardial necrosis and the "time-dependent" effects of coronary perfusion in limiting myocardial damage, paved the way for pharmacologic (fibrinolysis) and mechanical (coronary angioplasty, bypass grafting) reperfusion strategies that currently represent standards of care.[25–27] Efforts at the national level designed to reduce MI-related mortality have focused on education, early recognition, and prompt evidence-based intervention.

Low Molecular Weight Heparin

The contribution of coagulation proteins, including factor Xa and thrombin, to cardiovascular thrombosis stimulated interest in safe and effective antagonists. In acute coronary syndromes, as well as in acute venous thromboembolism, low molecular weight heparin (LMWH) has shown great promise and is rapidly becoming an accepted therapy.[27–32]

Platelet Glycoprotein-IIb/IIIa Receptor Antagonists

Given that the platelet is a pivotal component of arterial thrombosis, and that a congenital disorder is characterized by the absence of a platelet surface receptor and a bleeding tendency (Glanzmann thrombasthenia), platelet glycoprotein (GP)-IIb/IIIa receptor antagonists have, through intense investigation, become a mainstay in the treatment of high-risk patients with acute coronary syndromes and those undergoing percutaneous coronary intervention.[33]

Combination Pharmacotherapy

Astute observations made over the past two decades regarding thrombosis, fibrinolysis, anticoagulants, and platelet antagonists will undoubtedly lead to their combined administration in clinical practice.[34] This effort will focus on establishing doses that will attenuate thrombosis while maintaining vascular and hemostatic integrity.

CORONARY ATHEROGENESIS

After monocytes attach to the morphologically intact but dysfunctional vascular endothelium, a net directed migration of cells occurs through the endothelium to the subendothelial space, where they undergo differentiation. The phenomenon of "monocyte activation and differentiation" plays an important role in atherosclerosis, particularly with regard to plaque remodeling and lesion progression. This complex process proceeds through at least two mechanisms: (1) the generation of reactive oxygen species (free radicals); and (2) the phenotypic modulation and expression of a scavenger receptor or family of receptors. The chemical modification of low-density lipoprotein (LDL) results in its avid uptake by blood monocytes (now considered tissue macrophages) and subsequent transformation to foam cells. The specific receptor responsible for the uptake of modified LDL fails to effectively downregulate; as a result, a substantial amount of intracellular LDL cholesterol accumulates. When the influx of LDL particles exceeds the capacity of the macrophage scavenger receptors to remove them from the intracellular space, oxidized LDL particles accumulate within the arterial intima; this event irreversibly injures endothelial cells, smooth muscle cells, and macrophages. Disruption of relatively fragile macrophage-derived foam cells ensues, leading to the release of cytotoxic lipid material into the extracellular compartment of the intima and the formation of a cholesteryl ester–rich atheromatous core.[35–37]

CORONARY ARTERIAL THROMBOGENESIS

The clinical expression of atherosclerotic vascular disease is determined by pathologic events that lead to coronary thrombosis (or thromboembolism). In this regard, two factors are key: (1) the propensity of plaques to rupture, and (2) the thrombogenicity of exposed plaque components.

The morphologic characteristics of plaques destined to rupture have been determined through careful analyses of lesions that exhibit disruption. Observational studies of necropsy and atherectomy tissue samples have shown

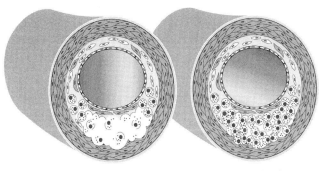

Vulnerable plaque   Nonvulnerable plaque

Figure 20-1 Vulnerable plaques are characterized by a prominent lipid core, a thin fibrous cap, and an active state of inflammation. In contrast, nonvulnerable plaques are fibrotic and are less likely to disrupt (provoking thrombosis).

convincingly that plaques associated with intraluminal thrombosis are rich in extracellular lipid, and that the lipid core of these "vulnerable or rupture-prone" plaques occupies a large proportion of the overall plaque volume. The degree of cross-sectional narrowing of the vessel lumen is typically less than 50%.[38] In addition to a large lipid core, vulnerable plaques are characterized by a thin fibrous cap and high macrophage density.[39] Whereas most individuals with atherosclerotic coronary artery disease exhibit a diversity of plaque types, most have a preponderance of one specific type (vulnerable or nonvulnerable) (Fig. 20-1). The genetic and acquired determinants of plaque type and predisposition to disruption are subjects of intense investigation.

Under normal physiologic conditions, cellular blood components interact with the vessel wall for the purpose of normal vascular repair. Exposure of circulating blood to disrupted or dysfunctional surfaces initiates a series of complex yet orderly steps that give rise to the rapid deposition of platelets, erythrocytes, leukocytes, and insoluble fibrin, which, if poorly regulated, establishes a mechanical barrier to blood flow (Fig. 20-2).

Thrombosis that occurs within the arterial circulatory system involves platelets and fibrin in a relatively small, tightly packed network. By contrast, venous thrombi consist of a more loosely woven, larger network of erythrocytes, leukocytes, and fibrin.

The process of vascular thrombosis, particularly in the coronary arterial bed, is dynamic, with clot formation and dissolution occurring almost simultaneously. The overall extent of thrombosis and ensuing circulatory compromise is therefore determined by the predominant force that "shifts" the delicate balance in one direction or another. If local thrombotic stimuli exceed the vessel's own thromboresistant capacity, thrombosis will occur. If, on the other hand, the stimulus is not particularly strong and the intrinsic defenses are intact, clot formation of clinical importance is unlikely. In many circumstances, systemic factors contribute to or "magnify" local prothrombotic factors, shifting the balance toward thrombosis.

Overall, the site, size, and composition of thrombi forming within the heart and arterial circulatory system are determined by the following:

- Alterations in blood flow
- Thrombogenicity of vascular and endocardial surfaces
- Concentration and reactivity of plasma cellular components
- Preservation and functional capability of physiologic protective mechanisms.

Platelet Deposition

Platelets that attach to disrupted vascular surfaces adhere, activate, and aggregate to form a rapidly enlarging platelet mass. Under physiologic conditions, this represents the first or primary step in hemostasis. In contrast, pathologic thrombosis is characterized by a poorly regulated response to vessel wall injury that escalates to the point of circulatory compromise.

The biology of platelet deposition involves several processes:

- Platelet attachment to collagen or exposed surface adhesive proteins
- Platelet activation and intracellular signaling
- Expression of platelet receptors for adhesive proteins
- Platelet aggregation
- Platelet recruitment mediated by thrombin, thromboxane A$_2$, and adenosine diphosphate, as well as other biochemical agents.

Activation of Coagulation Factors

Thrombin is generated rapidly in response to vascular injury. It also plays a central role in platelet recruitment and formation of an insoluble fibrin network. The thrombotic process is localized, amplified, and modulated by a series

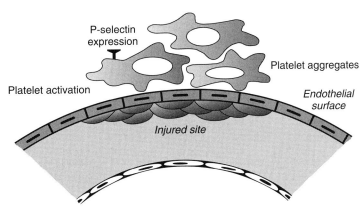

Figure 20-2 The initiating step in arterial thrombosis is both tissue factor and platelet dependent.

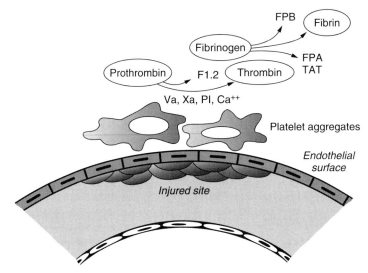

Figure 20-3 The growth phase of arterial thrombosis is coagulation protein dependent.

of biochemical reactions that are driven by the reversible binding of circulating proteins (coagulation factors) to damaged vascular cells, elements of exposed subendothelial connective tissue (especially collagen), platelets (which also express receptor sites for coagulation factors), and macrophages. These events lead to an assembly of enzyme complexes that increase local concentrations of procoagulant material; in this way, a relatively minor initiating stimulus can be greatly amplified to yield a thrombus (Fig. 20-3).

Fibrin Formation

The final phase of arterial thrombosis involves the generation of a stable fibrin network, which provides a structural scaffold for circulating cellular elements and vascular remodeling. In this pivotal process, thrombin cleaves two peptides, fibrinopeptide A and fibrinopeptide B, to form fibrin monomers, which, in turn, polymerize to form soluble fibrin strands. Orderly assembly and branching and lateral association of fibrillar strands follow, terminating with factor XIII–mediated covalent crosslinking to form a cohesive fibrin network or a mature thrombus.

ESTABLISHING A UNIFIED PLATFORM FOR THE DIAGNOSIS AND MANAGEMENT OF CARDIOVASCULAR THROMBOTIC DISORDERS

Cell-Based Model of Coagulation

The "waterfall" or "cascade" model of coagulation, proposed almost simultaneously by McFarland, Davie, and Ratnoff,[40] provided a biochemical basis for an understanding of coagulation reactions. However, its separation into intrinsic and extrinsic pathways and the omission of platelets (and other cellular elements) from the overall working framework limited the model's direct application to in vivo hemostasis and thrombosis.

Initiation takes place on cells or specialized particles (monocytes, macrophages, neutrophils, activated endothelial cells, smooth muscle cells, apoptotic cells, platelet particles, circulating vesicles) that bear the transmembrane glycoprotein

tissue factor (TF).[41] Exposed tissue factor binds and fully activates coagulation factor VII (FVIIa); subsequently, both FIX and FX are activated (which then activates FV), generating a small amount of thrombin from prothrombin (FII). In the amplification phase that follows, the small amount of generated thrombin activates platelets (causing release of α-granule contents) and factors V, XI, and VIII (cleaving the latter from von Willebrand factor [VWF]). FXIa generates additional FIXa (whose action is accelerated by FVIIIa), whereas FVa accelerates the enzymatic action of FXa. During the propagation phase, FIXa binds to activated platelets, causing further activation of FX. Complexing of FXa and FVa to membrane surfaces leads to a "burst" of thrombin generation. Major hemostatic roles of thrombin include conversion of soluble fibrinogen to a tri-dimensional network of fibrin (coagulation), activation of platelets through at least two different G-protein–coupled protease-activated receptors (PARs),[42] and nonphysiologic constriction of structurally or functionally impaired (at the endothelial level) vessels.

Thrombus growth in rapidly flowing blood is closely linked to the presence of soluble and surface-bound VWF.[43] This multimeric protein not only acts as a bridge for the initial tethering and translocation of platelets to subendothelial collagen (via platelet GP-Ib), it also induces the surface expression of platelet GP-IIb/IIIa (also referred to as $\alpha_{IIb}\beta_3$), leading to stable adhesion and subsequent aggregation of activated platelets.[44]

Idling Coagulation: Setting the Stage for Thrombotic Events

Traditional models of coagulation, although they underemphasize the functionality of cellular surfaces for determining biochemical and physiologic events, have underscored the importance of enzymatic amplification potential as a mechanism for "responsive coagulation."[45] "Idling coagulation systems," characterized by low circulating levels of active clotting proteins, require constant regulation to prevent activation thresholds from being reached. Under normal circumstances, modest stimuli do not activate coagulation, whereas strong stimuli provoke a full response. The "idling model" emphasizes the regulatory properties of enzymatic cofactors, such as

FVIII- and FIXa-mediated generation of FXa. The FIXa:VIIIa complex loses its activity through FVIIIa decay and inactivation by activated protein C. TF is regulated by tissue factor pathway inhibitor (TFPI). Thus, the functionality of both pivotal coagulation proteases is determined by their cofactors (and their varying inhibition kinetics).

Blood-Borne Propensity for Arterial, Venous, and Microcirculatory Thromboses

TF exists at high concentrations within atherosclerotic plaques, activated endothelial cells, fibroblasts, macrophages, and vascular smooth muscle cells; however, TF antigen can also be identified within the circulating blood of patients with coronary artery disease.[46] TF-containing neutrophils, monocytes, and microparticles circulating in peripheral blood can be delivered to sites of vascular injury, where they contribute directly to the initiation of thrombus formation and its subsequent propagation.[41,43] Adherent leukocytes enhance fibrin deposition through CD18-dependent capture of fibrin protofibrils that are flowing in plasma and through FXII-dependent thrombin generation. They also activate platelets, providing a fully functional platform for fibrin formation under flow conditions.[47]

A blood-borne propensity for thrombosis that is not entirely dependent on vascular disease provides a biologic explanation for the observed disparities between "degree" or "extent" of atherosclerosis and risk of thrombotic events in the arterial vascular bed,[48] as well as for the propensity toward venous thrombosis noted with malignancy and after trauma or major surgery.

Cellular Interfacing in Cardiovascular Thrombosis

Several traditionally held views that warrant reconsideration for a fuller appreciation of the dynamic environment that characterizes vascular bed–specific thrombosis include the following: (1) circulating platelets adhere to exposed subendothelial tissues solely to prevent bleeding, (2) leukocytes respond to inflammatory stimuli solely to facilitate tissue repair, and (3) these two preceding events occur independently of one another.[43]

An emerging model of importance for an understanding of atherosclerosis and other thrombosis-prone disease states involves platelet and leukocyte adhesion to activated endothelial cells, leukocyte adhesion to activated platelets, and multicellular interactions among platelets, leukocytes, and endothelial cells on vascular surfaces.[43] Each event is supported by the engagement of cell surface receptors (selectins and integrins) with soluble or membrane-anchored ligands, which include VWF, fibrinogen, collagen, fibronectin, P-selectin, CD40 ligand, GP-Ib-IX-V complex, GP-IIb/IIIa, GP-$\alpha_2\beta_1$ and GP-$\alpha_5\beta_1$, P-selectin, GP ligand-1, neutrophil Mac-1, CD40, and a variety of other intercellular and vascular adhesion molecules.[49]

ATHEROTHROMBOTIC VASCULAR DISEASE: CLINICAL PRACTICE

Management of atherothrombotic vascular disease involving the coronary, cerebral, and peripheral vascular beds includes an increasingly complex array of fibrinolytic and antithrombotic agents. It is important for the hematology consultant to become familiar with these commonly used agents, along with their mechanisms of action, pharmacology, and potential impact on hemostasis (Table 20-1, Figs. 20-4 and 20-5).[50,51]

PLATELET-DIRECTED THERAPIES

The pivotal role of platelets in atherothrombosis provides a biology-based platform for targeted approaches to drug development, clinical trial testing, and employment in patient care.[52]

20

Table 20-1 Antithrombotic Agents Used in Treating Atherothrombotic Cardiovascular Disease

Oral Antiplatelet Therapy

Aspirin	Initial dose of 162–325 mg nonenteric formulation is followed by 75–325 mg/day of an enteric formulation.
Clopidogrel (Plavix)	75 mg/day; a loading dose of 4–8 tablets (300–600 mg) is frequently administered to initiate treatment.
Ticlopidine (Ticlid)	250 mg twice daily; a loading dose of 500 mg can be used when rapid onset of inhibition is required; assessment of platelet and white cell counts during treatment is required. Rarely used now.

Parenteral Anticoagulants

Dalteparin (Fragmin)	120 IU per kilogram subcutaneously every 12 hours (maximum, 10,000 IU twice daily)
Enoxaparin (Lovenox)	1 mg per kilogram SC every 12 hours; the first dose may be preceded by a 30-mg IV bolus (in ST segment elevation myocardial infarction [MI])
Heparin, unfractionated (UFH)	Bolus 60–70 U per kilogram (maximum, 4000 U) IV followed by infusion of 12–15 U/kg/hr (maximum, 1000 U per hour) titrated to partial thromboplastin time (PTT) 1.5–2.5× that of control
Fondaparinux (Arixtra)	2.5 mg subcutaneously every 24 hours

Intravenous Antiplatelet Therapy

Abciximab (ReoPro)	0.25 mg per kilogram bolus followed by infusion of 0.125 µg/kg/min (maximum, 10 µg per minute) for 12 hours
Eptifibatide (Integrilin)	180 µg per kilogram bolus ×2 followed by infusion of 2.0 µg/kg/min for 18 hours*
Tirofiban (Aggrastat)	0.4 µg per kilogram ×30 min, followed by infusion of 0.1 µg/kg/min for 12–24 hours

*Different dose regimens were tested in recent clinical trials before percutaneous interventions were provided.

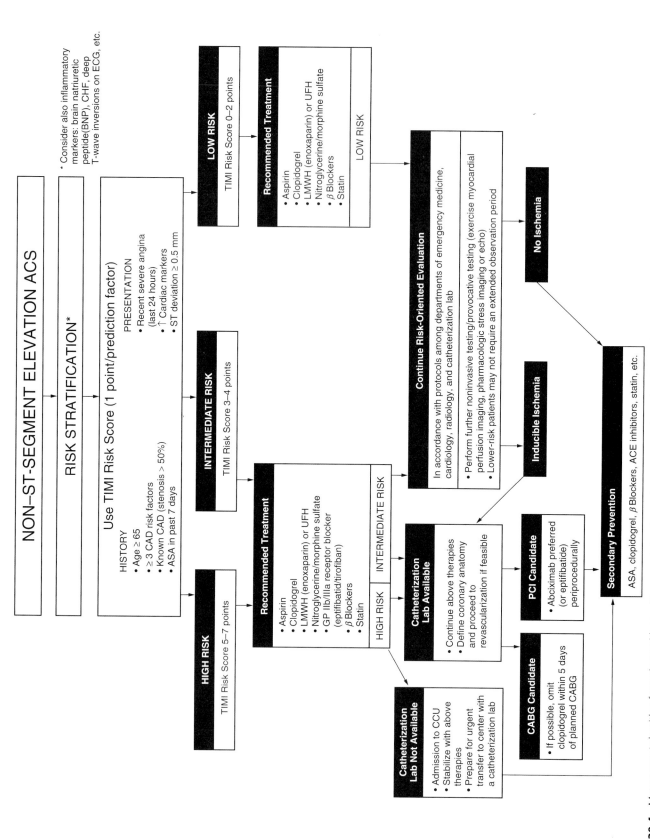

NON–ST-SEGMENT ELEVATION ACS

RISK STRATIFICATION*

* Consider also inflammatory markers: brain natriuretic peptide(BNP), CHF, deep T-wave inversions on ECG, etc.

Use TIMI Risk Score (1 point/prediction factor)

HISTORY
- Age ≥ 65
- ≥ 3 CAD risk factors
- Known CAD (stenosis > 50%)
- ASA in past 7 days

PRESENTATION
- Recent severe angina (last 24 hours)
- ↑ Cardiac markers
- ST deviation ≥ 0.5 mm

HIGH RISK
TIMI Risk Score 5–7 points

INTERMEDIATE RISK
TIMI Risk Score 3–4 points

LOW RISK
TIMI Risk Score 0–2 points

Recommended Treatment
- Aspirin
- Clopidogrel
- LMWH (enoxaparin) or UFH
- Nitroglycerine/morphine sulfate
- GP IIb/IIIa receptor blocker (eptifibatid/tirofiban)
- β Blockers
- Statin

HIGH RISK   INTERMEDIATE RISK

Recommended Treatment
- Aspirin
- Clopidogrel
- LMWH (enoxaparin) or UFH
- Nitroglycerine/morphine sulfate
- β Blockers
- Statin

LOW RISK

Catheterization Lab Not Available
- Admission to CCU
- Stabilize with above therapies
- Prepare for urgent transfer to center with a catheterization lab

Catheterization Lab Available
- Continue above therapies
- Define coronary anatomy and proceed to revascularization if feasible

Continue Risk-Oriented Evaluation
In accordance with protocols among departments of emergency medicine, cardiology, radiology, and catheterization lab
- Perform further noninvasive testing/provocative testing (exercise myocardial perfusion imaging, pharmacologic stress imaging or echo)
- Lower-risk patients may not require an extended observation period

Inducible Ischemia

No Ischemia

CABG Candidate
- If possible, omit clopidogrel within 5 days of planned CABG

PCI Candidate
- Abciximab preferred (or eptifibatide) periprocedurally

Secondary Prevention
ASA, clopidogrel, β Blockers, ACE inhibitors, statin, etc.

Figure 20-4 Management algorithm for patients with non–ST-segment elevation acute coronary syndrome (ACS). This information is based on Class I recommendations from the American College of Cardiology (ACC)/American Heart Association (AHA) 2002 Guideline Update for the Management of Patients with Unstable Angina and Non–ST-Segment-Elevation Myocardial Infarction. (From Braunwald E, Antman EM, Beasley JW, et al: ACC/AHA guidelines for the management of patients with unstable angina and non–ST-segment elevation myocardial infarction: A report of the American College of Cardiology/American Heart Association Task Force on Practice Guidelines (Committee on the Management of Patients with Unstable Angina). J Am Coll Cardiol 2000;36:970–1062. Reproduced with permission.)

Acute Ischemia Pathway

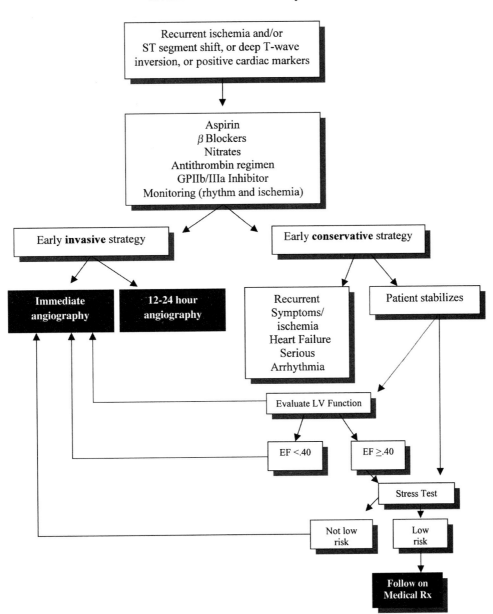

Figure 20-5 Management pathway for patients at high risk for myocardial infarction and cardiovascular death. An early aggressive approach is recommended for most patients. (From Boden WE, Pepine CJ: Introduction to "optimizing management of non–ST-segment elevation acute coronary syndromes:" Harmonizing advances in mechanical and pharmacologic intervention. J Am Coll Cardiol 41:S1–S6, 2003. Reproduced with permission.)

Aspirin

Aspirin has been available for more than a century and represents a mainstay in the prevention and treatment of vascular events, including stroke, MI, peripheral vascular occlusion, and sudden death. Accordingly, most patients with atherosclerotic vascular disease will receive aspirin.

Mechanism of Action

Aspirin irreversibly acetylates cyclo-oxygenase (COX), impairing prostaglandin metabolism and synthesis of thromboxane A_2 (TxA_2). As a result, platelet aggregation in response to collagen, adenosine diphosphate (ADP), thrombin (in low concentrations), and TxA_2 is attenuated[53] (Fig. 20-6).

Because aspirin more selectively inhibits COX-1 activity (found predominantly in platelets) than COX-2 activity

(expressed in tissues after an inflammatory stimulus), its ability to prevent platelet aggregation is achieved with relatively low doses, in contrast to the drug's potential anti-inflammatory effects, which require much higher doses.[54]

Pharmacokinetics

Aspirin is rapidly absorbed in the proximal gastrointestinal (GI) tract (stomach, duodenum), achieving peak serum levels within 15 to 20 minutes and significant platelet inhibition within 40 to 60 minutes. Enteric-coated preparations are less well absorbed, causing an observed delay in peak serum levels and significant platelet inhibition after 60 and 90 minutes, respectively. The antiplatelet effect occurs even before acetylsalicylic acid is detectable in peripheral blood, probably as a result of platelet exposure in the portal circulation.

20

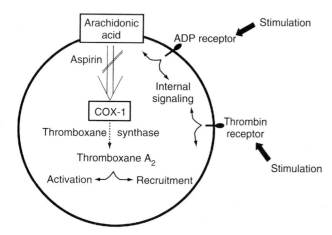

Figure 20-6 Aspirin is a potent, irreversible inhibitor of platelet cyclo-oxygenase (COX-1), reducing platelet activation and recruitment.

The plasma concentration of aspirin decays rapidly with a circulating half-life of approximately 20 minutes. Despite the drug's rapid clearance, platelet inhibition persists for the life span of the platelet (7 ± 2 days) because of aspirin's irreversible inactivation of COX-1. Because 10% of circulating platelets are replaced every 24 hours, platelet activity (primary hemostasis) returns toward normal ($\geq$50% of normal activity) within 5 to 6 days of the last aspirin dose.[55]

Adverse Effects

The adverse effect profile of aspirin in general and its associated risk for major hemorrhage in particular are determined largely by dose, duration of administration, associated structural defects (peptic ulcer disease, *Helicobacter pylori* infection), hemostatic abnormalities (inherited, acquired), and concomitant use of other antithrombotic agents.

Enteric coating of aspirin has *not* been shown to reduce the likelihood of adverse effects involving the GI tract. Patients with gastric erosions or peptic ulcer disease who require treatment with aspirin should concomitantly receive a proton pump inhibitor to minimize the risk of hemorrhage.

Aspirin Administration in Clinical Practice

The beneficial effects of aspirin are determined largely by the absolute risk of vascular events. Patients at low risk (healthy individuals without predisposing risk factors for vascular disease) derive minimal benefit, and those at high risk (unstable angina, prior MI, stroke) derive considerable benefit.[56] A risk-based approach to aspirin administration is recommended to avoid subjecting individuals who are unlikely to benefit from aspirin administration to its potential adverse effects.

PRIMARY PREVENTION OF VASCULAR EVENTS

Aspirin was tested in three primary prevention trials involving more than 30,000 healthy individuals.[57–59] Collective available data show strongly that aspirin reduces the risk of vascular events (Fig. 20-7).[54]

The Women's Health Study[60] randomly assigned 39,876 healthy women 45 years of age or older to receive 100 mg of aspirin on alternate days or placebo and followed them for 10 years. A 9% risk reduction in major cardiovascular events was reported among those who took aspirin. Women older than 65 years of age enjoyed the greatest benefit. The greatest overall impact was noted in the reduction of ischemic stroke (relative risk, 0.76). GI bleeding requiring transfusion was increased by 40% with aspirin.

SECONDARY PREVENTION OF VASCULAR EVENTS

The Antiplatelet Trialists' Collaboration,[61] which is based on a comprehensive evaluation of existing data, provides convincing evidence in support of aspirin's ability to prevent vascular events (vascular death, nonfatal MI, nonfatal stroke) in a wide variety of high-risk patients; overall, antiplatelet therapy (predominantly aspirin therapy) reduces nonfatal MI by one third, nonfatal stroke by one third, and vascular death by one quarter.

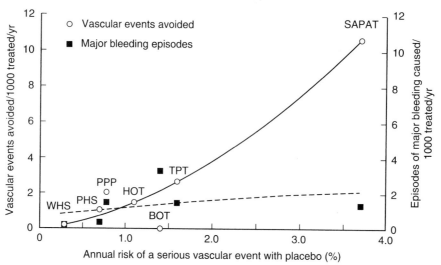

Figure 20-7 Benefits and risks of low-dose aspirin in primary prevention trials. The numbers of vascular events avoided and episodes of major bleeding caused per 1000 patients treated with aspirin per year are plotted from the results of individual placebo-controlled trials of aspirin in different patient populations characterized by varying degrees of cardiovascular risk, as noted on the abscissa. WHS denotes Women's Health Study; PHS, Physicians' Health Study; PPP, Primary Prevention Project; HOT, Hypertension Optimal Treatment study; BDT, British Doctors Trial; TPT, Thrombosis Prevention Trial; SAPAT, Swedish Angina Pectoris Aspirin Trial. (From Patrono C: Aspirin as an antiplatelet drug. N Engl J Med 330:1287–1294, 1994. Reproduced with permission.)

Aspirin Dosing

An updated meta-analysis of the Antiplatelet Trialists' Collaboration provides additional information on the effects of various doses of aspirin.[61] Overall, among 3570 patients included in three trials that directly compared doses of aspirin (≥75 mg daily vs <75 mg daily), significant differences in vascular events were observed (two trials compared 75 to 325 mg aspirin daily vs <75 mg daily, and one trial compared 500 to 1500 mg aspirin daily vs <75 mg daily). With direct and indirect comparisons of aspirin dose, the proportionate reduction in vascular events was 19% with 500 to 1500 mg daily, 26% with 160 to 325 mg daily, and 32% with 75 to 150 mg daily. The effects of antiplatelet drugs other than aspirin (vs control) were assessed in 166 trials that included 81,731 patients. Indirect comparisons provided no clear evidence of differences in reduction of serious vascular events (χ^2 for heterogenicity between any aspirin regimen and other antiplatelet drugs = 10.8; ns). Most direct comparisons assessed the effects of replacing aspirin with another antiplatelet agent.

The effect of adding another antiplatelet drug to an aspirin regimen (vs aspirin alone) has been assessed in 43 trials that included 39,205 patients. Overall, a 15% reduction in serious vascular events was observed ($P = .0001$). The benefits of adding an intravenous GP-IIb/IIIa receptor antagonist to aspirin were particularly evident among patients undergoing percutaneous coronary intervention (PCI).

Coronary Artery Bypass Grafting

More than 20 clinical trials have been conducted to determine the effectiveness of antiplatelet therapy in preventing early (≥10 days) and late (6 to 12 months) saphenous vein graft occlusion. Ten of these trials investigated aspirin in doses ranging from 100 mg to 975 mg daily. Several also assessed patients who were given internal mammary coronary bypass grafts.[62,63]

Considered collectively, and aided by the Antiplatelet Trialists' Collaboration overview, data reveal improved saphenous vein graft patency with aspirin administration. Although a direct benefit for internal mammary bypass grafts has not been established, treatment is recommended on the basis of the common coexistence of vascular disease (and the risk for thrombotic events).

Transient Ischemic Attacks/Stroke

The International Stroke Trial and the Chinese Acute Stroke Trial[64,65] evaluated the efficacy and safety of aspirin given at a daily dose of 300 mg and 160 mg, respectively, to nearly 40,000 patients with acute ischemic stroke. Treatment was initiated within 48 hours of symptom onset and continued for 2 to 4 weeks. Combined results suggest an absolute benefit of 10 fewer deaths or nonfatal strokes per 1000 patients during the first month of treatment. The risk of hemorrhagic stroke was also increased (two excess events per 1000 patients).

Long-term aspirin administration reduces the likelihood of stroke (and other vascular events) in patients with transient ischemic attacks (TIAs) and completed minor strokes. Although debate is ongoing within the neurology community regarding the optimal daily dose, 75 to 325 mg is considered an acceptable range.

The combination of aspirin (25 mg) and extended-release dipyridamole (200 mg twice daily) is more effective than aspirin alone for the prevention of stroke. Patients who are unable to take aspirin should be treated with clopidogrel (75 mg daily).

Percutaneous Coronary Intervention

PCI, including standard balloon angioplasty, rotational atherectomy, and laser angioplasty, with or without stent placement, is associated with vascular injury, atheromatous plaque disruption, platelet activation, and, at times, coronary thromboembolism. Several studies performed over the past decade have documented reduced periprocedural complications, including thrombus formation, abrupt closure, and MI, with antiplatelet therapy given prior to PCI (relative risk reduction [RRR], 60%).[66,67]

The current recommendations for PCI include aspirin (325 mg daily) for the secondary prevention of cardiovascular events; for patients unable to tolerate aspirin, pretreatment with clopidogrel (300 mg) followed by 75 mg daily is suggested.

Aspirin Response Variability

The ability of aspirin to inhibit platelet aggregation is discordant and is seen in upward of 30% of individuals who are nonresponders or who exhibit a paradoxical increase in platelet aggregation and activation after high-dose (325 mg) administration.

The ability of aspirin to reduce COX activity varies considerably among individuals; in addition, atherosclerosis is associated with increased TF level expression caused by cytokine-mediated induction. It is important to recognize that an acquired form of aspirin resistance may be induced by concomitant administration of ibuprofen.[68] Lastly, genetic polymorphisms and resulting gene expression of COX and thromboxane synthase may limit the effectiveness of aspirin.[69]

A classification scheme for aspirin resistance has been proposed[70,71] that includes three categories: type 1, inhibition of platelet TxA_2 formation in vitro but not in vivo; type 2, inability of aspirin to inhibit TxA_2 formation in vitro and in vivo; and type 3, TxA_2-independent platelet activation (pseudoresistance).

Clinical Impact of Aspirin Resistance and Failure

Despite its proved benefit, aspirin therapy has inherent limitations; the existing literature supports the conclusion that patients who are receiving aspirin can and do experience cardiovascular events. Accordingly, ongoing investigations are designed to better define aspirin failure and aspirin resistance.[72,73] A recent editorial calls into question both the existence and significance of aspirin resistance.[73a]

Clopidogrel

Clopidogrel, a thienopyridine derivative, is a platelet antagonist that is several times more potent than ticlopidine, yet is associated with fewer adverse effects. The important role of ADP-mediated platelet activation and aggregation in atherothrombotic vascular disease has made the surface P2Y12 receptor a favored target.

In Vitro and Ex Vivo Effects on Platelets

Clopidogrel, a prodrug, is extensively metabolized in the liver to an active compound with a plasma elimination half-life of 7.7 ± 2.3 hours. Dose-dependent inhibition of ADP-mediated platelet aggregation is observed several hours after a single oral dose of clopidogrel is given, with more significant inhibition achieved with loading doses (≥ 300 mg). A 600-mg oral loading dose achieves effective platelet inhibition in 2 to 3 hours. Repeated doses of 75 mg clopidogrel per day inhibit aggregation, and steady state is reached between days 3 and 7. At steady state, the average inhibition to ADP is between 40% and 60%.

Clopidogrel selectively inhibits the binding of ADP to its platelet receptor (P2Y12) and the subsequent G-protein–linked mobilization of intracellular calcium and activation of the GP-IIb/IIIa complex.[74]

Absorption

Clopidogrel is rapidly absorbed after oral administration, with peak plasma levels of the predominant circulating metabolite occurring approximately 60 minutes later.

Safety

Available information suggests that clopidogrel offers safety advantages over ticlopidine, particularly with regard to bone marrow suppression and other hematologic abnormalities. Although thrombotic thrombocytopenic purpura (TTP) has been reported with clopidogrel,[75] its occurrence (11 cases per 3 million patients treated) is rare, and it has not been reported in randomized clinical trials performed to date.

Clinical Experience

The well-documented benefits derived from platelet-directed therapy among patients with atherosclerotic vascular disease, coupled with a worrisome adverse effect profile associated with ticlopidine, have fostered the rapid development of clopidogrel as a potential alternative to existing therapies. The Clopidogrel versus Aspirin in Patients at Risk for Ischemic Events (CAPRIE) Study[76] was designed to test the hypothesis that clopidogrel (75 mg daily) would reduce vascular events in high-risk patients by approximately 15% compared with aspirin (325 mg daily). The study population consisted of patients with atherosclerotic vascular disease manifested as recent ischemic stroke, recent MI, or symptomatic peripheral arterial occlusive disease. A total of 19,185 patients were enrolled in the international trial. Mean duration of follow-up was 1.91 years. Patients treated with clopidogrel (by intention-to-treat analysis) had a 5.32% annual risk of ischemic stroke, MI, or vascular death compared with 5.83% among aspirin-treated patients (RRR, 8.7%; 95% confidence interval [CI], 0.3 to 16.5; $P = .043$)

Although CAPRIE was not empowered to identify differences between specific subsets, for patients experiencing a stroke, the average event rate per year was 5.03% in the clopidogrel group compared with 4.84% in the aspirin group (relative risk increase, 3.7%; $P = .66$). In contrast, patients with peripheral vascular disease experienced a 3.71% annual event rate with clopidogrel and a 4.86% rate with aspirin (RRR, 23.8%; $P = .002$).

No major differences in safety were noted between treatment groups; however, a greater proportion of patients receiving aspirin had the study drug permanently discontinued because of GI hemorrhage, indigestion, nausea, or vomiting. Approximately 1 of every 1000 patients treated with clopidogrel experienced neutropenia (<1200 per microliter) (similar to outcomes with aspirin treatment).

In the CAPRIE study,[77] all-cause mortality, vascular death, MI, stroke, and rehospitalization were determined for 1480 patients who had previously undergone bypass grafting. Those randomly assigned to clopidogrel had a 31.2% RRR in events compared with those given aspirin treatment. Considering the composite end point used in the main CAPRIE trial—vascular death, MI, or ischemic stroke—a 36.3% relative reduction was seen with clopidogrel (5.8% per year) compared with aspirin (9.1% per year) ($P = .004$).

The trial design employed in CAPRIE could not provide an answer to the important question of dual platelet inhibition (aspirin plus clopidogrel). Accordingly, an additional study was undertaken. The CHARISMA (Clopidogrel for High Atherothrombotic Risk and Ischemic Stabilization, Management, and Avoidance) study[78] randomly assigned 15,603 patients with clinically evident cardiovascular disease or multiple risk factors to receive low-dose aspirin. Patients were subsequently followed for a median of 28 months, with a primary efficacy end point of the composite of MI, stroke, or clopidogrel plus aspirin reported in 7.3% with placebo plus aspirin (relative risk, 0.93; 95% CI, 0.83 to 1.05; $P = .22$). Respective rates for the principal secondary end point, which included hospitalization for ischemic events, were 16.7% and 17.9% (relative risk, 0.92; 95% CI, 0.86 to 0.995; $P = .04$). Rates of severe bleeding were 1.7% and 1.3%, respectively. Among patients with clinically evident atherothrombosis, the secondary end point primarily occurred in 6.9% of patients receiving combination therapy versus 7.9% of those given aspirin alone (relative risk, 0.88; 96% CI, 0.77 to 0.998; $P = .046$). In contrast, patients with multiple risk factors (but not documented atherothrombotic disease) experienced a primary end point rate of 6.6% with combination therapy versus 5.5% with aspirin alone (relative risk, 1.2; 95% CI, 0.91 to 1.59; $P = .20$). The rate of death from cardiovascular causes was higher with combination therapy (3.9% vs 2.2%; $P = .01$).

On the basis of available data from CHARISMA, one could conclude that the combination of clopidogrel plus aspirin is not more effective than aspirin alone in reducing the rate of MI, stroke, or death from cardiovascular causes among patients with stable cardiovascular disease or multiple cardiovascular risk factors. In contrast, benefit has been noted among individuals with symptomatic atherothrombotic disease. However, this observation requires further investigation.

Percutaneous Coronary Stenting

A multicenter, randomized, controlled trial, Clopidogrel Plus ASA vs Ticlopidine Plus ASA in Stent Patients Study (CLASSICS),[79] included 1020 patients undergoing coronary stent placement who received aspirin (325 mg once daily) plus ticlopidine (250 mg twice daily), aspirin plus clopidogrel (75 mg daily), or aspirin plus front-loaded clopidogrel (300 mg as an initial dose followed by 75 mg once daily). Treatment was continued for 28 days after stent placement. Intravenous GP-IIb/IIIa antagonists were not administered to patients enrolled in the trial. The primary safety end point was a composite of neutropenia, thrombocytopenia, bleeding, and drug discontinuation for adverse events (noncardiac). The secondary efficacy end point was a composite of MI, target vessel revascularization, and cardiovascular death.

The primary end point occurred in 9.1% of ticlopidine-treated patients, 6.3% of clopidogrel-treated patients (75 mg), and 2.9% of front-loaded clopidogrel–treated patients. Early drug discontinuation was reported in 8.2%, 5.1%, and 2.0% of patients, respectively. The most commonly observed adverse effects that prompted drug discontinuation were allergic reactions, GI distress, and skin rash. Secondary cardiovascular end points were reached by 0.9%, 1.5%, and 1.3% of patients, respectively.

The importance of adequate platelet inhibition preceding and following PCI (with stenting) was confirmed in the Percutaneous Coronary Intervention–Clopidogrel in Unstable Angina to Prevent Recurrent Events (PCI-CURE) study.[80] A total of 2658 patients undergoing PCI were randomly assigned to double-blind treatment with clopidogrel or placebo (aspirin alone) for, on average, 6 days before the procedure followed by 4 weeks of open-label thienopyridine (after which the study drug was resumed for 8 months). The primary end point (cardiovascular death, MI, or urgent target vessel revascularization within 30 days) was reached in 4.5% of clopidogrel-treated patients and 6.4% of placebo-treated patients (30% RRR) Long-term administration of clopidogrel was associated with a lower rate of death, MI, or any revascularization and no increase in bleeding complications.

Intracoronary radiation therapy is an available method for treating patients with in-stent restenosis; however, late total occlusion and thrombosis are serious complications, with rates approaching 10% to 15%. Accumulating evidence suggests that prolonged treatment with clopidogrel and aspirin (≥6 months) is more effective in preventing late thrombosis when compared with an abbreviated course (1 month).[81]

At least 3 months of clopidogrel treatment are recommended after a sirolimus (Cypher; Johnson and Johnson, New Brunswick, NJ) drug-eluting stent (DES) is placed; 6 months are required for those receiving a paclitaxal (Taxus; Boston Scientific, Natick, MA) DES.

Acute Coronary Syndromes

The benefits of therapy with aspirin and clopidogrel were considered in the Clopidogrel in Unstable Angina to Prevent Recurrent Events (CURE) trial.[82] A total of 12,562 patients experiencing an acute coronary syndrome without ST segment elevation received clopidogrel (300 mg immediately, 75 mg daily) plus aspirin (75 to 325 mg daily) or aspirin alone for 3 to 12 months. The composite of death, MI, or stroke occurred in 9.3% and 11.4% of patients, respectively (RRR, 20%). In hospital refractory ischemia, congestive heart failure and revascularization procedures were also less likely to occur in clopidogrel-treated patients. Although a greater risk of major hemorrhage was observed with combination therapy (3.7% vs 2.7%; relative risk, 1.38), life-threatening bleeding and hemorrhagic stroke occurred at similar rates across groups.

Pretreatment with Clopidogrel and Clinical Benefit

The CREDO (Clopidogrel for the Reduction of Events During Observation) trial[83] evaluated the long-term benefit (12 months) of treatment with clopidogrel after PCI, as well as the potential benefits of initiating clopidogrel with a preprocedural loading dose (in addition to aspirin therapy). A total of 2116 patients scheduled for elective PCI were randomly assigned to receive clopidogrel (300 mg) or placebo beginning 3 to 24 hours before PCI. All patients were given aspirin (325 mg). More than two thirds of patients had experienced a recent MI or unstable angina as an indication for PCI. Thereafter, all patients received clopidogrel (75 mg daily) through day 28. From day 29 through 12 months, patients in the loading dose group were given clopidogrel (75 mg daily) or placebo. Both groups continued to receive standard therapy, including aspirin (81 to 325 mg daily). Pretreatment with clopidogrel was associated with a nonsignificant 18.5% RRR for the combined end point of death, MI, or target vessel revascularization at 28 days. It is biologically conceivable that larger loading doses (600 mg) or more prolonged pretreatment may yield enhanced benefit.

Two recent trials—the Clopidogrel as Adjunctive Reperfusion Therapy (CLARITY)-Thrombolysis in Myocardial Infarction (TIMI) 28 trial[84] and the Clopidogrel and Metoprolol in Myocardial Infarction Trial/Second Chinese Cardiac Study (COMMIT/CCS-2-Clopidogrel)[85]—suggested a role for clopidogrel in the treatment of patients with ST segment elevation MI. In the CLARITY-TIMI 28 trial, the addition of clopidogrel (300 mg loading dose, then 75 mg per day) to a regimen of aspirin plus thrombolysis before angiography improved the patency rate of the infarct-related artery and reduced ischemic complications in patients who presented within 12 hours of onset of ST segment elevation MI. The primary efficacy end point (a composite of infarct-related arterial occlusion [TIMI grade 0/1], death, or recurrent MI before angiography) was reduced by 36% with clopidogrel, and effects were driven predominantly by a reduction in arterial occlusion; no increase in major bleeding or intracranial hemorrhage occurred.

Approach to Patients Receiving Long-Term Clopidogrel Therapy

Two series of 20 consecutive patients with coronary artery disease received 600 mg of clopidogrel. The first patient group had not received clopidogrel previously; the second group had taken 75 mg previously for at least 30 days. Six hours after loading, platelet aggregation in response to ADP (20 μmol per liter) was inhibited by 31% and 51%, respectively. Clopidogrel inhibited ADP-induced expression of platelet GP-IIb/IIIa and P-selectin receptors as well.[86]

Clopidogrel Response Variability

Although the incidence rates and mechanism likely differ, clopidogrel and aspirin resistance may have cumulative clinical relevance. Available evidence suggests that clopidogrel resistance (<10% inhibition of ADP-mediated platelet aggregation) occurs in upward of 20% of patients after a 300 mg loading dose[87] and may reveal patients who are at risk for coronary arterial events.[88] Patients with heightened platelet activity (prior to treatment) appear to be at greatest risk for clopidogrel resistance.[89] Although the mechanism(s) underlying clopidogrel resistance have not been elucidated, alterations in cytochrome P450 metabolism activity (conversion of prodrug to active drug), polymorphisms of the platelet ADP receptor, or individual differences in post–receptor signaling pathways are likely contributors.

PLATELET GLYCOPROTEIN (GP)-IIB/IIIA RECEPTOR ANTAGONISTS

The GP-IIb/IIIa receptor (totaling 50,000 to 70,000 copies per platelet) represents a common pathway for platelet aggregation in response to a wide variety of biochemical and mechanical stimuli. Accordingly, it represents an attractive target for pharmacologic inhibition that can be applied to patients with acute coronary syndromes.

INTRAVENOUS PLATELET GP-IIB/IIIA RECEPTOR ANTAGONISTS

The evolution of GP-IIb/IIIa receptor antagonists began with murine monoclonal antibodies and recently has focused on small peptide or nonpeptide molecules that have structural similarities to fibrinogen. Three intravenous GP-IIb/IIIa receptor antagonists have been approved by the U. S. Food and Drug Administration: abciximab (ReoPro; Centocor, Leiden, The Netherlands), tirofiban (Aggrastat; Merck & Co., Inc., Whitehouse Station, NJ), and eptifibatide (Integrilin; Millennium Pharmaceuticals, Inc., Cambridge, Mass).

ABCIXIMAB

Abciximab (ReoPro) is the Fab fragment of the chimeric human-murine monoclonal antibody c7E3.

Pharmacokinetics

After an intravenous bolus has been administered, free plasma concentrations of abciximab decrease rapidly with an initial half-life of less than 10 minutes and a second-phase half-life of 30 minutes, representing rapid binding to the platelet GP-IIb/IIIa receptor. Abciximab remains in the circulation for 10 or more days in the platelet-bound state.

Pharmacodynamics

Intravenous administration of abciximab in doses ranging from 0.15 mg/kg to 0.3 mg/kg produces a rapid dose-dependent inhibition of platelet aggregation in response to ADP. At the highest dose, 80% of platelet GP-IIb/IIIa receptors are occupied within 120 minutes, and platelet aggregation, even in response to 20 mM ADP, is inhibited

completely. Sustained inhibition is achieved with prolonged infusions (12 to 24 hours), and low-level receptor blockade is present for up to 10 days after cessation of the infusion: however, platelet pharmacodynamics during infusions beyond 24 hours has not been fully characterized. Platelet aggregation in response to 5 mM ADP returns to more than 50% of baseline within 24 hours of drug cessation.

Clinical Experience

In nearly 2100 patients undergoing balloon coronary angioplasty or atherectomy who were at high risk for ischemic (thrombotic) complications, abciximab (0.25 mg per kilogram bolus) followed by 12-hour continuous infusion (10 μg per minute) reduced by 35% the occurrence of death or MI or the need for an urgent intervention (repeat angioplasty, stent placement, balloon pump insertion, or bypass grafting).[90] At 6 months,[91] the absolute difference between patients with a major ischemic event and those with elective revascularization was 8.1% among patients who received abciximab (bolus plus infusion) compared with those administered placebo (35.1% vs 27.0%; 23% relative reduction). At 3 years,[92] the composite end point occurred in 41.1% of those who were given an abciximab bolus plus infusion, 47.4% of those receiving an abciximab bolus *only*, and, 47.2% of those to whom placebo was given.

The Evaluation in PTCA (Percutaneous Transluminal Coronary Angioplasty) to Improve Long-term Outcome with Abciximab GPIIb/IIIa Blockade (EPILOG) study[93] included 2792 patients who were undergoing elective or urgent percutaneous coronary revascularization and who received abciximab with standard, weight-adjusted unfractionated heparin (UFH; initial bolus, 100 U per kilogram; target activated clotting time [ACT] ≥300 seconds) or placebo along with standard-dose, weight-adjusted heparin. At 30 days, the composite event rate was observed in high-risk and low-risk patients.

The c7E3 Fab Antiplatelet Therapy in Unstable Refractory Angina (CAPTURE) study[94] was designed to investigate whether abciximab, infused for 18 to 24 hours prior to coronary angioplasty, could improve outcomes in patients with refractory (myocardial ischemia despite nitrates, heparin, and aspirin) unstable angina. A total of 1265 patients were randomly assigned to abciximab or placebo. Within 30 days, the primary end point (death, MI, urgent revascularization) occurred in 11.3% of abciximab-treated patients and 15.9% of placebo-treated patients (n = 0.012). The rate of MI was lower *before* and *during* coronary interventions with abciximab administration.

Patients who participated in the Global Use of Strategies to Open Occluded Arteries in Acute Coronary Syndromes trial (GUSTO-IV-ACS)[95] had chest pain and ST segment depression or elevated troponin levels. They were randomly assigned to receive placebo, abciximab for 24 hours, or abciximab for 48 hours with recommended avoidance of revascularization during the initial 48 hours. Neither abciximab group fared better than the placebo group with respect to death or MI at 30 days. In addition, early mortality rates were higher with prolonged abciximab infusion, suggesting a prothrombotic (or other adverse) effect.

The Abciximab Before Direct Angioplasty and Stenting in Myocardial Infarction Regarding Acute and Long-Term

Follow-Up (ADMIRAL) trial[96] included 300 patients with PCI (plus stenting) who were infused with abciximab or placebo. At 30 days, a composite of death, reinfarction, or urgent revascularization (target vessel) had occurred in 6% of abciximab-treated and 14.6% of placebo-treated patients; at 6 months, the corresponding figures were 7.4% and 15.9%, respectively. Early administration of abciximab improved coronary patency before stenting, success rates of the procedures, and rate of patency 6 months after the procedure.

In the GUSTO V study,[97] 16,588 patients with acute ST segment elevation MI received reteplase (standard dose) or half-dose reteplase plus abciximab. Although 30-day mortality rates did not differ significantly, fewer nonfatal ischemic complications of MI occurred with reteplase plus abciximab compared with reteplase alone. Intracranial hemorrhage rates did not differ between treatments; however, moderate to severe bleeding was more likely with combined therapy, and patients >75 years of age were at increased risk for hemorrhagic stroke (odds ratio [OR], 1.91). All patients in GUSTO V received UFH and aspirin therapy.

TIROFIBAN

Tirofiban (Aggrastat; Merck & Co., Inc., Whitehouse Station, NJ), a tyrosine derivative with a molecular weight of 495 kd, is a nonpeptide inhibitor (peptidomimetic) of the platelet GP-IIb/IIIa receptor.

Pharmacodynamics

Tirofiban, like other nonpeptides, mimics the geometric, stereotactic, and charge characteristics of the RDG sequence (of fibrinogen), thus interfering with platelet aggregation.

Three doses of tirofiban were evaluated in a phase 1 study of patients undergoing coronary angioplasty who received one of three regimens intravenously with a bolus dose of 5, 10, or 15 µg per kilogram and a continuous (16- to 24-hour) infusion of 0.05, 0.10, or 0.15 µg/kg/min.[98] Dose-dependent inhibition of ex vivo platelet aggregation was observed within minutes of bolus administration and was sustained during the continuous infusion.

Clinical Experience

The Randomized Efficacy Study of Tirofiban Outcomes and Restenosis (RESTORE) trial[99] was a randomized, double-blind, placebo-controlled trial of tirofiban in patients with ACS who were undergoing PCI.

Patients (n = 2139) received tirofiban as a 10 µg per kilogram intravenous bolus over a 3-minute period and a continuous IV infusion of 0.15 µg/kg/min over 36 hours. All patients received UFH and aspirin therapy. The primary composite end point (death, MI, angioplasty, failure requiring bypass surgery or unplanned stent placement, recurrent ischemia requiring repeat angioplasty) at 30 days was reduced from 12.2% in the placebo group to 10.3% in the tirofiban group (16% relative reduction).

The Platelet Receptor Inhibition in Ischemic Syndrome Management (PRISM) trial[100] included 3231 patients with non–ST segment elevation acute coronary syndrome (ACS).

All patients received aspirin and were randomly assigned to treatment with UFH or tirofiban, given as a loading dose of 0.6 µg/kg/min over 30 minutes followed by a maintenance infusion of 0.15 µg/kg/min for 48 hours (angiography/revascularization was discouraged during the infusion period). The primary composite end point (death, MI, refractory ischemia) at 48 hours was attained in 3.8% of tirofiban-treated patients and 5.6% of placebo (aspirin/heparin)-treated patients (risk reduction, 33%). Benefit was maintained but overall was more modest at 7 and 30 days.

The PRISM in Patients Limited by Unstable Signs and Symptoms (PLUS) trial[101] included 1915 patients with non–ST segment elevation ACS who were treated with aspirin and UFH and were subsequently randomly assigned to tirofiban (0.4 µg/kg/min IV for 30 min, then 0.1 µg/kg/min for a minimum of 48 hours and a maximum of 108 hours) or placebo (UFH). Angiography and revascularization were performed at the discretion of the treating physician. Tirofiban-treated patients had a lower composite event rate over 7 days than the placebo group (12.9% vs 17.9%; risk reduction, 34%). This benefit was mainly due to a reduced incidence of MI (47% risk reduction) and refractory ischemia (30% risk reduction). Benefit was maintained at 30 days (22% risk reduction in composite event rate) and at 6 months. The trial originally included a tirofiban alone arm (no heparin) that was dropped because of excess mortality at 7 days.

The importance of early PCI among patients with non–ST segment elevation ACS was underscored in the Treat Angina With Aggrastat and Determine Cost of Therapy With an Invasive or Conservative Strategy (TACTICS)–Thrombolysis in Myocardial Infarction (TIMI) 18 trial,[102] as was the benefit of aggressive pharmacologic therapy (GP-IIb/IIIa receptor antagonist) in combination with PCI for patients at greatest risk for adverse ischemic outcomes (prior MI, ST segment changes, elevated cardiac biomarkers).

EPTIFIBATIDE

Eptifibatide (Integrilin; Millennium Pharmaceuticals, Inc., Cambridge, Mass) is a nonimmunogenic cyclic heptapeptide with an active pharmacophore that is derived from the structure of barbourin, a platelet GP-IIb/IIIa inhibitor from the venom of the southeastern pigmy rattlesnake.[103]

Pharmacokinetics

The plasma half-life of eptifibatide is 10 to 15 minutes, and clearance is predominantly renal (75%) and to a lesser degree hepatic (25%). The antiplatelet effect has a rapid onset of action and causes a rapid decline in activity.

Pharmacodynamics

In a pilot study of PCI, patients were randomly assigned to one of four eptifibatide dosing schedules: 180 µg/kg bolus, 1 µg/kg/min infusion; 135 µg/kg IV bolus, 0.5 µg/kg/min IV infusion; 90 µg/kg IV bolus, 0.75 µg/kg/min IV infusion; and 135 µg/kg IV bolus, 0.75 µg/kg/min IV infusion.

All patients received aspirin and UFH and were continued on study drug for 18 to 24 hours. The two highest bolus doses produced >80% inhibition of ADP-mediated platelet aggregation within 15 minutes of administration in most patients (>75%). A constant IV infusion of 0.75 μg/kg/min maintained the antiplatelet effect, whereas an infusion of 0.50 μg/kg/min IV allowed gradual recovery of platelet function. In all dosing groups, platelet function returned to >50% of normal from baseline within 4 hours of termination of the infusion.[104]

Clinical Experience

The Integrilin to Minimize Platelet Aggregation and Coronary Thrombosis (IMPACT-II) trial[105] enrolled 4010 patients undergoing elective, urgent, or emergent PCI. Patients were assigned to placebo, a IV bolus of 135 μg per kilogram eptifibatide followed by an IV infusion of 0.5 μg/kg/min for 20 to 24 hours, or a 135 μg per kilogram bolus followed by a 0.75 μg/kg/min infusion. Within 30 days, the composite end point (death, MI, unplanned revascularization, stent placement for abrupt closure) occurred in 11.4%, 9.2%, and 9.9% of patients, respectively. Although the benefits of treatment were maintained at 6 months, differences between groups were not statistically significant.

The IMPACT-After Myocardial Infarction (AMI) Study[106] was designed to determine the effects of eptifibatide on coronary arterial patency when used adjunctively with tissue plasminogen activity (tPA). A total of 132 patients with MI received tPA, heparin, and aspirin and were randomly assigned to receive a bolus and continuous infusion of one of six eptifibatide doses or placebo. Doses ranged from 36 to 180 μg per kilogram (bolus) to 0.2 to 0.75 μg/kg/min (IV infusion). Study drug was started within 24 hours. The highest-dose eptifibatide groups had more complete reperfusion (TIMI grade 3 flow) and shorter mean time to ST segment recovery than placebo-treated patients. The composite clinical event rate (death, reinfarction, revascularization, heart failure, hypertension, stroke) was relatively high in all groups: 44.8% in eptifibatide-treated patients and 41.8% in placebo-treated patients.

The Platelet Glycoprotein IIb/IIIa in Unstable Angina Receptor Suppression Using Integrilin Therapy (PURSUIT) trial[107] included patients with non–ST segment elevation ACS with symptoms within 24 hours and electrocardiographic changes within 12 hours (of ischemia). A total of 10,948 patients were randomly assigned to eptifibatide, 180 μg per kilogram bolus plus 1.3 μg/kg/min infusion; eptifibatide, 180 μg per kilogram IV bolus plus 2.0 μg/kg/min IV infusion; or placebo for up to 3 days (in addition to UFH [in most patients] and aspirin). The 30-day event rate of death or nonfatal MI was 14.2% with eptifibatide and 15.7% with placebo (1.5% absolute reduction). Reduction in MI or death (composite) with eptifibatide was observed at later time points.

The Enhanced Suppression of the Platelet GPIIb/IIIa Receptor with Integrilin Trial (ESPRIT) was designed to test the hypothesis that a minimum threshold of 80% GP-IIb/IIIa receptor blockade was required for benefit.[108] A total of 2064 patients received eptifibatide (180 μg per kilogram IV boluses [×3] 10 minutes apart, followed by continuous IV infusion of 2.0 μg/kg/min for 18 to 24 hours) or placebo prior to PCI. The trial was terminated early for efficacy because patients receiving eptifibatide had a 4.0% absolute reduction in death, MI, urgent target vessel revascularization, or "bail out" GP-IIb/IIIa antagonist use within 48 hours compared with placebo. Major events were significantly fewer at 30 days as well.

GP-IIB/IIIA RECEPTOR ANTAGONISTS AND DIABETES MELLITUS

Patients with diabetes mellitus experience increased mortality in the setting of ACS. A meta-analysis of diabetic populations enrolled in six large-scale clinical trials (n = 6458 patients) revealed a 30-day mortality reduction with GP-IIb/IIIa receptor antagonist use from 6.2% to 4.6% (26% RRR). Benefit was greatest in those undergoing PCI (70% RRR).[108]

Agent-Specific Characteristics

Although considered collectively as GP-IIb/IIIa receptor antagonists, abciximab, tirofiban, and eptifibatide differ at several levels, including molecular weight, binding characteristics, route of clearance, plasma half-life, platelet-bound and biologic half-lives, potential reversibility, approved indications, and use in clinical practice (Table 20-2).

The duration of platelet inhibition after drug discontinuation and the potential for reversing pharmacologic effects are particularly important properties in cases of emergent surgery and major hemorrhagic complications. In general, return of platelet function toward a physiologic state (≥50% inhibition) occurs within 4 hours after cessation of tirofiban and eptifibatide treatment. In contrast, cessation of 12 hours are required for return of platelet function following abciximab (Fig. 20-8). Some of the

Table 20-2 Agent-Specific Characteristics for Glycoprotein (GP)-IIB/IIIA Receptor Antagonists

Characteristic	Abciximab	Eptifibatide	Tirofiban
Type	Antibody	Peptide	Nonpeptide
Molecular weight, daltons	≈50,000	≈800	≈500
Platelet-bound half-life	Long	Short	Short
Plasma half-life	Short (min)	Extended (2 hr)	Extended (2 hr)
Drug/GP-IIb/IIIa receptor ratio	1.5–2.0	250–2500	>250
50% return of platelet function (without transfusion)	12 hr	≈4 hr	≈4 hr
Route of clearance	RES	Renal/hepatic	Renal
Dose adjustment required with renal insufficiency	No	Yes	Yes

RES, reticuloendothelial system.

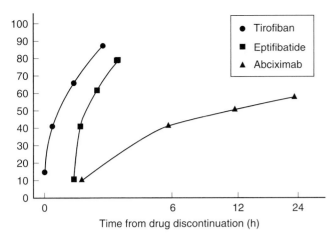

Figure 20-8 The biologic half-life for the small molecule glycoprotein (GP)-IIb/IIIa antagonists (eptifibatide, tirofiban) is relatively brief compared with that for abciximab. The vertical scale is percentage of normal platelet function.

delayed return of physiologic platelet function that occurs after abciximab termination may be counterbalanced by its low free plasma concentrations and drug/receptor ratio. These properties are consistent with the observed return of hemostatic potential after platelet transfusion (and may also limit platelet-inhibiting potential with marked mobilization of GP-IIb/IIIa receptors from intraplatelet storage pools). In contrast, high plasma concentrations observed with small-molecule inhibitors limit the effectiveness of platelet transfusions. Fibrinogen supplementation (fresh frozen plasma, cryoprecipitate) is the logical choice for restoration of hemostatic potential, given the competitive nature of binding and the relative availability of platelet GP-IIb/IIIa receptors.[109]

Do Platelet GP-IIb/IIIa Receptor Antagonists Achieve a Mortality Reduction?

When considering the potential benefits of treatment, a clinician must carefully consider the inherent risk for adverse outcomes. A meta-analysis of 19 randomized, placebo-controlled trials that included more than 20,000 patients with ACS (ST elevation and non-ST ACS) reported a 31% risk reduction (for mortality) at 30 days and 21% at 6 months in those patients given a platelet GP-IIb/IIIa receptor antagonist (vs those not treated) in the setting of PCI.[110] Major bleeding was increased only in trials in which anticoagulant therapy (UFH) was continued after the procedure (relative risk, 1.70).

Aggrenox

The dipyridamole component of Aggrenox and cilostazol, both phosphodiesterase inhibitors, are used predominantly in patients with peripheral vascular and cerebrovascular disease.

Aggrenox (Boehringer Ingelheim Pharmaceuticals Inc., Ridgefield, Conn) is a combination platelet antagonist that includes aspirin (25 mg) and dipridamole (200 mg extended-release preparation). It is typically administered twice daily.

Mechanisms of Action

The mechanism of action of aspirin has been discussed previously. Dipyridamole inhibits cyclic adenosine monophosphate (cAMP)-phosphodiesterase (PDE) and cyclic-3′,5′-GMP-PDE.[111]

Pharmacokinetics

The pharmacokinetic profile of aspirin has been summarized previously. Peak dipyridamole levels in plasma are achieved within several hours of oral administration (50 mg aspirin and 400 mg dose of Aggrenox). Extensive metabolism via conjugation with glucuronic acid occurs in the liver. No significant pharmacokinetic interactions have been reported between aspirin and dipyridamole coadministered as Aggrenox.

Pharmacodynamics

Dipyridamole inhibits platelet aggregation through two distinct mechanisms. First, it attenuates adenosine uptake into platelets (as well as endothelial cells and erythrocytes). The resulting increase elicits a rise in cellular adenylate cyclase concentrations, resulting in elevated cAMP levels, which inhibit platelet activation to several stimuli, including ADP, collagen, and platelet-activating factor. Dipyridamole also inhibits PDE. The subsequent increase in cAMP elevates nitric oxide concentration, facilitating platelet inhibitory potential.[112]

Adverse Effects

The ESPS (European Stroke Prevention Study)-2[113] reported that 79.9% of patients experienced at least one on-treatment adverse event. The most common adverse effects were GI complaints and headache.

Dipyridamole has vasodilatory effects and should be used with caution in patients with severe coronary artery disease, in whom episodes of angina pectoris may increase. Patients receiving Aggrenox should not be administered adenosine for myocardial perfusion studies.

Administration in Older Patients

Plasma concentrations of dipyridamole are nearly 40% higher in patients older than 65 years of age compared with younger individuals.

Clinical Experience

Aggrenox has not been studied in patients with ACS. The ESPS-2[113] included 6602 patients with ischemic stroke (76% of the total population) or transient ischemic attack who were randomly assigned to receive Aggrenox, dipyridamole alone, aspirin alone, or placebo. Aggrenox reduced the risk of stroke by 22.1% compared with aspirin, and by 24.4% compared with dipyridamole. Both differences were statistically significant ($P = .008$ and $P = .002$, respectively). Aggrenox is not considered interchangeable with its individual components, particularly aspirin, which may be required in larger doses among patients with coronary artery disease (CAD). In addition, the vasodilatory effects of dipyridamole may cause coronary "steal" and angina pectoris. Accordingly, Aggrenox should be used cautiously, if at all, in the setting of advanced CAD.

Cilostazol

Cilostazol is a guinolinone derivative that inhibits cellular PDE.

Mechanism of Action

Cilostazol inhibits PDE III, reducing cAMP degradation. The resulting increase within platelets and endothelial cells impairs platelet aggregation and leads to vasodilation.

Pharmacokinetics

Cilostazol is well absorbed after oral administration, particularly when given with a high-fat meal. Metabolism occurs via the hepatic cytochrome P450 enzymes, and most metabolites are excreted in the urine (75% of overall clearance). One of two active metabolites is responsible for more than 50% of PDE III inhibition. The elimination half-life of cilostazol (and its metabolites) is approximately 12 hours.

Pharmacodynamics

Increasing cAMP concentrations within endothelial cells cause vasodilation, whereas elevated levels within platelets impair their ability to aggregate.

Adverse Effects

The adverse effect most commonly associated with cilostazol administration is headache. Other relatively frequent causes of drug discontinuation include palpitations and diarrhea.

Several PDE III inhibitors have been associated with decreased survival in patients with class III/IV congestive heart failure. Accordingly, cilostazol should *not* be administered to patients with congestive heart failure (of any severity).

Use in Older Patients

The clearance of cilostazol (and its metabolites) has not been determined in patients older than age 65.

Use in Patients with Renal Insufficiency

Moderate to severe renal impairment increases cilostazol metabolite levels and alters protein binding of the parent compound. Patients with advanced renal insufficiency have not been studied.

Clinical Experience

Cilostazol is approved for the treatment of patients with intermittent claudication. Across eight clinical trials, improvement in walking distance (compared with placebo) was approximately 40% to 50%.[114] Although experience with cilostazol after coronary arterial stenting has been reported,[115] its long-term administration to patients with CAD has not been studied. Short-term coadministration with aspirin reduced ADP-mediated platelet aggregation by 30% to 40% (compared with aspirin alone). No randomized clinical trials of cilostazol in ACS have been conducted; however, it has been used for thromboprophylaxis after coronary arterial stenting.[116–119]

Cilostazol is recommended for patients with disabling claudication, particularly when revascularization cannot be offered. Although it has platelet-inhibiting properties, cilostazol should not be considered a substitute for aspirin or clopidogrel in patients with ACS who have concomitant peripheral vascular disease.

Hemorrhagic Complications Associated with Platelet-Directed Therapy

The contribution of platelets to the clinical expression of atherosclerotic vascular disease and the well-documented benefits derived from their pharmacologic attenuation provide a strong rationale for use in daily practice. Although the risk of drug-related complications must be considered in terms of all treatment strategies, this effort is particularly important for agents that impair hemostasis. It is not uncommon in current clinical practice for several platelet antagonists to be administered concomitantly.

A meta-analysis of 50 randomized clinical trials,[120] which included a total of 338,191 patients with atherothrombotic vascular disease, found a very low risk of hemorrhagic stroke (0.2%) with aspirin (≤325 mg daily), thienopyridines, and intravenous GP-IIb/IIIa receptor antagonists. The risk of major hemorrhage was greater, ranging from 1.7% with aspirin to 3.6% in those given intravenous GP-IIb/IIIa receptor antagonists (Fig. 20-9). Incidences of combined major and minor hemorrhagic events were 3.6% for low-intensity aspirin (<100 mg daily), 9.1% for moderate-intensity aspirin (100 to 325 mg daily), and 8.5% for clopidogrel.

Nonsteroidal Anti-inflammatory Drugs

Nonsteroidal anti-inflammatory drugs (NSAIDs) are among the most commonly used pharmaceutical agents in the United States. Although the potential cardiovascular risk associated with their use, particularly when taken over prolonged periods of time, has not yet been defined, most physicians recommend short courses of therapy at the lowest effective dose. A listing of NSAIDs that emphasizes their platelet-inhibiting properties and biologic half-lives appears in Table 20-3.

Anticoagulants

The participation of coagulation proteases, particularly factor Xa and factor IIa (thrombin), in several phases of cell-based coagulation forms the basis for the routine use of pharmacologic therapy in patients with thrombotic disorders of the arterial circulatory system. Among hospitalized patients, thrombin-inhibiting drugs (UFH, LMWH, pentasaccharide [fondaparinux]) and direct thrombin inhibitors (DTIs) are used frequently, often in combination with platelet-directed antagonists, creating substantial pertubations in hemostasis.

Unfractionated Heparin

Unfractionated heparin is a heterogeneous, negatively charged mucopolysaccharide consisting of approximately 18 to 50 saccharide units (molecular weight, 5000 to 30,000 daltons). Antithrombin III (ATIII) neutralizes thrombin and other activated serine proteases (factors Xa, IXa, XIa, and XIIa)—a reaction that is increased 10^3- to 10^4-fold by binding of heparin to ATIII.

After IV administration, heparin binds to a variety of plasma proteins, endothelial cells, and macrophages, explaining, in part, the wide variability in anticoagulant effects

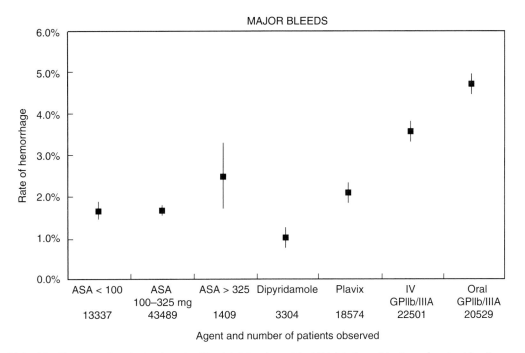

Figure 20-9 Major bleeding according to treatment with platelet antagonists. Weighted combination of major bleeding events with 95% confidence interval (CI) across treatment group. (From Patrono C: Aspirin as an antiplatelet drug. N Engl J Med 330:1287–1294, 1994.)

Table 20-3 Platelet-Inhibiting Properties of Nonsteroidal Anti-Inflammatory Drugs

Drug	Site of Action	Route	Biologic $t_{\{1/2\}}$	Recommended Time off Therapy*
Piroxicam	COX-1, -2	PO	50 hr	10 days
Indomethacin	COX-1, -2	PO/PR	5 hr	2 days
Ketorolac	COX-1, -2	PO/IV	7 hr	2 days
Ibuprofen	COX-1, -2	PO	2 hr	1 day
Naproxen	COX-1, -2	PO	13 hr	2 days
Diclofenac	COX-1, -2	PO	2 hr	1 day
Celecoxib	COX-2	PO	10–17 hr†	None

*Prior to invasive procedures.
†$t_{\{1/2\}}$ increases with dose.
$t_{\{1/2\}}$, half-life; COX, cyclo-oxygenase.

observed for a given dose. It is cleared from the circulation through a rapid saturable mechanism and a slower first-order mechanism. The result is a dose-dependent half-life that ranges from 60 minutes after an IV dose of 100 U per kilogram to 180 minutes for a dose of 400 U per kilogram.[121,122]

Adverse Effects

Heparin-induced thrombocytopenia (HIT) (see Chapter 25) and hemorrhage are the most feared complications of heparin administration. Another adverse effect is osteopenia (with long-term administration).

Clinical trials have been conducted to compare the benefits of heparin and aspirin among patients with unstable angina and non–ST segment elevation MI. The first trial, performed by Théroux and colleagues,[123] compared aspirin (325 mg twice daily), heparin (5000 U bolus, 1000 U per hour by intravenous infusion), their combination, and placebo in 479 patients. This is the only study that compared heparin (alone) and aspirin (alone), as well as their combination. Refractory angina occurred in 8.5%, 16.5%, and

10.7% of patients, respectively (0.47 relative risk for heparin compared with aspirin [95% CI, 0.21 to 1.05; $P = .06$]). MI occurred in 0.9%, 3.3%, and 1.6% of patients, respectively (0.25 relative risk [95% CI, 0.03 to 2.271; $P = .18$]), and any event was observed in 9.3%, 16.5%, and 11.5% of patients, respectively (0.52 relative risk [95% CI, 0.24 to 1.14; $P = .10$]). Serious bleeding, defined as a fall in hemoglobin concentration of 2 g or more, or the need for a transfusion, occurred in 1.7%, 1.7%, and 3.3% of patients, respectively. Most events were followed by cardiac catheterization.

Remaining trials investigated the potential advantages of combination therapy (heparin plus aspirin) over aspirin monotherapy. Although these treatments were not statistically different, consistent trends observed across each study favored combined pharmacotherapy and its ability to reduce death or MI (combined end point). Pooled analysis of the Antithrombotic Therapy in Acute Coronary Syndromes (ATACS) trial, the Research Group on Instability in Coronary Artery Disease in Southeast Sweden (RISC) study, and the Théroux and colleagues trial yielded a relative risk of 0.44 (95% CI, 0.21 to 0.93) for death/MI, in favor of combination therapy.[124–128]

Therapeutic Levels of Anticoagulation

Although the pathobiology of non–ST segment ACS is fundamentally understood, the required intensity of anticoagulation remains poorly defined. The challenge is multifactorial but likely relates to inherent complexities in the pharmacokinetics and pharmacodynamics of heparin, the dynamic nature of coronary arterial thrombosis, and the use of coagulation tests designed primarily to assess hemostatic potential. In essence, current laboratory-based tests are oriented more toward the drug (and its potential to cause bleeding) than the disease.

Available evidence supports a weight-adjusted dosing regimen with heparin therapy as a means of providing a more predictable and constant level of systemic anticoagulation. An initial bolus of 60 to 70 U per kilogram (maximum, 5000 U; initial infusion, 12 to 15 U/kg/hr IV [maximum, 1000 U per hour]) titrated to a target partial thromboplastin time (PTT) of 50 to 75 seconds is recommended, assuming the pretreatment PTT is normal.[128–130]

A "weaning" schedule at the time of treatment completion may reduce the occurrence of rebound thrombin generation and ischemic/thrombotic events.[130]

Indirect, Selective Factor Xa Inhibitors

Synthetic Pentasaccharide

Fondaparinux (Arixtra; GlaxoSmithKline, Research Triangle Park, NC) is a synthetic pentasaccharide that requires ATIII for selective FXa binding.[131] Different from heparin compounds, fondaparinux does not interact with platelets (or platelet-derived proteins). After subcutaneous administration in healthy volunteers, fondaparinux is nearly 100% bioavailable, and absorption is rapid (maximum plasma concentration [C_{max}] within 2 hours).[132] Clearance occurs through renal mechanisms with a terminal half-life of 17 ± 3 hours (slightly longer in elderly volunteers). Overall, drug clearance is 25% slower in patients with mild renal impairment (creatine clearance [CrCl], 50 to 80 mL per minute), approximately 40% slower with moderate renal impairment (CrCl, 30 to 50 mL per minute), and 55% slower in the setting of severe renal impairment (CrCl, <30 mL per minute).

The OASIS (Organization to Assess Strategies in Acute Ischemic Syndromes)-5 Study[133] assigned 20,078 patients with ACS to receive fondaparinux (2.5 mg daily SQ) or enoxaparin (1 mg per kilogram of body weight twice daily SQ) for a mean of 6 days and evaluated death, MI, or refractory ischemia at 9 days (the primary outcome measure), as well as major bleeding and a combination of the two. The numbers of patients with primary outcome events were similar in the two groups (fondaparinux, 5.8%, vs enoxaparin, 5.7%; hazard ratio in the fondaparinux group, 1.01; 95% CI, 0.90 to 1.13), satisfying the noninferiority criteria. The rate of major bleeding at 9 days was markedly lower with fondaparinux than with enoxaparin (2.2% vs 4.1%; hazard ratio, 0.52; $P < .001$). A composite of the primary outcome measure in major bleeding at 9 days favored fondaparinux (7.3% vs 9%; hazard ratio, 0.81; $P < .001$).

Fondaparinux was always associated with a significant reduction in the number of patients with fatal bleeding and TIMI major bleeding. Regardless of treatment, patients who had major bleeding during hospitalization had significantly higher rates of death, reinfarction, or stroke at 30 days and at 180 days than did patients without major or minor bleeding. These higher event rates associated with bleeding persisted after adjustments were made for a number of clinical characteristics that are commonly associated with bleeding. Accordingly, almost the entire difference in mortality between fondaparinux- and enoxaparin-treated patients at the end of the study could be attributed to the lower rate of bleeding associated with fondaparinux.

In a subgroup analysis, benefits and risks were found to be consistently in favor of fondaparinux. Rates of bleeding were consistently lower with fondaparinux, regardless of whether UFH was administered before randomization. The proportions of patients undergoing PCI (39.5% in the fondaparinux group and 39.5% in the enoxaparin group) and coronary arterial bypass grafting (15.3% and 14.5%, respectively) were similar in the two groups. Rates of the combination of death, MI, and refractory ischemia were similar at 9 days, at 30 days, and at the end of the study. An increase in guiding catheter thrombus formation was observed with fondaparinux (0.9% vs 0.3%); however, rates of other complications, including pseudoaneruysm formation, large hematomas, major bleeding, and complications involving the vascular access site, were all less common with fondaparinux than with enoxaparin. Collectively, the rate of death, MI, stroke, major bleeding, or any procedural complication at 9 days was 16.6% with fondaparinux as compared with 20.6% with enoxaparin (relative risk, 0.81; 95% CI, 0.73 to 0.90; $P < .001$).

The OASIS-6 study[134] was a randomized double-blind comparison of fondaparinux 2.5 mg once daily versus placebo for up to 8 days in 12,092 patients with ST segment elevation MI. The composite of death or reinfarction at 30 days served as the primary outcome measure, with secondary assessments at 9 days and at final follow-up (3 to 6 months). Death or reinfarction at 30 days was significantly reduced from 11.2% in the control group to 9.7% among patients receiving fondaparinux (hazard ratio, 0.86; 95% CI, 0.77 to 0.9; $P = .008$). These benefits were observed at 9 days and at study completion. Mortality was significantly reduced throughout the study in patients receiving fondaparinux; in a comparison of patients receiving fondaparinux versus those given UFH, fondaparinux was found to be superior in preventing death or reinfarction at 30 days (hazard ratio, 0.82; 95% CI, 0.66 to 1.02; $P = .08$) and at study end (hazard ratio, 0.77; 95% CI, 0.64 to 0.93; $P = .008$). Significant benefit was observed among patients receiving fibrinolytic therapy (hazard ratio, 0.79; $P = .003$) and those not given reperfusion therapy. No benefit was noted in patients undergoing primary PCI. Rates of death, MI, and severe bleeding were significantly lower at day 9 with fondaparinux (hazard ratio, 0.83; 95% CI, 0.73 to 0.94; $P = .003$), as they were at study completion. The composite outcome of death, MI, or stroke was reduced at all three time points.

The use of a single fixed dose (2.5 mg once daily SQ) of fondaparinux without monitoring or dose adjustment for weight across a broad range of creatinine levels, coupled with simplicity, safety, and efficacy in ACS, will likely facilitate its use and may transfer, with further investigation, to prehospital and possibly posthospital settings among carefully selected patients. The apparent lack of HIT associated with fondaparinux use is also attractive.

Low Molecular Weight Heparin

LMWH is prepared by the depolymerization of porcine heparin. A variety of processes are used, yielding distinctive products whose molecular weights range from 4000 to 6500 days.[135] Similar to heparin, approximately one third of LMWH polysaccharide chains contain the pentasaccharide sequence necessary for binding to ATIII. The LMWH/ATIII complex (consisting of a predominance of shorter chain polysaccharides) has relatively weak thrombin inhibitory activity but retains the ability to inactivate factor Xa. The ratio of anti-Xa activity to anti-IIa activity ranges from 2:1 to 4:1. Similar to heparin, LMWH is not able to inhibit thrombin bound to fibrin.

Pharmacokinetics

When LMWH is administered in fixed or weight-adjusted doses by the subcutaneous route, more than 90% of the dose is absorbed. In contrast to heparin, LMWH has minimal binding to cells or plasma proteins, resulting in persistence of free drug in the circulation and a longer plasma half-life of activity. Although the half-life of heparin averages about 90 minutes, the plasma half-life of LMWH averages about 180 minutes (the half-lives of three LMWHs range from 90 to 260 minutes). However, because LMWH is nearly always administered subcutaneously, the functional half-life may be considerably longer.

Antibodies directed against complexes of LMWH and platelet factor 4 may develop but at a rate lower than is experienced with heparin therapy. Full-blown HIT may occur. Equally rare is necrosis at the site of skin injection with LMWH, which may represent a form of local HIT. LMWH cannot be administered as a substitute for heparin in patients with HIT.

Clinical Experience

Original experiences with LMWH[136] involved 205 patients with unstable angina who were randomly assigned to aspirin (200 mg daily), aspirin (200 mg daily) plus heparin (5000 U bolus, 400 U/kg/day IV infusion), or high-dose nadroparin (214 IU per kilogram twice daily by subcutaneous injection) plus aspirin (200 mg daily). Patients underwent continuous ST segment monitoring during the first 48 hours of treatment. Overall, 73% of patients receiving LMWH were free from ischemic events, compared with 39% of those given heparin and 40% of patients given aspirin alone. Fewer silent ischemic events occurred in the LMWH group (18%) compared with those receiving heparin (29%) or aspirin alone (34%). Recurrent angina occurred in 95%, 26%, and 19% of patients, respectively, and MIs were not reported in LMWH-treated patients (compared with 1% in the heparin and 6% in the aspirin alone groups). Major bleeding occurred infrequently in all treatment groups.

A larger study (FRagmin during InStability in Coronary artery disease [FRISC]-1)[137] included 1506 patients with unstable angina and non–ST segment elevation MI who were randomly assigned to LMWH (dalteparin, 120 IU per kilogram of body weight subcutaneously [maximum 10,000 IU] twice daily for 6 days, then 7500 IU once daily for 35 to 45 days) or placebo. All patients received SQ PO aspirin (300 mg first dose, 75 mg daily thereafter). Accordingly, FRISC-1 investigated the combination of LMWH plus aspirin versus aspirin alone. The risk of death or MI was reduced by 63% at day 6. The probability of death or MI and the need for revascularization remained lower in LMWH-treated patients at 40 days; however, little difference between groups was observed beyond the treatment period.

In the FRIC (FRagmin In unstable Coronary artery disease) study,[138] 1482 patients with unstable angina and non–ST segment elevation MI were assigned twice-daily weight-adjusted SC injections of LMWH (dalteparin 120 IU per kilogram SQ) or dose-adjusted (target PTT, 1.5× control) IV heparin for 6 days (acute treatment phase). Patients randomly assigned to UFH received a continuous infusion for at least 48 hours and were given the option of continuing the infusion or changing to a SQ regimen (12,500 U every 12 hours). In the double-blind comparison that took place from days 6 to 45 (prolonged treatment phase), patients received LMWH (dalteparin, 7500 IU SQ once daily) or placebo. Aspirin (75 to 165 mg/day) was started in all patients as early as possible after hospital admission and was continued throughout the study. During the first 6 days, rates of death, recurrent angina, and MI were 7.6% in heparin-treated patients and 9.3% in LMWH-treated patients (relative risk, 1.18; 95% CI, 0.84 to 1.66). Revascularization was required in 5.3% and 4.8% (CI, 0.57 to 1.35). Between days 6 and 45, the composite end point was reached by 12.3% of patients in the LMWH and placebo groups.

The ESSENCE (Efficacy and Safety of Subcutaneous Enoxaparin in Non–Q Wave Coronary Events) trial[139] randomly assigned 3171 patients with angina at rest or non–ST segment elevation MI to LMWH (enoxaparin, 1 mg per kilogram SQ twice daily) or IV heparin (target PTT, 55 to 85 seconds). Therapy was continued for a minimum of 48 hours (maximum, 8 days). All patients received aspirin (100 to 325 mg daily). Median duration of therapy for both groups was 2.6 days. At 14 days, the risk of death, recurrent angina, or MI was 16.6% among patients receiving LMWH and 19.8% in those given heparin (16% risk reduction). A similar risk reduction (15.0%) for the composite outcome was observed at 30 days. The benefit of LMWH treatment was maintained at 1 year.[140]

The TIMI-11B study compared enoxaparin and heparin in 3910 patients with unstable angina and non–ST segment elevation MI.[141] This trial design had several unique features that differentiated it from the ESSENCE design. First, enoxaparin therapy was initiated with a 30 mg IV bolus, followed by 1.0 mg per kilogram SQ twice daily. Second, heparin treatment was given according to a weight-adjusted dosing strategy (a 70 U per kilogram bolus, followed by 15 U/kg/h IV infusion to a target PTT 1.5 to 2.5× control). Finally, an out-of-hospital treatment phase compared enoxaparin and placebo for approximately 6 weeks (patients ≥65 kg received 60 mg SQ twice daily; those <65 kg were given 45 mg SQ twice daily for a total of 43 days). Treatment with enoxaparin was associated with

357

a significant reduction in the composite outcome of death, MI, or urgent revascularization compared with heparin at day 14 (14.2 vs 16.7%; RRR, 15%; P = .03). Continued treatment beyond the initial hospital phase did not provide added benefit (17.3 vs 19.7%; RRR, 12%; P = .051).

A meta-analysis of the ESSENCE and TIMI-IIB trials, totaling 7081 patients with non–ST segment elevation ACS, revealed a 20% reduction in the risk of any ischemic event,[142] favoring enoxaparin over heparin. Differences were statistically significant at 48 hours and 43 days. The combined end point of death or MI was reduced by 20% at 48 hours (P = .02) and by 18% at 43 days (P = .02). A significant treatment benefit for enoxaparin on rate of death, nonfatal MI, or urgent revascularization was observed at 1 year (hazard ratio, 0.88; P = .008; absolute difference, 2.5%). A progressively greater treatment benefit was observed as the level of patient risk at baseline increased.

Combined Pharmacology and Interventional Strategies

FRISC-2 (FRagmin and fast revascularization during InStability in Coronary artery disease)[143] included 2267 patients with unstable coronary disease who received 5 days of dalteparin (120 IU per kilogram SQ every 12 hours) and were then randomly assigned to an invasive or conservative treatment strategy. In a separate randomization, patients received dalteparin (5000 to 7500 IU SQ every 12 hours) or placebo injections for 3 months. By 30 days, a significant reduction in death or MI favored dalteparin-treated patients (3.1 vs 5.9%; P = .002). This benefit decayed over the next 2 months. An invasive strategy (coronary angiography and revascularization) was associated with a significant reduction in death or MI at 6 months compared with ischemia-driven revascularization (9.4% vs 12.1%; P = .03). Mortality rates were 1.9% and 2.9%, respectively. At the 24-month follow-up, reductions in mortality (3.7% vs 12.7%; risk ratio, 0.72; P = .005) and in the composite end point of death or MI (12.1 vs 16.3%; risk ratio, 0.74; P = .003) were noted in the invasive rather than the noninvasive group. The need for repeat hospitalizations and late revascularization procedures was reduced with an early invasive strategy as well.

The RITA (Randomized Intervention Trial of unstable Angina) study randomly assigned 1810 patients with non–ST segment elevation ACS who received enoxaparin (1 mg per kilogram SQ twice daily for 2 to 8 days) and aspirin to an early intervention or conservative strategy.[144] At 4 months, 9.6% of patients randomly assigned to early intervention had died, experienced an MI, or experienced refractory angina compared with 14.5% in the conservative group (risk ratio, 0.66; 95% CI, 0.51 to 0.85; P = .001). Death or MI was similar in both treatment groups at 1 year (7.6% vs 8.3%, respectively; risk ratio, 0.91; 95% CI, 0.67 to 1.25; P = .58). Fewer patients undergoing early intervention experienced symptoms of angina or required antianginal medications.

In the SYNERGY (Superior Yield of the New Strategy of Enoxaparin, Revascularization and Glycoprotein IIb/IIIa Inhibitors) trial,[145] 10,027 high-risk patients were randomly assigned to heparin or enoxaparin. Overall, 92% of patients underwent coronary angiography, 47% had PCI (in hospital), and 57% received GP-IIb/IIIa antagonists. The primary end point of death or nonfatal MI at 3 days occurred in 14.5% of patients assigned to heparin and 14.0% of those given enoxaparin (OR, 0.956; 95% CI, 0.869 to 1.063),

fulfilling the noninferiority criteria. No differences in ischemic events during PCI occurred among the various thrombin inhibitors. Major bleeding was modestly increased with enoxaparin; however, transfusion rates did not differ, and a relationship between advancing age, reduced creatinine clearance, and risk of hemorrhage was noted.

The SYNERGY trial supports enoxaparin as an alternative to heparin in high-risk patients who are treated aggressively. The impact of age and renal insufficiency on bleeding risk is important and should stimulate further investigation of preferred dosing strategies.

In the ExTRACT (Enoxaparin and Thrombolysis Reperfusion for Acute Myocardial Infarction Treatment)-TIMI 25 study,[146] 20,506 patients with ST segment elevation MI who were scheduled to undergo fibrinolysis received enoxaparin throughout the index hospitalization or heparin for at least 48 hours. The primary efficacy end point, death or nonfatal recurrent MI through day 30, occurred in 12% of patients in the heparin group and 9.9% of those in the enoxaparin group (17% reduction in relative risk; P < .001). Nonfatal reinfarction occurred in 4.5% of patients receiving heparin and 3% of those who were given enoxaparin (33% reduction in relative risk; P < .001). A nonstatistically significant reduction in death occurred (7.5% vs 6.9%, respectively; P = .11). Major bleeding occurred in 1.4% and 2.1% of patients, respectively. The composite of death, nonfatal reinfarction, or nonfatal intracranial hemorrhage (a measure of net clinical benefit) occurred in 12.2% of patients administered heparin and 10.1% of those given enoxaparin (P < .001).

LMWH and Platelet GP-IIb/IIIa Receptor Antagonist Combination Therapy

The effective level of factor Xa inhibition has not been determined for patients with ACS who are receiving LMWH. Available information, derived from clinical trials of PCI, shows that anti-Xa activity >0.5 IU per milliliter is associated with a low incidence of ischemic/thrombotic and hemorrhagic events.[147] Attenuative coagulation tests, including traditional PTT and activated clotting time (ACT) assays, may provide some insight into LMWH preparations characterized by low anti-Xa/anti-IIa activity.[148]

The potential benefits of enoxaparin (1 mg per kilogram IV every 12 hours) and the platelet GP-IIb/IIIa receptor antagonist tirofiban (10 µg/kg IV bolus over 3 min, followed by 0.1 µg/kg/min IV for 48 to 108 hours) versus weight-adjusted UFH and tirofiban were investigated in the A to Z trial[149]—a prospective, open-label, randomized study of 3987 patients with non–ST segment elevation ACS. Death, recurrent MI, or refractory ischemia at 7 days occurred in 8.4% of enoxaparin-treated patients and 9.4% of those receiving heparin (hazard ratio, 0.88) (criteria for noninferiority satisfied). Risk reductions were of greater magnitude (favoring enoxaparin) among patients at highest risk and those treated conservatively. Major bleeding was more common in patients receiving enoxaparin (0.9% vs 0.4% with heparin; one excess major hemorrhagic event for every 200 patients treated); however, transfusion rates were low overall (0.9%) and did not differ between groups.

A systematic evaluation of clinical trials comparing enoxaparin and heparin for the treatment of patients with ACS was conducted by Petersen and colleagues.[150] A total of 6 trials that included 21,946 patients were analyzed; a statistically significant reduction in the combined

30-day end point of death or MI favored enoxaparin (10.1% vs 11.0%; OR, 0.91). Patients who were receiving no pretreatment anticoagulant therapy were found to derive a particularly robust benefit from enoxaparin (8.0% vs 9.4%; OR, 0.81). Major hemorrhage and blood transfusion rates did not differ between treatment groups.

In the ACUITY (Acute Catheterization and Urgent Triage Strategy) trial[151] (presented at the Amercian College of Cardiology National Meeting, Atlanta, GA, 2006), 13,819 patients with ACS randomly received bivalirudin plus a GP-IIb/IIIa receptor angatonist, heparin (heparin or enoxaparin) plus a GP-IIb/IIIa receptor antagonist, or bivalirudin alone. The primary outcome, which consisted of all-cause mortality, MI, or unplanned revascularization for ischemia at 30 days, did not differ significantly between groups. Bivalirudin alone was associated with a 50% reduction in major bleeding complications. On the basis of findings from ACUITY, bivalirudin use in hospitalized patients increased, necessitating greater familiarity with its properties among consulting hematologists.

Influence of Renal Function

Factor Xa inhibition pharmacokinetics was studied in 445 patients receiving enoxaparin (1.0 to 1.25 mg per kilogram SQ every 12 hours).[152] Mean apparent clearance, distribution volume, and plasma half-life were 0.733 L per hour, 5.24 L, and 5 hours, respectively. CrCl emerged as the most important factor affecting apparent clearance, area under the curve, and anti-Xa activity. Clearance was reduced by 22% in patients with CrCl <40 mL per minute (compared with patients with normal renal performance [CrCl >80 mL per minute]). These patients had higher peak and trough anti-Xa activity and were more likely to experience major hemorrhagic events. Renal performance may not influence pharmacokinetics after single-dose intravenous administration of enoxaparin. Studies designed to evaluate appropriate dosing and possible dose titration in patients with end-stage renal disease must be undertaken to provide guidance in ways to approach optimal patient care.

Direct Thrombin Inhibitors

The pivotal role of thrombin in all phases of coagulation, cellular proliferation, and cellular interactions involved centrally in inflammatory processes provides an attractive target for pharmacologic inhibition. Because these agents directly inhibit thrombin independently of ATIII, they are referred to as a class of direct thrombin inhibitors (DTIs). The development of DTIs has evolved rapidly to include intravenous and oral preparations.

Hirudin. Hirudin is extracted from the parapharyngeal gland of the medicinal leech *Hirudo medicinalis*. Several derivatives and recombinant preparations have been developed, including the most widely used agent lepirudin (Refludan; ZLB Behring GmbH, Marburg, Germany).

Hirudin binds to the catalytic and fibrinogen-binding sites of thrombin and thus is considered a bivalent inhibitor.

Pharmokinetics. The plasma half-life of hirudin is 50 to 65 minutes, and it has a biologic half-life of 2 hours.[153] Properties of heparins, hirudin, and bivalirudin are highlighted in Table 20-4. The predominant renal clearance of hirudin must be emphasized for safe clinical use.

Hirudin forms a tight complex with thrombin, inhibiting the conversion of fibrinogen to fibrin and thrombin-induced platelet aggregation. These actions are independent of ATIII. Thrombin bound to fibrin is also complexed and inhibited. On the downside, the ability of thrombin to complex with thrombomodulin and activating protein C is also inhibited. Hirudin does not bind to platelet factor 4, nor does it elicit antibodies that induce platelet and endothelial cell activation; thus, it can be safely administered to patients with HIT. Hirudin has weak immunogenicity, so that diminished (or rarely increased) responsiveness after repeated dosing is possible. The use of hirudin in the management of heparin-induced thrombocytopenia is discussed in Chapter 25.

Clinical Use. In the GUSTO IIb trial,[154] patients with non–ST segment elevation ACS received heparin or hirudin (0.1 mg per kilogram IV bolus; 0.1 mg/kg/h IV infusion). At 24 hours, the risk of death or nonfatal MI was reduced in hirudin-treated patients (1.3% vs 2.1%; P = .001). The primary end point of death or nonfatal MI at 30 days was reached in 8.9% and 9.8% of patients, respectively (OR, 0.89; P = .006). The risk of moderate bleeding was increased with hirudin treatment (8.8% vs 7.7%; P = .03).

The OASIS-1 study[155] included 909 patients with unstable angina or suspected MI without ST segment elevation who were randomly assigned to receive heparin (5000 U bolus IV; infusion of 1000 to 1200 U per hour), low-dose hirudin (0.2 mg per kilogram bolus; IV infusion of 0.1 mg/kg/hr), or moderate-dose hirudin (0.4 mg per kilogram IV bolus; infusion of 0.15 mg/kg/hr IV). Doses of heparin

Table 20-4 Properties of Heparins, Bivalirudin, and Hirudin

Property	Heparin	LMWH	Fondaparinux	Bivalirudin and Hirudin
Thrombin inhibition	Requires ATIII	Requires ATIII	Requires ATIII	Directly inhibited
Clot-bound thrombin	Not inhibited	Not inhibited	Not inhibited	Inhibited
Thrombocytopenia	Yes	Yes	Not reported	No
Immunogenicity	Yes	Yes	Not reported	Rare
Effects on PTT	Yes	No	No	Yes
Effects on PT	Minimal, some at high doses	No	No	Moderate*
Metabolism	Cellular and renal binding	Renal	Renal	Renal
Antidote	Protamine	Protamine partially	None	None

*Greater effect with bivalirudin.
PTT, activated partial thromboplastin time; ATIII, antithrombin III; LMWH, low molecular weight heparin; PT, prothrombin time.

and hirudin were titrated to a target PTT of 60 to 100 seconds. Hirudin, compared with heparin, reduced the composite incidence of cardiovascular death, MI, or refractory angina at 7 days (OR, 0.57; 95% CI, 0.32 to 1.02), as well as a composite of death, MI, or refractory/severe angina requiring revascularization at 7 days (OR, 0.49; 95% CI, 0.27 to 0.86). Overall event rates were lowest in the moderate-dose hirudin group.

Favorable results in OASIS-1 prompted a large phase 3 trial, OASIS-2,[156] which randomly assigned 10,141 patients with non–ST segment elevation ACS to a 72-hour infusion of moderate-dose hirudin (as defined in OASIS-1) or heparin. The primary outcome (composite of death or MI at 7 and 35 days) was reported in 3.6% and 4.2% of patients (OR, 0.87; 95% CI, 0.75 to 1.01), respectively. Although statistically significant differences between groups were not observed, the combined OASIS-1 and OASIS-2 experience revealed a significant reduction in the likelihood of death or MI at 35 days among hirudin-treated patients (OR, 0.86; 95% CI, 0.74 to 0.99).

Hirudin is almost exclusively excreted through the kidneys; as a result of this fact, renal function must be considered carefully prior to administration. Most clinical trials excluded patients with a serum creatinine of 2.0 mg per deciliter or greater. It is important to acknowledge that even in the setting of mild renal impairment (CrCl, 50 to 80 mL per minute), excessive levels of systemic anticoagulation (and accompanying risk for hemorrhage) may occur without dosing modification. If hirudin is administered to patients with renal insufficiency, frequent PTT monitoring is highly recommended.

Bivalirudin. Bivalirduin (Angiomax; The Medicines Company, Parsippany, NJ) is an intravenous DTI that acts by binding to the catalytic and anion-binding exosite. It prolongs thrombin time, PTT, and prothrombin time (PT) in a concentration-dependent manner.

Pharmacokinetics. After a 1 mg per kilogram IV bolus is given, peak concentrations are achieved rapidly, and a plasma half-life of 25 minutes is seen among patients with normal renal function. Drug elimination is reduced by 20% in the setting of moderate renal impairment, by 50% in severe renal impairment, and by 80% in dialysis-dependent patients. Pharmacokinetic characteristics translate to half-lives of 34 minutes, 57 minutes, and 3.5 hours, respectively.

Bivalirudin is U. S. Food and Drug Administration (FDA) approved for use in patients with non–ST segment elevation ACS who are undergoing PCI. The basis for approval stems from several large-scale clinical trials.[157] Among 4312 patients with new-onset, severe, accelerating, or resting angina undergoing PCI, a 22% reduction in death, MI, or urgent revascularization at 7 days was observed in those given bivalirudin compared with heparin (6.2 vs 7.9%; P = .03). Absolute and relative differences were maintained at 90 days. A marked reduction (62%) in bleeding complications was reported among bivalirudin-treated patients.

In the REPLACE-1 (Randomized Evaluation in Percutaneous coronary intervention Linking Angiomax to reduced Clinical Events) trial,[158] 1020 patients received bivalirudin (0.75 mg per kilogram IV bolus; infusion of 1.75 mg/kg/hr IV) or heparin. Prior treatment with aspirin and a thienopyridine was encouraged in anticipation of stenting. A platelet GP-IIb/IIIa receptor antagonist was administered to 71% of patients. Bivalirudin was associated with a 19% reduction in the clinical end point of death, MI, urgent revascularization, and bleeding complications (minor, major, transfusions) at 48 hours.

REPLACE-2[159] randomly assigned 6010 patients undergoing urgent or elective PCI to bivalirudin plus a provisional GP-IIb/IIIa receptor antagonist (abciximab or eptifibatide) or to UFH plus a GP-IIb/IIIa receptor antagonist. Aspirin and clopidogrel pretreatment were recommended. Approximately 45% of patients had unstable angina or MI (within the prior 7 days). The composite of death, MI, and urgent revascularization at 30 days occurred in 7.1% of heparin-treated patients and in 7.6% of those treated with bivalirudin (OR, 0.917; 95% CI, 0.772 to 1.089; P = .32). Major bleeding was documented in 4.1% and 2.4% of patients, respectively (P = .001). Minor bleeding (25.7% vs 13.4%; P = .001) and thrombocytopenia (<100,000 per microliter) (1.7% vs 0.7%; P < .001) were also less common with bivalirudin treatment. GP-IIb/IIIa receptor antagonist therapy was given to 7.2% of bivalirudin-treated patients.

Impact of Renal Insufficiency. Patients with moderate and severe renal impairment have reductions in bivalirudin clearance: however, analyses of data derived from 4312 patients with unstable angina showed increased bleeding risk for bivalirudin- and heparin-treated patients with progressive degrees of renal insufficiency. The incidence of major bleeding was, however, consistently less for bivalirudin than heparin at all levels of renal impairment.[157]

Overall data suggest that a bivalirudin dose adjustment is indicated for patients with moderate or severe renal impairment. Encouraging results from REPLACE-2 may provide guidance for reducing hemorrhagic risk in patients with renal insufficiency by virtue of the short infusion length for bivalirudin administration and provisional use of GP-IIb/IIIa receptor antagonists (which may themselves increase the risk of hemorrhage in this high-risk patient subset).[159]

The use of bivalirudin among individuals with and those at risk for HIT who require PCI is favored (over argatroban) by many interventional cardiologists on the basis of experience in the angioplasty suite and comparative analyses among patients with ACS.

Argatroban. Argatroban (Glaxo-SmithKline) is a synthetic DTI derived from L-arginine that acts by binding reversibly to the active site of thrombin. A linear relationship has been noted between argatroban plasma levels and prolongations of thrombin time, PTT, and PT.

Pharmacokinetics. Peak concentrations of argatroban are reached rapidly after IV injection, and the plasma half-life ranges between 39 and 51 minutes. Metabolism occurs in the liver by hydroxylation and aromatization via CYP3A4/5.

Clinical Use. Argatroban is approved for use among patients with HIT, including those with current HIT and previous HIT and/or those with heparin-dependent antibodies.

Comparative Benefits of Direct Thrombin Inhibitors. A meta-analysis of clinical trials was performed to obtain additional information and precise estimates of DTIs in the management of ACS.[160] A total of 11 randomized trials that included 35,970 patients were identified. Compared with heparin, DTIs were associated with a lower risk of death or MI at the end of treatment (up to 7 days) (4.3% vs 5.1%; OR, 0.85; 95% CI, 0.77 to 0.94; $P = .001$) and at 30 days (7.4% vs 8.2%; OR, 0.91; 95% CI, 0.84 to 0.99; $P = .02$). Seven trials studied 30,154 patients who had an ACS (unstable angina or non–ST segment elevation MI) or were undergoing PCI. In those with ACS, treatment with a DTI was associated with a reduction in death or MI compared with UFH (3.7% vs 4.6%; OR, 0.80; 95%, CI, 0.70 to 0.92). Similar reductions were observed in PCI trials (3.0% vs 3.8%; OR, 0.79; 95% CI, 0.59 to 1.06). A statistically insignificant increased rate of major bleeding with DTIs was seen in trials of ACS (1.6% vs 1.4%; OR, 1.11; 95% CI, 0.93 to 1.34), but a significant difference was noted in PCI trials (3.7% vs 7.6%; OR, 0.46; 95% CI, 0.36 to 0.59). No differences in rates of intracranial hemorrhage were noted.

Risk reduction in death or MI at the end of treatment was similar in trials comparing hirudin or bivalirudin with UFH, but a slight excess was seen with univalent inhibitors (4.7% vs 3.5%; OR, 1.35; 95% CI, 0.89 to 2.05). When major bleeding outcomes were analyzed by specific DTIs, hirudin was associated with an excess of major bleeding compared with heparin (1.7% vs 1.3%; OR, 1.28; 95% CI, 1.06 to 1.55), whereas both bivalirudin (4.2% vs 9.0%; OR, 0.55; CI, 0.34 to 0.56) and univalent inhibitors (0.7% vs 1.3%; OR, 0.55; 95% CI, 0.25 to 1.20) were associated with lower rates of major bleeding.

CURRENT GUIDELINES FOR ANTITHROMBOTIC THERAPY IN CARDIOVASCULAR DISEASE

Several national and international task forces, assembled by the American Heart Association, American College of Cardiology, American College of Chest Physicians, and Society for Cardiovascular Angiography and Interventions, have established guidelines for the management of ACS.[161–163] Recommendations for the use of antithrombotic therapy are summarized in Tables 20-5, 20-6, and 20-7.

Special Clinical Settings

The hematology consultant may be confronted with a variety of conditions for which antithrombotic therapy is recommended.

Mural Thrombosis and Embolic Events

Left ventricular mural thrombosis is a potential complication of acute MI,[164] particularly in cases involving the wall and the apex.

A meta-analysis performed by Vaitkus and Barnathorn[165] highlights the risk of cardioembolism among patients with mural thrombosis diagnosed by transthoracic echocardiography, along with the beneficial impact of anticoagulant therapy in reducing events.[165]

Atheromas of the Ascending Aorta

The consistently high incidence of "cryogenic stroke" in most stroke registries and databases led to further consideration of alternative causes beyond carotid artery disease, atrial fibrillation, and left heart cardioembolism. The development of transesophageal echocardiography and its use in the assessment of patients experiencing acute ischemic stroke have provided much needed insight.[166,167] Atheromas of the ascending aorta are present in upward of 25% of patients with stroke and/or peripheral embolism. In this setting, the incidence of recurrent events is high, approaching 15% to 25% within 1 year of the original event. Features associated with an increased incidence of embolic events (atheroemboli, thromboemboli) include plaque thickness greater than 4 mm,[168] absence of calcification, ulceration,

Table 20-5 Recommended Antithrombotic Agents

Antiplatelets

Class I

1. Aspirin 162 to 325 mg should be given PO on day 1 of ST elevation myocardial infarction (STEMI); in the absence of contraindications, it should be continued indefinitely on a daily basis thereafter at a dose of 75 to 162 mg PO. (Level of Evidence: A)
2. A thienopyridine (preferably clopidogrel) should be orally administered to patients who are unable to take aspirin because of hypersensitivity or major gastrointestinal intolerance. (Level of Evidence: C)
3. For patients taking clopidogrel for whom coronary artery bypass grafting (CABG) is planned, if possible, the drug should be withheld for at least 5 days, preferably for 7, unless the urgency for revascularization outweighs the risks of bleeding. (Level of Evidence: B)
4. For patients who have undergone diagnostic cardiac catheterization and for whom percutaneous coronary intervention (PCI) is planned, clopidogrel should be started and continued for at least 1 month after bare metal stent implantation and for several months after drug-eluting stent implantation (3 months for sirolimus, 6 months for paclitaxel) and up to 12 months in patients who are not at high risk for bleeding. (Level of Evidence: B)

Anticoagulants

Class I

1. Intravenous unfractionated heparin (UFH; bolus, 60 U per kilogram; maximum, 4000 U IV; initial infusion, 12 U per kilogram per hour; maximum, 1000 U per hour) or LMWH should be used in patients after STEMI who are at high risk for systemic emboli (large or anterior myocardial infarction [MI], atrial fibrillation, previous embolus, known LV thrombus, or cardiogenic shock). (Level of Evidence: C)

Class IIa

1. It is reasonable that STEMI patients not undergoing reperfusion therapy who do not have a contraindication to anticoagulation should be treated with intravenous or subcutaneous UFH or with subcutaneous LMWH for at least 48 hours. In patients whose clinical condition necessitates prolonged bed rest and/or minimized activities, it is reasonable that treatment should be continued until the patient is ambulatory. (Level of Evidence: C)

Class IIb

1. Prophylaxis for deep venous thrombosis (DVT) with subcutaneous LMWH (dosed appropriately for specific agent) or with subcutaneous UFH, 7500 U to 12500 U twice per day until completely ambulatory; may be useful, but the effectiveness of such a strategy is not well established in the contemporary era of routine aspirin use and early mobilization. (Level of Evidence: C)

Table 20-6 Acute Management of Non–ST Elevation Acute Coronary Syndrome (NSTE ACS)

Antiplatelet Therapies

Aspirin

For all patients who present with NSTE ACS, without a clear allergy to aspirin, we recommend immediate aspirin, 75 to 325 mg PO, and then daily, 75 to 162 mg PO (Grade 1A).

Thienopyridines

For all NSTE ACS patients with an aspirin allergy, we recommend immediate treatment with clopidogrel, 300 mg dose PO, followed by 75 mg per day PO indefinitely (Grade 1A).

In all NSTE ACS patients in whom diagnostic catheterization will be delayed or when coronary bypass surgery will not occur until >5 days after coronary angiography, we recommend that clopidogrel should be administered immediately as PO therapy (300 mg), followed by 75 mg per day PO for 9 to 12 months, in addition to aspirin (Grade 1A).

Glycoprotein (GP)-IIb/IIIa Inhibitors

In moderate- to high-risk patients who present with NSTE ACS, we recommend IV eptifibatide or tirofiban for initial (early) treatment, in addition to treatment with aspirin and heparin (Grade 1A). In these moderate- to high-risk patients who are also receiving clopidogrel, we recommend eptifibatide or tirofiban as additional initial treatment (Grade 2A).

For patients who present with NSTE ACS, we recommend **against** abciximab as initial treatment, except when coronary anatomy is known and percutaneous coronary intervention (PCI) is planned within 24 hours (Grade 1A).

Antithrombin Therapies

Unfractionated Heparin (UFH)

For patients who present with NSTE ACS, we recommend IV UFH over no heparin therapy for short-term use with antiplatelet therapies (Grade 1A). We recommend weight-based dosing of UFH and maintenance of partial thromboplastin time (PTT) at between 50 sec and 75 sec (Grade 1C+).

For the acute treatment of patients with NSTE ACS, we recommend SQ LMWH over UFH (Grade 1B).

We recommend against routine monitoring of the anticoagulant effects of LMWH (Grade 1C).

We suggest that LMWH should be continued during PCI treatment of the NSTE ACS patient when it has been started as the "upstream" anticoagulant (Grade 2C).

For patients who receive glycoprotein (GP)-IIb/IIIa inhibitors as upstream treatment for NSTE ACS, we suggest LMWH over UFH as the anticoagulant of choice (Grade 2B).

Direct Thrombin Inhibitors (DTIs)

In patients who present with NSTE ACS, we recommend **against** the use of DTIs as routine initial antithrombotic therapy (Grade 1B).

Underlying values and preferences: This recommendation acknowledges the limitations of individual trials of DTIs in NSTE ACS, as well as the complexities of using DTIs rather than UFH or LMWH.

Post–Myocardial Infarction (MI) and Post–ACS

In patients with ACS with and without ST segment elevation, the following apply:

We recommend aspirin given in initial doses of 160 to 325 mg PO, and then indefinite therapy, 75 to 162 mg/day PO (Grade 1A).

For patients with a history of aspirin-induced bleeding or with risk factors for bleeding, we recommend lower doses (≤100 mg) of aspirin (Grade 1C+).

For patients in whom aspirin is contraindicated or is not tolerated, we recommend clopidogrel, 75 mg per day PO, for long-term administration (Grade 1A).

and superimposed thrombi (particularly with a mobile component).[169,170]

Treatment of patients with atheromas involving the ascending aorta includes meticulous atherosclerotic vascular disease risk factor modification and use of hydroxymethylglutaryl–coenzyme A (HMG-CoA) reductase inhibitors. Patients with cerebrovascular events and mobile thrombus seen on transesophageal echocardiography should receive anticoagulant therapy with an oral vitamin K antagonist to a target international normalized ratio (INR) of 2.5 (range, 2.0 to 3.0).[171–173] All other patients should receive platelet-directed therapy with aspirin.

Ventricular Assist Devices

Chronic left ventricular heart failure, the end result of advanced ischemic heart disease and nonischemic cardiomyopathy, is the leading cause of death in the United States and developed countries, affecting nearly 10 per 1000 individuals 65 years of age and older.[174] The development of left ventricular assist devices (LVADs) and the start of the artificial heart program in 1964 provide a much needed "bridge" to transplantation and, in some instances, a successful temporizing measure for clinical stabilization of recovery, referred to as "destination therapy."

LVADs receive blood from the left ventricle by means of an inflow cannula and subsequently pump it to the aorta via an outflow cannula. Early-generation devices used an external drive pump and vent, predisposing to infection and limited patient mobility. Later devices employed a powerpack placed subcutaneously and internal venting systems of various designs.[175]

Cardiac devices currently used for cardiac mechanical support are summarized in Table 20-8. Most require anticoagulant therapy because of a recognized risk for thrombosis and thromboembolism, which, in the early experience, approached 20% to 30% of patients.[176,177] The HeartMate device (Thoratec Corporation, Pleasanton, CA) is associated with a lower reported incidence of thromboembolism[178]; as a result, platelet-directed therapy with aspirin may, in select patients, provide adequate thromboprophylaxis. Nevertheless, thrombosis/thromboembolism remains a constant concern in patients with mechanical ventricular assist devices.[179,180]

Dosing Dilemmas: An Opportunity for Improved Safety

In a prospective observational analysis of 30,136 patients with non–ST segment elevation ACS, 42% received an initial dose of heparin, LMWH, or LMWH or a GP-IIb/IIIa receptor antagonist outside the recommended range of dosing (Table 20-9). Patient characteristics associated with excess drug dosing included older age, female sex, low body weight, renal insufficiency, diabetes mellitus, and congestive heart failure. Excess antithrombotic drug dosing was associated with major bleeding complications, increased length of hospital stay, and higher rates of mortality.[181]

An Evolving View of Blood Transfusion

The frequency of anemia among hospitalized patients has led to the liberal use of blood (erythrocyte) transfusions. Current clinical practice still acknowledges (and follows) the age-old "10/30" rule, first proposed in 1942.[182] This

Table 20-7 Antiplatelet and Antithrombotic Adjunctive Therapies for Percutaneous Coronary Intervention (PCI)

Class I

1. Patients already taking daily long-term aspirin therapy should take 75 to 325 mg of aspirin PO before the PCI procedure is performed. (Level of Evidence: A)
2. Patients who are not already taking daily long-term aspirin therapy should be given 300 to 325 mg of aspirin PO at least 2 hours and preferably 24 hours before the PCI procedure is performed. (Level of Evidence: C)
3. After the PCI procedure has been completed, in patients with no aspirin resistance, allergy, or increased risk of bleeding, aspirin 325 mg daily PO should be given for at least 1 month after bare metal stent implantation, 3 months after sirolimus eluting stent implantation, and 6 months after paclitaxel eluting stent implantation, after which daily long-term PO aspirin use should be continued indefinitely at a dose of 75 to 162 mg PO. (Level of Evidence: B)
4. A loading dose of clopidogrel should be administered before PCI is performed. (Level of Evidence: A) An oral loading dose of 300 mg, administered at least 6 hours before the procedure is begun, has the best established evidence of efficacy. (Level of Evidence: B)
5. In patients who have undergone PCI, clopidogrel 75 mg PO daily should be given for at least 1 month after bare metal stent implantation (unless the patient is at increased risk of bleeding; then it should be given for a minimum of 2 weeks), 3 months after sirolimus stent implantation, and 6 months after paclitaxel stent implantation, and ideally up to 12 months in patients who are not at high risk of bleeding. (Level of Evidence: B)

Class IIa

1. If clopidogrel is given at the time the procedure is performed, supplementation with glycoprotein (GP)-IIb/IIIa receptor antagonists may be more beneficial than clopidogrel alone in facilitating earlier platelet inhibition. (Level of Evidence: B)
2. For patients with an absolute contraindication to aspirin, it is reasonable to give a 300-mg oral loading dose of clopidogrel, administered at least 6 hours before PCI, and/or GP-IIb/IIIa antagonists, administered at the time of PCI. (Level of Evidence: C)
3. When a loading dose of clopidogrel is administered, a regimen greater than 300 mg PO is reasonable for achieving higher levels of antiplatelet activity more rapidly, but efficacy and safety compared with a 300 mg PO loading dose are less well established. (Level of Evidence: C)
4. It is reasonable that patients who undergo brachytherapy should be given daily clopidogrel 75 mg PO indefinitely and daily aspirin 75 to 325 mg PO indefinitely, unless the risk of bleeding is significant. (Level of Evidence: C)

Class IIb

In patients in whom subacute thrombosis may be catastrophic or lethal (unprotected left main, bifurcating left main, or last patent coronary vessel), platelet aggregation studies may be considered, and the dose of clopidogrel increased to 150 mg PO per day, if less than 50% inhibition of platelet aggregation is demonstrated. (Level of Evidence: C)

60-year-old study demonstrated an increase in cardiac output when hematocrit was below 30%—a response that was believed to be maladaptive. In 2003 to 2004, 3500 patients received erythrocyte transfusions each day in U.S. hospital intensive care unit (ICU) settings, totaling 1.25 million transfusions per year in the ICU alone.[183] However, few hard data are available to support this "reflex transfusion response." A retrospective case-controlled study showed that elderly patients who presented with acute MI experienced a lower 30-day mortality rate when erythrocyte transfusions were administered to achieve hematocrit greater than 30%.[184] Whether these data provide definitive support for transfusion practices has been questioned because of the study's lack of randomization, unequal numbers in case and control groups, and low overall frequency of transfusion.

In contrast, a prospective, randomized, multicenter trial of 357 critically ill patients with underlying cardiovascular disease failed to show mortality reduction with liberal transfusion; only a trend toward fewer deaths was observed in a relatively small subgroup of patients (n = 77) characterized by severe ischemic heart disease (unstable angina or acute MI).[185]

Rao and colleagues[186] examined the potential impact of erythrocyte transfusion in 24,111 patients with ACS. Several surprising observations were reported from the post hoc analysis. First, significantly higher 30-day all-cause mortality and 30-day death or MI rates were described among patients who received transfusions. Second, this increased risk persisted after adjustment was made for potentially confounding clinical variables (adjusted hazard ratio, 3.94) and after several statistical methods were used to adjust for bias. Third, 30-day mortality was particularly high when transfusions were given for hematocrit levels of 25% or above (compared with hematocrit less than 25%).

Hebert and colleagues[187] enrolled 838 critically ill patients with euvolemia after initial treatment who had hemoglobin levels lower than 9.0 g per deciliter within 72 hours of ICU admission and randomly assigned them to a restrictive strategy of transfusion (red cells transfused if hemoglobin <7.0 g per deciliter) or a liberal strategy (transfusion if hemoglobin fell to below 10.0 g per deciliter). Rates of 30-day mortality were similar in the two groups (18.7% vs 23.3%; $P = .11$), with an exception noted among patients younger than 55 years of age and those with an Acute Physiology and Chronic Health Evaluation (APACHE) II score of less than 20, in whom rates were lower with a restrictive strategy of transfusion. Cardiac events, including pulmonary edema and MI, were more frequent in the liberal strategy group than in the restricted strategy group during the ICU stay; however, no significant differences in rates of cardiac events (or infectious complications) were reported among those who died during the 48 hours preceding death. Similarly, no significant differences in mortality were observed between treatment groups in the modestly sized subgroup of patients with a primary or secondary diagnosis of cardiac disease (20.5% in the restrictive strategy group and 22.9% in the liberal strategy group). Finally, transfusion emerged as a risk factor for poor outcomes in patients with trauma who experienced a higher mortality rate during hospitalization when blood products were administered (after control was provided for the degree of anemia and shock).[188]

Table 20-8 Comparison of Available Cardiac Devices

Pulsatile Pumps
Thoratec

Indications	Right, left, or biventricular support
Advantages	Fits in a wide range of patient sizes (body surface area, 0.73 to 2.5 m²)
	Pump can be changed without invasive surgery
	Can replace the entire function of the supported ventricle
Disadvantages	Requires strict anticoagulation with risks of bleeding and thromboembolism
	High risk of infection
	Limited patient mobility
	Not approved for home use

HeartMate

Indications	Left ventricular support
Advantages	No need for anticoagulation
	Portability of controller and batteries permits good patient mobility and hospital discharge
	Can replace the entire function of the supported ventricle
Disadvantages	Drive line crossing the skin poses a risk of infection
	Left ventricle support only
	Not suitable for patients with body surface area ≤1.5 m²

Novacor

Indications	Left ventricular support
Advantages	Portability of controller and batteries permits patient mobility and hospital discharge
Disadvantages	Need for strict anticoagulation with higher risk of bleeding or thromboembolism
	Drive line crossing the skin poses a high risk of infection
	Left ventricle support only
	Not suitable for patients with body surface area ≤1.5 m²

Continuous Flow Pumps

Indications	Left ventricular support
Advantages	Small size permits patient mobility
	Quiet
	Suitable for wide range of patient body habitus
Disadvantages	Need for anticoagulation; risks of bleeding and thromboembolism unknown
	May not replace the entire function of the supported ventricle
	Nonpulsatile flow
	Still in early clinical trials

Modified from Nemeh HW, Smedira NG: Mechanical treatment of heart failure: The growing role of LVADs and artificial hearts. Cleveland Clin J Med 3:223–233, 2003.

Data derived predominantly from retrospective and modestly sized prospective studies raise the suspicion that an association between transfusion and morbidity or mortality may exist, yet questions remain about whether the relationship is causal and how contributing factors may differ (or may manifest differently) on the basis of coexisting illness and accompanying conditions.

Table 20-9 Dosing Recommendations and Categories of Antiplatelet and Antithrombin Agents for Non–ST Segment Elevation Acute Coronary Syndrome*

	Dosing Recommendations
Unfractionated heparin	IV bolus of 60–70 U per kilogram followed by an infusion of 12–15 U/kg/hr IV. Elderly patients (>60 years) may require lower heparin doses.
Low molecular weight heparin	Enoxaparin: 1 mg/kg SQ every 12 hours. Dose is reduced by 50% by increasing intervals to every 24 hours if creatinine clearance <30 mL per minute. Elderly patients at high risk of bleeding. Dalteparin: Use caution in elderly patients with low body weight or predisposed to renal insufficiency.
Glycoprotein-IIb/IIIa inhibitors[†]	Eptifibatide: Bolus 180 µg per kilogram IV and infusion of 2.0 µg/kg/min IV for 72–96 hours. Reduce infusion rate by 50% to 1 µg/kg/min if creatinine clearance is ≤30 mL per minute or serum creatinine is 2 to 4 mg per deciliter. Tirofiban: IV bolus 0.4 µg per kilogram per minute and infusion of 0.1 µg per kilogram per minute IV for 48 to 96 hours. Reduce bolus and infusion by 50% to 0.05 µg/kg/min IV if creatinine clearance ≤30 mL per minute. Systeme Internationale (SI) conversions: To convert creatinine clearance to mL per second, multiply by 0.0167; serum creatinine to µmol per liter, multiply by 88.4.

*Dosing recommendations from guidelines and product labels. Mild and major excess categories are subgroups of excess dosing catergories.

Defining Hemorrhagic Risk

Risk of hemorrhage associated with antithrombotic therapy, in addition to its intrinsic effects on primary hemostasis, secondary hemostasis, and intensity of effect, is influenced strongly by patient characteristics. Advanced age, renal insufficiency, presence of hypertension, and combined drug therapy contribute to the overall risk of hemorrhagic events, including central nervous bleeding.[189] Table 20-10 suggests some treatment pathways (in addition to time) for hemorrhagic complications associated with these agents.

GI hemorrhage is second only to mucocutaneous bleeding as a source of major bleeding and as a source of major events among patients receiving platelet-directed therapy. In a large case-controlled study,[190] relative risks of upper GI bleeding associated with long-term administration were as follows: aspirin, 4.0; clopidogrel, 2.3; dipyridamole, 0.9; indobufen, 3.8; and ticlopidine, 3.1. Available evidence suggests that risk is increased when aspirin and clopidogrel are used in combination. Although protein pump inhibitors reduce the likelihood of aspirin-related recurrent GI bleeding among patients with treated peptic ulcer disease,[191]

Table 20-10 Agent-Specific Approach to Hemorrhagic Complications

Agent	Category	Mechanism of Action	Antidote	Available Substrate for Attenuating Effects
Aspirin	Platelet antagonist	Cyclo-oxygenase inhibition	DDAVP	Platelet transfusion
Clopidogrel	Platelet antagonist	ADP receptor inhibition	None	Platelet transfusion
Ticlopidine	Platelet antagonist	ADP receptor inhibition	None	Platelet transfusion
Abciximab	Platelet antagonist	GP-IIb/IIIa receptor inhibition	None	Platelet transfusion, FFP, Cryoprecipitate
Tirofiban	Platelet antagonist	GP-IIb/IIIa receptor inhibition	None	Cryoprecipitate, FFP, platelet transfusion
Eptifibatide	Platelet antagonist	GP-IIb/IIIa receptor inhibition	None	Cryoprecipitate, FFP, platelet transfusion
UFH	Anticoagulant	Anti-IIa and -Xa via ATIII	Protamine	None
LMWH	Anticoagulant	Anti-IIa and -Xa via ATIII	Protamine (60% effective)	None
Fondaparinux	Anticoagulant	Anti-Xa via ATIII	None	None
Lepirudin	Anticoagulant	Anti-IIa (direct)	None	FFP, plasmapheresis
Argatroban	Anticoagulant	Anti-IIa (direct)	None	FFP, plasmapheresis
Danaparoid	Anticoagulant	Anti-IIa (direct)	None	Plasmapheresis

DDAVP, 1-deamino-8-D-arginine vasopressin; ADP, adenosine diphosphate; GP, glycoprotein; UFH, unfractioned heparin; LMWH, low molecular weight heparin; FFP, fresh frozen plasma.

their protective effects with clopidogrel have not been established.[192]

Minimizing Surgical Bleeding Risk

The recommended approach for minimizing major hemorrhage in the surgical setting begins with a thorough understanding of antithrombotic drugs that includes their pharmaceutical pharmacodynamics, biologic half-lives, preoperative dosing and antidotes, and neutralizing agents or potential removal strategies, as clinical circumstances and the risk/benefit relationship dictate.[193] The timing of surgery and the specific technique used must also be considered carefully. Hospitalized patients with an ACS are particularly prone and unnecessarily disadvantaged at the time of surgery if they receive excessive doses of antithrombotic therapy over the days leading up to surgery (of if emergent surgery is required).[181]

Antifibrinolytic agents such as aprotinin[194] have been used during cardiac surgery to reduce blood loss, transfusion requirements, and the proinflammatory state that accompanies cardiopulmonary bypass.[195] Aprotinin has also been shown to reduce postoperative blood loss among clopidogrel-treated patients, including those given the platelet antagonist within 5 days of surgery.[196] Emerging data that suggested that the use of alternative antifibrinolytic agents such as ε-aminocaproic acid and tranexamic acid may be safer than administration of aprotinin and require further evaluation.[197]

Recombinant factor VIIa, a hemostatic agent licensed for the treatment of bleeding episodes among patients with hemophilia and inhibitors, may also have a place in the management of bleeding associated with platelet disorders,[198] including the coagulopathy induced by cardiac surgery.[199] In vitro studies suggest a factor Xa/thrombin-dependent mechanism of platelet activation.[200] As with any and all treatments given with the intent of shifting the hemostatic balance toward thrombosis, potential risks must be weighed carefully against benefits.[201]

REFERENCES

1. American Heart Association: Statistics. Available at: heart.org Statistics.
2. In Jewett B (ed): The Dialogues of Plato, 3rd ed. New York, Macmillan, 1892, pp 339–543.
3. Lee HDP(translator): Aristotle: Meterologica. Loeb Classical Library. Cambridge, Harvard University Press, 1952.
4. Pettit JL: Dissertation sur la manie're d'arrester le sang dans les hemorrhagies. Mem Acad R Sci 1:85–102, 1731.
5. Forester JM (translator): Milpighi M: De Polypo Cordis, 1686. Uppsala, Almquiest & Wiksels, 1956.
6. Babington BG: Some considerations with respect to the blood founded on one or two very simple experiments on that fluid. Med Chir Trans 16:293–319, 1930.
7. Buchanan A: On the coagulation of the blood and other fibriniferous liquids. Lond Med Gaz 1845; 1:617. Reprinted in J Physiol (Lond) 2:158–168, 1879–1880.
8. Schmidt A: Zur Blutlehre. Leipzig, Bogel, 1803.
9. Otto JC: An account of an hemorrhagic disposition existing in certain families. Med Repos 6:1–4, 1803.
10. Hay J: Account of a remarkable haemorrhagic disposition, existing in many individuals of the same family. N Engl J Med 2:221–225, 1813.
11. Thackrah CT: An Inquiry into the Nature and Properties of the Blood. London, Cox and Sons, 1819.
12. De Blainville HMD: Injection de matiére cerebrale dans les veins. Gaz Med Paris 2:524, 1834.
13. Howell WH: The nature and action of the thromboplastin (zymoplastic) substance of the tissues. Am J Physiol 31:1–21, 1912.
14. Mills CA: Chemical nature of tissue coagulants. J Biol Chem 46:135–165, 1921.
15. Donné A: De l'origine des globules du sang, de leur mode de formation et leur fin. CR Acad Sci (Paris) 14:366–368, 1842.
16. Osler W: An account of certain organisms occurring in the liquor sanguinis. Proc Roy Soc Lond 22:391–398, 1874.
17. Hayem G: Sur le méhanisme de l'arret des hemorrhagies. CR Acad Sci 95:18–21, 1885.
18. Konttinen YP: Fibrinolysis: Chemistry, Physiology, Pathology and Clinics. Tampere, Finland, Oy Star Ab, 1968.
19. Hedin SG: On the presence of a proteolytic enzyme in the normal serum of the ox. J Physiol (Lond) 30:195–201, 1904.
20. Christensen LR, MacLeod CM: Proteolytic enzyme of serum: Characterization, activation, and reaction with inhibitors. J Gen Physiol 23:559–583, 1945.
21. Gratia A (quoted by Kontinnen YP): Fibrinolysis: Chemistry, Physiology, Pathology and Clinics. Finland, Tampere, Oy Star Ab, 1968.
22. Tillett WS, Garner RL: The fibrinolytic activity of hemolytic streptococci. J Exp Med 58:485–502, 1933.

23. Sherry S, Fletcher A, Akljaersig N: Fibrinolysis and fibrinolytic activity in man. Physiol Rev 39:343–381, 1959.

24. ISIS-2 (Second International Study of Infarct Survival) Collaborative Group: Randomized trial of intravenous streptokinase, oral aspirin, both, or neither among 17,187 cases of suspected acute myocardial infarction: ISIS-2. Lancet 2:349–360, 1988.

25. Lambrew CT: The National Heart Attack Alert Program: Overview and mission. J Thromb Thrombol 3:247–248, 1996.

26. Hand M: Educational strategies to prevent prehospital delay in patients at high risk for acute myocardial infarction: A report by the National Heart Attack Alert Program. J Thromb Thrombol 6:47–61, 1998.

27. Hand M, Brown C, Horan M, et al: The National Heart Attack Alert Program: Progress at 5 years in educating providers, patients and the public: Future directions. J Thromb Thrombol 6:9–17, 1998.

28. Antman E, for the TIMI 11B Investigators: Enoxaparin prevents death and cardiac ischemic events in unstable angina–non-Q-wave MI: Results of the TIMI 11b trial. Circulation 100:1593–1601, 1999.

29. Cohen M, Demers C, Gurfinkel EP, for the ESSENCE Investigators: A comparison of low-molecular-weight heparin with unfractionated heparin for unstable coronary artery disease. N Engl J Med 337:447–452, 1997.

30. The FRISC Study Group: Low molecular weight heparin during instability in coronary artery disease. Lancet 347:561–568, 1996.

31. Klein W, Buchwald A, Hillis SE, et al: Comparison of low molecular weight heparin with unfractionated heparin acutely and with placebo for 6 weeks in the management of unstable coronary artery disease. Fragmin in Unstable Coronary Artery Disease Study (FRIC). Circulation 96:61–68, 1997.

32. FRISC II Investigations: Long-term low-molecular mass heparin in unstable coronary artery disease: FRISC II prospective randomized multicentre study. Lancet 354:701–707, 1999.

33. Kong DF, Califf RM, Miller DP, et al: Clinical outcomes of therapeutic agents that block the platelet glycoprotein IIb/IIIa integrin in ischemic heart disease. Circulation 98:2829–2835, 1998.

34. Antman EM, for the TIMI 14 Investigators: Abciximab facilitates the rate and extent of thrombolysis: Results of the TIMI 14 trial. Circulation 99:2720–2732, 1999.

35. Jaucherm JR, Lopez M, Sprague EA, et al: Mononuclear cell chemoattractant activity from cultured arterial smooth muscle cells. Exp Mol Pathol 37:166–174, 1982.

36. Schwartz CJ, Valente AJ, Sprague EA, et al: Atherosclerosis as an inflammatory process: The roles of monocyte-macrophage. Ann N Y Acad Sci 454:115–120, 1985.

37. Goldstein JL, Ho YK, Basu SK, et al: Binding site on macrophages that mediates uptake and degradation of acetylated low density lipoprotein, producing massive cholesterol deposition. Proc Natl Acad Sci U S A 76:333–337, 1979.

38. Little WC, Constantinescu M, Applegate RJ, et al: Can coronary angiography predict the site of a subsequent myocardial infarction in patients with mild-to-moderate coronary artery disease? Circulation 78:1157–1166, 1988.

39. Davies MJ, Thomas AC: Plaque fissuring: The cause of acute myocardial infarction, sudden ischemic death and crescendo angina. Br Heart J 53:363–373, 1985.

40. Davie EW: A brief historical review of the waterfall/cascade of blood coagulation. J Biol Chem 278:50819–50832, 2003.

41. Giesen PL, Rauch U, Bohrmann B, et al: Blood-borne tissue factor: Another view of thrombosis. Proc Natl Acad Sci U S A 96:2311–2315, 1999.

42. De Cristofaro R, De Candia E: Thrombin domains: Structure, function and interaction with platelet receptors. J Thromb Thrombol 15:151–163, 2003.

43. McEver RP: Adhesive interactions of leukocytes, platelets, and the vessel wall during hemostasis and inflammation. Thromb Haemost 86:746–756, 2001.

44. Savage B, Sixma JJ, Ruggeri ZM: Functional self-association of von Willebrand factor during platelet adhesion under flow. Proc Natl Acad Sci U S A 99:425–430, 2005.

45. Jesty J, Beltrami E: Positive feedbacks of coagulation: Their role in threshold regulation. Arterioscler Thromb Vasc Biol 25:2463–2469, 2005.

46. Falciani M, Gori AM, Fedi S, et al: Elevated tissue factor and tissue factor pathway inhibitor circulating levels in ischemic heart disease patients. Thromb Haemost 79:495–499, 1998.

47. Goel MS, Diamond SL: Neutrophil enhancement of fibrin deposition under flow through platelet-dependent and -independent mechanism. Arterioscler Thromb Vasc Biol 21:2093–2098, 2001.

48. Karnicki K, Owen WG, Miller RS, McBane RD II: Factors contributing to individual propensity for arterial thrombosis. Arterioscler Thromb Vasc Biol 22:1495–1499, 2002.

49. Weber C, Springer TA: Neutrophil accumulation on activated, surface-adherent platelets in flow is medicated by interaction of Mac-1 with fibrinogen bound to alphaIIbbeta3 and stimulated by platelet-activating factor. J Clin Invest 100:2085–2093, 1997.

50. Braunwald E, Antman EM, Beasley JW, et al: ACC/AHA guidelines for the management of patients with unstable angina and non-ST-segment elevation myocardial infarction: A report of the American College of Cardiology/American Heart Association Task Force on Practice Guidelines (Committee on the Management of Patients with Unstable Angina). J Am Coll Cardiol 36:970–1062, 2000.

51. Boden WE, Pepine CJ: Introduction to "optimizing management of non–ST-segment elevation acute coronary syndromes:" Harmonizing advances in mechanical and pharmacologic intervention. J Am Coll Cardiol 41:S1–S6, 2003.

52. Freedman JE: Molecular regulation of platelet-dependent thrombosis. Circulation 112:2725–2734, 2005.

53. Roth GJ, Majerus PW: The mechanism of the effect of aspirin on human platelets I. Acetylation of a particular fraction protein. J Clin Invest 56:624–632, 1975.

54. Patrono C: Aspirin as an antiplatelet drug. N Engl J Med 330:1287–1294, 1994.

55. O'Brien JR: Effects of salicylates on human platelets. Lancet 1:779–783, 1968.

56. Awtry EH, Loscalzo J: Aspirin. Circulation 101:1206–1218, 2000.

57. Steering Committee of the Physician's Health Study Research Group: Final report on the aspirin component of the ongoing Physician's Health Study. N Engl J Med 321:129–135, 1989.

58. The Medical Research Council's General Practice Research Framework: Thrombosis prevention trial: Randomized trial of low intensity oral anticoagulation with warfarin and low-dose aspirin in the primary prevention of ischemic heart disease in men at increased risk. Lancet 351:233–241, 1998.

59. Peto R, Gray R, Collins R, et al: Randomized trial of prophylactic daily aspirin in British male doctors. Br Med J 926:313–316, 1988.

60. Ridker PM, Cook NR, Lee IM, et al: A randomized trial of low-dose aspirin in the primary prevention of cardiovascular disease in women. N Engl J Med 352:1293–1304, 2005.

61. Antiplatelet Trialists' Collaboration: Collaborative meta-analysis of randomized trials of antiplatelet therapy for prevention of death, myocardial infarction, and stroke in high risk patients. BMJ 324:71–86, 2002.

62. Lorenz RL, Schacky CV, Weber M, et al: Improved aortocoronary by pass patency by low-dose (100 mg daily): Effects of platelet aggregation and thromboxane formation. Lancet 1:1261–1264, 1984.

63. Goldman S, Copeland J, Moritz T, et al: Internal mammary artery and saphenous vein graft patency: Effects of aspirin. Circulation 82:IV237–IV242, 1990.

64. International Stroke Trial Collaborative Group, The International Stroke Trial (IST): A randomized trial of aspirin, subcutaneous heparin, both or neither among 19,435 patients with acute ischemic stroke. Lancet 349:1569–1581, 1997.

65. CAST (Chinese Acute Stroke Trial) Collaborative Group (CAST): Randomized placebo controlled trial of early aspirin use in 20,0000 patients with acute ischemic stroke. Lancet 349:1641–1649, 1997.

66. Barnathan ES, Schwartz JS, Taylor L, et al: Aspirin and dipyridamole in the prevention of acute coronary thrombosis complicating coronary angioplasty. Circulation 76:125–134, 1987.

67. Schwartz L, Bourassa MG, Lesperance J, et al: Aspirin and dipyridamole in the prevention of restenosis after percutaneous transluminal coronary angioplasty. N Engl J Med 318:1714–1749, 1988.

68. Catelle-Lawson F, Reilly MP, Kapoor SC, et al: Cyclooxygenase inhibitors and antiplatelet effects of aspirin. N Engl J Med 345:1809–1817, 2001.

69. Nair GV, Davis DJ, McKenzi ME, et al: Aspirin in patients with coronary artery disease: Is it simply irresistible? J Thromb Thrombol 11:117–126, 2001.

70. Weber A-A, Przytukski B, Schanz A, et al: Towards definition of aspirin resistance: A typological approach. Platelets 13:37–40, 2002.

71. Patrono C: Aspirin resistance: Definition, mechanisms and clinical read-outs. J Thromb Haemost 1:1710–1713, 2003.

72. Gum PA, Kottke-Marchant K, Welsch PA, et al: A prospective, blinded determination of the natural history of aspirin resistance among stable patients with cardiovascular disease. J Am Coll Cardiol 41:961–965, 2003.

73. Eikelboom JW, Hirsh J, Weitz JI, et al: Aspirin resistant thromboxane biosynthesis and the risk of myocardial infarction, stroke or cardiovascular death in patients at high risk for cardiovascular events. Circulation 105:1650–1655, 2002.

73a. Dalen JE: Aspirin resistance: Is it real? Is it clinically significant? Am J Med 120:1–4, 2007.

74. Gachet C, Savi P, Ohlmann P, et al: ADP receptor induced activation of guanine nucleotide binding proteins in rat platelet membranes: An effect selectively blocked by the thienopyridine clopidogrel. Thromb Haemost 68:79–83, 1992.

75. Bennett CL, Connors JM, Carwile JM, et al: Thrombotic thrombocytopenia purpura associated with clopidogrel. N Engl J Med 342:1773–1777, 2000.

76. CAPRIE Steering Committee: A randomised, blinded trial of clopidogrel versus aspirin in patients at risk for ischaemic events (CAPRIE). Lancet 348:1329–1339, 1996.

77. Bhatt DL, Chew DP, Hirsch AT, et al: Superiority of clopidogrel versus aspirin in patients with prior cardiac surgery. Circulation 103:363–368, 2001.

78. Pfeffer M, Jarcho J: The charisma of subgroups and the subgroups of CHARISMA. N Engl J Med 354:1744–1746, 2006.

79. Bertrand ME: Double-blind study of the safety of clopidogrel with and without a loading dose in combination with aspirin compared with ticlopidine in combination with aspirin after coronary stenting: The Clopidogrel Aspirin Stent International Cooperative Study (CLASSICS). Circulation 102:624–629, 2000.

80. Mehta SR, Yusuf S, Peters RJ, for the CURE Investigators: Effects of pretreatment with clopidogrel and aspirin followed by long-term therapy in patients undergoing percutaneous coronary intervention: The PCI-CURE Study. Lancet 358:527–533, 2001.

81. Waksman R, Ajani AE, White RL, et al: Prolonged antiplatelet therapy to prevent late thrombosis after intracoronary radiation in patients with restenosis: Washington Radiation for In-Stent restenosis Trial plus 6 months of clopidogrel (WRIST PLUS). Circulation 103:2332–2335, 2001.

82. The Clopidogrel in Unstable Angina to Prevent Recurrent Events Trial Investigators: Effects of clopidogrel in addition to aspirin in patients with acute coronary syndromes without ST-segment elevation. N Engl J Med 345:494–502, 2001.

83. Steinhubl SR, Berger PB, Mann JT III, et al: Early and sustained dual oral antiplatelet therapy following percutaneous coronary intervention: A randomized controlled trial. JAMA 288:2411–2420, 2002.

84. Sagbatine MS, Cannon CP, Gibson CM, et al: CLARITY-TIMI 28 Investigators: Addition of clopidogrel to aspirin and fibrinolytic therapy for myocardial infractin with ST-segment elevation. N Engl J Med 352:1179–1189, 2005.

85. Chen Z: Randomized, placebo-controlled trial of adding clopidogrel to aspirin in 46,000 acute myocardial infarction patients (COMMIT/CCS-2-Clopidogrel). Presented at: American College of Cardiology Annual Scientific Session; Orlando, Fla; March 6–9, 2005, Available at www.acc05online.acc.org/highlights/keyLectures.aspz?sessioID=7989&&date=9. Accessed November 29, 2005.

86. Kastrati A, von Beckerath N, Joost A, et al: Loading with 600 mg clopidogrel in patients with coronary artery disease with and without chronic clopidogrel therapy. Circulation 110:1916–1919, 2004.

87. Gurbel PA, Bliden KP: Interpretation of platelet inhibition by clopidogrel and the effect of non-responders. J Thromb Haemost 1:1318–1319, 2003.

88. Matetzky S, Shenkman B, Guetta V, et al: Clopidogrel resistance is associated with increased risk of recurrent atherothrombotic events in patients with acute myocardial infarction. Circulation 109:3171–3175, 2004.

89. Gurbel PA, Bliden KP, Hiatt BL, O'Connor CM: Clopidogrel for coronary stenting: Response variability, drug resistance, and the effect of pretreatment platelet reactivity. Circulation 107:2908–2913, 2003.

90. Evaluation of Platelet IIb/IIIa Inhibition for Prevention of Ischemic Complications (EPIC) Investigators: Use of a monoclonal antibody directed against the platelet glycoprotein IIb/IIIa receptor in high-risk coronary angioplasty. N Engl J Med 330:956–961, 1994.

91. Topol EJ, Califf RM, Weisman HF, et al, for the EPIC Investigators: Randomized trial of coronary intervention with antibody against platelet IIb/IIIa integrin for reduction of clinical restenosis: Results at six months. Lancet 343:881–886, 1994.

92. Topol EJ, Ferguson JJ, Weisman HF, et al: Long-term protection from myocardial ischemic events in a randomized trial of brief integrin beta3 blockade with percutaneous coronary intervention. JAMA 278:479–484, 1997.

93. EPILOG Investigators: Platelet glycoprotein IIb/IIIa receptor blockade and low-dose heparin during percutaneous coronary revascularization. N Engl J Med 336:1689–1696, 1997.

94. CAPTURE Investigators: Randomized placebo-controlled trial of abciximab before and during coronary intervention in refractory unstable angina: The CAPTURE study. Lancet 349:1429–1435, 1997.

95. The Gusto IV Investigators: Effect of glycoprotein IIb/IIIa receptor blocker abciximab on outcome in patients with acute coronary syndromes without early coronary revascularization: The GUSTO IV-ACS randomized trial. Lancet 357:1915–1924, 2001.

96. Montalescot G, Barrgan P, Wittenberg O, et al, for the ADMIRAL Investigators: Platelet glycoprotein IIb/IIIa inhibition with coronary stenting for acute myocardial infarction. N Engl J Med 344:1895–1903, 2001.

97. Topol EJ, the GUSTO V Investigators: Reperfusion therapy for acute MI with fibrinolytic therapy or combination reduced fibrinolytic therapy and platelet glycoprotein IIb/IIIa inhibition: The GUSTO V randomised trial. Lancet 357:1905–1914, 2001.

98. Kereiakes DJ, Kleiman NS, Ambrose J, et al: Randomized double-blind, placebo-controlled dose-ranging study of tirofiban (MK-383) platelet IIb/IIIa blockade in high risk patients undergoing coronary angioplasty. J Am Coll Cardiol 27:356–542, 1996.

99. Randomized Efficacy Study of Tirofiban for Outcomes and Restenosis (RESTORE) Investigators: Effects of platelet glycoprotein IIb/IIIa blockade with tirofiban on adverse cardiac events in patients with unstable angina or acute myocardial infarction undergoing coronary angioplasty. Circulation 96:1445–1453, 1997.

100. Platelet Receptor Inhibition in Ischemic Syndrome Management (PRISM) Study Investigators: A comparison of aspirin plus tirofiban with aspirin plus heparin for unstable angina. N Engl J Med 338:1498–1505, 1998.

101. Platelet Receptor Inhibition in Ischemic Syndrome Management in Patients Limited by Unstable Signs and Symptoms (PRISM PLUS) Study Investigators: Inhibition of platelet glycoprotein IIb/IIIa receptor with tirofiban in unstable angina and non–Q wave myocardial infarction. N Engl J Med 338:1488–1497, 1998.

102. Cannon CP, Weintraub WS, Demopoulos LA, et al: for the TACTICS-TIMI 18 Investigators: Comparison of early invasive and conservative strategies for patients with unstable coronary syndromes treated with the glycoprotein IIb/IIIa inhibitor tirofiban. N Engl J Med 344:1879–1887, 2001.

103. Philips DR, Scarborough RM: Clinical pharmacology of eptifibatide. Am J Cardiol 80:11B–20B, 1997.

104. Harrington RA, Kleiman NS, Kottke-Marchant K, et al: Immediate and reversible platelet inhibition after intravenous administration of a peptide glycoprotein IIb/IIIa inhibitor during percutaneous coronary intervention. Am J Cardiol 76:1222–1227, 1995.

105. Integrilin to Minimize Platelet Aggregation and Coronary Thrombosis (IMPACT)-II Investigators: Randomised placebo-controlled trial of effect of eptifibatide on complications of percutaneous coronary intervention: IMPACT-II. Lancet 349:1422–1428, 1997.

106. Ohman EM, Kleiman NS, Gacioch G, et al: for the IMPACT-AMI Investigators: Combined accelerated tissue-plasminogen activator and platelet glycoprotein IIb/IIIa integrin receptor blockade with integrilin in acute myocardial infarction: Results of a randomized, placebo-controlled, dose-ranging trial. Circulation 95:846–854, 1997.

107. The Platelet Glycoprotein IIb/IIIa in Unstable Angina: Receptor Suppression Using Integrilin Therapy (PURSUIT) Trial Investigators: Inhibition of platelet glycoprotein IIb/IIIa with eptifibatide in patients with acute coronary syndromes. N Engl J Med 339:436–443, 1998.

108. Roffi M, Chew DP, Mukherjee D, et al: Platelet glycoprotein IIb/IIIa inhibitors reduce mortality in diabetic patients with non–ST segment elevation acute coronary syndromes. Circulation 104:2767–2771, 2001.

109. Li YF, Becker RC, Spencer FA: Comparative efficacy of fibrinogen and platelet supplementation on the in vitro reversibility of competitive glycoprotein IIa/IIIb (alphaIIb/beta3) receptor–directed platelet inhibition. Am Heart J 412:204–210, 2001.

110. Karvouni E, Katritsis DG, Ioannidis JPA: Intravenous glycoprotein IIb/IIIa receptor antagonists reduce mortality after percutaneous coronary interventions. J Am Coll Cardiol 41:26–32, 2003.

111. Bunag RD, Douglas CR, Imai S, Berne RM: Influence of a pyrimido-pyrimidine derivative on deamination of adenosine by blood. Circ Res 15:83–88, 1964.

112. Eisert WG: Near-field amplification of antithrombotic effects of dipyridamole through vessel wall cells. Neurology 57 (5 suppl 2): S20–S23, 2001.

113. Diener HC, Cunha L, Forbes C, et al: European Stroke Prevention Study-2: Dipyridamole and acetylsalicylic acid in the secondary prevention of stroke. J Neurol Sci 143:1–13, 1996.

114. Dawson DL, Cutler BS, Meissner MH, et al: Cilostazol has beneficial effects in treatment of intermittent claudication: Results from a multicenter, randomized, prospective, double-blind trial. Circulation 98:678–686, 1998.

115. Kozuma K: Effects of cilostazol on late lumen loss and repeat revascularization after Palmaz-Schatz coronary stent implantation. Am Heart J 141:124–130, 2001.

116. Lee SW, Park SW, Hong MK, et al: Comparison of cilostazol and clopidogrel after successful coronary stenting. Am J Cardiol 95:859–862, 2005.

117. Lee SW, Park SW, Hong MK, et al: Triple versus dual antiplatelet therapy after coronary stenting: Impact on stent thrombosis. J Am Coll Cardiol 46:1833–1837, 2005.

118. Douglas JS Jr, Holmes DR Jr, Kereiakes DJ, et al: Cilostazol for Restenosis Trail (CREST) Investigators: Coronary stent restenosis in patients treated with cilostazol. Circulation 112:2826–2832, 2005.

119. Han Y, Wang S, Li Y, et al: Cilostazol improves long-term outcomes after coronary stent implantation. Am Heart J 150:568, 2005.

120. Serebruany VL, Malinin AI, Eisert RM, Sane DC: Risk of bleeding complications with antiplatelet agents: Meta-analysis of 338,191 patients enrolled in 50 randomized controlled Trials. Am J Hematol 74:40–47, 2004.

121. Lam LH, Silbert JE, Rosenberg RD: The separation of active and inactive forms of heparin. Biochem Biophys Res Commun 69:570–577, 1976.

122. Beguin S, Lindhout T, Hemker HC: The mode of action of heparin in plasma. Thromb Haemost 60:457–462, 1988.

123. Théroux P, Ouimet H, McCans J, et al: Aspirin, heparin or both to treat acute unstable angina. N Engl J Med 319:1105–1111, 1988.

124. Cohen M, Adams PC, Hawkins L, et al: Usefulness of antithrombotic therapy in resting angina pectoris or non–Q-wave myocardial infarction in preventing death and myocardial infarction (a pilot study from the Antithrombotic Therapy in Acute Coronary Syndromes Study Group). Am J Cardiol 66:1287–1292, 1990.

125. Cohen M, Adams PC, Parry G, et al: Combination antithrombotic therapy in unstable rest angina and non–Q-wave infarction in non prior aspirin users: Primary end points analysis from the ATACS trial: Antithrombotic Therapy in Acute Coronary Syndromes Research Group. Circulation 89:81–88, 1994.

126. The RISC Group: Risk of myocardial infarction and death during treatment with low dose aspirin and intravenous heparin in men with unstable coronary artery disease: The RISC Group. Lancet 336:327–330, 1990.

127. Holdright D, Patel D, Cunningham D, et al: Comparison of the effect of heparin and aspirin versus aspirin alone on transient myocardial ischemia and in-hospital prognosis in patients with unstable angina. J Am Coll Cardiol 24:39–45, 2004.

128. Allison O, Whooley MA, Oler J, Grady D: Adding heparin to aspirin reduces the incidence of myocardial infarction and death in patients with unstable angina: A meta-analysis. JAMA 276:811–815, 1996.

129. Raschke RA, Reilly BM, Guidry JR, et al: The weight-based heparin dosing nomogram compared with a standard care nomogram. Ann Intern Med 119:874–881,1993.

130. Becker RC, Ball SP, Eisenberg P, for the Antithrombotic Therapy Consortium Investigators: Randomized, multicenter trial of weight-adjusted intravenous heparin dose titration and point-of-care coagulation monitoring in hospitalized patients with active thromboembolic disease. Am Heart J 137:59–71, 1999.

131. Petitou M, Lormeau JC, Choay J: Chemical synthesis of glycosaminoglycans: A new approach to antithrombotic drugs. Nature 350 (suppl): 30–33, 1991.

132. Donat F, Duret JP, Santoni A, et al: The pharmacokinetics of fondaparinux sodium in healthy volunteers. Clin Pharmakinet 41 (suppl 2): 1–9, 2002.

133. The Fifth Organization to Assess Strategies in Acute Ischemic Syndromes Investigators: Comparison of fondaparinux and enoxaparin in acute coronary syndromes. N Engl J Med 354:1464–1476, 2006.

134. The OASIS-6 Trial Group: Effects of fondaparinux on mortality and reinfarction in patients with acute ST-segment elevation myocardial infarction: The OASIS-6 randomized trial. JAMA 295:1519–1530, 2006.

135. Hirsh J, Levin M: Low molecular weight heparin. Blood 79:1–17, 1992.

136. Gurfinkel EP, Manos EJ, Mejail RI, et al: Low molecular weight heparin versus heparin or aspirin in the treatment of unstable angina and silent ischemia. J Am Coll Cardiol 26:313–318, 1995.

137. The FRISC Study Group: Low molecular weight heparin during instability in coronary artery disease. Lancet 347:561–568, 1996.

138. Klein W, Buchwald A, Hillis SE, et al: Comparison of low molecular weight heparin with unfractionated heparin acutely and with placebo for 6 weeks in the management of unstable coronary artery disease. Fragmin in Unstable Coronary Artery Disease Study (FRIC). Circulation 96:61–68, 1997.

139. Cohen M, Demers C, Gurfinkel EP, for the ESSENCE Investigators: A comparison of low-molecular weight heparin with unfractionated heparin for unstable coronary artery disease. N Engl J Med 337:447–452, 1997.

140. Antman EM, Cohen M, McCabe C, et al: Enoxaparin is superior to unfractionated heparin for preventing clinical events at 1-year follow-up of TIMI 11B and ESSENCE. Eur Heart J 23:264–268, 2002.

141. Antman EM, for the TIMI IIB Investigators: Enoxaparin prevents death and cardiac ischemic events in unstable angina, non–Q wave MI: Results of the TIMI 11B Trial. Circulation 100:1593–1601, 1999.

142. Antman EM, Cohen M, Bradley D, et al: Assessment of the treatment effect of enoxaparin for unstable angina/non–Q-wave myocardial infarction: TIMI 11B-ESSENCE meta-analysis. Circulation 100: 1602–1608, 1999.

143. FRISC II Investigators: Prolonged low molecular mass heparin (dalteparin) in unstable coronary artery disease: A prospective randomized multicenter trial. Lancet 354:701–707, 1999.

144. Fox KAA, Poole-Wilson PA, Henderson RA, et al: Interventional versus conservative treatment for patients with unstable angina or non–ST-elevation myocardial infarction: The British Heart Foundation RITA 3 randomised trial. Lancet 360:743–751, 2002.

145. SYNERGY Trial Investigators: Enoxaparin vs unfractionated heparin in high-risk patients with non–ST-segment elevation acute coronary syndromes managed with an intended early invasive strategy: Primary results of the SYNERGY randomized trial. JAMA 292:45–54, 2004.

146. Antman EM, Morrow D, McCabe C, et al: for the ExTRACT-TIMI 25 Investigators: Enoxaparin versus unfractionated heparin with fibrinolysis for ST-elevation myocardial infarction. N Engl J Med 354:1477–1488, 2006.

147. Collet JP, Montalescot G, Lison L, et al: Percutaneous coronary intervention after subcutaneous enoxaparin pretreatment in patients with unstable angina pectoris. Circulation 103:658–663, 2001.

148. Marmur JD, Anand SX, Bagga RS, et al: The activated clotting time can be used to monitor the low molecular weight heparin dalteparin after intravenous administration. J Am Coll Cardiol 41:394–402, 2003.

149. Blazing MA, de Lemons JA, White HD, et al, for the A to Z Investigators: Safety and efficacy of enoxaparin vs unfractionated heparin in patients with non–ST-segment elevation acute coronary syndromes who receive tirofiban and aspirin: A randomized controlled trial. JAMA 292:55–64, 2004.

150. Petersen JL, Mahaffey KW, Hasselblad V, et al: Efficacy and bleeding complications among patients randomized to enoxaparin or unfractionated heparin for antithrombin therapy in non–ST-segment elevation acute coronary syndromes: A systematic overview. JAMA 292:89–96, 2004.

151. Stone GW, McLaurin BT, Cox DA, et al: Bivalirudin for patients with acute coronary syndromes. N Engl J Med 355:2203–2216, 2006.

152. Becker RC, Spencer FA, Gibson M, Rust JE: Influence of patient characteristics and renal function on factor Xa inhibition pharmacokinetics and pharmacodynamics after enoxaparin administration in non–ST-segment elevation acute coronary syndromes. Am Heart J 143:753–759, 2002.

153. Verstaeta M, Nurmohamed M, Klenast J, et al: Biologic effects of recombinant hirudin (CGP 39.9) in human volunteers. European Hirudin in Thrombosis Group. J Am Coll Cardiol 22:1080–1088, 1993.

154. The Global Use of Strategies to Open Occluded Coronary Arteries (GUSTO) IIB Investigators: A comparison of recombinant hirudin with heparin for the treatment of acute coronary syndromes. N Engl J Med 335:775–782, 1996.

155. Organization to Assess Strategies for Ischemic Syndromes (OASIS) Investigators: Comparison of effects of two doses of recombinant hirudin compared with heparin in patients with acute myocardial ischemia without ST elevation: A pilot study. Circulation 96: 769–777, 1997.

156. Organization to Assess Strategies for Ischemic Syndromes (OASIS-2) Investigators: Effects of recombinant hirudin (lepirudin) compared with heparin on death, myocardial infarction, refractory angina, and revascularization procedures in patients with acute myocardial

ischaemia without ST elevation: A randomised trial. Lancet 353:429–438, 1999.

157. Bittl JA, Strony J, Brinker JA, et al, for the Hirulog Angioplasty Study Investigators: Treatment with bivalirudin (hirulog) as compared with heparin during coronary angioplasty for unstable or postinfarction angina. N Engl J Med 333:764–769, 1995.

158. Lincoff AM, Bittl JA, Kleiman NS, et al: The REPLACE 1 Trial: A pilot study of bivalirudin versus heparin during percutaneous coronary intervention with stenting and GP IIb/IIIa blockade. J Am Coll Cardiol 39 (suppl A): 16A, 2002.

159. Lincoff AM, Bittl JA, Harrington RA, et al, for the REPLACE-2 Investigators: Bivalirudin and provisional glycoprotein IIb/IIIa blockade compared with heparin and planned glycoprotein IIb/IIIa blockade during percutaneous coronary intervention: REPLACE-2 randomized trial. JAMA 289:853–863, 2003.

160. The Direct Thrombin Inhibitor Trialists' Collaborative Group: Direct thrombin inhibitors in acute coronary syndromes: Principal results of a meta-analysis based on individual patients' data. Lancet 359:294–302, 2002.

161. ACC/AHA Guidelines for the Management of Patients with ST-Elevation Myocardial Infarction—Executive Summary: A report of the American College of Cardiology/American Heart Association Task Force on Practice Guidelines (Writing Committee to Revise the 1999 Guidelines for the Management of Patients With Acute Myocardial Infarction). J Am Coll Cardiol 44:671–719, 2004.

162. Hirsh J, Guyatt G, Albers G, Schünemann H: The Seventh ACCP Conference on Antithrombotic and Thrombolytic Therapy: Evidence-based guidelines. Chest 126:172S–173S, 2004.

163. Smith S, Feldman T, Hirshfeld J, et al: ACC/AHA/SCAI 2005 guideline update for percutaneous coronary intervention: A report of the American College of Cardiology/American Heart Association Task Force on Practice Guidelines (ACC/AHA/SCAI Writing Committee to Update the 2001 Guidelines for Percutaneous Coronary Intervention. 2005). Available at:www.acc.org, www.americanheart.org or www.scai.org.

164. Visser CA, Kan G, Meltzer RS, et al: Embolic potential of left ventricular thrombus after mycardial infarction. J Am Coll Cardiol 5:1276–1280, 1985.

165. Vaitkus PT, Barnathom ES: Embolic potential, prevention and management of mural thrombus complicating anterior myocardial infarction: A meta-analysis. J Am Coll Cardiol 22:100–109, 1993.

166. Tunick PA, Kronzon I: Atheromas of the thoracic aorta: Clinical and therapeutic update. J Am Coll Cardiol 35:545–554, 2000.

167. Victor G, Dávila-Román MD, Murphy SF, et al: Atherosclerosis of the ascending aorta is an independent predictor of long-term neurologic events and mortality. J Am Coll Cardiol 33:1308–1316, 1999.

168. Amarenco P, Cohen A, Tzouri C, et al: Atherosclerotic disease of the aortic arch and the risk of ischemic stroke. N Engl J Med 331:1474–1479, 1994.

169. Maarenco P, Duyckaerts C, Tzourio C, et al: The prevalence of ulcerated plaques in the aortic arch in patients with stroke. N Engl J Med 326:221–225, 1992.

170. Khatibzadeh M, Mitusch R, Stierle U, et al: Aortic atherosclerotic plaques as a source of systemic embolism. J Am Coll Cardiol 27:664–669, 1996.

171. The Stroke Prevention in Atrial Fibrillation Investigators Committee on Echocardiography: Transesophageal echocardiography correlates of thromboembolism in high-risk patients with nonvalvular atrial fibrillation. Ann Intern Med 128:639–647, 1998.

172. Dressler FA, Craig WR, Castello R, et al: Mobile aortic atheroma and systemic emboli: Efficacy of anticoagulation and influence of plaque morphology on recurrent stroke. J Am Coll Cardiol 31:134–138, 1998.

173. Ferrari E, Vidal R, Chevallier T, et al: Atherosclerosis of the thoracic aorta and aortic debris as a marker of poor prognosis: Benefit of oral anticoagulants. J Am Coll Cardiol 33:1317–1322, 1999.

174. Jessup M: Mechanical cardiac-support devices: Dreams and devilish details. N Engl J Med 345:1490–1493, 2001.

175. Kumpati GS, McCarthy PM, Hoercher KJ: Left ventricular assist device as a bridge to recovery: Present status. J Cardiol Surg 16:294–301, 2001.

176. Wagner W, Johnson P, Kromos R, Griffity B: Evaluation of bioprosthetic valve–associated thrombus in ventricular assist device patients. Circulation 88:2023–2029, 1993.

177. Mehta S, Aufier T, Pae W, et al: Combined registry for clinical use of mechanical ventricular assist pumps and the total artificial heart in conjunction with heart transplantation: Sixth official report—1994. J Heart Lung Transplant 14:585–593, 1995.

178. Slater J, Rose E, Levin H, et al: Low thrombotic risk without anticoagulation using advanced-design left ventricular assist devices. Ann Thorac Surg 62:1321–1328, 1996.

179. Reilly M, Wiegers S, Cucchiara A, et al: Frequency, risk factors and clinical outcomes of left ventricular assist device–associated ventricular thrombus. Am J Cardiol 86:1156–1159, 2000.

180. Delgado R, Frazier O, Myers T, et al: Direct thrombolytic therapy for intraventricular thrombosis in patients with the Jarvik 2000 left ventricular assist device. J Heart Lung Transplant 24:231–233, 2005.

181. Alexander K, Chen A, Roe M, et al, for the CRUSADE Investigators: Excess dosing of antiplatelet and antithrombin agents in the treatment of non–ST-segment elevation acute coronary syndromes. JAMA 294:3108–3116, 2005.

182. Adam RC, Lunch JS: Anesthesia in cases of poor risk: Some suggestion for decreasing the risk. Surg Gynecol Obstet 74:1011–1101, 1942.

183. Corwin HL, Gettinger A, Pearl RG, et al, for the CRIT Study: Anemia and blood transfusion in the critically ill—Current clinical practice in the United States. Crit Care Med 20:159–178, 2004.

184. Wu WC, Rathore SS, Wang Y, et al: Blood transfusion in elderly patients with acute myocardial infarction. N Engl J Med 345:1230–1236, 2001.

185. Hebert PC, Yetisir E, Martin C, et al, Transfusion Requirements in Critical Care Investigators for the Canadian Critical Trials Group: Is a low transfusion threshold safe in critically ill patients with cardiovascular disease? Crit Care Med 29:227–234, 2001.

186. Rao SV, Jollis JG, Harrington RA, et al: Relationship of blood transfusion and clinical outcomes in patients with acute coronary syndromes. JAMA 292:1555–1562, 2004.

187. Hebert PC, Wells G, Blajchman MA, et al: A multicenter, randomized, controlled clinical trial of transfusion requirements in critical care. Transfusion Requirements in Critical Care Investigators, Canadian Critical Care Trials Group. N Engl J Med 340:409–417, 1999.

188. Malone DL, Dunne J, Tracy JK, et al: Blood transfusion, independent of shock severity, is associated with worse outcome in trauma. J Trauma 54:898–907, 2003.

189. Hart R, Tonarelli SB, Pearce LA: Avoiding central nervous system bleeding during antithrombotic therapy: Recent data and ideas. Stroke 36:1588–1593, 2005.

190. Ibanex L, Vidal X, Vendrell L, et al: Spanish-Italian Collaborative Group for the Epidemiology of Gastrointestinal Bleeding: Upper gastrointestinal bleeding associated with antiplatelet drugs. Aliment Pharmacol Ther 23:235–242, 2006.

191. Chan FK, Ching JY, Hung LC, et al: Clopidogrel versus aspirin and esomeprazole to prevent recurrent ulcer bleeding. N Engl J Med 352:238–244, 2005.

192. Liberopoulos EN, Elisaf MS, Tselepis AD, et al: Upper gastrointestinal hemorrhage complicating antiplatelet treatment with aspirin and/or clopidogrel: Where are we now? Platelets 17:1–6, 2006.

193. Harder S, Klinkhardt U, Alvarez JM: Avoidance of bleeding during surgery in patients receiving anticoagulant and/or antiplatelet therapy: Pharmacokinetic and pharmacodynamic considerations. Clin Pharmacokinet 43:963–981, 2004.

194. Sodha NR, Boodhwant M, Bianchi C, et al: Aprotinin in cardiac surgery. Expert Rev Cardiovasc Ther 4:151–160, 2004.

195. Levy JH: Massive transfusion coagulopathy. Semin Hematol 43:S59–S63, 2006.

196. van der Linden J, Lindvall G, Sartipy U: Aprotinin decreased postoperative bleeding and number of transfusions in patients on clopidogrel undergoing coronary artery bypass graft surgery: A double-blind, placebo-controlled, randomized clinical trial. Circulation 112:1276–1280, 2005.

197. Mangano DT, Tudor IC, Dietzel C: Multicenter Study of Perioperative Ischemia Research Group; Ischemia Research and Education Foundation: The risk associated with aprotinin in cardiac surgery. N Engl J Med 354:353–365, 2006.

198. Ozele MC, Svirin P, Larina L: Use of recombinant factor Viia in the management of severe bleeding episodes in patients with Bernard-Soulier syndrome. Ann Hematol 84:816–822, 2005.

199. Romagnoli S, Bevilacqua S, Gelsomino S, et al: Small dose recombinant activated factor VII (NovoSeven) in cardiac surgery. Anesth Analg 102:1320–1326, 2006.

200. Wilbourn B, Harrison P, Mackie IJ, et al: Activation of platelets in whole blood by recombinant factor VIIa by a thrombin-dependent mechanism. Br J Haematol 122:651–661, 2003.

201. Basso IN, Keeling D: Myocardial infarction following recombinant activated factor VII in a patient with type 2A von Willebrand disease. Blood Coagul Fibrinolysis 6:503–504, 2004.

Chapter 21

Risk Factors for Cardiovascular Disease and Arterial Thrombosis

Mary Cushman, MD, MSc • Barbara M. Alving, MD

INTRODUCTION

The hematologist, working in concert with cardiologists and vascular surgeons, may play an important role in guiding the effective and appropriate assessment of the patient who has sustained or is at risk for arterial thrombosis. This chapter reviews established risk factors and newer markers, such as C-reactive protein (CRP), that are used to determine risks for atherosclerosis and arterial events. Tests determined not to be helpful through evidence-based methods are also listed, and discussion of future areas of needed research is provided.

Major established risk factors for coronary heart disease (CHD) that are used to identify treatments for lowering low-density lipoprotein (LDL) cholesterol have been extensively reviewed in the third report of the National Cholesterol Education Program Adult Treatment Panel III (ATP III) on the detection, evaluation, and treatment of adults with high blood cholesterol.[1,2] This report focuses on level of risk and appropriate treatment for the primary prevention of CHD and for prevention of progression and acute events in those with established CHD. The first step in risk assessment is to calculate a 10-year predicted risk of CHD with the use of a tool such as the Framingham Risk Score.[3] Online calculators are available to assist clinicians (http://hp2010.nhlbihin. net/atpiii/calculator.asp). Accepted major risk factors include cigarette smoking, hypertension, high levels of LDL cholesterol, low levels of high-density lipoprotein (HDL) cholesterol, history of premature CHD in first-degree relatives, and patient age and gender (Table 21-1). Diabetes and other manifestations of arterial disease (e.g., peripheral artery disease, stroke) are considered CHD equivalents. In these settings, and when multiple risk factors are present that would confer a greater than 20% 10-year risk of CHD, treatment given to lower LDL cholesterol levels to <70 mg per deciliter is recommended. Among those with a 10-year predicted risk of 10% to 20%, benefits of lipid-lowering drugs are sometimes uncertain, and in this group, new risk factors might be considered.

Major risk factors have been validated in populations of various ethnicities.[4] Furthermore, prospective trials have found that 80% to 90% of patients with CHD have one or more of these conventional risk factors.[5] Between 87% and 100% of patients with fatal CHD have a history of at least one major risk factor.[6] Thus, the challenge of validating risk factors that provide additional value above that provided by those already recognized is great.[7,8]

NEWER MARKERS FOR ASSESSING ARTERIAL THROMBOSIS

Optimal assessment of new biomarkers of vascular risk should be conducted in prospective studies in which evaluation of the exposure of interest is done at baseline in apparently healthy individuals at risk for future cardiovascular disease (CVD). When the clinician considers application of these markers to treat a patient with a potentially new risk factor, several criteria must be met (Table 21-2). Measurement of the potential new risk marker must enhance the clinician's ability to predict risk compared with established traditional risk factors[9,10]; this value must be generalizable to a diverse population and should provide information that will guide the clinician in selecting a prevention strategy. Optimally, the risk factor that is assessed ought to be modifiable, or at least, its assessment should reveal an appropriate treatment that might not otherwise be administered. The analyte of interest must be measurable with an assay that is easy to apply to the population, is cost effective, and has appropriate sensitivity and specificity.[11]

C-Reactive Protein

Epidemiologic studies of new plasma and genetic markers for coronary risk have focused on three major domains: reduced fibrinolytic potential, increased thrombotic potential, and inflammation. CRP, one of the most extensively studied inflammation markers, appears to provide additional value in selected settings. CRP is synthesized by hepatocytes and rises several hundred-fold in response to circulating cytokines induced by acute injury. In the absence of acute inflammation, CRP levels tend to be stable within individuals over long periods, and they provide an index of underlying low-grade inflammation.

Many biologic roles have been described for CRP in relation to atherosclerosis.[12] Whether CRP has a direct role in thrombus formation is not clear, although its circulating level is directly correlated with levels of some hemostatic factors,[13] and experimental evidence has shown that CRP can induce monocyte tissue factor expression.[14] CRP colocalizes with complement in atherosclerotic plaques[15]; it can activate complement[16] and may regulate adhesion molecule expression by endothelial cells.[17] Further, CRP is chemotactic for monocytes within plaques.[18]

Many prospective epidemiologic studies have linked baseline levels of CRP to future risks of myocardial infarction,

Table 21-1 Risk Factors for Arterial Thrombosis

Major Risk Factors for Coronary Heart Disease (CHD)*

Cigarette smoking
Hypertension (blood pressure ≥140/90 mm Hg or patient receiving antihypertensive medication)
Low high-density lipoprotein (HDL) cholesterol and high low-density lipoprotein (LDL) cholesterol
Diabetes mellitus
Other forms of atherosclerosis (i.e., peripheral arterial disease)
Family history of premature CHD in first-degree relatives (males <55 years of age; females <65 years of age)

Other Markers for Consideration

C-reactive protein (CRP) (measured as high sensitivity-CRP [hs-CRP])
Lipoprotein-associated phospholipase A2 (Lp-PLA₂)
Cardiolipin antibody and lupus anticoagulant
Genetic markers for Fabry disease (stroke)

Tests Not Proved to Add Clinical Value

Fibrinogen levels
Homocysteine levels
Methylenetetrahydrofolate reductase (MTHFR) polymorphisms

Markers of Fibrinolysis

Tissue-type plasminogen activator (tPA) levels
Plasminogen activator inhibitor-1 (PAI-1) levels

Markers for Venous Thrombosis Risk (examples)

Factor V Leiden
Prothrombin 20210
Protein C
Lipoprotein(a) levels
D-Dimer levels

*Adapted from reference 1.

Table 21-2 Criteria for Consideration in Evaluation of Biochemical Risk Markers

Clinically applicable assay
High sensitivity and specificity
High within-person reproducibility
Significant population variability
Generalizability to diverse populations
Data obtained through valid epidemiologic study designs
Additive to predictive capacity of established risk factors
Cost-effectiveness
Assessment has the potential to result in a treatment or prevention strategy that would not otherwise have been used

stroke, and coronary heart disease mortality among individuals free of known cardiovascular disease.[19] The first report that linked elevated CRP (measured as high-sensitivity [hs]-CRP) with risk of future vascular events included patients with unstable angina.[20] In this study, higher levels of hs-CRP were associated with the development of recurrent acute coronary syndromes. In 1996, this finding was extended when a report from the Multiple Risk Factor Intervention Trial (MRFIT) showed that baseline hs-CRP was associated with future fatal coronary heart disease among male smokers who had other cardiac risk factors.[21] In that study, hs-CRP was measured in blood samples drawn 5 to 17 years before the onset of clinical events, pointing out

the potential for discriminating very long-term risk, and suggesting that hs-CRP measurement did not simply reflect generalized illness. In a larger study of apparently healthy middle-aged American men followed for 8 years, those with hs-CRP levels in the highest quartile at baseline had a twofold increase in the risk of future stroke, a threefold increase in the risk of myocardial infarction, a fourfold increase in the risk of undergoing surgery for peripheral vascular disease compared with study participants with lower levels of hs-CRP, but no increased risk of venous thrombosis.[22,23] These effects were additive to those of total cholesterol and HDL cholesterol in terms of risk prediction.[24]

Similar data confirming these observations have been reported in many prospective observational studies that studied other types of populations, such as women[25] and the elderly.[26] A meta-analysis reported that hs-CRP concentrations in the top one third of the population distribution were associated with a twofold increased risk of myocardial infarction.[27] Among individuals with stable and unstable coronary syndromes, and in those who have a prior history of myocardial infarction, hs-CRP may be useful for developing a prognosis and for choosing treatment.[20,28–32]

hs-CRP assays, along with World Health Organization standards for calibration, are commercially available for use in the clinic.[33,34] Standard clinical assays for CRP do not have adequate sensitivity and accuracy to detect levels in the range that is relevant for coronary risk prediction; accordingly, hs-CRP assays are required. Current guidelines (published in 2003) prepared by a group convened by the Centers for Disease Control and Prevention and the American Heart Association state that hs-CRP is the best marker of inflammation in assessment of risk for CVD (Table 21-3).[33] The guideline report and subsequently published studies indicate that measurement of hs-CRP may be useful in directing prevention of first CHD events for those individuals determined to be at intermediate risk for CHD (10% to 20% predicted risk over 10 years). Relative risk categories, which were derived on the basis of hs-CRP levels (as averaged from two measurements taken 2 weeks apart) are as follows: low risk, <1 mg per liter; average risk, 1 to 3 mg per liter; high risk, >3 mg per liter. In the current guideline report, it is suggested that values >10 mg per liter should prompt a workup for clinical inflammatory conditions; however, 5% to 10% of apparently healthy individuals have levels in this range, and two studies published subsequently showed that these values are

Table 21-3 Recommendations for Testing for High-Sensitivity C-Reactive Protein (hs-CRP) in Clinical Practice

- hs-CRP level may be useful in directing primary prevention of coronary heart disease (CHD) for individuals at intermediate predicted risk (10%–20% over 10 years).
- hs-CRP might be useful in those without known heart disease to encourage improvement in lifestyle risk factors.
- hs-CRP can be used in patients with stable CHD or acute coronary syndromes as an independent marker of prognosis for recurrent events (e.g., myocardial infarction, restenosis after percutaneous coronary intervention).
- The benefits of measuring hs-CRP in the clinical settings described above have not been established.

Adapted from reference 33.

associated with an even higher risk of CHD,[26,34] so they may have meaning as well in risk prediction. In the general population, about one third of people have CRP >3 mg per liter, although this proportion may be higher in some groups, such as women and some nonwhite ethnic groups.[35]

Once elevated levels of hs-CRP have been detected, interventions may be selected that may reduce those levels. Because levels are correlated with risk factors such as smoking, obesity, fitness, and physical inactivity, knowledge of the level may be motivational in encouraging patients to improve their lifestyles (although this has not been studied specifically). Statin therapy also lowers hs-CRP; some studies in primary and secondary prevention settings suggest that those with higher hs-CRP may derive benefit from therapy, regardless of LDL level.[31,36,37]

Although high levels of hs-CRP provide an independent marker for risk of CHD, the clinical benefit of measurement of hs-CRP is debated. Levels of hs-CRP in patients with stable coronary disease or acute coronary syndromes are an independent marker of prognosis for recurrent events, such as myocardial infarction or restenosis after precutaneous coronary intervention.[33] Two large trials reported that the lower the concentration of hs-CRP from intensive statin therapy 30 days after an acute coronary syndrome, the lower the risk of subsequent vascular events, regardless of statin dose.[31,37] In primary prevention settings, it remains unresolved whether patients with desirable lipid levels and elevated hs-CRP will derive benefit from initiation of statin therapy, although one study did suggest this.[36] An ongoing large prevention trial will address this question.[38]

For the practicing hematologist who sees patients with established arterial disease, if hs-CRP is elevated (>3 mg per liter on more than one occasion), statin therapy would currently be indicated (essentially, all patients with established arterial disease should be treated anyway with the goal of attaining a target LDL cholesterol <70 mg per deciliter). Optimal blood pressure control (<120/80 mm Hg) should be recommended, regardless of hs-CRP. The accuracy of monitoring hs-CRP to tailor the statin dose has not been substantiated, but it has been suggested that the lower the hs-CRP value, the lower the subsequent risk of vascular events. In primary prevention settings (where a hematologist is less likely to be involved), if a nondiabetic patient with a 10-year predicted CHD risk of 10% to 20% has hs-CRP >3 mg per liter on more than one occasion, lifestyle changes are indicated regarding smoking cessation, weight loss, increased physical activity, and a prudent diet. If LDL cholesterol is in the borderline range, indicating statin therapy by current guidelines, the practitioner may elect earlier introduction of treatment.

MARKERS FOR STROKE

Lipoprotein-associated phospholipase A2 (Lp-PLA$_2$), an enzyme synthesized by monocytes and macrophages, hydrolyzes oxidized phospholipids, thereby generating lysophosphatidylcholine and oxidized fatty acids, which have proinflammatory properties in atherosclerotic plaque. This enzyme, which is bound mainly to LDL cholesterol in the circulation, has been assessed in a prospective observational study, the Atherosclerosis Risk in Communities (ARIC) study, which involved more than 15,000 healthy middle-aged men and women.[39] Investigators in this study found that measurements of Lp-PLA$_2$ and hs-CRP may be useful beyond assessment of traditional risk factors (smoking, systolic hypertension, lipid levels, and diabetes) for risk prediction of stroke. Those who had the highest tertile of hs-CRP or Lp-PLA$_2$ were about twice as likely to have an ischemic stroke as those in the lowest tertile.[39] On the basis of these and other findings, the U.S. Food and Drug Administration approved a test that measures Lp-PLA$_2$. This test, known as the PLAC test (diaDexus, San Francisco, Calif), is available at reference laboratories and has been associated with risk of myocardial infarction and stroke in other studies.[40–42] The exact clinical role of Lp-PLA$_2$ testing remains to be defined, and specific inhibiting drugs are currently under development.

Two additional markers for stroke risk include appropriate tests to rule out antiphospholipid syndrome (see Chapter 19) and testing for Fabry disease. One-time laboratory tests for antiphospholipid antibodies after acute stroke were not helpful in determining long-term treatment in one clinical trial,[43] emphasizing the need for proper diagnosis. According to a report on persons between the ages of 18 and 55 years with unexplained acute cerebrovascular events, 4.9% of men and 2.4% of women had a biologically significant α-galactosidase gene mutation. Deficient α-galactosidase induces endothelial dysfunction and results in the phenotypic expression of Fabry disease.[44]

MARKERS OF UNPROVED OR INSIGNIFICANT VALUE IN CLINICAL PRACTICE

None of the hemostatic factor gene polymorphisms that have been studied in CHD provides increased value in risk prediction over traditional risk factors.[45] These include factor V Leiden, prothrombin 20210, and the plasminogen activator inhibitor-1 (PAI-1) 4G/5G variant (which results in elevated PAI-1 levels). Few population-based data are available on association of the rarer thrombophilic disorders with arterial disease (e.g., deficiency of protein C, protein S, or antithrombin III).

Epidemiologic studies that related hemostatic gene polymorphisms to arterial disease have been inconsistent and largely negative.[45–50] Although in some subgroups, such as young women, these factors may be associated with myocardial infarction,[51,52] optimal treatment approaches for such patients and the role of anticoagulant therapy, compared with aspirin or control of conventional risk factors, is not known. Because of this, assessment must be individualized. Standard guidelines do not exist.

Total Plasma Homocysteine

Homocysteine, a sulfhydryl amino acid, plays a major role in the metabolism of methionine. Patients with rare inherited deficiencies in the enzymes methionine synthase, methylenetetrahydrofolate reductase (MTHFR), and, in particular, cystathione beta-synthase may have marked plasma elevations of homocysteine and often

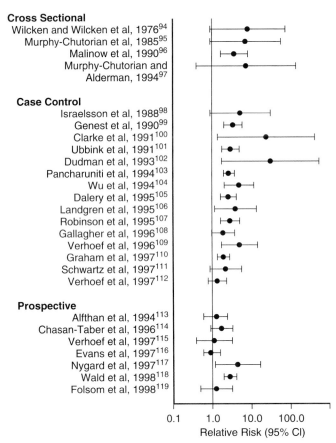

Figure 21-1 Prospective studies of homocysteine as a risk factor for future cardiovascular disease in populations free of clinical disease. (From Christen WG, Ajani VA, Glyun RJ, et al: Blood levels of homocysteine and increased risks of cardiovascular disease: Causal or casual? Arch Intern Med 160:422–434, 2000, with permission.)

experience premature atherothrombosis or venous thrombosis. Several mechanisms may link severe hyperhomocysteinemia (plasma concentration >100 μmol per liter) to vascular damage, including direct endothelial toxicity, induction of vascular smooth muscle proliferation, impairment of endothelially derived relaxing factor, and accelerated oxidation of LDL cholesterol.[53] On a population basis, severe hyperhomocysteinemia is rare. Mild to moderate hyperhomocysteinemia (plasma concentration >15 μmol per liter) is present in up to 10% of individuals; however, this prevalence has decreased dramatically in countries that have instituted fortification of grain with folic acid because the usual cause of mild to moderate hyperhomocysteinemia is low dietary folate intake. Folic acid, cyanocobalamin (vitamin B_{12}), and pyridoxine (vitamin B_6) are all involved in the regulation of methionine metabolism; several studies have detected inverse associations between homocysteine concentration and plasma levels of these vitamins. Administration of folic acid in doses between 0.5 and 5.0 mg per day produces a reduction in homocysteine levels.

Screening for hyperhomocysteinemia among asymptomatic individuals to determine risk is controversial and is not currently recommended by the American College of Cardiology or the American Heart Association.[54] Published reports on the relative risk of CHD with elevated homocysteine are shown in Figure 21-1; this illustration shows the differences between retrospective and prospective studies,

as well as among prospective studies. Several possible reasons have been proposed for conflicting results among prospective studies. Studies may be too heterogeneous in terms of methods or population source to be comparable with one another. Larger associations are evident in studies with shorter versus longer follow-up periods. Adjustment for potential confounders, such as vitamin intake, varies widely. Conflicting data suggest that the magnitude of any increased risk associated with hyperhomocysteinemia is likely to be modest and may be limited to those relatively few individuals with substantial elevations in total plasma homocysteine.

Four clinical trials of B vitamin supplementation published since 2004 have shown no benefit of homocysteine lowering for arterial vascular events. A trial of 3749 patients with acute myocardial infarction showed no benefit of various combinations of folic acid, vitamin B_{12}, and vitamin B_6 in terms of recurrent cardiovascular events; it was suggested that harm may result from triple-vitamin therapy.[55] Another trial randomly assigned 5522 patients 55 years of age and older with established CVD or diabetes to triple therapy with 2.5 mg folic acid, 50 mg vitamin B_6, and 1 mg vitamin B_{12} daily or placebo; results showed no overall benefit in reduction of cardiovascular events or death from CVD, with the exception of a 25% reduction in stroke (95% confidence interval [CI], 0.59 to 0.97).[56] However, another large, randomized trial of 3680 patients with stroke compared high-dose vitamin B supplementation (25 mg vitamin B_6, 0.4 mg vitamin B_{12}, 2.5 mg folic acid daily) with low doses found in multivitamins (200 μg vitamin B_6, 6 μg vitamin B_{12}, and 20 μg folic acid daily); no clinical benefit of plasma homocysteine lowering was discerned in the prevention of recurrent stroke or other end points.[57] A smaller study of high-dose folate (15 mg daily) or placebo in patients with chronic renal failure showed no effect on measures of atherosclerosis or clinical events.[58] Although only the last study specifically included patients with elevated plasma homocysteine levels, on the basis of these findings, homocysteine testing to define vascular risk does not seem appropriate at this time, given the lack of availability of an effective intervention. Genetic testing for the thermolabile variant of MTHFR is similarly not indicated.

Lipoprotein(a)

Lipoprotein(a) (Lp[a]) is composed of an apo B–containing lipoprotein structure that is virtually identical to that of LDL; it is attached by a single disulfide bond to a long, carbohydrate-rich protein designated apolipoprotein(a) (apo[a]). Apo(a) is highly homologous with plasminogen,[59] and it has been hypothesized that Lp(a) competes with plasminogen for binding sites on fibrin and endothelial cell surfaces, thus inhibiting fibrinolysis. Several lines of evidence support a biologic role for Lp(a) in atherothrombosis, including in vitro inhibition of plasminogen binding to fibrin and inhibition of tissue-type plasminogen activator (tPA)-catalyzed fibrinolysis.[60–62] A role in atherogenesis is suggested by other data: Lp(a) is more likely to accumulate in plaques from patients with unstable compared with stable angina, and it colocalizes with macrophages in unstable plaques.[63] Lp(a) also induces monocyte chemoattractant activity in human vascular endothelial cells.[64]

The clinical role of Lp(a) as a marker of risk for future coronary events is controversial. To date, more than a dozen prospective studies of Lp(a) have been published; many, but not all, have reported positive associations. For example, in three large studies, no association between baseline plasma concentration of Lp(a) and subsequent vascular risk was reported.[65–67] In contrast, four other studies reported positively graded associations between plasma Lp(a) level and risk of CHD.[68–71] A meta-analysis of prospective studies reported a relative risk of 1.7 (95% CI, 1.4 to 1.9) for Lp(a) in the top one third compared with the bottom one third of the distribution.[72]

Most guideline authorities do not recommend that Lp(a) evaluation be included in general screening programs. One reason not to recommend inclusion of Lp(a) evaluation in general screening programs is that Lp(a) levels vary among different racial cohorts, and at least one study has found no association between Lp(a) and vascular disease among African Americans.[73] Further, conflicting data in women suggest that findings in men cannot easily be generalized.[74] In a cohort of initially healthy women, very high levels (>90th percentile) were associated with increased risk for CVD in those women who also had high levels of LDL cholesterol.[75] Thus, the predictive value of Lp(a) may be limited to those with underlying hyperlipidemia—a relationship attenuated by LDL cholesterol reduction.[76] Additionally, lack of uniformity has been noted in methods used for testing for Lp(a).[77] In part, the tandem-repeat structure of apo(a) has made commercial assays difficult to calibrate—an issue that may be overcome by developing assays that make use of apo(a) monoclonal antibodies specific for unique epitopes of the Lp(a) molecule. However, whether such specific antibodies will improve the predictive value of Lp(a) testing remains uncertain.

Fibrinogen

Fibrinogen directly affects blood clotting, plasma rheology, platelet aggregation, and endothelial function. Further, plasma fibrinogen plays a major role in monocyte adhesion, and both fibrinogen and fibrin degradation products have been shown to stimulate smooth muscle proliferation. Thus, through hemostatic and inflammatory mechanisms, plasma fibrinogen level is closely related to thrombus formation.[78] Of the major novel markers for coronary artery disease, fibrinogen was the earliest to undergo extensive epidemiologic evaluation. Prospective data from many studies[45,79–81] all confirm that higher plasma fibrinogen levels are associated with risk of future myocardial infarction, stroke, or cardiovascular death, and in some studies, with non-CVD mortality. In a pooled analysis involving more than 150,000 participants from 31 prospective studies, after adjustment was made for conventional risk factors, each 1 g per liter higher fibrinogen increment was associated with a 1.8-fold higher risk of vascular events.[82] In some studies[83,84] but not in others, evidence has been presented that assessment of plasma fibrinogen levels adds to the predictive value of lipid screening. At the present time, because it is not clear how one should intervene for patients with higher fibrinogen levels, and because of assay standardization problems, no convincing evidence supports the value of measuring plasma levels of fibrinogen levels as a marker of CVD risk.

Fibrinolysis

The balance between plasminogen activators, primarily tPA and its main inhibitor, PAI-1, determines the overall activity of the fibrinolytic system. Fibrinolytic proteins may be detected in plasma with the use of sensitive assays for antigen and activity levels. In general, an increased PAI-1 concentration is associated with impaired fibrinolysis, which may lead to reduced plasmin, accumulation of fibrin and activation of metalloproteinase activity.[85] Determination of plasma fibrinolytic activity, however, has not provided additional predictive power in the establishment of risk for CVD.

Some of the difficulties associated with assessment of plasma fibrinolytic activity might be overcome by assessment of genetic markers of fibrinolytic function; genetic variations associated with PAI-1 and tPA production have been described. However, studies of an insertion–deletion polymorphism in the promotor region of the PAI-1 gene and of an Alu-repeat insertion–deletion polymorphism in the tPA gene have been inconsistent regarding relation to risk of CVD.

Hemostatic Activation Markers

D-Dimer is formed by the degradation of crosslinked fibrin by plasmin; therefore, plasma levels of D-dimer reflect ongoing fibrin formation and breakdown. Epidemiologic studies suggest that D-dimer may have predictive power for first and recurrent vascular events.[11,86–91] However, little evaluation has been conducted of the clinical usefulness of D-dimer measurement, and its generalizability remains uncertain.

FUTURE DIRECTIONS IN CORONARY RISK PREDICTION

In the future, cardiovascular risk reduction will involve the development of interventions that stabilize plaques and that incorporate evolving genetic approaches. Some of these interventions may be based on studies of the novel risk factors mentioned in this chapter. Novel therapeutic targets currently in development include new anti-inflammatory drugs, as well as antithrombotics and drugs that interfere with cytokine function, metalloproteinase activity, and nuclear receptor/transcription factors.[92]

Genetic screening is likely to represent a dramatic paradigm shift in coronary disease prevention in the future. Although it is clear that family history is a determinant of the risk of myocardial infarction, the net impact of family history on risk is modest. Although association of single-gene polymorphisms with atherothrombosis has so far been disappointing,[93] the advent of high-throughput multilocus gene screening should provide a more robust approach to cardiovascular risk prediction.

REFERENCES

1. Executive Summary of the Third Report of the National Cholesterol Education Program (NCEP): Expert Panel on Detection, Evaluation, and Treatment of High Blood Cholesterol in Adults (Adult Treatment Panel III). JAMA 285:2486–2497, 2001.
2. Third Report of the National Cholesterol Education Program (NCEP): Expert Panel on Detection Evaluation, and Treatment of High Blood Cholesterol in Adults (Adult Treatment Panel III) Final Report. Circulation 106:3143–3421, 2002.
3. Wilson PW, D'Agostino RB, Levy D, et al: Prediction of coronary heart disease using risk factor categories. Circulation 97:1837–1847, 1998.
4. D'Agostino RB, Grundy S, Sullivan L, Wilson P: Validation of the Framingham coronary heart disease prediction scores. JAMA 286:180–187, 2001.
5. Khot UN, Khot MB, Bajzer CT, Sapp SK, et al: Prevalence of conventional risk factors in patients with coronary heart disease. JAMA 290:898–904, 2003.
6. Greenland P, Knoll MD, Stamlev J, et al: Major risk factors as antecedents of fatal and nonfatal coronary heart disease events. JAMA 290:891–897, 2003.
7. Wang TJ, Gona P, Larson MG, et al: Multiple biomarkers for the prediction of the first major cardiovascular events and death. N Engl J Med 355:2631–2639, 2006.
8. Folsom AR, Chambless LE, Ballantyne CM, et al: An assessment of incremental coronary risk prediction using C-reactive protein and other novel risk markers: The Atherosclerosis Risk in Communities Study. Arch Intern Med 166:1368–1373, 2006.
9. Ridker PM: Evaluating novel cardiovascular risk factors: can we better predict heart attacks? Ann Intern Med 130:933–937, 1999.
10. Greenland P, O'Malley PG: When is a new prediction marker useful? A consideration of lipoprotein-associated phospholipase A_2 and C-reactive protein for stroke risk. Arch Intern Med 165:2454–2456, 2005.
11. Shiplander MT, Moore EG: Rapid, fully automated measurement of plasma homocyst(e)ine with the Abbott Imx Analyzer. Clin Chem 41:991–995, 1995.
12. Verma S, Devaraj S, Jialal I: Is C-reactive protein an innocent bystander or proatherogenic culprit? C-reactive protein promotes atherothrombosis. Circulation 113:2135–2350, 2006; discussion, 2150.
13. Cushman M, Lemaitre RN, Kuller LH, et al: Fibrinolytic activation markers predict myocardial infarction in the elderly: The Cardiovascular Health Study. Arterioscler Thromb Vasc Biol 19:493–498, 1999.
14. Cermak J, Key N, Bach R, et al: C-reactive protein induces human peripheral blood monocytes to synthesize tissue factor. Blood 82:513–520, 1993.
15. Torzewski J, Torzewski M, Bowyer DE, et al: C-reactive protein frequently colocalizes with the terminal complement complex in the intima of early atherosclerotic lesions of human coronary arteries. Arterioscler Thromb Vasc Biol 18:1386–1392, 1998.
16. Bhakdi S, Torzewski M, Klouche M, et al: Complement and atherogenesis: binding of CRP to degraded, nonoxidized LDL enhances complement activation. Arterioscler Thromb Vasc Biol 19:2348–2354, 1999.
17. Pasceri V, Willerson JT, Yeh ETH: Direct proinflammatory effect of C-reactive protein on human endothelial cells. Circulation 102:2165–2168, 2000.
18. Torzewski M, Rist C, Mortensen RF, et al: C-reactive protein in the arterial intima: Role of C-reactive protein receptor–dependent monocyte recruitment in atherogenesis. Arterioscler Thromb Vasc Biol 20:2094–2099, 2000.
19. Ridker PM, Haughie P: Prospective studies of C-reactive protein as a risk factor for cardiovascular disease. J Invest Med 46:391–395, 1998.
20. Liuzzo G, Biasucci LM, Gallimore R, et al: The prognostic value of C-reactive protein and serum amyloid, a protein, in severe unstable angina. N Engl J Med 331:417–424, 1994.
21. Kuller LH, Tracy RP, Shaten J, et al: Relation of C-reactive protein and coronary heart disease in the MRFIT nested case-control study. Am J Epidemiol 144:537–547, 1996.
22. Ridker PM, Cushman M, Stampfer MJ, et al: Inflammation, aspirin, and the risk of cardiovascular disease in apparently healthy men. N Engl J Med 336:973–979, 1997.
23. Ridker PM, Cushman M, Stampfer MJ, et al: Plasma concentration of C-reactive protein and risk of developing peripheral vascular disease. Circulation 97:425–428, 1998.
24. Ridker PM, Glynn RJ, Hennekens CH: C-reactive protein adds to the predictive value of total and HDL cholesterol in determining risk of first myocardial infarction. Circulation 97:2007–2011, 1998.
25. Ridker PM, Hennekens CH, Buring JE, et al: C-reactive protein and other markers of inflammation in the prediction of cardiovascular disease in women. N Engl J Med 342:836–843, 2000.
26. Cushman M, Arnold AM, Psaty BM, et al: C-reactive protein and the 10-year incidence of coronary heart disease in older men and women: The Cardiovascular Health Study. Circulation 112:25–31, 2005.
27. Danesh J, Whincup P, Walker M, et al: Low grade inflammation and coronary heart disease: Prospective study and updated meta-analysis. BMJ 321:199–204, 2000.
28. Haverkate F, Thompson SG, Pyke SDM, et al: Production of C-reactive protein and risk of coronary events in stable and unstable angina. Lancet 349:462–466, 1997.
29. Morrow D, Rifai N, Antman E, et al: C-reactive protein as a potent predictor of mortality independently and in combination with troponin T in acute coronary syndromes. J Am Coll Cardiol 31:1460–1465, 1998.
30. Ridker PM, Rifai N, Pfeffer MA, et al: Inflammation, pravastatin, and the risk of coronary events after myocardial infarction in patients with average cholesterol levels. Circulation 98:839–844, 1998.
31. Ridker PM, Cannon CP, Morrow D, et al: C-reactive protein levels and outcomes after statin therapy. N Engl J Med 352:20–28, 2005.
32. Nissen SE, Tuzcu EM, Schoenhagen P, et al: Statin therapy, LDL cholesterol, C-reactive protein, and coronary artery disease. N Engl J Med 352:29–38, 2005.
33. Pearson TA, Mensah GA, Alexander W, et al: Markers of inflammation and cardiovascular disease: Application to clinical and public health practice: A statement for healthcare professionals from the Centers for Disease Control and Prevention and the American Heart Association. Circulation 107:499–511, 2003.
34. Ridker PM, Cook N: Clinical usefulness of very high and very low levels of C-reactive protein across the full range of Framingham risk scores. Circulation 109:1955–1959, 2004.

35. Lakoski SG, Cushman M, Criqui M, et al: Gender and C-reactive protein: data from the Multiethnic Study of Atherosclerosis (MESA) cohort. Am Heart J 152:593–598, 2006.

36. Ridker PM, Rifai N, Clearfield M, et al: For the Air Force/Texas Coronary Atherosclerosis Prevention Study Investigators: Measurement of C-reactive protein for the targeting of statin therapy in the primary prevention of acute coronary events. N Engl J Med 344:1959–1965, 2001.

37. Morrow DA, de Lemos JA, Sabatine MS, et al: Clinical relevance of C-reactive protein during follow-up of patients with acute coronary syndromes in the Aggrastat-to-Zocor trial. Circulation 114:281–288, 2006.

38. Ridker PM: Rosuvastatin in the primary prevention of cardiovascular disease among patients with low levels of low-density lipoprotein cholesterol and elevated high-sensitivity C-reactive protein: Rationale and design of the JUPITER trial. Circulation 108:2292–2297, 2003.

39. Ballantyne CM, Hoogeveen RC, Bang H, et al: Lipoprotein-associated phospholipase A$_2$, high-sensitivity C-reactive protein, and risk for incident ischemic stroke in middle-aged men and women in the Atherosclerosis Risk In Communities (ARIC) study. Arch Intern Med 165:2479–2484, 2005.

40. Koenig W, Khuseyinova N, Lowel H, et al: Lipoprotein-associated phospholipase A2 adds to risk prediction of incident coronary events by C-reactive protein in apparently healthy middle-aged men from the general population: Results from the 14-year follow-up of a large cohort from southern Germany. Circulation 110:1903–1908, 2004.

41. Packard CJ, O'Reilly DS, Caslake MJ, et al: Lipoprotein-associated phospholipase A2 as an independent predictor of coronary heart disease. West of Scotland Coronary Prevention Study Group. N Engl J Med 343:1148–1155, 2000.

42. Oei HH, van der Meer IM, Hofman A, et al: Lipoprotein-associated phospholipase A2 activity is associated with risk of coronary heart disease and ischemic stroke: The Rotterdam study. Circulation 111:570–575, 2005.

43. Levine SR, Brey RL, Tilley BC, et al: Antiphospholipid antibodies and subsequent thrombo-occlusive events in patients with ischemic stroke. JAMA 291:576–584, 2004.

44. Rolfs A, Bottcher T, Nzchiesche M, et al: Prevalence of Fabry disease in patients with cryptogenic stroke: A prospective study. Lancet 366:1794–1796, 2005.

45. Ye Z, Liu EHC, Higgins JPT, et al: Seven haemostatic gene polymorphisms in coronary disease: Meta-analysis of 66,155 cases and 91,307 controls. Lancet 367:651–658, 2006.

46. Folsom AR, Wu KK, Rosamond WD, et al: Prospective study of hemostatic factors and incidence of coronary heart disease: The Atherosclerosis Risk in Communities (ARIC) study. Circulation 96:1102–1108, 1997.

47. Ridker PM, Hennekens CH, Lindpaintner K, et al: Mutation in the gene encoding for coagulation factor V and the risk of myocardial infarction, stroke, and venous thrombosis in apparently healthy men. N Engl J Med 332:912–917, 1995.

48. Cushman M, Rosendaal F, Cook E, et al: Factor V Leiden does not increase cardiovascular risk in the elderly. Thromb Haemost 79:912–915, 1998.

49. Ridker PM, Hennekens CH, Miletich JP: G20210A mutation in prothrombin gene and risk of myocardial infarction, stroke, and venous thrombosis in a large cohort of U.S. men. Circulation 99:999–1004, 1999.

50. Cushman M: Hemostatic risk factors for cardiovascular disease. In Schechter GP, Hoffman R, Schrier SL (eds): Hematology 1999. Washington, DC, The American Society of Hematology, 1999, pp 236–242.

51. Rosendaal FR, Siscovick DS, Schwartz SM, et al: A common prothrombin variant (20210 G to A) increases the risk of myocardial infarction in young women. Blood 90:1747–1750, 1997.

52. Doggen CJM, Manger Cats V, Bertina RM, et al: Interaction of coagulation defects and cardiovascular risk factors: Increased risk of myocardial infarction associated with factor V Leiden or prothrombin 20210A. Circulation 97:1037–1041, 1998.

53. Welch GN, Loscalzo J: Mechanisms of disease: Homocysteine and therothrombosis. N Engl J Med 338:1042–1050, 1998.

54. Malinow MR, Bostom AG, Krauss RM: Homocyst(e)ine, diet, and cardiovascular disease: A statement for healthcare professionals from the Nutrition Committee, American Heart Association. Circulation 99:178–182, 1999.

55. Bonaa KH, Njolstad I, Ueland PM, et al: Homocysteine lowering and cardiovascular events after acute myocardial infarction. N Engl J Med 354:1578–1588, 2006.

56. Lonn E, Yusuf S, Arnold MJ, et al: Homocysteine lowering with folic acid and B vitamins in vascular disease. N Engl J Med 354:1567–1577, 2006.

57. Toole JF, Malinow MR, Chambless LE, et al: Lowering homocysteine in patients with ischemic stroke to prevent recurrent stroke, myocardial infarction, and death: the Vitamin Intervention for Stroke Prevention (VISP) randomized controlled trial. JAMA 291:565–575, 2004.

58. Zoungas S, McGrath BP, Branley P, et al: Cardiovascular morbidity and mortality in the Atherosclerosis and Folic Acid Supplementation Trial (ASFAST) in chronic renal failure: A multicenter, randomized, controlled trial. J Am Coll Cardiol 47:1108–1116, 2006.

59. McLean JW, Tomlinson JE, Kuang WJ, et al: cDNA sequence of human apolipoprotein(a) is homologous to plasminogen. Nature 330:132–137, 1987.

60. Hajar KA, Gavish D, Breslow JL, et al: Lipoprotein(a) modulation of endothelial cell surface fibrinolysis and its potential role in atherosclerosis. Nature 339:303–305, 1989.

61. Harpel PC, Gordon BR, Parker TS: Plasmin catalyzes binding of lipoprotein(a) to immobilized fibrinogen and fibrin. Proc Natl Acad Sci U S A 86:3847–3851, 1989.

62. Loscalzo J, Weinfeld M, Fless G, et al: Lipoprotein (a), fibrin binding, and plasminogen activation. Arteriosclerosis 10:240–245, 1990.

63. Dangas G, Mehran R, Harpel PC, et al: Lipoprotein(a) and inflammation in human coronary atheroma: Association with severity of clinical presentation. J Am Coll Cardiol 32:2035–2042, 1998.

64. Poon M, Zhang X, Dunsky KG, et al: Apolipoprotein(a) induces monocyte chemotactic activity in human vascular endothelial cells. Circulation 96:2514–2519, 1997.

65. Jauhiainen M, Koskinen P, Ehnholm C, et al: Lipoprotein(a) and coronary heart disease risk: A nested case-control study of the Helskinki Heart Study participants. Atherosclerosis 89:59–67, 1991.

66. Ridker PM, Hennekens CH, Stampfer MJ: A prospective study of lipoprotein (a) and the risk of myocardial infarction. JAMA 270:2195–2199, 1993.

67. Cantin B, Gagnon F, Moorjani S, et al: Is lipoprotein(a) an independent risk factor for ischemic heart disease in men? The Quebec Cardiovascular Study. J Am Coll Cardiol 31:519–525, 1998.

68. Schaefer EJ, Lamon-Fava S, Jenner JL, et al: Lipoprotein(a) levels and risk of coronary heart disease in men. The Lipid Research Clinics Coronary Primary Prevention Trial. JAMA 271:999–1003, 1994.

69. Cremer P, Nagel D, Labrot B, et al: Lipoprotein(a) as a predictor of myocardial infarction in comparison to fibrinogen, LDL cholesterol and other risk factors: results from the prospective Gottingen Risk Incidence and Prevalence Study (GRIPS). Eur J Clin Invest 24:444–453, 1994.

70. Wald NJ, Law M, Watt HC, et al: Apolipoproteins and ischaemic heart disease: Implications for screening. Lancet 343:75–79, 1994.

71. Wild SH, Fortmann SP, Marcovina SM: A prospective case control study of lipoprotein(a) levels and apo(a) size and risk of coronary heart disease in Stanford five-city project participants. Arterioscler Thromb Vasc Biol 17:239–245, 1997.

72. Danesh J, Collins R, Peto R: Lipoprotein(a) and coronary heart disease: A meta-analysis of prospective studies. Circulation 102:1082–1085, 2000.

73. Moliterno DJ, Jokinen EV, Miserez AR, et al: No association between plasma lipoprotein(a) concentrations and the presence or absence of coronary atherosclerosis in African-Americans. Arterioscler Thromb Vasc Biol 15:850–855, 1995.

74. Sunayama S, Daida H, Mokuno H, et al: Lack of increased coronary atherosclerotic risk due to elevated lipoprotein(a) in women 55 years of age. Circulation 94:1263–1268, 1996.

75. Danik JS, Rifai N, Buring JE, Ridker PM: Lipoprotein(a), measured with an assay independent of apolipoprotein(a) isoform size, and risk of future cardiovascular events among initially healthy women. JAMA 296:1363–1370, 2006.

76. Maher VM, Brown BG, Marcovina SM, et al: Effects of lowering elevated LDL cholesterol on the cardiovascular risk of lipoprotein(a). JAMA 274:1771–1774, 1995.

77. Tate JR, Rifai N, Berg K, et al: International Federation of Clinical Chemistry standardization project for measurement of lipoprotein(a). Phase 1. Evaluation of analytical performance of lipoprotein(a) assay systems and commercial calibratorss. Clin Chem 44:1629–1640, 1998.

78. Ernst E, Resch KL: Fibrinogen as a cardiovascular risk factor: A meta-analysis and review of the literature. Ann Intern Med 118:956–963, 1993.

21

79. Tracy RP, Arnold AM, Ettinger W, et al: The relationship of fibrinogen and factors VII and VIII to incident cardiovascular disease and death in the elderly: Results from the Cardiovascular Health Study. Arterioscler Thromb Vasc Biol 19:1776–1783, 1999.

80. Danesh J, Collins R, Appleby P, et al: Association of fibrinogen, C-reactive protein, albumin, or leukocyte count with coronary heart disease: Meta-analyses of prospective studies. JAMA 279:1477–1482, 1998.

81. Ma J, Hennekens CH, Ridker PM, et al: A prospective study of fibrinogen and risk of myocardial infarction in the Physicians' Health Study. J Am Coll Cardiol 33:1347–1352, 1999.

82. Danesh J, Lewington S, Thompson SG, et al: Plasma fibrinogen level and the risk of major cardiovascular diseases and nonvascular mortality: An individual participant meta-analysis. JAMA 294:1799–1809, 2005.

83. Heinrich J, Balleisen L, Schulte H, et al: Fibrinogen and factor VII in the prediction of coronary risk: Results from the PROCAM study in healthy men. Arterioscler Thromb 14:54–59, 1994.

84. Thompson S, Kienast J, Pyke S, et al: Hemostatic factors and the risk of myocardial infarction or sudden death in patients with angina pectoris. N Engl J Med 332:635–641, 1995.

85. Collen D, Lijnen HR: Basic and clinical aspects of fibrinolysis and thrombolysis. Blood 78:3114–3124, 1991.

86. Ridker PM, Hennekens CH, Cerskus A, et al: Plasma concentration of cross-linked fibrin degradation product (D-dimer) and the risk of future myocardial infarction among apparently healthy men. Circulation 90:2236–2240, 1994.

87. Fowkes FGR, Lowe GDO, Housely E, et al: Cross-linked fibrin degradation products, progression of peripheral arterial disease, and risk of coronary heart disease. Lancet 342:84–86, 1993.

88. Lowe GDO, Yarnell JWG, Sweetnam PM, et al: Fibrin D-dimer, tissue plasminogen activator, plasminogen activator inhibitor, and the risk of major ischemic heart disease in the Caerphilly Study. Thromb Haemost 79:129–133, 1998.

89. Folsom AR, Aleksic N, Park E, et al: Prospective study of fibrinolytic factors and incident coronary heart disease: The Atherosclerosis Risk in Communities (ARIC) study. Arterioscler Thromb Vasc Biol 21:611–617, 2001.

90. Pradhan AD, LaCroix AZ, Langer RD, et al: Tissue plasminogen activator antigen and D-dimer as markers for atherothrombotic risk among healthy postmenopausal women. Circulation 110:292–300, 2004.

91. Smith A, Patterson C, Yarnell J, et al: Which hemostatic markers add to the predictive value of conventional risk factors for coronary heart disease and ischemic stroke? The Caerphilly study. Circulation 112:3080–3087, 2005.

92. Libby P: Molecular basis of acute coronary syndromes. Circulation 91:2844–2850, 1995.

93. Ridker PM, Stampfer MJ: Assessment of genetic markers for coronary thrombosis: Promise and precaution. Lancet 353:687–688, 1999.

94. Wilcken DEL, Wilcken B: The pathogenesis of coronary artery disease: A possible role for methionine metabolism. J Clin Invest 57:1079–1082, 1976.

95. Murphy-Chutorian DR, Wexman MP, Grieco AJ, et al: Methionine intolerance: A possible risk factor for coronary artery disease. J Am Coll Cardiol 6:725–730, 1985.

96. Malinow MR, Sexton G, Averbuch M, et al: Homocyst(e)inemia in daily practice: Levels in coronary artery disease. Coron Art Dis 1:215–220, 1990.

97. Murphy-Chutorian D, Alderman EL: The case that hyperhomocysteinemia is a risk factor for coronary artery disease. Am J Cardiol 73:705–707, 1994.

98. Israelsson B, Brattstrom LE, Hultberg BL: Homocysteine and myocardial infarction. Atherosclerosis 71:227–233, 1988.

99. Genest JJ Jr, McNamara JR, Salem DN, et al: Plasma homocyst(e)ine levels in men with premature coronary artery disease. J Am Coll Cardiol 16:1114–1119, 1990.

100. Clarke R, Daly L, Robinson K, et al: Hyperhomocysteinemia: An independent risk factor for vascular disease. N Engl J Med 324:1149–1155, 1991.

101. Ubbink JB, Vermaak WJH, Bennett JM, et al: The prevalence of homocysteinemia and hypercholesterolemia in angiographically defined coronary artery disease. Klin Wochenschr 69:627–534, 1991.

102. Dudman NPB, Wilcken DEL, Wang J, et al: Disordered methionine/homocysteine metabolism in premature vascular disease. Arterioscler Thromb Vasc Biol 13:1253–1260, 1993.

103. Pancharuniti N, Lewis CA, Sauberlich HE, et al: Plasma homocyst(e)ine, folate, and vitamine B12 concentrations and risk for early-onset coronary artery disease. Am J Clin Nutr 59:940–948, 1994.

104. Wu LL, Wu J, Hunt SC, et al: Plasma homocyst(e)ine as a risk factor for early familial coronary artery disease. Clin Chem 40:552–561, 1994.

105. Dalery K, Lussier-Cacan S, Selhub J, et al: Homocysteine and coronary artery disease in French Canadian subjects: Relation with vitamins B₁₂, B₆, pyridoxal phosphate, and folate. Am J Cardiol 75:1107–1111, 1995.

106. Landgren F, Israelsson B, Lindgren A, et al: Plasma homocysteine in acute myocardial infarction: Homocysteine-lowering effect of folic acid. J Intern Med 237:381–388, 1995.

107. Robinson K, Mayer EL, Miller DP, et al: Hyperhomocysteinemia and low pyridoxal phosphate: Common and independent reversible risk factors for coronary artery disease. Circulation 92:2825–2830, 1995.

108. Gallagher PM, Meleady R, Shields DC, et al: Homomcysteine and risk of premature coronary heart disease: Evidence for a common gene mutation. Circulation 94:2154–2158, 1996.

109. Verhoef P, Stampfer MJ, Buring JE, et al: Homocysteine metabolism and risk of myocardial infarction: Relation with B₁₂, B₆, and folate. Am J Epidemiol 143:845–859, 1996.

110. Graham IM, Daly LE, Refsum HM, et al: Plasma homocysteine as a risk factor for vascular disease: The European Concerted Action Project. JAMA 277:1775–1781, 1997.

111. Schwartz SM, Siscovick DS, Malinow MR, et al: Myocardial infarction in young women in relation to plasma total homocysteine folate, and a common variant in the methylenetetrahydrofolate reductase gene. Circulation 96:412–417, 1997.

112. Verhoef P, Kok FJ, Kruyssen ACM, et al: Plasma total homocysteine, B vitamins, and risk of coronary atherosclerosis. Arterioscler Thromb Vasc Biol 17:989–995, 1997.

113. Alfthan G, Pekkanen J, Jauhiainen M, et al: Relation of serum homocysteine and lipoprotein(a) concentrations to atherosclerotic disease in a prospective Finnish popluation-based study. Atherosclerosis 106:9–19, 1994.

114. Chasan-Taber L, Selhub J, Rosenberg IH, et al: A prospective study of folate and vitamin B6 and risk of myocardial infarction in US physicians. J Am Coll Nutr 15:136–143, 1996.

115. Verhoef P, Hennekens CH, Allen RH, et al: Plasma total homocysteine and risk of angina pectoris with subsequent coronary artery bypass surgery. Am J Cardiol 79:799–801, 1997.

116. Evans RW, Shaten BJ, Hempel JD, Cutler JA, Kuller LH, for the MRFIT Research Group. Homocyst(e)ine and risk of cardiovascular disease in the Multiple Risk Factor Intervention Trial. Arterioscler Thromb Vasc Biol 17:1947–1953, 1997.

117. Nygard O, Nordrehaug JE, Refsum H, et al: Plasma homocysteine levels and mortality in patients with coronary artery disease. N Engl J Med 337:230–236, 1997.

118. Wald NJ, Watt HC, Law MR, et al: Homocysteine and ischemic heart disease: Results of a prospective study with implications regarding pervention. Arch Intern Med 158:862–867, 1998.

119. Folsom AR, Nieto J, McGovern PG, et al: Prospective study of coronary heart disease incidence in relation to fasting total homocysteine, related genetic polymorphisms, and B vitamins. Circulation 98:204–210, 1998.

Chapter 22

Peripheral Arterial Disease

William R. Hiatt, MD

INTRODUCTION

Peripheral arterial disease (PAD) of the lower extremities is one of the major manifestations of systemic atherosclerosis. The disease affects from 4% to 12% of adults (depending on the population studied).[1,2] Risk factors are typical of those for atherosclerosis and include advanced age, cigarette smoking, diabetes mellitus, hyperlipidemia, hypertension, and inflammation; the most important are diabetes and smoking.[1,3]

Clinical manifestations of PAD range from asymptomatic in 20% to 50%, atypical leg pain in 40% to 50%, typical claudication in 10% to 35% and critical leg ischemia (CLI) in 1% to 2% (Fig. 22-1). Asymptomatic patients with PAD have severely limited limb function, including limited walking distance and speed.[4] Therefore, from a functional perspective, all patients with PAD have symptomatic limitations.

Claudication is pain in the legs on walking, primarily in the calves, which does not go away with continued walking and is relieved by rest. Among patients with claudication, symptom severity follows a stable course over 5 years in 70% to 80%, with only 10% to 20% developing worsening claudication and 1% to 2% experiencing the onset of CLI, which is the most severe manifestation of PAD.[5] Patients with CLI have severe arterial occlusive disease, usually involving multiple segments. Clinical evidence of CLI includes ischemic pain in the distal foot, ischemic ulceration, or gangrene. Patients with CLI are at high risk of limb loss.

PAD is highly associated with critical coronary and carotid artery diseases, and it predisposes patients with these conditions to markedly increased risks of myocardial infarction, ischemic stroke, and vascular death.[6] For example, in patients with PAD, adjusted cardiovascular mortality is increased sixfold.[7] This risk is approximately equal between men and women, and it is elevated even if the patient has had no prior clinical evidence of cardiovascular disease.[8] With increasing severity of PAD, as measured by the ankle-brachial index (ABI), come concomitant increased risks of myocardial infarction, ischemic stroke, and vascular death.[9] After 5 years, 20% of patients experience a nonfatal myocardial infarction or stroke, and 15% to 30% die (see Fig. 22-1). Therefore, the initial goals of management are to recommend changes in lifestyle, to identify and modify cardiovascular risk factors, and to administer antiplatelet drugs to reduce the risk of cardiovascular events. These treatments may also slow the progression of atherosclerosis in the peripheral circulation and may inhibit clinical progression of disease.

In patients with claudication, the goal of treatment is to improve exercise performance, community-based walking ability, and quality of life. In patients with CLI, the goals of therapy are to prevent limb loss, to heal ischemic ulcers, to relieve pain at rest, and to improve functional status. For patients with claudication, approaches used to treat symptoms include supervised exercise rehabilitation, administration of cilostazol, and select use of revascularization procedures. In contrast, no effective medical therapy for CLI is available, as these patients require restoration of blood flow to heal wounds, relieve ischemic pain, and prevent limb loss.

DIAGNOSIS

All patients at risk for arterial disease (age >50 years with a history of smoking or diabetes, and all persons >70 years of age)[10] should undergo history and physical examination for assessment of symptoms of claudication or CLI. Palpation of arterial pulses should be performed, with focus on the brachial, femoral, and pedal arteries (posterior tibial and dorsalis pedis). Absence of a femoral pulse indicates inflow disease of the aorta or iliac arteries; in patients with a palpable femoral pulse but no pedal pulse, disease is confined to the arteries in the leg. Patients with CLI develop pain in the distal foot at rest that can progress to ischemic ulceration and gangrene. The ulcers are painful, do not bleed when manipulated, and often have a dark necrotic base.

Any patient with reduced or absent pulses in the leg should be suspected of having PAD and should undergo measurement of the ABI, which is also a class 1 recommendation. The ABI is the ratio of systolic blood pressure in the ankle divided by systolic blood pressure in the arm. A Doppler ultrasound instrument is required to detect pulse, and typically, pressures in both arms and each tibial vessel in both ankles are measured. The standard calculation is based on the highest pressure in each ankle and the highest arm pressure. Each leg receives an independent ABI measurement, and a value <0.90 in either leg indicates PAD.[11,12]

Vascular Laboratory and Imaging

Although the ABI is an accurate screening test for PAD, it does have limitations (Table 22-1). In a few patients with diabetes or renal disease, the tibial vessels become calcified and incompressible. With incompressible vessels, ankle pressure is often >200 to 250 mm Hg, leading to an ABI

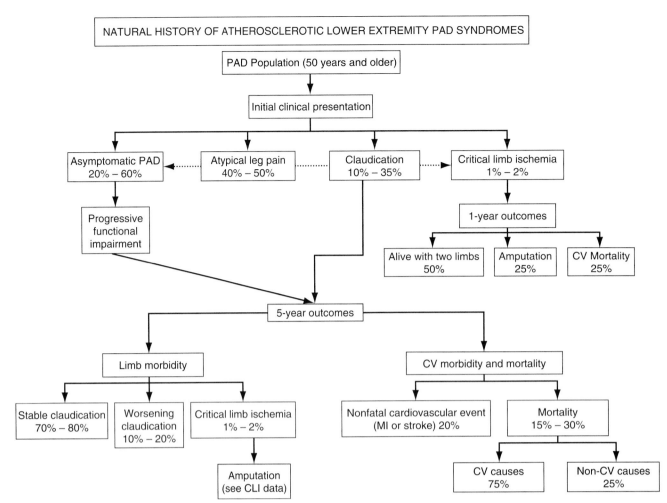

Figure 22-1 Natural history of peripheral arterial disease. CLI = critical leg ischemia. (From Hirsch AT, Haskal ZJ, Hertzer NR, et al: ACC/AHA 2005 guidelines for the management of patients with peripheral arterial disease (lower extremity, renal, mesenteric, and abdominal aortic): Executive summary, a collaborative report from the American Association for Vascular Surgery/Society for Vascular Surgery, Society for Cardiovascular Angiography and Interventions, Society for Vascular Medicine and Biology, Society of Interventional Radiology, and the ACC/AHA Task Force on Practice Guidelines (Writing Committee to Develop Guidelines for the Management of Patients with Peripheral Arterial Disease) endorsed by the American Association of Cardiovascular and Pulmonary Rehabilitation; National Heart, Lung, and Blood Institute; Society for Vascular Nursing; TransAtlantic Inter-Society Consensus; and Vascular Disease Foundation. J Am Coll Cardiol 47:1239–1312, 2006.)

value >1.40. In these patients, additional testing followed by results from the vascular laboratory may help the clinician to make an accurate diagnosis of PAD. These tests include toe pressures and pulse volume recordings. In some patients with claudication, the ABI may be falsely normal with an iliac artery stenosis and no other occlusive disease distal to the iliac lesion. In this situation, the stenosis is not hemodynamically significant at rest, but a pressure drop can be induced with exercise. A resting ABI is obtained in each ankle, and then the patient is asked to walk on a treadmill for up to 5 minutes. Exercise may also consist of toe raises until claudication pain occurs. The ABI is repeated immediately after exercise; a 20% decrease from rest is diagnostic of PAD.[13] Additional diagnostic tests include transcutaneous measurements of tissue oxygen content. These evaluations may provide information on the potential for ulcer healing in patients with CLI.

The vascular laboratory can also provide information on localization and severity of arterial lesions. Anatomic localization can be achieved with noninvasive imaging tests. The decision to proceed to this stage of evaluation is predicated on the need for revascularization as the next step in treatment. Therefore, indications for revascularization must be considered before additional testing is performed. These indications include lifestyle-limiting claudication that has not responded to medical therapy (i.e., lifestyle modification, exercise training, and/or drug therapy), CLI (including management of ischemic rest pain and ischemic ulcers), and prevention of limb loss. Tests used for disease localization include segmental limb pressure, pulse volume recording, Doppler segmental waveform, arterial duplex ultrasonography, magnetic resonance angiography (MRA), and computed tomographic angiography (CTA).

With the use of sequential limb blood pressure cuffs placed on the upper and lower thigh, calf, and ankle, segmental limb arterial blood pressures may be obtained. Each pressure measurement is compared with the cuff above and the contralateral limb. For example, pressure obtained in the proximal thigh cuff is normally >30 mm Hg higher than the brachial pressure. Lower pressures suggest the presence of inflow aortoiliac artery disease. Pressure in each cuff should be no greater than 20 mm Hg lower than that in the pressure cuff proximal to that level. Disease localization occurs one segment proximal to the cuff with the lower

Table 22-1 Vascular Laboratory and Imaging Tests

Vascular Laboratory Examination	Information Obtained	Limitations
Segmental limb pressure	Localizes arterial disease to specific vascular segments	Inaccurate in patients with noncompressible arteries
	May aid in predicting wound healing potential	Special cuffs required
	Used to monitor the results of revascularization	Proximal thigh cuff occasionally uncomfortable for patient
Pulse volume recording	Localizes arterial disease	Semiquantitative
	Monitors results of revascularization	Requires a skilled technologist
	Predicts wound healing	
	Accurate even when ankle vessels are noncompressible	
Duplex ultrasound	Provides anatomic localization of arterial lesions	Requires a skilled technologist
	Defines severity of focal stenosis	Limited when aorta and iliac vessels are evaluated in some patients
	Aids in decisions regarding revascularization	Limited with arterial calcification
	Used for graft surveillance after surgery	
Magnetic resonance angiography	Provides disease localization throughout lower extremity arterial circulation	Overestimation of degree of stenosis
	Aids in decisions regarding revascularization	Inaccurate in arteries with metal clips
	Avoids iodinated contrast	
Computed tomographic angiography	Provides disease localization throughout lower extremity arterial circulation	Requires iodinated contrast
	Aids in decisions regarding revascularization	Requires multislice detectors
		Accuracy not fully determined

pressure. Therefore, if the pressure in the lower thigh cuff is 30 mm Hg lower than that in the high thigh cuff, superficial femoral artery occlusive disease is suggested.

Pulse volume recordings are plethysmographic measurements that provide semiquantitative hemodynamic information. The same cuffs are used as for segmental limb pressure, but they are inflated to pressures that do not occlude flow. Each arterial pulse displaces volume in the cuff, which is recorded as an arterial waveform. With increasing arterial occlusive disease, the pulse volume recording changes in amplitude and contour. These tests require a highly trained technologist, along with a vascular physician, for interpretation of results. The test is particularly useful in patients with calcified, noncompressible tibial vessels. In this situation, the pulse waveform can still be interpreted, and this information may be used to rule PAD in or out.

Arterial duplex ultrasonography provides accurate arterial imaging and grading of arterial stenoses. Current methods use both color imaging and Doppler velocity to determine the location and severity of arterial disease. A doubling in peak systolic velocity suggests stenosis greater than 50%. Arterial duplex ultrasonography requires a highly skilled technologist, is time intensive, and requires a vascular physician for interpretation of results.

MRA is the preferred noninvasive imaging modality in many centers.[14] It is safe and provides high-resolution, three-dimensional imaging of the major vessels from the abdomen to the feet. MRA is useful for treatment planning before intervention and for assessing the suitability of lesions for endovascular approaches. MRA avoids the use of iodinated contrast, which is relatively contraindicated in patients with contrast allergy or renal insufficiency. Its limitations include that it is contraindicated in patients with implanted defibrillators, spinal cord stimulators, and certain arterial stents. In particular, Nitinol stents (Cordis Corporation, Miami Lakes, Fla) produce the least artefact. Also, heavily calcified arteries can be evaluated by MRA but not by CTA.

CTA is also highly accurate for evaluating the location and extent of arterial disease; accuracy is greater than that of duplex imaging, particularly when multislice detectors are used.[15] Multislice CTA enables rapid imaging of the abdominal, pelvic, and lower extremity vessels with significant resolution. Major limitations of CTA involve the use of iodinated contrast, radiation exposure, and loss of accuracy in heavily calcified vessels. Arterial stents may cause significant artefact, possibly precluding adequate evaluation.

Contrast angiography remains the primary arterial imaging modality; it is often done in the same setting as angioplasty. The test carries risks for severe reaction to contrast (approximately 0.1%) and similarly low risks of mortality. Other complications include arterial dissection, atheroemboli, contrast-induced renal failure, and access site complications (e.g., pseudoaneurysm, arteriovenous fistula, hematoma).

TREATMENT

Cardiovascular Risk Reduction Therapies

Patients with PAD have multiple cardiovascular risk factors that require aggressive management to individual target goals. Evidenced-based therapies are summarized in Table 22-2.

Smoking Cessation

Cigarette smoking is associated with a markedly increased risk for cardiovascular events, progression of leg arterial disease, amputation, and worsened patency of revascularization procedures. Given these associations, smoking cessation has been a cornerstone in the management of PAD. Although advice to stop smoking is associated with modest quit rates, the addition of nicotine replacement and behavior programs is associated with reasonable quit rates at 5 years and a survival advantage over the long term.[16] Pharmacologic therapy, including nicotine replacement and antidepressant drug therapy, can be helpful in smoking cessation.[17] The drug bupropion has been shown to be effective in many smokers.[18] Thus, a practical approach would be to combine behavior modification, nicotine replacement therapy, and bupropion to achieve the best quit rates.

The role of smoking cessation in relieving the symptoms of claudication is not clear, and studies have not consistently

Table 22-2   Evidence-Based Drug Therapy for Peripheral Arterial Disease

Indication	Drug	Dose	Duration	Efficacy	Safety
Cardiovascular Prevention	Aspirin	81 mg/day	Life	• 25% CV risk reduction over placebo in patients with history of MI or stroke • 18% nonsignificant risk reduction in PAD without prior MI or stroke	Peptic ulcer disease UGI bleed
	Clopidogrel	75 mg/day	Life	• 24% risk reduction over aspirin 325 mg/day	Rash Pruritus
	Ramipril	10 mg/day	Life	• 20% CV risk reduction over placebo	Cough Renal insufficiency
	Simvastatin	40 mg/day	Life	• 24% CV risk reduction over placebo • Effective even in PAD with no prior history of MI or stroke • Effective even when baseline LDL cholesterol level <116 mg/dL	Rare myositis Rare hepatocellular toxicity
	Bisoprolol	5–10 mg/day	Perioperative period	• Reduced risk of perioperative MI and cardiac death with vascular surgery	Asthma exacerbation
Graft Patency	Aspirin	81–325 mg/day	Life	• 43% risk reduction in graft occlusion compared with placebo • Effective in prosthetic grafts	As above
	Warfarin	INR ≈3.0	Up to 2 years	• Effective in vein grafts	Higher bleeding risk
Claudication	Pentoxifylline	400 mg TID	Years	• 0%–25% improvement in ACD	Nausea
	Cilostazol	50 to 100 mg BID	Years	• 50% improvement in ACD	Headache Diarrhea No increase in CV death Avoid in heart failure

CV, cardiovascular events, including myocardial infarction (MI), stroke (cerebrovascular accident [CVA]), and vascular death; PAD, peripheral arterial disease; UGI, upper gastrointestinal; LDL, low-density lipoprotein; INR, International Normalized Ratio; ACD, absolute (maximal) walking distance on a treadmill. (From Hirsch AT, Haskal ZJ, Hertzer NR, et al: ACC/AHA 2005 guidelines for the management of patients with peripheral arterial disease (lower extremity, renal, mesenteric, and abdominal aortic): Executive summary, a collaborative report from the American Association for Vascular Surgery/Society for Vascular Surgery, Society for Cardiovascular Angiography and Interventions, Society for Vascular Medicine and Biology, Society of Interventional Radiology, and the ACC/AHA Task Force on Practice Guidelines (Writing Committee to Develop Guidelines for the Management of Patients with Peripheral Arterial Disease) endorsed by the American Association of Cardiovascular and Pulmonary Rehabilitation; National Heart, Lung, and Blood Institute; Society for Vascular Nursing; TransAtlantic Inter-Society Consensus; and Vascular Disease Foundation. J Am Coll Cardiol 47:1239–1312, 2006.)

shown that smoking cessation is associated with improved walking distance.[19,20] Therefore, patients should be encouraged to stop smoking primarily to reduce their systemic risk and their risk of progression to amputation, but they should not be promised improved symptoms immediately on cessation.

Hyperlipidemia

Current recommendations for the management of lipid disorders in PAD are to achieve a low-density lipoprotein (LDL) cholesterol level of less than 100 mg/dL and to modulate the increased triglyceride and low high-density lipoprotein (HDL) pattern.[21] More recent guidelines recommend that high-risk patients with PAD reduce their LDL cholesterol level to less than 70 mg/dL.[22] Subgroup analyses of previous trials in patients with coronary artery disease showed that aggressive lipid lowering was associated with a decreased risk of claudication or an absent femoral pulse.[23]

The most direct evidence for statin therapy in PAD comes from the Heart Protection Study.[24] This study enrolled more than 20,500 subjects at high risk for cardiovascular events, including 6748 patients with PAD. Many of the patients with PAD had not had a previous cardiovascular event. Overall, simvastatin 40 mg/day was associated with a 12% reduction in total mortality, 17% reduction in vascular mortality, and 24% reduction in coronary heart disease (CHD) events. Similar results were obtained in the PAD subgroup, independent of the baseline prevalence of coronary artery disease. This is the first large, randomized trial of statin therapy to show that aggressive lipid modification can significantly improve outcomes in the PAD population.

Hypertension

Hypertension is an independent risk factor for PAD that requires aggressive therapy to reduce cardiovascular risk. Current guidelines recommend achieving a blood pressure lower than 140/90 mm Hg, except in patients with diabetes or renal insufficiency, for whom the goal is a blood pressure lower than 130/80 mm Hg.[25] Regarding specific drug choice, β-adrenergic blocking agents have previously been contraindicated in PAD because of the possibility of worsening claudication symptoms.[26] However, this concern has not been borne out by randomized trials; thus, β-adrenergic blocking agents can be used in patients with claudication.[27] In particular, patients with PAD who also have concomitant coronary disease may receive additional cardioprotection from β-adrenergic blocking agents. Therefore, this should be considered a viable drug class for these patients.

Angiotension-converting enzyme (ACE) inhibitor drugs have shown benefit beyond blood pressure lowering in high-risk groups. Specific results were derived from the HOPE (Heart Outcomes Prevention Evaluation) study of 4046 patients with PAD.[28] In this subgroup, a 22% risk reduction was observed in patients randomly assigned to ramipril compared with placebo, which was independent of blood pressure lowering. On the basis of this finding, ramipril received approval for cardiovascular risk reduction. Thus, as a drug class, ACE inhibitors would certainly be recommended in these patients.

Diabetes

Diabetes, the most potent risk factor for PAD, is associated with peripheral neuropathy that, when combined with arterial insufficiency, greatly increases the risks of foot ulceration and limb loss. Several studies of patients with type 1 and type 2 diabetes have shown that aggressive blood sugar lowering can prevent microvascular complications (particularly retinopathy) but not cardiovascular disease or PAD.[29,30] A more recent study in which pioglitazone was used in patients with diabetes and cardiovascular disease showed a reduction in risks of myocardial infarction, stroke, and vascular death as a secondary end point of the study.[31] Additional studies will be needed to confirm this cardiovascular benefit of the drug class. The current American Diabetes Association–recommended goal for treatment of patients with diabetes is a hemoglobin (Hb)$_{A1C}$ of 7%. However, it is not clear whether achieving that goal with current medications will have a cardiovascular protective effect.

Additional PAD Risk Factors

Elevated plasma homocysteine levels are an independent risk factor for PAD, but information on the clinical benefit of lowering homocysteine levels with folate is lacking.[32] C-reactive protein (CRP) is an independent risk factor for PAD. Measurement of CRP may guide lipid therapy in that statin drugs lower CRP levels, and reduction in CRP levels may contribute to the benefits of statin drugs.[33] Alterations in coagulation are not typically associated with PAD, and no evidence suggests that anticoagulant therapy prevents the development of PAD or claudication.

Antiplatelet Drug Therapy

Aspirin is a well-established antiplatelet drug for the secondary prevention of cardiovascular events in patients with known cardiovascular disease. The Antithrombotic Trialists' Collaboration meta-analysis showed a 25% odds reduction in subsequent cardiovascular events with the use of low-dose aspirin (75 to 160 mg/day).[34] In patients with PAD who have not had a cardiovascular event, no conclusive evidence has proved that aspirin is beneficial.[35] In the more recent meta-analysis, when PAD data were combined with those from trials in which not only aspirin but more effective agents such as clopidogrel and picotamide were given, a significant 23% odds reduction in ischemic events occurred.[34] Thus, although antiplatelet drugs are clearly indicated in the overall management of PAD, aspirin does not have U.S. Food and Drug Administration (FDA) approval for use in patients with PAD who do not have other clinical evidence of cardiovascular disease (e.g., prior myocardial infarction, stroke).[36]

Thienopyridines are adenosine diphosphate (ADP) antagonists that have been well studied in patients with cardiovascular disease. Ticlopidine has been evaluated in several trials in patients with PAD and has shown benefit in reducing the risks of myocardial infarction, stroke, and vascular death.[37] Clopidogrel also has been shown to reduce the risk of myocardial infarction, ischemic stroke, and vascular death in patients with PAD. The overall benefit of clopidogrel in PAD was a 24% risk reduction over the use of aspirin, with a highly acceptable safety profile.[38] Thus, current American Heart Association/American College of Cardiology (AHA/ACC) guidelines recommend both aspirin and clopidogrel as acceptable antiplatelet drugs for the PAD population.[22]

Hypercoagulable States

Abnormalities of coagulation are commonly associated with the development of venous thrombosis and thromboembolism, yet they play a negligible role in arterial events. Arterial and venous thrombosis has been associated with elevations in homocysteine levels. However, known inherited hypercoagulable states have been less well evaluated in patients with PAD. In one study, presence of the lupus anticoagulant was associated with peripheral atherosclerosis.[39] Also, markers of platelet activation, such as increased β-thromboglobulin levels, are also associated with PAD.[40] Hypercoagulability has been associated with decreased long-term patency of bypass grafts.[41] Routine testing for hypercoagulability is not indicated in the evaluation of PAD.

Treatment of Claudication

Figure 22-2 provides an overview of the treatment of claudication.

Exercise Rehabilitation

A supervised exercise rehabilitation program is a safe and effective treatment approach for patients with claudication.[42] A walking- or treadmill-based training program conducted in a cardiac rehabilitation or other supervised setting produces the best results.[43] Patients should be monitored by a skilled nurse or technician. A typical supervised exercise program begins with 30 minutes of intermittent exercise and increases to 60 minutes as tolerated. The initial workload of the treadmill is set to a speed and grade combination that brings on claudication pain within 3 to 5 minutes. Patients walk at this work rate until they achieve claudication of moderate severity. They rest until the claudication abates, and then they resume exercise. On a weekly basis, patients should be reassessed clinically as they are able to walk farther and farther at their chosen workload. The typical duration of an exercise program is 3 months. On completion of the exercise program, similar evaluations are performed to define improvements in treadmill walking distance and questionnaire end points.[44] Mechanisms of benefit include improvements in walking efficiency and adaptations in skeletal muscle metabolism and microcirculation.[45]

Claudication Drug Therapy

The goals of claudication therapy are to enhance walking speed and distance, exercise performance, and the physical aspects of quality of life. A number of drugs have not been shown to be effective in the treatment of patients with claudication. Examples include vasodilators, prostaglandins, and serotonin receptor antagonists.[46-48] Pentoxifylline has been approved for the treatment of claudication, with early trials suggesting a modest improvement in maximum treadmill walking distance.[49] However, in a recent study, pentoxifylline was no more effective than placebo and was inferior to cilostazol.[50] A meta-analysis concluded that the drug produced modest increases in treadmill walking distance over placebo, but the overall clinical benefits were questionable.[51]

Cilostazol provides the best evidence for efficacy among currently available drugs for claudication. This drug is a phosphodiesterase type 3 inhibitor that has favorable effects on HDL cholesterol metabolism, produces vasodilation, and exhibits antiplatelet properties. In a number of studies, cilostazol improved pain-free and maximum walking distance as compared with placebo.[52-54] In these same studies, cilostazol improved the physical domains of quality of life—a finding confirmed through a meta-analysis of six trials.[55] The most common adverse effects of cilostazol include headache, transient diarrhea, palpitations, and dizziness. Cilostazol should not be given to patients with claudication who also have heart failure; this recommendation is based on previous concerns about increased mortality risk with this class of drugs in patients with heart failure.[56] Safety data have been gathered from more than 2700 patients treated with cilostazol and followed for up to 6 months. Total cardiovascular morbidity and all cause mortality were 6.5% for cilostazol 200 mg/day, 6.3% for cilostazol 100 mg/day, and 7.7% for placebo.[57] These data do not show an increased cardiovascular mortality risk with cilostazol, yet this drug has an FDA "black box" warning stating that its use should be avoided in patients with PAD who also have clinical evidence of heart failure.

Additional drugs are now being studied in clinical trials for their potential use in patients with claudication. Propionyl-L-carnitine is a metabolic agent that has been shown to improve treadmill performance and quality of life in patients with claudication.[58,59] Angiogenic agents also are potentially valuable and are currently under study.

Revascularization

The decision to proceed to revascularization, whether endovascular or surgical, should be based on a lack of response to overall medical management that includes a supervised exercise program or claudication drug therapy. Patients considered for revascularization should have a severe physical disability, defined as inability to conduct work or other ambulatory activities. Patients should be carefully evaluated to ensure that no other significant comorbidity is present that would continue to limit the patient's physical capacity. These limitations may include arthritis or pulmonary and cardiac disease that limits activity to a greater extent than claudication does. In this situation, even successful treatment of claudication would not be expected to provide overall benefit to the patient if other medical conditions are more limiting. In addition, vascular laboratory and imaging modalities must confirm the presence of a suitable lesion for treatment, and the patient should not be at high risk to undergo an invasive procedure. In general, specific decisions about which procedure to perform (angioplasty or vascular surgery) should be based on the current TransAtlantic Inter-Society Consensus (TASC) and AHA/ACC guidelines.[22,60]

Angioplasty

Percutaneous transluminal angioplasty (PTA) to treat peripheral arterial stenoses or occlusions has been an accepted therapy for patients with severe intermittent claudication or CLI. Patients who benefit the most from PTA are those with proximal aortoiliac stenosis or occlusions or short segment femoropopliteal stenosis or occlusion.[61,62] For iliac stenosis or occlusion, 1-year patency rates range from 60% to 80%, and for those with a stent, those rates increase to 70% to 90%.[22] Femoropopliteal angioplasty has a 1-year patency rate

III

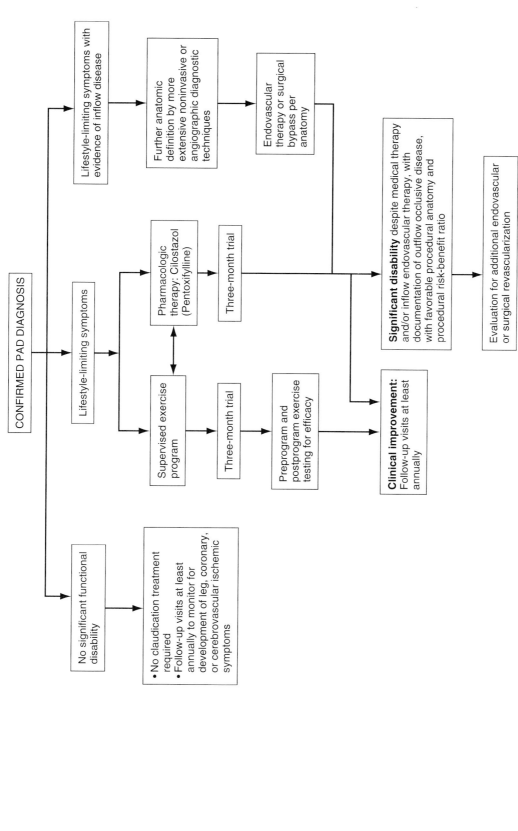

Figure 22-2 Treatment algorithm for claudication. (From Hirsch AT, Haskal ZJ, Hertzer NR, et al: ACC/AHA 2005 guidelines for the management of patients with peripheral arterial disease (lower extremity, renal, mesenteric, and abdominal aortic): Executive summary, a collaborative report from the American Association for Vascular Surgery/Society for Vascular Surgery, Society for Cardiovascular Angiography and Interventions, Society for Vascular Medicine and Biology, Society of Interventional Radiology, and the ACC/AHA Task Force on Practice Guidelines (Writing Committee to Develop Guidelines for the Management of Patients with Peripheral Arterial Disease) endorsed by the American Association of Cardiovascular and Pulmonary Rehabilitation; National Heart, Lung, and Blood Institute; Society for Vascular Nursing; TransAtlantic Inter-Society Consensus; and Vascular Disease Foundation. J Am Coll Cardiol 47:1239–1312, 2006.)

ranging from 50% to 89%, and with the addition of a stent, the range is 60% to 80%.[22]

Percutaneous revascularization procedures are generally safe, but they may be associated with low rates of such adverse effects as arterial dissection, bleeding, hematoma, thrombosis, atheroembolism, and contrast nephropathy. Patients who have complex lesions that require prolonged procedures and many catheter manipulations are at greatest risk of severe complications. The severe complication rate from PTA for intermittent claudication is approximately 1% to 2%.

Vascular Surgery

Surgical revascularization is rarely required to treat intermittent claudication because of the strong likelihood that medical therapy and angioplasty will be successful. Vascular surgery also is associated with significant perioperative morbidity and mortality. Therefore, clinicians must carefully weigh the risks and benefits of surgery before recommending it to patients with intermittent claudication. In particular, a failed bypass graft may lead to the development of CLI (due to the loss of collaterals) in a patient who may not have ever been at risk for this complication. In contrast, patients with CLI should be considered for revascularization. Again, the critical issues are vascular disease anatomy, availability of conduit material (vein is preferred), and patient comorbidities.

With aortoiliac and aortofemoral bypass surgery, the perioperative mortality rate is 1% to 3%, but 5-year patency rates range from 85% to 90%. Vein-to-below knee femoropopliteal bypass has a perioperative mortality rate of 1% to 6% and a patency rate of 65% at 5 years. However, with prosthetic material, the patency rate drops to 33% at 5 years.[63] Femoral-to-tibial bypass with vein (often used for limb salvage) has a patency rate of up to 75% at 5 years.

Drug Therapy to Reduce Cardiac Risk in Vascular Surgery

Patients with PAD who undergo vascular surgery are at high risk of cardiovascular complications. Previous attempts to address this risk through risk stratification prior to vascular surgery relied on clinical assessment and cardiac imaging.[64] Clinical risk factors for major vascular surgery include age greater than 70 years, angina, and history of myocardial infarction, heart failure, or stroke.[65] Although clinical and imaging strategies can be used to identify high-risk patients for vascular surgery, the benefit derived from coronary revascularization prior to vascular surgery remains unproved. A recent study randomly assigned 5859 patients scheduled for vascular surgery (elective aortic or leg bypass surgery) to coronary artery revascularization or best medical therapy.[66] The coronary revascularization strategy did not improve long-term outcomes. Therefore, evaluation of the coronary or carotid circulation prior to peripheral vascular surgery should not be a routine matter, and it should be considered only in patients with symptoms in that regional circulation that merit further study.

An alternative method of reducing cardiac risk in patients undergoing vascular surgery is to provide perioperative β-adrenergic blockade. For example, oral metoprolol prior to vascular surgery reduced cardiac ischemia during surgery.[67] The best evidence is seen with bisoprolol (a selective β₁-adrenergic blocker) given to high-risk patients undergoing vascular surgery.[68] In a study of high-risk vascular patients defined as having cardiac risk factors and a positive dobutamine stress echocardiogram, bisoprolol prevented nonfatal myocardial infarction and cardiac death at 30 days. At 2-year follow-up of the same patients, the incidence of a cardiac event was 12% in the treated group and 32% in the placebo group ($P = .025$; number needed to treat is 5).[69] A meta-analysis of all studies to date confirms the cardioprotective effects of β-adrenergic blockade in patients with PAD undergoing vascular surgery.[70] Thus, the use of a β-adrenergic blocker was associated with short- and long-term reductions in cardiac events after major vascular surgery.

Drug Therapy for Graft Patency

Aspirin has provided good evidence for the prevention of graft occlusion after peripheral vascular surgical bypass.[71] Ticlopidine has also been shown to promote vein graft patency.[72] Anticoagulation has been recommended as an adjuvant to maintain surgical graft patency, but its use remains controversial. Aspirin has been compared with oral anticoagulation in the Dutch Bypass Oral Anticoagulants or Aspirin study in 2690 patients undergoing infrainguinal bypass.[73] The primary end point of graft patency was equal between groups after 21 months of follow-up. However, when patients were divided into subgroups according to type of graft material used, anticoagulation maintained vein graft patency better than aspirin but with a higher risk of bleeding complications. In contrast, aspirin maintained prosthetic graft patency better than anticoagulation. These results were robust and therefore suggest that patients receiving vein grafts should be preferentially treated with warfarin, and those treated with prosthetic material should be treated with aspirin.

CONCLUSIONS

Peripheral arterial disease is a common manifestation of atherosclerosis. Early detection is easily achieved with the ABI, and additional noninvasive testing can be performed in the vascular laboratory. Given the systemic nature of atherosclerosis, all patients with PAD, whether they have a prior history of coronary disease or not, should be considered for secondary prevention strategies. These include aggressive management of smoking, reduction of LDL cholesterol to <100 mg/dL (<70 mg/dL in high-risk patients), reduction of blood pressure, and treatment for diabetes to target goals. Drugs shown to have particular benefit in these patients include the statins for LDL reduction, ACE inhibitors to treat blood pressure, and β blockers in the perioperative setting. In addition, all patients should be given an antiplatelet drug; clopidogrel is known to produce greater benefit than aspirin in the PAD population.

Treatment for claudication includes a formal exercise rehabilitation program and cilostazol as a medical option. A trial of exercise or drug therapy should continue for at least 3 months so that efficacy can be determined. Primary revascularization options for claudication consist of angioplasty, and for CLI, angioplasty and vascular bypass surgery for limb salvage.

Acknowledgments

Dr. Hiatt has received honoraria and grant support through a Bristol-Myers Squibb–Sanofi-Aventis partnership.

REFERENCES

1. Hiatt WR, Hoag S, Hamman RF: Effect of diagnostic criteria on the prevalence of peripheral arterial disease: The San Luis Valley diabetes study. Circulation 91:1472–1479, 1995.

2. Selvin E, Erlinger TP: Prevalence of and risk factors for peripheral arterial disease in the United States: Results from the National Health and Nutrition Examination Survey,1999–2000. Circulation 110:738–743, 2004.

3. Newman AB, Siscovick DS, Manolio TA, et al, for the Cardiovascular Health Study Collaborative Research Group: Ankle-arm index as a marker of atherosclerosis in the Cardiovascular Health Study (CHS) Collaborative Research Group. Circulation 88:837–845, 1993.

4. McGrae MM, Greenland P, Liu, K, et al: Leg symptoms in peripheral arterial disease: Associated clinical characteristics and functional impairment. JAMA 286:1599–1606, 2001.

5. Weitz JI, Byrne J, Clagett GP, et al: Diagnosis and treatment of chronic arterial insufficiency of the lower extremities: A critical review. Circulation 94:3026–3049, 1996.

6. Ness J, Aronow WS: Prevalence of coexistence of coronary artery disease, ischemic stroke, and peripheral arterial disease in older persons, mean age 80 years, in an academic hospital-based geriatrics practice. J Am Geriatr Soc 47:1255–1256, 1999.

7. Criqui MH, Langer RD, Fronek, A, et al: Mortality over a period of 10 years in patients with peripheral arterial disease. N Engl J Med 326:381–386, 1992.

8. Newman AB, Shemanski L, Manolio TA, et al, for the Cardiovascular Health Study Group: Ankle-arm index as a predictor of cardiovascular disease and mortality in the Cardiovascular Health Study. Arterioscler Thromb Vasc Biol 19:538–545, 1999.

9. Vogt MT, McKenna M, Anderson, SJ, et al: The relationship between ankle-arm index and mortality in older men and women. J Am Geriatr Soc 41:523–530, 1993.

10. Hirsch AT, Criqui MH, Treat-Jacobson D, et al: Peripheral arterial disease detection, awareness, and treatment in primary care. JAMA 286:1317–1324, 2001.

11. Hiatt WR: Medical treatment of peripheral arterial disease and claudication. N Engl J Med 344:1608–1621, 2001.

12. Fowkes FGR: The measurement of artherosclerotic peripheral arterial disease in epidemiological surveys. Int J Epidemiol 17:248–254, 1988.

13. Raines JK, Darling RC, Buth, J, et al: Vascular laboratory criteria for the management of peripheral vascular disease of the lower extremities. Surgery 79:21–29, 1976.

14. Koelemay MJ, Lijmer JG, Stoker, J, et al: Magnetic resonance angiography for the evaluation of lower extremity arterial disease: A meta-analysis. JAMA 285:1338–1345, 2001.

15. Willmann JK, Wildermuth S: Multidetector-row CT angiography of upper- and lower-extremity peripheral arteries. Eur Radiol 15 (suppl 4): D3–D9, 2005.

16. Anthonisen NR, Skeans MA, Wise, RA, et al: The effects of a smoking cessation intervention on 14.5-year mortality: A randomized clinical trial. Ann Intern Med 142:233–239, 2005.

17. Daughton D, Susman J, Sitorius M, et al, for The Nebraska Primary Practice Smoking Cessation Trial Group: Transdermal nicotine therapy and primary care: Importance of counseling, demographic, and participant selection factors on 1-year quit rates. Arch Fam Med 7: 425–430, 1998.

18. Tonstad S, Farsang C, Klaene, G, et al: Bupropion SR for smoking cessation in smokers with cardiovascular disease: A multicentre, randomised study. Eur Heart J 24:946–955, 2003.

19. Jonason T, Bergstrom R: Cessation of smoking in patients with intermittent claudication. Acta Med Scand 221:253–260, 1987.

20. Quick, CRG, Cotton, LT: The measured effect of stopping smoking on intermittent claudication. Br J Surg 69 (suppl): S24–S26, 1982.

21. Executive Summary of the Third Report of the National Cholesterol Education Program (NCEP) Expert Panel on Detection, Evaluation, and Treatment of High Blood Cholesterol in Adults (Adult Treatment Panel III). JAMA 285:2486–2497, 2001.

22. Hirsch AT, Haskal ZJ, Hertzer NR, et al: ACC/AHA 2005 guidelines for the management of patients with peripheral arterial disease (lower extremity, renal, mesenteric, and abdominal aortic): Executive summary, a collaborative report from the American Association for Vascular Surgery/Society for Vascular Surgery, Society for Cardiovascular Angiography and Interventions, Society for Vascular Medicine and Biology, Society of Interventional Radiology, and the ACC/AHA Task Force on Practice Guidelines (Writing Committee to Develop Guidelines for the Management of Patients with Peripheral Arterial Disease) endorsed by the American Association of Cardiovascular and Pulmonary Rehabilitation; National Heart, Lung, and Blood Institute; Society for Vascular Nursing; TransAtlantic Inter-Society Consensus; and Vascular Disease Foundation. J Am Coll Cardiol 47:1239–1312, 2006.

23. Pedersen TR, Kjekshus J, Pyorala, K, et al: Effect of simvastatin on ischemic signs and symptoms in the Scandinavian simvastatin survival study (4S). Am J Cardiol 81:333–335, 1998.

24. MRC/BHF Heart Protection Study of cholesterol lowering with simvastatin in 20,536 high-risk individuals: A randomised placebo-controlled trial. Lancet 360:7–22, 2002.

25. Chobanian AV, Bakris GL, Black, HR, et al: Seventh report of the Joint National Committee on Prevention, Detection, Evaluation, and Treatment of High Blood Pressure. Hypertension 42:1206–1252, 2003.

26. Frohlich ED, Tarazi RC, Dustan HP: Peripheral arterial insufficiency: A complication of beta-adrenergic blocking therapy. JAMA 208: 2471–2472, 1969.

27. Radack K, Deck C: Beta-adrenergic blocker therapy does not worsen intermittent claudication in subjects with peripheral arterial disease: A meta-analysis of randomized controlled trials. Arch Intern Med 151:1769–1776, 1991.

28. The Heart Outcomes Prevention Evaluation Study Investigators: Effects of an angiotensin-converting enzyme inhibitor, ramipril, on cardiovascular events in high-risk patients. N Engl J Med 342: 145–153, 2000.

29. Effect of intensive diabetes management on macrovascular events and risk factors in the Diabetes Control and Complications Trial. Am J Cardiol 75:894–903, 1995.

30. UK Prospective Diabetes Study (UKPDS) Group: Intensive blood-glucose control with sulphonylureas or insulin compared with conventional treatment and risk of complications in patients with type 2 diabetes (UKPDS 33). Lancet 352:837–853, 1998.

31. Dormandy JA, Charbonnel B, Eckland, DJ, et al: Secondary prevention of macrovascular events in patients with type 2 diabetes in the PROactive Study (PROspective pioglitAzone Clinical Trial In macroVascular Events): A randomised controlled trial. Lancet 366:1279–1289, 2005.

32. Jacques PF, Selhub J, Bostom, AG, et al: The effect of folic acid fortification on plasma folate and total homocysteine concentrations. N Engl J Med 340:1449–1454, 1999.

33. Ridker PM, Cannon CP, Morrow, D, et al: C-reactive protein levels and outcomes after statin therapy. N Engl J Med 352:20–28, 2005.

34. Collaborative meta-analysis of randomised trials of antiplatelet therapy for prevention of death, myocardial infarction, and stroke in high risk patients. BMJ 324:71–86, 2002.

35. Antiplatelet Trialists' Collaboration: Collaborative overview of randomised trials of antiplatelet therapy—I: Prevention of death, myocardial infarction, and stroke by prolonged antiplatelet therapy in various categories of patients. BMJ 308:81–106, 1994.

36. U.S. Food and Drug Administration: Internal analgesic, antipyretic, and antirheumatic drug products for over-the-counter human use: Final rule for professional labeling of aspirin, buffered aspirin, and aspirin in combination with antacid drug products. Federal Register 63:56802–56819, 1998.

37. Janzon L, Bergqvist D, Boberg, J, et al: Prevention of myocardial infarction and stroke in patients with intermittent claudication: Effects of ticlopidine. Results from STIMS, the Swedish Ticlopidine Multicenter Study. J Int Med 227:301–308, 1990.

38. CAPRIE Steering Committee: A randomised, blinded, trial of clopidogrel versus aspirin in patients at risk of ischaemic events (CAPRIE). Lancet 348:1329–1339, 1996.

39. Donaldson MC, Weinberg DS, Belkin, M, et al: Screening for hypercoagulable states in vascular surgical practice: A preliminary study. J Vasc Surg 11:825–831, 1990.

40. Catalano M, Russo U, Libretti A: Plasma beta-thromboglobulin levels and claudication degrees in patients with peripheral vascular disease. Angiology 37:339–342, 1986.

41. Curi MA, Skelly CL, Baldwin, ZK, et al: Long-term outcome of infrainguinal bypass grafting in patients with serologically proven hypercoagulability. J Vasc Surg 37:301–306, 2003.

42. Nehler MR, Hiatt WR: Exercise therapy for claudication. Ann Vasc Surg 13:109–114, 1999.

43. Hiatt WR, Wolfel EE, Meier RH, Regensteiner JG: Superiority of treadmill walking exercise vs. strength training for patients with peripheral arterial disease: Implications for the mechanism of the training response. Circulation 90:1866–1874, 1994.

44. Regensteiner JG, Steiner JF, Hiatt WR: Exercise training improves functional status in patients with peripheral arterial disease. J Vasc Surg 23:104–115, 1996.

45. Stewart KJ, Hiatt WR, Regensteiner JG, Hirsch AT: Exercise training for claudication. N Engl J Med 347:1941–1951, 2002.

46. Coffman JD: Vasodilator drugs in peripheral vascular disease. N Engl J Med 300:713–717, 1979.

47. Mohler ER III, Hiatt WR, Olin, JW, et al: Treatment of intermittent claudication with beraprost sodium, an orally active prostaglandin I2 analogue: A double-blinded, randomized, controlled trial. J Am Coll Cardiol 41:1679–1686, 2003.

48. Hiatt WR, Hirsch AT, Cooke, JP, et al: Randomized trial of AT-1015 for treatment of intermittent claudication: A novel 5-hydroxytryptamine antagonist with no evidence of efficacy. Vasc Med 9:18–25, 2004.

49. Porter JM, Cutler BS, Lee, BY, et al: Pentoxifylline efficacy in the treatment of intermittent claudication: Multicenter controlled double-blind trial with objective assessment of chronic occlusive arterial disease patients. Am Heart J 104:66–72, 1982.

50. Dawson DL, Cutler BS, Hiatt, WR, et al: A comparison of cilostazol and pentoxifylline for treating intermittent claudication. Am J Med 109:523–530, 2000.

51. Girolami B, Bernardi E, Prins, MH, et al: Treatment of intermittent claudication with physical training, smoking cessation, pentoxifylline, or nafronyl: A meta-analysis. Arch Intern Med 159:337–345, 1999.

52. Beebe HG, Dawson DL, Cutler, BS, et al: A new pharmacological treatment for intermittent claudication: Results of a randomized, multicenter trial. Arch Intern Med 159:2041–2050, 1999.

53. Money SR, Herd JA, Isaacsohn, JL, et al: Effect of cilostazol on walking distances in patients with intermittent claudication caused by peripheral vascular disease. J Vasc Surg 27:267–274, 1998.

54. Dawson DL, Cutler BS, Meissner MH, Strandness DEJ: Cilostazol has beneficial effects in treatment of intermittent claudication: Results from a multicenter, randomized, prospective, double-blind trial. Circulation 98:678–686, 1998.

55. Regensteiner JG, Ware JE Jr, McCarthy WJ, et al: Effect of cilostazol on treadmill walking, community-based walking ability, and health-related quality of life in patients with intermittent claudication due to peripheral arterial disease: Meta-analysis of six randomized controlled trials. J Am Geriatr Soc 50:1939–1946, 2002.

56. Packer M, Carver JR, Rodeheffer RJ, et al, for the PROMISE Study Research Group: Effect of oral milrinone on mortality in severe chronic heart failure. N Engl J Med 325:1468–1475, 1991.

57. Pratt CM: Analysis of the cilostazol safety database. Am J Cardiol 87:28D–33D, 2001.

58. Hiatt WR, Regensteiner JG, Creager, MA, et al: Propionyl-L-carnitine improves exercise performance and functional status in patients with claudication. Am J Med 110:616–622, 2001.

59. Brevetti G, Perna S, Sabba, C, et al: Propionyl-L-carnitine in intermittent claudication: Double-blind, placebo-controlled, dose titration, multicenter study. J Am Coll Cardiol 26:1411–1416, 1995.

60. Dormandy JA, Rutherford RB, for the TASC Working Group: Management of peripheral arterial disease (PAD). J Vasc Surg 31:S1–S296, 2000.

61. Hunink MG, Wong JB, Donaldson, MC, et al: Revascularization for femoropopliteal disease: A decision and cost-effectiveness analysis. JAMA 274:165–171, 1995.

62. Bosch JL, Haaring C, Meyerovitz, MF, et al: Cost-effectiveness of percutaneous treatment of iliac artery occlusive disease in the United States. Am J Roentgenol 175:517–521, 2000.

63. Szilagyi DE, Elliott JP Jr, Smith RF, et al: A thirty-year survey of the reconstructive surgical treatment of aortoiliac occlusive disease. J Vasc Surg 3:421–436, 1986.

64. Eagle KA, Brundage BH, Chaitman, BR, et al: Guidelines for perioperative cardiovascular evaluation for noncardiac surgery. Report of the American College of Cardiology/American Heart Association Task Force on Practice Guidelines. Committee on Perioperative Cardiovascular Evaluation for Noncardiac Surgery. Circulation 93:1278–1317, 1996.

65. Boersma E, Poldermans D, Bax, JJ, et al: Predictors of cardiac events after major vascular surgery: Role of clinical characteristics, dobutamine echocardiography, and beta-blocker therapy. JAMA 285:1865–1873, 2001.

66. McFalls EO, Ward HB, Moritz, TE, et al: Coronary-artery revascularization before elective major vascular surgery. N Engl J Med 351:2795–2804, 2004.

67. Pasternack PF, Grossi EA, Baumann, FG, et al: Beta blockade to decrease silent myocardial ischemia during peripheral vascular surgery. Am J Surg 158:113–116, 1989.

68. Poldermans D, Boersma E, Bax JJ, et al: The effect of bisoprolol on perioperative mortality and myocardial infarction in high-risk patients undergoing vascular surgery. for the Dutch Echocardiographic Cardiac Risk Evaluation Applying Stress Echocardiography Study Group. N Engl J Med 341:1789–1794, 1999.

69. Poldermans D, Boersma E, Bax JJ, et al: Bisoprolol reduces cardiac death and myocardial infarction in high-risk patients as long as 2 years after successful major vascular surgery. Eur Heart J 22:1353–1358, 2001.

70. Schouten O, Shaw LJ, Boersma, E, et al: A meta-analysis of safety and effectiveness of perioperative beta-blocker use for the prevention of cardiac events in different types of noncardiac surgery. Coron Artery Dis 17:173–179, 2006.

71. Collaborative overview of randomised trials of antiplatelet therapy—II: Maintenance of vascular graft or arterial patency by antiplatelet therapy. Antiplatelet Trialists' Collaboration. BMJ 308:159–168, 1994.

72. Becquemin JP: Effect of ticlopidine on the long-term patency of saphenous-vein bypass grafts in the leg. N Engl J Med 337:1726–1731, 1997.

73. Efficacy of oral anticoagulants compared with aspirin after infrainguinal bypass surgery (The Dutch Bypass Oral Anticoagulants or Aspirin Study): A randomised trial. Lancet 355:346–351, 2000.

Chapter 23

Thrombosis and Cancer

Frederick R. Rickles, MD, FACP • Mark Levine, MD, MSc

INTRODUCTION

Patients with cancer are highly susceptible to venous thromboembolism (VTE), a complication that may contribute significantly to the morbidity and mortality of the disease. All mechanisms for the production of the hypercoagulable state characteristic of cancer are not well defined. Those mechanisms that are known seem to interdigitate the biology of cancer with the major regulatory pathways that mediate blood coagulation, platelet–vessel wall interaction, fibrinolysis, and inflammatory cytokine production. Thus, the events responsible for thrombosis in cancer appear to be a result, in part, of an overexuberant host response in an attempt to delimit tumor growth.

Although many parallels exist between the host response to tumor growth and other biologic processes such as inflammation (e.g., cancer viewed by the pathologist as a "wound that will not heal"),[1] the close-knit relationship between thrombosis and cancer appears unique from the view of the epidemiologist, as follows. First, an association exists between idiopathic VTE and occult malignancy. The increased risk for a new cancer diagnosis within 6 to 12 months of the diagnosis of an episode of idiopathic VTE (including pulmonary embolism) is supported by data from retrospective analyses of large numbers of unselected patients; population-based, retrospective cohort analyses from large registries; and, more recently, by the results of well-designed, prospective studies. Odds ratios favoring the risk of cancer in idiopathic VTE from these studies range from a four- to sevenfold increased risk. Second, cancer survival is significantly worse in patients in whom the diagnosis of VTE is established concurrently with or soon after the diagnosis of cancer, as compared with patients without cancer. Third, the risk that VTE will complicate cancer is substantially higher than in patients without cancer. In surgical patients with known cancer, for example, the odds ratio for an episode of postoperative VTE is approximately 2, when compared with a control group of patients without cancer subjected to the same procedures. A similar odds ratio of approximately 2 to 3 exists for the relative risk for recurrence of VTE in the first 3 months after an initial episode of acute VTE in patients with cancer whose VTE were treated with unfractionated heparin and warfarin, compared with patients without cancer.

Therefore, patients with idiopathic VTE are at increased risk for harboring occult cancer and patients with cancer are at increased risk for VTE and recurrent VTE. Indeed, patients with cancer are considered among the highest-risk patients for VTE and, therefore, should routinely receive prophylaxis prior to surgery. Less clear are appropriate recommendations regarding anticoagulant prophylaxis for the prevention of thrombosis of central venous catheters, or during radiotherapy and/or chemotherapy. Unfortunately, bleeding complications in anticoagulated patients with cancer also occur with increased frequency. Several randomized, controlled studies have now been completed and suggest better strategies for anticoagulant management of these patients.

EPIDEMIOLOGY

Idiopathic Venous Thromboembolism and Occult Cancer

The close relationship between tumor growth and activation of blood coagulation has been known since the days of Professor Armand Trousseau, who first described the clinical association between idiopathic VTE and occult malignancy,[2] and has been reviewed recently.[3–5] Migratory thrombophlebitis as a presenting manifestation of cancer, which has come to be known as Trousseau syndrome, is rather uncommon. However, several prospective studies have shown that patients with carefully defined idiopathic or primary VTE are at significantly higher risk for the subsequent diagnosis of malignancy than are patients who present with secondary VTE (i.e., VTE due to known causes, including congenital thrombophilia, use of oral contraceptives, pregnancy, immobilization, and so forth) (Fig. 23-1).[4,5]

Even though several studies have suggested that idiopathic VTE may be a sign of an occult malignancy,[4–8] it remains unclear whether rigorous investigation of such patients for an occult tumor will prove cost effective. The results of a small randomized trial evaluating extensive screening versus no screening in patients who present with idiopathic VTE have been published.[9] The battery of tests used in the extensively screened group included ultrasound and computed tomography of the abdomen and pelvis, a hemoccult test, gastroscopy, colonoscopy, sputum cytology, mammography, pelvic examination, prostate examination, and tumor markers. Of 99 patients in the extensively screened group, cancers were detected initially in 13, compared with none of 102 patients in the control group. However, 10 patients in the control group and 1 in the screened group developed cancer during the 2-year follow-up period. No statistically significant difference was detected in cancer-related mortality in the two groups (3.9% vs 2%, respectively). Given such results, it is premature to recommend

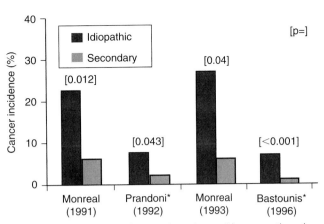

Figure 23-1 Incidence of cancer in patients with venous thrombo-embolism.

*True prospective studies (in the studies reported by Monreal and associates, data were collected prospectively, but analyses were performed retrospectively).[4,5] (From Rickles FR, Levine MN: Epidemiology of thrombosis in cancer. Acta Haematol 106:6–12, 2001, with permission.)

extensive screening in patients who present with idiopathic VTE, particularly because many of the cancers detected by screening cannot be cured by currently available therapy. Often a complete history, physical examination, chest x-ray, and rectal examination can provide clues as to the presence of an underlying cancer. This approach is supported by the retrospective cohort study reported by Cornuz and colleagues.[10] A decision analysis of screening, however, suggested possible gains in life expectancy with targeted screening for prostate, colon, and bladder cancers in men and for colon, breast, and endometrial cancers in women.[11]

Venous Thromboembolism as a Complication of Cancer

Thromboembolism is a frequent finding in autopsy series of patients with cancer,[2–4] but the true incidence of VTE in these patients is difficult to determine from the literature.

Incidence of Thrombosis in Patients with Malignancy

The incidence of thrombosis in patients with cancer can be gleaned from several different sources. Large epidemiologic studies specifically examining the incidence of VTE in patients with cancer had been lacking until recently. In the general population, the incidence of a first episode of deep vein thrombosis (DVT) or pulmonary embolism (PE) was recorded in Olmsted County, Minnesota, from 1966 through 1990.[12] During this period, the overall age- and sex-adjusted annual incidence of VTE was 117 per 100,000. A dramatic rise in incidence rates occurred among patients older than 65 years, with rates almost doubling for each subsequent decade of age. This study population was composed of patients with cancer and patients without cancer. Observed incidence rates may represent a very conservative estimate of the incidence of VTE in a cancer population. In a nested case-controlled study of 625 patients with a first episode of VTE from this database, risk factors for thrombosis were examined.[13] Malignancy was associated with an odds ratio of 6.5 for the occurrence of VTE.

In another population-based study, Levitan and colleagues[14] examined the discharge diagnoses of more than 7000 Medicare patients (>65 years of age) admitted to the hospital with a diagnosis of malignancy and either DVT or PE. The ratio of the number of patients with a particular type of cancer who had VTE to the number of patients with that type of malignancy provided an estimate of which cancers were most likely to lead to thrombosis. Highest rates were found with cancer of the ovary (120 per 10,000 patients), brain tumor (117 per 10,000 patients), and cancer of the pancreas (110 per 10,000 patients). In a recently reported case-controlled study of more than 3000 consecutive patients with a first episode of VTE, Blom and colleagues[15] reported an overall sevenfold increased risk of VTE in patients with malignancy (odds ratio, 6.7; confidence interval [CI], 5.2 to 8.6] versus persons without malignancy (Fig. 23-2).[15,16] Patients with hematologic malignancies had the highest risk, adjusted for age and sex (odds ratio, 28.0; CI, 4.0 to 199.7), followed by lung and gastrointestinal cancers. Risk was highest in the first few months after the cancer was diagnosed, and those with distant metastases had a higher risk compared with patients without metastases (adjusted odds ratio, 19.8; CI, 2.6 to 149.1). Similar results to those of the Levitan study were reported more recently by Blom and colleagues[17] on the basis of a linkage analysis of the complete databases of the Cancer Registry of the Western Netherlands (86,151 subjects) and of the anticoagulation clinics of Leiden and The Hague (157,482 subjects). In this latter study, overall cumulative incidence of VTE in the first 6 months was 12.3 of 1000 patients with cancer (95% CI, 11.5 to 13.0), and patients with tumors of the bone, ovary, brain, and pancreas had the highest cumulative incidence of VTE. The different representation of tumors with high incidence of VTE in the two Blom studies most likely reflects the different methods used. In the more recent study, the use of much larger databases may have facilitated a more accurate assessment of VTE with a relatively low incidence of tumors.

Although VTE has been reported at autopsy in up to 30% of patients with cancer,[18] the optimal study design for determining the true incidence of clinical VTE in patients with cancer is a prospective cohort study, which has not been described. Alternatively, the incidence of thrombosis may be derived from prospective clinical trials of systemic therapy in women with early breast cancer (Table 23-1).[4]

The rate of thrombosis over a 5-year period in women with axillary node–negative breast cancer on tamoxifen therapy was approximately 0.9%. It was recognized early that tamoxifen therapy was thrombogenic in women with breast cancer. The Breast Cancer Prevention Trial conducted by the National Surgical Adjuvant Breast and Bowel Project (NSABP) provided an opportunity to examine prospectively this relationship and to estimate the thrombogenic effects of tamoxifen alone. In this trial, healthy women at risk for developing breast cancer were randomly assigned to tamoxifen or placebo for 5 years. The risk of DVT was increased in the tamoxifen-treated group compared with the placebo group: 0.13% per year versus 0.084% per year. Corresponding rates for PE were 0.069% and 0.023%, respectively. The highest rates of thrombosis associated with the use of tamoxifen were observed in women older than 50 years of age; with tamoxifen, the risk of stroke was increased while no increase was observed in the risk for myocardial infarction.

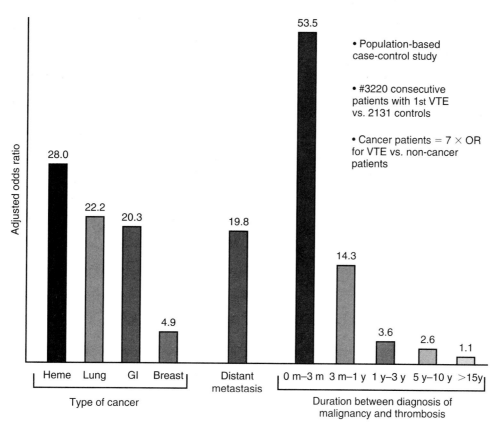

Figure 23-2 Effects of Malignancy on Risk of Venous Thrombosis. Figure adapted from a review of the original paper.[15,16] (Reproduced with permission from the publisher.)

Table 23-1 Incidence of Thrombosis in Early-Stage Breast Cancer

Study	Treatment	No. of Patients	% of Patients with Thrombosis
Node-Negative			
Fisher, 1989	T	1318	0.9
	Placebo	1326	0.15
Fisher, 1997	CMFT	768	4.2
	T	771	0.8
Node-Positive			
Levine, 1988	CMFVP	102	8.8
	CMFVP + AT	103	4.9
Pritchard, 1996	CMF + T	353	9.6
	T	352	1.4
Clahsen, 1994	Perioperative FAC	1292	2.1
	No Rx	1332	0.8
Rivkin, 1994	CMFVP + T	303	3.6
	CMFVP	300	1.3
	T	295	0
Fisher, 1990	ACT	383	3.1
	T	367	1.6
Weiss, 1981	CMFVP	143	6.3
	CMF	144	3.5

A, adriamycin; C, cyclophosphamide; F, fluorouracil; M, methotrexate; P, prednisone; T, tamoxifen; V, vincristine. (NOTE: Full citations for these studies can be found in References 3 and 4; adapted from Levine M, Lee AYY, Kakkar AK: Cancer and Thrombosis. In: Hemostasis and Thrombosis, 5th Ed. (eds.) RW Colman, VJ Marder, A Clowes, et al. Lippincott Williams & Wilkins, Philadelphia, Chapter 85, pp. 1251–1262, 2005, with permission.)

Rates of thrombosis in women with node-positive breast cancer on chemotherapy ranged between 1% and 9%, with the highest rates of thrombosis observed in postmenopausal women. In these trials, groups of women receiving chemotherapy plus tamoxifen showed an increased risk of thrombosis over chemotherapy alone. Rates of thrombosis in women with metastatic breast cancer vary. In a case series reported by Goodnough and colleagues (see Table 23-1),[19] the rate of thrombosis in patients receiving chemotherapy for metastatic breast cancer was 17.5%, although in a randomized trial reported by Levine and associates,[20] the rate was only 4.5% (see Table 23-1). Clinicians are often faced with the scenario of a patient with a past history of VTE who develops breast cancer and requires therapy with a hormonal agent. On the basis of results from recent trials, aromatase inhibitors appear to have a much lower risk of thrombosis when compared with tamoxifen (see Chapter 34). Even in women with advanced breast cancer, thrombosis rates of only 2% to 4% were reported with these agents.[21,22]

Data on the incidence of thrombosis in other patient groups are limited and are summarized in Table 23-2. Another group of patients discovered to be at high risk for thrombosis were those with brain tumors, who are on extended follow-up. In a review by Marras and coworkers,[23] rates of symptomatic VTE as high as 18% per year were described in a single study,[24] in which the authors reported an overall risk rate of 24% (see Table 23-2). Among patients with germ cell tumors, 8.4% of 179 patients given platinum-based chemotherapy developed VTE. Reported rates of VTE in other solid tumors include

Table 23-2 Incidence of Thrombosis in Different Tumors

Study	Tumor Type*	Patients	Thrombosis, %
Brandes	Malignant glioma	75	24.0
Weijl	Germ cell	179	8.4
Blom	Lung	537	4.4
Solit	Prostate	30	17.0
Von Tempelhoff	Ovarian	47	10.6
Wun	Cervix (cisplatin, radiation, w/ erythropoietin [epo])	75	22.6
Wun	Cervix (cisplatin, radiation w/o epo)	72	2.7
Lavey	Cervix (cisplatin, radiation w/epo)	53	13.0
Ottinger	Non-Hodgkin lymphoma	593	6.6
Seifter	Hodgkin lymphoma	177	6.0
DeStefano	Leukemia	379	6.3

*Patients with advanced cancer receiving chemotherapy. (From Levine M, Lee AYY, Kakkar AK: Cancer and Thrombosis. In: Hemostasis and Thrombosis, 5th Ed. (eds.) RW Colman, VJ Marder, A Clowes, et al. Lippincott Williams & Wilkins, Philadelphia, Chapter 85, pp. 1251–1262, 2005, with permission.)

the following: 4.4% per year in patients with lung cancer, 10.6% in women with advanced ovarian cancer receiving chemotherapy, 17% in men with prostate cancer receiving chemotherapy, and 3% in women with carcinoma of the cervix receiving concurrent chemotherapy and radiation. Of particular interest in the latter study, erythropoietin (EPO) appeared to increase thrombotic risk to 23%.

Emerging evidence suggests that this erythroid hormone increases thrombotic risk, particularly among patients with cancer. In a study of women with advanced cervical cancer receiving radiation, cisplatin chemotherapy, and EPO, the rate of thrombosis was 13%.[24] A randomized trial that evaluated EPO in women with advanced breast cancer was stopped early, when four of 14 patients (28.5%) in the EPO arm developed thrombosis compared with none of 13 women in the control arm.[25] See Update on Erythropoietin Therapy at the end of this chapter.

Other hematopoietic growth factors have not been well studied. Barbui and colleagues[26] conducted a meta-analysis of studies in which patients with cancer were treated with hematopoietic growth factors. Although the analysis was not conclusive, the authors suggested that an increased risk of thrombosis was associated with the use of granulocyte-macrophage colony stimulating factor (GM-CSF). Multiple mechanisms for an increased risk of thrombosis associated with the use of hematopoietic growth factors have been postulated, including reduced blood flow associated with simple elevation of hematocrit as expected with EPO use, direct effects of EPO on the vessel wall, leukocyte stasis in response to GM-CSF, and so forth, but few specific data are available to shed light on this important area of research.

Reports from most trials in patients with colorectal cancer receiving chemotherapy have not included rates of thrombosis. The explanation for this is unclear, but it is possible that it is due to underreporting.[27] A careful audit of early deaths in a randomized trial of irinotecan, 5-fluorouracil (5-FU), and leucovorin versus 5-FU/leucovorin as adjuvant therapy in colon cancer, however, noted an excessive number of vascular deaths (arterial and venous) in the former arm (1.9% vs 0.6%, respectively).[28] In a trial of irinotecan plus 5-FU/leucovorin versus 5-FU/leucovorin in patients with metastatic colorectal cancer, a statistically significant increased rate of thromboembolic events was

reported in patients given the three-drug regimen versus 5-FU/leucovorin (5% vs <1%, respectively).[27] Thrombosis rates of 5% to 10% have been reported in patients with Hodgkin or non-Hodgkin lymphoma who were receiving chemotherapy, along with a rate of 6.3% in adult patients with acute leukemia; the highest rates were reported in patients with acute promyelocytic leukemia.

Interest in the thrombogenicity of anticancer agents has been rekindled among medical oncologists and hematologists, in part because of the unexpectedly high rate of VTE among patients with cancer receiving novel anticancer agents aimed at specific molecular targets within the cancer cell, often shared by the tumor vascular endothelium. For example, drugs that target the vascular endothelial growth factor (VEGF) receptor or VEGF itself, including thalidomide, have been shown to increase the risk of thrombosis, particularly when used in association with traditional chemotherapy drugs (Table 23-3).[27–37] Kuenen and colleagues[33] conducted a phase 1 study of cisplatin, gemcitabine, and SU5416 in patients with solid tumors. SU5416 inhibited the autophosphorylation of the VEGF receptor that followed the interaction of the receptor with VEGF, thereby blocking the intracellular signaling pathway. This trial was stopped early because 8 of 19 patients experienced thrombosis. It is likely that chemotherapy combined with the antiangiogenic agent leads to thrombin generation and endothelial cell activation, resulting in a net shift toward a prothrombotic state.[38]

The anti-VEGF agent bevacizumab (Avastin; Genentech, Inc., South San Francisco, Calif) has been evaluated in a number of randomized clinical trials (see Table 23-3). In the first trial, which was reported by Kabbinavar and colleagues,[35] patients with metastatic colon cancer were treated with 5-FU plus leucovorin compared with these agents plus bevacizumab. A statistically significant increase in VTE was observed among patients who received the anti-VEGF agent. In addition, an increase in bleeding complications was noted. In a later trial conducted by Hurwitz and colleagues,[37] chemotherapy was compared with chemotherapy plus bevacizumab; no difference was detected in the rate of VTE between treatment groups. Bevacizumab has been evaluated in two randomized trials in women with metastatic breast cancer.[39,40] In one trial, capecitabine was compared with

Table 23-3   Incidence of Thrombosis with Antiangiogenesis Agents

Study	Tumor	Patients	Thrombosis, %
Zangari, 2001	*Myeloma:*		
	Chemotherapy plus thalidomide	87	35.0
	Chemotherapy alone	134	15.0
Kabbinavar, 2003	*Colorectal cancer:*		
	5-FU + leucovorin (L)	36	2.9
	5-FU + L + bevacizumab (5 mg/kg)	35	14.2
	5-FU + L + bevacizumab (10 mg/kg)	33	6.2
Hurwitz, 2004	5-FU + L	411	16.2
	5-FU + L + bevacizumab	402	19.4
Miller, 2005	*Metastatic breast cancer:*		
	Capecitabine	215	5.6
	Capecitabine + bevacizumab	229	7.4
Miller, 2005	Paclitaxel	330	0.3
	Paclitaxel + bevacizumab	342	1.2

(NOTE: Adapted and updated from Levine M, Lee AYY, Kakkar AK: Cancer and Thrombosis. In: Hemostasis and Thrombosis, 5th Ed. (eds.) RW Colman, VJ Marder, A Clowes, et al. Lippincott Williams & Wilkins, Philadelphia, Chapter 85, pp. 1251–1262, 2005, with permission.)

capecitabine plus bevacizumab. In the second trial, paclitaxel plus bevacizumab was compared with paclitaxel alone. No increase in VTE was observed in patients treated with bevacizumab. In a trial reported by Johnson and associates,[41] patients with non–small cell lung cancer were randomly assigned to carboplatinum and paclitaxel versus the same agents plus two different doses of bevacizumab.[41] No difference was detected between the groups in terms of VTE rate, but a statistically significant increase in bleeding was associated with bevacizumab. It is unclear why increased VTE was observed in the first randomized trial of bevacizumab in patients with colon cancer, but not in subsequent trials.

Recently, thalidomide has been widely used in the treatment of patients with multiple myeloma, and the risk for VTE has been reported to be increased (see Table 23-3). Although thalidomide therapy *alone* has not been associated typically with a particularly high risk of thrombosis in patients with advanced or refractory myeloma (1%),[42] when combined with chemotherapy, Zangari and colleagues[30] reported that 14 of 50 patients (28%) developed VTE, compared with only 2 of 50 patients (4%) given chemotherapy and dexamethasone without thalidomide. Thalidomide in combination with dexamethasone also appears to be associated with an increased risk of thrombosis, as reported in 6 of 50 patients (12%) newly diagnosed with myeloma.[43] The increased incidence of VTE in the thalidomide plus dexamethasone arm persisted (17% vs 3% in the dexamethasone alone arm) when the cohort doubled in size, as was reported recently by these same authors.[44] Of interest, this combination did not result in an increased rate of VTE in a recently published series of 31 patients with amyloidosis, in which only one case of VTE was reported.[45] As might be expected, risk of VTE rises when hematopoietic cell transplantation is added into the equation, as was shown recently by the 30% rate in the series reported by Barlogie and colleagues.[46]

Finally, patients with cancer with indwelling central venous catheters (CVC) are believed to be at increased risk for thrombosis of the axillary-subclavian vein, with incidence rates of up to 35% reported in the older literature.[47,48] In addition, the catheters themselves are prone to thrombotic occlusion, despite the use of routine heparin

flushes. As will be noted subsequently, however, the risk of thrombosis in more recent randomized, controlled trials has been substantially lowered (e.g., 4% to 5%), perhaps because of improved local measures in the care of CVC and/or improved biocompatibility of catheter materials (see Chapter 32).

Cancer Survival and Thromboembolism

Patients with cancer who develop VTE have a short life expectancy. In a population-based study reported by Silverstein and colleagues,[12] the presence of cancer was an independent predictor of worse survival in patients who presented with acute VTE. Similarly, Sorensen and colleagues[49] showed that patients with cancer who present concurrently with clinically apparent VTE had a worse survival rate than those with cancer without VTE. Levitan and associates[14] reported after analysis of the Medicare database, that the mortality rate for patients with VTE and malignant disease was substantially increased compared with that for malignant disease alone.[14]

Increased Risk of Venous Thromboembolism in Patients With Cancer Subjected to Surgery

Patients with cancer who undergo surgery are at an approximate twofold increased risk of postoperative thrombosis compared with noncancer patients subjected to the same operations.[50,51] The risk of VTE in patients with cancer who undergo specific types of surgery can be derived from the "no treatment" control arms of trials undertaken to evaluate prophylactic measures in surgery.[52] The outcome measured typically in these studies was thrombosis, as detected by fibrinogen leg scanning; approximate rates were as follows: general surgery, 29%; gynecologic surgery, 20%; urologic surgery, 41%; orthopaedic surgery, 50% to 60%; and neurosurgery, 28%. However, many of these thrombi were asymptomatic, and some studies included patients without cancer. On the basis of these data, however, patients with cancer have been stratified by the 2004 Consensus Conference of the American College of Chest Physicians into their highest risk category,[53] compelling the routine use of "short-term" anticoagulant therapy as prophylaxis against VTE in preparation for surgery.

We will discuss this in greater detail in a subsequent section.

Tumors Associated With Thrombosis

Sack and colleagues[54] compiled a series of case reports from the literature and reported that the cancers most commonly associated with thrombosis were pancreas, lung, and stomach.[54] Lieberman and coworkers, in a retrospective series,[55] reported that lung and pancreas were the most common cancers associated with thrombosis in men, and that gynecologic, colorectal, and pancreas were the most common sites associated with thrombosis in women.[55] However, it is likely that the distribution of specific cancers associated with thrombosis follows the frequency of cancer in the general population.[56] This is best observed in patients entered into prospective clinical trials of antithrombotic agents. In a study by Levine and associates,[57] which evaluated outpatient therapy with low molecular weight heparin (LMWH) for proximal DVT, 103 of 500 patients had cancer. The most common anatomic sites in men were the prostate, colorectal, brain, and lung, and the most common sites in women were the breast, ovary, and lung.

PATHOGENESIS OF VENOUS THROMBOEMBOLISM IN CANCER

Virchow Triad

Patients with cancer have multiple reasons to develop VTE, which can be classified according to the pathophysiologic mechanisms first proposed by Virchow in 1856.[58] Patients with cancer often experience stasis, which is caused by prolonged bed rest or obstruction of vascular flow from extrinsic compression or direct vascular invasion by tumor. Vascular damage may occur as the result of direct invasion by tumor, and more subtle vascular injury often occurs because of the frequent use of central venous access devices, aggravated by the administration of cancer chemotherapy drugs. Indeed, virtually all commonly used intravenous cancer chemotherapy agents have been shown to be capable of activating blood coagulation in vivo, presumably through induction of vascular injury.[59] Finally, patients with cancer have a primary hypercoagulable state, the pathogenesis of which is exceedingly complex[3,60]; this is summarized diagrammatically in Figure 23-3 and discussed below.

Tumor Procoagulants

Tumor cells themselves possess a variety of procoagulant properties, including tissue factor (TF) and cancer procoagulant (CP), both of which directly activate clotting, as well as procoagulant cytokines such as interleukin (IL)-1β, tumor necrosis factor (TNF)-α, IL-8, and VEGF, which indirectly activate clotting via their proinflammatory properties particularly targeted to the endothelium. Tumor cell VEGF is chemotactic for macrophages and endothelial cells; it activates TF in both cells. Tumor cells also activate platelets and polymorphonuclear leukocytes and, via integrin expression, they form adhesive interactions with platelets and the endothelium of blood vessels. Tumor cell interaction with the vessel wall reduces endothelial cell secretion of tissue plasminogen activator (tPA) and expression of the angiogenesis inhibitor thrombomodulin

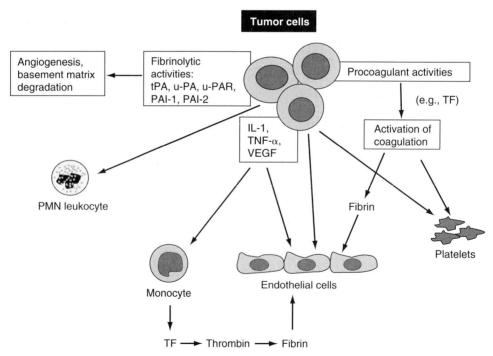

Figure 23-3 Principal pathways of tumor cell interaction with the hemostatic system. TF, tissue factor; PAI, plasminogen activator inhibitor; u-PAR, urokinase-type plasminogen activator receptor; u-PA and tPA, urokinase-type plasminogen activator and tissue plasminogen activator; IL-1, interleukin-1; TNF-α, tumor necrosis factor alpha; VEGF, vascular endothelial growth factor. (From Falanga A, Rickles FR: The pathogenesis of venous thromboembolism in cancer. N Oncol Thromb 1:9–16, 2005, with permission.)

(TM), and enhances endothelial cell synthesis of plaminogen activator inhibitor-1 (PAI-1). Finally, substantial experimental evidence supports the presence of increased numbers of activated monocytes/macrophages in the circulation of patients with cancer in proximity to growing tumors.[61] These antigen-processing cells express TF on their surface, presumably as part of the host immune response to the tumor and/or in response to secretion of tumor products. Tumor-associated macrophages have been shown to assemble the entire coagulation cascade and form cross linked fibrin (XLF) on their surface in apposition to growing tumor.[3,61] The activation of coagulation in the tumor microenvironment, which routinely spills into the circulation of patients with cancer (vide infra), may be a primitive effort on the part of the host to limit the spread of tumor cells.

Coagulation Activation, Fibrin Generation, and Tumor Angiogenesis

Interleukin-8, previously known as melanoma growth factor, is a potent proangiogenic cytokine elaborated by a variety of cells, including the endothelial cell itself. XLF formed on the surface of vascular endothelial cells (VECs) can upregulate the gene for IL-8 and induce the synthesis and release of IL-8 from endothelial cells in a dose-dependent fashion. Therefore, it seems likely that multiple products of blood coagulation, including both thrombin and fibrin, can stimulate the activation and migration of endothelial cells (perhaps via IL-8 release) and induce a self-perpetuating system for further activation of blood coagulation (by induction of TF).[62,63] In addition, however, expression of the proangiogenic cytokine, VEGF, by human tumor cells is regulated by transfection of the cells with the gene for TF.[64] Once transplanted into a xenogeneic murine recipient, human breast and melanoma tumor cells expressing high levels of the TF gene are capable of inducing a significant increase in angiogenesis in the animal. TF and VEGF have been colocalized to tumor cells in patients with breast or lung cancer,[61] and TF likely induces cell signaling that results in enhanced VEGF synthesis.

These results suggest a new role for TF in the stimulation of angiogenesis, independent of its role in blood coagulation,[63,64] and might result ultimately in a novel therapeutic approach to cancer therapy. Indeed, other groups have successfully targeted TF in tumor cells and VECs in experimental approaches to model tumors[65–67]; phase 1 studies are under way to explore the treatment of human tumors through the use of several different hybrid antitumor agents designed to target the neovascular response of growing tumors—so-called vascular targeting agents.[68] At the molecular level, it has now been shown in several tumor models that oncogene expression activates TF, influences systemic blood coagulation, modulates other regulators of hemostasis, and triggers angiogenesis.[69–71] Therefore, effective targeting of TF may prove useful in limiting tumor growth and reducing the hypercoagulability characteristics of cancer.[68,72,73] In the meantime, more effective strategies for reducing the risk of VTE are under development, particularly because any cancer therapy that perturbs the highly prothrombotic tumor angiogenic endothelium may result in an increased risk of VTE.

VENOUS THROMBOEMBOLISM PROPHYLAXIS IN PATIENTS WITH CANCER

Primary Prophylaxis

Surgical Patients

Clinical trials have shown the efficacy of low-dose, unfractionated heparin (UFH) in preventing deep vein thrombosis and PE in patients undergoing major surgery.[51,74] In these studies, many of the patients had cancer. Standard UFH can be depolymerized to low molecular weight fragments.[75,76] LMWH has a more predictable anticoagulant response than UFH, a longer plasma half-life, and better bioavailability when administered subcutaneously (less nonspecific binding to plasma proteins and circulating blood cells). In addition, in laboratory studies, LMWH preparations cause less bleeding with equivalent antithrombotic effects. Standard UFH is usually given three times a day, whereas LMWH can be administered once a day. Recent studies have shown equal efficacy and enhanced safety for LMWH compared with UFH in high-risk major surgery.[77,78] In 2001, Mismetti and colleagues[79] published a meta-analysis of trials that compared LMWH with UFH in high-risk major surgery. In their analysis, which included patients undergoing surgery for cancer, no differences were detected in rates of asymptomatic DVT, clinical PE, death, or major bleeding between LMWH and UFH. Mechanical methods of thromboprophylaxis have also been shown to be effective in surgical patients,[51] although these are less effective than anticoagulation, and when used alone are particularly ineffective in patients with cancer. Thus, in the patient with cancer who is undergoing surgery, prophylaxis should consist of low-dose UFH or LMWH, together with graduated compression stockings. Regarding the duration of prophylaxis, the definition of "short-term" anticoagulant therapy as prophylaxis against VTE in cancer remains an open question. Berqvist and colleagues[80] demonstrated a significantly lower rate of VTE when cancer patients were treated with prophylactic doses of LMWH for at least 1 month after surgery. These results are supported by data from a more recent open-label trial by Rasmussen and associates,[81] in which 343 patients undergoing major abdominal surgery were randomly assigned to receive 7 days of standard thromboprophylaxis with 5000 IU of the LMWH dalteparin once daily or extended prophylaxis with the same dose for 3 additional weeks. Patients had mandatory bilateral venography at day 28. The cumulative incidence of VTE was reduced from 16.3% with short-term prophylaxis to 7.3% after prolonged prophylaxis ($P = 0.01$; relative risk reduction [RRR], 55%). The number needed-to-treat to prevent one case of VTE was 12, and no significant difference was noted between groups with regard to bleeding events.

Medical Patients

Fewer data are available on prophylaxis in ambulatory patients with cancer. Levine and associates[82] conducted a trial that showed that very low dose warfarin is safe and effective for the prevention of VTE in patients with metastatic breast cancer receiving chemotherapy. The warfarin dose was 1 mg daily for 6 weeks; it was adjusted so that an International Normalized Ratio (INR) could be maintained at between 1.3 and 1.9. An economic analysis of this trial showed the cost-effectiveness of the approach.[83] Despite this study, oncologists do not routinely use prophylaxis in patients with cancer who are receiving chemotherapy with oral anticoagulants. The most likely reasons are concern for bleeding and the logistics of laboratory monitoring and dose adjustment. An alternative is to reserve prophylaxis for high-risk situations (e.g., previous history of VTE, a pelvic mass that causes poor venous drainage from the lower limbs), but clearly, more research is needed in these high-risk groups. In addition, patients with cancer who are bedridden are at risk for thrombosis, which occurs often in the setting of an acute hospitalization for a complication related to cancer (e.g., pain crisis, infection, hypercalcemia). Patients with advanced cancer are also admitted to the hospital on occasion for palliative care. Low-dose UFH and LMWH have been found to be effective in patients hospitalized with acute medical illness.[84,85] It would seem reasonable, therefore, for practitioners to institute prophylaxis with low-dose UFH or LMWH for patients with advanced malignancy when admitted to the hospital.

Venous Catheters

Strategies for the prevention of venous catheter–associated thrombosis in patients with cancer have also been reported, as noted previously (see Chapter 32). Studies of very low dose warfarin (1 mg/day) or LMWH (e.g., dalteparin sodium at 2500 IU/day) have shown significant reduction in the incidence of catheter-related thrombosis.[47,48] In these earlier trials, many thrombotic events were asymptomatic. Despite the results of these trials, substantial variation characterizes the use of antithrombotic prophylaxis in standard practice. Further, it should be noted that 1 mg per day of warfarin, which was originally believed to not significantly prolong the prothrombin time, may lead to substantial elevation of the INR in patients with colorectal cancer given infusional 5-FU.[86] Recently, the results of four randomized trials in patients with central vein catheters were reported.[87–90] In the trial by Reichardt and colleagues,[87] patients with cancer were randomly assigned to dalteparin (5000 U once daily) or placebo.[87] Screening ultrasonography was done at the end of the study. Rates of thrombosis were very low in both groups, at about 3%. In the trial by Couban and colleagues,[88] patients with cancer received 1 mg of warfarin or placebo.[88] No difference was detected in symptomatic thrombosis, and rates were low in both groups, at approximately 4%. In an Italian trial reported by Verso and coworkers,[89] patients with cancer were randomly assigned to enoxaparin LMWH or placebo.[89] Patients underwent venography, which detected thrombosis in 18% of the placebo-treated group and 14% of the LMWH group. This difference was not statistically significant. Rates of symptomatic thrombosis were low in both groups (3.1% vs 1%, respectively). Results of the most recent trial were reported by Young and colleagues from the United Kingdom.[90] Patients with cancer with central vein catheters were randomly assigned to warfarin 1 mg daily, or no prophylaxis if the physician was uncertain about the efficacy of prophylaxis. If the physician was certain about prophylaxis, patients were randomly assigned

to 1 mg of warfarin or warfarin adjusted to an INR of 1.5. The overall rate of symptomatic catheter-associated thrombosis was only 5%. In the first stratum, warfarin did not reduce thrombosis (odds ratio, 0.94) and was associated with increased major bleeding (2% vs 0.2%). In the second stratum, the rate of thrombosis was reduced with adjusted-dose warfarin (3% vs 7%; odds ratio, 0.43), but major bleeding was increased (4% vs 2%). A recent cohort study also reported low rates of thrombosis in patients with cancer with central vein catheters.[91] The reason for the observed low rates of thrombosis in these trials is unclear, although both the availability of new generations of catheters with better biocompatibility and improved catheter care have been implicated. Further research is required. At this juncture, the weight of the evidence would not support the routine use of antithrombotic prophylaxis in such patients, although selected high-risk patients may be an exception.

Secondary Prophylaxis

Patients with cancer who have established VTE are more likely to develop recurrent VTE during oral anticoagulation than are patients without cancer.[92,93] In a trial reported by Levine and associates,[94] patients with proximal DVT were randomly assigned to UFH by continuous intravenous infusion in the hospital or to LMWH given subcutaneously at home. Both groups received 3 months of oral anticoagulant therapy. No difference was detected in the rate of recurrent thromboembolism between treatment groups. However, the rate of recurrent VTE in 103 patients with cancer was 14% compared with 4% among 317 noncancer patients ($P = .001$).[94] Prandoni and coworkers[92] reported data from long-term follow-up of a large series of patients with proximal DVT, who received at least 3 months of oral anticoagulant therapy. The frequency of recurrent VTE was 10.3% in 58 patients with cancer compared with 4.7% among 297 noncancer patients ($P = .12$). This difference achieved statistical significance for the subgroup of patients in the therapeutic range (i.e., INR, 2 to 3; 8.6% vs 1.3%; $P < .01$). In a more recent update of these data, this important observation was validated for all patients.[93] In the trial reported by the Columbus investigators,[95] which compared LMWH with UFH for proximal DVT, rates of recurrent thromboembolism were 8.6% in patients with cancer and 4.1% in noncancer patients. Therefore, patients with cancer were at higher risk for recurrence of VTE in that study, suggesting that they may be relatively resistant to treatment with oral anticoagulants.

Several, large, prospective, randomized clinical trials comparing the relative efficacy of extended LMWH therapy versus oral anticoagulation as secondary prophylaxis in patients with cancer patients have been completed recently.

Results of the CLOT (Comparison of Low molecular weight heparin versus Oral anticoagulant Therapy for prevention of recurrent venous thromboembolism in patients with cancer) study were reported by Lee and colleagues[96]; they confirmed the superiority of LMWH over warfarin for long-term secondary prophylaxis in patients with cancer. These results have established at least 6 months of LMWH as the new standard of care for patients with cancer with VTE.[53]

TREATMENT OF PATIENTS WITH ESTABLISHED VENOUS THROMBOEMBOLISM

The objectives of treating patients with VTE are to prevent death from pulmonary embolism, to reduce morbidity from the acute event, to minimize postphlebitic symptoms, and to prevent thromboembolic pulmonary hypertension. The physician is often confronted with the issue of whether VTE in a patient with terminal malignant disease should be treated. Treatment may be useful for palliation of symptoms of acute VTE, including reduction of painful swelling of the leg from DVT and reversal of dyspnea and chest pain in pulmonary embolism. The decision to treat with anticoagulants is particularly difficult in a patient with a very short life expectancy.

Initial Treatment

Treatment of acute venous thrombosis should be initiated with heparin followed by oral anticoagulant therapy.[78] LMWH has largely replaced UFH as initial therapy for acute venous thrombosis. Historically, patients required hospital admission to receive UFH by continuous intravenous infusion, and the infusion rate was adjusted so that a target partial thromboplastin time (PTT) could be maintained. LMWH is administered subcutaneously and does not typically require monitoring by a laboratory test of coagulation.

In several randomized trials, LMWH has been shown to be as safe and effective as UFH for the treatment of hospitalized patients with acute proximal DVT. Three large randomized clinical trials in patients with acute proximal DVT compared intravenous UFH in the hospital with LMWH administered at home.[94,95,97] In a subgroup analysis of these three studies, consisting of 405 patients with cancer, no difference was detected in recurrent VTE between treatment groups—a finding confirmed in two more recent cohort studies.[98,99] These results show that LMWH can be used safely and effectively to treat patients with acute VTE (including uncomplicated pulmonary embolism) in the home setting and should reassure the treating physician that home therapy of VTE with LMWH is a reasonable alternative for selected patients with cancer.

Secondary Prevention—Best Choice of Anticoagulant and Appropriate Duration of Therapy

Patients with DVT who are treated with an initial course of heparin therapy require continual anticoagulant therapy to prevent recurrence. Vitamin K antagonists have been shown to be effective in preventing recurrent thrombosis in patients with established VTE.[78] The risk of clinical bleeding for patients with INR in the therapeutic range is relatively low (approximately 2% per year in recent clinical trials).[100] Once again, however, this rate is based primarily on studies of patients *without* cancer, and conventional wisdom suggests that patients with cancer are at higher risk of hemorrhagic complications while receiving oral anticoagulant drugs. The results of two previous prospective cohort studies had been reassuring, with rates of major

bleeding similar in anticoagulated patients with cancer (3.4%) to those in patients without cancer (3%),[92] or 0.004 event per patient-month of treatment versus 0.003 event per patient-month of treatment, respectively.[101] A more recent prospective 11-year study by Prandoni and colleagues,[93] however, reports a significant, twofold increased risk of major bleeding in anticoagulated patients with cancer versus patients without cancer.

It is common practice to continue oral anticoagulant therapy for 3 months after a first episode of proximal DVT or PE. The patient with active malignant disease who has had an episode of established thrombosis is likely to be at continuing risk of recurrent VTE, even after 3 months of warfarin.[80,81] Although no clinical trials have yet examined prospectively as the primary end point the appropriate length of oral anticoagulant therapy in patients with cancer and VTE, three studies have considered the issue of duration of anticoagulant therapy in patients with idiopathic DVT—a group considered to be at continuing risk of thromboembolism.[102-104] Schulman and colleagues[102] randomly assigned patients with idiopathic proximal DVT to 6 weeks or 6 months of oral anticoagulant therapy after initial heparin therapy. Patients who received 6 months of treatment had a significant reduction in the rate of recurrent thromboembolism. Investigators then randomly assigned patients with a second episode of DVT to 6 months or indefinite duration of oral anticoagulant therapy. Patients who received treatment of longer duration had a significant reduction in recurrent thromboembolism and a small increase in bleeding.[103] Kearon and coworkers[104] reported the results of a trial in which patients with idiopathic DVT were randomly assigned to receive 3 months or 2 years of oral anticoagulant therapy. A significant reduction in recurrence favored patients who received anticoagulant therapy of longer duration. On the basis of the results of these trials, it would seem prudent to continue anticoagulant therapy beyond 3 months while these patients remain at high risk for VTE recurrence. In the patient at particularly high risk for bleeding, the dose of warfarin can be lowered to maintain an INR close to 2.0; the efficacy of maintaining the patient's INR between 1.5 and 2.0, however, remains controversial.[105,106]

Warfarin therapy is particularly complicated in the patient with cancer for a number of reasons. It is often difficult to maintain the INR within the therapeutic range because patients with cancer experience anorexia and vomiting, limiting their dietary intake of vitamin K. In addition, drug interactions (e.g., chemotherapy/antibiotics) can influence the anticoagulant effects of vitamin K–dependent anticoagulants (in either direction). Interruption of oral anticoagulant therapy occurs commonly in patients with cancer because of the development of thrombocytopenia, or for the performance of diagnostic or therapeutic procedures such as thoracentesis and abdominal paracentesis. Reversal of the anticoagulant effect with vitamin K may be required. Subsequently, it may require days to weeks to achieve the target therapeutic range after reintroduction of warfarin. Finally, frequent blood sampling is required for monitoring the INR, and venous access may be difficult to attain in these patients.

Therefore, certain features of long-term anticoagulant therapy with LMWH are attractive for patients with cancer. For example, LMWH does not require laboratory monitoring and can be administered subcutaneously once or twice daily on the basis of body weight. Clinical experience suggests that LMWH may be effective in warfarin failure.[107] Finally, on the basis of preclinical data and meta-analyses, the potential for less bleeding exists. In several small trials, long-term oral anticoagulant therapy has been compared with long-term LMWH[108–114]; regrettably, very few patients with cancer were studied. Several recent randomized trials have provided new information on the long-term treatment of patients with cancer with VTE.

In the trial reported by Meyer and colleagues,[115] patients with cancer with acute VTE were randomly assigned to 3 months of enoxaparin or warfarin at a targeted INR of 2.0 to 3.0. The primary outcome measure was a composite of major bleeding and recurrent VTE. In 71 patients who received warfarin, the outcome event rate was 21%, compared with 10.5% in 67 patients who received LMWH ($P = .09$). This observed difference, which was not statistically significant, was attributed primarily to the rates of major bleeding in the two groups: 16.9% in patients given warfarin versus 7.5% in those given LMWH. Lee and associates (the CLOT trial),[96] as noted in the previous section, randomly assigned cancer patients to long-term dalteparin versus long-term oral anticoagulant therapy. Over the 6-month study period, 27 of 336 patients in the dalteparin group compared with 53 of 336 patients in the oral anticoagulant group experienced recurrent VTE. The probability of VTE at 6 months was reduced from 17.4% in the oral anticoagulant group to 8.8% in the dalteparin group; the hazard ratio was 0.48 ($P = .0017$). No statistically significant difference was detected in major bleeding between groups (3.6% and 5.6%, respectively). The rate of any bleeding (major plus minor) was 18.5% in the oral anticoagulant group compared with 13.6% in the dalteparin group ($P = .09$). On the basis of the results of these trials, long-term therapy with LMWH should be viewed as an important advance in the management of patients with cancer and acute VTE. Therapy with LMWH substantially reduces the rate of recurrent VTE without an increase in bleeding, thereby improving the quality of life of patients with cancer. Long-term use of LMWH also simplifies the management of such patients. It avoids the need for laboratory monitoring, which is advantageous for both the patient and the physician. If a patient requires an urgent procedure, the LMWH is simply discontinued; it is not necessary to reverse the anticoagulant effect.

In general, the duration of long-term treatment of patients with VTE is based on the individual patient's risks for recurrent thrombosis and bleeding. In patients with malignancy, the risk of recurrent thrombosis depends on the usual thrombotic risk factors (e.g., surgery, bed rest), as well as factors specific to cancer, such as stage or activity of cancer and the use of chemotherapy and hormonal agents.

Currently, the recommendation from the American College of Chest Physicians (ACCP) for patients with cancer who experience an acute thromboembolic event is to treat them for a minimum of 3 to 6 months with LMWH, then with "anticoagulant therapy indefinitely or until the cancer is resolved."[116] However, as in patients without cancer, the exact duration of therapy should be tailored individually. In patients with metastatic disease, anticoagulant therapy should be continued indefinitely, or until

a contraindication to anticoagulation develops. In those who have active but nonmetastatic disease, anticoagulant therapy should be given for at least 6 months and as long as cancer is evident, or while the patient is receiving chemotherapy. In patients with cancer who have no evidence of active cancer and who have developed a thrombotic event in association with a strong risk factor such as surgery, a minimum of 3 months of anticoagulant treatment is probably reasonable, especially if relative contraindications are evident for continuing anticoagulation.

Patients at Particular Risk of Hemorrhage

In patients with a "relative" contraindication to anticoagulation therapy (e.g., those with metastatic brain or pericardial tumor with intense vascularity, such as melanoma, renal, and so forth), it is reasonable to use LMWH as initial treatment for acute VTE and then to use either adjusted-dose UFH or LMWH to reduce the bleeding risk associated with long-term oral anticoagulant therapy. Alternatively, an inferior vena cava (IVC) filter can be placed electively in patients at high risk for bleeding to avoid the need for long-term anticoagulant therapy. Although it is not without complications (e.g., leg edema, recurrent or remote [visceral or cerebral] DVT), the overall rate of pulmonary embolism in this high-risk group in whom a filter is used is low (≈2%).[117]

Inferior Vena Cava Filters

Placement of an inferior vena cava filter should be reserved for patients who have active bleeding, those at high risk for bleeding, and those who develop recurrent VTE despite adequate anticoagulation therapy (defined by appropriate laboratory test results) (see Chapter 31). If a filter is inserted concurrently with administration of anticoagulant therapy, the risk of pulmonary embolism is reduced initially. However, in the absence of concurrent anticoagulant therapy, a very high percentage of patients develop venous hypertension after filter placement and are far more likely to develop recurrent DVT over the long term (see Chapter 31); the protective effects of IVC filters are much diminished beyond the short term (e.g., 2 to 6 weeks). The recent availability of removable IVC filters makes it possible to use these filters for at least 2 to 6 weeks.[118,119] Indeed, early results of small, observational studies, most of which have included a significant percentage of patients with cancer, are encouraging in that removal may be possible after up to 6 months or even longer.[120–122] However, the absence of randomized, controlled trials or even rigorous, prospective cohort studies makes it difficult to adequately assess the cost/benefit ratio of these new devices. Cautious optimism is warranted, but better studies are needed and long-term follow-up is essential.

Central Vein Thrombosis

As was noted previously in the section on prevention, central vein catheters, which are used commonly in patients with cancer, particularly for the administration of chemotherapy and the provision of long-term supportive care (e.g., antibiotics, blood products, growth factors), present a particular problem for the oncologist. Although the rate of thrombosis has been reduced presumably by improved biocompatibility of the catheters and enhanced local care, thrombosis still occurs with sufficient frequency to represent an impediment to good care. Catheter-related thrombi may involve the tip of the catheter alone or the length of the catheter (i.e., with formation of a "fibrin sheath"), or they may extend to involve the veins of the upper limbs, neck, and mediastinum.[122] The usual treatment for catheter tip thrombosis is low-dose thrombolytic therapy with streptokinase, urokinase, or tPA.[123] Recommended treatment of patients with symptomatic upper limb vein thrombosis related to use of a catheter is full-dose anticoagulant therapy with heparin (UFH or LMWH given initially) followed by oral anticoagulant therapy. Available data are insufficient to reveal whether thrombolytic therapy and/or catheter removal should be used in the setting of catheter-associated upper limb thrombosis, in which full-dose anticoagulant therapy is used. At present, considerable variation in common practice has been noted; therefore, this issue needs to be resolved, if possible, through appropriately designed clinical trials.

ANTICOAGULATION THERAPY AND SURVIVAL IN CANCER

Since the publication in 1981 of the results of the first randomized trial of warfarin as an adjuvant to chemotherapy in patients with small cell carcinoma of the lung (SCCL),[124] an old theory that anticoagulation may enhance survival in cancer has been revitalized. In the Veterans Administration Cooperative Studies Program trial (CSP #75), patients with SCCL and no clinical evidence of VTE were treated with the same chemotherapy regimen but were randomly assigned to receive standard doses of warfarin or no anticoagulation therapy. Survival was twice as long in the warfarin group (50 weeks vs 24 weeks; $P = .03$); this could not be accounted for by protection against clinically apparent VTE or serious bleeding.[124] These results, which were replicated in a trial conducted by the Cancer and Leukemia Group B,[125] together with the results of a cancer subset analysis of several large, randomized clinical trials of LMWH versus UFH therapy in patients with acute proximal DVT,[126] have stimulated a renewed interest in the potential anticancer effects of antithrombotic agents.

In the trial reported by Hull and colleagues,[127] the overall mortality rate for patients with cancer was 9.6% in hospitalized patients receiving standard UFH compared with 4.7% in patients treated with LMWH ($P = .05$). In a trial reported by Prandoni and colleagues,[128] the overall mortality rate for patients with cancer in the UFH-treated group was 12% compared with 7% among LMWH-treated patients (not statistically significant). In 1995, Lensing and coworkers[129] conducted a meta-analysis of trials of LMWH versus standard UFH for the treatment of patients with DVT. The overall mortality rate was 3.9% for patients treated with LMWH versus 7.1% for those treated with standard UH—a relative risk reduction of 47% ($P < .04$). In 195 patients with cancer in the studies subjected to meta-analysis, mortality risk reduction was 64% in favor of LMWH ($P < .01$). Two more recent meta-analyses have confirmed these findings.[130,131] These findings suggest that LMWH might exert an inhibitory

effect on tumor growth that is superior to that observed with standard UFH, although it remains difficult to explain how short-term therapy (e.g., 7 days) with LMWH can influence the natural history of a malignant tumor that has existed for many months.

Several clinical trials evaluating longer-term administration of LMWH to patients with cancer with and without VTE have recently been completed (e.g., FAMOUS [Fragmin for Advanced Malignancy Outcome Study], CLOT, MALT [Malignancy And Low molecular weight Treatment trial]) and have provided additional support for the antineoplastic properties of LMWH. In the CLOT study,[132] for example, 12-month cumulative mortality was 20% and 35% for patients with cancer without metastasis at the time of presentation with VTE, who received LMWH or warfarin, respectively (hazard ratio, 0.50; 95% CI, 0.27 to 0.95; $P = .03$; Fig. 23-4). However, both the CLOT study and the FAMOUS trial[133] demonstrated through post hoc analyses survival advantages for patients with limited-stage disease. In view of the limitations of post hoc subgroup analysis, both reports must be viewed principally as hypothesis-generating studies. However, two additional studies provided prospective data that are supportive. Altinbas and colleagues[134] recently published the results of LMWH therapy (18 weeks) as an adjunct to chemotherapy in patients with small cell lung cancer without VTE, and Klerk and associates (the MALT trial)[135] treated patients with a variety of advanced cancers (also without VTE) with LMWH or placebo for 6 weeks. Both studies showed statistically significant survival advantages for LMWH-treated patients, regardless of initial stage of disease. Additional studies are needed to confirm these encouraging results. However, evidence is accumulating that supports adoption of the routine clinical practice of recommending lifelong anticoagulation for patients with active cancer and VTE disease.

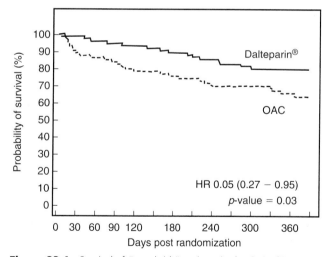

Figure 23-4 Survival of "good-risk" patients in the CLOT (Comparison of Low molecular weight heparin versus Oral anticoagulant Therapy for prevention of recurrent venous thromboembolism in patients with cancer) Study. Post hoc analysis of patients with cancer with no evidence of distant metastasis at the time of presentation treated with oral anticoagulants (OAC) or low molecular weight heparin (dalteparin) for a concurrent venous thromboembolic event. (From Lee AY, Rickles FR, Julian J, et al, for the CLOT Investigators: Impact of dalteparin low-molecular-weight heparin (LMWH) on survival: Results of a randomized trial in cancer patients with venous thromboembolism (VTE). J Clin Oncol 23:2123–2129, 2005, with permission.)

UPDATE ON ERYTHROPOIETIN THERAPY

One approach in managing anemia in cancer patients is to use recombinant human erythropoietin (EPO). There are several different erythropoietin stimulating agents (ESAs) which include epoetin alfa, darbopoetin alfa, and epoetin beta. Multiple trials in cancer patients have shown that treatment with ESAs increases hemoglobin levels and decreases the need for erythrocyte transfusions. It is unclear however, whether ESAs improve the quality of life of cancer patients. In recent years there has been considerable discussion about the thrombogenic potential of ESAs and whether they are associated with tumor growth.[136–138]

Three randomized trials in cancer patients reported an increased risk of thrombotic and cardiovascular events associated with ESAs and were prematurely stopped.[139] A recent meta-analysis conducted by the Cochrane Institute demonstrated a 1.67 increased risk of thrombosis associated with ESAs.[140] The etiology of thrombosis related to ESAs is unclear but likely to be multifactorial in cancer and other ill patients already prone to thrombosis.

The Food and Drug Administration (FDA) issued a recent public health advisory (March 9, 2007), describing "an increased risk of death, blood clots, strokes and heart attacks in patients with chronic renal failure when ESAs were administered at higher than recommended doses. In other studies, more rapid tumor growth occurred in patients with head and neck cancer who received these higher doses."[141] In the 1,400 subject CHOIR study of patients with CRF,[142] the composite end point of death and all cardiovascular events was significantly more frequent in the group with a target hemoglobin of 13.5 g/dL than in the group with a target hemoglobin of 11.3 g/dL ($p = 0.03$ by log rank test with a hazard ratio of 1.3; 95% CL 1.03–1.74). In the Danish Head and Neck Cancer Study Group trial (DAHANCA 10), the 3-year loco-regional control in patients treated with an ESA was significantly worse than for those not receiving the ESA ($p = 0.01$) and there was a non-significant trend toward worse overall survival.[143] The risk for deep vein thrombosis in elective spinal surgery patients randomized to receive an ESA preoperatively for hemoglobin values > 10 and ≤ 13 g/dL was 4.7%, more than twice that of patients who received usual blood conservation care (2.1%).[141] These FDA warnings support to "adjust the ESA dose to maintain the lowest hemoglobin level needed to avoid transfusions" . . . in those patients with appropriate indications (e.g., anemia of chronic renal failure, cancer with anemia caused by chemotherapy, major surgery to reduce potential blood transfusions and for anemia due to zidovudine therapy in HIV patients).

A second FDA Oncology Drug Advisory Committee meeting on the safety of erythropoietin was held in May 2007.[144] Concern was expressed regarding the safety of ESAs in terms of thromboembolism and tumor growth and the panel recommended more restrictions on labeling and more studies exploring safety. Meanwhile it seems prudent to be judicious in the use of ESAs in cancer patients (limiting it to those on chemotherapy) and in most if not all patients in general. The ESA-stimulated hemoglobin level should not exceed the recommended indication, currently 12 gms/dL.

SUMMARY AND CONCLUSIONS

Patients with idiopathic VTE are at higher risk for the development of cancer, and patients with cancer are at higher risk for the development of VTE. The risk of clinically important VTE after surgery is at least twofold greater in patients with cancer than in those without cancer, and the risk for recurrent VTE in patients with cancer is two- to threefold greater than in patients without cancer, in spite of therapeutic levels of oral anticoagulation. Patients with cancer are at high risk for VTE because they are often immobilized and exposed to prothrombotic challenges (e.g., chemotherapy, use of central venous catheters), and because they are intrinsically hypercoagulable. The hypercoagulable state in cancer is multifactorial, mediated by the potent direct procoagulant properties of tumor cells and the indirect procoagulant effects of tumor cells on the host immune response and the vascular endothelium. Angiogenic blood vessels are particularly susceptible to thrombosis because, in contrast to normal blood vessels, the VECs of tumor blood vessels express TF de novo. For all these reasons, primary prophylaxis is absolutely indicated for patients with cancer who are undergoing surgery, and it should be strongly considered for high-risk patients with central venous catheters and for those receiving chemotherapy—particularly in the treatment of those with mucin-secreting adenocarcinoma, brain tumor, and other high-risk malignancies. Secondary prophylaxis should be considered and should last as long as the cancer is active. LMWH has proven superior to oral anticoagulants for secondary prophylaxis of VTE in some patients with cancer, and it may contribute to increased survival through as yet undefined mechanisms.

REFERENCES

1. Dvorak H: Tumors: Wounds that do not heal. N Engl J Med 315:1650–1659, 1986.
2. Trousseau A: Phlegmasia alba dolens. In Clinique Medicale de l'Hotel Dieu de Paris.Paris, JB Balliere et Fils, 1865, pp 654–712.
3. Dvorak HB, Rickles FR: Malignancy and hemostasis. In Colman RW, Marder VJ, Clowes A, et al (eds): Hemostasis and Thrombosis, 5th ed. Philadelphia, Lippincott Williams & Wilkins, 2005, pp 851–876.
4. Levine M, Lee AYY, Kakkar AK: Cancer and thrombosis. In Colman RW, Marger VJ, Clowes A, et al (eds): Hemostasis and Thrombosis, 5th ed. Philadelphia, Lippincott Williams & Wilkins, 2005, pp 1251–1262.
5. Rickles FR, Levine MN: Epidemiology of thrombosis in cancer. Acta Haematol 106:6–12, 2001.
6. Monreal M, Fernandez-Llamazares J, Perandreu J, et al: Occult cancer in patients with venous thromboembolism: Which patients, which cancers? Thromb Haemost 78:1316–1318, 1997.
7. Sorensen HT, Mellemkjaer L, Steffensen FH, et al: The risk of a diagnosis of cancer after primary deep venous thrombosis or pulmonary embolism. N Engl J Med 338:1169–1173, 1998.
8. Baron JA, Gridley G, Weiderpass E, et al: Venous thromboembolism and cancer. Lancet 351:1077–1080, 1998.
9. Piccioli A, Lensing AWA, Prins MH, et al: Extensive screening for occult malignant disease in idiopathic venous thromboembolism: A prospective clinical trial. J Thromb Haemost 2:884–889, 2004.
10. Cornuz J, Pearson SD, Creager MA, et al: Importance of findings on the initial evaluation for cancer in patients with symptomatic idiopathic deep venous thrombosis. Ann Intern Med 125:785–793, 1996.
11. Barosi G, Marchetti M, Dazzi L, Quaglini S: Testing for occult cancer in patients with idiopathic deep vein thrombosis: A decision analysis. Thromb Haemost 78:1319–1326, 1997.
12. Silverstein MD, Heit JA, Mohr DN, et al: Trends in the incidence of deep vein thrombosis and pulmonary embolism: A 25-year population-based study. Arch Intern Med 158:585–593, 1998.

13. Heit JA, Silverstein MD, Mohr DN, et al: Predictors of survival after deep vein thrombosis and pulmonary embolism: A population-based, cohort study. Arch Intern Med 159:445–453, 1999.

14. Levitan N, Dowlati A, Remick SC, et al: Rates of initial and recurrent thromboembolic disease among patients with malignancy versus those without malignancy: Risk analysis using Medicare claims data. Medicine (Baltimore) 78:285–291, 1999.

15. Blom JW, Doggen CJM, Osanto S, Rosendaal FR: Malignancies, pro-thrombotic mutations, and the risk of venous thrombosis. JAMA 293:715–722, 2005.

16. Silver S: Cancer and clotting: Understanding the risks. The Hematologist 2:1–2, 2005.

17. Blom JW, Vanderschoot JPM, Oostindier MJ, et al: Incidence of venous thrombosis in a large cohort of 66,329 cancer patients: Results of a record linkage study. J Thromb Haemost 4:529–535, 2006.

18. Shen VS, Pollak EW: Fatal pulmonary embolism in cancer patients: Is heparin prophylaxis justified? South Med J 73:841–843, 1980.

19. Goodnough LT, Saito H, Manni A, et al: Increased incidence of thromboembolism in stage IV breast cancer patients treated with a five-drug chemotherapy regimen: A study of 159 patients. Cancer 54:1264–1268, 1984.

20. Levine MN, Gent M, Hirsh J, et al: The thrombogenic effect of anti-cancer drug therapy in women with stage II breast cancer. N Engl J Med 318:404–407, 1988.

21. Bonneterre J, Thurlimann B, Robertson JFR, et al: Anastrozole versus tamoxifen as first-line therapy for advanced breast cancer in 668 postmenopausal women: Results of the tamoxifen or arimidex randomized group efficacy and tolerability study. J Clin Oncol 22:3748–3757, 2000.

22. The ATAC Group: Anastrozole alone or in combination with tamoxifen versus tamoxifen alone for adjuvant treatment of postmenopausal women with early breast cancer: First results of the ATAC randomised trial. Lancet 359:2131–2139, 2002.

23. Marras LC, Geerts WH, Perry JR: The risk of venous thromboembolism is increased throughout the course of malignant glioma: An evidence-based review. Cancer 89:640–646, 2000.

24. Lavey RS, Liu PY, Greer BE, et al: Recombinant human erythropoietin as an adjunct to radiation therapy and cisplatin for Stage IIB-IVA carcinoma of the cervix: A Southwest Oncology Group study. Gynecol Oncol 95:145–151, 2004.

25. Rosenzweig MQ, Bender CM, Lucke JP, et al: The decision to prematurely terminate a trial of R-HuEPO due to thrombotic events. J Pain Symptom Manage 27:185–190, 2004.

26. Barbui T, Finazzi G, Grassi A, Marchioli R: Thrombosis in cancer patients treated with hematopoietic growth factors: A meta-analysis. Thromb Haemost 75:368–371, 1996.

27. Bleiberg H, Di Leo A, Rothenberg ML, et al: Mortality associated with irinotecan plus bolus fluorouracil/leucovorin. J Clin Oncol 20:1145–1146, 2002.

28. Rothenberg ML, Meropol NJ, Poplin EA, et al: Mortality associated with irinotecan plus bolus fluorouracil/leucovorin: Summary findings of an independent panel. J Clin Oncol 19:3801–3807, 2001.

29. Marx GM, Steer CB, Harper P, et al: Unexpected serious toxicity with chemotherapy and antiangiogenic combinations: Time to take stock! J Clin Oncol 20:1446–1448, 2002.

30. Zangari M, Anaissie E, Barlogie B, et al: Increased risk of deep-vein thrombosis in patients with multiple myeloma receiving thalidomide and chemotherapy. Blood 98:1614–1615, 2001.

31. Osman K, Comenzo R, Rajkumar SV: Deep venous thrombosis and thalidomide therapy for multiple myeloma. N Engl J Med 344:1951–1952, 2001.

32. Urbauer E, Kaufmann H, Nosslinger T, et al: Thromboembolic events during treatment with thalidomide. Blood 99:4247–4248, 2002.

33. Kuenen BC, Rosen L, Smit EF: Dose-finding and pharmacokinetic study of cisplatin, gemcitabine and SU5416 in patients with solid tumors. J Clin Oncol 20:1657–1667, 2002.

34. Cropp GF, Hannah AL: SU5416, a molecularly targeted novel antiangiogenic drug: Clinical pharmacokinetics and safety review. Clin Cancer Res 6:95, 2002.

35. Kabbinavar F, Hurwitz HI, Fehrenbacher L, et al: Phase II, randomized trial comparing bevacizumab plus fluorouracil (FU)/leucovorin (LV) with FU/LV alone in patients with metastatic colorectal cancer. J Clin Oncol 21:60–65, 2003.

36. Zangari M, Barlogie B, Anaissie E, et al: Deep vein thrombosis in patients with multiple myeloma treated with thalidomide and chemotherapy: Effects of prophylactic and therapeutic anticoagulation. Br J Cancer 126:715–721, 2004.

37. Hurwitz H, Fehrenbacher L, Novotny W, et al: Bevacizumab plus irinotecan, fluorouracil, and leucovorin for metastatic colorectal cancer. N Engl J Med 350:2335–2342, 2004.

38. Ma L, Francia G, Viloria-Petit A, et al: In vitro procoagulant activity induced in endothelial cells by chemotherapy and antiangiogenic drug combinations: Modulation by lower dose chemotherapy. Cancer Res 65:5365–5373, 2005.

39. Miller KD, Chap LI, Holmes FA, et al: Randomized phase III trial of capecitabine compared with bevacizumab plus capecitabine in patients with previously treated metastatic breast cancer. J Clin Oncol 23:792–799, 2005.

40. Miller KD, Wang M, Galow J, et al: E2100: A randomized phase III trial of paclitaxel versus paclitaxel plus bevacizumab as first-line therapy for locally recurrent or metastatic breast cancer. Presented at: 41st Annual Meeting of the American Society of Clinical Oncology; May 13–17 2005; Orlando, Fla. Available at:http://www.asco.org/ac/1,_12-003046.00asp. Accessed January 19, 2006.

41. Johnson MJ, Sproule MW, Paul J: The prevalence and associated variables of deep venous thrombosis in patients with advanced cancer. Clin Oncol 11:105–110, 1999.

42. Barlogie B, Desikan R, Eddlemon P, et al: Extended survival in advanced and refractory multiple myeloma after single-agent thalidomide: Identification of prognostic factors in a phase 2 study of 169 patients. Blood 98:492–494, 2001.

43. Rajkumar SV, Hayman S, Gertz MA, et al: Combination therapy with thalidomide plus dexamethasone for newly diagnosed myeloma. J Clin Oncol 20:4319–4323, 2002.

44. Rajkumar SV, Blood E, Vesole D, et al: Phase III clinical trial of thalidomide plus dexamethasone compared with dexamethasone alone in newly diagnosed multiple myeloma: A clinical trial coordinated by the Eastern Cooperative Oncology Group. J Clin Oncol 24: 431–436, 2006.

45. Palladini G, Perfetti V, Perlini S, et al: The combination of thalidomide and intermediate-dose dexamethasone is an effective but toxic treatment for patients with primary amyloidosis (AL). Blood 105:2949–2951, 2005.

46. Barlogie B, Tricot G, Anaissie E, et al: Thalidomide and hematopoietic-cell transplantation for multiple myeloma. N Engl J Med 354:1021–1030, 2006.

47. Bern MM, Lokich JJ, Wallach SR, et al: Very low doses of warfarin can prevent thrombosis in central vein catheters: A randomized prospective trial. Ann Intern Med 112:423–428, 1990.

48. Monreal M, Alastrue A, Rull M, et al: Upper extremity deep vein thrombosis in cancer patients with venous access devices: Prophylaxis with a low molecular weight heparin (fragmin). Thromb Haemost 75:251–253, 1996.

49. Sorensen HT, Mellemkjaer L, Olsen JH, Baron JA: Prognosis of cancers associated with venous thromboembolism. N Engl J Med 343:1846–1850, 2000.

50. Kakkar VV, Howe CT, Nicolaides AN, et al: Deep vein thrombosis of the leg: Is there a high risk group? Am J Surg 120:527–531, 1970.

51. Claggett GP, Reisch JS: Prevention of venous thromboembolism in general surgical patients. Ann Surg 208:227–240, 1988.

52. Levine MN: Cancer patients. In Goldhaber S (ed): Prevention of Venous Thromboembolism, New York, Marcel Dekker, 1993, pp 463–483.

53. Geerts WH, Pineo GF, Heit JA, et al: Prevention of venous thromboembolism: The Seventh ACCP Conference on Antithrombotic and Thrombolytic Therapy. Chest 126:338S–400S, 2004.

54. Sack GH, Levin J, Bell WR: Trousseau's syndrome and other manifestations of chronic disseminated coagulopathy in patients with neoplasms. Medicine 56:1–37, 1977.

55. Lieberman JS, Borrero J, Urdoncta E, Wright IS: Thrombophlebitis and cancer. JAMA 177:542–545, 1961.

56. Rickles FR, Edwards RL: Activation of blood coagulation in cancer: Trousseau's syndrome revisited. Blood 62:14–31, 1983.

57. Levine M, Gent M, Hirsh J, et al: A comparison of low molecular weight heparin administered primarily at home with unfractionated heparin administered in the hospital for proximal deep vein thrombosis. N Engl J Med 334:677–681, 1996.

58. Virchow R: Gesammelte Abhaldungen zur Wissensdiafflichem Medicine. Frankfurt Meidinger Sohn, 1856.

59. Edwards RL, Klaus M, Matthews E, et al: Heparin abolishes the chemotherapy-induced increase in plasma fibrinopeptide A levels. Am J Med 89:25–28, 1990.

60. Rickles FR, Falanga A: Molecular basis for the relationship between thrombosis and cancer. Thromb Res 102:V215–V224, 2001.

(Updated:Falanga A, Rickles FR: The pathogenesis of venous thromboembolism in cancer. N Oncol Thrombosis 1:9–16, 2005.)

61. Shoji M, Hancock WW, Abe K, et al: Activation of coagulation and angiogenesis in cancer: Immunohistochemical localization in situ of clotting proteins and VEGF in human cancers. Am J Pathol 152:399–411, 1998.

62. Shoji M, Abe K, Nawroth PP, Rickles FR: Molecular mechanisms linking thrombosis and angiogenesis in cancer. Trends Cardiovasc Med 7:52–59, 1997.

63. Rickles FR, Shoji M, Abe K: The role of the hemostatic system in tumor growth, metastasis and angiogenesis: Tissue factor is a bifunctional molecule capable of inducing both fibrin deposition and angiogenesis in cancer. Int J Hematol 73:145–150, 2001.

64. Abe K, Shoji M, Chen J, et al: Regulation of vascular endothelial growth factor production and angiogenesis by the cytoplasmic tail of tissue factor. Proc Nat Acad Sci U S A 96:8663–8668, 1999.

65. Zhang Y, Deng Y, Werndt T, et al: Intravenous somatic gene transfer with antisense tissue factor restores blood flow by reducing tumor necrosis factor–induced tissue factor expression and fibrin deposition in mouse meth A sarcomas. J Clin Invest 97:2213–2224, 1996.

66. Huang X, Molema G, King S, et al: Tumor infarction in mice by antibody-directed targeting of tissue factor to tumor vasculature. Science 275:547–555, 1997.

67. Hu Z, Sun Y, Garen A: Targeting tumor vasculature endothelial cells and tumor cells for immunotherapy of human melanoma in a mouse xenograft model. Proc Nat Acad Sci U S A 96:8161–8166, 1999.

68. Thorpe PE, Chaplin DJ, Blakey DC: The First International Conference on vascular targeting agents. Cancer Res 63:1144–1147, 2003.

69. Boccaccio C, Sabatino G, Medico E, et al: The *Met* oncogene drives a genetic programme linking cancer to haemostasis. Nature 434:396–400, 2005.

70. Rong Y, Post DE, Pieper RO, et al: PTEN and hypoxia regulate tissue factor expression and plasma coagulation in glioblastoma. Cancer Res 65:1406–1413, 2005.

71. Yu JL, May L, Lhotak V, et al: Oncogenic events regulate tissue factor expression in colorectal cancer cells: Implications for tumor progression and angiogenesis. Blood 105:1734–1741, 2005.

72. Rickles FR, Patierno SR, Fernandez P: Tissue factor, thrombin and cancer. Chest 124:58S–68S, 2003.

73. Fernandez P, Patierno SR, Rickles FR: Tissue factor and fibrin in tumor angiogenesis. Semin Thromb Haemost 30:31–44, 2004.

74. Collins R, Scrimgeour A, Yusuf S, Peto R: Reduction in fatal pulmonary embolism and venous thrombosis by perioperative administration of subcutaneous heparin. N Engl J Med 318:1162–1173, 1988.

75. Weitz JI: Drug therapy: Low-molecular weight heparins. N Engl J Med 337:688–698, 1997.

76. Hirsh J, Levine MN: Low molecular weight heparin. Blood 79:1–17, 1992.

77. Nurmohamed MT, Rosendaal FR, Buller HR, et al: Low molecular weight heparin versus standard heparin in general and orthopedic surgery: A meta-analysis. Lancet 340:152–155, 1992.

78. Ginsberg JS: Management of venous thromboembolism. N Engl J Med 335:1816–1824, 1996.

79. Mismetti P, Laporte S, Darmon JY, et al: Meta-analysis of low molecular weight heparin in the prevention of venous thromboembolism in general surgery. Br J Surg 88:913–930, 2001.

80. Bergqvist D, Agnelli G, Cohen AT, et al, for the ENOXACAN II investigators: Duration of prophylaxis against venous thromboembolism with enoxaparin after surgery for cancer. N Engl J Med 346:975–980, 2002.

81. Rasmussen MS, Jorgensen LN, Wille-Jorgensen P, et al: Prolonged prophylaxis with dalteparin to prevent late thromboembolic complications in patients undergoing major abdominal surgery: A multicenter randomized open-label study. J Thromb Haemost 4:2384–2390, 2006.

82. Levine M, Hirsh J, Gent M, et al: Double blind trial of very low dose warfarin for prevention of thromboembolism in stage IV breast cancer. Lancet 343:886–889, 1994.

83. Rajan R, Gafni A, Levine M, et al: Very low dose warfarin prophylaxis to prevent thromboembolism in women with metastatic breast cancer receiving chemotherapy: An economic evaluation. J Clin Oncol 13:42–46, 1995.

84. Geerts WH, Heit JA, Clagett GP, et al: Prevention of venous thromboembolism. Chest 119:132S–175S, 2001.

85. Samama MM, Cohen AT, Darmon JY, et al: A comparison of enoxaparin with placebo for the prevention of venous thromboembolism in acutely ill medical patients: Prophylaxis in Medical Patients with Enoxaparin Study Group. N Engl J Med 341:793–800, 1999.

86. Masci G, Magagnoli M, Zucali PA, et al: Minidose warfarin prophylaxis for catheter-associated thrombosis in cancer patients: Can it be safely associated with fluorouracil-based chemotherapy? J Clin Oncol 21:736–739, 2003.

87. Reichardt P, Kretzschmar A, Biakhov M, Irwin D: A phase III double-blind, placebo-controlled study evaluating the efficacy and safety of daily low-molecular-weight heparin (dalteparin sodium, fragmin) in preventing catheter-related complications in cancer patients with central venous catheters. Proc Am Soc Clin Oncol 21:1474, 2002. Abstract.

88. Couban S, Goodyear M, Burnell M, et al: Randomized placebo-controlled study of low dose warfarin for the prevention of central venous catheter–associated thrombosis in patient with cancer. J Clin Oncol 23:4063–4069, 2005.

89. Verso M, Agnelli G, Bertoglio S, et al: Enoxaparin for the prevention of venous thromboembolism associated with central vein catheter: A double-blind, placebo-controlled, randomized study in cancer patients. J Clin Oncol 23:4057–4062, 2005.

90. Young AM, Begum G, Billingham AI, et al: WARP: A multicentre prospective randomized controlled trial (RCT) of thrombosis prophylaxis with warfarin in cancer patients with central venous catheters (CVCs). Proc Am Soc Clin Oncol 24:8004, 2005. Abstract.

91. Walshe LJ, Malak SF, Eagan J, Sepkowitz KA: Complication rates among cancer patients with peripherally inserted central catheters. J Clin Oncol 20:3276–3281, 2002.

92. Prandoni P: Antithrombotic strategies in patients with cancer. Thromb Haemost 78:141–144, 1997.

93. Prandoni P, Lensing AW, Piccioli A, et al: Recurrent venous thromboembolism and bleeding complications during anticoagulant treatment in patients with cancer and venous thrombosis. Blood 100:3484–3488, 2002.

94. Levine M, Gent M, Hirsh J, et al: A comparison of low molecular weight heparin administered primarily at home with unfractionated heparin administered in the hospital for proximal deep vein thrombosis. N Engl J Med 334:677–681, 1996.

95. The Columbus Investigators: Low molecular weight heparin in the treatment of patients with venous thromboembolism. N Engl J Med 337:657–662, 1997.

96. Lee AYY, Levine MN, Baker R, et al, for the CLOT Investigators: Low-molecular-weight heparin versus a coumarin for the prevention of recurrent venous thromboembolism in patients with cancer. N Engl J Med 349:146–153, 2003.

97. Koopman MMW, Prandoni P, Piovella F, et al: Treatment of venous thrombosis with intravenous unfractionated heparin administered in the hospital as compared with subcutaneous low molecular weight heparin administered at home. N Engl J Med 334:682–687, 1996.

98. Harrison L, Mcginnis J, Crowther M, et al: Assessment of outpatient treatment of deep vein thrombosis with low molecular weight heparin. Arch Intern Med 158:2001–2003, 1998.

99. Wells P, Kovacs MJ, Bormanis J, et al: Expanding eligibility for outpatient treatment of deep vein thrombosis and pulmonary embolism with low molecular weight heparin. Arch Intern Med 158:1809–1812, 1998.

100. Levine MN, Raskob GE, Bleyth RJ, et al: Hemorrhagic complications of anticoagulant treatment: The Seventh ACCP Conference on Antithrombotic and Thrombolytic Therapy. Chest 126:287S–310S, 2004.

101. Bona RD, Sivjee KY, Hickey AD, et al: The efficacy and safety of oral anticoagulation in patients with cancer. Thromb Haemost 74:1055–1058, 1995.

102. Schulman S, Rhedin AS, Lindmarker P: A comparison of six weeks with six months of oral anticoagulant therapy after a first episode of venous thromboembolism. N Engl J Med 332:1661–1665, 1995.

103. Schulman S, Granqvist S, Holmstrom M, et al, for the Duration of Anticoagulation Trial Study Group: The duration of oral anticoagulant therapy after a second episode of venous thromboembolism. N Engl J Med 336:393–398, 1997.

104. Kearon C, Gent M, Hirsh J, et al: A comparison of three months of anticoagulation with extended anticoagulation for a first episode of idiopathic venous thromboembolism. N Engl J Med 340:901–907, 1999.

105. Kearon C, Ginsberg JS, Kovacs MJ, et al, for the ELATE Investigators: Comparison of low-intensity warfarin therapy with conventional-intensity warfarin therapy for long-term prevention of recurrent venous thromboembolism. N Engl J Med 349:631–639, 2003.

106. Ridker PM, Goldhaber SZ, Danielson E, et al: Long-term, low-intensity warfarin therapy for the prevention of recurrent venous thromboembolism. N Engl J Med 348:1425–1434, 2003.

107. Luk C, Wells PS, Anderson D, Kovacs MJ: Extended outpatient therapy with low molecular weight heparin for the treatment of recurrent

III

venous thromboembolism despite warfarin therapy. Am J Med 111:270–273, 2001.

108. Pini M, Aiello S, Manotti C, et al: Low molecular weight heparin versus warfarin in the prevention of recurrences after deep vein thrombosis. Thromb Haemost 72:191–197, 1994.

109. Das SK, Cohen AT, Edmondson RA, et al: Low-molecular-weight heparin versus warfarin for prevention of recurrent venous thromboembolism: A randomized trial. World J Surg 20:521–526, 1996.

110. Lopaciuk S, Bielska-Falda H, Noszczyk W, et al: Low molecular weight heparin versus acenocoumarol in the secondary prophylaxis of deep vein thrombosis. Thromb Haemost 81:26–31, 1999.

111. Gonzalez-Fajardo JA, Arreba E, Castrodeza J, et al: Venographic comparison of subcutaneous low-molecular weight heparin with oral anticoagulant therapy in the long-term treatment of deep venous thrombosis. J Vasc Surg 30:283–292, 1999.

112. Veiga F, Escriba A, Maluenda MP, et al: Low molecular weight heparin (enoxaparin) versus oral anticoagulant therapy (acenocoumarol) in the long-term treatment of deep venous thrombosis in the elderly: A randomized trial. Thromb Haemost 84:559–564, 2000.

113. Hull RD, Pineo GF, Brant RF, et al: Long-term low-molecular-weight heparin versus usual care in proximal-vein thrombosis patients with cancer. Am J Med 119:1062–1072, 2006.

114. Lorio A, Guercini F, Pini M: Low molecular weight heparin for the long-term treatment of symptomatic venous thromboembolism: Meta-analysis of the randomized comparisons with oral anticoagulants. J Thromb Haemost 1:1906–1913, 2003.

115. Meyer G, Marjanovic Z, Valcke J, Lorcerie B: Comparison of low-molecular-weight heparin and warfarin for the secondary prevention of venous thromboembolism in patients with cancer. Arch Intern Med 162:1729–1735, 2002.

116. Buller HR, Agnelli G, Hull RD, et al: Antithrombotic therapy for venous thromboembolic disease: The Seventh ACCP Conference on Antithrombotic and Thrombolytic Therapy. Chest Suppl 126:401S–428S, 2004.

117. Schwarz RE, Marrero AM, Conlon KC, Burt M: Inferior vena cava filters in cancer patients: Indication and outcome. J Clin Oncol 14:652–657, 1996.

118. Decousus H, Leizorovicz A, Parent F, et al: A clinical trial of vena caval filters in the prevention of pulmonary emboblism in patients with proximal deep-vein thrombosis. Prevention du Risque d'Emblie Pulmonaire par Interruption Cave Study Group. N Engl J Med 338:409–415, 1998.

119. Milward SF, Oliva VL, Bell SD, et al: Gunther-Tulip retrievable vena cava filter: Results from the registry of the Canadian Interventional Radiology Association. J Invest Radiol 12:1053–1058, 2001.

120. Pieri S, Agresti M, Morucci M, De'Medici L: Optional vena cava filters: Preliminary experience with a new vena cava filter. Radiol Med 105:56–62, 2003.

121. Imberti D, Bianchi M, Farina A, et al: Clinical experience with retrievable vena cava filters: Results of a prospective observational multicenter study. J Thromb Haemost 3:1370–1375, 2005.

122. Hull RD: Changes in the technology of inferior vena cava filters promise improved benefits to the patient with less harm, but a paucity of evidence exists. J Thromb Haemost 3:1368–1369, 2005.

123. Bona RD: Thrombotic complications of central venous catheters in cancer patients. Semin Thromb Hemost 25:147–157, 1999.

124. Zacharski LR, Henderson WG, Rickles FR, et al: Effect of sodium warfarin on survival in small cell carcinoma of the lung: VA Cooperative Study #75. JAMA 245:831–835, 1981.

125. Chahinian AP, Propert KJ, Ware JH, et al: A randomized trial of anticoagulation with warfarin and alternating chemotherapy in extensive small cell lung cancer by the Cancer and Leukemia Group B. J Clin Oncol 7:993–1002, 1989.

126. Green D, Hull RD, Brant R, Pineo GF: Lower mortality in cancer patients treated with low molecular weight versus standard heparin. Lancet 339:1476, 1992. Letter.

127. Hull RD, Raskob GL, Pineo GF: Subcutaneous low molecular weight heparin compared with continuous intravenous heparin in the treatment of proximal vein thrombosis. N Engl J Med 326:975–982, 1992.

128. Prandoni P, Lensing AWA, Buller HR: Comparison of subcutaneous low molecular weight heparin with intravenous standard heparin in proximal deep vein thrombosis. Lancet 339:441–445, 1992.

129. Lensing AW, Prins MH, Davidson BL, Hirsh J: Treatment of deep venous thrombosis with low molecular weight heparins: A meta-analysis. Arch Intern Med 155:601–607, 1995.

130. Siragussa S, Cosmi B, Piovella F, et al: Low molecular weight heparins and unfractionated heparin in the treatment of patients with acute venous thromboembolism: Results of a meta-analysis. Am J Med 100:269–277, 1996.

131. Hettiaranchchi RJK, Prins MH, Buller HR, Prandoni P: Undiagnosed malignancy in patients with deep-vein thrombosis: Incidence, risk indicators, and diagnosis. Cancer 83:180–185, 1998.

132. Lee AY, Rickles FR, Julian J, et al, for the CLOT Investigators: Impact of dalteparin low-molecular-weight heparin (LMWH) on survival: Results of a randomized trial in cancer patients with venous thromboembolism (VTE). J Clin Oncol 23:2123–2129, 2005.

133. Kakkar AK, Levine MN, Kadziola Z, et al: Low molecular weight heparin, therapy with daleparin, and survival in advanced cancer: The Fragmin Advanced Malignancy Outcome Study (FAMOUS). J Clin Oncol 22:1944–1948, 2004.

134. Altinbas M, Coskun HS, Er O, et al: A randomized clinical trial of combination chemotherapy with and without low-molecular-weight heparin in small cell lung cancer. J Thromb Haemost 2:1266–1271, 2004.

135. Klerk CPW, Smorenburg SM, Otten JM MB, et al: The effect of low molecular weight heparin on survival in patients with advanced malignancy. J Clin Oncol 23:2130–2135, 2005.

136. Leyland-Jones B, Semiglazov V, Pawlicki M, et al: Maintaining normal hemoglobin levels with epoetin alfa in mainly nonanemic patients with metastatic breast cancer receiving first-line chemotherapy: A survival study. J Clin Oncol 23:5960–5972, 2005.

137. Henke M, Laszig R, Rübe C, et al: Erythropoietin to treat head and neck cancer patients with anaemia undergoing radiotherapy: Randomised, double-blind, placebo-controlled trial. The Lancet 362:1255–1260, 2003.

138. Wright J, Ung Y, Julian JA, et al: Randomized, double-blind, placebo-controlled trial of erythropoietin in non-small-cell lung cancer with disease-related anemia. J Clin Oncol 25:1027–1032, 2007.

139. Luksenburg H, Weir A, Wager R: FDA Briefing Document for May 4, 2004 ODAC meeting (http://www.fda.gov/ohrms/dockets/ac/cder04.html#Oncologic).

140. Bohlius J, Wilson J, Seidenfeld J, et al: Erythropoietin or darbepoetin for patients with cancer (review). The Cochrane Library 2007, Issue 2.

141. FDA News. FDA Strengthens Safety Information for Erythropoiesis-Stimulating Agents (ESAs). http://www.fda.gov/bbs/topics/NEWS/2007/NEW01582.html. Accessed March 23, 2007.

142. Singh AK, Szczech L, Tang KL, et al, for the CHOIR Investigators: Correction of anemia with Epoetin Alfa in chronic kidney disease. N Engl J Med 355:2085–2098, 2006.

143. Overgaard J: Interim analysis of DAHANCA 10. Study of the importance of Novel Erythropoiesis Stimulating Protein (Aranasep®) for the effect of radiotherapy with primary squamous cell carcinoma of the head and neck. http://conman.au.dk/dahanca. December 1, 2006. Accessed March 23, 2007.

144. FDA Briefing Document for May 10, 2007 ODAC meeting (http://www.fda.gov/ohrms/dockets/ac/07/briefing/2007-4301b2-00-index.htm).

Chapter 24

Thrombotic Thrombocytopenic Purpura

Joel L. Moake, MD

INTRODUCTION

Thrombotic thrombocytopenic purpura (TTP) is the most extensive and dangerous intravascular platelet clumping disorder. For about 55 years after the disease was first recognized, almost everyone with TTP died quickly. Physicians were fascinated by the dramatic clinical presentations and were horrified by the near 100% mortality rate. Many hematologists, even those with limited experience in trying to manage this rarely encountered patient, believed intuitively that an understanding of the mechanism of systemic intravascular platelet aggregation in TTP would provide important insights into the pathophysiology of common, localized forms of arterial platelet thrombosis (e.g., heart attack, stroke).

Until the 1970s and 1980s, most physicians had never seen a case of TTP. Hematologists, even after years in practice, could recall one or two patients, at most, who had been given this diagnosis. Then, for unknown reasons, the disease increased in prevalence. Probably about 2000 new cases of acute acquired idiopathic TTP now occur annually in North America. At the Texas Medical Center in Houston, about 30 to 50 patients newly diagnosed with TTP are admitted each year (compared with 0 to 2 per year in the 1970s). This is likely to represent a true increase in acute acquired idiopathic TTP, and not simply improvement in recognition of a disorder with long-established clinical and laboratory characteristics. Furthermore, several drugs in common use during the 1990s (e.g., ticlopidine) were found to induce, in a fraction of the many exposed patients, a type of TTP that is clinically indistinguishable from the acute acquired idiopathic type. Therefore, the remark several years ago in reference to paroxysmal nocturnal hemoglobinuria made by Dr. Wendell Rosse of the Duke University Medical Center that "more people study the disease than have it" no longer applies to TTP.

HISTORICAL REVIEW

Eli Moschcowitz was born in Hungary in 1879 and was brought to the United States at the age of 2 years. He received his doctor of medicine degree from the College of Physicians and Surgeons of Columbia University in 1900 and was subsequently trained in surgery and histopathology in New York City and Berlin.[1] On September 15, 1923, Dr. Moschcowitz admitted "Patient KZ," a 16-year-old girl, to the Beth Israel Hospital in New York City. She had experienced abrupt onset of petechiae, anemia, and pallor; these

were followed rapidly by paralysis, coma, and, on September 20, 1923, death. Moschcowitz believed that he had observed a new disease and reported the tragic course of his young patient in 1924 in the *Proceedings of the New York Pathological Society*.[2] Terminal arterioles and capillaries in the unlucky teenager were occluded by hyaline thrombi, later determined to be composed mostly of platelets, without perivascular inflammation or endothelial desquamation. Moschcowitz suspected a "powerful poison which had both agglutinative and hemolytic properties"[2,3] as the cause of this frightening new disease, now known as thrombotic thrombocytopenic purpura (TTP).

Before researchers had any inkling of the pathophysiology of TTP, Byrnes and Khurana[4] reported in 1977 that relapses in chronic TTP could be prevented or reversed by the infusion of only a few units of fresh frozen plasma (FFP) or its cryoprecipitate-poor fraction (cryosupernatant) without concurrent plasmapheresis. It was also discovered by Byrnes and Khurana[4] and Bukowski and colleagues[5] (and subsequently confirmed by studies in several hundred patients[6,7]) that plasma infusion combined with plasmapheresis (plasma exchange) allows most patients to survive an episode of TTP. In most of these patients, the disorder neither recurs nor produces persistent overt organ damage.[6]

In 1982, "unusually large" von Willebrand factor (VWF) multimers found in the plasma of patients with the rarest subtype of the disorder, chronic relapsing TTP, were proposed by Moake and coworkers[8] as the agglutinative substance. Unusually large VWF multimers are: (1) more immense and more adhesive to platelets than the largest VWF multimeric species normally circulating in plasma[9]; (2) secreted in long strings by human endothelial cells[10]; (3) designed to entangle (after retrograde secretion by endothelial cells) with subendothelial fibrous components, to maximize VWF-mediated platelet adhesion onto subendothelium exposed by vascular damage; and (4) eliminated rapidly through a vigilant processing activity[8,11] that occurs in normal plasma. The 1982 report concluded that "patients with chronic relapsing TTP have a defect in the processing of very large VIII:VWF multimers [as the VWF component of the factor VIII was then known] after synthesis and secretion by endothelial cells, and . . . this defect makes patients susceptible to periodic relapses."[8]

In 1997 and 1998, Furlan and associates[12–14] and Tsai and Lian[15] reported that the "VWF processing activity" is a VWF-cleaving metalloprotease enzyme that is absent in patients with familial TTP and is transiently inhibited in many patients with acquired idiopathic TTP. This VWF-cleaving metalloprotease was soon thereafter characterized as a member of a large array of structurally related enzymes known as the "ADAMTS" family (defined later).[16–18]

CLINICAL MANIFESTATIONS

Severe thrombocytopenia and hemolytic anemia with one or several fragmented red cells (schistocytes) in many 1000-power, immersion oil fields of the blood smear (i.e., >1% of total red cells),[19] along with neurologic symptoms and signs, constitute the characteristic clinical triad. Neurologic disorders may range in severity from transient bizarre mentation and, behavior to sensorimotor deficits, aphasia, seizures, or coma. The peripheral blood smear typically shows increased reticulocytes (polychromatic large erythrocytes) and, often, nucleated red blood cells, in response to intense hemolysis. Fever and/or renal dysfunction occurs in a minority of patients. Renal abnormalities may include proteinuria and hematuria, as well as azotemia. Symptoms and signs of ischemia in the retinal (visual defects), coronary (conduction abnormalities), and abdominal circulation (abdominal pain) may be noted. Microvascular occlusions that cause ischemia of the sinoatrial or atrioventricular node, or of the bundle of His or the Purkinje conduction system, may cause sudden death.[20–22] Abdominal manifestations, sometimes resembling pancreatitis, have been more commonly recognized during the past few years. Perhaps 5% to 10% of TTP episodes may now begin with abdominal symptoms.[23]

Early, evolving, and overt manifestations of an acute acquired idiopathic TTP episode and of the therapeutic actions triggered are summarized in Table 24-1. A patient may appear in the emergency department or the physician's office at any stage of the disorder.

LABORATORY FINDINGS

The degree of thrombocytopenia in TTP reflects the extent of intravascular platelet clumping. Platelet counts are often less than 20,000 per microliter during acute episodes of TTP. Erythrocyte fragmentation occurs as red blood cells attempt to bypass at high flow rates microvascular platelet aggregates, producing characteristic schistocytes on peripheral blood films (Fig. 24-1). Occasionally, schistocytes do not appear until one or several days after the initial clinical presentation. Hemolysis is predominantly intravascular and, along with tissue damage, contributes to increased serum levels of lactate dehydrogenase (LDH).[23] Thrombo-

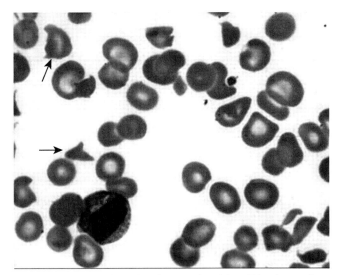

Figure 24-1 (*See also Color Plate 24-1.*) Peripheral blood smear from a patient with TTP. Notice that several red blood cells are schistocytes, which result from mechanical hemolysis. Some resemble apples from which a large bite has been taken.

cytopenia, hemolytic anemia, schistocytosis, and LDH elevations are often less extreme in diarrhea-associated acute renal failure of the hemolytic-uremic syndrome (HUS) than in TTP.

Coagulation studies are characteristically normal during the early stages of a TTP episode.[23] If considerable tissue necrosis occurs, however (as during an especially severe or protracted episode of TTP), secondary disseminated intravascular coagulation (DIC) may also occur as a result of overactivation of the coagulation pathway. This overactivation follows the binding of factor VIIa to exposed tissue factor on injured tissue cells. The ominous development of secondary DIC can be detected by the appearance of elevated levels of D-dimers or fibrin degradation products, prolongation of prothrombin or partial thromboplastin time, and decreased fibrinogen levels.

TYPES OF THROMBOTIC THROMBOCYTOPENIC PURPURA

Since plasma therapy has been generally applied, many patients have survived episodes of TTP. It has become apparent that several conditions are associated with the disorder, which may have more than one cause (Table 24-2).[23] About two thirds of adult patients with the relatively

---

Table 24-1 Real-Time Considerations in Thrombotic Thrombocytopenic Purpura

	Early	Evolving	Overt
Thrombocytopenia	75,000–100,000 μL	30,000–75,000 μL	<30,000 μL
Schistocytes	Occasional	Some	Many
Increased LDH	Slight	Several-fold	Extreme
CNS abnormalities	No	+/–	Usually
GI abnormalities	No	+/–	+/–
Renal abnormalities	No	+/–	+/–
Action	Observe	Glucocorticoids	Glucocorticoids
	Evaluate for other diagnosis	Plasma exchange	Plasma exchange

LDH, lactate dehydrogenase; CNS, central nervous system; GI, gastrointestinal.

Table 24-2 Clinical Types of Thrombotic Thrombocytopenic Purpura

Familial (chronic relapsing)
Acquired idiopathic (+/– recurrence)
  Drugs: Thienopyridine-associated
    Ticlopidine (Ticlid)
    Clopidogrel (Plavix)
Thrombotic microangiopathies that resemble TTP (or HUS)
  Drugs: Mitomycin, cyclosporine, tacrolimus, quinine, combination chemotherapy, gemcitabine, total body irradiation
  Bone marrow/stem cell transplantation
  Solid organ transplantation

TTP, thrombotic thrombocytopenic purpura; HUS, hemolytic-uremic syndrome.

common acquired idiopathic TTP ("out-of-the-blue" TTP) have a single episode that never recurs (presuming that treatment is successful). About one third of adult patients who recover from an initial TTP episode have recurrences at irregular intervals, often commencing within the first year after the initial episode. TTP occasionally occurs during pregnancy, especially in the last trimester.[24]

In a less common type of the disease, familial (or congenital) TTP, frequent episodes may occur at regular ($\approx$3- to 4-week) intervals. This entity, which has also been called chronic relapsing TTP, is usually (but not always) seen initially in infants and children.[8,12,25]

During the past few years, the structurally similar platelet function inhibitors ticlopidine (Ticlid; Roche Pharmaceuticals, Nutley, NJ, USA)[26,27] and clopidogrel (Plavix; Bristol-Myers Squibb/Sanofi Pharmaceuticals Partnership, New York, NY, USA)[28] have been associated with the induction of TTP in a fraction of exposed patients. These two drugs, which differ from each other by a single carboxymethyl group, inhibit a platelet adenosine diphosphate (ADP) receptor site and are used to suppress arterial platelet thrombosis. A fraction of patients with human immunodeficiency virus-1 (HIV-1) infection also develop TTP.

Mitomycin C, quinine, cyclosporine FK506 (tacrolimus), chemotherapeutic agents in combination, gemcitabine, and total body irradiation have been associated with the subsequent development of thrombotic microangiopathy.[29–38] This syndrome often more closely resembles HUS than TTP and usually develops weeks to months after exposure.[34] Patients who have been treated for various illnesses with bone marrow/stem cell transplantation make up a relatively large subgroup.[34] Thrombotic microangiopathy has also been reported after solid organ transplantation (i.e., kidney, liver, heart, and lung).[33]

CAUSES AND PATHOPHYSIOLOGY OF THROMBOTIC THROMBOCYTOPENIC PURPURA

Early vascular lesions in TTP consist almost exclusively of platelet thrombi without evidence of perivascular inflammation or other overt vessel wall disease.[39,40] Microvascular ("hyaline") occlusions are seen in most organs, including the lungs and the eyes. Most frequently involved are the brain, heart, spleen, kidneys, pancreas, and adrenals.

Histopathologic and clinical findings in TTP suggest that organ ischemia and thrombocytopenia may be caused by direct, potentially reversible platelet adhesion/aggregation in the microcirculation of multiple organs concurrently. Immunohistochemical studies of TTP thrombi reported in 1985 by Asada and coworkers[40] revealed an abundance of VWF with little fibrinogen/fibrin, supporting the 1982 suggestion[8] that VWF is involved in the microvascular platelet adhesion/aggregation that characterize the disorder.

von Willebrand Factor, ADAMTS13, and Thrombotic Thrombocytopenic Purpura

Monomers of VWF (280,000 daltons) are linked together by disulfide bonds into multimers with varying molecular masses that range into the millions of daltons.[41] Multimers of VWF are constructed within megakaryocytes and endothelial cells and are stored within platelet α granules and endothelial cell Weibel-Palade bodies. Most plasma VWF multimers are derived from endothelial cells. Both endothelial cells and platelets produce VWF multimers that are larger than the multimers in normal plasma.[41] These ultra-large (or "unusually large")von Willebrand factor (ULVWF) multimers bind more efficiently than the largest plasma VWF multimers to the glycoprotein (GP)-Ibα components of the platelet GP-Ib-IX-V receptors.[9,42] The initial attachment of ULVWF multimers to GP-Ibα receptors,[42] and subsequently to activated platelet integrin αIIbβ3 (GP-IIb/IIIa complexes), induces platelet adhesion and aggregation in vitro in the presence of elevated levels of fluid shear stress.[9,43] After retrograde secretion by endothelial cells, ULVWF multimers become entangled in subendothelial collagen, thereby maximizing VWF-mediated adhesion of blood platelets to any subendothelium exposed by vascular damage and endothelial cell desquamation. An efficient "processing activity"[8,11] in normal plasma prevents the highly adhesive ULVWF multimers, which are also secreted antegrade into the vessel lumen, from persisting in the bloodstream.

The VWF processing activity is now known to be a specific VWF-cleaving metalloprotease in normal plasma that prevents persistence in the circulation of ULVWF multimers.[12,14,15] The enzyme degrades ULVWF multimers by cleaving 842Tyr-843Met peptide bonds in susceptible A2 domains of VWF monomeric subunits.[44–46] The VWF-cleaving metalloprotease is number 13 in a family of 18 distinct ADAMTS-type enzymes identified to date that share structural similarities.[16,17] ADAMTS13 (a *d*isintegrin *a*nd *m*etalloproteinase with *t*hrombo*s*pondin components) has eight thrombospondin-1–like domains. More precisely, plasma ADAMTS13 is composed of an aminoterminal reprolysin-type metalloprotease domain followed by the following: a disintegrin domain; a thrombospondin-1–like domain; a cysteine-rich domain that contains an arginine-glycine-aspartate (RGD) sequence: a spacer domain; seven additional thrombospondin-1–like domains; and two nonidentical CUB-type domains at the carboxylterminal end of the molecule (Fig. 24-2). CUB domains contain peptide sequences similar to *c*omplement subcomponents C1r/C1s, embryonic sea *u*rchin protein egf, and *b*one morphogenic protein-1.[47] ADAMTS13 is a Zn^{2+}- and Ca^{2+}-requiring

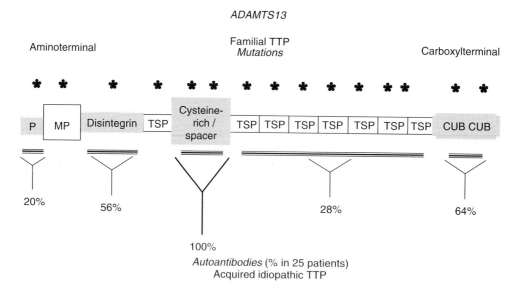

Figure 24-2 Domain structure of ADAMTS13 (*a di*sintegrin *a*nd *m*etalloproteinase *w*ith *th*rombospondin components), the plasma von Wille-brand Factor (VWF)–cleaving metalloprotease. P, propeptide; MP, metalloprotease (proteolytic) domain; TSP, thrombospondin-1–like domain (eight are present); CUB, two nonidentical domains that contain peptide segments similar to complement components, C1r/C1s, a sea urchin protein, and a *b*one morphogenic protein. *Indicates the location of mutations in patients with familial TTP that affect secretion or function of ADAMTS13 (above enzyme structure). The percentages of polyclonal autoantibodies directed against specific domains of ADAMTS13 in 25 patients with acquired idiopathic TTP are indicated below the enzyme structure.[70]

190,000-dalton glycosylated protein that is encoded on chromosome 9q34 and is produced predominantly in the liver. ADAMTS13 is inhibited in vitro by ethylenediamine-tetraacetic acid (EDTA); therefore, functional assays of the enzyme are usually performed with the use of citrate plasma.[12,14–17,44–46,48,49] Plasma anticoagulated with heparin, chloromethylketones (e.g., phenylalanine-proline-aspartate-chloromethylketone [PPACK]), hirudin, and other direct thrombin inhibitors would also probably be satisfactory for testing.

ULVWF multimers are cleaved by ADAMTS13 as they are secreted in long "strings" from stimulated endothelial cells (Fig. 24-3).[10,50] ULVWF multimeric strings may be anchored in the endothelial cell membrane to P-selectin molecules that are secreted concurrently with ULVWF multimers from Weibel-Palade bodies.[51] Included among the agents that stimulate endothelial cells to secrete ULVWF multimers are the proinflammatory cytokines, tumor necrosis factor (TNF)-α, interleukin (IL)-8, and IL-6 (in complex with the IL-6 receptor),[52] as well as the Shiga toxins (discussed later). One of the repeated CUB domains at the carboxylterminal end of each ADAMTS13 enzyme, along with the cysteine-rich/spacer region, may modulate the binding of ADAMTS13 to ULVWF multimers as they are secreted by endothelial cells.[53–55] Specifically, ADAMTS13 enzymes may attach under flowing conditions to accessible A3 domains in the monomeric subunits of ULVWF multimers[50]; they then cleave 842Tyr-Met0843 peptide bonds in adjacent A2 domains (see Fig. 24-3). Partial unfolding of emerging ULVWF multimers through fluid shear stress may increase the efficiency of ADAMTS13 attachments to ULVWF multimers, followed by ULVWF cleavage.[10,44] The VWF A1 domain may exert a negative steric influence on VWF cleavage by ADAMTS13, because platelet GP-Ibα binding to the VWF A1 domain renders the adjacent VWF A2 domain more susceptible to proteolysis by ADAMTS13.[56]

Failure to degrade ULVWF multimers has long been suspected to cause familial and acquired idiopathic types of TTP, or to predispose an individual to these disorders (see Fig. 24-3).[8,57] Critical experiments conducted to verify this concept were reported in 1997 and 1998. Four patients were described with chronic relapsing TTP who had a deficiency of VWF-cleaving protease activity (ADAMTS13) in plasma.[12] Because no inhibitor of the enzyme was detected, this deficiency was ascribed to an abnormality in production, survival, or function of the protease. During the following year, the pathogenesis of the more common acquired idiopathic type of TTP was elucidated.[13–15] Patients with acquired idiopathic TTP had little, if any, plasma VWF–cleaving protease activity during acute episodes; however, this activity increased toward normal on recovery. Although the plasma assays in these studies were "nonphysiologic," they were, nonetheless, innovative and informative. Immunoglobulin (Ig)G autoantibodies against components of the enzyme probably accounted for the lack of protease activity in most patients with acquired idiopathic TTP.[13–15] The reasons for this transient immune dysregulation, as well as for the selective antigenic targeting of the VWF-cleaving protease, are not yet known.

Patients with familial chronic relapsing TTP frequently have ULVWF multimers in their plasma.[8,57] ULVWF multimers are also detected using a sensitive gel electrophoresis method in some patient plasma samples during acute episodes of acquired idiopathic TTP, but not after recovery.[57] These findings were explained by investigators[12–15] who discovered a chronic absence from plasma of the VWF-cleaving protease (ADAMTS13) in familial chronic relapsing TTP, as well as transient inhibition of the enzyme during acute episodes of acquired idiopathic TTP.

Most patients with familial TTP have less than about 5% of normal ADAMTS13 activity in their plasma, regardless of whether plasma is obtained during or after

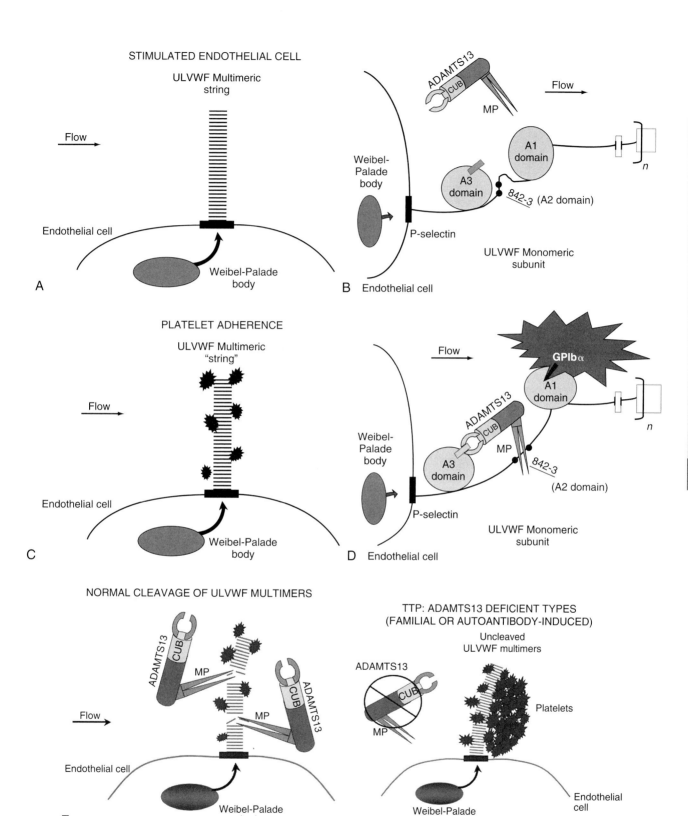

Figure 24-3 (Legend appears on next page)

Figure 24-3 *(See also Color Plate 24-3.)* Proposed mechanism of ultra-large von Willebrand factor (ULVWF) multimeric string cleavage by ADAMTS13 (a *d*isintegrin *a*nd *m*etalloproteinase with *t*hrombospondin components). **A,** Stimulation of endothelial cells causes secretion of long ULVWF multimeric strings. **B,** "Close-up" of one of the many monomeric subunits that make up a ULVWF multimeric string. ULVWF multimeric strings may be anchored in the endothelial cell membrane to P-selectin molecules that are secreted concurrently with ULVWF multimers from Weibel-Palade bodies. The A1, A2 (with the 842Tyr-843Met ADAMTS13 proteolytic cleavage site), and A3 domains are shown. Adequate quantities of ADAMTS13 enzymes are present in the plasma of normal individuals. The carboxylterminal CUB region (two nonidentical domains that contain peptide segments similar to complement components, C1r/C1s, a sea *u*rchin protein, and a *b*one morphogenic protein) is indicated, and the proteolytic metalloprotease domain (MP) is drawn as a pincer-like structure on the aminoterminal portion of the enzyme. **C,** Platelets from flowing blood adhere to the long ULVWF multimeric strings immediately after string secretion. **D,** Platelet adherence (via platelet glycoprotein [GP]-Ibα) to the A1 domain of ULVWF monomeric subunits increases the exposure of neighboring A2 842Tyr-843Met peptide bonds in ULVWF multimeric strings. ADAMTS13 molecules attach via one of their CUB domains to the A3 domain of ULVWF monomeric subunits, and then cleave the adjacent (and now exposed) 842Tyr-843Met bond. **E,** ADAMTS13 cleavage through this mechanism occurs in various monomers along the length of ULVWF multimeric strings. The smaller VWF forms that circulate after cleavage do not induce the adhesion and aggregation of platelets during normal blood flow. **F,** Absent or severely reduced activity of ADAMTS13 in the plasma of patients with TTP prevents the timely cleavage of ULVWF multimeric strings as they are secreted from endothelial cells. Uncleaved ULVWF multimers induce the adhesion and subsequent aggregation of platelets in flowing blood. TTP may be caused by familial deficiencies of ADAMTS13 secretion or activity caused by ADAMTS13 gene mutations, or they may result from acquired autoantibody-induced defects of ADAMTS13 activity (or survival).

acute episodes (provided that they have not recently received plasma infusions). Most patients with acquired idiopathic types of TTP have less than about 5% of normal ADAMTS13 activity in their plasma only during acute TTP episodes.[12–15,23,58] Severe deficiency of ADAMTS13 activity in plasma from patients with TTP correlates with failure to cleave ULVWF multimers as they emerge from the surfaces of endothelial cells (see Fig. 24-3).[10] As a consequence, ULVWF multimers secreted by endothelial cells remain anchored to these cells in long strings (Fig. 24-4).[10] This anchoring may occur via P-selectin molecules that have transmembrane domains and are secreted along with ULVWF multimers from the Weibel-Palade bodies of endothelial cells.[51] (P-selectin molecules are predominantly retained in the cell membrane as the Weibel-Palade contents are secreted.) Passing platelets adhere via their GP-Ibα receptors to these long, uncleaved ULVWF multimeric strings.[10] (Platelets do not adhere to the smaller VWF forms that circulate after cleavage of ULVWF multimers.[41]) Many additional platelets subsequently aggregate under flowing conditions, probably via activated GP-IIb/IIIa, onto the ULVWF multimeric strings to form large, potentially occlusive platelet thrombi (see Fig. 24-3).[10,59]

ULVWF multimeric strings are capable of detaching from endothelial cells in the absence of ADAMTS13 activity and in the presence of fluid shear stress and with the increasing torque generated as platelets adhere and aggregate onto ULVWF strings.[10] The detached ULVWF–platelet strings may "embolize" to microvessels downstream and contribute to organ ischemia. The formation of ULVWF–platelet thrombi and emboli may account for the following observations: (1) ULVWF multimers are chronically detected in the plasma of familial TTP patients, as well as in the plasma of some patients with acquired idiopathic TTP, during acute episodes[8,11,23,57]; (2) increased VWF antigen is found, through flow cytometry, on platelets during episodes of familial or acquired TTP[60]; and (3)

STIMULATED HUMAN ENDOTHELIAL CELLS (HISTAMINE; FLOW)

Anti-VWF-FITC   Anti-VWF-FITC + propidium iodide

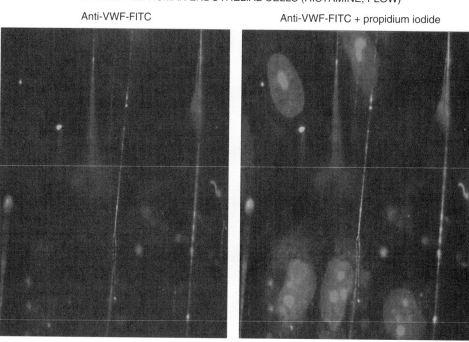

Figure 24-4 *(See also Color Plate 24-4.)* Unusually large (UL) VWF multimeric strings, secreted by human umbilical vein endothelial cells stimulated by histamine under flowing conditions, were stained green by rabbit anti-human VWF IgG + goat anti-rabbit-fluorescein isothyocyanate (FITC) in the absence *(left)* or presence *(right)* of the red nuclear stain, propidium iodide.

abundant VWF antigen (but not fibrinogen) is observed by immunohistochemistry on platelet occlusive lesions in TTP.[40]

Plasma ADAMTS13 activity is almost always absent or severely reduced in patients with familial TTP,[12,61,62] as a consequence of homozygous (or doubly heterozygous) mutations in each of the two ADAMTS13 *9q34* genes.[18,23,24,58,63] Mutations in familial TTP have been detected all along the gene in regions that encode different domains (see Fig. 24-2).[18,23,24,58,63] With severe familial deficiency of ADAMTS13 activity, episodes of TTP usually commence during infancy or childhood. In some patients, however, overt TTP episodes do not develop for years (e.g., during a first pregnancy),[24] if ever. This latter observation suggests that in vivo ADAMTS13 cleavage of ULVWF multimers that are emerging from stimulated endothelial cells may exceed plasma enzyme activity measured through in vitro nonphysiologic assays. Additionally, or alternatively, accentuated secretion of ULVWF multimers by endothelial cells induced by estrogen or proinflammatory cytokines[52] may be required to provoke TTP episodes in some patients with severe plasma ADAMTS13 deficiency.

In some infants with <5% ADAMTS13 and neonatal onset of familial chronic relapsing TTP, transient or progressive renal failure is a prominent component of the disorder.[64] These patients clinically resemble two patients described in 1960 by Schulman and colleagues[8,65] and in 1978 by Upshaw[8,66]; consequently, this pediatric subgroup is sometimes said to have "Upshaw-Schulman syndrome."

Many patients with acquired idiopathic TTP have absent or severely reduced plasma ADAMTS13 activity during an initial episode, as well as during later recurrences.[13-15] ADAMTS13 activity increases in these patients after recovery from a single, or recurrent, episode. IgG antibodies (presumably autoantibodies) that inhibit plasma ADAMTS13 activity can be detected in 44% to 94% of patients through the nonphysiologic techniques that are currently available.[13-15,24,67,68] These results suggest the presence of a transient, or intermittently recurrent, defect in immune regulation in many patients who have acquired idiopathic TTP associated with transient, or recurrent, ADAMTS13 deficiency. Antibodies that inhibit plasma ADAMTS13 have also been identified in a few patients with ticlopidine- or clopidogrel-associated TTP.[28,69] It is not yet known whether a transient, severe defect in ADAMTS13 production or survival occurs in patients with acquired TTP who do not have detectable autoantibodies against the enzyme. Alternatively, failure to detect autoantibodies in some patients may reflect the limited sensitivity of the test systems that are currently in use.

In one recent study of polyclonal autoantibodies against ADAMTS13 in 25 patients with acquired TTP,[70] epitope targets always included the cysteine-rich/spacer domain sequence, and antibodies were exclusively directed against the cysteine-rich/spacer domain sequence in 3 of the 25 patients. The other 22 autoantibodies reacted with the cysteine-rich/spacer domain sequence plus the CUB domains (64%), the metalloprotease/disintegrin-like/first thrombospondin-1–like domain sequence (56%), or the second-to-eighth thrombospondin-1–like domain sequence (28%) (see Fig. 24-2). The propeptide region was also identified by 20% of autoantibodies,[70] indicating that removal of the propeptide is not required for secretion of active enzyme.[71] Autoantibodies inhibit the activity of ADAMTS13 or decrease its survival.

The propensity to produce ADAMTS13 autoantibodies is almost certainly genetically determined. This is emphasized by the recent discovery in twin sisters of acquired idiopathic TTP caused by IgG autoantibodies against ADAMTS13.[72]

Relapses occur in 23% to 44% of patients with acquired idiopathic TTP,[24,67,73,74] often during the first year after the initial episode.[24] These relapsing patients usually have acquired idiopathic TTP with severe plasma ADAMTS13 deficiency that is often due to the presence of autoantibodies against ADAMTS13.[24]

In a few instances, pregnancy-related episodes of TTP have been caused by autoantibodies against ADAMTS13.[24] The risk of recurrent TTP during any subsequent pregnancies is controversial, with estimates of possible recurrence (per woman) ranging from 26% to 73%.[24]

Plasma ADAMTS13 activity in healthy adults ranges from approximately 50% to 178% with the use of currently available static, nonphysiologic assays. Activity is often reduced to below normal levels in liver disease, disseminated malignancies,[75] chronic metabolic and inflammatory conditions, and pregnancy, as well as in newborns.[76] With the exception of those peripartum women who develop overt TTP,[24,67] ADAMTS13 activity observed in patients with these conditions is not reduced to the extremely low values (<5% of normal) found in most patients with familial or acquired idiopathic TTP.

OTHER OBSERVATIONS

About twice as many women as men develop acquired idiopathic TTP. Most patients are in the 20- to 60-year age range; no racial or seasonal predisposition is obvious, and case clustering is rare. Most patients who develop acute idiopathic TTP have no identifiable associated risk factor, although TTP during pregnancy or the postpartum period accounts for a small percentage of cases. Neame[77] suggested that abnormal immune modulation might contribute to its onset under these circumstances. Indeed, a specific defect in immune regulation is likely to be the basis for the "escape" of autoantibody production against ADAMTS13 in most patients with acute idiopathic TTP. How ticlopidine or clopidogrel might promote this anti-ADAMTS13 "escape" in occasional patients is not currently known.

The possibility that immunologic events are involved in acute idiopathic TTP is supported by studies that suggest macrophage/lymphocyte activation in some patients.[78,79] Elevated levels of IL-1, IL-6, the soluble IL-2 receptor, TNF-α, and transforming growth factor-β (TGF-β) have been reported in the disorder. Evidence also suggests that patients who lack the class II major histocompatibility locus antigen, DR53, may be susceptible to thrombotic microangiopathy.[80]

Acquired idiopathic TTP has been associated occasionally with diseases characterized by autoimmune or other types of abnormal immune responses, including systemic lupus erythromatosus (SLE),[81] autoimmune "idiopathic" thrombocytopenic purpura (ITP),[82] and the acquired immunodeficiency syndrome (AIDS).[83-85]

REPRESENTATIVE CASES OF TTP

Case 1

A 3-month-old girl became pale and jaundiced and had several transient episodes of hemiparesis. Physical examination findings were normal. Hemoglobin was 8.4 g per deciliter, platelets were 11,000/μL, and reticulocytes (polychromatophilic red cells) and 3+/4+ schistocytes were seen on her peripheral blood film. Serum LDH level was elevated five-fold, and unconjugated bilirubin was increased. Computed tomography of the brain showed ischemic changes.

Several days after admission, it was determined that ADAMTS13 activity was not detectable in a citrate plasma sample obtained prior to any therapy, and that the sample did not contain a detectable inhibitor directed against ADAMTS13.

Packed red blood cells and FFP were administered; this was followed by rapid clinical and hematologic remission over 2 days. Neurologic recovery was complete.

A regimen of periodic FFP infusions was tentatively planned (10 mL per kilogram every 3 weeks) for her probable familial (congenital) chronic relapsing TTP.

Case 2

A 22-year-old man developed headache and confusion. He had been healthy previously and was taking no medicine. His hemoglobin was 6.7 g per deciliter, and platelets were 5000/μL. Schistocytes (4+/4+) and reticulocytes were prominent on his peripheral blood film. Serum LDH level was 10 times normal. Computed tomography showed no intracerebral hemorrhage.

The admission citrate plasma sample obtained before treatment was later found to have no detectable ADAMTS13 activity; a high-titer inhibitor to ADAMTS13 was found in this sample.

The patient was given high-dose methylprednisolone, packed red blood cells, immediate FFP infusion, and 3 days of plasma exchange (with FFP) commencing on the night of admission. On day 4, he became comatose, and cryosupernatant was substituted for FFP in the daily exchanges. He awakened on day 7, and neurologic symptoms disappeared by day 8. On day 10, platelets were 43,000/μL; by day 17, platelets were 203,000/μL, and LDH levels were normal. Plasma exchange with cryosupernatant was continued for 5 additional days and was then stopped. Glucocorticoids were tapered over a period of weeks. The patient has not had a recurrence of the acute acquired idiopathic TTP episode over the subsequent several years.

OTHER THROMBOTIC MICROANGIOPATHIES

Some patients develop the characteristic clinical manifestations of thrombotic microangiopathy without overt associated conditions or plasma ADAMTS13 deficiency (at least as measured by techniques currently available).[67,73,74,86,87] The cause of the disorder in this subgroup of patients, who have a higher mortality rate than patients with severe ADAMTS13 deficiency, is unknown. In some of these patients, any possible relationship with ADAMTS13

deficiency is clouded by the transfusion of normal blood products that contain ADAMTS13 before testing of patient plasma for enzyme activity.[24]

Neither bone marrow/stem cell transplantation–associated thrombotic microangiopathy nor diarrhea-associated HUS (caused by Shiga toxin–producing enterohemorrhagic *Escherichia coli*) is usually associated with absence or severely reduced levels of plasma ADAMTS13 activity.[14,26,73,88,89] The explanation for VWF abnormalities in the plasma of some patients with chemotherapy/transplant-associated thrombotic microangiopathy is unknown.[32] (See also section on "Types of TTP.")

DIFFERENTIAL DIAGNOSIS OF THROMBOTIC THROMBOCYTOPENIC PURPURA

The constellation of thrombocytopenia, hemolysis, and schistocytosis also occurs (to an extent that is usually less extreme than in TTP) in HUS, DIC, preeclampsia/eclampsia, the HELLP syndrome (preeclampsia-associated *H*emolysis, *E*levated *L*iver function tests, and *L*ow *P*latelets), malignant hypertension, severe vasculitis, scleroderma with associated hypertension and renal failure, and Evans syndrome (concurrent autoimmune thrombocytopenia and direct Coombs test–positive autoimmune hemolysis); in patients with a malfunctioning prosthetic cardiac valve; and, occasionally, after cocaine use (Table 24-3).[23,90]

Of these, the most frequently troublesome diagnostic dilemma is TTP versus either HUS or DIC. The other types of thrombotic microangiopathy are usually quickly suspected on the basis of the patient's recent medical history.

Of all the conditions mentioned here, only TTP is associated with absent or severely reduced plasma ADAMTS13 levels. Absence and/or severe reduction in ADAMTS13 is always present in familial TTP, but it occurs only during episodes of acquired idiopathic TTP.

DISTINCTION BETWEEN THROMBOTIC THROMBOCYTOPENIC PURPURA AND HEMOLYTIC-UREMIC SYNDROME

Platelet adhesion/aggregation on uncleaved ULVWF multimeric strings in the microcirculation in TTP produce fluctuating ischemia or infarction in various organs, including

Table 24-3 Differential Diagnosis of Thrombotic Thrombocytopenic Purpura
Hemolytic-uremic syndrome
Disseminated intravascular coagulation
Evans syndrome*
Malignant hypertension
Malfunctioning prosthetic cardiac valve
Severe vasculitis
Pregnancy
Preeclampsia/eclampsia
HELLP syndrome†

*Autoimmune thrombocytopenia and autoimmune hemolysis.
†*H*emolysis, *E*levated *L*iver function tests, and *L*ow *P*latelets.

the brain, in 50% to 71% of episodes.[6,7] In the closely related HUS, initially reported by Gasser and colleagues in 1955,[91] ischemia is predominantly renal and occurs as a consequence of platelet adhesion/aggregation and fibrin polymer formation atop glomerular endothelial cells. Thrombocytopenia, erythrocyte fragmentation, and increased serum levels of LDH are usually less extreme in HUS (Table 24-4). However, the variability of organ dysfunction in TTP (including renal abnormalities in 50% to 75% of episodes)[7] and the extrarenal manifestations that may complicate HUS can make the two syndromes difficult to distinguish.[6,7,23,92] Furthermore, clinical presentations that resemble TTP or HUS are sometimes associated with similar conditions (e.g., transplantation, chemotherapy/total body irradiation).

HUS consists of the triad of thrombocytopenia, acute renal failure, and intravascular hemolytic anemia with schistocytosis and elevated serum LDH. Renal dysfunction is severe in HUS, in contrast to most cases of TTP, and often requires dialysis. Oliguria, anuria, chronic renal failure, and hypertension sometimes complicate HUS; however, this is uncommon in patients who recover from episodes of TTP. Although the microvascular thrombi in HUS are usually predominantly renal, other organs are sometimes involved.[23,92,93]

Especially in children, HUS is frequently preceded by hemorrhagic enterocolitis caused by cytotoxin-producing serotypes of *E coli* (e.g., 0157:H7) or *Shigella* species.[23,92,94,95] Shiga toxin (Stx)-1 and Stx-2 produced by enterohemorrhagic *E coli* usually cause diarrhea-associated HUS. This relatively common disorder is characterized by obstruction of the glomerular microvasculature by platelet–fibrin thrombi, acute renal failure, thrombocytopenia, intravascular hemolytic anemia, elevated plasma VWF antigen, and plasma levels of ADAMTS13 activity that are within a broad normal range.[14,23,26] This latter finding may partially explain the poor response of these patients to plasma infusion or exchange.

It has recently been shown[96] that either Stx-1 or Stx-2 stimulates the rapid and profuse secretion of unusually large ULVWF multimeric strings from human endothelial cells, including glomerular microvascular endothelial cells. Perfused normal human platelets immediately adhere to the secreted ULVWF multimeric strings, and the rate of ULVWF–platelet string cleavage by ADAMTS13 is delayed in the presence of Stx-1 or Stx-2. Studies suggest that Stx-induced formation of ULVWF strings and impairment

of ULVWF–platelet string cleavage by ADAMTS13 explain the initial platelet adhesion that is noted atop Stx-stimulated glomerular endothelial cells in diarrhea-associated HUS. These findings may explain glomerular microvascular occlusion and acute renal failure in diarrhea-associated HUS.[96]

Truly recurrent episodes of acquired idiopathic TTP are distinct from a single protracted episode with brief intervening periods of incomplete remission.[6] Recurrence of acquired idiopathic TTP occurs in at least 11% to 36% of patients with TTP.[6,7,24] HUS usually occurs as a single episode, except in rare individuals who have a familial, recurrent type of a the disease. In these latter patients (often children), the level of a plasma complement control protein, factor H, may be abnormally low. The result is overactivation of complement component 3 (C3) to C3b whenever the alternative complement pathway is activated.[97,98] A similar clinical syndrome results from deficiency in another alternative complement pathway control substance, membrane cofactor protein (MCP),[98] or from deficiency of C3b-cleaving protease (factor I).[99]

In adults, a thrombotic microangiopathy (TMA) that clinically more often resembles HUS than TTP may occur after: (1) the administration of mitomycin, cyclosporine, or quinine; (2) bone marrow or solid organ transplantation; (3) total body irradiation; or (4) the use of gemcitabine or multiple chemotherapeutic agents.[34,92,100] Plasma ADAMTS13 levels are within a broad normal range, and the pathophysiology is currently unknown.[23,88]

TTP and HUS are clinical diagnoses. Tissue obtained from a biopsy specimen of bone marrow, gingiva, or kidney may be taken at a time when only a few (or no) arterial thrombi are found in the microvessels of the area sampled. This may account for the finding of characteristic microvascular hyaline thrombi in only about 50% of gingival biopsy specimens from patients considered on the basis of clinical evidence to have TTP.[101] Biopsy samples are infrequently useful acutely in diagnosis. In severely thrombocytopenic patients, the procedure may be unsafe.

TTP and HUS are manifestations of excessive microvascular platelet adhesion/aggregation. If the platelet adhesion/aggregation is systemic and extensive, and especially if the central nervous system is involved, the disorder is called TTP. If platelet adhesion/aggregation (and fibrin formation) is relatively less extensive and predominantly involves the kidneys, the patient is considered to have HUS. Severe renal involvement in a patient with TTP or extrarenal manifestations in a patient with HUS can hopelessly obfuscate clinical boundaries between the two syndromes. This situation will persist until rapid, trustworthy, and accessible clinical laboratory tests become available to detect plasma ADAMTS13 activity. Furlan and colleagues[14] initially reported in 1998 that patients given a diagnosis of TTP had little or no plasma VWF–cleaving metalloproteinase (now ADAMTS13) activity, whereas plasma activity was normal (or nearly so) in patients considered to have acquired HUS. These provocative findings, verified since that time by other investigators,[26,58] may eventually provide the basis for more precise differentiation of the two entities and probably explain why plasma therapy, which is frequently so effective in TTP, is often disappointing in acquired HUS.

Table 24-4 Distinction Between Thrombotic Thrombocytopenic Purpura and Hemolytic-Uremic Syndrome

Thrombocytopenia/schistocytosis/LDH elevation is usually more severe in TTP
Renal ischemia/injury is usually more severe in HUS
Nonrenal organ ischemia/injury is usually more severe in TTP
Plasma ADAMTS13 activity is often absent/severely reduced in TTP; within a broad normal range in HUS

LDH, lactate dehydrogenase; TTP, thrombotic thrombocytopenic purpura; HUS, hemolytic-uremic syndrome; ADAMTS13, a *d*isintegrin and *m*etalloproteinase with *t*hrombospondin domains.

TREATMENT OF PATIENTS WITH THROMBOTIC THROMBOCYTOPENIC PURPURA

The demonstration by Byrnes and Khurana in 1977[4] that TTP relapses could be prevented or reversed by the infusion of FFP or cryosupernatant (plasma depleted of VWF-rich cryoprecipitate, fibrinogen, fibronectin, and IgM) was followed in 1985 by the observation that the processing of ULVWF multimers was restored in patients with familial chronic relapsing TTP through the transfusion of FFP, cryosupernatant,[11,102] or solvent/detergent-treated plasma.[25] These plasma products were effective alone, in quantities ranging from one to several units, without the need for concurrent plasmapheresis. Tsai and Lian[15] and Furlan and associates[14] proved in 1998 that these plasma products contain functionally active ADAMTS13.

Infants and young children with familial TTP produce inadequate quantities, or functionally defective forms, of ADAMTS13.[12,23,61] The reason why the infusion of normal ADAMTS13 only about every 3 weeks prevents TTP episodes in these patients is unknown. The plasma half-life of infused ADAMTS13 activity is relatively long ($\approx$2 days).[61] The functional half-life of the enzyme may be even longer because ADAMTS13 docks and cleaves one ULVWF multimeric string after another as each string is secreted from endothelial cells.[50,54]

Adults and older children with acquired idiopathic TTP episodes associated with ADAMTS13 deficiency require daily plasma exchange (Table 24-5). Plasma exchange combines plasmapheresis (which may remove circulating ULVWF–platelet strings, agents that stimulate endothelial cells to secrete ULVWF multimers, and autoantibodies against ADAMTS13) with the infusion of FFP or cryosupernatant (both of which contain uninhibited ADAMTS13). Solvent/detergent-treated plasma and methylene blue/light-treated plasma[103] (for inactivation of lipid envelope viruses) also contain active ADAMTS13; however, protein S activity is below normal in solvent/detergent plasma.[103]

Skipping even one day before complete remission may lead to rapid relapse. More than one exchange per day has not been proved to be beneficial. Infusion of normal FFP at a rate of about 30 mL/kg/day can be provided initially until plasma exchanges are arranged. This should occur as quickly as practical but often requires a few to many hours. Plasma infusion alone is less effective in acquired

idiopathic TTP than is plasma exchange,[7] and it may result in volume overload. Patients with TTP who experience coma, cardiac failure, or severe renal dysfunction should begin to receive plasma exchange as soon as possible (see Chapter 30).

Cryosupernatant is at least as effective as FFP in plasma exchange procedures,[4,104,105] and it is certainly no less effective. If a patient with TTP responds minimally within the first few days of therapy, or actually deteriorates, cryosupernatant can be substituted for FFP in the plasma exchange procedures.[105] Adult patients with TTP who are refractory to FFP exchanges may respond better to exchanges with cryosupernatant.[105]

The process of treating plasma with a solvent and detergent to inactivate lipid envelope viruses (HIV-1, hepatitis B and C viruses) also removes large VWF multimers. Both solvent/detergent-treated plasma[15,103] and methylene blue/light-treated plasma[103] (which also inactivates lipid envelope viruses) contain active ADAMTS13. Although solvent/detergent-treated plasma is effective in treating patients during episodes of TTP,[25] its production and use has declined because the manufacturing process results in protein S activity that is below the levels of untreated normal plasma.[103]

Plasma exchange with FFP or cryosupernatant allows about 80% to 90% of patients with acquired, "out-of-the-blue" TTP to survive an episode.[6,7,24] Patients with acquired idiopathic TTP who have severe ADAMTS13 deficiency often respond more effectively and rapidly to this procedure than do patients with normal levels of ADAMTS13 who are given a diagnosis of TTP. This was shown in a recent study of 38 consecutive patients at one hospital who were diagnosed with TTP.[106] Of 10 patients who did not respond to daily plasma exchange, 8 had normal plasma ADAMTS13 (activity was absent in the other 2). In contrast, of 28 patients who responded to plasma exchange, 25 had absent or severely reduced plasma ADAMTS13 (activity was normal in the other 3). Of 25 patients with severe ADAMTS13-deficient TTP who responded to plasma exchange, 15 required only 7 exchanges to attain platelet counts above 150,000/μL and normal serum LDH values.

Lower titers of plasma ADAMTS13 autoantibodies may be associated with better response to plasma exchange procedures than are higher levels of anti-ADAMTS13 antibodies produced for longer periods.[74,107,108] In association with plasma exchange, production of ADAMTS13 autoantibodies may be suppressed by high-dose glucocorticoids,[6] four to eight weekly doses of rituximab (monoclonal antibody against CD20 on B lymphocytes),[109–112] rituximab combined with cyclophosphamide,[24,113] or (most radically) splenectomy.[114–116]

Recovery from TTP is not usually associated with persistent, overt organ damage[6,7]; however, some compromise of cognitive function may be subsequently detectable through careful testing.[24] Although almost all TTP recurrences can be quickly recognized by blood counts and LDH measurements, several disturbing exceptions have been reported. For example, three women who had recovered from previous episodes of TTP subsequently experienced symptoms of stroke without thrombocytopenia, but with absent ADAMTS13 yet with symptomatic response to plasma exchange.[112,117]

Table 24-5 Treatment of Patients with Thrombotic Thrombocytopenic Purpura

Immediate infusion of FFP (30 mL/kg/day)
Daily plasma exchange with FFP or cryosupernatant*
    (3–4 L/day)
Glucocorticoids (e.g., intravenous prednisolone at
    200 mg/day)
Red blood cells as needed
Platelets only for life-threatening events, including
    intracerebral or GI hemorrhage, or before invasive
    procedures with high bleeding risk

*Cryosupernatant = plasma depleted of VWF-rich cryoprecipitate. FFP, fresh frozen plasma; GI, gastrointestinal; VWF, von Willebrand factor.

If a patient who is experiencing a TTP episode is taking ticlopidine or clopidogrel, or any other suspicious drug (e.g.,mitomycin, cyclosporine, quinine), then this medicine should be stopped immediately.

Although many adult patients have recovered from TTP episodes without receiving glucocorticoids, in one large series, a subset of patients with TTP recovered after receiving glucocorticoid therapy alone.[6] On the basis of this study by Bell and colleagues,[6] it is probably prudent to institute glucocorticoid therapy—in association with plasma exchange—in all adult patients with initial or recurrent TTP episodes, unless a strong contraindication is present. The usefulness of glucocorticoids may reflect the proposed autoimmune pathogenesis in most adult patients (e.g., glucocorticoids may suppress the production of autoantibodies against ADAMTS13). Bell and coworkers[6] administered prednisolone intravenously immediately after diagnosis was confirmed at a dosage of about 200 mg per day and continued this regimen until the patients recovered.

Depending on the hemoglobin level and intensity of hemolysis, red blood cell transfusions may be required. If the platelet count is very low and bleeding is a primary problem, or if intracranial bleeding is noted on computed tomography scanning or magnetic resonance imaging, then transfusion of platelets will be necessary. (Anecdotal observations suggest that this might be done at a slow rate, to avoid infusion of a large bolus of platelets in only a few minutes.) With some exceptions (Table 24-5), it is probably better to withhold platelet transfusions because they have been temporally associated with exacerbation of the microcirculatory thrombotic process within the central nervous system.[39,118]

Plasma exchange should be continued for longer than three days[6] after patients attain complete remission (i.e., a normal neurologic status, a platelet count of 150,000 to 200,000/μL, a rising hemoglobin value, and a normal serum LDH level). Schistocytes in declining numbers often persist for many days on peripheral blood films, and so these cannot be used as a reliable marker for remission. With only three additional post-remission exchanges, incomplete response with rapid relapse is likely.[6] At least five additional post-remission exchanges are currently used empirically in some centers (e.g., the Texas Medical Center hospitals in Houston). The procedure should then be stopped, and the glucocorticoid dosage tapered and discontinued over a period of several weeks. Decreasing frequency of plasma exchanges over days or weeks has not been shown to provide additional benefit in most patients. Platelet counts should be monitored regularly so that incipient relapse can be detected. If TTP does recur, the same treatment program (i.e., glucocorticoids/plasma exchange) that has previously induced remission should be repeated.

Many adult patients with acquired idiopathic TTP who turn out to have recurrent episodes will have their first recurrence during the year after the initial episode.[24] In others, episodes do not recur for months to years after an initial episode. A small study of a few patients (before the availability of rituximab) suggests that frequent relapses may be controlled by splenectomy.[115]

In patients who achieve only a partial response, or whose condition worsens during therapy, plasma exchanges should be continued for a period of a few to many additional days in an effort to achieve complete remission. In these patients, concomitant heparin-associated thrombocytopenia (HIT) or

bacterial infection (e.g., from the plasma exchange catheter) should be suspected (Tables 24-6 and 24-7). HIT is especially likely if platelets begin to decrease without a concomitant increase in the LDH values that have decreased progressively toward normal during therapy. In the latter situation, exposure of the patient to heparin should be eliminated (including via keep-open intravenous lines or indwelling catheters, during dialysis, or on the tips of Swan-Ganz catheters). It is not known whether any treatment other than heparin removal (e.g., hirudin, argatroban) is required in patients with HIT who are also undergoing plasma exchange for TTP. In the absence of evidence to the contrary, the addition of hirudin or argatroban during therapy for TTP is probably too dangerous in most patients.

First-line treatment does not work in some patients with acquired idiopathic TTP episodes. Other forms of therapy may be added if plasma exchanges with FFP or cryosupernatant, glucocorticoids, and rituximab are unsuccessful or are only partially successful (see Table 24-6). Treatment options include the addition of vincristine,[119] which depolymerizes platelet microtubules and may alter the availability of GP-Ibα-IX-V or GP-IIb/IIIa receptors for VWF on platelet surfaces; splenectomy[114] (removal of immunologic cells involved in ADAMTS13 autoantibody production); and the addition of other immunosuppressive agents in an attempt to suppress production of these autoantibodies (e.g., azathioprine [Imuran; Burroughs-Wellcome, Phoenix, Ariz., USA][120] or cyclophosphamide [Cytoxan; Bristol-Myers Squibb, Princeton, NJ, USA][113]).

Table 24-6 Treatment Options for Patients with Refractory Acquired Idiopathic Thrombotic Thrombocytopenic Purpura

Continuation of daily plasma exchange with cryosupernatant (3–4 L/day)
Rituximab (375 mg/kg weekly for 4–8 weeks)
Elimination of heparin from catheter lines and ports
Search for and management of catheter (or other) infections
Vincristine (no more than 2 mg on day 1; then, 1 mg on days 4, 7, and 10)
Splenectomy
Azathioprine (Imuran; 50–150 mg/day) or cyclophosphamide (Cytoxan; 1 g/m²)

Table 24-7 Relapse After Partial Remission During Plasma Exchange Therapy for Acquired Idiopathic TTP

Possible Explanations
Failure to perform uninterrupted series of *daily* exchanges
Premature discontinuation of daily exchange before durable remission
Infection (e.g., of vascular access catheter) or inflammation*
Heparin-induced thrombocytopenia (HIT)†
Undiagnosed mimicking disorder (e.g., disseminated malignancy)

*Infection or inflammation may provoke secretion of ULVWF multimeric strings by cytokine-mediated stimulation of endothelial cells.
†HIT during TTP therapy may resemble a TTP relapse. In superimposed HIT, however, the falling platelet count may not be accompanied by another increase in serum LDH.

The use of aspirin during TTP episodes is controversial.[121,122] Platelet adhesion/aggregation onto uncleaved ULVWF multimeric strings under arterial flowing conditions is the underlying pathophysiology of the ADAMTS13-deficient types of TTP. Aspirin would not be expected to impair this process because blockade of cyclooxygenase-mediated platelet thromboxane A_2 generation by aspirin does not inhibit shear-induced platelet adhesion/aggregation in vitro.[123] Aspirin may actually exacerbate hemorrhagic complications in some patients,[121] especially those who are severely thrombocytopenic.

TREATMENT OF PATIENTS WITH OTHER TYPES OF THROMBOTIC MICROANGIOPATHY (TMA)

This group of disorders often more closely resembles HUS than TTP. They usually occur weeks to months after exposure to mitomycin C, cyclosporine FK506 (tacrolimus), chemotherapeutic agents in combination, gemcitabine, total body irradiation, bone marrow/stem cell transplantation, or solid organ transplantation. Recent exposure to quinine induces a similar syndrome.

Discontinuation of any putative disease-inducing drug should occur immediately. Patients in this "pathogenesis unknown" category of thrombotic microangiopathy, as well as those with diarrhea-associated HUS, often respond poorly to plasma exchange.[23,34] It has been shown recently, however, that some patients improve in association with exchange.[67] It is, therefore, appropriate to commence daily plasma exchange procedures and continue them for a sufficient period so that effectiveness can be determined.

Several patients with HUS-like thrombotic microangiopathy after solid organ transplantation have been reported to respond to plasma exchange plus intravenous immune globulin (IVIg).[124,125] Plasma adsorption over staphylococcal protein A columns has been reported to be useful in thrombotic microangiopathy that results from mitomycin C exposure.[126]

Creative ideas about the causes and treatments of these disorders are urgently needed.

NEW APPROACHES TO THERAPY

As testing for plasma ADAMTS13 has become increasingly available, results of testing during remission have allowed new observations and have generated thoughtful speculation (Table 24-8).

The sequence of the 190,000-dalton ADAMTS13 has been determined, and the enzyme has been partially purified from normal human plasma fractions.[16,17,46] Recombinant, active ADAMTS13 has also been prepared[127] and may soon be produced in therapeutic quantities through the use of insect or mammalian cells (capable of ADAMTS13 glycosylation) or bacteria (incapable of glycosylating ADAMTS13; problem with endotoxin contamination). As a consequence, purified or recombinant ADAMTS13 may soon be developed for therapeutic use in TTP. A plasma level of ADAMTS13 of only about 5% of normal is sufficient to prevent or truncate TTP episodes in most patients.[23,48,58,62,73] Gene therapy, consequently, may eventually offer a practical approach to

attaining more lasting remissions in children with familial chronic relapsing TTP.

It may also be possible to produce active, altered forms of recombinant ADAMTS13 that have less binding affinity for ADAMTS13 autoantibodies. These types of ADAMTS13 may prove useful in the treatment of patients with acquired idiopathic TTP.[128]

New additives to blood products capable of destroying viruses, both with and without lipid envelopes (e.g., parvovirus B19), may become available to supplant the solvent/detergent combination that eliminates HIV, hepatitis B and C viruses, and other lipid envelope viruses from plasma.[25] These additives may be useful if they have little or no negative effects on ADAMTS13 in plasma or cryosupernatant, or on purified or recombinant enzyme preparations.

Efficient techniques for removing ADAMTS13 autoantibodies (e.g., new types of protein A or protein G immunoadsorption columns), combined with infusion of concentrates of purified or recombinant ADAMTS13, may eventually prove useful. This type of therapy may be especially helpful in patients who have allergic reactions to other plasma components. Removal of ADAMTS13 autoantibodies by whatever technique will remain difficult because most autoantibodies identified to date have been IgG,[15] which has an extensive extravascular distribution.

Table 24-8 Recent Clinical Insights/Speculations

Familial vs. Acquired Idiopathic TTP:

- Familial TTP may present later in life (even in middle age) more frequently than previously anticipated.
- Some patients with an initial TTP episode in childhood or adolescence may have familial TTP.
- Relapses in familial TTP may be intermittent, irregular, and occur at unpredictable intervals (i.e., less frequent and regular episodes than previously anticipated).
- Familial TTP patients are probably included in most published series on "acquired" TTP therapy and are likely to respond more quickly to plasma manipulation than patients with autoantibody-mediated acquired idiopathic TTP.

TTP Testing and Therapy:

- A TTP patient of any age with extremely low ADAMTS13 activity or antigen levels *during remission* has familial TTP, and may respond rapidly to plasma infusion alone during subsequent relapse.
- If plasma infusion alone does not induce remission in a familial TTP patient within a few days, especially if the episode has been induced by infection (cytokine-stimulation of endothelial cell ULVWF string secretion), then it may be appropriate to proceed to plasma exchange.*
- Some doubt remains about the superiority of plasma exchange over plasma infusion alone for the treatment of all (unclassified) adult TTP patients.†
- Avoidance or reversal of fluid overload is a major advantage of plasma exchange (which has more iatrogenic complications).

*Poorly responsive infection-induced episodes of TTP *may* occasionally be an indication for *twice daily* plasma exchange (Kitchens CS, personal communication, 2006)
†Coppo P, et al: High-dose plasma infusion versus plasma exchange as early treatment of thrombotic thrombocytopenic purpura/hemolytic-uremic syndrome. Medicine 82:27–38, 2003.

COST CONTAINMENT

The treatment of patients with acute episodes of acquired idiopathic TTP is labor intensive, prolonged, and usually requires the services of hematologists and transfusion medicine specialists. Large volumes of FFP or the more expensive cryosupernatant are consumed. Cost reduction of consequence with the use of presently effective therapeutic options is unlikely. On the contrary, if purified or recombinant ADAMTS13 is ultimately used in place of FFP and cryosupernant, costs are likely to increase.

MEDICAL-LEGAL IMPLICATIONS

TTP is no longer a rare disorder; therefore, the diagnosis must be considered in every patient whose initial complete blood cell count shows thrombocytopenia and the presence of schistocytes. Under this circumstance, a serum LDH value should be obtained immediately, and if it is considerably elevated, physicians should mobilize to begin treatment for TTP. Until physicians develop a heightened—almost reflex—wariness about the increasing possibility of TTP in patients who present to general and emergency medicine settings, the burgeoning cottage industry in TTP-related malpractice claims will continue to thrive.

If the constellation of severe thrombocytopenia, schistocytosis and an elevated LDH level indicates that the diagnosis of TTP is likely, or even possible, then the treating physician should make this presumptive diagnosis and proceed with therapy on an emergency basis. Procrastination is unwise and dangerous. FFP infusion as temporary therapy, accompanied (if possible) by high-dose glucocorticoid administration, should commence as soon as possible. This should be followed by the insertion of a large-bore catheter and initiation of plasma exchange. These latter procedures may require from a few to many hours, sometimes up to 24, to implement. The daunting logistic difficulties are compounded if the patient must be transferred from an admitting hospital that lacks plasmapheresis equipment and personnel to another facility that has the capacity to perform plasma exchange procedures.

Before any severely thrombocytopenic patient who is not exsanguinating is transfused with platelets, the treating physician should specifically determine if either schistocytosis or an elevated serum LDH value is present.

Even with rapid diagnosis and proper therapy, perhaps 10% to 20% of patients die during TTP episodes. Under these circumstances, it is essential that health care practitioners help family members understand how a previously healthy individual can succumb "out of the blue" to an unpronounceable, incomprehensible disorder. Many patients continue to die unexpectedly from TTP, even when exceptional care is provided. Family members (and their lawyers) often blame physicians, when the true culprit is usually the confusing, dangerous, increasingly common, not-always-treatable disease that has been killing young people for more than 80 years.

If explanations are not thorough and thoughtful, a frequent next step is to presume that the tragic outcome must be the fault of the treating physicians and hospital. The likelihood is near 100% that some malpractice attorney will be eager to agree.

CONSULTATIVE CONSIDERATIONS

Disorders characterized by thrombocytopenia, hemolysis, schistocytosis, and LDH elevation are summarized in Table 24-3. HIT (see Chapter 25), which often causes progressive thrombocytopenia and thrombosis, is not usually accompanied by schistocytes.

The consulting hematologist should review quickly and personally the peripheral blood smear and then should rapidly focus on the likely diagnosis on the basis of patient examination findings and the results of a few additional laboratory studies done on an emergency basis (i.e., prothrombin time, partial thromboplastin time, D-dimer, fibrinogen, direct Coombs test, and creatinine).

If the differential diagnosis in an adult patient is believed to be TTP or HUS, then the patient should be presumed to have TTP, and steps to initiate therapy should be taken immediately.

REFERENCES

1. Marcus A: Eli Moschcowitz. In Hemolytic-Uremic Syndrome and Thrombotic Thrombocytopenic Purpura: Kaplan B, Trompeter RS, Moake JL (editors); New York, Marcel Dekker, 1992, pp. 19–27.
2. Moschcowitz E: Hyaline thrombosis of the terminal arterioles and capillaries: A hitherto undescribed disease. Proc NY Pathol Soc 24:21–24, 1924.
3. Moschcowitz E: An acute febrile pleiochromic anemia with hyaline thrombosis of the terminal arterioles and capillaries. Arch Intern Med 36:89–93, 1925.
4. Byrnes JJ, Khurana M: Treatment of thrombotic thrombocytopenic purpura with plasma. N Engl J Med 297:1386–1389, 1977.
5. Bukowski RM, Hewlett JS, Reimer RR, et al: Therapy of thrombotic thrombocytopenic purpura: An overview. Semin Thromb Hemost 7:1–8, 1981.
6. Bell WR, Braine HG, Ness PM, Kickler TS: Improved survival in thrombotic thrombocytopenic purpura–hemolytic-uremic syndrome clinical experience in 108 patients. N Engl J Med 325:398–403, 1991.
7. Rock G, Sumak K, Buskard N, et al: Comparison of plasma exchange with plasma infusion in the treatment of thrombotic thrombocytopenic purpura. N Engl J Med 325:393–397, 1991.
8. Moake JL, Rudy CK, Troll JH, et al: Unusually large plasma factor VIII:von Willebrand factor multimers in chronic relapsing thrombotic throbocytopenic purpura. N Engl J Med 307:1432–1435, 1982.
9. Moake JL, Turner NA, Stathopoulos NA, et al: Involvement of large plasma von Willebrand factor (vWF) multimers and unusually large vWF forms derived from endothelial cells in shear stress-induced platelet aggregation. J Clin Invest 78:1456–1461, 1986.
10. Dong J-F, Moake JL, Nolasco L, et al: ADAMTS-13 rapidly cleaves newly secreted ultralarge von Willebrand factor multimers on the endothelial surface under flowing conditions. Blood 100:4033–4039, 2002.
11. Moake JL, Byrnes JJ, Troll JH, et al: Effects of fresh-frozen plasma and its cryosupernatant fraction on von Willebrand factor multimeric forms in chronic relapsing thrombotic thrombocytopenic purpura. Blood 65:1232–1236, 1985.
12. Furlan M, Robles R, Solenthaler M, et al: Deficient activity of von Willebrand factor–cleaving protease in chronic relapsing thrombotic thrombocytopenic purpura. Blood 89:3097–3103, 1997.
13. Furlan M, Robles R, Solenthaler M, Lammle B: Acquired deficiency of von Willebrand factor–cleaving protease in a patient with thrombotic thrombocytopenic purpura. Blood 91:2839–2846, 1998.
14. Furlan M, Robles R, Galbusera M, et al: von Willebrand factor–cleaving protease in thrombotic thrombocytopenic purpura and hemolytic-uremic syndrome. N Engl J Med 339:1578–1584, 1998.
15. Tsai HM, Lian EC-Y: Antibodies of von Willebrand factor cleaving protease in acute thrombotic thrombocytopenic purpura. N Engl J Med 339:1585–1594, 1998.
16. Fujikawa K, Suzuki H, McMullen B, Chung D: Purification of von Willebrand factor–cleaving protease and its identification as a new member of the metalloproteinase family. Blood 98:1662–1666, 2001.

17. Zheng X, Chung C, Takayama TK, et al: Structure of von Willebrand factor cleaving protease (ADAMTS13), a metalloprotease involved in thrombotic thrombocytopenic purpura. J Biol Chem 276: 41059–41063, 2001.

18. Levy GA, Nichols WC, Lian EC, et al: Mutations in a member of the ADAMTS gene family cause thrombotic thrombocytopenic purpura. Nature 413:488–494, 2001.

19. Burns ER, Lou Y, Pathak A: Morphologic diagnosis of thrombotic thrombocytopenic purpura. Am J Hematol 75:18–21, 2004.

20. James TN, Monto RW: Pathology of the cardiac conduction system in thrombotic thrombocytopenic purpura. Ann Intern Med 65: 37–43, 1966.

21. Ridolfi RL, Hutchins GM, Bell WR: The heart and cardiac conduction system in thrombotic thrombocytopenic purpura: A clinico-pathologic study of 17 autopsied patients. Ann Intern Med 91: 357–363, 1979.

22. Bell MD, Barnhart JS, Martin JM: Thrombotic thrombocytopenic purpura causing sudden unexpected death: A series of eight patients. J Forensic Sci 35:601–613, 1990.

23. Moake JL: Thrombotic microangiopathies. N Engl J Med 347:589–600, 2002.

24. Sadler JE, Moake JL, Miyata T, George JN: Recent advances in thrombotic thrombocytopenic purpura. Hematology 1:407–423, 2004.

25. Moake J, Chintagumpala M, Turner N, et al: Solvent/detergent-treated plasma suppresses shear-induced platelet aggregation and prevents episodes of thrombotic thrombocytopenic purpura. Blood 84:490–497, 1994.

26. Tsai H-M, Chandler WL, Sarode R, et al: von Willebrand factor and von Willebrand factor–cleaving metalloprotease activity in *Escherichia coli* 0157:H7–associated hemolytic uremic syndrome. Pediatr Res 49:653–659, 2001.

27. Bennett CL, Weinberg PD, Rozenberg B-DK, et al: Thrombotic thrombocytopenic purpura associated with ticlopidine: A review of 60 cases. Ann Intern Med 128:541–544, 1998.

28. Bennett CL, Connors JM, Carwile JM, et al: Thrombotic thrombocytopenic purpura associated with clopidogrel. N Engl J Med 342:1773–1777, 2000.

29. Rabadi SJ, Khandekar JD, Miller HJ: Mitomycin-induced hemolytic uremic syndrome: Case presentation and review of literature. Cancer Treat Rep 66:1244–1247, 1982.

30. Atkinson K, Biggs JC, Hayes J, et al: Cyclosporin A associated nephrotoxicity in the first 100 days after allogeneic bone marrow transplantation: Three distinct syndromes. Br J Haematol 54:59–67, 1983.

31. Mach-Pascual S, Samii K, Beris P: Microangiopathic hemolytic anemia complicating FK506 (tacrolimus) therapy. Am J Hematol 52:310–312, 1996.

32. Charba D, Moake JL, Harris MA, Hester JP: Abnormalities of von Willebrand factor multimers in drug-associated thrombotic microangiopathies. Am J Hematol 42:268–277, 1993.

33. Singh N, Gayowski T, Marino IR: Hemolytic uremic syndrome in solid-organ transplant recipients. Transplant Int 9:68–75, 1996.

34. Moake JL, Byrnes JJ: Thrombotic microangiopathies associated with drugs and bone marrow transplantation. Hematol/Oncol Clin North Am 10:485–497, 1996.

35. Venat-Bouvet L, Ly K, Szelag JC, et al: Thrombotic microangiopathy and digital necrosis: Two unrecognized toxicities of gemcitabine. Anticancer Drugs 14:829–832, 2003.

36. Kojouri K, Vesely S, George JN: Quinine-associated thrombotic thrombocytopenic purpura–hemolytic uremic syndrome: Frequency, clinical features, and long-term outcomes. Ann Intern Med 135:1047–1051, 2001.

37. Gottschall JL, Elliot W, Lianos E, et al: Quinine-induced immune thrombocytopenia associated with hemolytic-uremic syndrome: A new clinical entity. Blood 77:306–310, 1991.

38. Humphreys BD, Sharman JP, Henderson JM, et al: Gemcitabine-associated thrombotic microangiopathy. Cancer 100:2664–2670, 2004.

39. Harkness D, Byrnes JJ, Lian EC-Y, et al: Hazard of platelet transfusion in thrombotic thrombocytopenic purpura. JAMA 246:1931–1933, 1981.

40. Asada Y, Sumiyoshi A, Hayashi T, et al: Immunochemistry of vascular lesions in thrombotic thrombocytopenic purpura, with special reference to factor VIII related antigen. Thromb Res 38:469–479, 1985.

41. Ruggeri ZM: Developing basic and clinical research on von Willebrand factor and von Willebrand disease. Thromb Haemost 84:147–149, 2000.

42. Arya M, Anvari B, Romo GM, et al: Ultra-large multimers of von Willebrand factor form spontaneous high-strength bonds with the platelet GP Ib-IX complex: studies using optical tweezers. Blood 99:3971–3977, 2002.

43. Moake JL, Turner NA, Stathopoulos NA, et al: Shear-induced platelet aggregation can be mediated by vWF released from platelets, as well as by exogenous large or unusually large vWF multimers, requires adenosine diphosphate, and is resistant to aspirin. Blood 71: 1366–1374, 1988.

44. Tsai HM, Sussman II, Nagel RL: Shear stress enhances the proteolysis of von Willebrand factor in normal plasma. Blood 83:2171–2179, 1994.

45. Tsai HM: Physiologic cleavage of von Willebrand factor by a plasma protease is dependent on its conformation and requires calcium ion. Blood 87:4235–4244, 1996.

46. Furlan M, Robles R, Lammle B: Partial purification and characterization of a protease from human plasma cleaving von Willebrand factor to fragments produced by in vivo proteolysis. Blood 87: 4223–4234, 1996.

47. Bork P, Beckmann G: The CUB domain: A widespread module in developmentally regulated proteins. J Molec Biol 231:530–545, 1993.

48. Barbot J, Costa E, Guerra M, et al: Ten years of prophylactic treatment with fresh-frozen plasma in a child with chronic relapsing thrombotic thrombocytopenic purpura as a result of a congenital deficiency of von Willebrand factor–cleaving protease. Br J Haematol 113:649–651, 2001.

49. Chung DW, Fujikawa K: Processing of von Willebrand factor by ADAMTS-13. Biochemistry 41:11065–11070, 2002.

50. Dong J-F, Moake JL, Bernardo A, et al: ADAMTS-13 metalloprotease interacts with the endothelial cell–derived ultra-large von Willebrand factor. J Biol Chem 278:29633–29639, 2003.

51. Padilla A, Moake JL, Bernardo A, et al: P-selectin anchors newly released ultralarge von Willebrand factor multimers to the endothelial cell surface. Blood 103:2150–2156, 2004.

52. Bernardo A, Ball C, Nolasco L, et al: Effects of inflammatory cytokines on the release and cleavage of the endothelial cell–derived ultra-large von Willebrand factor multimers under flow. Blood 104:100–106, 2004.

53. Bernardo A, Nolasco L, Ball C, et al: Peptides from the C-terminal regions of ADAMTS-13 specifically block cleavage of ultra-large von Willebrand factor multimers on the endothelial surface under flow. J Thromb Haemost, July 2003, Abstract #OC405.

54. Tao Z, Peng Y, Bernardo A, et al: Recombinant CUB-1 domain polypeptide inhibits the cleavage of ULVWF strings by ADAMTS13 under flow conditions. Blood 106:4139–4145, 2005.

55. Majerus EM, Anderson PJ, Sadler JE: Binding of ADAMTS13 to von Willebrand factor. J Biol Chem 280:21773–21778, 2005.

56. Nishio K, Anderson PJ, Zheng XL, Sadler JE: Binding of platelet glycoprotein Ibalpha to von Willebrand factor domain A1 stimulates the cleavage of the adjacent domain A2 by ADAMTS13. Proc Natl Acad Sci U S A 101:10578–10583, 2004.

57. Moake JL, McPherson PD: Abnormalities of von Willebrand factor multimers in thrombotic thrombocytopenic purpura and hemolytic-uremic syndrome. Am J Med 87:9N–15N, 1989.

58. Bianchi V, Robles R, Alberio L, et al: Von Willebrand factor–cleaving protease (ADAMTS13) in thrombotic thrombocytopenic disorders: A severely deficient activity is specific for thrombotic thrombocytopenic purpura. Blood 100:710–713, 2002.

59. Bernardo A, Ball C, Nolasco L, et al: Platelets adhered to endothelial cell-bound ultra-large von Willebrand factor strings support leukocyte tethering and rolling under high shear stress. J Thromb Haemost 3:562–570, 2005.

60. Chow TW, Turner NA, Chintagumpala M, et al: Increased von Willebrand factor binding to platelets in single episode and recurrent types of thrombotic thrombocytopenic purpura. Am J Hematol 57:293–302, 1998.

61. Furlan M, Robles R, Morselli B, et al: Recovery and half-life of von Willebrand factor–cleaving protease after plasma therapy in patients with thrombotic thrombocytopenic purpura. Thromb Haemost 81:8–13, 1999.

62. Allford SL, Harrison P, Lawrie AS, et al: Von Willebrand factor–cleaving protease in congenital thrombotic thrombocytopenic purpura. Br J Haematol 111:1215–1222, 2000.

63. Pimanda JE, Maekawa A, Wind T, et al: Congenital thrombotic thrombocytopenic purpura in association with a mutation in the second CUB domain of ADAMTS13. Blood 103:627–629, 2004.

64. Veyradier A, Obert B, Haddad E, et al: Severe deficiency of the specific von Willebrand factor–cleaving protease (ADAMTS 13) activity in a subgroup of children with atypical hemolytic uremic syndrome. J Pediatr 142:310–317, 2003.

65. Schulman I, Pierce M, Lukens A, Currimbhoy Z: Studies on thrombopoiesis I. A factor in normal human plasma required for platelet production: Chronic thrombocytopenia due to its deficiency. Blood 16:943–957, 1960.

66. Upshaw JD Jr: Congenital deficiency of a factor in normal plasma that reverses microangiopathic hemolysis and thrombocytopenia. N Engl J Med 298:1350–1352, 1978.

67. Vesely SK, George JN, Lammle B, et al: ADAMTS13 activity in thrombotic thrombocytopenic purpura–hemolytic uremic syndrome: Relation to presenting features and clinical outcomes in a prospective cohort of 142 patients. Blood 102:60–68, 2003.

68. Veyradier A, Girma JP: Assays of ADAMTS-13 activity. Semin Hematol 41:41–47, 2004.

69. Tsai H-M, Rice L, Sarode R, et al: Antibody inhibitors to von Willebrand factor metalloproteinase and increased von Willebrand factor–platelet binding in ticlopidine-associated thrombotic thrombocytopenic purpura. Ann Intern Med 132:794–799, 2000.

70. Klaus C, Plaimauer B, Studt JD, et al: Epitope mapping of ADAMTS13 autoantibodies in acquired thrombotic thrombocytopenic purpura. Blood 103:4514–4519, 2004.

71. Majerus EM, Zheng X, Tuley EA, Sadler JE: Cleavage of the ADAMTS13 propeptide is not required for protease activity. J Biol Chem 278:46643–46648, 2003.

72. Studt JD, Hovinga JA, Radonic R, et al: Familial acquired thrombotic thrombocytopenic purpura: ADAMTS-13 inhibitory autoantibodies in identical twins. Blood 103:4195–4197, 2004.

73. Veyradier A, Obert B, Houllier A, et al: Specific von Willebrand factor–cleaving protease in thrombotic microangiopathies: A study of 111 cases. Blood 98:1765–1772, 2001.

74. Zheng XL, Kaufman RM, Goodnough LT, Sadler JE: Effect of plasma exchange on plasma ADAMTS13 metalloprotease activity, inhibitor level, and clinical outcome in patients with idiopathic and non-idiopathic thrombotic thrombocytopenic purpura. Blood 103:4043–4049, 2004.

75. Oleksowicz L, Bhagwati N, DeLoen-Fernandez M: Deficient activity of von Willebrand's factor–cleaving protease in patients with disseminated malignancies. Cancer Res 59:2244–2250, 1999.

76. Mannucci PM, Canciani MT, Forza I, et al: Changes in health and disease of the metalloprotease that cleaves von Willebrand factor. Blood 98:2730–2735, 2001.

77. Neame PD: Immunologic and other factors in thrombotic thrombocytopenic purpura (TTP). Semin Thromb Hemost 6:416–429, 1980.

78. Wada H, Kaneko T, Ohiwa M, et al: Plasma cytokine levels in thrombotic thrombocytopenic purpura. Am J Hematol 40:167–170, 1992.

79. Zauli G, Gugliotta L, Catani L, et al: Increased serum levels of transforming growth factor beta-1 in patients affected by thrombotic thrombocytopenic purpura (TTP): Its implications on bone marrow haematopoiesis. Br J Haematol 84:381–386, 1993.

80. Joseph G, Smith KJ, Hadley TJ, et al: HLA-DR53 protects against thrombotic thrombocytopenic purpura/adult hemolytic uremic syndrome. Am J Hematol 47:189–193, 1994.

81. Nesher G, Hanna VE, Moore TL, et al: Thrombotic microangiographic hemolytic anemia in systemic lupus erythematosus. Semin Arthritis Rheum 24:165–172, 1994.

82. Zacharski LR, Lusted D, Glick JL: Thrombotic thrombocytopenic purpura in a previously splenectomized patient. Am J Med 60:1061–1063, 1976.

83. Yospur LS, Sun NC, Figueroa P, Niihara Y: Concurrent thrombotic thrombocytopenic purpura and immune thrombocytopenic purpura in an HIV-positive patient: Case report and review of the literature. Am J Hematol 51:73–78, 1996.

84. Nair JM, Bellevue R, Bertoni M, Dosik H: Thrombotic thrombocytopenic purpura in patients with the acquired immunodeficiency syndrome (AIDS)-related complex: A report of two cases. Ann Intern Med 109:209–212, 1988.

85. Leaf AN, Laubenstein LJ, Raphael B, et al: Thrombotic thrombocytopenic purpura associated with human immunodeficiency virus type 1 (HIV-1) infection. Ann Intern Med 109:194–197, 1988.

86. Raife T, Atkinson B, Montgomery R, et al: Severe deficiency of VWF-cleaving protease (ADAMTS13) activity defines a distinct population of thrombotic microangiopathy patients. Transfusion 44:146–150, 2004.

87. Mori Y, Wada H, Gabazza EC, et al: Predicting response to plasma exchange in patients with thrombotic thrombocytopenic purpura with measurement of vWF-cleaving protease activity. Transfusion 42:572–580, 2002.

88. van der Plas RM, Schiphorst ME, Huizinga EG, et al: von Willebrand factor proteolysis is deficient in classic, but not in bone marrow transplantation–associated thrombotic thrombocytopenic purpura. Blood 93:3798–3802, 1999.

89. Elliott MA, Nichols WL, Plumhoff EA, et al: Posttransplantation thrombotic thrombocytopenic purpura: A single-center experience and a contemporary review. Mayo Clin Proc 78:421–430, 2003.

90. Volcy J, Nzerue CM, Oderinde A, Hewan-Iowe K: Cocaine-induced acute renal failure, hemolysis, and thrombocytopenia mimicking thrombotic thrombocytopenic purpura. Am J Kidney Dis 35:E3, 2000.

91. Gasser C, Gautier E, Steck A, et al: [Hemolytic-uremic syndrome: Bilateral necrosis of the renal cortex in acute acquired hemolytic anemia.]. Schweiz Med Wochenschr 85:905–909, 1955.

92. Moake JL: Haemolytic-uraemic syndrome: Basic science. Lancet 343:393–397, 1994.

93. Kaplan BS, Proesmans W: The hemolytic uremic syndrome of childhood and its variants. Semin Hematol 24:148–160, 1987.

94. Karmali MA, Petric M, Lim C, et al: The association between idiopathic hemolytic uremic syndrome and infection by verotoxin-producing *Escherichia coli*. J Infect Dis 151:775–782, 1985.

95. Karmali MA: Infection by Shiga toxin–producing *Escherichia coli*: An overview. Mol Biotechnol 26:117–122, 2004.

96. Nolasco L, Turner N, Bernardo A, et al: Hemolytic–uremic syndrome–associated Shiga toxins promote endothelial cell secretion and impair ADAMTS-13 cleavage of unusually large von Willebrand factor multimers. Blood 106:4199–4209, 2005.

97. Warwicker P, Goodship THJ, Donne RL, et al: Genetic studies into inherited and sporadic hemolytic uremic syndrome. Kidney Int 53:836–844, 1998.

98. Bonnardeaux A, Pichette V: Complement dysregulation in haemolytic uraemic syndrome. Lancet 362:1514–1515, 2003.

99. Fremeaux-Bacchi V, Dragon-Durey MA, Blouin J, et al: Complement factor I: A susceptibility gene for atypical haemolytic uraemic syndrome. J Med Genet 41:e84, 2004.

100. Byrnes JJ, Moake JL: Thrombotic thrombocytopenic purpura and the hemolytic-uremic syndrome: Evolving concepts of pathogenesis and therapy. Clin Haematol 15:413–442, 1986.

101. Goodman A, Ramos R, Petrelli M, et al: Gingival biopsy in thrombotic thrombocytopenic purpura. Ann Intern Med 89:501–504, 1978.

102. Frangos JA, Moake JL, Nolasco L, et al: Cryosupernatant regulates accumulation of unusually large vWF multimers from endothelial cells. Am J Physiol 256:H1635–H1644, 1989.

103. Yarranton H, Lawrie AS, Purdy G, et al: Comparison of von Willebrand factor antigen, von Willebrand factor–cleaving protease and protein S in blood components used for treatment of thrombotic thrombocytopenic purpura. Transfus Med 14:39–44, 2004.

104. Rock G, Shumak KH, Sutton DM, et al: Cryosupernatant as replacement fluid for plasma exchange in thrombotic thrombocytopenic purpura. Members of the Canadian Apheresis Group. Br J Haematol 94:383–386, 1996.

105. Byrnes JJ, Moake JL, Klug P, Periman P: Effectiveness of the cryosupernatant fraction of plasma in the treatment of refractory thrombotic thrombocytopenic purpura. Am J Hematol 34:169–174, 1990.

106. Abassi E, Yawn D, Leveque C, et al: Correlation of ADAMTS-13 activity with response to plasma exchange in patients diagnosed with thrombotic thrombocytopenic purpura. Blood 104:242a, 2004. Abstract #3921.

107. Tsai HM: High titers of inhibitors of von Willebrand factor–cleaving metalloproteinase in a fatal case of acute thrombotic thrombocytopenic purpura. Am J Hematol 65:251–255, 2000.

108. Tsai HM, Li A, Rock G: Inhibitors of von Willebrand factor–cleaving protease in thrombotic thrombocytopenic purpura. Clin Lab 47:387–392, 2001.

109. Gutterman LA, Kloster B, Tsai HM: Rituximab therapy for refractory thrombotic thrombocytopenic purpura. Blood Cell Mol Dis 28:385–391, 2002.

110. Chemnitz J, Draube A, Scheid C, et al: Successful treatment of severe thrombotic thrombocytopenic purpura with the monoclonal antibody rituximab. Am J Hematol 71:105–108, 2002.

111. Reff M, Carner K, Chambers K, et al: Depletion of B cells in vivo by a chimeric mouse human monoclonal antibody to CD20. Blood 83:435–445, 1994.

112. Tsai HM, Shulman K: Rituximab induces remission of cerebral ischemia caused by thrombotic thrombocytopenic purpura. Eur J Haematol 70:183–185, 2003.

113. Zheng X, Pallera AM, Goodnough LT, et al: Remission of chronic thrombotic thrombocytopenic purpura after treatment with cyclophosphamide and rituximab. Ann Intern Med 138:105–108, 2003.

114. Thompson CE, Damon LE, Ries CA, Linker CA: Thrombotic microangiopathies in the 1980s: Clinical features, response to treatment, and the impact of the human immunodeficiency virus epidemic. Blood 80:1890–1895, 1992.

115. Crowther MA, Heddle N, Hayward CPM, et al: Splenectomy done during hematologic remission to prevent relapse in patients with thrombotic thrombocytopenic purpura. Ann Intern Med 125:294–296, 1996.

116. Kremer Hovinga JA, Studt JD, Demarmels Biasiutti F, et al: Splenectomy in relapsing and plasma-refractory acquired thrombotic thrombocytopenic purpura. Haematologica 89:320–324, 2004.

117. Downes KA, Yomtovian R, Tsai HM, et al: Relapsed thrombotic thrombocytopenic purpura presenting as an acute cerebrovascular accident. J Clin Apheresis 19:86–89, 2004.

118. Gordon LI, Kwaan HC, Rossi EC: Deleterious effects of platelet transfusions and recovery thrombocytosis in patients with thrombotic microangiopathy. Semin Hematol 24:194–201, 1987.

119. Gutterman LA, Stevenson TD: Treatment of thrombotic thrombocytopenic purpura with vincristine. JAMA 247:1433–1436, 1982.

120. Moake JL, Rudy CK, Troll JH, et al: Therapy of chronic relapsing thrombotic thrombocytopenic purpura with prednisone and azathioprine. Am J Hematol 20:73–79, 1985.

121. Rosove MH, Ho WG, Goldfinger D: Ineffectiveness of aspirin and dipyridamole in the treatment of thrombotic thrombocytopenic purpura. Ann Intern Med 96:27–33, 1982.

122. del Zoppo GJ: Antiplatelet therapy in thrombotic thrombocytopenic purpura. Semin Hematol 24:130–139, 1987.

123. Hardwick RA, Hellums JD, Moake JL, et al: Effects of antiplatelet agents on platelets exposed to shear stress. Trans Am Soc Artif Intern Organs 26:179–184, 1980.

124. Banerjee D, Kupin W, Roth D: Hemolytic uremic syndrome after multivisceral transplantation treated with intravenous immunoglobulin. J Nephrol 16:733–735, 2003.

125. Gatti S, Arru M, Reggiani P, et al: Successful treatment of hemolytic uremic syndrome after liver-kidney transplantation. J Nephrol 16:586–590, 2003.

126. Korec S, Schein PS, Smith FP, et al: Treatment of cancer-associated hemolytic-uremic syndrome with staphylococcal protein A immunoperfusion. J Clin Oncol 4:210–215, 1986.

127. Plaimauer B, Zimmermann K, Volkel D, et al: Cloning, expression, and functional characterization of the von Willebrand factor–cleaving protease (ADAMTS13). Blood 100:3626–3632, 2002.

128. Zhou W, Dong L, Ginsburg D, et al: Enzymatically active ADAMTS13 variants are not inhibited by anti-ADAMTS13 autoantibodies: A novel therapeutic strategy? J Biol Chem 280:39934–39941, 2005.

III

Chapter 25

Heparin-Induced Thrombocytopenia

Theodore E. Warkentin, MD

HISTORICAL OVERVIEW[1]

In 1958, a vascular surgeon, Rodger Weismann, and his resident, Richard Tobin, reported ten patients from whom they had extracted unusual platelet–fibrin thrombi that formed during a 1- to 2-week treatment course with heparin. These physicians suspected a causal relationship with heparin, perhaps via heparin-induced embolization of thrombus from the proximal aorta (the paucity of red cells in the thrombi argued against a cardiac origin). It was not until 1973, however, that another vascular surgeon (Donald Silver), a resident (R. H. Dixon), and a medical student (Glen R. Rhodes) recognized the concurrence of thrombocytopenia in similar patients. They observed that heparin rechallenge soon after platelet count recovery caused abrupt recurrence of thrombocytopenia. Moreover, patient plasma and heparin added to normal platelets in vitro caused platelet aggregation, suggesting that a patient-dependent factor such as immunoglobulin G (IgG) was responsible. In 1977, Silver and colleagues described eight patients with thrombocytopenia that complicated heparin use, noting thrombotic complications (usually affecting arteries) in seven of the patients. Drawing on the similar clinical profile depicted by Weismann and Tobin almost two decades before, Silver proposed the existence of a heparin-induced, antibody-mediated prothrombotic disorder with a paradoxical association with thrombocytopenia and a predilection for causing arterial thromboembolism.

Over the next two decades, the clinical and pathologic features of this distinct syndrome—now known as heparin-induced thrombocytopenia (HIT)—gradually emerged.[1–3] The presence of heparin-dependent, platelet-activating IgG antibodies became the laboratory hallmark of this syndrome, and sensitive and specific platelet activation assays were developed to detect the antibodies.[4,5] In 1992, Jean Amiral and associates identified the target antigen of HIT—a multimolecular complex between platelet factor 4 (PF4) and heparin.[6] This breakthrough led to the development of a new class of antigen assays that could be used to detect pathogenic "HIT antibodies." Over time, it became apparent that the spectrum of thrombosis complicating HIT included venous thrombosis; indeed, deep venous thrombosis (DVT) and pulmonary embolism appeared to occur even more often than arterial thrombosis.[3,7–9] The importance of venous thrombosis in HIT was underscored by the recognition in 1997 of an iatrogenic syndrome of limb loss in HIT—venous limb gangrene—in which warfarin treatment was implicated as the cause for progression of DVT to limb necrosis.[10] This study also found marked in vivo thrombin generation in HIT, giving rise to the concept that parallel activation of coagulation—rather than platelet activation alone—was central to the prothrombotic nature of HIT. This new concept coincided with the recognition that effective treatments for HIT consist of agents that reduce thrombin generation or directly inhibit thrombin.[2]

TERMINOLOGY

Most patients who develop thrombocytopenia during heparin treatment do not have HIT. Accordingly, various terms have been developed to distinguish HIT from other explanations for thrombocytopenia (Table 25-1).[2] The widely used term *heparin-induced thrombocytopenia* generally refers to the antibody-mediated syndrome and is used in this context in this chapter. Sometimes, however, *HIT type II* is used to indicate the immune-mediated syndrome. Although heparin may contribute to mild thrombocytopenia via nonimmune platelet–activating mechanisms (sometimes designated *HIT type I*), from a practical standpoint, this phenomenon usually cannot be distinguished from other clinical explanations for thrombocytopenia. Thus, the recommended term for these patients is *nonimmune heparin–associated thrombocytopenia*. Sometimes, such a patient's clinical picture so strongly resembles HIT that the term *pseudo-HIT* may be appropriate (vide infra).[11] *Subclinical seroconversion* refers to the situation in which anti-PF4/heparin antibodies may be detected but are not believed to be causing adverse clinical events such as thrombocytopenia or thrombosis. For example, a patient with septicemia-associated thrombocytopenia who has received heparin and who has detectable anti-PF4/heparin antibodies of the (nonpathogenic) IgM class has subclinical seroconversion.

PATHOGENESIS

The main pathologic event in HIT is formation of heparin-dependent antibodies of the IgG class that activate platelets via platelet FcγIIa receptors.[12,13] These antibodies recognize multimolecular complexes between a positively charged platelet α-granule protein, PF4 (member of the C-X-C subfamily of chemokines), and heparin.[6,14,15] Antigens formed appear on one or more sites of PF4 that have been conformationally modified because of binding to heparin.[16–19] Certain negatively charged substances other than

Table 25-1   Terminology of Thrombocytopenia Complicating Heparin Treatment

Terminology	Comment
Heparin-Induced Thrombocytopenia (HIT)	*Recommended term:*[2] widely used and denotes role of heparin in inducing thrombocytopenia
HIT type II	Popular term first used by Chong[1]
Heparin-associated thrombocytopenia (HAT)	Confusing, as term is used for both immune and nonimmune thrombocytopenias
Heparin-induced thrombocytopenia/ thrombosis syndrome (HITT or HITTS)	Sometimes used to denote that the patient with HIT has developed thrombosis
White clot syndrome	Indicates that the patient has platelet-rich thrombi in the artery(ies)
Delayed-onset HIT	Indicates HIT that begins after heparin exposure has been stopped
Nonimmune Heparin–Associated Thrombocytopenia (Nonimmune HAT)	*Recommended term:*[2] makes explicit the lack of immune causes, as well as the uncertain relationship between platelet count fall and heparin
HIT type I	Popular term first used by Chong[1]
Pseudo-HIT	Clinical situation that strongly mimics HIT
Subclinical seroconversion	Anti–platelet factor 4 (PF4)/heparin antibodies detected but not believed to be responsible for thrombocytopenia or other clinical events

heparin also support antigenic modification of PF4. For example, platelet-associated chondroitin sulfate can support binding of PF4,[20] which may explain the occurrence or persistence of HIT in some patients after heparin has been stopped. The highly sulfated anticancer agent pentosan polysulfate can induce thrombocytopenia and thrombosis caused by antibodies indistinguishable from those generated in HIT.[21] Also, PF4 complexed with polyvinyl sulfonate binds HIT antibodies[22]; this provides the basis for a commercial antigen assay for HIT.

Ultra-large PF4/heparin complexes are more efficiently formed by unfractionated heparin (UFH) rather than by low molecular weight heparin (LMWH),[23] which perhaps helps to explain why the former heparin type is more likely to cause HIT.[7,8] Heparin chains must be at least 12 to 14 saccharide units in length to form the HIT antigen, together with PF4.[22,24] However, recent studies[25] suggest that the thrombin inhibitor pentasaccharide, fondaparinux, can induce anti-PF4/heparin antibodies at a frequency similar to that of LMWH; ironically, these antibodies bind poorly to PF4/fondaparinux.[25,26] These observations suggest that immunogenicity (formation of antibody) and cross-reactivity (binding of antibodies to PF4/polyanion complexes) of polysaccharide anticoagulants are dissociated.[27] (See also section on prevention of HIT at the end of this chapter.)

Figure 25-1 summarizes the pathogenesis of HIT and emphasizes the central role of thrombin generation.[28] Levels of thrombin/antithrombin complexes (a marker of in vivo thrombin generation) are far greater in patients with HIT than in control subjects.[10,29] At least two factors probably contribute to increased thrombin generation. First, Fc receptor–mediated platelet activation by HIT/IgG antibodies causes formation of procoagulant, platelet-derived microparticles that accelerate coagulation reactions.[30–32] Second, PF4 released from platelets neutralizes the anticoagulant effects of heparin. In addition, it is possible that HIT antibodies effect procoagulant changes to endothelium[33] and monocytes,[34] as well as aggregation of polymorphonuclear leukocytes.[35] Such pancellular activation may help to explain the dramatic nature of some HIT-associated thrombi, such as white clots in large arteries. However, it remains uncertain whether activa-tion of cells other than platelets results from direct binding of HIT antibodies, or whether it occurs via inter-mediaries such as activated platelets or their products (microparticles).[36,37]

No clear genetic predisposition to HIT has been identified. Unlike some other immune-mediated thrombocytopenic disorders, no human leukocyte antigen (HLA) association has been identified.[38] Although an Arg_{131}/His_{131} $Fc\gamma RIIa$ receptor polymorphism is known to influence antibody-induced platelet activation, evidence conflicts regarding whether one of the genotypes is significantly more likely to be associated with HIT.[39] Recently, an $Fc\gamma RIIIa$ receptor polymorphism—Phe_{158}/Val_{158}—was shown to influence risk of HIT among patients in whom anti-PF4/heparin antibodies had formed: the concept proposed was that the homozygous Val_{158} predisposes to HIT by leading to greater platelet clearance by the phagocytic system.[40] Finally, the surprising observation was reported that repeated heparin exposure in patients with a previous history of HIT does not usually cause recurrence of HIT antibodies.[41] A related observation is that HIT antibodies are transient and are usually not detectable several weeks or months after an episode of HIT (mean time to antibody nondetectability, 50 to 80 days, depending on the assay performed).[41] Perhaps, absence of long-lasting immunologic memory explains these unusual clinical features of HIT.

Only a few of the patients in whom anti-PF4/heparin antibodies form during heparin treatment develop thrombocytopenia.[7,8,42] High-titer antibodies of the IgG class[43] that are detectable through sensitive platelet activation assays[44] are most likely to cause thrombocytopenia. Although anecdotal reports suggest that IgM and/or IgA antibodies may cause HIT,[45] this remains to be confirmed and seems unlikely.[46,47] Besides formation of pathogenic antibodies, some platelet-dependent factors, such as high $Fc\gamma IIa$ receptor numbers[48] and high platelet-associated PF4 levels,[20] may also be important.

Coexisting clinical factors strongly influence localization of thrombosis in HIT. For example, postoperative orthopaedic patients with HIT are much more likely to develop venous thrombosis, including pulmonary embolism, than arterial thrombotic events.[7,8] In contrast,

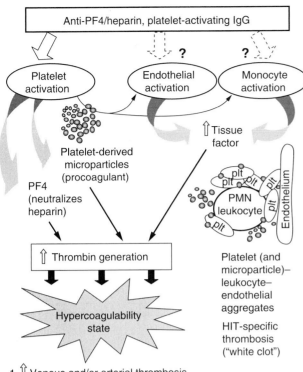

Figure 25-1 Pathogenesis of heparin-induced thrombocytopenia (HIT): a central role for thrombin generation. This figure illustrates two explanations for thrombosis in HIT. (1) Activation of platelets (Plt) by anti–platelet factor 4 (PF4)/heparin immunoglobulin (Ig)G antibodies (HIT antibodies), leading to formation of procoagulant, platelet-derived microparticles and neutralization of heparin by PF4 released from activated platelets, leads to marked increases in thrombin ("hypercoagulability state") that are characterized by increased risk for venous and arterial thrombosis and coumarin-induced venous limb gangrene. (2) However, it is also possible that unique pathogenetic mechanisms operative in HIT may explain unusual thromboses, such as arterial "white clots." For example, HIT antibodies have been shown to activate endothelium and monocytes (leading to cell surface tissue factor expression), although this stimulation may be largely "indirect" because of poorly defined mechanisms involving platelet activation and, possibly, formation of platelet-derived microparticles. Further, aggregates of platelets and polymorphonuclear (PMN) leukocytes have been described in HIT. To what extent these cooperative interactions between platelets, platelet-derived microparticles, PMN leukocytes, monocytes, and endothelium may lead to arterial (or venous) thrombotic events in HIT in large or small vessels remains unclear. (From Warkentin TE: An overview of the heparin-induced thrombocytopenia syndrome. Semin Thromb Hemost 30:273–283, 2004, with permission.[28])

post–cardiac surgery and medical patients are about as likely to develop arterial thrombosis as venous events.[42] Injury to blood vessels, such as that caused by indwelling catheters, is strongly associated with thrombosis in the affected vein or artery.[49,50]

FREQUENCY

The type of heparin preparation, the duration of treatment, the definition of thrombocytopenia used, and the patient population to whom heparin is given are among the factors that influence the frequency of HIT.[42] UFH causes HIT far more often than does LMWH (by at least an order of magnitude).[7,8,42,51–53] A meta-analysis found that heparin obtained from bovine lung is more likely to cause HIT than is heparin derived from porcine gut[42]; another study reported a higher rate of antibody formation with bovine compared with porcine UFH.[54] Greater immunogenicity and increased risk of HIT with bovine UFH likely reflect a longer chain length and a greater degree of sulfation, compared with porcine UFH.[42]

Because HIT typically begins after 5 or more days of heparin use, limiting heparin use to less than 5 days, when appropriate, should theoretically reduce the frequency of HIT. However, this approach may fail on occasion because even a brief exposure to heparin occasionally triggers formation of potent HIT antibodies that may cause thrombocytopenia and thrombosis, beginning several days after heparin has been stopped, so-called delayed-onset HIT.[50,55–58]

Sometimes, the "standard" platelet count threshold that indicates thrombocytopenia (150,000/µL) is inappropriate for use in defining HIT. For example, transient thrombocytosis is common 1 to 2 weeks after major surgery is performed. In such patients, an otherwise unexpected fall in platelet count during heparin treatment that exceeds 50% from the postoperative peak strongly suggests HIT.[8,50] When this definition of thrombocytopenia is used, the frequency of HIT is about 3% to 5% in postoperative orthopaedic patients who are administered UFH prophylaxis for 2 weeks.[8,52] Some investigators have used a lower proportionate platelet count decline of 30%[52,59] or 40%[60] to define thrombocytopenia.

Some patient populations are at greater risk for HIT (Fig. 25-2).[42,44] For example, cardiac surgical patients are most likely to form anti-PF4/heparin antibodies (approximate 50% to 70% risk[42,44,61]), but less than 5% of antibody-positive patients develop HIT (overall frequency of HIT, 1% to 2%). In contrast, although IgG antibodies form that are detectable by antigen assay in only 15% to 30% of orthopaedic patients who are administered UFH, as many as one sixth to one third of these patients develop HIT (overall frequency of HIT, 3% to 5%) (see Fig. 25-2).[42,44,46] HIT is less common in medical than in surgical patients and is rare during pregnancy.[42] Women are somewhat more likely than men to develop HIT.[62]

Platelet Count Monitoring for Heparin-Induced Thrombocytopenia

In recent years, recommendations to guide platelet count monitoring for HIT have taken into account the risk of HIT in various clinical situations.[5,63] Table 25-2 summarizes these recommendations. Platelet count should also be measured within a day of heparin initiation in a patient who has recently received this drug (within the past 100 days),[63] or in any patient who presents with thrombosis or other sequelae of HIT during or soon after receiving heparin therapy.

CLINICAL FEATURES

Table 25-3 lists the typical clinical features of HIT.

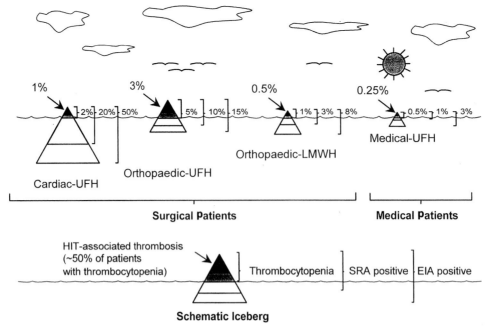

Figure 25-2 Multiple-iceberg model of heparin-induced thrombocytopenia (HIT). A schematic "iceberg," shown on the lower "water line," illustrates relations among HIT-associated thrombosis, thrombocytopenia, HIT antibodies detected by serotonin release assay (SRA), and HIT antibodies detected by platelet factor 4 (PF4)/polyanion enzyme immunoassay (EIA). Above, the relative sizes of the various icebergs reflect the relative frequency of HIT antibody formation, thrombocytopenia, and HIT-associated thrombosis among several different patient populations. Note that unfractionated heparin (UFH) is more likely than low molecular weight heparin (LMWH) to cause HIT among post–orthopaedic surgery patients. However, patient population–dependent effects are also evident (e.g., although cardiac surgical patients are more likely to form HIT antibodies, among patients who form HIT antibodies, orthopaedic patients are most likely to develop HIT). (From Lee DH, Warkentin TE: Frequency of heparin-induced thrombocytopenia. In Warkentin TE, Greinacher A [eds]: Heparin-Induced Thrombocytopenia, 3rd ed. New York, Marcel Dekker, 2004, pp 107–148, with permission.)

Table 25-2   Platelet Count Monitoring for Heparin-Induced Thrombocytopenia

Risk of HIT	Frequency of Platelet Count Monitoring
High (>1%): postoperative patients receiving UFH thromboprophylaxis; patients receiving therapeutic doses of UFH	At least alternate day platelet counts from day 4 to day 14 (if still receiving heparin)
Moderate (0.1%–1%): postoperative patients receiving LMWH; medical patients receiving UFH	Minimum, 2 or 3 platelet counts between day 4 and day 14 (if still receiving heparin)
Low (<0.1%): e.g., medical or pregnant patients receiving LMWH	Routine platelet count monitoring *not* recommended

This table summarizes recommendations found elsewhere.[5,63]
UFH, unfractionated heparin; LMWH, low molecular weight heparin.

Temporal Profile

The hallmark of HIT is a platelet count fall that begins between days 5 and 10 after heparin is started (first day of heparin use = day zero) (Fig. 25-3).[41] Such a "typical" onset is observed in about 70% of patients with HIT. In the remaining patients, a "rapid" onset of HIT occurs. Generally speaking, this situation is characterized by a patient who has recently received heparin (within the past 5 to 100 days), and in whom resumption of heparin causes an abrupt fall in the platelet count. This profile is caused by acute platelet activation in a patient with circulating, pre-existing HIT antibodies, formed in relation to recent heparin exposure, rather than rapid regeneration of HIT

antibodies because of an "anamnestic" (immune memory) response.[41,64]

Severity of Thrombocytopenia

Mild to moderate severity of thrombocytopenia is characteristic of HIT; the median platelet count nadir is about 60,000/μL,[65] and the platelet count falls to below 15,000/μL in only 5% of patients (Fig. 25-4). Remarkably, even when a patient with HIT develops such severe thrombocytopenia, petechiae usually are not seen. This clinical profile differs strikingly from that of patients with drug-induced immune thrombocytopenic purpura caused by quinine, quinidine, and sulfa antibiotics, in which the platelet count

Table 25-3   Clinical Features of Heparin-Induced Thrombocytopenia

Timing of Thrombocytopenia

Typical onset: between days 5 and 10 after heparin initiation (first day of immunizing heparin exposure = day 0)
Rapid onset: <1 day after resumption of heparin (in a patient recently exposed to heparin, and who therefore has residual circulating HIT antibodies)

Severity of Thrombocytopenia

Platelet count nadir: 15,000 to 150,000/μL in about 90% of patients (median nadir, about 50,000 to 60,000/μL in large patient series); sometimes, a platelet count decline that does not fall below 150,000/μL occurs in HIT; platelet count <15,000/μL occurs in only 5% of patients

Thrombosis is Common

>50% develop new thrombosis
Venous thrombosis: DVT > pulmonary embolism > warfarin-induced venous limb gangrene > adrenal hemorrhagic necrosis* > cerebral sinus thrombosis
Arterial thrombosis: limb artery thrombosis > stroke syndrome > myocardial infarction > mesenteric artery thrombosis > other arterial thromboses

Absence of Petechiae (even when platelets <15,000/μL)

Skin Lesions at Heparin Injection Sites

Severity ranges from erythematous plaques to skin necrosis

Acute Systemic (Anaphylactoid) Reactions After Intravenous Bolus Heparin

Acute inflammatory or cardiorespiratory signs, or neurologic (headache, transient global amnesia) or miscellaneous (e.g., flushing, diarrhea) signs and symptoms associated with abrupt platelet count fall

*Evidence suggests that adrenal hemorrhage complicating HIT is associated with adrenal infarction related to adrenal vein thrombosis.
HIT, heparin-induced thrombocytopenia; DVT, deep venous thrombosis.

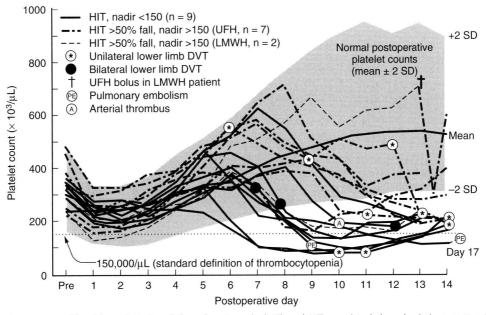

Figure 25-3   Platelet count profile of heparin-induced thrombocytopenia (HIT) and HIT-associated thrombosis in a post–orthopaedic surgery population. The bold line and shaded area indicate the geometric mean (±2 SD) platelet count in normal post–orthopaedic patients. Eighteen patients developed HIT (≥50% fall in platelet count between postoperative days 4 and 14): 9 patients had a platelet count nadir of less than 150,000/μL, and 9 patients had a platelet count nadir equal to or above 150,000/μL. Overall, 18 thrombotic events occurred in 13 of 18 patients with HIT. Note: Bilateral deep venous thrombosis (DVT) is counted as two thrombotic events, and pulmonary embolism (PE) is also counted as a thrombotic event. (This figure is a composite of two previous published figures from the following: Warkentin TE, Levine MN, Hirsh J, et al: Heparin-induced thrombocytopenia in patients treated with low-molecular-weight heparin or unfractionated heparin. N Engl J Med 332:1330–1335, 1995, with permission[7]; and Warkentin TE, Roberts RS, Hirsh J, Kelton JG: An improved definition of immune heparin-induced thrombocytopenia in postoperative orthopedic patients. Arch Intern Med 163:2518–2524, 2003, with permission.[8])

nadir is below 15,000/μL in most patients, and mucocutaneous hemorrhage is characteristic.

Venous Thrombosis

Venous thrombosis is the most common thrombotic complication.[3,9,50] As many as 50% of patients with HIT develop symptomatic DVT, and about half of these patients develop pulmonary embolism.[50,66] Some patients with DVT experience severe limb ischemia, including phlegmasia cerulea dolens and venous limb gangrene (vide infra). Adrenal vein thrombosis is believed to be the explanation for adrenal hemorrhagic necrosis, which occurs in about 3% to 5% of patients with HIT.[50] Bilateral adrenal hemorrhage causes

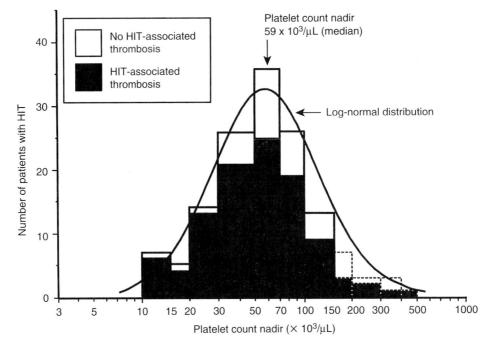

Figure 25-4 Platelet count nadirs of 142 patients with heparin-induced thrombocytopenia (HIT). A log-normal distribution of platelet count nadirs is seen (median platelet count nadir, 59,000/μL). HIT-associated thrombosis occurred in most patients with HIT, irrespective of the platelet count nadir. (From Warkentin TE: Clinical presentation of heparin-induced thrombocytopenia. Semin Hematol 35(suppl 5):9–16, 1998, with permission.[65])

acute and/or chronic adrenal failure, and prompt recognition of this complication, with institution of cortisol replacement, can be lifesaving.[67] Cerebral sinus thrombosis is another unusual life-threatening venous thrombotic event that is associated with HIT.[57,58,68]

Arterial Thrombosis

Arterial thrombosis was the first complication identified as a feature of HIT.[1] Characteristic pale thrombi extracted by surgeons led to the term *white clot syndrome* that is still sometimes used to indicate HIT. The typical location of thrombi in HIT, namely, lower limb artery occlusion > stroke syndrome > myocardial infarction, is the converse of that observed in (non-HIT) atherothrombosis (myocardial infarction > stroke syndrome > lower limb artery occlusion).[50]

Limb Ischemic Syndromes

Several explanations may be offered for limb-threatening ischemia in a given patient with HIT:[50] (1) occlusion of the distal aorta or iliofemoral or other large limb arteries by occlusive platelet-rich thromboemboli; (2) microembolization to small arteries/arterioles, or in situ formation of small thrombi within the microcirculation (distal limb ischemia despite palpable or Doppler-identifiable pulses); (3) severe DVT progressing to phlegmasia cerulea dolens; and (4) warfarin-induced venous limb gangrene. The last syndrome was the most common explanation for limb loss in one series.[10] Overt (decompensated) disseminated intravascular coagulation (DIC) manifest as hypofibrinogenemia, elevated international normalized ratio (INR), or red cell fragmentation is sometimes observed in patients with limb ischemia associated with microvascular thrombosis.[50]

Microvascular Thrombotic Complications of Warfarin

Table 25-4 summarizes two syndromes of tissue necrosis that may complicate coumarin (warfarin) therapy in patients with HIT:[10,29,69–73] venous limb gangrene and classic skin necrosis. In both syndromes, a profound disturbance in procoagulant/anticoagulant balance, namely, a failure of the protein C natural anticoagulant pathway to downregulate increased thrombin in the microvasculature, is believed to be present (Fig. 25-5).[10,69,70] Of the two syndromes, HIT is more likely to be complicated by venous limb gangrene.

Venous limb gangrene reportedly occurred in 8 of 66 (12%) patients with acute DVT complicating HIT in whom treatment included warfarin.[10] In some patients, concomitant use of a defibrinogenating snake venom, ancrod, may have contributed to this complication by increasing thrombin generation.[74] Although the frequency of this syndrome may be less than 5% to 10% in patients administered warfarin alone,[75] it is prudent to avoid warfarin anticoagulation in acute HIT until the patient is well anticoagulated with a parenteral agent that reduces thrombin generation, and until thrombocytopenia has substantially or, preferably, completely recovered.[63,76,77] Further, if HIT is diagnosed in a patient who is receiving warfarin, vitamin K should be promptly administered.[63,76–78]

Warfarin-induced venous limb gangrene has a distinct feature: a supratherapeutic INR that coincides with progression of DVT to distal limb necrosis. This characteristic elevation in INR is caused by a severe reduction in factor VII that parallels a severe reduction in protein C,[10] that is, the high INR is a surrogate marker for a low protein C level.[79] Early recognition of this syndrome and reversal of

Table 25-4 Warfarin-Induced Necrosis Syndromes: Venous Limb Gangrene Versus Classic Skin Necrosis

	Warfarin-Induced Venous Limb Gangrene	Classic Warfarin-Induced Skin Necrosis (WISN)
Clinical Picture	Necrosis of acral tissues in limb(s) affected by DVT during warfarin therapy that results in a supratherapeutic INR (typically, >3.5); this syndrome may follow a prodrome of phlegmasia cerulea dolens	Necrosis of skin and subdermal tissues, especially in central sites (e.g., breasts, buttocks, abdomen, thighs, calves) that begins 3 to 7 days after warfarin is begun
Predisposing Disorders	(1) Acute HIT; (2) adenocarcinoma associated with DIC	(1) Congenital deficiency of natural anticoagulant: (protein C > protein S > antithrombin III); (2) factor V Leiden; (3) acute HIT
Pathogenesis	Acquired severe deficiency of protein C, usually during initiation of warfarin therapy; at the same time, warfarin fails to downregulate increased thrombin generation associated with the underlying disorder (HIT or adenocarcinoma)	Unknown; believed to be caused in some patients by acquired severe deficiency of protein C related to preexisting congenital deficiency and rapid further fall in protein C levels on starting warfarin treatment (because of short half-life for protein C)

DVT, deep venous thrombosis; INR, international normalized ratio; HIT, heparin-induced thrombocytopenia; DIC, disseminated intravascular coagulation.

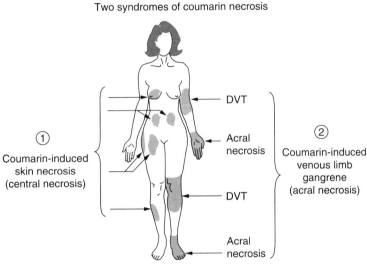

Figure 25-5 Two syndromes of coumarin (warfarin)-induced necrosis. (1) Coumarin-induced skin necrosis (central necrosis) and (2) coumarin-induced venous limb gangrene. Coumarin-induced skin necrosis most commonly affects the breasts, abdomen, thighs, buttocks, and calves and is often symmetrical; it is usually associated with congenital or acquired abnormalities in the protein C natural anticoagulant pathway. In contrast, venous limb gangrene occurs in patients with disseminated intravascular coagulation (DIC) associated with heparin-induced thrombocytopenia (HIT) or adenocarcinoma. This syndrome is characterized by microvascular thrombosis in a limb affected by deep venous thrombosis (DVT) that leads to acral (distal extremity) ischemic necrosis. (Reprinted, with modifications and with permission, from Warkentin TE: Heparin-induced thrombocytopenia: IgG-mediated platelet activation, platelet microparticle generation, and altered procoagulant/anticoagulant balance in the pathogenesis of thrombosis and venous limb gangrene complciating heparin-induced thrombocyopenia (HIT). Transfus Med Rev 10:249–258, 1996.[70])

warfarin anticoagulation with intravenous vitamin K and fresh frozen plasma may be limb saving.[10] Uncontrolled DIC associated with adenocarcinoma is another clinical situation that has been associated with limb gangrene during warfarin therapy.[11,79,80]

Heparin-Induced Skin Lesions

Inflammatory plaque–like or necrotic lesions that begin 6 or more days after subcutaneous injections of UFH or LMWH are begun are a manifestation of the HIT syndrome.[50,81,82] For unknown reasons, only a minority of patients who develop HIT during subcutaneous heparin usage develop injection site skin lesions. Many patients with heparin-induced skin lesions do not develop concomitant thrombocytopenia, even when HIT antibodies are detected by sensitive antigen or activation assays. Platelet counts should continue to be monitored for a few days in all patients with heparin-induced skin lesions; thrombocytopenia and thrombosis sometimes occur after heparin therapy has been discontinued.[83]

Neurologic Syndromes

Stroke syndromes caused by arterial (or even venous) thrombi are relatively common in HIT.[50] Cerebral sinus thrombosis[57,68,84] is suggested by headache, a decreased level of consciousness, and focal neurologic defects. Transient global amnesia is a rare complication of HIT that may follow an intravenous bolus of heparin.[50,85] Lower limb paralysis associated with infarction of the spinal cord or lumbosacral plexus has been reported.

Cardiac Syndromes

Besides myocardial infarction, other cardiac complications of HIT include intraventricular and intra-atrial thrombus formation that may lead to peripheral or pulmonary embolism. Cardiopulmonary arrest occurring shortly after intravenous heparin bolus administration is another manifestation of HIT.[50,86]

Outpatient Presentation of Heparin-Induced Thrombocytopenia (Delayed-Onset HIT)

HIT is often viewed as a diagnosis that affects hospital inpatients. However, some patients can develop potent platelet-activating antibodies after a brief course of heparin that results in thrombocytopenia and thrombosis, beginning several days *after* cessation of heparin.[50,55–58] With a diagnosis of *delayed-onset HIT*, such patients typically have very strong positive test results for HIT antibodies by immunoassay or platelet activation assay.[55] Platelet activation in the absence of heparin is another feature that is exhibited by some sera.

Heparin-Induced Thrombocytopenia in Children

HIT has been reported in children.[87–89] However, the frequency is less than that seen in adults. Although neonates develop HIT rarely, if at all,[90] older infants and children are at risk, particularly after cardiac surgery[88,91] or during treatment of thrombosis with UFH.[88] The ratio of venous to arterial thrombosis may be even higher in pediatric than in adult HIT.[88] Experience in treating children with HIT has been limited.[87–89,92]

DIFFERENTIAL DIAGNOSIS

Thrombocytopenia occurs commonly in hospitalized patients; most patients who develop a platelet count fall during heparin therapy do not have HIT. Indeed, in the intensive care unit, the estimated frequency of HIT (about 0.3% to 0.5%) is 100 times less than the frequency of thrombocytopenia from any cause (30% to 50%).[93–95] When thrombocytopenia occurs early during heparin treatment (within the first 4 days), the explanation usually rests with the patient's reason for hospitalization (e.g., hemodilution and platelet consumption after surgery, septicemia, DIC). However, HIT should be suspected in a patient with early-onset thrombocytopenia when the degree of platelet count fall is greater than would be expected for the patient's clinical situation and when the patient has recently been exposed to heparin (past few weeks or months). Indeed, such a rapid onset of thrombocytopenia occurs in about 25% of all patients in whom HIT is diagnosed.[41]

Pseudo-HIT refers to the condition diagnosed in patients whose clinical profile appears to suggest HIT, but in whom HIT antibodies cannot be detected by sensitive assays (Table 25-5).[11] For example, Figure 25-6 shows the courses of two patients with very similar platelet count profiles: one patient had pulmonary embolism–associated thrombocytopenia, and the other had HIT-associated pulmonary embolism.[11,96] For the former patient with pseudo-HIT, increased doses of heparin (to overcome heparin "resistance") resulted in platelet count and clinical recovery (see Fig. 25-6A).

CLINICAL SCORING SYSTEM

In evaluating a patient for possible HIT, the use of a clinical scoring system might be helpful. In one system, the 4 T's[97] (Table 25-6), the clinician assesses the likelihood of HIT on the basis of (1) magnitude of thrombocytopenia, (2) timing of thrombocytopenia, (3) presence of thrombosis (or other sequelae of HIT), and (4) whether other plausible explanations for thrombocytopenia or thrombosis are present. A low score (≤3 points) makes HIT unlikely (<2%)[98,99] (i.e., high negative predictive value). In some clinical settings, a high score indicates a high probability of HIT.[98,99]

Table 25-5 Pseudo-HIT Disorders: Thrombocytopenia and Thrombosis

Pseudo-HIT Disorder	Pathogenesis of Thrombocytopenia and Thrombosis
Adenocarcinoma	DIC secondary to procoagulant material(s) produced by neoplastic cells; platelet fall often occurs *after* heparin is stopped
Pulmonary embolism	Platelet activation by clot-bound thrombin*
Diabetic ketoacidosis	Hyperaggregable platelets in ketoacidosis
Antiphospholipid syndrome	Multiple mechanisms described, including platelet activation by antiphospholipid antibodies
Thrombolytic therapy	Platelet activation by thrombin bound to fibrin degradation products
Septicemia-associated purpura fulminans	Symmetrical peripheral gangrene resulting from DIC with depletion of protein C and antithrombin III
Infective endocarditis	Infection-associated thrombocytopenia; ischemic events caused by septic emboli
Paroxysmal nocturnal hemoglobinuria	Platelets susceptible to complement-mediated damage; platelet hypoproduction
Posttransfusion purpura (PTP)	"Pseudospecific" alloantibody-mediated platelet destruction (exception: bleeding, not thrombosis)

These "pseudo-HIT" disorders may mimic HIT by causing thrombocytopenia and thrombosis in association with heparin treatment. An exception is PTP, which causes bleeding but not thrombosis; however, PTP may resemble HIT in that both disorders usually occur about a week after major surgery requiring blood and postoperative heparin.
HIT, heparin-induced thrombocytopenia; DIC, disseminated intravascular coagulation.
*See Figure 25-6A for an example of thrombocytopenia associated with pulmonary embolism.
From Warkentin TE: Pseudo-heparin-induced thrombocytopenia. In Warkentin TE, Greinacher A (eds): Heparin-Induced Thrombocytopenia, 3rd ed. New York, Marcel Dekker, 2004, pp 313–334, with permission.

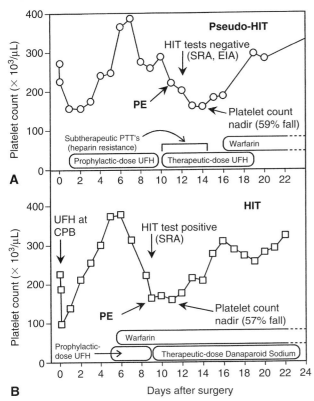

Figure 25-6 Two patients with pulmonary embolism (PE): Pseudo–heparin-induced thrombocytopenia (HIT) versus HIT. **A,** Platelet count fell by 59% (387,000 to 159,000/μL) during unfractionated heparin (UFH) therapy complicated by PE. Testing for HIT antibodies by serotonin release assay (SRA) and platelet factor 4 (PF4)/heparin enzyme immunoassay (EIA) was negative. Increase in heparin dose to overcome heparin "resistance" led to resolution of thrombocytopenia. Platelet count fell by 57% (378,000 to 161,000/μL) during UFH therapy after cardiopulmonary bypass (CPB) surgery complicated by PE. Testing for HIT antibodies was strongly positive. Substitution of heparin by danaparoid led to resolution of thrombocytopenia. Similar platelet count profiles in these two patients with postoperative PE illustrate how difficult it may be to diagnose HIT on clinical grounds alone. (From Warkentin TE: Pseudo–heparin-induced thrombocytopenia. In Warkentin TE, Greinacher A [eds]: Heparin-Induced Thrombocytopena, 3rd ed. New York, Marcel Dekker, 2004, pp 313–334, with permission.)

In addition to the physician's estimate of the pretest probability of HIT, results of laboratory testing for HIT antibodies (vide infra) are important because they may be associated with a high likelihood ratio (strong positive test result) or a very low likelihood ratio (negative testing by one or more sensitive assays).[100] Thus, in a clinicopathologic disorder such as HIT, the physician must carefully integrate clinical and laboratory data to arrive at the diagnosis (see "Interpretation of HIT Antibody Test Results").

LABORATORY TESTING

Two major classes of assays detect HIT antibodies: platelet activation (functional) and PF4/polyanion antigen assays.[4,5,101] Platelet activation assays, which include aggregation of platelets in citrate-anticoagulated platelet-rich plasma (developed in the 1970s), as well as assays that use washed platelets (developed in the 1980s), implicate the presence of HIT antibodies via their platelet-activating properties.[4] In contrast, PF4/polyanion antigen assays, which were developed in the 1990s,[6] detect HIT antibodies on the basis of their reactivity with PF4 complexed to heparin or other polyanions. Thus, laboratory testing for HIT parallels another hypercoagulable state, the antiphospholipid syndrome, in which both functional ("lupus anticoagulant" testing) and antigen (anticardiolipin antibody) assays are used for diagnosis (see Chapter 19).

Platelet Activation Assays

Platelet activation assays detect HIT antibodies of the IgG class via their ability to crosslink platelet FcγIIa receptors in the presence of heparin, causing platelet activation.[12] Because platelet activation is a nonspecific end point, care must be taken to distinguish HIT antibodies from thrombin, immune complexes, or other platelet activators.[4,101]

Washed Platelet Activation Assays

Washed platelet activation assays that use platelets resuspended in calcium-containing buffer are reliable assays for HIT, provided that platelets are handled properly; for example, the use of apyrase (an enzyme that degrades adenine nucleotides) during platelet washing is important for maintaining sensitivity of platelets to subsequent stimulation by adenosine diphosphate (ADP), an important potentiating factor in HIT.[4,102]

The platelet serotonin release assay (SRA) quantitates the release of ^{14}C-labeled serotonin from platelets as a marker of platelet activation.[103,104] The clinical usefulness of this assay has been validated: a positive test result was strongly associated with thrombocytopenia beginning on or after 5 days of heparin therapy (indicating probable HIT) in a large study (odds ratio, approximately 80).[8] Use of a flow cytometer to detect platelet-derived microparticles involves similar platelet handling methods but avoids a radioisotope.[105]

The heparin-induced platelet activation (HIPA) assay[106–108] assesses aggregation of washed platelets incubated with patient serum and heparin in U-bottomed polystyrene microtiter wells containing two stainless steel spheres, under conditions of platelet stirring. At 5-minute intervals, the wells are examined against an indirect light source: a change in appearance of the reaction mixture from turbidity (nonaggregated platelets) to transparency (aggregated platelets) indicates platelet activation.

Advantages of washed platelet activation assays include (1) their high sensitivity for detecting clinically significant HIT antibodies; (2) their (relatively) low sensitivity for detecting clinically insignificant HIT antibodies, compared with antigen assays; and (3) their ability to permit batch evaluation of many patient samples under several reaction conditions, thereby enhancing test specificity. Because washed platelets are activated by IgG (but not by IgA and/or IgM) HIT antibodies, washed platelet activation assays have greater specificity for clinical HIT compared with antigen assays that detect antibodies of all three antibody classes.[46,47]

Disadvantages include the technically demanding nature of these assays[108] (including requirement for fresh platelets from normal platelet donors) and the need for radiolabeling (SRA), expensive equipment (flow cytometer), and a

Table 25-6 Estimating the Pretest Probability of HIT: "4 T'S" Scoring System

	2	1	0
Thrombocytopenia (acute)	>50% platelet count fall to nadir ≥20,000/μL	30%–50% platelet count fall (or >50% directly resulting from surgery); or nadir 10,000–19,000/μL	<30% platelet count fall; or nadir <10,000/μL
Timing* of platelet count fall, thrombosis, or other sequelae of HIT (first day of heparin course = day 0)	Day 5–10 onset; or day 1 (if recent heparin exposure within past 5–30 days)	Consistent with day 5–10 fall, but not clear (e.g., missing platelet counts); or day 1 (heparin exposure within past 31–100 days); or platelet fall after day 10	Platelet count fall ≤4 days without recent heparin exposure
Thrombosis or other sequelae (e.g., skin lesions, ASR)	Proved new thrombosis; or skin necrosis; or post–intravenous heparin bolus ASR	Progressive or recurrent thrombosis; erythematous skin lesions; or suspected thrombosis (not proved)	None
oTher cause for thrombocytopenia	No explanation for platelet count fall is evident	Possible other cause is evident	Definite other cause is present

Pretest probability score: 6–8 = high; 4–5 = intermediate; 0–3 = low.
Points: 0, 1, or 2 for each of 4 categories: maximum possible score = 8.
HIT, heparin-induced thrombocytopenia; ASR, acute systemic reaction.
*First day of immunizing heparin exposure considered day 0 (the most immunizing exposure should be considered first, e.g., unfractionated heparin [UFH] received during cardiac surgery is more immunogenic than UFH or low molecular weight heparin given for acute coronary syndrome); the day the platelet count begins to fall is considered the day of onset of thrombocytopenia (it generally takes 1 to 3 more days before an arbitrary threshold that defines thrombocytopenia is passed).
From Warkentin TE, Heddle NM: Laboratory diagnosis of immune heparin-induced thrombocytopenia. Curr Hematol Rep 2:148–157, 2003.[97]
Reprinted, with modifications, with permission.

subjective observer-dependent end point (HIPA). Further, the laboratory must maintain a panel of positive control sera. Test serum also must first undergo controlled heat treatment (to inactivate thrombin), which sometimes causes ex vivo formation of IgG immune complexes, yielding an indeterminate test result (activation of platelets at all heparin concentrations).[4,101] Platelet-activating anti-HLA alloantibodies may also yield an indeterminate result.

Quality control involves selecting blood donors whose platelets respond well to HIT sera, as well as testing various strong and weak positive control sera. Because HIT sera and washed platelets exhibit variable reactivity in a hierarchical manner,[104] a positive result with the use of a "weak" positive HIT serum control ensures that platelet handling was adequate to permit accurate interpretation of test results.

Platelet Aggregation Assays that Use Platelet-Rich Plasma

Aggregation assays that use platelet-rich plasma are the most widely used activation assays for detecting HIT antibodies because they require the ubiquitous platelet aggregometer and involve relatively simple methods.[109,110] The aggregation response of platelets (prepared as citrated platelet-rich plasma from a normal donor) to platelet-poor plasma obtained from the patient, in the presence of therapeutic heparin levels (0.5 to 1.0 U per milliliter), is assessed and compared with reactivity in the presence of buffer control and high heparin concentrations (100 U/μL). Unfortunately, these aggregation assays are relatively insensitive for diagnosing HIT: As few as 33% to 50% of samples that test positive in a washed platelet assay yield a positive aggregation assay result.[107] Another problem is that nonspecific platelet activation may occur more commonly than with washed platelet methods, increasing the chance of a false-positive result.[4]

PF4/Polyanion Immunoassays

Solid Phase Enzyme Immunoassays

Antigen assays use enzyme immunoassay (EIA) methods to detect binding of HIT antibodies to their PF4-containing antigen target, which is usually immobilized to a solid phase. Two antigen assay kits are available commercially. One assay (Asserachrom HPIA; Diagnostica Stago, Paris, France) uses PF4/heparin complexes, whereas the other test (available from Genetic Testing Institute, Waukesha, Wis, USA) uses PF4 bound to polyvinyl sulfonate (PVS).[22] Both commercial tests detect HIT antibodies of the three major immunoglobulin classes (IgG, IgA, IgM). However, this might not provide an advantage over antigen assays that detect only IgG antibodies: Our laboratory found that an "in-house" EIA that detected only IgG anti-PF4/heparin antibodies[111] yielded positive results in all 15 patients identified with HIT in prospective clinical trials (high sensitivity).[44] Further, the assay was more specific for HIT than were commercial EIAs,[46] yielding superior operating characteristics (i.e., sensitivity/specificity tradeoff at any given cutoff between negative and positive results).

Fluid Phase Enzyme Immunoassays

A fluid phase PF4/heparin EIA was developed by investigators in Australia.[112] Through this method, patient serum or plasma reacts with biotin–PF4/heparin complexes in a fluid phase, prior to capture of IgG antibodies—and any bound antigen—with staphylococcal protein A. Biotinylated antigen/antibody complexes, now bound to protein G sepharose via the Fc moieties of HIT IgG, are separated from unbound antigen by centrifugation and washing. Streptavidin-conjugated peroxidase is used to quantitate biotin–PF4/heparin/IgG complexes (streptavidin binds to biotin). This method may result in a lower false-positive rate because it avoids denaturation of the antigen caused by binding to a solid phase, and it detects only anti-PF4/heparin antibodies of the IgG class. It also permits the detection of in vitro cross-reactivity of HIT antibodies against various heparins and heparinoids.[112]

Rapid Immunoassays

A particle gel immunoassay uses PF4/heparin complexes bound to red, high-density polystyrene beads; after patient serum or plasma is added, anti-PF4/heparin antibodies bind to antigen-coated beads.[113] However, IgG class antibodies do not agglutinate polystyrene beads well; therefore, a secondary anti–human immunoglobulin antibody is added into the sephacryl gel. The rationale behind this (and other gel centrifugation assays) is that on centrifugation, agglutinated beads (indicating the presence of anti-PF4/heparin antibodies) do not migrate through the sephacryl gel, whereas nonagglutinated beads (indicating absence of antibodies) pass through the gel, thus forming a red band at the bottom. This method is available to blood banks that use a gel centrifugation technology system. Currently, particle gel immunoassay is available in Europe and Canada and is under investigation in the United States.

Limited assessment suggests sensitivity and specificity for HIT that are intermediate between washed platelet activation assays and standard solid-phase EIA.[114,115] Operating characteristics of the assay may be improved by determination of the titer of the blood sample that produces a positive result; a titer of 4 or greater appears to be of greater clinical significance than a positive result with neat or 1 in 2 diluted sera.[115]

Recently, another rapid immunoassay—the Health-TEST Heparin/Platelet Factor 4 Antibody Assay (Akers Biosciences, Inc., Thorofare, NJ, USA)—received U.S. Food and Drug Administration (FDA) approval for use in detecting anti-PF4/heparin antibodies. This assay uses a system known as Particle ImmunoFiltration Assay (PIFA), wherein patient serum is added to a reaction well that contains dyed particles coated with PF4 (*not* PF4/heparin). Lack of requirement for heparin presumably reflects formation of HIT antigens through close approximation of PF4 tetramers[26] (achieved under conditions of PF4 binding to particles). Subsequently, only nonagglutinated particles will migrate through the membrane filter. Thus, a negative test is shown by a blue color in the result well, whereas no color indicates a positive test. Operating characteristics of this assay remain largely undefined.

Interpretation of HIT Antibody Test Results

Interpretation of HIT antibody test results is complicated by the fact that only a minority of patients who develop anti-PF4/heparin antibodies experience thrombocytopenia.[7,8,46,116] A corollary to this is that a positive HIT test result may not therefore actually indicate HIT, particularly if a weak positive result is obtained and another convincing explanation for the thrombocytopenia can be provided.[4,46] Thus, tests for HIT should be interpreted in the clinical context of pretest probability. Further, the magnitude of a positive test result should be considered, with a "strong" test result indicating a greater likelihood for HIT than is suggested by a "weak" result.[46,100] Because antigen assays are more likely than activation assays to detect clinically insignificant HIT antibodies,[25,44,117] one algorithmic approach involves screening for HIT antibodies with a commercial antigen assay, but performing further confirmatory testing with a washed platelet activation assay if the clinical situation suggests another more plausible diagnosis despite a positive EIA. However, because existing antigen and washed platelet activation assays are extremely sensitive in detecting clinically significant HIT antibodies, negative results in one or (especially) both classes of assay provide strong evidence against HIT, irrespective of the patient's clinical course. Occasionally, when an unexpected negative test result is obtained with use of an antigen assay, referral for further testing by activation assay may be needed in that anecdotal evidence that a false-negative EIA event may result is rarely caused by antibodies directed against "minor" antigens other than PF4/heparin (e.g., interleukin-8, neutrophil-activating peptide-2); in such patients, sensitive activation assays yield positive results.[118]

By the time of discharge from the hospital, it is usually clear whether a patient had HIT or some imitator. The final diagnosis should be clearly stated in the discharge summary in order to minimize confusion in the future as patients may well be readmitted and given consideration for heparin exposure again.

TREATMENT OF PATIENTS WITH HIT-ASSOCIATED THROMBOSIS

Overall, about 50% to 75% of patients with a diagnosis of clinical HIT supported by a positive SRA develop new, progressive, or recurrent thrombosis during or soon after their episode of thrombocytopenia.[42,66] Thus, an alternative, rapidly acting, nonheparin anticoagulant must be used frequently for patients with strongly suspected (or confirmed) HIT. Two major FDA-approved options are available in the United States: lepirudin and argatroban. Both of these are direct thrombin inhibitors (DTIs). A third option, danaparoid, is available in some other countries (e.g., Canada, European Union). Oral anticoagulants, also known as vitamin K antagonists (VKAs), are *contra*indicated during acute HIT but may be used for long-term management of thrombosis following an episode of HIT. Table 25-7 lists some recommendations of the American College of Chest Physicians (ACCP) that may be helpful in the management of HIT.[63,119]

Lepirudin

Lepirudin (Refludan) is a derivative of hirudin—a DTI that is synthesized naturally by the salivary glands of the medicinal leech and is manufactured through recombinant technology.[120–122] The 65 amino acid polypeptide (6980 Da; Ki for thrombin, 60 fmol per liter) differs minimally in structure from its natural counterpart. Hirudin and its synthetic derivatives form noncovalent but irreversible complexes with thrombin, binding to two sites on thrombin (active site cleft and fibrinogen-binding site). Differing from heparin, hirudin acts independently of the plasma cofactors

Table 25-7 Recommendations of the Seventh Conference of the American College of Chest Physicians on Antithrombotic and Thrombolytic Therapy[63]

Nonheparin Anticoagulants for HIT

- For patients with strongly suspected (or confirmed) HIT, whether or not complicated by thrombosis, we recommend use of an alternative, nonheparin anticoagulant in therapeutic doses, such as lepirudin (grade 1C+), argatroban (grade 1C), bivalirudin (grade 2C), or danaparoid (grade 1B), over further UFH or LMWH therapy, and over no further anticoagulation (with or without vena caval filter).

Ultrasonography of Lower Limb Veins

- For patients with strongly suspected (or confirmed) HIT, whether or not clinical evidence of lower limb DVT is noted, we recommend routine ultrasonography of lower limb veins for investigation of DVT over not performing routine ultrasonography (grade 1C).

Vitamin K Antagonists (VKAs; Coumarins)

- For patients with strongly suspected (or confirmed) HIT, we recommend **against** the use of vitamin K antagonist (coumarin) therapy until after the platelet count has been substantially increased (e.g., to at least 100,000/µL and preferably 150,000/µL); that the VKA should be administered only during overlapping alternative anticoagulation (minimum, 5-day overlap) and should be begun with low maintenance doses (maximum, 5 mg warfarin; 6 mg phenprocoumon); that the alternative anticoagulant should not be stopped until the platelet count has reached a stable plateau and during at least the last 2 days, the INR is within the target therapeutic range (all grade 1C).
- For patients receiving VKAs at the time of diagnosis of HIT, we recommend use of vitamin K (grade 2C).

LMWH

- For patients with strongly suspected HIT, whether or not complicated by thrombosis, we recommend **against** the use of LMWH (grade 1C+).

Prophylactic Platelet Transfusions

- For patients with strongly suspected or confirmed HIT who do not have active bleeding, we suggest that prophylactic platelet transfusions should **not** be administered (grade 2C).

The implications of the grades of recommendation shown above are as follows:[119]

Grade of Recommendation	Clarity of Risk/Benefit	Methodologic Strength of Supporting Data	Implications
1C+	Clear	No RCTs, but strong RCT results may be unequivocally extrapolated, or overwhelming evidence can be obtained from observational studies	Strong recommendation; may apply to most patients in most circumstances
1B	Clear	RCTs with important limitations (inconsistent results, methodologic flaws)	Strong recommendation, likely to apply to most patients
1C	Clear	Observational studies	Intermediate-strength recommendation; may change when stronger evidence becomes available
2C	Unclear	Observational studies	Very weak recommendation; other alternatives may be equally reasonable

HIT, heparin-induced thrombocytopenia; UFH, unfractionated heparin; LMWH, low molecular weight heparin; DVT, deep venous thrombosis; RCT, randomized controlled trial.

From Warkentin TE, Greinacher A: Heparin-induced thrombocytopenia: Recognition, treatment, and prevention. The Seventh ACCP Conference on Antithrombotic and Thrombolytic Therapy. Chest 26(suppl):311S–337S, 2004, with permission.[63]

antithrombin III and heparin cofactor II. Hirudin also differs from heparin in terms of its greater ability to inhibit clot-bound thrombin. Thus, dependable thrombin neutralization may occur, even in the procoagulant milieu of HIT.

In normal subjects, the half-life of lepirudin is about 1.3 hours. However, this agent is renally excreted, and the half-life can rise substantially (by as much as 2 days) in patients with renal failure, leading to high risk for drug accumulation and bleeding. Lepirudin is usually monitored with the use of partial thromboplastin time (PTT), which reveals a fair correlation with plasma drug levels in many (but not all) situations. The target therapeutic range is 1.5 to 2.5 times the patient's nonanticoagulated baseline PTT (if known), or 1.5 to 2.5 times the mean of the laboratory normal range.[29] Although interpatient differences in lepirudin metabolism are known to occur, most patients show stable anticoagulation during lepirudin treat-

ment. However, the high frequency with which antilepirudin antibodies develop (which paradoxically enhances the anticoagulant response to lepirudin in some patients) means that daily PTT monitoring should be performed.[123] No antidote for lepirudin exists.

Anaphylaxis has been reported after intravenous bolus injection of lepirudin.[124,125] This event is likely related to high levels of antihirudin antibodies, in that patients with fatal reactions usually had received lepirudin over the previous few weeks or months.

Two prospective cohort studies[126,127] (with historical controls) of lepirudin for the treatment of patients with HIT-associated thrombosis and given according to a pre-specified dosing schedule led to its approval for this indication both in the European Union (March 1997) and in the United States (March 1998). The first study[126] showed a significantly reduced frequency of a composite end point of mortality, limb amputation, and new thromboembolic complications compared with outcomes in controls (cumulative frequency, 10% vs 23% at day 7 follow-up, and 25% vs 52% at day 35 follow-up, respectively; $P = .014$). The second study[127] found a trend in favor of lepirudin (cumulative frequency of composite end point, 31% vs 52%; $P = .12$). A meta-analysis[29] of these two studies found that a subtherapeutic PTT ratio (<1.5) was associated with an increased risk for thrombosis, whereas a therapeutic PTT ratio above the therapeutic range (>2.5) was associated with increased bleeding and no further reduction in antithrombotic efficacy. However, even for patients within the target therapeutic range, bleeding was increased significantly compared with outcomes in historical controls (relative risk = 3.21 [95% confidence interval, 1.7 to 6.0]; $P < .001$). Thus, more recent recommendations consist of avoiding the initial bolus in most situations and beginning with a lower maintenance rate (0.10 mg/kg/hr), with PTT monitoring provided at 4-hour intervals until stable PTT levels within the therapeutic range are documented (Table 25-8).[63,76,122,128,129]

A third prospective study (HAT-3 [Heparin-Associated Thrombocytopenia])[128] found that the frequency of the composite end point (categorical analysis) assessed on the basis of diagnosis of HIT among 205 study patients was 29.8%; the individual end point of new thrombosis was 13.7%. If events that occurred only after initiation of study drug are included, corresponding rates are 21.0 and 5.4%, respectively.

When findings from all three prospective studies (HAT-1, HAT-2, and HAT-3) are combined[128] and analysis is performed from the start of treatment, highly statistically significant ($P < .0001$) differences between lepirudin-treated patients and historical controls are seen for new thromboses (7.4% vs 25.0%, respectively) and for the composite end point (20.3% vs 43.3%, respectively). A trend toward reduced mortality (11.7 vs 17.5%; $P = .095$) is also seen. However, limb amputation rates were similar between lepirudin-treated patients and controls (5.5 vs 6.7%; $P = .618$). Major bleeding rates, ranging from 4% to 33% (for serum creatinine levels <50 μmol per liter and >90 μmol per liter), varied greatly in keeping with creatinine levels. Overall, 17.6% of lepirudin-treated patients—about 1 in 6—experienced a major bleeding event. The authors noted that because serum creatinine levels do not adequately reflect impaired renal function in the elderly and in critically ill patients, and because the overall mean maintenance dose

of lepirudin in the HAT-3 study was only 0.11 mg/kg/hr, an initial maintenance dose of 0.10 mg/kg/hr is appropriate in most situations with normal renal function.[128]

Results of a postmarketing study[130] of the use of lepirudin for the treatment of patients with HIT-associated thrombosis (n = 496 patients) revealed rates of new thrombosis (5.2%), death (10.9%), limb amputation (5.8%), and major bleeding (6.5%) that were similar to or lower than those reported in the three HAT trials. The mean maintenance dose (0.12 mg/kg/hr) also supports the use of a lower initial maintenance dose of up to 0.10 mg/kg/hr.

Table 25-9 summarizes the outcomes of lepirudin[29,128,130] and argatroban[131,132] treatment for HIT-associated thrombosis in prospective cohort studies (historical controls).

Argatroban

Argatroban (Novastan in some countries; marketed as Argatroban in the United States [GlaxoSmithKline, Research Triangle Park, NC, USA]) is a small-molecule DTI (527 Da; Ki for thrombin, 40 nmol per liter) that was associated with a lower thrombotic event rate in two prospective cohort treatment studies[131–133] that used a historical control group. Patients received argatroban at an initial dose of 2 μg/kg/min (no initial bolus) for an average of 6 days. The half-life of argatroban is relatively short (40 to 50 minutes).[134] Argatroban is primarily excreted into the hepatobiliary system; thus, the dose should be reduced by 75% in patients with impaired liver function. Table 25-10 provides an argatroban dosing schedule for the treatment or prevention of thrombosis in HIT.[134–139] As with lepirudin, postapproval experience indicates that lower initial dosing (e.g., 0.5–1 μg/kg/min) may be appropriate in some situations (e.g., critically ill patients,[136,137] those who are renally impaired[138,139]). No antidote for argatroban exists.

On June 30, 2000, argatroban was approved by the U.S FDA for the treatment of patients with HIT-associated thrombosis; it was launched for use in the United States in mid-November of the year 2000. Because clinical studies included patients with isolated HIT, argatroban also received this second indication from the FDA (prevention of HIT-associated thrombosis). Identical (therapeutic) doses are recommended for patients with isolated HIT and for those with HIT-associated thrombosis. Recently, argatroban was approved for use in anticoagulation during percutaneous coronary intervention (PCI) in patients in whom heparin

---

Table 25-8   Dosing Schedule for Lepirudin (Recombinant Hirudin)

For Rapid Intravenous Therapeutic Dose Anticoagulation:

Loading dose: ±0.4 mg per kilogram IV bolus*
Maintenance: 0.10 mg/kg/hr IV,†‡ with adjustments to maintain PTT at 1.5 to 2.5 times the mean of the normal
   laboratory range

*Avoid bolus except in situations of life- or limb-threatening ischemia in which immediate anticoagulation is desired.
†Although the U.S. Food and Drug Administration (FDA)-approved initial dosing is 0.15 mg/kg/hr, it is recommended[63,76,122,128,129] that the initial maintenance level be reduced to 0.10 mg/kg/hr (and even lower with documented renal insufficiency‡), and that monitoring be provided at 4-hour intervals until stable PTT values are documented (then once daily).
‡Reduce initial lepirudin infusion rate in patients with renal insufficiency, as follows (subsequent dose adjustments by PTT):[120] (1) normal renal function (serum creatinine [sCr], <1.0 mg per deciliter [<90 μmol per liter]): 0.10 mg/kg/hr; (2) mild renal dysfunction (sCr, 1.0–1.6 mg per deciliter [90–140 μmol per liter]): 0.05 mg/kg/hr; (3) moderate renal dysfunction (sCr, 1.7–4.5 mg per deciliter [140–400 μmol per liter]): 0.01 mg/kg/hr; (4) severe renal dysfunction (sCr, >4.5 mg per deciliter [>400 μmol per liter]): 0.005 mg/kg/hr or intermittent boluses of 0.005 mg/kg.

Table 25-9 Treatment Outcomes of HIT-Associated Thrombosis: Comparison of Two DTIs

Anticoagulant	Dosing (Duration of DTI Treatment, Mean Days)	N*	Study Design (Control Group)	% New Thrombosis (Controls)	% Limb Amputation (Controls)	% Composite End Point‡ (Controls)	% Major Bleeds (Controls)	Comment
Lepirudin[29]	Bolus, 0.4 mg per kilogram; 0.15 mg/kg/hr‡ (13.3)	113	Prospective (historical controls)	10.1% (27.2%)§ RRR = 63%	6.5% (10.4%) RRR = 38%	21.3% (47.8%)§ RRR = 55%	18.8% (7.1%)§	Meta-analysis of two prospective (historical control) studies (HAT-1[126], HAT-2[127]); all patients tested positive for HIT-Abs
Lepirudin[128]	See above (14.0)	98	Prospective	5.1%	6.1%	18.3%	20.4%	Extension study (HAT-3) performed awaiting regulatory approval; all patients tested positive for HIT-Abs
Lepirudin[130]	See above (12.1)	496	Postmarketing study	5.2%	5.8%	21.9%¶	5.4%	77% of patients tested positive for HIT-Abs; thrombotic death rate = 1.8%
Argatroban[131]	2μg/kg/min¶ (no bolus) (5.9)	144	Prospective (historical controls)	19.4% (34.8%)§ RRR = 44%	11.8% (10.9%)** RRR = -8%	43.8%†† (56.5%) RRR = 22%	11.1% (2.2%)	Positive testing for HIT-Abs not required for study entry (65% of patients shown to have HIT-Abs)
Argatroban[132]	See above (7.1 days)	229	Prospective (historical controls)	13.1%§ RRR = 62%	14.8% RRR = -36%	41.5%†† RRR = 27%	6.1%	Positive testing for HIT-Abs not required for study entry (number testing positive not reported)

End points shown represent time-to-event analysis (day 35) for meta-analysis of HAT-1 and HAT-2 lepirudin studies, categorical analysis for other lepirudin studies shown, and categorical analysis (day 37) for argatroban.

*The denominator, N, indicates the number of patients treated with DTI; controls, N = 75 (lepirudin) and N = 46 (argatroban).

†Composite end point: all-cause mortality, all-cause limb amputation, and/or new thrombosis (each patient counted only once), unless otherwise indicated.

‡PTT (partial thromboplastin time) adjusted to 1.5 to 2.5 times patient's baseline PTT (or mean laboratory normal range if the patient's baseline PTT is unavailable); indicated dosing given to 105 of 113 patients (remaining 8 patients received 0.2 mg per kilogram IV bolus in conjunction with thrombolytic therapy).

§Statistically significant difference (P < .05).

¶Composite end point likely overestimated, as some patients may have had more than one end point.

**PTT adjusted to 1.5 to 3.0 times patient's baseline PTT.

##One additional patient each is included in the DTI and control groups (compared with original publication[131]), as these two patients died and sustained limb amputation (personal communication, Dr. M. Hursting).

††P values not significant by categorical analysis, but P = .014 (hazard ratio = 0.57) and P = .008 (hazard ratio = 0.56) for Arg-911 and Arg-915 studies, respectively, with the use of time-to-event analysis.

DTI, direct thrombin inhibitor; HIT-Abs, heparin-induced thrombocytopenia antibodies; RRR, relative risk reduction (compared with historical controls); HAT, Heparin-Associated Thrombocytopenia trial.

Table 25-10 Dosing Schedule for Argatroban

For Rapid Intravenous Therapeutic Dose Anticoagulation:
Initial dose: 2 μg/kg/min IV*†
Maintenance: Above initial dose adjusted to maintain PTT 1.5
  to 3.0 times the initial baseline value
  (not to exceed 100 sec)

For Percutaneous Coronary Intervention (PCI):
Initial dose: 350 μg per kilogram (IV over 3–5 min)
Maintenance: 25 μg/kg/min (adjusted to maintain activated
  clotting time [ACT] between 300–450 sec; additional bolus
  doses of 150 μg per kilogram may be given as needed)

*Reduce starting dose to 0.5 μg/kg/min in a patient with hepatic
dysfunction.
†Literature[136–139] supports starting at a lower initial dose
(e.g., 0.5–1 μg/kg/min) in critically ill or renally compromised patients.
IV, intravenous; PTT, partial thromboplastin time.

is contraindicated because of acute HIT or a history of HIT.[135]

The primary adverse effect is bleeding. Argatroban is not immunogenic,[140] and (in contrast to lepirudin) anaphylaxis has not been reported with its use.

Monitoring is provided with use of the PTT, targeted at 1.5 to 3.0 times the patient's baseline value (maximum, 100 sec). Argatroban prolongs the INR to a greater extent than the other DTIs[121] (Fig. 25-7)—an issue that must be considered when warfarin treatment is overlapped (see "Direct Thrombin Inhibitor–Warfarin Overlap").

In prospective trials of DTI therapy for HIT-associated thrombosis, duration of argatroban therapy was only about half that of lepirudin treatment (6 to 7 days vs 13 to 14 days, respectively).[141] Given that a median of 4 days is needed for a platelet count of 150,000/μL to be reached (at which point initiation of warfarin therapy can be considered[63]), and that at least 5 days of DTI–warfarin overlap is required, it seems likely that patients with confirmed HIT who are treated with argatroban usually require a longer duration of treatment than was used in the prospective trials. Indeed, most thrombi that occurred during argatroban treatment of venous thromboembolism occurred soon *after* this agent was stopped, suggesting that the duration of DTI therapy had been too brief.[142]

Bivalirudin

Bivalirudin (Angiomax; The Medicines Company, Parsippany, NJ, USA) is a hirulog, that is, an analogue of hirudin. It is a 20 amino acid peptide (2180 Da) that is made through solid phase peptide synthesis.[121,143,144] Bivalirudin unites a C-terminal segment of 12 amino acids derived from native hirudin (residues 53 to 64) to an active site-binding tetrapeptide sequence (D-Phe-Pro-Arg-Pro) at its N-terminus, bridged by four glycine residues. The aminoterminal segment has high affinity and specificity for binding to the active site of thrombin, and the C-terminal domain binds to the fibrin(ogen) recognition site of thrombin. One difference between bivalirudin and hirudin is that the binding of bivalirudin to the active site of thrombin is transient, whereas with lepirudin, irreversible thrombin/hirudin complexes are formed. Its affinity for human thrombin (Ki = 2 nmol per liter) is somewhat

greater than that of the univalent DTI, argatroban (Ki = 40 nmol per liter), but it is much less than that of hirudin (Ki~0.0001 nmol per liter).[121]

In theory, bivalirudin has several pharmacologic advantages over other DTIs,[145] including a shorter half-life (25 to 30 minutes), predominant nonorgan (80% enzymic) clearance with only minor renal excretion (20%), minimal prolongation of the INR, and minimal (if any) immunogenicity. However, only anecdotal experience in the treatment of HIT has been reported,[146,147] and appropriate dosing for HIT remains unknown. One approach is to begin with an initial infusion rate of between 0.15 and 0.25 mg/kg/hr (initial bolus of 0.1 to 0.75 mg/kg) adjusted to a PTT of 1.5 to 2.5 times baseline.[145]

Bivalirudin was recently approved by the FDA for use in patients with, or at risk of, HIT or HIT-associated thrombosis who are undergoing PCI (see "Percutaneous Coronary Intervention").[148]

Direct Thrombin Inhibitor–Warfarin Overlap

Although all DTIs may prolong the INR, relative effects at therapeutic concentrations vary considerably, as follows: argatroban ≈ (xi)melagatran > bivalirudin > lepirudin (see Fig. 25-7).[121,149] Interestingly, when expressed in molar terms, lepirudin exhibits the greatest INR-prolonging effect (see Fig. 25-7, inset).[149] However, its high affinity for thrombin and low molar dosing requirements mean that it has the least effect compared with other DTIs given in clinically relevant doses.

Careful attention to overlap of DTI and warfarin is required to avoid adverse events such as recurrent thrombosis (including microvascular thrombosis) due to vitamin K antagonism and severe protein C depletion. In the argatroban trials, approximately 10% of patients developed thrombosis during the argatroban–warfarin overlap period; it is interesting to note that several of these patients had supratherapeutic INR levels (potentially indicating protein C depletion) at the time of thrombosis.[150]

As a general rule, warfarin should not be started until the patient has been satisfactorily anticoagulated with a parenteral anticoagulant and the platelet count has substantially recovered, usually to ≥150,000/μL.[63] Because of the marked effects of argatroban in prolonging the INR, the target therapeutic range during argatroban–warfarin cotherapy is approximately 3.0 to 5.0 when a relatively sensitive thromboplastin reagent (international sensitivity index [ISI] = 0.88) is used to determine the INR, and even higher (≈4.0 to 6.0) when an insensitive thromboplastin reagent (ISI = 1.31 or higher) is used.[134,151] Such high INR values do not appear to be associated with an increased risk of bleeding.[152] The potential risk of warfarin-associated microvascular thrombosis is an important reason why warfarin overlap should not be commenced until substantial resolution of thrombocytopenia has been attained and any symptomatic thrombosis is noted to be clinically stable or improving.

For patients in whom HIT is not diagnosed until treatment with warfarin has commenced, it is suggested that warfarin should be antagonized by vitamin K (≥5 mg), preferably given by slow intravenous infusion (over a minimum of 30 minutes). One reason for this approach is that warfarin prolongs both the PT and the PTT; therefore,

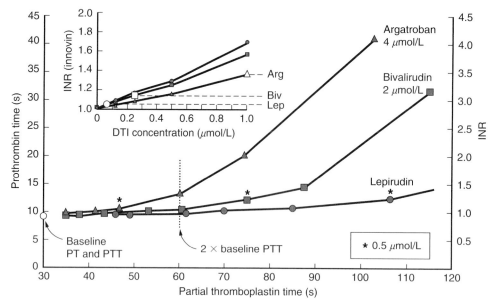

Figure 25-7 Prolongation of prothrombin time (PT) and international normalized ratio (INR) by direct thrombin inhibitors (DTIs). Three DTIs differ in their relative ability to prolong PT and INR with a given increase in partial thromboplastin time (PTT), as follows: argatroban > bivalirudin > lepirudin.[121] However, as is shown in the inset, when INR is plotted against molarity, it can be seen that the relative effects of the DTIs differ, as follows: lepirudin > bivalirudin > argatroban.[149] The explanation for this apparent paradox is that relative therapeutic concentrations of DTIs—when expressed in molar concentrations (μmol per liter)—differ markedly: The approximate therapeutic concentration of lepirudin (e.g., when estimated by the concentration that doubles the PTT) is about 0.0625 μmol per liter, whereas the corresponding concentration is about 0.25 μmol per liter for bivalirudin, and 1.0 μmol per liter for argatroban. This hierarchy presumably reflects the different affinities of the DTIs for thrombin, which can be ranked as follows: lepirudin (Ki = 0.0001 nmol per liter) > bivalirudin (Ki = 2 nmol per liter) > argatroban (Ki = 40 nmol per liter). Data shown in the figure are based on addition of DTIs to pooled normal human plasma; PT (INR) values were obtained with a sensitive thromboplastin reagent (international sensitivity index [ISI] = 1.0). If an insensitive thromboplastin had been used, the relatively greater prolongation of the INR by argatroban would have been even more marked. (From Warkentin TE: Bivalent direct thrombin inhibitors: Hirudin and bivalirudin. Best Pract Res Clin Haematol 17:105–125, 2004[121]; and Warkentin TE, Greinacher A, Craven S, et al: Differences in the clinically effective molar concentrations of four direct thrombin inhibitors explain their variable prothrombin time prolongation. Thromb Haemost 94:958–964, 2005, with permission.[149])

suboptimal anticoagulation with lepirudin or argatroban may result when PTT-based monitoring is provided.[78] Another reason why this approach should be used is that it reduces the risk of warfarin-induced microvascular thrombosis resulting from severe depletion in protein C activity.[10,71,72]

Danaparoid

Danaparoid sodium (Orgaran; Organon, Oss, The Netherlands) is a mixture of anticoagulant glycosaminoglycans, predominantly heparan sulfate (84%), dermatan sulfate (12%), and chondroitin sulfate (4%).[153,154] Heparan sulfate provides most of the anti–factor Xa activity of danaparoid, which is mediated via binding to antithrombin III. Dermatan sulfate, by binding to heparin cofactor II, provides some antithrombin III (anti-IIa) activity. However, the anti-Xa/anti-IIa ratio of danaparoid is at least 22, which is much higher even than that of LMWH (usual ratio, approximately 2 to 4). Danaparoid exhibits minimal nonspecific binding to plasma proteins; thus, resistance to its anticoagulant effects due to elevated acute phase reactants is usually not seen.

Danaparoid is well absorbed after subcutaneous administration, with peak levels reached 4 to 5 hours post injection. The near-100% bioavailability makes it easy for clinicians to determine the appropriate subcutaneous dosage for a stably anticoagulated patient who is receiving intravenous danaparoid. For example, 190 U per hour by intravenous infusion is approximately equal to 2250 U given twice daily by subcutaneous injection (both provide about 4500 U per 24 hours). Despite the long half-life of its anti–factor Xa activity (≈25 hours), the drug should be given intravenously or (at least) twice daily via the subcutaneous route, as the half-life for antithrombin III activity is about 2 to 4 hours. Danaparoid is renally metabolized, and the dose should be reduced somewhat (by about one third) for patients with renal failure. No antidote is available for danaparoid.

Danaparoid prolongs neither the PTT nor the PT, which facilitates assessment of overlapping warfarin therapy. Monitoring of the anticoagulant effects of danaparoid, when needed, is done by measuring plasma anti–factor Xa activity through chromogenic assay. This is similar to monitoring of LMWH, except that the standard calibration curve must be constructed with the use of danaparoid (if an LMWH standard curve is used, danaparoid concentrations will be overestimated). Anti–factor Xa monitoring for danaparoid is not widely available, but because danaparoid produces predictable anticoagulant effects, monitoring is often not necessary when a standard dose is given (Table 25-11). Patients in whom monitoring should be considered include those with substantial renal impairment, unusually low or high body weight, or life- or limb-threatening thrombosis; those in whom unexpected bleeding occurs should also be monitored. The usual target therapeutic range for danaparoid is 0.5 to 0.8 anti-Xa U/μL, although a higher level (about 1 U/μL) in a patient with severe thrombosis is appropriate.

Table 25-11   Dosing Schedule for Danaparoid

For Rapid Intravenous Therapeutic Dose Anticoagulation:
Loading dose: 2250 U IV bolus,* followed by 400 U per hour for 4 hours, and 300 U per hour for 4 hours; then, maintenance: 150–200 U per hour, aiming for anti–factor Xa level of 0.5–0.8 U/mL.

*Adjust initial intravenous bolus for body weight: <60 kg, 1500 U; 60–75 kg, 2250 U; 75–90 kg, 3000 U; >90 kg, 3750 U.

In contrast to the DTIs, danaparoid has no effect on the INR and the PTT; thus, monitoring of overlapping warfarin therapy remains unchanged. Because the half-life of danaparoid is relatively long, this drug usually can be stopped after 4 or 5 days of warfarin treatment, once the INR has reached the lower therapeutic range. For all these situations, it is prudent to start with expected maintenance doses of warfarin, rather than an initial loading dose.

Theoretically, the recommendation to give vitamin K to a patient who is receiving warfarin when HIT is diagnosed might not be applicable if treatment with danaparoid is planned, given the lack of interference by danaparoid with the INR. Figure 25-6B shows an example of a situation in which warfarin therapy was continued in a patient with HIT-associated thrombosis, although bridge therapy with therapeutic doses of danaparoid was provided until platelet count recovery occurred.

A randomized open-label clinical trial[155] found a higher frequency of complete clinical recovery from thrombosis (the primary end point) in patients treated with danaparoid and warfarin, compared with dextran and warfarin (56% vs 14%; P = .02). For the secondary end point of complete or partial clinical recovery, corresponding results were 86% versus 53%. Venous thrombotic events were almost three times more likely to show complete clinical recovery than were arterial thrombotic events.

A retrospective historical cohort study that compared outcomes in patients treated with danaparoid (with or without coumarin) versus outcomes in controls (ancrod [defibrinogenating snake venom], coumarin, or both) reported reduction in the day 35 efficacy end point (composite of thrombosis, thrombotic death, or limb amputation) in danaparoid-treated patients compared with controls (12 of 62 = 19.4% vs 24 of 56 = 42.9%; P = .0088).[156] Major bleeding occurred significantly less often in danaparoid-treated patients than in controls (11.3 vs 28.6%; P = .0211). Retrospective uncontrolled case series also support the efficacy of danaparoid as a treatment for patients with HIT-associated thrombosis.[157–159]

Danaparoid has been approved for DVT prophylaxis after hip replacement surgery (750 U two or three times daily by subcutaneous injection). This low-dose regimen would be appropriate for a patient with previous HIT who requires postoperative thromboprophylaxis. However, for patients with acute HIT, with or without thrombosis, a therapeutic regimen should be given (see Table 25-11).[160,161] In April 2002, danaparoid was withdrawn from the U.S. market, although it remains available (and widely used) in Canada and Europe.[154]

In vitro cross-reactivity against danaparoid can be detected in some HIT sera.[112] However, this cross-reactivity is generally weak and does not predict adverse clinical outcomes. In the author's opinion, treatment should not be delayed so that in vitro cross-reactivity studies can be conducted, nor is detectable in vitro cross-reactivity a contraindication to the use of danaparoid.

Fondaparinux

Fondaparinux is a sulfated pentasaccharide anticoagulant that catalyzes antithrombin III–mediated inhibition of factor Xa (but not thrombin). It has been approved in the United States for post–orthopaedic and abdominal surgery thromboprophylaxis (2.5 mg once daily, given subcutaneously) and for treatment of patients with DVT and pulmonary embolism (7.5 mg once daily, given subcutaneously [5.0 and 10.0 mg once daily subcutaneously for body weight <50 kg and >100 kg, respectively]).[162–164] Although use of fondaparinux in post–orthopaedic surgery thromboprophylaxis has been reported to be associated with formation of anti-PF4/heparin antibodies[25,165] at a frequency similar to that of LMWH,[25] the absence of cross-reactivity of these antibodies and of antibodies within HIT serum[166] for PF4/fondaparinux suggests that fondaparinux likely will have a lower (perhaps negligible) frequency of HIT, compared with LMWH (see section on the prevention of HIT).[27] To date, only one case of fondaparinux-associated HIT has been reported.[166a] Fondaparinux is an attractive anticoagulant option for patients with a history of HIT who require prophylactic or therapeutic doses of anticoagulation.

Some anecdotal experience with fondaparinux has been reported for the treatment of patients with acute HIT (with or without thrombosis).[167–169] Given the negligible in vitro cross-reactivity of HIT antibodies for PF4/fondaparinux complexes, fondaparinux may be considered a promising treatment option for acute HIT. However, caveats include uncertainty as to optimal dosing and minimal experience with this use thus far.

Choice of Parenteral Anticoagulant

The choice of parenteral anticoagulant depends on several factors, including patient renal and hepatic function, anticipated need to reverse anticoagulation quickly, monitoring methods used, drug availability/cost, and physicians' experience with a given agent.

Adjunctive Treatments

Adjunctive treatments can be useful in select patients with HIT.[76] Surgical thromboembolectomy can be limb saving in patients with acute occlusion of large limb arteries by platelet-rich thromboemboli. Lepirudin, argatroban, or danaparoid can be used for intraoperative anticoagulation during vascular surgery.[170] Thrombolytic therapy with streptokinase or tissue plasminogen activator may be tried in highly select patients, but issues such as the optimal choice and dose of concomitant parenteral anticoagulant remain unresolved (thrombolytic agents increase thrombin generation because thrombin bound to fibrin degradation products is relatively protected from inhibition by antithrombin III[171]). High-dose intravenous γ globulin can inhibit HIT antibody–mediated platelet activation[172] and may therefore be a useful treatment adjunct in patients with severe thrombocytopenia, DIC, or microvascular ischemia.[173] Antiplatelet agents, such as aspirin, can be tried in patients at high risk for arterial thrombosis, but issues such as bleeding when combined with antithrombotic drugs have not yet been resolved. (Notably, HIT may occur even in patients given combined antiplatelet therapy consisting of aspirin and clopidogrel.[174])

CAVEATS IN THE MANAGEMENT OF HEPARIN-INDUCED THROMBOCYTOPENIA

Physicians must be vigilant to ensure that heparin is not inadvertently given to patients with acute HIT. Because heparin is often given routinely (e.g., via "flushes" to indwelling catheters, or as heparin bonded to pulmonary artery catheters), a simple order to "discontinue heparin" may not necessarily result in removal of all heparin sources. Also, it is now recognized that certain treatments that might have intuitive appeal can actually worsen treatment outcomes in HIT:

- Warfarin-induced phlegmasia, venous limb gangrene, and skin necrosis syndromes. As discussed earlier, vitamin K antagonists can cause precipitous severe deficiency of protein C while at the same time not adequately reducing thrombin generation in acute HIT. Thus, during acute HIT, warfarin should be considered **contraindicated**. After substantial recovery of thrombocytopenia (preferably, >150,000/μL), and an alternative anticoagulant (e.g., lepirudin, argatroban, danaparoid, bivalirudin, fondaparinux) is being given, warfarin may be commenced at low maintenance doses (maximum initial dose, 5 mg), with at least 5 days of overlapping anticoagulation occurring before the parenteral anticoagulant is stopped. Sometimes, a patient is recognized as having HIT after several days of warfarin have already been given. In these situations, it is suggested that the coumarin effect should be reversed with vitamin K.[63] This is appropriate for two reasons: first, it reduces the risk of warfarin-induced venous limb gangrene (which can evolve quickly) because DTIs are usually monitored with the use of PTT, and second, warfarin-induced PTT prolongation may lead to underdosing of the DTI in a patient who is receiving warfarin.
- LMWH is less likely than UFH to cause HIT antibody formation[7,8,42,51–53]; unfortunately, this does not mean that it is an acceptable treatment for HIT. Through the use of sensitive activation assays, it has been determined that HIT antibodies are just as capable of activating platelets in the presence of LMWH as with UFH,[7,175] and clinical experience suggests that the risk for new, progressive, or recurrent thrombosis during treatment for HIT with LMWH approaches 50%.[176] Thus, LMWH should be considered **contraindicated** as treatment for HIT.[63]
- Platelet transfusions are relatively contraindicated for prophylaxis of bleeding in patients with acute

HIT.[63,177] This is so because petechiae and other signs of bleeding are usually not clinical features of HIT, despite even severe thrombocytopenia.[50] Further, platelet transfusions have been associated with thrombotic events in anecdotal reports.[178,179] However, if bleeding caused by anatomic or other factors complicates HIT, therapeutic platelet transfusions in this clinical context may be appropriate.
- Vena caval filters are not recommended by the author because they likely predispose to inferior vena cava or lower limb thrombosis,[76,180,181] and their deployment and use may encourage discontinuation or avoidance of further anticoagulation.
- Fasciotomies are sometimes performed in patients with ischemic limbs associated with HIT. Physicians should consider whether limb ischemia may be due to evolving microvascular thrombosis due to warfarin therapy and/or DIC, which might be better treated by intravenous vitamin K and aggressive anticoagulation.[170,182]

TREATMENT OF PATIENTS WITH ISOLATED HEPARIN-INDUCED THROMBOCYTOPENIA

Stopping heparin is an important step in managing proved or suspected HIT. However, several studies[66,183–185] indicate that cessation of heparin alone is ineffective therapy for patients with HIT, including those in whom HIT was diagnosed on the basis of thrombocytopenia alone (isolated HIT). A retrospective cohort study[66] estimated the risk for thrombosis as 10% at follow-up of 2 days, 40% at 7 days, and about 50% at 30 days. Other investigators reported[184] a 38% thrombotic event rate despite stopping of heparin; it is surprising that the frequency of thrombosis was not lower in patients in whom the heparin had been stopped soon (<48 hours) after onset of HIT, compared with patients in whom the diagnosis was made later (45% vs 34%; $P = .26$). A recent study by Zwicker and colleagues[185] found a frequency of 38% among patients with suspected isolated HIT in whom the diagnosis was supported by an EIA with an optical density greater than 1.0 U.

Tardy and colleagues[186] systematically performed compression ultrasonography or contrast venography in patients with isolated HIT. They thereby identified subclinical DVT in 8 of 16 consecutive patients with isolated HIT. These eight patients were treated with therapeutic doses of danaparoid, and the remaining eight patients without thrombosis received danaparoid in prophylactic doses. One death from fatal thrombosis was observed using this treatment approach. The high frequency of subclinical DVT at first recognition of HIT may explain the high risk for development of clinically evident venous thrombosis (40% to 50%) when patients are treated with heparin cessation alone.

Given this unfavorable natural history of isolated HIT, the Consensus Conference of the ACCP recommends that physicians consider giving a rapidly acting alternative anticoagulant for strongly suspected (or serologically confirmed) isolated HIT[63] (see Table 25-7). The author recommends that *therapeutic* doses of an alternative nonheparin agent (e.g., lepirudin, argatroban, danaparoid) should be given in this setting because standard *prophylactic* doses may not suffice in a clinical setting such as acute HIT.[161] (Note that lepirudin commenced at an initial infusion rate of 0.05 to 0.10 mg/kg/hr and without an initial bolus loading dose is considered to be a therapeutic dosing regimen because the intent is to attain a "therapeutic" PTT of 1.5 to 2.5 times baseline.[130]) However, use of prophylactic doses may be a reasonable approach if subclinical DVT has been excluded by imaging studies, or if the patient is judged to be at high risk for bleeding, or if confidence in the diagnosis of HIT is not high.[63] Nonheparin anticoagulant regimens that provide "prophylactic dose" anticoagulation include lepirudin 15 mg given subcutaneously twice daily (assumes normal renal function), fondaparinux 2.5 mg given subcutaneously daily, or danaparoid 750 U given subcutaneously twice or three times daily.[63]

Reported outcomes (end point of new thrombosis) for patients with isolated HIT have ranged from 4.4% (lepirudin)[187] to about 7%[132-134] (argatroban), which were substantially lower rates than those seen in controls (≈15% and 24%, respectively). Major bleeding rates were approximately 14% (lepirudin) and 4% (argatroban).

REEXPOSURE TO HEPARIN AFTER PREVIOUS HEPARIN-INDUCED THROMBOCYTOPENIA

Subsequent use of heparin is generally considered contraindicated in patients with a history of proven or suspected HIT. However, evidence suggests that it may be safe to use heparin again—at least for a brief period—in patients who have recovered from an episode of HIT.[41,76,188-190]

This is so because HIT antibodies are transient and are usually not detectable a few weeks or months after HIT has been resolved.[41] Moreover, HIT antibodies may not recur quickly (or at all) upon reexposure to heparin, requiring at least 5 days before clinically significant levels are attained.[41]

From a practical point of view, however, such deliberate reuse of heparin in patients with previous HIT is performed only in exceptional circumstances (e.g., patients who require cardiac surgery),[41,188-190] for which ideal alternative anticoagulants do not exist. Even in this situation, heparin would be given only for cardiopulmonary bypass itself. Use of heparin should be avoided in the preoperative and postoperative periods; alternative agents should be given for anticoagulation during heart catheterization or for postoperative anticoagulation.

SPECIALIZED CLINICAL SITUATIONS

Cardiac Surgery

The management of acute HIT in patients requiring cardiac surgery poses special problems. Table 25-12 lists various anticoagulant options when routine UFH use for cardiac surgery is contraindicated because of acute HIT or because of recent HIT in which platelet-activating anti-PF4/heparin antibodies remain detectable (subacute HIT).[145,188-191] In general, it is preferable to defer surgery whenever possible pending resolution of HIT, given the risk of coronary revascularization or valve replacement during an acute hypercoagulable state. Moreover, the oftentimes rapid disappearance of HIT antibodies within a few weeks or months after an episode of HIT[41,188] makes possible the subsequent use of heparin. For patients in whom

---

Table 25-12 Recommendations of the Seventh Conference of the American College of Chest Physicians on Antithrombotic and Thrombolytic Therapy for Cardiac Patients with HIT[63]

Patients with Previous HIT Undergoing Cardiac or Vascular Surgery
- For patients with a history of HIT who are HIT antibody negative and require cardiac surgery, we recommend the use of UFH over a nonheparin anticoagulant (grade 1C).
  Remark: Preoperative and postoperative anticoagulation, if indicated, should be administered with a nonheparin anticoagulant.

Patients with Acute or Subacute HIT Undergoing Cardiac Surgery
- For patients with acute HIT (thrombocytopenic, HIT antibody positive) who require cardiac surgery, we recommend one of the following alternative anticoagulant approaches (in descending order of preference): delaying surgery (if possible) until HIT antibodies are negative (see above) (grade 1C); using bivalirudin for intraoperative anticoagulation during cardiopulmonary bypass (if ecarin clotting time [ECT] available*) (grade 1C) or during off-pump cardiac surgery (grade 1C+); using lepirudin for intraoperative anticoagulation (if ECT available and patient has normal renal function) (grade 1C); using UFH plus the antiplatelet agent, epoprostenol (if ECT monitoring not available or renal insufficiency precludes lepirudin use) (grade 2C); using UFH plus the antiplatelet agent, tirofiban (grade 2C); or using danaparoid for intraoperative anticoagulation (if anti–factor Xa levels are available) (grade 2C).
- For patients with subacute HIT (platelet count recovery, but continuing HIT antibody positive), we recommend delaying surgery (if possible) until HIT antibodies are negative, then using heparin (see above) (grade 1C). Alternatively, we suggest the use of a nonheparin anticoagulation (see above) (grade 2C).

Percutaneous Coronary Interventions (PCIs)
- For patients with acute or previous HIT who require cardiac catheterization or PCI, we recommend use of an alternative anticoagulant, such as argatroban (grade 1C), bivalirudin (grade 1C), lepirudin (grade 1C), or danaparoid (grade 2C), over the use of heparin.

*A recent protocol for bivalirudin anticoagulation during cardiopulmonary bypass employs the activating clotting time (ACT), rather than the ECT, for intraoperative anticoagulant monitoring.[145,192]
HIT, heparin-induced thrombocytopenia; UFH, unfractionated heparin.

UFH is contraindicated, bivalirudin is emerging as a major nonheparin anticoagulant option[145] on the basis of its pharmacology (e.g., short half-life, predominant enzymatic metabolism), the potential for monitoring with the use of activated clotting time (ACT), growing experience in patients with HIT, and satisfactory outcomes in a randomized trial versus UFH for surgery requiring cardiopulmonary bypass (non-HIT patients).[192] However, the cardiac surgeon, anesthesiologist, and perfusionist must be aware of important technical issues, such as the need to avoid stagnant blood (because ongoing proteolysis of bivalirudin may lead to loss of its anticoagulant effect).[145]

Percutaneous Coronary Intervention

Both argatroban and bivalirudin have been approved in the United States for use in PCI when heparin is contraindicated because of acute HIT or a history of HIT. The recommended dose of bivalirudin is an initial intravenous bolus of 0.75 mg per kilogram, followed by a continuous infusion of 1.75 mg/kg/hr for the duration of the procedure.[145] Recommended argatroban dosing is shown in Table 25-9.

With both DTIs, procedural success in at least 95% of patients has been observed.[135,148]

Hemodialysis

Protocols have been published for the use of argatroban,[193–195] lepirudin,[193,194] or danaparoid[154,193,194] for anticoagulation during hemodialysis (HD) or hemofiltration (HF) in patients for whom heparin is contraindicated because of HIT. HD can also be performed in some patients with the use of saline. Anticoagulation of the ports after HD can be achieved with a nonheparin anticoagulant (e.g., danaparoid 750 U in 500 mL saline, with 5 to 10 mL of this solution inserted into each port; or hirudin 5 mg per milliliter per port, with just enough solution injected into each port to fill the lumen only [this must be aspirated prior to the next HD session]).[193]

Argatroban is an attractive nonheparin anticoagulant that may be used in HD or HF because it undergoes hepatic rather than renal excretion. No consensus has been reached as to the ideal dosing regimen, however. For HD, O'Shea and colleagues[193] reported the use of an initial pre-HD argatroban bolus of 100 µg per kilogram, followed

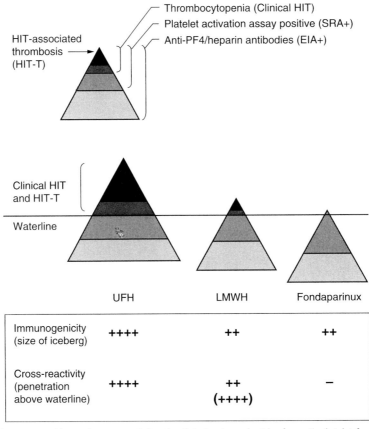

Figure 25-8 Dissociation of immunogenicity and cross-reactivity of sulfated polysaccharides for anti–platelet factor 4 (PF4)/polyanion antibodies. Of the three sulfated polysaccharide anticoagulants listed, unfractionated heparin (UFH) is most immunogenic (largest iceberg), whereas low molecular weight heparin (LMWH) and fondaparinux exhibit similar immunogenicity. However, in contrast to UFH and LMWH, which can form well with PF4 the antigens recognized by anti-PF4/heparin antibodies, fondaparinux forms these antigens poorly with PF4. It is uncertain whether the fondaparinux iceberg protrudes above the waterline (i.e., whether it might cause a syndrome resembling heparin-induced thrombocytopenia [HIT] or not). Note that the symbols indicate that cross-reactivity profile of LMWH differs in vivo (++) and in vitro (++++). EIA, enzyme immunoassay; HIT-T, HIT-associated thrombosis; SRA, serotonin release assay. (Reprinted, with permission, from Warkentin TE: HIT: Lessons learned. Pathophysiol Haemost Thromb 35:50–57, 2006.[27])

by a continuous infusion of 100 to 200 µg/kg/hr (1.7 to 3.3 µg/kg/min), to maintain the PTT at 1.5 to 3.0 times the normal mean PTT. In contrast, Murray and coworkers[195] reported the use of a somewhat higher initial argatroban bolus (250 µg per kilogram) but a similar infusion rate (2 µg/kg/min); observed PTT values were approximately 2 times those at baseline when this regimen was used. For HF, argatroban can be commenced at 0.5 to 1.0 µg/kg/min, with subsequent dose adjustments made by PTT (target, 1.5 to 2.0 times the normal mean PTT).[193,194]

Lepirudin anticoagulation for intermittent HD (every second day) can be achieved by a pre-HD bolus ranging from 0.08 to 0.15 mg/kg, with a target PTT of about 2.0 to 2.5 times the normal mean PTT (see Table 25-8).[193,194] For HF, an initially low-dose infusion rate (0.005 to 0.01 mg/kg/hr) with PTT monitoring (target, 1.5 to 2.0 times the normal mean PTT) is recommended, but careful attention to the PTT is warranted because gradual lepirudin accumulation may occur over time.[193,194]

Danaparoid anticoagulation for intermittent HD (every second day) can be achieved by administration of 3750 anti–factor Xa U before dialysis is begun.[154,193,194] Because of the long half-life of danaparoid, by the time of the third and fourth HD sessions, smaller pre-HD boluses (e.g., 3000 and 2250 U, respectively) should be given, preferably guided by measurement of anti–factor Xa levels (target, <0.4 U per milliliter pre-HD; >0.5 U per milliliter during HD). Recommended dosing for HF includes an initial bolus of 2250 U for an average-size patient, followed by 600 U per hour for 4 hours, then 400 U per hour for 4 hours, then infusion of between 200 and 400 U per hour based on anti–factor Xa levels (target, 0.5 to 1.0 U per milliliter).

PREVENTION OF HEPARIN-INDUCED THROMBOCYTOPENIA

Compared with UFH, use of LMWH is associated with a 50% lower risk that anti-PF4/heparin antibodies will be formed,[46] but an even greater reduction (≈90%) of HIT.[7,8,42,51–53] Whether the lower risk of HIT with LMWH, which has been established in post–orthopaedic surgery thromboprophylaxis, applies to other surgical patients is unclear. For example, intraoperative use of UFH during cardiac or vascular surgery may result in the production of HIT antibodies that can cause HIT even if a "safer" LMWH is used during the postoperative period (although one nonrandomized study[60] suggests that HIT risk is reduced by LMWH after cardiac surgery). In addition, data are conflicting as to whether risk of HIT is reduced by LMWH compared with UFH in medical patients.[42,196–198]

An apparent dissociation between immunogenicity and cross-reactivity of sulfated polysaccharides has been noted (Fig. 25-8).[27] Whereas UFH and LMWH both exhibit strong cross-reactivity with HIT antibodies in vitro, UFH is much more immunogenic than LMWH. In contrast, whereas LMWH and fondaparinux exhibit similar immunogenicity, fondaparinux exhibits negligible cross-reactivity with HIT antibodies. Thus, fondaparinux might convey a very low (perhaps negligible) risk that a syndrome resembling HIT will be induced. In addition, although the use of UFH or LMWH for venous thromboembolism after surgery may occasionally result in rapid-onset HIT (in a patient sensitized by recent perioperative use of heparin), this complication would not be expected to occur with fondaparinux.

REFERENCES

1. Warkentin TE: History of heparin-induced thrombocytopenia. In Warkentin TE, Greinacher A (eds): Heparin-Induced Thrombocytopenia, 4th ed. New York, Informa Healthcare USA, 2007, pp 1–19.
2. Warkentin TE, Chong BH, Greinacher A: Heparin-induced thrombocytopenia: Towards consensus. Thromb Haemost 79:1–7, 1998.
3. Warkentin TE: Heparin-induced thrombocytopenia: Pathogenesis and management. Br J Haematol 121:535–555, 2003.
4. Warkentin TE, Greinacher A: Laboratory testing for heparin-induced thrombocytopenia. In Warkentin TE, Greinacher A (eds): Heparin-Induced Thrombocytopenia, 4th ed. New York, Informa Healthcare USA, 2007, pp 227–260.
5. Warkentin TE: Platelet count monitoring and laboratory testing for heparin-induced thrombocytopenia: Recommendations of the College of American Pathologists. Arch Pathol Lab Med 126:1415–1423, 2002.
6. Amiral J, Bridey F, Dreyfus M, et al: Platelet factor 4 complexed to heparin is the target for antibodies generated in heparin-induced thrombocytopenia [Letter]. Thromb Haemost 68:95–96, 1992.
7. Warkentin TE, Levine MN, Hirsh J, et al: Heparin-induced thrombocytopenia in patients treated with low-molecular-weight heparin or unfractionated heparin. N Engl J Med 332:1330–1335, 1995.
8. Warkentin TE, Roberts RS, Hirsh J, Kelton JG: An improved definition of immune heparin-induced thrombocytopenia in postoperative orthopedic patients. Arch Intern Med 163:2518–2524, 2003.
9. Nand S, Wong W, Yuen B, et al: Heparin-induced thrombocytopenia with thrombosis: Incidence, analysis of risk factors, and clinical outcomes in 108 consecutive patients treated at a single institution. Am J Hematol 56:12–16, 1997.
10. Warkentin TE, Elavathil LJ, Hayward CPM, et al: The pathogenesis of venous limb gangrene associated with heparin-induced thrombocytopenia. Ann Intern Med 127:804–812, 1997.
11. Warkentin TE: Pseudo–heparin-induced thrombocytopenia. In Warkentin TE, Greinacher A (eds): Heparin-Induced Thrombocytopenia, 4th ed. New York, Informa Healthcare USA, 2007, pp 261–282.
12. Kelton JG, Sheridan D, Santos A, et al: Heparin-induced thrombocytopenia: Laboratory studies. Blood 72:925–930, 1988.
13. Chong BH, Fawaz I, Chesterman CN, Berndt MC: Heparin-induced thrombocytopenia: Mechanism of interaction of the heparin-dependent antibody with platelets. Br J Haematol 73:235–240, 1989.
14. Greinacher A, Pötzsch B, Amiral J, et al: Heparin-associated thrombocytopenia: Isolation of the antibody and characterization of a multimolecular PF4-heparin complex as the major antigen. Thromb Haemost 71:247–251, 1994.
15. Visentin GP, Ford SE, Scott JP, Aster RH: Antibodies from patients with heparin-induced thrombocytopenia/thrombosis are specific for platelet factor 4 complexed with heparin or bound to endothelial cells. J Clin Invest 93:81–88, 1994.
16. Newman PM, Chong BH: Further characterization of antibody and antigen in heparin-induced thrombocytopenia. Br J Haematol 107:303–309, 1999.
17. Ziporen L, Li ZQ, Park KS, et al: Defining an antigenic epitope on platelet factor 4 associated with heparin-induced thrombocytopenia. Blood 92:3250–3259, 1998.
18. Li ZQ, Liu W, Park KS, et al: Defining a second epitope for heparin-induced thrombocytopenia/thrombosis antibodies using KKO, a murine HIT-like monoclonal antibody. Blood 99:1230–1236, 2002.
19. Suh JS, Aster RH, Visentin GP: Antibodies from patients with heparin-induced thrombocytopenia/thrombosis recognize different epitopes on heparin:platelet factor 4. Blood 91:916–922, 1998.
20. Rauova L, Zhai L, Kowalska MA, et al: Role of platelet surface PF4 antigenic complexes in heparin-induced thrombocytopenia pathogenesis: Diagnostic and therapeutic implications. Blood 107:2346–2353, 2006.
21. Goad KE, Horne MK III, Gralnick HR: Pentosan-induced thrombocytopenia: Support for an immune complex mechanism. Br J Haematol 88:803–808, 1994.

25

22. Visentin GP, Moghaddam M, Beery SE, et al: Heparin is not required for detection of antibodies associated with heparin-induced thrombocytopenia/thrombosis. J Lab Clin Med 138:22–31, 2001.

23. Rauova L, Poncz M, McKenzie SE, et al: Ultralarge complexes of PF4 and heparin are central to the pathogenesis of heparin-induced thrombocytopenia. Blood 105:131–138, 2005.

24. Greinacher A, Alban S, Dummel V, et al: Characterization of the structural requirements for a carbohydrate based anticoagulant with a reduced risk of inducing the immunological type of heparin-associated thrombocytopenia. Thromb Haemost 74:886–892, 1995.

25. Warkentin TE, Cook RJ, Marder VJ, et al: Anti-platelet factor 4/heparin antibodies in orthopedic surgery patients receiving antithrombotic prophylaxis with fondaparinux or enoxaparin. Blood 106:3791–3796, 2005.

26. Greinacher A, Gopinadhan M, Günther JU, et al: Close approximation of two platelet factor 4 tetramers by charge neutralization forms the antigens recognized by HIT antibodies. Arterioscler Thromb Vasc Biol 26:2386–2393, 2006.

27. Warkentin TE: HIT: Lessons learned. Pathophysiol Haemost Thromb 35:50–57, 2006.

28. Warkentin TE: An overview of the heparin-induced thrombocytopenia syndrome. Semin Thromb Hemost 30:273–283, 2004.

29. Greinacher A, Eichler P, Lubenow N, et al: Heparin-induced thrombocytopenia with thromboembolic complications: Meta-analysis of two prospective trials to assess the value of parenteral treatment with lepirudin and its therapeutic aPTT range. Blood 96:846–851, 2000.

30. Warkentin TE, Hayward CPM, Boshkov LK, et al: Sera from patients with heparin-induced thrombocytopenia generate platelet-derived microparticles with procoagulant activity: An explanation for the thrombotic complications of heparin-induced thrombocytopenia. Blood 84:3691–3699, 1994.

31. Warkentin TE, Sheppard JI: Generation of platelet-derived microparticles and procoagulant activity by heparin-induced thrombocytopenia IgG/serum and other IgG platelet agonists: A comparison with standard platelet agonists. Platelets 10:319–326, 1999.

32. Hughes M, Hayward CPM, Warkentin TE, et al: Morphological analysis of microparticle generation in heparin-induced thrombocytopenia. Blood 96:188–194, 2000.

33. Cines DB, Tomaski A, Tanenbaum S: Immune endothelial-cell injury in heparin-associated thrombocytopenia. N Engl J Med 316:581–589, 1987.

34. Pouplard C, Iochmann S, Renard B, et al: Induction of monocyte tissue factor expression by antibodies to heparin-platelet factor 4 complexes developed in heparin-induced thrombocytopenia. Blood 97:3300–3302, 2001.

35. Khairy M, Lasne D, Amelot A, et al: Polymorphonuclear leukocyte and monocyte activation induced by plasma from patients with heparin-induced thrombocytopenia in whole blood. Thromb Haemost 92:1411–1419, 2004.

36. Herbert JM, Savi P, Jeske WP, Walenga JM: Effect of SR121566A, a potent GP IIb-IIIa antagonist, on the HIT serum/heparin-induced platelet mediated activation of human endothelial cells. Thromb Haemost 80:326–331, 1998.

37. Greinacher A, Warkentin TE: Heparin-induced thrombocytopenia. In Aird WC (ed): Endothelial Biomedicine, Cambridge, Cambridge University Press, 2007, pp 1344–1351.

38. Greinacher A, Mueller-Eckhardt G: Heparin-associated thrombocytopenia: No association of immune response with HLA. Vox Sang 65:151–153, 1993.

39. Denomme GA: Platelet and leukocyte Fcγ receptors in heparin-induced thrombocytopenia. In Warkentin TE, Greinacher A (eds): Heparin-Induced Thrombocytopenia, 4th ed. New York, Informa Healthcare USA, 2007, pp 187–208.

40. Gruel Y, Pouplard C, Lasne D, et al: The homozygous FcγRIIIa-158V genotype is a risk factor for heparin-induced thrombocytopenia in patients with antibodies to heparin-platelet factor 4 complexes. Blood 104:2791–2793, 2004.

41. Warkentin TE, Kelton JG: Temporal aspects of heparin-induced thrombocytopenia. N Engl J Med 344:1286–1292, 2001.

42. Lee DH, Warkentin TE: Frequency of heparin-induced thrombocytopenia. In Warkentin TE, Greinacher A (eds): Heparin-Induced Thrombocytopenia, 4th ed. New York, Informa Healthcare USA, 2007, pp 67–116.

43. Suh JS, Malik MI, Aster RH, Visentin GP: Characterization of the humoral immune response in heparin-induced thrombocytopenia. Am J Hematol 54:196–201, 1997.

44. Warkentin TE, Sheppard JI, Horsewood P, et al: Impact of the patient population on the risk for heparin-induced thrombocytopenia. Blood 96:1703–1708, 2000.

45. Amiral J, Wolf M, Fischer AM, et al: Pathogenicity of IgA and/or IgM antibodies to heparin-PF4 complexes in patients with heparin-induced thrombocytopenia. Br J Haematol 92:954–959, 1996.

46. Warkentin TE, Sheppard JI, Moore JC, et al: Laboratory testing for the antibodies that cause heparin-induced thrombocytopenia: How much class do we need? J Lab Clin Med 146:341–346, 2005.

47. Juhl D, Eichler P, Lubenow N, et al: Incidence and clinical significance of anti-PF4/heparin antibodies of the IgG, IgM, and IgA class in 755 consecutive patient samples referred for diagnostic testing for heparin-induced thrombocytopenia. Eur J Haematol 76:420–426, 2006.

48. Chong BH, Pilgrim RL, Cooley MA, Chesterman CN: Increased expression of platelet IgG Fc receptors in immune heparin-induced thrombocytopenia. Blood 81:988–993, 1993.

49. Hong AP, Cook DJ, Sigouin CS, Warkentin TE: Central venous catheters and upper-extremity deep-vein thrombosis complicating immune heparin-induced thrombocytopenia. Blood 101:3049–3051, 2003.

50. Warkentin TE: Clinical picture of heparin-induced thrombocytopenia. In Warkentin TE, Greinacher A (eds): Heparin-Induced Thrombocytopenia, 4th ed. New York, Informa Healthcare USA, 2007, pp 21–66.

51. Gruel Y, Pouplard C, Nguyen P, et al: Biological and clinical features of low-molecular-weight heparin–induced thrombocytopenia. Br J Haematol 121:786–792, 2003.

52. Greinacher A, Eichler P, Lietz T, Warkentin TE: Replacement of unfractionated heparin by low-molecular-weight heparin for post-orthopedic surgery antithrombotic prophylaxis lowers the overall risk of symptomatic thrombosis because of a lower frequency of heparin-induced thrombocytopenia [Letter]. Blood 106:2921–2922, 2005.

53. Martel N, Lee J, Wells PS: Risk for heparin-induced thrombocytopenia with unfractionated and low-molecular-weight heparin thromboprophylaxis: A meta-analysis. Blood 106:2710–2715, 2005.

54. Francis JL, Palmer GP III, Moroose R, Drexler A: Comparison of bovine and porcine heparin in heparin antibody formation after cardiac surgery. Ann Thorac Surg 75:17–22, 2003.

55. Warkentin TE, Kelton JG: Delayed-onset heparin-induced thrombocytopenia and thrombosis. Ann Intern Med 135:502–506, 2001.

56. Rice L, Attisha WK, Drexler A, Francis JL: Delayed-onset heparin-induced thrombocytopenia. Ann Intern Med 136:210–215, 2002.

57. Warkentin TE, Bernstein RA: Delayed-onset heparin-induced thrombocytopenia and cerebral thrombosis after a single administration of unfractionated heparin [Letter]. N Engl J Med 348:1067–1069, 2003.

58. Levine RL, Hursting MJ, Drexler A, et al: Heparin-induced thrombocytopenia in the emergency department. Ann Emerg Med 44:511–515, 2004.

59. Greinacher A, Farner B, Kroll H, et al: Clinical features of heparin-induced thrombocytopenia including risk factors for thrombosis: A retrospective analysis of 408 patients. Thromb Haemost 94:132–135, 2005.

60. Pouplard C, May MA, Iochmann S, et al: Antibodies to platelet factor 4-heparin after cardiopulmonary bypass in patients anticoagulated with unfractionated heparin or a low-molecular-weight heparin: Clinical implications for heparin-induced thrombocytopenia. Circulation 99:2530–2536, 1999.

61. Warkentin TE, Sheppard JI: No significant improvement in diagnostic specificity of an anti-PF4/polyanion immunoassay with use of high heparin confirmatory procedure [Letter]. J Thromb Haemost 4:281–282, 2006.

62. Warkentin TE, Sheppard JI, Sigouin CS, et al: Gender imbalance and risk factor interactions in heparin-induced thrombocytopenia. Blood 108:2937–2941, 2006.

63. Warkentin TE, Greinacher A: Heparin-induced thrombocytopenia: Recognition, treatment, and prevention. The Seventh ACCP Conference on Antithrombotic and Thrombolytic Therapy. Chest 126 (suppl): 311S–337S, 2004.

64. Lubenow N, Kempf R, Eichner A, et al: Heparin-induced thrombocytopenia: Temporal pattern of thrombocytopenia in relation to initial use or reexposure to heparin. Chest 122:37–42, 2002.

65. Warkentin TE: Clinical presentation of heparin-induced thrombocytopenia. Semin Hematol 35 (suppl 5): 9–16, 1998.

66. Warkentin TE, Kelton JG: A 14-year study of heparin-induced thrombocytopenia. Am J Med 101:502–507, 1996.

67. Ernest D, Fisher MM: Heparin-induced thrombocytopaenia complicated by bilateral adrenal haemorrhage. Intensive Care Med 17:238–240, 1991.

68. Meyer-Lindenberg A, Quenzel E-M, Bierhoff E, et al: Fatal cerebral venous sinus thrombosis in heparin-induced thrombotic thrombocytopenia. Eur Neurol 37:191–192, 1997.

69. Warkentin TE, Sikov WM, Lillicrap DP: Multicentric warfarin-induced skin necrosis complicating heparin-induced thrombocytopenia. Am J Hematol 62:44–48, 1999.

70. Warkentin TE: Heparin-induced thrombocytopenia: IgG-mediated platelet activation, platelet microparticle generation, and altered procoagulant/anticoagulant balance in the pathogenesis of thrombosis and venous limb gangrene complicating heparin-induced thrombocytopenia. Transfus Med Rev 10:249–258, 1996.

71. Smythe MA, Warkentin TE, Stephens JL, et al: Venous limb gangrene during overlapping therapy with warfarin and a direct thrombin inhibitor for immune heparin-induced thrombocytopenia. Am J Hematol 71:50–52, 2002.

72. Srinivasan AF, Rice L, Bartholomew JR, et al: Warfarin-induced skin necrosis and venous limb gangrene in the setting of heparin-induced thrombocytopenia. Arch Intern Med 164:66–70, 2004.

73. Warkentin TE: Coumarin-induced skin necrosis and venous limb gangrene. In Colman RW, Marder VJ, Clowes AW, et al, (eds): Hemostasis and Thrombosis: Basic Principles and Clinical Practice, 5th ed. Philadelphia, Lippincott Williams & Wilkins, 2006, pp 1649–1661.

74. Warkentin TE: Limitations of conventional treatment options for heparin-induced thrombocytopenia. Semin Hematol 35 (suppl 5): 17–25, 1998.

75. Wallis DE, Quintos R, Wehrmacher W, et al: Safety of warfarin anticoagulation in patients with heparin-induced thrombocytopenia. Chest 116:1333–1338, 1999.

76. Greinacher A, Warkentin TE: Treatment for heparin-induced thrombocytopenia: An overview. In Warkentin TE, Greinacher A (eds): Heparin-Induced Thrombocytopenia, 4th ed. New York, Informa Healthcare USA, 2007, pp 283–317.

77. Warkentin TE: Heparin-induced thrombocytopenia: Diagnosis and management. Circulation 110:e454–e458, 2004.

78. Warkentin TE: Should vitamin K be administered when HIT is diagnosed after administration of coumarin? [Letter] J Thromb Haemost 4:894–896, 2006.

79. Warkentin TE: Venous limb gangrene during warfarin treatment of cancer-associated deep venous thrombosis. Ann Intern Med 135:589–593, 2001.

80. Klein L, Galvez A, Klein O, Chediak J: Warfarin-induced limb gangrene in the setting of lung adenocarcinoma. Am J Hematol 76:176–179, 2004.

81. Warkentin TE: Heparin-induced skin lesions. Br J Haematol 92: 494–497, 1996.

82. Wütschert R, Piletta P, Bounameaux H: Adverse skin reactions to low molecular weight heparins: Frequency, management and prevention. Drug Saf 20:515–525, 1999.

83. Warkentin TE: Heparin-induced thrombocytopenia, heparin-induced skin lesions, and arterial thrombosis [Abstract]. Thromb Haemost 77 (suppl): 562, 1997.

84. Pohl C, Klockgether T, Greinacher A, et al: Neurological complications in heparin-induced thrombocytopenia [Letter]. Lancet 353:1678–1679, 1999.

85. Warkentin TE, Hirte HW, Anderson DR, et al: Transient global amnesia associated with acute heparin-induced thrombocytopenia. Am J Med 97:489–491, 1994.

86. Ansell JE, Clark WP Jr, Compton CC: Fatal reactions associated with intravenous heparin. Drug Intell Clin Pharm 20:74–75, 1986.

87. Klenner AF, Lubenow N, Raschke R, Greinacher A: Heparin-induced thrombocytopenia in children: 12 new cases and review of the literature. Thromb Haemost 91:719–724, 2004.

88. Klenner AF, Greinacher A: Heparin-induced thrombocytopenia in children. In Warkentin TE, Greinacher A (eds): Heparin-Induced Thrombocytopenia, 4th ed. New York, Informa Healthcare USA, 2007, pp 503–517.

89. Risch L, Fischer JE, Herklotz R, Huber AR: Heparin-induced thrombocytopenia in paediatrics: Clinical characteristics, therapy and outcomes. Intensive Care Med 30:1615–1624, 2004.

90. Klenner AF, Fusch C, Rakow A, et al: Benefit and risk of heparin for maintaining peripheral venous catheters in neonates: A placebo-controlled trial. J Pediatr 143:741–745, 2003.

91. Boning A, Morschheuser T, Blase U, et al: Incidence of heparin-induced thrombocytopenia and therapeutic strategies in pediatric cardiac surgery. Ann Thorac Surg 79:62–65, 2005.

92. Hursting MJ, Dubb J, Vermey-Gibboney CN: Argatroban anticoagulation in pediatric patients: A literature analysis. J Pediatr Hematol Oncol 28:4–10, 2006.

93. Warkentin TE, Cook DJ: Heparin, low molecular weight heparin, and heparin-induced thrombocytopenia in the ICU. Crit Care Clin 21:513–529, 2005.

94. Crowther MA, Cook DJ, Meade MO, et al: Thrombocytopenia in medical-surgical critically ill patients: Prevalence, incidence, and risk factors. J Crit Care 20:348–353, 2005.

95. Verma AK, Levine M, Shalansky SJ, et al: Frequency of heparin-induced thrombocytopenia in critical care patients. Pharmacotherapy 23:745–753, 2003.

96. Kitchens CS: Thrombocytopenia due to acute venous thromboembolism and its role in expanding the differential diagnosis of heparin-induced thrombocytopenia. Am J Hematol 76:69–73, 2004.

97. Warkentin TE, Heddle NM: Laboratory diagnosis of immune heparin-induced thrombocytopenia. Curr Hematol Rep 2:148–157, 2003.

98. Lo GK, Juhl D, Warkentin TE, et al: Evaluation of pretest clinical score (4 T's) for the diagnosis of heparin-induced thrombocytopenia in two clinical settings. J Thromb Haemost 4:757–758, 2006.

99. Lillo-Le Louët A, Boutouyrie P, Alhenc-Gelas M, et al: Diagnostic score for heparin-induced thrombocytopenia after cardiopulmonary bypass. J Thromb Haemost 2:1882–1888, 2004.

100. Warkentin TE: New approaches to the diagnosis of heparin-induced thrombocytopenia. Chest 127:35S–45S, 2005.

101. Warkentin TE, Sheppard JA: Laboratory testing for heparin-induced thrombocytopenia (HIT) antibodies. Transfus Med Rev 20:259–272, 2006.

102. Polgár J, Eichler P, Greinacher A, Clemetson KJ: Adenosine diphosphate (ADP) and ADP receptor play a major role in platelet activation/aggregation induced by sera from heparin-induced thrombocytopenia patients. Blood 91:549–554, 1998.

103. Sheridan D, Carter C, Kelton JG: A diagnostic test for heparin-induced thrombocytopenia. Blood 67:27–30, 1986.

104. Warkentin TE, Hayward CPM, Smith CA, et al: Determinants of platelet variability when testing for heparin-induced thrombocytopenia. J Lab Clin Med 120:371–379, 1992.

105. Lee DP, Warkentin TE, Denomme GA, et al: A diagnostic test for heparin-induced thrombocytopenia: Detection of platelet microparticles using flow cytometry. Br J Haematol 95:724–731, 1996.

106. Greinacher A, Michels I, Kiefel V, Mueller-Eckhardt C: A rapid and sensitive test for diagnosing heparin-associated thrombocytopenia. Thromb Haemost 66:734–736, 1991.

107. Greinacher A, Amiral J, Dummel V, et al: Laboratory diagnosis of heparin-associated thrombocytopenia and comparison of platelet aggregation test, heparin-induced platelet activation test, and platelet factor 4/heparin enzyme-linked immunosorbent assay. Transfusion 34:381–385, 1994.

108. Eichler P, Budde U, Haas S, et al: First workshop for detection of heparin-induced antibodies: Validation of the heparin-induced platelet activation (HIPA) test in comparison with a PF4/heparin ELISA. Thromb Haemost 81:625–629, 1999.

109. Nguyèn P, Lecompte T: Groupe d'Etude sur l'Hémostase et la Thromboses (GEHT) de la Société Française d'Hématologie: Heparin-induced thrombocytopenia: A survey of tests employed and attitudes in haematology laboratories. Nouv Rev Fr Hematol 36:353–357, 1994.

110. Chong BH, Burgess J, Ismail F: The clinical usefulness of the platelet aggregation test for the diagnosis of heparin-induced thrombocytopenia. Thromb Haemost 69:344–350, 1993.

111. Horsewood P, Warkentin TE, Hayward CPM, Kelton JG: The epitope specificity of heparin-induced thrombocytopenia. Br J Haematol 95:161–167, 1996.

112. Newman PM, Swanson RL, Chong BH: Heparin-induced thrombocytopenia: IgG binding to PF4-heparin complexes in the fluid phase and cross-reactivity with low molecular weight heparin and heparinoid. Thromb Haemost 80:292–297, 1998.

113. Meyer O, Salama A, Pittet N, Schwind P: Rapid detection of heparin-induced platelet antibodies with particle gel immunoassay (ID-HPF4). Lancet 354:1525–1526, 1999.

114. Eichler P, Raschke R, Lubenow N, et al: The new ID-heparin/PF4 antibody test for rapid detection of heparin-induced antibodies in

comparison with functional and antigenic assays. Br J Haematol 116:887–891, 2002.

115. Alberio L, Kimmerle S, Baumann A, et al: Rapid determination of anti-heparin/platelet factor 4 antibody titers in the diagnosis of heparin-induced thrombocytopenia. Am J Med 114:528–536, 2003.

116. Amiral J, Bridey F, Wolf M, et al: Antibodies to macromolecular platelet factor 4-heparin complexes in heparin-induced thrombocytopenia: A study of 44 cases. Thromb Haemost 73:21–28, 1995.

117. Bauer TL, Arepally G, Konkle BA, et al: Prevalence of heparin-associated antibodies without thrombosis in patients undergoing cardiopulmonary bypass surgery. Circulation 95:1242–1246, 1997.

118. Amiral J, Marfaing-Koka A, Wolf M, et al: Presence of auto-antibodies to interleukin-8 or neutrophil-activating peptide-2 in patients with heparin-associated-thrombocytopenia. Blood 88:410–416, 1996.

119. Guyatt G, Schunëmann H, Cook D, et al: Applying the grades of recommendation for antithrombotic and thrombolytic therapy. The Seventh ACCP Conference on Antithrombotic and Thrombolytic Therapy. Chest 126 (suppl): 179S–187S, 2004.

120. Greinacher A: Lepirudin for the treatment of heparin-induced thrombocytopenia. In Warkentin TE, Greinacher A (eds): Heparin-Induced Thrombocytopenia, 4th ed. New York, Informa Healthcare USA, 2007, pp 345–378.

121. Warkentin TE: Bivalent direct thrombin inhibitors: Hirudin and bivalirudin. Best Pract Res Clin Haematol 17:105–125, 2004.

122. Greinacher A: Lepirudin: A bivalent direct thrombin inhibitor for anticoagulation therapy. Exp Rev Cardiovasc Ther 2:339–357, 2004.

123. Eichler P, Friesen HJ, Lubenow N, et al: Antihirudin antibodies in patients with heparin-induced thrombocytopenia treated with lepirudin: Incidence, effects on aPTT, and clinical relevance. Blood 96:2373–2378, 2000.

124. Greinacher A, Lubenow N, Eichler P: Anaphylactic and anaphylactoid reactions associated with lepirudin in patients with heparin-induced thrombocytopenia. Circulation 108:2062–2065, 2003.

125. Badger NO, Butler K, Hallman LC: Excessive anticoagulation and anaphylactic reaction after rechallenge with lepirudin in a patient with heparin-induced thrombocytopenia. Pharmacotherapy 24:1800–1803, 2004.

126. Greinacher A, Völpel H, Janssens U, et al: for the HIT Investigators Group: Recombinant hirudin (lepirudin) provides safe and effective anticoagulation in patients with heparin-induced thrombocytopenia: A prospective study. Circulation 99:73–80, 1999.

127. Greinacher A, Janssens U, Berg G, et al, for the Heparin-Associated Thrombocytopenia Study (HAT) Investigators: Lepirudin (recombinant hirudin) for parenteral anticoagulation in patients with heparin-induced thrombocytopenia. Circulation 100:587–593, 1999.

128. Lubenow N, Eichler P, Lietz T: for the HIT Investigators Group: Lepirudin in patients with heparin-induced thrombocytopenia—Results of the third prospective study (HAT-3) and a combined analysis of HAT-1, HAT-2, and HAT-3. J Thromb Haemost 3:2428–2436, 2005.

129. Hacquard M, De Maistre E, Lecompte T: Lepirudin: Is the approved dosing schedule too high? [Letter] J Thromb Haemost 3:2593–2596, 2005.

130. Lubenow N, Eichler P, Greinacher A: Results of a large drug monitoring program confirms the safety and efficacy of Refludan (lepirudin) in patients with immune-mediated heparin-induced thrombocytopenia [Abstract]. Blood 100 (suppl): 502a, 2002.

131. Lewis BE, Wallis DE, Berkowitz SD, et al, for the ARG-911 Study Investigators: Argatroban anticoagulant therapy in patients with heparin-induced thrombocytopenia. Circulation 103:1838–1843, 2001.

132. Lewis BE, Wallis DE, Leya F, et al: Argatroban anticoagulation in patients with heparin-induced thrombocytopenia. Arch Intern Med 163:1849–1856, 2003.

133. Lewis BE, Wallis DE, Hursting MJ, et al: Effects of argatroban therapy, demographic variables, and platelet count on thrombotic risks in heparin-induced thrombocytopenia. Chest 129:1407–1416, 2006.

134. Lewis BE, Hursting MJ: Argatroban therapy in heparin-induced thrombocytopenia. In Warkentin TE, Greinacher A (eds): Heparin-Induced Thrombocytopenia, 4th ed. New York, Informa Healthcare USA, 2007, pp 379–408.

135. Lewis BE, Matthai WH Jr, Cohen M, et al: Argatroban anticoagulation during percutaneous coronary intervention in patients with heparin-induced thrombocytopenia. Catheter Cardiovasc Interv 57:177–184, 2002.

136. Williamson DR, Boulanger I, Tardif M, et al: Argatroban dosing in intensive care patients with acute renal failure and liver dysfunction. Pharmacotherapy 24:409–414, 2004.

137. Kiser TH, Jung R, MacLaren R, Fish DN: Evaluation of diagnostic tests and argatroban or lepirudin therapy in patients with suspected heparin-induced thrombocytopenia. Pharmacotherapy 25:1736–1745, 2005.

138. Arpino PA, Hallisey RK: Effect of renal function on the pharmacodynamics of argatroban. Ann Pharmacother 38:25–29, 2004.

139. Smythe MA, Stephens JL, Koerber JM, Mattson JC: A comparison of lepirudin and argatroban outcomes. Clin Appl Thromb Hemost 11:371–374, 2005.

140. Walenga JM, Ahmad S, Hoppensteadt D, et al: Argatroban therapy does not generate antibodies that alter its anticoagulant activity in patients with heparin-induced thrombocytopenia. Thromb Res 105:401–405, 2002.

141. Warkentin TE: Management of heparin-induced thrombocytopenia: A critical comparison of lepirudin and argatroban. Thromb Res 110:73–82, 2003.

142. Begelman SM, Hursting MJ, Aghababian RV, McCollum D: Heparin-induced thrombocytopenia from venous thromboembolism treatment. J Intern Med 258:563–572, 2005.

143. Bartholomew JR: Bivalirudin for the treatment of heparin-induced thrombocytopenia. In Warkentin TE, Greinacher A (eds): Heparin-Induced Thrombocytopenia, 4th ed. New York, Informa Healthcare USA, 2007, pp 409–439.

144. Maraganore JM, Bourdon P, Jablonski J, et al: Design and characterization of hirulogs: A novel class of bivalent peptide inhibitors of thrombin. Biochemistry 29:7095–7101, 1990.

145. Warkentin TE, Koster A: Bivalirudin: A review. Expert Opin Pharmacother 6:1349–1371, 2005.

146. Francis JL, Drexler A, Gwyn G, Moroose R: Successful use of bivalirudin in the treatment of patients suspected, or at risk of, heparin-induced thrombocytopenia [Abstract]. Blood 104 (suppl): 105b, 2004.

147. Chamberlin JR, Lewis B, Leya F, et al: Successful treatment of heparin-associated thrombocytopenia and thrombosis using Hirulog. Can J Cardiol 11:511–514, 1995.

148. Mahaffey KW, Lewis BE, Wildermann NM, et al: The Anticoagulant Therapy with Bivalirudin to Assist in the performance of percutaneous coronary intervention in patients with heparin-induced Thrombocytopenia (ATBAT) study: Main results. J Invasive Cardiol 15:611–616, 2003.

149. Warkentin TE, Greinacher A, Craven S, et al: Differences in the clinically effective molar concentrations of four direct thrombin inhibitors explain their variable prothrombin time prolongation. Thromb Haemost 94:958–964, 2005.

150. Hursting MJ, Lewis BE, Macfarlane DE: Transitioning from argatroban to warfarin therapy in patients with heparin-induced thrombocytopenia. Clin Appl Thromb Hemost 11:279–287, 2005.

151. Sheth SB, DiCicco RA, Hursting MJ, et al: Interpreting the international normalized ratio (INR) in individuals receiving argatroban and warfarin. Thromb Haemost 85:435–440, 2001.

152. Bartholomew JR, Hursting MJ: Transitioning from argatroban to warfarin in heparin-induced thrombocytopenia: An analysis of outcomes in patients with elevated international normalized ratio (INR). J Thromb Thrombolysis 19:183–188, 2005.

153. Meuleman DG, Hobbelen PMJ, Van Dedem G, Moelker HCT: A novel anti-thrombotic heparinoid (Org 10172) devoid of bleeding inducing capacity: A survey of its pharmacological properties in experimental animal models. Thromb Res 27:353–363, 1982.

154. Chong BH, Magnani HN: Danaparoid for the treatment of heparin-induced thrombocytopenia. In Warkentin TE, Greinacher A (eds): Heparin-Induced Thrombocytopenia, 4th ed. New York, Informa Healthcare USA, 2007, pp 319–343.

155. Chong BH, Gallus AS, Cade JF, et al: Prospective randomised open-label comparison of danaparoid with dextran 70 in the treatment of heparin-induced thrombocytopenia with thrombosis: A clinical outcome study. Thromb Haemost 86:1170–1175, 2001.

156. Lubenow N, Warkentin TE, Greinacher A, et al: Results of a systematic evaluation of treatment outcomes for heparin-induced thrombocytopenia in patients receiving danaparoid, ancrod, and/or coumarin explain the rapid shift in clinical practise during the 1990s. Thromb Res 117:507–515, 2006.

157. Magnani HN: Heparin-induced thrombocytopenia (HIT): An overview of 230 patients treated with orgaran (Org 10172). Thromb Haemost 70:554–561, 1993.

158. Magnani HN: Orgaran (danaparoid sodium) use in the syndrome of heparin-induced thrombocytopenia. Platelets 8:74–81, 1997.

159. Tardy-Poncet B, Tardy B, Reynaud J, et al: Efficacy and safety of danaparoid sodium (ORG 10172) in critically ill patients with heparin-associated thrombocytopenia. Chest 115:1616–1620, 1999.

160. Farner B, Eichler P, Kroll H, Greinacher A: A comparison of danaparoid and lepirudin in heparin-induced thrombocytopenia. Thromb Haemost 85:950–957, 2001.

161. Warkentin TE: Heparin-induced thrombocytopenia: Yet another treatment paradox? Thromb Haemost 85:947–949, 2001.

162. Turpie AG, Bauer KA, Eriksson BI, Lassen MR: Fondaparinux vs enoxaparin for the prevention of venous thromboembolism in major orthopedic surgery: A meta-analysis of 4 randomized double-blind studies. Arch Intern Med 162:1833–1840, 2002.

163. Buller HR, Davidson BL, Decousus H, et al: Fondaparinux or enoxaparin for the initial treatment of symptomatic deep venous thrombosis: A randomized trial. Ann Intern Med 140:867–873, 2004.

164. Buller HR, Davidson BL, Decousus H, et al: Subcutaneous fondaparinux versus intravenous unfractionated heparin in the initial treatment of pulmonary embolism. N Engl J Med 349:1695–1702, 2003.

165. Pouplard C, Couvret C, Regina S, Gruel Y: Development of antibodies specific to polyanion-modified platelet factor 4 during treatment with fondaparinux. J Thromb Haemost 3:2813–2815, 2005.

166. Savi P, Chong BH, Greinacher A, et al: Effect of fondaparinux on platelet activation in the presence of heparin-dependent antibodies: A blinded comparative multicenter study with unfractionated heparin. Blood 105:139–144, 2005.

166a. Warkentin TE, Maurer BT, Aster RH: Heparin-induced thrombocytopenia associated with fondaparinux [Letter]. N Engl J Med 356:2653–2654, 2007.

167. Kovacs MJ: Successful treatment of heparin-induced thrombocytopenia (HIT) with fondaparinux. Thromb Haemost 93:999–1000, 2005.

168. Kuo KH, Kovacs MJ: Fondaparinux: A potential new therapy for HIT. Hematology 10:271–275, 2005.

169. Harenberg J, Jorg I, Fenyvesi T: Treatment of heparin-induced thrombocytopenia with fondaparinux. Haematologica 89:1017–1018, 2004.

170. Warkentin TE: Heparin-induced thrombocytopenia and vascular surgery. Acta Chir Belg 104:257–265, 2004.

171. Weitz JI, Leslie B, Hudoba M: Thrombin binds to soluble fibrin degradation products where it is protected from inhibition by heparin-antithrombin but susceptible to inactivation by antithrombin-independent inhibitors. Circulation 97:544–552, 1998.

172. Greinacher A, Liebenhoff U, Kiefel V, et al: Heparin-associated thrombocytopenia: The effects of various intravenous IgG preparations on antibody mediated platelet activation—A possible new indication for high dose i.v. IgG. Thromb Haemost 71:641–645, 1994.

173. Frame JN, Mulvey KP, Phares JC, Anderson MJ: Correction of severe heparin-associated thrombocytopenia with intravenous immunoglobulin. Ann Intern Med 111:946–947, 1989.

174. Selleng K, Selleng S, Raschke R, et al: Immune heparin-induced thrombocytopenia can occur in patients receiving clopidogrel and aspirin. Am J Hematol 78:188–192, 2005.

175. Greinacher A, Michels I, Mueller-Eckhardt C: Heparin-associated thrombocytopenia: Antibody is not heparin-specific. Thromb Haemost 67:545–549, 1992.

176. Ranze O, Eichner A, Lubenow N, et al: The use of low-molecular-weight heparins in heparin-induced thrombocytopenia (HIT): A cohort study [Abstract]. Ann Hematol 79 (suppl 1): P198, 2000.

177. Contreras M: The appropriate use of platelets: An update from the Edinburgh Consensus Conference. Br J Haematol 101 (suppl 1): 10–12, 1998.

178. Babcock RB, Dumper CW, Scharfman WB: Heparin-induced thrombocytopenia. N Engl J Med 295:237–241, 1976.

179. Cimo PL, Moake JL, Weinger RS, et al: Heparin-induced thrombocytopenia: Association with a platelet aggregating factor and arterial thromboses. Am J Hematol 6:125–133, 1979.

180. Rice L: Heparin-induced thrombocytopenia: Myths and misconceptions (that will cause trouble for you and your patient). Arch Intern Med 164:1961–1964, 2004.

181. Ishibashi H, Takashi O, Hosaka M, et al: Heparin-induced thrombocytopenia complicated with massive thrombosis of the inferior vena cava after filter placement. Int Angiol 24:387–390, 2005.

182. Warkentin TE: The diagnosis and management of heparin-induced thrombocytopenia. In Bergan JJ (ed): The Vein Book, Amsterdam, Elsevier, 2007, pp 395–403.

183. Boon DMS, Michiels JJ, Stibbe J, et al: Heparin-induced thrombocytopenia and antithrombotic therapy [Letter]. Lancet 344:1296, 1994.

184. Wallis DE, Workman DL, Lewis BE, et al: Failure of early heparin cessation as treatment for heparin-induced thrombocytopenia. Am J Med 106:629–635, 1999.

185. Zwicker JI, Uhl L, Huang WY, et al: Thrombosis and ELISA optical density values in hospitalized patients with heparin-induced thrombocytopenia. J Thromb Haemost 2:2133–2137, 2004.

186. Tardy B, Tardy-Poncet B, Fournel P, et al: Lower limb veins should be systematically explored in patients with isolated heparin-induced thrombocytopenia [Letter]. Thromb Haemost 82:1199–1200, 1999.

187. Lubenow N, Eichler P, Lietz T, et al: Lepirudin for prophylaxis of thrombosis in patients with acute isolated heparin-induced thrombocytopenia: An analysis of 3 prospective studies. Blood 104:3072–3077, 2004.

188. Pötzsch B, Klovekorn WP, Madlener K: Use of heparin during cardiopulmonary bypass in patients with a history of heparin-induced thrombocytopenia [Letter]. N Engl J Med 343:515, 2000.

189. Koster A, Pötzsch B, Madlener K: Management of intraoperative anticoagulation in patients with heparin-induced thrombocytopenia undergoing cardiovascular surgery. In Warkentin TE, Greinacher A (eds): Heparin-Induced Thrombocytopenia, 4th ed. New York, Informa Healthcare USA, 2007, pp 487–502.

190. Warkentin TE, Greinacher A: Heparin-induced thrombocytopenia and cardiac surgery. Ann Thorac Surg 76:2121–2131, 2003.

191. Magnani HN, Beijering RJR, ten Cate JW, Chong BH: Orgaran anticoagulation for cardiopulmonary bypass in patients with heparin-induced thrombocytopenia. In Pifarré R (ed): New Anticoagulants for the Cardiovascular Patient. Philadelphia, Hanley & Belfus, 1997, pp 487–500.

192. Dyke CM, Smedira NG, Koster A, et al: A comparison of bivalirudin to heparin with protamine reversal in patients undergoing cardiac surgery with cardiopulmonary bypass: The EVOLUTION-ON study. J Thorac Cardiovasc Surg 131:533–539, 2006.

193. O'Shea SI, Ortel TL, Kovalik EC: Alternative methods of anticoagulation for dialysis-dependent patients with heparin-induced thrombocytopenia. Semin Dial 16:61–67, 2003.

194. Fischer KG: Hemodialysis in heparin-induced thrombocytopenia. In Warkentin TE, Greinacher A (eds): Heparin-Induced Thrombocytopenia, 4th ed. New York, Informa Healthcare USA, 2007, pp 463–485.

195. Murray PT, Reddy BV, Grossman EJ, et al: A prospective comparison of three argatroban treatment regimens during hemodialysis in end-stage renal disease. Kidney Int 66:2446–2453, 2004.

196. Pohl C, Kredteck A, Bastians B, et al: Heparin-induced thrombocytopenia in neurologic patients treated with low-molecular-weight heparin. Neurology 64:1285–1287, 2005.

197. Girolami B, Prandoni P, Stefani PM, et al: The incidence of heparin-induced thrombocytopenia in hospitalized medical patients treated with subcutaneous unfractionated heparin: A prospective cohort study. Blood 101:2955–2959, 2003.

198. Prandoni P, Siragusa S, Girolami B, Fabris F: and the Belzoni Investigators Group: The incidence of heparin-induced thrombocytopenia in medical patients treated with low-molecular-weight heparin: A prospective cohort study. Blood 106:3049–3054, 2005.

FURTHER READING

Warkentin TE, Greinacher A, eds: Heparin-Induced Thrombocytopenia, 4th ed. New York: Informa Healthcare, USA, 2007.

Part IV

Therapeutic Measures

Chapter 26

Antithrombotic Agents

Charles W. Francis, MD

INTRODUCTION

Antithrombotic drugs are among the most frequently used drugs in medicine. They include potent agents that affect hemostasis and are used to prevent or treat thrombotic disease. Knowledge of their properties and skill in therapeutic application are necessary to achieve maximum benefit and limit the frequency of bleeding complications. This chapter focuses on practical issues in the use of commonly used antithrombotic drugs and describes several new agents that have been introduced into clinical practice.

ORAL ANTICOAGULANTS

Historical Perspective

The development of vitamin K antagonists as oral anticoagulants is one of the most interesting stories in medicine. It began in the 1920s with investigation of a hemorrhagic disease in cattle, the cause of which was eventually found to be moldy hay that led to hypoprothrombinemia and a bleeding disorder. Additional studies ensued, and a coumarin derivative that inhibited vitamin K was eventually purified and introduced into clinical practice in the 1940s. Early studies showed that it was effective in treating patients with thrombosis, but bleeding complications were frequent, and a high degree of biologic variability in response was acknowledged. Several laboratory tests were investigated as approaches to improving anticoagulant control and outcomes, and eventually, the prothrombin time (PT) was widely adopted. Current therapy emphasizes the regulation of anticoagulant control with the international normalized ratio (INR), a derivative of the PT that normalizes test results on the basis of variability in potency of the thromboplastin used. Clinical outcomes have also greatly improved through application of modern clinical research methods to define the optimum therapeutic range, the most effective duration of treatment, and the patient populations most likely to benefit. Anticoagulation with vitamin K antagonists remains a challenging clinical problem because of the narrow therapeutic margin and high biologic variability; this limitation is counterbalanced by the high degree of efficacy of warfarin use in most of its indications. Intense efforts are under way to develop safe and effective alternative oral anticoagulants.

Mechanism and Pharmacology

The oral anticoagulants include several coumarins that act as competitive inhibitors of vitamin K and thereby inhibit the carboxylation reactions required for synthesis of several coagulation proteins, including factors II, VII, IX, and X.[1,2] Proteins C and S, which are involved in the inhibitory regulation of hemostasis, are also vitamin K dependent, and their levels also decrease during oral anticoagulation. The synthesis of all these vitamin K–dependent proteins is inhibited to a similar extent, and steady state levels during long-term therapy are reduced to the same degree. The initial rate of decrease, however, varies because of differences in plasma half-lives. Therefore, factor VII with a half-life of 6 hours declines rapidly, whereas prothrombin with a half-life of 72 hours decreases slowly after treatment has been initiated.

In North America, the most commonly used coumarin is warfarin (Coumadin; Bristol-Myers Squibb, Princeton, NJ). Warfarin is nearly completely absorbed after oral administration, and treatment is administered orally, although an intravenous preparation is available for use in circumstances in which oral intake is precluded. It does not work faster, however, than oral warfarin. Drug metabolism is complicated by binding to plasma proteins, including albumin, and also by hepatic metabolism, resulting in a variable plasma half-life. A number of drugs interact with warfarin by altering protein binding or hepatic metabolism. Because warfarin is a competitive vitamin K antagonist, its biologic action is further complicated by variability in dietary vitamin K intake. Polymorphisms in the hepatic microsomal P450 enzyme responsible for metabolism also affect individual dose response.[3,4] Together, these effects result in wide biologic variability in response to warfarin, so that close laboratory monitoring is required.

Administration and Monitoring

After therapy has begun, the onset of action is delayed as levels of vitamin K–dependent proteins decrease. Usually between 4 and 7 days of treatment is required for comparably decreased levels of vitamin K–dependent factors to be attained. The anticoagulant effect is monitored through measurement of PT, which is sensitive to decreases in vitamin K–dependent factors; this approach is further standardized by conversion to the INR. This reporting is now standard because different thromboplastins used to determine the PT vary in their sensitivity to the anticoagulant effect. Therefore, the degree of prolongation of the PT is variable with the use of different thromboplastins, but the INR is independent of the thromboplastin used. Administration of a large initial dose ("loading") results in rapid prolongation of the PT—an effect due largely to an initial rapid decrease in factor VII, which has a short half-life.

Table 26-1 Hints for the Successful Long-Term Use of Warfarin

Do not needlessly start and stop therapy (e.g., for biopsies or dental work). Low therapeutic international normalized ratios (INRs) (range, 2.0 to 2.2) will not result in excessive bleeding. Additionally, following this hint will minimize the risk of warfarin skin necrosis on reinitiation of warfarin therapy.

It is helpful to think of a patient's warfarin dose in terms of a cumulative weekly quantity, and then to make adjustments in daily doses of warfarin, which are small (i.e., only ±10% to 15%) in most cases. Skipping a day of therapy itself represents a 14% change in weekly dosage. Too frequently, changes are excessive, with undesirable results.

When changing doses, do not expect reliable changes in INR before 4 to 7 days. Doing so often results in misleading information and therapeutic overcompensation.

Do not be frustrated by INRs such as 1.8 or 3.3 in patients who have a desired INR range of 2.0 to 3.0, which is actually a very narrow range that is achievable only about 75% of the time under the best of circumstances.

Significant variances (e.g., INRs <1.5 or >6.0) nearly always have an explanation, such as missed or double doses, an intercurrent illness, significant changes in diet, and especially, the addition or substitution of some new drug or over-the-counter agent.

Instruct patients not to take or discontinue any medications, over-the-counter drugs, drug samples, alternative medicines, or drugs from friends or family without your knowledge.

If a new drug or therapy is added or diet is significantly changed, recheck the INR at day 4 to 5 to observe effects. This is better than relying on long lists of drug interactions or on one's memory.

The agents most commonly used to greatly increase (i.e., at least double or triple) the INR include amiodarone, metronidazole, and cimetidine. Those that greatly decrease the INR include dietary supplements (e.g., Ensure) and multivitamin pills that contain vitamin K.

In reversing the anticoagulant effects of warfarin, recall that warfarin's action occurs through its anti–vitamin K action. Accordingly, vitamin K therapy is usually the most logical, cheapest, safest, fastest, and most enduring therapy. Even INRs greater than 20 are normalized within 6 to 8 hours after slow IV infusion of vitamin K. Fresh frozen plasma is slow, expensive, and cumbersome, and it represents a major fluid challenge (6 to 8 U) in patients with very high INRs; its effects last only for the half-lives of the replaced factors (i.e., on the order of only 6 to 8 hours).

For long-term management, patients should become involved with their physicians in decision making. Use of a "warfarin diary" maintained by the patient greatly helps with recording of drugs and INRs and helps the patient realize that noticeable changes in INR may occur in association with changes in lifestyle and dietary alterations.

Warfarin clinics, which are often run by a health care provider or a physician who is dedicated to running such a clinic, greatly facilitate long-term warfarin therapy. This is accomplished, if by no other way, by INRs performed on site with notification of the patient within minutes. Accordingly, the duration of overanticoagulation or underanticoagulation intensity is enormously minimized.

Provide patients with a prescription for a small quantity of vitamin K tablets to be taken in case of an excessively elevated INR. This may help prevent a trip to the emergency department.

This is, however, not an adequate reflection of true antithrombotic effectiveness, which depends on a balanced reduction of all vitamin K–dependent factors. Such treatment may result in excessive factor VII reduction, which may produce bleeding, or it may cause a profound early decrease in the anticoagulant protein C, which may produce an unfavorable balance of antithrombotic and prothrombotic effects.[5,6] Anticoagulation should be initiated with a dose close to the expected daily maintenance requirement, which is usually between 5 and 10 mg. Lower doses should be used for small, elderly, or poorly nourished patients or those with an increased bleeding risk, and higher doses should be used for patients at low risk of bleeding who are younger and larger. Effects should be monitored at least every other day during initiation of treatment and less frequently during long-term therapy, depending on the stability of anticoagulation. Self-monitoring with a portable device may lead to excellent results in select patients (see Chapter 40).

Problems with therapy include variability in the anticoagulant response, which is frequently due to drugs that can increase or decrease the effects or to changes in the vitamin K content of the diet.[7] Patients should be advised to report any changes in medications to their physicians and to maintain a stable diet, particularly with respect to the content of foods high in vitamin K, including green vegetables, and dietary supplements that contain vitamin K (see Chapter 33). Variability in anticoagulation may also result from changes in absorption due to gastrointestinal illness, poor compliance, excessive use of alcohol, or over-the-counter alternative medications (Table 26-1).

Indications

Warfarin is used for prophylaxis of venous and arterial thromboembolism. It is highly effective in the primary prevention of venous thromboembolism in patients at high risk, such as orthopaedic patients undergoing hip or knee replacement. Short-term postoperative administration for a period of 7 to 14 days at an INR of 2 to 3 is effective in reducing the risk of venous thrombosis (Table 26-2). Oral anticoagulation is also highly effective as secondary prophylaxis in preventing recurrence after an initial episode of deep venous thrombosis or pulmonary embolism. After initial acute treatment with heparin or low molecular

Table 26-2 Recommended INR Values During Oral Anticoagulant Therapy

Condition	Target INR (Range)
Deep venous thrombosis treatment	2.5 (2.0–3.0)
Pulmonary embolism treatment	2.5 (2.0–3.0)
Deep venous thrombosis prophylaxis	2.5 (2.0–3.0)
Atrial fibrillation	2.5 (2.0–3.0)
Cardiac valve replacement	
Tissue valves	2.5 (2.0–3.0)
Mechanical valves	3.0 (2.5–3.5)
Acute myocardial infarction	2.5 (2.0–3.0)

INR, international normalized ratio.

weight heparin (LMWH) is provided, oral anticoagulation is continued on a long-term basis at an INR of 2 to 3 for variable periods depending on the risk of recurrence in the individual patient. Oral anticoagulation also is indicated for prophylaxis of arterial thromboembolism in patients with atrial fibrillation (currently or in past) or with artificial heart valves who are at risk of systemic embolization and stroke. In patients with mechanical heart valves, anticoagulation to a higher intensity of an INR of 2.5 to 3.5 is recommended. After an acute myocardial infarction (MI) occurs, oral anticoagulation is also indicated to prevent systemic embolization or recurrent MI.

Adverse Effects

The most serious and common complication of oral anticoagulation is bleeding, and its risk is related primarily to patient characteristics, intensity of the anticoagulation, and length of therapy.[8–10] Older age has been related to bleeding risk in several studies. The risk of bleeding is increased with surgery or significant trauma during oral anticoagulation. Similarly, a history of gastrointestinal bleeding, particularly if recent, is a major risk; renal insufficiency, hypertension, and a history of cerebrovascular disease may also be related to bleeding risk. Alcoholism and poor compliance are common causes of poor control and poor outcomes. The intensity of anticoagulation as reflected by the INR is the most important predictor of bleeding risk, which is low in the usual therapeutic range but begins to increase above INR 4.0. The cumulative risk of bleeding increases with longer duration of treatment, whereas the absolute risk appears greatest early, possibly because of unmasking of asymptomatic pathologic lesions. Overall, the total risk of bleeding with a 3-month course of anticoagulation for venous thromboembolism is between 3% and 5%, and in patients anticoagulated for prosthetic heart valves or atrial fibrillation, the yearly rate of major bleeding is also between 3% and 5%.

Warfarin skin necrosis is a rare complication of warfarin therapy that usually, but not always, occurs early in the course of anticoagulation or on reinitiation of treatment after a hiatus in therapy. Initial complaints typically consist of burning and tingling at the affected site, such as the breast, buttock, or thigh, or at another location with significant underlying adipose tissue. Painful hemorrhagic full-thickness skin infarction develops; it heals slowly and frequently requires skin grafting (see Fig. 11-22). Histopathology shows thrombosis in dermal and subdermal venules, and it is hypothesized that this is due to disproportionate rapid reduction of anticoagulant proteins C and S, predisposing to thrombosis. A recent publication pictorally demonstrates these changes well.[10a] The reason for its occurrence at anatomic sites with extensive subcutaneous fat is unknown.

Oral anticoagulation is avoided in pregnancy because warfarin crosses the placenta, and exposure during organogenesis in the first trimester can lead to fetal embryopathy with significant cranial bone malformations.[11] Anticoagulation later during pregnancy increases bleeding complications. Oral anticoagulants may be considered during the second trimester, but they are generally avoided because heparin, LMWH, and fondaparinux are reasonable alternatives.

Reversal of Oral Anticoagulation

Frequently, anticoagulation is reversed because of bleeding, surgery, trauma, or, especially, overdose. For patients with excessively prolonged INRs (e.g., greater than 6) without bleeding, appropriate interventions consist of holding warfarin doses, administering low doses of vitamin K, and increasing the frequency of monitoring (Table 26-3).[12,13] Serious bleeding or major warfarin overdose (e.g., INR >10) requires factor replacement and/or larger vitamin K doses that may need to be given intravenously. Anticoagulated patients who need invasive procedures represent a challenging management problem (Table 26-4).[14,15] Clinical decisions should be based on the need to balance the risk of thromboembolism with that of bleeding (see Chapter 38).

The goal of warfarin treatment is to induce anticoagulation and thereby avoid thromboembolism. It is important to note that the baseline risk of thromboembolism further increases during the immediate postoperative period.

Table 26-3 Reversal of Warfarin Therapy

Indication	Plan
INR <6	Lower or hold dose
INR 6–10	Give vitamin K 1–2 mg PO*; recheck INR 12–24 hours later
INR >10	Give vitamin K 2–4 mg PO*; recheck INR 12–24 hours later
Serious bleeding or major overdose	Give vitamin K 5–10 mg IV, plus, occasionally, fresh frozen plasma or prothrombin complex concentrate, rarely rFVIIa.

*Can also be given subcutaneously, but response is slower.
INR, international normalized ratio.
rFVIIa, recombinant activated factor VII.

Table 26-4 Reversing Warfarin Anticoagulation for Surgery

Low risk of thrombotic recurrence: Hold warfarin 4 to 5 days preoperatively. Check the INR 1 day before surgery, and perform surgery if it is 1.5 or less. Warfarin can be started postoperatively.

Moderate risk of thrombotic recurrence: Hold warfarin 4 to 5 days preoperatively. Check INR 1 day before surgery is performed to confirm it is below 1.5. Start unfractionated heparin or LMWH in prophylactic doses preoperatively, and continue until warfarin effect is in the therapeutic range after postoperative initiation.

High risk of thrombotic recurrence: Effective anticoagulation must be maintained. Warfarin should be stopped 4 to 5 days preoperatively. When INR is below 2.0, heparin or LMWH should be begun in therapeutic doses given intravenously or subcutaneously, respectively. Heparin should be held 6 hours and subcutaneous LMWH 24 hours preoperatively. Start heparin or LMWH in therapeutic doses postoperatively as soon as the bleeding risk is decreased and acceptable. Restart warfarin. Stop heparin when a therapeutic INR is achieved.

INR, international normalized ratio; LMWH, low molecular weight heparin.

26

In general, the bleeding risk is highest during surgery and begins to decrease toward baseline levels after approximately 1 week. Most surgery can be done with minimal bleeding risk in patients receiving warfarin with an INR near 1.5, although studies documenting an ideal INR or values of INR at which surgery is unsafe do not yet exist. After acute thrombosis, the risk of recurrence is high initially and declines over time. For example, recurrent venous thromboembolism occurs often during the first 1 to 2 weeks after diagnosis but is much less frequent after 8 to 12 weeks. Elective surgery and other invasive procedures associated with a high bleeding risk should be postponed if possible during the first several months after thrombosis is reported.

HEPARIN

Historical Perspective

Heparin derives its name from its original identification in approximately 1920 within an aqueous extract of liver that exhibited anticoagulant activity in vitro. It was not until approximately 1940, however, that heparin was used successfully as a treatment for thrombosis. Its use expanded subsequently as thrombotic disease was recognized more commonly and as extracorporeal and prosthetic vascular conduits came into use. Heparin is a biologic tissue extract that is highly heterogeneous. It was recognized early that most molecules in therapeutic preparations had no anticoagulant activity. The search for heparin derivatives with improved properties led to the introduction of LMWH in the 1990s. These preparations are derived from heparin through biologic or enzymatic degradation, and they exhibit improved pharmacologic properties. The culmination of these efforts led to identification of the five-saccharide sequence that mediates binding of heparin to antithrombin III, leading to its anticoagulant effects. Fondaparinux, a pentasaccharide based on this sequence, represents the newest addition as a therapeutic agent and the newest chapter in this long history.

Mechanism and Pharmacology

Heparin, a mixture of sulfated glycosaminoglycans, is a commonly used, rapidly acting parenteral anticoagulant.[16] It is extracted from the lungs and intestinal tissue of cows and swine, and it is assayed biologically. Heparin has no direct anticoagulant effects, but it acts through antithrombin III, a plasma serine protease inhibitor. Antithrombin III inhibits thrombin, factor Xa, and other coagulation enzymes in a reaction that is relatively slow but is accelerated more than 1000-fold in the presence of heparin. Heparin is not absorbed after oral ingestion, so it must be given subcutaneously or intravenously. Heparin interacts with proteins and cells in the blood, resulting in complex pharmacokinetics characterized by rapid equilibration and slower clearance. Heparin causes release of endothelial cell–bound tissue factor pathway inhibitor (TFPI), and this may contribute to its therapeutic actions. Plasma half-life increases with higher doses and is variable among individuals. After subcutaneous administration, bioavailability may be less than 50% and peak plasma levels occur after 30 to 60 minutes.

Administration and Monitoring

Heparin is usually given intravenously for full anticoagulation, and clinical studies have shown a reduced occurrence of bleeding complications with continuous intravenous rather than intermittent bolus therapy. The anticoagulant effect is immediate, but laboratory monitoring is needed because of variability in response among patients. This is most conveniently done with partial thromboplastin time (PTT). The appropriate PTT range for heparin therapy is usually between 1.5 and 2.5 times the mean of the normal range, but this varies depending on laboratory reagent and instrumentation, and each laboratory should establish a therapeutic range that is based on appropriate correlation with heparin levels. Clinically useful nomograms for treating patients with venous thromboembolism are available for use in adjusting heparin dose (Table 26-5).[17,18] Alternatively, heparin can be monitored with the use of anti-Xa levels, and this approach is useful when the PTT cannot be relied on, such as in patients with baseline prolongation of the PTT due to lupus anticoagulant. Other indications for using such heparin levels are listed in Table 26-6. The therapeutic range with a chromogenic anti-Xa assay is 0.3 to 0.7 U per milliliter. Somewhat lower heparin doses are recommended for patients with acute coronary syndromes. In patients with unstable angina and non–ST segment MI, an initial bolus of 60 to 70 U per kilogram (up to 5000 U) followed by an infusion of 12 to 15 U/kg/hr (up to 1000 U per hour) is recommended.[19] For patients who undergo thrombolysis with tissue plasminogen activator (tPA), a bolus of 60 U per kilogram (up to 4000 U) followed by an infusion of 12 U per kilogram (up to 1000 U per hour) is suggested.[20] Maintenance of levels in the therapeutic range provides an adequate antithrombotic level and limits bleeding. For prophylaxis of venous thromboembolic disease, heparin is administered subcutaneously in doses of 5000 U every 8 to 12 hours, with the 8-hourly regimen more appropriate in patients at higher risk. Minor prolongation of the PTT may occur, but monitoring is neither recommended nor required. When very high doses are administered, as occurs during cardiopulmonary bypass, on-site monitoring is provided with the use of activated clotting time (ACT).

Heparin Resistance

Causes of heparin resistance include increased heparin clearance during pregnancy and antithrombin III deficiency. Acquired antithrombin III deficiency may be seen in patients with extensive thrombosis or disseminated intravascular coagulation (DIC) or during cardiopulmonary bypass. Treatment with antithrombin III concentrates or recombinant human antithrombin III has been shown to restore heparin sensitivity in patients undergoing renal replacement therapy[21] or cardiac surgery with cardiopulmonary bypass.[22] Some patients appear to respond poorly to heparin, with inadequate prolongation of the PTT despite apparently adequate or even high heparin dosages (Table 26-7). This is often referred to as "heparin resistance," and it is due rarely to antithrombin III deficiency; more commonly, it is due to the acute phase response, which results in high levels of procoagulant proteins, particularly factor VIII and fibrinogen. The antithrombotic effects of heparin correlate best with plasma heparin levels,

Table 26-5 Intravenous Heparin Dosing Nomograms

Fixed-Dose Nomogram*[17]

PTT, sec[†]	Bolus Dose, U	Stop Infusion, min	Change in Infusion Rate[‡]	Time of Repeat PTT
<50	5000	0	+3 mL/hr	6 hours
50–59	0	0	+3 mL/hr	6 hours
60–85	0	0	0	Next morning
86–95	0	0	−2 mL/hr	Next morning
96–120	0	30	−2 mL/hr	6 hours
>120	0	60	−4 mL/hr	6 hours

Weight-Based Nomogram[18]

The initial dose is 80 U/kg given as a bolus, then 18 U/kg/hr. The following dose adjustments are based on PTT values obtained every 6 hours.

PTT, sec[§]	Bolus, U/kg	Infusion, U/kg/hr
<35	80	Increase rate by 4
35–45	40	Increase rate by 2
46–70	0	No change
71–90	0	Decrease rate by 2
>90	0	Decrease rate by 3

Dose Adjustment

*These modifications occurred after initial heparin loading and maintenance infusion.
[†]Reference range is 35 to 37 seconds. Therapeutic range is 60 to 85 seconds, corresponding to a plasma heparin level approximating 0.3 to 0.7 U per milliliter by anti–factor Xa activity.
[‡]1 mL/hr equals 40 U per hour.
[§]Reference range, 20 to 30 seconds.
PTT, partial thromboplastin time.

Table 26-6 Clinical Situations in which Measurement of Heparin Levels is Appropriate

Some clinical conditions are associated with prolonged PTT before heparin is administered. These include inherited factor deficiencies, severe liver deficiency, and antiphospholipid syndrome. Accordingly, monitoring of heparin dosage via PTT is greatly obfuscated. Check baseline PTT, begin heparin therapy at a reasonable dose, and confirm heparin levels with an anti-Xa assay to establish that the heparin level is in the therapeutic range.

In some cases, the clinical situation is such that one wishes, on the one hand, to treat a severe thrombotic episode with adequate heparin; on the other hand, one would not like to have excessive heparin levels. These would include situations in which the patient is bleeding, has recently had surgery or a stroke, or is given a diagnosis of severe thrombocytopenia.

Treatment of patients with massive thrombosis occasionally is complicated by heparin resistance. As more and more heparin is administered in an attempt to achieve a therapeutic PTT, one becomes concerned. It is comforting to determine the heparin level when one is giving massive doses such as ≥40,000 U of standard heparin per day. In these cases, the dose can be titrated until an anti-Xa level of 0.3 to 0.7 U per milliliter is achieved.

When LMWH or fondaparinux is used, determination of anti–factor Xa activity is useful in all cases described above, as well as when the clinician is uncertain regarding dosages in patients who are massively obese, or in those who are renally insufficient. Should a patient have a bleeding episode while receiving what one had considered to be appropriate doses of these agents, it is of value to confirm the level at which the adverse effect took place.

Obtaining heparin levels to rule out the presence of heparin when a patient theoretically had not been administered heparin is useful. One such clinical situation is postoperative bleeding with a very long PTT, which strongly suggests the possibility of heparin. This can also be useful when an unexpectedly prolonged PTT is detected in a patient with an indwelling heparinized central line, for whom the sample could be contaminated with heparin. Establishing that heparin was present or absent can help to narrow diagnostic considerations.

PTT, partial thromboplastin time; LMWH, low molecular weight heparin.

which may be adequate in these circumstances despite an apparent subtherapeutic PTT. Therefore, for patients who require more than 1500 U per hour, periodic monitoring with an anti-Xa assay is appropriate and provides a better indication of plasma levels.[23]

Indications

Heparin is commonly used in the prevention and treatment of venous thromboembolic disease. Treatment is initiated with an IV bolus followed by a constant infusion to maintain desired anticoagulant effects for a minimum of 5 days; this is followed by a longer period of oral anticoagulation. Heparin is also used in the treatment of patients with acute coronary syndromes and is effective in the short-term treatment of those with unstable angina and MI, as an adjunct to thrombolytic therapy, and in preventing acute reocclusion after angioplasty or stenting (see Chapter 20). It is used to maintain vascular patency during vascular surgery and in high doses and high levels

Table 26-7 Heparin Resistance

Definition: Inadequate prolongation of PTT or ACT despite administration of high doses of heparin (e.g., >1500 U/hr for treatment of venous thromboembolism, or 400 U/kg during cardiopulmonary bypass).

Causes: High levels of factor VIII and fibrinogen; antithrombin III deficiency; increased clearance during pregnancy.

Management: Measure antithrombin III levels. If low (e.g., <70%), consider giving antithrombin III to increase levels to 100%. If antithrombin III deficiency is not present, monitor heparin therapy with anti-Xa levels.

PTT, partial thromboplastin time; ACT, activated clotting time.

(e.g., approximately 3 U/mL) to permit extracorporeal circulation during cardiopulmonary bypass. In patients with DIC, heparin can be used in attempts to reduce hemostatic activation, prevent microvascular occlusion, and improve overall hemostasis (see Chapter 12).

Heparin is often used for anticoagulation during pregnancy (see Chapter 36).[11] Short-term treatment is administered as in the nonpregnant patient, and long-term anticoagulation may be provided with subcutaneous administration. Heparin is often the anticoagulant of choice during pregnancy because warfarin is associated with risks for fetal defects. For full anticoagulation, subcutaneous doses of 17,000 U or more every 12 hours may be required, with monitoring provided to maintain the PTT in the therapeutic range 4 to 6 hours after administration. Heparin requirements may increase during pregnancy, particularly in the third trimester. Heparin does not cross the placenta and exerts no anticoagulant effect in the fetus. It can, however, increase bleeding during delivery, and heparin may be discontinued briefly at the beginning of labor or prior to planned operative delivery.

Adverse Effects

The most frequent complication of heparin administration is bleeding that is related to the dose and intensity of treatment and to patient characteristics. Given the wide range of patients in whom heparin is used, it is difficult to state an average bleeding risk. However, in large groups of patients who receive heparin for treatment of venous thromboembolic disease, approximately 3% may have a major bleeding complication. Lower doses, such as those used for thromboprophylaxis, are rarely the sole or chief cause of hemorrhage.

Heparin-induced thrombocytopenia (HIT) (see Chapter 25) is immune-mediated platelet consumption caused by an antibody directed against a complex of heparin and platelet factor 4.[16,24,25] Platelets can fall to low levels associated with bleeding, yet HIT is more often associated with severe arterial or venous thromboembolic complications. HIT, when defined as a 50% reduction in baseline platelet count or a platelet count lower than 150,000 per microliter during therapy, occurs in about 3% of patients. In patients administered heparin for the first time, HIT usually occurs after 5 days, but thrombocytopenia may develop earlier if prior exposure has occurred. Platelet counts should be monitored during treatment and heparin discontinued if thrombocytopenia occurs. If a rapidly acting parenteral anticoagulant is needed, a direct thrombin inhibitor or fondaparinux can be used as an alternative.

Long-term heparin therapy causes radiographic evidence of bone loss in more than 15% of women receiving prolonged treatment during pregnancy. Symptomatic vertebral fractures occur in approximately 2%. Bone loss resolves after heparin is discontinued,[26,27] and risks with short-term use are not appreciable.

Reversal of Effect

A major advantage of heparin is its short half-life. Anticoagulant effect is eliminated within 2 to 3 hours after discontinuation of an intravenous infusion. Therefore, stopping the infusion and taking local measures are usually adequate to control bleeding (Table 24-8). In major or life-threatening bleeding, the anticoagulant effects of heparin may be neutralized with protamine sulfate, which is a basic polypeptide that binds tightly to the acidic heparin molecule. The usual dose of protamine is 1 mg, given to neutralize 100 U of heparin. The dose to be administered is based on an estimate of the amount of heparin remaining in the circulation. Protamine is routinely used to neutralize heparin after cardiopulmonary bypass with the use of standard formulas and ACT monitoring. Fresh frozen plasma has no role in reversing the effects of heparin.

LOW MOLECULAR WEIGHT HEPARIN

Mechanism and Pharmacology

Significant clinical problems with heparin include unpredictable absorption and bioavailability after subcutaneous administration and variable binding to plasma proteins and cells. When these problems occur simultaneously, heparin therapy must be monitored with coagulation tests and doses adjusted. Bleeding is a serious complication, osteoporosis may develop with prolonged use, and HIT occurs in approximately 3% of patients. These limitations led to studies of structural and functional relationships with heparin and eventually to the development of LMWHs. Preparations are produced through chemical or enzymatic treatment of heparin to decrease the size of the polysaccharide chains, yielding a product with a restricted molecular weight distribution with a mean of approximately 4000 to 5000 daltons.[16] Similar to heparin, LMWH exerts its antithrombotic effects through interaction with antithrombin III. In the presence of LMWH, antithrombin III inactivates factor Xa, as does unfractionated heparin, but it is less able to inactivate thrombin because of the shorter polysaccharide length. A comparison of the important clinical properties of heparin, LMWH, and fondaparinux is presented in Table 26-9. Several LMWH preparations are available, and they share many clinical and pharmacologic properties. Also, effectiveness and safety have proved similar in clinical trials. However, because each is produced by a different method and has some unique properties, pharmacologic properties and clinical results may vary.

LMWH preparations can be administered intravenously but are usually given subcutaneously because of their nearly complete absorption and obviously enhanced convenience. This is a clear benefit over unfractionated heparin, which exhibits variable and dose-dependent absorption after subcutaneous administration. Moreover, different from

Table 26-8 Approach to Hemorrhaging Patients Receiving Heparin

Questions	Considerations	Actions
Is bleeding due to heparin?	Do not assume that hemorrhage is necessarily due to heparin. Consider and evaluate for structural defects such as a tumor, ulcer, or nonligated vessel. Consider other inherited or acquired problems.	Apply local pressure, if possible. Correct structural bleeding. Ligate vessels.
Are aggravating factors present?	Rule out contribution to hemorrhage by thrombocytopenia, antiplatelet agents such as aspirin or NSAIDs, thrombolytic agents, oral anticoagulants, or acquired vitamin K deficiency.	Administer DDAVP for antiplatelet agent reversal and vitamin K for that deficiency. Transfuse platelets for thrombocytopenia.
Is the concentration of heparin unacceptably high if actions thus far implicate heparin?	Identify time and dose (confirmed by discussion with pharmacy and nursing) of last heparin administration. Estimate half-life of remaining heparin. Check heparin level.	Cease heparin administration. Attempt protamine reversal in exceptional cases. Do not administer FFP.
Is the indication for continuing anticoagulation stronger than the contraindication?	Failure to treat patients with thromboembolic indications with heparin is usually much more dangerous than the very rare hemorrhaging fatality caused by the use of heparin.	Lower the dose of heparin, and transfuse as necessary. Consider IVC devices in exceptional cases to prevent PE.

NSAIDs, nonsteroidal anti-inflammatory drugs; DDAVP, 1-deamino-8-D-arginine vasopressin; desmopressin; FFP, fresh frozen plasma; IVC, inferior vena cava; PE, pulmonary embolism.

Table 26-9 Comparisons Among Heparin, LMWH, and Fondaparinux

	Heparin	LMWH	Fondaparinux
Bioavailability after subcutaneous injection	Dose dependent, low	High	High
Half-life	1–2 hours	3–5 hours	17 hours
Need for monitoring	Routine	Occasional	Not yet known
Cost	Negligible	High	High
Prolongation of PTT	Dose dependent	Minimal	Minimal/none

LMWH, low molecular weight heparin; PTT, partial thromboplastin time.

heparin, LMWH exhibits much less binding to plasma proteins and cells. Consequently, blood levels and anticoagulant effects are more predictable after LMWH is administered. Also, LMWH preparations have a longer plasma half-life than does unfractionated heparin—a desirable effect in the absence of bleeding. Together, these properties make possible once- or twice-daily subcutaneous LMWH regimens that are practical for prophylaxis and therapy. LMWH preparations have significant renal clearance, and high plasma levels can rapidly accumulate after repeated doses are given to patients with reduced renal function. Therefore, monitoring of anti-Xa levels and dose adjustments are needed in patients with renal impairment. Markedly obese patients also represent a difficult group, in that dosing regimens have not been specifically tested in these patients and very high levels can result from weight-based dosing. Many experts "cap" the dose at the equivalent of approximately 12,500 U twice daily. Accordingly, in select cases, monitoring levels is very useful when combined with LMWH therapy (see Table 26-6).

Clinical Uses

The use of LMWH has expanded to encompass many applications for which heparin has been used traditionally.

The findings of extensive clinical studies are now available to guide prophylaxis and therapy of venous thromboembolic disease. Dosing regimens for LMWH preparations approved for use in North America and Europe are listed in Table 26-10. As of the date of this writing, enoxaparin (Lovenox; Aventis Pharmaceuticals Inc., Bridgewater, NJ, USA), dalteparin (Fragmin; Pfizer Inc., New York, NY, USA), and tinzaparin (Innohep; Pharmion Corporation, Boulder, Colo, USA) have been approved by the U.S. Food and Drug Administration (FDA) for use in the United States. Each is marketed for specific indications and labeling differs, with some assayed in anti-Xa units and some in milligrams. In general, 1 mg is approximately equivalent to 100 anti-Xa U. For details regarding indications and dosages, specific prescribing information should be reviewed.

For prophylaxis in surgery, regimens vary according to the risk of thrombosis.[28] Lower doses are recommended for low-risk patients, and increased doses are given to higher-risk patients, such as those undergoing surgery for active malignancy. Patients undergoing orthopaedic surgery are at particularly high risk, and increased daily or twice-daily doses are recommended. Generally, high doses are given the night before or postoperatively rather than immediately preoperatively to decrease the risk of surgical

THERAPEUTIC MEASURES

Table 26-10 Treatment Regimens with LMWH

	Drug*	Regimen
Prophylaxis		
General surgery		
Low risk	Dalteparin	2500 U, 1–2 hr preop and qd
	Enoxaparin	20 mg, 1–2 hr preop and qd
	Tinzaparin	3500 U, 2 hr preop and qd
High risk	Dalteparin	5000 U, 10–12 hr preop and qd
	Enoxaparin	40 mg, 10–12 hr preop and qd
Orthopaedic surgery	Dalteparin	5000 U, 8–12 hr preop and qd
	Enoxaparin	30 mg q12h starting 12–24 hr postop or 40 mg qd starting 12 hr preop
	Tinzaparin	50 U/kg, 2 hr preop and qd or 75 U/kg qd starting 12–24 hr postop
Spinal injury	Enoxaparin	30 mg q12h
Multiple trauma	Enoxaparin	30 mg q12h
Medical patients	Enoxaparin	20 mg qd (40 mg qd more effective in high-risk patients)
	Dalteparin	5000 U qd
Treatment		
Venous thromboembolism	Enoxaparin	1 mg/kg q12h or 1.5 mg/kg qd
	Dalteparin	100 U/kg q12h or 200 U/kg qd
	Tinzaparin	175 U/kg qd
Unstable angina	Enoxaparin	1 mg/kg q12h
	Dalteparin	100 U/kg q12h

*Brand names: dalteparin, Fragmin; enoxaparin, Lovenox; tinzaparin, Innohep.
LMWH, low molecular weight heparin.

bleeding. In patients who are given epidural anesthesia, the catheter should be placed prior to administration of LMWH or at the time of anticipated trough level. Additional doses are usually held for at least 2 hours after catheter insertion, withdrawal, or manipulation because of the risk of bleeding into the spinal canal.[29] LMWH is also effective in high-risk patients after spinal injury or multiple trauma. It can be used for prophylaxis in medical patients, and large prospective studies suggest that 40 mg of enoxaparin is more effective than 20 mg once daily in medical patients with acute illnesses.[30] Administration of dalteparin 5000 U once daily was also effective in acutely ill medical patients in a recent study.[31]

The pharmacokinetic properties of LMWH preparations make them suitable for treatment of patients with acute deep venous thrombosis and pulmonary embolism through subcutaneous administration; clinical studies have established the efficacy and safety of this approach.[32–34] High-dose regimens are used, and once- or twice-daily administration has been effective. Similar doses are used for treatment of those with acute coronary syndromes; evidence from clinical trials shows improved outcomes in patients with unstable angina who are treated acutely with LMWH as compared with unfractionated heparin. LMWH does not cross the placenta and has been used successfully for prophylaxis and treatment of pregnant patients with venous thromboembolic disease. Because of changes that may occur in weight and renal function, occasional monitoring with anti-Xa levels is advisable.

Adverse Effects

The primary complication of LMWH is bleeding. Minor bruising at injection sites is common and annoying but of little clinical consequence. Major bleeding occurs at approximately the same frequency as it does with unfractionated heparin when used in similar patient groups for the same indication. HIT is much less common with LMWH, occurring only 10% to 15% as often as with heparin, suggesting that HIT may be reduced by 80% through the use of LMWH. However, cross-reactivity of the antibody occurs, and LMWH is *not* an acceptable choice for continued anticoagulation in patients with HIT. Animal studies suggest that osteoporosis may be uncommon with LMWH; few clinical data are available.

Choice of Heparin Versus LMWH

Factors that govern the selection of heparin or LMWH include effectiveness, safety, convenience, and cost. Differences in characteristics (Tables 26-9 and 26-11) among these agents are exploited for the benefit of specific needs of each patient's situation; one drug is not "better" than the others. For prophylaxis in most surgical and medical patients, evidence indicates that heparin and LMWH are equally effective, and the lower cost of heparin makes it an attractive choice. In orthopaedic patients, LMWH is more effective than heparin and is therefore preferable. For treatment of those with venous thromboembolic disease, the safety and effectiveness of LMWH have been reported to be superior to those of unfractionated heparin. Subcutaneous regimens of LMWH offer enhanced patient convenience, and outpatient home treatment is the preference of most patients. Outpatient therapy requires intensive patient education, adequate medical supervision, and considerations of drug costs, insurance coverage, and adequate follow-up. The overall cost of outpatient therapy is much less than the cost of inpatient intravenous heparin treatment.

IV

456

In some specific circumstances, however, unfractionated heparin may be preferable.

In patients who may require an invasive procedure on an urgent basis, the short half-life of heparin administered intravenously is attractive. Also, patients with renal insufficiency have an increased bleeding risk, and decreased LMWH clearance may lead to high levels; intravenous heparin offers some advantages. LMWH is only incompletely reversed by protamine sulfate, making it difficult to use for bypass surgery. The use of LMWH for acute coronary syndromes is rapidly evolving and involves consideration of combination therapy, including potent antiplatelet agents and mechanical interventions. Some studies indicate greater effectiveness of LMWH in the treatment of patients with acute coronary syndromes.[35,36] A recent analysis has questioned the appropriateness of heparin dosing in several trials in which heparin and LMWH were compared for safety and efficacy.[37]

Fondaparinux

Fondaparinux is a completely synthetic heparin–like molecule with selective anti–factor Xa activity.[38] Its structure is based on the heparin sequence that interacts specifically with antithrombin III. It binds reversibly and with high affinity to antithrombin III, resulting in a conformational change that makes it effective in inhibiting factor Xa. However, its pentasaccharide chain is not long enough to interact with thrombin. Consequently, it has no appreciable thrombin inhibitory activity, and its mechanism of action involves reducing thrombin generation. Fondaparinux does not induce allergic responses because it is produced synthetically and contains no animal products.

After subcutaneous administration, peak plasma levels are reached after approximately 2 hours, and the elimination half-life is approximately 17 hours. Bioavailability is nearly complete after subcutaneous or intravenous administration. Intrasubject and intersubject availability is low, and little accumulation is noted after multiple daily doses. Fondaparinux plasma levels can be measured with the anti–factor Xa assay, and little effect is seen with the use of other coagulation tests, including PT, PTT, and thrombin time (TT).

Clinical studies have evaluated fondaparinux in the prevention and treatment of venous thromboembolism.[39–41] It has been approved by the FDA for the prevention of venous thromboembolism after major orthopaedic surgery at a dose of 2.5 mg administered subcutaneously once daily. This dose is effective for thromboprophylaxis in a variety of medical and surgical patients. It is also effective and has been approved for the treatment of those with deep vein thrombosis and pulmonary embolism when used at a dose of 7.5 mg subcutaneously once daily. Fondaparinux is available in therapeutic doses of 5 mg for smaller patients and 10 mg for larger patients.

Bleeding is the principal adverse affect, and frequency and severity of this effect have been similar to those observed with LMWH. Because the drug is excreted in the urine, elevated levels may be observed with renal insufficiency. Caution should be used in administering fondaparinux to patients with renal compromise.

No cross-reactivity with antibodies causing HIT has been reported; thus, fondaparinux has been used for (off-label) anticoagulation in patients with HIT. HIT has not yet been reported in patients given fondaparinux. This agent may be a particularly good choice in those who require subcutaneous administration. Although it has not yet been approved for the treatment of patients with HIT, many have used fondaparinux in this difficult situation.

LEPIRUDIN

Mechanism and Pharmacology

Hirudin, the anticoagulant that is present in the salivary glands of the medicinal leech, *Hirudo medicinalis*, is a highly specific direct inhibitor of thrombin (see Table 26-11). The biosynthetic polypeptide molecule called lepirudin is composed of 65 amino acids and is identical to natural hirudin, except for substitution of leucine for isoleucine at the N-terlecule and the absence of a sulfate group on tyrosine 63. Lepirudin (Refludan; Berlex, Montville, NJ, USA) binds tightly and nearly irreversibly to the catalytic site of thrombin,

Table 26-11	**Comparison of Properties of Anticoagulant Agents**					
	UFH	**LMWH**	**Fondaparinux**	**Lepirudin**	**Argatroban**	**Bivalirudin**
Size	Very large	Large	Small	Small	Very small	Small
MW, daltons	15,000	5000	1728	7000	527	2180
Thrombin inhibition	Indirect	Indirect	None	Direct	Direct	Direct
Thrombin binding affinity	++	+	None	+++	++	++
Route of administration	IV, SC	SC, IV	SC	IV, SC	IV	IV
Onset	Rapid	Rapid	Rapid	Rapid	Rapid	Rapid
Reversibility	Rapid	Slower	Slow	Slow	Rapid	Rapid
Clearance	Hepatic	Renal	Renal	Renal	Hepatic	Renal; proteolysis
Inhibition of clot bound	No	No	No	Yes	Yes	Yes
Tests for monitoring	PTT, Anti-Xa	Anti-Xa	Anti-Xa	PTT, ACT	PPT, ACT	PTT, ACT

UFH, unfractionated heparin; LMWH, low molecular weight heparin; MW, molecular weight; PTT, partial thromboplastin time; ACT, activated clotting time; IV, intravenous; SC, subcutaneous.

which imparts a prolonged duration of action. Lepirudin is renally excreted and so may accumulate in patients with renal impairment and potentially increase the risk of bleeding. The half-life appears to be 1 to 3 hours in normal volunteers but may be as long as 2 days in dialysis-dependent patients.

Administration and Monitoring

Lepirudin must be administered parenterally, which results in dose-dependent prolongation of PTT, PT, and TT. The usual dose is a bolus of 0.4 mg per kilogram given intravenously, followed by 0.15 mg/kg/hr given as a continuous infusion. Therapy is monitored, and the dose is adjusted on the basis of PTT, with a target range 1.5 to 2.5 times the mean control range. Because lepirudin is cleared by the kidneys, high plasma levels may result in patients with renal dysfunction; dose adjustments are required.

Indications and Clinical Use

Lepirudin is approved for anticoagulation in patients with HIT and associated thromboembolic disease to prevent additional thromboembolic complications. It has been used successfully in clinical trials for the treatment of patients with deep venous thrombosis and those with acute coronary syndromes. This direct thrombin inhibitor has no structural homology with heparin and thus no cross-reactivity with HIT antibodies. Two clinical trials of lepirudin use in patients with HIT have been completed.[42,43] In the Heparin-Associated Thrombocytopenia (HAT)-1 trial, lepirudin was associated with rapid and sustained recovery of platelet counts and adequate anticoagulation as assessed by PTT.[42] In HAT-2, a follow-up study, investigators showed that hirudin successfully prevented death, limb amputation, and new thromboembolic complications in patients with HIT.[35] Several patients in the HAT trials were treated with lepirudin and underwent successful percutaneous coronary intervention.[42,43]

Adverse Effects

Primary adverse effects have involved bleeding. Formation of antihirudin antibodies has been observed in about 40% of patients with HIT who were treated with lepirudin, which may decrease drug clearance and thus *increase* anticoagulant effects, possibly through delayed renal elimination of lepirudin/antihirudin complexes, which retain anticoagulant properties.[44]

Reversal of Effect

Lepirudin has no known antidote. If overdosage or excessive bleeding occurs, infusion should be discontinued immediately, PTT and other coagulation measurements obtained as appropriate, and the patient's hemoglobin concentration with preparations for blood transfusion assessed. Case reports suggest that hemofiltration or hemodialysis (with high-flux dialysis membranes with a cutoff point of 50,000 daltons) may be useful. Studies in pigs have shown reductions in bleeding with infusion of von Willebrand factor.

ARGATROBAN

Mechanism and Pharmacology

Argatroban is a small-molecule synthetic derivative of arginine that reversibly binds directly to the catalytic site of the thrombin molecule (see Table 26-11).[45,46] It has no homology with heparin and thus no cross-reactivity. The primary route of metabolism involves the liver, and the terminal elimination half-life is 39 to 51 minutes.

Administration and Monitoring

The recommended initial dose of argatroban for adult patients without hepatic impairment is 2 μg/kg/min, administered as a continuous infusion. Therapy is monitored through monitoring of the PTT. Steady state levels as determined by tests of anticoagulant effects (e.g., PTT) typically occur within 1 to 3 hours after argatroban therapy is initiated. Dose adjustment may be required to maintain the target PTT. Thus, the PTT should be assessed 2 hours after therapy is begun, to confirm that PTT is within the desired therapeutic range. The dose is then adjusted as clinically indicated ($\leq$10 μg/kg/min) until the steady state PTT is 1.5 to 3 times the initial baseline value ($\leq$100 seconds). The package insert should be reviewed before the patient's dose is determined.

Indications and Clinical Use

Argatroban recently received FDA approval as an anticoagulant for the prophylaxis or treatment of thrombosis in patients with HIT.[47] In two series, argatroban has been evaluated in patients with HIT who underwent coronary angioplasty.[48,49] A total of 50 patients were assessed. Procedural success was achieved in 98% of patients; complications included one retroperitoneal hematoma and one abrupt vessel closure. The anticoagulant effect of the drug is often difficult to predict in the catheterization laboratory, and no effective reversal agent has been identified.[48-50]

Adverse Effects

Hemorrhagic signs and symptoms and allergic reactions are the most commonly reported adverse effects.

Reversal of Effect

No specific antidote to argatroban has been identified. Excessive anticoagulation, with or without bleeding, may be controlled by decreasing the infusion rate or discontinuing argatroban. In clinical studies at therapeutic levels, anticoagulation parameters generally return to baseline within 2 to 4 hours after discontinuation of the drug. Reversal of anticoagulant effects may take longer in patients with hepatic impairment. If overdosage or excessive bleeding occurs, the infusion should be discontinued immediately, PTT and other coagulation parameters obtained as appropriate, and the patient's hemoglobin concentration made with preparations for blood transfusion assessed.

BIVALIRUDIN

Mechanism and Pharmacology

Bivalirudin (Angiomax; BenVenue Laboratories, Bedford, OH, USA) (see Table 26-11) is a 20 amino acid molecule that is engineered from naturally occurring hirudin to consist of only two amino acid sequences of hirudin that are important in binding to and inhibiting thrombin, which is connected by a bridge of four glycine residues. This bridge permits easy cleavage of the molecule, providing a more reversible interaction with the catalytic site of thrombin than hirudin, and resulting in a significantly lower bleeding risk. The half-life is relatively short (24 to 45 minutes) and administration results in rapid, dose-dependent prolongation of the ACT. Elimination of bivalirudin occurs primarily via the liver. Approximately 20% of standard doses are recovered in the urine. Bivalirudin has no structural similarity to heparin.

Administration and Monitoring

For reducing ischemic complications in patients with unstable or postinfarction angina who are undergoing coronary angioplasty, bivalirudin has been given intravenously at a dose of 1 mg per kilogram as an initial bolus, followed by a continuous infusion of 2.5 mg/kg/hr for 4 hours, then 0.2 mg/kg/hr for 14 to 20 hours. Bivalirudin was initiated immediately before angioplasty was performed, and aspirin (300 to 325 mg PO) was also given to all patients.[51] The package insert should be reviewed before the patient dose is determined.

Indications and Clinical Use

Bivalirudin is FDA approved as an anticoagulant in patients with unstable angina who are undergoing percutaneous transluminal coronary angioplasty (PTCA). In two clinical trials, bivalirudin was shown to be a safe substitute for heparin in patients without HIT undergoing percutaneous coronary intervention.[51,52] In an open-label, dose-finding trial of 258 patients, bivalirudin was used as an alternative to heparin.[52] Bivalirudin was associated with reduced bleeding complications, including retroperitoneal hemorrhage, a decreased need for transfusion, and less frequent occurrences of major hemorrhage than with heparin.

Adverse Effects

Bleeding is the most common adverse effect. Because of its small size and secondary structure, bivalirudin would not be expected to induce strong antibody responses on readministration, in contrast to larger molecules that have more significant secondary structures (such as hirudin). Antibivalirudin antibodies have not been detected during or up to 4 weeks after intravenous bivalirudin therapy in several studies. No allergic phenomena have been reported to date.

Reversal of Effect

No specific antidote to bivalirudin is available. Excessive anticoagulation, with or without bleeding, may be controlled by decreasing or discontinuing the infusion of bivalirudin. If overdosage or excessive bleeding occurs, the infusion should be discontinued immediately, PTT and other coagulation measurements obtained as appropriate, and the patient's hemoglobin concentration made with preparations for blood transfusion assessed.

REFERENCES

1. Ansel J, Hirsh J, Poller L, et al: The pharmacology and management of the vitamin K antagonists. Chest 126(suppl):204–233, 2004.
2. Schulman S: Clinical practice: Care of patients receiving long-term anticoagulant therapy. N Engl J Med 349:675–683, 2003.
3. D'Andrea G, D'Ambrosio R, Di Perna P, et al: A polymorphism in the VKORC1 gene is associated with an interindividual variability in the dose-anticoagulant effect of warfarin. Blood 105:645–649, 2005.
4. Rieder M, Reiner A, Gage B, et al: Effect of VKORC1 haplotypes on transcriptional regulation and warfarin dose. N Engl J Med 352:2285–2293, 2005.
5. Harrison L, Johnson M, Massicotte MP, et al: Comparison of 5-mg and 10-mg loading doses in initiation of warfarin therapy. Ann Intern Med 126:133–136, 1997.
6. Crowther M, Ginsberg J, Kearon C, et al: A randomized trial comparing 5-mg and 10-mg wargarin loading doses. Arch Intern Med 159:46, 1999.
7. Holbrook M, Pereira J, Labiris R, et al: Systematic overview of warfarin and its drug and food interactions. Arch Intern Med 165:1095, 2005.
8. Levine M, Raskob G, Beyth R, et al: Hemorrhagic complications of anticoagulant treatment. Chest 126(suppl):287–310, 2004.
9. Fitzmaurice D, Blann A, Lip G: Bleeding risks of antithrombotic therapy. BMJ 325:828, 2002.
10. Fang R, Chang Y, Hylek E, et al: Advanced age, anticoagulation intensity, and risk for intracranial hemorrhage among patients taking warfarin for atrial fibrillation. Ann Intern Med 141:745–752, 2004.
10a. Ayirookuzhi SJ, Chintapalli N, Gu X, et al: A gut reaction? Am J Med 120:143–145, 2007.
11. Bates S, Greer I, Hirsh J, et al: Use of antithrombotic agents during pregnancy. Chest 126(suppl):627–644, 2004.
12. Lubetsky A, Yonath H, Olchovsky D, et al: Comparison of oral vs intravenous phytonodione (vitamin K1) in patients with excessive anticoagulation: A prospective randomized controlled study. Arch Intern Med 163:2469, 2003.
13. Crowther M, Douketis J, Schnurr T, et al: Oral vitamin K lowers the international normalized ratio more rapidly than subcutaneous vitamin K in the treatment of warfarin-associated coagulopathy: A randomized controlled trial. Ann Intern Med 137:251, 2002.
14. Douketis J: Perioperative anticoagulation management in patients who are receiving oral anticoagulant therapy: A practical guide for clinicians. Thromb Res 108:3–13, 2003.
15. Kearon C, Hirsh J: Management of anticoagulation before and after elective surgery. N Engl J Med 336:1506–1511, 1997.
16. Hirsh J, Raschke R: Heparin and low-molecular-weight heparin. Chest 126(suppl):188–203, 2004.
17. Cruickshank MK, Levine MN, Hirsh J, et al: A standard heparin nomogram for the management of heparin therapy. Arch Intern Med 151:333–337, 1991.
18. Raschke R, Reilly B, Guidry J, et al: The weight-based heparin dosing nomogram compared with a "standard care" nomogram: A randomized controlled trial. Ann Intern Med 119:874–881, 1993.
19. Antman EM, Beasley J, Calitt R, et al: ACC AHA guidelines for the management of patients with unstable angina and non–ST-segment elevation myocardial infarction: A report of the American College of Cardiology American Heart Association Task Force on Practice Guidelines Committee on the Management of Patients With Unstable Angina. J Am Coll Cardiol 36:970–1062, 2000.
20. Ryan T, Antman EM, Brooks N, et al: 1999 update: ACC AHA guidelines for the management of patients with acute myocardial infarction: A report of the ACC AHA Task Force on Practice Guidelines Committee on Management of Acute Myocardial Infarction. J Am Coll Cardiol 34:890–911, 1999.
21. de Cheyron D, Bouchet B, Bruel C, et al: Antithrombin supplementation for anticoagulation during continuous hemofiltration in critically ill patients with septic shock: A case-control study. Crit Care 10:R45, 2006.
22. Avidan MS, Levy JH, Scholz J, et al: A phase III double-blind, placebo-controlled, multicenter study on the efficacy of recombinant human

antithrombin in heparin-resistant patients scheduled to undergo cardiac surgery necessitating cardiopulmonary bypass. Anesthesiology 102:276–284, 2005.

23. Levine J, Hirsh J, Gent M, et al: A randomized trial comparing activated thromboplastin time with heparin assay in patients with acute venous thromboembolism requiring large daily doses of heparin. Arch Intern Med 154:49–56, 1994.

24. Kaplan K, Francis D: Heparin-induced thrombocytopenia. Blood Rev 13:1–17, 1999.

25. Warkentin T, Greinacher A: Heparin-induced thrombocytopenia: Recognition, treatment, and prevention. Chest 126(suppl):311–337, 2004.

26. Dahlman T, Lindvall N, Helgren M: Osteopenia in pregnancy during long-term heparin treatment: A radiological study postpartum. Br J Obstet Gynaecol 97:221–228, 1990.

27. Dahlman T: Osteoporotic fractures and the recurrence of thromboembolism during pregnancy and the puerperium in 184 women undergoing thromboprophylaxis with heparin. Am J Obstet Gynecol 168:1265–1270, 1993.

28. Geerts W, Pineo G, Heit J, et al: Prevention of venous thromboembolism. Chest 126(suppl):338–400, 2004.

29. Horlocker T, Heit J: Low-molecular-weight heparin: Biochemistry, pharmacology, perioperative prophylaxis regimens, and guidelines for regional anesthetic management. Anesth Analg 85:874–885, 1997.

30. Samama M, Cohen A, Darmon J-Y, et al: A comparison of enoxaparin with placebo for the prevention of venous thromboembolism in acutely ill medical patients. N Engl J Med 341:793–800, 1999.

31. Leizorovicz A, Cohen A, Turpie A, et al: Randomized, placebo-controlled trial of dalteparin for the prevention of venous thromboembolism in acutely ill medical patients. Circulation 110:874–879, 2004.

32. Koopman M, Prandoni P, Piovella F, et al: Treatment of venous thrombosis with intravenous unfractionated heparin administered in the hospital as compared with subcutaneous low-molecular-weight heparin administered at home. N Engl J Med 334:682–687, 1996.

33. Levine M, Gent M, Hirsh J, et al: A comparison of low-molecular-weight heparin administered primarily at home with unfractionated heparin administered in the hospital for proximal deep-vein thrombosis. N Engl J Med 334:677–681, 1996.

34. van Dongen C, van den Belt A, Prins J, et al: Fixed dose subcutaneous low molecular weight heparins versus adjusted dose unfractionated heparin for venous thromboembolism. Cochrane Database Syst Rev 2004;CD001100:2004.

35. Wong G, Giugliano R, Antman EM: Use of low-molecular-weight heparins in the management of acute coronary artery syndromes and percutaneous coronary intervention. JAMA 289:331–342, 2003.

36. Petersen J, Mahaffrey K, Hasselblad V, et al: Efficacy and bleeding complications among patients randomized to enoxaparin or unfractionated heparin for antithrombin therapy in non–ST-segment elevation acute coronary syndromes. JAMA 292:89–96, 2004.

37. Raschke R, Hirsh J, Guidry JR: Suboptimal monitoring and dosing of unfractionated heparin in comparative studies with low-molecular-weight heparin. Ann Intern Med 138:720–723, 2003.

38. Samama M, Gerotziafas G: Evaluation of the pharmacological properties and clinical results of the synthetic pentasaccharide (fondaparinux). Thromb Res 109:1–11, 2003.

39. Turpie A, Bauer K, Eriksson B, et al: Fondaparinux vs. enoxaparin for the prevention of venous thromboembolism in major orthopedic surgery: A meta-analysis of 4 randomized double-blind studies. Arch Intern Med 162:1833–1840, 2002.

40. Buller H, Davidson B, Decousus H, et al: Subcutaneous fondaparinux versus intravenous unfractionated heparin in the initial treatment of pulmonary embolism. N Engl J Med 349:1695–1702, 2003.

41. Buller H, Davidson B, Decousus H, et al: Fondaparinux or enoxaparin for the initial treatment of symptomatic deep venous thrombosis: A randomized trial. Ann Intern Med 140:867–873, 2004.

42. Greinacher A, Volpel H, Janssen U, et al: Recombinant hirudin (lepirudin) provides safe and effective anticoagulation in patients with heparin-induced thrombocytopenia: A prospective study. Circulation 99:73–80, 1999.

43. Greinacher A, Janssens U, Berg G, et al: Lepirudin (recombinant hirudin) for parenteral anticoagulation in patients with heparin-induced thrombocytopenia. Heparin-Associated Thrombocytopenia Study (HAT) Investigators. Circulation 100:587–593, 1999.

44. Schiele G, Vuillemenot A, Kramarz P, et al: Use of recombinant hirudin as antithrombotic treatment in patients with heparin induced thrombocytopenia. Am J Hematol 50:20–25, 1995.

45. Hursting MJ, Alford KL, Becker JP, et al: Novastan (brand of argatroban): A small molecule, direct thrombin inhibitor. Semin Thromb Hemost 23:503–516, 1997.

46. Lewis BE, Walenga JM, Wallis DE: Anticoagulation with Novastan (argatroban) in patients with heparin induced thrombocytopenia and thrombosis syndrome. Semin Thromb Hemost 23:197–202, 1997.

47. Lewis BE, Wallis DE, Berkowitz SD, et al: Study Investigators for the ARG-911 Study: Argatroban anticoagulant therapy in patients with heparin-induced thrombocytopenia: A prospective, historical controlled study. Circulation 163:1838–1843, 2001.

48. Matthai WH: Use of argatroban during percutaneous coronary interventions in patients with heparin induced thrombocytopenia. Semin Thromb Hemost 25(suppl 1):57–60, 1999.

49. Lewis BE, Matthai W, Grassman ED, et al: Results of phase 2/3 trial of argatroban anticoagulation during PTCA of patients with heparin induced thrombocytopenia. Circulation 96:1–217, 1997.

50. Lewis BE, Ferguson JS, Grassman ED, et al: Successful coronary interventions performed with argatroban in patients with heparin induced thrombocytopenia and thrombosis syndrome. J Invas Cardiol 8:410–417, 1996.

51. Bittl JA, Strony J, Brinker JA, et al: Treatment with bivalirudin (hirulog) as compared with heparin during coronary angioplasty for unstable or post-infarction angina. for the Hirulog Angioplasty Study Investigators. N Engl J Med 333:764–769, 1995.

52. Topol EJ, Bonan R, Jewitt D, et al: Use of a direct antithrombin, hirulog, in place of heparin during coronary angioplasty. Circulation 87:1622–1629, 1993.

Chapter 27

Blood Component and Pharmacologic Therapy of Hemostatic Disorders

Charles D. Bolan, MD • Harvey G. Klein, MD

SYNOPSIS

Patients with disordered hemostasis present one of the greatest challenges to blood banks and transfusion practitioners. Early intervention with appropriate directed therapy can provide adequate hemostasis for a variety of bleeding conditions; however, the rapidly hemorrhaging patient can deplete the transfusion service's inventory and have a major impact on the hospital and the community. With the advent of potent agents such as recombinant factor VIIa (rFVIIa) therapy for use in a wide variety of disorders, the issues of cost, efficacy, adverse effects, monitoring, and optimal integration of pharmacologic treatment with blood transfusion therapies have achieved a highly prominent and visible role in patient care. This chapter addresses various blood-derived biologics, non–blood derived drugs, and strategies to prevent hemorrhage and manage hemostatic disorders. These biologics, pharmacologic agents, and other therapies and their use are discussed in this chapter and, where indicated, elsewhere in the text (Table 27-1).

INTRODUCTION AND HISTORICAL OVERVIEW

The evolution of the treatment of bleeding disorders with transfusions and pharmacologic therapy both parallels and differs from developments in traditional pharmacology. Early pharmaceutical preparations, such as digitalis, insulin, and vitamin B_{12}, were crude extracts that have been replaced by purer preparations or even by recombinant products. Similarly, the early use of whole blood transfusion to treat patients with conditions such as hemophilia and thrombotic thrombocytopenic purpura (TTP) has been supplanted by recombinant clotting factors, specific blood component therapy, and U.S. Pharmacopeia (USP)-standardized antidotes such as vitamin K to treat warfarin toxicity.[1,2] As progress in pharmacology has depended on an improved understanding of disease pathophysiology, so has progress in transfusion medicine depended on a detailed understanding of the mechanisms involved in hemostasis and the development of diagnostic laboratory assays to monitor management. To some extent, rational transfusion management remains impeded by the lack of widely accessible assays to measure platelet function, assess components of the fibrinolytic system, and measure the impact of hemostatic therapies at the site of cellular injury.

Several sentinel discoveries have played critical roles in blood transfusion and pharmacologic therapies for bleeding patients. Landsteiner's discovery of blood groups at the turn of the century allowed pretransfusion testing to be performed to avert reactions due to ABO-incompatible whole blood transfusion. Blood group compatibility remains of critical importance in red blood cell transfusion therapy and may exert significant impact when plasma, apheresis platelets, or manufactured plasma fractions that contain red blood cell antibodies are used. With the development of citrate anticoagulant for blood storage, whole blood transfusion was successfully adapted during the First World War, ultimately leading to the birth of the modern blood bank. The advent of the sterile plastic interconnected bag system has made component therapy possible.

Costs of the new safer blood components and fractions have risen dramatically. Likewise, the costs of pharmaceuticals and recombinant biologics are substantial. At the same time, the emergence of strategies for using pharmacologic agents to control bleeding associated with surgery may reduce the need for reoperation, improve overall mortality, reduce requirements for transfusion, and decrease exposure to allogeneic donors. Further, such agents may reduce the cost of therapy and may provide superior hemostasis when compared with traditional blood components. The promise of new agents, such as rFVIIa, is tempered by issues of cost, monitoring, and safety. Further, these agents have not yet undergone the same degree of scrutiny that revealed lower than expected efficacy or higher than expected toxicity during more extensive follow-up with previous agents such as 1-deamino-8-D-arginine vasopressin (DDAVP) or aprotinin. Despite these costs and uncertainties, the treating physician now has a variety of choices and a variety of considerations when faced with a hemorrhaging patient or one who is being prepared for procedures that are likely to challenge the hemostatic system.[3]

TRADITIONAL BLOOD COMPONENTS

The blood bank can now provide a wide range of blood components and plasma fractions, each with characteristic hemostatic properties and toxicities. Available products include those obtained by traditional single donation and by centrifugal separation of whole blood or donor aphere-

Table 27-1 Blood Components, Blood Products, and Pharmaceutical Agents

Traditional blood components
   Red blood cells (RBCs)
   Platelets
   Fresh frozen plasma (FFP)
   Cryoprecipitate
   Plasma fractions
Recombinant coagulation factors (also see Chapter 4)
Recombinant factor VIIa (rFVIIa)
Pharmaceutical agents
   DDAVP (1-deamino-8-D-arginine vasopressin)
   Lysine analogue antifibrinolytics
   Aprotinin
   Vitamin K
Estrogens
Protamine

Pharmacologic Agents Covered in Other Chapters

Antiplatelet agents (aspirin [ASA] and clopidogrel)
   (see Chapter 20)
Platelet glycoprotein IIb/IIIa inhibitor (abciximab, tirofiban,
   and eptifibatide) (see Chapter 20)
Warfarin (see Chapter 26)
Unfractionated heparin (see Chapter 26)
Low molecular weight heparin (LMWH) (see Chapter 26)
Fondaparinux (see Chapter 26)
Direct thrombin inhibitors (DTIs) (lepirudin, argatroban, and
   bivalirudin) (see Chapter 26)
Fibrinolytic agents (see Chapter 28)

sis, as well as those obtained from fractions of pooled products processed from collections from tens of thousands of donors, such as prothrombin complex concentrates (PCCs). Recombinant blood proteins such as rFVIIa, although not blood derived, may be considered interchangeably with their plasma-derived relatives or may be considered as a pharmacologic agent. The hemostatic properties and toxicities of these products are intimately related to the preparation processes. Increasingly, recombinant proteins have replaced virus-inactivated pooled plasma products for management of hemophilia A and B, and intermediate purity factor VIII (FVIII) preparations have replaced cryoprecipitate in the treatment of von Willebrand disease (VWD). Cryoprecipitate remains the mainstay of treatment for fibrinogen and factor XIII deficiencies, and fresh frozen plasma (FFP) may be used to provide replacement for deficiencies of other coagulation factors (factors XI, X, V, and II). Platelet concentrates and FFP are the blood components most frequently used for hemostasis; however, red blood cells and granulocytes, as well as other preparations, may have important hemostatic effects related to their plasma content or other properties.

Red Blood Cells

Red blood cells (RBCs), commonly referred to as "packed cells," may be prepared by whole blood donation or through aphereis procedures. Although not typically considered a hemostatic component, RBCs may contribute to normal clot formation, or perhaps more accurately, a decrease in RBCs may contribute to a bleeding tendency. Template bleeding time is prolonged as hematocrit falls, and RBC transfusions alone have been shown to improve hemostasis in patients with uremia[4] and chronic anemia.[5] The mechanism for this effect is not known but may involve

movement of platelets toward the vessel wall with increasing intravascular RBC mass,[6] or the action of RBC surface proteins that function as adhesion molecules.[7] RBC adhesion to endothelial cells plays a prominent pathologic role in malaria and sickle cell crisis, although the possible beneficial role of RBC adhesion during surgery or other conditions of compromised hemostasis is not known.

The adverse association of hematocrit with bleeding is greatest at hemoglobin concentrations <6 g per deciliter[5]; RBC transfusions may produce rapid hemostatic effects while restoring oxygen-carrying capacity. RBC transfusions provided to maintain hemoglobin concentrations greater than 9 g per deciliter produce no significant increment in hemostasis. Transfusions given to patients to maintain hemoglobin concentrations above 9 g per deciliter may be associated with decreased survival in intensive care units when compared with that reported in patients maintained at hemoglobin concentrations between 7 and 9 g per deciliter.[8]

Administration of the erythroid lineage cytokine erythropoietin (EPO) has become standard therapy in the treatment of anemia and in raising hemoglobin concentration in patients with renal disease and chronic conditions. Although EPO administration may have some effects on platelet reactivity,[9] the improvement in baseline hematocrit that occurs during EPO administration may account for the reduced incidence of bleeding in patients with uremia.[10]

Exclusive reliance on RBC replacement in the rapidly bleeding patient may induce a hemostatic defect. Stored RBCs contain no functional platelets and include as little as 5% to 10% plasma, depending on the preservative solution and method of collection used. Serial testing for platelet count and screening coagulation assays such as prothrombin time (PT) and partial thromboplastin time (PTT) should be performed to guide component replacement when large numbers of RBC concentrates are transfused in trauma cases involving massive transfusion,[11] which is conventionally defined as transfusion that exceeds one blood volume within 24 hours. Early balanced transfusion therapy is vital for massively bleeding patients and may prevent the onset of microvascular hemorrhage.[12] A proactive approach from the transfusion service is warranted.

Platelets

Platelet concentrates may be prepared by pooling platelets obtained through centrifugation from individual units of whole blood. A "unit" of platelets has been defined as containing at least 5.5×10^{10} platelets—hence the term "six pack," which describes a standardly prescribed dose of 3.3×10^{11}. Recent trends in blood center collection procedures have resulted in the attainment of most platelet products by single-donor apheresis, with the "dose" expressed by dividing the measured platelet content of the product by 3.0×10^{11}. These are arbitrary designations. Assessment of clinical response according to the dose of platelets administered and a posttransfusion platelet count measured within 1 hour of transfusion should be performed in all patients as a guide to further therapy (see later).

Apheresis or "single-donor" collections result in fewer donor exposures for a given dose of platelets. Apheresis platelets may contain 200 to 250 mL of donor plasma, but heat-labile clotting factors decay rapidly at a storage temperature of 22°C. It has been surprisingly difficult to document an advantage of single-donor apheresis platelets over pooled random donor components, although one suspects that alloimmunization, bacterial contamination, and virus transmission should all be reduced.[13]

Platelets are transfused for prophylactic and therapeutic indications. Prophylactic transfusion triggers remain controversial. Previous recommendations of using 20,000/μL in stable patients were based on estimates of bleeding in children with leukemia, many of whom had received aspirin prior to our realization that aspirin is such a powerful antiplatelet agent.[14] Subsequent studies, while avoiding aspirin, indicate that even far lower numbers are safe.[15,16] Many clinicians now administer prophylactically to stable, nonbleeding patients with amegakaryocytic thrombocytopenia due to chemotherapy and/or leukemia platelet transfusions given at platelet counts less than 5000/μL.[17] A trigger of 20,000/μL may be more prudent for patients who are febrile, have rapidly falling counts, or have evidence of additional hemostatic defects. Platelet counts of at least 50,000/μL may be more reassuring to the clinician when invasive procedures such as endoscopy, lumbar puncture, and bronchoscopy are anticipated. Meager evidence suggests that higher counts reduce morbidity and mortality. Clinical indications for therapeutic platelet transfusions are controversial and should be based on the patient's clinical condition, the cause of bleeding, and the number and function of circulating platelets.[18]

Bleeding due to platelet defects acquired after cardiopulmonary bypass surgery or aspirin ingestion often responds to platelet transfusion; oozing related to uremia does not respond in this way because transfused platelets rapidly acquire the uremic defect.[19] Evolving algorithms for platelet transfusion in surgical settings based on point-of-care testing of platelet count and function have the potential to improve patient care and blood product utilization.[20]

Most platelet transfusions are administered to patients with defects in platelet production or function. However, some patients with immune-mediated thrombocytopenia may have satisfactory responses to platelet transfusions.[21] Platelet survival generally lasts no longer than a few hours. Therefore, patients rarely benefit from prophylactic transfusions, although therapeutic transfusions may be lifesaving. Platelet transfusions are ordinarily considered to be contraindicated in patients with thrombotic platelet destruction, such as those with TTP, heparin-induced thrombocytopenia, and possibly disseminated intravascular coagulation (DIC).

Platelet transfusions should be monitored through baseline and posttransfusion platelet counts. Some physicians prefer to standardize this evaluation by calculating a "corrected count increment" (CCI)[22] as follows:

$$CCI \text{ at } 1 \text{ hour} = \frac{(platelet \text{ count}_{post} - platelet \text{ count}_{pre}) \times body \text{ surface area}(m^2)}{number \text{ of units transfused}}$$

A CCI above 4000 to 5000/μL suggests an adequate response to platelet transfusion, although two consecutive poor CCIs in the absence of fever, splenomegaly, active bleeding, consumption, ABO incompatibility, or other causes associated with increased platelet destruction suggest refractoriness.[23] Development of platelet immune refractoriness presents a vexing clinical problem. Many patients can be treated well with platelets from human leukocyte antigen (HLA)-compatible relatives or even unrelated matched donors. When such donors are unavailable, treatment of refractory patients by HLA "best-matching" or platelet cross-matches should be tried, but this may be cumbersome, expensive, and not uniformly efficacious. A computer-assisted matching program is proving increasingly helpful.[24] Repeated platelet transfusion in the absence of documented increments exposes patients to the potential risks of transfusion without evidence for any benefit and depletes an often scarce and costly blood resource.

Fresh Frozen Plasma

FFP is prepared by freezing the plasma component of a unit of whole blood within 6 to 8 hours of collection. Hemostatic activity of the coagulation factors is maintained even after storage for 1 year or longer, depending on the storage temperature. Once thawed, the plasma can be stored at a refrigerated temperature for no longer than 24 hours. On average, 1 mL of FFP contains 1 unit of each coagulation factor. However, the volume of a "unit" of FFP, the concentration of coagulation factors, and the citrate anticoagulant concentration are variable, depending on the donor blood composition and the anticoagulant solution used. In one study of individual units collected from 51 regular plasma donors, the 5th and 95th percentiles for factor V concentrations ranged from 69 to 127 U per deciliter and for factor VII from 83 to 169 U per deciliter, and the fibrinogen concentration ranged from 180 to 370 mg per deciliter and antithrombin III from 92 to 129 U per deciliter.[25]

FFP remains the blood component of choice for patients with deficiencies of factors II, V, X, and XI who require treatment.[26] FFP is commonly used to treat bleeding patients with acquired deficiencies of multiple coagulation factors, such as those with DIC, liver disease, dilutional coagulopathy, and TTP. FFP may also be used for rapid yet temporary reversal of the coagulopathy induced by oral anticoagulants (see later); these patients may require vitamin K therapy for long-term control, and those with cerebral hemorrhage may benefit from the use of rFVIIa or the higher concentration of vitamin K–dependent factors contained in PCC.[27] FFP has also been employed for replacement of deficiencies of protein C or S or other anticoagulant proteins in patients with thrombophilia. Prophylactic administration of FFP has not been found to improve patient outcomes in the setting of massive transfusion unless bleeding is associated with documented coagulopathy; these patients should be followed with coagulation tests to guide replacement therapy.[28] Depending on the cause of the prolongation, mild prolongations of PT and PTT (<1.5 times midpoint of the normal laboratory range) do not mandate for FFP prophylaxis for trauma patients or for those scheduled to undergo elective invasive procedures[29,30] (see Chapter 37). FFP transfusion in critically ill patients has limited efficacy and is associated with significant morbidity, in particular, pulmonary edema and acute lung injury.[31] Indiscriminate transfusion of FFP for mild,

27

clinically insignificant prolonged PT may result in unnecessary allergic reactions and delays in diagnostic procedures.[3] No clinical benefit has been documented.

Solvent detergent (SD) plasma is FFP that has been pooled and treated to inactivate lipid-encapsulated viruses such as human immunodeficiency virus (HIV), hepatitis B virus (HBV), and hepatitis C virus (HCV). SD plasma is no longer available in the United States but is widely used in Europe. SD plasma has more uniform concentrations of coagulation factors and reduced concentrations of high molecular weight von Willebrand factor (VWF)— a potential advantage for therapy of TTP but a potential disadvantage in other hemostatic disorders.[32] SD plasma also has reduced concentrations of protein S and α_2-plasmin inhibitor.[32] Use of SD in stable patients and in critically ill neonates, in women with obstetric and gynecologic emergencies, and in patients with liver disease appears safe and improves laboratory indices of coagulopathy.[33] The advantages of a product that is free of the major class of transfusion-transmitted viruses must be weighed against the potential disadvantages of trading a relatively safe single-donor component for one made from larger pools that may contain nonencapsulated viruses such as hepatitis A and parvovirus B19.

Cryoprecipitate

Cryoprecipitate is the cold insoluble fraction formed when FFP is thawed at 4°C. "Cryo" is rich in FVIII, FXIII, VWF, and fibrinogen.[26,34] The product can be stored frozen at −20°C for up to a year. When resuspended in a plasma volume of 10 to 20 mL after preparation from single-donor plasma, cryoprecipitate contains 80 to 100 U of FVIII/VWF, representing 40% to 70% of the original amount in the plasma, 100 to 250 mg fibrinogen, and approximately 30% of the original amount of FXIII.[34] Because of its higher concentration of these factors compared with FFP, cryoprecipitate served for decades as the primary replacement therapy for patients with hemophilia A and VWD. Cryoprecipitate for first-line therapy has been replaced by DDAVP (see later) for most mild cases of either disease, and by virus-inactivated or recombinant preparations, and it should no longer be used for these purposes unless other therapies are not available. Similarly, the use of cryoprecipitate to treat uremic bleeding (10 U per treatment) has largely been supplanted by treatment with DDAVP, estrogen or RBC transfusion, and EPO.[10] The use of cryoprecipitate as the source of fibrinogen for "home brewed" "fibrin glue" preparations is expected to disappear with the advent of standardized commercial products that contain virus-inactivated human fibrinogen[35] (see Chapter 29).

Currently, cryoprecipitate is used primarily as replacement therapy in patients with hypofibrinoginemia that is congenital (rare) or acquired (i.e., after thrombolytic therapy, DIC, plasmapheresis, or massive transfusions).[11,26] When used for these indications, 10 to 20 units are normally pooled and infused, with repeat doses administered every 6 to 8 hours, depending on clinical status and measurements of laboratory tests of coagulation or fibrinogen concentration. Fibrinogen levels greater than 50 mg/dL are considered sufficient to support physiologic hemostasis, resulting in normal PT or PTT. Cryoprecipitate may also be useful for treatment of patients with FXIII deficiency, a rare

congenital deficiency, or an acquired disorder resulting from autoantibody formation.[26] Commercially prepared, virus-inactivated fibrinogen concentrates are not yet available in the United States.

ADVERSE EFFECTS OF BLOOD TRANSFUSION THERAPY

All single-donor components carry approximately equivalent risks for HIV, HBV, and HCV infection. In the United States, the most widely quoted estimate of the risk of HIV transmission is 1 in 2,135,000 U transfused; of human T-lymphotropic virus (HTLV), 1 in 2,993,000 U; of HCV, 1 in 1,935,000 U; and of HBV, 1 in 205,000 U from blood provided by repeat donors. Slightly higher risks are observed in blood obtained from first-time donors.[36] The overall risk of transmission of HIV or HCV from a blood unit is estimated to be on the order of 1 in 2,000,000.[36] New and emerging pathogens such as West Nile virus, babesia, and infectious prions continually threaten world blood supplies.[37] Thus, despite increasingly sophisticated testing and screening strategies, until activation procedures for cellular components become available, infections from current and emerging agents will prevent realization of a zero-risk blood supply.[38]

Other adverse events are presently much more common than transfusion-transmitted viral infection. The reactions most often associated with transfusion are febrile nonhemolytic transfusion reactions (FNHTRs) from RBC or platelet transfusions, and urticarial reactions associated with FFP or plasma transfusion. These reactions are not life-threatening but may cause apprehension in the patient and may lead to significant delays in procedures or diagnostic studies until the cause has been determined. FNHTRs typically occur in less than 1% of transfusions overall but are more common with platelet transfusions and are observed in as many as 6% to 12% of adults with hematologic malignancies and in pediatric patients.[39] Urticarial allergic reactions may occur in 1% to 3% of transfusions of RBCs, platelets or FFP; anaphylactic shock occurs once per 20,000 to 47,000 U of blood components transfused.[40] Severe hemolytic transfusion reactions are associated almost exclusively with incompatible red cells, but hemolysis related to antibodies in plasma or platelet concentrates remains an important cause of morbidity and mortality.[41] Acute hemolytic transfusion reactions due to intravascular hemolysis may occur in one in 25,000 U, and delayed hemolytic transfusion reactions occur 5 to 10 times more frequently.[41] Both acute and delayed hemolytic reactions are associated with mortality, with estimated risks of 1 in 630,000 and 1 in 1,150,000 U, respectively.[41] Errors that result in transfusion of ABO-incompatible units are responsible for most fatal acute hemolytic transfusion reactions.[42]

The incidence of bacterial contamination and related shock is of particular concern in platelet transfusion. This component must be stored at room temperature and thus is particularly susceptible to bacterial growth. The true risk of contamination and frequency of reactions are unknown but are probably underreported. A wide variety of Gram-positive and Gram-negative organisms are associated with platelet contamination, and *Yersinia* species and other cryophilic organisms are most frequently implicated in RBC transfusions.[43] An estimated 25% of cases of transfusion-related bacterial sepsis are severe, resulting in septic shock or death.[43]

Estimates from early prospective studies indicate that bacterial contamination occurs in 0.3 of every 10,000 red blood cell units, 0.5 to 23 of every 10,000 apheresis platelet concentrates, and 5 to 30 of every 10,000 pooled random donor platelet concentrates.[43] Screening strategies recently introduced to detect bacterial contamination in platelet-pheresis components can detect up to 75% to 90% of contaminated units prior to release, which increases transfusion safety.[44] Current screening tests reduce effective platelet shelf life by 24 to 48 hours and have less than 100% sensitivity and specificity; thus, significant efforts to develop new strategies to reduce bacterial contamination are ongoing.[44]

Less common but dramatic and more severe reactions may occur as the result of transfusion-related acute lung injury (TRALI),[45] posttransfusion purpura (PTP),[46] and transfusion-associated graft-versus-host disease (TAGVHD).[47] The former two reactions are caused by plasma-containing components, and TAGVHD is associated with transfusion of cellular elements. These reactions are likely underdiagnosed, but each may be associated with clinically significant reactions.

TRALI is a life-threatening complication that occurs with severe acute pulmonary edema and hypoxemia associated with normal cardiac filling pressures that is indistinguishable from adult respiratory distress syndrome, occurring within 1 to 6 hours (usually within 1 to 2 hours) of plasma-containing blood component transfusion.[48] Treatment is supportive. The mechanisms of TRALI are unknown but likely involve a combination of immunologic effects mediated by HLA-specific antibodies or leukagglutinins in donor plasma, particularly in plasma obtained from multiparous female donors, and a neutrophil priming activity that depends in part on the patient condition.[49] According to one hypothesis, most instances of TRALI occur in a two-event model: first, a priming step involving adherence of polymorphonuclear white blood cells to the activated pulmonary endothelium in "at-risk" patients; second, infusion of antibodies directed against white blood cell antigens and/or biologic response modifiers from the stored blood component. In this model, patients at highest risk for TRALI include those with recent surgery, infection, volume overload, and other factors capable of pulmonary endothelial activation.

Because of the preexisting patient condition, TRALI may remain unsuspected as a cause of worsening pulmonary function and may go underdiagnosed. The true incidence of TRALI is unknown but may be as high as 0.34% of transfusions. TRALI reactions have been implicated in up to 12% of all transfusion-related fatalities and may be the single most common cause of death due to transfusion. Diagnosis and reporting of TRALI are important, so that the transfusion service can make an appropriate donor evaluation, including possible deferral from future donation.

PTP is characterized by dramatic precipitous thrombocytopenia occurring within 3 weeks of blood transfusion in a patient with a history of prior transfusion or pregnancy.[46] The sera of patients characteristically reveal the presence of

a potent antibody directed against donor platelet antigens that the recipient lacks. Profound thrombocytopenia occurs because of a poorly characterized reaction, resulting in destruction of transfused *and* autologous (patient) platelets, referred to as an "innocent bystander effect." The syndrome is most common after RBC transfusions but may occur after infusion of single-donor plasma and platelet products. Patients are refractory to transfusion of antigen-negative or -positive platelets but may respond rapidly to intravenous immune globulin (IVIg) or plasmapheresis with albumin replacement. Steroid therapy is ineffective.

TAGVHD is far less common than TRALI, although the precise incidence remains unknown.[47] Its presentation mimics bone marrow transplant–related graft-versus-host disease, with the additional clinical finding of bone marrow aplasia, typically occurring 8 to 10 days (maximum of 4 weeks) after transfusion. TAGVHD occurs when immunocompetent donor T cells in the blood component engraft within the recipient. The most susceptible patients are those who receive transfusions from closely matched family members and those who are immunocompromised, including organ and bone marrow transplant recipients, premature infants, patients with particular neoplasms, and those receiving therapy with purine analogue agents for malignancy or for autoimmune disease.[50] Leukocyte reduction is not effective prophylaxis. Blood product irradiation prevents TAGVHD.[51] Once present, TAGVHD is almost always fatal; thus, it is imperative that treating clinicians recognize at-risk patients and request blood product irradiation from the transfusion service.

Commercial Plasma Fractions

A variety of products prepared through special processing of plasma pools are used to treat patients with hemostatic disorders. Among the earliest preparations are the so-called PCCs, which are impure mixtures of vitamin K–dependent proteins that are isolated by ion exchange chromatography from the cryoprecipitate supernatant of large plasma pools after removal of antithrombin III and factor XI.[52] Various processing techniques involving ion exchangers permit production of four-factor concentrates, which include factor VII, or three-factor concentrates which consist mainly of factors II, IX, and X. The PCCs are standardized according to their factor IX content.[52] During production, activated clotting factors are produced that are later inactivated through a variety of processes, including manipulation of pH and addition of heparin and/or antithrombin III. These products may be further adjusted to produce activated PCCs used for treatment of patients with acquired FVIII or IX inhibitors (see Chapter 6). PCCs are now treated to inactivate transfusion-transmitted viruses. Adverse events associated with PCCs include immediate allergic reactions, heparin-induced thrombocytopenia (for preparations containing heparin), and thromboembolic complications such as DIC, arguably the most important adverse effect.[52] PCC administration is indicated only when the desired increase in factor activity cannot be achieved through other therapeutic measures (see treatment of cerebral bleeding in excessive oral anticoagulation with vitamin K later). PCCs should not be used in the treatment of hemophilia B or congenital factor VII deficiency, with the exception of emergency situations when specific factor replacements are not available.[53]

Virus-inactivated, intermediate purity factor VIII preparations with high VWF content have replaced cryoprecipitate as the primary therapy for VWD.[54–56] One of these products, Humate P (Centeon LLC, Kanakee, Ill, USA), has been approved by the U.S. Food and Drug Administration (FDA) for the treatment of patients with VWD, and the package insert now provides the concentration of ristocetin cofactor activity required to facilitate dosing.

RECOMBINANTLY DERIVED PLASMA COAGULATION PROTEINS

Recombinantly derived coagulation factors, such as factor-VIII and IX preparations used to treat hemophilia A and B, are more expensive than virus-inactivated pooled products. However, these agents provide physicians and patients with a variety of products of high purity and safety and have become the mainstay of therapy for previously untreated patients and those newly identified with these disorders (see Chapter 4). Of special interest in the field of hemostasis and transfusion medicine has been the adaptation of rFVIIa, developed initially for the treatment of hemophilic patients with inhibitors,[57] to a much broader use in a wide variety of hemostatic disorders[58,59] (see Chapter 6).

Recombinant Factor VIIa (rFVIIa) (NovoSeven)

Background

Since the first startling reports of hemostatic response in trauma patients with uncontrolled hemorrhage,[59,60] a growing body of literature has addressed the use of rFVIIa in settings outside the therapy of hemophilic patients with high-titer inhibitors. Although treatment of hemophilic patients with inhibitors and, more recently, treatment of patients with congenital factor VII deficiency[61] remain the only approved indications for rFVIIa in the United States, a body of published trials and anecdotal evidence describes the diversity of applications for this agent, reflective of its widespread use in community practice. Despite its high cost, rFVIIa is used in a variety of hemostatic disorders. Efficacy for these conditions, as well as appropriate dosing and laboratory monitoring, has not been fully established. A complete assessment of the risk:benefit ratio of rFVIIa, in light of its potential efficacy and a small but real incidence of significant toxicity, is not possible at the present time. Whether or not rFVIIa will achieve the promise of a safe, effective, broadly applicable or "universal" hemostatic agent continues to be debated.[62,63] Until more information becomes available, this agent should be reserved for life-threatening or urgent bleeding not controlled by traditional methods or in situations in which compatible blood components are unavailable. An overview of rFVIIa is presented in Table 27-2.

Mechanism of Action

rFVIIa was developed to produce hemostatic "bypassing" activity, without the adverse events associated with the use of PCCs in the treatment of hemophilic patients with inhibitors.[64] Although the full spectrum of activity and the interrelated mechanisms responsible for its clinical

activity have not been fully elucidated,[64,65] evidence suggests that the effects of this agent extend beyond those that are measurable through traditional in vitro assessments of hemostasis. In a cell-based model of coagulation described by Roberts, Hoffman, and Monroe (Fig. 27-1), rFVIIa, in combination with tissue factor (TF) locally exposed on damaged cell surface and factors V and X, generates thrombin, which catalyzes a series of reactions on the platelet membrane involving factors XI, VIII, and IX to cause platelet activation, release of VWF, and yet a larger burst of thrombin that further augments hemostasis. In addition to coagulation and platelet activation effects, thrombin activates factor XIII, resulting in fibrin crosslinking. The high local concentrations of thrombin produce a stable clot structure that is relatively resistant to fibrinolysis[66] and further counteracts fibrinolysis through activation of the thrombin activatable fibrinolysis inhibitor (TAFI).[67]

Table 27-2 Overview of Recombinant Factor VIIa

Action

In combination with tissue factor expressed on the cell surface at sites of injury acts to initiate coagulation with a small burst of thrombin produced via the factor X/factor V complex, leading to thrombin-mediated platelet activation and generation of factor IXa, resulting in a much larger burst of thrombin generation. May produce a stronger clot that is relatively resistant to fibrinolysis.

Administration

Administered as an intravenous bolus after reconstitution (20 minutes) by pharmacy, at 90 µg per kilogram for hemophilic patients with inhibitors, which, along with congenital factor VII deficiency, is the only approved indication in the United States.

Doses in other settings are not well established. Smaller doses of 20 to 40 µg per kilogram may be effective in oral anticoagulant reversal. A vial-based dosing algorithm that uses patient weight and indication has been used by some experienced transfusion services.[73]

Repeat dose is based on clinical response within 2 hours. No widely applicable satisfactory monitoring algorithms have been developed. Excess dosing should be avoided.

General Use

Control of bleeding hemophilia with inhibitors to factor VIII, factor IX, and congenital factor VII deficiency, and von Willebrand disease with von Willebrand factor inhibitors.

Urgent hemostasis in factor XI deficiency, thrombocytopathy, refractory thrombocytopenia, diffuse alveolar hemorrhage, trauma, and massive transfusion.

May be useful in "blood avoidance surgery" for patients whose clinical conditions or religious beliefs are incompatible with blood component therapy.

Possible Contraindications

Unlikely to be effective in patients with severe thrombocytopenia and zero levels of fibrinogen, factor V or X.

Consider giving concomitantly with fresh frozen plasma or platelets.

Use cautiously in disseminated intravascular coagulation.

Toxicity

Associated with a slight but real increased background incidence of arterial and venous thromboembolic events that may increase with higher doses or repeated dosing.

Contraindicated in patients with known hypersensitivity to manufacturing components.

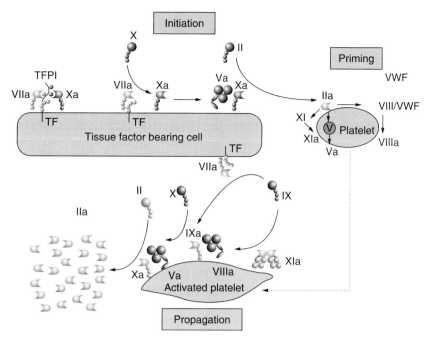

Figure 27-1 Hemostatic effects of recombinant factor VIIa, illustrated according to a cell-based model of coagulation. In combination with tissue factor expressed on the cell surface at sites of injury, recombinant factor VIIa acts to initiate hemostasis with a *small burst* of thrombin produced via the factor X/factor V complex. This leads to thrombin-mediated platelet activation and generation of factor IXa, resulting in coagulation caused by the much *larger burst* of thrombin generation. In addition to the effects on platelet activity and thrombin generation, this may result in a stronger clot that is relatively resistant to fibrinolysis. (Used with permission from HR Roberts 2006.)

Additional considerations for the clinical use of rFVIIa involve hypothermia and acidosis. Hypothermia inhibits platelet adhesion at mild temperatures (33°C to 37°C) and both platelet adhesion and coagulation at lower temperatures (below 33°C); acidosis further inhibits coagulation and can worsen hemorrhage.[68] Clinical anecdotal experience suggests that rFVIIa is effective in some hypothermic patients with acidosis; in vitro[68] and clinical studies indicate that activity is more significantly reduced by acidosis than by hypothermia.[69] The concomitant existence of hypothermia and acidosis complicates interpretation of the rFVIIa response, especially in trauma settings. Efforts to prevent hypothermia, maintain perfusion, and correct acidosis should be considered in the application of rFVIIa and in the interpretation of its response (see Chapter 46).

Dose and Administration

The appropriate dose of this agent has not been established outside of the recommendations given for patients with hemophilia. Dose drives costs to some extent for many aspects of medical therapy; at an average wholesale price of $1.60 per unit for rFVIIa in 2006, costs of $1908, $3816, and $7632 for available vial sizes of 1200, 2400, and 4800 μg, respectively, or $10,000 for a 70-kg individual treated at 90 μg per kilogram, are reminiscent of initial costs for recombinant FVIII therapy but involve an agent with a much broader and less clearly defined patient population.

rFVIIa has a short half-life in the circulation of 2 to 3 hours, and although circulating levels are not predictive of local response, the agent is given as an intravenous bolus every 2 to 3 hours until bleeding stops.[64,65] The package insert recommended dose is 90 μg per kilogram for hemophilic patients with inhibitors; effective doses of 20 to 25 μg per kilogram have been described in patients

with congenital factor VII deficiency.[65] Low doses in the range of 20 to 40 μg per kilogram have been effective for control of excessive oral anticoagulation[70] and as prophylaxis against surgical bleeding,[71] although higher doses are favored by some investigators.[72] In nonhemophilic patients, follow-up treatment schedules are problematic, and administration must be based on clinical response. After administration of the initial dose and formation of a stable clot at the site of bleeding in responding patients, repeat dosing may not provide further benefit and may result in increasing concentrations of rFVIIa at other nonbleeding sites with the potential for toxicity due to thrombosis. In patients who do not respond to the initial dose, repeated administration after a second dose may be a futile but costly approach. Issues of cost and vial wastage and lack of established dosing regimens have led transfusion services to develop vial-based dosing algorithms for rFVIIa based on the clinical condition and a broader range of patient weights.[73]

No laboratory monitoring tests have been clinically established to guide dosing or response,[74] and consideration of repeat dosing must be based on clinical response. This is not surprising given that the multiple interrelated mechanisms responsible for the activity of rFVIIa act at the site of tissue injury and may not be readily reflected in systemic circulation blood samples. In most patients, significant shortening of PT and PTT is observed, and the degree of shortening in trauma settings has been shown to correlate roughly with control of bleeding.[72] Preliminary studies indicate that rFVIIa may be futile in patients suffering from severe acidosis, or in those with markedly prolonged PT, poor prognosis trauma score, or elevated lactic acid levels.[69] Fibrinogen levels must be adequate (>40 to 50 mg per deciliter) to support clot formation. However, considerable overlap has been noted in these responses, and the results in practice are difficult to use to guide initial therapy. It has been proposed that more global assessments of hemostasis that more accurately reflect the kinetics of clot formation, such as the thromboelastogram (TEG), may provide a more reliable assessment of activity.[74] At the present time, these tests provide limited practical information but possibly may reassure clinicians that high-dose therapy has not produced a thrombogenic coagulation profile.[74]

Indications

Treatment of patients with hemophilia A or B who have developed inhibitors to factors VIII and IX, respectively, and, more recently, treatment of patients with congenital factor VII deficiency are the only FDA-approved indications for the use of rFVIIa in the United States[61]; however, in Europe, this treatment is also indicated for use in patients with Glanzmann thrombasthenia..[75] On the basis of its mechanism of action, rFVIIa would not be expected to provide hemostasis in patients without measurable levels of fibrinogen, factor V, or factor X, or in those with severe thrombocytopenia who have counts below 5000 per microliter,[65] in which case concomitant infusion of cryoprecipitate, FFP, or platelet concentrates has been attempted to provide a minimal level of substrates.[76]

Patients with coagulation factor deficiencies, thrombocytopenia, and qualitiative platelet defects have been successfully treated with rFVIIa.[64,65] In factor VII–deficient patients, doses of 15 to 20 µg per kilogram are administered every 2 to 3 hours, and in factor XI deficiency, doses ranged from 90 to 120 µg per kilogram given according to a similar schedule.[77,78] rFVIIa has been used in patients with both quantitative and qualitative platelet defects.[79,80] In one study of rFVIIa administration to patients with thrombocytopenia, shortening of the bleeding time by at least 2 minutes occurred after administration of 50 or 100 µg per kilogram of rFVIIa in 32% of patients with platelet counts lower than 20,000/µL, in 56% of those with counts of 21,000 to 39,000/µL, and in 68% of those with counts of at least 40,000/µL.[58] In this same study, full control was attained in 66%, and partial control in 33% of 9 bleeding episodes, which occurred in eight patients treated with rFVIIa; no association was observed between dose and response.[58] Similarly, in an international survey of responses to rFVIIa in Glanzmann thrombasthenia, responses were observed in 29 of 31 procedures and in 77 of 103 bleeding episodes, with "optimal" efficacy observed when a bolus of at least 80 µg per kilogram was repeated every 2.5 hours as needed.[80] As in the hemophilia setting, rFVIIa may be useful for patients with VWD who have developed antibodies against VWF or who have failed to respond to conventional therapy.[81]

Two recent placebo-controlled studies evaluated the use of rFVIIa in orthotopic liver transplantation (OLT), which may be associated with excessive blood loss from surgical causes, decreased concentrations of coagulation factors, hyperfibrinolysis, and thrombocytopenia. Planinsic and associates[82] randomly assigned 83 patients who were undergoing OLT for end-stage liver disease to treatment with placebo or a single bolus dose of 20, 40, or 80 µg per kilogram rFVIIa given 10 minutes before surgery, resulting in a significant reduction in requirement for FFP in the 80 µg per kilogram group.[82] A larger study compared

the efficacy and safety of doses of 60 µg per kilogram and 120 µg per kilogram rFVIIa given 10 minutes prior to skin incision, followed by repeat dosing every 2 hours until 30 minutes prior to the expected start of reperfusion of the transplanted liver.[83] Of the group of 179 patients who completed the observation period, 10% in the 60 µg per kilogram group avoided transfusion, as did 7% in the 120 µg per kilogram group and 0% of placebo-treated subjects ($P < .03$). No thromboembolic events or hepatic artery occlusions occurred in either of these studies. In patients with cirrhosis, rFVIIa shortened PT to normal or near normal values after doses of 5, 20, and 80 µg per kilogram without adverse effects.[84] In another study involving liver biopsy, rFVIIa dosed at 5, 20, 80, and 120 µg per kilogram resulted in a maximum reduction in PT values 30 minutes after dosing; a longer duration of shortening occurred with 80 and 120 µg per kilogram doses, and achievement of hemostasis occurred within 10 minutes of dosing in 74% of patients who were assessed by direct visualization via laparosopic biopsy, with no effects attributable to treatment dose.[85] In contrast to these studies, no beneficial effects compared with placebo were observed after rFVIIa infusion (20 or 40 µg per kilogram 5 minutes prior to infusion) in patients who underwent partial hepatectomy.[86]

rFVIIa has been increasingly applied for reversal of oral anticoagulation[87]—a setting in which responses frequently are observed at doses much lower than 90 µg per kilogram. In a group of volunteers pretreated with acenocoumarol in which the international normalized ratio (INR) was elevated to >2, and factor X and factor IX levels were reduced from between 9% and 46%, a single dose of rFVIIa given at 5 µg per kilogram normalized the INR within 12 hours, and doses of rFVIIa >120 µg per kilogram were found to correct INR for periods of 24 hours without signs of systemic coagulation.[88] In a clinical study of 13 patients with critically increased INR caused by warfarin-induced anticoagulation (including five in which the INR was >10, four who were at risk of clinical hemorrhage, and four who underwent procedures involving bleeding risk requiring immediate reversal), rFVIIa given at doses ranging from 15 to 90 µg per kilogram was associated with rapid and effective responses, with elevated INRs, and avoidance or reversal of bleeding.[70] In addition, in seven patients who experienced intracranial hemorrhage while receiving oral anticoagulants, doses of rFVIIa between 10 and 40 µg per kilogram were effective in augmenting hemostasis and in lowering the INR from pretreatment values of 1.7 to 6.6 down to less than 1.5 within 10 minutes.[89]

A recent double-blind, placebo-controlled study in patients with acute intracerebral hemorrhage who were not taking oral anticoagulants compared the effects of treatment with 40 µg per kilogram (108 patients), 80 µg per kilogram (92 patients), and 160 µg per kilogram (103 patients) of rFVIIa versus placebo (96 patients) given within 1 hour of diagnostic computed tomography (CT) (see Chapter 43).[90] Compared with a 29% growth in hematoma volume among placebo-treated patients, reduced growth at 24 hours was observed in the 40, 80, and 160 µg per kilogram rFVIIa treatment groups (16%, 14%, and 11%, respectively). Pooled data for all doses of rFVIIa indicated that treatment resulted in a 52% relative reduction in hemorrhage volume growth compared with placebo ($P = .01$). A 38% relative reduction in mortality at

3 months was reported for patients receiving rFVIIa (placebo 29% mortality vs 18% mortality for all doses of rFVIIa; $P = .02$), along with an absolute reduction in the risk of death or severe disability (death/disability: 69% placebo vs 53% for all doses of rFVIIa combined; $P = .004$ for all doses vs placebo). No dose response was associated with survival or disability; however, a significant increase in arterial thrombotic events was observed in rFVIIa-treated patients (see toxicity discussion later).

In spite of the dramatic response described in the initial report of successful use of rFVIIa for a rapidly exsanguinating patient with acidosis, hypothermia, and DIC due to a high-velocity gunshot injury,[59] it has been surprisingly difficult to clearly define the efficacy and optimal dose of rFVIIa in trauma settings.[69] Although recent placebo-controlled studies have revealed a trend toward improved survival and have pointed toward a reduced incidence of massive transfusion and reduction in RBC transfusion requirements in patients with blunt and penetrating trauma,[72] the overall benefits in randomized trials have not reflected the dramatic responses described in anecdotal reports or contained in the personal experience of many treating clinicians. Although human trials have not been powered to study survival end points,[72] results with animal models in the laboratory have yielded conflicting data, with favorable responses reported in some studies[91] and no effect described in others.[92] Although some trauma guidelines suggest an initial dose as high as 120 µg per kilogram,[93] even higher doses have been used,[72] while responses have been observed with doses as low as 20 µg per kilogram[94] or 60 µg per kilogram, as described in the initial report.[59] These clinical ambiguities are illustrated in a retrospective analysis of rFVIIa use in 40 patients with massive bleeding who were unresponsive to conventional therapy, in which 18 stopped bleeding completely and 14 experienced significant slowing of bleeding, for an overall response of 80% (Fig. 27-2). The median number of doses of rFVIIa used was two (range, 1 to 18), and individual doses ranged from 15 to 180 µg per kilogram. Only two patients had a history of trauma, and no evidence suggested a dose response in patients who achieved hemostasis or in those with thromboembolic complications (see toxicity discussion later).[94]

A large number of reports describe the use of rFVIIa in other settings. A small double-blind study of suprapubic prostatectomy that compared placebo (12 patients) with two different doses of rFVIIa (20 µg per kilogram [8 patients] and 40 µg per kilogram [16 patients]) found a significant dose-dependent reduction in perioperative blood loss (1235 mL and 1089 mL in the 20 and 40 µg per kilogram groups, respectively, vs 2688 mL in the placebo group [$P = .001$]), along with reduced operating room times for treated patients compared with controls.[71] No patients in the 40 µg per kilogram group received transfusions of any type, whereas more than half of those in the placebo group required allogenic RBC transfusion. This study is notable for the higher than expected RBC transfusion requirements in the placebo group, and it is similar in this respect to earlier randomized, blinded, placebo-controlled studies that pointed toward a beneficial effect of DDAVP on transfusion requirements in coronary artery bypass grafting.[95]

A more recent randomized, double-blind study of rFVIIa 90 µg per kilogram or placebo given to 48 patients who underwent semi-elective open reduction on traumatic pelvic and pelvic acetabular fractures reported only very modest results, with greater measured operative blood loss in rFVIIa-treated than in placebo-treated patients (2070 mL vs 1535 mL) and a trend over 48 hours that was not statistically significant toward reduced transfusion requirements (46% vs 67%) and reduced overall blood loss (2146 mL vs 2787 mL).[96] Similarly, no convincing efficacy

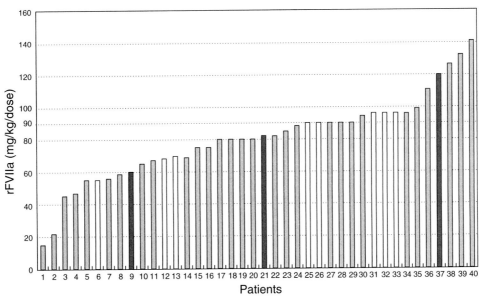

Figure 27-2 Individual responses according to control of bleeding and thromboembolic events in 40 patients (x axis) who received recombinant factor VIIa for intractable bleeding according to dose (y axis). Toxicity occurred in three patients (black bars)—two at the site of prior vascular manipulations and one with multiple pulmonary emboli in the setting of disseminated intravascular coagulation and occult lymphoma. Non-responding patients are shown as white bars. No relationship was noted between dose, response and toxicity in this retrospective study of data maintained on a nationwide registry. (Reproduced with permission from O'Connell NM, et al: Recombinant FVIIa in the management of uncontrolled hemorrhage. Transfusion 43:1711–1716, 2003.)

of rFVIIa therapy was observed in 100 patients with moderate or severe bleeding (lower or upper gastrointestinal tract; hemorrhagic cystitis; pulmonary, intracerebral, and other sites) that occurred 2 to 180 days after hematopoietic stem cell transplantation, as assessed in a double-blind design in which placebo was compared with 40, 80, or 160 μg per kilogram of rFVIIa administered every 6 hours for 36 hours.[97] Although patients who received the intermediate dose of 80 μg per kilogram were found to have reduced bleeding scores in a post hoc analysis, no significant reduction in transfusion requirements was observed among the treatment groups, and authors concluded that additional trials should be conducted to identify patients in this setting for whom rFVIIa is effective. Successful use of rFVIIa has also been described for control of bleeding in cardiac surgery,[98] pancreatitis,[99] refractory postpartum hemorrhage,[100] hemorrhage associated with low molecular weight heparin (LMWH),[101] and other conditions.[63] However, the use of rFVIIa in fit, healthy patients with normal laboratory results appears unwarranted during elective surgery in the absence of special circumstances that may justify its use.[96]

Toxicity

Initial assessments from clinical studies and registry data indicate a rate of serious complications of about 1%.[102] More recent data support an overall beneficial safety profile for patients with life-threatening hemorrhage associated with a small but real incidence of thrombotic events such as cerebrovascular accident, acute myocardial infarction, other arterial thrombosis, pulmonary embolism, and clotted devices in approximately 1% of 4520 estimated patients treated during the year 2004 (including 10 deaths).[61] Other non–life-threatening complications, such as rash, nausea, and allergic reactions, possibly related to the manufacturing process, may occur. Data collected in a smaller registry from the United Kingdom involving surgical and nonsurgical causes of bleeding revealed thrombotic complications in 3 of 40 (7.5%) evaluable patients, including two at sites of vascular manipulation and one with pulmonary emboli in a background of occult lymphoma, with no relationship noted between dosing and complications.[94] No data have established the safety or efficacy of rFVIIa in pregnancy, outside of anecdotal reports on postpartum hemorrhage and other obstetric complications.

More rigorous safety data in the setting of treatment for intracerebral hemorrhage were described by Mayer and colleagues,[90] who reported serious arterial thrombosis in 0 of 96 placebo-treated patients versus 16 (5%) of 303 rFVIIa-treated patients (including 6 of 108 [6%] at 40 μg per kilogram, 2 of 92 [2%] at 80 μg per kilogram, and 8 of 103 [8%] at 160 μg per kilogram; $P = .012$ for all rFVIIa groups vs placebo), as well as serious venous thrombosis in 2 (2%) placebo-treated patients versus 5 (2%) rFVIIa-treated patients (1% at 40 μg per kilogram, 2% at 80 μg per kilogram, and 2% at 160 μg per kilogram).[90] Overall survival and morbidity favored rFVIIa-treated patients; however, the manufacturer has released a safety warning as a result of this study to alert treating clinicians to the potential for thrombotic complications in "off-label" indications.[61]

The package insert also advises that thromboembolic risk may be increased in patients who have DIC, crush injury, and septicemia.[61] Despite this warning, a number of anecdotal reports describing safety in sepsis and DIC indicate that cautious use of rFVIIa may be beneficial in life-threatening bleeding in this setting,[102] without the degree of thrombosis that is associated with lysine analogue antifibrinolytic agents.[103] Similarly, although caution has also been advised when rFVIIa is used in conjunction with other hemostatic agents, anecdotal reports have described efficacy and safety when it is used concomitantly with antifibrinolytic agents[94,104] or after PCC use.[105] Thus, the appropriate application, dosing, and toxicity profile of rFVIIa are not yet fully known and remain areas of active clinical investigation.

PHARMACEUTICAL AGENTS

Pharmaceutical agents are occasionally used for replacement therapy but are more commonly used as adjunctive therapy along with blood products in the treatment of patients with hemostatic disorders.[10,106] A broad spectrum of agents is available. For example, DDAVP, a synthetic analogue of L-vasopressin, can be used for most mild forms of hemophilia A and VWD, and it is increasingly recognized to have multiple less well-defined effects that have been applied in a variety of hemostatic defects. Lysine analogues that inhibit fibrinolysis, such as ε-aminocaproic acid (EACA) and tranexamic acid (AMCA), are used systemically and locally for acquired and inherited defects in hemostasis and thrombocytopenia. Aprotinin, a bovine-derived serine protease inhibitor with potent antifibrinolytic activity, has been widely used to enhance surgical hemostasis after cardiopulmonary bypass. Vitamin preparations in the napthoquinone family (vitamin K) are used to prevent neonatal bleeding syndromes and to reverse warfarin anticoagulation or to treat patients who have ingested super-warfarin–like rodenticides. Other agents may be used as well, such as estrogens to treat uremic bleeding and protamine to reverse heparin-induced anticoagulation. With the rapid advent of rFVIIa therapy for diverse hemostatic disorders, the choice of optimal therapy in many settings has not been established, and this decision awaits the findings of future studies. An overview of selected hemostatic agents is provided in Table 27-3.

DDAVP

Background

The agent 1-deamino-8-D-arginine vasopressin (DDAVP), or desmopressin, is a synthetic analogue of the antidiuretic hormone L-vasopressin[107] that has been used to control bleeding in patients with mild congenital or acquired bleeding disorders for longer than 25 years.[108,109]

DDAVP may be self-administered by patients at home to prevent or treat bleeding episodes.[108] DDAVP is not a general hemostatic tonic reducing blood loss in all surgical settings.[110–112] It seems most efficacious in patients with prior aspirin ingestion[113] or possible platelet dysfunction from other causes.[114] An overview of DDAVP is presented in Table 27-4. Current uses of DDAVP in adults and children have been summarized in several comprehensive reviews.[108,115]

Table 27-3   Overview of Hemostatic Agents

Agent	Hemostatic Effects								
	Antifibrin-olysis	Activity of Vessel Wall	Localization to Injury	Platelet Function	Thrombin Generation	Speed of Onset	Ease of Monitoring	Cost	Toxicity
rFVIIa	+	+	++	++	++++	+++	−	++++	++
Amicar	++++	−	−	−	−	+++	−	+	+
Vitamin K (oral)	−	−	−	−	+	+	++	+	−
DDAVP	−	+	−	+	+	++	+	++	+

rFVIIa, recombinant factor VIIa; DDAVP, 1-deamino-8-D-arginine vasopressin.
Amicar (ε-aminocaproic acid) is manufactured by Wyeth Ayerst, Madison, NJ, USA.

Table 27-4   Overview of DDAVP

Action

Releases stored FVIII and VWF within 30 to 60 minutes; peak effect at 2 to 4 hours, lasts 6 to 12 hours. Has other hemostatic effects on platelets and endothelium.

Administration

Daily by intravenous, subcutaneous, and intranasal routes. Does not require concomitant use of antifibrinolytic agents. Tachyphylaxis may occur at more frequent dosing intervals or after several daily administrations.

General Use

Short-term control of various bleeding states. Initial efficacy usually preestablished with a test infusion.
Primary therapy for mild hemophilia A and VWD. More useful for type 1 than type 2 VWD, may be useful in some cases of severe type 3 VWD.
Widely used to control bleeding in acquired and congenital platelet defects, as well as in other conditions. Efficacy in this setting is less well defined because of the lack of appropriate tests to assess platelet function.
Use in surgical setting is not consistently associated with clinical improvement, except after aspirin ingestion.
Aprotinin and antifibrinolytics are superior in cardiac bypass. Efficacy may be improved for selected patients in whom platelet defects were identified by perioperative testing.

Possible Contraindications

Worsens thrombocytopenia in some patients with type 2B VWD.
Use cautiously in elderly patients and those with coronary artery disease.

Toxicity

Mild flushing and nausea are most common.
Water retention and hyponatremia which can be associated with seizures and headaches.
Possibly associated with myocardial infarction in the cardiac bypass setting.

DDAVP, 1-deamino-8-D-arginine vasopressin; FVIII, factor VIII; VWF, von Willebrand factor; VWD, von Willebrand disease.

Mechanisms of Action and Tachyphylaxis

The best characterized hemostatic activity of DDAVP involves its effect on raising circulating FVIII and VWF levels—an effect that appears to be due to its chemical similarity to vasopressin.[107,108] Compared with vasopressin, DDAVP has increased affinity for V-1 receptors that cause renal free water retention and rapid release of preformed FVIII and VWF from cellular stores, as well as markedly decreased affinity for V-2 receptors that mediate vasoconstriction.[107] In normal subjects, DDAVP increases FVIII and VWF levels within 30 minutes of infusion.[116] Levels peak at 300% to 400% of baseline in 1 to 2 hours and persist for 6 to 12 hours.[108]

DDAVP also induces a transient fivefold to sevenfold increase in tissue plasminogen activator (tPA) activity with resultant generation of plasmin, but the excess plasmin is rapidly counteracted by endogenous levels of α_2-plasmin inhibitor.[117] Adhesion of RBCs and platelets to endothelial cells is increased by DDAVP when studied in vitro.[118,119] These effects may be produced by direct action on the vessel wall,[119] or possibly by release of high molecular weight VWF at the endothelial cell surface.[120] In addition, shear stress at the vessel wall is decreased after DDAVP is infused in patients with congenital platelet defects, possibly as the result of higher circulating levels of high molecular weight multimers.[121–123] Other studies have shown that DDAVP may also (1) increase platelet microparticle formation,[124] (2) enhance the expression of TF on endothelial cells,[125] and (3) promote the expression of P-selectin[126] and the adhesive glycoprotein Ib on platelet membranes.[127] One or more of these or other unidentified effects may explain the observations that DDAVP shortens bleeding times in patients with severe VWD who have already received cryoprecipitate infusions[128] and in those with qualitative platelet disorders such as uremia,[129] liver disease,[130] or other acquired or congenital conditions[130–132] in which levels of FVIII and VWF are usually normal. In some studies, patients who had previously experienced severe bleeding during surgery attained adequate surgical hemostasis after they were given DDAVP.[132]

The mechanisms of action of DDAVP explain some important clinical observations. First, infusion in hemophilia A and VWD produces short-term increases in circulating FVIII and VWF, levels of which decrease after initial release from preformed cell stores.[108] DDAVP has been used alone in these conditions for brief minor surgical procedures, endoscopy, or dental work, but it is inadequate for procedures that require prolonged (i.e., >2 to 3 days) hemostasis. Second, repeat administration of DDAVP at less than 24-hour intervals or over several days is associated with tachyphylaxis caused by reduced laboratory and clinical responses.[133] The blunted response is presumably related to depletion of intracytoplasmic stores of FVIII and VWF. The pattern of tachyphylaxis is not predictable and is more marked in general for patients with hemophilia A compared with those with VWD. In one study of daily dosing, responses after a second dose were 30% of the first

Table 27-5 Hemostatic Preparations of DDAVP

Route	Concentration	Dose*	Volume	Cost[†]	Peak Response[‡]
Intravenous	4 µg/mL	21 µg (0.3 µg/kg)	5.25 mL (in 50 mL saline)	$116.00 per dose	30–60 minutes
Intranasal spray (Stimate)	1.5 mg/mL	One spray per nostril, 300 µg total	0.1 mL per spray	$46.00 per dose	90–120 minutes
Subcutaneous	4 µg/mL	21 µg (0.3 µg/kg)	5.25 mL	$116.00	90–120 minutes
Subcutaneous[§]	40 µg/mL[§]	21 µg (0.3 µg/kg)	0.52 mL	Not available in United States	90–120 minutes

*For a 70-kg adult.
[†]Average wholesale price.
[‡]For FVIII and VWF levels.
[§]This preparation is available only in Europe.
Stimate is manufactured by ZLB Behring LLC, King of Prussia, Pa, USA.

day response, but responses were not further reduced after the third and fourth doses.[133] In contrast to the diminished FVIII and VWF responses reported after repeated doses, fibrinolytic,[134] renal,[107] and platelet responses do not appear altered when doses are repeated frequently.[135] Although the hemostatic response to initial administration of DDAVP varies among patients, it is usually reproducible for a given patient.[133] Ideally, patients who may be given DDAVP should receive an initial test infusion at least several days prior to any planned invasive procedures to determine response.

Dose and Administration

DDAVP may be administered by intravenous, subcutaneous, and intranasal routes (Table 27-5). The intravenous dose is 0.3 µg per kilogram, administered over 30 minutes in 50 mL of normal saline for adults (and in 10 mL for children weighing less than 10 kg). The maximum response occurs at intravenous doses of 0.3 µg per kilogram. The subcutaneous dose is 0.3 to 0.4 µg per kilogram, and peak responses occur approximately 230% above baseline at 60 minutes after administration (slightly lower and later than the peak dose after intravenous administration). The intranasal dose is an order of magnitude higher than the intravenous or subcutaneous dose, generally 300 µg in adults. Higher doses do not enhance efficacy but may be associated with increased toxicity. A concentrated nasal spray formulation is available in the United States and in Europe. However, a concentrated preparation for subcutaneous use is not available in the United States, and the substantial volume required (7 mL for a 70-kg person) cannot be easily administered by subcutaneous injection. DDAVP is cleared by the liver and kidneys and has a plasma half-life of 124 minutes. Because many of its known hemostatic effects are caused indirectly, drug levels may be more relevant to renal effects and toxicity than to hemostasis.[136]

Indications

No controlled studies have evaluated the use of DDAVP compared with placebo or factor concentrates in patients with hemophilia A and VWD.[108] Because the bleeding tendency in hemophilia A, and to a lesser degree in VWD, correlates with measured blood levels of the deficient factor, the ability of DDAVP to transiently raise levels of FVIII and VWF has resulted in its approval for use in these disorders. DDAVP is now the treatment of choice for minor and even moderately invasive procedures in patients with these

disorders who respond to a test infusion. More recent data highlight the variable activity of DDAVP in patients with VWD, indicating that the frequency of responders is relatively low when strict criteria are used, which may be defined as increases in FVIII and VWF ristocetin cofactor activity of at least 30 IU per deciliter and threefold over baseline, and shortening of the bleeding time to 12 minutes or less (Fig. 27-3).[137] Although FVIII and VWF ristocetin cofactor activity responses occurred in most patients, a complete response, including shortening of the bleeding time, was observed in only 7 of 40 patients with type 1 VWD (18%), in 1 of 15 with type 2A (7%), in 3 of 21 with type 2M (14%), and in 3 of 4 with type 2N (75%).[137] In this study, VWD genotype was more predictive of response than was phenotype in types 2A and 2N, but not in type 1 VWD, underscoring the need for a test infusion and assessment of response in individual patients. This has caused some to question if shortening of the bleeding time is an appropriate objective.

The use of DDAVP in type IIB VWD is controversial in that patients may develop mild thrombocytopenia related to affinity of the VWF for platelets.[56] Infusion of DDAVP and release of endogenous VWF stores into the circulation may worsen thrombocytopenia. Nevertheless, several studies have reported improved hemostasis in type IIB VWD after infusion of DDAVP associated with little or only mild thrombocytopenia. Therefore, it is reasonable to consider the use of DDAVP in carefully selected patients with type IIB VWD.[138,139] Although most patients with severe VWD do not respond to DDAVP, a minority may achieve sufficient increases in FVIII levels to provide hemostasis for minor procedures.[140] In patients with severe hemophilia A, FVIII levels do not increase after DDAVP infusion; however, DDAVP may provide potential benefit by increasing VWF levels, resulting in an associated increased response in activity of infused FVIII concentrates.[141] DDAVP may also further shorten the bleeding time in patients with severe VWD who did not fully respond after cryoprecipitate infusion, possibly because of nonspecific effects on hemostasis.[128] Finally, DDAVP is useful in some mild cases of acquired VWD[142] but not when the disease is immune mediated, or when acquired VWD is associated with monocolonal gammopathy of uncertain significance.[143]

DDAVP augments hemostasis in a variety of acquired and congenital conditions with impaired hemostasis and limited treatment options.[108] In one double-blind, placebo-controlled study of patients with congenital platelet defects, DDAVP shortened the bleeding time most

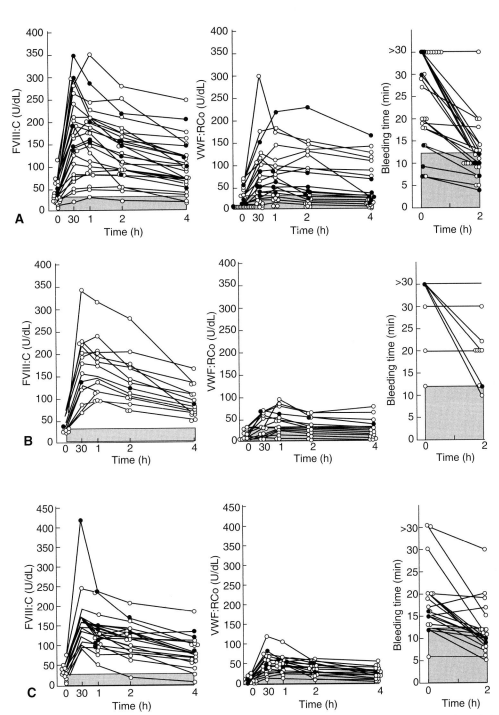

Figure 27-3 Biologic responses in factor VIII:C (*left*), ristocetin cofactor activity (*middle*), and bleeding time (*right*) after administration of DDAVP (1-deamino-8-D-arginine vasopressin) (0.3 μg per kilogram) to 26 patients with type 1 von Willebrand disease (VWD) (**A**), 15 patients with type 2A VWD (**B**), and 21 patients with type 2M VWD (**C**). A complete response, defined as at least a threefold increase in levels for factor VIIIC and ristocetin cofactor activity with a bleeding time of less than 12 minutes, was observed in only 27% of patients with type 1 VWD, as well as in 7% of those with type 2A, and 14% of patients with type 2M VWD. The variability of response underscores the importance of assessment of response after administration of a test dose of DDAVP in patients who have not previously been treated with this medication. (Reprinted with permission from Federici AB, Mazurier C, Berntorp E, et al: Biologic response to desmopressin in patients with severe type 1 and type 2 von Willebrand disease: Results of a multicenter European study. Blood 103:2032–2038, 2004.)

effectively in those with normal platelet–dense granule stores.[144] DDAVP has also reduced the bleeding time or has provided adequate surgical hemostasis in patients with storage pool defect,[131,145] Bernard-Soulier disease,[146] aspirin ingestion,[135] and other defects in platelet function.[108,132] DDAVP has been administered to patients with Ehlers-Danlos syndrome[147] and to those with mild factor XI

deficiency.[148] DDAVP shortens the bleeding time in some hemorrhagic diseases of multifactorial origin, such as hepatic cirrhosis and uremia. The usefulness of DDAVP in these conditions should be extrapolated with caution.

Except in surgical studies of transfusion requirements after aspirin ingestion, most studies have determined the efficacy of DDAVP by observing a shortening of the bleeding time and/or by assessing surgical hemostasis without controls and in only a small numbers of patients. Because bleeding time is a poor predictor of surgical bleeding, interpretation of these studies is problematic.[149] It may, however, be reasonable for the clinician to consider the use of DDAVP in these conditions when other treatments are not available, and after hemostasis has been maximized with the use of local measures, such as fibrin sealant or other agents.

Bleeding symptoms did not improve and may have worsened when DDAVP was combined with the vasoactive agent terlipressin for the treatment of acute variceal hemorrhage in patients with hepatic cirrhosis, perhaps because of competitive inhibition of drug activity.[150] Similarly, its use in uremia seems to be diminishing as increasing use of EPO and higher baseline hematocrits have decreased the frequency of uremic bleeding.[10] Other approaches may be useful in uremia; long-term control may be achieved with the use of estrogens, and patients with short-term bleeding may respond to RBC transfusions.[106]

Initial reports that DDAVP decreased blood loss and transfusion requirements after cardiac and spinal surgery have not been confirmed in follow-up studies.[108] A recent large meta-analysis revealed no reduction in bleeding after the use of DDAVP in cardiac surgery, in contrast to comparative studies with the lysine analogue antifibrinolytics and aprotinin.[151] Both aprotinin and antifibrinolytics were associated with a decreased need for repeat thoracotomy, and neither aprotinin nor antifibrinolytics increased the incidence of myocardial thrombosis. In contrast, DDAVP had no effect on repeat thoracotomy but was associated with a two- to fourfold increased risk of coronary thrombosis.[151] Although this study showed no beneficial reduction in blood loss after the use of DDAVP, average surgical blood loss was relatively small. Earlier analyses have suggested a potential benefit for the use of DDAVP in patients with greater blood loss.[152]

Methods that can be used to identify a subset of patients who might benefit from administration of DDAVP prior to surgery would be useful.[152] One such group appears to consist of patients with preoperative platelet defects, especially those who have been treated with aspirin. Blood loss was markedly reduced in patients with preoperative defects in platelet function identified by point-of-care testing who were given DDAVP compared with those who received placebo.[114] Three randomized, double-blinded, placebo-controlled trials have shown clinically significant reductions in blood loss and transfusion requirements after the use of DDAVP in patients who ingested aspirin before undergoing cardiac surgery.[113,153,154] DDAVP also reduced bleeding in an unblinded comparison with placebo in patients who ingested aspirin before cholecystectomy.[155] In addition, DDAVP has been shown to shorten bleeding time in normal volunteers after aspirin ingestion,[130] perhaps through its direct effects on platelets or increases in VWF.[135] rFVIIa has been reported to be used successfully in a case of aspirin-related bleeding,[156] and aprotinin has been shown to reduce bleeding in aspirin-treated patients who were undergoing cardiac bypass; however, these agents have not been compared directly with DDAVP.[157]

DDAVP has been used without adverse effects to control hemorrhage during pregnancy in a patient with Ehlers-Danlos syndrome[158]; however, little additional information is available on the safety of DDAVP or other hemostatic agents in pregnant women with bleeding disorders.[159] A review of the use of DDAVP to treat 53 pregnant women with diabetes insipidus found no risk to mother or child. However, the average daily dose of DDAVP in these cases—29 μg (range, 7.5 to 100 μg)—was significantly lower than that commonly used to augment hemostasis.[160]

Although some studies have indicated that DDAVP is not effective in patients with afibrinoginemia,[161] thrombocytopenia,[130] or Glanzmann disease,[130] other patients with Glanzmann disease or thrombocytopenia have reportedly responded.[162,163]

Toxicity

Most adverse effects associated with DDAVP are minor. Facial flushing, often marked, and minimal elevation in pulse rate or blood pressure are observed, more frequently with the intravenous than with the subcutaneous or intranasal route.[164] The most common clinically significant adverse event is hyponatremia, which results from the antidiuretic effects of this vasopressin analogue. Hyponatremic seizures have been observed in children 1 month to 8 years of age, especially when hypotonic fluids and multiple doses of DDAVP are administered in the surgical setting.[115] Less severe but significant symptoms of headache, nausea, and lethargy have been reported in adults after intranasal[165] or repeated intravenous and subcutaneous administration.[166] Careful monitoring of fluids, urine output, and electrolytes is therefore important, especially in children who are given DDAVP perioperatively and in older patients when mild renal insufficiency reduces their ability to excrete free water. Patients should be instructed to restrict fluid intake for 24 hours after receiving DDAVP.

Thrombosis is an obvious concern when drugs that enhance hemostasis are used. Isolated cases of thrombosis such as myocardial infarction, cerebral thrombosis, and unstable angina have been reported after use of DDAVP in patients at risk for thrombotic events.[167] In the surgical setting, one randomized, placebo-controlled study that was specifically designed to detect deep venous thrombosis in 50 patients undergoing hip surgery[168] and an early meta-analysis[169] did not detect an increased incidence of thrombosis after DDAVP therapy. A recent meta-analysis reported a two- to fourfold (95% confidence interval, 1.02 to 5.60) increased risk of myocardial infarction in patients undergoing cardiac surgery who received DDAVP.[151] Some experienced hemophilia centers do not routinely administer DDAVP to elderly patients or those with risk factors for coronary artery disease.[170] It therefore seems prudent to carefully evaluate patients who are receiving DDAVP for possible occult coronary artery disease and to avoid the concurrent use of antifibrinolytic agents in these patients.

Lysine Analogue Antifibrinolytic Agents

Background

Fibrinolysis occurs when plasmin that has been generated from plasminogen by plasminogen activators digests fibrin clots.[171] Both plasmin and plasminogen bind to fibrin through lysine-binding sites.[172] The synthetic lysine analogs AMCA and EACA delay fibrinolysis by competitively reducing the binding of plasminogen to fibrin.[172,173] These agents have been used for longer than 30 years to inhibit fibrinolysis and ensure clot stability.[173,174]

AMCA was developed within a few years of the development of EACA; it was noted to inhibit fibrinolysis more potently on a molar basis and to cause a reduced incidence of gastrointestinal problems at equivalent antifibrinolytic doses in healthy volunteers.[175] Much of the early use of antifibrinolytics in the United States involved EACA, whereas AMCA was used relatively more frequently in Europe.[173] Although AMCA and EACA have been considered as equivalent agents,[173] optimal dosing regimens have not been developed for either agent in most clinical settings, and reported toxicities vary.[176,177] Therefore, strict comparisons are difficult to make, and generalizations should be made cautiously when study findings are compared.

Lysine analogue antifibrinolytic drugs are effective and are clearly indicated in rare inherited conditions associated with excessive fibrinolysis, such as congenital α_2-plasmin inhibitor deficiency.[178] However, much of the recent enthusiasm for these drugs has focused on acquired disorders with evidence of excessive systemic fibrinolysis, especially cardiac bypass surgery and, to a lesser degree, orthopedic surgery performed with the use of tourniquets. It is important to note that either agent is useful when administered topically in areas with excessive local fibrinolysis, such as the oral cavity and the uterine cavity. In these instances, efficacy is well established and adverse effects are reduced compared with systemic administration.[10,106,179] AMCA and EACA are also frequently administered to reduce bleeding in such conditions as amegakaryocytic and peripheral immune-mediated thrombocytopenia, where the indication is less obvious and efficacy is presumably due to stabilization of fibrin clots.[180–183] As might be expected, there is less evidence of efficacy noted in these settings.[183] An overview of the use of these agents is given in Table 27-6.

Excessive thrombosis is a potentially devastating complication in clinical settings involving excessive procoagulant activity, such as DIC.[103,184] Thrombosis is not statistically increased with the use of AMCA or EACA in most settings other than DIC. However, the risk of this complication may have limited the more widespread application of these drugs in conditions such as menorrhagia or upper gastrointestinal hemorrhage, despite randomized studies that have shown benefit.[173,174]

Dose and Administration

Either agent may be administered orally, intravenously, or topically. EACA and AMCA are well absorbed orally and are cleared virtually unchanged by the kidneys.[172] These drugs are distributed widely throughout the body. AMCA crosses into the cerebrospinal fluid, semen, synovial fluid, and cord blood but is not secreted in saliva.[174] In the nonoperative setting, the half-life for both agents is approximately 1 to 2 hours in patients with normal renal function. The dose should be reduced in renal failure.[174,185] AMCA is approximately 6 to 10 times more potent than EACA on a molar basis[172]; however, few direct clinical pharmacokinetic and pharmacodynamic comparisons of the two agents have been performed.[174] A typical total daily oral dose for EACA is 10 to 24 g, administered as 2 to 4 g every 3 to 4 hours, and for AMCA, 3 to 4 g, administered as 1 g every 6 to 8 hours. Dosage in individual studies varies widely.[173] Studies have attempted to optimize dosing for these agents

---

Table 27-6 Overview of Lysine Analogue Antifibrinolytic Agents

Action

Clot stabilization by rapid inhibition of fibrinolysis associated with competition at lysine-binding sites of plasmin and plasminogen activators. Tranexamic acid is more potent on a molar basis than is ε-aminocaproic acid.

Administration

Every 4 to 8 hours by oral, intravenous, and topical routes. Dose should be reduced in kidney disease and has not been optimally determined in many conditions.

General Use

Short- and long-term control of various bleeding states. Consistent benefit in blinded, randomized studies of upper gastrointestinal bleeding and menorrhagia.

Effective topically, with decreased systemic effects in oral and cardiac surgery and ophthalmologic and other conditions, with excessive local fibrinolysis.

Wide use in thrombocytopenic states, with less consistent benefit noted.

Effective in rare acquired or congenital conditions characterized primarily by excessive fibrinolysis.

Effective in cardiac bypass surgery; less expensive and possibly less toxic than aprotinin at conventional doses.

Anecdotal use in conditions that lack effective and specific therapy.

Relative Contraindications

Disseminated intravascular coagulation (may be beneficial in those with primary fibrinolysis).

Urologic bleeding conditions.

Toxicity

Nausea, cramping, and diarrhea, more commonly with ε-aminocaproic acid.

Myonecrosis after longer-term oral use with ε-aminocaproic acid.

Thrombosis in settings requiring compensatory fibrinolysis, such as disseminated intravascular coagulation.

---

in conditions such as cardiac surgery, in which the clearance and distribution of these agents are altered.[185–187] Anecdotal and controlled studies have described improved control of bleeding with short-term, bolus,[188–190] and local or topical administration.[191–193] The optimal dose and route of administration may depend on the patient, the disease, or both.[174] In 2006, the average wholesale price for EACA was 7 cents per 250-mg oral tablet and $2.73 per 500-mg intravenous ampule; for AMCA, the wholesale price was $4.00 per 100-mg intravenous ampule (with the oral preparation not available through the U.S. government pharmacy in 2006).

Indications

Data on the efficacy of AMCA and EACA given to improve hemostasis in thrombocytopenic patients are conflicting and difficult to interpret. Two retrospective uncontrolled studies of 31 patients with thrombocytopenia, involving amegakaryocytic and immune-mediated origins, showed benefit with oral EACA.[180,181] A smaller study found that bleeding was controlled by EACA bolus infusion when platelet transfusions were unavailable or delayed,[189] and a larger, more recent retrospective analysis of 77 patients with mostly malignant hematology/oncology diseases and treatment-related thrombocytopenic bleeding described complete (66%) or partial (17%) cessation in bleeding and reduced platelet and RBC transfusion requirements after treatment with EACA given at a median 6 g per day for 8 days.[194]

A randomized, double-blinded, placebo-controlled study of AMCA administered to 38 patients to reduce bleeding in acute myeloid leukemia found a significant reduction in bleeding episodes and platelet transfusions during consolidation but not during induction therapy.[182] However, a smaller study of 8 patients with amegakaryocytic thrombocytopenia (7 with severe aplastic anemia and 1 with myelodysplasia) treated with AMCA in a placebo-controlled, double-blinded, crossover design found no improvement in bleeding. Only three patients were able to complete all phases of the study. Bleeding increased in patients who were receiving AMCA.[183] Such studies are extremely difficult to perform,[195] yet antifibrinolytic agents continue to be widely used for this indication.[10]

Lysine analogues are often used in cardiac bypass surgery, in which excessive bleeding and fibrinolysis are associated with the use of extracorporeal devices. Although early studies did not reveal a uniformly beneficial effect, antifibrinolytic use has increased recently as a cost-effective and perhaps safer alternative to aprotinin.[196] In contrast to DDAVP, these antifibrinolytic agents are administered prior to bypass and are associated with significant reductions in blood loss. A meta-analysis of placebo-controlled studies of antifibrinolytic agents in cardiac surgery that did not distinguish between AMCA and EACA showed lower rates of reexploration, improved mortality, and no significantly increased risk of myocardial infarction in the treatment group.[151] More recently, tranexamic use has been associated with decreased transfusion requirements in "off-pump" bypass grafting, indicating that activity is not limited to counteracting effects of the extracorporeal circulation.[197] In general, studies indicate that AMCA is more effective than EACA. However, these conclusions must be interpreted cautiously because the optimal dose of AMCA[186] or EACA[185] has yet to be determined.

Antifibrinolytic agents have also been shown to reduce bleeding in total knee arthroplasty, in which use of a tourniquet produces excessive fibrinolysis.[198,199]

When used in patients undergoing liver transplantation, antifibrinolytic agents reduced fibrinolysis[200] and showed efficacy similar to that of aprotinin.[201] Although individual studies do not uniformly document a reduction in transfusion requirements in these settings, meta-analyses[202] and critical reviews[203] support a positive effect. Studies that have attempted a cost/benefit analysis uniformly favor AMCA or EACA over aprotinin.[204–207] Although the issue of the optimal antifibrinolytic agent for use in bypass surgery is the subject of extensive and unresolved debate,[208–210] recent safety data appear to favor the use of lysine analogue agents over aprotinin.[196,211] On the basis of proposed mechanisms of action for efficacy and toxicity, some would favor these agents over aprotinin until similar safety data are obtained in other settings.[212]

Other applications of lysine analogues are increasingly supported by controlled studies, in contrast to the largely anecdotal use that previously characterized their use.[10,174] In a randomized, double-blinded, placebo-controlled study of 214 patients undergoing hepatectomy for tumor resection, preoperative intravenous administration of 500 mg AMCA followed by 250 mg every 6 hours for 72 hours was associated with significantly reduced blood loss and transfusion requirements (0% vs 16% of patients) and no thromboembolic complications.[213] Similarly, intraoperative and postoperative blood loss was significantly reduced in elective nasal surgery (endoscopic sinus surgery combined with septoplasty and conchotomy) in 200 patients who received AMCA (1 g orally every 8 hours, starting 2 hours before surgery and continuing for 5 days) compared with 200 patients who did not receive this agent; rebleeding requiring packing occurred in no AMCA patients and in 5 controls.[214] AMCA was associated with a reduced incidence of rebleeding and a 30% to 40% reduction in mortality in a meta-analysis that included 1200 patients from double-blinded, placebo-controlled trials of treatment in gastrointestinal hemorrhage.[215] A similar analysis found significant improvement in women with menorrhagia who received antifibrinolytic agents compared with hormonal methods and other treatment modalities.[216] Concern for thromboembolism has tempered the widespread use of these agents for excessive menstrual bleeding; however, studies have not shown an increased incidence of this complication to date.

AMCA reduced the incidence of rebleeding in patients with subarachnoid hemorrhage in two double-blinded, placebo-controlled studies; however, neurologic outcome was not improved.[217,218] Although uncontrolled studies have suggested that shorter courses of high-dose EACA[188] or lower-dose AMCA[219] might reduce rebleeding and prevent the complications associated with long-term use, the use of antifibrinolytic agents to treat patients with subarachnoid hemorrhage is not supported by recent evidence or practice recommendations.[220] In addition, a recent study reported no beneficial effect on hematoma enlargement when EACA was used to treat patients with intracerebral hemorrhage[221] (see Chapter 43).

Anecdotal reports indicate that antifibrinolytic agents may be successful in hereditary hemorrhagic telangiectasia (Osler-Weber-Rendu syndrome),[222] in disorders with excessive local fibrinolysis due to vascular malformations such as Klippel-Trénaunay[223] or Kasabach-Merritt syndrome,[224] and in rare instances in which hemorrhage is caused by excessive fibrinolysis, such as in the setting of prostate cancer.[225] Administration of antifibrinolytic agents to patients with excessive local coagulation due to vascular malformations was associated with thrombosis and obliteration of intravascular channels. Because of the potential for thrombosis in DIC, these drugs should be used with extreme caution, if at all, in this setting.

Topical or local administration of these drugs has been successful in a variety of clinical settings. Topical AMCA dramatically reduced the incidence of rebleeding after traumatic hyphema, with decreased systemic symptoms compared with oral administration, and it improved long-term outcomes compared with those seen in untreated controls.[193] Similarly, the usefulness of topical administration was illustrated in a double-blinded study of patients undergoing cardiac surgery in whom a solution of tranexamic acid (1 g in 100 mL saline) was poured into the pericardial cavity and over the mediastinal tissues before closure. Chest tube drainage but not transfusion requirements were significantly reduced, and AMCA blood levels were undetectable.[226] In mennorhagia associated with the use of an intrauterine device, local administration of AMCA or aprotinin reduced the pain and symptoms of bleeding.[191]

In the setting of dental surgery, antifibrinolytics are proposed to counteract excessive fibrinolysis in the oral cavity, which occurs because of the absence of endogenous fibrinolytic inhibitors.[227] Blinded placebo-controlled studies over 30 years ago showed reduced bleeding and decreased requirements for clotting factor concentrates in patients with hemophilia A and B who received systemic oral administration of EACA, 6 g four times daily for 7 to 10 days.[228] In a prospective, double-blinded study of 20 anticoagulated patients, AMCA mouthwash or placebo administered as 10 mL of a 4.8% aqueous solution was applied prior to sutures and as a 2-minute rinse four times a day for 7 days; 10 bleeding episodes occurred in 8 patients in the placebo group, and only one bleeding episode was reported in the treatment group. Only one patient had detectable blood levels of AMCA (2.5 μg per milliliter of plasma).[227] Since that time, topical administration of AMCA, along with the use of DDAVP and fibrin sealant, has become part of established multimodality therapy in hemophilia dental centers.[170]

Local measures to provide hemostasis are preferred to temporary discontinuation of warfarin in anticoagulated patients—a practice that may result in thromboembolism.[229] It is interesting to note that in one placebo-controlled trial of patients receiving oral anticoagulants, the addition of AMCA mouthwash offered no benefit over the use of local measures alone, such as gelatin sponge and fibrin glue.[230] Because placebo rinses may interfere with the formation of stable clot in the oral cavity, these early placebo-controlled studies should be evaluated in the context of studies in which improved local control measures were applied. Similar results have been observed in the treatment of epistaxis, in which no difference in efficacy was reported when gel impregnated with AMCA or placebo was used for treatment.[231]

Toxicity

The most common adverse effects of lysine analogue antifibrinolytic therapy consist of mild dose-dependent gastrointestinal symptoms such as nausea, cramping, and diarrhea. These symptoms are less frequently reported with AMCA than with EACA.[172–174] Myonecrosis, possibly due to inhibition of carnitine synthesis, has been described, although rarely, after long-term oral administration of EACA (therapy >4 weeks).[176,177] Myonecrosis has not been reported after AMCA administration, and some patients who have developed this complication while on EACA have been successfully treated for many months with AMCA.[174] Reversible visual impairment due to nonthrombotic malfunction of the pigmented retina has been described in a patient with renal failure who was receiving AMCA for control of a bleeding ulcer.[232] Administration of EACA, primarily through the intravenous route, has rarely been associated with hypotension and subsequent acute tubular necrosis; rapid infusion of this agent may result in bradyarrhythmia or tachyarrhythmia.[233]

These drugs do not appear to differ in their potential to cause thrombosis at usual clinical doses. Widespread thrombosis has occurred in DIC, in which increased fibrinolysis may mitigate organ ischemia.[184] Some studies have attempted to use antifibrinolytic therapy in conjunction with heparin anticoagulation in DIC and "excessive" fibrinolysis characterized by low levels of α_2-plasmin inhibitor. Although bleeding improved in most cases, some patients developed generalized organ system failure attributed to thrombosis.[184]

Renal complications associated with the use of lysine analogue antifibrinolytics, including ureteral obstruction, renal infarction, and electrolyte disturbances such as anion gap metabolic acidosis and hyperkalemia, may cause infrequent but clinically significant effects.[233] High-grade ureteral obstruction due to clot formation caused by inhibition of urokinase may occur when antifibrinolytics are used to treat patients with gross hematuria. No increased risk of this complication was observed in nine patients with macroscopic hematuria of various causes when EACA was given at divided oral doses (150 mg per kilogram total daily dose administered every 6 hours for up to 21 days)[234]; in a contrasting report, thrombosis occurred in patients who had evidence only of microscopic hematuria and who were treated with standard AMCA therapy (4 to 4.5 g total daily dose administered every 6 to 8 hours for 1 to 3 days).[235] Local therapy, administered by irrigation, has been successful for control of intractable urinary bleeding localized to the bladder.[192,236] Animal studies have indicated a possible teratogenic effect for EACA[237]; however, a review of AMCA use in pregnancy found no significant thrombosis or fetal injury.[238]

Aprotinin

Aprotinin is a bovine-derived protein that inhibits plasmin and multiple other human proteases.[239] Before its hemostatic applications were discovered, aprotinin had been widely used in Europe for the treatment of patients with pancreatitis and other inflammatory conditions.[210] During studies of aprotinin given to reduce neutrophil activation in cardiac bypass surgery,[240] investigators noted that the operative field was dry, and that transfusion requirements for patients undergoing repeat open heart surgery were markedly reduced.

The precise role of aprotinin in cardiac bypass surgery is not clear because this condition is associated with abnormal platelet function, decreased factor levels, activation of the fibrinolytic system, and coagulopathy related to heparin and protamine sulfate (see Chapter 37).[106,241] However, a series of studies have clearly established aprotinin as effective in reducing blood loss during open heart surgery.[151] Aprotinin may have similar activity in orthotopic liver transplantation, in which bleeding may also occur, in part because of excessive fibrinolysis.[242] Aprotinin is effective also in reducing blood loss in surgical patients who were recently treated with aspirin.[157] In a meta-analysis of pharmacologic strategies designed to reduce blood loss in cardiac surgery, aprotinin was the only agent associated with reduced mortality, and both aprotinin and lysine analogue antifibrinolytic agents reduced overall transfusion requirements and the need for reexploration.[151] However, serious concerns about the safety of aprotinin have been raised in two recent studies in which propensity scoring analysis was used. This is a retrospective technique that may be more suitable for detection of drug toxicity.[212]

In one study, the use of aprotinin (1295 patients), EACA (883 patients), or AMCA (822 patients) resulted in decreased blood loss compared with no agent (1295 patients); however, the use of aprotinin was associated with a greater than twofold increase in the risk of renal failure requiring dialysis in primary or complex surgery, as well as a 55% increase in the rate of myocardial infarction and a 181% increase in the risk of stroke or encephalopathy in complex surgery, with no associated increase in these values observed for EACA or AMCA.[196] In the second study, transfusion requirements and survival in patients undergoing cardiac bypass surgery who received aprotinin or AMCA were similar; however, a higher incidence of postoperative renal dysfunction or dialysis requirement was observed in the aprotinin group—an effect that was greatest in those who had impaired preoperative renal function.[211] Aprotinin is also significantly more expensive than lysine analogue antifibrinolytics, with an average wholesale price in 2006 of $314 for a 10 mL ampule of 10,000 KIU per milliliter. Although the cost-effectiveness and merits of aprotinin compared with lysine antifibrinolytics continue to be debated,[205,207,208] recent safety studies have raised concerns about the routine use of aprotinin versus these agents in coronary artery bypass surgery.[196,211]

Interpretation of such study findings remains complicated by methods used to assign weight to end points such as mortality and reexploration, total blood use, and long-term outcomes, as well as the effects of various dosing regimens.[206] Although aprotinin-mediated inhibition of plasmin may be the primary mode of action for reduction of blood loss,[239] inhibition of other enzymes and binding to renal vascular endothelium may be associated with its other effects.[151,196,210]

A unique toxicity of significant concern with aprotinin (a bovine protein) is anaphylaxis, which occurs in approximately 0.5% of initial exposures and up to 9% of repeat exposures and may result in shock and death.[243]

Vitamin K

Background

Vitamin K, *koagulationvitamin*, was discovered by Dam,[244] who demonstrated that chicks fed an ether-extracted diet developed a hemorrhagic diathesis that responded to a fat-soluble factor. He showed shortly thereafter that administration of vitamin K corrected the prolonged clotting tests of patients with obstructive jaundice, further noting that this correction occurred more rapidly after intramuscular than after subcutaneous administration.[245] Vitamin K was soon demonstrated to correct bleeding in hemorrhagic disease of the newborn.[244] With recognition that the bleeding in "spoiled sweet clover disease of cattle" was due to a compound (identified later as bishydroxycoumarin, or dicumoral) that interfered with vitamin K–dependent synthesis of active prothrombin, vitamin K subsequently acquired an established role in the management of excessive anticoagulation due to warfarin, super-warfarin rodenticides, and other orally active anticoagulants with similar mechanisms of action. Vitamin K is also indicated in acquired vitamin K deficiency, which occurs frequently in intensive care settings,[246,247] and it is effective in some cases of hepatic cirrhosis.[248]

Compounds with vitamin K activity exist in nature in two forms. Each possesses the 2-methyl-1,4-napthoquinone ring that is required for activity, but all differ in terms of the three-position side chain.[249] Vitamin K_1 phyllaquinones are synthesized by plants that possess the same phytyl side chain as chlorophyll, and they are the major dietary source of vitamin K. Vitamin K_1 content varies widely among foods, and diet is a major potential source of variation in response to oral anticoagulants. Absorption of dietary vitamin K occurs in the ileum and requires the formation of mixed micelles composed of bile salts and the products of pancreatic lipolysis.[249] Thus, oral absorption is impaired in conditions of bilary obstruction or pancreatic insufficiency. Vitamin K_2 menadiones are synthesized by gut bacteria and comprise a spectrum of molecular forms with side chains based on repeating unsaturated 5-carbon units. The physiologic importance of the large quantity of vitamin K_2 menadiones produced by bacterial flora of the large intestine is not clear.[249] Great numbers of menadiones, which are stored in the liver, may perform a reserve function of protecting against dietary vitamin K deficiency, which is rare in healthy adults. Whether slow, chronic, inefficient absorption of high concentrations of colonic vitamin K_2 is physiologically relevant compared with the highly efficient absorption of lower concentrations of intermittent dietary vitamin K_1 in the ileum remains a matter of debate.[249,250]

Mechanism of Action, Dose, and Administration

Vitamin K functions as an essential cofactor in the posttranslational gammacarboxylation of glutamic acid moieties in the N-terminal region of a series of proteins.[251] Originally recognized as essential for the synthesis of functional prothrombin, vitamin K later was identified as necessary for several normal functioning coagulation factors (II, VII, IX, and X), naturally occurring anticoagulant proteins (protein C and S), and, more recently, other proteins such as osteocalcin that are involved in bone metabolism.[250] Gammacarboxylation produces protein-constituent amino acids with stable divalent anionic charges that may interact with calcium ions by localizing clotting factors to appropriate areas of phospholipid membranes or by allowing formation of internal calcium channels.[251] Prior to participating in the carboxylation reaction, vitamin K must first be reduced to an active hydroquinone form. This carboxylation reaction produces a gammacarboxylic glutamic acid as the hydroquinone is converted to an inactive vitamin K epoxide. Vitamin K epoxide is reduced back to the active hydroquinone by vitamin K epoxide reductase, regenerating additional vitamin K to participate in carboxylation.[251] Thus, vitamin K is recycled in a process that involves 100 to 1000 times more vitamin K daily than is absorbed from dietary or colonic sources.[249] Descarboxylated, functionally inactive forms of vitamin K–dependent proteins (also called *proteins induced by vitamin K absence*, or *PIVKA*) may be detected in the circulation of patients on oral anticoagulant therapy or in those with vitamin K deficiency due to malabsorption or with functional vitamin K deficiency induced by liver disease.[252]

Enzymes that reduce and recycle vitamin K and vitamin K epoxide have different sensitivities to oral anticoagulant–induced inhibition.[251] This biochemical quirk explains why vitamin K functions as an antidote to excessive oral anticoagulation, and why patients on warfarin therapy who receive higher doses of vitamin K may appear resistant to reinstitution of warfarin therapy. The primary site of inhibition by warfarin is vitamin K epoxide reductase, which, under physiologic conditions, is the enzyme that reduces vitamin K to the active hydroquinone required for carboxylation.[251] A second reductase is present that is not inhibited by warfarin. This warfarin-insensitive reductase can reduce vitamin K to the active hydroquinone in the presence of high tissue concentrations of vitamin K. Thus, exogenous vitamin K can produce additional active vitamin K hydroquinone via this warfarin-insensitive step, bypassing the warfarin-induced inhibition of vitamin K epoxide reductase and reversing excessive anticoagulation.[251] If vitamin K levels accumulate, this same process may lead to warfarin resistance on resumption of anticoagulation.[253] Therefore, only small, if even incremental, doses of vitamin K should be administered to control excessive anticoagulation in patients who will require further antithrombotic therapy.

High oral doses of vitamin K do not affect the synthesis or raise the concentration of coagulation factors in normal, healthy subjects.[253] Lowered levels of vitamin K–dependent factors in patients on oral anticoagulants recover at the same rate during the first 8 hours after vitamin K administration; thereafter, recovery depends on the rate of synthesis of newly gammacarboxylated factors by the liver.[253] Levels of factor VII reconstitute most rapidly, followed by levels of factors IX and X, and finally by levels of prothrombin.[253] The differential rate of circulating factor levels after vitamin K administration has practical importance in monitoring recovery from anticoagulant therapy. Oral anticoagulation is most frequently monitored with the INR (and the PT, from which the INR is calculated); the INR is most sensitive to acute decreases in factor VII levels. The INR attempts to account for the variable sensitivity of different thromboplastin reagents by adjusting the degree of prolongation of the PT according to the International Sensitivity Index (ISI) provided for each reagent used to perform the test.[254] During stable anticoagulant therapy, the INR is determined on the basis of decreases in several vitamin K–dependent coagulant and anticoagulant protein levels, which remain in relatively constant ratios to one another. However, initial improvement of a markedly prolonged INR after administration of vitamin K for excessive anticoagulation may relate largely to a rapid increase in the factor VII level alone. In this setting, the slower recovery of factor IX may remain at clinically significant low levels, which may appear as a persistently prolonged PTT. Thus, the INR in this setting may be misleading and should not be used alone in interpreting levels attained during stable anticoagulation. If available, measurement of factor levels may be useful in predicting bleeding risk before invasive procedures are performed or in guiding further therapy.

Dose and Administration

Vitamins K_1 and K_2 are active when administered orally or intravenously. However, the only preparation currently available in the United States is a vitamin K_1 preparation, phytonadione (AquaMEPHYTON; Merck & Co., West Point, Pa, USA). A similar product (Konakion; Roche Colorado, Boulder, Colo, USA) for intravenous use is available in Europe and Australia. Both liquid preparations are prepared as a colloid solution, each milliliter containing 2 or 10 mg of phytonadione in a polyoxyethylated fatty acid derivative, which functions as a cremaphor to solubilize the vitamin K. The AquaMEPHYTON preparation is effective when administered intravenously, subcutaneously, intramuscularly, or orally. Intramuscular administration may cause hemorrhage in anticoagulated patients and should be used only for prophylaxis against hemorrhagic disease of the newborn. The adverse effects reported with intravenous administration (see later) have limited its use, even though intravenous administration is more rapid and reliable than the subcutaneous or oral route.[253,255,256] A colloidal system based on mixed micelles of lecithin and glycocholic acid that solubilize lipophilic vitamin K was developed to reduce the toxicity attributed to the cremaphor component of current preparations; however, significant symptoms were reported when this preparation was used, and it is no longer under development.[257] Scored tablets, containing 5 mg of phytonadione, are available; these permit a dose as low as 2.5 mg; therefore, administration of smaller doses of oral vitamin K requires the use of liquid preparations. Although injectable and oral preparations have been available for nearly half a century, the appropriate dose and route of administration remain controversial.[258] Despite careful pharmacodynamic studies, clinical guidelines have changed frequently[254,259–261] because of variability in patient responses and concerns regarding toxicity.[258] In 2006, average wholesale prices for vitamin K were 65 cents per 5-mg oral tablet and $3.61 per 1-mg intravenous ampule.

Indications

Vitamin K is used most often to reverse excessive anticoagulation caused by warfarin. Indications include patients with serious bleeding and those requiring only temporary control of therapeutic anticoagulation in preparation for surgical procedures. The goals of therapy are prompt control of bleeding without toxicity, prevention of resistance to reinstitution of warfarin, and avoidance of subtherapeutic anticoagulation.[262] The response to vitamin K administration may depend on the direction, rate of change, and degree of prolongation of clotting times; the time, dose, and type of anticoagulant administered; and the presence of concurrent liver disease, antibiotic use, or dietary factors.[263] Vitamin K and other effective therapies used to reduce the INR in patients receiving warfarin are listed in Table 27-7.

Anticoagulant reversal is more prompt with intravenous than with subcutaneous administration of vitamin K[255,256] (Fig. 27-4). In a prospective, randomized, single-blinded study of 22 patients, the INR decreased from a mean initial value of 8.0 down to 4.6 and 3.1 after 8 and 24 hours, respectively, in patients who received 1 mg intravenously, compared with a mean initial value of 8.5, which decreased down to 8.0 and 5.0 at the same times in patients who were given 1 mg SC.[256] Similarly, the response after oral ingestion of vitamin K, although less rapid than after intravenous vitamin K, is more rapid than after subcutaneous administration (Fig. 27-5). Oral vitamin K administration is also more rapid than that observed after simple discontinuation of warfarin,[258] which may be prolonged in elderly patients.[264] Oral doses as low as 0.5[27] to 2.0 mg[27,260] have been recommended in patients at risk for mild to moderate prolongation of the

Table 27-7 Effective Therapies in Reducing International Normalized Ratio (INR) in Patients Administered Warfarin

Method	Mechanism	Clinical Situation	Advantages	Drawbacks
Reduction of warfarin dosage	Deceases total warfarin dose	Outpatient INR 3–6; no bleeding	Safe, effective	Slow (days); possibly confusing to patient
Holding of warfarin dose 1–2 days	Decreases total warfarin dose	Outpatient INR 5–8; no bleeding	Safe, effective	Slow (days); often confusing to patient
Ingestion of spinach or salads	Increases vitamin K intake	Outpatient INR 5–8; no bleeding	Safe, probably effective	Slow (24 hours); never studied
Low dose (≈1 mg) vitamin K given orally	Increases vitamin K intake	Outpatient INR 6–12; no bleeding	Effective within 24 hours	Difficult dosage to obtain
Moderate dose (2–5 mg) vitamin K given orally	Increases vitamin K intake	Inpatient or outpatient INR 10–15; no bleeding or INR 5–10 with bleeding	Effective within 24 hours	Takes ≈24 hours to work; often results in subtherapeutic INR
Low dose (0.5–1 mg) vitamin K given intravenously	Increases vitamin K intake	Inpatient or outpatient INR 6–12 with or without bleeding or INR 2–5 prior to invasive procedure	Works within 6–8 hours; rarely results in subtherapeutic INR; useful for patients who wish to remain on warfarin	Slight risk of anaphylaxis
High dose (5–20 mg) vitamin K, given intravenously	Greatly increases vitamin K intake	Inpatient INR ≥ 8 with bleeding or accidental warfarin ingestion	Relatively safe; very rapid (6–8 hours) effect; inexpensive	Slight risk of anaphylaxis; often results in subtherapeutic INR
Fresh frozen plasma (FFP)	Supplies missing coagulation factors	Inpatient INR ≥ 8 with bleeding	Effective in 1–2 hours in actual practice*; effective "immediately" in theory	Cumbersome; short half-lives of factors, warfarin not reversed; risks of infusion include volume and infection
Prothrombin complex concentrates (PCCs)	Supplies missing coagulation factors	Inpatient INR ≥ 8 with bleeding; CNS bleeding	Effective in 1–2 hours in actual practice	Not always available; expensive; risks of thrombosis and DIC; short half-lives of factors, warfarin not reversed
Recombinant factor VIIa (NovoSeven)	Induces thrombin generation at site of injury with platelet activation	Inpatient; urgent reversal; INR > 8 with bleeding or CNS bleeding	Effective in 20 minutes; short half-life; must follow clinically	Very expensive; risk of thrombosis probably less than PCCs; warfarin not reversed

*Including time for diagnosis, thawing, procuring, and administration.
CNS, central nervous system; DIC, disseminated intravascular coagulation.
NovoSeven is manufactured by Novo Nordisk, Inc., Princeton, NJ, USA.

INR who are not bleeding. An algorithm has been developed for estimating an appropriate oral dose on the basis of the INR[265]; however, results should be confirmed by institutions that use the respective thromboplastin reagents.

Simple discontinuation of warfarin for excessive anticoagulation may have unanticipated adverse thrombotic effects.[266] The use of large oral and subcutaneous doses of vitamin K has been associated with thrombosis and subsequent warfarin resistance requiring heparin therapy.[267] Thrombosis may be related to attainment of subtherapeutic INR levels and more rapid recovery of factor VII and other coagulant enzymes compared with proteins C and S.[266] Smaller vitamin K doses of 0.5 to 1 mg given intravenously are frequently effective for reversal of excessive anticoagulation.[268–270] In patients scheduled to undergo minor procedures while they are maintained on a stable dose of warfarin, 1 mg intravenous vitamin K transiently

normalized INR, with the effect vanishing within several days.[271] In another study of healthy volunteers who were given stable doses of oral anticoagulants, the effect of 1 mg of vitamin K administered intravenously was detectable for several days, and the effects of 5 and 25 mg were detectable on laboratory tests for up to 1 and 2 weeks, respectively.[253] Similar results have been attained with the use of low-dose oral vitamin K.[265] The subcutaneous route produces a more prolonged effect than the oral or intravenous route and results in a higher frequency of subtherapeutic INR values[258]; in one study, INR values below 2.0 were observed in 5 of 22 subjects (23%) at 72 hours after intravenous treatment compared with 14 of 33 subjects (42%) after subcutaneous therapy.[255] The use of the subcutaneous route is rational for its depot effect in the long-term replenishment of vitamin K in malnourished patients.

In patients who require more rapid reversal of anticoagulation, plasma products produce results within minutes.

IV

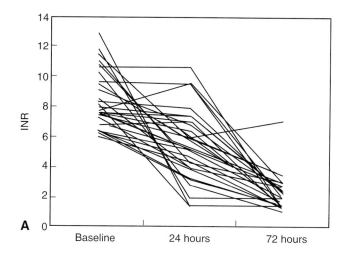

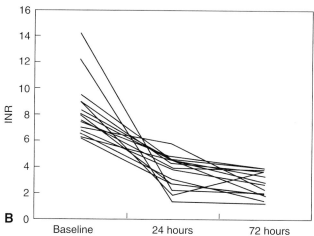

Figure 27-4 Individual values of the international normalized ratio (INR) at baseline and at 24 and 72 hours after vitamin K therapy following subcutaneous administration in 33 patients (**A**) and intravenous administration in 22 patients (**B**). Subjects with an INR between 6 and 10 received 0.5 mg (25 subcutaneous and 20 intravenous), and those with an INR between 6 and 10 received 3.0 mg (8 subcutaneous and 2 intravenous). (Adapted from Nee R, Doppenschmidt D, Donovan DJ, Andrews TC: Intravenous versus subcutaneous vitamin K₁ in reversing oral anticoagulation. Am J Cardiol 83:288, 1999. With permission from Excerpta Medica, Inc.)

continues to be inhibited by residual warfarin after FFP or PCC is used. The use of either product should be monitored and supplemented with vitamin K as appropriate. Infusion of PCC provides the most rapid infusion of all vitamin K–dependent factors and may provide a superior clinical outcome compared with FFP for patients with intracranial hemorrhage[273]; use of rFVIIa in this setting has also provided rapid control of hemostasis.[89] As with FFP, the factor content of PCC is variable, and a dose based on factor IX levels is often used. In such cases, the risks of thrombosis and DIC associated with PCC must be balanced against the risk of the clinical condition and the risk of slower response to treatments with less toxicity. Although infusion of vitamin K may surprisingly correct an astronomically prolonged INR rapidly in patients with good hepatic function,[274] rFVIIa or possibly PCC therapy should be also be used for patients with anticoagulant-associated intracerebral hemorrhage.

Vitamin K is established therapy for the prevention of hemorrhagic disease in the newborn because of transient vitamin K deficiency during the first week of life and onset of vitamin K deficiency weeks to months later.[275] Its effectiveness in other conditions is less well documented. Patients with cirrhosis[248] or liver cancer[276] may have circulating descarboxylated coagulation factors similar to those seen in vitamin K deficiency, which may be due to an acquired deficiency of the vitamin K decarboxylase. Although the mechanism was not described, administration of 10 mg vitamin K subcutaneously for 3 days as described in one report normalized prolonged PT values in 37% of patients with cirrhosis.[248] Vitamin K deficiency occurs commonly in malnourished patients in intensive care units, with or without concomitant antibiotic use,[277] accounting for four or five cases yearly in one tertiary care referral center[246] and for 20% of cases with prolongation of the PT (more than 1.5 times normal) in another.[247] Intravenous administration over 30 minutes of 5 to 25 mg vitamin K corrected the coagulopathy within 12 hours in these critically ill patients.[246,277] A much smaller dose of vitamin K—1 mg given intravenously—is effective within 24 hours when vitamin K deficiency is due to malabsorption in patients who are not critically ill, and the effect lasts 1 to 2 weeks.[253] Patients with severe hemorrhagic diathesis due to ingestion of the powerful super-warfarin rodenticide brodifacoum may require initial oral administration of 100 mg daily of vitamin K for 2 months, tapered slowly over 300 days because of the extremely prolonged half-life of the poison.[278] In contrast, prolonged PT values associated with the relatively weaker anticoagulant activity of some antibiotics (moxalactam, cefoperazone, cefamandole, cefotetan, and cefmetazole) that have the N-methylthiotetrazole (NMTT) side chain, respond rapidly to small doses in many cases.[279,280]

Toxicity

The major toxicity associated with administration of vitamin K is the rare but dramatic occurrence of anaphylaxis, which has been associated with fatalities.[281] Published studies have reported fatalities due to vitamin K administration only after intravenous administration of "relatively modest doses" of 10 mg, and data obtained via the U.S. Department of Health and Human Services Food and Drug Administration Spontaneous Reporting System Adverse Reactions

If one discounts the 30 to 45 minutes generally required to thaw FFP and the time for infusion, results with FFP or PCC occur more rapidly than with vitamin K alone, but they are transient and less durable because of the 6- to 7-hour half-life of infused factor VII. In one study, volunteer subjects who were therapeutically anticoagulated after four daily doses of 7.5 mg oral warfarin received 1 L of FFP over 100 minutes (mean dose, 12 mL per kilogram), resulting in a mean 0.12 IU per milliliter increase in factor VII levels and a mean 2-second decrease in PT at 15 minutes, followed by a return to pre-FFP infusion levels within 8 hours.[272] The very modest improvement in these patients with minimal prolongation of coagulation tests, along with other adverse effects associated with FFP use described earlier, indicates that the very large doses of FFP required to restore adequate levels of vitamin K–dependent factors in excessively anticoagulated patients may be clinically difficult or impossible to administer, particularly in elderly patients. Additionally, the synthesis of new factors

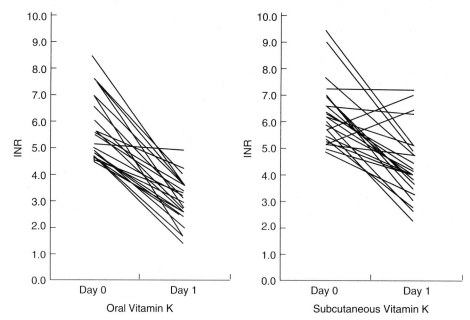

Figure 27-5 Individual values of the international normalized ratio (INR) at baseline and 1 day after 1 mg oral and 1 mg subcutaneous vitamin K. Oral vitamin K acted more quickly than subcutaneous vitamin K, and more patients had an INR between 1.8 and 3.2 after oral administration. (Adapted from Crowther MA, Douketis JD, Schnurr T, et al: Oral vitamin K lowers the international normalized ratio more rapidly than subcutaneous vitamin K in the treatment of warfarin-associated coagulopathy. Ann Intern Med 137:251–254, 2002, American College of Physicians, Philadelphia.)

describe very rare nonfatal anaphylaxis after oral or subcutaneous administration and fatal anaphylaxis after intramuscular and intravenous administration.[282] Symptoms of flushing and chest pain after intravenous administration of phytonadione were described as early as 1952, and cardiac irregularities in the 1960s were attributed to injections given more rapidly than 10 mg per minute or to the propylene glycol content of an older preparation that has since been withdrawn from the market.[283] Although these reactions have been attributed to the cremaphor excipient used in this preparation, severe anaphylaxis also occurred in a patient who received an intravenous injection of a mixed micelles vitamin K_1 preparation composed of glycoholic acid and lecithin that was designed to reduce anaphylaxis.[284] It is not clear whether the vitamin, the excipient, formation of a hapten between vitamin K and emulsifying agents, or nonimmunologic mechanisms led to this reaction.[284]

What is known about reactions after vitamin K administration may be summarized as follows: (1) anaphylactic reactions occur and are unpredictable; (2) repeated administration to the same patient does not necessarily carry the same risks; (3) slow injection does not prevent these reactions but permits interruption of the injection as soon as the onset of symptoms occurs[285] (although it is recommended that the rate of intravenous administration should not exceed 1 mg per minute, fatalities have occurred despite adherence to these guidelines[281]); (4) severe reactions have been reported most frequently in elderly patients who have received doses greater than 5 mg and after repeat dosing[281] (however, anaphylaxis has occurred in young patients even after the first administration); (5) some patients have reported no adverse events after subsequent administration following prior anaphylaxis[286]; (6) no dose dependency is evident in the frequency of reactions; however, reactions are rare when doses of 1 mg or less are used, and no fatalities have been reported at these doses[253,255,256,268–271,287]; (7) the cremaphor excipients in various preparations used in the United States and overseas are not identical but may carry the same risks[285]; and (8) shock occurs as the result of severe peripheral vasodilation, and treatment should be directed to counteract this effect.[286] One patient appeared to respond to an injection of high-dose steroids (100 mg dexamethasone).[288]

Caution should be exercised with intravenous vitamin K administration. However, when other routes are not feasible, or when rapid, reliable dosing is required, it seems prudent to dissolve the preparation in 125 mL of isotonic solution[285] and administer it carefully over 20 to 30 minutes.[288] Small doses usually suffice, and the infusion should be halted if flushing or hypotension occurs.

OTHER AGENTS

Estrogens

Conjugated estrogens, which have been used since the 1960s to augment hemostasis for a wide variety of conditions, also have hemostatic effects in uremia.[289,289–296] Livio and coworkers[292] demonstrated in a double-blinded, placebo-controlled study that conjugated estrogens given intravenously at a dose of 0.6 mg per kilogram daily shortened bleeding time in patients with uremia; this effect lasted 2 weeks and was manifest within 6 hours of the initial dose, with the maximum effect achieved at between 5 and 7 days. Additional studies in patients with uremia have confirmed the effectiveness of estrogens in shortening bleeding time with single, or repeated, intravenous doses of 0.6 mg per kilogram; administration of 0.3 mg per kilogram was ineffective.[297] A single dose of 25 mg of Premarin (Wyeth Pharmaceuticals Inc., Philadelphia, PA, USA) administered intravenously 2 hours prior to surgery produced no effect on hemostatic parameters and did not reduce blood loss.[298] Oral estrogens (50 mg daily of Premarin) also shorten bleeding time and may control bleeding symptoms in uremic patients after 7.0 ± 4.2 days of therapy.[299] Similarly, transdermal administration of estradiol at 50 or 100 µg per 24 hours every 3.5 days has been reported to shorten bleeding time in uremia and reduce transfusion requirements.[300]

Estrogens have also been used for patients with VWD. Three women who previously required blood product therapy for control of bleeding due to VWD were able to undergo successful surgical procedures after they were treated with oral estrogens administered as replacement therapy or for contraception for 2 years prior to surgery, followed by 5 mg of conjugated estrogens daily during postoperative recovery. Each patient had previously exhibited a decrease in VWD-related bleeding during pregnancy and subsequent normalization of coagulation tests during oral estrogen treatment; results of these same tests were abnormal when they were performed 8 weeks after treatment discontinuation.[290]

The mechanism of action for estrogen therapy has not been well characterized and may involve effects on the mucopolysaccharide content of the vessel wall, increased synthesis of VWF by endothelial cells, or other less clearly defined effects on hemostasis.[289,301,302] These actions may explain the efficacy of oral estrogens in patients with gastrointestinal bleeding due to Osler-Weber-Rendu syndrome or angiodysplasia.[295] Significant hemostatic toxicity has not been reported. Mild gynecomastia, weight gain, and dyspepsia have been reported in men.[295] Adverse effects in men and gynecologic symptoms in women are frequently not specifically addressed.

Protamine

Protamine sulfate is a polycationic, highly positively charged protein derived from salmon sperm protein, with a molecular weight of approximately 4500 daltons.[303] Protamine has been used to neutralize anticoagulation due to unfractionated heparin administration (UFH) after cardiac bypass surgery in more than 2,000,000 patients yearly.[303] The mechanism of action involves binding to the negatively charged heparin molecules, forming a stable complex, and displacing antithrombin III (ATIII) from the heparin:ATIII complex.[304] Protamine is the only effective available antidote to excessive anticoagulation produced by UFH; it is not nearly as effective against the anticoagulant activity of LMWH or fondaparinux; coagulation tests such as PTT are not useful in monitoring its action against these agents.[305] Although it has not been established by controlled studies or supported by animal models, anecdotal evidence suggests that rFVIIa (50 to 120 µg per kilogram) may be effective in controlling massive bleeding associated with LMWH.[101,156] Protamine possesses additional intrinsic anticoagulant activities (including induction of platelet clumping with resultant thrombocytopenia, and interference with the formation of fibrin by thrombin),[306] so that doses in excess of those calculated to neutralize UFH should be avoided. Protamine administration may be associated with other adverse effects during bypass surgery, including hypotension, increased pulmonary artery pressure, pulmonary neutrophil sequestration, and anaphylaxis, which are mediated by complement activation, histamine release,

thromboxane and nitric oxide production, and antibody production.[303] In one report, the frequency of allergic reactions may be increased in patients with a history of prior insulin use but probably not in those with a history of fish allergy or vasectomy.[303]

Protamine sulfate, which is administered by intravenous infusion, has an immediate onset and duration of action of about 2 hours. Dosing strategies to neutralize excessive anticoagulation induced by UFH are often based on the use of 1 mg of protamine to neutralize 80 to 100 USP U of heparin.[306] Because the action of protamine is shorter than that of heparin, follow-up coagulation tests should be performed to detect a "heparin rebound" effect. Ordinarily, the dosage should not exceed 100 mg given over 2 hours, unless blood coagulation tests indicate a need for larger doses.

Protamine is administered after completion of bypass surgery according to estimates of circulating heparin concentrations attained with dosing algorithms and measurement of the activated clotting time (ACT).[307] Monitoring protocols can markedly influence protamine doses used to neutralize UFH. In some but not all prospective studies, point-of-care hemostasis testing systems developed to replace traditional ACT-based empirical regimens have reduced protamine dosage and postoperative bleeding.[307] In addition to improved monitoring, UFH neutralization may be enhanced in the future by refinements in monitoring and by the use of new agents such as low molecular weight protamine,[304] recombinant platelet factor 4, or heparinase.[307] The usefulness of protamine in most outpatient settings has been greatly reduced by the use of LMWH instead of UFH for most nonprocedural indications.

MANAGEMENT OF PATIENTS WHO REFUSE OR ARE REFRACTORY TO BLOOD TRANSFUSION THERAPY

One of the most challenging clinical activities in transfusion medicine involves control of hemostasis or perioperative management for patients who refuse transfusion, or those whose clinical status renders them transfusion refractory or for whom compatible blood components are otherwise not available.[308] Examples of the former include those whose religious beliefs preclude the use of various blood-derived compounds; examples of the latter include those who have rare blood types with multiple red cell alloantibodies, thrombocytopenia with severe HLA alloimmunization, or multiple coagulation factor deficiencies in the setting of immunoglobulin (Ig)A deficiency and a history of anaphylaxis with prior plasma infusion.

In most settings, a careful approach coordinated through the hospital transfusion committee (Table 27-8) that consists of anesthesia, surgery, transfusion medicine, and hemostasis specialists may be useful in elective settings or in planned approaches to acute management. Information derived from surgery in Jehovah's Witnesses (see later) who undergo elective surgery without transfusion indicates that morbidity and mortality begin to rise sharply as postoperative hemoglobin falls to the range of 5 to 6 g per deciliter.[309] A variety of approaches involving the use of autotransfusion devices, normovolemic hemodilution, autologous donation, evaluation of anemia, and use of

Table 27-8 Collaborative Educational and Treatment Issues for Hospital Transfusion Committees

I. Transfusion of fresh frozen plasma (FFP)
  A. Evaluation of prothrombin time triggers
  B. Disease indications and contraindications
II. Transfusion of platelets and red cells
  A. Platelet thresholds and red cell transfusion triggers
  B. Platelet refractoriness
III. Transfusion of cryoprecipitate
IV. Plasma exchange therapy for thrombotic thrombocytopenic purpura (TTP), other diseases
V. Pharmaceutical agents—inventory and guidelines
  A. DDAVP (1-deamino-8-D-arginine vasopressin) for von Willebrand disease (VWD), hemophilia A, uremia, aspirin ingestion
  B. Antifibrinolytics for surgery, hyperfibrinolytic states, local application
  C. Recombinant factor VIIa for surgery, trauma, thrombocytopenia
  D. Guidelines for warfarin overdosage and administration of vitamin K
VI. Surgical support
  A. Massive transfusion guidelines
  B. Cell savers
  C. Autologous blood donation
  D. Point-of-care testing and collaborative treatment algorithms
VII. Treatment of patients who do not have available compatible blood components or who refuse blood component transfusions
  A. Jehovah's Witnesses
  B. True immunoglobulin (Ig)A deficiency with clinical anaphylaxis
  C. Thrombocytopenia or thrombocytopahy with severe human leukocyte antigen (HLA) alloimmunization or antiplatelet antibodies

IV

EPO therapy may be employed to augment red cell mass and minimize the need for RBC transfusion therapy[310]; the choice of hemostatic agents to optimize hemostasis should be tailored to the clinical condition (see Table 27-3).

Several additional caveats must be considered in the approach to patients who refuse blood transfusion because of religious beliefs, such as Jehovah's Witness patients.[311] As with beliefs involving diet or work habits, no single set of criteria that is uniformly adhered to by all followers of a religion, including Jehovah's Witness patients, can be used for transfusion support. Although most patients refuse transfusion with RBCs, platelets, or plasma, some may also refuse albumin, recombinant proteins, or the use of procedures in which their blood is physically separated from the body, such as preoperative autologous donation and some methods of acute normovolemic hemodilution. In these situations, it is prudent and essential to work carefully in advance with the patient and to include religious advisors and other church representatives if desired to define allowable therapies and review the planned approach. The application of a comprehensive approach for Jehovah's Witness patients undergoing liver transplantation (involving preoperative consent for refusal of transfusion and specific consent for therapeutic techniques, including cell salvage, acute normovolemic hemodilution, preoperative EPO therapy, and use of rFVIIa and antifibrinolytic agents) resulted in 100% survival after 19 living donor procedures and 75% survival in 8 deceased donor cases.[312]

484

SUMMARY

Research into and development of new blood products and pharmaceutical agents will continue to offer increasingly sophisticated approaches for the care and management of patients with disordered hemostasis.[313] Strategies for appropriate use may be best established, reviewed, and revised in collaborative settings such as with the hospital transfusion committee (see Table 27-8). For those patients with congenital hemostatic disorders, recombinant products and the advent of gene therapy promise additional safety and efficacy but will also be associated with the potential for increased costs of development. Improved laboratory testing and rapid identification of appropriate therapy in surgical and other settings based on point-of-care testing and collaboratively developed guidelines promise additional benefits for those patients with acquired disorders.[114]

REFERENCES

1. Ratnoff OD: Why do people bleed? In Wintrobe MM (ed): Blood, Pure and Eloquent, New York, McGraw-Hill, Inc., 1980, pp 601–658.
2. Diamond LK: A history of blood transfusion. In Wintrobe MM (ed): Blood, Pure and Eloquent, New York, McGraw-Hill, Inc., 1980, pp 659–690.
3. Alving B, Alcorn K: How to improve transfusion medicine: A treating physician's perspective. Arch Pathol Lab Med 123:492–495, 1999.
4. Livio M, Gotti E, Marchesi D, et al: Uraemic bleeding: role of anaemia and beneficial effect of red cell transfusions. Lancet 2:1013–1015, 1982.
5. Ho CH: The hemostatic effect of packed red cell transfusion in patients with anemia. Transfusion 38:1011–1014, 1998.
6. Turrito VT, Weiss HJ: Red blood cells: Their dual role in thrombus formation. Science 207:541–543, 1980.
7. Parsons SF, Spring FA, Chasis JA, Anstee DJ: Erythroid cell adhesion molecules: Lutheran and LW in health and disease. Baillieres Best Pract Res Clin Haematol 12:729–745, 1999.
8. Hebert PC, Wells G, Blajchman MA, et al: A multicenter, randomized, controlled clinical trial of transfusion requirements in critical care. Transfusion Requirements in Critical Care Investigators, Canadian Critical Care Trials Group. N Engl J Med 340:409–417, 1999.
9. Stohlawetz PJ, Dzirlo L, Hergovich N, et al: Effects of erythropoietin on platelet reactivity and thrombopoiesis in humans. Blood 95:2983–2989, 2000.
10. Mannucci PM: Hemostatic drugs. N Engl J Med 339:245–253, 1998.
11. Faringer PD, Mullins RJ, Johnson RL, Trunkey DD: Blood component supplementation during massive transfusion of AS-1 red cells in trauma patients. J Trauma 34:481–485, 1993.
12. Johansson PI, Hansen MB, Sorensen H: Transfusion practice in massively bleeding patients: Time for a change? Vox Sang 89:92–96, 2005.
13. Ness PM, Campbell-Lee SA: Single donor versus pooled random donor platelet concentrates. Curr Opin Hematol 8:392–396, 2001.
14. Gaydos LA, Freireich EJ, Mantel N: The quantitative relation between platelet count and hemorrhage in patients with acute leukemia. N Engl J Med 266:905–909, 1962.
15. Gmur J, Burger J, Schanz U, et al: Safety of stringent prophylactic platelet transfusion policy for patients with acute leukaemia. Lancet 338:1223–1226, 1991.
16. Rebulla P, Finazzi G, Marangoni F, et al: The threshold for prophylactic platelet transfusions in adults with acute myeloid leukemia. Gruppo Italiano Malattie Ematologiche Maligne dell'Adulto. N Engl J Med 337:1870–1875, 1997.
17. Beutler E: Platelet transfusions: The 20,000/microL trigger. Blood 81:1411–1413, 1993.
18. Schiffer CA, Anderson KC, Bennett CL, et al: Platelet transfusion for patients with cancer: Clinical practice guidelines of the American Society of Clinical Oncology. J Clin Oncol 19:1519–1538, 2001.
19. Fuse I: Disorders of platelet function. Crit Rev Oncol Hematol 22:1–25, 1996.

20. Despotis GJ, Skubas NJ, Goodnough LT: Optimal management of bleeding and transfusion in patients undergoing cardiac surgery. Semin Thorac Cardiovasc Surg 11:84–104, 1999.

21. Carr JM, Kruskall MS, Kaye JA, Robinson SH: Efficacy of platelet transfusions in immune thrombocytopenia. Am J Med 80: 1051–1054, 1986.

22. Vengelen-Tyler V: Blood transfusion practice. In Vengelen-Tyler V (ed): Technical Manual, Bethesda, Md, AABB Press, 1999, pp 451–481.

23. Slichter SJ, Davis K, Enright H, et al: Factors affecting posttransfusion platelet increments, platelet refractoriness, and platelet transfusion intervals in thrombocytopenic patients. Blood 105:4106–4114, 2005.

24. Nambiar A, Duquesnoy RJ, Adams S, et al: HLA Matchmaker-driven analysis of responses to HLA-typed platelet transfusions in alloimmunized thrombocytopenic patients. Blood 107:1680–1687, 2006.

25. Beeck H, Becker T, Kiessig ST, et al: The influence of citrate concentration on the quality of plasma obtained by automated plasmapheresis: A prospective study. Transfusion 39:1266–1270, 1999.

26. Alving BM: Beyond hemophilia and von Willebrand disease: Treatment of patients with other inherited coagulation factor and inhibitor deficiencies. In Alving BM (ed): Blood Components and Pharmacologic Agents in the Treatment of Congenital and Acquired Bleeding Disorders Bethesda, Md, AABB Press, 2000, pp 341–356.

27. Guidelines on oral anticoagulation: Third edition. Br J Haematol 101:374–387, 1998.

28. Ciavarella D, Reed RL, Counts RB, et al: Clotting factor levels and the risk of diffuse microvascular bleeding in the massively transfused patient. Br J Haematol 67:365–368, 1987.

29. Counts RB, Haisch C, Simon TL, et al: Hemostasis in massively transfused trauma patients. Ann Surg 190:91–99, 1979.

30. McVay PA, Toy PT: Lack of increased bleeding after liver biopsy in patients with mild hemostatic abnormalities. Am J Clin Pathol 94:747–753, 1990.

31. Gajic O, Dzik WH, Toy P: Fresh frozen plasma and platelet transfusion for nonbleeding patients in the intensive care unit: Benefit or harm? Crit Care Med 34 (5 suppl): S170–S173, 2006.

32. Klein HG, Dodd RY, Dzik WH, et al: Current status of solvent/detergent-treated frozen plasma. Transfusion 38:102–107, 1998.

33. Chekrizova V, Murphy WG: Solvent-detergent plasma: Use in neonatal patients, in adult and paediatric patients with liver disease and in obstetric and gynaecological emergencies. Transfus Med 16:85–91, 2006.

34. Poon MC: Cryoprecipitate: Uses and alternatives. Transfus Med Rev 7:180–192, 1993.

35. Jackson MR, Alving BM: Fibrin sealant in preclinical and clinical studies. Curr Opin Hematol 6:415–419, 1999.

36. Dodd RY, Notari EP, Stramer SL: Current prevalence and incidence of infectious disease markers and estimated window-period risk in the American Red Cross blood donor population. Transfusion 42:975–979, 2002.

37. Alter HJ: Emerging, re-emerging and submerging infectious threats to the blood supply. Vox Sang 87 (suppl 2): 56–61, 2004.

38. Klein HG: Will blood transfusion ever be safe enough? [Editorial] JAMA 284:238–240, 2000.

39. Heddle NM, Kelton JG: Febrile nonhemolytic transfusion reactions. In Popovsky MA (ed): Transfusion Reactions, Bethesda, Md, AABB Press, 1996, pp 45–80.

40. Vamvakas EC, Pineda AA: Allergic and anaphylactic reactions. In Popovsky MA (ed): Transfusion Reactions, Bethesda, Md, AABB Press, 1996, pp 81–125.

41. Davenport RD: Hemolytic transfusion reactions. In Popovsky MA (ed): Transfusion Reactions, Bethesda, Md, AABB Press, 1996, pp 1–44.

42. Linden JV, Wagner K, Voytovich AE, Sheehan J: Transfusion errors in New York State: An analysis of 10 years' experience. Transfusion 40:1207–1213, 2000.

43. Goldman M, Blajchman MA: Bacterial contamination. In Popovsky MA (ed): Transfusion Reactions, Bethesda, Md, AABB Press, 1996, pp 125–165.

44. Blajchman MA, Beckers EA, Dickmeiss E, et al: Bacterial detection of platelets: Current problems and possible resolutions. Transfus Med Rev 19:259–272, 2005.

45. Popovsky MA: Transfusion related acute lung injury (TRALI). In Popovsky MA (ed): Transfusion Reactions, Bethesda, Md, AABB Press, 2001, pp 155–170.

46. McFarland JG: Posttransfusion pupura. In Popovsky MA (ed): Transfusion Reactions, Bethesda, Md, AABB Press, 2001, pp 187–212.

47. Webb IJ, Anderson KC: Transfusion-associated graft-verus-host disease. In Popovsky MA (ed): Transfusion Reactions, Bethesda, Md, AABB Press, 2001, pp 171–186.

48. Goldman M, Webert KE, Arnold DM, et al: Proceedings of a consensus conference: Towards an understanding of TRALI. Transfus Med Rev 19:2–31, 2005.

49. Silliman CC, Boshkov LK, Mehdizadehkashi Z, et al: Transfusion-related acute lung injury: Epidemiology and a prospective analysis of etiologic factors. Blood 101:454–462, 2003.

50. Anderson K: Broadening the spectrum of patient groups at risk for transfusion-associated GVHD: Implications for universal irradiation of cellular blood components. Transfusion 43:1652–1654, 2003.

51. Leitman SF, Holland PV: Irradiation of blood products: Indications and guidelines. Transfusion 25:293–303, 1985.

52. Hellstern P: Production and composition of prothrombin complex concentrates: Correlation between composition and therapeutic efficiency. Thromb Res 95 (4 suppl 1): S7–S12, 1999.

53. Hellstern P, Halbmayer WM, Kohler M, et al: Prothrombin complex concentrates: Indications, contraindications, and risks: A task force summary. Thromb Res 95 (4 suppl 1): S3–S6, 1999.

54. Mannucci PM, Tenconi PM, Castaman G, Rodeghiero F: Comparison of four virus-inactivated plasma concentrates for treatment of severe von Willebrand disease: A cross-over randomized trial. Blood 79:3130–3137, 1992.

55. Chang AC, Rick ME, Ross PL, Weinstein MJ: Summary of a workshop on potency and dosage of von Willebrand factor concentrates. Haemophilia 4 (suppl 3): 1–6, 1998.

56. Montgomery RR, Coller BS: Von Willebrand disease. In Colman RW, Hirsh J, Marder VJ Salzman EW (eds): Hemostasis and Thrombosis: Basic Principles and Clinical Practice, 3rd ed. Philadelphia, Lippincott, 1994, pp 134–168.

57. Lusher J, Ingerslev J, Roberts H, Hedner U: Clinical experience with recombinant factor VIIa. Blood Coagul Fibrinolysis 9:119–128, 1998.

58. Kristensen J, Killander A, Hippe E, et al: Clinical experience with recombinant factor VIIa in patients with thrombocytopenia. Haemostasis 26 (suppl 1): 159–164, 1996.

59. Kenet G, Walden R, Eldad A, Martinowitz U: Treatment of traumatic bleeding with recombinant factor VIIa. [Letter] Lancet 354:1879, 1999.

60. Martinowitz U, Kenet G, Segal E, et al: Recombinant activated factor VII for adjunctive hemorrhage control in trauma. J Trauma 51:431–438, 2001.

61. O'Connell KA, Wood JJ, Wise RP, et al: Thromboembolic adverse events after use of recombinant human coagulation factor VIIa. JAMA 295:293–298, 2006.

62. Levi M: Recombinant factor VIIa: A general hemostatic agent? Not yet. J Thromb Haemost 2:1695–1697, 2004.

63. Roberts HR: Recombinant factor VIIa: A general hemostatic agent? Yes. J Thromb Haemost 2:1691–1694, 2004.

64. Hedner U, Erhardtsen E: Potential role for rFVIIa in transfusion medicine. Transfusion 42:114–124, 2002.

65. Roberts HR, Monroe DM, White GC: The use of recombinant factor VIIa in the treatment of bleeding disorders. Blood 104:3858–3864, 2004.

66. Wolberg AS, Allen GA, Monroe DM, et al: High dose factor VIIa improves clot structure and stability in a model of haemophilia B. Br J Haematol 131:645–655, 2005.

67. Bajzar L, Manuel R, Nesheim ME: Purification and characterization of TAFI, a thrombin-activable fibrinolysis inhibitor. J Biol Chem 270:14477–14484, 1995.

68. Meng ZH, Wolberg AS, Monroe DM III, Hoffman M: The effect of temperature and pH on the activity of factor VIIa: Implications for the efficacy of high-dose factor VIIa in hypothermic and acidotic patients. J Trauma 55:886–891, 2003.

69. Mohr AM, Holcomb JB, Dutton RP, Duranteau J: Recombinant activated factor VIIa and hemostasis in critical care: A focus on trauma. Crit Care 9 (suppl 5): S37–S42, 2005.

70. Deveras RA, Kessler CM: Reversal of warfarin-induced excessive anticoagulation with recombinant human factor VIIa concentrate. Ann Intern Med 137:884–888, 2002.

71. Friederich PW, Henny CP, Messelink EJ, et al: Effect of recombinant activated factor VII on perioperative blood loss in patients undergoing retropubic prostatectomy: A double-blind placebo-controlled randomised trial. Lancet 361:201–205, 2003.

72. Boffard KD, Riou B, Warren B, et al: Recombinant factor VIIa as adjunctive therapy for bleeding control in severely injured trauma

patients: Two parallel randomized, placebo-controlled, double-blind clinical trials. J Trauma 59:8–15, 2005.

73. Goodnough LT, Lublin DM, Zhang L, et al: Transfusion medicine service policies for recombinant factor VIIa administration. Transfusion 44:1325–1331, 2004.

74. Gabriel DA, Carr M, Roberts HR: Monitoring coagulation and the clinical effects of recombinant factor VIIa. Semin Hematol 41 (1 suppl 1): 20–24, 2004.

75. Grounds RM, Bolan C: Clinical experiences and current evidence for therapeutic recombinant factor VIIa treatment in nontrauma settings. Crit Care 9 (suppl 5): S29–S36, 2005.

76. Savani BN, Dunbar CE, Rick ME: Combination therapy with rFVIIa and platelets for hemorrhage in patients with severe thrombocytopenia and alloimmunization. Am J Hematol 81:218–219, 2006.

77. Poon MC: Use of recombinant factor VIIa in hereditary bleeding disorders. Curr Opin Hematol 8:312–318, 2001.

78. Salomon O, Zivelin A, Livnat T, et al: Prevalence, causes, and characterization of factor XI inhibitors in patients with inherited factor XI deficiency. Blood 101:4783–4788, 2003.

79. Goodnough LT: Experiences with recombinant human factor VIIa in patients with thrombocytopenia. Semin Hematol 41 (1 suppl 1): 25–29, 2004.

80. Poon MC, D'Oiron R, Von DM, et al: Prophylactic and therapeutic recombinant factor VIIa administration to patients with Glanzmann's thrombasthenia: Results of an international survey. J Thromb Haemost 2:1096–1103, 2004.

81. Ciavarella N, Schiavoni M, Valenzano E, et al: Use of recombinant factor VIIa (NovoSeven) in the treatment of two patients with type III von Willebrand's disease and an inhibitor against von Willebrand factor. Haemostasis 26 (suppl 1): 150–154, 1996.

82. Planinsic RM, van der MJ, Testa G, et al: Safety and efficacy of a single bolus administration of recombinant factor VIIa in liver transplantation due to chronic liver disease. Liver Transpl 11:895–900, 2005.

83. Lodge JP, Jonas S, Jones RM, et al: Efficacy and safety of repeated perioperative doses of recombinant factor VIIa in liver transplantation. Liver Transpl 11:973–979, 2005.

84. Bernstein DE, Jeffers L, Erhardtsen E, et al: Recombinant factor VIIa corrects prothrombin time in cirrhotic patients: A preliminary study. Gastroenterology 113:1930–1937, 1997.

85. Jeffers L, Chalasani N, Balart L, et al: Safety and efficacy of recombinant factor VIIa in patients with liver disease undergoing laparoscopic liver biopsy. Gastroenterology 123:118–126, 2002.

86. Lodge JP, Jonas S, Oussoultzoglou E, et al: Recombinant coagulation factor VIIa in major liver resection: A randomized, placebo-controlled, double-blind clinical trial. Anesthesiology 102:269–275, 2005.

87. Levi M, Bijsterveld NR, Keller TT: Recombinant factor VIIa as an antidote for anticoagulant treatment. Semin Hematol 41 (1 suppl 1): 65–69, 2004.

88. Erhardtsen E, Nony P, Dechavanne M, et al: The effect of recombinant factor VIIa (NovoSeven) in healthy volunteers receiving acenocoumarol to an International Normalized Ratio above 2.0. Blood Coagul Fibrinolysis 9:741–748, 1998.

89. Sorensen B, Johansen P, Nielsen GL, et al: Reversal of the International Normalized Ratio with recombinant activated factor VII in central nervous system bleeding during warfarin thromboprophylaxis: Clinical and biochemical aspects. Blood Coagul Fibrinolysis 14:469–477, 2003.

90. Mayer SA, Brun NC, Begtrup K, et al: Recombinant activated factor VII for acute intracerebral hemorrhage. N Engl J Med 352:777–785, 2005.

91. Martinowitz U, Holcomb JB, Pusateri AE, et al: Intravenous rFVIIa administered for hemorrhage control in hypothermic coagulopathic swine with grade V liver injuries. J Trauma 50:721–729, 2001.

92. Klemcke HG, Delgado A, Holcomb JB, et al: Effect of recombinant FVIIa in hypothermic, coagulopathic pigs with liver injuries. J Trauma 59:155–161, 2005.

93. Martinowitz U, Michaelson M: Guidelines for the use of recombinant activated factor VII (rFVIIa) in uncontrolled bleeding: A report by the Israeli Multidisciplinary rFVIIa Task Force. J Thromb Haemost 3:640–648, 2005.

94. O'Connell NM, Perry DJ, Hodgson AJ, et al: Recombinant FVIIa in the management of uncontrolled hemorrhage. Transfusion 43: 1711–1716, 2003.

95. Salzman EW, Weinstein MJ, Weintraub RM, et al: Treatment with desmopressin acetate to reduce blood loss after cardiac surgery: A double-blind randomized trial. N Engl J Med 314:1402–1406, 1986.

96. Raobaikady R, Redman J, Ball JA, et al: Use of activated recombinant coagulation factor VII in patients undergoing reconstruction surgery for traumatic fracture of pelvis or pelvis and acetabulum: A double-blind, randomized, placebo-controlled trial. Br J Anaesth 94: 586–591, 2005.

97. Pihusch M, Bacigalupo A, Szer J, et al: Recombinant activated factor VII in treatment of bleeding complications following hematopoietic stem cell transplantation. J Thromb Haemost 3:1935–1944, 2005.

98. von Heymann C, Hotz H, Konertz W, et al: Successful treatment of refractory bleeding with recombinant factor VIIa after redo coronary artery bypass graft surgery. J Cardiothorac Vasc Anesth 16:615–616, 2002.

99. Laffan MA, Tait RC, Blatny J, et al: Use of recombinant activated factor VII for bleeding in pancreatitis: A case series. Pancreas 30: 279–284, 2005.

100. Ahonen J, Jokela R: Recombinant factor VIIa for life-threatening post-partum haemorrhage. Br J Anaesth 94:592–595, 2005.

101. Hu Q, Brady JO: Recombinant activated factor VII for treatment of enoxaparin-induced bleeding. Mayo Clin Proc 79:827, 2004.

102. Roberts HR, Monroe DM III, Hoffman M: Safety profile of recombinant factor VIIa. Semin Hematol 41 (1 suppl 1): 101–108, 2004.

103. Ratnoff OD: Epsilon aminocaproic acid: A dangerous weapon. N Engl J Med 280:1124–1125, 1999.

104. Ingerslev J: Efficacy and safety of recombinant factor VIIa in the prophylaxis of bleeding in various surgical procedures in hemophilic patients with factor VIII and factor IX inhibitors. Semin Thromb Hemost 26:425–432, 2000.

105. Key NS, Christie B, Henderson N, Nelsestuen GL: Possible synergy between recombinant factor VIIa and prothrombin complex concentrate in hemophilia therapy. Thromb Haemost 88:60–65, 2002.

106. Bolan CD, Alving BM: Pharmacologic agents in the management of bleeding disorders. Transfusion 30:541–551, 1990.

107. Richardson DW, Robinson AG: Desmopressin. Ann Intern Med 103:228–239, 1985.

108. Mannucci PM: Desmopressin (DDAVP) in the treatment of bleeding disorders: The first 20 years. Blood 90:2515–2521, 1997.

109. Mannucci PM: Desmopressin: A nontransfusional form of treatment for congenital and acquired bleeding disorders. Blood 72:1449–1455, 1988.

110. Laupacis A, Fergusson D: Drugs to minimize perioperative blood loss in cardiac surgery: Meta-analyses using perioperative blood transfusion as the outcome. The International Study of Peri-operative Transfusion (ISPOT) Investigators. Anesth Analg 85:1258–1267, 1997.

111. Green D, Wong CA, Twardowski P: Efficacy of hemostatic agents in improving surgical hemostasis. Transfus Med Rev 10:171–182, 1996.

112. Janssens M, Hartstein G, David JL: Reduction in requirements for allogeneic blood products: Pharmacologic methods. Ann Thorac Surg 62:1944–1950, 1996.

113. Dilthey G, Dietrich W, Spannagl M, Richter JA: Influence of desmopressin acetate on homologous blood requirements in cardiac surgical patients pretreated with aspirin. J Cardiothorac Vasc Anesth 7:425–430, 1993.

114. Despotis GJ, Levine V, Saleem R, et al: Use of point-of-care test in identification of patients who can benefit from desmopressin during cardiac surgery: A randomised controlled trial. Lancet 354:106–110, 1999.

115. Sutor AH: DDAVP is not a panacea for children with bleeding disorders. Br J Haematol 108:217–227, 2000.

116. Mannucci PM, Canciani MT, Rota L, Donovan BS: Response of factor VIII/von Willebrand factor to DDAVP in healthy subjects and patients with haemophilia A and von Willebrand's disease. Br J Haematol 47:283–293, 1981.

117. Levi M, de Boer JP, Roem D, et al: Plasminogen activation in vivo upon intravenous infusion of DDAVP: Quantitative assessment of plasmin-alpha 2-antiplasmin complex with a novel monoclonal antibody based radioimmunoassay. Thromb Haemost 67:111–116, 1992.

118. Tsai HM, Sussman II, Nagel RL, Kaul DK: Desmopressin induces adhesion of normal human erythrocytes to the endothelial surface of a perfused microvascular preparation. Blood 75:261–265, 1990.

119. Barnhart MI, Chen S, Lusher JM: DDAVP: Does the drug have a direct effect on the vessel wall? Thromb Res 31:239–253, 1993.

120. Takeuchi M, Nagura H, Kaneda T: DDAVP and epinephrine-induced changes in the localization of von Willebrand factor antigen in endothelial cells of human oral mucosa. Blood 72:850–854, 1988.

121. Ruggeri ZM, Mannucci PM, Lombardi R, et al: Multimeric composition of factor VIII/von Willebrand factor following administration of DDAVP: Implications for pathophysiology and therapy of von Willebrand's disease subtypes. Blood 59:1272–1278, 1982.

122. Sakariassen KS, Cattaneo M, Berg A, et al: DDAVP enhances platelet adherence and platelet aggregate growth on human artery subendothelium. Blood 64:229–236, 1984.

123. Cattaneo M, Pareti FI, Zighetti M, et al: Platelet aggregation at high shear is impaired in patients with congenital defects of platelet secretion and is corrected by DDAVP: Correlation with the bleeding time. J Lab Clin Med 125:540–547, 1995.

124. Horstman LL, Valle-Riestra BJ, Jy W, et al: Desmopressin (DDAVP) acts on platelets to generate platelet microparticles and enhanced procoagulant activity. Thromb Res 79:163–174, 1995.

125. Galvez A, Gomez-Ortiz G, Diaz-Ricart M, et al: Desmopressin (DDAVP) enhances platelet adhesion to the extracellular matrix of cultured human endothelial cells through increased expression of tissue factor. Thromb Haemost 77:975–980, 1997.

126. Wun T, Paglieroni TG, Lachant NA: Desmopressin stimulates the expression of P-selectin on human platelets in vitro. J Lab Clin Med 126:401–409, 1995.

127. Sloand EM, Alyono D, Klein HG, et al: 1-Deamino-8-D-arginine vasopressin (DDAVP) increases platelet membrane expression of glycoprotein Ib in patients with disorders of platelet function and after cardiopulmonary bypass. Am J Hematol 46:199–207, 1994.

128. Cattaneo M, Moia M, Delle VP, et al: DDAVP shortens the prolonged bleeding times of patients with severe von Willebrand disease treated with cryoprecipitate: Evidence for a mechanism of action independent of released von Willebrand factor. Blood 74:1972–1975, 1989.

129. Mannucci PM, Remuzzi G, Pusineri F, et al: Deamino-8-D-arginine vasopressin shortens the bleeding time in uremia. N Engl J Med 308:8–12, 1983.

130. Mannucci PM, Vicente V, Vianello L, et al: Controlled trial of desmopressin in liver cirrhosis and other conditions associated with a prolonged bleeding time. Blood 67:1148–1153, 1986.

131. Kobrinsky NL, Israels ED, Gerrard JM, et al: Shortening of bleeding time by 1-deamino-8-D-arginine vasopressin in various bleeding disorders. Lancet 1:1145–1148, 1984.

132. Kentro TB, Lottenberg R, Kitchens CS: Clinical efficacy of desmopressin acetate for hemostatic control in patients with primary platelet disorders undergoing surgery. Am J Hematol 24:215–219, 1987.

133. Mannucci PM, Bettega D, Cattaneo M: Patterns of development of tachyphylaxis in patients with haemophilia and von Willebrand disease after repeated doses of desmopressin (DDAVP). Br J Haematol 82:87–93, 1992.

134. Vicente V, Estelles A, Laso J, et al: Repeated infusions of DDAVP induce low response of FVIII and vWF but not of plasminogen activators. Thromb Res 70:117–122, 1993.

135. Lethagen S, Olofsson L, Frick K, et al: Effect kinetics of desmopressin-induced platelet retention in healthy volunteers treated with aspirin or placebo. Haemophilia 6:15–20, 2000.

136. Pullan PT, Burger HG, Johnston CI: Pharmacokinetics of 1-desamino-8-D-arginine vasopressin (DDAVP) in patients with central diabetes insipidus. Clin Endocrinol (Oxf) 9:273–278, 1978.

137. Federici AB, Mazurier C, Berntorp E, et al: Biologic response to desmopressin in patients with severe type 1 and type 2 von Willebrand disease: Results of a multicenter European study. Blood 103:2032–2038, 2004.

138. Fowler WE, Berkowitz LR, Roberts HR: DDAVP for type IIB von Willebrand disease. [Letter] Blood 74:1859–1860, 1989.

139. McKeown LP, Connaghan G, Wilson O, et al: 1-Desamino-8-arginine-vasopressin corrects the hemostatic defects in type 2B von Willebrand's disease. Am J Hematol 51:158–163, 1996.

140. Castaman G, Lattuada A, Mannucci PM, Rodeghiero F: Factor VIII:C increases after desmopressin in a subgroup of patients with autosomal recessive severe von Willebrand disease. Br J Haematol 89:147–151, 1995.

141. Deitcher SR, Tuller J, Johnson JA: Intranasal DDAVP induced increases in plasma von Willebrand factor alter the pharmacokinetics of high-purity factor VIII concentrates in severe haemophilia A patients. Haemophilia 5:88–95, 1999.

142. Tefferi A, Nichols WL: Acquired von Willebrand disease: Concise review of occurrence, diagnosis, pathogenesis, and treatment. Am J Med 103:536–540, 1997.

143. Federici AB, Stabile F, Castaman G, et al: Treatment of acquired von Willebrand syndrome in patients with monoclonal gammopathy of uncertain significance: Comparison of three different therapeutic approaches. Blood 92:2707–2711, 1998.

144. Rao AK, Ghosh S, Sun L, et al: Mechanisms of platelet dysfunction and response to DDAVP in patients with congenital platelet function defects: A double-blind placebo-controlled trial. Thromb Haemost 74:1071–1078, 1995.

145. Schulman S, Johnsson H, Egberg N, Blomback M: DDAVP-induced correction of prolonged bleeding time in patients with congenital platelet function defects. Thromb Res 45:165–174, 1987.

146. Noris P, Arbustini E, Spedini P, et al: A new variant of Bernard-Soulier syndrome characterized by dysfunctional glycoprotein (GP) Ib and severely reduced amounts of GPIX and GPV. Br J Haematol 103:1004–1013, 1998.

147. Stine KC, Becton DL: DDAVP therapy controls bleeding in Ehlers-Danlos syndrome. J Pediatr Hematol Oncol 19:156–158, 1997.

148. Castaman G, Ruggeri M, Rodeghiero F: Clinical usefulness of desmopressin for prevention of surgical bleeding in patients with symptomatic heterozygous factor XI deficiency. Br J Haematol 94:168–170, 1996.

149. Lind SE: The bleeding time does not predict surgical bleeding. Blood 77:2547–2552, 1991.

150. de Franchis R, Arcidiacono PG, Carpinelli L, et al: Randomized controlled trial of desmopressin plus terlipressin vs. terlipressin alone for the treatment of acute variceal hemorrhage in cirrhotic patients: A multicenter, double-blind study. New Italian Endoscopic Club. Hepatology 18:1102–1107, 1993.

151. Levi M, Cromheecke ME, de Jonge E, et al: Pharmacological strategies to decrease excessive blood loss in cardiac surgery: A meta-analysis of clinically relevant endpoints. Lancet 354:1940–1947, 1999.

152. Cattaneo M, Harris AS, Stromberg U, Mannucci PM: The effect of desmopressin on reducing blood loss in cardiac surgery: A meta-analysis of double-blind, placebo-controlled trials. Thromb Haemost 74:1064–1070, 1995.

153. Gratz I, Koehler J, Olsen D, et al: The effect of desmopressin acetate on postoperative hemorrhage in patients receiving aspirin therapy before coronary artery bypass operations. J Thorac Cardiovasc Surg 104:1417–1422, 1992.

154. Sheridan DP, Card RT, Pinilla JC, et al: Use of desmopressin acetate to reduce blood transfusion requirements during cardiac surgery in patients with acetylsalicylic acid–induced platelet dysfunction. Can J Surg 37:33–36, 1994.

155. Flordal PA, Sahlin S: Use of desmopressin to prevent bleeding complications in patients treated with aspirin. Br J Surg 80:723–724, 1993.

156. Ng HJ, Koh LP, Lee LH: Successful control of postsurgical bleeding by recombinant factor VIIa in a renal failure patient given low molecular weight heparin and aspirin. Ann Hematol 82:257–258, 2003.

157. Flordal PA: Pharmacological prophylaxis of bleeding in surgical patients treated with aspirin. Eur J Anaesthesiol Suppl 14:38–41, 1997.

158. Weinbaum PJ, Cassidy SB, Campbell WA, et al: Pregnancy management and successful outcome of Ehlers-Danlos syndrome type IV. Am J Perinatol 4:134–137, 1987.

159. Kadir RA: Women and inherited bleeding disorders: Pregnancy and delivery. Semin Hematol 36 (3 suppl 4): 28–35, 1999.

160. Ray JG: DDAVP use during pregnancy: An analysis of its safety for mother and child. Obstet Gynecol Surv 53:450–455, 1998.

161. Castaman G, Rodeghiero F: Failure of DDAVP to shorten the prolonged bleeding time of two patients with congenital afibrinogenemia. Thromb Res 68:309–315, 1992.

162. DiMichele DM, Hathaway WE: Use of DDAVP in inherited and acquired platelet dysfunction. Am J Hematol 33:39–45, 1990.

163. Kobrinsky NL, Tulloch H: Treatment of refractory thrombocytopenic bleeding with 1-desamino-8-D-arginine vasopressin (desmopressin). J Pediatr 112:993–996, 1988.

164. Kohler M, Hellstern P, Miyashita C, et al: Comparative study of intranasal, subcutaneous and intravenous administration of desamino-D-arginine vasopressin (DDAVP). Thromb Haemost 55:108–111, 1986.

165. Dunn AL, Powers JR, Ribeiro MJ, et al: Adverse events during use of intranasal desmopressin acetate for haemophilia A and von Willebrand disease: A case report and review of 40 patients. Haemophilia 6:11–14, 2000.

166. Humphries JE, Siragy H: Significant hyponatremia following DDAVP administration in a healthy adult. Am J Hematol 44:12–15, 1993.

167. Mannucci PM, Lusher JM: Desmopressin and thrombosis. [Letter] Lancet 2:675–676, 1989.

168. Flordal PA, Ljungstrom KG, Fehrm A: Desmopressin and postoperative thromboembolism. Thromb Res 68:429–433, 1992.

169. Mannucci PM, Carlsson S, Harris AS: Desmopressin, surgery and thrombosis. [Letter] Thromb Haemost 71:154–155, 1994.

170. Federici AB, Sacco R, Stabile F, et al: Optimising local therapy during oral surgery in patients with von Willebrand disease: Effective results from a retrospective analysis of 63 cases. Haemophilia 6:71–77, 2000.

171. Collen D: On the regulation and control of fibrinolysis. Edward Kowalski Memorial Lecture. Thromb Haemost 43:77–89, 1980.

172. Verstraete M: Clinical application of inhibitors of fibrinolysis. Drugs 29:236–261, 1985.

173. Sherry S, Marder VJ: Therapy with antifibrinolytic agents. In Colman RW, Hirsh J, Marder VJ Salzman EW (eds): Hemostasis and Thrombosis: Basic Principles and Clinical Practice, Philadelphia, Pa, Lippincott, 1994, pp 335–352.

174. Dunn CJ, Goa KL: Tranexamic acid: A review of its use in surgery and other indications. Drugs 57:1005–1032, 1999.

175. Okamoto S, Sato S, Takada Y, Okamato U: An active stereoisomer (transform) of AMCHA and its antifibrinolytic (antiplasmic) action in vitro and in vivo. Keio J Med 13:177, 1964.

176. Kane MJ, Silverman LR, Rand JH, et al: Myonecrosis as a complication of the use of epsilon amino-caproic acid: A case report and review of the literature. Am J Med 85:861–863, 1988.

177. Seymour BD, Rubinger M: Rhabdomyolysis induced by epsilon-aminocaproic acid. Ann Pharmacother 31:56–58, 1997.

178. Aoki N, Saito H, Kamiya T, et al: Congenital deficiency of alpha 2-plasmin inhibitor associated with severe hemorrhagic tendency. J Clin Invest 63:877–884, 1979.

179. Nilsson IM: Local fibrinolysis as a mechanism for haemorrhage. Thromb Diath Haemorrh 34:623–633, 1975.

180. Gardner FH, Helmer RE: Aminocaproic acid: Use in control of hemorrhage in patients with amegakaryocytic thrombocytopenia. JAMA 243:35–37, 1980.

181. Bartholomew JR, Salgia R, Bell WR: Control of bleeding in patients with immune and nonimmune thrombocytopenia with aminocaproic acid. Arch Intern Med 149:1959–1961, 1989.

182. Shpilberg O, Blumenthal R, Sofer O, et al: A controlled trial of tranexamic acid therapy for the reduction of bleeding during treatment of acute myeloid leukemia. Leuk Lymphoma 19:141–144, 1995.

183. Fricke W, Alling D, Kimball J, et al: Lack of efficacy of tranexamic acid in thrombocytopenic bleeding. Transfusion 31:345–348, 1991.

184. Williams EC: Plasma alpha 2-antiplasmin activity: Role in the evaluation and management of fibrinolytic states and other bleeding disorders. Arch Intern Med 149:1769–1772, 1989.

185. Butterworth J, James RL, Lin Y, et al: Pharmacokinetics of epsilon-aminocaproic acid in patients undergoing aortocoronary bypass surgery. Anesthesiology 90:1624–1635, 1999.

186. Horrow JC, Van Riper DF, Strong MD, et al: The dose-response relationship of tranexamic acid. Anesthesiology 82:383–392, 1995.

187. Karski JM, Dowd NP, Joiner R, et al: The effect of three different doses of tranexamic acid on blood loss after cardiac surgery with mild systemic hypothermia (32 degrees C). J Cardiothorac Vasc Anesth 12:642–646, 1998.

188. Leipzig TJ, Redelman K, Horner TG: Reducing the risk of rebleeding before early aneurysm surgery: A possible role for antifibrinolytic therapy. J Neurosurg 86:220–225, 1997.

189. Chakrabarti S, Varma S, Singh S, Kumari S: Low dose bolus aminocaproic acid: An alternative to platelet transfusion in thrombocytopenia? [Letter] Eur J Haematol 60:313–314, 1998.

190. Ong YL, Hull DR, Mayne EE: Menorrhagia in von Willebrand disease successfully treated with single daily dose tranexamic acid. Haemophilia 4:63–65, 1998.

191. Tauber PF, Wolf AS, Herting W, Zaneveld LJ: Hemorrhage induced by intrauterine devices: Control by local proteinase inhibition. Fertil Steril 28:1375–1377, 1977.

192. Singh I, Laungani GB: Intravesical epsilon aminocaproic acid in management of intractable bladder hemorrhage. Urology 40:227–229, 1992.

193. Crouch ERJ, Williams PB, Gray MK, et al: Topical aminocaproic acid in the treatment of traumatic hyphema. Arch Ophthalmol 115:1106–1112, 1997.

194. Kalmadi S, Tiu R, Lowe C, et al: Epsilon aminocaproic acid reduces transfusion requirements in patients with thrombocytopenic hemorrhage. Cancer 107:136–140, 2006.

195. Bell WR: Platelets and coagulation factors. In Spivak J, Bell WR (eds): Yearbook of Hematology, Baltimore, Mosby, 1991, pp 245–246.

196. Mangano DT, Tudor IC, Dietzel C: The risk associated with aprotinin in cardiac surgery. N Engl J Med 354:353–365, 2006.

197. Wei M, Jian K, Guo Z, et al: Tranexamic acid reduces postoperative bleeding in off-pump coronary artery bypass grafting. Scand Cardiovasc J 40:105–109, 2006.

198. Hiippala ST, Strid LJ, Wennerstrand MI, et al: Tranexamic acid radically decreases blood loss and transfusions associated with total knee arthroplasty. Anesth Analg 84:839–844, 1997.

199. Orpen NM, Little C, Walker G, Crawfurd EJ: Tranexamic acid reduces early post-operative blood loss after total knee arthroplasty: A prospective randomised controlled trial of 29 patients. Knee 13:106–110, 2006.

200. Kaspar M, Ramsay MA, Nguyen AT, et al: Continuous small-dose tranexamic acid reduces fibrinolysis but not transfusion requirements during orthotopic liver transplantation. Anesth Analg 85:281–285, 1997.

201. Ickx BE, van der Linden PJ, Melot C, et al: Comparison of the effects of aprotinin and tranexamic acid on blood loss and red blood cell transfusion requirements during the late stages of liver transplantation. Transfusion 46:595–605, 2006.

202. Cid J, Lozano M: Tranexamic acid reduces allogeneic red cell transfusions in patients undergoing total knee arthroplasty: Results of a meta-analysis of randomized controlled trials. Transfusion 45:1302–1307, 2005.

203. Xia VW, Steadman RH: Antifibrinolytics in orthotopic liver transplantation: Current status and controversies. Liver Transpl 11:10–18, 2005.

204. Casati V, Guzzon D, Oppizzi M, et al: Hemostatic effects of aprotinin, tranexamic acid and epsilon-aminocaproic acid in primary cardiac surgery. Ann Thorac Surg 68:2252–2256, 1999.

205. Bennett-Guerrero E, Sorohan JG, Gurevich ML, et al: Cost-benefit and efficacy of aprotinin compared with epsilon-aminocaproic acid in patients having repeated cardiac operations: A randomized, blinded clinical trial. Anesthesiology 87:1373–1380, 1997.

206. Harmon DE: Cost/benefit analysis of pharmacologic hemostasis. Ann Thorac Surg 61 (2 suppl): S21–S25, 1996.

207. Munoz JJ, Birkmeyer NJ, Birkmeyer JD, et al: Is epsilon-aminocaproic acid as effective as aprotinin in reducing bleeding with cardiac surgery? A meta-analysis. Circulation 99:81–89, 1999.

208. Murkin JM: Con: Tranexamic acid is not better than aprotinin in decreasing bleeding after cardiac surgery. J Cardiothorac Vasc Anesth 8:474–476, 1994.

209. Guenther CR: Pro: Tranexamic acid is better than aprotinin in decreasing bleeding after cardiac surgery. J Cardiothorac Vasc Anesth 8:471–473, 1994.

210. Royston D: Aprotinin versus lysine analogues: The debate continues. Ann Thorac Surg 65 (4 suppl): S9–S19, 1998.

211. Karkouti K, Beattie WS, Dattilo KM, et al: A propensity score case-control comparison of aprotinin and tranexamic acid in high-transfusion-risk cardiac surgery. Transfusion 46:327–338, 2006.

212. Hunter D: First, gather the data. N Engl J Med 354:329–331, 2006.

213. Wu CC, Ho WM, Cheng SB, et al: Perioperative parenteral tranexamic acid in liver tumor resection: A prospective randomized trial toward a "blood transfusion"–free hepatectomy. Ann Surg 243:173–180, 2006.

214. Yaniv E, Shvero J, Hadar T: Hemostatic effect of tranexamic acid in elective nasal surgery. Am J Rhinol 20:227–229, 2006.

215. Henry DA, O'Connell DL: Effects of fibrinolytic inhibitors on mortality from upper gastrointestinal haemorrhage. BMJ 298:1142–1146, 1999.

216. Cooke I, Lethaby A, Farquhar C: Antifibrinolytics for heavy menstrual bleeding. Cochrane Database Syst Rev 2:CD000249, 2000.

217. Vermeulen M, Lindsay KW, Murray GD, et al: Antifibrinolytic treatment in subarachnoid hemorrhage. N Engl J Med 311:432–437, 1984.

218. Roos Y: Antifibrinolytic treatment in subarachnoid hemorrhage: A randomized placebo-controlled trial. STAR Study Group. Neurology 54:77–82, 2000.

219. Schisano G, Nina P: Antifibrinolytic therapy. [Letter] J Neurosurg 87:486–487, 1997.

220. Carley S, Sen A: Best evidence topic report: Antifibrinolytics for the initial management of subarachnoid haemorrhage. Emerg Med J 22:274–275, 2005.

221. Piriyawat P, Morgenstern LB, Yawn DH, et al: Treatment of acute intracerebral hemorrhage with epsilon-aminocaproic acid: A pilot study. Neurocrit Care 1:47–51, 2004.

222. Saba HI, Morelli GA, Logrono LA: Brief report: Treatment of bleeding in hereditary hemorrhagic telangiectasia with aminocaproic acid. N Engl J Med 330:1789–1790, 1994.

223. Poon MC, Kloiber R, Birdsell DC: Epsilon-aminocaproic acid in the reversal of consumptive coagulopathy with platelet sequestration in a

vascular malformation of Klippel-Trénaunay syndrome. Am J Med 87:211–213, 1989.

224. Ortel TL, Onorato JJ, Bedrosian CL, Kaufman RE: Antifibrinolytic therapy in the management of the Kasabach Merritt syndrome. Am J Hematol 29:44–48, 1988.

225. Cooper DL, Sandler AB, Wilson LD, Duffy TP: Disseminated intravascular coagulation and excessive fibrinolysis in a patient with metastatic prostate cancer: Response to epsilon-aminocaproic acid. Cancer 70:656–658, 1992.

226. De Bonis M, Cavaliere F, Alessandrini F, et al: Topical use of tranexamic acid in coronary artery bypass operations: A double-blind, prospective, randomized, placebo-controlled study. J Thorac Cardiovasc Surg 119:575–580, 2000.

227. Sindet-Pedersen S, Ramstrom G, Bernvil S, Blomback M: Hemostatic effect of tranexamic acid mouthwash in anticoagulant-treated patients undergoing oral surgery. N Engl J Med 320:840–843, 1989.

228. Walsh PN, Rizza CR, Matthews JM, et al: Epsilon-aminocaproic acid therapy for dental extractions in haemophilia and Christmas disease: A double blind controlled trial. Br J Haematol 20:463–475, 1971.

229. Wahl MJ: Dental surgery in anticoagulated patients. Arch Intern Med 158:1610–1616, 1998.

230. Blinder D, Manor Y, Martinowitz U, et al: Dental extractions in patients maintained on continued oral anticoagulant: Comparison of local hemostatic modalities. Oral Surg Oral Med Oral Pathol Oral Radiol Endod 88:137–140, 1999.

231. Tibbelin A, Aust R, Bende M, et al: Effect of local tranexamic acid gel in the treatment of epistaxis. ORL J Otorhinolaryngol Relat Spec 57:207–209, 1995.

232. Kitamura H, Matsui I, Itoh N, et al: Tranexamic acid–induced visual impairment in a hemodialysis patient. Clin Exp Nephrol 7:311–314, 2003.

233. Manjunath G, Fozailoff A, Mitcheson D, Sarnak MJ: Epsilon-aminocaproic acid and renal complications: Case report and review of the literature. Clin Nephrol 58:63–67, 2002.

234. Stefanini M, English HA, Taylor AE: Safe and effective, prolonged administration of epsilon aminocaproic acid in bleeding from the urinary tract. J Urol 143:559–561, 1990.

235. Schultz M, van der Lelie H: Microscopic haematuria as a relative contraindication for tranexamic acid. Br J Haematol 89:663–664, 1995.

236. Lakhani A, Raptis A, Frame D, et al: Intravesicular instillation of ε-aminocaproic acid for patients with adenovirus-induced hemorrhagic cystitis. Bone Marrow Transplant 24:1259–1260, 1999.

237. Johnson AL, Skoza L, Claus E: Observations on epsilon aminocaproic acid. Thromb Diath Haemorrh 7:203, 1962.

238. Lindoff C, Rybo G, Astedt B: Treatment with tranexamic acid during pregnancy, and the risk of thrombo-embolic complications. Thromb Haemost 70:238–240, 1993.

239. Longstaff C: Studies on the mechanisms of action of aprotinin and tranexamic acid as plasmin inhibitors and antifibrinolytic agents. Blood Coagul Fibrinolysis 5:537–542, 1994.

240. Royston D, Bidstrup BP, Taylor KM, Sapsford RN: Effect of aprotinin on need for blood transfusion after repeat open-heart surgery. Lancet 2:1289–1291, 1987.

241. van Oeveren W, Jansen NJ, Bidstrup BP, et al: Effects of aprotinin on hemostatic mechanisms during cardiopulmonary bypass. Ann Thorac Surg 44:640–645, 1987.

242. Porte RJ, Molenaar IQ, Begliomini B, et al: Aprotinin and transfusion requirements in orthotopic liver transplantation: A multicentre randomised double-blind study. EMSALT Study Group. Lancet 355:1303–1309, 2000.

243. Diefenbach C, Abel M, Limpers B, et al: Fatal anaphylactic shock after aprotinin reexposure in cardiac surgery. Anesth Analg 80:830–831, 1995.

244. Shampo MA, Kyle RA: Henrik Dam: Discoverer of vitamin K. Mayo Clin Proc 73:46, 1998.

245. Dam H, Glavind J: Vitamin K in human pathology. Lancet 1:720–721, 1938.

246. Alperin JB: Coagulopathy caused by vitamin K deficiency in critically ill, hospitalized patients. JAMA 258:1916–1919, 1987.

247. Chakraverty R, Davidson S, Peggs K, et al: The incidence and cause of coagulopathies in an intensive care population. Br J Haematol 93:460–463, 1996.

248. Spector I, Corn M: Laboratory tests of hemostasis: The relationship to hemorrhage in liver disease. Arch Intern Med 119:577–582, 1967.

249. Shearer MJ: Vitamin K metabolism and nutriture. Blood Rev 6:92–104, 1992.

250. Vermeer C, Schurgers LJ: A comprehensive review of vitamin K and vitamin K antagonists. Hematol Oncol Clin North Am 14:339–353, 2000.

251. Furie B, Bouchard BA, Furie BC: Vitamin K–dependent biosynthesis of gamma-carboxyglutamic acid. Blood 93:1798–1808, 1999.

252. Blanchard RA, Furie BC, Jorgensen M, et al: Acquired vitamin K–dependent carboxylation deficiency in liver disease. N Engl J Med 305:242–248, 1981.

253. Van der Meer J, Hemker HC, Loeliger EA: Pharmacological aspects of vitamin K$_1$: A clinical and experimental study in man. Thromb Diath Haemorrh Suppl 29:1–96, 1968.

254. Hirsh J, Dalen JE, Deykin D, et al: Oral anticoagulants: Mechanism of action, clinical effectiveness, and optimal therapeutic range. Chest 108 (4 suppl): 231S–246S, 1995.

255. Nee R, Doppenschmidt D, Donovan DJ, Andrews TC: Intravenous versus subcutaneous vitamin K$_1$ in reversing excessive oral anticoagulation. Am J Cardiol 83:286–287, 1999.

256. Raj G, Kumar R, McKinney WP: Time course of reversal of anticoagulant effect of warfarin by intravenous and subcutaneous phytonadione. Arch Intern Med 159:2721–2724, 1999.

257. Soedirman JR, De Bruijn EA, Maes RA, et al: Pharmacokinetics and tolerance of intravenous and intramuscular phylloquinone (vitamin K$_1$) mixed micelles formulation. Br J Clin Pharmacol 41:517–523, 1996.

258. Taylor CT, Chester EA, Byrd DC, Stephens MA: Vitamin K to reverse excessive anticoagulation: A review of the literature. Pharmacotherapy 19:1415–1425, 1999.

259. Third ACCP Consensus Conference on Antithrombotic Therapy. Chest 102 (suppl): 303S–549S, 1992.

260. Guyatt GH, Cook DJ, Sackett DL, et al: Grades of recommendation for antithrombotic agents. Chest 114 (5 suppl): 441S–444S, 1998.

261. Ansell J, Hirsh J, Poller L, et al: The pharmacology and management of the vitamin K antagonists: The Seventh ACCP Conference on Antithrombotic and Thrombolytic Therapy 1. Chest 126 (3 suppl): 204S–233S, 2004.

262. Hirsh J: Reversal of the anticoagulant effects of warfarin by vitamin K1. [Editorial] Chest 114:1505–1508, 1998.

263. Cosgriff SW: The effectiveness of an oral vitamin K$_1$ in controlling excessive hypoprothrombinemia during anticoagulant therapy. Ann Intern Med 45:14–22, 1956.

264. White RH, McKittrick T, Hutchinson R, Twitchell J: Temporary discontinuation of warfarin therapy: Changes in the international normalized ratio. Ann Intern Med 122:40–42, 1995.

265. Wentzien TH, O'Reilly RA, Kearns PJ: Prospective evaluation of anticoagulant reversal with oral vitamin K$_1$ while continuing warfarin therapy unchanged. Chest 114:1546–1550, 1998.

266. Palareti G, Legnani C: Warfarin withdrawal: Pharmacokinetic-pharmacodynamic considerations. Clin Pharmacokinet 30:300–313, 1996.

267. Lousberg TR, Witt DM, Beall DG, et al: Evaluation of excessive anticoagulation in a group model health maintenance organization. Arch Intern Med 158:528–534, 1998.

268. Perry DJ, Kimball DBJ: Low dose vitamin K for excessively anticoagulated prosthetic valve patients. Mil Med 147:836–837, 1982.

269. Shetty HG, Backhouse G, Bentley DP, Routledge PA: Effective reversal of warfarin-induced excessive anticoagulation with low dose vitamin K1. Thromb Haemost 67:13–15, 1992.

270. Brophy MT, Fiore LD, Deykin D: Low-dose vitamin K therapy in excessively anticoagulated patients: A dose-finding study. J Thromb Thrombolysis 4:289–292, 1997.

271. Andersen P, Godal HC: Predictable reduction in anticoagulant activity of warfarin by small amounts of vitamin K. Acta Med Scand 198:269–270, 1975.

272. Hambleton J, Wages D, Radu-Radulescu L, et al: Pharmacokinetic study of FFP photochemically treated with amotosalen (S-59) and UV light compared to FFP in healthy volunteers anticoagulated with warfarin. Transfusion 42:1302–1307, 2002.

273. Fredriksson K, Norrving B, Stromblad LG: Emergency reversal of anticoagulation after intracerebral hemorrhage. Stroke 23:972–977, 1992.

274. Kitchens CS: Efficacy of intravenous vitamin K in a case of massive warfarin overdosage. Thromb Haemost 86:719–720, 2001.

275. Andrews M, Schmidt B: Hemorrhagic and thrombotic complications in children. In Colman RW, Hirsh J, Marder VJ Salzman EW (eds): Hemostasis and Thrombosis: Basic Principles and Clinical Practice, Philadelphia, Lippincott, 1994, pp 989–1063.

276. Furukawa M, Nakanishi T, Okuda H, et al: Changes of plasma des-gamma-carboxy prothrombin levels in patients with hepatocellular carcinoma in response to vitamin K. Cancer 69:31–38, 1992.

277. Ansell JE, Kumar R, Deykin D: The spectrum of vitamin K deficiency. JAMA 238:40–42, 1977.

278. Weitzel JN, Sadowski JA, Furie BC, et al: Surreptitious ingestion of a long-acting vitamin K antagonist/rodenticide, brodifacoum: Clinical and metabolic studies of three cases. Blood 76:2555–2559, 1990.

279. Lipsky JJ: Antibiotic-associated hypoprothrombinaemia. J Antimicrob Chemother 21:281–300, 1988.

280. Breen GA, St. Peter WL: Hypoprothrombinemia associated with cefmetazole. Ann Pharmacother 31:180–184, 1997.

281. Rich EC, Drage CW: Severe complications of intravenous phytonadione therapy: Two cases, with one fatality. Postgrad Med 72:303–306, 1982.

282. Fiore LD, Scola MA, Cantillon CE, Brophy MT: Anaphylactoid reactions to vitamin K. J Thromb Thrombolysis 11:175–183, 2001.

283. Elenbaas JK: Phytonadione-induced cardiovascular collapse. Drug Consults 1988.

284. Havel M, Muller M, Graninger W, et al: Tolerability of a new vitamin K1 preparation for parenteral administration to adults: One case of anaphylactoid reaction. Clin Ther 9:373–379, 1987.

285. Labatut A, Sorbette F, Virenque C: [Shock states during injection of vitamin K (Letter)]. Therapie 43:58, 1988.

286. Barash P, Kitahata LM, Mandel S: Acute cardiovascular collapse after intravenous phytonadione. Anesth Analg 55:304–306, 1976.

287. Whitling AM, Bussey HI, Lyons RM: Comparing different routes and doses of phytonadione for reversing excessive anticoagulation. Arch Intern Med 158:2136–2140, 1998.

288. Lefrere JJ, Girot R: Acute cardiovascular collapse during intravenous vitamin K1 injection. [Letter] Thromb Haemost 58:790, 1987.

289. Verstraete M, Vermylen J, Tyberghein J: Double blind evaluation of the haemostatic effect of adrenochrome monosemicarbazone, conjugated oestrogens and epsilonaminocaproic acid after adenotonsillectomy. Acta Haematol 40:154–161, 1968.

290. Alperin JB: Estrogens and surgery in women with von Willebrand's disease. Am J Med 73:367–371, 1982.

291. Weinstein P: Treatment of ophthalmic hemorrhage by premarin. Int Z Klin Pharmakol Ther Toxikol 2:72–73, 1969.

292. Livio M, Mannucci PM, Vigano G, et al: Conjugated estrogens for the management of bleeding associated with renal failure. N Engl J Med 315:731–735, 1986.

293. Ambrus JL, Schimert G, Lajos TZ, et al: Effect of antifibrinolytic agents and estrogens on blood loss and blood coagulation factors during open heart surgery. J Med 2:65–81, 1971.

294. Pluss J: Hemostasis by premedication with estrogen in hair-transplant surgery. J Dermatol Surg Oncol 3:320–321, 1977.

295. van Cutsem E, Rutgeerts P, Vantrappen G: Treatment of bleeding gastrointestinal vascular malformations with oestrogen-progesterone. Lancet 335:953–955, 1990.

296. Frenette L, Cox J, Arnall M, et al: Effectiveness of conjugated estrogen in orthotopic liver transplantation. South Med J 91:365–368, 1998.

297. Vigano G, Gaspari F, Locatelli M, et al: Dose-effect and pharmacokinetics of estrogens given to correct bleeding time in uremia. Kidney Int 34:853–858, 1988.

298. Jacobs P, Jacobson J, Kahn D: Perioperative administration of a single dose of conjugated oestrogen to uraemic patients is ineffective in improving haemostasis. Am J Hematol 46:24–28, 1994.

299. Shemin D, Elnour M, Amarantes B, et al: Oral estrogens decrease bleeding time and improve clinical bleeding in patients with renal failure. Am J Med 89:436–440, 1990.

300. Sloand JA, Schiff MJ: Beneficial effect of low-dose transdermal estrogen on bleeding time and clinical bleeding in uremia. Am J Kidney Dis 26:22–26, 1995.

301. Harrison RL, McKee PA: Estrogen stimulates von Willebrand factor production by cultured endothelial cells. Blood 63:657–664, 1984.

302. Kroon UB, Tengborn L, Rita H, Backstrom AC: The effects of transdermal oestradiol and oral progestogens on haemostasis variables. Br J Obstet Gynaecol 104 (suppl 16): 32–37, 1997.

303. Carr JA, Silverman N: The heparin–protamine interaction: A review. J Cardiovasc Surg (Torino) 40:659–666, 1999.

304. Byun Y, Singh VK, Yang VC: Low molecular weight protamine: A potential nontoxic heparin antagonist. Thromb Res 94:53–61, 1999.

305. Dietrich CP, Shinjo SK, Moraes FA, et al: Structural features and bleeding activity of commercial low molecular weight heparins: Neutralization by ATP and protamine. Semin Thromb Hemost 25 (suppl 3): 43–50, 1999.

306. Ratnoff OD: Some therapeutic agents influencing hemostasis. In Colman RW, Hirsh J, Marder VJ Salzman EW (eds): Hemostasis and Thrombosis: Basic Principles and Clinical Practice, Philadelphia, Lippincott, 1994, pp 1104–1133.

307. Despotis GJ, Gravlee G, Filos K, Levy J: Anticoagulation monitoring during cardiac surgery: A review of current and emerging techniques. Anesthesiology 91:1122–1151, 1999.

308. Martinowitz U, Zaarur M, Yaron BL, et al: Treating traumatic bleeding in a combat setting: Possible role of recombinant activated factor VII. Mil Med 169 (12 suppl): 16–18, 2004.

309. Carson JL, Noveck H, Berlin JA, Gould SA: Mortality and morbidity in patients with very low postoperative Hb levels who decline blood transfusion. Transfusion 42:812–818, 2002.

310. Ford PA, Borghaei H, Henry DH: Treatment of patients who refuse blood components. In Alving BM (ed): Blood Components and Pharmacologic Agents in the Treatment of Congenital and Acquired Bleeding Disorders. Bethesda, Md, AABB Press, 2000, pp 61–81.

311. Mann MC, Votto J, Kambe J, McNamee MJ: Management of the severely anemic patient who refuses transfusion: Lessons learned during the care of a Jehovah's Witness. Ann Intern Med 117:1042–1048, 1992.

312. Jabbour N, Gagandeep S, Mateo R, et al: Transfusion free surgery: Single institution experience of 27 consecutive liver transplants in Jehovah's Witnesses. J Am Coll Surg 201:412–417, 2005.

313. Klein HG: Transfusion medicine: The evolution of a new discipline. JAMA 258:2108–2109, 1987.

Chapter 28

Thrombolytic Therapy

Victor J. Marder, MD

INTRODUCTION

Thrombolytic therapy represents an acute phase of a prolonged antithrombotic management plan; decisions regarding the risk:benefit ratio are related to this usually brief but aggressive approach to vascular occlusion.[1–4] This review describes the properties of thrombolytic agents, the physiopathology of thrombolysis and bleeding complications, and the effects of treatment on blood coagulation and fibrinolytic parameters.

PLASMINOGEN ACTIVATORS

All of the currently approved thrombolytic agents are plasminogen activators (PAs) that induce plasmin action on fibrin contained within a thrombus, yielding an associated greater or lesser degree of plasma fibrinogenolysis (lytic state). Degradation of fibrin has the beneficial effect of reducing thrombus size (thrombolysis), but at the same time, PAs may cause bleeding through lysis of hemostatic plugs[2,3] or through vascular matrix degradation (Table 28-1). Rethrombosis may follow initial reperfusion, generally as the result of a persistent vascular lesion and plasma hypercoagulability. Relationships of these biologic actions of thrombolysis, loss of vascular integrity, rethrombosis, and the plasma lytic state control the effectiveness and safety of thrombolytic treatment. Six PAs have been approved by the U.S. Food and Drug Administration (FDA)[5] for use in major thrombotic disease: streptokinase (SK), urokinase (UK), alteplase (man-made form of tissue plasminogen activator [tPA]), anistreplase (anisoylated plasminogen streptokinase [APSAC]), reteplase, and tenecteplase (TNK-tPA) (UK is no longer available in the United States, and anistreplase is rarely used). Recombinant forms of UK, saruplase (pro-UK, scu-PA), staphylokinase, and bat-PA (PA from the salivary gland of *Desmodus rotundus*), chimerics of tPA and pro-UK, bifunctional agents composed of antifibrin or antiplatelet antibodies complexed to PA, and a recombinant plasminogen that is activated by thrombin are at various stages of testing.[5]

Primary differences among PAs relate to their antigenicity, half-life, potential for inducing a lytic state, and hemorrhagic potential (Table 28-2). Those PAs that are derived from a human protein (UK, alteplase, reteplase, saruplase, tenecteplase, lanoteplase) are minimally antigenic

or nonantigenic, whereas those produced by a bacterial species (SK, anistreplase, staphylokinase) present a potential for allergic response that may preclude prolonged or follow-up administration. The half-life of each PA determines whether it can be administered as a bolus injection, short infusion, or continuous infusion. The most suitable agents for bolus injections are anistreplase (half-life, approximately 40 minutes),[6] reteplase,[7] and tenecteplase[8]; the least suitable is alteplase (half-life, 5 minutes),[9] which is best administered by continuous infusion. Clinical results suggest that some of the newer agents (e.g., tenecteplase) produce less of a plasma lytic state,[10] but to date, all PAs are associated with a significant bleeding risk. The rate of bleeding is roughly equivalent for all agents, except for the higher rate of intracranial hemorrhage (ICH) seen with tPA[4,5] or tPA mutant derivatives,[7] relative to results when SK is used. Anticipation of greater safety with a new PA on the basis of findings of biochemical studies must be considered cautiously; no agent has yet been shown to be free of hemorrhagic risk.[11]

DIRECT FIBRINOLYTIC AGENTS

An approach that was studied in the 1950s[12] has recently been reassessed as a potentially safe method of inducing therapeutic thrombolysis, namely, the use of direct thrombolytic enzymes, such as plasmin[13,14] or its recombinant

---

This chapter is adapted from Marder VJ: Foundations of thrombolytic therapy. In Colman RW, Marder VJ, Clowes AW, et al (eds): Hemostasis and Thrombosis: Basic Principles and Practice, 5th edition. Philadelphia, Lippincott Williams & Wilkins, 2006.

Table 28-1 Principal Biologic Effects of Thrombolysis Therapy

Clinical Result	Process	Cellular and Biochemical Events
Benefit	Thrombolysis	Degradation of fibrin and disruption of platelets in the thrombus
Adverse effect	Systemic lytic state	Plasma fibrinogenolysis and derangement of platelet function
Complications	Bleeding	Degradation of fibrin in hemostatic plugs and of matrix in abnormal vessels, plus blood hypocoagulability
	Rethrombosis	Persistent local vascular lesions plus permissive status of blood coagulation

Table 28-2 Comparison of Plasminogen Activators

Agent	Source	Antigenic	Half-life, min	Regimen	Lytic State	Bleeding
Streptokinase	*Streptococcus*	Yes	20	Infusion	4+	4+
Urokinase	Cell culture	No	15	Infusion	4+	4+
Alteplase	Recombinant	No	5	Infusion 2+	4+	4+
Anistreplase	*Streptococcus* + Plasma product	No	70	Bolus	4+	4+
Reteplase	Recombinant	No	15	Double bolus	3+	4+
Saruplase (scu-PA)	Recombinant	No	5	Infusion	1–3+	4+
Staphylokinase	Recombinant	Yes	6	Infusion	1+	4+
Tenecteplase	Recombinant	No	15	Bolus	1+	4+
Bat-PA	Recombinant	Minimal	17	Infusion	1+	Probable
Lanoteplase	Recombinant	No	30	Bolus	2+	4+

scu-PA, saruplase; bat-PA, plasminogen activator from the salivary gland of *Desmodus rotundus.*
1+, minimal; 2+, mild; 3+, moderate; 4+, marked.

derivatives,[15] and alfimeprase, a genetic modification of a snake venom extract (fibrolase).[16] The potential for safety is based on regional administration of the agent by catheter,[13] after which it is quickly neutralized by plasma inhibitors, thereby minimizing its generalized circulation and reducing bleeding at sites of vascular injury.[13,17,18] Animal studies supportive of this hypothesis show that more than fourfold the therapeutic dose of plasmin does not induce bleeding, whereas tPA causes bleeding at the therapeutic dose and at dosages as low as 25% of the optimal therapeutic amount.[19] Thrombolysis under conditions of limited plasminogen content (restricted blood flow) yields better results with plasmin than are attained with tPA[13]; only the latter requires a replenished supply of this plasminogen for continued thrombolytic action.[17] The safety and efficacy profile of this approach in animals suggests that clinical use of direct fibrinolytic agents will provide a treatment option that will be associated with a greatly reduced risk of bleeding.

ADJUNCTIVE ANTITHROMBOTIC AGENTS

Aspirin and Heparin

The first definitive demonstration of adjunctive antiplatelet efficacy involved the use of aspirin in addition to SK to reduce mortality after acute myocardial infarction (AMI).[20] In patients treated within 6 hours, aspirin reduced 35-day mortality by 23%, equal to the reduction achieved by SK alone; the two agents used together produced an additive effect that amounted to a 39% relative risk reduction. The GUSTO (Global Utilization of Streptokinase and Tissue Plasminogen Activator for Occluded Coronary Arteries) study[21] documented that early intravenous heparin is no more effective than delayed subcutaneous heparin in enhancing patient survival 30 days after AMI. Coronary artery patency studies show that intravenous heparin added to aspirin and SK increases bleeding without the benefit of improved vascular patency.[22] Although delayed subcutaneous heparin combined with aspirin is relatively safe, Collins and associates[23] concluded that "there is little evidence of any additional clinical advantage with subcutaneous or with intravenous heparin" added to PA therapy.

Although it is generally agreed that heparin does not contribute significantly to a regimen of SK plus aspirin in AMI,[23]

physicians in the United States continue to use intravenous heparin in concert with tPA and aspirin.[24] The recommendation of the Seventh American College of Chest Physicians (ACCP) Conference is to use weight-adjusted heparin in combination with tPA.[25] The ASSENT-3 PLUS (Assessment of the Safety and Efficacy of a New Thrombolytic 3 Plus) trial[26] showed advantages of low molecular weight heparin (LMWH) over unfractionated heparin (UFH) in the composite efficacy end point of mortality, reinfarction, and ischemia, but a higher rate of ICH was observed with LMWH. Subcutaneous heparin added to aspirin during PA infusion increases the risk slightly (0.6% vs 0.4%),[27] but the use of tPA is a most important predictor,[28] along with age greater than 65 years, weight less than 70 kg, hypertension on admission, and a prior history of transient ischemic attack or cerebrovascular accident (CVA). A retrospective comparison of SK (41,000 patients), anistreplase (21,000 patients), and tPA (41,000 patients) showed incidences of ICH of 0.2%, 0.6%, and 0.6%, respectively.[11] Recent observations of accelerated regimen tPA versus SK, reteplase, or double-bolus tPA showed an overall risk of approximately 0.8% for accelerated tPA, with a significantly higher risk (2.1%) noted in elderly patients (>75 years of age).[22,29,30]

Direct Thrombin Inhibitors and Platelet Glycoprotein-IIb-IIIa Antagonists

Pilot studies in patients with AMI showed encouraging increases in 90-minute patency rates with hirudin rather than heparin,[31] but the relatively high dosages of this anticoagulant therapy resulted in unacceptable rates of ICH.[32] With a scaled-back dosage regimen of anticoagulant in patients receiving tPA or SK along with aspirin, a large patient trial of 3002 patients (Thrombolysis and Thrombin Inhibition in Myocardial Infarction [TIMI-9B]) showed no significant difference in clinical outcome with the use of heparin or hirudin.[33] Bivalirudin (Hirulog) use showed higher reperfusion rates than were seen with heparin when used with SK for AMI,[34] but a study of 17,000 patients with AMI treated with bivalirudin plus SK showed no improvement in survival over SK plus heparin.[35] Other antithrombin strategies, such as dalteparin with SK, efegatran with SK, and argatroban with tPA, have been tested for effect on coronary artery patency, but no convincing data have suggested improved efficacy.[5]

Effective glycoprotein (GP)-IIb/IIIa inhibition can be achieved by the monoclonal antibody 7E3 (abciximab; Centocor, Inc., Malvern, Pa) and by small-molecule inhibitors that block fibrinogen binding to platelets and prevent the cascade of biochemical events leading to aggregation. A phase 2 trial that compared reteplase with low-dose reteplase plus abciximab showed enhanced TIMI 3 flow with the combination regimen, but major bleeding was increased.[36] The GUSTO-V trial showed no difference in mortality between low-dose reteplase plus abciximab versus standard reteplase, but a higher rate of ICH was noted in the combination therapy group in patients older than 75 years.[37] The ACCP guidelines recommend against reduced dosage regimens of tenecteplase or reteplase with abciximab, in comparison with standard dosages of these thrombolytic agents.[25]

Ultrasound

The mechanism whereby ultrasound may produce its accentuation of PA-mediated lysis is not known, but thrombolysis may be achieved locally at the same time that systemic hemorrhage is avoided. Percutaneous, transvascular ultrasonic disruption of a femoral artery thrombus[38] and ultrasound as adjunct to tPA administration have been assessed in patients with acute ischemic stroke, with short-term patency advantage, albeit with uncertain long-term clinical benefit.[39]

Catheter-Directed (Regional) Infusion

The rationale for regional therapy is compelling for peripheral arterial occlusions (PAOs) because the thrombus is usually localized to a single vessel downstream from the catheter tip. Regional treatment of arterial thrombi achieves better thrombolysis than systemic therapy, but the PA is not strictly localized. During the infusion, the lytic state may be comparable with that following systemic administration, and bleeding or ICH may complicate therapy.[40] Local therapy for venous thromboembolic disease has a less compelling rationale, but this approach achieves an impressive degree of vascular reperfusion[41]; again, bleeding complications, including ICH, are not avoided.[42] For the treatment of thrombotic stroke, most studies have used systemic treatment to save time, but a local approach has also been effective.[43] Widespread application of mechanical revascularization therapy may render obsolete the question of local coronary artery delivery of thrombolytic agents.[44] Regional treatment for slower-progressing illnesses that offer the luxury of time required for this approach is most applicable for dissolving thrombi in occluded catheters.

PLASMA PROTEOLYTIC ("LYTIC") STATE

The "lytic state" describes the effect of plasmin in the circulation,[45] the most physiologic definition of which is a true decrease in plasma fibrinogen (Table 28-3) rather than a laboratory artefact, caused, for example, by heparin. Free plasmin also decreases platelet aggregation[46] after an initial phase of hyperaggregability.[47] Thus, a patient may experience sequential hypercoagulability, hypocoagulability,

Table 28-3 Development of the Plasma Proteolytic (Lytic) State

Biochemical State	Laboratory Parameter
Circulating plasminogen activator	Short euglobulin lysis time
Plasminogen converted to plasmin	Decreased plasminogen
Antiplasmin neutralizing plasmin	Low antiplasmin, plasmin/antiplasmin complexes
Free plasmin	Decreased fibrinogen, increased degradation products (including D-dimer)
Action on platelets	Hyperfunction and/or hypofunction
Hypocoagulable state	Prolonged global coagulation tests (PTT) and bleeding time

PTT, partial thromboplastin time.

or even the simultaneous occurrence of both, depending on the phase of lytic state that exists.

According to the concept that the actions of PAs in the blood and on the thrombus are separate events,[3] thrombolysis or bleeding would not necessarily correlate with the degree of lytic state. However, a recurring assumption holds that a PA with fibrinogen-sparing properties would cause less bleeding because the induced lytic state is minimized. For example, UK or SK treatment of pulmonary embolus (PE) or DVT regularly induces the lytic state, but changes in fibrinogen concentration, plasminogen, or euglobulin lysis time are not significantly different in patients with or without a hemorrhagic complication.[48,49] Further, SK-treated patients in the TIMI trial, phase 1, showed significantly lower fibrinogen values than did those treated with tPA, but the incidence of bleeding complications was the same with both treatments.[50] Also, patients treated with tPA who suffered ischemic (thrombotic) or hemorrhagic CVA had the same nadir concentration of fibrinogen.[51] The template bleeding time is prolonged during thrombolytic therapy, but no distinction is made between patients with and without hemorrhagic complications.[52] The only predictive blood value for hemorrhagic complications during tPA treatment is plasma tPA concentration (3.4 µg per milliliter in bleeders vs 2.2 µg per milliliter; $P = .002$).[53] The higher value noted in those who bled suggests that tPA has a direct effect on susceptible hemostatic plugs or vascular sites, to a greater extent with higher concentrations, independent of changes in fibrinogen concentration. This effect helps to explain the higher rate of ICH that occurs with high therapeutic dosages of tPA[54] and supports the concept that bleeding occurs independent of PA effect on blood coagulation; it probably is the result of action at sites of vascular injury or malformation.[4] A retrospective analysis of more than 40,000 patients in the GUSTO-I study found that independent predictors of hemorrhage consisted of older age, lighter body weight, female sex, and African ancestry, rather than any known degree of laboratory derangement.[55]

Laboratory results also do not predict vascular reperfusion or degree of patency. When a large systemic dose of

UK was used to treat acute PE, no correlation was noted between laboratory results and decreased embolus size[48]; DVT trials also showed no correlation of fibrinogen concentration with venographic change.[49] Even intracoronary SK for AMI showed no difference in nadir plasma fibrinogen in patients who did or did not reperfuse,[56] and similar measurements in patients with AMI receiving tPA also failed to show a correlation with posttreatment coronary artery patency.[53] Although universal agreement has not been reached, the data do suggest that changes in blood coagulation or fibrinolytic assays after PA administration do not directly reflect degree of thrombolysis. A reasonable approach to noninvasive measurement of successful thrombolysis would be to measure plasma levels of crosslinked fibrin degradation products (FDPs), but the data thus far are not conclusive; some show high predictability for successful vascular reperfusion,[57] and others fail to document such a correlation.[58]

Laboratory Monitoring

Different from treatment regimens with thrombin inhibitory agents such as heparin, PA dosage regimens are standardized, so dosage regulation on the basis of laboratory findings is unwarranted. Once a lytic state has been attained, the dose of PA does not have to be regulated because alterations based on laboratory markers would neither improve the chance of thrombolysis nor decrease the risk of hemorrhagic complications. An exception to this rule involves the use of direct thrombolytic agents, for which a direct relationship of dose to plasma fibrinogen has been identified[19]; only when fibrinogen is totally depleted would hemostatic safety possibly be compromised.

COMPLICATIONS

Bleeding

Absolute contraindications to PA therapy are those that may result in ICH or massive, life-threatening hemorrhage; in decisions regarding PA use, this risk must be weighed against the potential benefits of accelerated thrombolysis (Table 28-4). Thus, some patients with life-threatening thrombotic disease, for example, massive PE with profound shock or a large anterior wall AMI, may require potentially life-saving thrombolytic therapy even in the face of "absolute" contraindications. Patients with relatively less threatening thrombotic disease such as limited DVT would reasonably not receive PA therapy if the history includes a transient ischemic attack, prior thrombotic stroke, or untreated hypertension; those with an increased risk of symptomatic but not serious bleeding, for example, with arteriotomy or venotomy, active menses, or minor surgical or biopsy procedures, might be administered a PA. The elderly patient with AMI has a greater risk of bleeding, especially from ICH, but also a higher risk of death from AMI than does the younger patient. Therefore, the survival benefit in patients older than age 70 is relatively greater than in those younger than 60 years (80 vs. 25 lives saved per 1000 treated).[20,59]

In patients with life-threatening bleeding or sudden emergencies that require surgical intervention, normal hemostasis can quickly be reestablished by the clinician who discontinues PA infusion, replenishes plasma fibrinogen with whole plasma or cryoprecipitate, and provides fresh platelets to correct dysfunctional platelets (Table 28-5). If the PA has not yet been cleared from the circulation, fibrinolytic activity can be neutralized with a fibrinolytic inhibitor such as ε-aminocaproic acid or aprotinin. Coronary artery bypass graft surgery may be performed after PAs are used (both SK and TPA), but such therapy carries a risk of bleeding, albeit with a greater need for blood transfusion if performed at 12 hours rather than at 18 to 48 hours.[60,61] This procedure may be used to replace a deficient or defective pool of plasma fibrinogen. One possible reason for bleeding as late as 24 hours after PA infusion is that is the time required for fibrinogen to be synthesized sufficient for surgery. It is reasonable to replenish fibrinogen with cryoprecipitate because essentially no normal fibrinogen is present during SK[62] or tPA infusion[63]; also, platelet function may be restored with fresh platelet transfusions given for up to 24 hours after PA administration. In addition, antifibrinolytic therapy should be administered prophylactically if PA continues to circulate—an expected situation for varying lengths of time after the infusion has been stopped.[64]

Unhealed vascular trauma sites are susceptible for about 10 days after trauma to fibrinolytic bleeding caused by PA exposure. Once the clinician plans to treat a patient with a PA, unnecessary trauma should be avoided. For example, medications should be administered by mouth or intravenously, rather than intramuscularly, phlebotomy sites should be compressed for 5 or 10 minutes, and unnecessary arteriotomy should be postponed or avoided. Bleeding that occurs during PA infusion should be managed with blood replacement and, if necessary, with discontinuation of the infusion. Depending on the half-life of the activator, a fibrinolytic inhibitor may or may not be required, but fresh fibrinogen replacement and platelet transfusion are usually required to ensure hemostasis, whether one has administered a long- or a short-acting agent and independent of whether the patient is in a potent or mild plasma lytic state.

Allergy and Embolism

Treatment may be terminated in the face of allergic or pyrogenic adverse effects, which may also require administration of corticosteroids, antihistamines, or adrenergic agents for anaphylaxis, and antipyretics for fever. Allergic reactions are three to five times more frequent with

Table 28-4	**Absolute Contraindications to Fibrinolytic Therapy**
Risk	**Condition**
Intracranial bleeding	Hemorrhagic cerebrovascular accident, known intracranial neoplasm, recent cranial surgery or trauma (within 10 days), uncontrolled severe hypertension
Massive hemorrhage	Major surgery of thorax or abdomen (within 10 days), prolonged cardiopulmonary resuscitation, current severe bleeding site (e.g., gastrointestinal tract)

Table 28-5   Resolution of Hypocoagulable State Induced by Plasminogen Activators

	During Treatment	Immediately After Treatment	6 to 36 Hours After Treatment
Plasma fibrinogen	Low	Nadir	Progressive recovery
Need for cryoprecipitate	Yes	Yes	Yes
Bleeding time	Long	Variable	Normal*
Need for platelets	Yes	Yes	No
Circulating activator	Present	Variable	Absent
Need for antifibrinolytics	Yes	Yes	Yes

*Unless aspirin is also administered, in which case the potential for bleeding may persist.

bacterially derived products than with tPA-type derivatives, but even the latter may induce an allergic reaction such as bronchospasm or angioneurotic edema.[65,66] Hypotension occurs in about 12% of patients with AMI exposed to SK and 7% of those exposed to tPA, in comparison with only 1.5% of patients not exposed to a PA.[67] Embolic phenomena of clinical importance are distinctly unusual in patients with venous thromboembolic disease. In the Urokinase PE Trial (UPET),[48] recurrent PE occurred in 15% of patients receiving UK or heparin, but release of a venous thrombus to function as a fatal pulmonary embolus during PA treatment is distinctly unusual. Distal systemic embolization from a cardiac source during PA treatment is unusual, but up to 20% of patients with PAO suffer sudden distal embolism and new ischemia of the extremity.[68] In this circumstance, the best treatment is continued local instillation of PA, which usually is successful in dissolving the new embolus.

CLINICAL APPLICATIONS

Table 28-6 summarizes the FDA-approved agents included in the major categories of vascular thrombotic disease, namely MI, PAO, DVT, PE, acute ischemic stroke (CVA), and catheter occlusion. These approvals are based on pivotal clinical trials, but actual practice may reflect an evolution of dosage schedules or mode of administration. Table 28-7 summarizes the clinical benefits anticipated with the use of PA in patients with major vessel occlusion.

Deep Venous Thrombosis

The typical patient with DVT manifests a generally benign course. However, an occasional patient experiences marked proximal extension of the thrombus and massive pulmonary embolization despite anticoagulant treatment; in addition, postphlebitic syndrome may occur in 25% of

Table 28-6   Current Clinical Usages of Available Plasminogen Activators*

Agent	Clinical Indication	FDA-Approved Regimen	Common Use
Urokinase (Abbokinase)	PE	12-hr IV infusion	Agent intermittantly available.
	Acute MI	Intracoronary only	
	PAO, DVT	Not approved	Widespread usage by regional and catheter-directed route. Agent currently available.
	Thrombosed central line or shunt	5000 U in 1 mL	
Streptokinase (Streptase)	Acute MI	IV or IC	Used primarily by intravenous route.
	PE	IV over 12 hr	Effective when given for shorter courses, even 2 hr.
	DVT	IV for up to 36 hr	Shorter infusions (e.g., over 18 hr) safer.
	PAO	IV	IV route not as effective as regional route.
	Thrombosed arteriovenous cannulas	Local instillation	
Reteplase (Retavase)	Acute MI	Two bolus injections 30 min apart	Approved in 1999.
	PAO	Not approved	Used regionally "off-label".
Alteplase (Activase)	Acute MI	3 hr or 90 min	Accelerated dosage used most often.
	Acute ischemic stroke	90 mg over 1 hr	Limited usage, as must be applied within 3 hr of onset of symptoms.
	PE	100 mg/2 hr	Urokinase over 2 hr, equal efficacy.
Anistreplase (Eminase)	Acute MI	30 U over 2–5 min	Infrequently used.
Tenecteplase (TNKase)	Acute MI	Single bolus, weight adjusted	Approved in 2000.

DVT, deep vein thrombosis; FDA, U.S. Food and Drug Administration; IV, intravenous; IC, intracardiac; MI, myocardial infarction; PAO, peripheral arterial occlusion; PE, pulmonary embolism.
*Based on Physicians' Desk Reference. Montvale, NJ, Medical Economics Co., 2000.

Table 28-7 Natural History and Anticipated Clinical Benefit of Thrombolytic Treatment for Acute Thrombosis

Thrombotic Disorder	Natural History (with Antithrombotics)	Potential Benefit of Thrombolytics	Clinical Decisions
DVT	Slow resolution, subclinical PE frequent, postphlebitic syndrome in 25%–50% with proximal thrombi.	Treatment within 7 days, complete lysis in one half of cases; decreased incidence of postphlebitic syndrome.	Treat large proximal thrombi, especially with coexistent PE. Catheter delivery (urokinase, alteplase, reteplase) in wide usage but still under study.
PE	Slow (1 wk) reduction of pulmonary hypertension. Overall mortality 7%, up to 30% with massive PE and hypotension.	Earlier treatment (within 48 hr) induces rapid thrombolysis and accelerates reversal of pulmonary hypertension. Possible increased survival in patients with clinical shock.	Thrombolytics for massive PA with shock, coexistent cardiopulmonary disease, or submassive PE, if no contraindications.
PAO	Major surgical intervention in 95%, cardiopulmonary complications in 50%, loss of limb in 20%, 1-yr mortality up to 40%.	Striking thrombolysis in 70%, surgery avoided in 35%, no change in limb salvage but potential for decrease in 1-yr mortality.	Catheter delivery of PA superior to systemic infusion. Thrombolytic treatment preferred over surgery for initial treatment for the ischemic but salvageable limb.
MI	Overall mortality 11.5% vs 8.0% for inferior MI, 17.0% for anterior MI.	Overall mortality reduced by 20%–50%, most striking in patients with anterior MI treated within 4 hr after symptom onset.	Indicated for most patients within 6 hr of symptoms; angioplasty offers advantages and is increasingly used.
CVA	Irreversible deficits and risk of death depending on location; hemorrhagic transformation relatively infrequent (3%).	Good results only if treatment initiated within 3 hr, reversal of neurologic deficit at a cost of increased parenchymal hematoma.	Clear-cut functional benefit without increased mortality risk if treatment before 3 hr, but with increased risk of hemorrhagic transformation.

CVA, cerebrovascular accident; DVT, deep vein thrombosis; MI, myocardial infarction; PA, plasminogen activator; PAO, peripheral arterial (or graft) occlusion; PE, pulmonary embolism.

patients[69] as a late, disabling sequela of proximal DVT. Both of these eventualities are rationales for thrombolytic treatment.[70] Venous thrombi are lysed more rapidly and effectively when a PA is used (concurrently with anticoagulation); complete lysis is achieved in 50% of patients versus 10% with heparin alone.[71] Effective thombolysis reduces the incidence of postphlebitic syndrome from about 40% to 10%,[72] presumably because of more rapid clot lysis, which preserves venous valve leaflet integrity. However, with systemic (intravenous) administration of a PA over an interval of 2 to 7 days, the period of continued risk of hemorrhage results in an incidence of ICH that approaches 1%.[73]

Over the past 10 years, a more aggressive approach to PA delivery has consisted of regional perfusion by catheter directly into the thrombus, often combined with stent placement. Impressive recanalization rates have been attained, with up to 90% complete and partial lysis, and in anecdotal cases, substantial benefit has been noted in patients with symptoms lasting longer than 4 weeks.[41,74–76] It is likely that the clinical impression that old thrombi are resistant to thrombolysis may in fact reflect a problem of inadequate intravenous delivery of PA to a fully occluded vessel—a situation that may be overcome by direct catheter delivery of PA to a thrombus that is still amenable to thrombolysis. Although outcomes when regional infusion is combined with stenting are impressive, no prospective comparison has been made with systemic treatment, and bleeding complications continue to occur in 11% of cases, and death due to PE or ICH is not eliminated.[77] Inferior vena caval (IVC) filters are reasonably used in the management of proximal DVT in those few patients with strong contraindications to thrombolytic therapy, and in those with serious, coexistent PE, but such devices preclude neither subsequent proximal thrombosis or recurrent PE nor subsequent chronic anticoagulant therapy[78] (see Chapter 31).

Pulmonary Embolism

The anticipated clinical course of patients with PE varies according to the size of the embolus and the existing cardiopulmonary reserve.[48,79,80] With routine heparin anticoagulation, the overall risk of mortality is 7% to 9%, and much higher mortality rates are seen in patients with massive PE and concomitant shock due to acute cor pulmonale. Thrombolytic therapy is beneficial in reversing cardiovascular compromise and preventing chronic pulmonary hypertension (see Chapter 45). Short-term improvement follows treatment with UK, SK, or tPA plus heparin compared with heparin alone, as reflected by rate of thrombolysis, pulmonary artery reperfusion, recovery of abnormal perfusion lung scans, decrease in pulmonary arterial pressure, and improved right ventricular function. These benefits are most pronounced in patients with acute symptoms of less than 48 hours duration.[48] In long-term follow-up studies (mean, 7.4 years), pulmonary vascular response to exercise suggests that thrombolytic therapy may prevent chronic sequelae such as pulmonary hypertension.[81]

In a comparison of 2 hours of tPA versus 12 hours of SK, thrombolysis was more rapid with tPA, but no difference was observed in pulmonary artery obstruction on follow-up at 1 day or 10 days.[82] Two-hour infusions of tPA or UK produced equal angiographic benefit,[83] and SK compared with tPA also produced equal benefit on pulmonary resistance.[84] Bolus reteplase demonstrated a decrease in pulmonary resistance that was comparable with that produced by 2 hours of tPA.[85] Thus, by extrapolation, a short course of any PA is expected to be effective for reducing pulmonary resistance in massive PE. Administration of PA directly into the pulmonary artery is not superior to treatment with systemic PA.[86]

Controlled trials of PA versus heparin in patients with massive, submassive, or small PE have not shown differences in mortality,[87] perhaps because of the small patient enrollment. Case series of tPA during cardiopulmonary resuscitation of patients after fulminant PE have demonstrated dramatic survival benefit,[88] and uncontrolled studies show that patients with massive PE and clinical shock have a better outcome with PA therapy than with thoracotomy and pulmonary embolectomy.[89] Given the risk of ICH, a limited time window for maximum therapeutic response, and unproved mortality benefit to date, patient selection for thrombolysis should be limited to the seriously ill patient who would benefit the most in the immediate short term and avoidance of those at highest risk for ICH.

Peripheral Arterial Occlusion

A combined radiologic and medical approach is superior to surgery as initial therapy for the acutely threatened but not irreversibly ischemic limb. However, protection from serious hemorrhage is no greater with regional delivery of PA, and generalized atherosclerosis, hypertension, and other manifestations of arterial disease make thrombolytic therapy more likely to cause bleeding complications than in patients with venous thromboembolic disease. Chronic arterial occlusions do not respond to systemic (intravenous) PA administration,[90] but acute occlusions are amenable if therapy is undertaken within hours of symptom onset, especially if occlusion is due to an embolus.[91] Occlusion of small distal arteries technically unapproachable by surgery also may be responsive to systemic PA infusion.

Dotter and colleagues[92] first reported success with an intra-arterial thrombolytic agent (SK) in 1974, and despite hypotheses to the contrary, this approach did not prevent a systemic lytic state or associated hemorrhage. Subsequent studies of regional administration validate that reperfusion can be attained in 50% to 80% of cases, although an underlying stenosis may require angioplasty or bypass surgery to prevent prompt reocclusion.[93,94]

A prospective randomized comparison of regional thrombolytic therapy versus surgical bypass grafting as initial management of patients with ischemic limbs caused by arterial occlusion was reported in 1994.[95] In this study of 114 patients, catheter-directed infusion of UK reperfused 70% of thrombosed grafts or vessels, one third of which required simple angioplasty or patch grafting for long-term patency. Although overall limb salvage and in-hospital mortality were the same for patients receiving intra-arterial UK and surgical repair, 1-year mortality was lower in the thrombolytic group (16% vs 42%) because of the lower incidence of cardiopulmonary complications.

This study design was duplicated with recombinant UK, which achieved patency in 70% of cases and reduced the need for major surgical procedures by 40% (313 vs 551)[96] but failed to demonstrate a survival benefit. Serious bleeding occurred in 13% of patients who were given

recombinant UK (vs 6% with surgery), and ICH occurred in 1.5% of patients, perhaps as a result of concomitant heparin use. In a similar trial of tPA and UK, no clinical advantage was noted for PA administration over surgery.[97]

Retrospective analyses show tPA or UK to be superior to SK in terms of thrombolytic revascularization of occluded arteries (80% vs 64%) and hemorrhagic complications (5% vs 25%).[98] However, no prospective comparison has been conducted between SK and tPA or UK. Only one study directly compared tPA with UK[97]; no difference in clinical outcomes was reported. The similar efficacy of various PAs in comparative trials of PE and acute MI suggests that all agents offer equivalent advantages relative to surgery in the treatment of the salvageable ischemic limb. Reteplase, which was evaluated in a small series, achieved complete dissolution of a high percentage of occlusions, but with a 9% risk of major hemorrhage.[99] Intra-arterial staphylokinase achieved complete revascularization in 83% of occlusions; amputation-free survival at 1 year was 90.2%, but fatal ICH occurred in 2.1% of cases.[100]

Myocardial Infarction

Systemic PA infusion reduces mortality after AMI by more than 40% when administered within 1 to 2 hours, and by 20% to 25% at 4 to 6 hours after onset of symptoms[27]— a survival advantage that persists for at least a decade.[101] Aspirin virtually doubles the survival benefit of PA alone,[102] and heparin is problematic as an adjunct for SK[103] but is still considered important for tPA usage.[104] The GISSI-2 and ISIS-3 studies[105,106] showed the same mortality with SK, tPA, and anistreplase, but the GUSTO trial[107] showed a small but significant mortality advantage in favor of accelerated tPA plus IV heparin over SK—6.3% versus 7.2%, representing a difference of 9 patients per 1000 treated. The incidence of ICH was significantly higher with tPA in all three trials (0.7% vs 0.35% to 0.5%), mitigating against a clear-cut advantage for tPA. Reteplase restores coronary patency (TIMI 3 flow) more effectively than accelerated tPA (60% vs 45%),[108] but no decrease in mortality was reported for reteplase over tPA (7.47% vs 7.24%),[109] or even over SK (9.02% vs 9.53%),[110] despite the prior advantage demonstrated for tPA over SK. Tenecteplase achieved equivalent 30-day mortality against accelerated tPA (6.18% vs 6.15%) and equivalent rates of ICH (about 0.9%).[111] A third mutant PA, lanoteplase, was tested against tPA and was found to have an equivalent mortality rate but a significantly higher rate of ICH (1.12% vs 0.64%),[112] which likely explains why this agent has not been approved by the FDA for this particular indication.

Improvements in PA efficacy, especially with regard to coagulation-related reocclusion, have been addressed by the use of alternatives to heparin and aspirin as adjunctive agents (see earlier). Tenecteplase (plus LMWH or UFH) compared with reduced-dose tenecteplase (plus lower dose UFH and abciximab)[113] showed no significant 30-day mortality benefit; the same rate of ICH was reported in all groups (0.9%). Similarly, low-dose reteplase plus abciximab showed no significant difference in 30-day mortality in comparison with standard reteplase (5.6% vs 5.9%). Although overall ICH was not increased (0.6%), the rate was higher in patients older than 75 years of age (2.1% vs 1.1%) in the group given reteplase plus abciximab.[114]

28

Direct thrombin inhibitors (DTIs) such as bivalirudin accelerate reperfusion when used with SK, but not tPA.[115] The HERO-2 (Hirulog and Early Reperfusion/Occlusion) study in 17,000 patients with MI showed no difference in 30-day mortality (10.8% vs 10.9%),[35] again illustrating a disparity between 90-minute patency and mortality benefit. ICH was slightly but not significantly higher with hirudin than with heparin (0.6% vs 0.4%). If only to avoid the excess risk of ICH, immediate angioplasty is a feasible approach for large centers with this technical capacity.

Ischemic Stroke

In the 1990s, six randomized, blinded trials of systemic (IV) PA investigated the treatment of patients with ischemic stroke; three studied the use of SK, and three evaluated the effectiveness of tPA.[11] The most important distinguishing factor between these trials was the time delay from onset of symptoms to treatment; only one trial limited entry to 3 hours.[116] The three SK trials were terminated before completion because of an excess in mortality at 10 days, generally attributed to ICH; a fourth study showed a trend for increased 30-day mortality ($P = .08$).[11] The only study that showed no increase in mortality at 30 days was conducted by the National Institute of Neurological Disorders and Stroke rtPA Stroke Study Group; this group assessed tPA in patients enrolled within 3 hours of symptom onset; higher rates of death and severe disability were reported when placebo was used versus tPA (21% vs 17%).[116] Whether this distinction between the SK and tPA studies is due to the agent or to the regimen that was applied (less than vs more than 3-hour delay) was assessed by subgroup analyses of the Australian Streptokinase Trial[117] and the ECASS (European Cooperative Acute Stroke Studies)[118] trials with tPA. All studies showed favorable functional outcomes in patients treated within 3 hours, without excess mortality. Further evidence of the critical nature of this 3-hour time window is reflected by the ATLANTIS (Alteplase Thrombolysis for Acute Noninterventional Therapy in Ischemic Stroke) study of tPA,[119] in which 547 patients were treated at between 3 and 5 hours after symptom onset. Greater neurologic improvement was described at 24 hours for tPA-treated patients (40% vs 21%), but functional improvement at 3 months was not different (34% vs 32%), and symptomatic ICH (7% vs 1.1%; $P < .001$), fatal ICH (3% vs 0.3%; $P < .001$) at 10 days, and higher mortality at 3 months (11% vs 6.9%; $P = .09$) were more common with tPA. A meta-analysis of thrombolytic therapy in acute ischemic stroke (17 trials; 5216 patients)[120] concluded that thrombolytic therapy administered up to 6 hours after ischemic stroke significantly reduced death or dependence at follow-up (55.2% vs 59.7%) by 44 patients per 1000 treated; for treatment within 3 hours, the advantage increased to 126, but at a risk of 70 additional episodes of ICH per 1000. Only tPA has been tested in sufficient numbers of patients within this "golden window" of opportunity[121]; no direct comparison of tPA with SK has been undertaken.

Direct intra-arterial thrombolysis has been tested in a controlled trial with the use of saruplase (recombinant pro-UK) in patients with middle cerebral artery occlusion who present within 6 hours of symptoms.[122] Recanalization was more frequent with active agent (66% vs 18%) and at 90 days; a greater number of saruplase-treated patients were functionally independent (40% vs 25%). However, 90-day mortality was the same for treatment and placebo groups, and ICH was more frequent with saruplase (10.9% vs 3.1%).[123] A small trial evaluated intra-arterial reteplase in 16 patients with acute ischemic stroke that affected varying arterial locations[124]; reperfusion was evident in 88% and neurologic improvement at 24 hours was observed in 44%, but ICH occurred in 25%, and the overall mortality rate was 56%. The direct-acting fibrinolytic agents (see earlier) have the potential for safer therapy than is provided by PAs, but studies have not yet been initiated.

REFERENCES

1. Verstraete M: Biochemical and clinical aspects of thrombolysis. Semin Hematol 15:35, 1978.
2. Marder VJ: The use of thrombolytic agents: Choice of patient, drug administration, laboratory monitoring. Ann Intern Med 90:802, 1979.
3. Marder VJ, Sherry S: Thrombolytic therapy: Current status. N Engl J Med 18:1512, 1988.
4. Simoons ML, Arnold AE: Tailored thrombolytic therapy: A perspective. Circulation 88:2556, 1993.
5. Marder VJ: Foundations of thrombolytic therapy. In Colman RW, Marder VJ, Clowes AW, et al(eds): Hemostasis and Thrombosis: Basic Principles and Clinical Practice, 5th edition. Philadelphia, Lippincott, Williams & Wilkins, 2006, p 1739.
6. Staniforth DH, Smith RAG, Hibbs M: Streptokinase and anisoylated streptokinase plasminogen complex: Their action on haemostasis in human volunteers. Eur J Clin Pharmacol 24:751, 1983.
7. Bode C, Smalling RW, Berg G, et al: Randomized comparison of coronary thrombolysis achieved with double-bolus reteplase (recombinant plasminogen activator) and front-loaded, accelerated alteplase (recombinant tissue plasminogen activator) in patients with acute myocardial infarction. The RAPID II Investigators. Circulation 94:891, 1996.
8. Modi NB, Eppler S, Breed J, et al: Pharmacokinetics of a slower clearing tissue plasminogen activator variant, TNK-t-PA, in patients with acute myocardial infarction. Thromb Haemost 79:134, 1998.
9. Korninger C, Matsuo O, Suy R, et al: Thrombolysis with human extrinsic (tissue-type) plasminogen activator in dogs with femoral vein thrombosis. J Clin Invest 69:573, 1982.
10. Cannon CP, McCabe CH, Gibson CM, et al: TNK-tissue plasminogen activator in acute myocardial infarction: Results of the Thrombolysis in Myocardial Infarction (TIMI) 10A dose-ranging trial. Circulation 95:351, 1997.
11. Marder VJ, Stewart D: Towards safer thrombolytic therapy. Semin Hematol 39:206, 2002.
12. Ambrus JL, Ambrus CM, Back N, et al: Clinical and experimental studies on fibrinolytic enzymes. Ann N Y Acad Sci 68:97, 1957.
13. Marder VJ, Landskroner K, Novokhatny V, et al: Plasmin induces local thrombolysis without causing hemorrhage: A comparison with tissue plasminogen activator in the rabbit. Thromb Haemost 86:739, 2001.
14. Novokhatny V, Taylor K, Zimmerman TP: Thrombolytic potency of acid-stabilized plasmin: Superiority over tissue-type plasminogen activator in an in vitro model of catheter-assisted thrombolysis. J Thromb Haemost 1:1034–1041, 2003.
15. Nagai N, De Mol M, Van Hoef B, et al: Depletion of circulating α2-antiplasmin by intravenous plasmin or immunoneutralization reduces focal cerebral ischemic injury in the absence of arterial recanalization. Blood 97:3086, 2001.
16. Toombs CF: Alfimeprase: Pharmacology of a novel fibrinolytic metalloproteinase for thrombolysis. Haemostasis 31:141, 2001.
17. Novokhatny VV, Jesmok GJ, Landskroner KA, et al: Locally delivered plasmin: Why should it be superior to plasminogen activators for direct thrombolysis? Trends Pharmacol Sci 25:72, 2004.
18. Ouriel K, Cynamon J, Weaver FA, et al: A phase I trial of alfimeprase for peripheral arterial thrombolysis. J Vasc Interv Radiol 16:1075, 2005.
19. Stewart D, Kong M, Novokhatny V, et al: Distinct dose-dependent effects of plasmin and TPA on coagulation and hemorrhage. Blood 101:3002, 2003.

20. ISIS-2 (Second International Study of Infarct Survival) Collaborative Group: Randomized trial of intravenous streptokinase, oral aspirin, both, or neither among 17,187 cases of suspected acute myocardial infarction. Lancet 2:349, 1988.

21. The GUSTO Investigators: An international randomized trial comparing four thrombolytic strategies for acute myocardial infarction. N Engl J Med 329:673, 1993.

22. O'Connor CM, Meese R, Carney R, et al: A randomized trial of intravenous heparin in conjunction with anistreplase (anisoylated plasminogen streptokinase activator complex) in acute myocardial infarction: The Duke University Clinical Cardiology Study (DUCCS) I. J Am Coll Cardiol 23:11, 1994.

23. Collins R, Peto R, Baigent C, Sleight P: Aspirin, heparin, and fibrinolytic therapy in suspected acute myocardial infarction. N Engl J Med 336:847, 1997.

24. Mahaffey KW, Granger CB, Collins R, et al: Overview of randomized trials of intravenous heparin in patients with acute myocardial infarction treated with thrombolytic therapy. Am J Cardiol 77:551, 1996.

25. Menon V, Harrington RA, Hochman JS, et al: Thrombolysis and adjunctive therapy in acute myocardial infarction. The Seventh ACCP Conference on Antithrombotic and Thrombolytic Therapy. Chest 126:549S, 2004.

26. Wallentin L, Goldstein P, Armstrong PW, et al: Efficacy and safety of tenecteplase in combination with the low-molecular-weight heparin enoxaparin or unfractionated heparin in the prehospital setting: The Assessment of the Safety and Efficacy of a New Thrombolytic Regimen (ASSENT)-3 PLUS randomized trial in acute myocardial infarction. Circulation 108:135, 2003.

27. Fibrinolytic Therapy Trialists Collaborative Group: Indications for fibrinolytic therapy in suspected acute myocardial infarction: Collaborative overview of early mortality and major morbidity results from all randomised trials of more than 1000 patients. Lancet 343:311, 1994.

28. Simoons ML, Maggioni AP, Knatterud G, et al: Individual risk assessment for intracranial haemorrhage during thrombolytic therapy. Lancet 342:1523, 1993.

29. The Continuous Infusion Versus Double-Bolus Administration of Alteplase (COBALT) Investigators: A comparison of continuous infusion of alteplase with double-bolus administration for acute myocardial infarction. N Engl J Med 337:1124, 1997.

30. The Global Use of Strategies to Open Occluded Coronary Arteries (GUSTO III) Investigators: A comparison of reteplase with alteplase for acute myocardial infarction. N Engl J Med 337:1118, 1997.

31. Cannon CP, McCabe CH, Henry TD, et al: A pilot trial of recombinant desulfatohirudin compared with heparin in conjunction with tissue-type plasminogen activator and aspirin for acute myocardial infarction: Results of the Thrombolysis in Myocardial Infarction (TIMI) 5 trial. J Am Coll Cardiol 23:993, 1994.

32. The Global Use of Strategies to Open Occluded Coronary Arteries (GUSTO) IIa Investigators: Randomized trial of intravenous heparin versus recombinant hirudin for acute coronary syndromes. Circulation 90:1631, 1994.

33. Antman EM: Hirudin in acute myocardial infarction. Thrombolysis and Thrombin Inhibition in Myocardial Infarction (TIMI) 9B Trial. Circulation 94:911, 1996.

34. Theroux P, Perez-Villa F, Waters D, et al: Randomized double-blind comparison of two doses of Hirulog with heparin as adjunctive therapy to streptokinase to promote early patency of the infarct-related artery in acute myocardial infarction. Circulation 98:2132, 1995.

35. White HD, Aylward PE, Frey MJ, et al: Randomized, double-blind comparison of Hirulog versus heparin in patients receiving streptokinase and aspirin for acute myocardial infarction (HERO). Hirulog Early Reperfusion/Occlusion (HERO) Trial Investigators. Circulation 96:2155, 1997.

36. Strategies for Patency Enhancement in the Emergency Department (SPEED) Group: Trial of abciximab with and without low-dose reteplase for acute myocardial infarction. Circulation 101:2788, 2000.

37. Antman EM, Giugliano RP, Gibson CM, et al: Abciximab facilitates the rate and extent of thrombolysis: Results of the thrombolysis in myocardial infarction (TIMI) 14 Trial. The TIMI 14 Investigators. Circulation 99:2720, 1999.

38. Rosenschein U, Rozenszajn LA, Kraus L, et al: Ultrasonic angioplasty in totally occluded peripheral arteries: Initial clinical, histological and angiographic results. Circulation 83:1976, 1991.

39. Alexandrov AV, Molina CA, Grotta JC, et al: Ultrasound-enhanced systemic thrombolysis for acute ischemic stroke. N Engl J Med 351:2170, 2004.

40. Ouriel K, Veith FJ, Sasahara AA: A comparison of recombinant urokinase with vascular surgery as initial treatment for acute arterial occlusion of the legs. N Engl J Med 338:1105, 1998.

41. Comerota AJ, Throm RC, Mathias SD, et al: Catheter-directed thrombolysis for iliofemoral deep venous thrombosis improves health-related quality of life. J Vasc Surg 32:130, 2000.

42. Ouriel K, Gray B, Clair DG, et al: Complications associated with the use of urokinase and recombinant tissue plasminogen activator for catheter-directed peripheral arterial and venous thrombolysis. J Vasc Interv Radiol 11:295, 2000.

43. Furlan A, Higashida R, Wechsler L, et al: Intra-arterial prourokinase for acute ischemic stroke. The PROACT II study: A randomized controlled trial. JAMA 282:2003, 1999.

44. Jacobs AK: Primary angioplasty for acute myocardial infarction: Is it worth the wait? N Engl J Med 349:798, 2003.

45. Sherry S, Fletcher AP, Alkjaersig N: Fibrinolysis and fibrinolytic activity in man. Physiol Rev 39:343, 1959.

46. Adelman B, Michelson AD, Loscalzo J, et al: Plasmin effect on platelet glycoprotein IB–von Willebrand factor interactions. Blood 65:32, 1985.

47. Rudd MA, George D, Amarante P, et al: Temporal effect of thrombolytic agents on platelet function in vivo and their modulation by prostaglandins. Circ Res 67:1175, 1990.

48. The Urokinase Pulmonary Embolism Trial: A national cooperative study. Circulation 47 (suppl II): 1, 1973.

49. Marder VJ, Soulen RL, Atichartakarn V, et al: Quantitative venographic assessment of deep vein thrombosis in the evaluation of streptokinase and heparin therapy. J Lab Clin Med 89:1018, 1977.

50. Rao AK, Pratt C, Berke A, et al: Thrombolysis in MI (TIMI) Trial—Phase I: Hemorrhagic manifestations and changes in plasma fibrinogen and the fibrinolytic system in patients treated with recombinant tissue plasminogen activator and streptokinase. J Am Coll Cardiol 11:1, 1988.

51. Gore JM, Sloan M, Price TR, et al: Intracerebral hemorrhage, cerebral infarction, and subdural hematoma after acute myocardial infarction and thrombolytic therapy in the thrombolysis in myocardial infarction study. Circulation 83:448, 1991.

52. Bernardi MM, Califf RM, Kleiman N, et al: Lack of usefulness of prolonged bleeding times in predicting hemorrhagic events in patients receiving the 7E3 glycoprotein IIb/IIIa platelet antibody. The TAMI Study Group. Am J Cardiol 72:1121, 1993.

53. Stump DC, Califf RM, Topol EJ, et al: Pharmacodynamics of thrombolysis with recombinant tissue-type plasminogen activator: Correlation with characteristics of and clinical outcomes in patients with acute myocardial infarction. Circulation 80:1222, 1989.

54. Carlson SE, Aldrich MS, Greenberg HS, Topol EJ: Intracerebral hemorrhage complicating intravenous tissue plasminogen activator treatment. Arch Neurol 45:1070, 1988.

55. Berkowitz SD, Granger CB, Pieper KS, et al: Incidence and predictors of bleeding after contemporary thrombolytic therapy for myocardial infarction. The Global Utilization of Streptokinase and Tissue Plasminogen Activator for Occluded Coronary Arteries (GUSTO) I Investigators. Circulation 95:2508, 1997.

56. White CW, Schwartz JL, Ferguson DW, et al: Systemic markers of fibrinolysis after unsuccessful intracoronary streptokinase thrombolysis for acute myocardial infarction: Does nonreperfusion indicate failure to achieve a systemic lytic state? Am J Cardiol 54:712, 1984.

57. Lawler CM, Bovill EG, Stump DC, et al: Fibrin fragment D-dimer and fibrinogen B beta peptides in plasma as markers of clot lysis during thrombolytic therapy in acute myocardial infarction. Blood 76:1341, 1990.

58. Brenner B, Francis CW, Fitzpatrick PG, et al: Relation of plasma D-dimer concentrations to coronary artery reperfusion before and after thrombolytic treatment in patients with acute myocardial infarction. Am J Cardiol 63:1179, 1989.

59. Gruppo Italiano per lo Studio Della Streptochinase Nell'infarto Miocardico: Effectiveness of intravenous thrombolytic treatment in acute myocardial infarction. Lancet 1:397, 1986.

60. Lee KF, Mandell J, Rankin JS, et al: Immediate versus delayed coronary grafting after streptokinase treatment: Post-operative blood loss and clinical results. J Thorac Cardiovasc Surg 95:216, 1988.

61. TIMI Research Group: Immediate vs delayed catheterization and angioplasty following thrombolytic therapy for acute MI: TIMI IIA results. JAMA 260:2849, 1988.

62. Mentzer RL, Budzynski AZ, Sherry S: High-dose, brief-duration intravenous infusion of streptokinase in acute myocardial infarction: Description of effects in the circulation. Am J Cardiol 57:1220, 1986.

28

63. Owen J, Friedman KD, Grossman BA, et al: Quantitation of fragment X formation during thrombolytic therapy with streptokinase and tissue plasminogen activator. J Clin Invest 79:1642, 1987.

64. Nunn B, Esmail R, Fears R, et al: Pharmacokinetic properties of anisoylated plasminogen streptokinase activator complex and other thrombolytic agents in animals and in humans. Drugs Suppl 3:88, 1987.

65. Goldhaber SZ, Heit J, Sharma GV RK, et al: Randomised controlled trial of recombinant tissue plasminogen activator versus urokinase in the treatment of acute pulmonary embolism. Lancet 2:293, 1988.

66. Francis CW, Brenner B, Leddy JP, Marder VJ: Angioedema during therapy with recombinant tissue plasminogen activator. Br J Haematol 77:562, 1991.

67. Third International Study of Infarct Survival Collaborative Group: ISIS-3: A randomized comparison of streptokinase vs aspirin alone among 41,299 cases of suspected acute myocardial infarction. Lancet 1:753, 1992.

68. Sicard GA, Schier JJ, Totty WG, et al: Thrombolytic therapy for acute arterial occlusion. J Vasc Surg 2:65, 1985.

69. Immelman EJ, Jeffery PC: The post-phlebitic syndrome: Pathophysiology, prevention and management. Clin Chest Med 5:537, 1984.

70. Hirsh J, Hoak J: Management of deep vein thrombosis and pulmonary embolism: A statement for healthcare professionals. Circulation 93:2212, 1996.

71. Francis CW, Marder VJ: Fibrinolytic therapy for venous thrombosis. Prog Cardiovasc Dis 34:193, 1991.

72. Turpie AGG, Levine MN, Hirsh J, et al: Tissue plasminogen activator vs heparin in DVT: Results of a randomized trial. Chest 97:172S, 1990.

73. Thrombolytic therapy in thrombosis: A National Institutes of Health consensus development conference. Ann Intern Med 93:141, 1980.

74. Schweizer J, Kirch W, Koch R, et al: Short- and long-term results after thrombolytic treatment of deep venous thrombosis. J Am Coll Cardiol 36:1336, 2000.

75. Semba CP, Dake MD: Iliofemoral deep venous thrombosis: Aggressive therapy with catheter-directed thrombolysis. Radiology 191:487, 1994.

76. Bjarnason H, Kruse JR, Azinger DA, et al: Iliofemoral deep vein thrombosis: Safety and efficacy outcome during 5 years of catheter-directed thrombolytic therapy. J Vasc Intervent Radiol 8:405, 1997.

77. Mewissen MW, Seabrook GR, Meissner MH, et al: Catheter-directed thrombolysis for lower extremity deep venous thrombosis: Report of a national multicenter registry. Radiology 211:39, 1999.

78. Decousus H, Leizorovicz A, Parent F, et al: A clinical trial of vena caval filters in the prevention of pulmonary embolism in patients with proximal deep vein thrombosis. N Engl J Med 338:409, 1998.

79. Dalen JE, Alpert JS: Natural history of pulmonary embolism. Prog Cardiovasc Dis 17:259, 1975.

80. Goldhaber SZ: Thrombolysis for pulmonary embolism. Prog Cardiovasc Dis 34:113, 1991.

81. Sharma GV, Folland ED, McIntyre KM, Sasahara AA: Long-term benefit of thrombolytic therapy in patients with pulmonary embolism. Vasc Med 5:91, 2000.

82. Meneveau N, Schiele F, Vuillemenot A, et al: Streptokinase versus alteplase in massive pulmonary embolus: A randomized trial assessing right heart hemodynamics and pulmonary vascular obstruction. Eur Heart J 18:1141, 1997.

83. Goldhaber SZ, Kessler CM, Heit JA, et al: Recombinant tissue-type plasminogen activator versus a novel dosing regimen of urokinase in acute pulmonary embolism: A randomized controlled multicenter trial. J Am Coll Cardiol 20:24, 1992.

84. Meneveau N, Schiele F, Metz D, et al: Comparative efficacy of a two-hour regimen of streptokinase versus alteplase in acute massive pulmonary embolism: Immediate clinical and hemodynamic outcome and one-year follow-up. J Am Coll Cardiol 31:1057, 1998.

85. Tebbe U, Graf A, Kamke W, et al: Hemodynamic effects of double bolus reteplase versus alteplase infusion in massive pulmonary embolism. Am Heart J 138:39, 1999.

86. Verstraete M, Miller GAH, Bounameaux H, et al: Intravenous and intrapulmonary recombinant tissue-type plasminogen activator in the treatment of acute massive pulmonary embolism. Circulation 77:353, 1988.

87. Urokinase Streptokinase Embolism Trial: Phase 2 results: A cooperative study. JAMA 229:1606, 1974.

88. Ruiz-Bailen M, Aguayo-de-Hoyos E, Serrano-Corcoles MC, et al: Thrombolysis with recombinant tissue plasminogen activator during cardiopulmonary resuscitation in fulminant pulmonary embolism: A case series. Resuscitation 51:97, 2001.

89. Urokinase Pulmonary Embolism trial: Phase 1 results: A cooperative study. JAMA 214:2163, 1970.

90. Martin M, Schoop W, Zietler E: Streptokinase in chronic arterial occlusive disease. JAMA 211:1169, 1970.

91. Amery A, Deloof W, Vermylen J, Verstraete M: Outcome of recent thromboembolic occlusions of limb arteries treated with streptokinase. Br Med J 4:639, 1970.

92. Dotter CT, Rosch J, Seaman AJ: Selective clot lysis with low-dose streptokinase. Radiology 111:31, 1974.

93. Hess H, Ingrisch H, Mietaschk A, et al: Local low-dose thrombolytic therapy of peripheral arterial occlusions. N Engl J Med 307:1627, 1982.

94. Sicard GA, Schier JJ, Totty WG, et al: Thrombolytic therapy for acute arterial occlusion. J Vasc Surg 2:65, 1985.

95. Ouriel K, Shortell CK, De Weese JA, et al: A comparison of thrombolytic therapy with operative revascularization in the initial treatment of acute peripheral arterial ischemia. J Vasc Surg 19:1021, 1994.

96. Ouriel K, Veith FJ, Sasahara AA, for the Thrombolysis or Peripheral Arterial Surgery (TOPAS) Investigators: A comparison of recombinant urokinase with vascular surgery as initial treatment for acute arterial occlusion of the legs. N Engl J Med 338:1105, 1998.

97. The STILE Investigators: Results of a prospective randomized trial evaluating surgery versus thrombolysis for ischemia of the lower extremity: The STILE trial. Ann Surg 220:251, 1994.

98. Belkin M, Belkin B, Bucknam CA, et al: Intra-arterial fibrinolytic therapy: Efficacy of streptokinase vs. urokinase. Arch Surg 121:769, 1986.

99. Ouriel K, Katzen B, Mewissen M, et al: Reteplase in the treatment of peripheral arterial and venous occlusions: A pilot study. J Vasc Interv Radiol 11:849, 2000.

100. Heymans S, Vanderschueren S, Verhaeqhe R, et al: Outcome and one year follow-up of intra-arterial staphylokinase in 191 patients with peripheral arterial occlusion. Thromb Haemost 83:666, 2000.

101. Franzosi MG, Santoro E, De Vita C, et al: Ten-year follow-up of the first megatrial testing thrombolytic therapy in patients with acute myocardial infarction: Results of the Gruppo Italiano per lo Studio della Sopravvivenza nell'Infarto-1 study. The GISSI Investigators. Circulation 98:2659, 1998.

102. ISIS-2 (Second International Study of Infarct Survival) Collaborative Group: Randomized trial of intravenous streptokinase, oral aspirin, both, or neither among 17,187 cases of suspected acute myocardial infarction. Lancet 2:349, 1998.

103. Collins R, Peto R, Baigent C, Sleight P: Aspirin, heparin, and fibrinolytic therapy in suspected acute myocardial infarction. N Engl J Med 336:847, 1997.

104. Mahaffey KW, Granger CB, Collins R, et al: Overview of randomized trials of intravenous heparin in patients with acute myocardial infarction treated with thrombolytic therapy. Am J Cardiol 77:551, 1996.

105. Gruppo Italiano per lo Studio Della Sopravvivenza nell'Infarto Miocardioco (GISSI): GISSI-2: A factorial randomized trial of alteplase versus streptokinase and heparin versus no heparin among 12,490 patients with acute myocardial infarction. Lancet 336:65, 1990.

106. The International Study Group: In-hospital mortality and clinical course of 20,891 patients with suspected acute myocardial infarction randomized between alteplase and streptokinase with or without heparin. Lancet 336:71, 1990.

107. The GUSTO Investigators: An international randomized trial comparing four thrombolytic strategies for acute myocardial infarction. N Engl J Med 329:673, 1993.

108. Smalling RW, Bode C, Kalbfleisch J, et al, for the RAPID Investigators: More rapid, complete and stable coronary thrombolysis with bolus administration of reteplase compared with alteplase infusion in acute myocardial infarction. Circulation 91:2725, 1995.

109. The Global Use of Strategies to Open Occluded Coronary Arteries (GUSTO III) Investigators: A comparison of reteplase with alteplase for acute myocardial infarction. N Engl J Med 337:1118, 1997.

110. International Joint Efficacy Comparison of Thrombolytics: Randomized, double-blind comparison of reteplase double-bolus administration with streptokinase in acute myocardial infarction (INJECT): Trial to investigate equivalence. Lancet 346:329–336, 1995.

111. Assessment of the Safety and Efficacy of New Thrombolytic Investigators: Single-bolus tenecteplase compared with front-loaded alteplase in acute myocardial infarction: The ASSENT-2 double-blind randomized trial. Lancet 354:716, 1999.

112. The InTIME-II Investigators: Intravenous NPA for the treatment of infarcting myocardium early: InTIME-II, a double-blind comparison of single-bolus lanoteplase vs accelerated alteplase for the treatment of patients with acute myocardial infarction. Eur Heart J 21:2005, 2000.

113. The Assessment of the Safety and Efficacy of a New Thrombolytic Regimen (ASSENT)-3 Investigators: Efficacy and safety of tenecteplase in combination with enoxaparin, abciximab, or unfractionated heparin: The ASSENT-3 randomized trial in acute myocardial infarction. Lancet 358:605, 2001.

114. Topol EJ, for The GUSTO V Investigators: Reperfusion therapy for acute myocardial infarction with fibrinolytic therapy or combination reduced fibrinolytic therapy and platelet glycoprotein IIb/IIIa inhibition: The GUSTO V randomized trial. Lancet 357:1905, 2001.

115. Metz BK, White HD, Granger CB, et al, for the Global Use of Strategies to Open Occluded Coronary Arteries in Acute Coronary Syndromes (GUSTO-IIb) Investigators: Randomized comparison of direct thrombin inhibition versus heparin in conjunction with fibrinolytic therapy for acute myocardial infarction: Results from the GUSTO-IIb Trial. J Am Coll Cardiol 31:1493, 1998.

116. The National Institute of Neurological Disorders and Stroke rt-PA Stroke Study Group: Tissue plasminogen activator for acute ischemic stroke. N Engl J Med 333:1581, 1995.

117. Donnan GA, Davis SM, Chambers BR, et al: Streptokinase for acute ischemic stroke with relationship to time of administration: Australian Streptokinase (ASK) Trial Study Group. JAMA 276:961, 1996.

118. Hacke W, Kaste M, Fieschi C, et al: Intravenous thrombolysis with recombinant tissue plasminogen activator for acute hemispheric stroke. The European Cooperative Acute Stroke Study (ECASS). JAMA 274:1017, 1995.

119. Clark WM, Wissman S, Albers GW, et al: Recombinant tissue-type plasminogen activator (alteplase) for ischemic stroke 3 to 5 hours after symptom onset. The ATLANTIS study: A randomized controlled trial. Alteplase Thrombolysis for Acute Noninterventional Therapy in Ischemic Stroke. JAMA 282:2019, 1999.

120. Wardlaw JM, del Zoppo G, Yamaguchi T: Thrombolysis for acute ischemic stroke. Cochrane Database Syst Rev 2:CD000213, 2000.

121. Wardlaw JM, Warlow CP, Counsell C: Systematic review of evidence of thrombolytic therapy for acute ischemic stroke. Lancet 350:607, 1997.

122. Furlan A, Higashida R, Wechsler L, et al: Intra-arterial prourokinase for acute ischemic stroke. The PROACT II study: A randomized controlled trial. JAMA 282:2003, 1999.

123. Kase CS, Furlan AJ, Wechsler L, et al: Cerebral hemorrhage after intra-arterial thrombolysis for ischemic stroke: The PROACT II trial. Neurology 57:1603, 2001.

124. Qureshi AI, Ali Z, Suri MF, et al: Intra-arterial third-generation recombinant tissue plasminogen activator (reteplase) for acute ischemic stroke. Neurosurgery 49:41, 2001.

28

Chapter 29

Topical Hemostatic Agents for Localized Bleeding

Mark R. Jackson, MD

INTRODUCTION

For many years, topical hemostatic agents have consisted primarily of various forms of animal collagen and gelatin. These commercially prepared products have been used by surgeons in the operating room as adjuncts to surgical hemostasis. Most of these products have limited, if any, inherent coagulation properties and merely serve as a scaffold for fibrin deposition. Newer products, such as fibrin sealant, are now available as commercial preparations. These materials are combinations of highly purified, virally inactivated human thrombin and fibrinogen, and as such, they provide the final step in the coagulation cascade. Other products include combinations of gelatin matrix with bovine thrombin that possess some of the properties of the older agents and provide some inherent coagulation properties. Newer still are hemostatic, nonthrombogenic products designed primarily as sealants and adhesives, which can serve such purposes as sealing vascular anastomoses.

These materials are best categorized into two groups—topical sponge and mesh materials, and sealant and adhesive materials. In this chapter, we review these products, their intended and potential future uses, and the clinical settings in which they are used.

INTRAOPERATIVE AND POSTOPERATIVE BLEEDING

The most common cause of significant intraoperative bleeding is inadequate surgical hemostasis, so-called "silk deficiency." No pharmacologic or blood bank products can be substituted for careful dissection and attention to technical detail. Application of digital pressure to an area of active bleeding is a useful maneuver while more definitive steps are in progress. Even apparently trivial bleeding from skin edges and subcutaneous tissue may cause up to 100 to 200 mL of blood loss, if unattended.[1] Dissection with the use of electrocautery rather than a scalpel reduces blood loss.[2,3]

Intraoperative disorders of hemostasis occur for a number of reasons. Coagulopathy in patients with vascular trauma is related more to hypotension and hypoperfusion than to dilutional factors.[4] Tissue hypoxia may cause release of plasminogen activators, thereby stimulating fibrinolysis. Hypothermia may be another contributing factor, particularly in the trauma patient. Dilutional thrombocytopenia can occur in the massively transfused patient, particularly after infusion of 20 or more units of banked or cell salvage blood.[5]

To successfully manage hemostasis at the local level, physicians in the operating room must first correct systemic attributes that contribute to coagulopathy. Hemodynamic stability and normal temperature must be restored. Dilutional coagulopathy should be addressed with platelet or factor replacement, as indicated by laboratory markers of hemostasis. Disorders of hemostasis caused by antiplatelet agents and anticoagulation introduce an additional layer of complexity in patients such as those undergoing cardiac or vascular surgery and for whom reversal of antithrombotic therapy might be undesirable or not practical. Topical hemostatic agents may provide a useful adjunct to securing adequate hemostasis in patients who have persistent local bleeding despite all reasonable efforts to restore systemic coagulation mechanisms, even with the use of sutures and electrocautery.

TOPICAL SPONGE AND MESH MATERIALS

Collagen-Based Materials

A number of absorbable bovine collagen products are available commercially for use as topical hemostatic agents (Table 29-1). These materials are often packaged as sheets that can be cut to various sizes once opened and placed on the sterile surgical field. These materials are somewhat stiff, so they often can be more easily used and manipulated if they are moistened with saline solution or blood from the wound. Also, when these materials are dry, they are somewhat "sticky" and are not as easily handled. Many surgeons moisten these products with solutions of bovine thrombin. Once moistened, these sheets have the consistency of wet felt and can be easily wrapped around a vascular anastomosis, or placed in a single layer on a relatively flat bleeding wound surface. Such materials may be useful for small capsular tears of the spleen, for example. Collagen-based topical agents are absorbable and therefore may remain in the wound if necessary.

Microfibrillar collagen has a consistency similar to sawdust and is packaged as a powder. Similar to other collagen products, it absorbs surrounding blood and basically functions as a mechanical template on which the patient's fibrin clot is formed. Microfibrillar collagen has a tendency to adhere to the surgeon's gloves and instruments, as well as

Table 29-1   Summary of Commonly Used Topical Hemostatic Agents Available in the United States

Agent	Manufacturer	Composition	Clinical Comments
Sealants and Adhesives			
Tisseel VH	Baxter	Human fibrin sealant	Purified, pasteurized human proteins. Component proteins mixed using "two-into-one" syringe. Preparation may require 20 minutes because of the need for warming of constituent protein solutions. Does not adhere well to some prosthetic vascular grafts.
CoSeal	Baxter	Polymerized polyethylene glycol	Newer product. Adheres well to prosthetic grafts; works well for suture line bleeding. Prepared from a "two-into-one" syringe, as with fibrin sealant. Prepared at room temperature.
BioGlue	Cryolife Inc.	Bovine serum albumin crosslinked with glutaraldehyde	Used most often in cardiac and thoracic aortic dissection surgery. Tenacious bonding properties.
Absorbable Sponge and Mesh Materials			
Surgicel	Ethicon, Johnson & Johnson	Oxidized regenerated cellulose	Applied in "sheets," meshlike consistency. Can be easily "rolled" for endoscopic use.
Surgicel Fibrillar	Ethicon, Johnson & Johnson	Oxidized regenerated cellulose	"Feltlike" consistency. Bulkier than Surgicel, which may be advantageous in deeper wounds.
FloSeal	Baxter	Collagen particles and bovine thrombin	"Slurry-like" consistency. Easily prepared.
Gelfoam	Upjohn & Pharmacia	Gelatin	Stiff, sheetlike consistency. Often moistened and used with bovine collagen.
Avitene	CR Bard	Microfibrillar collagen	Several preparations—sheets and powder. Powder form has a "sawdust" consistency. Clings tenaciously to wound and surgeon's fingers. Bulkiness is advantageous in deeper wounds and in "wetter" wounds.

to the wound. Because of its powder-like consistency, it can be placed easily within irregular surfaces and crevices of deep wounds.

Collagen materials have demonstrated hemostatic efficacy in preclinical and clinical studies.[6,7] Early preclinical studies of the hemostatic properties of microcrystalline collagen in a canine model of arterial injury reported a 93% rate of early hemostasis when collagen was applied to a carotid artery puncture made with a 17-gauge trocar.[6] Hemostasis was far superior with microcrystalline collagen than with oxidized cellulose or pressure alone. An interesting finding from these experiments involved the use of collagen in animals anticoagulated with intravenously administered heparin (300 IU per kilogram). Of this group, 24% had delayed bleeding during the 1-hour experiment, suggesting that intact coagulation mechanisms are instrumental in ensuring maximal effectiveness of these collagen topical agents.

Cellulose-Based Materials

Topical hemostatic agents composed of oxidized regenerated cellulose are also available as fabric-like and as fibrillar (powder-like) products. The cellulose fabric can be cut to conform to the wound or to wrap a vascular anastomosis. Because the material is softer than collagen and gelatin products, predeployment wetting is optional. The cellulose fabric is also thinner than most collagen products and is knitted in a manner that produces interstices. A potential advantage of cellulose over collagen and gelatin-based agents is that oxidized regenerated cellulose has exhibited antibacterial properties in vitro.[8,9] Similar to collagen, oxidized regenerated cellulose is absorbable and can remain in the wound. Cellulose products come in two configurations—a mesh material and a feltlike (fibrillar) material (see Table 29-1). Fibrillar cellulose is preferred by the author during open vascular surgery procedures for which a mass of thrombogenic material is desired for tamponade effect and when sealant properties are not required.

Gelatin-Based Materials

Purified gelatin of bovine origin is also used as a topical hemostatic agent. It is prepared as a thin, wafer-like sheet that has the consistency of styrofoam. Once moistened, it is pliable and easily conforms to the shape of a wound or a vascular anastomosis. Similar to collagen and cellulose-based agents, gelatin-based materials are absorbable and can remain in the wound after closure. Many surgeons use bovine thrombin as the wetting agent. Gelatin-based topical hemostatic agents have been compared with collagen-based agents in a number of animal models of hemostasis. Although some studies have shown superiority of the collagen products,[10,11] others have demonstrated equivalency.[12,13]

Recently, another gelatin-based hemostatic agent has been approved by the U.S. Food and Drug Administration (FDA) (FloSeal). This product is composed of bovine source gelatin granules and bovine thrombin. These two ingredients are mixed together and placed in a single-barrel syringe prior to use. The gelatin and thrombin mixture is then applied to the site of bleeding. The final product has a granular, gel-like consistency, and is easily applied with the accompanying syringe. Recently, investigators at Columbia University College of Physicians and Surgeons reported results of a cohort group of 93 patients who experienced hemorrhage in a multicenter, randomized clinical trial in which this hemostatic agent was evaluated in a total of 309 patients who were undergoing cardiac, vascular, and spinal surgery.[14] Patients were randomly assigned to receive FloSeal or bovine thrombin–soaked Gelfoam (Upjohn and Pharmacia, Kalamazoo, Mich, USA) applied at sites of bleeding that required topical hemostatic agents. Hemostasis at 10 minutes was achieved in 94% of patients with FloSeal, and in only 60% in the control group ($P = .001$). All patients were tested preoperatively and at 6 to 8 weeks for the development of antibodies to bovine thrombin and factor V. Although no evidence of antibody-related hemorrhage was noted in either group, bovine thrombin antibodies were detected by enzyme-linked immunosorbent assay in 9 patients treated with FloSeal and in 12 control patients ($P = .76$). Bovine factor V antibodies were detected in 11 patients treated with FloSeal and in 15 controls ($P = .43$).

FloSeal has been evaluated in a multicenter randomized clinical trial of hemostasis during peripheral vascular surgery and was found to be more effective than Gelfoam and bovine thrombin.[15] The primary end point, cessation of bleeding within 10 minutes of application, was met in 94% of FloSeal patients and in only 76% of controls ($P = .036$). Time to hemostasis was also superior in the FloSeal group at 2.5 minutes versus 6.5 minutes. Although these differences are statistically significant, differences in time to hemostasis are modest in the context of an operation that could take 2 or more hours, particularly in a setting with little need for blood transfusion.

SEALANTS AND ADHESIVES

Combinations of Thrombin and Fibrinogen

The use of fibrin-based topical hemostatic products was reported as early as 1909.[16] Subsequent developments allowed the purification of thrombin and fibrinogen, which eventually led to the development of fibrin sealant products in the 1970s. Because of concerns regarding transmission of viral blood-borne infection, the FDA revoked the license for commercial fibrinogen concentrates in 1978. Since then, careful donor selection and the development of a variety of viral inactivation methods have largely resolved the viral safety issue.

Until the recent approval of Tisseel VH (Baxter Healthcare Corporation, Deerfield, Ill, USA), the use of fibrin sealant in the United States was restricted to the so-called "home-brews" of bovine thrombin and human pooled cryoprecipitated plasma as sources of fibrinogen. With the availability of commercial fibrin sealant preparations and other newer hemostatic agents, such "home-brews" are used less often. Such preparations are also limited by the lack of viral inactivation methods. Single donor and autologous cryoprecipitates have also been used in an effort to minimize

infectious risk. Additional limitations of these preparations include a relatively low fibrinogen concentration and induction of antibodies against bovine factor V.[17–19] The bovine thrombin preparation with the lowest concentration of bovine factor V is produced by Jones Medical Industries (St. Louis, Mo, USA).[20]

Antibodies to bovine factor V and thrombin may produce coagulopathy and bleeding and are not merely a laboratory abnormality (see Chapter 6). The classic feature of such an acquired factor V deficiency caused by antibody formation is excessive bleeding that is not responsive to administration of vitamin K or fresh frozen plasma.[20] Laboratory findings include prolonged prothrombin time (PT) and partial thromboplastin time (PTT) that are not corrected by mixing patient and normal plasma in vitro and by reduced factor V activity (usually <30%).[20] Bleeding patients should be treated with fresh frozen plasma or platelet transfusion for factor V replacement. Immunosuppression with steroids has also been used effectively.[20] For patients who require continued anticoagulation, it should not be assumed that elevations in PT and PTT indicate a state of "autoanticoagulation."[21] Nonetheless, the probability of increased risk of bleeding with continued anticoagulation must be weighed against the risk of thrombosis; therefore, the decision for or against anticoagulation must be individualized for each patient. Cessation of pharmacologic anticoagulation through monitoring for thrombus by serial echocardiography has been used successfully in one such patient with a prosthetic aortic valve.[22]

Cryoprecipitate-based fibrin glue is prepared with equal volumes of thawed cryoprecipitated plasma as the source of fibrinogen and bovine thrombin with calcium chloride.[23] These solutions are placed in separate syringes and are mixed together to form a layer of fibrin polymer. The consistency of such home brews varies widely for two primary reasons. First, the fibrinogen concentration of cryoprecipitate varies considerably, ranging from approximately 4 mg per milliliter to 25 mg per milliliter.[24] Fibrinogen concentration has been shown to correlate with the tensile and adhesive strength of fibrin sealant.[16] Another limitation that may compromise the final material properties of the fibrin polymer is the method of fibrinogen/thrombin mixture used. The tensile strength of the fibrin polymer is less when incomplete or inadequate mixture occurs.[25] A dual-syringe delivery device similar to that used to apply the two components of epoxy glue is commercially available and can simplify the simultaneous administration and mixing of fibrinogen and thrombin solutions (Micromedics, Inc., St. Paul, Minn, USA). The two syringes are connected and are joined at their tips by a "Y" connector, through which the two solutions mix as they are applied to the wound. Catheter and spray tips are also available to allow the use of different delivery methods according to the nature of the bleeding site. Catheter tips work well when precise application is important, such as to the suture line of a vascular anastomosis. Spray tips are better suited for application over a large surface area, such as to the donor site in skin grafting procedures.

Commercially Prepared Fibrin Sealants

In processing their protein concentrates, most manufacturers of commercial fibrin sealant use two of six approved viral inactivation methods. These six processes include solvent/detergent treatment, two-step vapor heat, wet heat, dry heat, nanofiltration, and ultraviolet light.[26]

Although several commercial preparations are currently in use in clinical trials, Tisseel VH is the only product that has been approved in the United States. This two-component fibrin sealant product contains separate vials for a purified human fibrinogen concentrate and a purified human thrombin concentrate. In addition to several filtration steps and freeze drying, protein concentrates are subjected to a two-step vapor heat treatment for viral inactivation. Aprotinin, an antifibrinolytic agent of bovine origin, is present in the fibrinogen component of Tisseel VH. In addition to viral inactivation, advantages of commercial fibrin sealants over "home-brew" fibrin glue include higher fibrinogen concentration (50 to 150 mg per milliliter)[26] and ready availability, without the need for cryoprecipitate from the blood bank to be thawed. Most commercial preparations require warming to 37°C prior to use. Warming devices are available to facilitate this step.

A number of fibrin sealant products have been evaluated in prospective and retrospective studies. In a randomized clinical trial in which the hemostatic efficacy of human fibrin sealant was evaluated during cardiac reoperation, 92.6% of patients randomly assigned to receive fibrin sealant had complete hemostasis at 5 minutes, compared with only 12.4% of patients treated with conventional topical agents.[27] At 1 year of follow-up, no evidence of inflammation in response to fibrin sealant was apparent. A post hoc analysis of data showed improved survival, a shorter hospital stay, and less blood loss at 12 hours in the group treated with fibrin sealant.[28] In another randomized clinical trial, fibrin sealant prepared by the Scottish National Blood Transfusion Service was evaluated in vascular surgery procedures.[29] Seventeen patients who were about to undergo carotid endarterectomy with adjunctive polytetrafluoroethylene (PTFE) patch angioplasty were randomly assigned to receive fibrin sealant or nothing on PTFE patch suture holes. Suture holes in PTFE graft material have an inherent tendency to bleed and may be associated with hemorrhagic complications.[30] Fibrin sealant was prepared with the use of heat-treated fibrinogen from pooled donor plasma cryoprecipitate and solvent/detergent-treated human thrombin. The fibrinogen concentration ranged from 29 to 39 mg per milliliter. The fibrin sealant was administered through a dual-syringe technique. A statistically significant reduction was reported in time to achieve hemostasis in the fibrin sealant group (5.5 minutes) compared with controls (19 minutes; $P < .005$). No difference was noted in survival or measured blood loss. No thrombotic or neurologic complications occurred in patients treated with fibrin sealant. Another clinical trial comparing the hemostatic efficacy of human fibrin sealant with thrombin-soaked Gelfoam during PTFE carotid patch closure showed no differences between the two groups.[31] It was this author's observation that fibrin sealant did not adhere well to PTFE graft material.

Other studies support the hemostatic efficacy of fibrin sealant products in liver surgery and burn surgery. A randomized clinical trial comparing human fibrin sealant with standard topical hemostatic agents during liver resection surgery showed improved hemostasis at 10 minutes in the fibrin sealant group.[32] Hemostasis was achieved in 91% of fibrin sealant–treated patients compared with 70% of controls. In a multicenter clinical trial in which fibrin sealant was compared with no treatment at split-thickness skin graft donor sites, fibrin sealant was found to achieve hemostasis within 2.5 minutes compared with 7 minutes without treatment.[33] The relatively modest improvement in time to hemostasis and lack of a control treatment group made it difficult for investigators to recommend fibrin sealant for this clinical application.

Most of the attention focused on fibrin sealant products is related to issues of safety and hemostatic efficacy of the sealant itself. Although this is understandable and appropriate, the development of customized delivery devices that allow optimal application of fibrin sealant for different clinical uses is an important and sometimes overlooked issue. The standard dual-syringe technique is adequate for most applications; however, some limitations have been noted. For example, tips that attach to the "Y" connector frequently become plugged with fibrin, such that replacement is generally required for repeat administration from the same dual-syringe device. The current Tisseel VH Kit does not contain a spray tip, thus limiting the clinician's ability to apply a thin layer of sealant over a large surface area wound, such as a skin graft harvest site or a full-thickness burn tangential excision wound. Currently available catheter tips are not long enough to reach into deep wounds; when compared with the short tip, a longer single-channel tip might be more predisposed to plugging problems.

Another issue related to the importance of the delivery device is the cost of using large volumes of fibrin sealant. Considerable advantage is provided by a device that would allow efficient use of a limited volume of fibrin sealant to cover larger wounds. For example, a stellate liver fracture from blunt trauma would likely require multiple kits for complete application. The maximum total volume provided in the Tisseel VH Kit is 10 mL of sealant. Although this quantity or smaller amounts would be adequate for many indications, it is likely that several kits would be necessary for some wounds. The development of application devices that would release a finer spray might allow more cost-effective use of a given volume of sealant.

Fibrin sealant products are best used for diffuse, nonsurgical bleeding, such as suture hole bleeding at a vascular anastomosis, parenchymal bleeding after suture of vessels, and general oozing of blood from wound edges in patients with hemostatic defects. More significant bleeding sources should be sutured or treated with electrocautery, as appropriate. Although fibrin sealant appears to be a useful adjunct to surgical hemostasis, it is not a substitute. If fibrin sealant is applied to an actively bleeding wound, the sealant will usually "float off" the area of bleeding without achieving hemostasis. Moreover, current forms of liquid fibrin sealant make application of pressure, an often vital maneuver, somewhat problematic. Application of pressure may disrupt the adhesive bond of the sealant to the wound, causing the sealant to adhere more to the surgeon's glove or to gauze material, which may result in disruption of the sealant when pressure is removed. These material properties of liquid fibrin sealant limit its usefulness in wounds that are associated with significant or active bleeding.

The use of fibrin sealant incorporated into a dry dressing offers the potential of addressing some of the material property limitations associated with actively bleeding wounds. Commercially prepared fibrin sealant dressings consisting of a thin layer of lyophilized human thrombin and fibrinogen applied to one side of a sheet of equine collagen have been used clinically in Europe but currently are not approved for use in the United States. Clinical reports on the use of such fibrin sealant dressings are encouraging,[34] although randomized clinical trials are needed. A dry dressing of lyophilized fibrinogen and thrombin mounted on an absorbable backing delivers a higher concentration of fibrin to the wound and permits the application of pressure—a critically important adjunctive maneuver in surgical hemostasis. The mass effect of the backing material might also be important for maintaining contact of the fibrin sealant with the bleeding wound. Such materials are easy to handle; once they have become wet with blood in the wound, they can assume the contour of the wound surface.[35] Preclinical studies have reported superior hemostasis with fibrin sealant dressings compared with controls consisting of collagen fleece,[35] Silastic and immunoglobulin G,[36] and surgical gauze.[37,38] In a study in which the hemostatic efficacy of a fibrin sealant dressing was explored in a porcine model of femoral artery injury, a fibrin sealant dressing with 15 minutes of minimal pressure was effective in achieving complete hemostasis at femoral artery lacerations 4 mm in length.[36] It is unlikely that use of liquid fibrin sealant alone, particularly when used without adjunctive pressure application, would be effective with brisk arterial bleeding, as was encountered in this study.

Other Sealants

CoSeal is a surgical sealant formed by polymerization of two polyethylene glycols (PEGs). The two PEGs are mixed through a "Y-adapter" attached to two syringes, each containing one PEG material. This product received FDA approval in December of 2003. This material is well suited for sealing leaks such as those that occur at a vascular anastomosis. In the author's experience, this product appears to be more adherent to PTFE grafts than are fibrin sealant products. The Premarket Approval Application (PMA) submitted to the FDA in 2003 presented data showing superior efficacy of CoSeal for immediate sealing of vascular anastomoses compared with absorbable gelatin sponge/thrombin. Because this is a relatively new product, clinical reports describing hemostatic efficacy are limited.

BioGlue (CryoLife Inc., Kennesaw, Ga, USA), another surgical adhesive that can be used for vascular hemostasis, is an animal-based sealant made of bovine serum albumin cross-linked by glutaraldehyde. The two components are mixed in a predefined ratio and the enclosed delivery device is used. Polymerization begins within 30 seconds and is achieved at full strength within 2 minutes. This product forms a tenacious, firm bond. It is used most frequently by cardiac surgeons and appears to be particularly well suited for use as an adhesive agent during surgical repair of thoracic aortic dissection. BioGlue has been used successfully during cardiac surgery, as was reported in a registry of 115 consecutive patients.[39]

SUMMARY

Although topical hemostatic agents are no substitute for precise surgical technique in the treatment of patients with localized bleeding disorders, several products may serve as

useful adjuncts in these situations. Historically, collagen, cellulose, and gelatin-based products have been used most frequently in the United States as topical hemostatic agents, but with the recent FDA approval of fibrin sealant, this may change. As additional manufacturers bring fibrin sealant products to market, it is likely that newer application devices and fibrin sealant formulations will be developed that are more closely tailored to specific clinical needs. Newer agents with a gelatin and collagen base are now available, and additional agents are under development. These products will add choices to our present array of topical agents. Sealant agents such as CoSeal and BioGlue have strong adhesive properties that appear attractive for use with vascular anastomoses (both) and for aortic dissection repair (BioGlue). Clinical indications for these products will be determined in well-designed clinical trials. Better delivery devices for the application of these sealant materials are under development and will greatly improve the clinical usefulness of these hemostatic agents.

REFERENCES

1. Spence RK: Bleeding and the vascular surgery patient. Semin Vasc Surg 7:104–113, 1994.
2. Miller E, Paull DE, Morrissey K, et al: Scalpel versus electrocautery in modified radical mastectomy. Am Surg 54:284–286, 1988.
3. Pearlman NW, Stiegmann GV, Vance V, et al: A prospective study of incisional time, blood loss, pain and healing with carbon dioxide laser, scalpel and electrosurgery. Arch Surg 126:1018–1020, 1991.
4. Collins JA: Recent developments in the area of massive transfusion. World J Surg 11:75–81, 1987.
5. Leslie S, Toy P: Laboratory hemostatic abnormalities in massively transfused patients given red blood cells and crystalloid. Am J Clin Pathol 96:770–773, 1991.
6. Abbott WM, Austen WG: The effectiveness and mechanism of collagen-induced topical hemostasis. Surgery 78:723–729, 1975.
7. Morgenstern L: Microcrystalline collagen used in experimental splenic injury: A new surface hemostatic agent. Arch Surg 109:44–47, 1974.
8. Dineen P: Antibacterial activity of oxidized regenerated cellulose. Surg Gynecol Obstet 142:481–486, 1976.
9. Dineen P: The effect of oxidized regenerated cellulose on experimental infected splenotomies. J Surg Res 23:114–116, 1977.
10. Hanisch ME, Baum N, Beach PD, et al: A comparative evaluation of Avitene and gelfoam for hemostasis in experimental canine prostatic wounds. Invest Urol 12:333–336, 1975.
11. Coln D, Horton J, Ogden ME, et al: Evaluation of hemostatic agents in experimental splenic lacerations. Am J Surg 145:256–259, 1983.
12. Sanfilippo JS, Barrows GH, Yussman MA: Comparison of Avitene, topical thrombin, and gelfoam as sole hemostatic agent in tuboplasties. Fertil Steril 33:311–316, 1980.
13. Benoit PW, Hunt LM: Comparison of a microcrystalline collagen preparation and gelatin foam in extraction wounds. J Oral Surg 34:1079–1083, 1976.
14. Cosgrove DM, Badduke BR, Hill JD, et al: Controlled clinical trial of a novel hemostatic agent in cardiac surgery. The Fusion Matrix Study Group. Ann Thorac Surg 69:1376–1382, 2000.
15. Weaver FA, Hood DB, Zatina M, et al: Gelatin-thrombin–based hemostatic sealant for intraoperative bleeding in vascular surgery. Ann Vasc Surg 16:286–293, 2002.
16. Sierra DH: Fibrin sealant adhesive systems: A review of their chemistry, material properties and clinical applications. J Biomat Applicat 7:309–352, 1993.
17. Zehnder JL, Leung LLK: Development of antibodies to thrombin and factor V with recurrent bleeding in a patient exposed to topical bovine thrombin. Blood 76:2011–2016, 1990.
18. Banninger H, Hardegger T, Tobler A, et al: Frequent development of inhibitors of bovine thrombin and human factor V. Br J Haematol 85:528–532, 1993.
19. Nichols WL, Daniels TM, Fisher PK, et al: Antibodies to bovine thrombin and coagulation factor V associated with surgical use of topical bovine thrombin or fibrin "glue:" A frequent finding [Abstract]. Blood 82:59, 1993.

20. Christie RJ, Carrington L, Alving B: Postoperative bleeding induced by topical bovine thrombin: Report of two cases. Surgery 121:708–710, 1997.

21. Ortel TL, Charles LA, Keller FG, et al: Topical thrombin and acquired coagulation factor inhibitors: Clinical spectrum and laboratory diagnosis. Am J Hematol 45:128–135, 1994.

22. Zumberg MS, Waples JM, Kao KJ, et al: Management of a patient with a mechanical aortic valve and antibodies to both thrombin and factor V after repeat exposure to fibrin sealant. Am J Hematol 64:59–63, 2000.

23. Cohn SM, Feinstein AJ, Nicholas JM, et al: Recipe for a poor man's fibrin glue. J Trauma 44:907, 1998.

24. Ness PM, Perkins HA: Cryoprecipitate as a reliable source of fibrinogen replacement. JAMA 241:1690–1691, 1979.

25. Redl H, Schlag G, Dinges HP: Methods of fibrin seal application. Thorac Cardiovasc Surg 30:223–227, 1982.

26. Jackson MR, Alving BM: Fibrin sealant in preclinical and clinical studies. Curr Opin Hematol 6:415–419, 1999.

27. Rousou J, Levitsky S, Gonzalez-Lavin L, et al: Randomized clinical trial of fibrin sealant in patients undergoing resternotomy or reoperation after cardiac operations: A multicenter study. J Thorac Cardiovasc Surg 97:194–203, 1989.

28. Levitsky S: Randomized clinical trial of Immuno's fibrin sealant in patients undergoing resternotomy or reoperation after cardiac operations: A multicenter study [Letter]. Transfusion 36:845, 1996.

29. Milne AA, Murphy WG, Reading SJ, et al: Fibrin sealant reduces suture line bleeding during carotid endarterectomy: A randomised trial. Eur J Vasc Endovasc Surg 10:91–94, 1995.

30. McCready RA, Siderys H, Pittman JN, et al: Delayed postoperative bleeding from polytetrafluoroethylene carotid artery patches. J Vasc Surg 15:661–663, 1992.

31. Jackson MR, Gillespie DL, Longenecker EG, et al: Hemostatic efficacy of fibrin sealant (human) on expanded polytetrafluoroethylene carotid patch angioplasty: A randomized clinical trial. J Vasc Surg 30:461–466, 1999.

32. Schwartz M, Madariaga J, Hirose R, et al: Comparison of a new fibrin sealant with standard topical hemostatic agents. Arch Surg 139:1148–1154, 2004.

33. Nervi C, Gamelli RL, Greenhalgh DG, et al: A multicenter clinical trial to evaluate the topical hemostatic efficacy of fibrin sealant in burn patients. J Burn Care Rehabil 22:99–103, 2001.

34. Agus GB, Bono AV, Mira E, et al: Hemostatic efficacy and safety of TachoComb in surgery: Ready to use and rapid hemostatic agent. Int Surg 81:316–319, 1996.

35. Jackson MR, Taher MM, Burge JR, et al: Hemostatic efficacy of a fibrin sealant dressing in an animal model of kidney injury. J Trauma 45:662–665, 1998.

36. Jackson MR, Friedman SA, Carter AJ, et al: Hemostatic efficacy of a fibrin sealant–based topical agent in a femoral artery injury model: A randomized, blinded, placebo-controlled study. J Vasc Surg 26:274–280, 1997.

37. Larson MJ, Bowersox JC, Lim RC Jr, et al: Efficacy of a fibrin hemostatic bandage in controlling hemorrhage from experimental arterial injuries. Arch Surg 130:420–422, 1995.

38. Holcomb J, MacPhee M, Hetz S, et al: Efficacy of a dry fibrin sealant dressing for hemorrhage control after ballistic injury. Arch Surg 133:32–35, 1998.

39. Passage J, Jalali H, Tam RK, et al: BioGlue surgical adhesive: An appraisal of its indications in cardiac surgery. Ann Thorac Surg 74:432–437, 2002.

IV

Chapter 30

Therapeutic Apheresis

Chelsea A. Sheppard, MD • Christopher D. Hillyer, MD

INTRODUCTION

The hematologist, in his or her role as the admitting physician or as a consultant, invariably must consider, prescribe, or oversee a variety of procedures that remove or modify a portion of the circulating blood. These procedures are collectively called *apheresis*, from Greek *aphairesis* meaning "to take away by force, or withdraw." Apheresis is most often used in the treatment of patients; this use is called *therapeutic apheresis*. It is different from *donor apheresis*, which is used to collect platelets, granulocytes, or peripheral blood stem cells (PBSCs) from normal individual donors. To allow the primary or consulting hematologist to determine whether, if, how, and when therapeutic apheresis procedures and technologies are appropriately used, this chapter provides background, mechanical, and technical information; the use and complications of therapeutic apheresis in specific disease categories and entities are discussed (Fig. 30-1). Additionally, specialized applications, including the approach to pediatric patients, photopheresis, and liposorption technology, are detailed.

THERAPEUTIC APHERESIS— TERMINOLOGY

Therapeutic apheresis is a process in which whole blood is removed from a patient and separated by centrifugation into components, thus allowing a single element to be removed or modified while the remaining components are returned to the patient. The decision of whether plasma or cells are to be removed or modified leads to the two common subtypes of therapeutic apheresis: (1) *plasmapheresis*, and (2) *therapeutic cytapheresis*. Plasmapheresis is also called *therapeutic plasma exchange* (TPE). In TPE, the patient's plasma is removed and the plasma volume is replaced with saline, albumin, and/or fresh frozen plasma (FFP), thus maintaining volume and oncotic equilibrium. During therapeutic cytapheresis, pathologic or excess cells are separated from circulation and discarded, while remaining blood components are replaced. Generally, the addition of a prefix to -pheresis indicates which element is being removed, thus the terms *leukapheresis*, *platelet-pheresis*, and *erythrocytapheresis*. In leukapheresis and therapeutic plateletpheresis, excess and/or abnormal cells are removed and discarded; therefore, the terms stand alone. However, in erythrocytapheresis, abnormal or damaged red blood cells (RBCs) must be replaced with banked RBCs so that adequate oxygen delivery can be maintained;

the term *erythrocytapheresis* is used synonymously with the term *RBC exchange*. Historically, RBC exchange was used as a therapeutic modality, and the term has a treatment-related connotation. More recently, RBC exchange has been used in a prophylactic setting to allow for transfusion of patients with sickle cell anemia and removal of sickle hemoglobin blood, thus minimizing iron overload and preventing hyperviscosity. This procedure has come to be known as *prophylactic erythrocytapheresis*.

MECHANICAL AND TECHNICAL CONSIDERATIONS OF THERAPEUTIC APHERESIS

Most readers will appreciate that therapeutic apheresis is an automated procedure that is available in most tertiary care hospitals or is provided via contract services such as the local or regional blood or dialysis center. It is important to know, however, that apheresis can be performed manually by a hematologist, even in adults, through serial removal of 50-mL aliquots of venous whole blood and replacement of this with an equal amount of allogeneic banked packed RBCs and appropriate fluids. Indeed, manual leukapheresis can be lifesaving and easily accomplished in one sitting. Finally, manual plasmapheresis or cytapheresis is the procedure of choice in infants and children who are too small to tolerate the significant extracorporeal volume required by fully automated apheresis devices.

Automated Apheresis

In general, currently used automated apheresis devices separate plasma and cellular elements by centrifugation. Depending on the separation chamber configuration and whether the blood is batched and processed, or whether separation, removal, and return are ongoing simultaneously, these systems are classified as intermittent (also called discontinuous) or continuous flow. Detailed descriptions of the various devices that are available are beyond the scope of this chapter, and the reader is referred to another source.[1] As a general rule, high-flow automated devices (1) are primed to allow for removal of all air from the circuit and maintenance of the patient's volume, (2) require venous access for inflow to the machine and blood return to the patient, (3) have a significant extracorporeal volume (ECV), which approaches 500 mL for adult configurations, (4) are programmable with patient sex, height, weight, and hematocrit entered at a keypad, as well as the blood

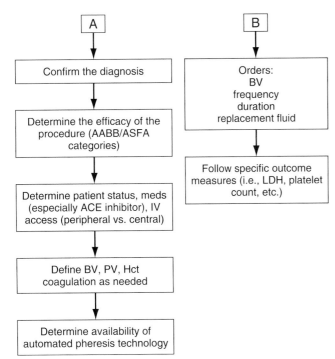

Figure 30-1 Flow diagram of initial apheresis steps for the consultant. AABB, American Association of Blood Banks; ASFA, American Society for Apheresis.

volume to be processed, (5) have decreasing efficiency in removal of the pathologic protein or formed element as the procedure progresses, and (6) require that an anticoagulant be added to the extracorporeal blood, usually citrate, so that clotting of blood in the apheresis tubing can be avoided. Each of these is discussed in greater detail in the following sections.

Priming

Machine tubing, or software, is most often primed with saline, and no residual air is left in the set. In anemic patients, bank blood may be used; this mitigates the dilution that the saline prime provides on machine startup. This is discussed further in the following section.

Venous Access

Any type of apheresis procedure requires adequate blood flow to and from the machine. This can be established via lines to peripheral or central veins or a combination of the two. However, placement of a central venous catheter increases the risks of infection and thrombosis and therefore should be used only when peripheral access is inadequate.[2] Frequently, peripheral access is attained through the large veins in the antecubital fossa. Ideally, the draw and return lines are located on different arms to prevent repeated processing of the same blood, or recirculation. Additionally, large-bore needles (i.e., 16- to 18-gauge) and draw lines capable of providing blood flow rates of up to 120 mL per minute are recommended. High hematocrit levels and plasma hyperviscosity may adversely affect flow rates. Large-bore, dual-lumen catheters designed for apheresis or hemodialysis can provide adequate flow and are recommended when central access is required. Peripherally inserted central venous catheters (PICCs), implantable ports, and standard double- and triple-lumen

catheters are generally considered inadequate and therefore should not be used.[3] For single events in emergency situations, femoral catheters may be used. Ultimately, a central venous catheter should be placed if apheresis is to be continued. Any disorder in which vascular tone is diminished may preclude the use of peripheral veins for access. Adverse effects related to vascular access are discussed in the following sections.

Extracorporeal Volume

Extracorporeal volume (ECV) is the volume of all blood elements removed from the body during the procedure. These consist of blood in the bowl or chamber, the tubing, and any other devices used during the procedure, including blood warmers or affinity columns. The ECV for each system is fixed and dependent on the type of equipment used and the type of procedure performed.[4] In asymptomatic adults and stable pediatric patients, extracorporeal blood volume should not exceed 15% of total blood volume (TBV), and intraprocedural extracorporeal hematocrit levels should be no less than 24% to avoid hypovolemia.[3] Usually, at these levels, no change is noted in cardiac output or oxygen consumption.[4,5] Anemic patients and small children, however, may be unable to tolerate this amount of extracorporeal red cell volume, although widely accepted criteria for preprocedural or intraprocedural transfusion in children are not available. Therefore, consideration must be given to the patient's condition, underlying cardiac and pulmonary disease, red cell volume (RCV), and chronicity of anemia. Several approaches, including priming of the machine with RBCs and preprocedural or intraprocedural transfusion, have been used to prevent intraprocedural hypovolemia and dilutional exacerbation of anemia. For patients in critical condition, cardiac monitoring may be warranted.

Programming and Input of Patient Values

Sex, height, weight, and hematocrit are entered on a keypad, as is the blood volume to be processed. This allows the machine to calculate the patient's TBV, RCV, and plasma volume. It is noteworthy that these algorithms used for the calculations may prove inaccurate for certain patient populations. Once started, automatic flow rate determination and time lead to display of processed blood volumes and predicted length of the procedure.

Total blood volume may be estimated by the consulting hematologist via several methods that are based on weight[6] or weight and height (Nadler's formula)[7]; however, these calculations may vary depending on the lean body mass of the individual and may overestimate an obese patient's blood volume and underestimate a muscular patient's blood volume.[3] Infants have greater blood volumes compared with adults, and men generally have greater blood volumes than equivalently sized women. Estimates of TBV that are based on patient age, sex, and weight have been published.[6] Red cell volume is directly related to the patient's hematocrit (RCV = TBV × pre-Hct %/100) and becomes more important in anemic patients. Additionally, it has been suggested that "intraprocedural hematocrit (assuming the patient is maintained in an isovolemic state during apheresis) may be more predictive of the patient's tolerance of temporary extracorporeal red cell loss than extracorporeal percentages."[3] In this circumstance, intraprocedural hematocrit may be calculated as

(RCV − Extracorporeal RCV)/TBV × 100. Total plasma volume (PV = TBV − RCV) is used to determine the appropriate apheresis dose, in milliliters to be processed. PV is generally underestimated in patients with large intravascular concentrations of paraproteins.[8–11]

Blood or Plasma Volume to be Processed and Apheresis Frequency

The amount of blood or plasma that should be processed in a single procedure is based on a balance between the amount of blood that must be processed to achieve a desired effect, the loss of efficiency that occurs as the procedure continues, and the extent of treatment that the patient can hemodynamically tolerate. In general, 1.5 blood or plasma volumes are processed per procedure, and procedures are ordered no more often than once per day. Procedure frequency and duration are disease specific and are noted below. Additionally, the patient's condition must be considered daily when aggressive daily apheresis is attempted. Further discussion is included in the individual disease sections.

Efficiency

TPE and cytapheresis remove patient plasma or cells, thus eliminating a part of the pathologic process and leading to clinical improvement. Because these procedures require large volume removal from the intravascular compartment, a replacement fluid (see later) is given to maintain intravascular volume, oxygen-carrying capacity, and other lost elements, such as normal coagulation proteins and immunoglobulins. This one-compartment model in essence suggests that the first aliquots of patient plasma or blood that are removed are completely of patient origin, whereas the later aliquots, with constant circulation and thus mixing, contain an ever increasing amount of normal replacement fluid and less of the pathologic component. Thus, with the first blood or plasma volume processed, a removal efficiency of approximately 60% can be considered as typical. With the second blood or plasma volume processed, approximately 25% efficiency can be sought, and for the third volume processed, efficiency is more toward 10%. This model and its development have been extensively reviewed.[12] If one assumes that the intravascular compartment is closed and the procedure is rapid (completed prior to intracompartment equilibration), as is the assumption in the one-compartment model, then substances predominantly located in the intravascular compartment (i.e., immunoglobulin [Ig]M and fibrinogen) are removed more efficiently than are those located predominantly in the extravascular compartment (i.e., IgG and albumin).[8,10,12,13] With this knowledge, different investigators have attempted to predict the efficiency of apheresis procedures through the use of several different mathematical models. Deriving the mathematical formulas that express the fractional rates of exchange during continuous and discontinuous flow procedures is beyond the scope of this chapter. However, Chopek and McCullough[8] used these formulas to plot a curve that predicts the fraction of a substance that remains in relation to the number of plasma volumes removed. When this curve is used, it appears that for removal of soluble substances, the most efficient and tolerable exchange consists of a 1.5 plasma volume.

The effectiveness of TPE and therapeutic cytapheresis depends not only on the relative volume of plasma or cells removed but also on their synthetic rate, biodistribution, and ongoing redistribution into the intravascular space.[12,14] This becomes especially important when one considers either the distribution within total body water of IgG synthesized by a malignant clone or the production of myeloblasts in acute leukemia.

Anticoagulation

Anticoagulation is a vital component of apheresis. Citrate, the most commonly used anticoagulant for maintaining extracorporeal blood in a fluid state, binds calcium, thereby inhibiting calcium-dependent clotting reactions. Several formulations, including ACD-A and ACD-B, are used in apheresis. Citrate is generally preferable to heparin, which can cause heparin-induced thrombocytopenia (HIT). As citrate chelates calcium, hypocalcemia may result; this can in turn lead to perioral tingling and even tetany. Some populations (including children) are at greater risk for citrate toxicity; therefore, heparin, or heparin combined with citrate, may be used.

Replacement Fluids

Many physicians choose colloid replacement fluid rather than crystalloid to prevent the complication of dependent edema due to hypoalbuminemia, as has been seen when saline alone is used as the replacement.[15] The two most commonly used replacement fluids are albumin and FFP. Albumin (5%) is considered the standard replacement fluid for most indications in TPE with rare exception; its use is not complicated, in general, by transmission of infectious diseases. Replacement with 5% albumin is superior to saline replacement in that it provides proteins and thus helps maintain oncotic pressure. However, this need is uncommon, and if 5% albumin is used, caution is advised.

FFP is the preferred replacement fluid when one wishes to infuse a component of FFP into the patient in addition to removing a pathologic substance. The two generally accepted diagnoses for which FFP is preferred are thrombotic thrombocytopenic purpura (TTP) and Refsum disease. FFP is associated with a 2 to 3 times higher incidence of adverse events, including allergic reactions and citrate toxicity, as compared with albumin.[16–18] Finally, after successive instances of TPE with albumin replacement, FFP may be used to replace depleted fibrinogen. This can be accomplished by ending the procedure with replacement of FFP rather than albumin. In this circumstance, the choice and amount of FFP used should be guided by measurements attained through regular laboratory-based coagulation tests.

Evaluation and Care of the Patient

Prior to the first procedure, baseline laboratory values, including hematocrit or hemoglobin, electrolytes, platelet count, prothrombin time (PT), partial thromboplastin time (PTT), and perhaps ionized calcium (if citrate anticoagulation is to be used), should be acquired. Cardiac, renal, and hepatic function should be evaluated in patients prior to their first procedure. Other tests, such as fibrinogen and specific factor levels, may be indicated prior to the procedure if patients have known coagulation disorders. Knowledge of these baseline values is necessary in planning fluid volume management, modifying the amount of anti-coagulation to be used, and determining the appropriate schedule for and frequency of the procedure.[19]

It is generally accepted that dehydration should be corrected in most patients before the procedure is performed. In patients who are volume sensitive (i.e., end-stage renal disease), the tendency is to avoid rehydration; however, these patients tend to have excessive extravascular rather than intravascular fluid and remain at risk for intravascular hypovolemia. Patients with hypoproteinemia are at greater risk for intraprocedural hypovolemia. Alternatively, patients with elevated serum protein levels (i.e., multiple myeloma) and thus expanded intravascular volumes may receive crystalloid solutions for replacement in order to decrease intravascular volume, thus allowing for more efficient removal of the offending immunoglobulin.[3]

Medications such as vasopressors may be continued during apheresis procedures provided patients do not develop hypertension or tachycardia.[3] Given the short half-lives of most pressors, drug removal due to the procedure has only minimal effects on therapeutic blood levels. Patients who have a history of transfusion reactions may be premedicated with antipyretics and/or antihistamines to reduce future events. Regularly prescribed medication regimens should be adjusted so that medication is taken after apheresis when possible. Protein-bound medications should be given after the procedure is performed, and levels should be monitored when appropriate. Angiotensin-converting enzyme (ACE) inhibitors ideally should be discontinued 72 hours prior to transfusion to reduce allergic reactions (discussed in greater detail later).

Logistics

Many medical centers do not have their own pheresis equipment, and such work is contracted out to other facilities or consignees. This practice often delays the actual implementation of pheresis.

Other logistic barriers to the initiation of pheresis therapy include confirmation of the suspected diagnosis, informed consent, inadequate venous access (particularly with inertia of placement, as is frequently caused by those who actually insert such devices with undue concern for thrombocytopenia), availability and thawing of FFP, and other considerations. These issues often result in the accumulation of several (5–8) hours between the decision to order pheresis and actual implementation of the procedure.

Frequently, a single clinical service (typically hematology) oversees this operation, providing the equipment, personnel, and technical support for all patients who need pheresis, including those with neurologic, renal, or transplant rejection indications. Along with informed consent, it is advised that clinicians should obtain documentation stating that although the hematology service may be providing the technique, decisions regarding frequency, timing, and duration of pheresis sessions are made under the guidance of the service that is providing clinical discernment.

THERAPEUTIC PLASMA EXCHANGE

In 1985, the American Medical Association (AMA), in an attempt to guide clinicians in medical decision making,

assembled a panel of experts to review all evidence regarding the efficacy of plasmapheresis for various indications. These guidelines have been updated and revised by several different agencies since that time, including the American Association of Blood Banks (AABB), the American Society for Apheresis (ASFA), and the American Academy of Neurology. These potential indications have been classified into four categories on the basis of the amount and quality of supporting evidence favoring their use. Category I is reserved for those indications for which plasmapheresis has proved effective as a primary or standard therapy in controlled trials. Category II includes those diseases or syndromes for which plasmapheresis is supportive or adjunctive to primary therapy, or for which uncontrolled case series or reports suggest a benefit. Category III includes those syndromes for which the data are insufficient to indicate whether TPE is beneficial, and Category IV diagnoses are those for which TPE has been shown in controlled trials to provide no benefit. In the sections that follow here, the indications and rationales for apheresis for hematologic disorders (Categories I and II) are presented, as are those for nonhematologic disorders (Category I only) (Table 30-1).

Hematologic Disorders

Thrombotic Thrombocytopenic Pupura

Thrombotic thrombocytopenic purpura (TTP), often classified as a thrombotic microangiopathy (TMA), is a microangiopathic hemolytic anemia that results from the absence or inhibition of von Willebrand–cleaving protease (VWF-cp) activity, which may lead to the accumulation of ultra-large von Willebrand factor (ULVWF) multimers in plasma (see Chapter 24). These multimers produce platelet clumping under high shear stress in the microvasculature, thus causing thrombocytopenia, renal dysfunction, brain ischemia, and intravascular fragmentation of red blood cells. The classic patient presentation consists of fever, renal impairment, thrombocytopenia, and central nervous system impairment; symptoms range from mental status alterations to seizures and coma.[20] In 1996, the VWF-cp was shown to be a plasma protease that is now called ADAMTS-13 (*a dis*integrin *a*nd *m*etalloprotease with *t*hrombospondin subunits); it cleaves VWF multimers at the 842Tyr-843Met peptide bond.[21,22] Patients with the congenital form of TTP lack a functional enzyme altogether because of mutations in the ADAMTS-13 gene.[23] However, idiopathic or acquired TTP is the result of an inhibitory autoantibody to the protease ADAMTS-13.[24–27]

RATIONALE FOR TPE

The presence of an antibody inhibitor of ADAMTS-13 and the accumulation of ULVWF multimers in the plasma suggest immediately that the removal of such pathologic entities would result in improvement in patients with TTP. It is interesting to note that in TTP, the use of FFP as the replacement fluid has the added benefit of infusing normal donor ADAMTS-13, which is also beneficial. Indeed, FFP was originally used to treat patients with all forms of TTP, and it may be infused if plasma exchange is not immediately available. In those patients without antibody to the cleaving protease (congenital TTP), only 10 to 15 mL/kg of FFP infused every 2 to 3 weeks can achieve remission;

Table 30-1 Indication Categories For Therapeutic Apheresis

Disease	Procedure	Indication Category
Renal and Metabolic Diseases		
Antiglomerular basement membrane antibody disease	Plasma exchange	I
Rapidly progressive glomerulonephritis	Plasma exchange	II
Hemolytic-uremic syndrome	Plasma exchange	III
Renal transplantation		
Rejection	Plasma exchange	IV
Sensitization	Plasma exchange	III
Recurrent focal glomerulosclerosis	Plasma exchange	III
Heart transplant rejection	Plasma exchange	III
	Photopheresis	III
Acute hepatic failure	Plasma exchange	III
Familial hypercholesterolemia	Selective adsorption	I
	Plasma exchange	II
Overdose or poisoning	Plasma exchange	III
Phytanic acid storage (Refsum) disease	Plasma exchange	I
Autoimmune and Rheumatic Diseases		
Cryoglobulinemia	Plasma exchange	II
Idiopathic thrombocytopenic purpura	Immunoadsorption	II
Raynaud phenomenon	Plasma exchange	III
Vasculitis	Plasma exchange	III
Autoimmune hemolytic anemia	Plasma exchange	III
Rheumatoid arthritis	Immunoadsorption	II
	Lymphoplasmapheresis	II
	Plasma exchange	IV
Scleroderma or progressive systemic sclerosis (PSS)	Plasma exchange	III
Systemic lupus erythematosus	Plasma exchange	III
Hematologic Diseases		
ABO-mismatched marrow transplant	RBC removal (marrow)	I
	Plasma exchange (recipient)	II
Erythrocytosis or polycythemia vera	Phlebotomy	I
	Erythrocytapheresis	II
Leukocytosis and thrombocytosis	Cytapheresis	I
Thrombotic thrombocytopenic purpura	Plasma exchange	I
Posttransfusion purpura	Plasma exchange	I
Sickle cell disease	RBC exchange	I
Myeloma, paraproteinemia, or hyperviscosity	Plasma exchange	II
Myeloma or acute renal failure	Plasma exchange	II
Coagulation factor inhibitors	Plasma exchange	II
Aplastic anemia or pure RBC aplasia	Plasma exchange	III
Cutaneous T-cell lymphoma	Photopheresis	I
	Leukapheresis	III
HDN	Plasma exchange	III
PLT alloimmunization and refractoriness	Plasma exchange	III
	Immunoadsorption	III
Malaria or babesiosis	RBC exchange	III
Neurologic Disorders		
Chronic inflammatory demyelinating polyradiculoneuropathy	Plasma exchange	I
Acute inflammatory demyelinating polyradiculoneuropathy	Plasma exchange	I
Lambert-Eaton myasthenic syndrome	Plasma exchange	II
Multiple sclerosis		
Relapsing	Plasma exchange	III
Progressive	Plasma exchange	III
	Lymphocytapheresis	III
Myasthenia gravis	Plasma exchange	I
Acute central nervous system inflammatory demyelinating disease	Plasma exchange	II
Paraneoplastic neurologic syndromes	Plasma exchange	III
	Immunoadsorption	III
Demyelinating polyneuropathy with IgG and IgA	Plasma exchange	I
	Immunoadsorption	III
Sydenham chorea	Plasma exchange	II
Polyneuropathy with IgM (with or without Waldenström macro-globulinemia)	Plasma exchange	II
	Immunoadsorption	III
Cryoglobulinemia with polyneuropathy	Plasma exchange	II
Multiple myeloma with polyneuropathy	Plasma exchange	III

(Continued)

Table 30-1 Indication Categories For Therapeutic Apheresis (Cont'd.)

Disease	Procedure	Indication Category
POEMS syndrome	Plasma exchange	III
Systemic (AL) amyloidosis	Plasma exchange	IV
Polymyositis or dermatomyositis	Plasma exchange	III
	Leukapheresis	IV
Inclusion body myositis	Plasma exchange	III
	Leukapheresis	IV
Rasmussen encephalitis	Plasma exchange	III
Stiff-man syndrome	Plasma exchange	III
PANDAS	Plasma exchange	II

ABO, blood type; HDN, hemolytic disease of the newborn; IgG, immunoglobulin G; IgA, immunoglobulin A; IgM, immunoglobulin M; PLT, platelet; PANDAS, pediatric autoimmune neuropsychiatric disorders; POEMS, polyneuropathy, organomegaly, endocrinopathy, M component, and skin changes; RBC, red blood cell.

patients with acquired TTP usually require total plasma exchange.[28,29] Several investigators have studied whether TPE is indicated in those patients with clinical features of the disease but without evidence of autoantibody-mediated severe ADAMTS-13 deficiency.[30-32] The authors of a recent review concluded that on the basis of limited available evidence, TPE was indicated for idiopathic TTP, regardless of ADAMTS-13 activity level.[33]

USE OF TPE

TPE is first-line therapy for idiopathic TTP and should be commenced at the time of diagnosis.[34,35] Plasma infusion at 30 mg/kg/day may be used while TPE is being arranged.[36] Additionally, evidence suggests that corticosteroids may be helpful in suppressing autoantibody formation; many authorities recommend daily doses of up to 200 mg of prednisone.[37] However, because evidence supporting their clinical efficacy is lacking, corticosteroids are typically adjunctive or are given to patients for whom primary therapy has failed.[38]

Studies have shown that clinical response to TPE generally occurs within approximately 1 week (mean, 7 to 8 days); three of four patients respond within 2 weeks, and 25% may require up to 4 weeks of therapy.[39-41] However, the rate of recurrence is high (20% to 50%).[39,42-44] In a recent comprehensive review, Willis and Banderenko[41] summarized the reasons (including scarcity of accepted definitions for recurrence and remission, lack of an adequate test for remission, variable times to response and to treatment) why physicians may have difficulty in determining disease resolution, which leads to confusion regarding when TPE should be discontinued.[41] The AABB and ASFA have suggested that TPE should be continued until the patient demonstrates a platelet count of 100,000–150,000/µL and normal lactate dehydrogenase (LDH) for 2 consecutive days.[41] Others have suggested that 1.5 plasma volume exchanges with FFP replacement should be performed daily until neurologic signs and symptoms have resolved and platelet count and LDH values have normalized (some have advocated continuation of TPE for 5 days after remission).[37,45] Still others use a regimen of 1.5 plasma volumes for the first 3 days followed by 1 plasma volume daily.[46] The transition from daily to every-other-day TPE ("tapering") has not proved effective[39,47] but is frequently used anyway, most likely reflecting uncertainty among physicians regarding when therapy should be discontinued.

Despite these measures, some patients do not respond to therapy or they relapse when TPE is discontinued. In such situations, many practitioners switch from FFP to cryosupernatant as the replacement fluid because the latter consists of reduced numbers of ULVWF multimers, although recent data suggest that no benefit may be derived from this practice.[48,49] Recently, several case series and reports have successfully employed rituximab, a chimeric monoclonal antibody directed at the CD20 antigen expressed on the surface of B lymphocytes, for the treatment of TPE-dependent patients who appear refractory to other immunosuppressive therapies (e.g., corticosteroids, azathioprine, cyclosporin A, splenectomy). Rituximab is typically given in weekly infusions of 375 mg per meter squared.

THROMBOTIC MICROANGIOPATHIES OTHER THAN IDIOPATHIC TTP AND TPE

Although the clinical manifestations of TTP and other TMAs such as AIDS-associated TTP, hemolytic-uremic syndrome (HUS), and drug-induced TTP may be similar, the use of TPE for management of these disorders is controversial, and the mechanisms of pathogenesis are likely to be different. In diarrhea-associated HUS, TPE has shown no clinical benefit.[50] Lämmle and associates[33] recently reviewed the arguments for and against TPE in cases in which the ADAMTS-13 level was normal or moderately decreased; they cited only one study in which it was shown that response to TPE, number of subsequent exacerbations, number of apheresis procedures needed to reach remission, and death rate were not different between those with and without severe ADAMTS-13 deficiency. However, the relapse rate was higher among severely deficient patients.[30] These facts may be due at least in part to the absence of a universally accepted and reproducible ADAMTS-13 assay.

Patients with TMAs associated with hematopoietic stem cell transplantation, malignancy, and anticancer drugs have demonstrated measurable ADAMTS-13 activity; pregnancy-associated TMA has been reported to involve severe ADAMTS-13 deficiency.[33] Therefore, the likelihood that TPE would be effective therapy in patients with the former indications is unlikely, although TPE may be beneficial for the treatment of pregnancy-induced TTP. No randomized clinical trials have addressed these indications.

TPE (in conjunction with highly active antiretroviral therapy [HAART] therapy) has been used to treat patients with HIV-associated TTP and has been shown in several

IV

case series to be beneficial.[51,52] In one case report, plasmapheresis was ineffective in treating a human immunodeficiency virus (HIV)-positive patient with TTP; however, when antiviral therapy was started, the patient clinically improved.[53] Because no randomized clinical trials have addressed this issue, it is unknown whether TPE provides added benefit over antiviral therapy alone.

Posttransfusion Purpura

Posttransfusion purpura (PTP) is a rare disorder that is characterized by severe thrombocytopenia (<10,000/μL) and destruction of the recipient's and the donor's transfused platelets 7 to 10 days after transfusion. In general, PTP is self limited but may result in bleeding; fatal intracranial hemorrhage has been reported in 10% of cases.[54,55] Previously nontransfused, multiparous women between the ages of 30 and 80 years are most frequently affected; however, cases have been reported in men as well.[56,57] The pathogenesis of PTP remains largely unknown; however, several hypotheses have addressed the destruction of recipient and donor platelets. These hypotheses have been extensively reviewed and summarized below.[58]

RATIONALE FOR TPE

In most cases, alloantibodies to platelet membrane antigens (most notably, HPA-1a) and human leukocyte antigens (HLAs) have been implicated.[57,59–67] Soluble antigen has been found in antigen-positive donors, and circulating immune complexes have been identified in a patient with PTP.[68,69] Finally, some have advocated that passive adsorption of platelet antigen onto recipient platelets is causative.[68] Each of these possibilities leads one to consider that TPE may be effective in the management of PTP. A good review of these mechanisms has been recently reported.[58]

USE OF TPE

Given current pathologic hypotheses that the platelet destruction observed in PTP may be antibody mediated, removal of the offending antibody by TPE emerged as a potential therapy. Anecdotally, TPE has been successful; however, no clinical trials have assessed the efficacy of TPE versus intravenous immune globulin (IVIg) in the treatment of patients with PTP. Although PTP is a Category I indication for TPE, it is generally reserved for those patients who are refractory to IVIg or steroids, or who are significantly hemorrhaging. Albumin is typically used as the replacement fluid; however, in coagulopathic patients, FFP may be used.

ABO-Incompatible Bone Marrow Transplantation

ABO-incompatible bone marrow transplantation (BMT) may result in acute hemolysis, renal failure, disseminated intravascular coagulation (DIC), or death at the time of marrow infusion.[55] Historically, plasmapheresis was used to reduce the recipient's isohemagglutinin titer prior to transplantation.[55,70–73] However, bone marrow processing now prepares progenitor cell concentrates from harvested bone marrow with minimal residual red cell contamination.[88] Thus, at present, TPE is rarely done for patients with ABO-incompatible transplants; this is considered a Category II indication by the ASFA and a Category III indication by the AABB.

Myeloma

Plasma cell myeloma is characterized by the abnormal production of monoclonal antibodies, skeletal destruction, and anemia. In all, 10% to 30% of patients with myeloma present with renal failure.[74–76] Of those with myeloma, 5% (50% with Waldenström macroglobulinemia) develop hyperviscosity syndrome, which may include shortness of breath, cutaneous or mucosal bleeding, blurred vision or diplopia, and neurologic symptoms ranging from headaches and dizziness to seizures and coma. These symptoms are due to the rheologic effects of the paraprotein, which may be removed through TPE.

RATIONALE FOR TPE

TPE and immunoadsorption (IA) columns have been used to remove the pathologic proteins in myeloma. TPE is considered first-line therapy for hyperviscosity syndromes and has been used with varying results for acute renal failure. Three randomized, control trials have evaluated the use of TPE in acute renal failure associated with myeloma.[76–78] The most recent and largest clinical trial found no difference in outcomes in death versus dialysis dependence, or in glomerular filtration rate (GFR), between those patients receiving TPE and controls (who were given chemotherapy and dialysis only).[76] For symptomatic hyperviscosity syndrome, immediate TPE followed by disease-directed therapy is generally considered appropriate. Mehta and Singhal[79] reported anecdotal success (i.e., relief of symptoms) after several (two or three) 3-liter exchanges involving 5% albumin replacement. Acute renal failure and hyperviscosity syndrome associated with myeloma are considered by the ASFA and AABB to be category II indications for TPE and IA.

Other Hematologic Diseases

The removal of coagulation factor inhibitors in patients with factor deficiencies due to preformed antibodies to transfused products is considered by the ASFA and AABB to be a category II indication for TPE. The role of TPE or IA is to quickly decrease high antibody titers, thereby improving response to other therapies such as IVIg, factor VIII concentrates, prednisone, cyclophosphamide, and rituximab. Several authors have advocated combination therapy for inducing tolerance in these patients; however, no controlled trials have been performed.[80–84]

Aplastic anemia/pure red cell aplasia, hemolytic disease of the newborn, and platelet alloimmunization and refractoriness are considered Category III indications. IA for the treatment of platelet alloimmunization and refractoriness is also considered a Category III indication for TPE. For these diseases, TPE (or IA in some cases) is used in conjunction with other therapies or when first-line therapies are contraindicated or are not technically feasible.[55] No controlled, randomized trials have been performed for these indications.

Renal and Metabolic Disorders—Category I

Rapidly Progressive Glomerulonephritis

Goodpasture disease (GPD; also called antiglomerular basement antibody disease), Wegener granulomatosis, and systemic vasculitis may result in rapidly progressive glomerulonephritis (RPGN), characterized by inflammation of the glomeruli with necrosis and a crescent-shaped appearance. In GPD, immunofluorescence reveals the presence of linear deposits of an IgG antiglomerular basement membrane antibody that targets a domain specific to type IV collagen. Patients experience deterioration in renal function over a period of weeks,[85] which may result in irreversible kidney damage. Pulmonary hemorrhage is another common symptom of GPD.[86] Other inflammatory glomerular diseases (e.g., Wegener syndrome) have similar clinical manifestations that include RPGN and pulmonary hemorrhage.

RATIONALE FOR TPE

Each disease that results in RPGN has a different pathogenic mechanism. In GPD, but not in other forms of RPGN, a circulating pathologic antibody is central to the disease. Because TPE is effective in antibody removal, many studies have shown that it offers a successful therapeutic approach.

USE OF TPE

GPD is considered a Category I indication for TPE; aggressive therapy, consisting of TPE with cyclophosphamide and pulse methylprednisolone, is advocated by most authorities.[87] Daily 4-liter exchanges have been used for 7 days as initial therapy.[88–92] This regimen is generally followed by daily or every other day exchanges for the second week, or alternatively, until antibody titers are suppressed or pulmonary hemorrhage has ceased. Albumin (5%) given alone or in combination with FFP is generally recommended, except in those patients with pulmonary hemorrhage or eminent or recent renal biopsy in whom albumin replacement may cause a dilutional coagulopathy and worsen bleeding.[85] TPE in conjunction with prednisone or cyclophosphamide has proved effective in treating all antibody-mediated forms of RPGN.[93,94] Because GPD is usually self limited, short-term therapy (<6 months) is generally all that is required. In addition, early treatment has been advocated by Levy and coworkers[95] after worse outcomes were noted in patients with higher creatinine levels at presentation.

Primary therapy for those forms of RPGN that are *not* antibody mediated, cytoplasmic antineutrophil cytoplasmic antibody (c-ANCA) mediated (e.g., Wegener syndrome), or immune complex mediated (e.g., cryoglobulinemia) is focused on treating the underlying disease[85]; the role of TPE is controversial. The AABB and the ASFA classify antiglomerular basement membrane–negative RPGN as a Category II indication for TPE. Some studies appear to show no benefit[96,97]; others advocate the use of TPE in a secondary role to immunosuppressive therapy or in patients who present with severe renal disease.[88–91,98–100] In a recent case report of diffuse alveolar hemorrhage in a patient with Wegener syndrome and a high-titer c-ANCA, the authors advocate the use of TPE and call for a reevaluation of Category II status for this indication.[101]

Protein A–based immunoadsorption columns are touted as a method of selective extraction of IgG antibodies; they differ from TPE in that non-IgG plasma proteins are returned to the patient along with other blood components, abrogating the need for replacement fluids. These are discussed in greater detail later. Case reports that describe the use of this method present conflicting data,

especially with regard to improvement in renal function.[102–104] Vasculitis presumably secondary to percutaneous acetic acid injection (PAA-I) therapy has been reported and should be considered prior to its use.[105]

Refsum Disease

Hereditary motor and sensory neuropathy type IV, or Refsum disease, is a rare autosomal recessive disorder that is characterized by the inability to oxidize phyantic acid; it is mentioned briefly because the AABB and the ASFA have classified it is a Category I indication for TPE. The defective enzyme is phytanoyl–coenzyme A hydroxylase, which catalyzes the breakdown of phytanic to pristanic acid. Because phytanic acid is found in a variety of foodstuffs, dietary restriction is the main therapy; however, TPE has been useful in quickly reducing phyantic acid levels, which may be desirable given that visual and hearing impairments may not respond to therapy.[106,107] Also, FFP is used as the replacement fluid; it may provide phytanoyl–coenzyme A hydroxylase, thus promoting symptom amelioration.

Neurologic Disorders—Category I

Guillain-Barré Syndrome/Acute Inflammatory Demyelinating Polyneuropathy

Guillain-Barré syndrome (GBS) occurs with an annual incidence of 0.6 to 2 cases per 100,000 population and is thus the most commonly occurring paralytic disorder.[108–113] A number of variants or subtypes of GBS, including acute inflammatory/demyelinating polyneuropathy (AIDP) and chronic inflammatory/demyelinating polyneuropathy (CIDP), have been classified (see later). AIDP, the most common subtype of GBS, is usually characterized as an acute peripheral neuropathy with features of weakness, hyporeflexia or areflexia, and increased cerebrospinal fluid (CSF) protein in the absence of a pleocytosis. Infections (e.g., *Campylobacter jejuni*) frequently precede AIDP[114]; these are believed to be caused by damage to neuronal axons caused by macrophages. Activated T cells cross the blood–brain barrier, where they encounter a cross-reactive antigen in the endoneurium and release cytokines that activate macrophages, which then invade myelin sheaths and denude neuronal axons.[115,116]

RATIONALE FOR TPE

Although the precise causes of GBS and AIDP remain unknown, an antibody-mediated mechanism appears likely; thus, the fact that TPE has been used in treating these disorders is understandable. Indeed, several large and small randomized, controlled trials have reported success in decreasing the severity of acute illness and reducing the length of hospital stay and recovery time with the use of TPE.[117–122]

USE OF TPE

At this time, experts advocate instituting TPE (usually, five to six 1.5 plasma volume procedures performed over 2 weeks) within 14 days of symptom onset.[119,122,123] Cessation of TPE prior to control of the active phase of the disease may increase the risk of relapse.[124] Albumin (5%) is commonly used for replacing removed plasma. Studies have shown better response rates with four 1.5-L volume exchanges for colloid replacement than with two; no further improvement has been noted with six exchanges.[121] Others, however, have shown no comparative difference in outcome whether patients are treated with IVIg or TPE.[125] Therefore, the American Academy of Neurology recommended in 2003 in a practice parameter that TPE or IVIg should be used to treat patients with GBS who have lost the ability to walk.[126] However, questions remain regarding treatment failure and whether therapy is effective if delayed.[116] Finally, Dada and Kaplan[127] reported four cases of GBS with axonal involvement in which patients failed IVIg therapy but improved with TPE.

Chronic Inflammatory Demyelinating Polyneuropathy

CIDP is a chronically progressive or relapsing symmetrical, sensorimotor disorder. Nerve conduction studies demonstrate a predominant process of demyelination.

RATIONALE FOR TPE

In two small, prospective, double-blind studies, TPE appeared to show short-term benefit that was reversed when treatment was stopped.[128,129] Dyck and colleagues[129] randomly assigned 29 patients with static or worsening disease to receive TPE or sham exchange. One third of those who received TPE were significantly improved, and one third showed a trend toward improvement. In a crossover study, Hahn and coworkers[130] analyzed 18 patients with chronic progressive or relapsing disease. They concluded that TPE with concurrent immunosuppressive therapy was beneficial in both types of CIDP. In addition, they found that patients who were nonresponsive to TPE were improved by treatment with prednisone. Four randomized, double-blind trials evaluated the use of IVIg.[130–133] These trials reported short-term improvement. Dyck and associates[134] described no difference in short-term improvement with the use of IVIg or TPE. Recently, a joint task force of the European Federation of Neurological Societies (EFNS) and the Peripheral Nerve Society (PNS) published new recommendations for the treatment of patients with CIDP.[135] These guidelines suggest that IVIg or prednisone should be used as first-line therapy. TPE should be reserved for patients who are nonresponsive to first-line therapy.

USE OF TPE

According to Hahn and colleagues,[128] two to three exchanges per week should be performed until improvement has been established. Then, exchanges may be tapered over several months.

Myasthenia Gravis

Myasthenia gravis (MG) is an autoimmune disorder that is characterized by the presence of IgG antibodies directed against a portion of the acetylcholine receptor, thereby inhibiting electrical stimulation via acetylcholine at the neuromuscular junction. It occurs at all ages, but similar to other autoimmune disorders, it has a female predominance when occurring at a younger age. Clinically, patients experience weakness of voluntary muscle groups that worsens with exercise. In most patients (85%), MG generalizes after only 3 years, affecting the limbs, the bulbar muscles, and the diaphragm.[136] Between 2% and 3% of patients with MG experience a crisis each year.[137]

RATIONALE FOR TPE

TPE can quickly reduce the quantity of circulating antibodies to the acetylcholine receptor and is usually prescribed in conjunction with immunosuppressive therapy.[138] TPE is especially important in treating severe exacerbations when disease involves the bulbar muscles and the diaphragm. Patients will generally present with difficulty swallowing, aspiration, and/or respiratory compromise.

USE OF TPE

Although cholinesterase inhibitors and steroid and nonsteroid immunosuppressants are typically the mainstay therapies for MG,[139] TPE should be used in situations in which response to pharmacologic therapy is insufficient, or during a myasthenic crisis. TPE, when used for the treatment of an acute myasthenic crisis, should be performed by removing 1.5 plasma volumes daily and replacing with 5% albumin until the patient has clinically improved.[140,141] Some clinicians suggest that tapering of schedules (TPE performed once or twice a month) may be beneficial until a stable response has been achieved.[138,142] Only a few clinical trials have compared the use of IVIg with TPE in MG crisis; the largest of these, conducted by Gajdos and associates, showed similar efficacy.[143] Recently, an extensive review of the literature regarding the efficacy of IVIg in the treatment of patients with neurologic disease (including comparisons with other therapies) was published.[144]

THERAPEUTIC CYTAPHERESIS

Plateletpheresis

Thrombocytosis may occur as the result of a reactive process or as a primary clonal hematologic disorder such as essential thrombocythemia (ET) and other myeloproliferative disorders (see Chapter 18). Patients with abnormally high platelet counts may be at risk for thrombotic and hemorrhagic complications. In fact, half of all patients with ET present with vasomotor, thrombotic, or hemorrhagic complications.[145] Thromboses occur in arterial and venous circulation and in the microvasculature, as well as in large arteries in the brain and heart.[146]

Erythromelalgia is an example of one such thrombotic complication. It is a presenting feature in nearly half of all cases of ET and is characterized as a painful, burning sensation in the palms and soles that is accompanied by redness and warmth, which occur as a result of platelet aggregation that leads to microvascular thrombosis of acral vessels.[147]

Rationale for Plateletpheresis

Studies have shown that the platelets in ET are morphologically and functionally abnormal.[147] However, neither the platelet count nor standard clinical laboratory tests such as platelet aggregation studies or bleeding time have been helpful in predicting who is at greater risk for thrombotic events.[146,148] Evidence indicates that patients over the age of 60 years and particularly those with a previous thrombosis are at increased risk for a future thrombosis.[145,149]

In these patients, it may be beneficial to attempt to lower the platelet count to prevent recurrent thrombosis.

Use of Plateletpheresis

The ASFA and AABB have classified thrombocytosis as a Category I indication for cytapheresis. The goal of TPE is simply to reduce the platelet count. Adami,[150] in a study of 132 patients who received plateletpheresis over a 15-year period, found that patients with ET and elevated platelet counts (greater than 1,500,000/μL) had a significantly greater number of symptoms than did those with lower platelet counts. Tefferi and associates[151] advocated the use of cytoreductive therapy in high-risk patients (those age 60 years or older and/or with a history of thrombosis) aimed at maintaining platelet levels below 400,000/μL. However, as Greist points out in her comprehensive review of the subject,[146] drug therapy may take days to weeks to achieve maximum effect. Therefore, she and others believe that plateletpheresis is acutely indicated in patients with ongoing life-threatening organ dysfunction from an acute bleed or thrombotic episode (e.g., cerebrovascular ischemia).[55,146,148,152]

No studies have determined the exact platelet count for which plateletpheresis is required. Also, it is not known what absolute platelet count leads to relief of clinical symptoms, or what an adequate postpheresis platelet count should be. General practice is to cytoreduce at >1,000,000/μL abnormal platelets; plateletpheresis is usually performed until clinical symptoms have resolved. Some authorities recommend the use of plateletpheresis at counts between 500,000 and 1,000,000/μL, depending on the rate of increase noted in measured platelet count. In one study, patients with elevated platelet counts (1,000,000 to 3,500,000/μL) attained a 35% to 50% reduction in platelet count after a single exchange of 1.25 blood volumes.[153]

The use of plateletpheresis in ET for indications other than acute events or for the prevention of a recurrent event is controversial. For instance, it is unclear whether platelet reduction is of benefit in the management of ET during pregnancy,[151,154–156] in the perioperative setting,[157,158] or for reactive or secondary thrombocytosis.[146] Evidence consists primarily of case reports and small case series.

Leukapheresis

Leukostasis is the term that is used to describe rheologic abnormalities that may occur in the cerebral and pulmonary microvasculature of patients with acute leukemia who present with high blast counts—usually >100,000 blasts/μL, or hyperleukocytosis (HL).[159–161] The incidence of hyperleukocytosis varies according to age at diagnosis and type of leukemia (i.e., acute myeloid leukemia [AML] or acute lymphocytic leukemia [ALL]). Occurrence ranges from 5% to 30%.[162] The clinical presentation also varies from exertional dyspnea to severe respiratory distress and stupor to coma. Vascular complications include retinal hemorrhage, retinal vein thrombosis, myocardial infarction, acute limb ischemia, and renal vein thrombosis.[163] DIC occurs in 15% to 40% of patients.[162] HL has been associated with a higher incidence of fatal hemorrhage during the first week of chemotherapy[164] and a shorter duration of complete remission. The pathogenesis leading to

the development of clinical manifestations is not entirely known. Data suggest that chemokine-induced interactions between leukemic cells and the target organ endothelium may be responsible for the vascular disruption that ultimately leads to the end organ damage observed. Porcu and associates[162] have described these potential mechanisms in a recent comprehensive review.

Rationale for Leukapheresis

The goal of leukapheresis in the setting of leukostasis, leukemia, and a high blast count is to remove circulating leukemic blasts from the peripheral blood; leukapheresis prior to induction therapy has been advocated. However, whether leukapheresis leads to improved survival and clinical outcomes is controversial. Some studies have shown that early death is more frequent when HL is present.[165,166] The presumed advantages of leukapheresis involve the removal of large numbers of circulating blasts and the recruitment of marginated leukemic cell aggregates away from the microvasculature and extramedullary sites and into the intravascular space. Other investigators have found evidence to suggest that leukoreduction may mitigate the tumor lysis syndrome and hemorrhage that may occur as a result of induction therapy.[167] Additionally, it is unknown when, how, and for how long leukapheresis may be used effectively.

Porcu and colleagues[168] studied early death after leukoreduction with a target postprocedural white blood cell (WBC) count of 50,000/μL. Although this level was achieved, no difference in WBC count was observed at the time of death, nor at discontinuation of leukapheresis, between those who died within 1 week of therapy and those who survived.[168] Therefore, investigators concluded that "the value of leukapheresis in the management of leukostasis (was) not established." Investigators, including Porcu and coworkers, have questioned whether qualitative changes in leukemic cells are more responsible for the disease than is the actual quantity of cells. However, leukapheresis for the indication of leukocytosis is still considered a Category I indication by the ASFA and the AABB.

Use of Leukapheresis

Practically, leukapheresis is a more complicated procedure than plateletpheresis because of the size of the cells and the rapid synthetic rate of the malignancy. The standard approach requires the processing of 8 to 10 liters of blood during the procedure[55,169] and measurement of the postprocedure count. Some clinicians prescribe daily cytapheresis until the blast count, or the WBC count, is <100,000/μL.

Erythrocytapheresis (Red Blood Cell Exchange)

Initially, red blood cell exchange (RCE) was indicated only for acute complications associated with hemoglobinopathies. In the treatment of patients with sickle cell disease, RCE is a Category I indication. RCE is also used in the treatment of infectious and metabolic diseases. The use of RCE for the treatment of protozoan infections (e.g., malaria and babesia) is considered a Category III indication; its use for erythrocytosis or polycythemia vera is considered a Category II indication. Current studies are exploring the use of RCE as prophylactic erythrocytapheresis to prevent iron accumulation, in lieu of chronic simple transfusions, in patients with sickle cell disease.

Sickle Cell Disease

Hemolytic anemia, pain crisis, and organ ischemia are classic features of sickle cell disease (SCD), which is caused by a single amino acid (Glu to Val) substitution in the β-globin gene of hemoglobin, leading to the formation of $β^S$ globin chains (see Chapter 47). Deoxygenated (and even poorly oxygenated) hemoglobin (Hb) S–containing cells are poorly deformable and have an increased propensity for polymerization, causing the characteristic shape change observed on peripheral smear—the sickle cell.[170,171] It was originally believed that the end organ damage observed in SCD was solely attributable to the polymerization of these cells, which made them less deformable and therefore apt to occlude the microvasculature. This would result in even further sickling caused by local stasis and hypoxia.[172] However, it is currently believed that the mechanism of tissue infarction is more complicated than just physical obstruction. Current theories and data suggest that a complex interaction occurs between these abnormal cells, inflammatory responses, and the activated endothelium that is very important in the adhesion of these cells to the endovasculature.[173–180] Furthermore, it is as yet unclear whether sickle cells that promote occlusion beget inflammatory responses, or whether inflammation triggers acute events, including stroke. Hebbel and associates[180] argue that multiple, overlapping factors are probably responsible; however, "the process of vaso-occlusion, regardless of its proximate cause, causes tissue ischemia and injury..."

RATIONALE OF TPE IN SCD

Because sickle cells are themselves pathologic, removal of those cells is advantageous. RCE makes it possible to remove these cells while replacing them with predominantly hemoglobin A–containing cells, thereby maintaining a net balance in iron accumulation. RCE has been used historically as first-line therapy in the management of acute sickle crisis to prevent end organ failure and for perioperative treatment of patients with SCD. Admixtures of Hb A and S improve overall solubility and reduce polymerization.

Replacement of sickle cells with Hb A–containing cells during a crisis has been shown to be clinically effective.[181,182] Additionally, evidence suggests that RCE improves the rheologic characteristics of the patient's blood.[172] Authorities in the field have published current indications for exchange transfusions, which include acute neurologic events, severe acute chest syndrome, acute multiorgan failure, preparation for major surgery, and long-term use (in lieu of simple transfusion) to avoid or reduce iron loading, as well as the management of acute priapism.[172,183,184] Finally, RCE may have some role in the management of SCD during pregnancy.

The use of transfusion therapy in acute chest syndrome (ACS) is well documented. RCE is generally recommended to decrease Hb S concentration to 30% or less when clinical deterioration (e.g., respiratory decompensation) or organ failure is evident.[183] Most experts agree that RCE should be performed immediately during an acute ischemic stroke. In high-risk children, as identified by transcranial Doppler (TCD) velocity, evidence supports maintenance of Hb S levels lower than 30% to prevent a first stroke[185] and long-term transfusion in children with previous strokes to prevent recurrence.[186–188] Some authorities have written that RCE should be considered only for high-risk procedures or in patients with underlying pulmonary disease.[183,189]

No randomized trials have examined clinical outcomes of pregnancy in transfused versus nontransfused patients. The evidence from nonrandomized trials is controversial. Prophylactic transfusion may reduce the incidence of pain crisis and thus may be indicated if painful episodes are increasing in frequency. Otherwise, most experts recommend that transfusion should be used in the same ways as it is for nonpregnant patients with SCD or prior to cesarean section.[183] Priapism is characterized by sickle cell occlusion in the corpora cavernosa. No clinical trials have evaluated the efficacy of transfusion therapy; however, in some case reports, long-term transfusion therapy and/or RCE has shown benefit in the treatment of patients with priapism.[190,191] Serious adverse events have been reported to occur as a result of transfusion therapy (more discussion later).

USE OF RCE IN SCD

The percentage of circulating sickle cells prior to RCE, the desired final hematocrit, and the hematocrit level of the replacement product are used to calculate the volume of red cells to be removed and replaced. The hematocrit level of the replacement unit is an estimate in that all units have slightly varying hematocrit levels. The generally accepted goal of RCE is to raise the level of Hb A to 70% while lowering the level of Hb S to less than 30%. It is important, however, to maintain the patient's hematocrit below 30% (or <110% to 120% of baseline) to prevent transient hyperviscosity and maintain adequate oxygen delivery.[181] In addition, an elevated postexchange hematocrit has been associated with the development of ASPEN syndrome (association of sickle cell disease, priapism, exchange transfusion, and neurologic events) or neurologic events (i.e., headaches, seizures, obtundation) that may occur after partial exchange transfusion associated with the release of vasoactive substances[192,193] in the setting of priapism.

Other Hematologic Diseases

Protozoan Infection

Plasmodia and *Babesia* are protozoa that infect human red blood cells. High plasmodium parasite levels have been associated with poor prognosis,[194] and the pathogenesis of malaria is incompletely understood. In a recent review, Weatherall and colleagues[195] refuted the notion that malaria is a disorder with a single organ target and attempted to shift the paradigm of thought toward that of a complex, multisystem disorder with several key pathogenic processes, including "rapid expansion of infected red cell mass, destruction of both infected and uninfected RBCs, microvascular obstruction, and inflammatory process," all of which may combine to compromise tissue perfusion.

RCE has been used to decrease parasite burden in heavily infected patients. Because no randomized, controlled clinical trials have been undertaken, it is difficult to assess the efficacy of this therapy. However, its proposed benefit is the rapid removal of nonsequestered, infected red cells and the possible removal of circulating toxins that may contribute to the pathogenesis of the disease. Riddle and coworkers[196] have questioned the efficacy of removing nonsequestered, infected cells when sequestered cells are more pathogenic and are not removed by RCE. In this recent meta-analysis, Riddle and colleagues evaluated eight case-controlled studies and found no significant overall survival benefit with adjuvant RCE (except potentially in patients with partial immunity, for whom a relatively higher level of parasitemia is common.) Some have advocated the use of RCE in critically ill patients with high levels of parasitemia (>20% for malaria, >5% for Babesia). Again, conclusive scientific evidence to support this practice does not exist. The AFSA and the AABB list malarial infection and babesiosis as Category III indications for erythrocytapheresis.

Polycythemia Vera

Erythrocytosis and polycythemia vera are terms that are characterized by increased red cell mass that occurs as the result of a clonal disease or a secondary reaction to chronic hypoxemia. These patients have an increased hematocrit (Hct), leading to an increase in blood viscosity. Symptoms of erythrocytosis can range from headache, hypertension, visual disturbances, and confusion to cerebral infarction or hemorrhage and thrombosis of the abdominal vessels.[55,197-199] In polycythemia vera (PV), life expectancy and quality of life are directly related to control of red cell mass.[55,198,199]

Removal of red cells is first-line therapy for patients with PV and is to be considered for secondary erythrocytosis.[198-201] Maintenance of Hct at <45% with the use of phlebotomy minimizes the risk for thromboembolic complications. Thus, this value should be the highest target of treatment; many hematologists maintain the Hct between 39% and 45%.[199-203] At a Hct level of 60%, whole blood viscosity is 2.5- to 3-fold that of blood with a Hct of 40%.[204] Signs of hemorrhage or infarction in conjunction with an elevated Hct require immediate red cell removal through erythrocytapheresis to decrease Hct levels. This usually leads to rapid improvement.[202] For this indication, saline or albumin is the recommended replacement fluid.[203]

COMPLICATIONS

A variety of infectious and noninfectious reactions seen with simple transfusion of FFP may also be seen when plasma is used as replacement during TPE (Table 30-2). In recent years, the risk of transfusion-transmitted infectious disease has been largely eliminated with the introduction of nucleic acid testing (NAT) for HIV and hepatitis C virus (HCV). The result has been a comparative increase in the percentage of fatalities related to noninfectious serious

Table 30-2 Infectious and Noninfectious Reactions Seen with Simple Transfusion of Fresh Frozen Plasma When Plasma is Used as Replacement During Total Parenteral Nutrition

Adverse Event	Causes	Signs and Symptoms	Management
Hypovolemia	Fluid shifts Inadequate fluid replacement Pump malfunction	Drop in blood pressure Tachycardia	Saline or red cell priming; consider transfusion
Allergic reaction	Antibody to donor plasma proteins	Hives Dyspnea and facial swelling Hypotension Tachycardia and bronchospasm	IV diphenhydramine; epinephrine or corticosteroid
Atypical reactions due to ACE inhibitors	Elevated bradykinin levels	Flushing, hypotension, dyspnea, and bradycardia	Stop ACE inhibitors 72 hr prior to transfusion; if emergent pheresis is required, use FFP as replacement fluid
Isovolemic hypotension	Vasovagal reaction	Hypotension Bradycardia Sweating	Put patient in Trendelenburg position; give saline bolus
Hypocalcemia	Citrate toxicity Albumin administration	In children: Acute abdominal pain, agitation, pallor, diaphoresis, tachycardia, and hypotension In adults: Circumoral paresthesias, chills, nausea, and a tremulous feeling in the chest; rarely, overt tetany, cardiac arrhythmias	Slow the rate of infusion; give IV or PO calcium; consider switching anticoagulant from citrate to heparin
Vascular access		Hematomas Venous sclerosis Thrombosis Pneumothorax Subcutaneous emphysema Infection	Use peripheral access when appropriate
Coagulopathy	Dilution with albumin replacement	Prolonged clotting assays Bleeding	Use FFP as partial or complete replacement

IV, intravenous; ACE, angiotensin-converting enzyme; FFP, fresh frozen plasma; PO, by mouth.

hazards of transfusion, including transfusion-related acute lung injury (TRALI).

Between May and December 1995, the Hemapheresis Committee of the AABB conducted a large, prospective, multicenter study to investigate the incidence and types of adverse events observed during apheresis procedures.[18] They found the overall rate of adverse events (N = 242) to be 4.75%. In addition, they found that the type of procedure, the type of instrument, and the patient's underlying disease were all specific factors that affected the incidence of adverse events. TPE with plasma replacement resulted in twice the number of adverse events as were seen with TPE without plasma replacement (7.8% and 3.4%, respectively). RCE yielded the largest percentage of adverse events (10.3%). Peripheral blood progenitor cell collection and selective extraction via immunoadsorption columns produced the lowest rates (1.66% and 1.19%, respectively). Citrate-related events occurred in 1.5% of procedures. Seven cases of tetany and seizure occurred during TPE procedures in which FFP was used for replacement. Vasovagal events occurred in 2.6% of procedures. In all, 1.6% of procedures were reported to have resulted in an adverse reaction that was caused by a transfused blood component; the overwhelming majority of these occurred during TPE with plasma replacement. Other studies have reported that patients with neurologic disease are more prone to hypotensive and/or vasovagal events.[205] Peripheral or perioral paresthesias and mild lightheadedness were regarded as physiologic events and were not counted. Additionally, vascular access problems that prevented completion of the procedure were excluded. A total of three deaths were reported; however, none could be attributed to the apheresis procedure. Hypotension during apheresis has been attributed to several factors, including hypovolemia, allergic reactions, the vasovagal reflex, and complement activation.[206]

Hypovolemia

Fluid shifts that occur during the procedure, inadequate fluid replacement, and pump malfunctions that abrogate return of the patient's blood may cause hypovolemia during apheresis.[3] Fluid shifts are usually tolerated by adults and older children. In standard procedures, saline is used to prime the extracorporeal circuit. First, whole blood is withdrawn from the patient, the saline prime is diverted into a waste collection bag, and replacement fluid is administered. Thus, a deficit fluid balance is maintained during the procedure. Young children, anemic patients, and those with heart disease or who are hemodynamically unstable for other reasons may be unable to tolerate the fluid shifts and hemodilution created by saline priming. These patients may require preprocedural or intraprocedural transfusions. Priming the circuitry with blood rather than saline is another technique that is used to maintain isovolemia during the procedure. In this instance, no final "rinseback" is needed.

Allergic Reactions

Allergic reactions characterized by a range of symptoms from hives, dyspnea, and facial swelling to hypotension, tachycardia, and bronchospasm have been associated with FFP, albumin, and plasma protein fraction and plasma expanders (e.g., hydroxyethyl starch [HES]). Ethylene oxide gas used to sterilize disposable apheresis kits has been associated with periorbital edema, conjunctival swelling, and tearing.[207] Those with mild reactions may be treated with intravenous diphenhydramine. More severe reactions may require epinephrine or corticosteroid treatment and respiratory support.

Atypical reactions have occurred in patients on ACE inhibitor therapy while they were undergoing hemodialysis, low-density lipoprotein apheresis, IgG affinity column apheresis, TPE, or desensitization immunotherapy.[208] In a retrospective study, atypical reactions characterized by flushing, hypotension, dyspnea, and bradycardia were observed in 100% (14 of 14) of patients who were receiving ACE inhibitor therapy at the time of apheresis. Only 7% (20 of 285) of patients who were not receiving ACE inhibitors developed atypical reactions. In all, 11% of patients had an atypical reaction, with 41% of all such reactions occurring in those individuals on ACE inhibitors.[208] One study showed that plasma bradykinin concentrations were higher in plasmapheresis donors on ACE inhibitors than they were in controls.[209] This may help substantiate the hypothesis that a patient taking ACE inhibitors, which decrease bradykinin catabolism, who subsequently receives a large volume of albumin that contains a low level of pre-kallikrein activator (an activator of bradykinin) may develop a "toxic concentration" of bradykinin.[210] Bradykinin activates endothelial cells, thereby causing vasodilatation, increased vascular permeability, production of nitric oxide, and mobilization of arachidonic acid.[211] As a general rule, ACE inhibitors are discontinued prior to apheresis procedures.

Vasovagal Reactions

Vasovagal reactions are the most common adverse reactions associated with donor apheresis; however, they are less likely to occur with whole blood donation.[212] According to one multicenter, case-controlled, retrospective study, female donors, young donors, and first-time donors are more likely to experience vasovagal reactions.[213] The patient's or donor's pulse generally slows down, thus distinguishing this type of reaction from a hypotensive reaction. Removal of blood should be slowed or discontinued as symptoms occur or progress. The patient should be placed in the Trendelenburg position and should be maintained in this position until the reaction has resolved. Vital signs should be monitored. Some clinicians advocate saline administration.[214]

Hypocalcemia and Citrate Toxicity

For a variety of reasons, ionized calcium levels may decrease during apheresis. Citrate, which binds calcium and is commonly used as an anticoagulant in blood products and during apheresis, may be infused, or calcium-free albumin, which also binds free calcium, may be used as the replacement fluid. Alternatively, citrate-rich FFP may be used as the replacement fluid. Approximately 1% of the body's calcium is found in the plasma; of this, only one half is free, or unbound.[215] Under normal physiologic circumstances, approximately 10% of plasma calcium is bound to small anions in the circulation (e.g., phosphate). However, the infusion of exogenous anions such as citrate leads to an increase in the anion-bound fraction at the expense of the ionized calcium fraction.

The amount of citrate used during the procedure is dependent on the amount of blood to be processed, the length of the procedure, and the flow rate required. Thus, procedures such as leukapheresis, which require a large volume of citrate to be infused and in which virtually all of the anticoagulant is returned to the patient, frequently require supplemental calcium infusions to prevent citrate toxicity.[216] Additionally, citrate is present in relatively large amounts in packed red cells and plasma. Therefore, hypocalcemia may result from citrate toxicity during TPE replacement with plasma. Finally, citrate is metabolized within the liver and to a lesser extent within the kidneys and skeletal muscle.[217] Thus, in patients with liver and kidney dysfunction, unmetabolized citrate may accumulate.

Several studies have shown that during donor platelet-pheresis, citrate causes a 20% to 30% decrease in ionized calcium levels.[218,219] An increase in parathormone levels occurs in response to dropping ionized calcium levels during these procedures.[19,220] However, an expected net calcium loss is sustained; thus, many physicians use calcium gluconate or calcium chloride prophylactically to prevent the occurrence of hypocalcemic reactions. No clinical trials support this practice.

Hypocalcemia presents differently in children than in adults. Children may experience signs and symptoms of acute abdominal pain, agitation, pallor, diaphoresis, tachycardia, and hypotension.[19] Adults typically experience circumoral paresthesias, chills, nausea, and a tremulous feeling in the chest. Adults rarely experience overt tetany, and although electrocardiographic changes may be demonstrated, cardiac arrhythmias are rare. Pearl and associates[221–223] described citrate-related alkalosis as another form of citrate toxicity in which patients with renal disease who are unable to effectively excrete bicarbonate become alkalotic after TPE with plasma replacement.

Adverse Effects Related to Vascular Access

As was previously mentioned, central venous access imposes greater risks than does peripheral access. Studies have shown that, except for a minority of cases and procedures, peripheral access is adequate.[2] Hematomas, venous sclerosis, thrombosis, pneumothorax, subcutaneous emphysema, and infection are not uncommon problems with indwelling catheters.[224] Catheter-related infections may result in sepsis. Catheter care and heparin flushes to prevent clots in the line should be performed regularly. If platelet count starts to precipitously drop, it is important for the clinician to consider the diagnosis of heparin-induced thrombocytopenia (HIT). Cases of HIT in which heparin flushes were the only source of heparin have been reported.[225–228]

Hypoglobulinemia and Infection

Normal immunoglobulin levels are known to decrease by approximately 60% from baseline after a single volume exchange.[12] Wing and associates,[229] in a small, nonrandomized, retrospective study, showed that patients with RPGN

who had intensive TPE combined with immunosuppressive therapy were more likely to acquire a life-threatening infection than were those treated with immunosuppressive therapy alone. However, in a larger, randomized study of patients with lupus nephritis who were given immunosuppressive therapy alone or in combination with TPE,[230] these finding were not well supported.[85] Still, with the use of regular TPE, measurement of IgG levels and coagulation parameters is recommended.

SPECIAL APPLICATIONS

Pediatrics

The indications and treatment protocols for apheresis in pediatric populations have been largely extrapolated from adult studies. However, the pathophysiology of a disease and response to treatment may differ in children.[4] Some technical considerations regarding the maintenance of adequate intravascular volume and vascular access limitations are specific to children. Studies of adult patients may underestimate adverse events in children who undergo similar procedures. The use of continuous flow apheresis machines is recommended in lieu of intermittent flow devices because ECV is minimized and isovolemic fluid balance is better maintained.[19] This is especially true for small, anemic, and/or hemodynamically unstable patients. In children who weigh less than 8 kg, manual exchange may be required.

Children are frequently unable to tolerate the fluid shifts and hemodilution that may occur with a saline prime. In these cases, priming the apheresis circuit with blood rather than with saline may be necessary and is recommended if the ECV exceeds 10% to 15% of the child's TBV, if the intraprocedural hematocrit decreases to below 20%, or if the child weighs 20 kg or less. Leukocyte-reduced RBCs are frequently used for this purpose; however, some advocate the use of reconstituted whole blood units for the purpose of priming in children who weigh less than 10 kg.[19] As was previously mentioned, correct calculation of TBV is extremely important for accurate estimation of intraprocedural ECV. TBV estimates calculated automatically with the use of apheresis instruments and popular formulas may be significantly discrepant, especially in pediatric patients.[4] Citrate anticoagulation is almost always used in conjunction with heparin or not at all in children because they are more susceptible to citrate toxicity. Several different methods for dosing have been described[4,216,231–234]

Photopheresis

Photopheresis (also called extracorporeal photochemotherapy, or ECP) is a procedure in which peripheral mononuclear cells are separated via apheresis, treated with a photoactivating agent (i.e., a psoralen compound) and ultraviolet A (UVA) light, and finally returned to the patient. In a photoconjugating reaction, DNA is cross-linked, causing strand breaks that result in inhibition of cellular proliferation and eventual apoptosis in exposed cells.[235] ECP is indicated for the palliative treatment of patients with cutaneous T-cell lymphoma (CTCL) but also has produced reported benefits in the treatment of various autoimmune diseases, solid organ allograft rejection, and graft-versus-host disease. The realization that these clinically heterogeneous diseases have similar pathophysiologic mechanisms and responses to immunosuppressive agents has led to the development of immunomodulatory hypotheses.[236] Two formulations of the psoralen compound, 8-MOP (methoxsalen, 8-methoxypsoralen), may be used. An oral formulation given 2 hours prior to leukapheresis shows variability in drug absorption and may require drug level measurements to ascertain that the level is adequate. The second formulation is a sterile solution (Uvadex; Therakos Inc., Exton, Pa, USA) that may be injected directly into the buffy coat of the collection bag prior to UVA exposure. This formulation has more predictable drug levels, eliminates the 2-hour incubation period needed for the oral formulation, and reduces the amount of total 8-MOP that the patient receives, thereby reducing adverse effects.[237] ECP is contraindicated in patients who have had previously documented reactions to psoralen or a history of porphyria cutanea tarda, erythropoietic protoporphyria, variegate porphyria, xeroderma pigmentosa, albinism, or other light-sensitive diseases.

CTCL

CTCL is a form of non-Hodgkin lymphoma (NHL) that is observed as CD4+ malignant T cells that typically manifest as skin patches and plaques located on the trunk. Treatment of CTCL is aimed at reducing symptoms and preventing secondary complications and progression of the disease, thereby affecting survival.[238] Clinical trials have shown complete and partial remissions in erythrodermic CTCL and Sézary syndrome with ECP.[239–241] The efficacy of ECP in the treatment of early-stage mycosis fungoides is a matter of controversy. Despite the advantages that ECP provides in terms of whole body photochemotherapy, versus PUVA (psoralen + long-wave ultraviolet radiation), one randomized clinical trial found that PUVA was superior to ECP in treating patients with skin disease at the plaque stage of mycosis fungoides.[242]

Graft-Versus-Host Disease

Graft-versus-host disease (GVHD) is a common and potentially fatal complication of bone marrow transplantation (BMT). Acute and chronic GVHD have different clinical presentations and a different temporal relationship to the transplant. Acute GVHD occurs during the first 100 days after BMT. Chronic GVHD usually presents with various features, including a dry, itching rash and jaundice. Patients with chronic GVHD who are unresponsive to one or more immunosuppressive agents are usually included in ECP protocols and studies.[243–245]

In the only prospective study, Foss and associates[246] examined 25 patients with chronic GVHD and found that ECP is beneficial in their treatment, regardless of type of transplant (matched unrelated versus matched related), Akpek score (a prognostic scoring system based on disease onset and degree of skin involvement and thrombocytopenia, in which a score of 2.5 or more has an inferior outcome), and duration of chronic GVHD. Their findings corroborated the findings of an earlier retrospective study.[247]

Selective Extraction of Lipoproteins

Low-density lipoprotein (LDL)-apheresis (LDL-A) is used as first-line treatment for patients with familial hypercholesterolemia (FH). FH is characterized by hypercholesterolemia from birth, subsequent development of xanthomas, and premature atherosclerosis, with increased risk of premature coronary artery disease.[248] The most common complications of homozygous FH are aortic valve fibrosis and stenosis.[249]

The goal of LDL-A therapy is to remove excess LDL while leaving high-density lipoprotein (HDL) in the circulation. Several methods, including immunoadsorption, dextran/sulfate cellulose adsorption (DSA), the heparin extracorporeal LDL precipitation system (HELP), and direct adsorption of lipoprotein through hemoperfusion (DALI), are currently used to extract lipoproteins. A full discussion of these methods is beyond the scope of this chapter; however, Naoumova and colleagues[250] have prepared a comprehensive review of current methods of management of familial hypercholesterolemia. All of these methods have been shown to reduce LDL cholesterol (LDL-C),[251] lipoprotein(a) (Lp[a]),[252–254] adhesion molecules,[255,256] and C-reactive protein,[257,258] while improving vascular endothelial function and hemorheology.[259,260] All of these factors are likely beneficial in arresting the development of atherosclerosis.[261]

The frequency, dose, and level of LDL-C reduction required to impede the progression of disease are unknown, but repetitive LDL-A is usually provided on a monthly or twice monthly basis. Naoumova and coworkers[250] advocate the use of apheresis combined with drug therapy to achieve the lowest LDL-C levels possible in the absence of guidelines based on randomized, controlled trials. Some authorities have recommended that the frequency of apheresis should be adjusted to the activity of the LDL receptors and other individual patient factors.[262] Selective apheresis has been used successfully to treat children with FH.[263–265] Pediatric tubing kits are available for DSA (Dextransulfat-Adsorption system; Kaneka, Osaka, Japan). Case reports of pheresis during pregnancy have shown success in control of hypercholesterolemia[264,266–268] and improvement in uterine and umbilical flow.[269]

REFERENCES

1. Burgstaler EA: Current instrumentation for apheresis. In McLeod BC, Price TH, Weinstein R (eds): Apheresis: Principles and Practice, Bethesda, Md, AABB Press, 2003, pp 95–130.
2. Noseworthy JH, Shumak KH, Vandervoort MK: Long-term use of antecubital veins for plasma exchange. The Canadian Cooperative Multiple Sclerosis Study Group. Transfusion 29:610–613, 1989.
3. Jones HG, Bamdarenko N: Management of the therapeutic apheresis patient. In McLeod BC, Price TH, Weinstein R (eds): Apheresis: Principles and Practice Bethesda, Md, AABB Press, 2003, pp 253–282.
4. Kim HC: Therapeutic pediatric apheresis. J Clin Apher 15:129–157, 2000.
5. Collins JA: Hemorrhage, shock, and burns. In Petz LD, Swisher SN (eds): Clinical Practice of Blood Transfusion., New York, Churchill Livingstone, Inc, 1981, pp 425–453.
6. Gilcher RO: Apheresis: Practice and principles. In Rossi EC, Simon TL, Moss GS, Gould SA (eds): Principles of Transfusion Medicine, Baltimore, Md, Williams and Wilkins, 1996, pp 537–545.
7. Mollison PL, Engelfriet CP, Conteras M: Blood Transfusion in Clinical Medicine 9th ed Oxford, England, Blackwell Scientific Publications, 1993, Appendix 5, pp 791–793.

8. Chopek M, McCullough J: Protein and biochemical changes during plasma exchange. In Berkman EM, Umlas J (eds): Therapeutic Hemapheresis. Washington, DC, AABB Press, 1980, pp 13–52.

9. Calabrese LH, Clough JD, Krakauer RS, Hoeltge GA: Plasmapheresis therapy of immunologic disease: Report of nine cases and review of the literature. Cleve Clin Q 47:53–72, 1980.

10. Berkman EM, Orlin JB: Use of plasmapheresis and partial plasma exchange in the management of patients with cryoglobulinemia. Transfusion 20:171–178, 1980.

11. Alexanian R: Blood volume in monoclonal gammopathy. Blood 49:301–307, 1977.

12. Weinstein R: Basic principles of therapeutic blood exchange. In McLeod BC, Price TH, Weinstein R (eds): Apheresis: Principles and Practice Bethesda, Md, AABB Press, 2003, pp 295–320.

13. Orlin JB, Berkman EM: Partial plasma exchange using albumin replacement: Removal and recovery of normal plasma constituents. Blood 56:1055–1059, 1980.

14. Jones JV, Clough JD, Klinenberg JR, Davis P: The role of therapeutic plasmapheresis in the rheumatic diseases. J Lab Clin Med 97:589–598, 1981.

15. Powell LC Jr: Intense plasmapheresis in the pregnant Rh-sensitized woman. Am J Obstet Gynecol 101:153–170, 1968.

16. Huestis DW: Mortality in therapeutic haemapheresis. Lancet 1:1043, 1983.

17. Sutton DM, Nair RC, Rock G: Complications of plasma exchange. Transfusion 29:124–127, 1989.

18. McLeod BC, Sniecinski I, Ciavarella D, et al: Frequency of immediate adverse effects associated with therapeutic apheresis. Transfusion 39:282–288, 1999.

19. Rogers RL, Cooling LLW: Therapeutic apheresis in pediatric patients. In McLeod BC, Price TH, Weinstein R (eds): Apheresis: Principles and Practice, Bethesda, Md, AABB Press, 2003, pp 477–492.

20. Amorosi EL, Ultmann JE: Thrombotic thrombocytopenic purpura: Report of 16 cases and a review of the literature. Medicine (Baltimore) 45:139–159, 1966.

21. Furlan M, Robles R, Lamie B: Partial purification and characterization of a protease from human plasma cleaving von Willebrand factor to fragments produced by in vivo proteolysis. Blood 87:4223–4234, 1996.

22. Tsai HM: Physiologic cleavage of von Willebrand factor by a plasma protease is dependent on its conformation and requires calcium ion. Blood 87:4235–4244, 1996.

23. Levy GG, et al: Mutations in a member of the ADAMTS gene family cause thrombotic thrombocytopenic purpura. Nature 413:488–494, 2001.

24. Furlan M, Robles R, Galbusera M, et al: von Willebrand factor–cleaving protease in thrombotic thrombocytopenic purpura and the hemolytic-uremic syndrome. N Engl J Med 339:1578–1584, 1998.

25. Furlan M, Robles R, Solenthaler M, Lammle B: Acquired deficiency of von Willebrand factor–cleaving protease in a patient with thrombotic thrombocytopenic purpura. Blood 91:2839–2846, 1998.

26. Tsai HM, Lian EC: Antibodies to von Willebrand factor–cleaving protease in acute thrombotic thrombocytopenic purpura. N Engl J Med 339:1585–1594, 1998.

27. Moake JL: Moschcowitz, multimers, and metalloprotease. N Engl J Med 339:1629–1631, 1998.

28. Furlan M, Lammle B: Aetiology and pathogenesis of thrombotic thrombocytopenic purpura and haemolytic uraemic syndrome: The role of von Willebrand factor–cleaving protease. Best Pract Res Clin Haematol 14:437–454, 2001.

29. Upshaw JD Jr: Congenital deficiency of a factor in normal plasma that reverses microangiopathic hemolysis and thrombocytopenia. N Engl J Med 298:1350–1352, 1978.

30. Vesely SK, George JN, Lammle B, et al: ADAMTS13 activity in thrombotic thrombocytopenic purpura–hemolytic uremic syndrome: Relation to presenting features and clinical outcomes in a prospective cohort of 142 patients. Blood 102:60–68, 2003.

31. Mori Y, Wada H, Gabazza EC, et al: Predicting response to plasma exchange in patients with thrombotic thrombocytopenic purpura with measurement of vWF-cleaving protease activity. Transfusion 42:572–580, 2002.

32. Zheng XL, Kaufman RM, Goodnough LT, Sadler JE: Effect of plasma exchange on plasma ADAMTS13 metalloprotease activity, inhibitor level, and clinical outcome in patients with idiopathic and nonidiopathic thrombotic thrombocytopenic purpura. Blood 103:4043–4049, 2004.

33. Lämmle B, Kremer Hovinga JA, Alberio L: Thrombotic thrombocytopenic purpura. J Thromb Haemost 3:1663–1675, 2005.

34. Blitzer JB, Granfortuna JM, Gottlieb AJ, et al: Thrombotic thrombocytopenic purpura: Treatment with plasmapheresis. Am J Hematol 24:329–339, 1987.

35. Pereira A, Mazzara R, Monteaguda J, et al: Thrombotic thrombocytopenic purpura/hemolytic uremic syndrome: A multivariate analysis of factors predicting the response to plasma exchange. Ann Hematol 70:319–323, 1995.

36. Lankford KV, Hillyer CD: Thrombotic thrombocytopenic purpura: New insights in disease pathogenesis and therapy. Transfus Med Rev 14:244–257, 2000.

37. Bell WR, Braine HG, Ness PM, Kickler TS: Improved survival in thrombotic thrombocytopenic purpura–hemolytic uremic syndrome: Clinical experience in 108 patients. N Engl J Med 325:398–403, 1991.

38. Cataland SR, Wu HM: Immunotherapy for thrombotic thrombocytopenic purpura. Curr Opin Hematol 12:359–363, 2005.

39. Bandarenko N, Brecher ME: United States Thrombotic Thrombocytopenic Purpura Apheresis Study Group (US TTP ASG): Multicenter survey and retrospective analysis of current efficacy of therapeutic plasma exchange. J Clin Apher 13:133–141, 1998.

40. Rock G, Shumak KH, Sutton DM, et al: Cryosupernatant as replacement fluid for plasma exchange in thrombotic thrombocytopenic purpura. Members of the Canadian Apheresis Group. Br J Haematol 94:383–386, 1996.

41. Willis MS, Bandarenko N: Relapse of thrombotic thrombocytopenic purpura: Is it a continuum of disease? Semin Thromb Hemost 31:700–708, 2005.

42. Sadler JE, Moake JL, Miyata T: Recent advances in thrombotic thrombocytopenic purpura. Hematology (Am Soc Hematol Educ Program) 407–423, 2004.

43. George JN: How I treat patients with thrombotic thrombocytopenic purpura–hemolytic uremic syndrome. Blood 96:1223–1229, 2000.

44. Shumak KH, Rock GA, Nair RC: Late relapses in patients successfully treated for thrombotic thrombocytopenic purpura. Canadian Apheresis Group. Ann Intern Med 122:569–572, 1995.

45. Moake JL, Chow TW: Thrombotic thrombocytopenic purpura: Understanding a disease no longer rare. Am J Med Sci 316:105–119, 1998.

46. Rock GA, Shumak JH, Buskard NA, et al: Comparison of plasma exchange with plasma infusion in the treatment of thrombotic thrombocytopenic purpura. Canadian Apheresis Study Group. N Engl J Med 325:393–397, 1991.

47. Hayward CP, Sutton DM, Carter WH Jr, et al: Treatment outcomes in patients with adult thrombotic thrombocytopenic purpura–hemolytic uremic syndrome. Arch Intern Med 154:982–987, 1994.

48. Zeigler ZR, Shadduck RK, Gryn JF, et al: Cryoprecipitate poor plasma does not improve early response in primary adult thrombotic thrombocytopenic purpura (TTP). J Clin Apher 16:19–22, 2001.

49. Rock G, Anderson D, Clark W, et al: Does cryosupernatant plasma improve outcome in thrombotic thrombocytopenic purpura? No answer yet. Br J Haematol 129:79–86, 2005.

50. Tarr PI, Gordon CA, Chandler WL: Shiga-toxin–producing Escherichia coli and haemolytic uraemic syndrome. Lancet 365:1073–1086, 2005.

51. Miller RF, Scully M, Cohen H, et al: Thrombotic thrombocytopaenic purpura in HIV-infected patients. Int J STD AIDS 16:538–542, 2005.

52. Novitzky N, Thomson J, Abrahams L, et al: Thrombotic thrombocytopenic purpura in patients with retroviral infection is highly responsive to plasma infusion therapy. Br J Haematol 128:373–379, 2005.

53. Gruszecki AC, Wehrli G, Ragland BD, et al: Management of a patient with HIV infection–induced anemia and thrombocytopenia who presented with thrombotic thrombocytopenic purpura. Am J Hematol 69:228–231, 2002.

54. Shulman NR, Reid DM: Platelet immunology. In Coleman RW (ed): Hemostasis and Thrombosis., Philadelphia, JB Lippincott, 1994, pp 1860–1862.

55. Grima KM: Therapeutic apheresis in hematological and oncological diseases. J Clin Apher 15:28–52, 2000.

56. Gabriel A, Lassnigg A, Kurz M, Panzer S: Post-transfusion purpura due to HPA-1a immunization in a male patient: Response to subsequent multiple HPA-1a–incompatible red-cell transfusions. Transfus Med 5:131–134, 1995.

57. Lucas GF, Pittman SJ, Davies S, et al: Post-transfusion purpura (PTP) associated with anti–HPA-1a, anti–HPA-2b and anti–HPA-3a antibodies. Transfus Med 7:295–299, 1997.

58. Drew MJ: Therapeutic plasma exchange in hematologic disease and dysproteinemias. In McLeod BC, Price TH, and Weinstein R (eds): Apheresis: Principles and Practice. Bethesda, Md, AABB Press, 2003, pp 345–374.

59. Taaning E, Morling N, Ovesen H, Svejgaard J: Post transfusion purpura and anti-Zwb (−P1A2). Tissue Antigens 26:143–146, 1985.

60. Taaning E, Svejgaard A: Post-transfusion purpura: A survey of 12 Danish cases with special reference to immunoglobulin G subclasses of the platelet antibodies. Transfus Med 4:1–8, 1994.

61. Evenson DA, Stroncek DF, Pulkrabek S, et al: Posttransfusion purpura following bone marrow transplantation. Transfusion 35:688–693, 1995.

62. Keimowitz RM, Collins J, Davis K, Aster RH: Post-transfusion purpura associated with alloimmunization against the platelet-specific antigen, Baka. Am J Hematol 21:79–88, 1986.

63. Kickler TS, Herman JH, Furihata K, et al: Identification of Bakb, a new platelet-specific antigen associated with posttransfusion purpura. Blood 71:894–898, 1988.

64. Simon TL, Collins J, Kunicki TJ, et al: Posttransfusion purpura associated with alloantibody specific for the platelet antigen, Pen(a). Am J Hematol 29:38–40, 1988.

65. Christie DJ, Pulkrabek S, Putnam JL, et al: Posttransfusion purpura due to an alloantibody reactive with glycoprotein Ia/IIa (anti-HPA-5b). Blood 77:2785–2789, 1991.

66. Bierling P, Godeau B, Fromont P, et al: Posttransfusion purpura-like syndrome associated with CD36 (Naka) isoimmunization. Transfusion 35:777–782, 1995.

67. Vaughan-Neil EF, Ardeman S, Bevan G, et al: Post-transfusion purpura associated with unusual platelet antibody (anti-Pl-B1). Br Med J 1:436–437, 1975.

68. Kickler TS, Ness PM, Herman JH, Bell WR: Studies on the pathophysiology of posttransfusion purpura. Blood 68:347–350, 1986.

69. Lillicrap DP, Ford PM, Giles AR: Prolonged thrombocytopenia in post-transfusion purpura (PTP) associated with changes in the crossed immunoelectrophoretic pattern of von Willebrand factor (vWF), circulating immune complexes and endothelial cell cytotoxicity. Br J Haematol 62:37–46, 1986.

70. Buckner CD, Clift RA, Sanders JE, et al: ABO-incompatible marrow transplants. Transplantation 26:233–238, 1978.

71. Gale RP, Feig S, Ho W, et al: ABO blood group system and bone marrow transplantation. Blood 50:185–194, 1977.

72. Berkman EM, Caplan S, Kim CS: ABO-incompatible bone marrow transplantation: Preparation by plasma exchange and in vivo antibody absorption. Transfusion 18:504–508, 1978.

73. Bensinger WI, Baker DA, Buckner CD, et al: Immunoadsorption for removal of A and B blood-group antibodies. N Engl J Med 304:160–162, 1981.

74. Blade J, Fernandez-Llama P, Bosch F, et al: Renal failure in multiple myeloma: Presenting features and predictors of outcome in 94 patients from a single institution. Arch Intern Med 158:1889–1893, 1998.

75. Knudsen LM, Hippe E, Hjorth M, et al: Renal function in newly diagnosed multiple myeloma: A demographic study of 1353 patients. The Nordic Myeloma Study Group. Eur J Haematol 53:207–212, 1994.

76. Clark WF, Stewart AK, Rock GA, et al: Plasma exchange when myeloma presents as acute renal failure: A randomized, controlled trial. Ann Intern Med 143:777–784, 2005.

77. Johnson WJ, Kyle RA, Pineda AA, et al: Treatment of renal failure associated with multiple myeloma: Plasmapheresis, hemodialysis, and chemotherapy. Arch Intern Med 150:863–869, 1990.

78. Zucchelli P, Pasquali S, Cagnoli L, Ferrari G: Controlled plasma exchange trial in acute renal failure due to multiple myeloma. Kidney Int 33:1175–1180, 1988.

79. Mehta J, Singhal S: Hyperviscosity syndrome in plasma cell dyscrasias. Semin Thromb Hemost 29:467–471, 2003.

80. Nilsson IM, Berntorp E, Zettervall O: Induction of immune tolerance in patients with hemophilia and antibodies to factor VIII by combined treatment with intravenous IgG, cyclophosphamide, and factor VIII. N Engl J Med 318:947–950, 1988.

81. Gjorstrup P, Berntorp E, Larsson L, Nilsson IM: Kinetic aspects of the removal of IgG and inhibitors in hemophiliacs using protein A immunoadsorption. Vox Sang 61:244–250, 1991.

82. Knobl P, Derfler K: Extracorporeal immunoadsorption for the treatment of haemophilic patients with inhibitors to factor VIII or IX. Vox Sang 77 (suppl 1): 57–64, 1999.

83. Fischer KG, Deschler B, Lubbert M: Acquired high-titer factor VIII inhibitor: Fatal bleeding despite multimodal treatment including rituximab preceded by multiple plasmaphereses. Blood 101:3753–3754, 2003; author reply 3754–3755.

84. Rivard GE, St. Louis J, Lacroix S, et al: Immunoadsorption for coagulation factor inhibitors: A retrospective critical appraisal of 10 consecutive cases from a single institution. Haemophilia 9:711–716, 2003.

85. Winters JL, Pineda AA, McLeod BC, Grima KM: Therapeutic apheresis in renal and metabolic diseases. J Clin Apher 15:53–73, 2003.

86. Kelly PT, Haponik EF: Goodpasture syndrome: Molecular and clinical advances. Medicine (Baltimore) 73:171–185, 1994.

87. Szczepiorkowski ZM: TPE in renal rheumatic and miscellaneous disorders. In McLeod BC, Price TH, Weinstein R (eds): Apheresis: Principles and Practice. Bethesda, Md, AABB Press, 2003, pp 375–410.

88. Pusey CD, Lockwood CM, Peters DK: Plasma exchange and immunosuppressive drugs in the treatment of glomerulonephritis due to antibodies to the glomerular basement membrane. Int J Artif Organs 6 (suppl 1): 15–18, 1983.

89. Glassock RJ: Intensive plasma exchange in crescentic glomerulonephritis: Help or no help? Am J Kidney Dis 20:270–275, 1992.

90. Kaplan AA: Therapeutic apheresis for renal disorders. Ther Apher 3:25–30, 1999.

91. Bolton WK: Goodpasture's syndrome. Kidney Int 50:1753–1766, 1996.

92. Savage CO, Pusey CD, Bowman C, et al: Antiglomerular basement membrane antibody mediated disease in the British Isles 1980–4. Br Med J (Clin Res Ed) 292:301–304, 1986.

93. Johnson JP, Moore J Jr, Austin HA III, et al: Therapy of anti–glomerular basement membrane antibody disease: Analysis of prognostic significance of clinical, pathologic and treatment factors. Medicine (Baltimore) 64:219–227, 1985.

94. Lockwood CM, Boulton-James JM, Lowenthal RM, et al: Recovery from Goodpasture's syndrome after immunosuppressive treatment and plasmapheresis. Br Med J 2:252–254, 1975.

95. Levy JB, Turner AN, Rees AJ, Pusey CD: Long-term outcome of anti–glomerular basement membrane antibody disease treated with plasma exchange and immunosuppression. Ann Intern Med 134:1033–1042, 2001.

96. Glockner WM, Sieberth HG, Wichmann HE, et al: Plasma exchange and immunosuppression in rapidly progressive glomerulonephritis: A controlled, multi-center study. Clin Nephrol 29:1–8, 1988.

97. Cole E, Cattran D, Magil A, et al: A prospective randomized trial of plasma exchange as additive therapy in idiopathic crescentic glomerulonephritis. The Canadian Apheresis Study Group. Am J Kidney Dis 20:261–269, 1992.

98. Frasca GM, Zoumparidis NG, Borgnino LC, et al: Plasma exchange treatment in rapidly progressive glomerulonephritis associated with anti-neutrophil cytoplasmic autoantibodies. Int J Artif Organs 15:181–184, 1992.

99. Glassock RJ, Hirschman GH, Striker GE: Workshop on the use of renal biopsy in research on diabetic nephropathy: A summary report. Am J Kidney Dis 18:589–592, 1991.

100. Levy JB, Pusey CD: Antiglomerular basement membrane disease. In Jamison RL, Wilkensson R (eds): Nephrology London, Chapman and Hall, 1997, pp 599–615.

101. Nguyen T, Martin MK, Indrikovs AJ: Plasmapheresis for diffuse alveolar hemorrhage in a patient with Wegener's granulomatosis: Case report and review of the literature. J Clin Apher 20:230–234, 2005.

102. Palmer A, Cairns T, Dische F, et al: Treatment of rapidly progressive glomerulonephritis by extracorporeal immunoadsorption, prednisolone and cyclophosphamide. Nephrol Dial Transplant 6:536–542, 1991.

103. Stegmayr BG, Almroth G, Berlin G, et al: Plasma exchange or immunoadsorption in patients with rapidly progressive crescentic glomerulonephritis: A Swedish multi-center study. Int J Artif Organs 22:81–87, 1999.

104. Matic G, Michelsen A, Hofmann D, et al: Three cases of C-ANCA–positive vasculitis treated with immunoadsorption: Possible benefit in early treatment. Ther Apher 5:68–72, 2001.

105. Deodhar A, Allen E, Daoud K, Wahba I: Vasculitis secondary to staphylococcal protein A immunoadsorption (*Prosorba column*) treatment in rheumatoid arthritis. Semin Arthritis Rheum 32:3–9, 2002.

106. Lou JS, Snyder R, Griggs RC: Refsum's disease: Long term treatment preserves sensory nerve action potentials and motor function. J Neurol Neurosurg Psychiatry 62:671–672, 1997.

107. Wills AJ, Manning NJ, Reilly MM: Refsum's disease. QJM 94:403–406, 2001.

108. Rees JH, Thompson RD, Smeeton NC, Hughes RA: Epidemiological study of Guillain-Barré syndrome in south east England. J Neurol Neurosurg Psychiatry 64:74–77, 1998.

109. Bogliun G, Beghi E: Incidence and clinical features of acute inflammatory polyradiculoneuropathy in Lombardy, Italy, 1996. Acta Neurol Scand 110:100–106, 2004.

110. Chio A, Cocito D, Leone M, et al: Guillain-Barré syndrome: A prospective, population-based incidence and outcome survey. Neurology 60:1146–1150, 2003.

111. Van Koningsveld R, Van Doorn PA, Schmitz PI, et al: Mild forms of Guillain-Barré syndrome in an epidemiologic survey in The Netherlands. Neurology 54:620–625, 2000.

112. Govoni V, Granieri E: Epidemiology of the Guillain-Barré syndrome. Curr Opin Neurol 14:605–613, 2001.

113. Govoni V, Granieri E, Manconi M, et al: Is there a decrease in Guillain-Barré syndrome incidence after bovine ganglioside withdrawal in Italy? A population-based study in the Local Health District of Ferrara, Italy. J Neurol Sci 216:99–103, 2003.

114. Ropper AH: The Guillain-Barré syndrome. N Engl J Med 326:1130–1136, 1992.

115. Kieseier BC, Kiefer R, Gold R, et al: Advances in understanding and treatment of immune-mediated disorders of the peripheral nervous system. Muscle Nerve 30:131–156, 2004.

116. Hughes RA, Cornblath DR: Guillain-Barré syndrome. Lancet 366:1653–1656, 2005.

117. Greenwood RJ, Newsom-Davis J, Hughes Ra, et al: Controlled trial of plasma exchange in acute inflammatory polyradiculoneuropathy. Lancet 1:877–879, 1984.

118. Osterman PO, Fagius J, Lundemo G, et al: Beneficial effects of plasma exchange in acute inflammatory polyradiculoneuropathy. Lancet 2:1296–1299, 1984.

119. Plasmapheresis and acute Guillain-Barré syndrome: The Guillain-Barré Syndrome Study Group. Neurology 35:1096–1104, 1985.

120. Efficiency of plasma exchange in Guillain-Barré syndrome: Role of replacement fluids. French Cooperative Group on Plasma Exchange in Guillain-Barré syndrome. Ann Neurol 22:753–761, 1987.

121. Appropriate number of plasma exchanges in Guillain-Barré syndrome: The French Cooperative Group on Plasma Exchange in Guillain-Barré Syndrome. Ann Neurol 41:298–306, 1997.

122. Plasma exchange in Guillain-Barré syndrome: One-year follow-up. French Cooperative Group on Plasma Exchange in Guillain-Barré Syndrome. Ann Neurol 32:94–97, 1992.

123. Randomised trial of plasma exchange, intravenous immunoglobulin, and combined treatments in Guillain-Barré syndrome: Plasma Exchange/Sandoglobulin Guillain-Barré Syndrome Trial Group. Lancet 349:225–230, 1997.

124. Ropper AE, Albert JW, Addison R: Limited relapse in Guillain-Barré syndrome after plasma exchange. Arch Neurol 45:314–315, 1988.

125. van der Meche FG, Schmitz PI: A randomized trial comparing intravenous immune globulin and plasma exchange in Guillain-Barré syndrome: Dutch Guillain-Barré Study Group. N Engl J Med 326:1123–1129, 1992.

126. Hughes RA, Wijdicks EF, Barohn R, et al: Practice parameter: Immunotherapy for Guillain-Barré syndrome. Report of the Quality Standards Subcommittee of the American Academy of Neurology. Neurology 61:736–740, 2003.

127. Dada MA, Kaplan AA: Plasmapheresis treatment in Guillain-Barré syndrome: Potential benefit over IVIg in patients with axonal involvement. Ther Apher Dial 8:409–412, 2004.

128. Hahn AF, Bolton CF, Pillay N, et al: Plasma-exchange therapy in chronic inflammatory demyelinating polyneuropathy: A double-blind, sham-controlled, cross-over study. Brain 119 (Pt 4): 1055–1066, 1996.

129. Dyck PJ, Daube J, O'Brien P, et al: Plasma exchange in chronic inflammatory demyelinating polyradiculoneuropathy. N Engl J Med 314:461–465, 1986.

130. Hahn AF, Bolton CF, Zochodne D, Feasby TE: Intravenous immunoglobulin treatment in chronic inflammatory demyelinating polyneuropathy: A double-blind, placebo-controlled, cross-over study. Brain 119(Pt 4):1067–1077, 1996.

131. Mendell JR, Barohn RJ, Freimer ML, et al: Randomized controlled trial of IVIg in untreated chronic inflammatory demyelinating polyradiculoneuropathy. Neurology 56:445–449, 2001.

132. van Doorn PA, Brand A, Strengers PF, et al: High-dose intravenous immunoglobulin treatment in chronic inflammatory demyelinating polyneuropathy: A double-blind, placebo-controlled, crossover study. Neurology 40:209–212, 1990.

133. Vermeulen M, van Doorn PA, Brand A, et al: Intravenous immunoglobulin treatment in patients with chronic inflammatory demyelinating polyneuropathy: A double blind, placebo controlled study. J Neurol Neurosurg Psychiatry 56:36–39, 1993.

134. Dyck PJ, Litchy WJ, Kratz KM, et al: A plasma exchange versus immune globulin infusion trial in chronic inflammatory demyelinating polyradiculoneuropathy. Ann Neurol 36:838–845, 1994.

135. European Federation of Neurological Societies/Peripheral Nerve Society: Guideline on management of chronic inflammatory demyelinating polyradiculoneuropathy: Report of a joint task force of the European Federation of Neurological Societies and the Peripheral Nerve Society. J Peripher Nerv Syst 10:220–228, 2005.

136. Romi F, Gilhus NE, Aarli JA: Myasthenia gravis: Clinical, immunological, and therapeutic advances. Acta Neurol Scand 111:134–141, 2005.

137. Berrouschot J, Baumann I, Kalischewski P, et al: Therapy of myasthenic crisis. Crit Care Med 25:1228–1235, 1997.

138. Dau PC, Lindstrom JM, Cassel CK, et al: Plasmapheresis and immunosuppressive drug therapy in myasthenia gravis. N Engl J Med 297:1134–1140, 1977.

139. Sieb JP: Myasthenia gravis: Emerging new therapy options. Curr Opin Pharmacol 5:303–307, 2005.

140. Weinstein R: Therapeutic apheresis in neurological disorders. J Clin Apher 15:74–128, 2000.

141. Yeh JH, Chiu HC: Plasmapheresis in myasthenia gravis: A comparative study of daily versus alternately daily schedule. Acta Neurol Scand 99:147–151, 1999.

142. McLeod BC: Therapeutic plasma exchange in neurologic disorders. In McLeod BC, Price TH, Weinstein R (eds): Apheresis: Principles and Practice. Bethesda, Md, AABB Press, 2003, pp 321–344.

143. Gajdos P, Chevret S, Clair B, et al: Clinical trial of plasma exchange and high-dose intravenous immunoglobulin in myasthenia gravis. Myasthenia Gravis Clinical Study Group. Ann Neurol 41:789–796, 1997.

144. Fergusson D, Hutton B, Sharma M, et al: Use of intravenous immunoglobulin for treatment of neurologic conditions: A systematic review. Transfusion 45:1640–1657, 2005.

145. Besses C, Cervantes F, Pereira A, et al: Major vascular complications in essential thrombocythemia: A study of the predictive factors in a series of 148 patients. Leukemia 13:150–154, 1999.

146. Greist A: The role of blood component removal in essential and reactive thrombocytosis. Ther Apher 6:36–44, 2002.

147. Mitus AJ, Schafer AI: Thrombocytosis and thrombocythemia. Hematol Oncol Clin North Am 4:157–178, 1990.

148. Schafer AI: Bleeding and thrombosis in the myeloproliferative disorders. Blood 64:1–12, 1984.

149. Tefferi A, Solberg LA, Silverstein MN: A clinical update in polycythemia vera and essential thrombocythemia. Am J Med 109:141–149, 2000.

150. Adami R: Therapeutic thrombocytapheresis: A review of 132 patients. Int J Artif Organs 16 (suppl 5): 183–184, 1993.

151. Tefferi A, Silverstein MN, Hoagland HC: Primary thrombocythemia. Semin Oncol 22:334–340, 1995.

152. Taft EG, Babcock RB, Scharfman WB, Tartaglia AP: Plateletpheresis in the management of thrombocytosis. Blood 50:927–933, 1977.

153. Hester J: Therapeutic cell depletion. In McLeod BC, Price TH, Weinstein R (eds): Apheresis: Principles and Practice. Bethesda, Md, AABB Press, 2003, pp 238–294.

154. Kaibara M, Kobayashi T, Matsumoto S: Idiopathic thrombocythemia and pregnancy: Report of a case. Obstet Gynecol 65(3 suppl): 18S–19S, 1985.

155. Falconer J, Pineo G, Blahey W, et al: Essential thrombocythemia associated with recurrent abortions and fetal growth retardation. Am J Hematol 25:345–347, 1987.

156. Beard J, Hillmen P, Anderson CC, et al: Primary thrombocythaemia in pregnancy. Br J Haematol 77:371–374, 1991.

157. Schott U: Essential thrombocythemia and coronary artery bypass surgery. J Cardiothorac Vasc Anesth 8:552–555, 1994.

158. Hsiao HT, Ou SY: Successful microsurgical tissue transfer in a patient with postsplenectomy thrombocytosis treated with platelet-phoresis. J Reconstr Microsurg 13:555–558, 1997.

159. Porcu P, Cripe LD, Ng EW, et al: Hyperleukocytic leukemias and leukostasis: A review of pathophysiology, clinical presentation and management. Leuk Lymphoma 39:1–18, 2000.

IV

160. Freireich EJ, Thomas LB, Frei E 3rd, et al: A distinctive type of intracerebral hemorrhage associated with "blastic crisis" in patients with leukemia. Cancer 13:146–154, 1960.

161. Fritz RD, Forkner CE Jr, Freireich EJ, et al: The association of fatal intracranial hemorrhage and blastic crisis in patients with acute leukemia. N Engl J Med 261:59–64, 1959.

162. Porcu P, Farag S, Marcucci G, et al: Leukocytoreduction for acute leukemia. Ther Apher 6:15–23, 2002.

163. Majhail NS, Lichtin AE: Acute leukemia with a very high leukocyte count: Confronting a medical emergency. Cleve Clin J Med 71:633–637, 2004.

164. Hug V, Keating M, McCredie K, et al: Clinical course and response to treatment of patients with acute myelogenous leukemia presenting with a high leukocyte count. Cancer 52:773–779, 1983.

165. Dutcher JP, Schiffer CA, Wiernik PH: Hyperleukocytosis in adult acute nonlymphocytic leukemia: Impact on remission rate and duration, and survival. J Clin Oncol 5:1364–1372, 1987.

166. Giles FJ, Shen Y, Kantarjian HM, et al: Leukapheresis reduces early mortality in patients with acute myeloid leukemia with high white cell counts but does not improve long-term survival. Leuk Lymphoma 42:67–73, 2001.

167. Maurer HS, Steinherz PG, Gaynon PS, et al: The effect of initial management of hyperleukocytosis on early complications and outcome of children with acute lymphoblastic leukemia. J Clin Oncol 6: 1425–1432, 1988.

168. Porcu P, Danielson CF, Orazi A, et al: Therapeutic leukapheresis in hyperleucocytic leukaemias: Lack of correlation between degree of cytoreduction and early mortality rate. Br J Haematol 98:433–436, 1997.

169. Smith JW, Weinstein R: Therapeutic apheresis: A summary of current indication categories endorsed by the AABB and the American Society for Apheresis. Transfusion 43:820–822, 2003.

170. Aidoo M, Terlouw DJ, Kolczak MS, et al: Protective effects of the sickle cell gene against malaria morbidity and mortality. Lancet 359:1311–1312, 2002.

171. Ingram VM: A specific chemical difference between the globins of normal human and sickle-cell anaemia haemoglobin. Nature 178:792–794, 1956.

172. Thurston GB, Henderson NM, Jeng M: Effects of erythrocytapheresis transfusion on the viscoelasticity of sickle cell blood. Clin Hemorheol Microcirc 30:83–97, 2004.

173. Capon SM, Goldfinger D: Acute hemolytic transfusion reaction, a paradigm of the systemic inflammatory response: New insights into pathophysiology and treatment. Transfusion 35:513–520, 1995.

174. Smith BD, La Celle PL: Erythrocyte-endothelial cell adherence in sickle cell disorders. Blood 68:1050–1054, 1986.

175. Kaul DK, Fabry ME, Nagel RL: Microvascular sites and characteristics of sickle cell adhesion to vascular endothelium in shear flow conditions: Pathophysiological implications. Proc Natl Acad Sci U S A 86:3356–3360, 1989.

176. Zipursky A, Chachula DM, Brown EJ: The reversibly sickled cell. Am J Pediatr Hematol Oncol 15:219–225, 1993.

177. Miller LH, Good MF, Milon G: Malaria pathogenesis. Science 264:1878–1883, 1994.

178. Smolinski PA, Offermann MK, Eckman JR, Wick TM: Double-stranded RNA induces sickle erythrocyte adherence to endothelium: A potential role for viral infection in vaso-occlusive pain episodes in sickle cell anemia. Blood 85:2945–2950, 1995.

179. Mosseri M, Bartlett-Pandite AN, Wenc K, et al: Inhibition of endothelium-dependent vasorelaxation by sickle erythrocytes. Am Heart J 126:338–346, 1993.

180. Hebbel RP, Osarogiagbon R, Kaul D: The endothelial biology of sickle cell disease: Inflammation and a chronic vasculopathy. Microcirculation 11:129–151, 2004.

181. Sharon BI: Transfusion therapy in congenital hemolytic anemias. Hematol Oncol Clin North Am 8:1053–1086, 1994.

182. Lane PA: Sickle cell disease. Pediatr Clin North Am 43:639–664, 1996.

183. Lottenberg R, Hassell KL: An evidence-based approach to the treatment of adults with sickle cell disease. Hematology (Am Soc Hematol Educ Prog) 58–65, 2005.

184. Vichinsky E: Consensus document for transfusion-related iron overload. Semin Hematol 38 (1 Suppl 1): 2–4, 2001.

185. Adams RJ, McKie VC, Hsu L, et al: Prevention of a first stroke by transfusions in children with sickle cell anemia and abnormal results on transcranial Doppler ultrasonography. N Engl J Med 339:5–11, 1998.

186. Wang WC, Kovnar EH, Tonkin IL, et al: High risk of recurrent stroke after discontinuance of five to twelve years of transfusion therapy in patients with sickle cell disease. J Pediatr 118:377–382, 1991.

187. Cohen AR, Martin MB, Silber JH, et al: A modified transfusion program for prevention of stroke in sickle cell disease. Blood 79:1657–1661, 1992.

188. Scothorn DJ, et al: Risk of recurrent stroke in children with sickle cell disease receiving blood transfusion therapy for at least five years after initial stroke. J Pediatr 140:348–354, 2002.

189. Vichinsky EP, Haberkern CM, Neumayr L, et al: A comparison of conservative and aggressive transfusion regimens in the perioperative management of sickle cell disease. The Preoperative Transfusion in Sickle Cell Disease Study Group. N Engl J Med 333:206–213, 1995.

190. Miller ST, Rao SP, Dunn EK, Glassberg KI: Priapism in children with sickle cell disease. J Urol 154 (2 Pt 2): 844–847, 1995.

191. Rifkind S, Waisman J, Thompson R, Goldfinger G: RBC exchange pheresis for priapism in sickle cell disease. JAMA 242:2317–2318, 1979.

192. Rackoff WR, Ohene-Frempong K, Month S, et al: Neurologic events after partial exchange transfusion for priapism in sickle cell disease. J Pediatr 120:882–885, 1992.

193. Siegel JF, Rich MA, Brock WA: Association of sickle cell disease, priapism, exchange transfusion and neurological events: ASPEN syndrome. J Urol 150 (5 Pt 1): 1480–1482, 1993.

194. Field JW: Blood examination and prognosis in acute falciparum malaria. Trans R Soc Trop Med Hyg 43:33–48, 1949.

195. Weatherall DJ, Miller LH, Baruch DI, et al: Malaria and the red cell. Hematology (Am Soc Hematol Educ Prog) 35–57, 2002.

196. Riddle MS, Jackson JL, Sanders JW, Blazes DL: Exchange transfusion as an adjunct therapy in severe *Plasmodium falciparum* malaria: A meta-analysis. Clin Infect Dis 34:1192–1198, 2002.

197. Gerson SL, Lazarus HM: Hematopoietic emergencies. Semin Oncol 16:532–542, 1989.

198. Conley CL: Polycythemia vera. JAMA 263:2481–2483, 1990.

199. Perloff JK, Rosove MH, Child JS, Wright GB: Adults with cyanotic congenital heart disease: Hematologic management. Ann Intern Med 109:406–413, 1988.

200. Murphy S: Polycythemia vera. In Williams WJ, Beutler E, Erslev AJ, Litchman MA (eds): Hematology. New York, McGraw-Hill, 1990, pp 193–202.

201. Brittenham GM: Disorders in iron metabolism: Iron deficiency and overload. In Hoffman R, Benz EJ, Shattil SJ, et al (eds): Hematology: Basic Principles and Practice. New York, Churchill Livingstone, 1995, pp 492–523.

202. Valbonesi M, Bruni R: Clinical application of therapeutic erythrocytapheresis (TEA). Transfus Sci 22:183–194, 2000.

203. Zarkovic M, Kwaan HC: Correction of hyperviscosity by apheresis. Semin Thromb Hemost 29:535–542, 2003.

204. Kwaan HC, Bongu A: The hyperviscosity syndromes. Semin Thromb Hemost 25:199–208, 1999.

205. Ciavarella D, Wuest D, Strauss RG, et al: Management of neurologic disorders. J Clin Apher 8:242–257, 1993.

206. Shiga Y, Fujihara K, Onodera H, et al: Complement activation as a cause of transient hypotension during plasmapheresis. Artif Organs 22:1067–1079, 1998.

207. Leitman SF, Boltansky H, Alter HJ, et al: Allergic reactions in healthy plateletpheresis donors caused by sensitization to ethylene oxide gas. N Engl J Med 315:1192–1196, 1986.

208. Owen HG, Brecher ME: Atypical reactions associated with use of angiotensin-converting enzyme inhibitors and apheresis. Transfusion 34:891–894, 1994.

209. Perseghin P, Capra M, Baldini V, Sciorelli G: Bradykinin production during donor plasmapheresis procedures. Vox Sang 81:24–28, 2001.

210. Alving BM, Hojima Y, Pisano JJ, et al: Hypotension associated with prekallikrein activator (Hageman-factor fragments) in plasma protein fraction. N Engl J Med 299:66–70, 1978.

211. Kaplan AP, Joseph K, Silverberg M: Pathways for bradykinin formation and inflammatory disease. J Allergy Clin Immunol 109:195–209, 2002.

212. McLeod BC, Price TH, Owen H, et al: Frequency of immediate adverse effects associated with apheresis donation. Transfusion 38:938–943, 1998.

213. Trouern-Trend JJ, Cable RG, Badon SJ, et al: A case-controlled multicenter study of vasovagal reactions in blood donors: Influence of sex, age, donation status, weight, blood pressure, and pulse. Transfusion 39:316–320, 1999.

30

214. Randels MJ: Selection and care of apheresis donors. In McLeod BC, Price TH, Weinstein R (eds): Apheresis: Principles and Practice. Bethesda, Md, AABB Press, 2003, pp 131–142.

215. Roberts WH, Domen RE, Walters MI: Changes in calcium distribution during therapeutic plasmapheresis. Arch Pathol Lab Med 108:881–883, 1984.

216. Gorlin JB, Humphreys D, Kent P, et al: Pediatric large volume peripheral blood progenitor cell collections from patients under 25 kg: A primer. J Clin Apher 11:195–203, 1996.

217. Kramer L, Bauer E, Joukhadar C, et al: Citrate pharmacokinetics and metabolism in cirrhotic and noncirrhotic critically ill patients. Crit Care Med 31:2450–2455, 2003.

218. Hester JP, Ayyar R: Anticoagulation and electrolytes. J Clin Apher 2:41–51, 1984.

219. Bolan CD, Greer SE, Cecco SA, et al: Comprehensive analysis of citrate effects during plateletpheresis in normal donors. Transfusion 41:1165–1171, 2001.

220. Silberstein LE, Naryshkin S, Haddad JJ, Strauss JF 3rd: Calcium homeostasis during therapeutic plasma exchange. Transfusion 26:151–155, 1986.

221. Dzik WH, Kirkley SA: Citrate toxicity during massive blood transfusion. Transfus Med Rev 2:76–94, 1988.

222. Kelleher SP, Schulman G: Severe metabolic alkalosis complicating regional citrate hemodialysis. Am J Kidney Dis 9:235–236, 1987.

223. Pearl RG, Rosenthal MH: Metabolic alkalosis due to plasmapheresis. Am J Med 79:391–393, 1985.

224. Spindler JS: Subclavian vein catheterization for apheresis access. J Clin Apher 1:202–205, 1983.

225. Rizzoni WE, Miller K, Rick M, Lotze MT: Heparin-induced thrombocytopenia and thromboembolism in the postoperative period. Surgery 103:470–476, 1988.

226. Ling E, Warkentin TE: Intraoperative heparin flushes and subsequent acute heparin-induced thrombocytopenia. Anesthesiology 89:1567–1569, 1998.

227. Mayo DJ, Cullinane AM, Merryman PK, Horne MK 3rd: Serologic evidence of heparin sensitization in cancer patients receiving heparin flushes of venous access devices. Support Care Cancer 7:425–427, 1999.

228. Kadidal VV, Mayo DJ, Horne MK: Heparin-induced thrombocytopenia (HIT) due to heparin flushes: A report of three cases. J Intern Med 246:325–329, 1999.

229. Wing EJ, Bruns FJ, Fraley DS, et al: Infectious complications with plasmapheresis in rapidly progressive glomerulonephritis. JAMA 244:2423–2426, 1980.

230. Pohl MA, Lan SP, Berl T: Plasmapheresis does not increase the risk for infection in immunosuppressed patients with severe lupus nephritis. The Lupus Nephritis Collaborative Study Group. Ann Intern Med 114:924–929, 1991.

231. Fosburg M, Dolan M, Propper R, et al: Intensive plasma exchange in small and critically ill pediatric patients: Techniques and clinical outcome. J Clin Apher 1:215–224, 1983.

232. Kevy SV, Fosburg M: Therapeutic apheresis in childhood. J Clin Apher 5:87–90, 1990.

233. Diaz MA, Vicent MG, Garcia-Sanchez F, et al: Long-term hematopoietic engraftment after autologous peripheral blood progenitor cell transplantation in pediatric patients: Effect of the CD34+ cell dose. Vox Sang 79:145–150, 2000.

234. Gorlin JB: Therapeutic plasma exchange and cytapheresis. In Nathan DG, Orkin SH, Oski FA (eds): Nathan and Oski's Hematology of Infancy and Childhood. Philadelphia, WB Saunders, 1998, pp 1827–1838.

235. Gasparro FP, Dall'Amico R, Goldminz D, et al: Molecular aspects of extracorporeal photochemotherapy. Yale J Biol Med 62:579–593, 1989.

236. Maeda A, Schwarz A, Kernebeck K, et al: Intravenous infusion of syngeneic apoptotic cells by photopheresis induces antigen-specific regulatory T cells. J Immunol 174:5968–5976, 2005.

237. Foss FM: Photopheresis. In McLeod BC, Price TH Weinstein R (eds): Apheresis: Principles and Practice. Bethesda, Md, AABB Press, 2003, pp 623–642.

238. Lundin J, Osterborg A: Therapy for mycosis fungoides. Curr Treat Options Oncol 5:203–214, 2004.

239. Edelson R, Berger C, Gasparro F, et al: Treatment of cutaneous T-cell lymphoma by extracorporeal photochemotherapy: Preliminary results. N Engl J Med 316:297–303, 1987.

240. Heald P, Rook A, Perez M, et al: Treatment of erythrodermic cutaneous T-cell lymphoma with extracorporeal photochemotherapy. J Am Acad Dermatol 27:427–433, 1992.

241. Fraser-Andrews E, Seed P, Whittaker S, Russell-Jones R: Extracorporeal photopheresis in Sezary syndrome: No significant effect in the survival of 44 patients with a peripheral blood T-cell clone. Arch Dermatol 134:1001–1005, 1998.

242. Child FJ, Mitchell TJ, Whittaker SJ, et al: A randomized cross-over study to compare PUVA and extracorporeal photopheresis in the treatment of plaque stage (T2) mycosis fungoides. Clin Exp Dermatol 29:231–236, 2004.

243. Child FJ, Ratnavel R, Watkins P, et al: Extracorporeal photopheresis (ECP) in the treatment of chronic graft-versus-host disease (GVHD). Bone Marrow Transplant 23:881–887, 1999.

244. Greinix HT, Volc-Platzer B, Knobler RM: Extracorporeal photochemotherapy in the treatment of severe graft-versus-host disease. Leuk Lymphoma 36:425–434, 2000.

245. Fimiani M, Di Renzo M, Rubegni P: Mechanism of action of extracorporeal photochemotherapy in chronic graft-versus-host disease. Br J Dermatol 150:1055–1060, 2004.

246. Foss FM, DiVenuti GM, Chin K, et al: Prospective study of extracorporeal photopheresis in steroid-refractory or steroid-resistant extensive chronic graft-versus-host disease: Analysis of response and survival incorporating prognostic factors. Bone Marrow Transplant 35:1187–1193, 2005.

247. Apisarnthanarax N, Donato M, Korbling M, et al: Extracorporeal photopheresis therapy in the management of steroid-refractory or steroid-dependent cutaneous chronic graft-versus-host disease after allogeneic stem cell transplantation: Feasibility and results. Bone Marrow Transplant 31:459–465, 2003.

248. Muller C: Angina pectoris in hereditary xanthomatosis. Arch Intern Med 64:675–700, 1939.

249. Thompson GR: Familial hypercholesterolemia. In Wass JAH, Shalet EM (eds): Oxford Textbook of Endocrinology and Diabetes. Oxford, Oxford University Press, 2002, pp 1545–1552.

250. Naoumova RP, Thompson GR, Soutar AK: Current management of severe homozygous hypercholesterolaemias. Curr Opin Lipidol 15:413–422, 2004.

251. Thompson GR, Maher VM, Matthews S, et al: Familial hypercholesterolaemia regression study: A randomised trial of low-density-lipoprotein apheresis. Lancet 345:811–816, 1995.

252. Knisel W, Pfohl M, Muller M, et al: Comparative long-term experience with immunoadsorption and dextran sulfate cellulose adsorption for extracorporeal elimination of low-density lipoproteins. Clin Investig 72:660–668, 1994.

253. Schuff-Werner P, Schultz E, Seyde WC, et al: Improved haemorheology associated with a reduction in plasma fibrinogen and LDL in patients being treated by heparin-induced extracorporeal LDL precipitation (HELP). Eur J Clin Invest 19:30–37, 1989.

254. Julius U, Siegert G, Gromeier S: Intraindividual comparison of the impact of two selective apheresis methods (DALI and HELP) on the coagulation system. Int J Artif Organs 23:199–206, 2000.

255. Empen K, Otto C, Brodl UC, Parhofer KG: The effects of three different LDL-apheresis methods on the plasma concentrations of E-selectin, VCAM-1, and ICAM-1. J Clin Apher 17:38–43, 2002.

256. Motohashi K, Yamane S: The effect of apheresis on adhesion molecules. Ther Apher Dial 7:425–430, 2003.

257. Kojima S, Shida M, Yokoyama H: Changes in C-reactive protein plasma levels during low-density lipoprotein apheresis. Ther Apher Dial 7:431–434, 2003.

258. Napoli C, Ambrosio G, Scarpato N, et al: Decreased low-density lipoprotein oxidation after repeated selective apheresis in homozygous familial hypercholesterolemia. Am Heart J 133:585–595, 1997.

259. Kizaki Y, Ueki Y, Yoshida K, et al: Does the production of nitric oxide contribute to the early improvement after a single low-density lipoprotein apheresis in patients with peripheral arterial obstructive disease? Blood Coagul Fibrinolysis 10:341–349, 1999.

260. Aengevaeren WR, Kroon AA, Stalenhoef AF, et al: Low density lipoprotein apheresis improves regional myocardial perfusion in patients with hypercholesterolemia and extensive coronary artery disease. LDL-Apheresis Atherosclerosis Regression Study (LAARS). J Am Coll Cardiol 28:1696–1704, 1996.

261. Keller C: Indication of low-density lipoprotein apheresis in severe hypercholesterolemia and its atherosclerotic vascular complications: Dextran sulfate cellulose low-density lipoprotein apheresis. Ther Apher Dial 7:345–349, 2003.

262. Al-Shaikh AM, Abdullah MH, Barclay A, et al: Impact of the characteristics of patients and their clinical management on outcomes in children with homozygous familial hypercholesterolemia. Cardiol Young 12:105–112, 2002.

263. Makino H, Harada-Shiba M: Long-term effect of low-density lipoprotein apheresis in patients with homozygous familial hypercholesterolemia. Ther Apher Dial 7:397–401, 2003.

264. Thompson GR: LDL apheresis. Atherosclerosis 167:1–13, 2003.

265. Stefanutti C, Vivenzio A, Colombo C, et al: Treatment of homozygous and double heterozygous familial hypercholesterolemic children with LDL-apheresis. Int J Artif Organs 18:103–110, 1995.

266. Kroon AA, Swinkels DW, van Dongen PW, Stalenhoef AF: Pregnancy in a patient with homozygous familial hypercholesterolemia treated with long-term low-density lipoprotein apheresis. Metabolism 43:1164–1170, 1994.

267. Klingel R, Gohlen B, Schwarting A, et al: Differential indication of lipoprotein apheresis during pregnancy. Ther Apher Dial 7: 359–364, 2003.

268. Teruel JL, Lasuncion MA, Navarro JF, et al: Pregnancy in a patient with homozygous familial hypercholesterolemia undergoing low-density lipoprotein apheresis by dextran sulfate adsorption. Metabolism 44:929–933, 1995.

269. Beigel Y, Hod M, Fuchs J, et al: Pregnancy in a homozygous familial hypercholesterolemic patient treated with long-term plasma exchange. Am J Obstet Gynecol 162:77–78, 1990.

30

Chapter 31

Vena Caval Filters

Christine L. Hann, MD, PhD • Michael B. Streiff, MD

INTRODUCTION

Deep venous thrombosis (DVT) and pulmonary embolism (PE) occur in approximately 500,000 patients in the United States each year.[1] The vast majority of these episodes can be effectively managed with conventional anticoagulation, which is associated with a low incidence of recurrent thrombotic events (0.6 to 1.5 events per 100 patient-years) and major bleeding during therapy ($\approx$0.9 to 4.6 events per 100 patient-years).[2–4] Nonetheless, the increasing complexity of hospitalized patients ensures that all clinicians will have to treat patients with acute thrombosis for whom anticoagulation may be contraindicated. Modifications in vena caval filter technology and increased ease of insertion have prompted a number of authors to propose broadened indications for filter insertion.[5–18] Perhaps as a consequence of these changes, the number of vena caval filters inserted annually in the United States has increased 25-fold since the 1970s, such that almost 50,000 filters (178 filters per million population) were placed in the United States in 1999.[19] In comparison, only 20 to 30 vena caval filters are inserted annually in Sweden (3 filters per million inhabitants), an industrialized nation with a comparable quality of health care.[20] This 60-fold disparity warrants scrutiny. The purpose of this chapter is to review the available literature regarding vena caval filters and traditional and proposed indications for their use and to determine whether available data support current practices.

HISTORICAL PERSPECTIVE

The intellectual foundation of vena caval filtration as a means to prevent PE can be traced historically to two of the 19th century's greatest physicians, Rudolf Virchow and Armand Trousseau. In 1846, Virchow proposed the concept that pulmonary thrombi were in fact emboli that originated primarily in the veins of the lower extremities.[21] Two decades later, in his lectures at the Hotel Dieu in Paris, Trousseau suggested that a physical barrier to the migration of emboli might be an effective preventive measure.[22] In the 1930s, Homans popularized femoral vein ligation for the prevention of PE.[23] Although this procedure was effective in preventing emboli from the ipsilateral extremity, femoral vein ligation was associated with significant postthrombotic complications in the affected limb and did not provide protection from clots that may emanate from the contralateral extremity. Consequently, an impressive array of surgical procedures and devices focusing on vena caval interruption were developed over the subsequent four decades. Surgical inferior vena caval ligation was associated with an operative mortality of 12%, with 4% of patients experiencing recurrent PE and 22% developing postphlebitic syndrome.[24] However, some clinical series documented recurrent PE in 20% to 50% of patients after long-term follow-up.[25,26] To preserve caval blood flow, surgical plication was proposed to replace complete caval ligation. However, surgical plication of the vena cava proved to be technically demanding, so a variety of externally applied clips (Moretz, Miles, Adams, and Adams-DeWeese clips) were developed to reduce its complexity. Unfortunately, clinical results with these devices did not prove to be a major improvement (operative mortality, 10%; recurrent PE, 4%; postthrombotic syndrome, 16%)[24] but these experiences led to the development of intraluminal devices. The first widely used intraluminal device for vena caval interruption was the Mobin-Uddin umbrella filter. Although initial reports were favorable when the device was compared with caval plication (operative mortality, 0.6%; recurrent PE, 1.7%; venous stasis, 6.5%),[27] subsequent patient series noted higher rates of PE (7.8%), occlusion of the inferior vena cava (IVC) (53%), venous stasis (75%), and occasional episodes of cardiopulmonary migration.[28–30] These problems and the introduction of the stainless steel Greenfield filter precipitated removal of the Mobin-Uddin filter from the market in 1977.

The introduction of the stainless steel Kimray-Greenfield filter (SSGF; Boston Scientific, Natick, Mass, USA) in 1972 revolutionized the field of vena caval interruption. The preservation of many of its engineering features in subsequent devices is a testament to its revolutionary design. The filter consists of a cone constructed of stainless steel wire affixed to a central apical cap. The filtration area is maximized by having each of the six wire legs make alternating right and left hand bends. At the caudal terminus, each wire ends in a hook that serves to anchor the device within the vena cava (Fig. 31-1). The funnel shape of the filter is designed such that the cross-sectional area of the IVC is reduced by only 50% when the filter is filled to a two-thirds level with thrombus, theoretically providing the body's fibrinolytic system the opportunity to lyse retained clots.[31] Since its introduction in 1972, the Greenfield filter has been implanted in more than 120,000 patients.[32]

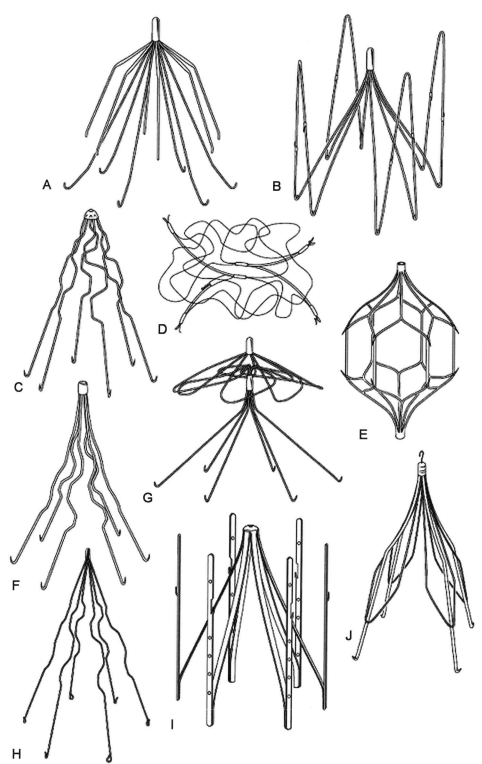

Figure 31-1 Vena caval filters. **A,** Bard G2 filter; **B,** Vena Tech LP filter; **C,** Stainless steel Greenfield filter; **D,** Bird's Nest filter; **E,** Nitinol TrapEase/OptEase filter; **F,** Percutaneous stainless steel Greenfield filter; **G,** Simon Nitinol filter; **H,** Titanium Greenfield filter; **I,** VenaTech filter; **J,** Günther Tulip filter.

CURRENTLY AVAILABLE VENA CAVAL FILTERS

Permanent Filters

Although placed percutaneously beginning in 1984, the original SSGF was too inflexible for easy insertion.[33]

It required a 29-French (Fr) (outer diameter, OD) introducer catheter, which was felt to be partially responsible for the high incidence of insertion site thrombosis (IST) (45%) that had been noted in some studies.[34] Consequently, Greenfield and colleagues[35] developed the titanium Greenfield filter (TGF) (Boston Scientific, Natick, Mass, USA), which was introduced in 1988 and received U.S. Food and Drug Administration (FDA) approval in 1989. Its conical design and the configuration of its six struts with terminal hooks were similar to those of the original SSGF (see Fig. 31-1). The titanium alloy (Beta II titanium alloy) allowed for greater flexibility, such that the filter could be introduced via a 12-Fr catheter (14.3-Fr OD). It was anticipated that reduction in catheter diameter would lead to a lower incidence of IST.[35] Because titanium is nonferromagnetic, the filter also would be at lower risk for migration during magnetic resonance (MR) imaging and may cause minimal MR imaging artefact.[36] Preliminary clinical studies with the TGF revealed a high rate of distal slippage and penetration of the caval wall[37]; therefore, modifications of the hook design and base diameter were made, resulting in the modified-hook titanium Greenfield filter (MHTGF) (Boston Scientific, Natick, Mass, USA), which was introduced in 1991 (see Fig. 31-1; Table 31-1).[38]

Although migration and penetration were largely improved in the MHTGF, tilting remained an occasional problem. To remedy this situation, the stainless steel percutaneous Greenfield filter (PGF) (Boston Scientific, Natick, Mass, USA) was developed. Similar to the SSGF in design, its apical hub differs in that it has a central hole that allows placement over a guidewire to prevent filter tilting and asymmetry. Its design gives it increased flexibility, allowing insertion via a small 12-Fr (15-Fr OD) catheter. The filter comprises six stainless steel struts, which are fitted into a cylindrical hub (see Fig. 31-1; Table 31-1). Once deployed, the filter is 49 mm in length and 32 mm in base diameter. The PGF can be used in patients with IVC diameters of 28 mm or less. To prevent migration, the anchor hooks are positioned bidirectionally, with four directed superiorly and two directed inferiorly.[39,40] Although the filter appears to be MR safe, its stainless steel composition causes significant image artefact.[40] In 2005, all PGFs manufactured before March 10, 2004, were recalled from the market because of eight reports of detachment of the filter carrier capsule at the bond with the insertion catheter, which, in two instances, led to serious patient injury, including one death.

The Bird's Nest filter (Cordis Corporation, Miami Lakes, Fla, USA), introduced in 1982, has a unique structure and comprises four stainless steel wires 25 cm long that are folded over several times and attached to two V-shaped struts. These struts have hooks on the end that affix the filter within the vena cava (see Fig. 31-1; Table 31-1).[41] It can be inserted via a 14-Fr OD catheter. Because the Bird's Nest filter expands up to a diameter of 60 mm, it is the filter of choice for patients with vena caval diameters greater than 30 mm.[42] The original version of the Bird's Nest filter was associated with several fatal episodes of migration, a flaw that has been remedied through the introduction of a new version with stiffer anchor struts.[43,44] The Bird's Nest filter generates the largest MR artefact of any filter because of its stainless steel construction, yet it appears to be stable in magnetic fields up to 1.5 Tesla (T).[45]

The LGM or VenaTech filter (B. Braun/VenaTech, Evanston, Ill, USA) is made of Phynox (pacemaker lead material) with six struts arranged in a conical fashion, similar to the Greenfield filter models. Side rails attached to the filter struts anchor the filter within the vena cava (see Fig. 31-1; Table 31-1).[46] The VenaTech filter received FDA approval in 1989 and is MR compatible.[47] It is inserted with a 12-Fr sheath (14-Fr OD) and can be placed in venae cavae up to 28 mm in

diameter.[48] The original VenaTech filter is now no longer available on the U.S. market and has been replaced by the VenaTech Low-Profile (LP) Filter (B. Braun/VenaTech, Evanston, Ill, USA), which was approved by the FDA in 2001. In contrast to its predecessor, the VenaTech LP filter uses eight Phynox wires shaped in a conical fashion that fuse caudally in pairs to form side rails that secure the filter to the vena caval wall. Each side rail has a hook that is oriented superiorly or inferiorly (see Fig. 31-1). It can be introduced by a 7-Fr sheath and, once deployed, is 43 mm in height and 40 mm in diameter. Its use is limited to IVC diameters of 28 mm or less, and it is MR compatible.[49]

The Simon Nitinol filter (Bard Peripheral Vascular, Tempe, Ariz, USA) is composed of a nickel/titanium alloy (Nitinol) that possesses thermal memory properties. At 4°C, the filter exists as a set of straight wires that automatically unfold at body temperature to form an umbrella filter with seven petals. Six hooked struts anchor the filter within the vena cava (see Fig. 31-1; Table 31-1). The FDA approved the filter in 1990, and it is designed for IVC diameters of 28 mm or less.[50–52]

The G2 filter system (Bard Peripheral Vascular, Tempe, Ariz, USA) is a 12-legged conical filter constructed of Nitinol wires that gained FDA approval for permanent placement in November of 2005. The conical array of six short and six long curved Nitinol wires creates two planes of caval filtration and has a maximal deployment length of 41 mm. The maximal caval diameter for placement is 28 mm. The flexibility afforded by its Nitinol construction allows placement with a 7-Fr (internal diameter) catheter system from a jugular or femoral venous access site (see Fig. 31-1; Table 31-1).

The TrapEase filter (Cordis Corporation, Miami Lakes, Fla, USA) is also composed of Nitinol and consists of two conical filter baskets—one facing cranially, the other caudally—that are connected to create two levels of caval filtration (see Fig. 31-1; Table 31-1). When viewed in cross section, the filter baskets form a filtration plane composed of six diamond-shaped flow corridors. Six struts with proximal and distal hooks anchor the baskets within the vena cava. The TrapEase filter was approved for clinical use by the FDA in 2000. It can be placed through a 6-Fr sheath in patients with IVC diameters of up to 30 mm. The filter's nickel titanium alloy ensures MR compatibility and produces minimal image artefact.[53,54]

The Günther Tulip filter (Cook, Inc., Bloomington, Ind, USA) is constructed of conichrome, an MR-compatible alloy similar to Phynox that is composed of cobalt, chromium, nickel, iron, molybdenum, and manganese. It has been in use in Europe since 1992 and first became available for use in the United States in 2001. In 2003, it received FDA approval for use as a retrievable filter. The filter basket is formed by four struts that are stabilized by wire loops that extend three quarters down the length of each strut. Hooks on the end of each strut attach the filter to the vena caval wall. A hook on the filter apex facilitates retrieval (see Fig. 31-1; Table 31-1). It can be introduced via an 8.5-Fr sheath (11-Fr OD) through a femoral or jugular approach and can be removed via a jugular approach.[55–57]

Nonpermanent Filters

Given the long-term complications of permanent filters, development of a safe and effective nonpermanent filter

31

Table 31-1 Specifications of Currently Available Permanent and Nonpermanent Vena Caval Filters

Filter	Recommended Caval Diameter (mm)	Length (mm)	Catheter ID (mm)	MRI Compatible	Material	Approach	FDA Approval (year)	Company	Maximum Recommended Dwell Time
Permanent Vena Caval Filters									
Titanium Greenfield filter (TGF)	28	50	12	Yes	Beta III Titanium Alloy	Jugular/femoral	1987	Boston Scientific	
Modified-hook Titanium Greenfield filter (MHTGF)	30	47	12	Yes	Titanium	Jugular/femoral	1990	Boston Scientific	
12-F Over-the-Wire Stainless Steel Greenfield filter (PGF)	28	50	12	Yes*	Surgical Stainless Steel	Jugular/femoral	1997	Boston Scientific	
Bird's Nest filter	40	80	12	Yes*	Biocompatible Stainless Steel	Jugular/femoral	1989	Cook Incorporated	
VenaTech LGM filter	28	38	10	Yes	Phynox Plate	Jugular/femoral	1989	B. Braun/VenaTech	
VenaTech LP filter	28	43	7	Yes	Phynox Wire	Jugular/femoral	2001	B. Braun/VenaTech	
Simon Nitinol filter	28	38	7	Yes	Nitinol	Jugular/femoral/antecubital	1990	Bard Peripheral Vascular	
G2	28	41	7	Yes	Nitinol	Jugular/femoral	2005	Bard Peripheral Vascular	
TrapEase filter	30	50	6	Yes	Nitinol	Jugular/femoral/antecubital	2000	Cordis Endovascular	
Günther Tulip filter	30	50	Jugular: 7 Femoral: 8.5	Yes	Conichrome	Jugular/femoral	2000	Cook Incorporated	
OptEase filter	30	54	6	Yes	Nitinol	Jugular/femoral/antecubital	2002	Cordis Endovascular	
Recovery filter	28	41	7	Yes	Nitinol	Femoral		Bard Peripheral Vascular	
Retrievable Vena Caval Filters									
Günther Tulip filter	30	50	Jugular: 7 Femoral: 8.5	Yes	Conichrome	Jugular/femoral	2003	Cook Incorporated	10–14 days
OptEase filter	30	54	6	Yes	Nitinol	Jugular/femoral/antecubital	2004	Cordis Endovascular	<12 days

* causes significant image artefact.

would be of great benefit to patients who have experienced an acute episode of venous thromboembolism (VTE) and have a short-term contraindication to anticoagulation. Nonpermanent filters can be divided into three categories: temporary, retrievable, and convertible. As their name suggests, temporary filters are designed only for short-term insertion and are held in place by a catheter or wire that is anchored to the insertion site. One temporary filter, the Tempo filter (B. Braun, Melsungen, Germany), was investigated in a clinical trial in the United States. Although initial results were promising,[58] subsequent episodes of catheter buckling and atrial migration halted further U.S. development.[59,60] Currently, no temporary filters are approved for use in the United States.

Retrievable filters resemble permanent filters in that they are anchored within the IVC by tethering hooks. These anchoring hooks, however, gradually become incorporated in the wall of the IVC, such that most retrievable filters can be left in place only for a limited time before they must be removed. However, if the need for prolonged, indefinite vena caval interruption arises, these filters may be left in place to function as permanent filters. Two filters have been approved for retrieval by the FDA: the Günther Tulip filter and the OptEase filter (Cordis Corporation, Miami Lakes, Fla, USA) (Table 31-1). A third, the Bard Recovery filter, was approved for retrieval until 2005, at which point it was replaced by the Recovery G2 filter (Bard Peripheral Vascular, Tempe, Ariz, USA), which at present is approved only for permanent use.

The Günther Tulip filter was approved for use as a retrievable filter in 2003 and is described earlier in the section on permanent filters. Although the manufacturer recommends that the Günther Tulip filter be removed within 10 to 14 days of placement, several investigators have successfully retrieved filters that have been implanted as long as 126 days.[55-57,61,62] Some have extended the caval life span by periodic filter repositioning.[63,64] In a cohort of 90 patients with Günther Tulip filters, Millward and associates[56] removed 51 of 52 devices successfully after a mean insertion time of 9 days. The only complication reported was filter occlusion, which occurred in two patients. De Gregorio and colleagues[63] had similar success retrieving 69 of 72 filters (96%) in which retrieval was attempted. Among a series of 53 filters, 16 of 19 filters (84%) were successfully retrieved after a median implantation time of 34 days (range, 7 to 126 days).[61] In contrast, Wicky and coworkers[62] were unable to remove 14 of 49 (19%) Günther Tulip filters because of large trapped thrombi.

In accordance with the TrapEase filter design, the OptEase retrievable vena caval filter is composed of Nitinol and has a double-basket design. Its six struts have superior barbs to provide resistance to migration. It can be placed through a 6-Fr sheath in patients with IVC diameters of up to 30 mm and is MR compatible (see Fig. 31-1). The OptEase filter was approved for use as a retrievable filter in 2004. The manufacturer recommends retrieval within 12 days of placement. In a multicenter study of 27 patients, 21 (78%) had their filters removed a mean of 11 days (range, 5 to 14 days) after implantation. Follow-up was available for 19 of 21 patients (91%). One patient's DVT extended through the access site for filter placement; no other adverse events occurred.[65] Rosenthal and associates[66] reported 94 trauma patients who had had OptEase filters

placed by intravascular ultrasound for prevention of PE. Placement-related complications included one IST (1%), two insertion site hematomas (2%), and three misplacements (3%) that were replaced within 24 hours. Mean implantation time was 19 days (range, 5 to 25 days). Retrieval was attempted in 34 patients (36%) and was successful in 31 (91% of attempts). In three instances, retained clot in the filter precluded retrieval. One patient (3%) experienced a PE post filter retrieval. No PE occurred during the period of filter implantation.[66] The follow-up period in patients whose filters were not retrieved was not reported. Although the collective experience is extremely limited, the OptEase filter, thus far, appears to have comparable performance with the Günther Tulip filter.

In 2002, Asch[67] reported an initial experience with the Bard Recovery filter in 32 patients (see Table 31-1). The mean implantation period was 53 days, and the longest duration was 134 days. Filter retrieval was successful in all 24 patients in whom it was attempted. No symptomatic episodes of PE, IVC, or insertion site thrombosis were noted. One filter with trapped clot migrated 4 cm from its implantation site. Grande and colleagues[68] reported a series of 106 patients. Three patients (3%) presented with a symptomatic PE after placement. One was fatal (1%). No symptomatic caval migration or thrombosis occurred. Retrieval, which was attempted in only 15 patients (14%) was successful in 14 (93%) at a mean of 150 days (range, 0 to 419 days). Subsequent reports of several symptomatic migrations of the Bard Recovery filter have resulted in its discontinuation as a retrievable filter. The redesigned filter, the Bard G2 filter, is not currently FDA approved for retrieval.

The concept of a convertible filter has also been proposed and patented. This type of filter would be constructed in such a way that in the filter position, wire elements of the device would form one or two filtration planes. If caval filtration were no longer necessary, the filter could be converted into a caval stent through manipulation of a built-in release mechanism. At present, no convertible filters have been approved by the FDA.

STUDIES ON THE EFFICACY OF INFERIOR VENA CAVAL FILTERS

The only purpose for placing an IVC filter is to prevent PE. Therefore, it is essential that every physician become familiar with data supporting the effectiveness of filters in this task and with their adverse effects. Unfortunately, the vast majority of data on vena caval filters has been derived from unrandomized case series. Substantial differences exist between studies regarding subject populations (and their risk of recurrent VTE) and the intensity, comprehensiveness, and duration of follow-up. Therefore, combined results of these studies (presented in Table 31-2 and Figs. 31-2 through 31-4) should be interpreted in light of these limitations. Nevertheless, in the absence of randomized comparisons of filters, these data are the principal available means by which filter efficacy and safety can be assessed. As is shown in Table 31-2 and Figure 31-2, most available filters are roughly equivalent to one another but are somewhat less effective than anticoagulation in the prevention of PE. Several more recently approved and/or less extensively studied filter models (Günther Tulip, VenaTech LP, TrapEase,

Table 31-2 Vena Caval Filter Outcomes: Compilation of Vena Caval Filter Studies

Filter Type	Study No.	Patient No.	F/U Duration (in months)	PE	DVT	IST	IVCT	Postthrombotic Syndrome
Stainless Steel Greenfield	42	3636	18 (1–60)	104 of 3038 (3.4%) (range, 0%–9%) Fatal, 38 (1.3%)	96 of 1634 (5.9%) (range, 0%–18%)	97 of 1131 (8.6%) (range, 1%–47%) 50 of 217 (23%)*	89 of 2529 (3.5%) (range, 0%–18%)	254 of 1353 (19%) (range, 0%–47%)
Titanium Greenfield	10	649	5.8 (0–81)	19 of 556 (3.4%) (range, 0%–4.4%) Fatal, 10 (1.8%)	5 of 22 (22.7%) (range, 0%–36%)	35 of 267 (13.1%) (range, 2%–39%) 23 of 82 (28%)*	16 of 364 (4.4%) (range, 1%–31%)	34 of 236 (14.4%) (range, 9%–20%)
Percutaneous stainless steel Greenfield	5	740	20.6 (8.5–26)	9 of 372 (2.4%) Fatal, 1 (0.3%)	41 of 305 (13.4%)	20 of 305 (6.6%)	8 of 267 (3%)	62 of 231 (27%)
Bird's Nest	18	1742	14.2 (0–60)	49 of 1441 (3.4%) (range, 0%–7.1%) Fatal, 22 (1.5%)	27 of 448 (6%) (range, 0%–20%)	31 of 417 (7.4%) (range, 0%–33%) 23 of 101 (23%)*	38 of 1334 (2.8%) (range, 0%–15%)	37 of 267 (14%) (range, 4%–41%)
VenaTech	16	1353	17.3 (0–65)	45 of 1266 (3.6%) (range, 0%–6.3%) Fatal, 12 (0.9%)	8 of 25 (32%) (range, 32%)	40 of 261 (15.3%) (range, 8%–44%) 16 of 44 (36%)*	102 of 1074 (9.5%) (range, 0%–28%)	95 of 232 (41%) (range, 24%–59%)
Simon Nitinol	12	1022	15 (0–62)	30 of 967 (3.1%) (range, 0%–5.3%) Fatal, 17 (1.8%)	11 of 123 (8.9%) (range, 8%–11%)	22 of 191 (11.5%) (range, 0%–64%) 11 of 36 (31%)*	48 of 945 (5.1%) (range, 0%–50%)	16 of 124 (12.9%) (range, 6%–44%)
Nitinol TrapEase	4	426	6.2 (4–15)	1 of 426 (0.2%) (range, 0%–0.5%) Fatal, 0	3 of 254 (1.2%) (range, 1.1%–1.5%)	1 of 254 (0.4%)	11 of 426 (2.6%) (range, 1.6%–4.6%)	NA
Günther Tulip	12	601	6.6 (1–29)	5 of 601 (0.8%) (range, 0%–3.6%) Fatal, 1 (0.2%)	6 of 601 (1%) (range, 0%–8.6%)	2 of 52 (3.8%) (range, 0%–8%)	9 of 138 (6.5%) (range, 0%–33%)	NA
VenaTech LP	2	91	2.3	0	3 of 91 (3.2%) (range, 0%–10%)	NA	2 of 61 (3.2%)	NA
Nitinol OptEase	2	121	1	0	0	1 of 121 (0.8%) (range, 0%–1.1%)	3 of 121 (2.5%) (range, 0%–3.1%)	NA
Recovery	2	138	4.1 (3–6)	4 of 138 (2.9%) Fatal, 1 (0.7%) (range, 2.8%–3.2%)	0	0	1 of 132 (0.8%) (range, 0%–0.9%)	NA

*Indicates IST rate in studies with routine radiographic/duplex surveillance.
F/U, follow up; PE, pulmonary embolism; DVT, deep venous thrombosis; IST, insertion site thrombosis; IVCT, inferior vena caval thrombosis.

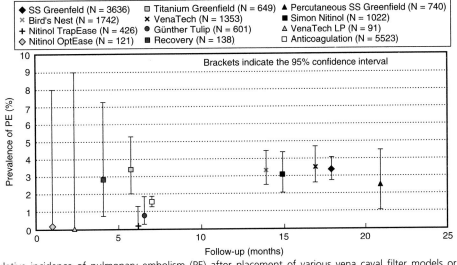

Figure 31-2 Cumulative incidence of pulmonary embolism (PE) after placement of various vena caval filter models or treatment with anticoagulation. (Derived from the meta-analysis of Douketis, Kearon et al., 1998.)

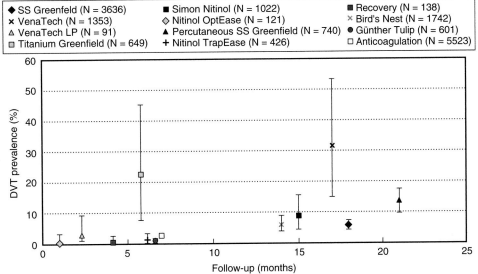

Figure 31-3 Cumulative incidence of deep venous thrombosis (DVT) after placement of various vena caval filter models or treatment with anticoagulation. (Derived from the meta-analysis of Douketis, Kearon et al., 1998.)

OptEase) appear to have lower PE event rates. However, small study populations, short durations of follow-up, and wide 95% confidence intervals suggest that these estimates are fairly imprecise and may change as patient numbers and surveillance time increase. No follow-up data for the Bard G2 Recovery filter have been published.

Although randomized comparisons of various filter models have not been performed, a single randomized trial of vena caval filters in the management of VTE has been published.[69,70] Investigators randomly assigned 400 patients with proximal DVT with or without PE who were judged to be at high risk for PE in a two-by-two factorial design to receive a vena caval filter or no filter and unfractionated heparin or enoxaparin. The subject population was clearly at high risk for adverse outcomes: 60% had idiopathic VTE, 35% had a previous history of VTE, 40% had iliac (37%) or vena caval (3%) thrombosis, and 14% had cancer. Four different types of vena caval filters were used: the VenaTech filter (56% of patients randomly assigned to the filter group), the titanium Greenfield filter

(27%), the Cardial filter (Bard, Saint-Etienne, France—not available in the United States), and the Bird's Nest filter (15.5%). Filters were placed within 48 hours of random assignment, and all patients were treated with unfractionated heparin or enoxaparin. Ventilation/perfusion scans were performed at baseline and after 8 to 12 days of anticoagulation. Warfarin was started on day 4, and heparin or enoxaparin was continued until the international normalized ratio (INR) was 2 or greater for 2 consecutive days. Ninety-nine percent of patients were discharged while on anticoagulation. Ninety-four percent received anticoagulant therapy for at least 3 months. Only 62% of filter patients and 64% of the group without filters received anticoagulation beyond 3 months. Thirty-eight percent of patients were still on oral anticoagulation at 2 years, and 35% received anticoagulation over the entire 8-year follow-up, with no significant differences noted between groups. After 12 days of treatment, vena caval filters were associated with a significant decrease in the incidence of (symptomatic and asymptomatic) PE compared with

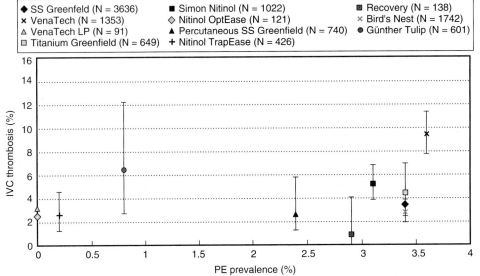

Figure 31-4 Cumulative incidence of inferior vena caval (IVC) thrombosis and pulmonary embolism (PE) after placement of various vena caval filter models.

anticoagulation alone (1.1% vs 4.8%; $P = .03$). When only symptomatic PEs were considered, differences between the filter and no filter groups were no longer significant (1% vs 3%). At 2 years, symptomatic PE tended to be less frequent among filter recipients than among those who had received anticoagulation alone (3% vs 6%), although this difference was not significant ($P = .16$).

Fatal emboli were also more common in patients treated solely with anticoagulation (0.5% vs 2.5%). However, vena caval filters were associated with significantly more recurrent DVT than was observed with anticoagulation alone (21% vs 12%; $P = .02$). No difference in bleeding or mortality was documented. Sixteen of 37 patients (43%) with vena caval filters who had recurrent DVT also had IVC thrombosis. At 8 years, outcome data on 99% of patients became available, and 198 patients (50%) were found to be alive. The occurrence of symptomatic PE was less frequent in filter recipients than in those treated with anticoagulation alone (6% vs 15%; $P = .008$). Fifty percent of PEs in the no filter group occurred during the first 2 years of follow-up. DVT was more frequent among filter patients (36% vs 28%; $P = .042$). Sixty-five percent of DVT occurred among filter patients within the first 2 years of follow-up. Symptomatic filter thrombosis occurred in 13% after 8 years. Postthrombotic syndrome (PTS) was observed in 70% of patients in both the filter and no filter groups. No difference in overall survival was reported.[70] These data indicate that filters, when used in conjunction with anticoagulation, offer a short-term reduction in the total number of PEs at the cost of a long-term increase in recurrent DVT with no reduction in mortality. Unfortunately, because 94% of patients received anticoagulation for at least 3 months, these data offer no insight into the outcome of the typical patient who has had a vena caval filter placed, namely, those who are believed to have contraindications to anticoagulant therapy. In addition, although it was not routine at the time the study was performed, extended duration anticoagulant therapy is commonly recommended for high-risk patients, as in the PREPIC (Prévention du Risque d'Embolie Pulmonaire

par Interruption Cave) study population. Therefore, it is likely that the benefits associated with filter placement in this study would be considerably less with currently recommended durations of anticoagulation for VTE.

Additional valuable information about the efficacy of vena caval filters can be found in the population-based observational study conducted by White and coworkers.[71] Using the linked California Patient Discharge Data Set, which tracks discharge diagnoses and procedures performed in all nonfederal hospitals in California, the researchers analyzed the outcomes of patients admitted from January 1991 to December 1995 for VTE. During this 5-year period, 3632 patients received a vena caval filter for VTE and 64,333 patients did not receive a filter. Filter recipients were more likely to have had major bleeding, surgery, cancer, stroke, myocardial infarction, chronic lung disease, or congestive heart failure within 3 to 6 months of their VTE diagnosis. For purposes of comparison, filter and control patients were subdivided into groups with 0, 1, or 2 or more previous hospitalizations for VTE.

Even after adjusting for risk factors for recurrent VTE, investigators found that patients who received vena caval filters were just as likely as nonrecipients to be readmitted for a PE. Similar to the results of the Decousus study,[69] White and associates[71] noted that filter placement was associated with a twofold increase in the risk of subsequent venous thrombosis, although only among patients with an initial episode of PE. Filters did not seem to have a short-term protective benefit against PE as the time course of recurrent PE was similar between filter recipients and nonrecipients. Filter recipients also were more likely to die during follow-up than were control patients. Because it is unlikely that filter placement alone is responsible for this mortality difference, the potential limitations of this type of analysis are underscored—that unidentified comorbidities may have been responsible in part for the inferior outcomes of filter recipients. Despite this limitation, the White study[71] provided valuable information that should be considered by any physician who contemplates the use of a vena caval filter for the treatment of patients with VTE.

FILTER COMPLICATIONS

Permanent Filters

Complications of IVC filters may occur at the time of insertion or months to years later.[72] Acute procedure-related complications include misplacement (1.3% of insertions), pneumothorax (0.02%), hematoma (0.6%), air embolism (0.2%), inadvertent carotid artery puncture (0.04%), and arteriovenous (AV) fistula (0.02%). According to the published case series, fatal complications of placement are rare, occurring in only 0.13% of insertions. Among various individual filter models, the published fatal complication rate is highest for the Bird's Nest filter (0.34%) compared with the original stainless steel Greenfield filter (0.11%), the titanium Greenfield filter (0.15%), and the VenaTech filter (0.07%). No fatal complications have been reported in the published literature for the PGF, the Simon Nitinol filter, the Günther Tulip filter, the Nitinol TrapEase, OptEase filters, or the Bard G2 filter,[73] although fatal events for several of these filters have been reported in the Manufacturer and User Facility Device Experience database, which is available through the FDA. The higher fatal complication rate associated with the Bird's Nest filter reflects primarily the results of a single study, which documented four episodes of fatal IVC thrombosis.[73] If one considers this experience as isolated, the fatal complication rate associated with the Bird's Nest filter is comparable with other filter models.

A common early postprocedural complication of filter placement is insertion site thrombosis (IST).[34,74–79] IST is a DVT that develops at the venous insertion site. Given the process of filter insertion and the patient population served by it, it is not surprising that nonocclusive and occasionally occlusive thrombi develop at the venous access site. IST appears to be less common with balloon dilation as opposed to the use of serial fixed diameter dilators for site preparation.[77] Counterintuitively, the literature does not support the notion that filters requiring larger introducer catheters are at higher risk for thrombosis.[74,75] One possible explanation for this observation may be that all introducer systems result in sufficient local endothelial trauma to precipitate VTE. Alternatively, the apparent absence of a difference in IST rates between insertion catheters of various sizes may reflect the limited number of patients investigated to date.

Delayed complications of filter placement include recurrent DVT, IVC thrombosis, filter migration, IVC penetration, and filter disruption. Because filters are often placed in patients with a VTE who cannot at least initially receive anticoagulation, recurrent DVT in this patient population is not an unexpected event. Case series data on the frequency of DVT after filter placement suggest that DVT may be more common with the titanium Greenfield filter and the VenaTech filter (see Table 31-2; Fig. 31-3). However, differences in follow-up and patient populations may be more responsible for these outcome differences than filter design. Ultimately, randomized comparisons are needed to determine whether important differences exist between filters. Consistent with the results of Decousus and White and colleagues, the rate of recurrent DVT among patients treated with anticoagulation as derived from a pooled analysis of randomized anticoagulation trials in the treatment of VTE is approximately half that identified in most case series of vena caval filters (see Fig. 31-3).[69–71,80]

IVC thrombosis, although substantially less problematic for contemporary filter models than for the Mobin-Uddin umbrella filter and IVC clips, remains a common event among filter recipients. Possible sequelae of IVC thrombosis include phlegmasia cerulea dolens, venous gangrene, recurrent DVT, and a heightened risk of postthrombotic syndrome and recurrent PE due to thrombi that extend proximally to the thrombosed filter. Case series data suggest that IVC thrombosis occurs in 2% to 10% of filter recipients (see Table 31-2).[81] Thirteen percent of filter recipients in the PREPIC study experienced symptomatic IVC thrombosis over 8 years of follow-up.[70] Although one might predict that filters associated with a higher frequency of IVC thrombosis would be associated with fewer PEs, case series data do not support this conclusion (Fig. 31-4). One conceivable explanation for this seemingly contradictory result may be the contribution to episodes of PE made by thrombi that have propagated *proximal* to thrombosed filters. Important differences in the use and sensitivity of screening procedures for IVC thrombosis and follow-up of patients for PE also are likely to be important contributors to this paradoxical outcome.

With regard to the frequency of IVC thrombosis, a study conducted by Crochet and associates is particularly enlightening.[82] In this study, routine radiographic surveillance, including abdominal radiography, duplex scanning, and venacavography, was performed in 142 patients who received VenaTech filters. IVC occlusion was identified in 22% and 33% of patients after 5 and 9 years of follow-up, respectively. Among the subgroup of patients with PE and anticoagulant therapy failure, the caval occlusion rate was 65%. Anticoagulation did not appear to favorably influence the rate of caval occlusion. Fifty percent of patients with caval occlusion experienced lower extremity swelling.

This study offers several important lessons. First, it strongly suggests that the frequency of IVC thrombosis is underestimated in many of the published case series. Although this study focused exclusively on the VenaTech filter, pooled data on IVC occlusion do not suggest that significant differences exist between filter types (see Fig. 31-4). Second, it suggests that trapped emboli rather than in situ thrombosis in the filter are primarily responsible for IVC thrombosis. In the past, thrombus trapping and in situ thrombosis of the filter due to its effect on blood flow have been proposed as reasons for IVC thrombosis. Patients who present with PE are more likely to experience recurrent PE than are patients with an initial DVT.[80,83] The fact that patients with PE and failure of anticoagulation constitute the only subgroup with a higher risk of IVC occlusion supports the premise that thrombus trapping is a major contributor to IVC occlusion.

Crochet and colleagues[82] found that anticoagulant therapy did not significantly reduce the incidence of vena caval occlusion. Two factors may have contributed to this result. The subgroup with the highest incidence of IVC occlusion comprised patients with previous anticoagulation failure and PE. The impact of this subgroup with anticoagulation resistance may have diminished the impact of anticoagulation on IVC occlusion. Unfortunately, no subgroup analysis has been performed to investigate this possibility. In addition, data on mean achieved anticoagulation intensity are not presented. Therefore, subtherapeutic anticoagulation may have substantially contributed to thrombotic complications in this study. A prior investigation found no evidence of enhanced prothrombin activation among filter recipients compared with patients without filters who were on long-term anticoagulation.[84] Consequently, it may be premature to consider anticoagulation ineffective in preventing thrombotic complications associated with vena caval filters.

Postthrombotic syndrome (PTS) is a common complication among patients after they have experienced VTE. In a consecutive series of 528 patients treated with conventional anticoagulation, cumulative incidences of PTS at 2, 5, and 8 years of follow-up were 25%, 30%, and 30%, respectively. The risk of PTS was strongly associated with recurrent ipsilateral DVT.[85] Pooled data from case series indicate a roughly similar incidence among filter recipients (see Table 31-2; Fig. 31-5). Nevertheless, the association of vena caval filters with recurrent VTE and the established association of recurrent ipsilateral DVT with subsequent PTS would tend to suggest that these case series data may underestimate the frequency of PTS among filter recipients.[69,71,85] In the PREPIC study, a similar proportion of filter recipients (70%) and those who received no filter (70%) experienced PTS within 8 years.[70] The high rate of PTS reflects the high-risk nature of the subject population (36% had a history of previous VTE) and the significant proportion of patients who had PTS at baseline (filter, 23%; no filter, 24%). The severity of preexisting venous insufficiency at baseline may account for the absence of any difference in PTS between groups. Alternatively, it is also possible that the ability of anticoagulant therapy to preserve valve function is insufficient to produce measurable protection against PTS. Because compression

stockings have been shown to reduce the incidence of PTS by 50%, routine use of compression stockings should be strongly encouraged among all filter patients (see Chapter 17).[86]

Filter migration was a significant problem with the Mobin-Uddin filter—a fact that resulted in several deaths.[27,29] Improved anchoring technology has made this event distinctly unusual among recipients of contemporary permanent filters (0.3%).[81] One unavoidable consequence of using hooks to reduce filter mobility is IVC penetration. Penetration occurs when filter components traverse the IVC wall and enter the pericaval space. Limited penetration of the IVC wall is desired and necessary if the filter is to be anchored at its intended location. Rarely, however, filter components penetrate into adjacent structures and produce clinical consequences (0.3%).[81] Small bowel obstruction,[87] duodenal perforation,[88,89] and retroperitoneal hemorrhage[72,90] due to penetration of the abdominal aorta or iliac artery are among the reported consequences of IVC penetration by filter components. Concomitant anticoagulation has been associated with several instances of bleeding and conceivably may enhance this risk.[90,91] Therefore, IVC filters should be placed cautiously during anticoagulation, and the development of abdominal pain in this setting warrants prompt abdominal imaging.

Filter tilting and strut fracture theoretically may contribute to impaired filtration efficiency and thus reduced filter performance in PE prevention.[92-94] Only a fraction of filter case series have documented tilting (5.3%) and strut fracture (2.7%).[81] However, clinical studies investigating possible adverse consequences of these events remain inconclusive.[95,96]

A recently recognized potential long-term source of complications associated with IVC filters is entrapment of guidewires used to place vascular access catheters.[97-99] Forceful attempts to remove guidewires have led to a

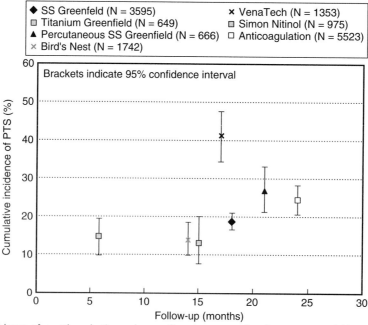

Figure 31-5 Cumulative incidence of postthrombotic syndrome after placement of various vena caval filter models or treatment with anticoagulation. (Estimate derived from Prandoni, Villalta et al., 1997.)

number of filter displacements that in some instances have required filter removal or placement of a second device.[98,100–103] One patient died from a cerebrovascular accident following anticoagulation after such an event.[104] Case reports and one experimental study suggest that VenaTech and Greenfield filters are more likely to result in guidewire entrapment.[105,106] In vitro tests indicate that the TrapEase filter may also entrap 3-mm and 1.5-mm J-tipped wires. Design modifications in the VenaTech LP make it much less likely to entrap guidewires and catheters.[106] Simple precautionary measures that may reduce the frequency of guidewire entrapment include prominent documentation of IVC filter placement in the medical record and provision of identification bracelets to patients with filters. Use of straight-tipped guidewires, which are less likely to become entrapped than J-tipped wires and limiting insertion of guidewires to 18 cm (the mean distance to the SVC:right atrial junction), minimizes the chances of this complication.[105–107] If a guidewire does become entrapped, physicians should immediately contact an interventional radiologist or vascular surgeon for safe removal of the wire under fluoroscopic guidance.

Filter-Specific Data from the Manufacturer and User Facility Device Experience (MAUDE) Database

Permanent Filters

The Manufacturer and User Facility Device Experience (MAUDE) database is a collection of adverse event reports associated with FDA-approved medical devices.[108] These voluntary reports have been collected since 1991. Although reports do not constitute a comprehensive dataset for all complications associated with vena caval filters, this database does provide narratives on commonly encountered events associated with vena caval filter implantation and use. Data on filters that received FDA approval after 1991 were collected and summarized as described below.

Between August 1996 and March 2006, 333 reports on the PGF were filed in the MAUDE database. Most reports were listed as difficulty in deployment (232 of 333; 70%). Failure to open completely was the most common reason for difficulty in deployment and was listed in 169 reports. Difficulty in guidewire removal was reported on 40 occasions. Central line guidewire entrapment was reported 8 times (2%). Filter migration was reported on 42 occasions (13%); 19 of these incidents were related to failure of the filter to open completely. Perforation was reported 10 times, and two of these cases were directly attributable to user error. In total, nine deaths were reported among patients who received a PGF; three of these appeared to be unrelated to PGF use.

Since its approval in 2000, 174 adverse events have been reported with the TrapEase filter. The most commonly reported event was filter thrombosis or occlusion (29% of reports), followed by difficulty with deployment (19%) and migration (14%). Filter or strut fracture was reported in 23 instances (13%). Perforation was reported in 9 cases (5%). Overall, 19 deaths attributable to the presence of the TrapEase filter were reported.

Since 2002, 34 reports have been filed in the MAUDE database on the VenaTech LP filter. Most of these were listed as difficulty in deployment or failure to open (21 of 34; 62%). Filter migration was reported on 18 occasions (53%); one third of cases occurred in conjunction with failure to open. Perforation was reported once. One death attributable to placement of a VenaTech LP filter has been reported to the MAUDE database.

Fifty-two reports on the G2 filter have been filed in the MAUDE database. Most reports were listed as difficulty or failure of filter deployment (35 of 53; 66%). Filter migration was reported in 19% of cases, and perforation and tilt were described to occur at a rate of 9% each. One death was reported in a patient who received a G2 filter; however, details of this event are not available.

Nonpermanent Filters

Sixty-nine complications involving the Günther Tulip filter have been reported to the MAUDE database since its approval as a retrievable device (December 2002 to March 2006). The most commonly reported complications were related to difficulty in filter deployment 48%; in five cases, the user commented that the filter legs appeared crossed. Migration was reported in 15% and device breakage in 4%. Difficulty in retrieval was reported in 4%. Post–filter placement thrombotic events, including PE, DVT, and filter thrombosis, were reported in 6% of patients; two of these thrombotic events resulted in death. Overall, death was the listed outcome in six reports; two cases were attributed to hemorrhage caused by the filter, and two deaths were a consequence of filter migration.

With respect to the OptEase filter, 39 complications were submitted to the MAUDE database since its approval as a retrievable device (period between December 2003 and March 2006). The most commonly reported complications were strut or filter fracture (23%) and difficulty with deployment (23%), although most of the latter events appeared to be due to user error. Filter migration was also frequently reported (15%). Post–filter placement thrombotic events, including PE, DVT, and filter thrombosis, were reported in 13%. Death was the listed outcome in two of these reports, although neither event was attributed by the user to the filter.

SHOULD PATIENTS WITH PERMANENT VENA CAVAL FILTERS RECEIVE PROPHYLACTIC ANTICOAGULATION?

As was outlined in previous sections, vena caval filters have been associated with several thrombotic complications, including IST, recurrent DVT, and IVC thrombosis. Therefore, should all patients with a vena caval filter receive long-term prophylactic anticoagulation to prevent these thrombotic complications? Anticoagulant therapy with vitamin K antagonists is known to be effective in the prevention of recurrent thromboembolism; however, this protection comes at the cost of increases in hemorrhagic morbidity and mortality, even when anticoagulation is managed by specialized anticoagulation clinics. Although anticoagulant therapy is often managed by anticoagulation clinics in the United Kingdom and Europe, management by individual practitioners remains the predominant mode of care in the United States. Therefore, the risks of major bleeding associated with any program of prophylactic anticoagulation in filter recipients in the United States are likely to be closer to 7% to 8% per patient-year of therapy, rather than the 2% to 3% per patient-year commonly reported by anticoagulation clinics.[109] Although anticoagulant therapy has been reported to reduce prothrombin activation in filter recipients,[84] it remains to be seen whether anticoagulant therapy would prevent clinical events or reduce mortality in patients with filters. In the PREPIC study, 35% of patients in both groups received anticoagulant therapy during the entire 8-year study follow-up period. Although indefinite anticoagulant therapy among all filter recipients may have prevented excessive thrombotic complications, it remains unclear whether the benefits of this approach would have exceeded the associated risks, because 26 filter recipients (15%) experienced major bleeding during the study period. Because no difference in mortality was observed between groups at the study conclusion, it seems unlikely that indefinite anticoagulant therapy among all filter recipients will be associated with a mortality benefit.

The case fatality rate of major bleeding in patients with VTE has been estimated to be 13%; the case fatality rate for recurrent DVT is approximately 5%.[80,110] This hemorrhagic mortality risk translates to an absolute fatal bleeding risk of 0.3% to 1% per patient-year, depending on the mode of anticoagulation management used (individual practitioner vs anticoagulant therapy management clinic). In contrast, according to the data from Decousus and coworkers, the absolute excess risk of recurrent DVT among filter recipients is on the order of 5% per patient-year, corresponding to a maximal excess risk of thrombotic mortality of 0.25% per patient-year (because filters are effective in the prevention of PE, this estimate of thrombotic mortality based on patients without filters is likely to be an overestimate).[69] Therefore, even with optimal anticoagulant therapy control, it is doubtful whether indefinite anticoagulation for filter recipients would result in net benefit, particularly in the setting of individual practitioner management. Furthermore, because the risk of recurrent VTE declines over time while the risk of bleeding with anticoagulant therapy remains constant, it is likely that the risk:benefit ratio is likely to worsen as time passes.[111,112] In the near future, anticoagulants with improved safety profiles may become clinically available, which should favorably alter the risk:benefit ratio for long-term anticoagulant therapy for many indications.[113] Until that time, available data indicate that anticoagulant therapy for patients with IVC filters should be guided by the thrombotic history of the patient (i.e., filter placed for prophylaxis only or as part of treatment of VTE), and not solely by the presence of a filter.

CAN PATIENTS WITH VENA CAVAL FILTERS UNDERGO MAGNETIC RESONANCE IMAGING?

Magnetic resonance (MR) imaging has become an increasingly important clinical imaging modality. Therefore, patients with vena caval filters are likely to require MR imaging at some point during their medical care. Thus far, no reports of filter migration as a result of MR imaging have been published. Ferromagnetic alloys such as stainless steel, as used in the original stainless steel Greenfield filter,

the percutaneous Greenfield filter, and the Bird's Nest filter, produce artefacts on MR imaging. The greatest artefact is seen with the SSGF and the Bird's Nest filter and much less is seen with the percutaneous Greenfield filter, nonetheless, stainless steel filter components have been shown to be stable at field strengths up to 1.5 T.[40,45,114]

Simon Nitinol, Nitinol TrapEase and OptEase, VenaTech, VenaTech LP, Günther Tulip, Bard G2, and titanium Greenfield filters are all composed of low ferromagnetic alloys, which do not cause significant MR image deterioration.[36,50,114–117] MR imaging as early as 1 week after placement was not associated with any consequences in a small series of patients in whom the Simon Nitinol filter was used.[50] Although it is likely that other low ferromagnetic devices will behave similarly, data on other filter models should prove useful for clinical decision making.

POTENTIAL INDICATIONS FOR IVC FILTER PLACEMENT (TABLE 31-3)

Since improved percutaneous techniques have been developed for filter placement, the number of indications cited for vena caval filter placement and the number of filters placed have increased dramatically. One report on IVC filter use revealed a fivefold increase in the number of caval filters placed at a single institution from 1980 to 1996.[118] These single-center data are corroborated by a recent analysis of U.S. national trends in filter use. Using the National Hospital discharge database, Stein and associates[19] documented a 25-fold increase in vena caval filter use between 1979 and 1999, despite a relatively relatively stable incidence of VTE during this period. Coincident with this trend has been increasing use of IVC filters for prophylactic indications, despite the absence of compelling data showing their efficacy in these situations.[19] In the following sections, we review data that support the use of vena caval filters for these extended indications (see Table 31-3).

CONTRAINDICATION TO ANTICOAGULATION

Although the vast majority of patients with VTE can be managed with anticoagulation, in a small subset of patients, anticoagulant therapy seems contraindicated. Because patients with an acute episode of VTE are at substantial risk for recurrence in the absence of anticoagulation,[119,120] vena caval filters represent a valuable treatment option for those who should not receive anticoagulation.

FAILURE OF ANTICOAGULANT THERAPY

Prevention of recurrent VTE is commonly proposed as an indication for vena caval filter placement. Although episodes of VTE do occur in patients who are therapeutically anticoagulated, these instances are unusual. Therefore, any patient with recurrent VTE despite anticoagulation should be carefully evaluated before vena caval filter placement is entertained so that potential therapeutic catastrophes can be avoided. First, it is important to determine whether the patient has been consistently therapeutic

Table 31-3 Putative Indications for Placement of Inferior Vena Caval Filters

(see text for details)

Indications	Comments
Contraindications to adequate anticoagulant therapy	Probably greatly inflated, given risk:benefit ratio of treatment in acute VTE. Seems appropriate for fresh (e.g., <3–4 days) neurosurgery; active hemorrhage of the GI tract, retroperitoneum, CNS, and pulmonary tree; known CNS metastases* or significant CNS trauma. Treatment for patients with severe coagulopathy or severe thrombocytopenia must be individualized.
Failure of ongoing anticoagulant therapy	Very rare; far more often, prior therapy is found to be inadequate or punctuated. Trousseau syndrome is the most common exception.
Pulmonary thromboendarterectomy	Uncertain benefit but prevalent practice.
Trauma	Rational, given the high morbidity and mortality of VTE in trauma patients. Randomized studies are urgently needed to resolve this question.
Free-floating venous thrombus	This previously widely held indication has been disproved.
Thrombolytic therapy for DVT	No firm indication.
Unsubstantiated indications	
Cancer patients	No firm indication.
High-risk orthopedic patients	No firm indication.
Bariatric surgery	No firm indication.
Other	

*Particularly hemorrhagic metastases or metastases from melanoma or choriocarcinoma.
VTE, venous thromboembolism; GI, gastrointestinal; CNS, central nervous system; DVT, deep venous thrombosis.

during the period preceding the recurrent thrombotic event. If such is not the case, it is appropriate to redouble efforts to maintain the patient in the therapeutic range and perhaps increase the target INR from 2 to 3 up to 2.5 to 3.5, rather than place a vena caval filter that may thrombose and promote morbidity if subtherapeutic anticoagulant therapy continues. In the setting of a substantial pulmonary circulatory clot burden, thrombolysis followed by anticoagulation may be more appropriate than filter placement. If the patient has been clearly therapeutic, hypercoagulable syndromes that require more intensive or alternative forms of anticoagulation should be excluded before a filter is placed. Although many patients with the antiphospholipid antibody syndrome are safely managed with conventional intensity warfarin anticoagulation (INR, 2 to 3),[121] a subset of these patients require high-intensity warfarin (INR, 3 to 4) to prevent thrombotic events (see Chapter 19).[122] A panel of coagulation assays sensitive to the presence of antiphospholipid antibodies, as well as immunoassays for antiphospholipid binding protein antibodies (anticardiolipin antibodies, anti–β_2-glycoprotein I antibodies), should be performed to diagnose this condition.[123]

Another hypercoagulable state that is strongly associated with resistance to warfarin anticoagulation of conventional intensity is Trousseau syndrome (see Chapter 12). First recognized by Armand Trousseau 140 years ago, Trousseau syndrome is a malignancy-associated hypercoagulable state that is characterized by arterial and/or venous thromboembolism (often migratory and involving superficial veins), nonbacterial thrombotic endocarditis, disseminated intravascular coagulation, and warfarin resistance.[124] Because this condition is a systemic hypercoagulable state, regional approaches to prevent thromboembolism such as vena caval filters are never adequate and, in the authors' anecdotal experience, are often associated with substantial thrombotic morbidity and mortality. This condition is best treated with heparin anticoagulants.

Heparin-induced thrombocytopenia (HIT) is a common early cause of anticoagulation failure (see Chapter 25). In 1% to 5% of patients, treatment with unfractionated heparin (0.3% among low molecular weight heparin [LMWH] recipients) for at least 4 days precipitates a prothrombotic immune thrombocytopenia. Although HIT typically results in thrombocytopenia (50% decline from baseline) 5 to 10 days after initiation of heparin therapy, patients less commonly develop thrombocytopenia within 24 hours in the setting of preformed HIT antibodies that result from heparin exposure within the previous 120 days. Even less common is delayed HIT, in which patients develop thrombocytopenia several weeks after heparin exposure. Patients typically present after a recent hospitalization with new moderate thrombocytopenia and a new thrombotic event. Use of heparin in this setting can result in worsening thrombocytopenia and progressive thrombosis. Although each of these presentations can result in recurrent thrombosis despite adequate heparin therapy and may be interpreted as a failure of anticoagulation, use of a vena caval filter in this setting is counterproductive and has resulted in worsening thrombosis. The only effective therapy is to discontinue all forms of heparin exposure and initiate therapy with a direct thrombin inhibitor (lepirudin or argatroban) or perhaps fondaparinux.

Recurrent events in the same location should prompt consideration of vascular abnormalities such as the May-Thurner syndrome or the Paget-Schrötter syndrome (thoracic outlet syndrome), both of which are underrecognized reasons for recurrent VTE (see Chapter 16). The May-Thurner syndrome is characterized by deformation and stenosis of the left iliac vein as a consequence of the overlying right iliac artery. Resulting stenosis precipitates recurrent episodes of left iliofemoral DVT. Thrombolysis and stenting of the affected vein segment may result in long-lasting resolution.[125] Occurrence of an upper extremity DVT without clear risk factors should prompt investigation for the Paget-Schrötter syndrome, a venous manifestation of thoracic outlet syndrome. In affected individuals, the subclavian vein is compressed by local anatomic structures (e.g., anterior scalene muscle, cervical ribs). Vascular wall damage and stasis may result in thrombosis. Historically, patients may relate a recent history of heavy lifting or exertion that involves the affected extremity. Venography of the upper limb vessels in stress positions (e.g., abduction, external rotation) is useful for demonstrating functional compression of the subclavian vein.[126,127] Therapy for the Paget-Schrötter syndrome consists of catheter-directed thrombolysis followed by surgical correction of the anatomic abnormality and anticoagulation.

PULMONARY THROMBOENDARTERECTOMY

In most patients, PE resolves with treatment such that no permanent clinically apparent physiologic sequelae occur. In a subset of patients (3.8%), these emboli may persist, or multiple subclinical episodes of PE may occur such that patients develop chronic thromboembolic pulmonary hypertension (CTEPH) (see Chapter 45).[128,129] Pulmonary thromboendarterectomy has proved to the most effective treatment for patients with CTEPH.[130] Although no randomized, controlled trials have been performed, vena caval filters are commonly placed preoperatively in these patients, and one small case series identified inadequate caval filtration as a common characteristic of patients who required repeat pulmonary thromboendarterectomy.[131] Although data supporting the usefulness of filters in this capacity are limited, the severity of the condition and limited treatment options for patients with CTEPH, as well as the difficulty associated with conducting a randomized trial in this patient population, indicate that indefinite anticoagulant therapy and filters should be strongly considered in all patients who undergo pulmonary thromboendarterectomy. This operation should not be confused with acute embolectomy for acute PE.

TRAUMA

VTE is a common complication of major trauma. In a prospective cohort study in which routine DVT surveillance was used with impedance plethysmography and contrast venography, 58% of trauma patients developed a DVT during the first few weeks of hospitalization in the absence of DVT prophylaxis.[132] Eighteen percent had a proximal DVT, and 1% experienced a symptomatic PE; half of these cases were fatal. Only 3 of 201 patients with adequate venography (1.5%) had a clinically apparent DVT. In a subgroup analysis, the authors found that patients with lower extremity orthopedic injuries (69%) and spinal trauma (62%) were at particularly high risk for DVT prophylaxis.[132] Using routine contrast spiral computed tomography (CT) scan surveillance, Schultz and colleagues[133] identified asymptomatic PE in 24% (22 of 90) of trauma patients, including 4 patients with a major clot burden, 1 of whom had a saddle embolism.[133] Standard methods of VTE prophylaxis, including subcutaneous unfractionated heparin and/or mechanical prophylaxis with sequential compression devices, are not entirely protective against VTE in trauma patients.[134,135] Although several studies have shown the effectiveness of LMWH with or without mechanical VTE prophylaxis,[136–139] concerns about bleeding complications have limited the use of LMWH among high-risk trauma patients and have led to a dramatic increase in vena caval filter use in this population.[140] One retrospective review noted an increase in prophylactic vena caval filter insertion in trauma patients— from 3% during the five year period 1991–1996 to 57% for the five year period 1996–2001.[141]

Does the literature support the use of vena caval filters in this capacity? More than two dozen unrandomized cohort published studies have assessed the usefulness of vena caval filters in the prevention of PE in high-risk trauma patients.[10,12,13,15,16,66,142–159] Compared with high-risk historical controls (symptomatic PE, 121 of 5765, 2.1%; fatal PE, 47 of 5765, 0.8%), permanent vena caval filters have demonstrated superior protection against PE (symptomatic PE, 12 of 1890, 0.6%; fatal PE, 2 of 1890, 0.1%). A lower frequency of events was seen among prospective controls (PE, 84 of 36,258, 0.2%; fatal PE, 9 of 36,258, 0.02%); however, these subjects were clearly at lower risk than were concurrent filter recipients (Fig. 31-6). Although many

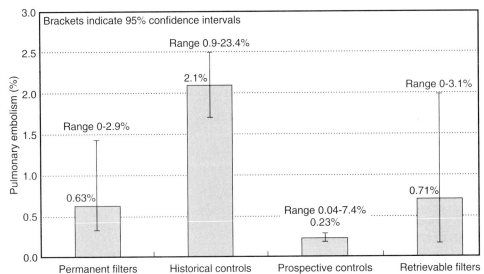

Figure 31-6 Incidence of pulmonary embolism among trauma patients treated with or without a prophylactic inferior vena caval (IVC) filter.

studies focused on the initial hospitalization, longer-term follow-up data were provided by nine studies, in which 61% of the subject population was followed for a mean of 29.1 months. Ten percent of patients (166 of 1546) had a DVT and 3.2% (22 of 708) developed IVC thrombosis during follow-up. Migration occurred in only six patients (0.8%).

A survey of trauma centers revealed that the perceived risk of complications associated with permanent vena caval filters has tempered the enthusiasm of trauma surgeons for the routine use of filters in high-risk trauma patients. In addition, investigators found that the availability of a retrievable filter would significantly increase the number of practitioners (from 29% to 53%) who would use prophylactic filters in trauma patients.[160] If they functioned similarly to permanent vena caval filters, retrievable filters theoretically could provide optimal mechanical PE prophylaxis in patients with transient contraindications to pharmacologic prophylaxis, while avoiding the long-term adverse effects of permanent filters. Indeed, the predicted enthusiasm for retrievable filters among providers has been borne out by a recent single-center study that documented a threefold increase in filter placement in trauma patients since the advent of retrievable filters.[143] Although only six studies of retrievable filters (Bard Recovery, Günther Tulip, and OptEase filters) with limited follow-up have been conducted in trauma patients, preliminary results suggest that retrievable and permanent devices may have similar efficacy (see Fig. 31-6).[66,142,143,146–148] Nevertheless, increased use of retrievable filters has not automatically translated into reduced rates of PE or filter-related complications among trauma patients.[143] These authors noted an equivalent incidence of symptomatic PE (0.2% vs 0.2%) and filter-related complications (1.8% vs 2.5%) before and after the advent of retrievable filters. The latter finding may reflect the low retrieval rate of these filters. In trauma studies of retrievable filters, only a minority (152 of 421; 36%) were retrieved. Furthermore, several reports have documented the occurrence of PE after retrieval of vena caval filters.[66,142,146,161] Therefore, it remains unclear whether retrievable filters will, once again, fulfill their initial promise as a useful form of mechanical PE prophylaxis for trauma patients. Clearly, demonstration of the true value of vena caval filters in the prevention of VTE in trauma patients awaits the execution of randomized trials.

FREE-FLOATING VENOUS THROMBUS

The presence of free-floating venous thrombus has been variably held to be associated with an increased risk of PE.[162–168] This observation has prompted some to suggest that IVC filters should be placed in all patients with free-floating thrombi.[165] Nevertheless, for several reasons, we believe it is unwise to recommend such a policy. First, the single well-executed prospective study found no evidence that free-floating clots were associated with a higher incidence of PE.[166] Second, in two of the previously cited studies, most PEs occurred prior to the diagnosis of free-floating DVT.[162,168] Therefore, changes in therapeutic approach would have had no impact on the clinical course of these patients. Furthermore, no study has shown that the addition of an IVC filter to adequate anticoagulant

therapy would improve clinical outcome. Therefore, until such data are available, no firm recommendations can be made to support the value, let alone the mandate, for IVC filters in the treatment of patients in this situation.

THROMBOLYSIS FOR PROXIMAL DEEP VENOUS THROMBOSIS

The principal complications of DVT are PE and PTS. Although thrombolysis does not reduce the risk of PE associated with DVT, studies of systemic and catheter-directed thrombolysis suggest that this approach may reduce the incidence of PTS.[169–172] However, systemic thrombolysis of proximal DVT (particularly iliofemoral or IVC thrombi) has been associated with several cases of fatal and nonfatal PE.[173,174] Therefore, prophylactic placement of vena caval filters has been proposed as a strategy for preventing PE in patients undergoing thrombolysis. When a variety of temporary filters were used during systemic thrombolysis, however, a European multicenter registry noted four cases of fatal PE (2.1%) and three cases of nonfatal PE (1.6%) despite filter protection.[175] Conversely, only one fatal pulmonary embolus (0.3%) occurred during a multicenter registry of catheter-directed thrombolysis without routine filter use.[172] Although they are far from conclusive, these data suggest that catheter-directed thrombolysis may be associated with a lower risk of PE compared with systemic thrombolysis. Furthermore, if thrombolysis were attempted in a patient deemed to be at high risk for embolization (e.g., poorly adherent IVC, iliac thrombi) or mortality from PE (e.g., patients with concomitant PE, those with limited cardiopulmonary reserve), the experience of Lorch and coworkers[175] would suggest that retrievable filters might be a better option.

UNSUBSTANTIATED INDICATIONS

Patients with Cancer

Malignancy is a well-documented independent risk factor for the development of VTE. In a prospective registry study of 5451 patients with objectively confirmed DVT, cancer was present in 32% of patients.[176] Early studies of anticoagulant therapy in cancer patients with VTE noted a high incidence of hemorrhagic complications (as great as 50% in one series) and recurrent thrombosis, which generated considerable interest in the routine use of vena caval filters in the treatment of patients with cancer who had VTE.[177–179] Case series of IVC filters in patients with cancer indicate that filters may be effective in the prevention of PE (pooled frequency of symptomatic PE, 23 of 1120, 2.0%; fatal PE, 9 of 1120, 0.8%), although the duration (7.5 months) and intensity of follow-up were limited.[6,14,174,178,180–189] However, nonrandomized comparisons with anticoagulant therapy have found greater thrombotic morbidity among filter recipients and no improvement in survival (Fig. 31-7).[7,177,190–193] In one single-institution retrospective study of 166 patients with cancer who had VTE, serious, life- or limb-threatening VTE complications occurred in 17% of filter recipients.[190] Therefore, despite the greater hemorrhagic morbidity of long-term anticoagulant therapy in patients with cancer, its risk:benefit profile appears to

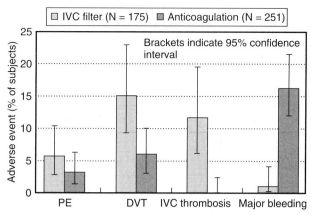

Figure 31-7 Frequency of adverse clinical events in studies of vena caval filter placement or anticoagulation for the treatment of patients with cancer with venous thromboembolism (VTE).

be more favorable than that associated with IVC filter use.[194,195] Recent studies of LMWH in the treatment of malignancy-associated VTE and clinical trials of new antithrombotic agents indicate that aggressive and adequate pharmacologic approaches, not mechanical approaches, will continue to be the preferred therapy for most patients with cancer who have VTE.[113,196]

High-Risk Orthopedic Patients

Patients undergoing orthopedic surgery such as total knee arthroplasty (TKA) or total hip arthroplasty (THA) are considered to be at very high risk for the development of VTE because of a number of factors that contribute to venous stasis, such as position on the operating table, use of thigh tourniquets during knee arthroplasty to provide a "bloodless" field, postoperative immobility, and vascular injury. In the absence of prophylaxis, the risk of proximal DVT in this patient population is 10% to 20%.[197] Several case series attest to the efficacy of IVC filters in the prevention of PE in orthopedic patients.[8,198–200] However, none of these studies incorporated random or masked treatment assignment or masked outcome assessment, and follow-up was of limited intensity and duration. Furthermore, many advances in orthopedic VTE prophylaxis (e.g., LMWH, fondaparinux) and anticoagulation monitoring (INR) have occurred since the time of publication of these studies. Therefore, with the availability of modern methods of VTE prophylaxis, it is doubtful whether IVC filter placement represents a useful option for the vast majority of orthopedic patients. Until well-designed studies have proved the usefulness of vena caval filters for this purpose, this indication for filter placement should be considered one that is primarily of historical significance. As with any major surgical procedure, IVC filters, in particular, retrievable filters, remain a useful option for patients who develop VTE during the immediate perioperative period, when full-dose anticoagulant therapy might be contraindicated.[118]

Bariatric Surgery

PE is considered the leading cause of perioperative death in bariatric surgical patients.[201] Although the reported

incidence of VTE during the immediate (30 days) postoperative period is 0% to 3%, nearly one third of patients who develop PE die.[202] This finding may reflect the lack of cardiac and pulmonary reserves in those who may have cor pulmonale resulting from obesity hypoventilation syndrome.[201] A survey of the members of the American Society of Bariatric Surgery found that of the 31% who responded, 95% routinely used VTE prophylaxis. The most commonly used method was low-dose heparin (50%), followed by sequential compression devices (SCDs) (33%), LMWH (13%), and other methods (4%). Thirty-eight percent of respondents used two or more methods in combination. Despite this practice, 48% of respondents reported at least one patient death that was due to PE.[203] As a result, placement of IVC filters has become a popular prophylaxis strategy among some bariatric surgeons.

Nevertheless, few data exist to support this practice or any VTE prophylaxis strategy in this patient population. In a prospective study of 106 consecutive Roux-en-Y gastric bypass patients, Prystowsky and associates[204] performed bilateral lower extremity duplex scans preoperatively and postoperatively. All patients were given 5000 U of heparin subcutaneously every 12 hours, as well as SCDs, and were ambulatory on postoperative day 1. Patients with a prior history of DVT received temporary vena caval filters. Of 100 patients without a history of DVT, 1 patient was found to have a DVT on a duplex scan performed on postoperative day 14. In contrast, 2 of 6 patients with a prior history of DVT developed a new thrombus DVT postoperatively. Although duplex ultrasonography represents a suboptimal study for assessing the incidence of DVT in an asymptomatic patient population, this study suggests that low-dose heparin combined with SCDs may represent a useful approach to DVT prevention in this patient population. Given that the mean body mass index of the subject population was greater than 51 kg/m², one wonders whether more intensive pharmacologic DVT prophylaxis would be even more effective and thus would obviate the use of IVC filters in high-risk bariatric surgery patients. One observational cohort study found that enoxaparin administered at 40 mg twice daily was significantly more effective than enoxaparin 30 mg given twice daily.[205]

At the present time, no firm recommendations for VTE prophylaxis can be made for this patient population. Until appropriate clinical trials are performed to address this deficiency in the literature, methods of VTE prophylaxis used for other high-risk populations, such as orthopedic surgery patients, should be used. Given the influence of weight on total blood volume and consequently on plasma heparin concentrations, higher dose regimens (e.g., enoxaparin 40 mg subcutaneously given every 12 hours) or doses adjusted by measured drug levels should be considered to reduce the chances of prophylaxis failure in this challenging patient population.

Other Indications

Vena caval filter placement has been proposed for the treatment of pregnant patients with VTE. Intrinsic (reductions in protein S activity, increases in factor VIII, fibrinogen, and von Willebrand factor activity) and environmental (reduced activity, IVC compression) factors make pregnancy a high-risk period for thrombotic events (see Chapter 36).[206-208] Several case series and case reports have documented the use of vena caval filters during pregnancy.[209-214] Although some researchers have claimed that anticoagulant therapy alone may be insufficient therapy for pregnant patients with VTE, substantial evidence indicates that appropriately monitored anticoagulant therapy is effective for the vast majority of patients.[215,216] Therefore, IVC filters should be reserved strictly for situations in which anticoagulation is contraindicated. In these instances, retrievable filters should be strongly considered, given the young age of potential recipients and thus the prolonged duration of time during which they will be at risk for complications associated with permanent filters.

Small clinical series have described the use of vena caval filters in pediatric patients,[217,218] transplant recipients,[219,220] and those with severe chronic obstructive pulmonary disease.[221] Because none of these conditions intrinsically precludes anticoagulant therapy, the use of filters in these populations should be restricted to patients who have absolute contraindications to anticoagulant therapy or those enrolled in well-designed studies. Prophylactic IVC filter placement has been described in a small number of thermally injured patients.[222] Further research to determine the efficacy of conventional VTE prophylactic methods and to identify the subsets of the burn patient population at highest risk for VTE should be performed before wider application of IVC filters is considered for this indication.

APPROPRIATE PREVENTIVE HEALTH CARE AND FOLLOW-UP FOR PATIENTS WITH PERMANENT VENA CAVAL FILTERS

Vena caval filters are associated with an increased incidence of DVT and IVC thrombosis[70]; therefore, routine clinical and objective radiologic follow-up evaluations have been recommended by consensus guidelines.[223] Clinical evaluation should include an assessment of subsequent episodes of VTE, physical findings of PTS, and current use of anticoagulant therapy, as well as any complications resulting in the discontinuation of anticoagulation. Useful objective radiologic studies include abdominal radiographs to determine placement stability, duplex ultrasound examination of the lower extremities to identify recurrent DVT or chronic venous insufficiency, and CT or MR imaging to identify extracaval filter extension and caval thrombosis. In addition, all patients with lower extremity DVT and a vena caval filter should be prescribed graduated compression stockings (30 to 40 mm Hg) to reduce the incidence of PTS. Anticoagulation should be continued for as long as dictated by the underlying thrombotic event. The benefits of indefinite anticoagulant therapy should be weighed against the risk of hemorrhagic complications, and a decision must be made on a case-by-case basis. Ideally, patients should carry identification to alert physicians to the presence of the filter, so that episodes of guidewire entrapment can be avoided.

CONCLUSIONS

Despite improvements in VTE prophylaxis and increasing acceptance of its importance among physicians, the incidence of VTE remains relatively stable. Therefore, the treatment of patients with VTE will remain an important issue for many physicians. An unprecedented number of new antithrombotic medications are under development or are currently in clinical trials. Although it is likely that these new medications will provide even safer and more effective pharmacologic options for the treatment of VTE, patients with firmly established contraindications to anticoagulant therapy will remain a challenge for medical and surgical practitioners. For these patients, IVC filters will remain an important therapeutic alternative. Similar to the evolution of pharmacologic antithrombotic therapy, IVC filter technology has advanced dramatically. In addition to a wide assortment of permanent IVC filters, several promising retrievable filters are now available for clinical use. If these devices prove to be as efficacious as permanent filters and are actually removed, they will likely represent the future of IVC filters, providing the clinician with greater flexibility to meet the demands of a broad array of different clinical situations. Ideally, these filters will offer the benefits of permanent filters without their long-term thrombotic consequences. Published clinical evaluations of filter performance up to the present, however, have consisted almost exclusively of clinical case series, which lack the rigor required to establish clinical efficacy. It is the fervent hope of the authors of this chapter that a serious effort will be made to rigorously evaluate these new devices to establish their true benefits and risks. Without these studies, IVC filters are destined to remain a subject of clinical controversy.

REFERENCES

1. Stein PD, Beemath A, Olson RE: Trends in the incidence of pulmonary embolism and deep venous thrombosis in hospitalized patients. Am J Cardiol 95:1525–1526, 2005.
2. Kearon C, Gent M, Hirsh J, et al: A comparison of three months of anticoagulation with extended anticoagulation for a first episode of idiopathic venous thromboembolism. N Engl J Med 340:901–907, 1999.
3. Kearon C, Ginsberg JS, Kovacs MJ, et al: Comparison of low-intensity warfarin therapy with conventional-intensity warfarin therapy for long-term prevention of recurrent venous thromboembolism. N Engl J Med 349:631–639, 2003.
4. Schulman S, Granqvist S, Holmstrom M, et al: The duration of oral anticoagulant therapy after a second episode of venous thromboembolism. The Duration of Anticoagulation Trial Study Group. N Engl J Med 336:393–398, 1997.
5. Britt LD, Zolfaghari D, Kennedy E, et al: Incidence and prophylaxis of deep vein thrombosis in a high risk trauma population. Am J Surg 172:13–14, 1996.
6. Cantelmo NL, Menzoian JO, Logerfo FW, et al: Clinical experience with vena caval filters in high-risk cancer patients. Cancer 50:341–344, 1982.
7. Cohen JR, Tenenbaum N, Citron M: Greenfield filter as primary therapy for deep venous thrombosis and/or pulmonary embolism in patients with cancer. Surgery 109:12–15, 1991.
8. Emerson RH Jr, Cross R, Head WC: Prophylactic and early therapeutic use of the Greenfield filter in hip and knee joint arthroplasty. J Arthroplasty 6:129–135, 1991.
9. Goluke PJ, Garrett WV, Thompson JE, et al: Interruption of the vena cava by means of the Greenfield filter: Expanding the indications. Surgery 103:111–117, 1988.

31

547

10. Gosin JS, Graham AM, Ciocca RG, Hammond JS: Efficacy of prophylactic vena cava filters in high-risk trauma patients. Ann Vasc Surg 11:100–105, 1997.

11. Jones TK, Barnes RW, Greenfield LJ: Greenfield vena caval filter: Rationale and current indications. Ann Thorac Surg 42 (6 suppl): S48–S55, 1986.

12. Khansarinia S, Dennis JW, Veldenz HC, et al: Prophylactic Greenfield filter placement in selected high-risk trauma patients. J Vasc Surg 22:231–235, 1995; discussion 235–236.

13. Leach TA, Pastena JA, Swan KG, et al: Surgical prophylaxis for pulmonary embolism. Am Surg 60:292–295, 1994.

14. Muchmore JH, Dunlap JN, Culicchia F, Kerstein MD: Deep vein thrombophlebitis and pulmonary embolism in patients with malignant gliomas. South Med J 82:1352–1356, 1989.

15. Rodriguez JL, Lopez JM, Proctor MC, et al: Early placement of prophylactic vena caval filters in injured patients at high risk for pulmonary embolism. J Trauma 40:797–802, 1996; discussion 802–804.

16. Rogers FB, Shackford SR, Wilson J, et al: Prophylactic vena cava filter insertion in severely injured trauma patients: Indications and preliminary results. J Trauma 35:637–641, 1993; discussion 641–642.

17. Rohrer MJ, Scheidler MG, Wheeler HB, Cutler BS: Extended indications for placement of an inferior vena cava filter. J Vasc Surg 10:44–49, 1989; discussion 49–50.

18. Sarasin FP, Eckman MH: Management and prevention of thromboembolic events in patients with cancer-related hypercoagulable states: A risky business. J Gen Intern Med 8:476–486, 1993.

19. Stein PD, Kayali F, Olson RE: Twenty-one–year trends in the use of inferior vena cava filters. Arch Intern Med 164:1541–1545, 2004.

20. Bergqvist D: The role of vena caval interruption in patients with venous thromboembolism. Prog Cardiovasc Dis 37:25–37, 1994.

21. Virchow RLK: Thombosis and Emboli. 1st ed. Canton, OH, Science History Publications, 1998.

22. Trousseau A: Phlegmasia alba dolens. In Trousseau A, (ed): Clinique Medicale de l'Hotel-Dieu de Paris. Paris, Balliere, 1865, pp 654–712.

23. Homans J: Thrombosis of deep veins of lower leg, causing pulmonary embolism. N Engl J Med 211:993–997, 1934.

24. Mansour M, Chang AE, Sindelar WF: Interruption of the inferior vena cava for the prevention of recurrent pulmonary embolism. Am Surg 51:375–380, 1985.

25. Gurewich V, Thomas DP, Rabinov KR: Pulmonary embolism after ligation of the inferior vena cava. N Engl J Med 274:1350–1354, 1966.

26. Piccone VA Jr, Vidal E, Yarnoz M, et al: The late results of caval ligation. Surgery 68:980–998, 1970.

27. Mobin-Uddin K, Utley JR, Bryant LR: The inferior vena cava umbrella filter. Prog Cardiovasc Dis 17:391–399, 1975.

28. Adelson J, Steer ML, Glotzer DJ, et al: Thromboembolism after insertion of the Mobin-Uddin caval filter. Surgery 87:184–189, 1980.

29. Cimochowski GE, Evans RH, Zarins CK, et al: Greenfield filter versus Mobin-Uddin umbrella: The continuing quest for the ideal method of vena caval interruption. J Thorac Cardiovasc Surg 79:358–365, 1980.

30. Wingerd M, Bernhard VM, Maddison F, Towne JB: Comparison of caval filters in the management of venous thromboembolism. Arch Surg 113:1264–1271, 1978.

31. Greenfield LJ, McCurdy JR, Brown PP, Elkins RC: A new intracaval filter permitting continued flow and resolution of emboli. Surgery 73:599–606, 1973.

32. Hann CL, Streiff MB: The role of vena caval filters in the management of venous thromboembolism Blood Rev. 19:179–202, 2005.

33. Tadavarthy SM, Castaneda-Zuniga W, Salomonowitz E, et al: Kimray-Greenfield vena cava filter: Percutaneous introduction. Radiology 151:525–526, 1984.

34. Kantor A, Glanz S, Gordon DH, Sclafani SJ: Percutaneous insertion of the Kimray-Greenfield filter: Incidence of femoral vein thrombosis. AJR Am J Roentgenol 149:1065–1066, 1987.

35. Greenfield LJ, Cho KJ, Pais SO, Van Aman M: Preliminary clinical experience with the titanium Greenfield vena caval filter. Arch Surg 124:657–659, 1989.

36. Teitelbaum GP, Ortega HV, Vinitski S, et al: Low-artifact intravascular devices: MR imaging evaluation. Radiology 168:713–719, 1988.

37. Teitelbaum GP, Jones DL, van Breda A, et al: Vena caval filter splaying: Potential complication of use of the titanium Greenfield filter. Radiology 173:809–814, 1989.

38. Greenfield LJ, Cho KJ, Proctor M, et al: Results of a multicenter study of the modified hook-titanium Greenfield filter. J Vasc Surg 14:253–257, 1991.

39. Cho KJ, Greenfield LJ, Proctor MC, et al: Evaluation of a new percutaneous stainless steel Greenfield filter. J Vasc Interv Radiol 8:181–187, 1997.

40. Johnson SP, Raiken DP, Grebe PJ, et al: Single institution prospective evaluation of the over-the-wire Greenfield vena caval filter. J Vasc Interv Radiol 9:766–773, 1998.

41. Roehm JO Jr, Gianturco C, Barth MH, Wright KC: Percutaneous transcatheter filter for the inferior vena cava: A new device for treatment of patients with pulmonary embolism. Radiology 150:255–257, 1984.

42. Reed RA, Teitelbaum GP, Taylor FC, et al: Use of the Bird's Nest filter in oversized inferior venae cavae. J Vasc Interv Radiol 2:447–450, 1991.

43. Ferris EJ, McCowan TC, Carver DK, McFarland DR: Percutaneous inferior vena caval filters: Follow-up of seven designs in 320 patients. Radiology 188:851–856, 1993.

44. Roehm JO Jr, Johnsrude IS, Barth MH, Gianturco C: The bird's nest inferior vena cava filter: Progress report. Radiology 168:745–749, 1988.

45. Watanabe AT, Teitelbaum GP, Gomes AS, Roehm JO Jr: MR imaging of the bird's nest filter. Radiology 177:578–579, 1990.

46. Ricco JB, Crochet D, Sebilotte P, et al: Percutaneous transvenous caval interruption with the "LGM" filter: Early results of a multicenter trial. Ann Vasc Surg 2:242–247, 1988.

47. Millward SF, Peterson RA, Moher D, et al: LGM (VenaTech) vena caval filter: Experience at a single institution. J Vasc Interv Radiol 5:351–356, 1994.

48. Taylor FC, Awh MH, Kahn CE Jr, Lu CT: Vena Tech vena cava filter: Experience and early follow-up. J Vasc Interv Radiol 2:435–440, 1991.

49. Kinney TB: Update on inferior vena cava filters. J Vasc Interv Radiol 14:425–440, 2003.

50. Grassi CJ, Matsumoto AH, Teitelbaum GP: Vena caval occlusion after Simon nitinol filter placement: Identification with MR imaging in patients with malignancy. J Vasc Interv Radiol 3:535–539, 1992.

51. Poletti PA, Becker CD, Prina L, et al: Long-term results of the Simon nitinol inferior vena cava filter. Eur Radiol 8:289–294, 1998.

52. Simon M, Athanasoulis CA, Kim D, et al: Simon nitinol inferior vena cava filter: Initial clinical experience: Work in progress. Radiology 172:99–103, 1989.

53. Rousseau H, Perreault P, Otal P, et al: The 6-F nitinol TrapEase inferior vena cava filter: Results of a prospective multicenter trial. J Vasc Interv Radiol 12:299–304, 2001.

54. Schutzer R, Ascher E, Hingorani A, et al: Preliminary results of the new 6F TrapEase inferior vena cava filter. Ann Vasc Surg 17:103–106, 2003.

55. Millward SF, Bhargava A, Aquino J Jr, et al: Günther Tulip filter: Preliminary clinical experience with retrieval. J Vasc Interv Radiol 11:75–82, 2000.

56. Millward SF, Oliva VL, Bell SD, et al: Günther Tulip retrievable vena cava filter: Results from the Registry of the Canadian Interventional Radiology Association. J Vasc Interv Radiol 12:1053–1058, 2001.

57. Neuerburg JM, Günther RW, Vorwerk D, et al: Results of a multicenter study of the retrievable Tulip vena cava filter: Early clinical experience. Cardiovasc Intervent Radiol 20:10–16, 1997.

58. Bovyn G, Gory P, Reynaud P, Ricco JB: The Tempofilter: A multicenter study of a new temporary caval filter implantable for up to six weeks. Ann Vasc Surg 11:520–528, 1997.

59. Kelly IM, Boyd CS: Buckling of the tethering catheter causes migration of a temporary caval filter to the right atrium. Clin Radiol 54:398–401, 1999.

60. Rossi P, Arata FM, Bonaiuti P, Pedicini V: Fatal outcome in atrial migration of the Tempofilter. Cardiovasc Intervent Radiol 22:227–231, 1999.

61. Terhaar OA, Lyon SM, Given MF, et al: Extended interval for retrieval of Günther Tulip filters. J Vasc Interv Radiol 15:1257–1262, 2004.

62. Wicky S, Doenz F, Meuwly JY, et al: Clinical experience with retrievable Günther Tulip vena cava filters. J Endovasc Ther 10:994–1000, 2003.

63. de Gregorio MA, Gamboa P, Gimeno MJ, et al: The Günther Tulip retrievable filter: Prolonged temporary filtration by repositioning within the inferior vena cava. J Vasc Interv Radiol 14:1259–1265, 2003.

64. Tay KH, Martin ML, Fry PD, et al: Repeated Günther Tulip inferior vena cava filter repositioning to prolong implantation time. J Vasc Interv Radiol 13:509–512, 2002.

65. Oliva VL, Szatmari F, Giroux MF, et al: The Jonas study: Evaluation of the retrievability of the Cordis OptEase inferior vena cava filter. J Vasc Interv Radiol 16:1439–1445, 2005; quiz 1445.

66. Rosenthal D, Wellons ED, Levitt AB, et al: Role of prophylactic temporary inferior vena cava filters placed at the ICU bedside under intravascular ultrasound guidance in patients with multiple trauma. J Vasc Surg 40:958–964, 2004.

67. Asch MR: Initial experience in humans with a new retrievable inferior vena cava filter. Radiology 225:835–844, 2002.

68. Grande WJ, Trerotola SO, Reilly PM, et al: Experience with the recovery filter as a retrievable inferior vena cava filter. J Vasc Interv Radiol 16:1189–1193, 2005.

69. Decousus H, Leizorovicz A, Parent F, et al: A clinical trial of vena caval filters in the prevention of pulmonary embolism in patients with proximal deep-vein thrombosis: Prevention du Risque d'Embolie Pulmonaire par Interruption Cave Study Group. N Engl J Med 338:409–415, 1998.

70. PREPIC Study Group: Eight-year follow-up of patients with permanent vena cava filters in the prevention of pulmonary embolism: The PREPIC (Prevention du Risque d'Embolie Pulmonaire par Interruption Cave) randomized study. Circulation 112:416–422, 2005.

71. White RH, Zhou H, Kim J, Romano PS: A population-based study of the effectiveness of inferior vena cava filter use among patients with venous thromboembolism. Arch Intern Med 160:2033–2041, 2000.

72. Ray CE Jr, Kaufman JA: Complications of inferior vena cava filters. Abdom Imaging 21:368–374, 1996.

73. Mohan CR, Hoballah JJ, Sharp WJ, et al: Comparative efficacy and complications of vena caval filters. J Vasc Surg 21:235–245, 1995; discussion 245–246.

74. Aswad MA, Sandager GP, Pais SO, et al: Early duplex scan evaluation of four vena caval interruption devices. J Vasc Surg 24:809–818, 1996.

75. Blebea J, Wilson R, Waybill P, et al: Deep venous thrombosis after percutaneous insertion of vena caval filters. J Vasc Surg 30:821–828, 1999.

76. Dorfman GS, Cronan JJ, Paolella LP, et al: Iatrogenic changes at the venotomy site after percutaneous placement of the Greenfield filter. Radiology 173:159–162, 1989.

77. Mewissen MW, Erickson SJ, Foley WD, et al: Thrombosis at venous insertion sites after inferior vena caval filter placement. Radiology 173:155–157, 1989.

78. Molgaard CP, Yucel EK, Geller SC, et al: Access-site thrombosis after placement of inferior vena cava filters with 12–14-F delivery sheaths. Radiology 185:257–261, 1992.

79. Tobin KD, Pais SO, Austin CB: Femoral vein thrombosis following percutaneous placement of the Greenfield filter. Invest Radiol 24:442–445, 1989.

80. Douketis JD, Kearon C, Bates S, et al: Risk of fatal pulmonary embolism in patients with treated venous thromboembolism. JAMA 279:458–462, 1998.

81. Streiff MB: Vena caval filters: A review for intensive care specialists. J Intensive Care Med 18:59–79, 2003.

82. Crochet DP, Brunel P, Trogrlic S, et al: Long-term follow-up of Vena Tech-LGM filter: Predictors and frequency of caval occlusion. J Vasc Interv Radiol 10 (2 Pt 1): 137–142, 1999.

83. Murin S, Romano PS, White RH: Comparison of outcomes after hospitalization for deep venous thrombosis or pulmonary embolism. Thromb Haemost 88:407–414, 2002.

84. Halbmayer WM, Haushofer A, Toth E, Fischer M: Inferior vena caval filters and systemic prothrombin activation in orally anticoagulated patients. Lancet 340:853, 1992.

85. Prandoni P, Villalta S, Bagatella P, et al: The clinical course of deep-vein thrombosis: Prospective long-term follow-up of 528 symptomatic patients. Haematologica 82:423–428, 1997.

86. Brandjes DP, Buller HR, Heijboer H, et al: Randomised trial of effect of compression stockings in patients with symptomatic proximal-vein thrombosis. Lancet 349:759–762, 1997.

87. Kupferschmid JP, Dickson CS, Townsend RN, Diamond DL: Small-bowel obstruction from an extruded Greenfield filter strut: An unusual late complication. J Vasc Surg 16:113–115, 1992.

88. Appleberg M, Crozier JA: Duodenal penetration by a Greenfield caval filter. Aust N Z J Surg 61:957–960, 1991.

89. Bianchini AU, Mehta SN, Mulder DS, et al: Duodenal perforation by a Greenfield filter: Endoscopic diagnosis. Am J Gastroenterol 92:686–687, 1997.

90. Woodward EB, Farber A, Wagner WH, et al: Delayed retroperitoneal arterial hemorrhage after inferior vena cava (IVC) filter insertion: Case report and literature review of caval perforations by IVC filters. Ann Vasc Surg 16:193–196, 2002.

91. Howerton RM, Watkins M, Feldman L: Late arterial hemorrhage secondary to a Greenfield filter requiring operative intervention. Surgery 109(3 Pt 1):265–268, 1991.

92. Greenfield LJ, Proctor MC: Experimental embolic capture by asymmetric Greenfield filters. J Vasc Surg 16:436–443, 1992; discussion 443–444.

93. Katsamouris AA, Waltman AC, Delichatsios MA, Athanasoulis CA: Inferior vena cava filters: In vitro comparison of clot trapping and flow dynamics. Radiology 166:361–366, 1988.

94. Thompson BH, Cragg AH, Smith TP, et al: Thrombus-trapping efficiency of the Greenfield filter in vivo. Radiology 172(3 Pt 2): 979–981, 1989.

95. Greenfield LJ, Proctor MC, Cho KJ, Wakefield TW: Limb asymmetry in titanium Greenfield filters: Clinically significant? J Vasc Surg 26:770–775, 1997.

96. Kinney TB, Rose SC, Weingarten KE, et al: IVC filter tilt and asymmetry: Comparison of the over-the-wire stainless-steel and titanium Greenfield IVC filters. J Vasc Interv Radiol 8:1029–1037, 1997.

97. Andrews RT, Geschwind JF, Savader SJ, Venbrux AC: Entrapment of J-tip guidewires by VenaTech and stainless-steel Greenfield vena cava filters during central venous catheter placement: Percutaneous management in four patients. Cardiovasc Intervent Radiol 21:424–428, 1998.

98. Dardik A, Campbell KA, Yeo CJ, Lipsett PA: Vena cava filter ensnarement and delayed migration: An unusual series of cases. J Vasc Surg 26:869–874, 1997.

99. Streib EW, Wagner JW: Complications of vascular access procedures in patients with vena cava filters. J Trauma 49:553–557, 2000; discussion 557–558.

100. Argiris A, Rademaker J, Mahmud M: Dislodgment of an inferior vena cava filter to the internal jugular vein. Intensive Care Med 23:1186–1187, 1997.

101. Browne RJ, Estrada FP: Guidewire entrapment during Greenfield filter deployment. J Vasc Surg 27:174–176, 1998.

102. Loesberg A, Taylor FC, Awh MH: Dislodgment of inferior vena caval filters during "blind" insertion of central venous catheters. AJR Am J Roentgenol 161:637–638, 1993.

103. Marelich GP, Tharratt RS: Greenfield inferior vena cava filter dislodged during central venous catheter placement. Chest 106:957–959, 1994.

104. Gibson MP, Chung RS, Husni EA, Kuivinen EP: Dislodgment and entrapment of a Greenfield filter. J Vasc Interv Radiol 10:378–379, 1999.

105. Kaufman JA, Thomas JW, Geller SC, et al: Guide-wire entrapment by inferior vena caval filters: In vitro evaluation. Radiology 198:71–76, 1996.

106. Stavropoulos SW, Itkin M, Trerotola SO: In vitro study of guide wire entrapment in currently available inferior vena cava filters. J Vasc Interv Radiol 14:905–910, 2003.

107. Andrews RT, Bova DA, Venbrux AC: How much guidewire is too much? Direct measurement of the distance from subclavian and internal jugular vein access sites to the superior vena cava–atrial junction during central venous catheter placement. Crit Care Med 28:138–142, 2000.

108. Center for Devices and Radiological Health: Manufacturer and User Facility Device Experience (MAUDE). Available at: http://www.fda.gov/cdrh/maude.html. Accessed January 2, 2007.

109. Ansell J, Hirsh J, Dalen J, et al: Managing oral anticoagulant therapy. Chest 119 (1 suppl): 22S–38S, 2001.

110. Linkins LA, Choi PT, Douketis JD: Clinical impact of bleeding in patients taking oral anticoagulant therapy for venous thromboembolism: A meta-analysis. Ann Intern Med 139:893–900, 2003.

111. Palareti G, Leali N, Coccheri S, et al: Bleeding complications of oral anticoagulant treatment: An inception-cohort, prospective collaborative study (ISCOAT). Italian Study on Complications of Oral Anticoagulant Therapy. Lancet 348:423–428, 1996.

112. van Dongen CJ, Vink R, Hutten BA, et al: The incidence of recurrent venous thromboembolism after treatment with vitamin K antagonists in relation to time since first event: A meta-analysis. Arch Intern Med 163:1285–1293, 2003.

113. Schulman S, Wahlander K, Lundstrom T, et al: Secondary prevention of venous thromboembolism with the oral direct thrombin inhibitor ximelagatran. N Engl J Med 349:1713–1721, 2003.

114. Teitelbaum GP, Bradley WG Jr, Klein BD: MR imaging artifacts, ferromagnetism, and magnetic torque of intravascular filters, stents, and coils. Radiology 166:657–664, 1988.

31

115. Bucker A, Neuerburg JM, Adam GB, et al: Real-time MR guidance for inferior vena cava filter placement in an animal model. J Vasc Interv Radiol 12:753–756, 2001.

116. Kim D, Edelman RR, Margolin CJ, et al: The Simon nitinol filter: Evaluation by MR and ultrasound. Angiology 43:541–548, 1992.

117. Kiproff PM, Deeb ZL, Contractor FM, Khoury MB: Magnetic resonance characteristics of the LGM vena cava filter: Technical note. Cardiovasc Intervent Radiol 14:254–255, 1991.

118. Athanasoulis CA, Kaufman JA, Halpern EF, et al: Inferior vena caval filters: Review of a 26-year single-center clinical experience. Radiology 216:54–66, 2000.

119. Douketis JD, Foster GA, Crowther MA, et al: Clinical risk factors and timing of recurrent venous thromboembolism during the initial 3 months of anticoagulant therapy. Arch Intern Med 160:3431–3436, 2000.

120. Kearon C, Hirsh J: Management of anticoagulation before and after elective surgery. N Engl J Med 336:1506–1511, 1997.

121. Crowther MA, Ginsberg JS, Julian J, et al: A comparison of two intensities of warfarin for the prevention of recurrent thrombosis in patients with the antiphospholipid antibody syndrome. N Engl J Med 349:1133–1138, 2003.

122. Khamashta MA, Cuadrado MJ, Mujic F, et al: The management of thrombosis in the antiphospholipid-antibody syndrome. N Engl J Med 332:993–997, 1995.

123. Wilson WA, Gharavi AE, Koike T, et al: International consensus statement on preliminary classification criteria for definite antiphospholipid syndrome: Report of an international workshop. Arthritis Rheum 42:1309–1311, 1999.

124. Sack GH Jr, Levin J, Bell WR: Trousseau's syndrome and other manifestations of chronic disseminated coagulopathy in patients with neoplasms: Clinical, pathophysiologic, and therapeutic features. Medicine (Baltimore) 56:1–37, 1977.

125. O'Sullivan G, Semba C, Bittner C, et al: Endovascular management of iliac vein compression (May-Thurner) syndrome. J Vasc Interv Radiol 11:515–518, 2000.

126. Kommareddy A, Zaroukian MH, Hassouna HI: Upper extremity deep venous thrombosis. Semin Thromb Hemost 28:89–99, 2002.

127. Prandoni P, Polistena P, Bernardi E, et al: Upper-extremity deep vein thrombosis: Risk factors, diagnosis, and complications. Arch Intern Med 157:57–62, 1997.

128. Pengo V, Lensing AW, Prins MH, et al: Incidence of chronic thromboembolic pulmonary hypertension after pulmonary embolism. N Engl J Med 350:2257–2264, 2004.

129. Jamieson SW, Nomura K: Indications for and the results of pulmonary thromboendarterectomy for thromboembolic pulmonary hypertension. Semin Vasc Surg 13:236–244, 2000.

130. Jamieson SW, Kapelanski DP, Sakakibara N, et al: Pulmonary endarterectomy: Experience and lessons learned in 1,500 cases. Ann Thorac Surg 76:1457–1462, 2003; discussion 1462–1464.

131. Mo M, Kapelanski DP, Mitruka SN, et al: Reoperative pulmonary thromboendarterectomy. Ann Thorac Surg 68:1770–1776, 1999; discussion 1776–1777.

132. Geerts WH, Code KI, Jay RM, et al: A prospective study of venous thromboembolism after major trauma. N Engl J Med 331:1601–1606, 1994.

133. Schultz DJ, Brasel KJ, Washington L, et al: Incidence of asymptomatic pulmonary embolism in moderately to severely injured trauma patients. J Trauma 56:727–731, 2004; discussion 731–733.

134. Upchurch GR Jr, Demling RH, Davies J, et al: Efficacy of subcutaneous heparin in prevention of venous thromboembolic events in trauma patients. Am Surg 61:749–755, 1995.

135. Velmahos GC, Nigro J, Tatevossian R, et al: Inability of an aggressive policy of thromboprophylaxis to prevent deep venous thrombosis (DVT) in critically injured patients: Are current methods of DVT prophylaxis insufficient? J Am Coll Surg 187:529–533, 1998.

136. Geerts WH, Jay RM, Code KI, et al: A comparison of low-dose heparin with low-molecular-weight heparin as prophylaxis against venous thromboembolism after major trauma. N Engl J Med 335:701–707, 1996.

137. Knudson MM, Morabito D, Paiement GD, Shackleford S: Use of low molecular weight heparin in preventing thromboembolism in trauma patients. J Trauma 41:446–459, 1996.

138. Norwood SH, McAuley CE, Berne JD, et al: A potentially expanded role for enoxaparin in preventing venous thromboembolism in high risk blunt trauma patients. J Am Coll Surg 192:161–167, 2001.

139. Schwarcz TH, Quick RC, Minion DJ, et al: Enoxaparin treatment in high-risk trauma patients limits the utility of surveillance venous duplex scanning. J Vasc Surg 34:447–452, 2001.

140. Devlin JW, Tyburski JG, Moed B: Implementation and evaluation of guidelines for use of enoxaparin as deep vein thrombosis prophylaxis after major trauma. Pharmacotherapy 21:740–747, 2001.

141. Carlin AM, Tyburski JG, Wilson RF, Steffes C: Prophylactic and therapeutic inferior vena cava filters to prevent pulmonary emboli in trauma patients. Arch Surg 137:521–525, 2002; discussion 525–527.

142. Allen TL, Carter JL, Morris BJ, et al: Retrievable vena cava filters in trauma patients for high-risk prophylaxis and prevention of pulmonary embolism. Am J Surg 189:656–661, 2005.

143. Antevil JL, Sise MJ, Sack DI, et al: Retrievable vena cava filters for preventing pulmonary embolism in trauma patients: A cautionary tale. J Trauma 60:35–40, 2006.

144. Duperier T, Mosenthal A, Swan KG, Kaul S: Acute complications associated with Greenfield filter insertion in high-risk trauma patients. J Trauma 54:545–549, 2003.

145. Greenfield LJ, Proctor MC, Michaels AJ, Taheri PA: Prophylactic vena caval filters in trauma: The rest of the story. J Vasc Surg 32:490–495, 2000; discussion 496–497.

146. Hoff WS, Hoey BA, Wainwright GA, et al: Early experience with retrievable inferior vena cava filters in high-risk trauma patients. J Am Coll Surg 199:869–874, 2004.

147. Morris CS, Rogers FB, Najarian KE, et al: Current trends in vena caval filtration with the introduction of a retrievable filter at a level I trauma center. J Trauma 57:32–36, 2004.

148. Offner PJ, Hawkes A, Madayag R, et al: The role of temporary inferior vena cava filters in critically ill surgical patients. Arch Surg 138:591–594, 2003; discussion 594–595.

149. Patton JH Jr, Fabian TC, Croce MA, et al: Prophylactic Greenfield filters: Acute complications and long-term follow-up. J Trauma 41:231–236, 1996; discussion 236–237.

150. Rogers FB, Shackford SR, Ricci MA, et al: Prophylactic vena cava filter insertion in selected high-risk orthopaedic trauma patients. J Orthop Trauma 11:267–272, 1997.

151. Rogers FB, Shackford SR, Ricci MA, et al: Routine prophylactic vena cava filter insertion in severely injured trauma patients decreases the incidence of pulmonary embolism. J Am Coll Surg 180:641–647, 1995.

152. Rogers FB, Strindberg G, Shackford SR, et al: Five-year follow-up of prophylactic vena cava filters in high-risk trauma patients. Arch Surg 133:406–411, 1998; discussion 412.

153. Rosenthal D, McKinsey JF, Levy AM, et al: Use of the Greenfield filter in patients with major trauma. Cardiovasc Surg 2:52–55, 1994.

154. Sekharan J, Dennis JW, Miranda FE, et al: Long-term follow-up of prophylactic Greenfield filters in multisystem trauma patients. J Trauma 51:1087–1090, 2001; discussion 1090–1091.

155. Webb LX, Rush PT, Fuller SB, Meredith JW: Greenfield filter prophylaxis of pulmonary embolism in patients undergoing surgery for acetabular fracture. J Orthop Trauma 6:139–145, 1992.

156. Wilson JT, Rogers FB, Wald SL, et al: Prophylactic vena cava filter insertion in patients with traumatic spinal cord injury: Preliminary results. Neurosurgery 35:234–239, 1994; discussion 239.

157. Winchell RJ, Hoyt DB, Walsh JC, et al: Risk factors associated with pulmonary embolism despite routine prophylaxis: Implications for improved protection. J Trauma 37:600–606, 1994.

158. Wojcik R, Cipolle MD, Fearen I, et al: Long-term follow-up of trauma patients with a vena caval filter. J Trauma 49:839–843, 2000.

159. Zolfaghari D, Johnson B, Weireter LJ, Britt LD: Expanded use of inferior vena cava filters in the trauma population. Surg Annu 27:99–105, 1995.

160. Quirke TE, Ritota PC, Swan KG: Inferior vena caval filter use in U.S. trauma centers: A practitioner survey. J Trauma 43:333–337, 1997.

161. Owings JT, Kraut E, Battistella F, et al: Timing of the occurrence of pulmonary embolism in trauma patients. Arch Surg 132:862–866, 1997; discussion 866–867.

162. Baldridge ED, Martin MA, Welling RE: Clinical significance of free-floating venous thrombi. J Vasc Surg 11:62–67, 1990; discussion 68–69.

163. Berry RE, George JE, Shaver WA: Free-floating deep venous thrombosis: A retrospective analysis. Ann Surg 211:719–722, 1990; discussion 722–723.

164. Monreal M, Ruiz J, Salvador R, et al: Recurrent pulmonary embolism: A prospective study. Chest 95:976–979, 1989.

165. Norris CS, Greenfield LJ, Herrmann JB: Free-floating iliofemoral thrombus: A risk of pulmonary embolism. Arch Surg 120:806–808, 1985.

166. Pacouret G, Alison D, Pottier JM, et al: Free-floating thrombus and embolic risk in patients with angiographically confirmed proximal deep venous thrombosis: A prospective study. Arch Intern Med 157:305–308, 1997.

167. Radomski JS, Jarrell BE, Carabasi RA, et al: Risk of pulmonary embolus with inferior vena cava thrombosis. Am Surg 53:97–101, 1987.

168. Voet D, Afschrift M: Floating thrombi: Diagnosis and follow-up by duplex ultrasound. Br J Radiol 64:1010–1014, 1991.

169. Arnesen H, Hoiseth A, Ly B: Streptokinase of heparin in the treatment of deep vein thrombosis: Follow-up results of a prospective study. Acta Med Scand 211:65–68, 1982.

170. Elliot MS, Immelman EJ, Jeffery P, et al: A comparative randomized trial of heparin versus streptokinase in the treatment of acute proximal venous thrombosis: An interim report of a prospective trial. Br J Surg 66:838–843, 1979.

171. Grossman C, McPherson S: Safety and efficacy of catheter-directed thrombolysis for iliofemoral venous thrombosis. AJR Am J Roentgenol 172:667–672, 1999.

172. Mewissen MW, Seabrook GR, Meissner MH, et al: Catheter-directed thrombolysis for lower extremity deep venous thrombosis: Report of a national multicenter registry. Radiology 211:39–49, 1999.

173. Grimm W, Schwieder G, Wagner T: [Fatal pulmonary embolism in venous thrombosis of the leg and pelvis during lysis therapy]. Dtsch Med Wochenschr 115:1183–1187, 1990.

174. Martin B, Martyak TE, Stoughton TL, et al: Experience with the Gianturco-Roehm Bird's Nest vena cava filter. Am J Cardiol 66:1275–1277, 1990.

175. Lorch H, Welger D, Wagner V, et al: Current practice of temporary vena cava filter insertion: A multicenter registry. J Vasc Interv Radiol 11:83–88, 2000.

176. Goldhaber SZ, Tapson VF: A prospective registry of 5,451 patients with ultrasound-confirmed deep vein thrombosis. Am J Cardiol 93:259–262, 2004.

177. Calligaro KD, Bergen WS, Haut MJ, et al: Thromboembolic complications in patients with advanced cancer: Anticoagulation versus Greenfield filter placement. Ann Vasc Surg 5:186–189, 1991.

178. Cohen JR, Grella L, Citron M: Greenfield filter instead of heparin as primary treatment for deep venous thrombosis or pulmonary embolism in patients with cancer. Cancer 70:1993–1996, 1992.

179. Moore FD Jr, Osteen RT, Karp DD, et al: Anticoagulants, venous thromboembolism, and the cancer patient. Arch Surg 116:405–407, 1991.

180. Greenfield LJ, Proctor MC, Saluja A: Clinical results of Greenfield filter use in patients with cancer. Cardiovasc Surg 5:145–149, 1997.

181. Hubbard KP, Roehm JO Jr, Abbruzzese JL: The Bird's Nest filter: An alternative to long-term oral anticoagulation in patients with advanced malignancies. Am J Clin Oncol 17:115–117, 1994.

182. Jarrett BP, Dougherty MJ, Calligaro KD: Inferior vena cava filters in malignant disease. J Vasc Surg 36:704–707, 2002.

183. Lossef SV, Barth KH: Outcome of patients with advanced neoplastic disease receiving vena caval filters. J Vasc Interv Radiol 6:273–277, 1995.

184. Rosen MP, Porter DH, Kim D: Reassessment of vena caval filter use in patients with cancer. J Vasc Interv Radiol 5:501–506, 1994.

185. Schwarz RE, Marrero AM, Conlon KC, Burt M: Inferior vena cava filters in cancer patients: Indications and outcome. J Clin Oncol 14:652–657, 1996.

186. Wallace MJ, Jean JL, Gupta S, et al: Use of inferior vena caval filters and survival in patients with malignancy. Cancer 101:1902–1907, 2004.

187. Walsh DB, Downing S, Nauta R, Gomes MN: Metastatic cancer: A relative contraindication to vena cava filter placement. Cancer 59:161–163, 1987.

188. Whitney BA, Kerstein MD: Thrombocytopenia and cancer: Use of the Kim-Ray Greenfield filter to prevent thromboembolism. South Med J 80:1246–1248, 1987.

189. Zerati AE, Wolosker N, Yazbek G, et al: Vena cava filters in cancer patients: Experience with 50 patients. Clinics 60:361–366, 2005.

190. Ihnat DM, Mills JL, Hughes JD, et al: Treatment of patients with venous thromboembolism and malignant disease: Should vena cava filter placement be routine? J Vasc Surg 28:800–807, 1998.

191. Levin JM, Schiff D, Loeffler JS, et al: Complications of therapy for venous thromboembolic disease in patients with brain tumors. Neurology 43:1111–1114, 1993.

192. Olin JW, Young JR, Graor RA, et al: Treatment of deep vein thrombosis and pulmonary emboli in patients with primary and metastatic brain tumors: Anticoagulants or inferior vena cava filter? Arch Intern Med 147:2177–2179, 1987.

193. Schiff D, DeAngelis LM: Therapy of venous thromboembolism in patients with brain metastases. Cancer 73:493–498, 1994.

194. Hutten BA, Prins MH, Gent M, et al: Incidence of recurrent thromboembolic and bleeding complications among patients with venous thromboembolism in relation to both malignancy and achieved international normalized ratio: A retrospective analysis. J Clin Oncol 18:3078–3083, 2000.

195. Prandoni P, Lensing AW, Piccioli A, et al: Recurrent venous thromboembolism and bleeding complications during anticoagulant treatment in patients with cancer and venous thrombosis. Blood 100:3484–3488, 2002.

196. Lee AY, Levine MN, Baker RI, et al: Low-molecular-weight heparin versus a coumarin for the prevention of recurrent venous thromboembolism in patients with cancer. N Engl J Med 349:146–153, 2003.

197. Geerts WH, Heit JA, Clagett GP, et al: Prevention of venous thromboembolism. Chest 119(1 suppl):132S–175S, 2001.

198. Bicalho PS, Hozack WJ, Rothman RH, Eng K: Treatment of early symptomatic pulmonary embolism after total joint arthroplasty. J Arthroplasty 11:522–524, 1996.

199. Vaughn BK, Knezevich S, Lombardi AV Jr, Mallory TH: Use of the Greenfield filter to prevent fatal pulmonary embolism associated with total hip and knee arthroplasty. J Bone Joint Surg Am 71:1542–1548, 1989.

200. Woolson ST, Harris WH: Greenfield vena caval filter for management of selected cases of venous thromboembolic disease following hip surgery: A report of five cases. Clin Orthop Relat Res 204:201–206, 1986.

201. Byrne TK: Complications of surgery for obesity. Surg Clin North Am 81:1181–1193, vii–viii, 2001.

202. Brolin RE: Gastric bypass. Surg Clin North Am 81:1077–1095, 2001.

203. Wu EC, Barba CA: Current practices in the prophylaxis of venous thromboembolism in bariatric surgery. Obes Surg 10:7–13, 2000.

204. Prystowsky JB, Morasch MD, Eskandari MK, et al: Prospective analysis of the incidence of deep venous thrombosis in bariatric surgery patients. Surgery 138:759–763, 2005; discussion 763–765.

205. Scholten DJ, Hoedema RM, Scholten SE: A comparison of two different prophylactic dose regimens of low molecular weight heparin in bariatric surgery. Obes Surg 12:19–24, 2002.

206. Cerneca F, Ricci G, Simeone R, et al: Coagulation and fibrinolysis changes in normal pregnancy: Increased levels of procoagulants and reduced levels of inhibitors during pregnancy induce a hypercoagulable state, combined with a reactive fibrinolysis. Eur J Obstet Gynecol Reprod Biol 73:31–36, 1997.

207. Clark P, Brennand J, Conkie JA, et al: Activated protein C sensitivity, protein C, protein S and coagulation in normal pregnancy. Thromb Haemost 79:1166–1170, 1998.

208. Gates S: Thromboembolic disease in pregnancy. Curr Opin Obstet Gynecol 12:117–122, 2000.

209. Aburahma AF, Boland JP: Management of deep vein thrombosis of the lower extremity in pregnancy: A challenging dilemma. Am Surg 65:164–167, 1999.

210. Aburahma AF, Mullins DA: Endovascular caval interruption in pregnant patients with deep vein thrombosis of the lower extremity. J Vasc Surg 33:375–378, 2001.

211. Banfield PJ, Pittam M, Marwood R: Recurrent pulmonary embolism in pregnancy managed with the Greenfield vena caval filter. Int J Gynaecol Obstet 33:275–278, 1990.

212. Narayan H, Cullimore J, Krarup K, et al: Experience with the Cardial inferior vena cava filter as prophylaxis against pulmonary embolism in pregnant women with extensive deep venous thrombosis. Br J Obstet Gynaecol 99:637–640, 1992.

213. Neill AM, Appleton DS, Richards P: Retrievable inferior vena caval filter for thromboembolic disease in pregnancy. Br J Obstet Gynaecol 104:1416–1418, 1997.

214. Owen RJ, Krarup KC: Case report: The successful use and removal of the Günther Tulip inferior vena caval filter in pregnancy. Clin Radiol 52:241–243, 1997.

215. Bates SM, Ginsberg JS: How we manage venous thromboembolism during pregnancy. Blood 100:3470–3478, 2002.

216. Greer IA: Prevention of venous thromboembolism in pregnancy. Best Pract Res Clin Haematol 16:261–278, 2003.

217. Cahn MD, Rohrer MJ, Martella MB, Cutler BS: Long-term follow-up of Greenfield inferior vena cava filter placement in children. J Vasc Surg 34:820–825, 2001.

218. Reed RA, Teitelbaum GP, Stanley P, et al: The use of inferior vena cava filters in pediatric patients for pulmonary embolus prophylaxis. Cardiovasc Intervent Radiol 19:401–405, 1996.

219. Kanda Y, Yamamoto R, Chizuka A, et al: Treatment of deep vein thrombosis using temporary vena caval filters after allogeneic bone marrow transplantation. Leuk Lymphoma 38:429–433, 2000.

220. Walker HS 3rd, Pennington DG: Inferior vena caval filters in heart transplant recipients with perioperative deep vein thromboses. J Heart Transplant 9:579–580, 1990.

221. Pomper SR, Lutchman G: The role of intracaval filters in patients with COPD and DVT. Angiology 42:85–89, 1991.

222. Still J, Friedman B, Furman S, et al: Experience with the insertion of vena caval filters in acutely burned patients. Am Surg 66:277–279, 2000.

223. Participants in the Vena Caval Filter Consensus Conference: Recommended reporting standards for vena caval filter placement and patient follow-up. Vena Caval Filter Consensus Conference. J Vasc Surg 30:573–579, 1999.

Chapter 32

Thrombosis Related to Venous Access Devices

McDonald K. Horne, III, MD • Richard Chang, MD

INTRODUCTION

Central venous access devices (VADs) are widely used to administer chemotherapy, blood components, and nutrition to patients, as well as for hemodialysis. These devices are typically inserted into the subclavian or internal jugular vein, either directly or after tunneling through subcutaneous tissue, or they may be threaded through peripheral arm veins. Less frequently, they are inserted into femoral veins or the inferior vena cava.[1] The catheters of most VADs are made of silicone rubber, which is highly flexible, although polyurethane, which is somewhat stiffer, is also used to prevent collapse of the lumen when particularly high flow is needed.[2] The most common complication associated with the use of VADs is infection. The second is thrombosis.

PATHOGENESIS AND INCIDENCE

VAD-related thrombus may be limited to the surface of the catheter itself or may involve the vein wall. Thrombogenesis at both sites starts soon after catheters are inserted and typically becomes clinically manifest within a few days or weeks.[3–6]

Catheters regularly begin accumulating a layer of fibrin as soon as they are inserted into a vein.[7] In particularly hypercoagulable patients, this initial "fibrin sheath" can become so robust at the catheter tip that it acts as a one-way valve to prevent withdrawal of blood through the lumen (Fig. 32-1).[8] In extreme cases, a sheath may encase the entire intravenous portion of the catheter from its tip to the venipuncture site.[9]

Thrombi involving the vein wall generally arise at two locations: the venipuncture site and anywhere that the catheter tip chronically rubs the venous endothelium. The venipuncture site is vulnerable because there the lumen of the vein is relatively narrow and may be significantly occluded by the catheter itself, leading to local venous stasis. Also present is the risk that the venipuncture itself will damage the venous wall sufficiently to make it prothrombotic. In a study of children, the incidence of VAD-related subclavian vein thrombosis was much greater when the catheter was inserted percutaneously (53% deep venous thrombosis [DVT]) than by the cut-down technique (17% DVT), presumably because the cut-down method was less traumatic to the vein.[10] Evidence of obstruction at the venipuncture site generally can be found by venography in about one third of catheterized subclavian veins, but usually only 5% to 10% of veins develop symptomatic occlusion.[3–5,10–12] The risk of thrombosis is greater when VADs are inserted into the femoral veins.[13,14]

The likelihood that a catheter will cause thrombus remote from the venipuncture site varies according to the location of its tip.[11,15,16] If the tip resides in the lower one third of the superior vena cava (SVC), repetitive trauma to the vein wall by the mobile catheter will be minimal, and the risk that a mural thrombus may develop is very low. If the tip remains in the upper part of the SVC, however, its movement may be restrained by the ipsilateral innominate vein, and the catheter may contact the SVC wall frequently and in the same location. This creates endothelial damage and a nidus for thrombosis and potential SVC occlusion (Fig. 32-2). Furthermore, a small risk of vascular erosion and perforation exists.[17] If the catheter tip does not advance out of the innominate vein, it will likely abrade this vein's wall, leading to thrombosis. Access through the right internal jugular vein into the SVC provides the straightest route for the catheter with the least risk of chronic venous wall trauma.[10,18]

CLINICAL PRESENTATION AND MANAGEMENT

Catheter Occlusion

The most common clinical manifestation of VAD-related thrombosis is the inability to withdraw blood from the catheter because of clot at its tip.[6,8] This problem must be distinguished from blockage caused when the catheter tip abuts against the vein wall. The latter blockage can usually be relieved by having the patient change position. When blood can be neither withdrawn nor infused through a catheter, the cause is more likely to be a kink in the tubing or intraluminal precipitation of medications rather than thrombus.[19,20]

Withdrawal occlusion related to thrombus is usually relieved by instillation of 2 mg (2 mL) of alteplase (recombinant tissue plasminogen activator; Genentech, South San Francisco, Calif, USA) that is left in for as long as 2 hours.[21] A similar regimen with urokinase is also effective.[22] If this treatment fails, it is wise to investigate the problem by injecting x-ray contrast material through the

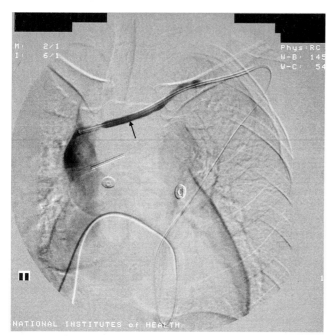

Figure 32-1 A fibrin sheath shown by injection of x-ray contrast material into the lumen of a vascular access device (VAD). The *arrow* indicates where the contrast has become trapped within the sheath that encases the catheter. Contrast does not extend to the tip of the catheter because the luminal opening is distal to the tip.

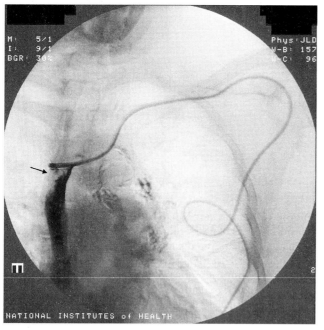

Figure 32-2 Thrombus *(arrow)* forming on the wall of the superior vena cava at a site where a poorly positioned catheter has chronically abraded the endothelium.

affected lumen while observing fluoroscopically. If a mural thrombus or a fibrin sheath is blocking the catheter tip, the problem can often be resolved by continuous infusion of a thrombolytic agent given at low doses for several hours. Successful regimens with urokinase and alteplase have been published.[23–25] We have used infusions of alteplase at 1 mg per hour for 6 to 12 hours (unpublished).

Occlusive Venous Thrombosis

This usually manifests as swelling and/or moderate pain in the shoulder, arm, or neck on the affected side. Rarely, the first sign will be symptoms of pulmonary emboli. Appropriate management of VAD-related thrombosis depends on the clinical state of the patient. Because VADs are used only in patients with major medical disorders, the risks of some available treatment options may be unacceptably large.

Goals of treatment include resolution of acute symptoms, prevention of pulmonary emboli, avoidance of long-term sequelae, and, in some cases, restoration of the vein so that it can be used again in the future for catheterization or hemodialysis. Simple removal of a VAD from a thrombosed vein usually relieves acute pain and swelling.[26] Before this is done, however, careful consideration must be given to the patient's current and future needs for central venous access. If these are nil, explantation of the catheter is the treatment of choice. A period of anticoagulation does not seem to be necessary for resolution of symptoms, but it is often prescribed.[26] Sometimes, because of concern about pulmonary emboli, anxiety is expressed about pulling a catheter through an occlusive thrombus. Although bits of thrombus are probably sheared off most catheters as they are removed, only one fatal embolus has been reported in this setting, and that occurred in a 1-year-old child.[27,28] Therefore, the practice of removing VADs through a thrombus rarely has adverse consequences.

If a VAD is still necessary for a patient's care, it does not need to be removed simply because it is in a thrombosed vein. Arm elevation alone will likely yield significant symptomatic relief.[29] Standard anticoagulation with unfractionated or low molecular weight heparin for 5 to 7 days may be even more effective.[26,30,31] This is followed by an extended period of prophylactic anticoagulation with warfarin (international normalized ratio [INR], 2 to 3) or low molecular weight heparin (e.g., 1 mg per kilogram enoxaparin per day).[32] Neither the optimal intensity nor the duration of prophylactic anticoagulation has been established in clinical trials; whether it is even necessary remains unknown. However, the presumption is that long-term anticoagulation reduces the risk of pulmonary emboli.[33,34] It may also prevent clot propagation into developing collateral veins and may reduce long-term symptoms. Therefore, it is reasonable to continue anticoagulation for the lifetime of the catheter, or at least until clinical circumstances make the risk of bleeding unacceptable.

The reported incidence of clinically apparent pulmonary embolus (PE) caused by VAD-related thrombosis is variable. Asymptomatic PEs are the most common. In one series, for example, four of 79 evaluable patients ($\approx$5%) with VAD-related DVT had symptoms of PE and positive lung scans.[35] Two of these patients died of PE despite heparin therapy. Nine other patients ($\approx$11%) had positive lung scans but no symptoms. In another report, symptomatic PEs were confirmed by imaging in 7 of 41 (17%) patients with catheter-related DVT.[36] However, in larger populations of patients at cancer centers, VAD-related PEs are rarely recognized.[26,29]

Chronic symptoms are uncommon in patients who develop acute VAD-related DVT.[26,37] However, even asymptomatic thrombosis, which is much more common than the symptomatic type, often permanently damages

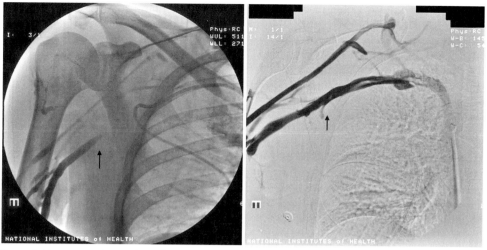

Figure 32-3 **Left panel,** Venogram shows thrombotic occlusion of the right axillary-subclavian vein (*arrow*). The intravenous catheter responsible for the thrombus can been seen proximally. **Right panel,** Venogram of the same patient after lysis of the thrombus with intraclot alteplase. The *arrow* shows the previously occluded axillary-subclavian vein. The vein that is more cephalad is the right cephalic vein.

an involved vein.[12,38,39] This outcome is clinically unimportant unless the vein is needed for a catheter at a later time, in which case reinsertion becomes difficult if not impossible. For patients who require multiple catheters over a long period, the loss of central venous access sites represents a significant clinical dilemma. Aggressive efforts to recanalize an acutely thrombosed vein are justified when a future need to recatheterize that vein is anticipated. The use of thrombolytic agents in combination with anticoagulation can produce satisfactory long-term results.[40–43]

Although thrombolytic therapy for VAD-related DVT is not standardized, we have developed a successful protocol by using recombinant tissue plasminogen activator (alteplase) in combination with anticoagulation (Fig. 32-3).[42,43] By "pulse-spraying" the drug directly into the thrombus, we achieve high local concentrations, and by choosing a thrombolytic agent that has binding affinity for fibrin, we maximize the chance that a significant amount of the drug will be retained in the thrombus.[44] Although we originally used alteplase in a concentration of 1 mg per milliliter and injected approximately 1 mL into each centimeter of clot, recently we reduced the concentration of alteplase to 100 µg per milliliter and injected no more than 4 mg into a thrombus associated with a VAD in the axillary-subclavian vein, regardless of its length. So far, our results are as good as those attained with higher doses (unpublished). We avoid treating thrombi that are known to have been symptomatic for over a month because these are relatively resistant to lysis. Usually, more acute thrombi partially lyse within 24 hours after the first treatment; then, we administer a second dose of alteplase. By the third day, antegrade flow typically has been well established. Throughout this time, we fully anticoagulate with unfractionated or low molecular weight heparin. We recommend removal of the catheter because in our experience, its continued presence increases the risk of rethrombosis. However, we always delay removal of the catheter until at least 24 hours after the last dose of alteplase is given. We are concerned that if we remove the catheter before giving the alteplase, the newly opened venipuncture wound in the region will bleed when high concentrations of thrombolytic

drug are deposited nearby. We continue prophylactic anticoagulation with warfarin or low molecular weight heparin for 6 weeks after the time the catheter is removed. In our experience, this regimen produces the greatest chance for long-term venous patency.

Although thrombolysis and anticoagulation generally produce good long-term venous patency, the addition of venous dilatation (angioplasty) and venous stents appears not to increase the benefit significantly. The need for repeated procedures is great.[45–47]

Superior Vena Cava Occlusion

A particularly distressing complication of VAD use is superior vena cava (SVC) occlusion, which originates at the site of trauma to the wall of the SVC (see Fig. 32-2). Rarely, if ever, does SVC obstruction result from propagation of clot from the subclavian veins. Symptoms of venous obstruction are often preceded by a period of catheter withdrawal occlusion that occurs as the catheter tip becomes embedded in mural thrombus.[48] Unless the bleeding risk is unacceptable, thrombolytic therapy, in combination with anticoagulation, is the treatment of choice.

Although peripheral intravenous administration of thrombolytic agents may be effective in lysing SVC thrombi, symptoms typically do not ameliorate before 12 to 72 hours, and the quantities of drug required produce hypofibrinogenemia and an increased risk of bleeding.[49,50] If the tip of the VAD catheter is embedded in the thrombus, as it often is, thrombolytic agents can also be delivered through the VAD itself directly into the thrombus.[51,52] If the tip of the VAD is not embedded in the thrombus, a second catheter must be inserted and positioned just distal to the obstruction so that the clot is bathed in the drug. Despite high local concentrations of a lytic agent, however, continuous infusions may be necessary for several days to remove the thrombus. If standard intravenous doses of drug are used (e.g., 4400 U/kg/hr urokinase), the patient will likely remain at an increased risk of bleeding for a protracted period. However, we have found that lower doses may be sufficient, and that treatment may be interrupted without rethrombosis, as long as anticoagulation is continued.[53] In theory, an agent with binding affinity for fibrin, such as alteplase, would be even more effective at low doses and could be given intermittently because it would not completely diffuse from the clot between treatments.[54] Alteplase 0.02 mg/kg/hr has been suggested for lysing of SVC thrombi.[55]

After maximal thrombolysis has been achieved, underlying stenosis of the SVC may be discovered. Although this can be relieved with balloon angioplasty, the benefit of this is usually temporary because of the elastic recoil of the vein.[56] Angioplasty followed by placement of metal venous stents is much more effective in preserving long-term patency.[55–57] However, a risk of rethrombosis is present because of small amounts of residual thrombus, and because the stents themselves are thrombogenic. Anticoagulants are usually prescribed for several months after stent placement, but the optimal duration and intensity of anticoagulation have not been established. Antiplatelet agents are also sometimes prescribed, although evidence suggesting that these are marginally antithrombotic in the venous circulation makes it unlikely that they are helpful.[57,58]

Right Atrial Thrombi

Although the optimal location for the tip of a VAD is the lower third of the SVC, precise placement of the catheter tip in that location is complicated by the fact that the catheter tip tends to move cephalad when a patient sits upright, thereby withdrawing into the upper SVC or even into the innominate vein.[15,59] One way to compensate for this is to purposely place the catheter tip in the right atrium (RA), but this practice remains controversial.[60] A U.S. Food and Drug Administration (FDA) bulletin from 1989 states that the catheter tip should not be intentionally inserted into the RA, nor positioned so that it might migrate there.[61] However, the FDA's major concern at the time appears to be catheter placement by improperly trained personnel; this worry is based on experience from the 1970s and 1980s before fluoroscopic guidance was routinely used during catheter insertion. Because the function of large bore, high-flow catheters used for dialysis and apheresis is better if their tips are located in the right atrium, the 2001 Kidney Disease Outcomes Quality Initiative Clinical Practice Guidelines advocate placement of the catheter tips at the SVC/right atrial junction or into the right atrium.[62] However, this is presumably why many reports of VAD complications involving the right heart describe patients on renal dialysis.

Wherever a catheter tip repetitively abrades the atrial endocardium, a mural thrombus is likely to develop.[63] Such a clot may remain sessile or may detach with motion of the heart and embolize or remain adherent to the catheter. By echocardiography, 6 of 13 adults and 13 of 55 children whose catheter tips were in the RA were seen to have developed RA thrombi that were attached to the atrial wall or that moved with the tip of the catheter.[64,65] In another study of children, the catheter tip in 31 of 85 patients (36%) was found in the RA, although only three RA thrombi were identified by echocardiography; all patients were asymptomatic.[10] Therefore, in general, the natural history of these thrombi is benign. They start to develop within a week of catheter placement; they then become

stabilized, without causing symptoms, and begin to calcify.[64,65] Incidental discovery of an RA thrombus does not necessarily mandate removal of the catheter. One option is to follow the thrombus with serial echocardiograms to be sure about whether it is enlarging; however, this usually causes significant anxiety for the patient and the medical staff. Therefore, anticoagulation (heparin followed by warfarin) is often prescribed for the lifetime of the catheter, with follow-up echocardiograms performed to confirm that the thrombus is stable or regressing.

If an RA thrombus is discovered during the course of investigation of pulmonary emboli or bacteremia or a new heart murmur, more aggressive management is required.[66–69] Similar to all thrombi, RA thrombi may become infected, thereby releasing clinically significant emboli. In addition, RA thrombi may impinge on the tricuspid valve or prolapse through it, in this way causing tricuspid regurgitation. In situations such as these, the catheter must be removed, but the concern involves whether this can be done without causing a significant embolus. If the thrombus moves with the atrial wall and is clearly adherent to it, there is little risk that it will dislodge when the catheter is retracted.[70] Once the catheter is out, the patient should be anticoagulated and treated with antibiotics, if appropriate, while the status of the thrombus is monitored periodically with the use of echocardiography. On the other hand, if the clot moves with the catheter and is clearly not attached to the atrial wall, it may be stripped off when the catheter is removed and may become an embolus. Removal of a large thrombus attached only to the catheter, therefore, requires surgery if it is likely to be infected or is damaging the tricuspid valve.[66] Otherwise, it also can be treated with anticoagulation followed by echocardiography.[70] Thrombolytic therapy is sometimes considered.[71] However, if this is delivered locally through the VAD, the clot may adhere to the catheter and may detach en masse, causing significant pulmonary artery obstruction. If thrombolytic therapy is given systemically, the usual risk of bleeding is associated.

PROPHYLAXIS AGAINST VENOUS ACCESS DEVICE–RELATED THROMBOSIS

Two types of prophylactic anticoagulation are used: periodic flushes of saline and heparin through the catheter lumina to prevent clot at the tip and catheter malfunction, and systemic anticoagulation to prevent thrombotic occlusion of the vein.

Although no evidence indicates that instillation of a catheter lumen with any concentration of heparin less than 500 U per milliliter is more effective than saline flushes alone in preventing catheter malfunction, lower concentrations are commonly used because, should multilumen catheters be flushed several times daily, the patient may achieve significant systemic anticoagulation.[72,73] Another problem with heparin flushes is that blood samples for reliable coagulation tests are difficult to obtain from a heparinized catheter, even after a discard.[74] A low risk of heparin-induced thrombocytopenia/thrombosis occurs, which may lead to thrombosis in the catheterized vein.[75–77] An alternative to heparin that appears to be at least modestly successful is the instillation of urokinase or alteplase into each lumen between catheter uses.[78,79]

Both warfarin and low molecular weight heparins have been tested in various regimens for their effectiveness in preventing catheter-induced vein thrombus. Bern and co-workers[80] published a randomized trial of 1 mg per day of warfarin to prevent symptomatic DVT related to subcutaneous ports in patients with cancer, about three quarters of whom had metastatic adenocarcinoma.[80] Four of 42 patients (9.5%) who were given warfarin and 13 of 40 patients (32.5%) who were given placebo developed symptomatic VAD-related DVT. However, this success was not reproduced in later studies in which the rate of symptomatic thrombosis in control groups (3%–12%) was substantially lower.[81–83] A randomized controlled trial of 1590 patients that is currently under way should clarify the role of warfarin in preventing VAD-related DVT.[84]

Impressive results were also published by Monreal and associates,[85] who used 2500 IU per day of dalteparin given systemically, although again the rate of symptomatic thrombosis in the control group was extraordinary (62%).[85] The efficacy of dalteparin seemed to be confirmed, however, in less thrombotic patients (14.6% symptomatic DVT in the control group, 1.9% in the treated group) in a subsequent, nonrandomized trial in which a larger dose of the drug (5000 IU per day) was used.[86] A recent randomized, placebo-controlled trial of 40 mg per day of enoxaparin for prophylaxis failed to significantly lower the risk of symptomatic DVT, but the incidence of this condition in the placebo group was only 3.1%.[87]

Therefore, use of the studied prophylactic anticoagulant regimens does not appear warranted in patient populations with a low rate of VAD-related DVT; however, in high-risk patients this may not be true. Because even the lowest dose regimens are not provided without bleeding risk in patients with advanced disease, our practice is to reserve prophylactic anticoagulation for patients with VAD who have previously had a catheter-related DVT. We prefer anticoagulant regimens (e.g., warfarin with an INR 1.5 to 2.0, 1 mg/kg/day enoxaparin) that have proved efficacious in other settings, and we accept the added rate of complication associated with patient care.

VASCULAR ACCESS FOR HEMODIALYSIS

Vascular access for hemodialysis must support flow rates of at least 400 mL per minute.[62,88] This is best achieved with an arteriovenous fistula (AVF) in the wrist (radial artery/cephalic vein) or, if the vessels are too small there, at the elbow (brachial artery/cephalic vein) or in the thigh (popliteal artery/saphenous vein).[62] Although AVFs have the best patency rates, about a quarter of them become occluded with a thrombus during the first year; this is usually promoted by the development of stenosis in the venous outflow.[89,90] When sites for AVFs have become depleted, arteriovenous grafts offer the next best prospect for hemodialysis, but these are even more prone to thrombose, again due to developing venous stenosis. Unfortunately, antiplatelet agents and warfarin do not improve the patency rates of grafts but are associated with excessive bleeding complications.[91,92] Venous catheters are the last choice for hemodialysis because the large

bore required is associated with a high rate of venous damage and thrombosis, but placement of the catheter in the right internal jugular vein maximizes the likelihood of long-term success.[93]

Hemodialysis flow rates are regularly measured. When they begin to fall, an x-ray contrast study (fistulogram) should be performed to assess venous stenosis which, if found, requires angioplasty. If thrombosis occurs despite regular monitoring, the problem must be addressed immediately so as not to delay dialysis.[94] Biding of time through insertion of a VAD is undesirable because of the high complication rate associated with this approach. A thrombosed AVF or graft can be treated with surgical thrombectomy or thrombolysis with percutaneous devices that mechanically break up and remove the clot, with or without the help of a thrombolytic drug, usually alteplase.[94–96] Thrombolysis is generally faster (lasting less than an hour), less traumatic for the patient, and less expensive than surgical thrombectomy. After the clot has been removed, any underlying venous stenosis must be dilated. Metallic stents can be used to maintain patency if dilatation alone fails, but maintaining long-term patency is difficult.[97,98]

REFERENCES

1. Gorman RC, Buzby GP: Difficult access problems. Surg Oncol Clin N Am 4:453–472, 1995.
2. Polderman KH, Girbes ARJ: Central venous catheter use. Part I: Mechanical complications. Intensive Care Med 28:1–17, 2002.
3. van Rooden CJ, Schippers EF, Barge RMY, et al: Infectious complications of central venous catheters increase the risk of catheter-related thrombosis in hematology patients: A prospective study. J Clin Oncol 23:2655–2660, 2005.
4. De Cicco M, Matovic M, Balestreri L, et al: Central venous thrombosis: An early and frequent complication in cancer patients bearing long-term silastic catheter. A prospective study. Thromb Res 86:101–113, 1997.
5. Cortelezzi A, Moia M, Falanga A, et al: Incidence of thrombotic complications in patients with haematological malignancies with central venous catheters: A prospective multicenter study. Br J Haematol 129:811–817, 2005.
6. Stephens LC, Haire WD, Kotulak GD: Are clinical signs accurate indicators of the cause of central venous catheter occlusion? J Parenter Enteral Nutr 19:75–79, 1995.
7. Raad II, Luna M, Khalil S-AM, et al: The relationship between the thrombotic and infectious complications of central venous catheters. JAMA 271:1014–1016, 1994.
8. Tschirhart JM, Rao MK: Mechanism and management of persistent withdrawal occlusion. Am Surg 54:326–328, 1988.
9. Mayo DJ, Pearson DC: Chemotherapy extravasation: A consequence of fibrin sheath formation around venous access devices. Oncol Nurs Forum 22:675–680, 1995.
10. Male C, Chait P, Andrew M, et al: Central venous line–related thrombosis in children: Association with central venous line location and insertion technique. Blood 101:4273–4278, 2003.
11. Caers J, Fontaine C, Vinh-Hung V, et al: Catheter tip position as a risk factor for thrombosis associated with the use of subcutaneous infusion ports. Support Care Cancer 13:325–331, 2005.
12. Horne MK, Mayo DJ, Alexander HR, et al: Venographic surveillance of tunneled venous access devices in adult oncology patients. Ann Surg Oncol 2:174–178, 1995.
13. Merrer J, De Jonghe B, Golliot F, et al: Complications of femoral and subclavian venous catheterization in critically ill patients. JAMA 286:700–707, 2001.
14. Trottier SJ, Veremakis C, O'Brien J, et al: Femoral deep vein thrombosis associated with central venous catheterization: Results from a prospective, randomized trial. Crit Care Med 23:52–59, 1995.
15. Cadman A, Lawrance JAL, Fitzsimmons L, et al: To clot or not to clot? That is the question in central venous catheters. Clin Radiol 59:349–355, 2004.

32

557

16. Petersen J, Delaney JH, Brakstad MT, et al: Silicone venous access devices positioned with their tips high in the superior vena cava are more likely to malfunction. Am J Surg 178:38–41, 1999.

17. Duntley P, Siever J, Korwes ML, et al: Vascular erosion by central venous catheters: Clinical features and outcome. Chest 10:1633–1638, 1992.

18. Lee SH, Hahn ST: Comparison of complications between transjugular and axillosubclavian approach for placement of tunneled, central venous catheters in patients with hematological malignancy: A prospective study. Eur Radiol 15:1100–1104, 2005.

19. Stephens LC, Haire WD, Kotulak GD: Are clinical signs accurate indicators of the cause of central venous catheter occlusion? J Parenter Enteral Nutr 19:75–79, 1995.

20. Holcombe BJ, Forloines-Lynn S, Garmhausen LW: Restoring patency of long-term central venous access devices. J Intraven Nurs 15:36–41, 1992.

21. Semba CP, Deitcher SR, Li X, et al: Treatment of occluded central venous catheters with alteplase: Results in 1064 patients. J Vasc Interv Radiol 13:1199–1205, 2002.

22. Haire WD, Deitcher SR, Mullane KM, et al: Recombinant urokinase for restoration of patency in occluded central venous access devices. Thromb Haemost 92:575–582, 2004.

23. Horne MK, Mayo DJ: Low-dose urokinase infusions to treat fibrinous obstructions of venous access devices in cancer patients. J Clin Oncol 15:2709–2714, 1997.

24. Savader SJ, Ehrman KO, Porter DJ, et al: Treatment of hemodialysis catheter–associated fibrin sheaths by rt-PA infusion: Critical analysis of 124 procedures. J Vasc Interv Radiol 12:711–715, 2001.

25. Bamgbola OF, del Rio M, Kaskel FJ, Flynn JT: Recombinant tissue plasminogen activator infusion for hemodialysis catheter clearance. Pediatr Nephrol 20:989–993, 2005.

26. Frank DA, Meuse J, Hirsch D, et al: The treatment and outcome of cancer patients with thromboses on central venous catheters. J Thromb Thrombolysis 10:271–275, 2000.

27. Brismar B, Hardstedt C, Jacobson S: Diagnosis of thrombosis by catheter phlebography after prolonged central venous catheterization. Ann Surg 194:779–783, 1981.

28. Rockoff MA, Gang DL, Vacanti JP: Fatal pulmonary embolism following removal of a central venous catheter. J Pediatr Surg 19:307–309, 1984.

29. Sabel MS, Smith JL: Principles of chronic venous access: Recommendations based on the Roswell Park experience. Surg Oncol 6:171–177, 1998.

30. Gould JR, Carloss HW, Skinner WL: Groshong catheter–associated subclavian venous thrombosis. Am J Med 95:419–423, 1993.

31. Savage KJ, Wells PS, Schulz V, et al: Outpatient use of low molecular weight heparin (dalteparin) for the treatment of deep vein thrombosis of the upper extremity. Thromb Haemost 82:1008–1010, 1999.

32. Horne MK: Secondary prophylaxis with low molecular weight heparin: The dose? Thromb Haemost 86:1129, 2001.

33. Becker DM, Philbrick JT, Walker FB: Axillary and subclavian venous thrombosis: Prognosis and treatment. Arch Intern Med 151:1934–1943, 1991.

34. Prandoni P, Polistena P, Bernardi E, et al: Upper-extremity deep vein thrombosis. Arch Intern Med 157:57–62, 1997.

35. Monreal M, Raventos A, Lerma R, et al: Pulmonary embolism in patients with upper extremity DVT associated to venous central lines: A prospective study. Thromb Haemost 72:548–550, 1994.

36. Kooij JDB, van der Zant FM, van Beek EJR, Reekers JA: Pulmonary embolism in deep venous thrombosis of the upper extremity: More often in catheter-related thrombosis. Nether J Med 50:238–242, 1997.

37. Donayre CE, White GH, Mehringer SM, Wilson ES: Pathogenesis determines late morbidity of axillosubclavian vein thrombosis. Am J Surg 152:179–184, 1986.

38. Axelsson ACK, Efsen F: Phlebography in long-term catheterization of the subclavian vein. Scand J Gastroenterol 13:933–938, 1978.

39. Kraybill WG, Allen BT: Preoperative duplex venous imaging in the assessment of patients with venous access. J Surg Oncol 52:244–248, 1993.

40. Fraschini G, Jadeja J, Lawson M, et al: Local infusion of urokinase for the lysis of thrombosis associated with permanent central venous catheters in cancer patients. J Clin Oncol 5:672–678, 1987.

41. Rodenhuis S, van't Hek LG FM, Vlasveld LT, et al: Central venous catheter associated thrombosis of major veins: Thrombolytic treatment with recombinant tissue plasminogen activator. Thorax 48:558–559, 1993.

42. Chang R, Horne MK, Mayo DJ, Doppman JL: Pulse-spray treatment of subclavian and jugular venous thrombi with recombinant tissue plasminogen activator. J Vasc Interv Radiol 7:845–851, 1996.

43. Horne MK, Mayo DJ, Cannon RO, et al: Intraclot recombinant tissue plasminogen activator in the treatment of deep venous thrombosis of the lower and upper extremities. Am J Med 108:251–255, 2000.

44. Horne MK, Chang R: Pharmacokinetics of pulse-sprayed recombinant tissue plasminogen activator for deep venous thrombosis. Thromb Res 111:111–114, 2003.

45. Beygui RE, Olcott C, Dalman RL: Subclavian vein thrombosis: Outcome analysis based on etiology and modality of treatment. Ann Vasc Surg 11:247–255, 1997.

46. Oderich GSC, Treiman GS, Schneider P, Bhirangi K: Stent placement for treatment of central and peripheral venous obstruction: A long-term multi-institutional experience. J Vasc Surg 32:760–769, 2000.

47. Sprouse LR, Lesar CJ, Meier GH, et al: Percutaneous treatment of symptomatic central venous stenosis angioplasty. J Vasc Surg 39:578–582, 2004.

48. Greenberg S, Kosinski R, Daniels J: Treatment of superior vena cava thrombosis with recombinant tissue type plasminogen activator. Chest 99:1298–1301, 1991.

49. Barclay GR, Allen K, Pennington CR: Tissue plasminogen activator in the treatment of superior vena caval thrombosis associated with parenteral nutrition. Postgrad Med 66:398–400, 1990.

50. Theriault RL, Buzdar AU: Acute superior vena caval thrombosis after central venous catheter removal: Successful treatment with thrombolytic therapy. Med Pediatr Oncol 18:77–80, 1990.

51. Gray BH, Olin JW, Graor RA, et al: Safety and efficacy of thrombolytic therapy for superior vena cava syndrome. Chest 99:54–59, 1991.

52. Morales M, Comas V, Trujillo M, Dorta J: Treatment of catheter-induced thrombotic superior vena cava syndrome: A single institution's experience. Support Care Cancer 8:334–338, 2000.

53. Mayo DJ, Pearson DC, Horne MK: Superior vena cava thrombosis associated with a central venous access device: A case report. Clin J Oncol Nurs 1:5–10, 1997.

54. Agnelli G, Buchanan MR, Fernandez F, et al: Sustained thrombolysis with DNA-recombinant tissue type plasminogen activator in rabbits. Blood 66:399–401, 1985.

55. Yim CD, Sane SS, Bjarnason H: Superior vena cava stenting. Interv Chest Radiol 38:409–424, 2000.

56. Rosenblum J, Leef J, Messersmith R, et al: Intravascular stents in the management of acute superior vena cava obstruction of benign etiology. J Parenter Enteral Nutr 18:362–366, 1994.

57. Sheikh MA, Fernandez BB, Gray BH, et al: Endovascular stenting of nonmalignant superior vena cava syndrome. Cath Cardiovasc Intervent 65:405–411, 2005.

58. Geerts WH, Pineo GF, Heit JA, et al: Prevention of venous thromboembolism. Chest 126:338S–400S, 2004.

59. Nazarian GK, Bjarnason H, Dietz CA, et al: Changes in tunneled catheter tip position when a patient is upright. J Vasc Interv Radiol 8:437–441, 1997.

60. Vesely TM: Central venous catheter tip position: A continuing controversy. J Vasc Interv Radiol 14:527–534, 2003.

61. Precautions necessary with central venous catheters FDA Drug Bulletin, July 1989.

62. National Kidney Foundation: K/DOQI clinical practice guidelines for vascular access, 2000. Am J Kidney Dis 37(suppl 1): S137–S181, 2001.

63. Fuchs S, Pollak A, Gilon D: Central venous catheter mechanical irritation of the right atrial free wall: A cause for thrombus formation. Cardiology 91:169–172, 1999.

64. Gilon D, Schechter D, Rein AJ JT, et al: Right atrial thrombi are related to indwelling central venous catheter position: Insights into time course and possible mechanism of formation. Am Heart J 135:457–462, 1998.

65. Korones DN, Buzzard CJ, Asselin BL, Harris JP: Right atrial thrombi in children with cancer and indwelling catheters. J Pediatr 128:841–846, 1996.

66. Ellis PK, Kidney DD, Deutsch L-S: Giant right atrial thrombus: A life-threatening complication of long-term central venous access catheters. J Vasc Interv Radiol 8:865–868, 1997.

67. Kingdon EJ, Holt SG, Davar J, et al: Atrial thrombus and central venous dialysis catheters. Am J Kidney Dis 38:631–639, 2001.

68. Ghani MK, Boccalandro D, Denktas AE, Barasch E: Right atrial thrombus formation associated with central venous catheter utilization in hemodialysis patients. Intensive Care Med 29:1829–1832, 2003.

69. Negulescu O, Coco M, Croll J, Mokrzycki MH: Large atrial thrombus formation associated with tunneled cuffed hemodialysis catheters. Clin Nephrol 59:40–46, 2003.

70. Shah A, Murray M, Nzerue C: Right atrial thrombi complicating use of central venous catheters in hemodialysis. Int J Artif Organs 27:772–778, 2004.

71. Cesaro S, Paris M, Corro R, et al: Successful treatment of a catheter-related right atrial thrombosis with recombinant tissue plasminogen activator and heparin. Support Care Cancer 10:253–255, 2002.

72. Rabe C, Gramann T, Sons X, et al: Keeping central venous lines open: A prospective comparison of heparin, vitamin C and sodium chloride sealing solutions in medical patients. Intensive Care Med 28:1172–1176, 2002.

73. Passannante A, Macik BG: Case report: The heparin flush syndrome: A cause of iatrogenic hemorrhage. Am J Med Sci 296:71–73, 1988.

74. Mayo DJ, Dimond E, Kramer W, Horne MK: Discard volumes necessary for clinically useful coagulation studies from heparinized Hickman catheters. Oncol Nurs Forum 23:671–675, 1996.

75. Kadidal VV, Mayo DJ, Horne MK: Heparin-induced thrombocytopenia (HIT) due to heparin flushes: A report of three cases. J Intern Med 246:325–329, 1999.

76. Mayo DJ, Cullinane AM, Merryman PK, Horne MK: Serologic evidence of heparin sensitization in cancer patients receiving heparin flushes of venous access devices. Support Care Cancer 7:425–427, 1999.

77. Hong AP, Cook DJ, Sigouin CS, Warkentin TE: Central venous catheters and upper-extremity deep-vein thrombosis complicating immune heparin-induced thrombocytopenia. Blood 101:3049–3051, 2003.

78. Dillon PW, Jones GR, Bagnall-Reeb HA, et al: Prophylactic urokinase in the management of long-term venous access devices in children: A children's oncology group study. J Clin Oncol 22:2718–2723, 2004.

79. Schenk P, Rosenkranz AR, Wolfl G, et al: Recombinant tissue plasminogen activator is a useful alternative to heparin in priming quinton permcath. Am J Kidney Dis 35:130–136, 2000.

80. Bern MM, Lokich JJ, Wallach SR, et al: Very low doses of warfarin can prevent thrombosis in central venous catheters. Ann Intern Med 112:423–428, 1990.

81. Bodner LJ, Nosher JL, Patel KM, et al: Peripheral venous access ports: Outcomes analysis in 109 patients. Cardiovasc Intervent Radiol 23:187–193, 2000.

82. Heaton DC, Han DY, Inder A: Minidose (1 mg) warfarin as prophylaxis for central vein catheter thrombosis. Intern Med J 32:84–88, 2002.

83. Couban S, Goodyear M, Burnell M, et al: Randomized placebo-controlled study of low-dose warfarin for the prevention of central venous catheter–associated thrombosis in patients with cancer. J Clin Oncol 23:1–7, 2005.

84. Young AM, Begum G, Billingham LJ, et al: WARP: A multicentre prospective randomized controlled trial (RCT) of thrombosis prophylaxis with warfarin in cancer patients with central venous catheters (CVCs). J Clin Oncol 23(suppl), 2005.

85. Monreal M, Alastrue A, Rull M, et al: Upper extremity deep venous thrombosis in cancer patients with venous access devices: Prophylaxis with a low molecular weight heparin (Fragmin). Thromb Haemost 75:251–253, 1996.

86. Lersch C, Eckel F, Sader R, et al: Initial experience with Healthport miniMax and other peripheral arm ports in patients with advanced gastrointestinal malignancy. Oncology 57:269–275, 1999.

87. Verso M, Agnelli G, Bertoglio S, et al: Enoxaparin for the prevention of venous thromboembolism associated with central vein catheter: A double-blind, placebo-controlled, randomized study in cancer patients. J Clin Oncol 23:4057–4062, 2005.

88. Beathard GA: Catheter thrombosis. Semin Dial 14:441–445, 2001.

89. Sparks SR, VanderLinden JL, Gnanadev DA, et al: Superior patency of perforating antecubital vein arteriovenous fistulae for hemodialysis. Ann Vasc Surg 11:165–167, 1997.

90. Revanur VK, Jardine AG, Hamilton DH, Jindal RM: Outcome for arterio-venous fistula at the elbow for haemodialysis. Clin Transplant 14:318–322, 2000.

91. Crowther MA, Clase CM, Margetts PJ, et al: Low-intensity warfarin is ineffective for the prevention of PTFE graft failure in patients on hemodialysis: A randomized controlled trial. J Am Soc Nephrol 13:2331–2337, 2002.

92. Kaufman JS, O'Connor TZ, Zhang JH, et al: Randomized controlled trial of clopidogrel plus aspirin to prevent hemodialysis access graft thrombosis. J Am Soc Nephrol 14:2313–2321, 2003.

93. Develter W, De Cubber A, Biesen WV, et al: Survival and complications of indwelling venous catheters for permanent use in hemodialysis patients. Artif Organ 29:399–405, 2005.

94. Beathard GA: Endovascular management of thrombosed dialysis access grafts. Am J Kid Dis 32:172–174, 1998.

95. Valji K: Transcatheter treatment of thrombosed hemodialysis access grafts. Am J Roentgenol 164:823–829, 1995.

96. Arbabzadeh M, Mepani B, Murray BM: Why do grafts clot despite access blood flow surveillance? Cardiovasc Intervent Radiol 25:501–505, 2002.

97. Pan H-B, Liang H-L, Lin Y-H, et al: Metallic stent placement for treating peripheral outflow lesions in native arteriovenous fistula hemodialysis patients after insufficient balloon dilatation. Am J Roentgenol 184:403–409, 2005.

98. Kolakowski S, Dougherty MJ, Calligaro KD: Salvaging prosthetic dialysis fistulas with stents: Forearm versus upper arm grafts. J Vasc Surg 38:719–723, 2003.

32

Chapter 33

Dietary Supplements and Hemostasis

Tieraona Low Dog, MD • Merry Jennifer Markham, MD

INTRODUCTION

Complementary and alternative medicine (CAM) consists of various medical therapies and health care products, including dietary supplements. In addition to natural products, other CAM treatments include prayer, hypnosis, chiropractic care, massage therapy, relaxation techniques, biofeedback, and acupuncture. This review focuses on the hemostatic effects of dietary supplements.

According to the Dietary Supplement Health and Education Act of 1994 (DSHEA), a dietary supplement is a product that is meant to supplement one's diet. Dietary supplements contain one or more of the following ingredients: a vitamin, a mineral, an herb or other botanical, an amino acid, or another dietary substance, or a combination of these ingredients or their extracts.[1] By definition, the dietary supplement is intended for ingestion in pill, capsule, tablet, or liquid form, but it is not for parenteral use.

DSHEA exempted this industry from the strict regulations of the U.S. Food and Drug Administration (FDA) for drug approval. Currently, no FDA regulations provide a minimum standard of practice for manufacturing; however, the FDA has developed guidelines for dietary supplement good manufacturing practices that are to be implemented in the future. These regulations focus on mandating practices to ensure the purity, quality, strength, and composition of supplements. Numerous articles in the literature have reported the presence in supplements of heavy metals, undeclared pharmaceuticals, and contaminants, and the inaccurate labeling of dietary ingredients. Accordingly, reviews of "drug effects" of unknown agents in unknown quantities containing unknown adulterants are essentially doomed to incompleteness and uncertainty.[2] Nonetheless, the ubiquitous use of these agents, often in conjunction with prescribed agents, justifies this effort. Note that the labels on these supplements are required to contain this disclaimer: "This product is not intended to diagnose, treat, cure, or prevent any disease."

A national survey conducted in 2002 found that 19% of adults in the United States had used natural products, including herbal and animal-based supplements (such as glucosamine) during the previous year.[3] Use of these products continues, although the specific agents used change in response to research, fad, popularity, and advertisements.[4] The top ten most commonly used supplements have been identified as echinacea, ginseng, ginkgo, garlic supplements, glucosamine, St. John's Wort, peppermint, fish oil or omega-3 fatty acids, ginger supplements, and soy supplements. The most likely user of natural products is a woman with an advanced education and a high income.[2] Although some of these agents have no known effects on coagulation, others have been associated with alterations in hemostasis (Table 33-1).

Most case reports suggesting a relationship between a hemorrhagic event and the use of a dietary supplemental agent do only that, as causation is difficult to prove and definitive studies are hard to find. The presence of the agent often gets the blame for the event. On the other hand, although it is highly unlikely that these supplemental agents produce hemostatic effects sufficient to cause clinical concern, they well may offer the "second hit" that, when combined with another hemostatic defect such as von Willebrand disease, thrombocytopenia, mild hemophilia, or anticoagulant use, may result in observable, even significant, laboratory or clinical changes. Accordingly, attempts to study these agents with the use of normal young volunteers who are taking no other drugs may not have been appropriately designed to detect such subtle alterations.

THE TEN MOST COMMONLY USED DIETARY SUPPLEMENT PRODUCTS

Echinacea

Echinacea (*Echinacea purpurea*, *Echinacea angustifolia*, *Echinacea pallida*) is commonly used for the prevention of colds and other respiratory tract infections. Orally, it is also used as an antiseptic, antiviral, and immune stimulant. It is frequently found in combination preparations with other vitamins, herbs, and minerals. Currently, no reports have documented effects of echinacea on hemostasis.

Ginseng

Another very popular dietary supplement, ginseng, may be found alone, in combination supplements, and in popular energy drinks. Two common species are available to consumers—American ginseng (*Panax quinquefolius*) and Asian or Chinese ginseng (*Panax ginseng*). Siberian ginseng (*Eleutherococcus senticosus*), also available on the market, is not a true ginseng (i.e., not of the *Panax* genus) but is reported to have similar health benefits. All three are used as a general tonic for promoting well-being, for increasing resistance to environmental stress, and for enhancing physical endurance. Siberian ginseng has not been reported to affect hemostasis or to interact with anticoagulant medications.

Table 33-1 The Ten Most Commonly Used Supplements and their Effects on Coagulation

Dietary Supplement	Effects on Coagulation
Echinacea	None reported
Ginseng	Possible antiplatelet activity May increase or decrease INR when taken with warfarin
Ginkgo biloba	Possible antiplatelet activity May increase risk of bleeding when taken with warfarin
Garlic	Possible antiplatelet activity May increase INR when taken with warfarin
Glucosamine	When taken alone, no reported effects on coagulation When combined with chondroitin, may increase INR when taken with warfarin
St. John's wort	May cause irregular menstrual bleeding when taken with oral contraceptives May decrease INR when taken with warfarin
Peppermint	None reported
Fish oils/omega-3 fatty acids	Possible antiplatelet activity May increase INR when taken with warfarin
Ginger	Possible antiplatelet activity May increase INR when taken with warfarin
Soy	Possible antiplatelet activity May decrease INR when taken with warfarin

INR, international normalized ratio.

When taken alone, American or Asian ginseng may increase the risk of bleeding through their antiplatelet activity.[5] When American or Asian ginseng is taken with warfarin, an altered international normalized ratio (INR) may result. Both a decrease and an increase in INR have been reported; however, the most commonly reported effect is a decrease in the effectiveness of warfarin.[6,7] In a randomized, controlled trial by Yuan and associates,[8] American ginseng administered for 2 weeks to subjects on warfarin significantly reduced the INR when compared with placebo. However, a pharmacokinetics study in rats revealed no alterations in warfarin levels and no impact on prothrombin time after *P. ginseng* was administered.[9] Although these herbs are related, they contain different constituents, which may, in part, account for the differences noted in laboratory data.

Ginkgo

Ginkgo biloba is commonly taken to improve dementia and memory loss, mood disturbances, difficulty concentrating, and sexual dysfunction. Ginkgo has been shown to decrease platelet function by inhibiting platelet aggregation.[10] Reports of four individual cases indicated that spontaneous bleeding may be associated with ginkgo use.[7,11] However, a prospective, double-blind, randomized, placebo-controlled study was carried out in 32 young, healthy male volunteers as a means of evaluating the effects of three dosages of ginkgo (120, 240, and 480 mg per day) on hemostasis, coagulation, and fibrinolysis. After 14 days of administration, ginkgo did not induce significant modifications in bleeding time, platelet function, or coagulation factors at any dosage when compared with placebo.[12] When combined with warfarin, an increased risk of bleeding is seen owing to the effect of the herb on platelet function. However, a recent study in healthy adults showed that ginkgo, when taken at recommended doses, did not alter the INR or the pharmacokinetics or pharmacodynamics of warfarin when patients were given a single large dose of

warfarin (25 mg) after 1 week of pretreatment with ginkgo.[13] Kohler and colleagues,[14] using 50 healthy male volunteers, were unable to find evidence suggesting any effect of ginkgo on these subjects' platelet function. At this time, the true effect of ginkgo on hemostasis or interaction with warfarin is not clear.

Garlic

Garlic (*Allium sativum*) is used as a flavoring ingredient in food preparations and is promoted as a dietary supplement for the treatment of patients with hypertension and hyperlipidemia, and for the prevention of cardiovascular disease. Garlic is used to prevent various cancers, including colorectal, gastric, breast, and prostate cancers. Garlic administration has been shown to inhibit platelet aggregation in several studies, possibly explaining the rationale for its use in the prevention of cardiovascular disease.[15–17] After 26 weeks of garlic consumption, roughly an 80% reduction was observed in serum thromboxane in healthy male volunteers who had eaten 3 g (roughly 1 clove) of fresh garlic daily.[18] Cooked garlic has a lower inhibitory effect on platelet aggregation than that attained with raw garlic.[19] Cases of postoperative bleeding during augmentation mammoplasty[20] and transurethral resection of the prostate[21] have been reported in patients taking garlic prior to surgery. Spontaneous spinal epidural hematoma has also been reported.[22] Evidence is lacking for a direct interaction of warfarin with garlic. A small, controlled study failed to find any significant change in INR values among patients stabilized on warfarin therapy (INR target, 2 to 3) who were started on 1200 mg of aged garlic extract (AGE) for 2 months in comparison with a placebo group.[23]

Glucosamine

Sometimes sold in combination with chondroitin sulfate, glucosamine is widely sold as an arthritis remedy; it is useful for osteoarthritis and temporomandibular joint arthritis. A meta-analysis supported the claims that glucosamine is at least modestly effective when used to relieve osteoarthritis symptoms.[24] Although no cases of spontaneous bleeding or interaction with antiplatelet drugs have been reported, one case report describes a possible interaction with warfarin.[25] A patient who had been on a stable dose of warfarin with therapeutic INR values developed supratherapeutic values after 4 weeks of taking a glucosamine-chondroitin supplement (3000 mg glucosamine and 2400 mg chondroitin daily).[23] It is possible that augmentation of the warfarin effect was due to the glucosamine, the chondroitin, or both, when taken at higher than recommended doses.[26] Recommended daily doses are 1500 mg per day of glucosamine and up to 1200 mg per day of chondroitin.[6]

St. John's Wort

St. John's wort (*Hypericum perforatum*) is taken for depression, anxiety, obsessive-compulsive disorder, attention deficit-hyperactivity disorder, and other mood disorders. Irregular menstrual bleeding and breakthrough bleeding have been reported in women who were taking St. John's wort concomitantly with oral contraceptives.[27] Clinical trials have confirmed this finding and suggest that the increase in breakthrough bleeding is due to an induction of cytochrome P450 3A enzyme activity, with resultant induction of the metabolism of the oral contraceptive and reduction in the contraceptive's effectiveness.[28,29] St. John's wort is known to reduce the effects of warfarin and is associated with decreased INRs. Warfarin binds to certain St. John's wort constituents in vitro, which may reduce the bioavailability of warfarin.[30] St. John's wort also induces the metabolism and clearance of warfarin by the cytochrome P450 system.[31] Reduction in INR in patients who are stable on warfarin suggests a possible induction of cytochrome P450 2C9.[32]

Peppermint

Peppermint leaf (*Mentha piperita* X) or oil is used for dyspepsia, colds, cough, nausea, irritable bowel syndrome, and tension headache. This herb has not been reported to alter hemostasis or to interact with anticoagulant or antiplatelet medications.

Fish Oils/Omega-3 Fatty Acids

Fish oil is taken orally for the treatment of patients with hypertriglyceridemia, coronary heart disease, hypertension, age-related maculopathy, bipolar disorder, obesity, stroke, rheumatoid arthritis, and various other disorders. Fish oil is typically derived from cold-water fish such as herring, mackerel, sardine, trout, or salmon. The oils have high concentrations of long-chain, polyunsaturated fats called omega-3 fatty acids. Fish oil–derived omega-3 fatty acids possess anti-inflammatory and antithrombotic properties because they compete with arachidonic acid in the cyclooxygenase and lipoxygenase pathways of platelet metabolism. Omega-3 fatty acids decrease platelet aggregation.[33,34] Some evidence suggests that excessive consumption of fish oils may increase the risk of hemorrhagic stroke.[35,36] A randomized, placebo-controlled study of 11 patients on chronic anticoagulation with warfarin found no alteration in INR values after they had taken 3 or 6 g of fish oil daily for 4 weeks.[37] Since the time of that trial, an increase in INR was reported after a patient on long-term warfarin anticoagulation doubled her dose of fish oil from 1000 mg to 2000 mg per day.[38]

Ginger

Orally, ginger (*Zingiber officinale*) is used for nausea, vertigo, dyspepsia, arthritis, loss of appetite, and migraine headache. Ginger is believed to decrease platelet aggregation via the arachadonic acid pathway.[11,39,40] One study reported a decrease in serum thromboxane B_2 when ginger was administered orally to rats.[41] Given this potential antithrombotic property, ginger should be used with caution in patients taking antiplatelet medications. When taken with warfarin, the herb may lead to an increased warfarin effect and elevated INR. A published case report describes a 76-year-old woman on long-term anticoagulation with warfarin who began having supratherapeutic INR values after she started to ingest raw ginger and tea made from ginger powder.[42] Her INR returned to stable values once she had discontinued the herb. An elevation in INR as a result of initiation of consumption of ginger products was documented in another patient on long-term phenprocoumon,[43] an oral vitamin K inhibitor in the coumarin class of drugs. In a recent clinical trial, 12 patients were pretreated with ginger for 1 week at recommended daily doses.[13] Patients were then administered a single 25-mg dose of warfarin. No association was found between consumption of ginger and INR or the pharmacokinetics and pharmacodynamics of warfarin.

Soy

Soybeans (*Glycine max*) are the most significant dietary source of isoflavones, which are naturally occurring plant compounds commonly referred to as "phytoestrogens" and named for their similarity in structure to the estrogen molecule and ability to bind to the estrogen receptor.[5,44] Phytoestrogens have been publicized as a therapeutic alternative for a variety of hormone-dependent conditions, including breast and prostate cancer, menopausal symptoms, osteoporosis, and cardiovascular disease.

Whether soy affects coagulation parameters is controversial. Dent and colleagues[45] found that 40 g of soy protein did not alter fibrinolytic or coagulation factors in perimenopausal women. In animal studies and in vitro, however, soy and soy isoflavones have been found to potentially inhibit platelet aggregation.[46-49] Schoene and Guidry[46] demonstrated that, when fed an isoflavone-rich soy protein (containing 1.45 mg per gram of the isoflavone genistein), rats developed alterations in their platelet function that could lead to decreased platelet activation and aggregation. When taken in combination with warfarin, soy may decrease anticoagulant effects and INR.[50]

COUMARIN-CONTAINING PLANTS

Coumarins belong to a group of compounds known as benzopyrones. They are fairly ubiquitous in the plant kingdom; more than 3400 naturally occurring coumarins have been identified. Some commonly ingested coumarin-containing foods include strawberries, apricots, and cherries, as well as spices such as cinnamon. Confusion seems to pervade the medical literature regarding the anticoagulant activity of this class of compounds. Although it is true that some coumarins have anticoagulant activity because of their chemical structure, the overall effect in vivo is quite weak. The parent compound, coumarin, does not possess any anticoagulant activity because it lacks a 4-hydroxy group with a carbon at the 3 position. Pharmacologic activities are all dependent on side chains and substitution around the central coumarin ring structure.

Part of the confusion may be in the very word itself. Ranchers in the northern United States reported an outbreak of lethal hemorrhage in their cattle during the 1920s. In 1922, Schofield, a Canadian veterinarian, determined that bleeding was due to a toxin from moldy feed made from sweet clover that acted as a potent anticoagulant. In 1939, Campbell and Link, two researchers working at the University of Wisconsin, identified that the toxin was bishydroxycoumarin (dicoumarol), which is formed when fungi in moldy sweet clover (*Melilotus officinalis*) oxidize coumarol to 4-hydroxycoumarin. The discovery of dicumarol led to the development of modern anticoagulant drugs such as warfarin. Because the base molecule for warfarin (Coumadin; Bristol-Myers Squibb, Princeton, NJ, USA) and related drugs is coumarin, these drugs are often referred to as coumarin drugs, although the parent molecule coumarin showed no anticoagulant activity in a human clinical trial.[51] Generalizations that warn physicians to be cautious about coumarins in foods and botanical remedies are not helpful.

MISCELLANEOUS SUPPLEMENTS

Many other popular dietary supplements have been the subjects of reports of altered hemostasis. Cranberry juice is used for the prevention and treatment of urinary tract infection. Several reports have documented interactions between warfarin and cranberry juice that led to elevations in INR values.[52] In one fatal case, a man's INR increased to greater than 50 after he began consuming an unknown quantity of cranberry juice.[53] Cranberry contains compounds that can be converted to salicylic acid in the body; thus, antiplatelet activity is possible. Duthie and coworkers[54] determined that consumption of cranberry juice was associated with a significant increase in salicylic acid in the urine, as well as elevated plasma levels.

Noni juice from *Morinda citrifolia* fruit is marketed as an immune booster, a digestive aid, and an antioxidant. At least one case report has described an interaction between Noni juice and warfarin that led to a decrease in INR.[55] Noni juice is reported to consist of multiple vitamins; however, it is unclear whether it contains vitamin K.

Quinine, a drug extracted from cinchona tree bark, has been marketed for several uses, including leg cramps, varicose veins, fever, and malaria. In the late 1990s, the FDA acted to limit the marketing of quinine on the basis of safety concerns, one of which includes drug-induced thrombocytopenia.[56,57] Several cases of rapid-onset thrombocytopenia caused by ingestion of quinine have been reported.[57,58]

Additionally, quinine is known to be associated with thrombotic thrombocytopenic purpura–hemolytic-uremic syndrome (TTP-HUS).[59]

Willow (*Salix* spp) has been used since ancient times to relieve pain. *Salix* species contain several prodrugs of salicylate, principally salicin, from which acetylsalicylic acid is derived to be marketed as aspirin. Although some impact has been noted on platelets, oral consumption of 240 mg per day of willow bark extract—the amount typically recommended for musculoskeletal pain—was found have a lesser effect on platelet aggregation than was observed with 100 mg per day of aspirin ($P = .001$).[60]

Coenzyme Q10 (also known as ubiquinone), flaxseed, and green tea have been reported to result in a decreased INR when taken with warfarin.[7,60] Dong quai, devil's claw, papaya, bromelain (an enzyme found in pineapple), cayenne, and feverfew may potentiate warfarin's effect.[61–64]

Vitamin E is taken for the treatment and prevention of Alzheimer disease and other dementias, macular degeneration, and cardiovascular disease. It is also used for cancer prevention and for the prevention of preeclampsia in pregnant women. Vitamin E is known to have an anticoagulant effect. This supplement inhibits platelet aggregation and adhesion,[65] as well as vitamin K–dependent clotting factors.[66,67] Given these properties, vitamin E may increase the risk of bleeding in patients taking other anticoagulants, including warfarin, and may enhance bleeding in patients with von Willebrand disease.

Patients on long-term anticoagulant therapy are sometimes told to avoid foods, such as broccoli and spinach. Schurges and colleagues[68] set out to study these foods in a vigorous and systematic way. Using healthy volunteers who were stabilized long term on warfarin to an INR of 2.0, investigators studied the effects of those foods taken with calculated incremental doses of vitamin K ranging from 50 μg to 500 μg. They deduced that no significant change in INR occurred until at least a total of 150 μg of available vitamin K was added to the diet; they further deduced that food supplements such as broccoli or spinach, which contain an aggregate of less than 100 μg per day of available vitamin K, do not significantly interfere with long-term oral anticoagulant therapy. They also studied the effects of a single large meal of vitamin K in the form of large quantities of broccoli or spinach containing 700 μg to 1500 μg of available vitamin K and found that each of those foods lowered the INR from a baseline of approximately 2.0 down to 1.6-1.7, but only for about 24 hours.

The applicability of these observations to patient care is not exactly clear in that these were all very young healthy patients who were taking no other medications. Additionally, the effects observed were at the lowest therapeutic INR target, namely, 2.0. The effect of a "therapeutic" menu of broccoli or spinach on an elevated INR such as 7 or 8 is unknown. It is clear that foodstuffs containing vitamin K can alter the INR. On the other hand, investigators found that a single meal of natto, a traditional Japanese soybean food, decreased the INR in volunteers for several days.[68] This finding probably is due to the fact that this food is moldy because of *Bacillus natto*, an organism on soy meal that produces significant amounts of vitamin K and presumably resides in the gut of those who eat this food, all the while elaborating vitamin K in the host's gastrointestinal tract.

Table 33-2   Unexpected Sources of Vitamin K that may Alter INR When Taken with Warfarin

Source	Amount of Vitamin K
Viactiv (McNeil Nutritionals LLC, Fort Washington, Pa, USA) soft calcium chews	40 μg per chew*
Boost (Novartis Nutrition Corporation, Fremont, Mich, USA)	30 μg per 8 fl oz*
Ensure (Abbott Laboratories, Abbott Park, Ill, USA)	30 μg per 8 fl oz*
Some energy or protein bars	40 to 65 μg per bar*
Olestra-containing "light" potato chips	80 μg per 1-ounce serving†
Natto (fermented soybean)	1000 μg per 100 g natto‡
Condiments such as mayonnaise	11 μg per 1 tablespoon
Soy bean emulsions (e.g., Intralipid 10% [Pharmacia & Upjohn AB, Sweden], Liposyn [Abbott Laboratories, Montreal, Canada]) and drugs (e.g., propofol) that use these emulsions or delivery vehicles	13 to 31 μg/dL§

*Johnson SR, Ernst ME, Graber MA: Commonly overlooked sources of vitamin K. Ann Pharmacother 37:302, 2003.
†Harrell CC, Kline SS: Vitamin K–supplemented snacks containing olestra: Implication for patients taking warfarin. JAMA 282:1133–1134, 1999.
‡Schurgers LJ, Shearer MJ, Hamulyak K, et al: Effect of vitamin K intake on the stability of oral anticoagulant treatment: Dose-response relationships in healthy subjects. Blood 104:2682–2689, 2004.
§Lennon C, Davidson KW, Sadowski JA, Mason JB: The vitamin K content of intravenous lipid emulsions. J Parenter Enteral Nutr 17:142–144, 1993.
INR, international normalized ratio.

Portions of these variables are due not only to the specific food and vitamin K contained in the food but to the bioavailability of vitamin K, which ranges from a few percentage points to a very high level. The authors concluded that consistency is probably more important than content in terms of dietary intake of vitamin K in patients anticoagulated on a long-term basis.

Table 33-2 lists some unexpected food sources of vitamin K that may interfere with therapeutic administration of warfarin.

RECOMMENDATIONS

Because the list of dietary supplements is long yet incomplete, and because even their alleged contents may be in dispute, it would be daunting to master lists of these agents and their potential effects on hemostasis. Probably a more functional approach would be to remember that these supplements may alter hemostasis; therefore, should such agents be encountered in patients, inquiry regarding them is clearly justified. More important in long-term care such as chronic anticoagulation therapy is stability of the use of supplements. Frequent starting and stopping of supplement use is likely to more be harmful than is consistent use.

REFERENCES

1. Dietary Supplement Health and Education Act of 1994. U.S. Food and Drug Administration, Center for Food Safety and Applied Nutrition. http://www.cfsan.fda.gov/~dms/dietsupp.html. Accessed February 24, 2007.
2. Wolsko PM, Solondz DK, Phillips RS, et al: Lack of herbal supplement characterization in published randomized controlled trials. Am J Med 118:1087–1093, 2005.
3. Barnes PM, Powell-Griner E, McFann K, Nahin RL: Complementary and Alternative Medicine Usage Among Adults: United States, 2002. Advance Data From Vital and Health Statistics. Publication no. 343. Hyattsville, Md, National Center for Health Statistics, 2004.
4. Kelly JP, Kaufman DW, Kelley K, et al: Recent trends in use of herbal and other natural products. Arch Intern Med 165:281–286, 2005.
5. Natural Medicines Comprehensive Database. Available at: www.naturaldatabase.com.
6. Stenton SB, Bungard TJ, Ackman ML: Interactions between warfarin and herbal products, minerals, and vitamins: A pharmacist's guide. Can J Hosp Pharm 54:186–192, 2001.
7. Fugh-Berman A: Herb–drug interactions. Lancet 355:134–138, 2000.
8. Yuan CS, Wei G, Dey L, et al: Brief communication: American ginseng reduces warfarin's effect in healthy patients: A randomized, controlled trial. Ann Intern Med 141:23–27, 2004.
9. Zhu M, Chan KW, Ng LS, et al: Possible influences of ginseng on the pharmacokinetics and pharmacodynamics of warfarin in rats. J Pharm Pharmacol 51:175–180, 1999.
10. Kudolo GB, Dorsey S, Blodgett J: Effect of ingestion of Ginkgo biloba extract on platelet aggregation and urinary prostanoid excretion in healthy and type 2 diabetic subjects. Thromb Res 108:151–160, 2002.
11. Vaes LPJ, Chyka PA: Interactions of warfarin with garlic, ginger, ginkgo, or ginseng: Nature of the evidence. Ann Pharmacother 34:1478–1482, 2000.
12. Bal Dit Sollier C, Caplain H, Drouet L: No alteration in platelet function or coagulation induced by EGb0761 in a controlled study. Clin Lab Haematol 25:251–253, 2003.
13. Jiang X, Williams KM, Liauw WS, et al: Effect of ginkgo and ginger on the pharmacokinetics and pharmacodynamics of warfarin in healthy subjects. Br J Clin Pharm 59:425–432, 2005.
14. Kohler S, Funk P, Kieser M: Influence of a 7-day treatment with Gingko biloba special extract EGb 761 on bleeding time and coagulation: A randomized, placebo-controlled, double-blind study in healthy volunteers. Blood Coagul Fibrinolysis 15:303–309, 2004.
15. Bordia A, Verma SK, Srivastava KC: Effect of garlic (Allium sativum) on blood lipids, blood sugar, fibrinogen and fibrinolytic activity in patients with coronary artery disease. Prostaglandins Leukot Essent Fatty Acids 58:257–263, 1998.
16. Rahman K, Billington D: Dietary supplementation with aged garlic extract inhibits ADP-induced platelet aggregation in humans. J Nutr 130:2662–2665, 2000.
17. Steiner M, Li W: Aged garlic extract, a modulator of cardiovascular risk factors: A dose-finding study on the effects of AGE on platelet functions. J Nutr 131:980S–984S, 2001.
18. Ali M, Thomson M: Consumption of a garlic clove a day could be beneficial in preventing thrombosis. Prostaglandins Leukot Essent Fatty Acids 53:211–212, 1995.
19. Ali M, Bordia T, Mustafa T: Effect of raw versus boiled aqueous extract of garlic and onion on platelet aggregation. Prostaglandins Leukot Essent Fatty Acids 60:43–47, 1999.
20. Burnham BE: Garlic as a possible risk for postoperative bleeding. Plast Reconstr Surg 95:213, 1995.
21. German K, Kumar U, Blackford HN: Garlic and the risk of TURP bleeding. Br J Urol 76:518, 1995.
22. Rose KD, Croissant PD, Parliament CF, Levin MB: Spontaneous spinal epidural hematoma with associated platelet dysfunction from excessive garlic consumption: A case report. Neurosurgery 26:880–882, 1990.

23. Rozenfeld V, Sisca TS, Callahan A, Crain J: Double-blind, randomized, placebo-controlled trial of aged garlic extract in patients stabilized on warfarin therapy [abstract]. Presented at: American Society of Health-System Pharmacists (ASHP) Midyear Clinical Meeting; December 3, 2000; Las Vegas, Nev.

24. McAlindon TE, LaValley MP, Gulin JP, Felson DT: Glucosamine and chondroitin for treatment of osteoarthritis: A systematic quality assessment and meta-analysis. JAMA 283:1469–1475, 2000.

25. Rozenfeld V, Crain JL, Callahan AK: Possible augmentation of warfarin effect by glucosamine-chondroitin. Am J Health-Syst Pharm 61:306–307, 2004.

26. Scott GN: Interaction of warfarin with glucosamine-chondroitin. Am J Health-Syst Pharm 61:1186, 2004.

27. Yue QY, Bergquist C, Gerdén B: Safety of St John's wort (Hypericum perforatum). Lancet 355:576–577, 2000.

28. Pfrunder A, Schiesser M, Gerber S, et al: Interaction of St. John's wort with low-dose oral contraceptive therapy: A randomized controlled trial. Br J Clin Pharm 56:683–690, 2003.

29. Hall SD, Wang Z, Huang SM, et al: The interaction of St John's wort and an oral contraceptive. Clin Pharmacol Ther 74:525–535, 2003.

30. Gröning R, Breitkreutz J, Müller RS: Physico-chemical interactions between extracts of Hypericum perforatum L. and drugs. Eur J Pharm Biopharm 56:231–236, 2003.

31. Jiang X, Williams KM, Liauw WS, et al: Effect of St. John's wort and ginseng on the pharmacokinetics and pharmacodynamics of warfarin in healthy subjects. Br J Clin Pharmacol 57:592–599, 2004.

32. Kaminsky LS, Zhang ZY: Human P450 metabolism of warfarin. Pharmacol Ther 73:67–74, 1997.

33. Connor WE: N-3 fatty acids from fish and fish oil: Panacea or nostrum? Am J Clin Nutr 74:415–416, 2001.

34. Leaf A: On the reanalysis of the GISSI-Prevenzione. Circulation 105:1874–1875, 2002.

35. Caicoya M: Fish consumption and stroke: A community case-control study in Asturias, Spain. Neuroepidemiology 21:107–114, 2002.

36. Pedersen HS, Mulvad G, Seidelin KN, et al: N-3 fatty acids as a risk factor for haemorrhagic stroke. Lancet 353:812–813, 1999.

37. Bender NK, Kraynak MA, Chiquette E, et al: Effects of marine fish oils on the anticoagulation status of patients receiving chronic warfarin therapy. J Thromb Thrombolysis 5:257–261, 1998.

38. Buckley M, Goff A, Knapp W: Fish oil interaction with warfarin. Ann Pharmacother 38:50–52, 2004.

39. Bordia A, Verma SK, Srivastava KC: Effect of ginger (Zingiber officinale Rosc.) and fenugreek (Trigonella foenumgraecum L.) on blood lipids, blood sugar and platelet aggregation in patients with coronary artery disease. Prostaglandins Leukot Essent Fatty Acids 56:379–384, 1997.

40. Koo KLK, Ammit AJ, Tran VH, et al: Gingerols and related analogues inhibit arachadonic acid–induced human platelet serotonin release and aggregation. Thromb Res 103:387–397, 2001.

41. Thomson M, Al-Qattan KK, Al-Sawan SM, et al: The use of ginger (Zingiber officinale Rosc.) as a potential anti-inflammatory and anti-thrombotic agent. Prostaglandins Leukot Essent Fatty Acids 67:475–478, 2002.

42. Lesho EP, Saullo L, Udvari-Nagy S: A 76-year-old woman with erratic anticoagulation. Cleveland Clin J Med 71:651–656, 2004.

43. Krüth P, Brosi E, Fux R, et al: Ginger-associated overanticoagulation by phenprocoumon. Ann Pharmacother 38:257–260, 2004.

44. Setchell KDR, Cassidy A: Dietary isoflavones: Biological effects and relevance to human health. J Nutr 129:758S–767S, 1999.

45. Dent SB, Peterson CT, Brace LD, et al: Soy protein intake by perimenopausal women does not affect circulating lipids and lipoproteins or coagulation and fibrinolytic factors. J Nutr 131:2280–2287, 1991.

46. Schoene NW, Guidry CA: Dietary soy isoflavones inhibit activation of rat platelets. J Nutr Biochem 10:421–426, 1999.

47. Schoene NW, Guidry CA: Genistein inhibits reactive oxygen species (ROS) production, shape change, and aggregation in rat platelets. Nutr Res 20:47–57, 2000.

48. Saxena R, Choudhry VP, Mishra DK, et al: Possible role of soyabean therapy in isolated platelet factor 3 (PF3) availability defect. Am J Hematol 60:170, 1999.

49. Anthony MS: Soy and cardiovascular disease: Cholesterol lowering and beyond. J Nutr 130:662S–663S, 2000.

50. Cambria-Kelly JA: Effect of soy milk on warfarin efficacy. Ann Pharmacother 36:1893–1896, 2002.

51. Kostering H, Bandura B, Merten HA, Wieding JU: The behavior of blood clotting and its inhibitors under long-term treatment with 5,6-benzo-alpha-pyrone (coumarin): A double-blind study. Arzneim Forsch 35:1303–1306, 1985.

52. Committee on Safety of Medicines and the Medicines and Healthcare Products Regulatory Agency: Possible interaction between warfarin and cranberry juice. Curr Probl Pharmacovigilance 29:8, 2003.

53. Suvarna R, Pirmohamed M, Henderson L: Possible interaction between warfarin and cranberry juice. BMJ 327:1454, 2003.

54. Duthie GG, Kyle JAM, Jenkinson AM, et al: Increased salicylate concentrations in the urine of human volunteers after consumption of cranberry juice. J Agric Food Chem 53:2897–2900, 2005.

55. Carr ME, Klotz J, Bergeron M: Coumadin resistance and the vitamin supplement "Noni." Am J Hematol 77:103–104, 2004.

56. Drug products containing quinine for the treatment and/or prevention of malaria for over-the-counter human use. Fed Reg 63: 13526–13529, 1998.

57. Brinker AD, Beitz J: Spontaneous reports of thrombocytopenia in association with quinine: Clinical attributes and timing related to regulatory action. Am J Hematol 70:313–317, 2002.

58. Reddy JC, Shuman MA, Aster RH: Quinine/quinidine-induced thrombocytopenia: A great imitator. Arch Intern Med 164:218–220, 2004.

59. Kojuri K, Vesely SK, George JN: Quinine-associated thrombotic thrombocytopenic purpura–hemolytic uremic syndrome: Frequency, clinical features, and long-term outcomes. Ann Intern Med 135:1047–1051, 2001.

60. Krivoy N, Pavlotzky E, Chrubasik S, et al: Effect of Salicis cortex extract on human platelet aggregation. Planta Med 67:209–212, 2001.

61. Wittkowsky AK: Drug interactions update: Drugs, herbs, and oral anticoagulation. J Thromb Thrombolysis 12:67–71, 2001.

62. Chan TK: Interaction between warfarin and danshen (Salvia miltiorrhiza). Ann Pharmacother 35:501–504, 2001.

63. Yu CM, Chan JCN, Sanderson JE: Chinese herbs and warfarin potentiation by 'Danshen.' J Intern Med 241:337–339, 1997.

64. Page RL, Lawrence JD: Potentiation of warfarin by dong quai. Pharmacotherapy 19:870–876, 1999.

65. Azzi A, Ricciarelli R, Zingg JM: Non-antioxidant molecular functions of α-tocopherol (vitamin E). FEBS Lett 519:8–10, 2002.

66. Booth SL, Golly I, Sacheck JM, et al: Effect of vitamin E supplementation on vitamin K status in adults with normal coagulation status. Am J Clin Nutr 80:143–148, 2004.

67. Dowd P, Zheng ZB: On the mechanism of the anticlotting action of vitamin E quinone. Proc Natl Acad Sci USA 92:8171–8175, 1995.

68. Schurges LJ, Shearer MJ, Hamulayák K, et al: Effect of vitamin K intake on the stability of oral anticoagulant treatment: Dose-response relationships in healthy subjects. Blood 104:2682–2689, 2004.

Part V

Issues Specific to Women

Chapter 34

Thrombotic Risk of Contraceptives and Other Hormonal Therapies

Suman Sood, MD • Steven Stein, MD • Barbara A. Konkle, MD

INTRODUCTION

Hormones are used in various forms for contraception, postmenopausal symptom management, treatment of patients with hormone-responsive cancers, and breast cancer risk reduction. This chapter focuses on the association of hormone therapy with thromboembolic disease. The benefits of these drugs are discussed in some detail. In deciding whether to prescribe hormone therapy, one must try to assess the risk:benefit ratio for that individual. Although much still needs elucidation, the goal of this chapter is to provide data on which clinicians can base these decisions.

BASIC SCIENCE

The increased risk of thrombosis in association with the use of hormones has been well established. In general, the effects of oral contraceptives (OCs) and hormone replacement therapy (HRT) on coagulation variables are modest, and reports suggest that the use of OCs induces changes in the procoagulant and anticoagulant pathways that may counterbalance each other.[1] Baseline epidemiologic studies in healthy women undergoing menopause have demonstrated increased levels of several coagulation factors, including factors VII and VIII and fibrinogen. These changes are due to estrogen status and to aging.[2]

Several studies have shown that estrogen activates the coagulation system. Caine and coworkers[3] showed that administration of 0.625 mg or 1.25 mg of conjugated equine estrogen to 29 healthy postmenopausal women (average age, 57 yr) for 3 months increased an index of thrombin generation (prothrombin fragments 1+2) in a dose-dependent manner. Thrombin activity, as indicated by the generation of fibrinopeptide A, was also increased. Furthermore, levels of inhibitors of thrombin generation (protein S) and activity (antithrombin III) were decreased relative to placebo. A similar study in which blood samples at baseline and after 3 months of therapy with unopposed estrogen therapy were tested versus placebo in 26 healthy postmenopausal women additionally showed significantly reduced concentrations of tissue factor pathway inhibitor (TFPI), an important inhibitor of the extrinsic pathway of coagulation.[4] These findings are similar in users of OCs, with increased levels of factors VII, VIII, and X and decreased antithrombin III and protein S levels contributing to an overall procoagulant state.[5]

One of estrogen's procoagulant mechanisms of action may occur through first-pass hepatic metabolism. Estrogen has been found to increase hepatic production of several plasma proteins involved in coagulation, including factor VII, factor X, and fibrinogen, and it has been implicated in the acquisition of a deficiency in plasma glucosylceramide levels, an activated protein C (APC) anticoagulant cofactor.[6] Moreover, use of OCs and HRT has been associated with higher levels of C-reactive protein (CRP).[7,8] Because it avoids first-pass hepatic metabolism, it has been suggested that transdermal hormone therapy may be a safer alternative to oral therapy in that it induces less activation of the coagulation system, including less APC resistance.[9–12] However, a decreased risk of thrombosis with the currently available transdermal contraceptive (norelgestromin/ethinyl estradiol) (Ortho Evra; Ortho-McNeil Pharmaceutical, Inc., Raritan, NJ, USA) has not been demonstrated.

Data about the effects of estrogen on the fibrinolytic system are conflicting, but on the whole, estrogen seems to induce heightened fibrinolytic activity.[13] This may be due at least in part to a decrease in fibrinogen and plasminogen activator inhibitor-1 (PAI-1) concentrations and increased plasminogen levels.[4] Levels of PAI-1, a critical inhibitor of fibrinolysis, are generally higher in postmenopausal women.[14] This hyperfibrinolysis may counterbalance the procoagulant effects of estrogen and may explain the low absolute risk of thromboembolism seen in women who are taking HRT.

Estrogens have both rapid and longer-term effects on the blood vessel wall. Estrogen influences the bioavailability of endothelially derived nitric oxide and causes relaxation of vascular smooth muscle cells.[15] The longer-term effects of estrogen are due, at least in part, to changes in vascular cell gene and protein expression, which may lead to inhibition of the response to vascular injury, reduced oxidation of low-density lipoprotein, and reduced levels of lipoprotein(a) (Lp[a]). However, the decrease in cholesterol levels seen with HRT has not been shown to correlate with a decreased risk of cardiovascular disease. Once atherosclerotic disease exists, estrogens may exacerbate the proinflammatory state by increasing CRP levels and matrix metalloproteinase activity.[16] In the future, genetic screening may play a role in determining who would benefit from estrogen therapy. Estrogen receptor polymorphisms in intron 1 have been associated with the magnitude of response of high-density lipoprotein cholesterol levels to estrogen or combination HRT, although the underlying mechanism remains unknown. It is unclear whether this population of women may benefit clinically from HRT.[17]

Recent data have shown a higher incidence of thrombotic risk in women who use third-generation combined oral contraceptives (e.g., desogestrel, gestodene, norgestimate, drospirenone) compared with second-generation progesterones (e.g., levonorgestrel, norethisterone).[18] It has been postulated that this may be explained by differential effects of progestins on plasma sensitivity to APC.[6,19] One explanation involves a differential increase in FVIII levels and a decrease in protein S activity (free protein S decreases with desogestrel and increases with levonorgestrel; the increase in free protein S with levonorgestrel may be due to a decrease in C4b-binding protein).[20,21] This suggests that the prothrombotic effects of estrogen may be inadequately counteracted by the lower androgenicity of the progestin component present in third-generation OCs but not in second-generation OCs, thus inducing APC resistance.

ORAL CONTRACEPTIVE USE AND THROMBOSIS

Venous Thromboembolism

Since their introduction, the use of OCs has been linked to an increased incidence of thromboembolic events.[22] First-generation OCs consisted of at least 50 µg of ethinyl estradiol or mestranol and a progestin, typically norethindrone. Because estrogen was suspected of increasing the risk for thromboemboli, contraceptives that contained less than 50 µg of estrogen and a new progestin, levonorgestrel, were introduced—second-generation OCs (see Table 34-1 for available combined hormonal contraceptives). Initial efforts to reduce the risk of venous thromboembolism (VTE) by reducing estrogen content have proved successful.[23–25] Bottiger and colleagues[24] noted a marked decline of approximately 80% in reports of nonfatal VTE per 100,000 users when low-dose estrogen OC replaced high-dose preparations. In the Oxford planning study, lower incidence rates were noted among users of low-dose contraceptives (39 per 100,000 person-years) compared with users of high-dose contraceptives (62 per 100,000 person-years).[25] Compared with non-OC users, women who take second-generation OCs have a risk of VTE that is increased about fourfold.[26]

The progestins desogestrel, gestodene, and norgestimate, in combination with no more than 35 µg of ethinyl estradiol, constitute third-generation OCs (see Table 34-1). Third-generation OCs increase the risk of VTE approximately twofold over second-generation products.[26] The risk of VTE with oral preparations for the newer progestins has been less well studied but should not be presumed to be less than that seen with third-generation products. VTE with OCs that contain drospirenone (Yasmin; Berlex, Montville, NJ, USA) or cyproterone acetate (Diane 35; Berlex, Pointe-Claire, Quebec, Canada, Estelle 35; Douglas, Auckland, New Zealand) has been reported,[27,28] and it produces acquired APC resistance similar to that found in women

taking third-generation products.[29] Because of the increased risk of thrombosis associated with cyproterone acetate–containing preparations, these are not recommended for routine contraception. On the basis of postmarketing adverse event reporting to the U.S. Food and Drug Admininstration (FDA), transdermal hormonal contraception (norelgestromin and ethinyl estradiol as Ortho Evra) cannot be assumed to carry a lower risk of VTE than is seen with oral preparations. The VTE risk associated with use of the vaginal ring (ethinyl estradiol and etonorgestrel) (NuvaRing; Organon Inc., Roseland, NJ, USA) is unknown.

The VTE-associated risk of progesterone-only containing contraceptives has been studied in eight case-controlled studies,[30–37] and none has shown a statistically significant increased risk of VTE in women who use these for contraception, although an increased risk has been found for other indications.[32]

Myocardial Infarction

Current use of OCs increases the risk of myocardial infarction, but most of the excess risk is attributable to an interaction with cigarette smoking.[38] Taken together, case-controlled and cohort studies suggest that current users of OCs who are younger than 40 years of age and who do not smoke have little or no increased risk for myocardial infarction. In general, young women (the primary users of OCs) have a low incidence of myocardial infarction. In the United States, the baseline annual risk for fatal ischemic heart disease ranges from 1 to 2 per 100,000 persons in women younger than 35 years of age to 4.1 per 100,000 persons in women 35 to 39 years of age, and to 10 to 21 per 100,000 persons for women in their 40s.[39] Thus, most studies have been too small to address whether the risk for myocardial infarction from OCs differs according to coronary risk factors other than smoking. The data consistently show that past use of OCs is not associated with increased risk. In a meta-analysis of 13 studies, Stampfer and coworkers[40] estimated that past users of OCs had a pooled relative risk for myocardial infarction of 1.01 (95% confidence interval [CI], 0.91 to 1.13). These findings suggest that any increase in risk for myocardial infarction due to OC use occurs only with current use and probably acts through an acute prothrombotic interaction with cigarette smoking. This statement is supported by the finding that angiographic studies of young women with myocardial infarction tend to show an absence of atherosclerosis in cases associated with current or recent use of OCs.[41]

Stroke

Prospective studies have not shown an increased risk for stroke among past users of OCs, and studies of stroke in current users have yielded inconsistent results.[38] Reported studies are often small, do not differentiate between hemorrhagic and thromboembolic strokes, and often do not control for other major risk factors. In studies that have shown an increased risk, the interaction with smoking does not seem to be as great as that associated with myocardial infarction.

The Nurses' Health Study[42] found no statistically significant increase in risk for stroke among past users of OCs (ischemic stroke and subarachnoid hemorrhage were

Table 34-1 Oral Contraceptives Available in the United States

Monophasic	Estrogen (µg)	Progestin (mg)
Genora 1/50, Nelova 1/50M, Norinyl 1+50, Ortho-Novum 1/50, Necon 1/50, Intercon	Mestranol (50)	Norethindrone (1)
Ovcon-50	Ethinyl estradiol (50)	Norethindrone (1)
Demulen 1/50, Zovia 1/50E	Ethinyl estradiol (50)	Ethynodiol (1)
Ovral	Ethinyl estradiol (50)	Norgestrel (0.5)
Genora 1/35, NEE 1/35, Nelova 1/35E, Norethrin 1/35E, Norinyl 1+35, Ortho-Novum 1/35, Intercon 1/35	Ethinyl estradiol (35)	Norethrindrone (1)
Brevicon, Modicon, Genora,	Ethinyl estradiol (35)	Norethindrone (0.5)
Nelova 0.5/35E, Necon 0.5/35	Ethinyl estradiol (35)	Norethindrone (0.5)
Ovcon-35	Ethinyl estradiol (35)	Norethindrone (0.4)
Ortho-Cyclen	Ethinyl estradiol (35)	Norgestimate (0.25)
Demulen 1/35, Zovia 1/35	Ethinyl estradiol (35)	Ethynodiol (1)
Loestrin 21 1.5/30, Loestrin Fe 1.5/30	Ethinyl estradiol (30)	Norethindrone (1.5)
Lo/Ovral	Ethinyl estradiol (30)	Norgestrel (0.3)
Desogen, Ortho-Cept	Ethinyl estradiol (30)	Desogestrel (0.15)
Levlen, Levora, Nordette	Ethinyl estradiol (30)	Levonorgestrel (0.15)
Seasonale*	Ethinyl estradiol (30)	Levonorgestrel (0.15)
Loestrin 21 1/20, Loestrin Fe 1/20	Ethinyl estradiol (20)	Norethindrone (1)
Alesse, Levlite	Ethinyl estradiol (20)	Levonorgestrel (0.1)
Progestin Only		
Micronor, Nor-QD	None	Norethindrone (0.35)
Ovrette	None	Norgestrel (0.075)
Triphasic		
Tri-Norinyl, Ortho-Novum 7/7/7, Necon 7/7/7	Ethinyl estradiol (35)	Norethindrone (0.5/0.75/1)
Tri-Levlen, Triphasil	Ethinyl estradiol (30/40/40)	Levonorgestrel (0.05/0.075/0.125)
OrthoTri-Cyclen	Ethinyl estradiol (35)	Norgestimate (0.18/0.215/0.25)
Ortho Tri-Cyclen Lo	Ethinyl estradiol (25)	Norgestimate (0.18/0.215/0.25)
Cyclessa	Ethinyl estradiol (25)	Norgestimate (0.1/0.125/0.150)
Other		
Yasmin	Ethinyl estradiol (30)	Drospirenone (3)
Estrostep, Estrostep Fe	Ethinyl estradiol (20/30/35)	Norethindrone (1)
Mircette	Ethinyl estradiol (20/0/10)	Desogestrel (0.15/0/0)

*13 wk active tablet/1 wk inert tablet.
Second-generation OC: Levonorgestrel and norethindrone containing.
Third-generation OC: Norgestimate and desogestrel containing.

combined in the study). In the Royal College of General Practitioners' Study,[43] past users who were smokers had an increased relative risk for stroke of 1.8 (95% CI, 1.1 to 2.8). The World Health Organization case-controlled study[44] also suggested that an interaction between smoking and contraceptives was associated with ischemic stroke.

Taken together, studies of low-dose OCs suggest that these drugs produce little increase in risk for ischemic stroke.[45] Occlusive stroke in young women occurs at an estimated annual rate of 5.4 per 100,000 person-years.[46] Fatal occlusive stroke is even rarer, with annual rates lower than 0.5 per 100,000 for women younger than 45 years of age.[39] Therefore, any attributable risk for death from occlusive stroke associated with the use of OCs is small at most, although smokers may be more susceptible. Current studies provide no persuasive evidence of any increase in risk for hemorrhagic stroke among young women without risk factors who use low-dose OCs.[38]

Hormonal Contraception and Thrombophilia

Inherited and acquired factors interact to modulate the risk of VTE in women who use OCs. Carriers of the factor V Leiden mutation have been studied most extensively. Early studies documented that the risk of VTE in women with FV Leiden who use OCs was greater than the additive risk of these two factors. Initial reports of VTE risk in women who use OCs described a greater than 30-fold increased risk,[47,48] although a pooled analysis of eight case-controlled studies found an odds ratio of 10.25 (95% CI, 5.69 to 18.45) for OC use in FV Leiden and of 7.14 (95% CI, 3.39 to 15.04) in women with the prothrombin 20210 mutation.[49] The risk appears to be greater in FV Leiden carriers who use third-generation OCs compared with second-generation products.[48] In a prospective cohort study of 236 asymptomatic female carriers of FV Leiden, almost all of whom were heterozygotes, the risk of VTE was 1.8% per year of OC use.[50]

Thrombophilic women are more likely to develop thrombosis early in their OC use, with a 19-fold (95% CI, 1.9 to 175.7) increase reported in the first 6 months, and an 11-fold (95% CI, 2.1 to 57.3) increase noted during the first year, based on a case-controlled study.[51] This study included women with a deficiency of protein C, protein S, or antithrombin III, or heterozygosity for the FV Leiden or prothrombin 20210 mutation.

Hormonal therapy and pregnancy have been associated with an increased risk of cerebral vein thrombosis. The use of OCs is strongly and independently associated with this disorder. The risk is increased in individuals with prothrombin 20210 and FV Leiden mutations.[52] A marked predominance in women with the prothrombin mutation who use OCs has been reported in two studies.[52,53] These findings are based on a small number of women, given that cerebral venous thrombosis is a rare event (see Chapter 16).

Other acquired or inherited factors modulate the risk of thrombosis in women who use OCs. In a case-controlled analysis, thrombophilic women who had a history of air travel of at least 8 hours duration had an increased risk of VTE (odds ratio [OR], 13.9; 95% CI, 1.7 to 117.5).[54] A synergistic effect of obesity (body mass index [BMI] > 25 kg/m^2) with OC use has been reported with tenfold increased risk.[55] Data from the Leiden Thrombophilia Study showed an increase in VTE risk with OC use in the setting of elevated factors II, V, and XI and with a decrease in factor XII.[56] Researchers did not find an increased risk with elevated FVIII levels, which has been shown to be a risk factor for initial and recurrent VTE in other settings.

COUNSELING THROMBOPHILIC WOMEN ON THE USE OF HORMONAL CONTRACEPTION

More and more people are undergoing testing to identify thrombophilic disorders related to family or personal medical issues. The physician is often asked about the use of hormonal contraception in women with thrombophilia. Combined hormonal contraception is believed to be contraindicated in women with a personal history of VTE. In such women, postmenopausal HRT is associated with an unacceptable risk of recurrent events.[57] Whether concomitant anticoagulation therapy decreases the risk sufficiently to compensate for this strategy is unknown, but such an approach is commonly used.

Information on the use of progestin-only contraceptives in this setting is limited. Conard and associates[58] evaluated the progestin chlormadinone acetate in 102 women, 71 of whom had a prior deep venous thrombosis (DVT) and 31 of whom had an identified thrombophilia. The occurrence of new or recurrent DVT was evaluated in a case-controlled manner in women with similar risk factors as controls. No significant difference in events was found.[58] Given these data, along with other data from women without diagnosed thrombophilia, progestin-only contraception may be an option in women with a low risk of recurrence, such as those with a past nonhormonal precipitated DVT.

A common consultation question involves the use of hormonal contraception in asymptomatic carriers of thrombophilic defects. In this setting, one must be sure that effective contraception is not refused as the result of an overestimation of VTE risk. Increases in the number of women seeking pregnancy termination have been noted after media-promoted fear of health risks associated with hormonal contraceptives.[59] When considering alternative contraception, one must take into account the efficacy of other methods, which is generally inferior, and the woman's acceptance of pregnancy termination if contraception should fail. Pregnancy itself is associated with an approximately fivefold increased risk of thrombosis. This risk is increased further in thrombophilic women, as are some pregnancy complications. It is assumed that women with inherited thrombophilias that carry a higher risk of VTE, such as antithrombin III deficiency, are at greater risk

Table 34-2 Estimated Risk of Venous Thromboembolism (VTE) per Year of Oral Contraceptive Use in Women Without Prior VTE*

	Age, 20 yr[†]	Age, 50 yr[†]
No defined thrombophilia[‡]	0.04%	0.4%
FV Leiden heterozygote	0.2%–0.7 %	2%–7 %
PT mutation heterozygote	0.1%–0.6 %	1%–6 %
FV/PT double heterozygote	0.2%–2.9 %	2%–29 %

*Odds ratio from Emmerich et al.[49]
[†]Underlying risk increases with age.[60]
[‡]Presume relative risk of VTE with OC use = 4.
FV, factor V; PT, prothrombin.

than those with milder defects, although this has not been proved in a clinical study.

The risk of DVT increases with increasing age. Women at age 20 have an approximately tenfold lower risk than women at age 50.[60] Thus, the absolute risk of developing a DVT in a young woman who uses OCs is significantly less than that in a woman who is approaching menopause, even with identical genetic risk factors (Table 34-2). Counseling must take this into account. In the Leiden Thrombophilia Study, a 1.8% per year risk of VTE was reported in asymptomatic carriers of FV Leiden who used OCs. This included all age groups, but the risk should be less in a young adult. The European Prospective Cohort on Thrombophilia Study evaluated the risk of first venous thrombosis in asymptomatic carriers of a familial thrombophilic defect.[61] It was found that fewer women with thrombophilia than controls used OCs, but VTE was only slightly more likely to occur in those with (0.5% per year [95% CI, 0.0 to 2.9]) than in those without thrombophilia (0.4% per year [95% CI, 0.1 to 0.9]).

Because VTE is a manifestation of multiple known and unknown genetic and environmental factors, family history may provide a clue as to thrombophilic tendency within the family, which may influence counseling. VTE-associated risk with hormonal contraception may be acceptable to many asymptomatic women with a low risk for thrombophilia when this and other factors are considered. Levonorgestrel-containing OCs produce the least APC resistance; thus, the least thrombogenic OC may be the one with the lowest estrogen dose and that includes levonorgestrel as the progestin.

HORMONE REPLACEMENT THERAPY AND THROMBOSIS

In the United States and other developed countries, more women die from cardiovascular disease than from any other disease. The Nurses' Health Study, among other observational studies, suggested that postmenopausal women who take estrogen therapy have fewer cardiovascular events (range, 40% to 50%) over time compared with untreated women.[62] After cessation of menses (menopause), average circulating estrogen levels eventually fall to less than 10% of premenopausal levels. This state of estrogen deficiency has been believed to contribute to the acceleration of several age-related health problems in women, including cardiovascular disease, osteoporosis, and possibly dementia. Despite a large and growing body of information, including the results of several well-conducted randomized trials on the risks and benefits of long-term HRT in preventing or treating some of the disorders associated with menopause, whether to take postmenopausal hormones remains a difficult decision and an area of therapeutic controversy.

HORMONE REPLACEMENT THERAPY AND CARDIOVASCULAR DISEASE

Atherosclerosis increases after menopause, especially among women who have undergone surgical oophorectomy.[63] More than 40 observational studies have suggested that HRT reduced cardiovascular morbidity and mortality in postmenopausal women.[64,65] Most of these studies were conducted in healthy postmenopausal women who used unopposed estrogen replacement therapy.

In the Heart and Estrogen/Progestin Replacement Study (HERS), the first large clinical trial undertaken to examine the effects of HRT on risk for cardiovascular disease, 2763 women with established coronary disease were randomly assigned to receive daily conjugated equine estrogen plus medroxyprogesterone acetate or placebo (Table 34-3).[66,100] After a mean of 4.1 years of follow-up, no differences were seen in the primary composite outcome of nonfatal myocardial infarction or death from coronary heart disease (HRT group, 179 events; placebo group, 182 events; relative hazard, 0.99 [95% CI, 0.81 to 1.22]) or any of the secondary clinical outcomes. This null result shook the foundation on which recommendations for widespread use of estrogen replacement had been built—that estrogen reduces a woman's risk for heart disease. On the basis of these results, assertions regarding secondary prevention of coronary heart disease could no longer be made with confidence. Initially, more detailed analysis of HERS results tantalizingly revealed that within the overall null effect, risk for coronary heart disease was reduced during years 3 to 5,

but this reduction was offset by the unexpected 50% increase in risk observed during year 1. However, data from 2.7 additional years of unblinded follow-up failed to show persistence of this promising trend in reducing cardiovascular risk despite the fact that 45% of women continued to take the original assigned therapy. At the end of 6.8 years, the relative hazard remained 1.00 (95% CI, 0.77 to 1.29).[67] In other secondary prevention trials, such as the placebo-controlled Estrogen Replacement for Atherosclerosis (ERA) trial, neither estrogen alone nor estrogen in combination with progestin affected the angiographically determined progression of coronary atherosclerosis in women with established coronary artery disease over a 3-year period.[68]

The National Institutes of Health (NIH)-sponsored Women's Health Initiative (WHI), a recent large-scale randomized, double-blinded trial of primary prevention of coronary heart disease, demonstrated an overall lack of benefit of long-term HRT. The WHI was a placebo-controlled long-term trial of HRT, calcium/vitamin D supplementation, and dietary modification that was conducted in 16,608 mostly healthy, ethnically diverse postmenopausal women; investigators explored the effects of these interventions on many end points, including the incidences of cardiovascular disease, osteoporotic fractures, and breast cancer.[69] Only 7.7% of participating women reported a prior history of cardiovascular disease. Women with an intact uterus at baseline were randomly assigned to receive daily conjugated equine estrogens plus medroxyprogesterone acetate versus placebo. The study was stopped early in 2002 by the Data Safety and Monitoring Board after an average follow-up time of 5.2 years because of an increase in coronary heart disease (CHD), stroke, and pulmonary embolism (PE), as well as evidence of breast cancer harm that outweighed the potential benefit of hormone use in terms of reducing fractures and preventing colon cancer. The estimated hazard ratio for CHD was 1.29 (95% CI, 1.02 to 1.63) with 286 total cases. The absolute risk excess per 10,000 women attributable to estrogen plus progestin was seven additional CHD events. As in the HERS trial, the difference between treatment groups began soon after randomization but in this trial was found to persist.

Clinical Event	HERS[66] (Estrogen + Progestin)	WHI[69] (Estrogen + Progestin)	WHI[70] (Estrogen alone)
CHD events	0.99 (0.80–1.22)	1.29 (1.02–1.63)	0.91 (0.75–1.12)
Stroke	1.23 (0.89–1.70)	1.41 (1.07–1.85)	1.39 (1.10–1.77)
Pulmonary embolism	2.79 (0.89–8.75)	2.13 (1.39–3.25)	1.34 (0.87–2.06)
DVT	2.80 (1.30–6.00)	2.07 (1.49–2.87)	1.47 (1.04–2.08)
Total VTE	2.70 (1.40–5.00)	2.11 (1.58–2.82)	1.33 (0.99–1.79)
Breast cancer	1.30 (0.77–2.19)	1.26 (1.00–1.59)	0.77 (0.59–1.01)
Colon cancer	0.69 (0.32–1.49)	0.63 (0.43–0.92)	1.08 (0.75–1.55)
Hip fracture	1.10 (0.49–2.50)	0.66 (0.45–0.98)	0.61 (0.41–0.91)
Death	1.08 (0.84–1.38)	0.98 (0.82–1.18)	1.04 (0.88–1.22)
Global index‡	–	1.15 (1.03–1.28)	1.01 (0.91–1.12)

Table 34-3   Risks of Thrombosis and Other Events from the HERS and WHI Studies*†

*Hazard ratios with 95% confidence intervals given.
†Data are based on the intent-to-treat analysis. For the primary CHD events outcome (myocardial infarction plus CHD death), the three trials had similar numbers of events and thus similar power. For other outcomes, the smaller HERS trial had fewer events and less precise hazard ratios.
‡The global index was composed of the first occurrence of any of the events listed in the table.
HERS, Heart and Estrogen/Progestin Replacement Study; WHI, Women's Health Initiative; CHD, coronary heart disease; DVT, deep venous thrombosis; VTE, venous thromboembolic events.

From Hulley SB, Grady D: The WHI estrogen-alone trial: Do things look any better? JAMA 291:1769–1771, 2004.

Conjugated equine estrogen is by far the most widely used estrogen in the United States, and it is the treatment for which epidemiologic data are most readily available. Because of the increased risks of endometrial hyperplasia and carcinoma associated with estrogen alone, most women who have not undergone hysterectomy are treated with a progestin in addition to estrogen. The addition of progestin provides a more nearly physiologic replacement regimen, but this agent may oppose some of the benefits of estrogen, particularly with respect to cardiovascular disease. In 10,739 women without a uterus, the WHI trial revealed that estrogen given alone did not increase CHD risk but failed to significantly reduce it.[70] The hazard ratio for CHD events was 0.91 (95% CI, 0.75 to 1.12) with an average of 6.8 years of follow-up. Without progestin, the effect of harm was less pronounced; this trend was especially noted in younger participants (hazard ratio [HR], 0.56; ages, 50 to 59 years vs HR, 1.04; ages 70 to 79 years).

As a result of these findings, thousands of women throughout the world have stopped taking HRT. Other prospective primary prevention trials, such as the United Kingdom–based Women's International Study of Long Duration Oestrogen after Menopause (WISDOM), were cancelled. However, the controversy about HRT continues. Many have argued that the methods used in observational studies were inherently confounded by a "healthy user bias," by which women for whom estrogens are prescribed are often healthier initially, and those who continue to take hormones tend to be free of disease. Thus, lower mortality among hormone users may have been attributed erroneously to the hormone itself.

Others have believed that it is the timing of the initiation of HRT that is the problem: most women in observational studies began to receive therapy at or near the menopausal transition, whereas in the WHI study, older women with a mean age of 62.7 years, averaging 12 years postmenopausal, were treated.[71] Theoretically, younger women have little to no atherosclerosis compared with the older cohort studied in the WHI; substantial preclinical data have suggested that the atheropreventive effects of estrogen exist before vascular damage occurs versus the possibility that adverse effects of estrogen in promoting thrombosis and inflammation are present once complex atheromas occur. The WHI found a nonsignificant trend toward lower risk with less passage of time since menopause; for women in whom menopause had begun less than 10 years previously, 10 to 19 years previously, and 20 or more years previously, the hazard ratios for CHD associated with postmenopausal hormone therapy compared with placebo were 0.89, 1.22, and 1.71, respectively.[72] Such findings are consistent with animal studies showing that the benefits of estrogen in preventing atherosclerosis were reversed in the presence of endothelial injury in rabbits.[73] Similarly, ovariectomized monkeys that began hormonal therapy at the time of surgery have a reduced incidence of atherosclerosis compared with monkeys that began therapy years after ovariectomy.[74] The Estrogen in the Prevention of Atherosclerosis (EPAT) trial, conducted in 222 healthy menopausal women without preexisting cardiovascular disease, found the average rate of progression of subclinical atherosclerosis, as measured by carotid intima media thickness (one of the earliest detectable anatomic changes in the development of atherosclerosis), to be lower in those taking unopposed estrogen versus those taking placebo (-0.0017 mm per year vs 0.0036 mm per year).[75] Of note, this protective effect disappeared in women placed on lipid-lowering medications. The question remains whether HRT initiated during the perimenopause may decrease the risk of coronary heart disease.

Other difficulties with earlier studies may have involved different formulations and schedules of HRT, incomplete follow-up and compliance, and other considerations such as the use of surrogate end points in trials that may have addressed the wrong mechanisms. Another area of controversy relates to the route of administration of estrogen. Some data suggest that transdermal patches are less likely to produce a hypercoaguable state because of reduced hepatic processing, inducing less production of various proinflammatory molecules, including CRP.[76] The Papworth Hormone-Replacement Therapy Atherosclerosis Trial, which compared transdermal estrogen given alone or in combination with norethindrone, also showed no cardiovascular benefit of HRT for secondary prevention in women with angiographically proved coronary heart disease, but no studies have been conducted as yet on primary prevention.[77]

To answer these lingering questions, trials such as the Kronos Early Estrogen Prevention Study (KEEPS) are currently recruiting subjects to study the effects of HRT in a younger population of women.[78] KEEPS is designed as a 5-year, randomized, placebo-controlled, double-blinded trial in 720 healthy perimenopausal women aged 42 to 58 years. Participants will have had cessation of menses after age 40 and no menses for 6 to 36 months prior to randomization. They will be divided into three groups and will receive transdermal estrogen, oral estrogen, or placebo. Women receiving estrogen will also be treated with a progestin. Participants will be followed for the development of atherosclerotic disease via carotid intimal medial thickness as a surrogate for cardiovascular end points. Studies such as these will be very helpful in elucidating the potential role of HRT in the prevention of coronary heart disease in perimenopausal women.

At this time, with the results of several large, well-conducted randomized trials suggesting a lack of net benefit and the presence of serious risk, it is recommended that HRT should not be initiated or continued in postmenopausal women for the purposes of primary or secondary prevention of coronary heart disease.[79]

HORMONE REPLACEMENT THERAPY AND STROKE

Data on increased risk of stroke with HRT have been clarified by the findings of recent large, randomized trials. A meta-analysis of nine observational primary prevention studies suggests that hormone therapy is associated with a small increase in stroke incidence (relative risk [RR], 1.12; 95% CI, 1.01 to 1.23), primarily caused by an increase in thromboembolic stroke (RR, 1.20; 95% CI, 1.01 to 1.40).[79,80] These results are consistent with findings from the WHI, which revealed an increased risk of stroke with a hazard ratio (HR) of 1.41 (95% CI, 1.07 to 1.85) in 212 cases. The absolute risk excess per 10,000 women attributable to estrogen plus progestin was small, at only eight additional strokes.[69] In contrast to CHD, excessive risk of stroke was not present in the first year, but it occurred during the second year and persisted. In the WHI study of women without a uterus who were receiving estrogen alone, the HR was 1.39 (95% CI, 1.10 to 1.77), suggesting that this adverse effect is attributable to the estrogen component of the hormone regimen.[70] It is interesting to note that in the WHI, 79.8% of strokes were ischemic. The adjusted HR for HRT versus placebo was significant for ischemic (HR, 1.44; 95% CI, 1.09 to 1.90) but not hemorrhagic or combined stroke, suggesting an increased risk for thromboembolic disease. In HERS, the risk of stroke was found to be nonsignificant with an HR of 1.23 (95% CI, 0.89 to 1.70).[81]

For secondary prevention, the Women's Estrogen for Stroke Trial (WEST) studied HRT provided after ischemic stroke and transient ischemic attacks (TIAs) among postmenopausal women. After a mean of 2.8 years of follow-up, no net benefit was found for the use of estrogen therapy in 664 women randomly assigned to unopposed estrogen or placebo. Secondary analysis revealed an increase in the risk of stroke-related death, along with evidence of an increased early risk of death. During the first 6 months after randomization, three fatal strokes and 18 nonfatal strokes were reported in the group assigned to estradiol, compared with one fatal stroke and eight nonfatal strokes in the placebo group (RR, 2.3; 95% CI, 1.1 to 5.0). Evidence also suggested that women randomly assigned to estradiol had more severe strokes. Among those with recurrent strokes, complete or near complete recovery was half as likely to occur among those randomly assigned to estrogen therapy.[82,83] On the basis of these results, HRT should not be initiated to reduce the risk of stroke or other cardiovascular disease in postmenopausal women.

HORMONE REPLACEMENT THERAPY AND VENOUS THROMBOEMBOLIC DISEASE

In general, observational studies have reported a two- to threefold increase in relative risk for thromboembolic events with the use of HRT.[84,85] This number has been confirmed by clinical trial data from the HERS[66] and WHI studies. In the HERS trial, confirmed venous thromboembolic events occurred in 34 women in the hormone group (6.2 per 1000 woman-years) and in 13 women in the placebo group (2.3 per 1000 woman-years). This translated to a relative HR of 2.7 (95% CI, 1.40 to 5.00) for users of the estrogen/progestin combination. The excess risk was 3.9 per 1000 woman-years (CI, 1.4 to 6.4 per 1000 woman-years), and the estimated number needed to treat for harm was one excess thromboembolic event for every 65 women taking hormones for 5 years. More women in the hormone group experienced deep venous thromboses (25 vs 9; relative hazard, 2.80; CI, 1.30 to 6.00; $P = .008$) and pulmonary emboli (11 vs 4; relative hazard, 2.79; CI, 0.89 to 8.75; $P = .08$); for three women, all in the hormone group, pulmonary embolism proved fatal. Similar to other studies, the risk appeared to be highest during the first 2 years of use and tended to decline with time (RR, 1.40; 95% CI, 0.64 to 3.05; $P = .08$).[79,86,87]

The WHI initially reported an overall HR for VTE of 2.11 (95% CI, 1.58 to 2.82), with 151 cases in treated participants versus 67 cases in the placebo group.[69] A slightly extended follow-up period revealed that venous thrombosis occurred in a total of 167 women who were taking estrogen plus progestin (3.5 per 1000 person-years) versus 76 women who were taking placebo (1.7 per 1000 person-years).[86] The HR for DVT was 2.07 (95% CI, 1.49 to 2.87) with 167 cases, and for PE, it was 2.13 (95% CI, 1.39 to 3.25) with 101 cases. The estimated excess number of events per 1000 women taking estrogen plus progestin for 10 years was 18. In women with a hysterectomy who received estrogen alone, the risk was attenuated, with an HR of 1.33 and a 95% CI of 0.99 to 1.79.[70] Only the increased risk of DVT reached statistical significance. The HR for DVT was 1.47 (95% CI, 1.04 to 2.08), and for PE, it was 1.34 (95% CI, 0.87 to 2.06).

An additional nested case-controlled study examining the association of various biomarkers, treatment assignment, and the risk of vascular outcomes was conducted during the WHI study.[86] All validated cases of VTE that occurred between randomization and a selected 2-year follow-up time point (n = 147) were paired with control cases matched for age, follow-up time, and baseline vascular disease. Analysis revealed that the risk associated with HRT increased with age: HR was 4.28 (95% CI, 2.38 to 7.72) in women aged 60 to 69 years and 7.46 (95% CI, 4.32 to 14.38) in women aged 70 to 79 years as compared with women aged 50 to 59 years who were taking placebo. The risk was also increased in overweight (BMI 25 to 30) and obese (BMI > 30) women with a HR of 3.80 (95% CI, 2.08 to 6.94) and 5.61 (95% CI, 3.12 to 10.11), respectively. Factor V Leiden positivity increased the hormone-associated risk of thrombosis by 6.69-fold over that reported in women on placebo without the mutation (95% CI, 3.09 to 14.49). A 2.6-fold increase was seen among heterozygotes and a 7.5-fold increase was noted among homozygotes, leading to an estimated absolute risk of VTE of 0.8% per year among women carrying an FV Leiden mutation and taking HRT. Estimates range from 795 unselected healthy women to 376 women with coronary heart disease who needed to be screened for FV Leiden mutations prior to initiation of HRT to prevent one episode of VTE over 5 years of treatment.[88] Different from users of OCs, other measured genetic variants, including prothrombin 20210, methylenetetrahydrofolate reductase mutation C677T, factor XIII Val34-Leu, PAI-1 4G/5G, and factor V HR2, were not found to modify the association of HRT with venous thrombosis. It is possible that the lower estrogen dose in HRT versus that in OCs explains this difference, rather than simply a higher baseline level of VTE in postmenopausal women compared with younger women that obscures the interaction.

Some data suggest that the mode of supplying estrogen may be crucial to the risk of VTE; it is intimated that transdermal estrogen may not be associated with an increased risk of thromboembolic events. In contrast to three very small prior case-controlled studies that showed a nonsignificant increased risk of VTE in users of transdermal HRT, Scarabin and colleagues[76] recently performed the hospital-based case-controlled Estrogen and Thromboembolism Risk (ESTHER) study in France to assess women with a first documented episode of idiopathic VTE. Overall, 32 patients (21%) and 27 controls (7%) were found to be current users of oral estrogen only replacement therapy versus 30 patients (19%) and 93 controls (24%) who were current users of transdermal HRT. The estimated risk of VTE in users of oral HRT was 3.5 (95% CI, 1.8 to 6.8); in users of transdermal HRT, it was 0.9 (95% CI, 0.5 to 1.6) compared with nonusers. When users of estrogen-only HRT were compared with users of transdermal HRT, the estimated risk of VTE was 4.0 (95% CI, 1.9 to 8.3).[76,85] This finding is biologically plausible in that oral but not transdermal estrogen has been found to enhance in vivo thrombin generation and induce an acquired resistance to protein C.[9,12] In addition, a lower antithrombin III concentration has been found in women on oral but not transdermal HRT.[89] It is possible that although oral HRT induces a procoagulant environment caused by an increase in general hepatic protein synthesis, transdermal estrogen replacement therapy has little effect on hemostasis. However, several confounding variables may exist in this observational study, including recall bias, preferential referral of cases, and in appropriateness of the selection of controls (they had more illnesses such as diabetes and were potentially unequally likely to be taking HRT). Data from large studies such as KEEPS will be instrumental in helping clinicians to prospectively determine the safety of transdermal estrogen therapy.

HRT is generally believed to be contraindicated in women with a history of DVT because of the unacceptable risk of recurrent events. Before the results of large trials such as HERS and WHI were known, Hoibraaten and coworkers[57] studied the risk of giving HRT to 140 postmenopausal women with a history of DVT or PE. The study was terminated prematurely for ethical reasons after the findings of the HERS trial were published. Despite the limited duration of the trial, a high incidence of recurrent VTE in women randomly assigned to hormonal therapy was found: eight women in the HRT group (10.7%) versus one woman in the placebo group (2.3%) developed VTE. Furthermore, all those in the HRT group experienced a thrombotic event within the first 261 days after inclusion in the study. Treatment groups were similar with regard to other risk factors for VTE, including time from previous VTE and rates of inherited thrombophilia (28% of women on HRT and 22% of women in the placebo group), suggesting that the bulk of the excess risk of thrombosis found in this study could be attributed to HRT. Few women with a prior history of VTE were enrolled in the WHI because of the eligibility criteria, but data also suggest an increased risk in this population: with HRT, HR 3.87 (95% CI, 0.45 to 33.34) versus those without a history of VTE, HR 2.06 (95% CI, 1.54 to 2.76).

In women who need to take HRT but who are at high risk of VTE, anticoagulation with warfarin or low molecular weight heparin may be considered, but no clinical trials have been performed to date to confirm the safety of this approach. This group includes women with a prior history of VTE, as well as those who carry an inherited thrombophilic state such as FV Leiden. In the HERS study, a trend toward the beneficial effects of baseline aspirin use was noted to attenuate the risk of thromboembolic disease (HR, 1.68; 95% CI, 0.96 to 2.92 for aspirin users vs HR, 4.23; 95% CI, 1.41 to 12.7 for nonusers),[87] although this was not seen in the WHI.

The decision regarding whether a woman should initiate or continue short-term hormonal therapy for menopausal symptom control must be made by weighing her individual risk:benefit ratio. The risk of VTE is unknown in women who take HRT for only a few months, although observational evidence suggests that the risk seems greatest during the first several months to 1 year after initiation of HRT. Phytoestrogens have also been used to relieve postmenopausal symptoms; the few prospective studies performed to date have not yet found any potential adverse effects of soy products on the coagulation system.[90]

SELECTIVE ESTROGEN RECEPTOR MODULATORS/SELECTIVE ESTROGEN RECEPTOR DOWN-REGULATORS, AROMATASE INHIBITORS, AND THROMBOSIS

Tamoxifen is one of the most effective treatments for patients with breast cancer because of its ability to antagonize estrogen-dependent growth by binding estrogen receptors and inhibiting proliferation of breast epithelial cells. However, tamoxifen has estrogenic agonist effects in other tissues such as bone and endometrium. Several novel anti-estrogenic compounds have been developed that have a reduced agonist profile in breast and gynecologic tissue; they thus offer the potential for enhanced efficacy and reduced toxicity compared with tamoxifen. In advanced breast cancer, clinical data are available for two groups of agents: selective estrogen receptor modulators (SERMs—further divided into "tamoxifen-like," namely, toremifene, droloxifene, and idoxifene, and "fixed-ring" compounds, namely, raloxifene, arzoxifene, and EM-800) and selective estrogen receptor down-regulators (SERDs—fulvestrant, SR 16234, and ZK 191703).

The estrogen agonist/antagonist tamoxifen is widely used in the management of breast cancer. Currently, this drug is used in the adjuvant setting after local therapy is provided for early-stage breast cancer that is hormone receptor positive, in the treatment of patients with metastatic breast cancer that is hormone receptor positive, and prophylactically in women deemed at high risk for the development of invasive breast cancer. In a meta-analysis of four major primary prevention trials of tamoxifen involving 28,406 subjects, the use of tamoxifen was associated with 118 serious VTEs versus 62 in the placebo group, with a relative risk of 1.9 (95% CI, 1.4 to 2.6), including six versus two cases of fatal pulmonary emboli. The risk of superficial thrombophlebitis was doubled with tamoxifen relative to placebo (68 vs 30 events).[91]

Saphner and associates[92] retrospectively analyzed the 10-year experience of 2673 women with breast cancer in multicenter trials conducted by the Eastern Cooperative Oncology Group (ECOG); an increase in VTE was associated with tamoxifen therapy alone, as well as with a substantial increase in patients allocated to combined treatment with tamoxifen plus chemotherapy compared with untreated controls or those who received chemotherapy alone. Specifically, the data showed that premenopausal patients who received chemotherapy and tamoxifen had a greater number of venous events than did those who received chemotherapy without tamoxifen (2.8% vs 0.8%; $P = .03$). Postmenopausal patients who received tamoxifen and chemotherapy had a greater number of venous thrombi than did those who were given tamoxifen alone (8.0% vs 2.3%; $P = .03$) or those who were observed (8.0% vs 0.4%; $P < .0001$). These findings and data from other studies suggest that chemotherapy contributes to thrombosis in patients with breast cancer.[93] A large United Kingdom–based General Practice Research Database study concluded that the relative risk estimate for VTE with current tamoxifen exposure, as compared with those who were never exposed and past use as a reference group, was 7.1 (95% CI, 1.5 to 33).[94]

In the breast cancer prevention trial, the National Surgical Adjuvant Breast and Bowel Project B-24 (NSABP P-1),[95] a randomized clinical trial of 13,388 women to evaluate the effectiveness of tamoxifen in the prevention of breast cancer in women considered to be at increased risk of the disease, the use of tamoxifen was associated with an increased risk of VTE. Pulmonary emboli were observed in almost three times as many women in the tamoxifen group as in the placebo group (18 vs 6; RR, 3.01; 95% CI, 0.15 to 9.27). A greater number of women who received tamoxifen developed DVT compared with women who received placebo (35 vs 22 cases, respectively). Average annual rates per 1000 women treated were 1.34 versus 0.84 (RR, 1.60; 95% CI, 0.91 to 2.86). (See Table 34-4 for a summary of tamoxifen breast cancer prevention studies.)[101–103]

In the NSABP B-24 randomized trial, in which the use of tamoxifen after lumpectomy and radiation therapy for ductal carcinoma in situ was compared with the use of placebo, one extra pulmonary embolism and seven extra deep venous thromboses were noted in the treatment arm.[96] A total of 891 women in the tamoxifen group had nine deep venous thromboses (1%) and two pulmonary emboli (0.2%). The placebo arm consisted of 890 women who had two deep venous thromboses (0.2%) and one pulmonary embolus (0.1%).

Relative risk estimates from studies published to date on the use of tamoxifen range from no effect up to a 7-times increased incidence of VTE. Most authorities in the field quote a 2- to 4-times increased relative risk for VTE with the use of tamoxifen versus that in patients who were not receiving the drug. Again, as has often been discussed in this chapter, the absolute risk of VTE in a patient on tamoxifen may be so low as to not influence the decision to use the agent in the management of any individual patient's breast cancer. Known thrombophilic mutations, such as FV Leiden and prothrombin 20210, do not appear

to interact with tamoxifen to impose an increased risk for VTE. A case-controlled study conducted by the National Surgical Adjuvant Breast and Bowel Project's Breast Cancer Prevention Project (BCPT) in 371 subjects compared the rate of FV Leiden and prothrombin 20210 mutations in women who experienced a VTE while receiving tamoxifen versus placebo. No statistical evidence of an additive effect of tamoxifen use to these two genetic mutations on the rate of thromboembolic events was found. They concluded that screening women at risk for breast cancer for FVL and/or prothrombin 20210 appears to offer no benefit in determining the risk of tamoxifen-associated thromboembolic events.[97]

Raloxifene hydrochloride is a SERM that is chemically distinct from tamoxifen and estradiol and that has antiestrogenic effects on breast and endometrial tissue and estrogenic effects on bone, lipid metabolism, and the coagulation system. Currently, raloxifene is FDA approved for the treatment of patients with postmenopausal osteoporosis. The Multiple Outcomes of Raloxifene Evaluation (MORE) study, which treated a total of 7705 postmenopausal women with osteoporosis, was the pivotal trial that led to the drug's approval.[98] In the MORE study, the use of raloxifene increased the risk of VTE (relative risk, 3.1; 95% CI, 1.5 to 6.2). After 40 months of follow-up, higher rates of DVT (38 cases) and PE (17 cases) were observed in the combined raloxifene groups (60-mg and 120-mg doses were used) than in the placebo groups (5 and 3 cases, respectively). One case of VTE occurred per 155 women treated with raloxifene for 3 years.

Raloxifene and tamoxifen both appear to increase the risk of VTE but to different degrees. The Study of Tamoxifen and Raloxifene (STAR) trial, one of the largest breast cancer prevention trials ever undertaken, randomized 19,747 postmenopausal women at high risk for breast cancer to receive either tamoxifen or raloxifene for 5 years. The investigators found no difference in the number of invasive breast cancers in each group, but fewer noninvasive breast cancers in the tamoxifen arm. Thromboembolic events occurred less often in the raloxifene group (RR, 0.70; 95% CI, 0.54 to 0.91). The cumulative incidence at 6 years was 21 per 1000 in the tamoxifen arm and 16 per 1000 in the raloxifene arm. PE and DVT occurred in 54 versus 35 women (RR, 0.64; 95% CI, 0.41–1.00) and in 87 versus 65 women (RR, 0.74; 95% CI, 0.53–1.03) assigned to tamoxifen and raloxifene, respectively. Fewer cases of uterine cancer and cataracts occurred in the raloxifene arm.

Table 34-4 Tamoxifen Breast Cancer Prevention Trials*

	Royal Marsden Trial[101]		NSABP P-1[95]		Italian Tamoxifen Study[102]		IBIS-1[103]		All Trials	
	T	P	T	P	T	P	T	P	T	P
Total patient no.	1238	1233	6681	6707	2700	2708	3573	3566	14192	14214
Breast cancers	62	75	124	244	34	45	69	101	289	465
DVT and PE	12	8	53	28	10	9	43	17	118	62
Superficial thrombophlebitis	8	5	NA		33	16	27	9	68	30

*The number of patients who experienced each end point is shown in the table.
DVT, deep venous thrombosis; IBIS-I, International Breast Cancer Intervention study I; Italian, Italian Tamoxifen Prevention study; Marsden, The Royal Marsden Hospital Tamoxifen Randomized Chemoprevention trial; NSABP P-1, National Surgical Adjuvant Breast and Bowel Project P-1 study; P, placebo; PE, pulmonary embolism; T, tamoxifen.

No differences were found in ischemic heart disease events, stroke, other invasive cancer sites, osteoporotic fractures, or mortality. At present, it is considered prudent not to prescribe either raloxifene or tamoxifen to a woman with a history of VTE, but this decision should be individualized on the basis of the woman's clinical history and known underlying risk factors. Consideration may be given to the use of DVT prophylaxis in combination with raloxifene or tamoxifen if the benefits of treatment are deemed greater than the associated risks.[98a]

AROMATASE INHIBITORS

At present, the treatment of postmenopausal women with hormone-responsive breast cancer is undergoing a shift toward the use of aromatase inhibitors instead of tamoxifen. In the United States, three aromatase inhibitors are clinically available: anastrazole (Arimidex; AstraZeneca Pharmaceuticals LP, Wilmington, DE, USA), letrozole (Femara; Novartis Pharmaceuticals Corporation, East Hanover, NJ, USA), and exemestane (Aromasin; Pfizer Inc, New York, NY, USA). The former two are nonsteroidal compounds with reversible binding properties, and the latter one is a steroidal compound with irreversible binding properties. Emerging data indicate that in terms of VTE risk, these agents are safer than tamoxifen. In the Arimidex, Tamoxifen, Alone or in Combination (ATAC) trial, patients experienced 73 total venous thromboembolic events on anastrazole (2%) versus 120 events on tamoxifen (4%), with an odds ratio of 0.60 (95% CI, 0.44 to 0.81).[99] Specifically, for deep venous thromboembolic events, patients on anastrazole experienced 40 events (1%) versus 60 events on tamoxifen (2%), with an odds ratio of 0.66 (95% CI, 0.43 to 1.00) In other words, anastrazole users experienced half the venous thromboembolic events that tamoxifen users reported, that is, 2% versus 4%.

Aromatase inhibitors are now the agents of choice in postmenopausal women with hormone-responsive breast cancer, both in the metastatic setting and alone or in sequence with tamoxifen in the early/adjuvant setting. They are currently being tested in breast cancer prevention trials, where the toxicity profiles of these agents have increased importance because of the otherwise healthy nature of the population.

SUMMARY

Although numerous studies have explored the thrombogenic potential of the agents discussed in this chapter, data in many areas are insufficient to confirm true risks of VTE. Often, the absolute risks for adverse events are so low that they do not affect the risk:benefit calculations that go into the decision of whether or not to use these agents. It is conceivable that in the future, more comprehensive pharmacogenomic studies will lead to individualization of hormonal contraception and HRT recommendations. As is almost always the case in clinical medicine, decisions must be highly individualized, because the benefits of these agents to the patient and to society may be large, and the risks may be small. With continued use of hormonal therapies, the need to better define risks for thrombotic

events in women with a remote history of thrombosis or a laboratory-defined thrombophilia is clear. Additionally, improved understanding of the pathogenesis of hormonally induced thrombosis would aid in the development of new therapies without this adverse effect.

REFERENCES

1. Speroff L, DeCherney A: Evaluation of a new generation of oral contraceptives. The Advisory Board for the New Progestins. Obstet Gynecol 81:1034–1047, 1993.
2. Meade TW, Haines AP, Imeson JD, et al: Menopausal status and haemostatic variables. Lancet 1:22–24, 1983.
3. Caine YG, Bauer KA, Barzegar S, et al: Coagulation activation following estrogen administration to postmenopausal women. Thromb Haemost 68:392–395, 1992.
4. Luyer MD, Khosla S, Owen WG, Miller VM: Prospective randomized study of effects of unopposed estrogen replacement therapy on markers of coagulation and inflammation in postmenopausal women. J Clin Endocrinol Metab 86:3629–3634, 2001.
5. Conard J: Biological coagulation findings in third-generation oral contraceptives. Hum Reprod Update 5:672–680, 1999.
6. Deguchi H, Bouma BN, Middeldorp S, et al: Decreased plasma sensitivity to activated protein C by oral contraceptives is associated with decreases in plasma glucosylceramide. J Thromb Haemost 3:935–938, 2005.
7. Kluft C, Leuven JA, Helmerhorst FM, Krans HM: Pro-inflammatory effects of oestrogens during use of oral contraceptives and hormone replacement treatment. Vascul Pharmacol 39:149–154, 2002.
8. Cushman M: Effects of hormone replacement therapy and estrogen receptor modulators on markers of inflammation and coagulation. Am J Cardiol 90:7F–10F, 2002.
9. Scarabin PY, Alhenc-Gelas M, Plu-Bureau G, et al: Effects of oral and transdermal estrogen/progesterone regimens on blood coagulation and fibrinolysis in postmenopausal women: A randomized controlled trial. Arterioscler Thromb Vasc Biol 17:3071–3078, 1997.
10. Post MS, Christella M, Thomassen LG, et al: Effect of oral and transdermal estrogen replacement therapy on hemostatic variables associated with venous thrombosis: A randomized, placebo-controlled study in postmenopausal women. Arterioscler Thromb Vasc Biol 23:1116–1121, 2003.
11. Vongpatanasin W, Tuncel M, Wang Z, et al: Differential effects of oral versus transdermal estrogen replacement therapy on C-reactive protein in postmenopausal women. J Am Coll Cardiol 41:1358–1363, 2003.
12. Oger E, Alhenc-Gelas M, Lacut K, et al: Differential effects of oral and transdermal estrogen/progesterone regimens on sensitivity to activated protein C among postmenopausal women: A randomized trial. Arterioscler Thromb Vasc Biol 23:1671–1676, 2003.
13. Scarabin PY, Plu-Bureau G, Zitoun D, et al: Changes in haemostatic variables induced by oral contraceptives containing 50 micrograms or 30 micrograms oestrogen: Absence of dose-dependent effect on PAI-1 activity. Thromb Haemost 74:928–932, 1995.
14. Gebara OC, Mittleman MA, Sutherland P, et al: Association between increased estrogen status and increased fibrinolytic potential in the Framingham Offspring Study. Circulation 91:1952–1958, 1995.
15. Joswig M, Hach-Wunderle V, Ziegler R, Nawroth PP: Postmenopausal hormone replacement therapy and the vascular wall: Mechanisms of 17 beta-estradiol's effects on vascular biology. Exp Clin Endocrinol Diabetes 107:477–487, 1999.
16. Zanger D, Yang BK, Ardans J, et al: Divergent effects of hormone therapy on serum markers of inflammation in postmenopausal women with coronary artery disease on appropriate medical management. J Am Coll Cardiol 36:1797–1802, 2000.
17. Herrington DM, Howard TD, Hawkins GA, et al: Estrogen-receptor polymorphisms and effects of estrogen replacement on high-density lipoprotein cholesterol in women with coronary disease. N Engl J Med 346:967–974, 2002.
18. Alhenc-Gelas M, Plu-Bureau G, Guillonneau S, et al: Impact of progestagens on activated protein C (APC) resistance among users of oral contraceptives. J Thromb Haemost 2:1594–1600, 2004.
19. Koenen RR, Christella M, Thomassen LG, et al: Effect of oral contraceptives on the anticoagulant activity of protein S in plasma. Thromb Haemost 93:853–859, 2005.

20. Kemmeren JM, Algra A, Meijers JC, et al: Effect of second- and third-generation oral contraceptives on the protein C system in the absence or presence of the factor V Leiden mutation: A randomized trial. Blood 103:927–933, 2004.

21. van Rooijen M, Silveira A, Hamsten A, Bremme K: Sex hormone–binding globulin: A surrogate marker for the prothrombotic effects of combined oral contraceptives. Am J Obstet Gynecol 190:332–337, 2004.

22. Jordan WM: Pulmonary embolism. Lancet 278:1146–1147, 1961.

23. Gerstman BB, Piper JM, Tomita DK, et al: Oral contraceptive estrogen dose and the risk of deep venous thromboembolic disease. Am J Epidemiol 133:32–37, 1991.

24. Bottiger LE, Boman G, Eklund G, Westerholm B: Oral contraceptives and thromboembolic disease: Effects of lowering oestrogen content. Lancet 1:1097–1101, 1980.

25. Vessey M, Mant D, Smith A, Yeates D: Oral contraceptives and venous thromboembolism: Findings in a large prospective study. Br Med J (Clin Res Ed) 292:526, 1986.

26. Vandenbroucke JP, Rosing J, Bloemenkamp KW, et al: Oral contraceptives and the risk of venous thrombosis. N Engl J Med 344: 1527–1535, 2001.

27. van Grootheest K, Vrieling T: Thromboembolism associated with the new contraceptive Yasmin. BMJ 326:257, 2003.

28. Vasilakis-Scaramozza C, Jick H: Risk of venous thromboembolism with cyproterone or levonorgestrel contraceptives. Lancet 358: 1427–1429, 2001.

29. van Vliet HA, Winkel TA, Noort I, et al: Prothrombotic changes in users of combined oral contraceptives containing drospirenone and cyproterone acetate. J Thromb Haemost 2:2060–2062, 2004.

30. Lidegaard O, Edstrom B, Kreiner S: Oral contraceptives and venous thromboembolism: A five-year national case-control study. Contraception 65:187–196, 2002.

31. Farmer RD, Lawrenson RA, Thompson CR, et al: Population-based study of risk of venous thromboembolism associated with various oral contraceptives. Lancet 349:83–88, 1997.

32. Vasilakis C, Jick H, del Mar Melero-Montes M: Risk of idiopathic venous thromboembolism in users of progestagens alone. Lancet 354:1610–1611, 1999.

33. Heinemann LA, Assmann A, DoMinh T, Garbe E: Oral progestogen-only contraceptives and cardiovascular risk: Results from the Transnational Study on Oral Contraceptives and the Health of Young Women. Eur J Contracept Reprod Health Care 4:67–73, 1999.

34. Lewis MA, Heinemann LA, MacRae KD, et al: The increased risk of venous thromboembolism and the use of third generation progestagens: Role of bias in observational research. The Transnational Research Group on Oral Contraceptives and the Health of Young Women. Contraception 54:5–13, 1996.

35. Cardiovascular disease and use of oral and injectable progestogen-only contraceptives and combined injectable contraceptives: Results of an international, multicenter, case-control study. World Health Organization Collaborative Study of Cardiovascular Disease and Steroid Hormone Contraception. Contraception 57:315–324, 1998.

36. Lidegaard O, Edstrom B, Kreiner S: Oral contraceptives and venous thromboembolism: A case-control study. Contraception 57: 291–301, 1998.

37. Poulter NR, Chang CL, Farley TM, Meirik O: Risk of cardiovascular diseases associated with oral progestagen preparations with therapeutic indications. Lancet 354:1610, 1999.

38. Chasan-Taber L, Stampfer MJ: Epidemiology of oral contraceptives and cardiovascular disease. Ann Intern Med 128:467–477, 1998.

39. Vital Statistics of the United States, 1992. v.1. Mortality, Part B. Hyattsville Md, US Dept of Health and Human Services, Centers for Disease Control and Prevention, National Center for Health Statistics, 1996, pp 24–27.

40. Stampfer MJ, Willett WC, Colditz GA, et al: Past use of oral contraceptives and cardiovascular disease: A meta-analysis in the context of the Nurses' Health Study. Am J Obstet Gynecol 163:285–291, 1990.

41. Jugdutt BI, Stevens GF, Zacks DJ, et al: Myocardial infarction, oral contraception, cigarette smoking, and coronary artery spasm in young women. Am Heart J 106:757–761, 1983.

42. Stampfer MJ, Willett WC, Colditz GA, et al: A prospective study of past use of oral contraceptive agents and risk of cardiovascular diseases. N Engl J Med 319:1313–1317, 1988.

43. Hannaford PC, Croft PR, Kay CR: Oral contraception and stroke: Evidence from the Royal College of General Practitioners' Oral Contraception Study. Stroke 25:935–942, 1994.

44. Ischaemic stroke and combined oral contraceptives: Results of an international, multicentre, case-control study. WHO Collaborative Study of Cardiovascular Disease and Steroid Hormone Contraception. Lancet 348:498–505, 1996.

45. Chan WS, Ray J, Wai EK, et al: Risk of stroke in women exposed to low-dose oral contraceptives: A critical evaluation of the evidence. Arch Intern Med 164:741–747, 2004.

46. Petitti DB, Sidney S, Bernstein A, et al: Stroke in users of low-dose oral contraceptives. N Engl J Med 335:8–15, 1996.

47. Vandenbroucke JP, Koster T, Briet E, et al: Increased risk of venous thrombosis in oral-contraceptive users who are carriers of factor V Leiden mutation. Lancet 344:1453–1457, 1994.

48. Bloemenkamp KW, Rosendaal FR, Helmerhorst FM, et al: Enhancement by factor V Leiden mutation of risk of deep-vein thrombosis associated with oral contraceptives containing a third-generation progestagen. Lancet 346:1593–1596, 1995.

49. Emmerich J, Rosendaal FR, Cattaneo M, et al: Combined effect of factor V Leiden and prothrombin 20210A on the risk of venous thromboembolism—Pooled analysis of 8 case-control studies including 2310 cases and 3204 controls. Study Group for Pooled-Analysis in Venous Thromboembolism. Thromb Haemost 86:809–816, 2001.

50. Middeldorp S, Meinardi JR, Koopman MM, et al: A prospective study of asymptomatic carriers of the factor V Leiden mutation to determine the incidence of venous thromboembolism. Ann Intern Med 135:322–327, 2001.

51. Bloemenkamp KW, Rosendaal FR, Helmerhorst FM, Vandenbroucke JP: Higher risk of venous thrombosis during early use of oral contraceptives in women with inherited clotting defects. Arch Intern Med 160:49–52, 2000.

52. Martinelli I, Sacchi E, Landi G, et al: High risk of cerebral-vein thrombosis in carriers of a prothrombin-gene mutation and in users of oral contraceptives. N Engl J Med 338:1793–1797, 1998.

53. de Bruijn SF, Stam J, Vandenbroucke JP: Increased risk of cerebral venous sinus thrombosis with third-generation oral contraceptives. Cerebral Venous Sinus Thrombosis Study Group. Lancet 351:1404, 1998.

54. Martinelli I, Taioli E, Battaglioli T, et al: Risk of venous thromboembolism after air travel: Interaction with thrombophilia and oral contraceptives. Arch Intern Med 163:2771–2774, 2003.

55. Abdollahi M, Cushman M, Rosendaal FR: Obesity: Risk of venous thrombosis and the interaction with coagulation factor levels and oral contraceptive use. Thromb Haemost 89:493–498, 2003.

56. van Hylckama Vlieg A, Rosendaal FR: Interaction between oral contraceptive use and coagulation factor levels in deep venous thrombosis. J Thromb Haemost 1:2186–2190, 2003.

57. Hoibraaten E, Qvigstad E, Arnesen H, et al: Increased risk of recurrent venous thromboembolism during hormone replacement therapy: Results of the randomized, double-blind, placebo-controlled estrogen in venous thromboembolism trial (EVTET). Thromb Haemost 84:961–967, 2000.

58. Conard J, Plu-Bureau G, Bahi N, et al: Progestogen-only contraception in women at high risk of venous thromboembolism. Contraception 70:437–441, 2004.

59. Goodyear-Smith F, Arroll B: Termination of pregnancy following panic: Stopping of oral contraceptives. Contraception 66:163–167, 2002.

60. Rosendaal FR: Venous thrombosis: A multicausal disease. Lancet 353:1167–1173, 1999.

61. Vossen CY, Conard J, Fontcuberta J, et al: Risk of a first venous thrombotic event in carriers of a familial thrombophilic defect. The European Prospective Cohort on Thrombophilia (EPCOT). J Thromb Haemost 3:459–464, 2005.

62. Stampfer MJ, Colditz GA, Willett WC, et al: Postmenopausal estrogen therapy and cardiovascular disease: Ten-year follow-up from the nurses' health study. N Engl J Med 325:756–762, 1991.

63. Colditz GA, Willett WC, Stampfer MJ, et al: Menopause and the risk of coronary heart disease in women. N Engl J Med 316:1105–1110, 1987.

64. Grodstein F, Stampfer M: The epidemiology of coronary heart disease and estrogen replacement in postmenopausal women. Prog Cardiovasc Dis 38:199–210, 1995.

65. Grodstein F, Stampfer MJ: Estrogen for women at varying risk of coronary disease. Maturitas 30:19–26, 1998.

66. Hulley S, Grady D, Bush T, et al: Randomized trial of estrogen plus progestin for secondary prevention of coronary heart disease in post-

menopausal women. Heart and Estrogen/Progestin Replacement Study (HERS) Research Group. JAMA 280:605–613, 1998.

67. Grady D, Herrington D, Bittner V, et al: Cardiovascular disease outcomes during 6.8 years of hormone therapy: Heart and Estrogen/Progestin Replacement Study follow-up (HERS II). JAMA 288:49–57, 2002.

68. Herrington DM, Reboussin DM, Brosnihan KB, et al: Effects of estrogen replacement on the progression of coronary-artery atherosclerosis. N Engl J Med 343:522–529, 2000.

69. Rossouw JE, Anderson GL, Prentice RL, et al: Risks and benefits of estrogen plus progestin in healthy postmenopausal women: Principal results from the Women's Health Initiative randomized controlled trial. JAMA 288:321–333, 2002.

70. Anderson GL, Limacher M, Assaf AR, et al: Effects of conjugated equine estrogen in postmenopausal women with hysterectomy: The Women's Health Initiative randomized controlled trial. JAMA 291:1701–1712, 2004.

71. Harman SM, Naftolin F, Brinton EA, Judelson DR: Is the estrogen controversy over? Deconstructing the Women's Health Initiative Study: A critical evaluation of the evidence. Ann N Y Acad Sci 1052:43–56, 2005.

72. Manson JE, Hsia J, Johnson KC, et al: Estrogen plus progestin and the risk of coronary heart disease. N Engl J Med 349:523–534, 2003.

73. Holm P, Andersen HL, Andersen MR, et al: The direct antiatherogenic effect of estrogen is present, absent, or reversed, depending on the state of the arterial endothelium: A time course study in cholesterol-clamped rabbits. Circulation 100:1727–1733, 1999.

74. Williams JK, Suparto I: Hormone replacement therapy and cardiovascular disease: Lessons from a monkey model of postmenopausal women. ILAR J 45:139–146, 2004.

75. Hodis HN, Mack WJ, Lobo RA, et al: Estrogen in the prevention of atherosclerosis: A randomized, double-blind, placebo-controlled trial. Ann Intern Med 135:939–953, 2001.

76. Scarabin PY, Oger E, Plu-Bureau G: Differential association of oral and transdermal oestrogen-replacement therapy with venous thromboembolism risk. Lancet 362:428–432, 2003.

77. Clarke SC, Kelleher J, Lloyd-Jones H, et al: A study of hormone replacement therapy in postmenopausal women with ischaemic heart disease: The Papworth HRT atherosclerosis study. Br J Obstet Gynaecol 109:1056–1062, 2002.

78. Harman SM, Brinton EA, Cedars M, et al: KEEPS: The Kronos Early Estrogen Prevention Study. Climacteric 8:3–12, 2005.

79. Hormone therapy for the prevention of chronic conditions in postmenopausal women: Recommendations from the U.S. Preventive Services Task Force. Ann Intern Med 142:855–860, 2005.

80. Humphrey LL, Chan BK, Sox HC: Postmenopausal hormone replacement therapy and the primary prevention of cardiovascular disease. Ann Intern Med 137:273–284, 2002.

81. Simon JA, Hsia J, Cauley JA, et al: Postmenopausal hormone therapy and risk of stroke: The Heart and Estrogen-Progestin Replacement Study (HERS). Circulation 103:638–642, 2001.

82. Brass LM: Hormone replacement therapy and stroke: Clinical trials review. Stroke 35:2644–2647, 2004.

83. Viscoli CM, Brass LM, Kernan WN, et al: A clinical trial of estrogen-replacement therapy after ischemic stroke. N Engl J Med 345:1243–1249, 2001.

84. Grodstein F, Stampfer MJ, Goldhaber SZ, et al: Prospective study of exogenous hormones and risk of pulmonary embolism in women. Lancet 348:983–987, 1996.

85. Gomes MP, Deitcher SR: Risk of venous thromboembolic disease associated with hormonal contraceptives and hormone replacement therapy: A clinical review. Arch Intern Med 164:1965–1976, 2004.

86. Cushman M, Kuller LH, Prentice R, et al: Estrogen plus progestin and risk of venous thrombosis. JAMA 292:1573–1580, 2004.

87. Hulley S, Furberg C, Barrett-Connor E, et al: Noncardiovascular disease outcomes during 6.8 years of hormone therapy: Heart and Estrogen/Progestin Replacement Study follow-up (HERS II). JAMA 288:58–66, 2002.

88. Herrington DM, Vittinghoff E, Howard TD, et al: Factor V Leiden, hormone replacement therapy, and risk of venous thromboembolic events in women with coronary disease. Arterioscler Thromb Vasc Biol 22:1012–1017, 2002.

89. Conard J, Samama M, Basdevant A, et al: Differential AT III: Response to oral and parenteral administration of 17 beta-estradiol. Thromb Haemost 49:252, 1983.

90. Teede HJ, Dalais FS, Kotsopoulos D, et al: Dietary soy containing phytoestrogens does not activate the hemostatic system in postmenopausal women. J Clin Endocrinol Metab 90:1936–1941, 2005.

91. Cuzick J, Powles T, Veronesi U, et al: Overview of the main outcomes in breast-cancer prevention trials. Lancet 361:296–300, 2003.

92. Saphner T, Tormey DC, Gray R: Venous and arterial thrombosis in patients who received adjuvant therapy for breast cancer. J Clin Oncol 9:286–294, 1991.

93. Levine MN, Gent M, Hirsh J, et al: The thrombogenic effect of anticancer drug therapy in women with stage II breast cancer. N Engl J Med 318:404–407, 1988.

94. Meier CR, Jick H: Tamoxifen and risk of idiopathic venous thromboembolism. Br J Clin Pharmacol 45:608–612, 1998.

95. Fisher B, Costantino JP, Wickerham DL, et al: Tamoxifen for prevention of breast cancer: Report of the National Surgical Adjuvant Breast and Bowel Project P-1 Study. J Natl Cancer Inst 90:1371–1388, 1998.

96. Fisher B, Dignam J, Wolmark N, et al: Tamoxifen in treatment of intraductal breast cancer: National Surgical Adjuvant Breast and Bowel Project B-24 randomised controlled trial. Lancet 353:1993–2000, 1999.

97. Abramson N, Costantino JP, Garber JE, et al: Effect of factor V Leiden and prothrombin G20210A mutations on thromboembolic risk in the National Surgical Adjuvant Breast and Bowel Project Breast Cancer Prevention Trial. J Natl Cancer Inst 98:904–910, 2006.

98. Ettinger B, Black DM, Mitlak BH, et al: Reduction of vertebral fracture risk in postmenopausal women with osteoporosis treated with raloxifene: Results from a 3-year randomized clinical trial. Multiple Outcomes of Raloxifene Evaluation (MORE) Investigators. JAMA 282:637–645, 1999.

98a. Vogel VG, Costantino JP, Wickerham DL, et al: Effects of tamoxifen vs raloxifene on the risk of developing invasive breast cancer and other disease outcomes: The NSABP study of tamoxifen and raloxifene (STAR) P-2 trial. JAMA 295:2727–2741, 2006.

99. Baum M, Budzar AU, Cuzick J, et al: Anastrozole alone or in combination with tamoxifen versus tamoxifen alone for adjuvant treatment of postmenopausal women with early breast cancer: First results of the ATAC randomised trial. Lancet 359:2131–2139, 2002.

100. Hulley SB, Grady D: The WHI estrogen-alone trial: Do things look any better? JAMA 291:1769–1771, 2004.

101. Powles T, Eeles R, Ashley S, et al: Interim analysis of the incidence of breast cancer in the Royal Marsden Hospital tamoxifen randomised chemoprevention trial. Lancet 352:98–101, 1998.

102. Veronesi U, Maisonneuve P, Costa A, et al: Prevention of breast cancer with tamoxifen: Preliminary findings from the Italian randomised trial among hysterectomised women. Italian Tamoxifen Prevention Study. Lancet 352:93–97, 1998.

103. Cuzick J, Forbes J, Edwards R, et al: First results from the International Breast Cancer Intervention Study (IBIS-I): A randomised prevention trial. Lancet 360:817–824, 2002.

Chapter 35

Management of Bleeding Disorders in Pregnancy

Stephanie Seremetis, MD • Victoria Afshani, MD

INTRODUCTION

Bleeding disorders during pregnancy and the puerperium pose specific and sometimes difficult management problems for the obstetrician and the consulting hematologist. Issues associated with diagnosis and management may be related to the mother and her unborn child. Various bleeding disorders can be categorized into several distinct categories. The first includes the inherited disorders, including the relatively common von Willebrand disease (VWD), the less common factor deficiencies, and inherited platelet disorders. The second category comprises acquired disorders that typically manifest prior to pregnancy, including immune thrombocytopenic purpura (ITP) and clotting factor inhibitors, but may also first occur in the context of pregnancy. Finally, disorders related directly to physical or pathophysiologic mechanisms may occur during pregnancy. Alterations in the normal hematologic responses to pregnancy that lead to dysregulation of the clotting cascade include disseminated intravascular coagulation (DIC) and *h*emolysis with *e*levated *l*iver function and *l*ow *p*latelets (HELLP) syndrome. Obstetric and anatomic causes include placental issues such as placenta previa, placenta accreta, and abruption, ectopic pregnancy, abortion and miscarriage, uterine atony due to twins or prolonged delivery, and retained products of conception. For management of these presentations, the reader is referred to textbooks on obstetrics and gynecology. Occasionally, medications are implicated when a bleeding tendency develops during pregnancy. The use of aspirin and heparin in women who have cardiac disease, including coronary artery disease and cardiac valve replacement with mechanical prostheses, as well as in women with systemic lupus erythematosus (SLE) with or without circulating anticoagulants or with known venous or arterial thromboses, have the potential to cause increased bleeding during pregnancy.

INHERITED DISORDERS OF BLEEDING IN PREGNANCY

Coagulation Factor Changes During Normal Pregnancy

Normal pregnancy is a relatively procoagulant state in that coagulation and fibrinolytic pathways undergo major changes that lead to a net increased propensity for hemostasis. Concentrations of some coagulation factors increase significantly, as do concentrations of plasminogen activation inhibitors, which reduce the activity of the fibrinolytic system. Both factor VIII and von Willebrand factor (VWF) increase steadily throughout gestation.[1–5] Factors VII and X and fibrinogen also rise significantly.[4,6] Other factors in the clotting cascade—factors II, IX, XII, and XIII—show no differences in levels throughout pregnancy.[6] Controversial data regarding factor XI levels have been published, with reports of either an increase or a fall in levels associated with advancing gestation.[6,7] Additionally, platelet count may decrease slightly during the third trimester because of dilution caused by hydremia during normal pregnancy but not to a degree that will pose a risk of bleeding during delivery.[8,9] Bleeding time, which reflects primary hemostasis, remains normal throughout pregnancy or may shorten, reflecting the increased platelet–endothelium interactions of pregnancy. Prothrombin time (PT) and partial thromboplastin time (PTT) may decrease to the lower limits of normal or may be slightly shortened in plasma from women in the third trimester, suggesting a low-grade process of intravascular coagulation.[9]

Coagulation Factor Changes in Inherited Bleeding Disorders

In pregnant women with inherited bleeding disorders, the data regarding coagulation factor levels are less certain. Women with type 1 VWD or who are carriers of hemophilia A sustain a significant rise in levels of factor VIII and in the antigen and activity of VWF during the second half of pregnancy. These women therefore rarely need hemostatic treatment later in pregnancy or during delivery. Factor IX levels, in contrast, remain relatively constant during gestation. Factor XI levels have not been measured prospectively during pregnancy in patients who are deficient in factor XI.

von Willebrand Disease

VWD is the most common inherited bleeding disorder, with prevalence in the general population estimated at 1% to 3%[4] (see Chapter 7 for a detailed discussion of VWD). The precise frequency of VWD is difficult to determine because there is considerable genotypic and clinical heterogeneity in this disorder. Most cases of VWD are inherited in an autosomal dominant pattern; thus, the implications for women of childbearing age are significant. The disorder is classified into three major types—types 1, 2, and 3—on the basis of the specific pathophysiologic mechanisms involved. The classification of VWD was recently the subject of a consensus committee of the International Society on Thrombosis and Haemostasis,[10] which proposed a revised system that retains the three major types of VWD and further classifies type 2 into four subtypes on the basis of laboratory and clinical data. Type 1 VWD, which accounts for 70% to 80% of all cases, usually causes only mild bleeding. Type 2 occurs in 10% of cases. Type 3 VWD, which is the only form that is inherited in an autosomal recessive pattern, accounts for an additional 10% of cases and causes the most severe bleeding manifestations. Correct determination of the specific subtype of VWD becomes important for counseling and therapy during pregnancy and delivery.[10,11]

Clinical Manifestations of VWD at Diagnosis

The clinical manifestations of VWD classically consist of mucocutaneaous hemorrhage, which contrasts with the deep-tissue hemorrhage associated with hemophilia A. Many cases, particularly of milder forms, remain undiagnosed until the pathways of coagulation are exposed to the stress of trauma, surgery, or administration of antiplatelet agents. Increasingly, menorrhagia has been identified as a sentinel symptom of an inherited coagulopathy in menstruating women.[12] Menorrhagia of long-standing duration, specifically from onset of menarche, recently has been shown to be a valuable predictor of a systemic bleeding disorder and may provide the first clue to milder forms of these disorders.[13] In one study, menorrhagia was defined objectively and was measured as a method of screening for bleeding disorders; 17% of women with this problem were subsequently diagnosed as having a coagulopathy. Conversely, almost 75% of women with a defined coagulopathy reported menorrhagia as a symptom.[12,13]

Changes in Factor Levels with Gestation

Among the original observations made by von Willebrand regarding the disease named for him was that obstetric patients with this disorder were at less risk of hemorrhage during pregnancy than at any other time. He also observed that these patients were at increased risk for postpartum bleeding episodes.[14] Type 1 VWD, which is a quantitative disorder that results from an absolute deficiency of VWF, typically has equivalently low plasma levels of all three aspects of the factor VIII complex: factor VIII coagulant activity (FVIII:C), VWF antigen (VWF:Ag), and VWF activity (VWF:Ac), usually in the range of 5 to 40 IU per deciliter. During pregnancy in type 1 patients, factor levels of VWF and factor VIII increase steadily, beginning in the second trimester, to levels that reach three to four times nonpregnant baseline levels by the time of delivery in most women. Levels may increase even further during active labor.[2] Immediately postpartum, levels begin to fall rapidly, and within several weeks, they reach prepregnancy status.

Type 2A VWD is a qualitative disorder caused by mutations in the VWF gene that result in a variable decrease in plasma VWF:Ag, a marked decrease in VWF:Ac measured as the VWF ristocetin cofactor (RcoF), and the absence of high and intermediate molecular weight VWF forms on gel electrophoresis.[15] The severity of the bleeding risk is proportionate with the level of vWF:RcoF.[16] VWF levels increase throughout pregnancy, but the abnormal multimers remain; thus, the benefit of this increase may not be as significant as for type 1 disease. Type 2B is further characterized by a mutation in the VWF gene that causes increased affinity for the platelet membrane glycoprotein Ib. Thrombocytopenia results from enhanced binding of platelets to VWF, and as VWF levels rise during pregnancy, thrombocytopenia may worsen.[17] Increased platelet aggregation, even in the setting of thrombocytopenia, may paradoxically predispose to thrombosis.

Type 3 VWD, the most severe and least common form, results from total absence of VWF:Ag and VWF:Ac caused by gross mutations of the VWF gene, with a resultant severe decrease (i.e., 2% to 5% of normal) in FVIII:C. Levels do not rise during pregnancy; therefore, pregnant women with this form of VWD remain at severe risk of hemorrhage throughout pregnancy, as well as during the postpartum period.

General experience suggests that low RcoF levels are the most important determinant of abnormal surgical or peripartum bleeding. Bleeding risk for most women with VWD appears to be greatest during the immediate postpartum or postabortion period, when factor VIII and VWF levels may drop precipitously.[3] Monitoring of factor levels should occur at least every 8 to 12 weeks, beginning at the confirmation of pregnancy and continuing for 6 to 8 weeks postpartum.[18] More frequent testing may be necessary during the puerperium. Factor levels of 50 IU per deciliter, which reflect the lower end of the normal range, generally are considered to be a safe threshold above which the risk of bleeding complications is not increased; they are the usual therapeutic goal for replacement therapy when such intervention is indicated.

First-trimester vaginal bleeding occurred in women with VWD at a rate of 33% in one study, which is twice the observed incidence of 16% in all pregnant women. However, the overall spontaneous miscarriage rate is the same (21%) in both groups, reflecting no evidence of increased pregnancy loss in this population. Increased documentation of even minor vaginal bleeding may reflect a reporting bias in women who have a heightened awareness of the significance of gestational bleeding in their circumstances. Furthermore, the incidence of antepartum hemorrhage was not increased in VWD.[5]

Therapy During Labor and Delivery

It is useful to recheck factor levels at 34 to 36 weeks gestation in preparation for delivery. At coagulation factor levels of 50 IU per deciliter and above, uncomplicated vaginal deliveries are unlikely to be associated with abnormal bleeding. If labor is prolonged, or if a cesarean section is planned or becomes necessary, factor levels should ideally exceed 50 IU per deciliter to minimize bleeding. A planned date of delivery by induction or by cesarean section may facilitate the timing of administration of factors. Many patients with type 1 VWD and some with type 2A do not require additional intervention prior to delivery because their factor levels have increased. Table 35-1 outlines therapies for various procedures that are performed during pregnancy or at parturition. Typically, factor concentrates such as Humate-P (ZLB Behring GmbH, Marburg, Germany), Alphanate (Grifols Biologicals, Inc., Los Angeles, Calif, USA), or

Table 35-1   Suggested Treatment During Pregnancy of Patients with Von Willebrand Disease

Type	1	2A	2B	3
Change expected with pregnancy	Usually normalize	May normalize	Von Willebrand factor rises, platelets fall	No change
Therapy for antenatal procedures (<50 IU per deciliter)	Humate-P, Alphanate, or Koate-DVI for 2–3 days	Humate-P, Alphanate, or Koate-DVI for 2–3 days	Humate-P, Alphanate, or Koate-DVI for 2–3 days	Humate-P, Alphanate, or Koate-DVI for 2–3 days
Vaginal delivery	No replacement if >50 IU per deciliter*	No replacement if >50 IU per deciliter*	Factor concentrate	Factor concentrate
Cesarean section	No replacement if >50 IU per deciliter*	No replacement if >50 IU per deciliter*	Factor concentrate for 7 days	Factor concentrate for 7 days
Postpartum	DDAVP/factor concentrate 3–4 days	DDAVP/factor concentrate 3–4 days	Factor concentrate for 3–4 days	Factor concentrate for 3–4 days

*If no factor replacement, monitor factor levels for 2 to 4 days after delivery.
Humate-P is manufactured by ZLB Behring GmbH, Marburg, Germany.
Alphanate is manufactured by Grifols Biologicals, Inc., Los Angeles, Calif, USA.
Koate-DVI is manufactured by Talecris Biotherapeutics, Inc., Research Triangle Park, NC, USA.

Koate-DVI (Talecris Biotherapeutics, Inc., Research Triangle Park, NC, USA),[19,20] which contain both factor VIII and VWF, are used to replace deficient factors in type 2B and type 3 VWD, as well as in those few patients with type 1 or 2A who do not reach acceptable factor levels. Parturient women with type 2B or type 3 VWD probably should receive factor replacement to a level greater than 50 IU per deciliter for at least 3 to 4 days to minimize hemorrhage. Specific dosing with clotting factor concentrates during pregnancy has not been established as distinct from other surgical prophylaxis in VWD. Data are available only from anecdotal reports and must be generalized from larger experience in the use of these clotting factor concentrates in surgery.[16] Dosing recommendations are made in terms of RcoF units, with the caution that only one of the currently available clotting factor concentrates that contain VWF (Humate-P) is labeled specifically with reference to RcoF units (see product insert, ZLB Behring). Delivery should be regarded as a moderate or severe challenge to hemostasis and should be treated by analogy as minor or major surgical episodes are treated. Thus, in major hemostatic challenge (e.g., cesarean section), a dose of 50 to 75 IU per kilogram VWF should be given, with subsequent dosing at 40 to 60 IU per kilogram every 8 to 12 hours for 3 days; the goal is to maintain the nadir level of RcoF at greater than 50 IU per deciliter.[16] Therapy can be changed to daily administration of 50 IU per kilogram for a total of up to 7 days of treatment. Again, it is difficult to establish clear norms for use of this intervention, in that very few to no data are available. It is widely assumed that cesarean section introduces the same stresses as a major surgical procedure, and episiotomy or a low-degree tear during delivery presents a minor surgical stress.

DDAVP in Pregnancy

Intravenous administration of 1-deamino-8-D-arginine vasopressin (DDAVP; desmopressin) increases FVIII:C and VWF concentrations by stimulating V-2 receptors. This elevation lasts for longer than 6 hours, and the biologic half-life is only marginally shorter than that of exogenous factor VIII and VWF from plasma concentrates.[21] DDAVP has also been shown to prevent bleeding in mild or moderate hemophilia or VWD. Some hematologists and obstetricians are reluctant to use it during pregnancy because of the risk of inducing uterine contractions and preterm labor. However, DDAVP is very specific to V-2 receptors and has little effect on smooth muscle V-1 receptors and consequently does not cause uterine contractions.[22] The other concern regarding antenatal use of DDAVP involves a possible decrease in blood flow from the placenta and subsequent intrauterine growth retardation; however, the vasopressor effect of DDAVP is weak.[22] Several publications have discussed the management of diabetes insipidus[23] and Ehlers-Danlos syndrome[24] in pregnant women with no harm to the fetus. Although the theoretical risk of uterine contraction may be a contraindication to use during pregnancy, this should not be a problem for a patient in labor. The use of DDAVP is indicated during the immediate postpartum period in type 1 and type 2A VWD, generally for a period of 3 to 4 days, to minimize the risk of postpartum hemorrhage, which has occurred in as many as 25% of parturients in some series.[25] When DDAVP is used during the postpartum period, hyponatremia has been reported; thus, serum sodium concentration should be monitored during DDAVP therapy. The use of hypotonic intravenous fluids should be minimized, and oral fluids should be somewhat restricted. Women who present with spontaneous miscarriage or elective termination are also at increased risk for hemorrhage and should empirically receive DDAVP therapy (if type 1 or 2A) or clotting factor concentrate for several days after the event. Women who exhibit evidence of bleeding despite DDAVP therapy should also receive a factor concentrate such as Humate-P.

Therapy During Prenatal Diagnostic Testing and for Anesthesia

Prenatal diagnosis of the fetus usually occurs within the first trimester of pregnancy, either by chorionic villous sampling or by amniocentesis. It is therefore possible, but less likely than would be the case later in pregnancy, that the coagulation factors involved will have increased to a safe range for invasive procedures. Measurement of maternal FVIII:C should be performed within 1 week of the procedure, and adequate therapy administered for factor VIII levels significantly below 50 IU per deciliter. Because this procedure represents a minor hemostatic challenge, correction should continue for 48 to 72 hours after it is

35

completed. Clotting factor concentrates may be used; in this instance, too, researchers disagree about the role of DDAVP. Anecdotes describe its use, and the literature provides no evidence of a specific contraindication in early pregnancy. It is our practice to have a comprehensive discussion with the patient about the risks and benefits of each of the approaches, and to individualize therapy.

The use of regional anesthesia must be considered for each woman because recommendations remain controversial. In one series, patients with type 1 or 2A VWD underwent epidural catheter placement when factor VIII levels measured 50 IU per deciliter or higher without untoward consequences.[26] Some centers recommend that bleeding time should also be checked, and they specify that if it is less than 15 minutes, the risk for hemorrhagic complications is not increased.

Hemophilias

Hemophilia A (factor VIII deficiency) and hemophilia B (factor IX deficiency) are both inherited in an X-linked recessive pattern. Women from hemophilia-affected families are most commonly asymptomatic carriers. However, 10% to 20% of female carriers may be at risk for significant bleeding complications caused by extreme lyonization and subsequent reduction of factor VIII or IX to levels below the minimal amount needed to maintain hemostatic equilibrium. Because only one chromosome is affected, hemophilia carriers would be expected on average to have factor levels that are 50% of normal, with normal defined as ranging from 50 to 150 IU per deciliter. However, levels as low as 5% have been reported to occur as a result of lyonization—the random inactivation of one of each pair of X chromosomes.[27] Factor levels below 30 IU per deciliter may lead to clinical bleeding analogous to that seen in mild hemophilia A.[28]

Two unusual conditions may result in factor VIII levels low enough to cause concern during pregnancy. The first, VWD type 2N (Normandy), consists of distinct missense mutations that inactivate the binding site of factor VIII on VWF. Platelet function and multimer patterns are normal, but FVIII:C levels are low—frequently less than 10%—which causes patients' laboratory results to resemble those of patients with mild hemophilia A. Because of the qualitative defect in the VWF protein, these patients have short-lived factor VIII response to DDAVP or to highly purified or recombinant factor VIII products. The agent of choice during pregnancy is a plasma-derived VWF product such as Humate-P, which contains normal VWF along with factor VIII.[29,30]

In the second condition, Turner syndrome (gonadal dysgenesis), the 45,X karyotype seen in 50% of cases produces streak gonads and infertility. However, 25% of affected individuals have (46,XX/45,X) mosaicism, and 25% have a (46,XX) structurally abnormal X chromosome.[31] A small number of these women have sufficient follicles to become pregnant, and if they are from hemophilia A–affected families, patients may exhibit severe factor deficiencies that must be managed appropriately during pregnancy.

The literature is limited regarding changes in clotting factors during pregnancy in patients with bleeding disorders. However, a significant rise in FVIII:C, vWF:Ag, and VWF:Ac has been reported in normal women, in carriers of hemophilia A, and, as previously discussed, in patients with VWD of various subtypes. These increases generally begin during the late first trimester, and gradually, levels continue to increase until the end of pregnancy. It is therefore extremely rare for women, even those who have low factor VIII levels at baseline as a consequence of extreme lyonization, to require treatment during late pregnancy or at parturition. However, prophylaxis for bleeding must be considered at the time of prenatal diagnostic testing; carriers with low factor VIII levels (whose levels may still be lower than 50 IU per deciliter at term) are at considerable risk of bleeding and require prophylactic treatment. In contrast to factor VIII and VWF, factor IX levels do not increase throughout pregnancy, although controversial results have been published regarding changes in this plasma protein. Hemostatic challenges of pregnancy, such as invasive prenatal diagnostic techniques, termination of pregnancy, spontaneous abortion, normal spontaneous vaginal delivery, and delivery by cesarean section, are all complicated by excessive and prolonged hemorrhage. Therefore, it is important that factor levels are checked before any of these procedures are undertaken, and that prophylactic treatment is arranged when factor levels are lower than 50 IU per deciliter for factors VIII and IX.[32] Because it may not be possible to measure factor levels in emergency situations, we recommend that these should be assayed at regular intervals during gestation—at least once per trimester. Usually, carriers of hemophilia A normalize factor VIII levels during pregnancy to well above 50 IU per deciliter and thus do not require therapeutic intervention. However, women who are carriers of factor IX deficiency often require prophylactic treatment with clotting factor concentrate because levels do not significantly change during pregnancy.

For women who are carriers of hemophilia A, DDAVP may be considered as an appropriate pharmacologic intervention to increase the level of factor VIII to above 50 IU per deciliter. Provisions regarding the use of this agent were outlined in the section on treatment of VWD during pregnancy and are not repeated here. If response to DDAVP is inadequate, or if the physician or the patient is uncomfortable about the use of DDAVP after the risks and benefits of this therapeutic approach have been comprehensively discussed, then treatment with recombinant factor VIII concentrates should be considered in the context of prophylaxis of excessive bleeding during invasive procedures or at the time of delivery (Table 35-2). Again, interventions at the time of prenatal diagnostic testing generally involve minor surgical procedures that require 3 days of therapy at levels that allow the attainment of a nadir of 50 IU per deciliter. Calculations of the dose to be administered are based on the baseline clotting factor available and the desired goals of therapy. Women who are carriers of hemophilia B are at increased risk of bleeding when diagnostic interventions are provided during pregnancy or at the time of labor and delivery. If the patient requires correction of the baseline concentration of factor IX, the use of recombinant factor IX concentrates is indicated (see Table 35-2). The goal is to maintain a nadir of 50 IU per deciliter or higher. Most diagnostic interventions are viewed as minor surgical procedures; cesarean section is considered a major surgical procedure.

Table 35-2 Suggested Factor Replacement for Selected Inherited Bleeding Disorders

	Prenatal Procedure/Labor and Delivery	Postpartum Care
Hemophilia A carrier	Factor >50 IU per deciliter: No therapy	No therapy
	Factor <50 IU per deciliter: DDAVP or rFVIII × 3 days	DDAVP or factor VIII concentrate for 3–4 days
Hemophilia B carrier	Factor >50 IU per deciliter: No therapy	No therapy
	Factor <50 IU per deciliter: rFIX concentrate × 3 days	rFIX concentrate 3–4 days
Factor VII deficiency	rFVIIa 15–30 mg per kilogram every 6 hours × 3 days	rFVIIa 15–30 mg per kilogram every 6 hours × 3 days
Factor XI deficiency	Factor XI concentrate to goal 40 IU per deciliter × 1 dose (10–15 mL per kilogram) or FFP	Factor XI concentrate every 48 hours × 3–5 days (10–15 mL per kilogram) or FFP
Factor XIII deficiency	Treatment throughout pregnancy with cryoprecipitate or factor XIII concentrate	3–4 days of cryoprecipitate or factor XIII concentrate

DDAVP, 1-deamino-8-D-arginine vasopressin; FFP, fresh frozen plasma; rFVIIa, recombinant factor VIIa; rFVIII, recombinant factor VIII; rFIX, recombinant factor IX.

Factor XI Deficiency

Factor XI deficiency is a genetic disorder that is prevalent among Ashkenazi Jews, with a heterozygous frequency of 8%.[33] Its frequency in non-Jews is unknown. The inheritance pattern is autosomal; severe deficiency occurs in homozygotes, and partial deficiency has been noted in heterozygotes. Normal plasma levels are 70 to 150 IU per deciliter. Homozygotes typically have factor levels below 15 IU per deciliter, and the range for heterozygotes is 15 IU per deciliter to the lower level of normal.[34] In contrast to those with VWD and hemophilia, factor XI–deficient patients do not have spontaneous pathologic bleeding but may experience significant hemorrhage after a hemostatic challenge. Menstruation may represent the first such challenge for women of childbearing age. A poor correlation between factor XI level and bleeding tendency has been noted,[34–36] and homozygotes with undetectable levels may have never experienced hemorrhage, even with surgery, trauma, or previous pregnancies. Such patients are usually discovered during family studies or through evaluation of a prolonged PTT. Additionally, the tendency to bleed after hemostatic challenge may vary over time in individuals with this deficiency. The presence of additional coagulation defects, the most common of which is VWD, in a factor XI–deficient patient can further influence bleeding risk.

Factor XI Deficiency in Pregnancy

Changes in plasma factor XI levels during pregnancy in factor XI–deficient women have not been studied extensively. Results in normal women have been conflicting, with some studies showing an increase[6] and others a fall in levels during pregnancy.[7,37] A single available study in which investigators studied factor XI–deficient women showed inconsistent changes during the second and third trimesters of pregnancy. Four women showed some increase and four exhibited a slight decrease from baseline in factor XI levels.[38] Prospective studies of changes in factor XI levels during pregnancy and the postpartum period are needed.

Therapy During Pregnancy

Conventional treatment for patients with factor XI deficiency includes the use of fresh frozen plasma. This therapy is potentially problematic in terms of the usual risks of transmission of infectious agents and volume challenge, the latter of which is partially balanced by the long half-life of infused factor XI (50 hours). Factor XI concentrate, currently in development but not available in the United States, permits correction of isolated factor deficiency with little risk of viral exposure.[39] Several case reports of factor XI–related thrombosis have been reported. This complication occurred only in a population with known preexisting thrombotic or vascular disease.[36,40] Although potential risk is due to the hypercoagulable state induced by pregnancy, no thrombotic complications have been reported in pregnant women who are deficient in factor XI. If factor XI replacement is prescribed, the goal of therapy should be to attain a factor level of approximately 40 IU per deciliter[38] to minimize bleeding; this should be sustained for a period of 3 to 4 days after a vaginal delivery and 4 to 5 days after a cesarean section (see Table 35-2). It is important that factor levels be maintained at levels as close as possible to the target level of 40 IU per deciliter, and that levels in excess of 100 IU per deciliter are avoided because levels this high theoretically may enhance thrombotic risk. The dose should not exceed 30 IU per kilogram.[39] When a woman has risk factors for a hypercoagulable state besides pregnancy (e.g., obesity, increased age, vascular disease), fresh frozen plasma should be used. In patients with no prior hemorrhagic history, regardless of factor XI level (even to 0% to 3%), it is reasonable to refrain from infusing any fresh frozen plasma or factor XI concentrate but to be prepared to do so should hemorrhage occur.

Preconception Counseling

Once the factor XI level has been discerned in a patient who is suspected of having factor XI deficiency, the probability of heterozygosity may be considered, and pedigree analysis should be performed to assess prior probability with the use of an available chart.[34] Prior to conception, patients from factor XI–deficient families may receive genetic counseling on the risks of vertical transmission of severe deficiency. Factor XI–deficient patients who are attempting to conceive should be counseled properly in advance about the risks of pregnancy and delivery, and they should be informed of the usefulness of hepatitis B vaccination should blood products become necessary. If pregnancy occurs prior to immunization, the vaccine can be given safely during pregnancy. Once a factor XI–deficient woman has become pregnant, the potential risks and benefits of prenatal testing must be addressed. Invasive procedures during pregnancy may be desirable for individual patients, but these must be evaluated on an individual patient basis because of the potential for significant accidental maternal, fetal, or placental bleeding.

Rare Inherited Bleeding Disorders

Rare inherited bleeding disorders include several other hereditary disorders of blood coagulation that may be associated with excessive bleeding in pregnancy. These include deficiencies in prothrombin, fibrinogen, and factors V, VII, X, and XIII (see Chapter 5). These disorders occur at a frequency of 1 to 2 per million persons and usually become manifest during childhood.[41] Because of the rarity of these conditions, experience in the specific management of obstetric problems in women with these bleeding disorders is very limited. Factor XIII–deficient women routinely spontaneously miscarry if they are not treated throughout pregnancy; thus, factor XIII seems necessary for successful and durable implantation of the fertilized ovum in the uterus. In addition, hereditary afibrinogenemia and hypofibrinogenemia (especially if the level is below 50 mg per deciliter), if untreated, also have been reported to be associated with recurrent pregnancy loss. Therapy for patients with rare inherited bleeding disorders is based on knowledge of the half-life and volume of distribution of the factor in question, as well as on the replacement therapy that is currently available. Factor VII–deficient patients may now be treated with recombinant factor VIIa. Dosing at 15 to 30 μg per kilogram given every 6 hours should be used during the peripartum and postpartum periods in those women with a significant bleeding history. Factor V–deficient patients, factor X–deficient patients, prothrombin-deficient patients, and those with factor XIII deficiency may be treated with fresh frozen plasma.[41] Cryoprecipitate is useful for the treatment of patients with hypofibrinogenemia, dysfibrinogenemia, or factor XIII deficiency; factor XIII concentrates, when available, may be used prophylactically throughout pregnancy and at the time of delivery (see Table 35-2).[42] Again, in none of these cases are specific recommendations available for the prophylaxis of bleeding during pregnancy and delivery. Therapeutic recommendations are based entirely on experience with the generic treatment of patients with these disorders during surgery and other bleeding episodes.

Preconception Counseling

Women from families with known inherited bleeding disorders should be assessed whenever possible prior to pregnancy to ascertain carrier status for the particular disease in question. The purpose of early identification is severalfold. First, the degree to which a woman is affected by a bleeding disorder is a major factor in decisions regarding the safety of conceiving and carrying a pregnancy to term, as well as in the development of appropriate and realistic expectations. Management of the disorder during pregnancy may require serial monitoring of factor levels, with baseline

levels attained prior to conception. Immunization against hepatitis A and B should be undertaken in patients who may require blood product transfusion during pregnancy or delivery. In certain disorders (e.g., VWD), it may be appropriate to treat patients and monitor response of plasma levels prior to pregnancy, to confirm the efficacy of therapy. Genetic counseling should be offered to all affected women and carrier women from affected families so that they may be given adequate information regarding inheritance to make decisions regarding pregnancy and prenatal diagnosis.

THROMBOCYTOPENIA

Normal platelet counts in nonpregnant women range from 150,000 to 300,000/μL. Relative thrombocytopenia is a normal physiologic response to pregnancy, and mean platelet count has been found to decrease successively at each trimester of normal, uncomplicated pregnancies. Maternal plasma volume expansion with increasing gestational age is believed to be the principal factor that causes a decrease in platelet count. In one study of healthy gravidas, mean platelet counts for successive trimesters were 322,000 ± 75,000, 298,000 ± 55,000, and 278,000 ± 75,000/μL.[43] Although mild relative thrombocytopenia is common and even expected in pregnancy, bleeding is rare with platelet counts above 50,000 to 75,000/μL, unless a qualitative platelet defect is also present. Generally, platelet counts below 100,000/μL should prompt a hematologic evaluation that is undertaken to exclude reversible or potentially life-threatening causes of thrombocytopenia.[43–45] Events and platelet counts of prior pregnancies very accurately predict the course of future pregnancies.

The most frequent cause of thrombocytopenia that occurs during pregnancy is incidental thrombocytopenia of pregnancy, also referred to as gestational thrombocytopenia. In one large series of pregnant women, 74% of patients with thrombocytopenia had incidental thrombocytopenia; the second most common cause was hypertensive disorders of pregnancy (in 21%). An immune disorder such as ITP or SLE was implicated in less than 5% of thrombocytopenic gravidas, and in less than 2%, DIC, thrombotic thrombocytopenic purpura (TTP), HELLP syndrome, or other related syndromes were found to be the cause of thrombocytopenia.[46]

Incidental thrombocytopenia of pregnancy was first described in 1988, when pregnant women considered to have ITP were distinguished from typical patients with ITP on the basis of their clinical course and that of their infants. In women for whom prepregnancy data were available, platelet counts were in the normal range. When platelet counts in these women were followed during the puerperium, counts returned to normal within 6 weeks of delivery,[47] consistent with normalization of plasma volume and other hemostatic factors that had been altered during pregnancy. The mechanism for decreased platelet count after pregnancy remains unknown, but it has been reported that mean platelet volumes are higher than in pregnant women with platelet counts in the normal range—a fact that suggests a nonimmunologic destructive process.[48]

Incidental thrombocytopenia of pregnancy typically is mild, with platelet counts usually ranging from 100,000 to 150,000/μL; counts as low as 70,000/μL are less commonly seen. The diagnosis is considered after a prior history of bleeding or known thrombocytopenia has been excluded, and in the absence of other hemostatic or systemic abnormalities that may alter platelet count. Laboratory studies that may be helpful include liver function tests, coagulation tests, and human immunodeficiency virus (HIV) testing. A recent normal platelet count that was obtained prior to conception or a mild thrombocytopenia that occurred during a prior pregnancy but resolved spontaneously in the postpartum period may be very useful in ascertaining the diagnosis of incidental thrombocytopenia. The definition of incidental thrombocytopenia that has been established is a platelet count of 70,000 to 150,000/μL in an otherwise healthy gravida.[47] It is recognized that platelet counts lower than 70,000/μL may represent incidental thrombocytopenia, and that patients with mild ITP may have platelet counts in the 70,000 to 100,000/μL range. The implications of confusion in the diagnosis of these two disorders are generally not clinically significant, in that obstetric management of the patient with mild ITP or gestational thrombocytopenia remains the same as that provided for a hematologically normal patient. Epidural anesthesia is not contraindicated for patients with platelet counts above 70,000/μL, and for these women, no benefit is derived from choosing cesarean section over vaginal delivery. Transfusion of platelets, likewise, is not indicated in the absence of overt bleeding.

The hypertensive disorders of pregnancy, which are the second most common cause of a low platelet count during pregnancy, are discussed in greater detail elsewhere in this chapter. Serial measurements of blood pressure (as well as tests of liver function and coagulation) should be attained at the time of diagnosis of thrombocytopenia, as well as at suitable intervals during the remainder of the pregnancy (determined by clinical course and the presence of continued platelet decline).

As with nonpregnant individuals, causes of thrombocytopenia in the gravida may be categorized as problems of decreased production, increased destruction, or sequestration. Initial evaluation of thrombocytopenia must include a review of the peripheral smear. The laboratory platelet count should be confirmed manually, and platelet and red blood cell morphology should be evaluated for clues to the cause of the thrombocytopenia. Pseudothrombocytopenia is a laboratory artefact that results from platelet clumping of normal platelets at the time of collection; it is of no clinical significance, except for the confusion and inappropriate treatment it may produce (see Chapters 9 and 10). The presence of megathrombocytes in the peripheral smear suggests compensation of the bone marrow for a state of increased peripheral removal of platelets. If the process is one of immune-mediated platelet removal, the red blood cell morphology is typically normal. Evidence of erythrocyte trauma in combination with decreased platelet counts may be indicative of a microangiopathic process, such as DIC, HELLP, or ITP. The presence of teardrop or nucleated red blood cells on the smear suggests a problem with primary bone marrow production. Leukocytes may also provide information on the cause of thrombocytopenia, suggesting a nutritional deficiency or a malignant process.

Initial corroborative laboratory studies that should be obtained in all pregnant women with confirmed thrombocytopenia include blood coagulation studies to evaluate for the presence of DIC. PT, PTT, fibrinogen, and fibrin split product (FSP) levels provide information that may help the clinician to rule out DIC. Liver function studies aid in the evaluation of the HELLP syndrome, which is discussed later in this chapter. Other laboratory evaluations that should be performed depend on the clinical history and may include tests for collagen vascular disease, including SLE and rheumatoid arthritis (RA), as well as testing for HIV infection.

A careful drug history may exclude possible toxic exposures. The possible offending agent should be discontinued and the platelet count monitored for recovery.

IMMUNE THROMBOCYTOPENIC PURPURA

Diagnosis

Immune thrombocytopenic purpura (ITP) is a relatively uncommon cause of thrombocytopenia in pregnancy; it occurs in less than 4% of thrombocytopenic gravidas, or in 1 to 2 per 1000 live births overall (see Chapter 9).[46] ITP is typically a chronic condition in adults. A long clinical history of easy bruising suggestive of a mild hemostatic impairment already may have led to the discovery of a mild thrombocytopenia that was diagnosed as ITP prior to pregnancy. Routine complete blood cell counts attained early in pregnancy identify most cases of ITP that were undiagnosed prior to pregnancy. The finding of a moderate asymptomatic thrombocytopenia as low as 50,000 to 70,000/μL in the absence of a hypertensive disorder of pregnancy during the first trimester is most likely to represent chronic ITP.[47] ITP is three times more prevalent in women than men, and it typically affects women during the second and third decades of life. Because ITP is a condition of young women, it is not an uncommon diagnosis during pregnancy. Practice guidelines recently set forth by the American Society of Hematology on the management of ITP include specific recommendations for the care of pregnant women and their newborn infants.[48] No reliable basis has been established for distinguishing ITP from incidental thrombocytopenia of pregnancy. The diagnosis is made on the basis of a review of clinical data for each patient. A history of thrombocytopenia or bleeding consistent with ITP (petechiae or epistaxis) prior to conception suggests the diagnosis of ITP. Platelet counts lower than 50,000/μL also are commonly found to be the result of ITP. Current recommendations of confirmatory testing include measurement of blood pressure and urinary protein to rule out preeclampsia, performance of liver function tests to exclude HELLP, and HIV testing. As in the case of nonpregnant women, the diagnosis of ITP rests on the exclusion of other systemic disorders as the cause of low platelets, the presence of normal white and red blood cell indices, the absence of splenomegaly, and the absence of toxic or drug exposures. Antiplatelet antibody testing is not routinely recommended because the assay has high rates of false-positive and false-negative results.

Management During Pregnancy

Management of ITP during pregnancy is distinguished from that provided to nonpregnant women in several ways.[48] First, attention must be paid to the potential adverse effects of standard ITP treatments on fetal development and on the course of pregnancy. Second, the incidence of thrombocytopenia is increased in newborns of mothers with documented ITP, which may affect obstetric management. The most commonly used initial therapy in nonpregnant individuals with a diagnosis of ITP is glucocorticoid administration, which is nonteratogenic to fetuses but may induce or exacerbate gestational diabetes mellitus and postpartum psychiatric disorders. Intravenous immunoglobulin (IVIg) is considered safe for the fetus but may cause maternal adverse effects. The use of immunosuppressive or cytotoxic agents, including cyclophosphamide, the vinca alkaloids, and azathioprine, is relatively contraindicated because effects on the fetus are unpredictable. As with any intra-abdominal surgical procedure, the use of splenectomy in refractory cases of ITP has been reported to increase preterm labor and loss of pregnancy during the first trimester; this procedure may be technically difficult to perform during the third trimester because of the size of the uterus. Last, adequate hemostasis is required at the time of delivery to reduce the risk of maternal postpartum bleeding complications.

Timing of Intervention

Gravidas with the diagnosis of ITP (confirmed as chronic or presumed to be a first presentation, given the timing of detection during the pregnancy and the absence of other causes) with platelet counts greater than 50,000/μL at any time during pregnancy and those with platelet counts of 30,000 to 50,000/μL during the first two trimesters and no evidence of bleeding should be observed. For women with platelet counts lower than 10,000/μL at any time during pregnancy, or with counts of 10,000 to 30,000/μL during the latter two trimesters, or with bleeding, intervention should be undertaken. The goal of therapy for the gravida with ITP is to maintain a safe (as distinct from normal) platelet count, particularly with regard to labor and delivery.

In gravidas who require treatment for thrombocytopenia, prednisone given at a dose of 1 mg/kg/day is the first choice of therapy when platelet counts are between 10,000 and 30,000/μL. The platelet count should rise to greater than 50,000/μL within approximately 1 week of initiation of therapy. The dose should then be tapered slowly to the minimum effective dose required to maintain platelet count in an acceptable range. Too rapid lowering of the steroid dose often results in recurrence of the thrombocytopenia. Women with severe thrombocytopenia (<10,000/μL) should receive IVIg as initial treatment, at a dose of 0.4 g/kg/day for 5 days or 1 g per kilogram daily for 2 days, and platelet transfusions should be administered if significant bleeding is present. IVIg often requires repeat administration every 2 to 4 weeks to maintain platelet count at an acceptable level, particularly near term. IVIg is also appropriate second-line treatment for women in whom glucocorticoid therapy has been unsuccessful. Splenectomy is rarely undertaken in gravidas because of the increased risks of surgery for both mother and fetus as compared with a nonpregnant individual. Current recommendations for the use of surgical intervention are the presence of ITP that is refractory to steroids and to IVIg, with platelet counts determined to be 10,000/μL in the second trimester and the occurrence of overt bleeding. When possible, pneumococcal vaccine should be administered 2 weeks prior to splenectomy.

Because of increased maternal and fetal risks associated with surgery, medical management recommendations for ITP in the pregnant woman differ from those for nongravidas in terms of the lower threshold required for the use of IVIg in pregnancy and the less frequent use of splenectomy.

Impact of Maternal Immune Thrombocytopenic Purpura on Fetal Platelet Count

Autoantibodies produced in ITP are of the immunoglobulin (Ig)G class; therefore, they readily cross the placenta. The manifestation of this phenomenon is variable in terms of fetal platelet count. The severity of maternal thrombocytopenia does not correlate with that of thrombocytopenia in the fetus[49,50]; moreover, the pharmacologic interventions used to raise maternal platelet count may not necessarily result in an elevated fetal platelet count.[51,52] Refractory severe maternal thrombocytopenia despite splenectomy and a previous history of delivery of a thrombocytopenic infant are predictors for neonatal thrombocytopenia in the current pregnancy.[53]

Currently, two methods are available by which fetal platelet counts can be determined (in utero), and both are problematic. Fetal scalp sampling, which involves removal of blood via a heparinized capillary tube from a small scalp laceration, requires that the woman must be in active labor and must have ruptured membranes and a dilated cervix. The fetal head must be engaged in the pelvis to allow access to the scalp. Platelet counts attained in this fashion may be grossly inaccurate because of contamination with amniotic fluid or maternal blood, or because of platelet clumping. Additionally, scalp hematoma may occur. A platelet count above 50,000/μL that is attained in this fashion is reassuring for a vaginal delivery. The second method, cordocentesis, or percutaneous umbilical blood sampling (PUBS), provides a more accurate platelet count but requires experience with the technique to minimize the potential risks to the fetus of postpuncture bleeding; this is usually self limited but may necessitate emergency cesarean section or may result in fetal death (in 1% of cases)—a figure similar to the fetal death rate without PUBS testing.[54] Risks to the fetus appear to be least problematic after 35 weeks gestation.[49] For women at term who have maintained a platelet count above 50,000/μL, cordocentesis may guide the decision to permit a vaginal delivery by ensuring that the fetal count is also adequate for that method of delivery. Infants born to mothers with ITP may experience further decline in platelet count during the first postpartum week.[49] If thrombocytopenia is severe, IVIg is recommended, along with the provision of platelet transfusional support with evidence of active bleeding.

ALLOIMMUNE THROMBOCYTOPENIA

Alloimmune thrombocytopenia (AIT) is a clinical entity that is distinct from ITP in that maternal platelet counts are usually normal or only mildly decreased, yet the fetus may experience a severe, life-threatening thrombocytopenia.[55] It results from maternal sensitization to fetal platelet antigens and may be considered the platelet equivalent to red blood cell Rh sensitization and hemolytic disease of the fetus and neonate. Fetal platelets apparently cross the placental barrier and are recognized as foreign by the maternal immune system. IgG antiplatelet antibodies are directed against platelet-specific antigens inherited from the father but absent from the mother's platelets. The incidence of this is approximately 1 in 1000 fetuses.[55] The abnormality that most frequently causes this disorder is an incompatibility in the polymorphism affecting the PLA (HPA-1) antigen encoded on the gene for platelet glycoprotein IIIa. Alloantibodies from a sensitized PLA1-negative mother cross the placenta and cause immune-mediated thrombocytopenia in a PLA1-positive fetus. The PLA antigen polymorphism also reportedly causes the most severe form of alloimmune thrombocytopenia.[56] The diagnosis is usually first made after the birth of a child with unexpected severe thrombocytopenia.

The chief complication of AIT is intracranial hemorrhage (ICH), which occurs in 10% to 20% of such severely affected neonates; 25% to 50% of cases occur in utero.[56] In contrast to Rh sensitization of red blood cells, AIT may occur during a first pregnancy. Efforts to screen mothers at risk to deliver affected infants are complicated by the fact that only 1 in 20 PLA1-negative mothers with antigen-incompatible partners ever become sensitized, despite repeated pregnancies. Thus, the incidence is not well predicted on the basis of antigen screening tests. However, once an affected fetus or neonate has been identified, the maternal risk of subsequent affected pregnancies ranges from 50% to 100%, dependent on the homozygosity or heterozygosity of the father for the allele, even with different mates. It is suggested that in cases of paternal heterozygosity for the PLA1 allele, amniocentesis should be performed at 15 to 18 weeks to allow platelet–antigen genotyping of the fetus. If the incompatible antigen is not present, fetal platelet count will be unaffected, and normal delivery may occur without further intervention. If the antigen is present, then PUBS at 20 to 24 weeks should be undertaken, with transfusion of maternal platelets provided to minimize risk to the fetus of hemorrhage during this procedure. If the fetus is found to be thrombocytopenic with a platelet count lower than 100,000/μL, maternal treatment with IVIg at a dose of 1 g/kg/wk should be instituted immediately and continued for the duration of the pregnancy; an increase or lack of further decrease in the fetal platelet count has been documented in 62% to 85% of affected fetuses when this therapy was provided.

Addition of low-dose steroid therapy has not been proved to increase response rates over those seen with IVIg alone. Repeat PUBS should be undertaken 3 to 6 weeks after therapy is begun, to document improvement in the platelet count. If the counts remain low, high-dose prednisone (60 mg/day) added to weekly IVIg will result in a rise in the platelet count in approximately half of remaining cases.[57] PUBS should again be performed in 3 to 6 weeks so that the platelet count can be determined. If the count remains below 50,000/μL, cesarean section should be performed. Delivery prior to 34 weeks for severe thrombocytopenia (<20,000/μL) is of questionable usefulness in that prematurity alone may also lead to ICH.

THE HELLP SYNDROME

The HELLP syndrome was first described in 1954 by Pritchard and coworkers, and it was given the acronym in 1982 by Weinstein on the basis of the three cardinal manifestations of the syndrome.[58] The "H" stands for *H*emolysis, the "EL" for *E*levated *L*iver enzymes, and the "LP" for *L*ow *P*latelets. It is considered in conjunction with disorders of preeclampsia and eclampsia to constitute a spectrum of heterogeneous hypertensive disorders that may occur during the latter half of pregnancy, and it is one of the leading causes of maternal morbidity and mortality in the Western world. The diagnosis of the HELLP syndrome is based on hematologic and serum chemistry abnormalities, but variation among centers regarding criteria that establish the diagnosis is ongoing. The University of Tennessee uses strict laboratory criteria, which include an abnormal peripheral smear with evidence of microangiopathic hemolytic anemia, total bilirubin above 1.2 mg per deciliter, lactate dehydrogenase (LDH) above 600 IU per liter, aspartate aminotransferase (AST) above 70 IU per liter, and platelet count below 100,000/μL.[59] A recent study of uncomplicated singleton pregnancies followed to delivery found that a small number of gravidas experienced an asymptomatic gradual decline in the platelet count to less than 150,000/μL. These women were more than seven times as likely to develop AST elevation as were those without thrombocytopenia; this suggests that the fall in platelets precedes the elevation in liver enzyme test results.[60]

The earliest clinical signs and symptoms of this disorder are protean; thus, it may be mistaken for other conditions, ranging from the benign to the life-threatening. This diagnosis may often be delayed if symptoms, including shoulder, neck, and upper body pain, malaise, nausea, vomiting, and headache, are attributed to a viral syndrome, gastritis, or a musculoskeletal problem. The disorder, in its more severe presentation, may be difficult to distinguish from other severe hepatic or hematologic syndromes seen in pregnancy. Severe preeclampsia, hemolytic-uremic syndrome (HUS), TTP, SLE, and acute fatty liver of pregnancy all may produce clinical manifestations and laboratory studies similar to those seen with the HELLP syndrome. Target organs in all the diseases listed here include the kidneys, the liver, and the vascular endothelium. Because it is possible for two syndromes to occur in the same individual, the diagnosis can be extremely difficult to confirm. Subtle differences between these conditions can be used to guide diagnosis of the correct clinical entity; correct diagnosis is essential because management of the condition during pregnancy may be significantly different for each disorder.

Table 35-3 Differentiation of HELLP from Similar Diseases*

	Platelets	PT/PTT	LDH	Bilirubin	Glucose	SBP	Proteinuria
HELLP	↓↓	N	↑↑↑	N	N	N/↑	↑
AFLP	↓	↑↑	N/↑	↑↑↑	↓	N	N
Preeclampsia	N	N	N	N	N	↑↑	↑↑
TTP	↓↓	N	↑↑	N	N	N	↑
HUS	N	N	↑	N	N	↑	↑↑

*Early in disease course.
AFLP, acute fatty liver of pregnancy; HELLP, *H*emolysis, *E*levated *L*iver Tests, *L*ow *P*latelets; HUS, hemolytic-uremic syndrome; LDH, lactate dehydrogenase; N, normal or no change; PT, prothrombin time; PTT, partial thromboplastin time; SBP, systemic blood pressure; TTP, thrombotic thrombocytopenic purpura. ↑, implies mild change, ↑↑, moderate change, ↑↑↑, severe change.

Several key characteristics have been identified for each of these disorders that may be useful in differentiation of the various syndromes. These features are presented in Table 35-3.[61] Thrombocytopenia is the earliest and most common hemostatic abnormality associated with the HELLP syndrome; it is seen in all gravidas with this diagnosis. Abnormalities of the coagulation cascade, manifested by elevated PT and PTT and decreased fibrinogen, and derangement of liver enzymes do not occur until very late in the course. LDH is frequently elevated much earlier than any liver abnormalities become apparent, suggesting that the initial source of the problem is hemolyzed red cells. In contrast, acute fatty liver of pregnancy typically displays high serum bilirubin concentrations, prolongation of PT and PTT, hypoglycemia, and only modestly diminished platelet counts. Both TTP and HUS can imitate HELLP in many of its clinical features. All three syndromes share microangiopathic hemolytic anemia, thrombocytopenia, proteinuria, increased serum LDH, and renal compromise. However, TTP typically does not cause marked derangement of hepatic function as manifested by elevations in AST and alanine aminotransferase (ALT). In HELLP, the degree of renal dysfunction is usually correlated with the level of hepatic impairment, whereas in HUS, renal failure is elevated to an extent that is out of proportion to the liver enzyme levels. Both TTP and HUS are managed through plasma exchange.

Preeclampsia is a well-defined clinical triad of hypertension, proteinuria, and nondependent edema; it can be mild or severe. The criteria for mild and severe disease have recently been established by the American College of Obstetrics and Gynecology.[61] The presence of grand mal seizures is classified as eclampsia, which is a life-threatening condition that is associated with a high risk of maternal and fetal mortality. The most efficacious treatment is prevention in a woman with identified preeclampsia. Immediate delivery of the fetus is mandatory once the syndrome has progressed to eclampsia. Measures that may be used to mitigate the sequelae of preeclampsia include control of blood pressure with intravenous hydralazine at doses of 5 to 10 mg given every 30 minutes, or labetalol, or less commonly, sodium nitroprusside, because of concern for fetal cyanide toxicity at doses above 10 μg/kg/min.[61] Seizure prophylaxis should be initiated in patients with preeclampsia who are in active labor and in patients with HELLP who are in labor, or at any time that epigastric pain is present. Intravenous magnesium sulfate administered as a bolus and then by continuous infusion is the treatment of choice; toxicity is monitored with the use of patellar reflexes and serum magnesium levels. Infusion may need to continue into the postpartum period until evidence indicates that the hypertensive disorder has been resolved.[61]

Once the diagnosis of the HELLP syndrome has been considered, some centers find it useful to further classify the disorder by severity to assist in prognosis and management during the peripartum period. A three-class system, based on maternal platelet count nadir, was devised. Class 1 is a platelet count below 50,000/μL, class 2 includes platelet counts between 50,000 and 100,000/μL, and class 3 consists of platelet counts above 100,000 but less than 150,000/μL. Regardless of the course during pregnancy and the immediate peripartum period, HELLP syndrome may further worsen during the postpartum period, resulting in pathologic thrombosis. Prophylactic administration of heparin is probably reasonable at this time in most cases of HELLP syndrome; no articles have documented the use of low molecular weight heparin in this clinical situation.

REFERENCES

1. Bennett B, Oxnard SC, Douglas AS, et al: Studies on antihemophilic factor (AHF, factor VIII) during labor in normal women, in patients with premature separation of the placenta, and in a patient with von Willebrand's disease. J Clin Lab Med 84:851–860, 1974.
2. Bennett B, Ratnoff OD: Changes in antihemophilic factor (AHF, factor VIII) procoagulant activity and AHF-like antigen in normal pregnancy, and following exercise and pneumoencephalography. J Clin Lab Med 80:256–263, 1972.
3. Conti M, Mari D, Conti E, et al: Pregnancy in women with different types of von Willebrand disease. Obstet Gynecol 68:282–285, 1986.
4. Economides DL, Kadir RA, Lee CA: Inherited bleeding disorders in obstetrics and gynecology. Br J Obstet Gynaecol 106:5–13, 1999.
5. Kadir RA, Lee CA, Sabin CA, et al: Pregnancy in women with von Willebrand's disease or factor XI deficiency. Br J Obstet Gynaecol 105:314–321, 1998.
6. Condie RG: A serial study of coagulation factors XII, XI, and X in plasma in normal pregnancy and in pregnancy complicated by pre-eclampsia. Br J Obstet Gynaecol 93:636–639, 1976.
7. Hilgartner MW, Smith CH: Plasma thromboplastin antecedent (factor XI) in the neonate. J Paediatr 66:747–752, 1965.
8. Burrows RF, Kelton JG: Thrombocytopenia at delivery: A prospective survey of 6715 deliveries. Am J Obstet Gynecol 162:731–734, 1990.
9. Forbes CD, Greer JA: Physiology of haemostasis and the effect of pregnancy. In Greer IA, Turpie AG, Forbes CD (eds): Haemostasis and Thrombosis in Obstetrics and Gynaecology, London, UK, Chapman & Hall, 1992, pp 1–26.
10. Sadler JE: A revised classification of von Willebrand disease. Thromb Haemost 71:520–525, 1994.
11. Mannucci PM: Treatment of von Willebrand's disease. N Engl J Med 357:683–694, 2004.

12. Lee CA: Women and inherited bleeding disorders: Menstrual issues. Semin Hematol 36 (suppl 4): 21–27, 1999.
13. Kadir RA, Economides DL, Sabin CA, et al: Frequency of inherited bleeding disorders in women with menorrhagia. Lancet 351:485–489, 1998.
14. von Willebrand E: Hereditar pseudo-hemofili. Finska Lakarsallskapets Handl 67:7–112, 1926.
15. Lyons SE, Bruck NE, Bowie EJ, Ginsburg D: Impaired intracellular transport produced by a subset of type IIa von Willebrand disease mutations. J Biol Chem 267:4424–4430, 1992.
16. Phillips MD, Santhouse A: von Willebrand disease: Recent advances in pathophysiology and treatment. Am J Med Sci 316:77–86, 1998.
17. Rick ME, Williams SB, Sacher RA, et al: Thrombocytopenia associated with pregnancy in a patient with type IIB von Willebrand's disease. Blood 69:786–789, 1987.
18. Walker ID: Investigation and management of haemorrhagic disorders in pregnancy. J Clin Pathol 47:100–108, 1994.
19. Metzner HJ, Hermentin P, Cuesta-Linker T, et al: Characterization of factor VIII/von Willebrand factor concentrates using a modified method of von Willebrand factor multimer analysis. Haemophilia 4 (suppl 3): 25–32, 1998.
20. Dobrkovska A, Krzensk U, Chediak JR: Pharmacokinetics, efficacy and safety of Humate-P in von Willebrand disease. Haemophilia 4 (suppl 3): 33–39, 1998.
21. Mannucci PM, Canciani MT, Rota L, et al: Response of factor VIII/von Willebrand factor to DDAVP in healthy subjects and patients with haemophilia A and von Willebrand's disease. Br J Haematol 47:283–293, 1981.
22. Mannucci PM: Desmopressin: A nontransfusional form of treatment for congenital and acquired bleeding disorders. Blood 72:1449–1455, 1988.
23. Burrow GN, Wassenaar W, Robertson GL, et al: DDAVP treatment of diabetes insipidus during pregnancy and the post-partum period. Acta Endocrinol (Copenh) 97:23–25, 1981.
24. Rochelson B, Caruso R, Davenport D, et al: The use of prophylactic desmopressin (DDAVP) in labor to prevent hemorrhage in a patient with Ehlers-Danlos syndrome. N Y State J Med 91:268–269, 1991.
25. Greer IA, Lowe GD, Walker JJ, et al: Haemorrhagic problems in obstetrics and gynaecology in patients with congenital coagulopathies. Br J Obstet Gynaecol 98:909–918, 1991.
26. Sage DJ: Epidurals, spinals and bleeding disorders in pregnancy: Review. Anaesth Intensive Care 18:319–326, 1990.
27. Lyon M: Sex chromatin and gene action in the mammalian X chromosome. Am J Hum Genet 14:135–148, 1962.
28. Bunschoten EPM, van Houwelingen JC, Visser SE JM, et al: Bleeding symptoms in carriers of hemophilia A and B. Thromb Haemost 59:349–352, 1988.
29. Sadler JE, Blinder M: von Willebrand disease: Diagnosis, classification, and treatment. In Colman RW, Hirsh J, Marder VJ, et al (eds): Hemostasis and Thrombosis, 4th ed. Philadelphia, Lippincott Williams & Wilkins, 2001, pp 825–837.
30. Nishino M, Nishino S, Sugimoto M, et al: Changes in factor VIII binding capacity of von Willebrand factor and factor VIII coagulant activity in two patients with type 2N von Willebrand disease after hemostatic treatment and during pregnancy. Int J Hematol 64:127–134, 1996.
31. Wilson JD, Griffin JE: Disorders of sexual differentiation. In Fauci AS, Braunwald E, Isselbacher KJ, et al (eds): Harrison's Principles of Internal Medicine, 14th ed. New York, McGraw-Hill, 1998, pp 2119–2131.
32. Yang MY, Ragni MV: Clinical manifestations and management of labor and delivery in women with factor IX deficiency. Haemophilia 10:483–490, 2004.
33. Seligsohn U: Factor XI deficiency. Thromb Haemost 70:68–71, 1993.
34. Bolton-Maggs PHB, Young Wan-Nin B, McCraw AH, et al: Inheritance and bleeding in factor XI deficiency. Br J Haemotol 69:521–528, 1988.
35. Kitchens CS: Factor XI: A review of its biochemistry and deficiency. Semin Thromb Hemost 17:55–72, 1991.
36. Bolton-Maggs PHB, Colvin BJ, Satchi G, et al: Thrombogenic potential of factor XI concentrate. Lancet 344:748–749, 1994.
37. Nossel HL, Lanzkowsky P, Levy S, et al: A study of coagulation factor levels in women during labour and in their newborn infants. Thromb Diath Haemorrh 16:185–197, 1966.
38. Kadir RA, Economides DL, Lee CA: Factor XI deficiency in women. Am J Hematol 60:48–54, 1999.
39. Kadir RA: Women and inherited bleeding disorders: Pregnancy and delivery. Semin Hematol 36 (suppl 4): 28–35, 1999.
40. Collins PW, Lilley P, Guldman E, et al: Clinical experience of factor XI deficiency: The use of fresh frozen plasma and factor XI concentrate. Thromb Haemost 73:1441, 1995(2070a).
41. Lusher J: Women and inherited bleeding disorders. Semin Hematol 36 (suppl 4): 10–20, 1999.
42. Inbal A, Muszbek L: Coagulation factor deficiencies and pregnancy loss. Semin Thromb Hemost 29:171–174, 2003.
43. Pitkin RM, Witte DL: Platelet and leukocyte counts in pregnancy. JAMA 242:2696–2698, 1979.
44. Pritchard JA, Weisman R Jr, Ratnoff OD, Vasburgh GJ: Intravascular hemolysis, thrombocytopenia, and other hematologic abnormalities associated with severe toxemia of pregnancy. N Engl J Med 250:89–98, 1954.
45. Cines DB, Blanchette VS: Immune thrombocytopenic purpura. N Engl J Med 346:995–1008, 2002.
46. Burrows RF, Kelton JG: Fetal thrombocytopenia and its relation to maternal thrombocytopenia. N Engl J Med 329:1463–1466, 1993.
47. Shehata N, Burrows RF, Kelton JG: Gestational thrombocytopenia. Clin Obstet Gynecol 42:327–334, 1999.
48. George JN, Woolf SH, Raskob GE, et al: Idiopathic thrombocytopenic purpura: A practice guideline developed by explicit methods for the American Society of Hematology. Blood 88:3–40, 1996.
49. Kelton JG: Management of the pregnant patient with idiopathic thrombocytopenic purpura. Ann Intern Med 99:796–800, 1983.
50. Kelton JG: Idiopathic thrombocytopenia purpura complicating pregnancy. Blood Rev 16:43–46, 2002.
51. McCrae KR, Samuels P, Schreiber AD: Pregnancy-associated thrombocytopenia: Pathogenesis and management. Blood 80:2697–2714, 1992.
52. Kaplan C, Daffos F, Forestier F, et al: Fetal platelet counts in thrombocytopenic pregnancy. Lancet 336:979–982, 1990.
53. Sharon R, Tatarsky I: Low fetal morbidity in pregnancy associated with acute and chronic idiopathic thrombocytopenic purpura. Am J Hematol 46:87–90, 1994.
54. Moise KJ Jr, Carpenter RJ Jr, Cotton DB, et al: Percutaneous umbilical cord sampling in the evaluation of fetal platelet counts in pregnant patients with autoimmune thrombocytopenic purpura. Obstet Gynecol 72 (3 Pt 1): 346–350, 1988.
55. Hohlfeld P, Forestier F, Kaplan C, et al: Fetal thrombocytopenia: A retrospective survey of 5,194 fetal blood samplings. Blood 84:1851–1856, 1994.
56. Bussel JB, Zabusky MR, Berkowitz RL, et al: Fetal alloimmune thrombocytopenia. N Engl J Med 337:22–26, 1997.
57. Skupski DW, Bussel JB: Alloimmune thrombocytopenia. Clin Obstet Gynecol 42:335–348, 1999.
58. Weinstein L: Syndrome of hemolysis, elevated liver enzymes, and low platelet count: A severe consequence of hypertension in pregnancy. Am J Obstet Gynecol 142:159–167, 1982.
59. Sibai BM: The HELLP syndrome (hemolysis, elevated liver enzymes, and low platelets): Much ado about nothing? Am J Obstet Gynecol 162:311–316, 1990.
60. Minakami H, Sato I: HELLP syndrome. JAMA 281:703–704, 1999.
61. Magann EF, Martin JN: Twelve steps to optimal management of HELLP syndrome. Clin Obstet Gynecol 42:532–550, 1999.

35

Chapter 36

Management of Thrombophilia and Antiphospholipid Syndrome During Pregnancy

Jody L. Kujovich, MD • Barbara M. Alving, MD

INTRODUCTION

Thromboembolic events that occur during pregnancy or during the postpartum period present unique diagnostic and therapeutic challenges that may affect both mother and fetus. Such events are not rare; venous thromboembolism (VTE) occurs in approximately 1 in 1000 pregnancies, and pulmonary embolism is a leading cause of maternal death.[1-4] This chapter discusses the prevention, diagnosis, and treatment of VTE in pregnant women, the role of inherited and acquired thrombophilia (i.e., antiphospholipid syndrome [APLS]) in inducing VTE and other complications that affect fetal development, and treatment approaches to pregnancy-related stroke. Benefits and risks of anticoagulant therapy in these different clinical settings are also reviewed.

Pregnancy is a prothrombotic state that involves all three components of Virchow's triad: venous stasis, endothelial damage, and alteration of circulating coagulation factors (Table 36-1). Venous stasis results from a hormonally induced increase in venous distensibility and obstruction of venous flow by the enlarging uterus. Pelvic vascular endothelial injury may occur at the time of delivery or as a result of venous hypertension. Pregnant women may have increased levels of several procoagulant factors, a progressive fall in protein S levels, acquired resistance to activated protein C, and impaired fibrinolysis.[1,3,5-10]

Evidence for thrombophilia is found in more than 50% of women with pregnancy-related VTE. The most common inherited thrombophilic disorders include factor V Leiden (FV Leiden), prothrombin 20210 gene mutation, and deficiencies of antithrombin III, protein C, or protein S. The most common acquired thrombophilic disorder is immune-mediated APLS. Elevated levels of homocysteine, which may be associated with an increased risk for thrombosis, may be due to environmental factors and/or to an underlying gene polymorphism (e.g., methylenetetrahydrofolate reductase [MTHFR] 677).

VENOUS THROMBOEMBOLISM IN PREGNANCY

The risk of VTE is four- to tenfold higher in pregnant than in nonpregnant women of similar age (Table 36-2).[3,11] This increased risk, which begins during the first trimester and continues throughout pregnancy, is greatest during the postpartum period.[3,12-15] According to one meta-analysis, more than 50% of cases of VTE that develop during pregnancy occur in the first two trimesters, and the risk for VTE is increased by 15-fold during the postpartum period.[15]

THROMBOPHILIA AND VENOUS THROMBOEMBOLISM DURING PREGNANCY

The risk of VTE during pregnancy is greater in women with thrombophilia than in those without this condition and is exacerbated by additional prothrombotic factors. FV Leiden is associated with a 5- to 16-fold increased thrombotic risk during pregnancy and the puerperium over that seen in nonpregnant women without thrombophilia (see Table 36-2).[16-20] Heterozygous carriers of the prothrombin 20210 mutation have a 3- to 15-fold higher risk of pregnancy-associated VTE than do unaffected women.[16,17,19,21] The widely varying prevalences and risks that have been reported may reflect the relatively small sample sizes and different cut-off levels used to define a deficiency. In a single family study, antithrombin III-deficient women had a nearly 50-fold higher risk of VTE during pregnancy and the puerperium than was noted in nonpregnant women, with the highest risk reported during the postpartum period.[22] In the absence of prophylactic anticoagulation, postpartum VTE occurred in 15% of previously asymptomatic deficient women, and in 50% of those with a prior history of VTE.

Homozygosity for the common MTHFR 677 mutation predisposes to mild hyperhomocysteinemia, usually in the setting of suboptimal folate levels. No consistent evidence suggests that the MTHFR 677 mutation increases the risk of VTE, independent of homocysteine levels. Therefore, laboratory testing for this gene mutation is not indicated. Hyperhomocysteinemia and high levels of several clotting factors are independent thrombotic risk factors, but their contributions to VTE during pregnancy are not well defined. High FVIII levels (>170% of normal) may also serve as a risk factor for thrombosis during pregnancy.[17]

Women with multiple or homozygous thrombophilic defects have the greatest risk of pregnancy-associated VTE.

Table 36-1   Risk Factors for Pregnancy-Related Venous Thromboembolism

Physiologic Changes During Pregnancy

Venous stasis
  Obstruction of venous return by enlarging uterus
  Increase in venous distensibility due to hormonal effects

Pelvic vascular injury due to venous hypertension or delivery

Alteration of circulating coagulation factors
  Increased procoagulant factors
  Decreased protein S levels
  Acquired resistance to activated protein C
  Impaired fibrinolysis

Risk Factors

Advanced maternal age
Obesity
Immobilization
Multiple gestations
High parity
Preeclampsia
Cesarean section
Prior venous thrombosis
Thrombophilia

This risk is increased 20- to 40-fold in homozygous FV Leiden women.[11,17] In one study, the risk of pregnancy-associated VTE was increased ninefold in women who were heterozygous for FV Leiden and 15-fold in those who were heterozygous for the prothrombin 20210 mutation. In contrast, this risk was increased >100-fold in women with both mutations, illustrating the dramatic increase in overall risk when thrombophilic mutations are combined.[16] In another retrospective study, VTE occurred in 18% of pregnancies in double heterozygous carriers of FV Leiden and the prothrombin 20210 mutation, compared with 6% of those with only the prothrombin 20210 mutation, suggesting that the combination of the two mutations confers a nearly threefold greater risk than is conferred by the prothrombin 20210 mutation alone.[23] In studies of thrombophilic families, VTE complicated 4% of pregnancies in double heterozygous carriers of

FV Leiden and the prothrombin 20210 mutation and 16% of pregnancies in women with homozygous FV Leiden, compared with 0.5% of pregnancies in unaffected relatives.[11,24,25] A recent meta-analysis found that the risk of pregnancy-related VTE was increased 34-fold and 26-fold in homozygous patients of FV Leiden and the prothrombin 20210 mutation, respectively.[26]

Although thrombophilia increases the relative risk of pregnancy-associated VTE, the absolute risk in asymptomatic carriers has not been well defined. Retrospective observational data and studies of thrombophilic families probably overestimate the risk in unselected asymptomatic women. Two prospective studies of unselected pregnant women screened for FV Leiden reported very low rates of VTE in heterozygous carriers (1% and 0%, respectively).[27,28] No thrombotic complications occurred during pregnancy or the puerperium among a large cohort of FV Leiden carriers identified by general population screening.[29] Several retrospective studies estimated the probability of VTE in FV Leiden carriers in the range of 2.5 to 3 per 1000 pregnancies.[2,16,17] This risk in women with the prothrombin 20210 mutation is approximately 1 in 200 to 300 pregnancies.[17] These estimates suggest that asymptomatic women with a single thrombophilic defect and no other predisposing factors have a relatively low absolute risk. In contrast, women with homozygous or combined thrombophilia have a much higher probability of VTE—in the range of 10 to 50 per 1000 pregnancies.[11,17] Women with antithrombin III deficiency also are at greater risk, although estimates range from 1 in 3 to 1 in 250 pregnancies, depending on the type and severity of deficiency.[2,16]

DIAGNOSIS OF VENOUS THROMBOEMBOLISM DURING PREGNANCY

Signs and symptoms of deep venous thrombosis (DVT), such as lower extremity pain and edema, and of pulmonary embolism (PE), such as dyspnea and tachypnea,

Table 36-2   Thrombophilia and Risk of Pregnancy-Associated Venous Thromboembolism

Thrombophilic Disorder	Prevalence in Women with Pregnancy-Associated VTE	Risk of Pregnancy-Associated VTE (odds ratio)*	Probability of Pregnancy-Associated VTE[†] (VTE/1000 pregnancies)
None	<50%	4–10	1
FV Leiden (heterozygous)	20%–46%	5–16	2–3
FV Leiden (homozygous)	2%–4%	20–40	40
PGM 20210 heterozygotes	6%–26%	3–15	3–5
PGM 20210 homozygotes	NA	26	NA
FVL/PGM (double heterozygotes)	7%–9%	9–107	10–50
ATIII deficiency[‡]	1%–19%	7–64	4–333
PC deficiency[§]	2%–14%	4–7	1–9
PS deficiency[¶]	1%–12%	2–3	1–3
High FVIII levels**	18%	4–5	2–3

*Risks relative to nonpregnant women without thrombophilia.
[†]Assuming baseline incidence of 1 VTE per 1000 to 1500 pregnancies.
[‡]Variably defined as <60% or <80% of normal activity.
[§]Variably defined as <50% or <70% of normal activity.
[¶]<53% to 55% of normal activity.
**>170% of normal activity.
VTE, venous thromboembolism; FV Leiden, factor V Leiden; PGM, prothrombin gene mutation; ATIII, antithrombin III; PC, protein C; PS, protein S; FVIII, factor VIII; NA, not applicable (data not sufficient).

may be attributed to pregnancy, thus causing a delay in diagnosis.[30] Approximately 80% to 85% of DVT sites in pregnant women are found in the left lower extremity; most involve the iliofemoral veins, which are associated with an enhanced likelihood of PE. Isolated calf vein DVT is uncommon, accounting for <10% of cases.[12,14,15] The striking predilection for the left leg is believed to be due to compression of the left iliac vein by the right iliac artery, which is exacerbated by the enlarging uterus. The risk for isolated iliac vein thrombosis is increased during pregnancy, although its true incidence is unknown. More than 66% of women with a pregnancy-related DVT exhibit symptoms of a post-thrombotic syndrome, perhaps reflecting the high frequency of iliofemoral vein involvement.[31,32]

In nonpregnant patients, the combination of a negative D-dimer assay and a low clinical probability safely rules out VTE. However, no studies have established the negative predictive value of D-dimer testing during pregnancy. The role of D-dimer testing is limited during pregnancy in that concentration increases with gestational age.[33] By the third trimester, D-dimer levels exceed conventional cut-off values for excluding VTE in nearly all women, and they do not return to normal levels until 4 to 5 weeks after delivery.[34] Higher D-dimer levels are found in women with preterm labor, placental abruption, and preeclampsia.

Because of the unreliability of clinical assessment and the uncertainty of D-dimer testing, an objective diagnosis is required in pregnant patients with suspected VTE. Compression ultrasound is the first-line diagnostic test for DVT because it does not involve radiation exposure. Ultrasound is highly sensitive and specific for proximal DVT in nonpregnant patients, but it is not known whether available data are applicable to pregnant women. Because a normal ultrasound does not reliably exclude calf vein DVT, serial testing over 7 to 14 days is recommended to rule out propagation of undetected calf vein thrombosis.[35–37] Compression ultrasound is inadequate for diagnosis of isolated iliac vein thrombosis and may not detect extension of proximal DVT into the iliac vein or inferior vena cava (IVC). Because of its high sensitivity and specificity for thrombosis in this location, magnetic resonance venography is recommended when clinical suspicion of iliac vein involvement is high.[38] Because of an uncertain natural history of superficial vein thrombosis below the knee during pregnancy, serial ultrasounds should be considered to exclude extension into the deep venous system.

The diagnosis of pulmonary embolism during pregnancy is complicated by concerns about fetal exposure to ionizing radiation. Most experts agree that the risks of undiagnosed PE far outweigh the theoretical risks of radiation exposure from diagnostic imaging.[35–37] With appropriate precautions, radiation exposure resulting from radionuclide lung or helical computed tomography (CT) scans is far below the threshold associated with an increased risk of teratogenesis.[37,39,40] A lower extremity ultrasound examination is appropriate for women with suspected PE in that a diagnosis of DVT allows treatment and thus avoids the need for further imaging. However, lower extremity DVT is detected in less than 50% of women with PE during pregnancy.[13] If the initial ultrasound examination is negative or nondiagnostic, a ventilation/perfusion (V/Q) or helical CT scan should be performed. The distribution of results of V/Q

scanning in pregnant women with suspected PE differs from that in nonpregnant women; a much higher prevalence of normal scans and fewer high-probability and non-diagnostic studies are noted.[36] An initial perfusion scan with reduced dose reduces the radiation exposure in that a normal study excludes PE, obviating the need for a ventilation scan. Limited available evidence suggests that withholding anticoagulation in pregnant women with a normal perfusion scan is safe. The accuracy of helical CT scanning has not been evaluated in pregnant women with suspected PE. Although the role of helical CT in pregnancy is not addressed in published guidelines, it is emerging as the first-line imaging study for use in patients with suspected PE.[41] Pulmonary angiography is rarely performed because it is invasive and requires a significantly higher radiation dose; it is not more accurate than helical CT scans.[37]

MANAGEMENT OF THROMBOSIS AND THROMBOPHILIA DURING PREGNANCY

Antithrombotic Therapy During Pregnancy

Because of the paucity of well-controlled trials, guidelines for anticoagulation during pregnancy are based largely on case series and studies in nonpregnant patients.[42] Although unfractionated heparin (UHF) or low molecular weight heparin (LMWH) is recommended during pregnancy, LMWH has generally replaced UFH in the management of VTE, on the basis of data that have established its safety and efficacy.[35,42–45] Despite widespread endorsement in consensus guidelines, LMWH has not yet been approved by the U.S. Food and Drug Administration (FDA) for use during pregnancy. LMWH has several advantages over UFH, including a more predictable dose response (obviating the need for frequent laboratory monitoring), a longer half-life (allowing once- or twice-daily dosing), and an improved safety profile with a probable lower risk of osteoporosis and heparin-induced thrombocytopenia (HIT). Because LMWH does not cross the placenta, no risk of fetal bleeding or teratogenicity is present, although bleeding at the uteroplacental junction may occur rarely. Potential maternal complications include bleeding, osteoporosis, HIT, and allergic skin reactions. One review of LMWH use during 2777 pregnancies found that rates of VTE and bleeding were comparable with those reported in nonpregnant patients.[44] Recurrent VTE occurred in <1% and major bleeding in approximately 2% of women who were given LMWH for prophylaxis or treatment during pregnancy. The rate of postpartum hemorrhage was similar to that reported in women who were not receiving anticoagulants, and most cases of bleeding were associated with an obstetric cause.[44,46]

Osteoporosis

Osteoporosis is a particular concern for pregnant women who may require LMWH (or UFH) over the course of gestation. In two studies, prolonged treatment with UFH reduced bone mineral density in up to 30% of patients and resulted in vertebral fracture in 2% to 3% of women receiving long-term prophylaxis during pregnancy.[47,48] Convincing evidence from animal models and clinical studies suggests that LMWH use is associated with a significantly lower risk of osteoporosis than is use of UFH.[49,50] One study measured bone mineral density at various time points after delivery in women randomly assigned to prophylactic doses of UFH or LMWH during pregnancy. Women who received UFH had significantly lower bone mineral density up to 3 years postpartum, consistent with animal data suggesting that adverse effects may not be reversible. In contrast, no difference in bone mineral density was observed between women who received LMWH and a group of untreated control women.[50] Other data also suggest that long-term treatment with LMWH, at least in prophylactic doses, does not adversely affect bone mineral density.[51] The effects of higher therapeutic doses have not been adequately studied.

Heparin-Induced Thrombocytopenia

HIT is extremely rare in pregnant women, even among those receiving long-term UFH.[52,53] The estimated incidence of HIT is <0.1% in obstetric patients who are given LMWH.[44] Recent American College of Chest Physicians (ACCP) guidelines suggest that platelet count monitoring is not required in pregnant women who are treated exclusively with LMWH.[54]

Skin Reactions

Allergic skin reactions to UFH and LMWH may complicate the management of pregnant women who require anticoagulation. Allergic skin reactions are reported in 0.6% to 29% of pregnant women given LMWH for prophylaxis or treatment of VTE.[43,44,55] The wide range in reported incidence likely reflects the varying types and severity of skin reactions described. Although several types of allergic reactions may occur, delayed type IV hypersensitivity reactions are the most common and show a striking predilection for women.[56] These reactions are characterized by erythematous plaques that are often pruritic. Such plaques typically develop at the sites of subcutaneous injection 10 days after initiation of therapy; however, they may also occur after several months of heparin administration.[55] When these plaques first appear, the patient should be evaluated for possible HIT because similar-appearing isolated skin lesions may progress to skin necrosis as a rare but documented manifestation of this condition.[57] Severe HIT-associated skin reactions may occur in the absence of thrombocytopenia.[58]

Allergic skin reactions to LMWH require a change in therapy in most cases.[55] Heparin-like compounds should be avoided in patients with HIT, skin necrosis, or type I immediate hypersensitivity reactions. Delayed type IV hypersensitivity reactions may resolve with a change in preparation, although cross-reactivity with other LMWHs is common. Cutaneous testing is occasionally useful in confirming the diagnosis and in screening for cross-reactivity with other LMWH preparations.[56]

Warfarin

In contrast to heparins, warfarin and other coumarin derivatives cross the placenta with the potential for fetal bleeding and teratogenicity.[42] Although warfarin may be safe during the first 6 weeks, the risk of embryopathy is highest between 6 and 12 weeks gestation.[42] Embryopathy, which is estimated to occur in the fetuses of 2.4% to 6.4% of

women receiving coumarin derivatives during the first trimester,[59–61] is characterized by nasal and limb hypoplasia, stippled epiphyses, and vertebral abnormalities.[42,59] Central nervous system abnormalities due to fetal intracerebral hemorrhage may occur after warfarin exposure at any time during pregnancy. Therapeutic maternal levels of anticoagulation may produce supratherapeutic effects on the fetus, caused in part by immaturity of the fetal liver. Fetal bleeding may occur at any time, especially at the time of birth, because of the combination of the anticoagulant effect and the trauma of delivery.[60] Children exposed in utero to warfarin during the second and third trimesters are reported to have a higher incidence of long-term neurodevelopmental problems.[62]

Women who receive warfarin therapy should be counseled prior to pregnancy about potential fetal risks.[42] Two strategies are recommended for women on long-term warfarin who are contemplating pregnancy. One option is to continue warfarin with frequent pregnancy testing, substituting LMWH or UFH as soon as pregnancy has been confirmed. Testing must be performed prior to the sixth week of gestation to minimize the risk of warfarin-induced embryopathy. Alternatively, the patient may be switched to LMWH prior to attempts at conception. Because warfarin is probably safe during the first 4 to 6 weeks of gestation, the former approach may be more convenient in reliable patients.[42] Personal preference and medicolegal concerns may also factor into the decision.

Other Antithrombotic Agents

Treatment options for pregnant women who are unable to receive heparin are limited. Danaparoid, which is not available in the United States, has low cross-reactivity with heparin-induced antibodies and has been used safely in pregnant women.[42] It does not appear to cross the placenta, and on the basis of measurements of anti-FXa levels in fetal cord blood and breast milk in a small number of women, it is believed to be safe for breastfeeding mothers.[63]

Direct thrombin inhibitors, such as lepirudin and argatroban, do not cross-react with heparin-induced antibodies and are recommended for nonpregnant patients with HIT.[54] A few case reports have described lepirudin use during pregnancy without maternal or fetal complications.[64,65] However, lepirudin and argatroban have not been adequately evaluated in pregnant women, and the extent of placental transfer is unknown.

Fondaparinux is a synthetically derived pentasaccharide that binds to antithrombin III, potentiating antithrombin III–mediated inactivation of factor Xa. It does not cross-react with HIT antibodies in vitro and is a potentially useful therapeutic agent for HIT, although it has not yet been approved for this indication.[66] Anecdotal reports have described the successful use of fondaparinux in pregnant women who were unable to receive heparin.[67,68] Fondaparinux was used in a small number of pregnant women with severe cutaneous reactions to LMWH without evidence of cross-reactivity or other adverse effects.[67] An ex vivo model in which perfused placentas were used indicated that fondaparinux was not transferred across the placenta.[69] A clinical study involving five pregnant women who were given prophylactic doses reported that fondaparinux activity was detectable in cord blood samples in concentrations that were approximately one tenth of those in maternal plasma.[67] Although these concentrations are not likely to be clinically significant, the extent of placental transfer with higher therapeutic doses is unknown.

At present, clinical experience with lepirudin or fondaparinux is insufficient to confirm their safety during pregnancy or breastfeeding. The use of these newer antithrombotic agents should be reserved for women for whom no other therapeutic alternatives are available. In these situations, the physician should discuss the risks and benefits of therapy in detail with the patient and her family. This discussion should be well documented in the medical records. Danaparoid, lepirudin, argatroban, and fondaparinux are classified as FDA pregnancy risk category B, meaning that no well-controlled studies in pregnant women have validated the findings of studies that were done with animals.

Laboratory Monitoring

In pregnant women receiving treatment doses of UFH, the partial thromboplastin time (PTT) may not reflect the true degree of anticoagulation, in part because of elevated levels of factor VIII.[70] Monitoring the anticoagulant activity of heparin with the use of the PTT in pregnant women may result in administration of inappropriately high doses, leading to an increased risk of bleeding for the patient. Measurement of anti-FXa activity levels is recommended for patients who appear to be "heparin resistant."[35] Doses of subcutaneous UFH are adjusted so that a midinterval anti-FXa level in the therapeutic range of 0.3 to 0.7 U per milliliter is achieved.[35]

For women receiving LMWH, a chromogenic anti-FXa assay is used to monitor the anticoagulant effect, although no consistent evidence suggests that anti-FXa levels correlate with efficacy or bleeding.[46,71] Currently, no consensus has been reached regarding laboratory monitoring of LMWH during pregnancy. Some experts recommend periodic checking of anti-FXa levels (e.g., shortly after initiation, and then every 1 to 3 months) when treatment doses are used in pregnant women.[42,72–74] Peak anti-FXa levels are measured approximately 4 hours after a subcutaneous injection is given. LMWH doses are adjusted to maintain levels in the therapeutic range for nonpregnant patients receiving twice-daily doses (0.5 to 1.2 U per milliliter).[42] The therapeutic range for once-daily dosing is less well defined but likely exceeds 1.0 U per milliliter for most LMWHs.[71] Measurement of anti-FXa levels is usually unnecessary when LMWH is administered in prophylactic doses.[46]

Primary Prophylaxis of Venous Thromboembolism in Asymptomatic Women

Because the probability of VTE during pregnancy is low, prophylactic anticoagulation is not routinely recommended for asymptomatic women with a single thrombophilic defect (Table 36-3). Clinical surveillance with prompt investigation of signs and symptoms of VTE may be adequate in low-risk women without other risk factors.[42] However, risk assessment must be individualized. Thrombophilic women should be counseled on the increased thrombotic risk during pregnancy and on the need for prompt evaluation of signs or symptoms suspicious for VTE. Women who do not receive antepartum anticoagulation should be offered a 4- to 6-week course of warfarin postpartum because the highest risk of VTE (especially PE) occurs during this period.[3,42] Prophylactic LMWH (or UFH) during pregnancy followed by 4 to 6 weeks of postpartum anticoagulation is recommended for women who are homozygous for FV Leiden or the prothrombin 20210 mutation, who are doubly heterozygous for both mutations, who may be deficient in antithrombin III, or who have been identified as having other combined thrombophilic defects.[42,74] The indications for prophylaxis are stronger in women with coexisting risk factors.

Table 36-3 Recommended Prophylaxis Against Venous Thromboembolism for Pregnant Women

Primary Prophylaxis—Asymptomatic Women	Antepartum	Postpartum
Low risk thrombophilia (single defect, no other risk factors)	Clinical surveillance	6 wk warfarin
Homozygous FV Leiden or prothrombin 20210 FV Leiden/prothrombin 20210 Antithrombin III deficiency Multiple thrombophilic defects	Prophylactic dose* LMWH	6 wk warfarin
Secondary prophylaxis—Women with previous VTE		
Single provoked VTE, no thrombophilia	Clinical surveillance	6 wk warfarin
Prior estrogen-related VTE ± thrombophilia	Prophylactic dose* LMWH	6 wk warfarin
Prior unprovoked VTE, no thrombophilia	Prophylactic dose* LMWH or clinical surveillance	6 wk warfarin
Prior VTE and thrombophilia (not on long-term warfarin)	Prophylactic* or intermediate dose† LMWH	6 wk warfarin
Prior VTE and thrombophilia (on long-term warfarin)	Adjusted dose‡ LMWH	Resume long-term warfarin

*Prophylactic dose = enoxaparin 40 mg SC q 24 hr or dalteparin 5000 U SC q 24 hr.
†Intermediate dose = enoxaparin 40 mg SC q 12 hr or dalteparin 5000 U SC q 12 hr.
‡Adjusted dose = enoxaparin 1 mg/kg SC q 12 hr or dalteparin 100 U/kg SC q 12 hr.
FV Leiden, factor V Leiden; VTE, venous thromboembolism; LMWH, low molecular weight heparin.

Secondary Prophylaxis in Women with Previous Thrombosis

The risk for VTE in pregnancy and especially during the postpartum period is generally increased for women with a prior history of VTE, although according to published studies, recurrence rates range from 0% to 15%. This risk appears to be higher in women with a prior unprovoked event and/or other coexisting inherited or acquired thrombotic risk factors.[75] The risk of recurrent VTE is increased after miscarriage and terminations and is particularly high after stillbirth.[76] This risk also appears to be increased for women with a prior estrogen-related thrombosis.[76]

When considering therapy for a patient who is currently pregnant, the physician should review the numbers and types of previous episodes (spontaneous or provoked by a transient risk factor), the requirements for long-term anticoagulation, thrombophilic defects, and concurrent risk factors, such as obesity, immobilization, and multiple gestation.[42,72]

Management options during pregnancy include clinical surveillance or active prophylaxis with LMWH or UFH (see Table 36-3). LMWHs are preferred for prophylaxis during pregnancy, although no consensus has been reached on the optimal dosing regimen. The use of UFH requires more frequent injections, and standard prophylactic doses (e.g., 5000 U every 12 hours) may be inadequate in women with a high-risk pregnancy. Thus, higher doses (7500 to 10,000 U every 12 hours) and/or doses that provide detectable prophylactic anti-FXa levels (0.1 to 0.3 U per milliliter) are often recommended.[42] Although no randomized controlled trials have confirmed efficacy during pregnancy, low recurrence rates were reported in all studies in which LMWH was used for prophylaxis of VTE.[44] Prophylaxis, when indicated, should be initiated as soon as pregnancy is confirmed.[13–15]

Available evidence suggests that women with a single prior provoked VTE who do not have thrombophilia or other persistent risk factors have a low rate of recurrence during pregnancy and may be safely followed without antepartum anticoagulation.[75] Prophylaxis during pregnancy should be considered, however, in women with a prior estrogen-related VTE.[42] Women with a history of VTE who do not receive prophylactic anticoagulation during pregnancy should be given a postpartum course of warfarin. Graduated elastic compression stockings are recommended for all women with a prior DVT.[42]

Women with a prior unprovoked VTE who do not have thrombophilia and who are not receiving long-term anticoagulation therapy may be treated with prophylactic LMWH (or UFH) or clinical surveillance. LMWH should particularly be considered for women with a prior PE because the risk of recurrence in these patients is relatively high.[77,78]

Women with a history of VTE and confirmed thrombophilia who are not receiving long-term anticoagulation should be given prophylactic LMWH during pregnancy, followed by a 6-week postpartum course of warfarin. Standard prophylactic doses (e.g., enoxaparin 40 mg every 24 hours) or intermediate doses (enoxaparin 40 mg twice daily) are appropriate, depending on the thrombophilic profile. For example, although prophylactic doses are adequate for most women with heterozygous FV Leiden, an intermediate dose of LMWH is recommended for those

with homozygous or combined defects, antithrombin III deficiency, or APLS.[42] Women with a prior VTE who are on long-term anticoagulant therapy usually require adjusted therapeutic doses of LMWH during pregnancy, followed by resumption of warfarin postpartum.[42]

The pentasaccharide fondaparinux has been successfully used for this indication.[68]

Treatment of Acute Thrombosis During Pregnancy

Women who develop acute VTE during pregnancy should receive therapeutic doses of LMWH or UFH. LMWHs are preferable because of their ease of administration, more predictable antithrombotic effects, and excellent safety profile.[42] Because of the increased clearance rate of LMWH during pregnancy, twice-daily regimens provide a more consistent anticoagulant effect than is attained with once-daily dosing. If UFH is administered, the initial dose is given intravenously as a bolus, followed by a continuous infusion adjusted to prolong the mid-interval PTT into the therapeutic range for at least 5 days. Adjusted subcutaneous doses of UFH or LMWH are substituted for the remainder of pregnancy. Multiple randomized trials and meta-analyses have confirmed that LMWH is at least as safe and effective as UFH for the treatment of nonpregnant patients with acute DVT and PE.[79–81]

Therapeutic doses of LMWH are usually continued throughout pregnancy because of the high risk of recurrent thrombosis. It is unknown whether the dose of LMWH can be safely reduced after an initial period of full anticoagulation because no studies have compared different dosing regimens in pregnant women. However, lowering of the dose of LMWH after an initial phase of therapeutic anticoagulation was effective in patients with malignancy, who are also at high risk for recurrence.[82] Therapeutic doses of LMWH should be continued for at least 4 to 6 weeks after diagnosis of acute VTE. Switching to an intermediate dose for the remainder of pregnancy may reduce the risks of bleeding and osteoporosis. Until evidence-based guidelines become available, decisions about dosing should be based on assessment of the risks of recurrence and adverse effects in each individual case.

Delivery

In general, therapeutic doses of LMWH or subcutaneous UFH should be discontinued 24 hours prior to elective induction of labor or cesarean section so that the risk of hemorrhage may be reduced and safe epidural anesthesia provided (Table 36-4).[42] Therapeutic doses of subcutaneous UFH may cause a persistent anticoagulant effect at the time of delivery.[83] Preliminary data suggesting that LMWH may be safely discontinued 12 hours before delivery of epidural anesthesia require confirmation in larger groups of women receiving therapeutic doses.[84] Reinitiation of LMWH should be delayed for at least 2 hours after the epidural catheter is removed. Women who are given LMWH should be instructed to discontinue their injections at the onset of spontaneous labor. If an unacceptable anticoagulant effect is expected at the time of delivery on the basis of the timing of the last dose or current anti-FXa levels, epidural anesthesia should be avoided. Protamine sulfate may partially reverse

Table 36-4   Management of Peripartum Antithrombotic Therapy

Discontinue LMWH 24 hours before elective induction or cesarean section or at onset of spontaneous labor.

High-risk women with recent VTE:
- Consider substituting IV UFH until 4 to 6 hours before expected time of delivery and/or retrievable IVC filter.
- Avoid epidural anesthesia if last dose LMWH within 12 hours or detectable anti-FXa levels.
- Consider protamine for excessive anticoagulation or bleeding at delivery if last dose of LMWH within preceding 8 hours.
- Consider antithrombin III replacement for antithrombin III–deficient women. First dose prior to delivery. Maintain antithrombin III level at 80% to 120% of normal until restarting LMWH postpartum

Postpartum
- Start LMWH and warfarin as soon as hemostasis is confirmed after delivery (within 12 hr).
- Delay at least 2 hours after epidural catheter removal.
- Continue LMWH until warfarin therapy adequate (INR 2–3 for 48 hr).

LMWH, low molecular weight heparin; VTE, venous thromboembolism; IVC, inferior vena caval; FXa, factor Xa; INR, international normalized ratio.

excessive anticoagulation at the time of delivery, especially if LMWH has been administered within the preceding 8 hours.[35,71] In women at very high risk of recurrence, intravenous UFH may be substituted and discontinued 4 to 6 hours before the expected time of delivery, to minimize the period of subtherapeutic anticoagulation.[42,85] Women with inherited antithrombin III deficiency might be considered for peripartum replacement therapy with purified antithrombin III concentrates. An initial dose of 50 U per kilogram is given prior to delivery. Plasma antithrombin III levels should be maintained in the optimal range of 80% to 120% until LMWH therapy is reinitiated postpartum. The shorter half-life of antithrombin III during pregnancy (approximately 29 hours) may necessitate daily dosing.

Postpartum Treatment

LMWH (or UFH) should be restarted postpartum as soon as adequate hemostasis has been confirmed, optimally within 12 hours after an uncomplicated delivery. Warfarin can be started at the same time. LMWH/UFH should be continued until the international normalized ratio (INR) is within the therapeutic range (2–3) for at least 48 hours. Postpartum anticoagulation should be continued for at least 6 weeks, or until a minimum total 3-month course is completed in cases of VTE occurring late in pregnancy.[42] The optimal duration of anticoagulation after pregnancy-related VTE is unknown. The decision regarding treatment duration should be based on the extent and timing of VTE during pregnancy, thrombophilic defects, prior thrombotic history, and coexisting risk factors. Women with APLS or antithrombin III deficiency are at high risk for recurrence and usually require long-term anticoagulation. LMWH, UFH, fondaparinux, and warfarin are not secreted into breast milk and are safe for women who plan to breast-feed.[42]

Inferior Vena Caval Filters

Indications for placement of filters in the IVC during pregnancy are the same as in nonpregnant patients, that is, acute VTE with a strong contraindication to anticoagulation, recurrent VTE despite adequate anticoagulation, and selected critically ill patients at high risk of recurrent fatal PE (see Chapter 31). Filter insertion into the IVC appears to be technically safe during pregnancy, as noted in case reports and case series.[86] The newer retrievable filters are as effective as permanent filters and have a similar complication rate.[87] Continued anticoagulation while the filter is in place is recommended unless the risk for bleeding outweighs the risk of thrombosis. Although the use of retrievable filters during pregnancy has not been systematically studied, multiple case reports describe their efficacy and the lack of associated maternal or fetal complications.[88] A retrievable filter inserted into the IVC prior to delivery provides protection against PE in high-risk women with proximal DVT who are given a diagnosis near term; the filter can be removed postpartum.

Thrombolytic Therapy

Current data on the use of thrombolytic therapy in pregnant women are limited to case reports and case series.[89–91] Thrombolytic agents have been used safely in small numbers of pregnant women with massive PE, thrombosed cardiac valves, acute stroke, large DVTs and renal vein thrombosis.[90–93] Information on their use has recently been collected and reviewed.[93] Systemic thrombolysis and local catheter-directed thrombolysis have both been performed successfully in pregnant women. Maternal hemorrhage and fetal loss are estimated to occur in approximately 6% of pregnant women receiving systemic thrombolysis, although the complication rate has not been well defined.[91]

Thrombolytic therapy should be reserved for pregnant women with life-threatening VTE (e.g., unstable PE with circulatory compromise) who require rapid clot lysis. When thrombolysis is required, recombinant tissue plasminogen activator and streptokinase are favored over urokinase because both are large molecules that do not cross the placenta in significant amounts.[91,93,94]

ANTIPHOSPHOLIPID ANTIBODIES AND THE ANTIPHOSPHOLIPID SYNDROME

Antiphospholipid antibodies (APLAs) comprise a heterogeneous group of autoantibodies directed against proteins bound to phospholipid. APLAs are found in 1% to 10% of healthy individuals, 4% to 14% of patients who present with VTE, and approximately 30% of those with lupus. Patients with APLA identified on two occasions of testing are given a diagnosis of APLS if they also have a history of arterial, venous, and/or small vessel thrombosis, or a history of pregnancy morbidity. Adverse pregnancy outcomes that are diagnostic of the syndrome include three or more unexplained spontaneous miscarriages before 10 weeks, one or more unexplained fetal deaths at or after 10 weeks, and premature birth (before 35 weeks) due to severe preeclampsia or placental insufficiency.[95] Women with APLS may have obstetric complications in the absence of a history of arterial or venous thrombosis. Laboratory criteria require demonstration of moderate or high levels of immunoglobulin (Ig)G or IgM anticardiolipin antibodies or a lupus inhibitor on two occasions at least 6 weeks apart. Lupus inhibitors and high-titer IgG anticardiolipin antibodies are most strongly associated with thrombotic complications of the syndrome.[96] A lupus inhibitor may also be a strong predictor of thrombosis during pregnancy.[97] It is unclear whether measurement of anti–β_2-glycoprotein (GP) I antibodies provides additional information about pregnancy complications beyond that attained through anticardiolipin antibody and lupus inhibitor testing.[98]

Implications of a Positive Test for APLA

The prevalence of APLA in unselected obstetric populations is similar to that in healthy nonpregnant individuals; it ranges from 2% to 9%.[99,100] APLAs are found in up to 20% of women with recurrent pregnancy loss (RPL); they are risk factors for fetal loss and other pregnancy complications.[101] In several studies, consistently lower live birth rates have been noted in low-risk women with APLA compared with women without these antibodies.[100,102–104] The association between APLA and fetal loss is strongest for unexplained losses that occur during the second or third trimester.[105,106] However, a recent meta-analysis reported a significant overall threefold increased risk of early and late pregnancy loss.[26] Pregnancy is assumed to markedly increase the risk of VTE in patients with APLA, but no large studies have estimated the risk. This assumption is based on the marked increase in overall thrombotic risk that occurs when multiple predisposing factors are combined. A small case-controlled study found that APLAs occurred in 27% of women with pregnancy-associated VTE compared with 3% of control women with uneventful pregnancies.[107]

Management During Pregnancy

During pregnancy, women with APLS are at risk for thrombosis, fetal loss, and possibly other maternal and fetal complications. Women with APLA should be counseled regarding potential thrombotic and obstetric complications. High-risk women should be evaluated prior to conception so that a plan for management during pregnancy can be formulated. Testing for other thrombophilic disorders should be considered, especially if patients report a prior history of VTE.[108] Coexisting prothrombotic risk factors enhance the risk for thrombosis in patients with APLA, underscoring the importance of a careful assessment in each individual case.[109] Pregnant women with APLS require close maternal and fetal monitoring, including frequent surveillance of fetal growth and development and periodic platelet counts, especially if they have had a history of thrombocytopenia. However, serial measurement of APLA is unnecessary because fluctuations in titer will not affect management.

Primary Prophylaxis in Asymptomatic Women

Treatment for asymptomatic women with APLA and no prior history of thrombosis or fetal loss is controversial (Table 36-5). Therapeutic strategies include clinical surveillance or low-dose aspirin given alone or in combination

Table 36-5 Management of Pregnant Women With Antiphospholipid Antibodies (APLA) in the Presence or Absence of Antiphospholipid Syndrome (APLS)

Monitoring
  Monitor fetal growth and development as well as maternal platelet count

Primary prophylaxis: Asymptomatic women with APLA
  Antepartum: Clinical surveillance or low-dose aspirin (80–100 mg/d) and/or prophylactic dose LMWH or UFH*
  Postpartum: Warfarin (INR 2–3) for 6 weeks

Secondary prophylaxis: Women with APLS (prior thrombosis)
  Women receiving long-term warfarin
    Antepartum: Adjusted dose LMWH or UFH ± low-dose aspirin (80–100 mg/d)
    Postpartum: Resume long-term warfarin (INR 2–3)
  Women not receiving warfarin
    Antepartum: Prophylactic or intermediate dose LMWH or UFH ± low-dose aspirin (80–100 mg/d)
    Postpartum: Warfarin (INR 2–3) for 6 weeks or longer

Secondary prophylaxis: Women with APLS (prior recurrent or late fetal loss)
  Antepartum: Prophylactic dose LMWH or UFH and low-dose aspirin (80–100 mg/d)
  Postpartum: Warfarin (INR 2–3) for 6 weeks

Treatment of acute thrombosis
  Antepartum: Adjusted dose LMWH or UFH throughout pregnancy
  Postpartum: Warfarin (INR 2–3) for extended period

*Heparin doses are defined in Table 36-3.
LMWH, low molecular weight heparin; UFH, unfractionated heparin; INR, international normalized ratio.

with prophylactic doses of heparin. No prospective trials have been conducted to evaluate prophylactic anticoagulation in women with APLA without clinical manifestations of the syndrome. In the absence of evidence-based recommendations, some experts suggest low-dose aspirin,[98] whereas others favor withholding of pharmacologic therapy because of the high probability of a successful pregnancy outcome.[110] The guidelines of the ACCP endorse surveillance, prophylactic doses of heparin (LMWH or UFH) and/or low doses of aspirin for asymptomatic women with persistent APLA.[42] The same approach is appropriate for women with one or two prior early pregnancy losses (before 10 weeks gestation). Treatment decisions should take into account the APLA profile and other thrombotic risk factors. In asymptomatic women with persistent APLA, a 6-week course of warfarin might be considered postpartum.

Secondary Prophylaxis in Women with Prior Thrombosis

Women with APLS based on persistent APLA and a history of thrombosis should receive prophylactic anticoagulation throughout pregnancy and during the postpartum period. Most experts favor low-dose aspirin given in combination with heparin, despite the lack of evidence of additional benefit.[42,98] Indications for aspirin may be stronger in women with prior arterial thrombosis and/or pregnancy complications. It is unknown whether a history of thrombosis enhances the risk of an adverse pregnancy outcome. The dose of heparin depends on previous thrombotic history and indications for long-term therapy. Therapeutic doses of LMWH or UFH are recommended for women on long-term anticoagulation prior to pregnancy, followed by resumption of warfarin postpartum. Women with APLA and a single prior VTE episode who are not receiving long-term anticoagulation may be treated with prophylactic or intermediate doses of LMWH (or UFH), followed by a 6-week postpartum course of warfarin.[42] LMWH is restarted after delivery, along with warfarin, and is continued until a therapeutic INR is attained.[2,3]

Secondary Prophylaxis in Women with Previous Fetal Loss

Women with APLS who have a history of recurrent and/or late fetal loss may require antithrombotic therapy during subsequent pregnancies. Available evidence suggests that aspirin alone is ineffective in preventing pregnancy loss in this population.[111] Two small, randomized trials showed that low-dose aspirin and prophylactic doses of UFH reduced the risk of pregnancy loss by 54%, compared with aspirin alone. Live birth rates were 71% and 80% with combination therapy, compared with 42% and 44% with aspirin alone.[111–113] Live birth rates were similar with high (16,000 to 40,000 U per day) and low (10,000 to 25,000 U per day) doses of UFH (80% and 76%, respectively).[114] The superiority of aspirin given together with heparin has established combination therapy as the standard of care for women with APLS characterized by APLA and fetal loss.

No large randomized trials have compared LMWH with UFH in the prevention of pregnancy complications in women with APLS. Prophylactic LMWH given alone or in combination with aspirin produced live birth rates ranging from 84% to 93% in several small comparative trials and prospective cohort studies.[97,115–118] A uniform treatment protocol tailored to the complete spectrum of APLA-associated obstetric complications resulted in the highest live birth rate (93%), underscoring the value of clinical pathways and comprehensive multidisciplinary care.[97] Despite the lack of randomized trials, most experts favor the use of LMWH because of its multiple advantages over UFH and evidence of equivalent efficacy in all other settings studied.[42,110] ACCP and other consensus guidelines recommend low-dose aspirin and prophylactic doses of heparin (LMWH or UFH) throughout pregnancy for women with APLS who have a history of two or more early miscarriages, or one or more late fetal losses, preeclampsia, fetal growth restriction (FGR), or placental abruption.[42,98,119] Aspirin therapy is started prior to conception or at the time of a positive pregnancy test. LMWH (or UFH) should be started as soon as pregnancy has been confirmed.[110] A postpartum course of anticoagulation is also recommended because women with APLA and fetal loss have an increased risk of subsequent thrombosis.[42,98,120] Women with previous thrombosis and pregnancy loss usually require higher adjusted doses of LMWH (or UFH) in combination with aspirin. No role for immunomodulatory agents (e.g., corticosteroids or IVIg) in the treatment of pregnant women with APLS has been established.[118]

Treatment of Acute Thrombosis

Pregnant women with APLS who develop acute thromboembolism require therapeutic doses of LMWH (or UFH)

throughout pregnancy, followed by a minimum 6-week course of warfarin postpartum. Reevaluation of APLA status postpartum is useful in newly diagnosed women because persistent APLAs are an indication for long-term anticoagulation. The general consensus favors indefinite anticoagulation on the basis of evidence that patients with APLS are at high risk for recurrent thrombosis if anticoagulation is stopped.[121,122] Two randomized trials showed that moderate-intensity warfarin (INR, 2 to 3) is as effective as high-intensity warfarin (INR, 3 to 4.5) in preventing recurrent thrombosis in patients with APLS.[123,124]

APLA and Other Pregnancy Complications

The association of APLA with other obstetric complications such as preeclampsia, FGR, and placental abruption is controversial, with conflicting results reported in different studies. High rates of preeclampsia and FGR (up to 50% and 30% of pregnancies, respectively) were reported in a series of women with known APLS that included a substantial number of women with lupus and/or prior thrombosis.[125,126] Unselected low-risk pregnant women with APLA identified by first-trimester screening had a higher incidence of preeclampsia in some[102,104,127] but not all studies.[101,103] APLAs were not associated with mild, severe, or early onset of preeclampsia in several series of unselected women who presented with the disorder,[128,129] and they did not predict a recurrence during a subsequent pregnancy.[130] However, in a recent meta-analysis, APLAs were associated with a nearly threefold increased risk of preeclampsia.[26] APLAs were associated with FGR or low-birthweight infants in several[104] but not other studies.[103]

Despite evidence of an improved live birth rate for women with APLS, it remains unclear whether the frequency of other pregnancy complications is reduced by antithrombotic therapy. No association has been found between the antithrombotic regimen and the frequency of preeclampsia, prematurity, or FGR in randomized trials of prophylaxis in women with fetal loss. Despite the higher live birth rates achieved with heparin and aspirin, a substantial number of successful pregnancies were complicated by preeclampsia, prematurity, and low-birthweight infants.[131,132] No trials have evaluated the efficacy of antithrombotic therapy in preventing these other complications in pregnant woman with APLS. Expert opinion and consensus guidelines suggest that antepartum low-dose aspirin and LMWH (or UFH) should be used for pregnant women with APLA and prior severe or recurrent preeclampsia, abruption, or FGR.[42,133]

PREGNANCY-ASSOCIATED STROKE

The estimated incidence of ischemic stroke associated with pregnancy is in the range of 4 to 18 events per 100,000 deliveries.[134–136] The time of greatest risk is the postpartum period.[135–138]

Most cases of embolic stroke are associated with a cardiac source in women with damaged or prosthetic valves. Peripartum cardiomyopathy, a rare complication of pregnancy, may result in a left ventricular thrombus and embolic stroke in up to 10% of cases.[139] Arterial thromboembolism may occur "paradoxically" through a patent foramen ovale (PFO) in patients with venous thrombosis.[140–142] Predisposition to venous thrombosis and hemodynamic changes associated with pregnancy may make paradoxical embolism through a PFO likely, especially with intense Valsalva maneuvers during labor and delivery (see Chapter 44). Cerebral vein thrombosis is another potential cause of pregnancy-related stroke.[134,138] Preeclampsia is the most common pregnancy-associated risk factor for stroke.[135,137]

The contribution of thrombophilia to pregnancy-related stroke is unclear; hyperhomocysteinemia and APLS are established risk factors for arterial thrombosis in nonpregnant patients. Inherited thrombophilic disorders are not major risk factors for stroke, and the cause remains unknown in as many as 22% to 32% of reported cases.[134,135]

Diagnostic evaluation of suspected stroke during pregnancy is similar to that performed in nonpregnant patients, although cerebral vein thrombosis and paradoxical embolism warrant special consideration. Routine head CT scanning with abdominal shielding results in an acceptably low fetal radiation exposure, and magnetic resonance imaging (MRI) is considered safe, especially in later trimesters.[139] Evaluation of pregnancy-related stroke should include an echocardiogram to look for a cardiac source of embolism and a PFO. Patients with a PFO and/or known thrombophilia should be evaluated for DVT, which is an indication for anticoagulation. Paradoxical emboli may also originate from pelvic veins in pregnant and postpartum women. The diagnosis of cerebral vein thrombosis requires a high index of suspicion; it is confirmed by MR venography because routine CT is so frequently falsely negative.

No controlled studies have investigated thrombolytic therapy during pregnancy, and pregnant women were excluded from the stroke trials. Although thrombolytic agents are generally avoided because of the risk of maternal and fetal complications, multiple reports have described their successful use in pregnant women with acute stroke.[92,93,143] Anticoagulation with LMWH or UFH is recommended for cerebral vein thrombosis, even in the presence of hemorrhagic infarction[144,145] (see Chapter 16).

No randomized trials of antithrombotic therapy have explored stroke prevention in pregnant women. Low-dose aspirin is recommended for women with a history of non-cardioembolic stroke with no other risk factors.[145] Available evidence suggests that low-dose aspirin given during the second and third trimesters is safe for mother and fetus.[42] Other antiplatelet agents should be avoided because their safety during pregnancy has not been confirmed. LMWH or UFH throughout pregnancy is suggested for women with a history of ischemic stroke and known thrombophilia or with a potential cardiac source of embolism.[145] Women with mechanical heart valves are at high risk for arterial thromboembolism and frequently require therapeutic dose anticoagulation throughout pregnancy. Adjusted doses of LMWH or UFH with laboratory monitoring are favored over second- and third-trimester warfarin, although the optimal antithrombotic regimen is controversial.[42] LMWH or UFH is also recommended for women who have had a recurrent transient ischemic attack (TIA), or who have sustained a stroke despite receiving aspirin therapy.

No consensus has been attained regarding the treatment of women with a history of stroke and APLS during pregnancy. Clinical studies in nonpregnant patients have shown that patients with APLS have a high risk of recurrent thrombosis, which tends to occur in the same vascular distribution as the original event. Thus, LMWH or UFH, with or without low-dose aspirin, should be considered for pregnant women with high-titer antibodies and multiple complications of APLS.

Women with a history of stroke may seek counseling regarding the risks associated with pregnancy. Extremely limited data are available on maternal and fetal outcomes of subsequent pregnancies in women with prior stroke. Two retrospective series have reported a low risk of recurrent stroke during subsequent pregnancies (0% and 1% of pregnancies, respectively).[146,147] None of the women with an initial pregnancy-related stroke experienced recurrence during subsequent pregnancies. The risk of recurrent stroke was increased during the postpartum period (relative risk, 9.7), but not during pregnancy itself.[147] Although these results should be interpreted with caution, the observed low risk of recurrence suggests that a history of stroke is not a contraindication to a future pregnancy.

THROMBOPHILIA AND OBSTETRIC COMPLICATIONS

Serious obstetric complications, including RPL, preeclampsia, FGR, and placental abruption, occur in 1% to 5% of pregnant women and are believed to involve impaired placental perfusion. Thrombophilia may enhance susceptibility to placental thrombosis and gestational vascular complications. In addition to APLS, most inherited thrombophilic disorders have been linked to fetal loss and other complications. Thrombophilic defects were identified in 49% to 65% of women with obstetric complications, compared with 18% to 22% of women with normal pregnancies, suggesting a three- to eightfold increase in risk (Table 36-6).[148,149]

Available evidence suggests that FV Leiden is a risk factor for recurrent pregnancy loss. A large number of case-controlled studies found a high prevalence of FV Leiden in women with unexplained RPL (up to 30%), compared with 1% to 10% of control subjects, with odds ratios ranging from 2 to 5.[150–154] Several other studies, however, found no association.[155–157] Most of these studies were smaller and primarily included women with first-trimester fetal losses that are often caused by nonthrombophilic factors.

The prothrombin 20210 mutation was linked to fetal loss in some but not all studies. This mutation was found in 4% to 9% of women with RPL (most during the first trimester), compared with 1% to 2% of those with uncomplicated pregnancies, with odds ratios ranging from 2 to 9.[150,158–162] A large case-controlled study identified FV Leiden and the prothrombin 20210 mutation as independent risk factors for a first unexplained fetal loss after 10 weeks gestation, with odds ratios of 3.5 and 2.6, respectively.[150] Two other studies found the prothrombin 20210 mutation in 9% to 13% of women with a first unexplained third-trimester loss, compared with 2% to 3% of control subjects, suggesting a two- to threefold increase in risk.[153,161] Several other studies found no significant association with fetal loss.[151,154] In several meta-analyses, FV Leiden and the prothrombin 20210 mutation each conferred

Table 36-6 Thrombophilia and Risk of Pregnancy Loss*

Thrombophilic Disorder	Prevalence in Women with Fetal Loss	Prevalence in Controls	Risk of Fetal Loss (odds ratio)
Factor V Leiden	8%–30%	1%–10%	2–5
Prothrombin 20210	4%–13%	1%–2%	2–9
Antithrombin III deficiency	0%–2%	0%–1.4%	2–5
Protein C deficiency	6%	0%–2.5%	2–3
Protein S deficiency	5%–8%	0%–0.2%	3–40
Hyperhomocysteinemia	17%–27%	5%–16%	3–7
Combined thrombophilia	8%–25%	1%–5%	5–14
APLA	20%	5%	3–5

*Variably defined as first or recurrent early and/or late pregnancy loss.
APLA, antiphospholipid antibody.

a two- to threefold increased risk of recurrent first-trimester and later fetal loss.[163–165]

Deficiencies in the natural anticoagulant proteins C, S, and antithrombin III increased the risk of fetal loss according to most,[166,167] but not all, of the limited number of studies.[154,160] These conflicting results may reflect the relative rarity of these disorders and the small numbers of women studied. In a report on thrombophilic families, 22% of pregnancies in women who were deficient in protein C, protein S, or antithrombin III ended in fetal loss, compared with 11% of those in unaffected family members, suggesting a twofold increase in risk.[167] An increased risk of stillbirth was reported in women with antithrombin III or protein S deficiency but not in those with protein C deficiency.[166] A prospective cohort study found no significant increase in risk of fetal loss, but only a small number of women were included in the trial.[168]

Hyperhomocysteinemia was found in 17% to 27% of women with first or recurrent fetal loss, compared with 5% to 16% of control women, with odds ratios ranging from 3 to 7.[169–171] Interpretation of these studies is complicated by varying definitions of hyperhomocysteinemia, timing and method of testing, and use of supplemental vitamins. One study suggested that homocysteine levels have a graded effect on risk, with levels greater than 15 μmol per liter conferring a sevenfold increased risk of a first fetal loss at 8 to 9 weeks gestation.[169] A meta-analysis found a three- to fourfold increased risk of recurrent early pregnancy loss in women with hyperhomocysteinemia.[172] In contrast, no convincing evidence suggests that a homozygous MTHFR 677 mutation is a risk factor for pregnancy complications independent of homocysteine levels. This mutation was not associated with an increased risk of early or late fetal loss in a large number of observational studies, a prospective study of primigravid women, and a large meta-analysis.[151,153,154,163,173]

Women with multiple thrombophilic defects have approximately a ninefold to 14-fold increased risk of late pregnancy loss compared with a fourfold higher risk with only a single defect.[151,166,174] Although most pregnancy losses occur during the first trimester, evidence suggests that thrombophilic women may have a higher risk of loss at later stages of gestation.[175] Multiple studies, including two meta-analyses, have suggested that FV Leiden carriers have a greater risk of late pregnancy loss than early first-trimester loss.[150,163,166,176] Other data suggest that women

with other thrombophilic defects also have a greater risk of late pregnancy loss.[151,166] One possible explanation is that late pregnancy loss reflects thrombosis of placental vessels, in contrast to first-trimester losses, which are more commonly due to other causes. However, thrombophilia also increases the risk of an early first-trimester fetal loss.[162,163,169,177]

Although preeclampsia, FGR, and placental abruption may also involve impaired placental perfusion, their association with thrombophilia remains controversial. This may reflect the varying diagnostic and selection criteria, different ethnic groups, and small number of cases included. Multiple case-controlled studies have found at least one thrombophilic defect in 40% to 72% of women with preeclampsia, compared with 8% to 20% of control women with normal pregnancies.[148,178,179] In contrast, other studies have not demonstrated an association.[157,180,181] The prevalence of FV Leiden was significantly higher in women with preeclampsia than in women with normal pregnancies, with odds ratios ranging from 2 to 6.[148,178,182,183] Several other studies found no difference in prevalence of the mutation between preeclamptic and control women.[157,180,181] A FV Leiden mutation did not increase the risk of preeclampsia in three prospective studies of unselected pregnant women who were screened during the first trimester.[27,28,173] Several large meta-analyses found an overall twofold to threefold increased risk of preeclampsia.[184–186]

The role of other thrombophilias in the pathogenesis of preeclampsia remains uncertain. Most studies, including two meta-analyses, have found no association with the prothrombin 20210 mutation.[157,181,185,187] A large number of studies have suggested that hyperhomocysteinemia increases the risk of preeclampsia. Women with second-trimester homocysteine levels greater than 5 to 10 μmol per liter had a three- to fourfold greater risk of developing preeclampsia, suggesting that hyperhomocysteinemia may reveal a high-risk group.[188,189] Most studies found no association between a homozygous MTHFR 677 mutation and preeclampsia, underscoring once again the importance of measuring homocysteine levels rather than MTHFR genotypes.[157,173] Conflicting results reported may be due at least in part to major differences in the severity of preeclampsia.[181,182] Thrombophilic women with severe preeclampsia may have a higher risk of serious maternal complications and adverse perinatal outcomes than those

36

without thrombophilia.[179,182] Thrombophilia was also linked to an earlier onset of severe preeclampsia in several studies.[182,187]

Data on the risk of FGR and placental abruption are more limited but also conflicting. In a recent meta-analysis, FV Leiden and the prothrombin 20210 mutation were both found to be associated with a significant two- to threefold increased risk of FGR.[190] In contrast, two larger case-controlled studies found no association between maternal or fetal thrombophilia and FGR.[191]

FV Leiden, the prothrombin 20210 mutation, and hyperhomocysteinemia were associated with an increased risk of placental abruption in some[148,192–194] but not other studies.[157,195]

Antithrombotic Therapy for Preventing Obstetric Complications

The high prevalence of thrombophilia in women with gestational vascular complications and the tendency for recurrence provide a rationale for trials of prophylactic anticoagulation to improve pregnancy outcomes. Current data on antithrombotic therapy in women with hereditary thrombophilia and pregnancy loss are limited to several observational studies and two randomized trials. In one study, 50 thrombophilic women with recurrent pregnancy loss received enoxaparin throughout 61 subsequent pregnancies. The live birth rate was 75% with enoxaparin prophylaxis, compared with 20% in prior untreated pregnancies.[196] Another study reported a similar live birth rate of 70% with enoxaparin prophylaxis compared with 44% in untreated historical control women.[197] A prospective randomized trial compared prophylactic doses of enoxaparin with low doses of aspirin in women with the prothrombin 20210 mutation, FV Leiden or protein S deficiency, and a single unexplained fetal loss. Enoxaparin prophylaxis was associated with a significantly higher live birth rate of 86% compared with 29% with aspirin, suggesting a 15-fold greater likelihood of a successful outcome.[198] The LIVE-ENOX trial randomly assigned thrombophilic women with a history of recurrent pregnancy loss to two different doses of enoxaparin. Prophylactic doses (40 mg per day and 80 mg per day) resulted in similar high live birth rates of 84% and 78%, respectively. These rates were substantially higher than the 23% live birth rate reported in prior untreated pregnancies.[199] No prospective randomized trials included an untreated control group, confirming the benefit of LMWH in this setting. However, the concordant results of these studies strongly suggest that anticoagulation therapy may improve pregnancy outcomes in thrombophilic women. Until additional studies are completed, antithrombotic prophylaxis should be considered in selected thrombophilic women with unexplained recurrent pregnancy loss after an informed discussion of the risks and potential benefits. The evolving consensus in favor of prophylactic anticoagulation is reflected by recent ACCP guidelines, which recommend prophylactic doses of LWMH or UFH and low doses of aspirin for thrombophilic women who have had recurrent pregnancy loss or a single loss during the second or third trimester.[42]

It is unknown whether lowering high homocysteine levels with supplemental vitamins will improve pregnancy outcome. In a small, uncontrolled series, 20 of 22 women with a history of hyperhomocysteinemia and RPL had a subsequent successful pregnancy after their homocysteine levels were normalized with folic acid and vitamin B6.[200] ACCP guidelines recommend supplemental folic acid throughout pregnancy for women who are homozygous for the MTHFR 677 mutation.[42] High homocysteine levels should be lowered with folic acid (1 to 2 mg per day), optimally given prior to conception.

Few data support the benefit of antithrombotic therapy in thrombophilic women with other pregnancy complications. A few uncontrolled studies of thrombophilic women with preeclampsia, FGR, or placental abruption reported improved pregnancy outcomes with UFH or LMWH given with or without aspirin.[201–203] However, these studies were small (total, 71 cases), and preeclampsia recurred in 38% of treated women in one study.[202] In the LIVE-ENOX study, incidences of preeclampsia, placental abruption, and FGR were substantially lower with enoxaparin prophylaxis than in prior untreated pregnancies.[204] A study of thrombophilic women with prior fetal loss who received enoxaparin or aspirin during a subsequent pregnancy showed that those who were given enoxaparin had newborns with significantly higher birth weights, and fewer were classified as small for gestational age.[198] However, neither study was designed to evaluate these complications as primary outcomes. ACCP guidelines recommend low doses of aspirin and prophylactic doses of LMWH or UFH for thrombophilic women with a history of severe or recurrent preeclampsia or placental abruption.[42] Decisions about antithrombotic therapy should be based on an individual risk:benefit assessment. Assessment of maternal thrombotic risk during pregnancy should also be incorporated into the clinical decision.

SCREENING FOR THROMBOPHILIA

It is widely agreed that routine laboratory screening for thrombophilia in pregnant women or women who might become pregnant is not warranted. Most experts favor a risk-stratified approach to testing—a strategy that is also cost effective.[42,74,205] Evaluation for thrombophilia is recommended in women with a personal history of VTE. Testing should also be considered in asymptomatic women with a family history of thrombophilia and/or thrombosis, particularly if a positive result will affect management.[42,74] Thrombophilic defects are found in up to 20% of women with normal pregnancies, suggesting that additional risk factors are required for the development of VTE or other complications. Selective thrombophilia screening requires an accurate patient history, focused on personal and family histories of thrombosis and prior exposure to circumstantial risk factors such as oral contraceptives.

Thrombophilic women have an increased risk of fetal loss and possibly other obstetric complications. Because the probability of a successful pregnancy outcome remains high, universal screening of pregnant women is not recommended. Women with unexplained fetal loss (≥3 miscarriages, intrauterine fetal death, or stillbirth), severe or recurrent preeclampsia, FGR, or placental abruption should be screened for APLAs. Recent ACCP guidelines also suggest that testing should be performed to identify inherited thrombophilias in light of accumulating evidence that prophylactic anticoagulation therapy may improve pregnancy outcomes.[42] Screening of women with a history of recurrent fetal loss or other unexplained severe pregnancy complications is reasonable after the implications of a positive test have been discussed, especially when a trial of LMWH is under consideration. Because of the risk of VTE, thrombophilic women may benefit from prophylaxis and counseling about present and future thrombotic risks.

Testing for patients with suspected thrombophilia includes a DNA assay for FV Leiden and for the prothrombin 20210 mutation, antithrombin III and protein C activity assays, free protein S antigen or activity assay, anticardiolipin antibody assay, multiple clotting tests for a lupus inhibitor, and measurement of plasma homocysteine level. Laboratory evaluation for thrombophilia can be performed during pregnancy with several caveats. Protein S antigen and activity levels decline during normal pregnancy (by $\geq 40\%$), making it difficult for clinicians to confirm or reliably exclude the diagnosis of an inherited deficiency. Homocysteine levels also decrease, especially with folic acid supplementation. Levels of antithrombin III, protein C, and protein S obtained immediately after an acute VTE may be misleadingly low, as has been noted in nonpregnant patients. DNA-based assays are reliable during pregnancy and acute thrombotic episodes; these are not affected by anticoagulant therapy. A complete laboratory evaluation should be performed, even after a single defect has been identified because combined thrombophilias are common.

PAROXYSMAL NOCTURNAL HEMOGLOBINURIA (PNH)

Paroxysmal nocturnal hemoglobinuria (PNH) is a special thrombophilic disorder that presents particular problems during pregnancy. PNH with and without pregnancy is discussed in Chapter 14.

REFERENCES

1. Lindqvist P, Dahlback B, Marsal K: Thrombotic risk during pregnancy: A population study. Obstet Gynecol 94:9, 1999.
2. McColl MD, Ramsay JE, Tait RC, et al: Risk factors for pregnancy associated venous thromboembolism. Thromb Haemost 78:1183–1188, 1997.
3. Heit JA, Kobbervig CE, James AH, et al: Trends in the incidence of venous thromboembolism during pregnancy or postpartum: A 30-year population-based study. Ann Intern Med 143:697–706, 2005.
4. Callaghan WM, Berg CJ: Pregnancy-related mortality among women aged 35 years and older, United States, 1991–1997. Obstet Gynecol 102 (5 Pt 1): 1015–1021, 2003.
5. Comp PC, Thurnau GR, Welsh J, Esmon CT: Functional and immunologic protein S levels are decreased during pregnancy. Blood 68:881–885, 1986.
6. Clark P, Brennand J, Conkie JA, et al: Activated protein C sensitivity, protein C, protein S and coagulation in normal pregnancy. Thromb Haemost 79:1166–1170, 1998.
7. Bremme K, Ostlund E, Almqvist I, et al: Enhanced thrombin generation and fibrinolytic activity in normal pregnancy and the puerperium. Obstet Gynecol 80:132–137, 1992.
8. Ros HS, Lichtenstein P, Bellocco R, et al: Pulmonary embolism and stroke in relation to pregnancy: How can high-risk women be identified? Am J Obstet Gynecol 186:198–203, 2002.
9. Melis F, Vandenbrouke JP, Buller HR, et al: Estimates of risk of venous thrombosis during pregnancy and puerperium are not influenced by diagnostic suspicion and referral basis. Am J Obstet Gynecol 191:825–829, 2004.
10. Danilenko-Dixon DR, Heit JA, Silverstein MD, et al: Risk factors for deep vein thrombosis and pulmonary embolism during pregnancy or

post partum: A population-based, case-control study. Am J Obstet Gynecol 184:104–110, 2001.
11. Martinelli I, Legnani C, Bucciarelli P, et al: Risk of pregnancy-related venous thrombosis in carriers of severe inherited thrombophilia. Thromb Haemost 86:800–803, 2001.
12. Ginsberg JS, Brill-Edwards P, Burrows RF, et al: Venous thrombosis during pregnancy: Leg and trimester of presentation. Thromb Haemost 67:519–520, 1992.
13. Gherman RB, Goodwin TM, Leung B, et al: Incidence, clinical characteristics, and timing of objectively diagnosed venous thromboembolism during pregnancy. Obstet Gynecol 94 (5 Pt 1): 730–734, 1999.
14. James AH, Tapson VF, Goldhaber SZ: Thrombosis during pregnancy and the postpartum period. Am J Obstet Gynecol 193:216–219, 2005.
15. Ray JG, Chan WS: Deep vein thrombosis during pregnancy and the puerperium: A meta-analysis of the period of risk and the leg of presentation. Obstet Gynecol Surv 54:265–271, 1999.
16. Gerhardt A, Scharf RE, Beckmann MW, et al: Prothrombin and factor V mutations in women with a history of thrombosis during pregnancy and the puerperium. N Engl J Med 342:374–380, 2000.
17. Gerhardt A, Scharf RE, Zotz RB: Effect of hemostatic risk factors on the individual probability of thrombosis during pregnancy and the puerperium. Thromb Haemost 90:77–85, 2003.
18. Lensen RP, Bertina RM, de Ronde H, et al: Venous thrombotic risk in family members of unselected individuals with factor V Leiden. Thromb Haemost 83:817–821, 2000.
19. Martinelli I, De Stefano V, Taioli E, et al: Inherited thrombophilia and first venous thromboembolism during pregnancy and puerperium. Thromb Haemost 87:791–795, 2002.
20. Meglic L, Stegnar M, Milanez T, et al: Factor V Leiden, prothrombin 20210G → A, methylenetetrahydrofolate reductase 677C → T and plasminogen activator inhibitor 4G/5G polymorphism in women with pregnancy-related venous thromboembolism. Eur J Obstet Gynecol Reprod Biol 111:157–163, 2003.
21. Simioni P, Sanson BJ, Prandoni P, et al: Incidence of venous thromboembolism in families with inherited thrombophilia. Thromb Haemost 81:198–202, 1999.
22. van Boven HH, Vandenbroucke JP, Briet E, Rosendaal FR: Gene–gene and gene–environment interactions determine risk of thrombosis in families with inherited antithrombin deficiency. Blood 94:2590–2594, 1999.
23. Samama MM, Rached RA, Horellou MH, et al: Pregnancy-associated venous thromboembolism (VTE) in combined heterozygous factor V Leiden (FVL) and prothrombin (FII) 20210 A mutation and in heterozygous FII single gene mutation alone. Br J Haematol 123: 327–334, 2003.
24. Martinelli I, Bucciarelli P, Margaglione M, et al: The risk of venous thromboembolism in family members with mutations in the genes of factor V or prothrombin or both. Br J Haematol 111:1223–1229, 2000.
25. Middeldorp S, Libourel EJ, Hamulyak K, et al: The risk of pregnancy-related venous thromboembolism in women who are homozygous for factor V Leiden. Br J Haematol 113:553–555, 2001.
26. Robertson L, Wu O, Langhorne P, et al: Thrombophilia in pregnancy: A systematic review. Br J Haematol 132:171–196, 2006.
27. Lindqvist PG, Svensson PJ, Marsaal K, et al: Activated protein C resistance (FV:Q506) and pregnancy. Thromb Haemost 81:532–537, 1999.
28. Dizon-Townson D, Miller C, Sibai B, et al: The relationship of the factor V Leiden mutation and pregnancy outcomes for mother and fetus. Obstet Gynecol 106:517–524, 2005.
29. Heit JA, Sobell JL, Li H, Sommer SS: The incidence of venous thromboembolism among Factor V Leiden carriers: A community-based cohort study. J Thromb Haemost 3:305–311, 2005.
30. Refuerzo JS, Hechtman JL, Redman ME, Whitty JE: Venous thromboembolism during pregnancy: Clinical suspicion warrants evaluation. J Reprod Med 48:767–770, 2003.
31. Bergqvist A, Bergqvist D, Lindhagen A, Matzsch T: Late symptoms after pregnancy-related deep vein thrombosis. Br J Obstet Gynaecol 97:338–341, 1990.
32. McColl MD, Ellison J, Greer IA, et al: Prevalence of the post-thrombotic syndrome in young women with previous venous thromboembolism. Br J Haematol 108:272–274, 2000.
33. Kline JA, Williams GW, Hernandez-Nino J: D-dimer concentrations in normal pregnancy: New diagnostic thresholds are needed. Clin Chem 51:825–829, 2005.
34. Epiney M, Boehlen F, Boulvain M, et al: D-dimer levels during delivery and the postpartum. J Thromb Haemost 3:268–271, 2005.

36

35. Bates SM, Ginsberg JS: How we manage venous thromboembolism during pregnancy. Blood 100:3470–3478, 2002.

36. Chan WS, Ginsberg JS: Diagnosis of deep vein thrombosis and pulmonary embolism in pregnancy. Thromb Res 107:85–91, 2002.

37. Scarsbrook AF, Evans AL, Owen AR, Gleeson FV: Diagnosis of suspected venous thromboembolic disease in pregnancy. Clin Radiol 61:1–12, 2006.

38. Fraser DG, Moody AR, Morgan PS, et al: Diagnosis of lower-limb deep venous thrombosis: A prospective blinded study of magnetic resonance direct thrombus imaging. Ann Intern Med 136:89–98, 2002.

39. Ginsberg JS, Hirsh J, Rainbow AJ, Coates G: Risks to the fetus of radiologic procedures used in the diagnosis of maternal venous thromboembolic disease. Thromb Haemost 61:189–196, 1989.

40. Winer-Muram HT, Boone JM, Brown HL, et al: Pulmonary embolism in pregnant patients: Fetal radiation dose with helical CT. Radiology 224:487–492, 2002.

41. Schuster ME, Fishman JE, Copeland JF, et al: Pulmonary embolism in pregnant patients: A survey of practices and policies for CT pulmonary angiography. AJR Am J Roentgenol 181:1495–1498, 2003.

42. Bates SM, Greer IA, Hirsh J, Ginsberg JS: Use of antithrombotic agents during pregnancy: The Seventh ACCP Conference on Antithrombotic and Thrombolytic Therapy. Chest 126 (3 suppl): 627S–644S, 2004.

43. Sanson BJ, Lensing AW, Prins MH, et al: Safety of low-molecular-weight heparin in pregnancy: A systematic review. Thromb Haemost 81:668–672, 1999.

44. Greer IA, Nelson-Piercy C: Low-molecular-weight heparins for thromboprophylaxis and treatment of venous thromboembolism in pregnancy: A systematic review of safety and efficacy. Blood 106:401–407, 2005.

45. Lepercq J, Conard J, Borel-Derlon A, et al: Venous thromboembolism during pregnancy: A retrospective study of enoxaparin safety in 624 pregnancies. Br J Obstet Gynaecol 108:1134–1140, 2001.

46. Greer I, Hunt BJ: Low molecular weight heparin in pregnancy: Current issues. Br J Haematol 128:593–601, 2005.

47. Dahlman TC: Osteoporotic fractures and the recurrence of thromboembolism during pregnancy and the puerperium in 184 women undergoing thromboprophylaxis with heparin. Am J Obstet Gynecol 168:1265–1270, 1993.

48. Douketis JD, Ginsberg JS, Burrows RF, et al: The effects of long-term heparin therapy during pregnancy on bone density: A prospective matched cohort study. Thromb Haemost 75:254–257, 1996.

49. Muir JM, Hirsh J, Weitz JI, et al: A histomorphometric comparison of the effects of heparin and low-molecular-weight heparin on cancellous bone in rats. Blood 89:3236–3242, 1997.

50. Pettila V, Leinonen P, Markkola A, et al: Postpartum bone mineral density in women treated for thromboprophylaxis with unfractionated heparin or LMW heparin. Thromb Haemost 87:182–186, 2002.

51. Carlin AJ, Farquharson RG, Quenby SM, et al: Prospective observational study of bone mineral density during pregnancy: Low molecular weight heparin versus control. Hum Reprod 19:1211–1214, 2002.

52. Warkentin TE, Levine MN, Hirsh J, et al: Heparin-induced thrombocytopenia in patients treated with low-molecular-weight heparin or unfractionated heparin. N Engl J Med 332:1330–1335, 1995.

53. Fausett MB, Vogtlander M, Lee RM, et al: Heparin-induced thrombocytopenia is rare in pregnancy. Am J Obstet Gynecol 185: 148–152, 2001.

54. Warkentin TE, Greinacher A: Heparin-induced thrombocytopenia: Recognition, treatment, and prevention: The Seventh ACCP Conference on Antithrombotic and Thrombolytic Therapy. Chest 126 (3 suppl): 311S–337S, 2004.

55. Bank I, Libourel EJ, Middeldorp S, et al: High rate of skin complications due to low-molecular-weight heparins in pregnant women. J Thromb Haemost 1:859–861, 2003.

56. Wutschert R, Piletta P, Bounameaux H: Adverse skin reactions to low molecular weight heparins: Frequency, management and prevention. Drug Saf 20:515–525, 1999.

57. Warkentin TE: Heparin-induced thrombocytopenia: Pathogenesis and management. Br J Haematol 121:535–555, 2003.

58. Myers B, Westby J, Strong J: Prophylactic use of danaparoid in high-risk pregnancy with heparin-induced thrombocytopaenia-positive skin reaction. Blood Coagul Fibrinolysis 14:485–487, 2003.

59. Blickstein D, Blickstein I: The risk of fetal loss associated with warfarin anticoagulation. Int J Gynaecol Obstet 78:221–225, 2002.

60. Hall JG, Pauli RM, Wilson KM: Maternal and fetal sequelae of anticoagulation during pregnancy. Am J Med 68:122–140, 1980.

61. Chan WS, Anand S, Ginsberg JS: Anticoagulation of pregnant women with mechanical heart valves: A systematic review of the literature. Arch Intern Med 160:191–196, 2000.

62. Wesseling J, Van Driel D, Heymans HS, et al: Coumarins during pregnancy: Long-term effects on growth and development of school-age children. Thromb Haemost 85:609–613, 2001.

63. Lindhoff-Last E, Kreutzenbeck HJ, Magnani HN: Treatment of 51 pregnancies with danaparoid because of heparin intolerance. Thromb Haemost 93:63–69, 2005.

64. Mehta R, Golichowski A: Treatment of heparin induced thrombocytopenia and thrombosis during the first trimester of pregnancy. J Thromb Haemost 2:1665–1666, 2004.

65. Aijaz A, Nelson J, Naseer N: Management of heparin allergy in pregnancy. Am J Hematol 67:268–269, 2001.

66. Parody R, Oliver A, Souto JC, Fontcuberta J: Fondaparinux (Arixtra) as an alternative anti-thrombotic prophylaxis when there is hypersensitivity to low molecular weight and unfractionated heparins. Haematologica 88:ECR32, 2003.

67. Dempfle CE: Minor transplacental passage of fondaparinux in vivo. N Engl J Med 350:1914–1915, 2004.

68. Mazzolai L, Hohlfeld P, Spertini F, et al: Fondaparinux is a safe alternative in case of heparin intolerance during pregnancy. Blood 108:1569–1570, 2006.

69. Lagrange F, Vergnes C, Brun JL, et al: Absence of placental transfer of pentasaccharide (fondaparinux, Arixtra) in the dually perfused human cotyledon in vitro. Thromb Haemost 87:831–835, 2002.

70. Chunilal SD, Young E, Johnston MA, et al: The APTT response of pregnant plasma to unfractionated heparin. Thromb Haemost 87:92–97, 2002.

71. Hirsh J, Raschke R: Heparin and low-molecular-weight heparin: The Seventh ACCP Conference on Antithrombotic and Thrombolytic Therapy. Chest 126 (3 suppl): 188S–203S, 2004.

72. Ginsberg JS, Bates SM: Management of venous thromboembolism during pregnancy. J Thromb Haemost 1:1435–1442, 2003.

73. McColl MD, Greer IA: Low-molecular-weight heparin for the prevention and treatment of venous thromboembolism in pregnancy. Curr Opin Pulm Med 10:371–375, 2004.

74. Barbour LA: ACOG practice bulletin: Thrombembolism in pregnancy. Int J Gynaecol Obstet 75:203–212, 2001.

75. Brill-Edwards P, Ginsberg JS, Gent M, et al: Safety of withholding heparin in pregnant women with a history of venous thromboembolism: Recurrence of clot in this pregnancy study group. N Engl J Med 343:1439–1444, 2000.

76. Pabinger I, Grafenhofer H, Kaider A, et al: Risk of pregnancy-associated recurrent venous thromboembolism in women with a history of venous thrombosis. J Thromb Haemost 3:949–954, 2005.

77. Douketis JD, Kearon C, Bates S, et al: Risk of fatal pulmonary embolism in patients with treated venous thromboembolism. JAMA 279:458–462, 1998.

78. Murin S, Romano PS, White RH: Comparison of outcomes after hospitalization for deep venous thrombosis or pulmonary embolism. Thromb Haemost 88:407–414, 2002.

79. Quinlan DJ, McQuillan A, Eikelboom JW: Low-molecular-weight heparin compared with intravenous unfractionated heparin for treatment of pulmonary embolism: A meta-analysis of randomized, controlled trials. Ann Intern Med 140:175–183, 2004.

80. Gould MK, Dembitzer AD, Doyle RL, et al: Low-molecular-weight heparins compared with unfractionated heparin for treatment of acute deep venous thrombosis: A meta-analysis of randomized, controlled trials. Ann Intern Med 130:800–809, 1999.

81. Merli G, Spiro TE, Olsson CG, et al: Subcutaneous enoxaparin once or twice daily compared with intravenous unfractionated heparin for treatment of venous thromboembolic disease. Ann Intern Med 134:191–202, 2001.

82. Lee AY, Levine MN, Baker RI, et al: Low-molecular-weight heparin versus a coumarin for the prevention of recurrent venous thromboembolism in patients with cancer. N Engl J Med 349:146–153, 2003.

83. Anderson DR, Ginsberg JS, Burrows R, Brill-Edwards P: Subcutaneous heparin therapy during pregnancy: A need for concern at the time of delivery. Thromb Haemost 65:248–250, 1991.

84. Maslovitz S, Many A, Landsberg JA, et al: The safety of low molecular weight heparin therapy during labor. J Matern Fetal Neonatal Med 17:39–43, 2005.

85. Clark SL, Porter TF, West FG: Coumarin derivatives and breast-feeding. Obstet Gynecol 95 (6 Pt 1): 938–940, 2000.

86. Aburahma AF, Mullins DA: Endovascular caval interruption in pregnant patients with deep vein thrombosis of the lower extremity. J Vasc Surg 33:375–378, 2001.

87. Hann CL, Streiff MB: The role of vena caval filters in the management of venous thromboembolism. Blood Rev 19:179–202, 2005.

88. Kawamata K, Chiba Y, Tanaka R, et al: Experience of temporary inferior vena cava filters inserted in the perinatal period to prevent pulmonary embolism in pregnant women with deep vein thrombosis. J Vasc Surg 41:652–656, 2005.

89. Bechtel JJ, Mountford MC, Ellinwood WE: Massive pulmonary embolism in pregnancy treated with catheter fragmentation and local thrombolysis. Obstet Gynecol 106 (5 Pt 2): 1158–1160, 2005.

90. Song JY, Valentino L: A pregnant patient with renal vein thrombosis successfully treated with low-dose thrombolytic therapy: A case report. Am J Obstet Gynecol 192:2073–2075, 2005.

91. Ahearn GS, Hadjiliadis D, Govert JA, Tapson VF: Massive pulmonary embolism during pregnancy successfully treated with recombinant tissue plasminogen activator: A case report and review of treatment options. Arch Intern Med 162:1221–1227, 2002.

92. Johnson DM, Kramer DC, Cohen E, et al: Thrombolytic therapy for acute stroke in late pregnancy with intra-arterial recombinant tissue plasminogen activator. Stroke 36:e53–e55, 2005.

93. Leonhardt G, Gaul C, Nietsch HH, Buerke M: Thrombolytic therapy in pregnancy. J Thromb Thrombolysis 21:271–276, 2006.

94. Stone SE, Morris TA: Pulmonary embolism during and after pregnancy. Crit Care Med 33 (10 suppl): S294–S300, 2005.

95. Wilson WA, Gharavi AE, Koike T, et al: International consensus statement on preliminary classification criteria for definite antiphospholipid syndrome: Report of an international workshop. Arthritis Rheum 42:1309–1311, 1999.

96. Galli M, Luciani D, Bertolini G, Barbui T: Lupus anticoagulants are stronger risk factors for thrombosis than anticardiolipin antibodies in the antiphospholipid syndrome: A systematic review of the literature. Blood 101:1827–1832, 2003.

97. Stone S, Hunt BJ, Khamashta MA, et al: Primary antiphospholipid syndrome in pregnancy: An analysis of outcomes in a cohort of 33 women treated with a rigorous protocol. J Thromb Haemost 3:243–245, 2005.

98. Tincani A, Branch W, Levy RA, et al: Treatment of pregnant patients with antiphospholipid syndrome. Lupus 12:524–529, 2003.

99. Lim W, Crowther MA, Eikelboom JW: Management of antiphospholipid antibody syndrome: A systematic review. JAMA 295:1050–1057, 2006.

100. Lockwood CJ, Romero R, Feinberg RF, et al: The prevalence and biologic significance of lupus anticoagulant and anticardiolipin antibodies in a general obstetric population. Am J Obstet Gynecol 161:369–373, 1989.

101. Lynch A, Byers T, Emlen W, et al: Association of antibodies to beta2-glycoprotein 1 with pregnancy loss and pregnancy-induced hypertension: A prospective study in low-risk pregnancy. Obstet Gynecol 93:193–198, 1999.

102. Pattison NS, Chamley LW, McKay EJ, et al: Antiphospholipid antibodies in pregnancy: Prevalence and clinical associations. Br J Obstet Gynaecol 100:909–913, 1993.

103. Lynch A, Marlar R, Murphy J, et al: Antiphospholipid antibodies in predicting adverse pregnancy outcome: A prospective study. Ann Intern Med 120:470–475, 1994.

104. Yasuda M, Takakuwa K, Tokunaga A, Tanaka K: Prospective studies of the association between anticardiolipin antibody and outcome of pregnancy. Obstet Gynecol 86 (4 Pt 1): 555–559, 1995.

105. Rai RS, Clifford K, Cohen H, Regan L: High prospective fetal loss rate in untreated pregnancies of women with recurrent miscarriage and antiphospholipid antibodies. Hum Reprod 10:3301–3304, 1995.

106. Levine JS, Branch DW, Rauch J: The antiphospholipid syndrome. N Engl J Med 346:752–763, 2002.

107. Ogunyemi D, Cuellar F, Ku W, Arkel Y: Association between inherited thrombophilias, antiphospholipid antibodies, and lipoprotein A levels and venous thromboembolism in pregnancy. Am J Perinatol 20:17–24, 2003.

108. Galli M, Finazzi G, Duca F, et al: The G1691 → A mutation of factor V, but not the G20210 → A mutation of factor II or the C677 → T mutation of methylenetetrahydrofolate reductase genes, is associated with venous thrombosis in patients with lupus anticoagulants. Br J Haematol 108:865–870, 2000.

109. Hansen KE, Kong DF, Moore KD, Ortel TL: Risk factors associated with thrombosis in patients with antiphospholipid antibodies. J Rheumatol 28:2018–2024, 2001.

110. Derksen RH, Khamashta MA, Branch DW: Management of the obstetric antiphospholipid syndrome. Arthritis Rheum 50:1028–1039, 2004.

111. Empson M, Lassere M, Craig JC, Scott JR: Recurrent pregnancy loss with antiphospholipid antibody: A systematic review of therapeutic trials. Obstet Gynecol 99:135–144, 2002.

112. Rai R, Cohen H, Dave M, Regan L: Randomised controlled trial of aspirin and aspirin plus heparin in pregnant women with recurrent miscarriage associated with phospholipid antibodies (or antiphospholipid antibodies). BMJ 314:253–257, 1997.

113. Kutteh WH: Antiphospholipid antibody–associated recurrent pregnancy loss: Treatment with heparin and low-dose aspirin is superior to low-dose aspirin alone. Am J Obstet Gynecol 174:1584–1589, 1996.

114. Kutteh WH, Ermel LD: A clinical trial for the treatment of antiphospholipid antibody–associated recurrent pregnancy loss with lower dose heparin and aspirin. Am J Reprod Immunol 35:402–407, 1996.

115. Farquharson RG, Quenby S, Greaves M: Antiphospholipid syndrome in pregnancy: A randomized, controlled trial of treatment. Obstet Gynecol 100:408–413, 2002.

116. Noble LS, Kutteh WH, Lashey N, et al: Antiphospholipid antibodies associated with recurrent pregnancy loss: Prospective, multicenter, controlled pilot study comparing treatment with low-molecular-weight heparin versus unfractionated heparin. Fertil Steril 83:684–690, 2005.

117. Ruffatti A, Favaro M, Tonello M, et al: Efficacy and safety of nadroparin in the treatment of pregnant women with antiphospholipid syndrome: A prospective cohort study. Lupus 14:120–128, 2005.

118. Triolo G, Ferrante A, Ciccia F, et al: Randomized study of subcutaneous low molecular weight heparin plus aspirin versus intravenous immunoglobulin in the treatment of recurrent fetal loss associated with antiphospholipid antibodies. Arthritis Rheum 48:728–731, 2003.

119. ACOG Practice Bulletin: Management of recurrent pregnancy loss. Number 24, February 2001. (Replaces Technical Bulletin Number 212, September 1995). American College of Obstetricians and Gynecologists. Int J Gynaecol Obstet 78:179–190, 2002.

120. Erkan D, Merrill JT, Yazici Y, et al: High thrombosis rate after fetal loss in antiphospholipid syndrome: Effective prophylaxis with aspirin. Arthritis Rheum 44:1466–1467, 2001.

121. Buller HR, Agnelli G, Hull RD, et al: Antithrombotic therapy for venous thromboembolic disease: The Seventh ACCP Conference on Antithrombotic and Thrombolytic Therapy. Chest 126 (3 suppl): 401S–428S, 2004.

122. Schulman S, Svenungsson E, Granqvist S: Anticardiolipin antibodies predict early recurrence of thromboembolism and death among patients with venous thromboembolism following anticoagulant therapy. Duration of Anticoagulation Study Group. Am J Med 104:332–338, 1998.

123. Finazzi G, Marchioli R, Brancaccio V, et al: A randomized clinical trial of high-intensity warfarin vs. conventional antithrombotic therapy for the prevention of recurrent thrombosis in patients with the antiphospholipid syndrome (WAPS). J Thromb Haemost 3:848–853, 2005.

124. Crowther MA, Ginsberg JS, Julian J, et al: A comparison of two intensities of warfarin for the prevention of recurrent thrombosis in patients with the antiphospholipid antibody syndrome. N Engl J Med 349:1133–1138, 2003.

125. Branch DW, Silver RM, Blackwell JL, et al: Outcome of treated pregnancies in women with antiphospholipid syndrome: An update of the Utah experience. Obstet Gynecol 80:614–620, 1992.

126. Lima F, Khamashta MA, Buchanan NM, et al: A study of sixty pregnancies in patients with the antiphospholipid syndrome. Clin Exp Rheumatol 14:131–136, 1996.

127. Branch DW, Andres R, Digre KB, et al: The association of antiphospholipid antibodies with severe preeclampsia. Obstet Gynecol 73:541–545, 1989.

128. Dreyfus M, Hedelin G, Kutnahorsky R, et al: Antiphospholipid antibodies and preeclampsia: A case-control study. Obstet Gynecol 97:29–34, 2001.

129. Lee RM, Brown MA, Branch DW, et al: Anticardiolipin and anti–beta2-glycoprotein-I antibodies in preeclampsia. Obstet Gynecol 102:294–300, 2003.

36

130. Branch DW, Porter TF, Rittenhouse L, et al: Antiphospholipid antibodies in women at risk for preeclampsia. Am J Obstet Gynecol 184:825–832, 2001; discussion 832–834.

131. Backos M, Rai R, Baxter N, et al: Pregnancy complications in women with recurrent miscarriage associated with antiphospholipid antibodies treated with low dose aspirin and heparin. Br J Obstet Gynaecol 106:102–107, 1999.

132. Bats AS, Lejeune V, Cynober E, et al: Antiphospholipid syndrome and second- or third-trimester fetal death: Follow-up in the next pregnancy. Eur J Obstet Gynecol Reprod Biol 114:125–129, 2004.

133. Branch DW, Khamashta MA: Antiphospholipid syndrome: Obstetric diagnosis, management, and controversies. Obstet Gynecol 101:1333–1344, 2003.

134. Jaigobin C, Silver FL: Stroke and pregnancy. Stroke 31:2948–2951, 2000.

135. Kittner SJ, Stern BJ, Feeser BR, et al: Pregnancy and the risk of stroke. N Engl J Med 335:768–774, 1996.

136. Sharshar T, Lamy C, Mas JL: Incidence and causes of strokes associated with pregnancy and puerperium: A study in public hospitals of Ile de France. Stroke in Pregnancy Study Group. Stroke 26:930–936, 1995.

137. James AH, Bushnell CD, Jamison MG, Myers ER: Incidence and risk factors for stroke in pregnancy and the puerperium. Obstet Gynecol 106:509–516, 2005.

138. Jeng JS, Tang SC, Yip PK: Stroke in women of reproductive age: Comparison between stroke related and unrelated to pregnancy. J Neurol Sci 221:25–29, 2004.

139. Helms AK, Kittner SJ: Pregnancy and stroke. CNS Spectr 10:580–587, 2005.

140. Agostoni P, Gasparini G, Destro G: Acute myocardial infarction probably caused by paradoxical embolus in a pregnant woman. Heart 90:e12, 2004.

141. Kozelj M, Novak-Antolic Z, Grad A, Peternel P: Patent foramen ovale as a potential cause of paradoxical embolism in the postpartum period. Eur J Obstet Gynecol Reprod Biol 84:55–57, 1999.

142. Giberti L, Bino G, Tanganelli P: Pregnancy, patent foramen ovale and stroke: A case of pseudoperipheral facial palsy. Neurol Sci 26:43–45, 2005.

143. Elford K, Leader A, Wee R, Stys PK: Stroke in ovarian hyperstimulation syndrome in early pregnancy treated with intra-arterial rt-PA. Neurology 59:1270–1272, 2002.

144. Albers GW, Amarenco P, Easton JD, et al: Antithrombotic and thrombolytic therapy for ischemic stroke: The Seventh ACCP Conference on Antithrombotic and Thrombolytic Therapy. Chest 126 (3 suppl): 483S–512S, 2004.

145. Sacco RL, Adams R, Albers G, et al: Guidelines for prevention of stroke in patients with ischemic stroke or transient ischemic attack: A statement for healthcare professionals from the American Heart Association/American Stroke Association Council on Stroke. Co-sponsored by the Council on Cardiovascular Radiology and Intervention. (The American Academy of Neurology affirms the value of this guideline.) Stroke 37:577–617, 2006.

146. Coppage KH, Hinton AC, Moldenhauer J, et al: Maternal and perinatal outcome in women with a history of stroke. Am J Obstet Gynecol 190:1331–1334, 2004.

147. Lamy C, Hamon JB, Coste J, Mas JL: Ischemic stroke in young women: Risk of recurrence during subsequent pregnancies. French Study Group on Stroke in Pregnancy. Neurology 55:269–274, 2000.

148. Kupferminc MJ, Eldor A, Steinman N, et al: Increased frequency of genetic thrombophilia in women with complications of pregnancy. N Engl J Med 340:9–13, 1999.

149. Brenner B: Inherited thrombophilia and pregnancy loss. Thromb Haemost 82:634–640, 1999.

150. Lissalde-Lavigne G, Fabbro-Peray P, Cochery-Nouvellon E, et al: Factor V Leiden and prothrombin G20210A polymorphisms as risk factors for miscarriage during a first intended pregnancy: The matched case-control 'NOHA first' study. J Thromb Haemost 3:2178–2184, 2005.

151. Brenner B, Sarig G, Weiner Z, et al: Thrombophilic polymorphisms are common in women with fetal loss without apparent cause. Thromb Haemost 82:6–9, 1999.

152. Ridker PM, Miletich JP, Buring JE, et al: Factor V Leiden mutation as a risk factor for recurrent pregnancy loss. Ann Intern Med 128 (12 Pt 1): 1000–1003, 1998.

153. Martinelli I, Taioli E, Cetin I, et al: Mutations in coagulation factors in women with unexplained late fetal loss. N Engl J Med 343:1015–1018, 2000.

154. Gris JC, Quere I, Monpeyroux F, et al: Case-control study of the frequency of thrombophilic disorders in couples with late foetal loss and no thrombotic antecedent—The Nimes Obstetricians and Haematologists Study 5 (NOHA5). Thromb Haemost 81:891–899, 1999.

155. Volzke H, Grimm R, Robinson DM, et al: Factor V Leiden and the risk of stillbirth in a German population. Thromb Haemost 90:429–433, 2003.

156. Kutteh WH, Park VM, Deitcher SR: Hypercoagulable state mutation analysis in white patients with early first-trimester recurrent pregnancy loss. Fertil Steril 71:1048–1053, 1999.

157. Alfirevic Z, Mousa HA, Martlew V, et al: Postnatal screening for thrombophilia in women with severe pregnancy complications. Obstet Gynecol 97 (5 Pt 1): 753–759, 2001.

158. Foka ZJ, Lambropoulos AF, Saravelos H, et al: Factor V leiden and prothrombin G20210A mutations, but not methylenetetrahydrofolate reductase C677T, are associated with recurrent miscarriages. Hum Reprod 15:458–462, 2000.

159. Reznikoff-Etievan MF, Cayol V, Carbonne B, et al: Factor V Leiden and G20210A prothrombin mutations are risk factors for very early recurrent miscarriage. Br J Obstet Gynaecol 108:1251–1254, 2001.

160. Raziel A, Kornberg Y, Friedler S, et al: Hypercoagulable thrombophilic defects and hyperhomocysteinemia in patients with recurrent pregnancy loss. Am J Reprod Immunol 45:65–71, 2001.

161. Souza SS, Ferriani RA, Pontes AG, et al: Factor V leiden and factor II G20210A mutations in patients with recurrent abortion. Hum Reprod 14:2448–2450, 1999.

162. Pihusch R, Buchholz T, Lohse P, et al: Thrombophilic gene mutations and recurrent spontaneous abortion: Prothrombin mutation increases the risk in the first trimester. Am J Reprod Immunol 46: 124–131, 2001.

163. Rey E, Kahn SR, David M, Shrier I: Thrombophilic disorders and fetal loss: A meta-analysis. Lancet 361:901–908, 2003.

164. Kovalevsky G, Gracia CR, Berlin JA, et al: Evaluation of the association between hereditary thrombophilias and recurrent pregnancy loss: A meta-analysis. Arch Intern Med 164:558–563, 2004.

165. Dudding TE, Attia J: The association between adverse pregnancy outcomes and maternal factor V Leiden genotype: A meta-analysis. Thromb Haemost 91:700–711, 2004.

166. Preston FE, Rosendaal FR, Walker ID, et al: Increased fetal loss in women with heritable thrombophilia. Lancet 348:913–916, 1996.

167. Sanson BJ, Friederich PW, Simioni P, et al: The risk of abortion and stillbirth in antithrombin-, protein C–, and protein S–deficient women. Thromb Haemost 75:387–388, 1996.

168. Vossen CY, Preston FE, Conard J, et al: Hereditary thrombophilia and fetal loss: A prospective follow-up study. J Thromb Haemost 2:592–596, 2004.

169. Gris JC, Perneger TV, Quere I, et al: Antiphospholipid/antiprotein antibodies, hemostasis-related autoantibodies, and plasma homocysteine as risk factors for a first early pregnancy loss: A matched case-control study. Blood 102:3504–3513, 2003.

170. Fatini C, Gensini F, Battaglini B, et al: Angiotensin-converting enzyme DD genotype, angiotensin type 1 receptor CC genotype, and hyperhomocysteinemia increase first-trimester fetal-loss susceptibility. Blood Coagul Fibrinolysis 11:657–662, 2000.

171. Nelen WL, Blom HJ, Steegers EA, et al: Homocysteine and folate levels as risk factors for recurrent early pregnancy loss. Obstet Gynecol 95:519–524, 2000.

172. Nelen WL, Blom HJ, Steegers EA, et al: Hyperhomocysteinemia and recurrent early pregnancy loss: A meta-analysis. Fertil Steril 74:1196–1199, 2000.

173. Murphy RP, Donoghue C, Nallen RJ, et al: Prospective evaluation of the risk conferred by factor V Leiden and thermolabile methylenetetrahydrofolate reductase polymorphisms in pregnancy. Arterioscler Thromb Vasc Biol 20:266–270, 2000.

174. Alonso A, Soto I, Urgelles MF, et al: Acquired and inherited thrombophilia in women with unexplained fetal losses. Am J Obstet Gynecol 187:1337–1342, 2002.

175. Sarig G, Younis JS, Hoffman R, et al: Thrombophilia is common in women with idiopathic pregnancy loss and is associated with late pregnancy wastage. Fertil Steril 77:342–347, 2002.

176. Tormene D, Simioni P, Prandoni P, et al: The risk of fetal loss in family members of probands with factor V Leiden mutation. Thromb Haemost 82:1237–1239, 1999.

177. Tal J, Schliamser LM, Leibovitz Z, et al: A possible role for activated protein C resistance in patients with first and second trimester pregnancy failure. Hum Reprod 14:1624–1627, 1999.

178. Grandone E, Margaglione M, Colaizzo D, et al: Prothrombotic genetic risk factors and the occurrence of gestational hypertension with or without proteinuria. Thromb Haemost 81:349–352, 1999.

179. Kupferminc MJ, Fait G, Many A, et al: Severe preeclampsia and high frequency of genetic thrombophilic mutations. Obstet Gynecol 96:45–49, 2000.

180. De Maat MP, Jansen MW, Hille ET, et al: Preeclampsia and its interaction with common variants in thrombophilia genes. J Thromb Haemost 2:1588–1593, 2004.

181. Morrison ER, Miedzybrodzka ZH, Campbell DM, et al: Prothrombotic genotypes are not associated with pre-eclampsia and gestational hypertension: Results from a large population-based study and systematic review. Thromb Haemost 87:779–785, 2002.

182. Mello G, Parretti E, Marozio L, et al: Thrombophilia is significantly associated with severe preeclampsia: Results of a large-scale, case-controlled study. Hypertension 46:1270–1274, 2005.

183. Grandone E, Margaglione M, Colaizzo D, et al: Factor V Leiden, C > T MTHFR polymorphism and genetic susceptibility to pre-eclampsia. Thromb Haemost 77:1052–1054, 1997.

184. Kosmas IP, Tatsioni A, Ioannidis JP: Association of Leiden mutation in factor V gene with hypertension in pregnancy and pre-eclampsia: A meta-analysis. J Hypertens 21:1221–1228, 2003.

185. Lin J, August P: Genetic thrombophilias and preeclampsia: A meta-analysis. Obstet Gynecol 105:182–192, 2005.

186. Alfirevic Z, Roberts D, Martlew V: How strong is the association between maternal thrombophilia and adverse pregnancy outcome? A systematic review. Eur J Obstet Gynecol Reprod Biol 101:6–14, 2002.

187. Gerhardt A, Goecke TW, Beckmann MW, et al: The G20210A prothrombin-gene mutation and the plasminogen activator inhibitor (PAI-1) 5G/5G genotype are associated with early onset of severe preeclampsia. J Thromb Haemost 3:686–691, 2005.

188. Cotter AM, Molloy AM, Scott JM, Daly SF: Elevated plasma homocysteine in early pregnancy: A risk factor for the development of severe preeclampsia. Am J Obstet Gynecol 185:781–785, 2001.

189. Cotter AM, Molloy AM, Scott JM, Daly SF: Elevated plasma homocysteine in early pregnancy: A risk factor for the development of nonsevere preeclampsia. Am J Obstet Gynecol 189:391–394, 2003; discussion 394–396.

190. Howley HE, Walker M, Rodger MA: A systematic review of the association between factor V Leiden or prothrombin gene variant and intrauterine growth restriction. Am J Obstet Gynecol 192:694–708, 2005.

191. Infante-Rivard C, Rivard GE, Yotov WV, et al: Absence of association of thrombophilia polymorphisms with intrauterine growth restriction. N Engl J Med 347:19–25, 2002.

192. Wiener-Megnagi Z, Ben-Shlomo I, Goldberg Y, Shalev E: Resistance to activated protein C and the Leiden mutation: High prevalence in patients with abruptio placentae. Am J Obstet Gynecol 179 (6 Pt 1): 1565–1567, 1998.

193. Vollset SE, Refsum H, Irgens LM, et al: Plasma total homocysteine, pregnancy complications, and adverse pregnancy outcomes: The Hordaland Homocysteine study. Am J Clin Nutr 71:962–968, 2000.

194. Facchinetti F, Marozio L, Grandone E, et al: Thrombophilic mutations are a main risk factor for placental abruption. Haematologica 88:785–788, 2003.

195. Prochazka M, Happach C, Marsal K, et al: Factor V Leiden in pregnancies complicated by placental abruption. Br J Obstet Gynaecol 110:462–466, 2003.

196. Brenner B, Hoffman R, Blumenfeld Z, et al: Gestational outcome in thrombophilic women with recurrent pregnancy loss treated by enoxaparin. Thromb Haemost 83:693–697, 2000.

197. Carp H, Dolitzky M, Inbal A: Thromboprophylaxis improves the live birth rate in women with consecutive recurrent miscarriages and hereditary thrombophilia. J Thromb Haemost 1:433–438, 2003.

198. Gris JC, Mercier E, Quere I, et al: Low-molecular-weight heparin versus low-dose aspirin in women with one fetal loss and a constitutional thrombophilic disorder. Blood 103:3695–3699, 2004.

199. Brenner B, Hoffman R, Carp H, et al: Efficacy and safety of two doses of enoxaparin in women with thrombophilia and recurrent pregnancy loss: The LIVE-ENOX study. J Thromb Haemost 3:227–229, 2005.

200. Quere I, Mercier E, Bellet H, et al: Vitamin supplementation and pregnancy outcome in women with recurrent early pregnancy loss and hyperhomocysteinemia. Fertil Steril 75:823–825, 2001.

201. Grandone E, Brancaccio V, Colaizzo D, et al: Preventing adverse obstetric outcomes in women with genetic thrombophilia. Fertil Steril 78:371–375, 2002.

202. Riyazi N, Leeda M, de Vries JI, et al: Low-molecular-weight heparin combined with aspirin in pregnant women with thrombophilia and a history of preeclampsia or fetal growth restriction: A preliminary study. Eur J Obstet Gynecol Reprod Biol 80:49–54, 1998.

203. Kupferminc MJ, Fait G, Many A, et al: Low-molecular-weight heparin for the prevention of obstetric complications in women with thrombophilias. Hypertens Pregnancy 20:35–44, 2001.

204. Brenner B, Bar J, Ellis M, et al: Effects of enoxaparin on late pregnancy complications and neonatal outcome in women with recurrent pregnancy loss and thrombophilia: Results from the LIVE-ENOX study. Fertil Steril 84:770–773, 2005.

205. Wu O, Robertson L, Twaddle S, et al: Screening for thrombophilia in high-risk situations: A meta-analysis and cost-effectiveness analysis. Br J Haematol 131:80–90, 2005.

Part VI

Special Issues

Chapter 37

Surgery and Hemostasis

Craig S. Kitchens, MD

By observing and studying the effects of surgery and trauma on hemostasis—including physiologic as well as hypocoagulable and hypercoagulable situations—our understanding of the interrelationship between hemostasis and surgery has been advanced.

The following topics will be addressed in this chapter:

- Surgery for patients with congenital hemostatic defects
- The effects of surgery on hemostasis (with particular reference to cardiopulmonary bypass and orthotopic liver transplantation)
- Preoperative hemostatic testing
- Invasive procedures for patients with abnormal coagulation tests
- Invasive procedures for patients on anticoagulant therapy
- Consultation on patients with intraoperative or postoperative hemorrhage

Blood coagulation exists to halt excessive blood loss. It is paradoxical that surgery and trauma simultaneously represent major risk factors for both hemorrhagic and thrombotic complications. Although Kearon and Hirsh estimated that surgery and trauma increase the baseline risk of thrombosis up to a hundred-fold,[1] patients with mild hemophilia who have never bled from stresses of everyday life may bleed vigorously from surgical procedures.[2]

The history of the discovery of blood coagulation has been well reviewed by Ratnoff,[3] whereas the maturation of our understanding of and management of traumatic and surgical wounds has been reviewed thoroughly by Majno.[4] The concept of pressure dressings and ligature of blood vessels to control excessive bleeding was not described until 300 to 200 BC by physicians in Alexandria. It was not until the 18th century that the French surgeon Petit deduced that the clotting of blood had something to do with the control of hemorrhage following surgery; before that time, it was believed that constriction and retraction of vessels were the only mechanisms of hemostasis.[4] Not until the end of the 19th century did Wright observe that blood from hemophiliacs clotted more slowly than normal blood and that perhaps this observation was causally related to the hemorrhage characteristics of hemophilia.[3]

SURGERY FOR PATIENTS WITH CONGENITAL HEMOSTATIC DEFECTS

That hemophiliacs bleed abnormally has been known since antiquity.[5] Because uncontrolled bleeding occurred in the hemophiliac's daily life, surgical procedures were generally avoided. Any surgery that was performed on hemophiliacs was usually done as a heroic measure; the results were expectedly disastrous and many patients bled to death.

Transfusion science was essentially nonexistent until World War II. Whole blood was available for hemophiliacs but it is now clear that although whole blood improved the hematocrit value, it was unable to raise the level of either factor VIII or factor IX by more than about 10% to 20%. With the development of blood banking following World War II, acute surgical hemorrhagic mortality dropped from 50% before any blood banking to about 25%. Cryoprecipitate was discovered by Dr. Judith Pool in the 1960s, allowing factor VIII levels to reach briefly any level desired. Hemorrhagic mortality dropped to 2%. After factor VIII and factor IX concentrates became available in the 1970s, factor VIII and factor IX levels could be raised to any level desired, theoretically indefinitely, and surgical mortality approached zero.[6] Patients still experience nonfatal hemorrhage at an overall rate of approximately 18%.[6–9] Elective diagnostic procedures such as liver biopsy have been reported to be both safe and effective in directing subsequent therapeutic decision making.[10–12]

Extracorporeal shock-wave lithotripsy (ESWL) can be performed safely using factor replacement levels of 50% to 60% before the treatments and for 3 to 5 days posttreatment. As in normal patients undergoing ESWL, hematuria is common, but serious (capsular or retroperitoneal) hematomas were not encountered in a series of 11 hemophiliacs so managed.[13]

Factor levels should be maintained in the patient undergoing surgery as high and as long as indicated. The prescribed factor is infused the morning prior to surgery and the factor level is measured before anesthesia induction to confirm that the factor has been appropriately administered and that no unexpectedly low increment of factor resulted (i.e., less than about 60% calculated), which could be the first and only sign of an occult inhibitor.

For fairly minor surgical procedures (including procedures such as endoscopy with biopsy, arthroscopic surgery, skin or breast biopsies, lymph node biopsies, and complicated dental work), the factor level is customarily kept at a "trough" of approximately 30% and a "peak" of about 60% for 3 to 4 days, with longer amounts being necessary if there is significant traction along the incision line. For more invasive surgery such as open abdominal or orthopedic surgery and particularly cardiovascular or neurologic surgery, a targeted "trough" concentration of 80% with a "peak" of 150% is advised. Although these levels are clearly higher than physiologically required for hemostasis, the higher levels provide a cushion for missed doses or other logistic problems. "Peak and trough" levels are followed once a day for several days and can probably be gradually lowered as surgical hemostasis becomes more secure after about the fourth or fifth day. Most hemostatic wounds are well healed from a hemostatic point of view by the fourth or fifth day and, therefore, after that time factor levels can be allowed to drift down to about one half the levels required at the time of surgery. The most notable exceptions to these are procedures that are characterized by significant tension along the incision line such as open abdominal operations or operations through the muscles of posture (e.g., nephrectomy position). Therapy is often quite prolonged at a slightly lower level (50% to 60%) following major orthopedic surgery during rehabilitation and aggressive physical therapy. Otherwise, we rarely give factor longer than 7 to 10 days following surgical procedures. Table 37-1 provides general guidelines for surgical procedures in hemophiliacs.

If one wishes to use continuous infusion of factor concentrates, a more even level of factor concentration results with less severe peaks and troughs. Less factor administration is possible and overall costs are decreased as less factor is consumed. Therapeutic levels closer to 60% to 70% are sufficient accordingly.[14,15]

Cardiovascular surgery can be done successfully in hemophiliacs. Best results are obtained if the surgeons, anesthesiologists, and perfusion technicians all use their routine protocols based on the dictum that a hemophiliac with near 100% replacement therapy can and should undergo diagnostic and therapeutic cardiac catheterization receiving heparin, protamine, and aprotinin as would any other patient. Monitoring the appropriate factor concentration, probably best managed by the hematologist so that others can focus on their tasks, is the only difference.[16,17] An advantage of placing bioprosthetic heart valves in those patients requiring valve replacement is that the dilemma presented by the chronic use of warfarin postoperatively can be avoided. The use of aspirin chronically for ischemic heart disease is uncertain and must be approached on a case-by-case basis,[17] although its low-dose (81 mg/day orally) use following coronary artery bypass grafting (CABG) appears rational and safe.

In the rarer contact factor deficiencies (factor XII, high-molecular-weight kininogen, and prekallikrein), replacement therapy for surgery is not indicated. In order to monitor adequate heparin levels during cardiopulmonary bypass, the patient's baseline activated clotting time (ACT) cannot be used because it is 600 to 800 seconds before heparin infusion and is not "corrected" by factor replacement therapy. Davidson and coworkers successfully used heparin levels to monitor a patient with such a deficiency and also documented typical levels of thrombin generation during the CABG despite the inherited defect.[18] It is essential to discuss with the surgeon (or other clinicians) that during treatment, hemostasis will be normal and, therefore, the surgical procedure should be carried out as completely and fully as it would be in a normal patient.

Bleeding may be more obstinate following oral surgical procedures or following prostate surgery because of profibrinolytic agents in saliva and urine that bathe the wounds dissolving hemostatic clots. For patients undergoing either prostate or oral surgery, an antifibrinolytic agent (ϵ-aminocaproic acid, [EACA], 2 g every 8 hours orally, or tranexamic acid, 20 mg/kg orally every 8 hours for approximately a week) helps prevent otherwise stable clots from being lysed.[19] These agents can be administered intravenously for patients taking nothing by mouth.

Special attention may be required in patients with von Willebrand disease (VWD) (see Chapter 7) undergoing invasive procedures. In patients undergoing fairly minor procedures (such as dental procedures, colonoscopies, arthroscopic examinations, and most biopsies) DDAVP, 0.3 μg/kg intravenously, suffices for patients with type 1 VWD. This dose of DDAVP can be given daily or twice daily for about 3 days before the agent typically becomes ineffective because of tachyphylaxis. Hyponatremia can be troubling and can cause seizures; accordingly, free water intake must be minimized during DDAVP therapy. However, this brief period usually suffices for hemostasis with such procedures. Antifibrinolytic agents in doses mentioned earlier are advised concomitantly for mucosal procedures.

In patients with type 2 or type 3 VWD or in patients with type 1 VWD who are undergoing more extensive procedures requiring hemostatic control longer than the 3 days that can be provided by DDAVP, factor VIII concentrates (Alphanate or Humate P) containing von Willebrand factor (VWF) work well. Cryoprecipitate is an effective agent and should be considered in certain settings. Many clinicians have noticed that it is much easier to correct the factor VIII clotting activity or VWF level to desirable levels (i.e., 30% to 50% or higher) than it is to correct the bleeding time or platelet function assay (PFA). Most experts have deduced that it is preferable to monitor the factor VIII activity or VWF level rather than the bleeding time or PFA because typically neither of the latter two tests correct with otherwise appropriate therapy and failure of the bleeding time or PFA to correct does not predict bleeding.[20,21,22]

Table 37-1   Guidelines for Successful Surgery in Patients with Congenital Hemostatic Disorders

- Establish the correct hemostatic diagnosis
- Confirm the inhibitor, hepatitis, and human immunodeficiency virus status of the patient
- Assume that surgical indications are the same as those in hemostatically normal patients
- Develop and follow a surgical plan
- Consult with the blood bank concerning logistics
- Expose patient to minimal amount of factor lot numbers
- Consult with the anesthesiologist
- Prohibit intramuscular medications, especially preoperatively
- Avoid aspirin, aspirin-containing medications, and other platelet-inhibiting medications
- Determine and administer the appropriate preoperative clotting factor dosage, and measure the plasma level before induction of anesthesia
- Monitor appropriate hemostatic tests frequently
- Sustain a hemostatic level of the patient's deficient factor as long as needed by repeated intravenous infusions of the appropriate agent
- Consider whether adjunctive agents, e.g., antifibrinolytic drugs or hypotensive anesthesia, might enhance hemostasis

For patients with inhibitors who need surgery, it is advisable to be cautious, especially regarding elective surgery. Refer to Chapter 6 for general comments regarding hemorrhage in patients who have inhibitors. Porcine factor VIII has been effectively employed for hemostasis[23] as has activated prothrombin complex concentrate (FEIBA).[24] Typical doses are an initial IV bolus infusion of 100 IU/kg followed by 50 IU/kg every 8 to 12 hours. There is no laboratory test to monitor for efficacy. Recombinant factor VIIa (NovoSeven)[25] has proved effective for surgical procedures in patients with factor VIII or factor IX inhibitors, usually infused initially at 90 μg/kg intravenously every 2 to 3 hours for 48 hours followed by dose reduction during a total of 5 days of treatment.[26,27,28] No laboratory testing is agreed on as being highly effective to monitor therapy.

EFFECT OF SURGERY ON HEMOSTASIS

Large-vessel hemorrhage (in general, named arteries or veins) tends to require physical methods such as cautery, pressure, ligature, or tamponade to control blood loss, whereas microcirculatory hemorrhage depends on an intact hemostatic system. Tissue factor (TF) is released from damaged blood vessels and with native plasma activated factor VII vigorously initiates the extrinsic arm of the coagulation system.[29,30] Thrombin generation should be sufficient that enough platelets are stimulated to adhere to denuded areas of the open endothelium and then recruit, through release of their attractants, enough platelets to begin aggregation to breach the leak. Any compromise in this elaborate system, such as a factor deficiency, thrombocytopenia, or excessive anticoagulation therapy might well result in hemorrhage. This schema physiologically regains hemostatic control of an open vascular system, yet may potentially result in an equally devastating thrombotic condition if not properly controlled.

Thrombotic Signals as a Result of Surgery

Initiators of coagulation include TF and other cytokines, particularly tumor necrosis factor (TNF) and interleukin 6 (IL-6) if inflammation or infection are present.[31,32] These cytokines rapidly accelerate the extrinsic system. Tissue destruction and TF release also occur in medical situations such as myocardial infarction,[33] sepsis,[34] and malignancy (see Chapters 15 and 23). During the first several hours following surgery or significant trauma, there is an increase to approximately twice normal in circulating tissue plasminogen activator (tPA) levels and a rapid decrease toward normal levels by the end of the first 24 hours. Beginning approximately 2 hours after trauma, levels of plasminogen activator inhibitor type I (PAI-1) begin to rapidly rise, approaching levels 4 to 5 times normal, and then gradually decrease over a day or so—only to have a secondary peak at about day seven.[31,32,35,36] During that period, these high levels of PAI-1 dampen the fibrinolytic system, a process that has been termed "fibrinolytic shutdown."[35] Of interest, it has been observed that warfarin administration dampens the increase in the PAI-1 reflex and thus may attenuate fibrinolytic shutdown which could explain, in part, its net antithrombotic effect.[37]

While thrombin is being generated, antithrombin III is consumed as it neutralizes thrombin by forming thrombin: antithrombin (TAT) III complexes.[38] Antithrombin III levels acutely can become severely reduced during surgery, particularly with trauma and especially after burns.[39]

Levels of these mediators fluctuate rapidly and their degree of perturbation as measured by static laboratory tests will be a function not only of the type, degree, and duration of trauma, but also of the timing of blood sample collection. Experimental evidence in reproducible trauma in animals validates that graduated degrees of trauma result in graduated degrees of hypercoagulability.[40]

Shock and stasis often follow trauma. Stasis and venodilation may be induced in surgery by various anesthetic agents. General anesthetics cause more systemic venostasis than local anesthetics used in epidural anesthesia. General anesthesia is associated with higher levels of PAI-1 generation 24 hours after the surgery and a higher incidence of thrombosis when compared in a controlled manner with patients undergoing the same procedure using epidural anesthesia. These higher levels of PAI-1 correlated well with subsequent thrombosis.[41] Hamer and colleagues[41a] demonstrated that venous stasis is associated with hypoxia in venous valve pockets and may account in part for these pockets serving as loci of thrombosis generation. In endothelial cell cultures, hypoxia is associated with release of P-selectin from the endothelial cells, which may contribute to local inflammation.[41b] Comerota and colleagues[42] studied the degree of venodilation of arm veins in patients undergoing total hip replacement. In patients who experienced a postoperative DVT, the mean degree of venous dilation was 29% over presurgical diameters, whereas the mean dilation of those who did not experience DVT was only 12%. All patients who experienced more than 20% dilation of their arm veins experienced a DVT. Venodilation created "microtears" in the endothelial lining that exposed underlying collagen and may very well have served as the nidus or trigger for thrombosis associated with surgery.

One of the newer concepts in the initiation and perpetuation of thrombosis involves "microparticles." Microparticles (MP) are of ubiquitous origin, derived from the membranes of platelets, erythrocytes, leukocytes, and endothelial cells.[43] They are present in normal human blood but they increase in response to several disease states, trauma, and surgery.[44-47] By virtue of their high surface-to-volume ratios they act as effective portages for various mediators such as TF, components of platelet membrane receptors, VWF, and other constituents[47-49] that seem active in stimulation, proliferation, and apoptosis of various cells.[50] Our understanding of this new area in vascular physiology, disease, and injury will rapidly proliferate. These theories of surgically induced hypercoagulability are listed in Table 37-2.

Various other situations and events might have an impact on the effects of surgery on hemostasis and thrombosis. In major orthopedic surgery, epidural anesthesia seems to result in comparatively less hypercoagulability than does general anesthesia.[51,52] The use of tourniquets in total knee replacement seems to lessen the hypercoagulability while increasing the net fibrinolysis in that operation when compared with not using a tourniquet.[53] Boldt and colleagues[54] deduced that there was no net difference between use of normal saline or lactated Ringer's solution as replacement strategies with respect to input on hemostasis. Coronary artery bypass graft (CABG) appears less

Table 37-2 Putative Causes of Hypercoagulability in Surgery and Trauma

- Generation of large amounts of procoagulant factors
- Generation of high concentrations of PAI-1 ("fibrinolytic shutdown")
- Venous stasis with venous valve pocket hypoxia
- Pooling of blood
- Venous microtears
- Microparticles

PAI-1, plasminogen activator inhibitor-1.

hypercoagulable when performed on-pump rather than off-pump according to Quigley and colleagues.[55] The use of hetastarch was found to be associated with increased post-CABG hemorrhage in a dose-response manner.[56] Mild hypothermia (32° C to 36° C) did not affect hemostasis in one study[57] but more severe and prolonged hypothermia,[58] as well as acidosis, grossly impeded hemostasis (see Chapter 46). In a recent randomized trial, normothermic off-pump CABG resulted in less hemorrhage and fewer transfused blood products than did relative hypothermia.[59] It is of interest that harboring the gene for factor V Leiden mutation is correlated with decreased blood loss in cardiopulmonary bypass (CPB).[60]

White and associates[61] have prepared a useful database regarding varying degrees of apparent hypercoagulability of various surgical procedures, demonstrating the higher incidence of thrombosis following vascular, orthopedic, and central nervous system parenchymal surgeries compared with a lower incidence following minor orthopedic, urologic, and head and neck surgery cases.

Prophylaxis Against Thrombosis

Prophylaxis against DVT and pulmonary embolism (PE) are discussed thoroughly in Chapter 14, as well as in a recent consensus.[62] The role of mechanical and similar adjuncts in prophylaxis against venous thromboembolism (VTE) verifies their use. Westrich[63] demonstrated that intermittent pneumatic compression (IPC) in total knee replacement surgery was, in their hands, more effective than low molecular weight heparin (LMWH) and far more effective than aspirin alone in reducing both DVT and PE. However, they did note only a 33% compliance rate with patients for whom IPC was prescribed. Others have demonstrated not only the effectiveness of IPC and similar devices but the additive effect of this methodology with chemical (heparin) prophylaxis.[64,65] The efficacy is theoretically due to a decrease in cross-sectional area of capacitance veins, thus generating both an increase in linear blood flow as well as protection of venous valve competency. There are clinical data supporting the theory that IPCs work in part by release of endogenous tPA.[66] Additionally, because the vein wall is less distended, one might speculate a decrease in microtears in the venous wall.[65]

Whereas there has been a general and increasing acceptance of chemical prophylaxis in surgical patients, there remains a reticence on the part of neurosurgeons for understandable fear of possible additional risk of hemorrhage. For many indications, IPC is probably effective.[64–67] However, several recent analyses of VTE prophylaxis in neu-

rosurgical patients[68–70] have indicated that not only is LMWH itself safe but, when combined with IPC, it adds to the efficacy of VTE prophylaxis either without any additional risk of hemorrhage[68,69,71,72] or with such a small amount of increased risk that such risk of hemorrhage is easily absorbed by the decrease in overall morbidity and mortality from VTE.[72] In these studies, all prophylactic doses of LMWH were initiated postoperatively. In one small study involving only patients undergoing brain tumor surgery, LMWH was given preoperatively with an increased risk (5 of 46 patients) of intracranial hemorrhage.[73] rFVIIa has been employed in some neurosurgical cases with recalcitrant hemorrhage, although the risk:benefit ratio has not yet been determined.[74]

There is considerable debate regarding the need for VTE prophylaxis in patients undergoing laparoscopic surgery[75] with arguments for[76] it and against it.[77] In patients with prior VTE, prophylaxis seems indicated and rational. The reduction in net tissue damage afforded by laparoscopic surgery seems counterbalanced by the effects of the use of pneumoperitoneum and the Trendelenburg position.

The coagulation challenges associated with two surgical procedures, *cardiopulmonary bypass* and *orthotopic liver transplantation (OLT)*, are multiple with many various abnormalities noted; however, more likely than not the changes leading to significant hemorrhage are mediated by surges of endogenous tPA resulting in a brisk hyperfibrinolytic state.

Cardiopulmonary Bypass Surgery

The effects of CPB on blood have been thoroughly reviewed.[78–80] Whereas platelet defects have been ascribed to CPB,[81] these are mostly multiple, minor, and transient.[82,83] These aberrations are produced, in part, by partial activation of platelets coming in contact with the nonbiologic material of the CPB pump and oxygenator apparatus as well as binding and agglutination of platelets to such material. Platelet glycoprotein Ib (GpIb) is decreased on these platelets but it is doubtful whether this change itself is sufficient to cause a significant hemostatic challenge. Of interest, through some mechanisms differing from its antifibrinolytic effects, aprotinin seems to restore normal platelet activity.[84] Hemorrhage may be serious enough to result in re-exploration in 3% to 7%[85] of cases of CABG and is associated with a 30% increase in mortality.[78]

Patients with acute coronary syndrome (ACS) are frequently administered antiplatelet agents because of their efficacy. However, because of clinical uncertainty regarding the timing of necessary operative intervention, patients frequently may be taken to the surgery suite while being administered such agents. Exposure to clopidogrel within three days of CABG results in excessive postoperative bleeding and reoperation;[86] therefore, its use ideally should be withheld prior to elective or semi-elective CABG. Administration of ASA up to the time of CABG is common. Although blood loss in patients undergoing this procedure while on aspirin is statistically higher than for those patients stopping aspirin use a week before surgery (410 mL compared with 539 mL, $p = 0.01$), these differences are of questionable clinical importance and did not lead to more transfusions in the patients who were given aspirin.[87]

There is considerable growing opinion that the amount of bleeding encountered in CABG may be of less total clinical outcome significance than the total amount of blood products transfused, and, that increased use of blood products seems to be associated with less favorable long-term outcome.[82,87] For instance, in the above ASA study, although patients received ASA blood slightly more often, they were transfused the same amounts yet had better oxygenation and shorter ventilation times than patients off aspirin for the week preceding CABG surgery.[87]

When excessive hemorrhage in CPB patients was believed to be caused by acquired platelet defects, many studies examined the efficacy of routine use of DDAVP in managing those defects.[88,89] DDAVP was not uniformly efficacious in reducing mortality, re-exploration, and blood use, and may have even contributed to a twofold risk of perioperative acute myocardial infarction (Table 37-3). These data suggest that hemorrhage in the majority of CPB patients is not primarily due to a platelet defect or at least a platelet defect that could be reversed by the administration of DDAVP. DDAVP should not be used routinely in CPB patients but employed only when it is apparent that a patient is hemorrhaging and then it should be given in the routine dosage (0.3 µg/kg intravenously).[90,91] This approach may minimize hemorrhage in patients taking aspirin prior to their surgery.[92]

Similarly the routine nonspecific use of platelet transfusions, as well as fresh frozen plasma (FFP) infusion, is not indicated.[93,94] Indeed, using the large aprotinin database, Spiess and coauthors[95] demonstrated that use of platelet transfusions was associated with multiple types of poor outcome, including infection, vasopressor use, stroke, and death.

Meta-analysis of six studies found neither rationale for nor reduction in blood loss with routine prophylactic use of FFP in CABG.[96] Autotransfusion of shed blood during CABG using cell saver techniques was found in a randomized trial to be safe, resulting in no apparent clinical or laboratory aberrations while decreasing significantly the use of any homologous transfused blood or blood products.[97] Two studies comparing preoperative use of LMWH with UFH in ACS patients undergoing CABG demonstrated more re-exploratory surgery for hemorrhage[98] and a higher transfusion rate for those patients receiving LMWH.[99]

There is now general consensus that the majority of excessive bleeding following CPB is due to the surge of tPA that occurs during rewarming of the patient, which temporally correlates with coming off the CPB apparatus and closure of the mediastinum.[100,101] Until that time, circulating levels of tPA are not particularly high as the surge does not begin until the rewarming phase. Of interest, patients who undergo cardiothoracic surgery without CPB do not experience this tPA surge.[100] Patients undergoing "off-pump" CABG do not lose as much blood as those "on-pump"[102,103] and use of ASA off-pump did not increase shed blood.[104]

Pharmacologic agents block the effects of tPA. Aprotinin is a serpin isolated from bovine pancreas. It is a powerful inhibitor of plasmin and thus an effective blocker of fibrinolysis. It has little or no anti-tPA or platelet activity.[105,106] A meta-analysis of 72 trials including 8409 CPB patients concluded that of multiple hemostatic agents, aprotinin was associated with the greatest decrease in blood loss, mortality, rate of re-exploration, and overall blood use[89] whether the routine-dose aprotinin (2 million KIU as an IV bolus followed by 500,000 KIU IV every hour) or lower doses was employed. Others[79,107-112] have stated that other fibrinolytic agents are as good as and particularly less expensive than aprotinin.

Perioperative myocardial infarction occurred in 4% of patients receiving lower-dose aprotinin and in 8% of those receiving the conventional dose; however, the overall mortality rate was still half that of patients not receiving aprotinin. The overall perioperative myocardial infarction rate was essentially the same as placebo.[89]

Aprotinin has also been shown in both case reports and small studies to be efficacious in special situations requiring CPB such as patients undergoing hypothermic surgery,[113] heart transplantation,[114] aortic surgery,[115] CABG in patients with ITP,[116] or lung transplantation,[117] and in patients requiring a left ventricular assist device (LVAD) as a bridge while awaiting transplant.[118]

Re-exploration to assess hemorrhage is necessary in 3% to 7% of cases following CPB,[85] and 67% of the time a specific bleeding site responding to local measures is found.[78] Of interest, Pelletier[85] found for the 33% of cases in which they did not find a surgical or anatomic correctable reason for hemorrhage, most hemorrhage simply stopped as though the re-exploration itself had a net hemostatic effect. Studying their hypothesis, various coagulation components of mediastinal blood were measured and compared with

Table 37-3   Meta-Analysis of Efficacy of Hemostatic Agents Compared with Placebo for Perioperative Hemorrhage Associated with Cardiopulmonary Bypass Surgery

	Mean Decrease in Blood Loss, mL	Odds Ratio			
		Mortality	Re-exploration	Blood Product Use	Perioperative AMI[a]
Aprotinin[b]	446	0.55	0.37	0.37	1.13
Antifibrinolytic agents[c]	264	0.78	0.44	0.46	0.48
DDAVP[d]	114	1.02	0.67	0.79	2.4

[a]AMI, acute myocardial infarction.
[b]Either "conventional" or "low" dose.
[c]Either EACA or tranexamic acid.
[d]DDAVP, 1-deamino-8-D-arginine vasopressin. Data from Laupacis A, Fergusson D: Drugs to minimize perioperative blood loss in cardiac surgery: Meta-analyses using perioperative blood transfusions as the outcome. Anesth Analg 85:1258–1267; and Levi M, Cromheecke ME, deJonge E, et al: Pharmacological strategies to decrease excessive blood loss in cardiac surgery: Meta-analysis of clinically relevant endpoints. Lancet 354:1940–1947, 1999.

systemic levels in the same patient. The fibrinogen and α_2-plasmin inhibitor levels were both significantly lower ($p = 0.05$), whereas the levels of PAI-1 and fibrin degradation products (FDPs) were both significantly higher ($p = 0.05$) in the shed mediastinal blood than in systemic blood. They used these data as evidence for increased fibrinolytic activity primarily in the mediastinal cavity itself and that drainage via exploration may have eliminated self-perpetuating local hyperfibrinolysis. Khalil and colleagues have reproduced similar findings and additionally showed the efficacy of the installation of aprotinin into the pericardial sac.[119]

Although operative and postoperative hemorrhage experienced in modern CABG surgery is largely controlled by advances in technical skills, cell saver techniques, improved equipment, and the use of antifibrinolytic agents, occasionally hemorrhage can be significant. Several small series[120–124] have reported late use of "last-effort" recombinant human activated factor VII (rFVIIa) to control hemorrhage with apparent efficacy, although thrombotic events have been reported.[124–125] One consensus group recognized that off-label use of rFVIIa in cardiothoracic surgery patients was feasible as rescue therapy in actively hemorrhaging patients for whom all routine hemostatic measures have failed although the risk:benefit ratio has yet to be determined in any randomized trials.[126] A recent editorial[126a] has called into question these off-label uses citing the heavy reporting bias against experiences having negative results and major or fatal complications. A summary of the few available controlled trials with use of rFVIIa in these off-label situations suggests a less favorable outlook than that reached by the census group.

Aprotinin, EACA, and tranexamic acid[127,128] exert their primary procoagulant effects by blocking the action of plasmin, thereby greatly impeding fibrinolysis. Thrombotic events to include either arterial (myocardial infarction or stroke) or venous (DVT or PE) events do not appear increased using these agents.[101,129,130] Two recent publications[111,130a] have questioned the continued use of aprotinin in CABG surgery citing apparent acute and chronic complications (respectively) in patients who were administered aprotinin when compared with either control CABG patients or CABG patients administered EACA or tranexamic acid as alternative antifibrinolytic agents. An accompanying editorial[130b] reviews the latter report, pointing out the limitations of epidemiologic non-randomized studies. Before one reaches conclusions from these two publications, one has to also consider the multiple reports showing that aprotinin was associated with less blood loss, fewer transfusions of blood and blood products, and seemingly better outcomes.[79,87,89,95,112] This contentious area is rightfully under intense review and debate and will probably not be decided until head-to-head randomized studies are used in CABG patients comparing aprotinin with other antifibrinolytic agents for both short-term and long-term results.

Because aprotinin is prepared from bovine pancreas, it could be expected to cause immunologic reactions, including anaphylaxis.[131] Dietrich and colleagues[132] studied 248 cases of re-exposure to aprotinin and found a 3% incidence of adverse reactions, which typically occurred on initiation of aprotinin administration and were characterized by an acute fall in blood pressure. All survived the reaction. Only 1.5% of patients experienced adverse reaction on re-exposure if more than 6 months had lapsed since their last exposure. Patients who had had re-exposure within 6 months had a reaction rate of 4.5%.

Drugs that block the platelet glycoprotein IIb-IIIa (GP-IIb/IIIa) platelet receptor (see Chapter 20) are used in patients with ACS, a population that may undergo emergent CABG with CPB and attendant extra risk for hemorrhage. Following abciximab, the GP-IIb/IIIa receptor blocker with the longest half-life, a 12-hour hiatus after the last infusion is recommended.[133] Because abciximab is very tightly bound to platelet membranes with negligible amounts of unbound circulating abciximab in the plasma, use of platelet transfusions is rational for preparation of patients requiring emergent surgery before 12 hours have lapsed since the last abciximab infusion.

Hyperfibrinolysis following CPB is associated with a tPA surge that may occur in response to enhanced procoagulant activity. Dietrich and colleagues[134] operated on patients at risk for post-CPB hyperfibrinolysis by first treating them with warfarin to a mean international normalized ratio (INR) of 2.4; their control group had an INR of 1.1. Those patients undergoing CPB at the therapeutic INR required less heparin to reach appropriate anticoagulation as determined by the activated clotting time (ACT) and in particular required less heparin during the operation to maintain an appropriate ACT value. These data suggest that warfarin pretreatment resulted in less thrombin (and therefore less fibrin) generation during CPB with a subsequent diminished tPA surge. Blood loss at 6 and 12 hours with warfarin-treated patients was 381 and 505 mL, respectively, whereas the control group lost 472 and 527 mL, respectively—reaching statistical significance ($p < 0.05$). They noticed no correlation with blood loss even with patients at the highest INRs, including up to 6.0. They neither reversed the warfarin nor administered FFP during the operation.[134] Similarly, higher—as opposed to lower—heparin levels during CABG were found to be associated paradoxically with less blood loss. This enhanced anticoagulation is believed to result in decreased thrombin generation, which, in turn, translates into less thrombosis, less rebound hyperfibrinolysis, less bleeding, fewer transfusions, and better immediate and long-term outcomes.[79]

Orthotopic Liver Transplantation

Orthotopic liver transplantation (OLT) historically has been complicated by massive hemorrhage and heavy demands on the transfusion service. In the past several years our understanding of the hemorrhagic nature of OLT has increased to the point that effective therapy has greatly reduced both the incidence and severity of hemorrhage as well as impact on the blood bank (see Chapter 39).

OLT often is performed in patients with profound deterioration of their hemostatic system, even preoperatively, given the role of the liver in coagulation and fibrinolysis. The platelet count is often low because of hypersplenism. Accordingly, it previously had been regarded that these preoperative changes were the primary cause(s) of hemostatic failure in OLT.

Our understanding of hemostatic failure has been assisted by dividing OLT into four phases: the preoperative, anhepatic, and reperfusion phases with a convalescent phase occurring in the week or two following the transplantation.

The hemostatic changes characteristic of OLT have been described by many.[135–140]

In brief summary, the patient has impaired hemostasis that deteriorates during the anhepatic phase because there is not even an impaired liver attempting to clear activated coagulation products or any released tPA. During the reperfusion phase, the surge of tPA results from washout from the donor liver following anastomosis with the recipient. This release of tPA is enhanced by shock, acidemia, and probably hypothermia. It is also during this phase that hemorrhage can become excessive. Those using thromboelastography (TEG) were instrumental in the discovery of reperfusion hyperfibrinolysis.[135] In the convalescent period from postoperative days 1 through 14, procoagulant factors appear to replenish faster than anticoagulant factors. This may, in part, explain acute hepatic artery thrombosis that, if it happens, does so in this period.

Several groups infused aprotinin (using 2 million KIU as a loading dose followed by 500,000 KIU every hour until skin closure) at the time of reperfusion noting marked decreases in blood loss and transfusion requirements of red cells, FFP, and platelets.[141,142] Patients who did not require transfusion of any blood product increased from 17% in patients not receiving aprotinin to 39% in those who did receive aprotinin.[143] Although some studies have shown no benefit using the same aprotinin regimen,[143,144] a double-blind study[145] supports the use of aprotinin in OLT.

In OLT patients who experienced hemorrhage despite all surgical and pharmacologic corrective efforts, rFVIIa seemed effective in a small number of patients over a broad range of rFVIIa dosage.[146] However, rFVIIa was not effective in reducing blood loss when prophylactically administered to OLT patients.[147] One recent consensus study regarding off-label use of rFVIIa deemed its use "appropriate" following failure of all routine measures, although randomized studies are needed to determine the risk:benefit ratio.[126,126a]

Aprotinin use may also decrease blood loss and transfusion needs in patients undergoing total hip replacement,[148] total knee replacement,[149] orthopedic tumor surgery, or removal of infected orthopedic hardware.[150] Doses were less than those used with CPB or OLT—yet blood loss was decreased by 40% to 60% without a major increase in DVT (although all patients received LMWH for these procedures). Aprotinin has not gained universal acceptance in orthopedics, perhaps because blood loss usually is much less for these surgical procedures than with CPB or OLT and a majority of orthopedic blood loss can be recovered by use of cell savers.[151]

PREOPERATIVE HEMOSTATIC TESTING

Screening for Hemostatic Defects

Approximately 3% of all surgical procedures will be accompanied by a degree of hemorrhage deemed by the surgeon to be excessive. In their large meta-analysis of more than 50 randomized double-blinded studies comparing low-dose heparin with placebo in DVT prophylaxis, Collins and colleagues noted that among the 7486 controls receiving placebo, 3.3% of patients were judged to have bled excessively by the surgeon and that 0.1% succumbed to

bleeding.[152] Three papers[153–155] rendered a similar rate of hemorrhage among patients who are undergoing surgical procedures during studies of appropriateness of preoperative hemostatic testing. Of 4499 patients, 2% were deemed to bleed excessively. The sensitivity of hemostatic screening tests in these 4499 patients was 18%, the specificity was 90%, the positive predictive value was 3%, and the negative predictive value was 98%. There was no correlation between results of these preoperative screening tests for hemostatic competence and surgery-related hemorrhage. Of the 85 patients who bled,[153–155] 70% had completely normal tests. Of the 435 patients who had abnormal tests, only 15 bled, implying that 97% of patients potentially identified as those likely to bleed did not bleed. Nonetheless preoperative prothrombin time (PT), partial thromboplastin time (PTT), and platelet counts are almost as common as a routine admission order and their use seems to have become a habit.[156–158]

Approximately $30 billion are spent in the United States for preoperative testing of all types,[159] yet the clinical value of these tests is extremely limited. In studying over 1000 patients at the Mayo Clinic who underwent surgery without *any* preoperative tests, outcome analyses show that the death or major operative mortality rate was 0%. None required blood tranfusion.[160]

Multiple studies continue to support the agreed-on conclusion that obtaining routine preprocedural coagulation study is without merit. That abnormal hemostasis exists and is identifiable is irrefutable, but repeated studies fail to document the role of laboratory testing in identifying such patients because those with abnormal hemostasis are best discovered by a thorough history and physical examination. This is true for general surgical patients,[161] those undergoing tonsillectomy and adenectomy,[162] cataract surgery,[163] and neurosurgical procedures.[164]

To contrast with the dozen or so studies reaching exactly the same conclusions, there is no study offering contradictory evidence or opinion. Accordingly, the statistical weight garnered by this unanimous thrust is so considerable that further studies of the general population seem without merit. This conclusion was arrived at in four of four overviews[165–168] on this subject.

Why do physicians continue these practices? One reason is habit.[156,158] One survey[168] found habit offered as an explanation in 52% of such practices, whereas 45% used "defensive medicine" as their rationale.

The routine use of the bleeding time as a predictor of hemostatic competency in patients without a bleeding history is without foundation.[169] However, if patients do have a bleeding history, the bleeding time is held as worthwhile in sorting out whether the abnormal bleeding is associated with platelet:endothelial dysfunction. The bleeding time is not even effective to predict among patients taking aspirin preoperatively which patients are likely to bleed.[169] The platelet function assay (PFA) has replaced the bleeding time (see Chapter 41) for platelet function analysis, although a prolonged PFA does not necessarily imply enhanced hemorrhagic risk.

The best method to determine hemorrhagic risk with surgery is an adequate history and physical examination (Table 37-4).[160,169,170] What is the role of hemostatic testing among individuals who have undiagnosed disorders of hemostasis? This small group of patients may or may not

Table 37-4 **Appropriate Questions to Screen for Possible Abnormal Hemostasis**
• Have you or anyone in your family ever been labeled a "bleeder"? Has someone in the family ever sustained abnormal bleeding?
• Have you ever bled with surgery or following childbirth? What surgical procedures have you had, including major surgery, minor surgery, biopsies, and dental extractions?
• Did a surgeon or dentist ever have to re-explore the wound site or did you ever have to return to the operative suite for hemorrhagic control?
• Have you ever had excessive menstrual periods? How long do your periods last? How many pads or tampons are needed each day? Have you ever required iron supplementation for anemia due to a menstrual blood loss?
• Do you bruise excessively? Are these bruises multiple? Are they confined only to the outer thighs or other areas that are subject to trauma? Are any of these bruises palpable (i.e., are they true hematomas) or are they level with the surface of the skin?
• Do you have nosebleeds now or was there ever a time in your life when you did have spontaneous nosebleeds?
• Have you ever required a blood or plasma transfusion and, if so, why?
• Have you ever bruised or experienced hemorrhage following trauma, car accidents, falls, organized or unorganized sports, altercations, or any acts of violence?

show abnormal hemostatic testing. However, far more specific and sensitive is the history of bleeding. Three papers have examined the presentation of patients harboring mild hemophilia at risk for hemorrhage, perhaps even in a major fashion, following operative procedures.[2,171,172] The patients included in these papers are the very ones who are of concern to surgeons and other persons practicing invasive procedures, yet they represent substantially less than 1% of the population. Of the patients described in these three papers, patients who had undergone dental extraction and/or tonsillectomy without subsequent bleeding, did not harbor an underlying heritable hemorrhagic diathesis indicative of the history's ability to accurately predict adequate hemostasis. A positive medical history of bleeding was found to be 12.5 times more likely to predict the true hemorrhagic potential than any battery of laboratory tests. In using newer tests to identify patients with VWD, Biron and colleagues found that whereas 1% of the population tested true positive, 10% tested false positive.[173] Naturally, patients may acquire causes of bleeding such as severe or decompensated liver disease, administration of anticoagulant drugs, or the development of a spontaneous inhibitor of a coagulation factor (see Chapter 6).

What if hemostatic screening tests return abnormal? In one report,[153] abnormal studies were found in 1.9% of screened patients. When another sample was collected and the test was repeated before the surgical procedure, results of half of those abnormal tests returned normal, showing that specimen collection, laboratory error, or laboratory variability explained many abnormalities.

When the cause of persistently prolonged PTTs of unknown etiology[174] was determined, 67% of patients were not at actual risk for hemorrhage because the nature of the process leading to the prolongation (bad laboratory sample, laboratory error, lupus anticoagulant, and prelaboratory variability) would not be expected to result in

postoperative hemorrhage. However, the other 33% were at very clear risk to bleed; moreover, 81% of these 33% had already given a clear, positive history of a hemorrhagic diathesis even before the nature of their laboratory abnormality was determined. There was a lack of correlation between the degree of prolongation of the PTT and the risk of bleeding, a conclusion made by others[153]; the risk of bleeding rather is a function of the *cause* of the PTT prolongation, not the *degree* of prolongation. Of significant concern is the fact that often an abnormal result frequently is ignored or forgotten by the practitioner who ordered the tests.[157,175] One might question why such laboratory tests are unable to define precisely which patients are likely to bleed following an invasive procedure. Table 37-5 gives lines of reasoning why this is true.

Hemostatic tests should be ordered much less frequently than they customarily are. They are indicated in patients who answer affirmatively to any of the questions in Table 37-4. Others have stated that indications of screening tests as determined by the history and physical examination should include those with malabsorption, trauma, a history of active hemorrhage, a history of chemotherapy or radiotherapy, purpura, anemia, or the prior use of anticoagulants.[176] Some[177] have added patients with liver disease, operations characteristically associated with a blood loss of greater than 1500 mL, or highly invasive procedures such as those included in Table 37-6. It would seem rational to include those patients refusing to accept blood or blood product infusion. Using criteria similar to these, four studies indicated that screening was appropriate in 11%,[153] 8%,[155] 23%,[176] and 19%[178] of patients, giving a mean of 15%, implying that 85% of preoperative hemostatic testing

Table 37-5 **Why Hemostatic Testing is Not Usually Sufficient to Detect Those Likely to Experience Operative Hemorrhage**
• Patients suffering the worst hemorrhagic disorders, classic hemophilia A or B, are identified very early in life and have established diagnoses for life. Accordingly, preoperative screening is not effective or even warranted as the diagnosis is already known.
• The great majority of postoperative bleeding is not due to hemostatic failure but to a surgical or technical problem more appropriately corrected by surgical maneuvers. Exhaustive preoperative screening cannot predict operative errors.
• Traditional tests to screen for hemostatic disorders (PT, PTT, platelet count) were designed primarily to detect static disorders of hemostasis. As such, they do not reflect accurately ongoing changes in a situation as dynamic as trauma or surgery.
• The most flagrant examples of hemostatic failure—disseminated intravascular coagulation, hyperfibrinolysis, and thrombocytopenia—develop during an operation and cannot be predicted by tests performed before the operation.
• The PT and PTT are expected to give abnormal results approximately 2.3% of the time. If one is screening for mild defects in factor VIII or factor IX, these disorders occur in about 1:20,000 males and, therefore, the ratio of true positives to false positives is on the order of 1:500.*

*From Clarke JR, Eisenberg JM: A theoretical assessment of the value of the PTT as a preoperative screening test in adults. Med Decis Making 1:40–43, 1981, with permission.
PT, prothrombin; PTT, prothrombin time.

Table 37-6   A Schema for Preoperative Hemostatic Evaluation

Level of Risk*	Screening History		Proposed Surgery	Recommended Tests
Minimal	Negative ± prior surgery	and	Minor	None
Low	Negative with prior surgery	and	Major	Platelet count, PTT, or none
Moderate	Possible bleeding disorder	or	CNS, CPB, or Prostatectomy	Above tests *plus* BT (or PFA), PT
High	Highly suspicious or documented bleeding disorder	and	Major or minor	Above tests *plus* factors VIII, IX, and XI levels, TT If these are negative, pursue diagnosis

*Level of risk is estimated by the product of the risk of bleeding times the clinical consequence of bleeding.
BT, bleeding time; CNS, central nervous system; CPB, cardiopulmonary bypass; PTT, partial thromboplastin time; PT, prothrombin time; TT, thrombin time. The bleeding time may well be replaced by platelet function assays (PFA) (see Chapter 41).
Modified from Rapaport SI: Preoperative hemostatic evaluation: Which tests, if any? Blood 61:229–231, 1983; and Woodman RC, Harker LA: Bleeding complications associated with cardiopulmonary bypass. Blood 76:1680–1687, 1990, with permission.

is without merit. Table 37-6 offers a proposed schema for preoperative hemostatic evaluation that seems rational, defensible, and conscious of cost containment issues.

Screening for Thrombotic Disorders

Bleeding is not the only complication that can follow operative procedures. Venous thromboembolism (VTE) can be a major or fatal complication of a surgical procedure. Whereas risk stratification and prophylactic measures to reduce these risks are covered in Chapter 14, suffice it to say that a history of a VTE places the patient at 30 to 40 times the risk of the normal population to experience yet another VTE and that risk is still further exacerbated perhaps 100-fold by surgery.[1] These patients may well deserve screening for the more common thrombophilic abnormalities, particularly if laboratory findings may alter therapy.

Routine coagulation or special tests (e.g., factor V Leiden and prothrombin 20210 mutations) are not indicated to screen the general population solely for the possibility of VTE following surgery.[179] An abnormally short PTT (less than 23 seconds) has been suggested to predict for poor outcome, including death, thrombosis, or bleeding.[180]

In preparation to undergo certain procedures (as in hip or knee replacement, as well as renal transplantation) known to be at high risk for VTE, some[181–184] have questioned whether preoperative screening for thrombophilic conditions is warranted. Whereas the data are inconclusive, it must be recalled that because the relative risk (RR) of the main recognized thrombophilic disorders ranges only from about 2 (factor V Leiden) to 6 (antithrombin III deficiency), the RR of such surgery as this is closer to 100, bringing into focus the clinical application of the question being asked. As with patients prone to postoperative hemorrhage, an appropriately performed history and physical examination again is the best path to predict the possibility of thrombotic events.[185] Particular attention should be paid to cancer, heart failure, use of estrogens, and especially a history of VTE.[186] These risks are not simply additive but increasing risk factors implies even more rapid escalation of overall risk for VTE following surgery. More than 30 years ago Kakkar and colleagues[187] showed that the risk factors most predictive for VTE were a previous VTE, varicose veins, and operations on patients with a malignancy or patients over 60 years of age. For patients identified to be at very high risk for thrombosis, more aggressive thromboprophylaxis is indicated.[188]

Special heed should be paid to those patients who recently experienced a VTE. Sarasin and Bounameaux[189] have determined that patients who recently have had a VTE are at extreme risk for VTE recurrence following an invasive procedure during the first 20 weeks after their VTE with a gradual decrease in this very high rate after that 20-week period. They suggested that patients who are at such high risk for VTE that any elective procedures should be postponed for several months. Similar conclusions were rendered by Kearon and Hirsh.[1]

INVASIVE PROCEDURES IN PATIENTS WITH ABNORMAL COAGULATION TESTS

Those practicing invasive procedures typically assume a direct relationship between in vitro routine coagulation tests and the adequacy of in vivo hemostasis. There is little evidence to support this stance as suggested in the previous subchapter on preoperative screening tests. Nonetheless, many view coagulation tests to be touchstones of physiology. Multiple examples exist of abnormal hemostasis with normal routine coagulation tests as well as normal hemostasis in patients with substantially prolonged tests.[190]

In severe hepatic disease, the situation is even worse. Most routine coagulation tests are severely altered but hemostatic bleeding may be minimal as most visceral bleeding is from large vessels and due to hemodynamic rather than hemostatic defects. Recently Mannucci's group has shown that total thrombosis generation (probably the best predictor of physiologic hemostasis) is actually normal in those with cirrhosis, despite severe alteration in conventional coagulation tests.[191]

Invasive procedures such as bronchoscopy, endoscopy, lumbar punctures, paracentesis, and the insertion of lines for central venous access are part of modern medical practice. Although many patients needing these procedures have abnormal coagulation studies, published data underscore the safety and acceptable outcomes of such procedures in cancer patients, transplant patients, and patients in intensive care units. There is no published evidence for increased risks of procedure-related hemorrhage, and there is no controlled study that indicates at what levels the PT, PTT, and platelet count actually represent or predict contraindications to invasive procedures or that prophylactic replacement of blood products reduces risk of hemorrhage resulting from an invasive procedure.[192,192a–d]

General surgery in patients with thrombocytopenia from acute leukemia was far safer than the preconceived notions of hematologists or surgeons. Bishop and colleagues[193] performed 130 invasive procedures on patients whose platelet count was less than 50,000/μL (and usually remained less than 50,000/μL despite platelet transfusion therapy because of refractoriness to platelet transfusion). Only 7% required more than four units of packed red blood cells at the time of major surgery and none died secondary to the operation or from resultant bleeding. They concluded that major surgery or invasive procedures had a positive risk:benefit ratio in such patients. Studying laparoscopic splenectomy for refractory idiopathic thrombocytopenic purpura, Keidar and colleagues[194] deduced the procedure was hemostatically secure if patient counts were 20,000/μL or higher without a need for platelet transfusion. Those with platelet counts of less than 20,000/μL bled more and required more platelet and red blood cell transfusions, but all survived. In cancer patients, gastrointestinal endoscopies and biopsy for investigation of patients with gastrointestinal hemorrhage can be safely performed with platelet counts as low as 20,000/μL.[195] It is held that platelets in clinical conditions characterized by high platelet turnover (e.g., ITP) are more hemostatically efficient than platelets in conditions of low production (e.g., aplasia) so this matter can be factored into one's use of platelet transfusions.

Liver Biopsy

It is frequent practice to administer a few units of FFP prior to liver biopsy in patients with liver failure to decrease risk of hemorrhage. There are no data to support the three operative premises (1) that bleeding is likely; (2) that giving FFP improves the PT, and (3) that hemorrhagic risk is decreased by the administration of the FFP. In patients having PTs greater than 3 seconds above normal, administration of three units of FFP failed to correct the PT; however, subsequent liver biopsy did not result in hemorrhage.[196] In a larger study, McGill and colleagues performed 9212 liver biopsies over a 21-year period[197] if patients' ratio of the PT to control (i.e., the prothrombin time ratio [PTR]) was less than 1.5 (corresponding now to an INR of approximately 1.8) and the platelet count was 55,000/μL or higher. Among the 32 (0.03%) patients who experienced significant post-biopsy hemorrhage, there was no correlation between any coagulation test results and hemorrhage. McVay and Toy[198] performed a similar study in which they limited liver biopsy to patients whose PT ratio was below 1.5, (estimated INR of 1.8) PTT ratio below 1.5, and platelet count 50,000/μL or higher. They found that 6 of 175 (3.4%) patients were judged to have bled abnormally. They found no correlation between the hemorrhage and pre-procedure hemostatic results. Additionally, they showed that of their patients who did experience hemorrhage, the only positive predictor was the presence of liver malignancy. They concluded that the infusion of FFP and/or platelets within these variables was not warranted. Boberg and colleagues questioned whether a prolonged bleeding time heralded increased risk of hemorrhage following liver biopsy. In their study, they were unable to find that the risk of bleeding correlated with the bleeding time except, unex-

plainably, in patients who were bone marrow transplant patients. They also corroborated that there was no correlation between hemorrhage and platelet count, PT, or PTT.[199] Ewe[200] studied the "liver bleeding time," meaning that, following laparoscopic liver biopsy, the site was directly observed to determine duration of bleeding. In 200 patients, 10 experienced prolonged bleeding yet the pre-biopsy studies were unable to predict which of their patients would hemorrhage. These biopsies were performed on patients whose platelet counts were as low as 30,000/μL, PT ratios as high as 2.2 (implying an INR of at least 2.6), and whole blood clotting times markedly prolonged. Makris and colleagues[201] in a prospective study measured PT, PTT, TT, fibrinogen concentration, bleeding time, and platelet count prior to liver biopsy. All patients were prospectively screened by computed tomography (CT) scanning 24 hours after the biopsy. Over half the patients had at least one abnormal screening test and many had more than one with PTs as long as 19.5 seconds (INR of approximately 2.0), PTTs as long as 67 seconds (or almost twice their control), and bleeding times as long as 19 minutes with platelet counts as low as 52,000/μL. Only two patients out of 104 bled abnormally as determined by the CT scan and these patients had completely normal pre-biopsy screening tests. Bravo and colleagues[202] extensively reviewed liver biopsy. They pointed out that the mortality of liver biopsy was 1:10,000 and that the vast majority of such mortality occurred in patients with cirrhosis or, especially, tumors. Inexplicably they listed as absolute contraindicators those patients with PTs prolonged greater than 3 seconds, platelet counts less than 50,000/μL, and a bleeding time longer than 10 minutes. No data are offered to support these contentions.

Evidence-based methodology has failed thus far to establish cutoff values of hemostatic tests beyond which liver biopsy is unsafe; additionally, no trial has demonstrated that the administration of platelets or FFP before this procedure has clinical efficacy or rationale.[94,197,198] If one is concerned about hemostatic integrity, this is an indication for performing transvenous liver biopsy because bleeding would be directly into the vascular system.

Esophagogastroduodenoscopy and Colonoscopy

Concurrent aspirin or nonsteroidal anti-inflammatory drug (NSAID) administration increases the risk of minor bleeding following esophagogastroduodenoscopy (EGD) and colonoscopy with biopsy threefold, from 2.1% to 6.3%. However, major bleeding, defined as the need for hospitalization or for treatment directed toward the bleeding, occurred at the same rate, namely 0.6%, whether or not aspirin or a NSAID was used.[203] Guidelines promulgated by the American Society of Gastrointestinal Endoscopy do not suggest cessation of antiplatelet agents prior to endoscopic procedures.[204] This consensus panel endorsed the continuation of warfarin therapy for low-risk procedures (EGD or colonoscopy ± biopsy and biliary or pancreatic stent [without sphincterotomy]) provided the INR is not supratherapeutic. Patients having true high risk for thromboembolism yet requiring endoscopic procedures were not adequately addressed and recommendations for such patients have not been promulgated.[205]

Paracentesis and Thoracentesis

In 108 patients undergoing either paracentesis or thoracentesis and whose PT and PTT were at least twice normal and platelet counts were as low as 50,000/μ/L, 10% of patients received four units of FFP prior to procedure, while the other 90% did not. There was no correlation between hemorrhage as defined by hemoglobin concentration dropping at least 2 g/dL and any preoperative hemostatic tests or especially the infusion of FFP.[206] Similar findings were reported by Webster and colleagues.[207] Permanent peritoneal dialysis catheters may be safely inserted or removed in patients with end-stage renal disease without cessation of aspirin therapy.[208]

Bronchoscopy

Five studies are available regarding the safety of bronchoscopy with transbronchial biopsy in patients with abnormal hemostatic tests. Kozak and Brath[209] studied bleeding in such patients and were unable to show any correlation between hemostatic test results and the risk of hemorrhage. In a major bone marrow transplant unit where thrombocytopenia is common, Weiss and colleagues[210] performed 66 fiberoptic bronchoscopies and bronchioalveolar lavages; only four patients bled, with one event being major but not fatal. Thirteen of their patients underwent these studies with platelet counts less than 20,000/μ/L. Because a diagnosis was secured by their procedure in one half the cases, they concluded that the risk:benefit ratio is strongly in favor of the procedure. In a prospective study, Bjortuft and colleagues[211] performed 105 consecutive biopsies on patients monitoring the PT, PTT, bleeding time, and platelet count. They measured the actual blood loss by repeated suction and defined blood loss greater than 20 mL as worrisome. The mean blood loss for all patients was 7 mL but eight patients (8%) bled more than 20 mL; no losses were life threatening. Of interest, there was no correlation between the pre-biopsy test results and the ability to predict blood loss. They also noted that none of their 17 (16%) patients with bleeding times longer than 10 minutes experienced excessive hemorrhage. Diette and colleagues[212] determined that bronchoscopy in patients with lung transplants resulted in hemorrhage at a rate higher than in patients without transplants, but found that perturbations in the PT, PTT, or platelet count neither explained nor predicted those who bled. Herth and associates[213] reported that concomitant aspirin use was not associated with additional hemorrhage in patients undergoing transbronchial biopsy so pre-procedure cessation of aspirin was not justified.

Lumbar Puncture

Although lumbar puncture has been studied less thoroughly, Howard and colleagues[214] examined the safety of lumbar puncture, which was commonly done for diagnostic and therapeutic purposes in patients with leukemia and thrombocytopenia. They performed 5223 consecutive lumbar punctures on patients whose platelet counts were below 100,000/μL with 941 of those patients having platelet counts ranging from 0 to 50,000/μL (29 had counts below 10,000/μL). They observed no serious complications and correctly assumed that this procedure was indicated despite

thrombocytopenia because of its favorable risk:benefit ratio. They also concluded prophylactic platelet transfusions may not be indicated for a lumbar puncture if the platelet count is 10,000/μL or higher.

Central Venous Access Devices

Six studies have addressed the role of pre-procedure coagulation studies and outcome of insertion of central venous access devices, typically either subclavian vein (SC) or internal jugular vein (IJ) cannulation. Ray and Shenoy[215] divided a large cohort of patients into three groups—those having platelet counts of less than 50,000/μL, those with platelet counts between 50,000 and 100,000/μL, and patients whose platelet count was greater than 100,000/μL. They observed no differences in bleeding or other complication rates, although it was their practice to administer platelets routinely prior to insertion of such devices in patients with platelet counts less than 50,000/μL. Although the average platelet count increased by only 12,000/μL following transfusion, they proceeded with the cannulation, which caused them to question whether platelet transfusion improved the patient's risk-to-benefit ratio. Four patients having platelet counts less than 50,000/μL did not receive platelet transfusions yet did not experience abnormal bleeding.

Goldfarb and Lebrec[216] performed 1000 consecutive IJ cannulations in patients with "coagulopathies" and experienced a bleeding rate of 1%. Fisher and Mutimer[217] performed either IJ or SC cannulation in 658 patients with severe liver disease whose INR averaged greater than 1.5 (median 2.4, range 1 to 16) and/or had platelet counts less than 150,000/μL (median 10,000, range 9000 to 1,088,000/μL). Patients received neither prophylactic FFP nor platelet transfusions. Among these 658 patients, there was one major event (a hemothorax occurring in a patient whose INR was 1.5 and platelet count was 68,000/μL), which was deemed due to inadvertent laceration of the subclavian artery. The risk of local hematoma formation (which rarely requires any treatment other than pressure) was 6% in patients whose INR was 5 or less and 12% in patients whose INR was above 5. Four risk factors predicted minor bleeding: (1) the IJ site tended to bleed more than the SC site; (2) a procedure requiring more than one pass with the needle to cannulate the vein; (3) failure to easily insert the guidewire; and (4) patients whose INR was above 5. Values of the INR or other coagulation factors were not contraindications to a central line placement, particularly if it was deemed that such placement was beneficial for the patient's overall care.

Foster and colleagues[218] examined the advisability and safety of central venous catheterization insertion in 259 patients awaiting or having just undergone OLT. Their patients' mean platelet count was 47,000/μL (range 8000 to 79,000/μL), mean PTT of 97 seconds (range 78 to 100 seconds) and estimated mean INR 2.0 (range 1.5 to 8.0). They administered no pre-procedure FFP or platelets, yet noted no serious bleeding using their most experienced operator. They concluded that there are no data supporting fear of increased bleeding complications in central venous cannulation in patients with coagulopathy.

DeLoughery and colleagues[219] examined the outcome of central line placement as a function of hemostatic testing in critically ill patients. They performed 938 procedures with 41% of the patients having at least one abnormal test, 27% having several abnormalities, and 17% having undergone no testing prior to the procedure. Thirty-seven percent of their patients received some blood product prior to the procedure. They found that 16 (1.7%) of patients experienced minor bleeding and that only 2 (0.2%) experienced serious bleeding (neither was fatal). They concluded that laboratory data did not predict bleeding and that, in retrospect, the infusion of blood products, particularly FFP, was inappropriate.

Doerfler and colleagues[220] inserted 104 central lines in patients with abnormalities of coagulation. They judged that seven (6.5%) had some abnormal bleeding; all seven had a platelet count of 37,000/μL or less. They had not infused platelets into patients prior to the procedure but used their most experienced operator. There was no predictive value of routine coagulation testing.

In summary, all these studies show that there is no predictive value of routine tests prior to the insertion of central lines. FFP and platelets should not be administered routinely and the most experienced operator seems most appropriate to insert lines in these challenging cases. Thus, there is no reproducible laboratory value that serves as a cutoff for safe insertion and there is no value in delay caused by testing and costly, time-consuming infusion of blood or blood products. The bleeding rate appears to be extremely low, on the order of 1% to 2% and with no report of any fatality in these series. When one considers the benefit of such access, it is clear that the risk:benefit ratio favors performing the procedure. Especially noticeable is that no study has shown that the pre-procedure infusion of FFP or platelets decreases any real or hypothetical increase in hemorrhage.[219,220]

Arteriotomy

Examining the courses of 1000 cases of femoral artery puncture, Darcy and coworkers[221] reported that neither the pre-procedure PT nor the PTT was predictive for arterial hematoma formation in a cohort of patients undergoing femoral arteriotomy. They had arbitrarily limited the study to patients whose PTs were 18 seconds or less. Hematomas formed at a rate of 8% to 10% independent of any of these test results.

INVASIVE PROCEDURES FOR PATIENTS ON ANTICOAGULANT THERAPY

Many patients are receiving chronic oral anticoagulant therapy that was prescribed for clear indications. Accordingly it is not advisable for another practitioner preparing a patient for surgery or an invasive procedure to unilaterally stop warfarin therapy because of fear of bleeding. Should the risk of bleeding be considerably less than the operator perceives (which is almost always the case), then the risk:benefit ratio of withholding warfarin might very well be unfavorable for the patient's overall care. The risk of stopping anticoagulant therapy obviously varies from patient to patient with the risks of thrombosis being often at a fairly low risk (such as patients with atrial fibrillation who are on warfarin for primary prophylaxis of a stroke) to moderate risk (such as patients with modern prosthetic heart valves), to those with extremely high risk (such as patients who have had thromboses or have active antiphospholipid syndrome). There is substantial evidence[1,222] that a thromboembolic event (such as may result from withholding anticoagulants) has a 30-fold higher incidence for death or permanent sequelae than does a hemorrhagic event that may occur from continuing a patient on anticoagulant therapy for a procedure.

Kearon and Hirsh estimated that major surgery itself increases the risk of a thromboembolic event up to 100 times, a factor to be incorporated in estimating the risk: benefit ratio regarding the wisdom of stopping or continuing anticoagulant therapy for a procedure.[1] It is especially dangerous to perform any elective surgery in someone who has had a thrombotic event within the previous 20 weeks;[189] in nearly all such cases, elective invasive procedures should be withheld unless anticoagulation is carried out at the lowest therapeutic intensity. This topic is specifically addressed in Chapter 38, but some general comments seem appropriate in this chapter also.

A 1979 paper by Katholi and colleagues[223] is frequently cited claiming that for patients with older prosthetic heart valves undergoing noncardiac surgery while remaining on anticoagulant therapy (estimated INRs in that time period of 2 to 7) 50% experienced some bleeding, with 10% having serious bleeding, yet none fatal. However, they also reported that of 35 patients with prosthetic heart valves, for whom anticoagulants were withheld, there were two fatal thromboembolic events. Stopping anticoagulant therapy in this small cohort was unfavorable. The hemorrhagic rate of procedures done at modern therapeutic range INRs (2 to 3) has yet to be scientifically and thoroughly determined.

A survey of ophthalmologists[224] showed that although most of them unilaterally stopped anticoagulant therapy before lens implantation, there were no hemorrhagic consequences reported by those who did not stop anticoagulant therapy. However, among those ophthalmologists who did discontinue therapy, there were nine thromboembolic events, including two fatal events.

Until recently it was standard dentistry practice to stop anticoagulant therapy for extractions or similar procedures. This practice was reviewed by Weibert,[225] who concluded that modern therapy with INRs of 2 to 3 does not result in any appreciable increased bleeding or, that if any bleeding occurred, it was never serious and was easily controlled by local measures. In a recent study[226] of dental patients on warfarin therapy, all patients continued their medication. Patients were randomized to receive Gelfoam sponges and sutures, those two measures plus tranexamic acid, or all three of these efforts plus fibrin glue. All patients fared the same and none bled significantly. Because the first option, namely Gelfoam sponges and suture, was the easiest to carry out, that was the method recommended. This entire subject has been thoroughly reviewed by Wahl,[227] who concludes that the risk:benefit ratio of maintaining patients on oral anticoagulants for any oral procedure greatly favors the patient remaining on warfarin and the risk for bleeding is greatly exaggerated or misunderstood. Recent editorials in the dental literature support these tactics.[228]

Hip surgery for fractured hips or total hip replacement has always been an operation fraught with thromboembolism, which is the major cause of death in such patients.

In a very early (1959) controlled study, Sevitt and Gallagher[229] reported pinning fractured hips in patients on no anticoagulant therapy or on the vitamin K antagonist phenindione. One hundred fifty patients were in the control group and 150 patients received full-dose phenindione. Although it is impossible to precisely reconstruct what those patients' INRs were, they were likely in the range of 5 to 8. Whereas one could have predicted at such INRs some major bleeding would occur (five in the phenindione group and two in the control group), deaths from pulmonary embolism were decreased by 80%.

Later, in 1971, Salzman and colleagues[230] used warfarin anticoagulation to an estimated INR of 2.5 to 4.5 in a similar study and showed a 20% risk of bleeding, which was about the same as patients receiving aspirin or dextran as their control group yet with a decrease in VTE in the group on warfarin. In 1983, Francis and coworkers[231] began warfarin anticoagulant therapy to an estimated INR of 1.8 several days prior to total hip replacement or total knee replacement. Four percent of their patients bled, which was the same incidence as controls receiving dextran. Of the patients who were treated with warfarin compared with dextran, there was a 60% reduction in DVT and an 88% reduction in large proximal vein thrombosis. These papers showed that major surgery is feasible with very acceptable bleeding, with INRs that are not so high as to provoke bleeding but high enough to result in excellent prophylaxis of VTE in very high-risk patients.

In a cohort of 100 consecutive patients at high risk for thromboembolism who underwent major surgery, an INR of 1.8 ± 0.2 was associated with acceptable bleeding and a low risk of thromboembolism. Additionally, the time required for reconstituting a full therapeutic INR averaged only 2 days.[232] In a recent editorial, Sandset and Abildgaard[233] point out that surgical procedures are carried out in many European centers in patients on warfarin therapy with INRs up to 2.0 with acceptable bleeding risk. Torn and Rosendaal[234] found an odds ratio of only 1.3 when invasive procedures were carried out with INRs > 3.0 when compared with those procedures on patients whose INRs were <2.0.

These data appear highly consistent with the hypothesis that perceived hemorrhagic risks in patients operated on with INRs > 1.5 are greatly overestimated, and that although randomized controlled trials are lacking, that surgery with higher INRs is feasible, safe, and rational. Clearly each patient needs an individual estimate of their unique risk:benefit ratio depending on their risk and consequence for hemorrhage or thrombosis.

A growing list of varying procedures in addition to dental, ophthalmic, and hip surgery reveals no additional hemorrhagic risk for patients on warfarin, provided the INR is not supratherapeutic and, based on risk:benefit analysis, does not justify discontinuing warfarin for these procedures; this list includes hand surgery,[235] transrectal prostate biopsy,[236] and extensive cutaneous surgery.[237,238] The rigorous logic employed in the extensive review by Otley[238] is particularly clear and useful, even for those in disciplines different from cutaneous surgery and is strongly recommended reading for anyone wishing to frame a risk:benefit profile. Perhaps as important as the growing list of disciplines, procedures, and varying INRs in these referenced reports is the total unanimity of these opinions with no known studies suggesting otherwise.

If a patient on chronic oral anticoagulant therapy undergoes surgery without warfarin, many practitioners will use a "heparin bridge" to protect the patient during the brief period of subtherapeutic INR during the surgery and particularly after the surgery while the INR returns to therapeutic levels. LMWH may be used for this purpose (See Chapter 38).[239,240]

As more patients are administered chronic oral anticoagulation, it should be expected that more cases of trauma will occur in such patients. The fate of trauma patients who are on chronic oral anticoagulant therapy as a pre-injury condition has been addressed.[241–243] Surprisingly, there appears to be little if any extra morbidity or mortality in such patients when compared with similar trauma patients lacking the pre-injury condition of warfarin therapy, with the possible exception of those patients experiencing closed head injuries.[243]

Should a patient need emergent surgery (such as for trauma or an acute abdominal process), it may be advisable to reverse, or at least partially reverse, the effect of the warfarin prior to surgery. This can be done quite safely with very small doses of intravenous vitamin K, which will decrease the INR within 6 hours.[244] Intravenous administration is safe when small amounts, such as 0.5 to 1.0 mg, are administered in a diluted solution over approximately 30 minutes. Not only do higher doses far too often result in total reversal of the warfarin (which may not be desirable) but also doses greater than 1 to 2 mg frequently lead to warfarin resistance, making it difficult to re-achieve a therapeutic INR. When vitamin K is given intravenously it is safe while being faster and more reliable than giving it subcutaneously or orally.[245–247] Should one overshoot and the INR become unacceptably subtherapeutic, a heparin, LMWH, or pentasaccharide bridge method can be employed until the patient's INR returns to therapeutic range.

CONSULTATION ON PATIENTS WITH INTRAOPERATIVE OR POSTOPERATIVE HEMORRHAGE

Hematologists and transfusion medicine specialists are called by surgeons, anesthesiologists, and critical care personnel for the evaluation of bleeding either during an operation or afterward. Surgery or major trauma is the ultimate test of the hemostatic system. Accordingly, it is possible for patients who have never hemorrhaged to any significant degree to bleed excessively.

Nearly all reviews of intraoperative and early postoperative bleeding[78,248] point out that 75% to 90% of all such bleeding is technical in nature because of a structural problem such as an undone ligature, failed clamp, or partially secured vessel. It is very important to work with the surgeon because the cause of bleeding must be either surgical or hemostatic failure. Early in the consultation process it is advisable to have personnel draw blood samples for routine available coagulation tests. A sample of blood must be drawn from a fresh peripheral venipuncture. This may seem counterintuitive to the anesthesiologist, who may have several vascular devices from which blood could be drawn. Too frequently samples are adulterated by the infusion of heparin or even saline, erythrocytes, or plasma.[249]

Therefore, the very sample that one needs for critical decision-making must not be suspect from the very beginning. It is advisable to call the coagulation laboratory so that technicians can be alerted to both the seriousness of these particular tests as well as to work with the hematologist in a sequential manner regarding subsequent tests, the indications for which will unfold as the laboratory consultation progresses. Assessment of all patients experiencing substantial hemorrhage usually includes a PT, PTT, TT, platelet count, and measurements for D-dimer (or other FSPs). If the PT, PTT, and TT are all prolonged with decreased plasma fibrinogen levels and decreased platelets with positive assays for D-dimers, disseminated intravascular coagulation (DIC) is very high on the list for hemorrhage. If the FDPs are high but with the PT, PTT, and platelet count fairly well preserved with a very long TT, hyperfibrinolysis is strongly suggested. Conversely, if the TT is the sole test that is relatively the most prolonged, the culprit more often than not is excessive heparin either systemically administered or possibly from a contaminated sample from an intravenous line containing heparin. It must be recalled that neither LMWH nor the newer pentasaccharides prolong the PT, PTT, or TT so their involvement cannot be eliminated by those tests being normal.[250] The coagulation laboratory can set up a 1:1 mix of patient plasma with normal plasma to repeat the PT, PTT, and TT if any of these three tests are abnormal on initial testing of the patient's plasma. If the 1:1 mixture results in a previously abnormal test becoming normal, it strongly suggests a deficiency that can occur either congenitally, because of vitamin K deficiency or warfarin therapy, or from severe liver disease. Should the 1:1 mixture not correct the abnormal test(s), then an inhibitor, to include heparin, FDPs or D-dimers, or spontaneous acquired inhibitor,[251] is strongly suggested. The use of the thromboelastogram (TEG) by anesthesiologists has been discussed vigorously.[252,253] Whereas this test does not traditionally fit into hematologists' thinking, it clearly is one of the most accurate and rapid ways to detect hyperfibrinolysis especially in situations that are characterized by hyperfibrinolysis, namely CPB and OLT.

PFAs, especially at the point of care, would seem to be able to quickly reveal platelet dysfunction. Two studies[254,255] address this situation in CPB patients. In one study, although platelet dysfunction could be demonstrated, there was only a poor correlation between PFA abnormalities and hemorrhage following CPB and the PFA abnormalities were not substantiated by the more traditional but cumbersome platelet aggregation studies.[254] The other study failed to demonstrate significant PFA studies in post-CPB patients; some patients with mild platelet aggregation abnormalities did not experience abnormal hemostasis,[255] and TEG appeared to better predict bleeding and guide therapy. These findings are consistent with the notion that although platelet abnormalities are commonly detected following CPB, they are brief and of questionable overall importance. While agreeing that point-of-care testing was of marginal diagnostic significance, Avidan and associates[256] pointed out that its use within a protocol for hemorrhage following CPB patients resulted in more focused transfusion practice than in post-CABG hemorrhage patients whose care was under traditional clinical discretion, which overall resulted in overall fewer transfused blood products.

Next the consultant should ascertain if any preoperative coagulation tests were done and what the results were. Often preoperative tests were abnormal yet were either not seen or not acted on. A slight prolongation of the PTT could very well represent a mild, previously undetected deficiency of factor VIII, IX, or XI, or if the PT and PTT are both prolonged while the level of albumin is low and bilirubin is elevated, significant liver disease is suggested. If the preoperative and intraoperative coagulation tests mentioned are all normal, a local structural or technical problem is likely to be at fault.

Once laboratory studies are initiated, attention must be paid to the clinical features of hemorrhage. As Table 37-7 depicts, the nature of bleeding is very helpful. The concept that bleeding is due to a structural defect is greatly strengthened if there is bleeding from a single site while other potential sites are not bleeding. If bleeding is sudden and massive with bright red, pulsatile blood, arterial bleeding is probable. Clinical features that favor a basic hemostatic defect are multiple concurrent bleeding sites. Concomitant hemoglobinuria and hemoglobinemia strongly implicates transfusion reaction-induced DIC. Slow and persistent oozing, particularly several days after surgery, suggests a hemostatic defect. Table 37-8 lays out an overall evaluation. Appropriate questions asked of the treatment team and review of the chart or any pre-existing data often are the best sources of information.

Table 37-9 lists several hemostatic details that may or may not affect postoperative hemorrhage. Low-dose prophylactic use of heparin does not increase bleeding according to comprehensive meta-analyses.[152] Agents that may substantially impair platelet function are aspirin and NSAIDs (particularly ketorolac) in the postoperative period. Recalling that perhaps 1% of the population may have von Willebrand syndrome, it is highly possible that the addition of aspirin or NSAIDs is enough to expose the underlying nature of that heretofore stealth bleeding diathesis.[257] Increasingly, antiplatelet agents, not only clopidogrel but GP-IIb/IIIa inhibitors are used in clinical practice and may be associated with hemorrhage. Of the three GP-IIb/IIIa inhibitors, only abciximab-related hemorrhage is reversed by platelet transfusion owing to the extreme protein binding of abciximab. Platelet transfusions are not acutely effective due to extant plasma levels for both

---

Table 37-7 Clinical Features of Hemorrhage

Clinical Features Favoring Structural or Technical Defects
- Bleeding from a single site while other candidate sites are not bleeding
- Sudden onset of massive and/or rapid bleeding
- Bright red or pulsatile bleeding from an identifiable source

Clinical Features Favoring Hemostatic Defect
- Multiple simultaneous bleeding sites
  Surgical incision
  Vascular access sites
  Mucosal membranes
  Skin
  Hematuria
  Hemoglobinuria or hemoglobinemia
- Slow persistent ooze of blood from a non-identifiable source
- Delayed hemorrhage following adequate hemostasis

Table 37-8 Evaluation of Postoperative Hemorrhage

- Obtain fresh venipuncture sample of blood for:
  Thrombin time
  Prothrombin time
  Partial thromboplastin time
  1:1 mix with normal plasma of the above, if any are abnormal
  Blood smear for schistocytes and platelet count estimation Signs of sepsis such as leftward shift, toxic granulation, or vacuolization of granulocytes
- Note features of bleeding (see Table 37-7)
- Repeat directed history and physical examination
- Review patient's chart:
  Were preoperative liver and renal tests normal?
  Were preoperative coagulation screening tests normal?
  Were aspirin or NSAIDs administered?
- Is the patient septic?
- Was the patient transfused? With what? When?
- Was bovine thrombin or fibrin glue containing bovine thrombin used as hemostatic agent?
- What surgical procedure was performed?
- Was anesthesia time prolonged?
- Note type and rate of bleeding
- Estimate consequences of continued bleeding

NSAIDs, nonsteroidal anti-inflammatory drug(s).

Table 37-9 Details that Affect Intraoperative or Postoperative Hemorrhage

Does Not Affect
- Low-dose heparin prophylaxis
- Low-dose warfarin prophylaxis
- Osler-Weber-Rendu syndrome
- Mild thrombocytopenia ($\geq$60,000/μL)

Occasionally Affects
- Aspirin or NSAID administration
- Adjusted-dose heparin prophylaxis
- Poor metabolic/nutrition states*
- Moderate thrombocytopenia (30,000–60,000/μL)

Frequently Affects
- Ticlopidine, clopidogrel, or GP-IIb/IIIa inhibitors
- Platelet defects, especially with concomitant aspirin or NSAID administration
- Factor VIII or IX levels <30% of normal
- Fibrinogen <60 mg/dL
- Severe thrombocytopenia (<30,000/μL)
- Multiorgan failure

NSAID, nonsteroidal anti-inflammatory drug.
*Prolonged use of glucocorticosteroids, malnutrition, inanition, bedridden state from chronic illness, septicemia, and chronic renal or hepatic failure.

Table 37-10 Causes of Intraoperative or Postoperative Hemorrhage

*Intraoperative Hemorrhage**
- Structural/technical defects
- Disseminated intravascular coagulation
- Heparin overdosage
- Hyperfibrinolysis

*Early Postoperative (Days 0 to 2)**
- Structural/technical defects
- Thrombocytopenia
- Qualitative platelet disorders
- Mild/moderate hereditary coagulation disorder

*Delayed Postoperative Bleeding (Days 2 to 7)**
- Thrombocytopenia
- Aspirin or NSAID administration
- Vitamin K deficiency
- Multiorgan failure
- Antibodies to factor V following use of bovine thrombin in fibrin glue

NSAID, nonsteroidal anti-inflammatory drug.
*These times are those commonly encountered but are used only as approximations.

---

tically is very brisk but usually of short duration. In CPB and OLT in which the index of suspicion and prevalence is high, prompt administration of aprotinin or another fibrinolytic agent as discussed earlier in this chapter is strongly indicated. Thrombocytopenia that begins postoperatively and becomes worse, particularly if it is associated with thrombosis, is highly suggestive of heparin-induced thrombocytopenia (see Chapter 25). Vitamin K deficiency of an acquired nature is surprisingly common in intensive care situations, particularly if the patient has been ill for some time and, therefore, malnourished from the onset; after several days/weeks in the intensive care unit, one becomes depleted of vitamin K-dependent factors. One clinical hallmark of this situation is that the PT tends to prolong comparatively earlier than the PTT. Vitamin K deficiency is diagnosed and treated by the suspicion of this problem and the response of the patient to vitamin K administration.[264]

Table 37-11 offers several therapeutic options. Watching and waiting with the appropriate administration of red blood cells and fluid is often appropriate, particularly if the rate of bleeding seems to be decreasing. Re-exploration of the surgical site not only often will identify the bleeding site but also may be therapeutic in itself because it may remove thromboplastic as well as fibrinolytic agents released from large collections of clotted blood.[85] If a specific diagnosis is made, therapy obviously is addressed toward that cause.

Table 37-11 Therapeutic Options in Intraoperative or Postoperative Hemorrhage

- Acute volume and red cell administration as indicated
- Angiography with or without arterial embolization
- Watchful waiting
- Re-exploration of bleeding site
- Limited use of FFP, cryoprecipitate, and platelet transfusion, except for precise diagnoses and indications
- DDAVP
- Antifibrinolytic agents
- Use rFVIIa in select cases

DDAVP, 1-deamino-8-D-arginine vasopressin; FFP, fresh frozen plasma.

---

eptifibatide and pirofiban.[258] By far, the rarest abnormality is mild, previously undiagnosed hemophilia,[2] which is characterized by a slow ooze that usually starts on postoperative days 1 to 3 and is rarely of a brisk or alarming nature initially. Characteristically, hemostasis in mild hemophiliacs undergoing surgery is surprisingly normal for the first day or so during high levels of wound-induced TF generation. The nature of hemophilic bleeding has been described exquisitely in the older literature; the interested reader is referred to such descriptive papers.[259–263]

Table 37-10 presents various causes of postoperative bleeding. The differential diagnosis is, in part, a function of time from the operation. Hyperfibrinolysis, although not limited to patients undergoing CPB or OLT, characteris-

In desperate situations in which more traditional methods have failed and even without a specific diagnosis, many have employed rFVIIa reporting reasonable results. We are learning how to use this new and valuable tool in our therapeutic armamentarium. Consensus recommendations for use[126] and complications[125] exist but have yet to be verified with appropriately done studies, which are clearly needed. Dosage is usually initially 40 to 90 μg/kg which may be repeated every 2 hours for 8 to 12 hours total if hemostasis is not achieved earlier.

The use of topical surgical adjuvants including fibrin glue is covered thoroughly in Chapter 29. Bleeding that begins 4 to 14 days or even longer after surgery in which fibrin glue was employed raises the possibility of the induction of anti-bovine factor II and/or factor V, which may have cross-reactivity to their human counterparts. Management of such problems has been recently reviewed.[265]

The administration of DDAVP is effective for platelet dysfunction due to aspirin or NSAIDs. Administration of 0.3 μg/kg intravenously over 30 minutes is effective in bleeding due to platelet dysfunction.

The tempo, depth, and thoroughness of evaluation will be a function of the potential consequences of continued bleeding. A small amount of bleeding in a confined space on which pressure cannot be applied (such as the brain or internal organ) is obviously of more immediate concern than bleeding outside the body such as from a wound on an extremity. Accordingly, a more conservative approach may be indicated for the latter. Attempts at surgical techniques to stop true hemostatic defects are not successful; suturing to replace the hemostatic function of a missing coagulation factor will not work. In fact, the tighter one attempts to suture, the more inward the bleeding becomes, which continues and can dissect internally at an alarming rate and actually cause more damage than had the blood been allowed to escape the confines of the body.

Not all excessive hemorrhage is necessarily due to hemostatic failure. Bleeding in large, named vessels—particularly arteries—requires surgical repair. Bleeding from those vessels is rarely, if ever, due to a defect in the hemostatic system. Massive amounts of clotting factors, plasma, and platelets will not correct large structural lesions but can result in dilutional coagulopathy, which can mimic or actually result in DIC (See Chapter 46).[266,267] Table 37-12 offers some suggestions, if not hypotheses, regarding advice and hints on how to construct a reasoned risk:benefit stratification. There is much work to do. Studies providing data or answers to these points are needed.

Table 37-12 Observations Concerning Bleeding and Thrombosis in Risk:Benefit Stratification*

1. Evidence-based medicine (EBM) teaches us with statistical power what to expect from a population with a specific question, yet tells us little of what will happen to an individual patient within that population, given one's ultimate unique condition. Although EBM is a valuable guideline, final determinations are clinically based.
2. Given that either bleeding or thrombosis can be serious if not catastrophic, outcomes are nearly always better following a hemorrhagic event than a thrombotic event. In 21st-century medicine, far more patients experience thrombotic than hemorrhagic death.
3. Structural disorders, such as esophageal varices, tumors, and fresh postoperative sites, do not require the presence of anticoagulants to bleed, but any anticoagulants (heparin, warfarin, or antiplatelet agents) administered will invariably be blamed for any hemorrhage, regardless of its size, nature, or location.
4. Because bleeding is perceived as abnormal in 3–5% of all procedures, one should expect, and tolerate, a similar baseline occurrence for procedures carried out with concurrent anticoagulant therapy.
5. In patients experiencing macrovascular hemorrhage who have abnormal hemostatic tests, it is more important to address the cause or site (lacerated organs, unsuccessfully ligated vessels, or blunt trauma) than to spend time addressing and "correcting" the laboratory abnormalities with infusion of fresh frozen plasma (FFP), platelets, and the like.
6. True hemostatic failure with microvascular bleeding typified by classic hemophilia A or B patients inadvertently undergoing trauma or surgery without factor replacement is ONLY corrected by replacement of the missing factor—regardless of one's surgical expertise.
7. Microvascular bleeding is due to hemostatic failure resulting from inadequate thrombin generation, thrombocytopenia, or excessive fibrinolysis (disseminated intravascular coagulation [DIC], hyperfibrinolysis). Such bleeding is diffuse and typically oozes up from vascular beds without any clear physical site of origin, thereby largely eliminating the possibility of hemostatic success with a ligature or other physical measures. Macrovascular bleeding, on the other hand, typically emanates from lesions or vessels large enough to see the bleeding point. Such vessels are usually large enough to have been named. Classic hemostasis resulting in fibrin generation has little to offer; mechanical means such as pressure, suture, cautery, or ligation are the most effective.
8. To date, nearly all studies concerning invasive procedures for patients on chronic anticoagulant therapy begin with the premise that anticoagulant therapy must be stopped or modified, despite no evidence that demonstrates the correctness of that premise. No study has proved—or even strongly implied—at what INR patients on warfarin are statistically more likely to bleed than patients not on warfarin undergoing similar procedures. A few studies *suggest* that a cutoff INR is clearly above 2.0 and probably close to 3.5.
9. Determining risk:benefit ratio requires an accurate assessment of risk for bleeding with or without anticoagulant therapy, as well as the risk for thrombosis with or without concurrent anticoagulant therapy. This is not always apparent in the extant literature on this subject. For instance, some guidelines consider polypectomy or fine needle aspiration to be procedures of high risk for bleeding, whereas others deem brain tumor surgery or cardiothoracic surgery to be high-risk procedures. High-risk patients for one group may consist of mechanical heart valves in the mitral position, yet no mention is made of patients with much higher thrombotic risk, such as those with anticardiolipin syndrome, prior life-threatening thrombosis, thrombosis within 6 months of an invasive procedure, or patients who have already experienced thrombosis when anticoagulation has been held for a prior procedure.
10. Performing invasive procedures on patients with either severe thrombocytopenia or patients with therapeutic or anticoagulant therapy–induced prolongation of standard coagulation tests will occasionally be associated with hemorrhage, despite one's best efforts to construct a risk:benefit ratio as favorable as possible for an individual patient. Such events must not dissuade one from further efforts on behalf of our patients.

INR, International Normalized Ratio.
*See text for details.

REFERENCES

1. Kearon C, Hirsh J: Management of anticoagulation before and after elective surgery. N Engl J Med 336:1506–1511, 1997.
2. Kitchens CS: Occult hemophilia. Johns Hopkins Med J 146:255–259, 1980.
3. Ratnoff OD: Why do people bleed? In Wintrobe MM (ed): Blood, Pure and Eloquent. New York, McGraw-Hill, 1980, pp 600–657.
4. Majno G: The Healing Hand. Man and Wound in the Ancient World. Cambridge, Mass, Harvard University Press, 1975, pp 1–571.
5. Rosner F: Hemophilia in the Talmud and rabbinic writings. Ann Intern Med 70:833–837, 1969.
6. Kitchens CS: Surgery in hemophilia and related disorders: A prospective study of 100 consecutive procedures. Medicine 65:34–45, 1986.
7. Rudowski WJ, Scharf R, Ziemski JM: Is major surgery in hemophiliac patients safe? World J Surg 11:378–386, 1987.
8. Brown B, Steed DL, Webster MW, et al: General surgery in adult hemophiliacs. Surgery 99:154–159, 1986.
9. Kasper CK, Boylen AL, Ewing NP, et al: Hematologic management of hemophilia after surgery. JAMA 253:1279–1283, 1985.
10. Theodore D, Fried MW, Kleiner DE, et al: Liver biopsy in patients with inherited disorders of coagulation and chronic hepatitis C. Haemophilia 10:413–421, 2004.
11. Saab S, Cho D, Quon DVK, et al: Same day outpatient transjugular liver biopsies in haemophilia. Haemophilia 10:727–731, 2004.
12. Shin JL, Teitel J, Swain MG, et al: Canadian multicenter retrospective studies evaluating transjugular liver biopsy in patients with congenital bleeding disorders and hepatitis C: Is it safe and useful? Am J Hematol 78:85–93, 2005.
13. Czaplicki M, Jakubczyk T, Judycki J, et al: ESWL in hemophiliac patients. Eur Urol 38:301–302, 2000.
14. Mortinowitz U, Schulman S, Gitel H, et al: Adjusted dose continuous infusion of factor VIII in patients with haemophilia A. Br J Haematol 82:729–734, 1992.
15. Tagariello G, Davoli PG, Gaso GB, et al: Safety and efficacy of high-purity concentrates in haemophiliac patients undergoing surgery by continuous infusion. Haemophilia 5:426–430, 1999.
16. Palanzu DA, Sadr FS: Coronary artery bypass grafting in a patient with haemophilia B. Perfusion 10:265–270, 1995.
17. MacKinlay N, Taper J, Renisson F, et al: Cardiac surgery and catheterization in patients with haemophilia. Haemophilia 6:84–88, 2000.
18. Davidson SJ, Burman JF, Rutherford LC, et al: High molecular weight kininogen deficiency: A patient who underwent cardiac surgery. Thromb Haemost 85:195–197, 2001.
19. Zanon E, Martinelli F, Bacci C, et al: Proposal of a standard approach to dental extraction in hemophilia patients: A case-control study with good results. Haemophilia 6:533–536, 2000.
20. Hanna W, Bona RD, Zimmerman CE, et al: The use of intermediate and high purity factor VIII products in the treatment of von Willebrand disease. Thromb Haemost 71:173–179, 1994.
21. Foster P: A perspective on the use of FVIII concentrates and cryoprecipitate prophylactically in surgery or therapeutically in severe bleeding in patients with von Willebrand disease unresponsive to DDAVP: Results of an international study. Thromb Haemost 74:1370–1378, 1995.
22. Nitu-Whalley IC, Griffioen A, Harrington C, et al: Retrospective review of the management of elective surgery with desmopressin and clotting factor concentrates in patients with von Willebrand disease. Am J Hematol 66:280–284, 2001.
23. Scharf R, Kucharski W, Nowak T: Surgery in hemophilia A patients with factor VIII inhibitor: 10 Year experience. World J Surg 20:1171–1181, 1996.
24. Tjonnfjord GE, Brinch L, Gedde-Dahl T III, Brosstad FR: Activated prothrombin complex concentrate (FEIBA®) treatment during surgery in patients with inhibitors of FVIII/IX. Haemophilia 10: 174–178, 2004.
25. Quintana-Molina M, Martinez-Bahamonde F, Gonzalez-Garcia E, et al: Surgery in haemophilic patients with inhibitor: 20 Years of experience. Haemophilia 10 (Suppl 2): 30–40, 2004.
26. Rodriguez-Merchan EC: Orthopaedic surgery in persons with haemophilia. Thromb Haemost 89:34–42, 2003.
27. Habermann B, Hochmuth K, Hovy L, et al: Management of haemophilic patients with inhibitors in major orthopaedic surgery in immunoadsorption, substitution of factor VIII and recombinant factor VIIa (NovoSeven®): A single centre experience. Haemophilia 10:705–712, 2004.
28. Ludlam C: Identifying and managing inhibitor patients requiring orthopaedic surgery: The multidisciplinary team approach. Haemophilia 11 (Suppl 1): 7–10, 2005.
29. Blomback M, Eklund J, Hellgren M, et al: Blood coagulation and fibrinolytic factors as well as their inhibitors in trauma. Scand J Clin Lab Invest (Suppl) 178:15–23, 1985.
30. Boisclair MD, Lane DA, Philippou H, et al: Mechanisms of thrombin generation during surgery and cardiopulmonary bypass. Blood 82:3350–3357, 1993.
31. Koh SC, Pua HL, Tay DH, et al: The effects of gynaecological surgery on coagulation activation, fibrinolysis and fibrinolytic inhibitor in patients with and without ketorolac infusion. Thromb Res 79: 501–514, 1995.
32. Sorensen JV: Levels of fibrinolytic activators and inhibitors in plasma after severe trauma. Blood Coagul Fibrinol 5:43–49, 1994.
33. Moschos CB, Khan MI, Regan TJ: Thrombogenic properties of blood during early ischemic and nonischemic injury. Am J Physiol 220:1882–1884, 1971.
34. Voss R, Matthias FR, Borkowsk G, et al: Activation and inhibition of fibrinolysis in septic patients in an internal intensive care unit. Br J Haematol 75:99–105, 1990.
35. Kluft C, Verheijen JH, Jie AF, et al: The postoperative fibrinolytic shutdown: A rapidly reverting acute phase pattern for the fast acting inhibitor of tissue type plasminogen activator after trauma. Scand J Clin Lab Invest 45:605–610, 1985.
36. Kambayashi J, Sakon M, Yokota M, et al: Activation of coagulation and fibrinolysis during surgery, analyzed by molecular markers. Thromb Res 60:157–167, 1990.
37. McCallum PK, Thomson JM, Poller L: Effects of fixed minidose warfarin on coagulation and fibrinolysis following major gynaecological surgery. Thromb Haemost 64:511–515, 1990.
38. Kowal-Vern A, Gamelli RL, Walenga RJM, et al: The effect of burn wound size on hemostasis: A correlation of the hemostatic changes to the clinical state. J Trauma 33:50–57, 1992.
39. Gorman R, Gordan L, Zumberg M, Kitchens C: Successful use of argatroban as an anticoagulant in burn-related severe acquired antithrombin III deficiency after heparin failure. Thromb Haemost 86:1596–1597, 2001.
40. Borgstrom S, Gelin LE, Zederefeldt B: The formation of vein thrombi following tissue injury: An experimental study in rabbits. Acta Chir Scand 247:1–14, 1951.
41. Rosenfeld BA, Beattie C, Christopherson R, et al: The effects of different anesthetic regimens on fibrinolysis and the development of postoperative arterial thrombosis. Anesthesiology 79:435–443, 1993.
41a. Hamer JD, Malone PC, Silver IA: The PO2 in venous valve pockets: Its possible bearing on thrombogenesis. Br J Surg 68:166–170, 1981.
41b. Closse C, Seigneur M, Renard M, et al: Influence of hypoxia and hypoxia-reoxygenation on endothelial P-selectin expression. Thromb Res 85:159–164, 1997.
42. Comerota AJ, Stewart GJ, Alburger PD, et al: Operative venodilation: A previously unsuspected factor in the cause of postoperative deep vein thrombosis. Surgery 106:301–309, 1989.
43. Diamant M, Tushuizen ME, Sturk A, Nieuwland R: Cellular microparticles: New players in the field of vascular disease? Eur J Clin Invest 34:392–401, 2004.
44. Brodsky SV, Zhang F, Nasjletti A, Goligorsky MS: Endothelium-derived microparticles impair endothelial function in vitro. Am J Physiol Heart Circ Physiol 286:H1910–H1915, 2004.
45. Ikeda M, Iwamoto S, Imamura H, et al: Increased platelet aggregation and production of platelet-derived microparticles after surgery for upper gastrointestinal malignancy. J Surg Res 115:174–183, 2003.
46. Biro E, Sturk-Maquelin KN, Vogel GM, et al: Human cell-derived microparticles promote thrombus formation in vivo in a tissue factor-dependent manner. J Thromb Haemost 1:2561–2568, 2003.
47. Craft JA, Marsh NA: Increased generation of platelet-derived microparticles following percutaneous transluminal coronary angioplasty. Blood Coagul Fibrinolysis 14:719–728, 2003.
48. Jy W, Jimenez JJ, Mauro LM, et al: Endothelial microparticles induce formation of platelet aggregates via a von Willebrand factor/ristocetin dependent pathway, rendering them resistant to dissociation. J Thromb Haemost 3:1301–1308, 2005.
49. Butenas S, Bouchard BA, Brummel-Ziedins KE, et al: Tissue factor activity in whole blood. Blood 105:2764–2770, 2005.
50. Freyssinet JM: Cellular microparticles: What are they bad or good for? J Thromb Haemost 1:1655–1662, 2003.

51. Hollmann MW, Wieczorek KS, Smart M, Durieux ME: Epidural anesthesia prevents hypercoagulation in patients undergoing major orthopedic surgery. Reg Anesth Pain Med 26:215–222, 2001.

52. Kohro S, Yamakage M, Arakawa J, et al: Surgical/tourniquet pain accelerates blood coagulability but not fibrinolysis. Br J Anaesth 80:460–463, 1998.

53. Aglietti P, Baldini A, Vena LM, et al: Effect of tourniquet use on activation of coagulation in total knee replacement. Clin Orthop Relat Res 371:169–177, 2000.

54. Boldt J, Haisch G, Suttner S, et al: Are lactated Ringer's solution and normal saline solution equal with regard to coagulation? Anesth Analg 94:378–384, 2002.

55. Quigley RL, Fried DW, Pym J, Highbloom RY: Off-pump coronary artery bypass surgery may produce a hypercoagulable patient. Heart Surg Forum 6:94–98, 2003.

56. Avorn J, Patel M, Levin R, Winkelmayer WC: Hetastarch and bleeding complications after coronary artery surgery. Chest 124: 1437–1442, 2003.

57. Kettner SC, Sitzwohl C, Zimpfer M, et al: The effect of graded hypothermia (36 degrees C—32 degrees C) on hemostasis in anesthetized patients without surgical trauma. Anesth Analg 96:1772–1776, 2003.

58. Kermode JC, Zheng Q, Milner EP: Marked temperature dependence of the platelet calcium signal induced by human von Willebrand factor. Blood 94:199–207, 1999.

59. Hofer CK, Worn M, Tavakoli R, et al: Influence on body core temperature on blood loss and transfusion requirements during off-pump coronary artery bypass grafting: A comparison of 3 warming systems. J Thorac Cardiovasc Surg 129:838–843, 2005.

60. Donahue BS, Gailani D, Higgins MS, et al: Factor V Leiden protects against blood loss and transfusion after cardiac surgery. Circulation 107:1003–1008, 2003.

61. White RH, Zhou H, Romano PS: Incidence of symptomatic venous thromboembolism after different elective or urgent surgical procedures. Thromb Haemost 90:446–455, 2003.

62. Geerts WH, Pineo GF, Heit JA, et al: Prevention of venous thromboembolism. Chest 126:338S–400S, 2004.

63. Westrich GH: The role of mechanical and other adjuncts. Am J Knee Surg 12:55–60, 1999.

64. Hull RD, Pineo GF: Intermittent pneumatic compression for the prevention of venous thromboembolism. Chest 109:6–9, 1996.

65. Agu O, Hamilton G, Baker D: Graduated compression stockings in the prevention of venous thromboembolism. Br J Surg 86: 992–1004, 1999.

66. Kohro S, Yamakage M, Sato K, et al: Intermittent pneumatic foot compression can activate blood fibrinolysis without changes in blood coagulability and platelet activation. Acta Anaesthesiol Scand 49:660–664, 2005.

67. Epstein NE: Intermittent pneumatic compression stocking prophylaxis against deep venous thrombosis in anterior cervical spinal surgery: A prospective efficacy study in 200 patients and literature review. Spine 30:2538–2543, 2005.

68. Nurmohamed MT, van Riel AM, Henkens CMA, et al: Low molecular weight heparin and compression stockings in the prevention of venous thromboembolism in neurosurgery. Thromb Haemost 75:233–238, 1996.

69. Agnelli G, Piovella F, Buoncristiani P, et al: Enoxaparin plus compression stockings compared with compression stockings alone in the prevention of venous thromboembolism after elective neurosurgery. N Engl J Med 339:80–85, 1998.

70. Agnelli G: Prevention of venous thromboembolism after neurosurgery. Thromb Haemost 82:925–930, 1999.

71. Iorio A, Agnelli G: Low-molecular-weight and unfractionated heparin for prevention of venous thromboembolism in neurosurgery. Arch Intern Med 160:2327–2332, 2000.

72. Raabe A, Gerlach R, Zimmermann M, Seifert V: The risk of haemorrhage associated with early postoperative heparin administration after intracranial surgery. Acta Neurochir (Wien) 143:1–7, 2001.

73. Dickinson LD, Miller LD, Patel CP, et al: Enoxaparin increases the incidence of postoperative intracranial hemorrhage when initiated preoperatively for deep venous thrombosis prophylaxis in patients with brain tumors. Neurosurgery 43:1074–1081, 1998.

74. Park P, Fewel M, Garton H, et al: Recombinant activated factor VII for the rapid correction of coagulopathy in nonhemophilic neurosurgical patients. Neurosurgery 53:34–39, 2003.

75. Ageno W, Dentali F, Squizzato A: Prophylaxis of venous thromboembolism following laparoscopic surgery: Where is the evidence? J Thromb Haemost 3:214–215, 2005.

76. Tincani E, Piccoli M, Turrini F, et al: Video laparoscopic surgery: Is out-of-hospital thromboprophylaxis necessary? Always. J Thromb Haemost 3:216–220, 2005.

77. Ljungstrom K-G: Is there a need for antithrombotic prophylaxis during laparoscopic surgery? Not always. J Thromb Haemost 3:212–213, 2005.

78. Bevan DH: Cardiac bypass haemostasis: Putting blood through the mill. Br J Haematol 104:208–219, 1999.

79. Despotis GJ, Avidan MS, Hogue CW Jr: Mechanisms and attenuation of hemostatic activation during extracorporeal circulation. Ann Thorac Surg 72:S1821–S1831, 2001.

80. Whitlock R, Crowther MA, Ng HJ: Bleeding in cardiac surgery: Its prevention and treatment—an evidence-based review. Crit Care Clin 21:589–610, 2005.

81. Harker L, Malpass TW, Branson HE, et al: Mechanism of abnormal bleeding in patients undergoing cardiopulmonary bypass: Acquired transient platelet dysfunction associated with selective α-granule release. Blood 56:824–834, 1980.

82. Hertfelder JH, Bos M, Weber D, et al: Perioperative monitoring of primary and secondary hemostasis in coronary artery bypass grafting. Semin Thromb Hemost 31:426–440, 2005.

83. Wahba A, Videm V: Heart surgery with extracorporeal circulation leads to platelet activation at the time of hospital discharge. Eur J Cardiothorac Surg 23:1046–1050, 2003.

84. Bradfield JF, Bode AP: Aprotinin restores the adhesive capacity of dysfunctional platelets. Thromb Res 109:181–188, 2003.

85. Pelletier MP, Solymoss S, Lee A, et al: Negative reexploration for cardiac postoperative bleeding: Can it be therapeutic? Ann Thorac Surg 65:999–1002, 1998.

86. Englberger L, Faeh B, Berdat PA, et al: Impact of clopidogrel in coronary artery bypass grafting. Eur J Cardiothorac Surg 26:96–101, 2004.

87. Gerrah R, Elami A, Stamler A, et al: Preoperative aspirin administration improves oxygenation in patients undergoing coronary artery bypass grafting. Chest 127:1622–1626, 2005.

88. Laupacis A, Fergusson D: Drugs to minimize perioperative blood loss in cardiac surgery: Meta-analyses using perioperative blood transfusions as the outcome. Anesth Analg 85:1258–1267..

89. Levi M, Cromheecke ME, deJonge E, et al: Pharmacological strategies to decrease excessive blood loss in cardiac surgery: Meta-analysis of clinically relevant endpoints. Lancet 354: 1940–1947, 1999.

90. Cattaneo M, Harris A-S, Stromberg U, et al: The effect of desmopressin on reducing blood loss in cardiac surgery: A meta-analysis of double-blind, placebo-controlled trials. Thromb Haemost 74:1064–1070, 1995.

91. Czer LSC, Bateman TM, Gray RJ, et al: Treatment of severe platelet dysfunction and hemorrhage after cardiopulmonary bypass: Reduction in blood product usage with desmopressin. J Am Coll Cardiol 9:1139–1147, 1987.

92. Gratz I, Koehler J, Olsen D, et al: The effect of desmopressin acetate on postoperative hemorrhage in patients receiving aspirin therapy before coronary artery bypass operations. J Thorac Cardiovasc Surg 104:1417–1422, 1992.

93. NIH Consensus Conference: Platelet transfusion therapy. JAMA 257:1777–1780, 1987.

94. NIH Consensus Conference: Fresh-frozen plasma: Indications and risks. JAMA 253:551–553, 1985.

95. Spiess BD, Royston D, Levy JH, et al: Platelet transfusions during coronary artery bypass graft surgery are associated with serious adverse outcomes. Transfusion 44:1143–1148, 2004.

96. Casbard AC, Williamson LM, Murphy MF, et al: The role of prophylactic fresh frozen plasma in decreasing blood loss and correcting coagulopathy in cardiac surgery. A systematic review. Anaesthesia 59:550–558, 2004.

97. Murphy GJ, Allen SM, Unsworth-White J, et al: Safety and efficacy of perioperative cell salvage and autotransfusion after coronary artery bypass grafting: A randomized trial. Ann Thorac Surg 77: 1553–1559, 2004.

98. Jones HU, Muhlestein JB, Jones KW, et al: Preoperative use of enoxaparin compared with unfractionated heparin increases the incidence of re-exploration for postoperative bleeding after open-heart surgery in patients who present with an acute coronary syndrome: Clinical investigation and reports. Circulation 106 (12 Suppl 1): I19–I22, 2002.

99. Kincaid EH, Monroe ML, Saliba DL, et al: Effects of preoperative enoxaparin versus unfractionated heparin on bleeding indices in patients undergoing coronary artery bypass grafting. Ann Thorac Surg 76:124–128, 2003.

100. Hunt BJ, Parratt RN, Segal HC, et al: Activation of coagulation and fibrinolysis during cardiothoracic operations. Ann Thorac Surg 65:712–718, 1998.

101. Smith CR: Management of bleeding complications in redo cardiac operations. Ann Thorac Surg 65 (4 Suppl): S2–8, 1998.

102. Stassano P, Musumeci A, Santise G, et al: Can epsilon-aminocaproic acid balance the off-pump bleeding advantage? Cardiovasc Surg 11:219–223, 2003.

103. Nuttall GA, Erchul DT, Haight TJ, et al: A comparison of bleeding and transfusion in patients who undergo coronary artery bypass grafting via sternotomy with and without cardiopulmonary bypass. J Cardiothorac Vasc Anesth 17:447–451, 2003.

104. Srinivasan AK, Grayson AD, Pullan DM, et al: Effect of preoperative aspirin use in off-pump coronary artery bypass operations. Ann Thorac Surg 76:41–45, 2003.

105. Wahba A, Black G, Koksch M, et al: Aprotinin has no effect on platelet activation and adhesion during cardiopulmonary bypass. Thromb Haemost 75:844–848, 1996.

106. Ray MJ, Marsh NA: Aprotinin reduces blood loss after cardiopulmonary bypass by direct inhibition of plasmin. Thromb Haemost 78:1021–1026, 1997.

107. Casati V, Guzzon D, Oppizzi M, et al: Hemostatic effects of aprotinin, tranexamic acid and epsilon-aminocaproic in primary cardiac surgery. Ann Thorac Surg 68:2252–2256, 1999.

108. Munoz JJ, Birkmeyer NJ, Birkmeyer JD, et al: Is epsilon-aminocaproic acid as effective as aprotinin in reducing bleeding with cardiac surgery? A meta-analysis. Circulation 99:81–89, 1999.

109. Slaughter TF, Faghih F, Greenberg CS, et al: The effects of epsilon-aminocaproic acid on fibrinolysis and thrombin generation during cardiac surgery. Anesth Analg 85:1221–1226, 1997.

110. Chauhan S, Das SN, Bisoi A, et al: Comparison of epsilon aminocaproic acid and tranexamic acid in pediatric cardiac surgery. J Cardiothorac Vasc Anesth 18:141–143, 2004.

111. Mangano DT, Tudor IC, Dietzel C: The risk associated with aprotinin in cardiac surgery. N Engl J Med 354:353–365, 2006.

112. Henry DA, Moxey AJ, Carless PA, et al: Anti-fibrinolytic use for minimising perioperative allogeneic blood transfusion. The Cochrane Database of Systematic Reviews 1, 2006.

113. Rooney SJ, Bonser RS: The management of bleeding following surgery requiring hypothermic circulatory arrest. J Card Surg 12:238–242, 1997.

114. Prendergast TW, Furukaa S, Beye AJ 3rd, et al: Defining the role of aprotinin in heart transplantation. Ann Thorac Surg 62:670–674, 1996.

115. Okita Y, Takamoto S, Ando M, et al: Is use of aprotinin safe with deep hypothermic circulatory arrest in aortic stenosis? Investigations on blood coagulation. Circulation 94:177–181, 1996.

116. Whitten CW, Allison PM, Latson TW, et al: Management of the thrombocytopenic cardiac surgical patient: A role for aprotinin. Anesth Analg 79:796–800, 1994.

117. Gu YJ, de Haan J, Brenken UP, et al: Clotting and fibrinolytic disturbance during lung transplantation: Effect of low-dose aprotinin. Groningen Lung Transplant Group. J Thorac Cardiovasc Surg 112:599–606, 1996.

118. Goldstein DJ, Seldomridge JA, Chen JM, et al: Use of aprotinin in LVAD recipients reduces blood loss, blood use, and perioperative mortality. Ann Thorac Surg 59:1063–1067, 1995.

119. Khalil PN, Ismail M, Kalmar P, et al: Activation of fibrinolysis in the pericardial cavity after cardiopulmonary bypass. Thromb Haemost 92:568–574, 2004.

120. Razon Y, Erez E, Vidne B, et al: Recombinant factor VIIa (NovoSeven) as a hemostatic agent after surgery for congenital heart disease. Paediatr Anaesth 15:235–240, 2005.

121. Halkos ME, Levy JH, Chen E, et al: Early experience with activated recombinant factor VII for intractable hemorrhage after cardiovascular surgery. Ann Thorac Surg 79:1303–1306, 2005.

122. Hyllner M, Houltz E, Jeppsson A: Recombinant activated factor VII in the management of life-threatening bleeding in cardiac surgery. Eur J Cardiothorac Surg 28:254–258, 2005.

123. von Heymann C, Redlich U, Jain U, et al: Recombinant activated factor VII for refractory bleeding after cardiac surgery: A retrospective analysis of safety and efficacy. Crit Care Med 33:2241–2246, 2005.

124. Raivio P, Suojaranta-Ylinen R, Kuitunen AH: Recombinant factor VIIa in the treatment of postoperative hemorrhage after cardiac surgery. Ann Thorac Surg 80:66–71, 2005.

125. O'Connell KA, Wood JJ, Wise RP, et al: Thromboembolic adverse events after use of recombinant human coagulation factor VIIa. JAMA 295:293–298, 2006.

126. Shander A, Goodnough LT, Ratko T, et al: Consensus recommendations for the off-label use of recombinant human factor VIIa (NovoSeven®) therapy. P&T 30:644–658, 2005.

126a. Dzik WH: Off-label reports of new biologics: Exciting new therapy or dubious research? Examples from recombinant activated factor VII. J Intensive Care Med 21:54–59, 2006.

127. Slaughter TF, Greenberg CS: Antifibrinolytic drugs and perioperative hemostasis. Am J Hematol 56:32–36, 1997.

128. Dunn CJ, Goa KL: Tranexamic acid: A review of its use in surgery and other indications. Drugs 57:1005–1032, 1999.

129. Schmaier AH: Aprotinin: Can its benefits be offset by harmful effects? Transfusion 37:1105–1107, 1997.

130. Murkin JM: Attenuation of neurologic injury during cardiac surgery. Ann Thorac Surg 72:S1838–S1844, 2001.

130a. Mangano DT, Miao Y, Vuylsteke A, et al: Mortality associated with aprotinin during 5 years following coronary artery bypass graft surgery. JAMA 297:471–479, 2007.

130b. Ferguson TB: Aprotinin—are there lessons learned? JAMA 297:527–529, 2007.

131. Cohen DM, Norberto J, Cartabuke R, et al: Severe anaphylactic reaction after primary exposure to aprotinin. Ann Thorac Surg 67:837–838, 1999.

132. Dietrich W, Spath P, Ebell A, et al: Prevalence of anaphylactic reactions to aprotinin: Analysis of two hundred forty eight reexposures to aprotinin in heart operations. J Thorac Cardiovasc Surg 113:194–201, 1997.

133. Duke C, Grammie JS: Surgical implications of platelet glycoprotein IIb-IIIa inhibition. J Thorac Cardiovasc Surg 116:1083–1084, 1998.

134. Dietrich W, Dilthey G, Spannagl M, et al: Warfarin pretreatment does not lead to increased bleeding tendency during cardiac surgery. J Cardiothorac Vasc Anesth 9:250–254, 1995.

135. Sato M, Nasha B, Ringe B, et al: Coagulation disorder during liver transplantation. Blood Coagul Fibrinolysis 2:25–31, 1991.

136. Himmelreich G, Hundt K, Nevhaus P, et al: Decreased platelet aggregation after reperfusion in orthotopic liver transplantation. Transplantation 53:582–586, 1992.

137. Sato M, Nashan B, Grosse H, et al: Hemostatic studies of ex situ hepatic surgery. Jpn J Surg 21:561–565, 1991.

138. Grosse H, Lobbes W, Sato M, et al: Systemic fibrinogenolysis in liver transplantation. Transplant Proc 22:2303–2304, 1990.

139. Velasco F, Villalba R, Fernandez M, et al: Diminished anticoagulant and fibrinolytic activity following liver transplantation. Transplantation 53:1256–1261, 1992.

140. Grosse H, Lobbes W, Frambach M, et al: The use of high dose aprotinin in liver transplantation: The influence on fibrinolysis and blood loss. Thromb Res 63:287–297, 1991.

141. Llamas P, Cabrera R, Gomez-Arnau J, et al: Hemostasis and blood requirements in orthotopic liver transplantation with and without high-dose aprotinin. Haematologica 83:338–346, 1998.

142. Lentschener C, Benhamou D, Mercier FJ, et al: Aprotinin reduces blood loss in patients undergoing elective liver resection. Anesth Analg 84:875–881, 1997.

143. Kufner RP: Antifibrinolytics do not reduce transfusion requirements in patients undergoing orthotopic liver transplantation. Liver Transpl Surg 3:668–674, 1997.

144. Garcia-Huete L, Domenech P, Sabate A, et al: The prophylactic effect of aprotinin on intraoperative bleeding in liver transplantation: A randomized clinical study. Hepatology 26:1143–1148, 1997.

145. Porte RJ, Molenaar IQ, Begliomini B, et al: Aprotinin and transfusion requirements in orthotopic liver transplantation: A multicentre randomized double-blind study. Lancet 355:1303–1309, 2000.

146. Markiewicz M, Kalicinski P, Kaminski A, et al: Acute coagulopathy after reperfusion of the liver graft in children correction with recombinant activated factor VII. Transplant Proc 35:2318–2319, 2003.

147. Planinsic RM, van der Meer J, Testa G, et al: Safety and efficacy of a single bolus administration of recombinant factor VIIa in liver transplantation due to chronic liver disease. Liver Transpl 11:895–900, 2005.

148. D'Ambrosio A, Borghi B, Damato A, et al: Reducing perioperative blood loss in patients undergoing total hip arthroplasty. Int J Artif Organs 22:47–51, 1999.

149. Hiippala ST, Strid LJ, Wennerstrand MI, et al: Tranexamic acid radically decreases blood loss and transfusions associated with total knee arthroplasty. Anesth Analg 84:839–844, 1997.

150. Capdevia X, Calvet Y, Biboulet P, et al: Aprotinin decreases blood loss and homologous transfusions in patients undergoing major orthopedic surgery. Anesthesiology 88:50–57, 1998.

151. Kasper SM, Schmidt J, Rutt J: Is aprotinin worth the risk in total hip replacement? Anesthesiology 81:517–519, 1994.

37

152. Collins R, Scrimgeour A, Yusuf S, et al: Reduction in fatal pulmonary embolism and venous thrombosis by perioperative administration of subcutaneous heparin. Overview of results of randomized trials in general, orthopedic and urologic surgery. N Engl J Med 318: 1162–1173, 1988.

153. Burk CD, Muller L, Handler SD: Preoperative history and coagulation screening in children undergoing tonsillectomy. Pediatrics 89:691–695, 1992.

154. Haberman SD II, Shattuck TG, Dion NM: Is outpatient suction cautery tonsillectomy safe in a community hospital setting? Laryngoscope 100:551–555, 1990.

155. Suchman AL, Mushlin AL: How well does the activated partial thromboplastin time predict postoperative hemorrhage? JAMA 256:750–753, 1986.

156. Kitchens CS: Preoperative PT's, PTT's, cost-effectiveness, and health care reform: Radical changes that make good sense. Chest 106: 661–662, 1994.

157. Schein OD, Katz J, Bass EB, et al: The value of routine preoperative medical testing before cataract surgery. N Engl J Med 342:168–175, 2000.

158. Bryson GL: Has preoperative testing become a habit? Can J Anaesth 52:557–561, 2005.

159. Roizen MF: More preoperative assessment by physicians and less by laboratory tests. N Engl J Med 342:204–205, 2000.

160. Narr BJ, Warner ME, Schroeder DR, et al: Outcomes of patients with no laboratory assessment before anesthesia and a surgical procedure. Mayo Clin Proc 72:505–509, 1997.

161. Koscielny J, Ziemer S, Radtke H, et al: A practical concept for preoperative identification of patients with impaired primary hemostasis. Clin Appl Thromb Hemost 10:195–204, 2004.

162. Eberl W, Wendt I, Schroeder HG: Preoperative coagulation screening prior to adenoidectomy and tonsillectomy. Klin Padiatr 217:20–24, 2005.

163. Imasogie N, Wong DT, Luk K, Chung F: Elimination of routine testing in patients undergoing cataract surgery allows substantial savings in laboratory costs: A brief report. Can J Anaesth 50: 246–248, 2003.

164. Schramm B, Leslie K, Myles PS, Hogan CJ: Coagulation studies in preoperative neurosurgical patients. Anaesth Intensive Care 29: 388–392, 2001.

165. Chee YL, Greaves M: Role of coagulation testing in predicting bleeding risk. Hematol J 4:373–378, 2003.

166. Eckman MH, Erban JK, Singh SK, Kao GS: Screening for the risk for bleeding or thrombosis. Ann Intern Med 138:W15–W24, 2003.

167. Patel RI, DeWitt L, Hannallah RS: Preoperative laboratory testing in children undergoing elective surgery: Analysis of current practice. J Clin Anesth 9:569–575, 1997.

168. Toker A, Shvarts S, Perry ZH, et al: Clinical guidelines, defensive medicine, and the physician between the two. Am J Otolaryngol 25:245–250, 2004.

169. Peterson P, Hayes TE, Arkin CF, et al: The preoperative bleeding time lacks clinical benefits. Arch Surg 133:134–139, 1998.

170. Bowie EJW, Owen CA Jr: The significance of abnormal preoperative hemostatic tests. Prog Hemost Thromb 5:179–209, 1980.

171. Aggeler PM, Hoag MS, Wallerstein RO, et al: The mild hemophilias. Occult deficiencies of AHF, PTC and PTA frequently responsible for unexpected surgical bleeding. Am J Med 30:84–94, 1961.

172. Bachmann F: Diagnostic approach to mild bleeding disorders. Semin Hematol 17:292–305, 1980.

173. Biron C, Mahieu B, Rochette A, et al: Preoperative screening for von Willebrand disease type 1: Low yield and limited ability to predict bleeding. J Lab Clin Med 134:605–609, 1999.

174. Kitchens CS: Prolonged activated partial thromboplastin time of unknown etiology: A prospective study of 100 consecutive cases referred for consultation. Am J Hematol 27:38–45, 1988.

175. Golub R, Cantu R, Sorrento JJ, et al: Efficacy of preadmission testing in ambulatory surgical patients. Am J Surg 163:565–571, 1992.

176. Kaplan EB, Sheiner LB, Boeckmann AJ, et al: The usefulness of preoperative laboratory screening. JAMA 253:3576–3581, 1985.

177. Litaker D: Preoperative screening. Med Clin North Am 83:1565–1581, 1999.

178. Eisenberg JM, Clarke JR, Sussman SA: Prothrombin and partial thromboplastin times as preoperative screening test. Arch Surg 117:48–51, 1982.

179. Bauer KA: The thrombophilias: Well-defined risk factors with uncertain therapeutic implications. Ann Intern Med 135:367–373, 2001.

180. Reddy NM, Hall SW, MacKintosh FR: Partial thromboplastin time: Prediction of adverse events and poor prognosis by low abnormal values. Arch Intern Med 159:2706–2710, 1999.

181. Wahlander K, Larson G, Lindahl TL, et al: Factor V Leiden (G1691A) and prothrombin gene G20210A mutations as potential risk factors for venous thromboembolism after total hip or total knee replacement surgery. Thromb Haemost 87:580–585, 2002.

182. Andrassy J, Zeier M, Andrassy K: Do we need screening for thrombophilia prior to kidney transplantation? Nephrol Dial Transplant 19 (Suppl 4): iv64–iv68, 2004.

183. Mont MA, Jones LC, Rajadhyaksha AD, et al: Risk factors for pulmonary emboli after total hip or knee arthroplasty. Clin Orthop Relat Res 422:154–163, 2004.

184. Salvati EA, Della Valle AG, Westrich GH, et al: Heritable thrombophilia and development of thromboembolic disease after total hip arthroplasty. Clin Orthop Relat Res 441:40–55, 2005.

185. Christiansen SC, Cannegieter SC, Koster T, et al: Thrombophilia, clinical factors, and recurrent venous thrombotic events. JAMA 293:2352–2361, 2005.

186. Lowe GD: Prediction of postoperative deep-vein thrombosis. Thromb Haemost 78:47–52, 1997.

187. Kakkar VV, Howe CT, Nicolaides AN, et al: Deep vein thrombosis of the leg: Is there a "high risk" group? Am J Surg 120:527–530, 1970.

188. Caprini J, Arcelus JI, Reyna JJ: Effective risk stratification of surgical and nonsurgical patients for venous thromboembolic disease. Semin Hematol 39 (2 Suppl 5): 12–19, 2001.

189. Sarasin FP, Bounameaux H: Duration of oral anticoagulant therapy after proximal deep vein thrombosis in a decision analysis. Thromb Haemost 71:286–291, 1994.

190. Kitchens CS: To bleed or not to bleed? Is that the question for the PTT? J Thromb Haemost 3:2607–2611, 2005.

191. Tripodi A, Salerno F, Chantarangkul V, et al: Evidence of normal thrombin generation in cirrhosis despite abnormal conventional coagulation tests. Hepatology 41:553–558, 2005.

192. Dzik WH: Predicting hemorrhage using preoperative coagulation screening assays. Current Hematology Reports 3:324–330, 2004.

192a. Dara SI, Rana R, Afessa B, et al: Fresh frozen plasma transfusion in critically ill medical patients with coagulopathy. Crit Care Med 33:2667–2671, 2005.

192b. Gajic O, Dzik WH, Toy P: Fresh frozen plasma and platelet transfusion for nonbleeding patients in the intensive care unit: Benefit or harm? Crit Care Med 34:S170–S173, 2006.

192c. Abdel-Wahab OI, Healy B, Dzik WH: Effect of fresh-frozen plasma transfusion on prothrombin time and bleeding in patients with mild coagulation abnormalities. Transfusion 46:1279–1285, 2006.

192d. Holland LL, Brooks JP: Toward rational fresh frozen plasma transfusion: The effect of plasma transfusion on coagulation test results. Am J Clin Pathol 126:133–139, 2006.

193. Bishop JF, Schiffer CA, Aisner J, et al: Surgery in acute leukemia: A review of 167 operations in thrombocytopenic patients. Am J Hematol 26:147–155, 1987.

194. Keidar A, Feldman M, Szold A: Analysis of outcome of laparoscopic splenectomy for idiopathic thrombocytopenic purpura by platelet count. Am J Hemato 80:95–100, 2005.

195. Chu DZJ, Shivshanker K, Stroehlein JR, et al: Thrombocytopenia and gastrointestinal hemorrhage in the cancer patient: Prevalence of unmasked lesion. Gastrointest Endosc 29:269–272, 1983.

196. Gazzard BG, Henderson JM, Williams R: The use of fresh frozen plasma or a concentrate of factor IX as replacement therapy before liver biopsy. Gut 16:621–625, 1975.

197. McGill DB, Rakela J, Zinsmeister AR, et al: A 21-year experience with major hemorrhage after percutaneous liver biopsy. Gastroenterology 99:1396–1400, 1990.

198. McVay PA, Toy PT CY: Lack of increased bleeding after liver biopsy in patients with mild hemostatic abnormalities. Am J Clin Pathol 94:747–753, 1990.

199. Boberg KM, Brosstad F, Egeland T, et al: Is a prolonged bleeding time associated with an increased risk of hemorrhage after liver biopsy? Thromb Haemost 81:378–381, 1999.

200. Ewe K: Bleeding after liver biopsy does not correlate with indices of peripheral coagulation. Dig Dis Sci 26:388–393, 1981.

201. Makris M, Nakielny R, Toh CH, et al: A prospective investigation of the relationship between haemorrhagic complications of percutaneous needle biopsy of the liver and coagulation screening tests. Br J Haematol 81:51(abstr), 1992.

202. Bravo AA, Sheth SG, Chopra S: Liver biopsy. N Engl J Med 344: 495–500, 2001.

203. Shiffman ML, Farrel MT, Yee YS: Risk of bleeding after endoscopic biopsy or polypectomy in patients taking aspirin or other NSAIDs. Gastrointest Endosc 40:458–462, 1994.

204. American Society for Gastrointestinal Endoscopy: Guideline on the management of anticoagulation and antiplatelet therapy for endoscopic procedures. Gastrointest Endosc 55:775–779, 2002.

205. Blacker DJ, Eelco FM, Wijdicks EFM, McClelland RL: Stroke risk in anticoagulated patients with atrial fibrillation undergoing endoscopy. Neurology 61:964–968, 2003.

206. McVay PA, Toy PTCY: Lack of increased bleeding after paracentesis and thoracentesis in patients with mild coagulation abnormalities. Transfusion 31:164–171, 1991.

207. Webster ST, Brown KL, Luchey MR, Nostrank TT: Hemorrhagic complications of large-volume abdominal paracentesis. Am J Gastroenterol 91:366–368, 1996.

208. Shpitz B, Plotkin E, Spindel Z, et al: Should aspirin therapy be withheld before insertion and/or removal of a permanent peritoneal dialysis catheter? Am Surg 68:762–764, 2002.

209. Kozak EA, Brath LK: Do "screening" coagulation tests predict bleeding in patients undergoing fiberoptic bronchoscopy with biopsy? Chest 106:703–705, 1994.

210. Weiss SM, Hert RC, Gianola FJ, et al: Complications of fiberoptic bronchoscopy in thrombocytopenic patients. Chest 104:1025–1028, 1993.

211. Bjortuft O, Brosstad F, Boe J: Bronchoscopy with transbronchial biopsies: Measurement of bleeding volume and evaluation of the predictive value of coagulation tests. Eur Respir J 12:1025–1027, 1998.

212. Diette GB, Weiner CM, White P: The higher risk of bleeding in lung transplant recipients from bronchoscopy is independent of traditional bleeding risks: Results of a prospective cohort study. Chest 115:397–402, 1999.

213. Herth FJF, Becker HD, Ernst A: Aspirin does not increase bleeding complications after transbronchial biopsy. Chest 122:1461–1464, 2002.

214. Howard SC, Gajjar A, Ribeiro RC, et al: Safety of lumbar puncture for children with acute lymphoblastic leukemia and thrombocytopenia. JAMA 284:2222–2224, 2000.

215. Ray CE Jr, Shenoy S: Patients with thrombocytopenia: Outcome of radiologic placement of central venous access devices. Radiology 204:97–99, 1997.

216. Goldfarb G, Lebrec D: Percutaneous cannulation of the internal jugular vein in patients with coagulopathies: An experience based on 1000 attempts. Anesthesiology 56:321–323, 1982.

217. Fisher NC, Mutimer DJ: Central venous cannulation in patients with liver disease and coagulopathy: A prospective audit. Intensive Care Med 25:481–485, 1999.

218. Foster PF, Moore LR, Sankary HN, et al: Central venous catheterization in patients with coagulopathy. Arch Surg 127:273–275, 1992.

219. DeLoughery TG, Liebler JM, Simonds V, et al: Invasive line placement in critically ill patients: Do hemostatic tests matter? Transfusion 36:827–831, 1996.

220. Doerfler ME, Kaufman B, Goldenberg AS: Central venous catheter placement in patients with disorders of coagulation. Chest 110:185–188, 1996.

221. Darcy MD, Kanterman RY, Kleinhoffer MA, et al: Evaluation of coagulation tests as predictors of angiographic bleeding complications. Radiology 198:741–744, 1996.

222. Eckman MH, Beshansky JR, Durand-Zaleski I, et al: Anticoagulation for noncardiac procedures in patients with prosthetic heart valves: Does low risk mean high cost? JAMA 263:1513–1521, 1990.

223. Katholi RE, Nolan SP, McGuire LD: Living with prosthetic heart valves: Subsequent noncardiac operations and the risk of thromboembolism or hemorrhage. Am Heart J 92:162–167, 1976.

224. Stone LS, Kline OR Jr, Sklar C: Intraocular lenses and anticoagulation and antiplatelet therapy. Am Intra-ocular Implant Soc J 11:165–168, 1985.

225. Weibert RT: Oral anticoagulant therapy in patients undergoing dental surgery. Clin Pharm 11:857–864, 1992.

226. Blinder D, Manor Y, Martinowitz U, et al: Dental extractions in patents maintained on continued oral anticoagulant: Comparison of local hemostatic modalities. Oral Surg Oral Med Oral Pathol Oral Radiol Endod 88:137–140, 1999.

227. Wahl MJ: Dental surgery in anticoagulated patients. Arch Intern Med 158:1610–1616, 1998.

228. Alexander R, Ferretti AC, Sorensen JR: Stop the nonsense not the anticoagulants: A matter of life and death. NY State Dent J 68:24–26, 2002.

229. Sevitt S, Gallagher NG: Prevention of venous thrombosis and pulmonary embolism in injured patients: A trial of anticoagulant prophylaxis with phenindione in middle-aged and elderly patients with fractured necks of femur. Lancet 2:981–989, 1959.

230. Salzman EW, Harris WH, DeSanctis RW: Reduction in venous thromboembolism by agents affecting platelet function. N Engl J Med 284:1287–1292, 1971.

231. Francis CW, Marder VJ, Evarts CMC, et al: Two-step warfarin therapy. Prevention of postoperative venous thrombosis without excessive bleeding. JAMA 249:374–378, 1983.

232. Larson BG, Zumberg MS, Kitchens CS: A feasibility study of continuing dose-reduced warfarin for invasive procedures in patients with high thromboembolic risk. Chest 127:922–927, 2005.

233. Sandset PM, Abildgaard U: Perioperative management of oral anticoagulant therapy. Thromb Res 108:1–2, 2003.

234. Torn M, Rosendaal FR: Oral anticoagulation in surgical procedures: risks and recommendations. Br J Haematol 123:676–682, 2003.

235. Wallace DL, Latimer MD, Belcher HJ: Stopping warfarin therapy is unnecessary for hand surgery. J Hand Surg (Br) 29:203–205, 2004.

236. Ihezue CU, Smart J, Dewbury KC, et al: Biopsy of the prostate guided by transrectal ultrasound. Relation between warfarin use and incidence of bleeding complications. Clin Radiol 60:459–463, 2005.

237. Ah-Weng A, Natarajan S, Velangi S, Langtry JA: Preoperative monitoring of warfarin in cutaneous surgery. Br J Dermatol 149:386–389, 2003.

238. Otley CC: Continuation of medically necessary aspirin and warfarin during cutaneous surgery. Mayo Clin Proc 78:1392–1396, 2003.

239. Spandorfer JM, Lynch S, Weitz HH, et al: Use of enoxaparin for the chronically anticoagulated patient before and after procedure. Arch Intern Med 158:1610–1616, 1998.

240. Kovacs MJ, Kearon C, Rodger M, et al: Single-arm study of bridging therapy with low-molecular-weight heparin for patients at risk of arterial embolism who require temporary interruption of warfarin. Circulation 110:1658–1663, 2004.

241. Wojcik R, Cipolle MD, Seislove E, et al: Preinjury warfarin does not impact outcome in trauma patients. J Trauma 51:1147–1152, 2001.

242. Mina AA, Bair HA, Howells GA, Bendick PJ: Complications of preinjury warfarin use in the trauma patient. J Trauma 54:842–847, 2003.

243. Lavoie A, Ratte S, Clas D, et al: Preinjury warfarin use among elderly patients with closed head injuries in a trauma center. J Trauma 56:802–807, 2004.

244. Shetty HGM, Backhouse G, Bentley DP, et al: Effective reversal of warfarin-induced excessive anticoagulation with low dose vitamin K. Thromb Haemost 67:13–15, 1992.

245. Whitling AM, Bussey HI, Lyons RM: Comparing different routes and doses of phytonadione for reversing excessive anticoagulation. Arch Intern Med 158:2136–2140, 1998.

246. Raj G, Kumar R, McKinney WP: Time course of reversal of anticoagulant effect of warfarin by intravenous and subcutaneous phytonadione. Arch Intern Med 159:2721–2724, 1999.

247. Shields RC, McBaive RD, Kuiper JD, et al: Efficacy and safety of intravenous phytonadione (vitamin K_1) in patients on long-term oral anticoagulant therapy. Mayo Clin Proc 76:260–266, 2001.

248. Woodman RC, Harker LA: Bleeding complications associated with cardiopulmonary bypass. Blood 1680–1687, 1990.

249. Manco-Johnson MJ, Nuss R, Jacobson LJ: Heparin neutralization is essential for accurate measurement of factor VIII activity and inhibitor assays in blood samples drawn from implanted venous access devices. J Lab Clin Med 136:74–79, 2000.

250. Linkins LA, Julian JA, Rishcke J, et al: In vitro comparison of the effect of heparin, enoxaparin and fondaparinux on tests of coagulation. Thromb Res 107:241–244, 2002.

251. Rice L: Surreptitious bleeding in surgery: A major challenge in coagulation. Clin Lab Haematol 22 (Suppl1): 17–20, 2000.

252. Mallett SV, Cox DJ: Thromboelastography. Br J Anaesth 69:307, 1992.

253. Wang JS, Lin CY, Hung WT, et al: Thromboelastogram fails to predict postoperative hemorrhage in cardiac patents. Ann Thorac Surg 53:435, 1992.

254. Forestier F, Coiffic A, Mouton C, et al: Platelet function point-of-care tests in post-bypass cardiac surgery: Are they relevant? Br J Anaesth 89:715–721, 2002.

255. Hertfelder HJ, Bos M, Weber D, et al: Perioperative monitoring of primary and secondary hemostasis in coronary artery bypass grafting. Semin Thromb Hemost 31:426–440, 2005.

256. Avidan MS, Alcock EL, DaFonseca J, et al: Comparison of structured use of routine laboratory tests or near-patient assessment with clini-

cal judgement in the management of bleeding after cardiac surgery. Br J Anaesth 92:178–186, 2004.

257. Prim MP, De Deigo JI, Jimenez-Yuste V, et al: Analysis of the causes of immediate unanticipated bleeding after pediatric adenotonsillectomy. Int J Pediatr Otorhinolaryngol 67:341–344, 2003.

258. Merrit JC, Bhatt DL: The efficacy and safety of perioperative antiplatelet therapy. J Thromb Thrombolysis 17:21–27, 2004.

259. Edmonds AR: Death from respiratory obstruction in haemophilia. Med J Aust 1:227–228, 1951.

260. MacDonald AC, Robson JB, Waapshaw H: Haemophilia with respiratory obstruction. Br Med J 1:1144–1146, 1953.

261. Pappas AM, Barr JS, Salzman EW, et al: The problem of unrecognized "mild hemophilia." JAMA 187:772–774, 1964.

262. Coy J, Bivins BA, Belin RP: Surgical procedures in unsuspected hemophilia. Arch Surg 109:835–836, 1974.

263. Ghosh K, Madkaikar M, Jijina F, et al: Open heart surgery with mitral valve replacement: Ordeal of an undiagnosed haemophilia patient. Clin Lab Haematol 25:131–133, 2003.

264. Alperin JB: Coagulopathy caused by vitamin K deficiency in critically ill, hospitalized patients. JAMA 258:1916–1919, 1987.

265. Zumberg MS, Waples JM, Kao KJ, et al: Management of a patient with a mechanical aortic valve and antibodies to both thrombin and factor V after repeat exposure to fibrin sealant. Am J Hematol 64:59–63, 2000.

266. Miller RD, Robbins TO, Tong MJ, Barton SL: Coagulation defects associated with massive blood transfusions. Ann Surg 174:794–801, 1971.

267. Hardy JF, de Moerloose P, Samama CM: The coagulopathy of massive transfusion. Vox Sang 89:123–127, 2005.

Chapter 38

Anticoagulation in the Perioperative Period

Bundarika Suwanawiboon, MD ● Thomas L. Ortel, MD, PhD*

Hematologists are frequently consulted to evaluate patients who receive long-term oral anticoagulant therapy and may require temporary interruption of warfarin prior to surgery or an invasive procedure. In general, these patients are maintained on chronic anticoagulation for clinical conditions associated with an increased thrombotic risk, including mechanical prosthetic heart valves, chronic atrial fibrillation, or venous thromboembolism, making perioperative management problematic. On the one hand, disruption of oral anticoagulation will expose the patient to an increased risk of thromboembolism, but the degree of risk is clearly variable among such patients. On the other hand, there is a legitimate, but often exaggerated, risk of hemorrhagic complications if anticoagulant therapy is continued. Prior to formulating a management recommendation, these issues must be individually addressed using risk:benefit ratio formulations as best as possible. These considerations are best managed by a hematologist with experience in the management of antithrombotic therapy and perioperative hemorrhage.

Presently, there is little consensus on the optimal management of anticoagulant therapy in this particular scenario. In addition, there are no randomized prospective clinical studies to evaluate the efficacy and safety of different perioperative anticoagulation approaches. Most recommendations are based largely on empirical data and the extrapolation of anticoagulant benefit estimated from thrombotic and bleeding risks identified in certain procedures and patient groups, which may not be entirely applicable to patients in different clinical settings. This chapter provides a summary of currently available evidence and suggests a management framework concerning the perioperative and postoperative management of patients on chronic anticoagulation. Nevertheless, clinicians must keep in mind that the recommendation for each patient should be individualized to maintain a balance between efficacy of anticoagulant therapy in the prevention of thromboembolic events and safety of the treatment to minimize potential hemorrhagic complications.

When considering the rates at which complications occur, it is also important to bear in mind the clinical consequences of these complications. For example, approximately 20% of arterial thromboembolic events are fatal, and 40% result in serious permanent disability.[1] Additionally, up to 6% of recurrent venous thromboembolic events are fatal.[1] In contrast, several studies have demonstrated that ~3% of major postoperative bleeding events are fatal with most patients making a full recovery after hemorrhagic complications.[1] These observations suggest that a hemorrhagic complication may not be as devastating as a thromboembolic event, and should also be taken into consideration when making a recommendation for the individual patient.

PREOPERATIVE ASSESSMENT

Prior to considering discontinuation of oral anticoagulation and selecting an alternative anticoagulant agent, several issues need to be addressed: (1) Perioperative thromboembolic risk; (2) Perioperative and postoperative bleeding risk; and (3) Potential benefit of perioperative anticoagulation.

These issues will be discussed in more detail subsequently. Other variables that may play a role in the decision-making include patient preference and the cost of supplemental perioperative anticoagulation, particularly in the case of intravenous unfractionated heparin, which generally requires hospitalization for drug administration and laboratory monitoring.

Perioperative Thromboembolic Risk

The assessment of perioperative thromboembolic risk can be stratified based on the indication for anticoagulation. Most patients require long-term oral anticoagulant therapy because of a mechanical prosthetic heart valve, chronic atrial fibrillation, or venous thromboembolism. Specific patient populations will be considered separately.

Patients with a Mechanical Prosthetic Heart Valve

Long-term anticoagulant therapy is indicated in patients with a mechanical prosthetic heart valve because of the risk of systemic thromboembolism and valve thrombosis. In the absence of anticoagulant therapy, the incidence rates of prosthetic valve thrombosis and major embolism (resulting in death, residual neurologic deficit, or peripheral ischemia requiring surgery) are approximately 1.8% per patient-year and 4% per patient-year, respectively (derived from a meta-analysis of 46 studies including 13,088 patients, combining patients with prosthetic valves in the aortic and/or mitral

*TLO is supported by a cooperative agreement (U18 DD00014) with the Hematologic Diseases Branch, the Centers for Disease Control and Prevention.

positions, as well as all types of prosthetic valves, predominantly Starr-Edwards, Björk-Shiley, Medtronic-Hall, and St. Jude).[2] The rate of these complications decreased to 1% per patient-year with warfarin therapy.[2]

In general, a prosthetic valve in the mitral position is considered to have higher thrombogenicity and is associated with a greater risk for valve thrombosis and systemic embolization than a prosthetic valve in the aortic position[2,3] owing to increased vascular stasis around the mitral valve.[4] Risk of thrombotic complication is also affected by the design and construction materials of the valve prosthesis. The risk is highest in patients who have a caged-ball type of valve (e.g., Starr-Edwards), followed by the single-leaflet tilting disc type (e.g., Björk-Shiley, Medtronic-Hall) and the bileaflet tilting disc type (e.g., St. Jude, Carbomedics), which is the least thrombogenic.[2,4–6]

In patients who have more than one prosthetic valve, the risk for thromboembolic complication is higher than that of patients with a single valve prosthesis.[2–4] Furthermore, the presence of concomitant atrial fibrillation also increases the risk of thrombogenicity of a prosthetic valve.[2]

When anticoagulation therapy is transiently discontinued, the principal concern is the risk of thrombosis. However, it is difficult to estimate the daily risk of thromboembolism in the absence of anticoagulation therapy due to limited data and the fact that most studies involve patients with first-generation prosthetic heart valves. Recent data from patients with newer generation mechanical heart valves (e.g., St. Jude and Björk-Shiley valve prostheses) provide the estimation of an annualized risk of any thrombotic complication varying from 10% to 23%.[7] The summary of annual thrombotic risk associated with prosthetic heart valves in the absence of antithrombotic therapy is listed in Table 38-1.

Patients with Chronic Atrial Fibrillation

Patients with atrial fibrillation are at increased risk for systemic embolism. The risk is highest in patients with a prior transient ischemic attack or stroke, particularly if the embolic event occurred within the preceding month (high-risk group), with an incidence of 12% to 15% per year.[5,8,9] The thromboembolic risk is also modified by the presence of additional risk factors, including hypertension, diabetes mellitus, increasing age (age >65 years) and impaired left ventricular function (Table 38-2).[10–12]

Patients with lone atrial fibrillation who are 65 years in age or younger and have none of the additional stroke risk factors listed in Table 38-2 have the lowest risk of stroke, with an

Table 38-1 Thrombotic Risk Associated with Prosthetic Valves in the Absence of Antithrombotic Therapy

Prosthesis Type	Rate of Thrombosis (% per year)
Multiple (St. Jude) prosthetic valves	91
Dual-leaflet (St. Jude) mitral valve	22
Single-leaflet (Björk-Shiley) aortic valve	23
Dual-leaflet (St. Jude) aortic valve	10–12

Adapted from Ansell J, Hirsh J, Poller L, et al: The pharmacology and management of the vitamin K antagonists: The Seventh ACCP Conference on Antithrombotic and Thrombolytic Therapy. Chest 126:204S-233S, 2004.

Table 38-2 Additional Risk Factors for Stroke in Patients with Chronic Atrial Fibrillation

Condition	Relative risk*
Prior TIA/stroke	2.5–2.9
Left ventricular dysfunction	2.5
Hypertension[†]	1.6–2.0
Increasing age[‡]	1.6–1.8
Diabetes mellitus	1.6–1.7

Risk factors for stroke and efficacy of antithrombotic therapy in atrial fibrillation: Analysis of pooled data from five randomized controlled trials. Arch Intern Med 154:1449–1457, 1994.
*Relative to all patients with atrial fibrillation whose absolute risk for stroke is approximately 5%/year. Compiled from Hart RG, Pearce LA, McBride R, et al: Factors associated with ischemic stroke during aspirin therapy in atrial fibrillation: Analysis of 2012 participants in the SPAF I-III clinical trials. The Stroke Prevention in Atrial Fibrillation (SPAF) Investigators. Stroke 30:1223–1229, 1999.
[†]Hypertension is defined as systolic blood pressure >160 mm Hg
[‡]Age >65 years
Adapted from Douketis JD: Perioperative anticoagulation management in patients who are receiving oral anticoagulant therapy: A practical guide for clinicians. Thromb Res 108:3–13, 2002; and Heit JA: Perioperative management of the chronically anticoagulated patient. J Thromb Thrombolysis 12:81–87, 2001.

incidence of less than 1% per year.[5,11,13] Nevertheless, most patients with atrial fibrillation fall into a moderate-risk group (atrial fibrillation with the presence of stroke risk factors as listed in Table 38-2, but without history of stroke or transient ischemic attack [TIA]) with an incidence of stroke of 3% to 7% per year.[5,9] Unfortunately, the data concerning the perioperative thromboembolic risk during the temporary interruption of oral anticoagulation in patients with atrial fibrillation are sparse. Nonetheless, it has been estimated that the daily risk of systemic embolism, interpolating from the aforementioned data, are roughly 0.28% to 0.38% in the high-risk group, followed by 0.06% and 0.15% in the moderate-risk group, and 0.02% to 0.04% in the low-risk group.[5,11,12]

Patients with Venous Thromboembolism

The risk of additional thromboembolic complications is highest in patients who present with acute venous thromboembolism (within the preceding month), with an estimated thrombotic rate of 40% per year in the absence of anticoagulant therapy.[1,14,15] The risk of recurrent events then declines rapidly over the following 3 months to approximately 10% per year.[1,14] In patients with recurrent venous thromboembolism, an estimated risk of 15% per year is speculated if anticoagulant therapy is discontinued.[1,14] The risk of venous thromboembolism based on time of onset is summarized in Table 38-3.

There are no data regarding the risk of recurrent disease if oral anticoagulant therapy is temporarily interrupted.[5] The presence of additional independent risk factors also modifies the probability of disease recurrence. These factors include increasing age and body mass index, malignant neoplasm, chronic disease such as neurologic disease with extremity paresis, antiphospholipid syndrome, homozygosity for factor V Leiden polymorphism, and combined heterozygosity for the factor V Leiden and prothrombin 20210 polymorphism.[1,5,16–20] Furthermore, patients with previous postoperative venous thromboembolism will be more likely to develop recurrent disease after surgery, although there are no data to

Table 38-3 Thrombotic Risk Associated with Venous Thromboembolism Without Concomitant Anticoagulant Therapy

Clinical Presentation	Thrombotic Risk*
Acute Venous Thromboembolism	
Within first month	40%
Months 2 and 3	10%
Recurrent Venous Thromboembolism	15% per year

*Risk not including surgery associated risk of venous thromboembolism.
Adapted from Kearon C, Hirsh J: Management of anticoagulation before and after elective surgery. N Engl J Med 336:1506–1511, 1997.

Table 38-4 Risk Stratification for Perioperative Thromboembolism

High Risk of Thromboembolism

Recent (<3 months) history of venous or arterial thromboembolism
Mechanical valve in mitral position and/or older model of prosthetic valve (e.g., single-disc or caged-ball type)
Recent mechanical valve placement (<3 months)
Atrial fibrillation with history of systemic embolization
Atrial fibrillation in the presence of mechanical heart valve
Acute intracardiac thrombus confirmed by echocardiography
Rheumatic atrial fibrillation
Presence of hypercoagulable state
    Recurrent episodes of (≥2) arterial* or idiopathic venous thromboembolism
    Life threatening venous thromboembolism (e.g., mesenteric or cerebral vein thrombosis, Budd-Chiari syndrome)
    Protein C or protein S deficiency
    Antithrombin III deficiency
    Homozygous factor V Leiden mutation
    Antiphospholipid-antibody syndrome

Moderate Risk of Thromboembolism

Newer model of prosthetic valve (e.g., St. Jude) in mitral position
Older model of mechanical valve in aortic position
Cerebrovascular disease with multiple (≥2) strokes or transient ischemic attacks without risk factors for cardiac embolism
Atrial fibrillation with risk factors for cardiac embolism† but without history of stroke or transient ischemic attack

Low Risk of Thromboembolism

Remote history of venous thromboembolism (>3–6 months)
Atrial fibrillation without a history of stroke or other risk factors for cardiac embolism†
Bileaflet mechanical valve in aortic position

*Risk not including primary atherosclerotic events, e.g., stroke or myocardial infarction due to intrinsic cerebrovascular or coronary disease.
†Risk factors for cardiac embolism such as ejection fraction <40%, diabetes, hypertension, non-rheumatic valvular heart disease, transmural myocardial infarction within preceding month.
Adapted from Ansell J, Hirsh J, Poller L, et al: The pharmacology and management of the vitamin K antagonists: The Seventh ACCP Conference on Antithrombotic and Thrombolytic Therapy. Chest 126:204S-233S, 2004; and Jaffer AK, Brotman DJ, Chukwumerije N: When patients on warfarin need surgery. Cleve Clin J Med 70:973–984, 2003.

provide a reliable estimate of this risk.[5] Table 38-4 summarizes a risk stratification scheme for thromboembolism based on patient-related characteristics when assessing the need for perioperative anticoagulant therapy.

Preoperative and Postoperative Bleeding Risks

Risk of Bleeding Associated with Patient Characteristics

The first step to evaluate perioperative and postoperative bleeding risk is to obtain a thorough patient history to rule out the possibility of an underlying coagulopathy. Other pertinent information that will help determine the surgical bleeding risk includes history of aspirin, nonsteroidal anti-inflammatory drug (NSAID) or other antiplatelet therapy; history of blood transfusion; bleeding during previous invasive procedures, (e.g., dental cleaning/extraction, child-birth, surgery, or trauma), and other medical problems. Certain medical conditions may also increase the risk of bleeding. Examples include hepatic or renal insufficiency, dysproteinemias, myeloproliferative disorders, or malignancy/sepsis-associated disseminated intravascular coagulation. Preoperative laboratory screening tests should be obtained, if clinically indicated, to further evaluate for an underlying bleeding disorder.

Generally, a routine complete blood count is ordered to screen for anemia or thrombocytopenia, regardless of a bleeding history. Coagulation screening tests other than prothrombin time/INR on the morning of the procedure are seldom indicated.[16] It has been suggested that patients who undergo surgery with an INR > 1.5 have an increased risk of postoperative hemorrhagic complications.[5] Additional coagulation testing may be required in the patient who has a history of a bleeding diathesis, an underlying medical disease that may increase the risk of bleeding, and in patients with positive family history of abnormal bleeding.

Risk of Bleeding Associated with Type of Surgery or Procedure

Several procedure-specific factors significantly influence the perioperative and postoperative hemorrhagic outcomes and the decision for anticoagulant management. These include the location and extent of surgery and the accessibility of bleeding to compression or other physical means of control (e.g., packing, suturing, cautery, topical hemostatic or anti-fibrinolytic agent).[16,21] Procedures that appear to have a low risk of bleeding despite the continuation of oral anticoagulation include most outpatient dental procedures,[22–29] cataract extraction,[30–35] and most cutaneous surgery, including Mohs micrographic surgery.[36] Examples of moderate-risk procedures include major intra-abdominal surgery and orthopedic surgery.[5] High-risk procedures include cardiac and major vascular surgery,[37] prostatectomy,[38,39] bladder surgery,[5] and renal biopsy.[40]

The incidence of excessive perioperative blood loss in patients undergoing cardiac surgery with cardiopulmonary bypass is approximately 13% to 16% when abnormal bleeding is defined as more than 10 units of perioperative blood transfusion. This incidence drops to 5% to 7% if excessive bleeding is defined as greater than 2 L blood loss within the first 24 postoperative hours.[37,41] For

Table 38-5 Risk Stratification for Perioperative Hemorrhage

High Risk

Coronary artery bypass graft surgery
Cardiac valve replacement
Major vascular surgery
Neurosurgical procedure
Major cancer surgery
Prostatectomy or bladder surgery
Renal biopsy, bowel polypectomy

Moderate Risk

Major intrathoracic surgery
Major orthopedic surgery
Major intra-abdominal surgery
Pacemaker insertion
Hernia*
Laparoscopic cholecystectomy*

Low Risk

Most cutaneous surgery
Cataract surgery
Coronary angiography[†]
Outpatient dental procedures[‡]

---

*Low to moderate risk
[†]In an emergent or semi-emergent situation, cardiac catheterization can be performed with a patient taking warfarin but preferably the drug should be discontinued ~72 hours prior to the procedure (desired INR ≤ 1.5).[120]
[‡]Including single and multiple dental extractions and alveolectomy.
Adapted from Douketis JD: Perioperative anticoagulation management in patients who are receiving oral anticoagulant therapy: A practical guide for clinicians. Thromb Res 108:3–13, 2002.

Table 38-6 Hemorrhagic Risk Stratification for Endoscopic Procedures

High Risk

Polypectomy*
Biliary sphincterotomy (2.5–5%)
Pneumatic or bougie dilation
PEG placement
Endosonographic guided fine needle aspiration
Laser ablation and coagulation (<6%)
Treatment of varices

Low Risk

EGD ± biopsy
Flexible sigmoidoscopy ± biopsy
Colonoscopy ± biopsy
ERCP without sphincterotomy
Biliary/pancreatic stent without endoscopic sphincterotomy
Endosonography without fine needle aspiration
Enteroscopy

---

*Bleeding risk 1–2.5% in colonoscopic polypectomy and 4% in gastric polypectomy.
Adapted from Eisen GM, Baron TH, Dominitz JA, et al: Guideline on the management of anticoagulation and antiplatelet therapy for endoscopic procedures. Gastrointest Endosc 55:775–779, 2002.

patients undergoing an elective general or orthopedic surgery, results from a meta-analysis of 52 randomized controlled trials (29 in general surgery and 23 in orthopedic surgery) including a total of 2658 patients in the placebo-control groups demonstrated that the rate of major bleeding was approximately 4%.[42] This estimate of hemorrhagic complication is obtained from patients who did not receive any anticoagulant therapy and, therefore, can be regarded as a normal and baseline risk for major bleeding anticipated in any patient undergoing a general surgical procedure. A classification scheme of surgical bleeding risk related to the type of procedure is provided in Table 38-5.

Endoscopic Procedures

Among various elective gastrointestinal endoscopic procedures, diagnostic esophagogastroduodenoscopy (EGD), flexible sigmoidoscopy and colonoscopy with or without biopsy, diagnostic endoscopic retrograde cholangiopancreatography (ERCP), biliary stent insertion without endoscopic sphincterotomy, and endosonography (EUS), are categorized as low-risk procedures based on the 2002 guidelines on the management of anticoagulation and antiplatelet therapy for endoscopic procedures by the American Society for Gastrointestinal Endoscopy (ASGE).[43]

Procedures with an increased bleeding risk include colonoscopic or gastric polypectomy,[44,45] laser ablation and coagulation,[46,47] endoscopic sphincterotomy,[48] and those procedures where bleeding is inaccessible or uncontrollable by endoscopic means such as pneumatic or bougie dilation of benign or malignant strictures and EUS-guided fine needle

aspiration.[43] Table 38-6 summarizes the list of high- and low-risk endoscopic procedures according to the ASGE.

Potential Benefits of Perioperative Anticoagulation

Patients with a Mechanical Prosthetic Heart Valve

The rationale for bridging anticoagulant therapy with unfractionated heparin (UFH) or low molecular weight heparin (LMWH) during the period when oral anticoagulation is temporarily discontinued is to shorten the time when the patient is at risk for thromboembolic events because of subtherapeutic anticoagulation.[49–51]

Katholi and colleagues reported that there were no thromboembolic events among 25 patients with isolated aortic valve prostheses (Starr-Edwards Model 1200 and MaGovern) who received no perioperative anticoagulation before a procedure, compared with two fatal thromboembolic episodes in ten patients with mitral valve prostheses (Kay-Shiley disc, Starr-Edwards Model 6120 and MaGovern) (Table 38-7).[52] In contrast, nine patients who underwent noncardiac surgery and continued warfarin therapy, with estimated INRs of 2.5 to 7.0, sustained three major hemorrhages requiring "unanticipated" transfusion support.[52] Subsequently, a prospective cohort study was performed to evaluate the outcome of patients undergoing noncardiac procedures on two different perioperative anticoagulation protocols (45 procedures in 39 patients).[53] In patients with isolated mechanical aortic valves, warfarin was discontinued 3 to 5 days prior to the procedure without bridging anticoagulation. For patients with mitral valve prostheses, warfarin anticoagulation was rapidly reversed by parenteral vitamin K given within 24 hours prior to the surgery and intravenous UFH was initiated 12 hours preoperatively. There were no thromboembolic events in either patient group. However, there was one major bleeding event in a patient with a prosthetic mitral valve (see Table 38-7).

Table 38-7 Thromboembolic Events in Patients with Prosthetic Heart Valves Receiving Perioperative Anticoagulation with Unfractionated Heparin or Continued Warfarin

Author	Type of Study	No. of Patients (No. Procedures)	Valve Replaced[a]	Perioperative Therapy[b]	Thrombo-embolic Events	Bleeding Events
Katholi, et al, 1976[52]	Retrospective	36 (44)	A (n = 31) M+C (n = 13)	None[c] (n = 25) Warfarin[d] (n = 6) None (n = 10) Warfarin (n = 3)	0 0 2 0	3[e] 1[f]
Katholi, et al, 1978[53]	Prospective cohort	39 (45)[g]	A (n = 19) M+C (n = 26)	None (n = 18) IV UFH (n = 1) IV UFH[h]	0 0 0	1[i] 2[j]
Tinker & Tarhan, 1978[54]	Retrospective	159 (180)	A (n = 105) M (n = 57) T (n = 1) C (n = 17)	None (n = 155)[k] Warfarin (n = 23)	6[l]	42[m]
Madura, et al, 1994[49]	Retrospective	17 (17)	A (n = 8) M (n = 4) T (n = 1) C (n = 4)	IV UFH[n]	0	5[o]

A, aortic valve prosthesis; M, mitral valve prosthesis; T, tricuspid valve prosthesis; and C, combined prostheses; IV, intravenous; UFH, unfractionated heparin.

[a]The numbers in parentheses refer to the number of procedures performed for the different types of valves. For the first three studies, most patients had Starr-Edwards prosthetic valves. Other valves included the Smeloff-Cutter mitral valve, MaGovern aortic and mitral valves, and the Braunwald-Cutter aortic and mitral valves. The type of valve replacement was not reported in the fourth study.

[b]The numbers in parentheses refer to the number of procedures performed using a particular strategy.

[c]None indicates that anticoagulation was simply discontinued for 3 to 5 days prior to surgery.

[d]Warfarin anticoagulation was not discontinued for the surgical procedure.

[e]There were three major perioperative hemorrhages.

[f]"Significant bleeding" was noted in one patient in the postoperative setting (no description of bleeding nature).

[g]Twenty-three major operations (hysterectomy, 8; pulse generator change, 5; bowel resection, 4; cholecystectomy, 3; subtotal gastrectomy, 2; and craniotomy, 1). 22 Minor operations (biopsy or excision, 9; dental extraction, 5; arteriography, 4; mastectomy, 2; and hemorrhoidectomy, 2).

[h]Intravenous unfractionated heparin (unspecified dose) starting 12 hours postoperatively.

[i]Minor incisional hematoma; heparin was started early after operation (time of onset not specified).

[j]One patient with abdominal incisional hematoma and one patient with vaginal cuff bleeding, requiring blood transfusion.

[k]Anticoagulation discontinued 1 to 3 days prior to surgery in 113 operations and 4 or more days in 42 operations.

[l]Thromboembolic complications occurred from 12 months to more than 2 years after the surgery.

[m]Intraoperative difficulties with "hemostasis" were encountered in 24 patients; postoperative bleeding was "prominent" in 7 procedures; and hematomas occurred in 11 cases. Most of the bleeding complications were associated with an elevated prothrombin time at the time of surgery.

[n]IV UFH started after discontinuation of warfarin and stopped 6 to 12 hrs before surgery.

[o]Five bleeding complications; all required re-operation for control of bleeding or evacuation of hematoma.

Similar results were obtained by Tinker and Tarhan in a larger retrospective study. There were six episodes of thromboembolism among 159 patients with prosthetic heart valves undergoing 180 noncardiac operations in which anticoagulation was discontinued an average of 2.9 days preoperatively. The majority of patients had older generations of valve prostheses (Starr-Edwards) in the aortic position, but 36% of patients had mitral valve prostheses and 11% had multiple prostheses (see Table 38-7).[54]

The advantages of perioperative heparin administration have also been described in a small study performed by Madura and colleagues who found no thromboembolic events in 17 patients with prosthetic valves undergoing major surgery. All of the patients received bridging UFH infusions while warfarin was withheld. Five patients (29%) had bleeding complications and required re-operation, however (see Table 38-7).[49]

Carrel and colleagues examined three different approaches of perioperative anticoagulant therapy and outcomes in 235 patients with prosthetic heart valves who required noncardiac surgery. In this study, perioperative treatment included continuation of warfarin, or discontinuation of warfarin with and without intravenous or subcutaneous heparin administration.[5,55] Overall, the incidence of hemorrhagic complications was 8% (18 of 235 patients)

and that of thromboembolic events was 7% (16 of 235 patients). Interpretation of the results was limited by inadequate follow up information and the questionable adequacy of perioperative anticoagulation.[5,55]

Since the availability of LMWH, there has been increasing interest in examining the role of these agents in perioperative therapy when oral anticoagulation is discontinued. This option is appealing because LMWH offers a predictable anticoagulant effect and convenient route of drug administration that can be delivered in an outpatient setting. Traditional bridging anticoagulant therapy using intravenous UFH is more costly and labor intensive because it requires inpatient hospitalization for dose adjustment and laboratory monitoring.[56,57]

Currently, there are several studies evaluating the efficacy of LMWH as bridging therapy in chronically anticoagulated patients who require an invasive procedure. In these studies, mechanical valve patients represent the majority of the study population (50% to 100%). All but one of the studies[58] are prospective. Results from these studies have suggested that LMWH appears to be at least as effective as UFH in the perioperative setting if the proper dose is used with overall low incidence rates of both thromboembolic events and major bleeding that are comparable with those seen with UFH.[22,59] The summaries of

Table 38-8 Clinical Studies Using Low Molecular Weight Heparin as Perioperative Anticoagulation in Patients on Chronic Warfarin Anticoagulation

Author	Type of Study	No. Patients (% Valves)[a]	Type of LMWH	Dose	Thromboembolic events (%)	Bleeding events (%)
Kovacs et al[60]	Prospective cohort	224 (50%)	Dalteparin	200 IU/kg qD[b]	8 (3.6%)[c]	15 (6.7%)[d]
Spandorfer et al[61]	Prospective cohort	20 (60%)	Enoxaparin	1 mg/kg bid	0	3 (12.5%)[e]
Johnson & Turpie[62]	Prospective cohort	515 (41%)	Dalteparin or Enoxaparin	100 IU/kg bid (n = 372) 1 mg/kg bid (n = 143)	0	2 (0.4%)[f]
Ferreira et al[63]	Prospective cohort	20 (100%)	Enoxaparin or fraxiparin	variable[g]	0	Not provided
Galla and Fuhs[58]	Retrospective	60 (100%)	Enoxaparin	30 mg bid	0	3 (3.8%)
Tinmouth et al[65]	Prospective cohort	24 (50%)	Dalteparin	200 IU/kg qD	0	2 (7.7%)[h]
Ferreira et al[66]	Prospective cohort	82 (100%)[i]	Enoxaparin	1 mg/kg bid[j]	0	9 (11%)[k]
Douketis et al[59]	Prospective cohort	650 (33%)	Dalteparin	100 IU/kg bid	4 (0.6%)[l]	6 (0.9)[m]

[a]The percentage in parentheses represents the percentage of patients with prosthetic heart valves of the total number of patients studied.
[b]Dalteparin dose was reduced to 100 IU/kg on the morning before surgery (maximum, 9000 IU).
[c]Six of eight episodes of thromboembolism occurred in patients who had warfarin therapy deferred or withdrawn because of bleeding.
[d]Major hemorrhage (overt bleeding with a drop of hemoglobin >2 g/dL within a 24-hour period or transfusion of at least 2 units of blood; intracranial, intraspinal, intraocular, retroperitoneal, or pericardial bleeding; and fatal bleeding).
[e]Postprocedure bleeding, all soft tissue bleeding (2 minor bleeding and 1 patient had a drop of Hb of 2 g/dL but did not require blood transfusion).
[f]Two major bleeds (rectus muscle sheath hematoma and bleeding at incision); 17 minor bleeding episodes.
[g]Dosage used depended on the patient's weight and the INR before starting the treatment.
[h]Minor bleeding (hematuria and spotting after a cervical biopsy).
[i]Type of prosthesis; Sorin Bicarbon prosthesis (35%), Carbomedics (33%), Björk-Shiley (27%), Medtronic-Hall (4%), and Starr-Edwards (1%). Fifty-two percent of patients had prosthetic aortic valves.
[j]Enoxaparin dose was adjusted to the lowest dose to obtain an anti-Xa level above 0.4 IU/mL in patients with creatinine ≥1.5 mg/dL (≥133 μmol/L).
[k]Eight minor bleeding (only one patient required blood transfusion) and one major bleeding (intracranial bleeding).
[l]Mean follow up period = 13.8 days. Two deaths due to cardiac arrests possibly due to thromboembolism; one patient with stroke and one patient with TIA.
[m]All major bleeding events (nonfatal upper gastrointestinal tract bleeding, 4 wound hematomas, and a rectus abdominis sheath hematoma).

clinical studies using LMWH as a bridging anticoagulant therapy are shown in Table 38-8.[58–66]

Patients with Atrial Fibrillation

In patients with chronic atrial fibrillation who are undergoing elective surgery, there are no clinical trials directly assessing perioperative anticoagulation therapy and patient outcome.[16]

Patients with Venous Thromboembolism

Patients with a history of acute venous thromboembolism within the preceding month who require temporary interruption of oral anticoagulation should receive preoperative and postoperative intravenous UFH because of an estimated 1% absolute increase in the risk of recurrence per day without anticoagulation and the extremely high incidence of postoperative thromboembolism.[1,15] Postoperative intravenous UFH was felt to be justified despite doubling the rate of bleeding because of the net reduction in serious morbidity in these patients with perioperative anticoagulant therapy.[1] For patients who require an invasive procedure during the second and third months after an acute episode of venous thromboembolism, preoperative intravenous heparin is not suggested unless the patient has other risk factors for thromboembolism (e.g., hospitalization) because the risk of recurrent thromboembolic events is sufficiently

decreased. Nevertheless, postoperative administration of therapeutic doses of heparin is recommended owing to the expected 100-fold increase in the risk of developing venous thromboembolism after surgery.[1]

Three months after the initial presentation of a venous thromboembolic event, preoperative anticoagulation is generally not warranted, and the use of postoperative therapeutic intravenous UFH is debatable. However, exceptions may be considered in patients who have significant residual clot burden, who have had multiple prior thrombotic events, who have had life-threatening events such as mesenteric or cerebral vein thrombosis, or who are not at increased risk of hemorrhage. There is also a role for alternative postoperative venous thromboembolic prophylaxis with subcutaneous low doses of UFH or LMWH in patients with a low risk of bleeding.[1,67]

MANAGEMENT RECOMMENDATIONS

The following recommendations, divided into preoperative, perioperative, and postoperative settings, are based on previous study results and the Seventh American College of Chest Physicians Conference on Antithrombotic and Thrombolytic Therapy.[7] Nevertheless, it must be emphasized that there are guidelines and that the decision for perioperative and postoperative anticoagulation needs to be individualized and made on a case-by-case basis.

Preoperative Anticoagulation Management

Discontinuation of Warfarin Therapy

For procedures typically deemed to require a "normal" prothrombin time (INR < 1.2) at the time of surgery (i.e., for high-risk procedures listed in Tables 38-5 and 38-6), warfarin should be discontinued at least 3 to 4 days prior to the surgery (in patients with a target INR of 2.0 to 3.0) to allow the INR to return to normal or at least to a near normal range (INR = 1.2 to 1.4).[68,69] Warfarin might be withheld for an extra 1 to 2 days in patients who are normally maintained at a higher target INR (above 3.0) [1,5] Caution should be made in elderly patients who sometimes may require a longer time for the INR to normalize after warfarin is stopped.[5,68] The prothrombin time/INR can be tested on the day prior to the surgery to ensure that it has fallen into the desired target range that is assumed to be safe to perform the procedure. Other investigators also suggest checking the INR on the day warfarin therapy is stopped.[5]

For patients with a low risk of bleeding who are undergoing a low bleeding risk procedure (Tables 38-5 and 38-6), oral anticoagulation may be continued at the regular dose with no adjustments. An alternative strategy would be to slightly decrease the dose for several days prior to the procedure, to obtain a lower INR (although not a normal prothrombin time) at the time of the procedure.

Reversal of Oral Anticoagulation

If the INR is greater than 1.5 on the day before surgery, administration of low-dose oral vitamin K (2.5 mg) or intravenous vitamin K (e.g., 1.5 mg administered over 60 minutes) will likely normalize the INR without causing a delay in time to therapeutic oral anticoagulation when warfarin is resumed after surgery.[5,16] Intravenous vitamin K is reserved by some clinicians for patients with malabsorption who require an urgent procedure, and large doses should be avoided as they have been reported to cause anaphylactoid reactions.[16,70] Another alternative is to give a small dose of vitamin K (1 mg) subcutaneously, although this route of administration may result in erratic absorption.[70] In patients who need rapid reversal of oral anticoagulation owing to the need for urgent surgery, fresh frozen plasma (FFP) transfusion may be required. The required volume of transfused FFP can be calculated by estimating the plasma volume (plasma volume [in mL] is approximately 40 × body weight [in kg]) and determining the target net increase in plasma coagulant factor activity.[16] In general, average-sized individuals will require approximately 15 or 16 mL/kg of FFP (containing 100% activity of factor II) to significantly reverse a therapeutic INR.[16] The major limitation of FFP therapy is the risk of transfusion-related infection and intravascular volume overload. In addition, concomitant vitamin K therapy is required owing to the short half-life of factor VII in plasma (4 to 6 hours). An alternative for patients at risk of volume overload is prothrombin complex concentrate infusion; current preparations carry a low risk for thrombotic complications and very low incidence of transfusion-related infections.

Discontinuation of Antiplatelet Therapy

The risk of bleeding complications associated with antiplatelet therapy was recently reported by Serebruany and colleagues in a meta-analysis involving 338,191 patients who were receiving antiplatelet agents.[71] In this meta-analysis, the majority of patients had sustained acute coronary syndromes with 40% of the eligible studies involving percutaneous coronary interventions. Low-dose aspirin (<100 mg) and dipyridamole resulted in the lowest hemorrhagic complications with total bleeding rates of 3.6% and 6.7%, respectively.[71] The majority of these studies used the Thrombolysis in Myocardial Infarction (TIMI) study group criteria, with the total bleeding risk including major, minor, gastrointestinal bleeding, and stroke.[71] A relatively increased risk of bleeding (9.1% to 9.9%) was found to be associated with a higher dose of aspirin (≥100 mg), which was comparable with the risk observed in patients taking clopidogrel (8.5%). However, the incidence of hemorrhagic complications was highest among patients receiving intravenous and oral platelet surface glycoprotein IIb/IIIa inhibitors, with total bleeding rates of 49% and 44.6%, respectively.[71]

Controversy remains as to whether it is necessary to withhold antiplatelet therapy prior to the surgery, and, if so, when would be the optimal time to discontinue therapy. Theoretically, it would be prudent to discontinue aspirin and other antiplatelet agents at least 7 days prior to the procedure, given that aspirin, ticlopidine and clopidogrel irreversibly inhibit platelet function.[72,73] Nevertheless, clinical evidence supporting this common practice is sparse, and most of the data are from patients undergoing high bleeding risk procedures, such as cardiothoracic surgery. Furthermore, recent demonstration of considerable recovery of platelet function as early as 3 days after discontinuation of aspirin in cardiac surgery patients raises the question of whether early cessation of aspirin (>7 days before surgery) is necessary.[74] Data on this topic for other types of surgery are either limited or unavailable. Therefore, clinicians need to individualize their recommendations based on the consideration of risk:benefit ratio involved in the specific type of procedure and the patient's indication for antiplatelet therapy.

Earlier data from a number of studies, including prospective controlled trials, indicate that preoperative aspirin use (usually ≥75 mg/day, within 2 days before surgery) in patients undergoing coronary artery bypass graft surgery is associated with increased blood loss, transfusion requirements, and re-exploration for bleeding.[75–82] Recent evidence, however, suggests that preoperative aspirin within 5 to 7 days before surgery appears to be safe without a significant increase in adverse postoperative hemorrhagic complications.[83–88] On the contrary, the combination of clopidogrel and aspirin prior to bypass surgery has been shown to increase the risk of postoperative bleeding, particularly if higher doses of aspirin are used (200 to 325 mg/day).[89–92] To avoid excessive postoperative bleeding and transfusion, the American College of Cardiology/American Heart Association (ACC/AHA) task force has recommended cessation of aspirin and other antiplatelet inhibitors (excluding clopidogrel) 7 to 10 days prior to elective cardiac operation in certain clinical settings such as chronic stable angina and low-risk plaque morphology.[93] For clopidogrel, the ACC/AHA recommended that this medication be discontinued at least 5 days prior to elective bypass surgery.[93]

Despite the paucity of evidence, several published reports suggest that certain elective interventions may be performed safely on patients who are at low bleeding risk who are taking aspirin and/or other NSAIDs in standard doses without significant increases in the risk of hemorrhage.[43] These include EGD with biopsy, colonoscopy with biopsy, polypectomy, biliary sphincterotomy, and transbronchial biopsy.[48,94-96] In addition, several controlled studies demonstrated that there was no increase in severe bleeding complications in patients undergoing cutaneous surgery regardless of the continuation of aspirin and NSAIDs prior to the procedures (excluding procedures that involved deep tissue resection or dissection).[36,97-100] Therefore, it may be reasonable to continue aspirin in a low bleeding risk patient requiring antiplatelet therapy for a medically necessary reason (e.g., history of stroke, TIA, or coronary artery disease) who is scheduled for an elective procedure as mentioned earlier.

Perioperative Anticoagulation Management

Patients should be categorized into high-, intermediate-, or low-risk groups based on both personal and procedural thromboembolic and bleeding risks (see Tables 38-4 to 38-6).[5,16,101] For patients at high risk for thromboembolism, a therapeutic dose of UFH or LMWH should start within ~ 2 days after warfarin is stopped.[5,7] UFH can be given as a continuous intravenous infusion as an inpatient or as a subcutaneous injection as an outpatient. If continuous intravenous UFH is used, the drug should be titrated to achieve a targeted partial thromboplastin time (PTT) that correlates with therapeutic heparin levels (0.3 to 0.7 IU/mL by factor Xa inhibition).[102] Intravenous UFH is usually discontinued approximately 5 to 6 hours before surgery with the expectation that the anticoagulant effect (half-life about 1 hour) will have worn off at the time of surgery (providing that the PTT is not supratherapeutic at the time the anticoagulant therapy is stopped).[1,7,21] For patients taking therapeutic subcutaneous UFH, the last injection should be given 12 to 24 hours before surgery.[7]

Currently, there are several regimens for LMWH bridging therapy as listed in Table 38-9.[16] If once-daily LMWH (half-life about 5 to 6 hours) is used, it should be administered in the mornings, with the last dose given on the day prior to surgery (i.e., 24 hours before surgery).[5] An alternative strategy for once daily dosing regimen would be to reduce the last dose by 50%.[16] With either regimen (once-daily or twice-daily), LMWH therapy should be stopped 12 to 24 hours (or 20 to 24 hours) before surgery.[5,7] Importantly, in patients with renal insufficiency, LMWH therapy may need to be stopped more than 24 hours before surgery to allow for prolonged clearance of the drug.

In patients with a moderate risk of thromboembolism (see Table 38-4) undergoing a moderate or high bleeding risk procedure, a low dose of UFH (5000 units subcutaneous) or a prophylactic dose of LMWH can be given beginning approximately two days preoperatively after warfarin is discontinued.[7] Some investigators would recommend

Table 38-9 Perioperative Anticoagulant Regimens for Therapeutic Range Low Molecular Weight Heparin (LMWH)

LMWH	Dose	Time of Last Dose*
Enoxaparin sodium (Lovenox)	1 mg/kg SC q 12 hours,	12–24 hours
	or 1.5 mg/kg SC qd	24 hours
Dalteparin sodium (Fragmin)	100 anti-Xa IU/kg SC q 12 hours,	12–24 hrs
	or 200 anti-Xa IU/kg SC qd	24 hours
Tinzaparin sodium (Innohep)	175 anti-Xa IU/kg SC qd	24 hours
Ardeparin sodium (Normiflo)	130 anti-Xa IU/kg SC q 12 hours	12–24 hours

*Time to last dose given prior to surgery.
SC, subcutaneously.

a higher dose of UFH or a full dose of LMWH in this setting depending on the clinical situation.[7] For patients with low risk of thromboembolism, preoperative bridging anticoagulant therapy with full dose UFH or LMWH is generally not necessary.[1,5,7,16,101]

Role of Prophylactic Inferior Vena Cava Filter Placement

Prophylactic inferior vena cava (IVC) filter placement may be considered for patients who are at extremely high risk for recurrent venous thromboembolic disease, for instance, patients who have had an acute episode of pulmonary embolism or extensive proximal deep-vein thrombosis and who have received anticoagulant therapy for less than two weeks after the onset of the thromboembolic events. In addition, prophylactic IVC filter placement may be considered in patients who have a history of pulmonary embolism with limited cardiopulmonary reserve to tolerate another embolic insult, or in the very rare patient in whom anticoagulant therapy is contraindicated.[1,103] Such patients usually include neurosurgical patients operated on within a few days of a new thromboembolic event, or central nervous system bleeds only a few days old.

Because of the concerns about the possible long-term complications associated with permanent IVC filter placement (e.g., deep venous thrombosis [DVT] and IVC thrombosis at the insertion site),[104-106] retrievable IVC filters have been developed to provide an alternative to a permanent IVC filter for patients who require only short-term protection against pulmonary emboli while anticoagulant therapy is interrupted. These IVC filters are safe and effective in the prevention of pulmonary emboli.[107-109] Although there is no available clinical study dedicated to prospectively examining the role of prophylactic retrievable IVC filter in patients receiving chronic anticoagulation who undergo temporary disruption of anticoagulant therapy, previous studies have included subsets of patients with DVT and/or pulmonary embolism in whom anticoagulants were judged to be contraindicated due to planned surgeries.[107-109] Thus, this type of IVC filter would be ideal for use in the perioperative setting. See Chapter 31 for further discussion.

In patients who are receiving preoperative intravenous UFH, it is stated that anticoagulation should be discontinued at least 3 hours prior to filter insertion and restarted as soon as possible after insertion.[107] Whereas this might be correct, it is yet to be proved; some patients may choose this interval to thrombose again.

Postoperative Anticoagulation Management

Resumption of UFH or LMWH

In general, adequate postoperative hemostasis is usually achieved by 24 to 48 hours after surgical closure in patients who undergo intra-abdominal, intrathoracic, or orthopedic surgery.[5] However, patients who undergo surgical procedure for infection or malignancy may continue to have an increased risk of bleeding because of the difficulty to control bleeding or oozing from raw surfaces.[16]

If there is evidence of ongoing blood loss in the postoperative setting, postoperative anticoagulation should be withheld until the bleeding has subsided. On the contrary, if there is adequate postoperative hemostasis, the decision to resume full-dose anticoagulant therapy may be influenced by the risk of bleeding associated with the specific operation. For instance, in patients undergoing high bleeding risk procedures (see Tables 38-5 and 38-6), the resumption of therapeutic anticoagulation with LMWH should be deferred for 24 to 48 hours after surgery. However, in select types of surgery, for example neurosurgery and certain orthopedic procedure (e.g., total hip replacement), for which postoperative bleeding associated with anticoagulation can lead to devastating complications,[16] the decision to resume therapeutic dose of LMWH may be delayed to 48 to 72 hours after surgery even with adequate postoperative hemostasis and may not be given at all if there is concern for ongoing bleeding. If the bleeding risk in the postoperative setting is significant, the initial dose of LMWH could be started at a prophylactic dose beginning on the first or second day after surgery.

In patients undergoing moderate bleeding risk procedures, prophylactic dose of LMWH can usually be resumed on the evening after surgery (12 hours) and can be increased subsequently to therapeutic dose, starting 24 to 48 hours after surgery, if the patient tolerates the prophylactic treatment well without bleeding complications.[5]

If UFH is used for bridging anticoagulant therapy, the treatment can usually be resumed 12 to 24 hours after surgery when there is evidence of adequate hemostasis.[5,110] To minimize the risk of postoperative bleeding, it is recommended that UFH be started without a bolus, at no more than the expected maintenance infusion rate.[1,111] The PTT should be checked 12 hours after restarting therapy to allow time for a stable anticoagulant response.[1] Alternatively, UFH may be given subcutaneously as twice-daily injections.[112] This approach requires daily, mid-interval PTT testing to be performed to monitor the anticoagulant effect and adjust the dose as necessary. If patients develop hemorrhagic complications while receiving UFH, protamine sulfate can be given to reverse the anticoagulant effect.

Resumption of Postoperative Oral Anticoagulation

Warfarin therapy can be restarted the evening after surgery (same day) in the majority of patients, provided that there is no evidence of ongoing bleeding and adequate hemostasis has been achieved. The warfarin dose corresponding to the patient's usual dose on that day of the week can be used as an initial dose[5] and INR monitoring should be initiated after the first two or three doses of warfarin therapy.[7] If the patient had received a higher dose of vitamin K (e.g., 5 to 10 mg) in the preoperative setting, it has been suggested to increase the patient's warfarin dose (e.g., doubling) for two consecutive days after surgery, although there are no data supporting this recommendation.[5] Alternatively in this setting, one could manage the patient on LMWH after surgery as needed before attempting to convert back to warfarin.

Discontinuation of UFH or LMWH Postoperative Bridging Therapy

UFH and LMWH should be continued postoperatively until the INR has been in the therapeutic range for at least two consecutive days.[5,7]

Management of Specialized Clinical Settings

Patients with Spinal Anesthesia or Continuous Epidural Analgesia

Epidural hematoma is a rare but devastating complication in patients receiving anticoagulant therapy undergoing spinal anesthesia.[113,114] In patients who have non-traumatic placement of an epidural catheter followed by immediate removal after surgery, anticoagulant therapy may be resumed 12 hours after the operation. However, the resumption of postoperative anticoagulation should be postponed to at least 24 hours after surgery if there is history of trauma ("bloody tap") associated with epidural catheter placement. For patients who have an indwelling epidural catheter for analgesic administration, it has been recommended that anticoagulation should be withheld until the epidural catheter is removed.[5] Nevertheless, there are certain criteria that allow co-administration of LMWH and continuous epidural analgesia: (1) epidural catheter placement was non-traumatic; (2) low-dose LMWH is used (enoxaparin 30 mg twice-daily or dalteparin 5000 IU once-daily)[115]; (3) warfarin is not started until after the epidural catheter is removed; (4) the epidural catheter is removed during the trough anticoagulant effect of LMWH (i.e., 18 to 22 hours after the last dose, for daily dosing); and (5) antiplatelet therapy (e.g. aspirin or NSAIDs) is avoided until the removal of the epidural catheter.[5,115–117]

Patients with Renal Insufficiency

Nearly all of the clinical studies evaluating the role of LMWH as perioperative bridging anticoagulant therapy have excluded patients with renal insufficiency, defined by estimated creatinine clearance less than 30 mL/minute[61]; or serum creatinine greater than 1.4 mg/dL[65] or 2.0 mg/dL.[59] This is due to the fact that LMWH is primarily excreted by the kidney and significant bioaccumulation of these drugs can occur in patients with impaired renal function. In actual clinical practice, these patients are commonly encountered. In this regard, LMWH should be avoided in patients with severe renal insufficiency, and UFH would be the anticoagulant of choice.[102] If LMWH is used in this setting, an anti-factor Xa level should be measured to monitor the anticoagulant effect of LMWH. The level should be obtained four hours after the LMWH dose, with a targeted anti-factor Xa level of about 0.3–0.5 up to 1.0–1.2 u/mL (for twice daily dosing) if the intent is therapeutic dosing; prophylactic dosing would have a lower target range of about 0.1–0.3 µ/mL.[102] These patients will likely also require a longer time to eliminate the LMWH in the preoperative setting.

Patients with History of Heparin-Induced Thrombocytopenia

UFH and LMWH are typically avoided in patients with a history of heparin-induced thrombocytopenia (HIT). In this setting, perioperative or postoperative anticoagulant therapy can be attained by one of the following drugs: danaparoid sodium, lepirudin, or argatroban. (Of note, danaparoid sodium is no longer available in the United States). Clinicians must keep in mind that these anticoagulants are not reversible and caution must be used in patients undergoing high bleeding risk procedures. For patients with acute HIT, warfarin should be given when patients are adequately anticoagulated with a drug that reduces thrombin generation in HIT, such as lepirudin, argatroban, or danaparoid sodium because of the risk of causing venous limb gangrene if warfarin is used alone.[102] The role of pentasaccharide therapy in this situation appears to be very promising.

Patients with Particularly High Thromboembolic Risk

Recently, Larson and colleagues have shown that continuation of dose-reduced oral anticoagulation is feasible in patients with high thromboembolic risks (e.g., history of DVT within the past 6 months, prior postoperative DVT or pulmonary embolism, inherited thrombophilia, and antiphospholipid syndrome), who require an invasive procedure.[118] In this noncontrolled retrospective study, preoperative warfarin was continued and adjusted to maintain the target INR of 1.5 to 2.0. Heparin (LMWH or UFH) was given as a supplement only if the INR dropped below 1.5 and baseline warfarin dose was resumed on the evening of surgery. Among the 99 operations stratified by the Johns Hopkins Medical Institutions Surgical Classification System[119] (moderate risk 47%; major risk 10%; and critical risk 1%),[118,119] there were only two thromboembolic events (one symptomatic DVT and one fatal embolic stroke). The incidence of major and minor hemorrhagic complications was 2% and 4%, respectively, but nearly one half of the studied patients underwent low bleeding risk procedures. Despite several limitations of this study, it has demonstrated the feasibility of moderate intensity warfarin (INR 1.5 to 2.0) in the perioperative setting for patients at a particularly high-risk for thromboembolism.

REFERENCES

1. Kearon C, Hirsh J: Management of anticoagulation before and after elective surgery. N Engl J Med 336:1506–1511, 1997.
2. Cannegieter SC, Rosendaal FR, Briet E: Thromboembolic and bleeding complications in patients with mechanical heart valve prostheses. Circulation 89:635–641, 1994.
3. Cannegieter SC, Rosendaal FR, Wintzen AR, et al: Optimal oral anticoagulant therapy in patients with mechanical heart valves. N Engl J Med 333:11–17, 1995.
4. Vongpatanasin W, Hillis LD, Lange RA: Prosthetic heart valves. N Engl J Med 335:407–416, 1996.
5. Douketis JD: Perioperative anticoagulation management in patients who are receiving oral anticoagulant therapy: A practical guide for clinicians. Thromb Res 108:3–13, 2002.
6. Stein PD, Alpert JS, Bussey HI, et al: Antithrombotic therapy in patients with mechanical and biological prosthetic heart valves. Chest 119:220S–227S, 2001.
7. Ansell J, Hirsh J, Poller L, et al: The pharmacology and management of the vitamin K antagonists: The Seventh ACCP Conference on Antithrombotic and Thrombolytic Therapy. Chest 126:204S–233S, 2004.
8. Secondary prevention in non-rheumatic atrial fibrillation after transient ischaemic attack or minor stroke. EAFT (European Atrial Fibrillation Trial) Study Group. Lancet 342:1255–1262, 1993.
9. Albers GW, Dalen JE, Laupacis A, et al: Antithrombotic therapy in atrial fibrillation. Chest 119:194S–206S, 2001.
10. Laupacis A, Albers G, Dalen J, et al: Antithrombotic therapy in atrial fibrillation. Chest 114:579S–589S, 1998.
11. Risk factors for stroke and efficacy of antithrombotic therapy in atrial fibrillation: Analysis of pooled data from five randomized controlled trials. Arch Intern Med 154:1449–1457, 1994.
12. Hart RG, Pearce LA, McBride R, et al: Factors associated with ischemic stroke during aspirin therapy in atrial fibrillation: Analysis of 2012 participants in the SPAF I-III clinical trials. The Stroke Prevention in Atrial Fibrillation (SPAF) Investigators. Stroke 30:1223–1229, 1999.
13. Kopecky SL, Gersh BJ, McGoon MD, et al: The natural history of lone atrial fibrillation: A population-based study over three decades. N Engl J Med 317:669–674, 1987.
14. Coon WW, Willis PW 3rd. Recurrence of venous thromboembolism. Surgery 73:823–827, 1973.
15. Kearon C: Perioperative management of long-term anticoagulation. Semin Thromb Hemost 24(Suppl 1): 77–83, 1998.
16. Heit JA: Perioperative management of the chronically anticoagulated patient. J Thromb Thrombolysis 12:81–87, 2001.
17. Heit JA, Mohr DN, Silverstein MD, et al: Predictors of recurrence after deep vein thrombosis and pulmonary embolism: A population-based cohort study. Arch Intern Med 160:761–768, 2000.
18. Schulman S, Svenungsson E, Granqvist S: Anticardiolipin antibodies predict early recurrence of thromboembolism and death among patients with venous thromboembolism following anticoagulant therapy. Duration of Anticoagulation Study Group. Am J Med 104:332–338, 1998.
19. Lindmarker P, Schulman S, Sten-Linder M, et al: The risk of recurrent venous thromboembolism in carriers and non-carriers of the G1691A allele in the coagulation factor V gene and the G20210A allele in the prothrombin gene. DURAC Trial Study Group. Duration of Anticoagulation. Thromb Haemost 81:684–689, 1998.
20. De Stefano V, Martinelli I, Mannucci PM, et al: The risk of recurrent deep venous thrombosis among heterozygous carriers of both factor V Leiden and the G20210A prothrombin mutation. N Engl J Med 341:801–806, 1999.
21. Ansell J, Hirsh J, Dalen J, et al: Managing oral anticoagulant therapy. Chest 119:22S–38S, 2001.
22. Dunn AS, Turpie AG: Perioperative management of patients receiving oral anticoagulants: A systematic review. Arch Intern Med 163:901–908, 2003.
23. Wahl MJ: Dental surgery in anticoagulated patients. Arch Intern Med 158:1610–1616, 1998.
24. Anavi Y SA, Gutman D, Laufer D: Dental extractions during anticoagulant therapy. Isr J Dent Med 28:9–12, 1981.
25. Cone A: Dental abscess in an anticoagulated patient with ankylosing spondylitis. Br J Hosp Med 49:190, 1993.
26. Frank B, Dickhaus DW, Claus EC: Dental extractions in the presence of continual anticoagulant therapy. Ann Intern Med 59:911–913, 1963.
27. Greenberg M, Miller MF, Lynch MA: Partial thromboplastin time as a predictor of blood loss in oral surgery patients receiving coumarin anticoagulants. J Am Dent Assoc 84:583–587, 1972.
28. Martinowitz U, Mazar AL, Taicher S, et al: Dental extraction for patients on oral anticoagulant therapy. Oral Surg Oral Med Oral Pathol 70:274–277, 1990.

29. Ramstrom GS-PS, Hall G, Blomback M, Alander U: Prevention of postsurgical bleeding in oral surgery using tranexamic acid without dose modification of oral anticoagulants. J Oral Maxillofac Surg 51:1211–1216, 1993.

30. Hall DL, Steen WH Jr., Drummond JW, Byrd WA: Anticoagulants and cataract surgery. Ophthalmic Surg 19:221–222, 1998.

31. Gainey SP, Robertson DM, Fay W, Ilstrup D: Ocular surgery on patients receiving long-term warfarin therapy. Am J Ophthalmol 108:142–146, 1989.

32. Roberts CW, Woods SM, Turner LS: Cataract surgery in anticoagulated patients. J Cataract Refract Surg 17:309–312, 1991.

33. Carter K, Miller KM: Phacoemulsification and lens implantation in patients treated with aspirin or warfarin. J Cataract Refract Surg 24:1361–1364, 1998.

34. Robinson GA, Nylander A: Warfarin and cataract extraction. Br J Ophthalmol 73:702–703, 1989.

35. McMahon L: Anticoagulants and cataract surgery. J Cataract Refract Surg 14:569–571, 1988.

36. Otley CC, Fewkes JL, Frank W, Olbricht SM: Complications of cutaneous surgery in patients who are taking warfarin, aspirin, or nonsteroidal anti-inflammatory drugs. Arch Dermatol 132:161–166, 1996.

37. Despotis GJ, Skubas NJ, Goodnough LT: Optimal management of bleeding and transfusion in patients undergoing cardiac surgery. Semin Thorac Cardiovasc Surg 11:84–104, 1999.

38. Nielsen JD, Gram J, Holm-Nielsen A, et al: Post-operative blood loss after transurethral prostatectomy is dependent on in situ fibrinolysis. Br J Urol 80:889–893, 1997.

39. Chakravarti A, MacDermott S: Transurethral resection of the prostate in the anticoagulated patient. Br J Urol 81:520–522, 1998.

40. Hergesell O, Felten H, Andrassy K, et al: Safety of ultrasound-guided percutaneous renal biopsy-retrospective analysis of 1090 consecutive cases. Nephrol Dial Transplant 13:975–977, 1998.

41. Despotis GJ, Filos KS, Zoys TN, et al: Factors associated with excessive postoperative blood loss and hemostatic transfusion requirements: A multivariate analysis in cardiac surgical patients. Anesth Analg 82:13–21, 1996.

42. Leizorovicz A, Haugh MC, Chapuis FR, et al: Low molecular weight heparin in prevention of perioperative thrombosis. BMJ 305:913–920, 1992.

43. Eisen GM, Baron TH, Dominitz JA, et al: Guideline on the management of anticoagulation and antiplatelet therapy for endoscopic procedures. Gastrointest Endosc 55:775–779, 2002.

44. Waye JD: Colonoscopy. CA Cancer J Clin 42:350–365, 1992.

45. Remine S, Huges RW, Weiland LH: Endoscopic gastric polypectomy. Mayo Clin Proc 56:371–375, 1981.

46. Mathus-Vliegen E, Tytgat GN: Nd:YAG laser photocoagulation in colorectal adenoma: Evaluation of its safety, usefulness and efficacy. Gastroenterology 90:1865–1873, 1986.

47. Rutgeerts P, Vantrappen G, Broeckaert L, et al: Palliative Nd:YAG laser therapy for cancer of the esophagus and gastroesophageal junction: Impact on quality of remaining life. Gastrointest Endosc 34:87–90, 1988.

48. Cotton PB, Lehman G, Vennes J, et al: Endoscopic sphincterotomy complications and their management: An attempt at consensus. Gastrointest Endosc 37:383–393, 1991.

49. Madura JA, Rookstool M, Wease G: The management of patients on chronic coumadin therapy undergoing subsequent surgical procedures. Am Surg 60:542–546, 1994; discussion 546–547.

50. Busuttil WJ, Fabri BM: The management of anticoagulation in patients with prosthetic heart valves undergoing non-cardiac operations. Postgrad Med J 71:380–382, 1995.

51. Bryan AJ, Butchart EG: Prosthetic heart valves and anticoagulant management during non-cardiac surgery. Br J Surg 82:577–578, 1995.

52. Katholi RE, Nolan SP, McGuire LB: Living with prosthetic heart valves: Subsequent noncardiac operations and the risk of thromboembolism or hemorrhage. Am Heart J 92:162–167, 1976.

53. Katholi RE, Nolan SP, McGuire LB: The management of anticoagulation during noncardiac operations in patients with prosthetic heart valves: A prospective study. Am Heart J 96:163–165, 1978.

54. Tinker JH, Tarhan S: Discontinuing anticoagulant therapy in surgical patients with cardiac valve prostheses. Observations in 180 operations. JAMA 239:738–739, 1978.

55. Carrel TP, Klingenmann W, Mohacsi PJ, et al: Perioperative bleeding and thromboembolic risk during non-cardiac surgery in patients with mechanical prosthetic heart valves: An institutional review. J Heart Valve Dis 8:392–398, 1999.

56. Amorosi SL, Tsilimingras K, Thompson D, et al: Cost analysis of "bridging therapy" with low-molecular-weight heparin versus unfractionated heparin during temporary interruption of chronic anticoagulation. Am J Cardiol 93:509–511, 2004.

57. Spyropoulos AC, Frost FJ, Hurley JS, Roberts M: Costs and clinical outcomes associated with low-molecular-weight heparin vs unfractionated heparin for perioperative bridging in patients receiving long-term oral anticoagulant therapy. Chest 125:1642–1650, 2004.

58. Galla J, Fuhs BE: Outpatient anticoagulation protocol for mechanical valve recipients undergoing non-cardiac surgery. J Am Coll Cardiol 35:531A, 2000.

59. Douketis JD, Johnson JA, Turpie AG: Low-molecular-weight heparin as bridging anticoagulation during interruption of warfarin: Assessment of a standardized periprocedural anticoagulation regimen. Arch Intern Med 164:1319–1326, 2004.

60. Kovacs MJ, Kearon C, Rodger M, et al: Single-arm study of bridging therapy with low-molecular-weight heparin for patients at risk of arterial embolism who require temporary interruption of warfarin. Circulation 110:1658–1663, 2004.

61. Spandorfer JM, Lynch S, Weitz HH, et al: Use of enoxaparin for the chronically anticoagulated patient before and after procedures. Am J Cardiol 84:478–480, A410, 1999.

62. Johnson J, Turpie AGG: Temporary discontinuation of oral anticoagulants: Role of low molecular weight heparin. Thromb Haemost 86(Suppl): 662, 2001.

63. Ferreira I, Dos L, Tornos MP, et al: Is low-molecular-weight heparin a safe alternative to unfractionated heparin in patients with prosthetic mechanical heart valves who must interrupt antithrombotic therapy? Eur Heart J 21(Suppl): 301, 2000.

64. UPMC Health System. Home LMWH bridge therapy in cardiac valve replacement: Safe, effective, and cost saving. Formulary 35:990–991, 2000.

65. Tinmouth AH, Morrow BH, Cruickshank MK, et al: Dalteparin as periprocedure anticoagulation for patients on warfarin and at high risk of thrombosis. Ann Pharmacother 35:669–674, 2001.

66. Ferreira I, Dos L, Tornos P, et al: Experience with enoxaparin in patients with mechanical heart valves who must withhold acenocoumarol. Heart 89:527–530, 2003.

67. Geerts WH, Pineo GF, Heit JA, et al: Prevention of venous thromboembolism: The Seventh ACCP Conference on Antithrombotic and Thrombolytic Therapy. Chest 126:338S–400S, 2004.

68. White RH, McKittrick T, Hutchinson R, Twitchell J: Temporary discontinuation of warfarin therapy: Changes in the international normalized ratio. Ann Intern Med 122:40–42, 1995.

69. Palareti G, Legnani C: Warfarin withdrawal: Pharmacokinetic-pharmacodynamic considerations. Clin Pharmacokinet 30:300–313, 1996.

70. Whitling AM, Bussey HI, Lyons RM: Comparing different routes and doses of phytonadione for reversing excessive anticoagulation. Arch Intern Med 158:2136–2140, 1998.

71. Serebruany VL, Malinin AI, Eisert RM, Sane DC: Risk of bleeding complications with antiplatelet agents: Meta-analysis of 338,191 patients enrolled in 50 randomized controlled trials. Am J Hematol 75:40–47, 2004.

72. Patrono C, Coller B, FitzGerald GA, et al: Platelet-active drugs: The relationships among dose, effectiveness, and side effects: The Seventh ACCP Conference on Antithrombotic and Thrombolytic Therapy. Chest 126:234S–264S, 2004.

73. Patrono C, Coller B, Dalen JE, et al: Platelet-active drugs: The relationships among dose, effectiveness, and side effects. Chest 119:39S–63S, 2001.

74. Gibbs NM, Weightman WM, Thackray NM, et al: The effects of recent aspirin ingestion on platelet function in cardiac surgical patients. J Cardiothorac Vasc Anesth 15:55–59, 2001.

75. Goldman S, Copeland J, Moritz T, et al: Improvement in early saphenous vein graft patency after coronary artery bypass surgery with antiplatelet therapy: Results of a Veterans Administration Cooperative Study. Circulation 77:1324–1332, 1988.

76. Taggart DP, Siddiqui A, Wheatley DJ: Low-dose preoperative aspirin therapy, postoperative blood loss, and transfusion requirements. Ann Thorac Surg 50:424–428, 1990.

77. Torosian M, Michelson EL, Morganroth J, MacVaugh H 3rd: Aspirin- and coumadin-related bleeding after coronary-artery bypass graft surgery. Ann Intern Med 89:325–328, 1978.

78. Michelson EL, Morganroth J, Torosian M, Mac Vaugh H 3rd: Relation of preoperative use of aspirin to increased mediastinal

blood loss after coronary artery bypass graft surgery. J Thorac Cardiovasc Surg; 1978 76:694–697, 1978.

79. Ferraris VA, Ferraris SP, Lough FC, Berry WR: Preoperative aspirin ingestion increases operative blood loss after coronary artery bypass grafting. Ann Thorac Surg 45:71–74, 1988.

80. Sethi GK, Copeland JG, Goldman S, et al: Implications of preoperative administration of aspirin in patients undergoing coronary artery bypass grafting. Department of Veterans Affairs Cooperative Study on Antiplatelet Therapy. J Am Coll Cardiol 15:15–20, 1990.

81. Bashein G, Nessly ML, Rice AL, et al: Preoperative aspirin therapy and reoperation for bleeding after coronary artery bypass surgery. Arch Intern Med 151:89–93, 1991.

82. Kallis P, Tooze JA, Talbot S, et al: Pre-operative aspirin decreases platelet aggregation and increases post-operative blood loss: A prospective, randomised, placebo controlled, double-blind clinical trial in 100 patients with chronic stable angina. Eur J Cardiothorac Surg 8:404–409, 1994.

83. Cannon CP, Mehta SR, Aranki SF: Balancing the benefit and risk of oral antiplatelet agents in coronary artery bypass surgery. Ann Thorac Surg 80:768–779, 2005.

84. Bybee KA, Powell BD, Valeti U, et al: Preoperative aspirin therapy is associated with improved postoperative outcomes in patients undergoing coronary artery bypass grafting. Circulation 112:I286–I292, 2005.

85. Dacey LJ, Munoz JJ, Johnson ER, et al: Effect of preoperative aspirin use on mortality in coronary artery bypass grafting patients. Ann Thorac Surg 70:1986–1990, 2000.

86. Munoz JJ, Birkmeyer NJ, Dacey LJ, et al: Trends in rates of reexploration for hemorrhage after coronary artery bypass surgery. Northern New England Cardiovascular Disease Study Group. Ann Thorac Surg 68:1321–1325, 1999.

87. Tuman KJ, McCarthy RJ, O'Connor CJ, et al: Aspirin does not increase allogeneic blood transfusion in reoperative coronary artery surgery. Anesth Analg 83:1178–1184, 1996.

88. Vuylsteke A, Oduro A, Cardan E, Latimer RD: Effect of aspirin in coronary artery bypass grafting. J Cardiothorac Vasc Anesth 11:831–834, 1997.

89. Yende S, Wunderink RG: Effect of clopidogrel on bleeding after coronary artery bypass surgery. Crit Care Med 29:2271–2275, 2001.

90. Hongo RH, Ley J, Dick SE, Yee RR: The effect of clopidogrel in combination with aspirin when given before coronary artery bypass grafting. J Am Coll Cardiol 40:231–237, 2002.

91. Genoni M, Tavakoli R, Hofer C, et al: Clopidogrel before urgent coronary artery bypass graft. J Thorac Cardiovasc Surg 126:288–289, 2003.

92. Peters RJ, Mehta SR, Fox KA, et al: Effects of aspirin dose when used alone or in combination with clopidogrel in patients with acute coronary syndromes: Observations from the Clopidogrel in Unstable angina to prevent Recurrent Events (CURE) study. Circulation 108:1682–1687, 2003.

93. Eagle KA, Guyton RA, Davidoff R, et al: ACC/AHA 2004 guideline update for coronary artery bypass graft surgery: A report of the American College of Cardiology/American Heart Association Task Force on Practice Guidelines. Circulation 110:e340–e437, 2004.

94. Schiffman ML, Farrel MT, Yee YS: Risk of bleeding after endoscopic biopsy or polypectomy in patients taking aspirin or other NSAIDs. Gastrointest Endosc 40:458–462, 1994.

95. Freeman ML, Nelson DB, Sherman S, et al: Complications of endoscopic biliary sphincterotomy. N Engl J Med 335:909–918, 1996.

96. Herth FJ, Becker HD, Ernst A: Aspirin does not increase bleeding complications after transbronchial biopsy. Chest 122:1461–1464, 2002.

97. Billingsley EM, Maloney ME: Intraoperative and postoperative bleeding problems in patients taking warfarin, aspirin, and nonsteroidal antiinflammatory agents: A prospective study. Dermatol Surg 1997;23:381–383, discussion 384–385.

98. Bartlett GR: Does aspirin affect the outcome of minor cutaneous surgery? Br J Plast Surg 52:214–216, 1999.

99. Lawrence C, Sakuntabhai A, Tiling-Grosse S: Effect of aspirin and nonsteroidal antiinflammatory drug therapy on bleeding complications in dermatologic surgical patients. J Am Acad Dermatol 31:988–992, 1994.

100. Otley CC: Continuation of medically necessary aspirin and warfarin during cutaneous surgery. Mayo Clin Proc 78:1392–1396, 2003.

101. Jaffer AK, Brotman DJ, Chukwumerije N: When patients on warfarin need surgery. Cleve Clin J Med 70:973–984, 2003.

102. Hirsh J, Raschke R: Heparin and low-molecular-weight heparin: The Seventh ACCP Conference on Antithrombotic and Thrombolytic Therapy. Chest 126:188S–203S, 2004.

103. Kinney TB: Update on inferior vena cava filters. J Vasc Interv Radiol 14:425–440, 2003.

104. Langan EM 3rd, Miller RS, Casey WJ 3rd, et al: Prophylactic inferior vena cava filters in trauma patients at high risk: Follow-up examination and risk/benefit assessment. J Vasc Surg 30:484–488, 1999.

105. Greenfield LJ, Proctor MC, Michaels AJ, Taheri PA: Prophylactic vena caval filters in trauma: The rest of the story. J Vasc Surg 32:490–495, 2000; discussion 496–497.

106. Blebea J, Wilson R, Waybill P, et al: Deep venous thrombosis after percutaneous insertion of vena caval filters. J Vasc Surg 30:821–828, 1999.

107. Linsenmaier U, Rieger J, Schenk F, et al: Indications, management, and complications of temporary inferior vena cava filters. Cardiovasc Intervent Radiol 21:464–469, 1998.

108. de Gregorio MA, Gamboa P, Gimeno MJ, et al: The Gunther Tulip retrievable filter: Prolonged temporary filtration by repositioning within the inferior vena cava. J Vasc Interv Radiol 14:1259–1265, 2003.

109. Millward SF, Bormanis J, Burbridge BE, et al: Preliminary clinical experience with the Gunther temporary inferior vena cava filter. J Vasc Interv Radiol 5:863–868, 1994.

110. Cruickshank MK, Levine MN, Hirsh J, et al: A standard heparin nomogram for the management of heparin therapy. Arch Intern Med 151:333–337, 1991.

111. Hirsh J, Raschke R, Warkentin TE, et al: Heparin: Mechanism of action, pharmacokinetics, dosing considerations, monitoring, efficacy, and safety. Chest 108:258S–275S, 1995.

112. Prandoni P, Bagatella P, Bernardi E, et al: Use of an algorithm for administering subcutaneous heparin in the treatment of deep venous thrombosis. Ann Intern Med 129:299–302, 1998.

113. Horlocker TT: Low molecular weight heparin and neuraxial anesthesia. Thromb Res 101:V141–V154, 2001.

114. Lawton MT, Porter RW, Heiserman JE, et al: Surgical management of spinal epidural hematoma: Relationship between surgical timing and neurological outcome. J Neurosurg 83:1–7, 1995.

115. Douketis JD, Kinnon K, Crowther MA: Anticoagulant effect at the time of epidural catheter removal in patients receiving twice-daily or once-daily low-molecular-weight heparin and continuous epidural analgesia after orthopedic surgery. Thromb Haemost 88:37–40, 2002.

116. Horlocker TT, Wedel DJ: Spinal and epidural blockade and perioperative low molecular weight heparin: Smooth sailing on the Titanic. Anesth Analg 86:1153–1156, 1998.

117. Douketis J, Wang J, Cuddy K, et al: The saftey of co-administered continuous epidural analgesia and low-molecular-weight heparin after major orthopedic surgery: Assessment of a standardized patient management protocol. Thromb Haemost 96:387–389, 2006.

118. Larson BJ, Zumberg MS, Kitchens CS: A feasibility study of continuing dose-reduced warfarin for invasive procedures in patients with high thromboembolic risk. Chest 127:922–927, 2005.

119. Gross R, Babbott SF: Evaluation of healthy patients and ambulatory surgical patients. In Gross RJ and Caputo GM, (eds): Kammerer and Gross' Medical Consultation, Baltimore, Williams & Wilkins, 1998, pp 25–53.

120. Bonow RO, Carabello B, de Leon AC Jr., et al: Guidelines for the management of patients with valvular heart disease: Executive summary. A report of the American College of Cardiology/American Heart Association Task Force on practice guidelines. Circulation 98:1949–1984, 1998.

Chapter 39

Hemostatic Alterations in Liver Disease and Liver Transplantation

Marco Senzolo, MD • Andrew K. Burroughs, MD

The liver plays key roles in blood coagulation being involved in both primary and secondary hemostasis.[1] It is the site of synthesis of all coagulation factors, except for von Willebrand factor (VWF), and their inhibitors.[2] Liver damage is commonly associated with impairment of coagulation when liver function reserve is poor. The hemostatic system is in a delicate balance between prothrombotic and antithrombotic processes, aiming to prevent excessive blood loss from injured vessels and to prevent spontaneous thrombosis. Liver failure is accompanied by multiple changes in the hemostatic system because of reduced plasma levels of pro-coagulative and anti-coagulative clotting proteins synthesized by the intact liver.[3] Vitamin K deficiency may coexist, so that abnormal clotting factors are produced. Moreover, during liver failure, there is a reduced capacity to clear activated hemostatic proteins and protein inhibitor complexes from the circulation. Thus the global effect of liver disease with regard to hemostasis is complex, so that patients with advanced liver disease can experience severe bleeding or even thrombotic complications (Table 39-1). Finally, when marked portal hypertension develops with collateral circulation and secondary splenomegaly, thrombocytopenia develops due to splenic sequestration, but thrombocytopenia may also be due to decreased hepatic thrombopoietin synthesis. There is also impaired platelet function. These hemostatic abnormalities do not always lead to spontaneous bleeding, but the onset of complications of cirrhosis such as variceal bleeding or infection/sepsis may precipitate worsening of coagulation status. The presence of a consumptive coagulopathy, other than secondary to sepsis or other predisposing causes, is disputed.

Usually therapy for coagulation disorders in liver disease is needed only during bleeding or before invasive procedures. When end-stage liver disease occurs, liver transplantation is the only treatment available that can restore normal hemostasis and correct genetic defects, such as hemophilia or factor V Leiden mutation. During liver transplantation, hemorrhage may occur due to the preexisting hypocoagulable state, the collateral circulation caused by portal hypertension, and increased fibrinolysis which occurs during this surgery.

HEMOSTATIC FACTORS

Procoagulant Factors

The liver is the site of synthesis of fibrinogen and factors II, V, VII, IX, X, XI, XII, and XIII.[4] VWF is synthesized by the endothelium.[5] Factor VIII is synthesized mainly by the hepatic sinusoidal endothelial cells,[6,7] but also by endothelial and non-parenchymal cells in the kidney, spleen, lungs, and brain.[8] Thus, the plasma concentration of factor VIII is not decreased with liver disease, and may be increased, as many chronic liver diseases are associated with chronic inflammation.[9] This occurs because of increased endothelial synthesis or a reduced clearance via low-density lipoprotein receptor-related protein, which is synthesized by the liver.[5] However, the biologic activity of the synthesized molecule is lower than the plasma concentration.[10] Factor VIII is high in fulminant hepatic failure and low in disseminated intravascular coagulation (DIC)[11] but this differential diagnosis is seldom an issue in clinical practice.

Vitamin K is an essential cofactor for the production of biologically active forms of the coagulation factors II, VII, IX, and X. It promotes hepatic post-ribosomal conversion of certain glutamic acid residues in the protein precursors to γ-carboxyglutamic acid (Gla). These active forms of the clotting factors chelate calcium at the Gla site, resulting in effective hemostatic function. When γ-carboxylation is impaired due to deficiency or antagonism of vitamin K, inert precursors are synthesized, (known as Proteins Induced by Vitamin K Absence [PIVKA]) and released into the bloodstream.[12] The clinical significance of these precursors is not clear. In the case of prothrombin, a specific and sensitive immunoassay has been developed which is able to detect small decreases in Gla content of this incomplete PIVKA prothrombin before any changes occur in conventional coagulation tests.[13] In cholestasis, reduction of vitamin K absorption from the small intestine due to decreased bile salt production can be compensated with parenteral administration of vitamin K 10 mg daily for 24 to 48 hours; but in parenchymal liver disease, decreased levels of coagulation factors are dependent on a decreased synthesis—so there is no improvement with vitamin K administration.[14] Nevertheless, 25% of patients with acute liver injury have a subclinical deficit of vitamin K which may benefit from parenteral administration with corresponding improvement of the International Normalized Ratio (INR).[15]

In acute liver failure, the first factors in which plasma concentrations fall are those with the shortest half-lives, factors V and VII (12 hours and 4 to 6 hours, respectively), and levels of factors II, VII, and X will subsequently fall.[16] Factor VIII, together with VWF, is usually elevated, whereas

39

Table 39-1 Hemostatic Alterations Associated with Liver Disease

Favoring Hemorrhage	Favoring Thrombosis
Low platelet count	Elevated levels of factors VIII and VWF
Impaired platelet function and platelet-vessel wall interaction	Decreased levels of protein C, protein S, antithrombin III, α_2 macroglobulin
Enhanced platelet inhibition by nitric oxide (NO) and prostacyclin	Heparin cofactor II elevated
Decreased levels of coagulation factors (II, V, VII, IX, X, and XI)	Decreased levels of plasminogen
Quantitative and qualitative abnormalities of fibrinogen	
Low level of α_2-plasmin inhibitor, TAFI, histidine-rich glycoprotein	
Increased levels of tPA, with small increase of PAI-1 levels	

TAFI, thrombin activatable fibrinolytic inhibitor.

there is only a slight reduction of factors IX and X. The differential effects on clotting factors levels during acute liver failure occur because high levels of cytokines increase levels of tissue factor (TF) which activate factors II, V, VII, and X, whereas any thrombin generated is inhibited by antithrombin III, preventing activation of factors VIII, XI, and consequently XI, thus preserving their plasma levels.[9]

Higher plasma des-γ-carboxy (PIVKA) prothrombin concentrations are found in patients with hepatocellular carcinoma due to a local production by tumor cells. This abnormal prothrombin is believed to be a growth factor for this tumor and to be associated with a poor prognosis.[17]

Prothrombin gene mutation (20210) is the most common thrombophilic defect in patients with portal vein thrombosis without cirrhosis (extrahepatic portal hypertension), accounting for 22% of cases,[18] whereas, factor V Leiden mutation is the most common hereditary thrombophilic disorder associated with 20% of cases of hepatic vein thrombosis in Western countries,[19] and, less commonly, is encountered in patients with portal vein thrombosis.[20]

von Willebrand Factor

Plasma concentration of VWF is substantially increased in patients with acute liver failure owing to its increased synthesis as an acute phase reactant protein in response to tissue injury.[21–23] With liver injury this may also be secondary to endotoxemia associated with endothelial dysfunction.[5] In chronic liver disease, endothelial shear stress related to portal hypertension may also contribute to the high plasma levels of VWF via a nitric oxide (NO) stimulus.[24] A correlation between severity of liver disease and VWF plasma antigen levels has been documented. Unfortunately, studies on the function of VWF in patients with liver cirrhosis are conflicting with regard to normal[5] or reduced[22] platelet aggregation in response to ristocetin.

Fibrinogen

Plasma fibrinogen is an acute-phase reactant, and it remains normal or increased in patients with liver disease.[25] Lower levels due to decreased synthesis, yet above 100 mg/dL, have been reported only in patients with extremely severe liver disease.[26] However, the high fibrinogen concentrations found in patients with chronic hepatitis, cholestatic jaundice, and hepatocellular carcinoma do not result in increased ability to clot because this synthesized form is a nonfunctional dysfibrinogen. About 60% to 70% of patients with liver disease have this dysfibrinogen due to an increased activity of sialyltransferase expressed by immature hepatocytes generated during hepatic injury. This leads to a low molecular weight fibrinogen with abnormal α chains and higher sialic acid content.[27] Clinically, this results in an abnormal thrombin time (TT), despite almost normal PT and PTT, with an apparent normal concentration of total clottable fibrinogen. This abnormality is reversed following recovery of liver function.[28]

Platelets

Abnormalities in both number and function of platelets are common in patients with liver disease and contribute to the impaired hemostasis seen in these patients. About one third of patients with chronic liver disease develop thrombocytopenia, which is usually mild to moderate (70,000–90,000/μL), and worsens parallel to disease progression with associated increased hypersplenism, which furthers platelet sequestration.[29–31]

Thrombocytopenia has not been associated with an increased risk of bleeding from esophageal varices (i.e., structural bleeding) or other sources, although there are only a few studies evaluating this, but it has been shown to be correlated with blood loss during surgery (i.e., hemostatic bleeding).[32] A higher spleen diameter/platelet count ratio has been shown to have a high predictive value for the presence of esophageal varices in patients with liver cirrhosis.[33]

The issue of sequestration versus other causes of thrombocytopenia in cirrhosis has been evaluated recently by comparing platelet number in extrahepatic portal hypertension, with that of cirrhotics having a similar-sized spleen. This has shown a less severe thrombocytopenia in the non-cirrhotic patient.[34] Synthetic function of the liver is essential for platelet production via thrombopoietin (TPO), which regulates platelet production in the bone marrow.[35] Although TPO is increased in patients with thrombocytopenia owing to a homeostatic response,[36] this occurs to a lesser degree with severe or chronic liver diseases than in those subjects with a normal liver.[37] Lower TPO mRNA levels in cirrhotic liver tissue[38] have been shown, confirming impaired TPO synthesis. In addition, a low platelet production from the bone marrow in cirrhotic patients has been shown.[39]

Hepatitis C virus (HCV),[40] acute viral infection, alcohol abuse, and folate deficiency can all result in some myelosuppression[41]—further lowering platelet counts. Consumption coagulopathy is not common in cirrhosis and even if DIC is present at a chronic low level, it does not influence platelet count.[42,43] Thrombocytopenia may also be contributed to by immune-mediated mechanisms owing to an increased production from B cells of antibodies binding platelet surface antigen GPIIb/IIIa and GPIb/I, which has been shown in viral-induced cirrhosis B and C[44] and cholestatic liver diseases (primary biliary cirrhosis [PBC] and primary sclerosing cholangitis [PSC]).[45] Among 368 patients with viral-induced cirrhosis, elevated titers of platelet-associated immunoglobulin G were observed in 88% with HCV and 47% with HBV.[40]

Platelet function, as well as decreased platelet number, is impaired in patients with liver disease. Platelet aggregation in response to ADP, arachidonic acid, collagen, and thrombin is subnormal, probably owing to a defective signal transduction mechanism.[46] Intrinsic defects[47] and abnormal plasma factors[48] have also been shown to contribute to platelet function abnormalities. An abnormal content of arachidonic acid in platelet membranes is found in liver disease and induces less aggregation ability mediated by thromboxane A_2.[49] In plasma from cirrhotic patients, the presence of an abnormal high density lipoprotein (HDL) level may alter NO content in the cell, leading to abnormal aggregability.[50] Cholestatic liver diseases, which can demonstrate a normal or hypercoagulable state by thromboelastography,[51] have normal or hyperactive platelet function when assessed by platelet function assay (PFA-100) closure time and flow cytometry of receptors.[52] When the platelet number is too low, both cytometry or aggregation studies may be difficult to interpret; thromboelastography, which is a global test of clot formation and dissolution, measures both platelet function and number by maximum amplitude (ma) parameter,[53] and can be used to assess platelet function.

Splenectomy is generally contraindicated in patients with liver cirrhosis because of the high mortality rate and a risk of secondary portal vein thrombosis, leading to increased risk of bleeding from esophageal-gastric varices and more difficult surgery during subsequent liver transplantation.[54] Splenic embolization with 30% to 50% reduction in flow can normalize or significantly improve platelet number in some patients with liver cirrhosis[55] and may be helpful if invasive procedures, such as embolization of hepatocellular carcinoma or interferon therapy for viral hepatitis are required. Insertion of a transjugular intrahepatic portosystemic shunt (TIPS) has been shown to increase, but not to normalize, platelet number.[56,57]

ANTICOAGULANT FACTORS

Antithrombin III

Antithrombin III (ATIII) is a non–vitamin K-dependent glycoprotein synthesized by the liver but also by the endothelium.[58] It has low concentration in patients with liver disease, probably because of reduced synthesis and/or increased consumption due to hyperfibrinolysis.[59] Usually the ATIII deficit is mild and thrombosis as a complication is very rare, reported only sporadically.[60] ATIII replacement does not correct hyperfibrinolysis in patients with liver cirrhosis.

Protein C and Protein S

Proteins C and S are vitamin K–dependent glycoproteins synthesized mainly by hepatocytes.[61] Therefore, during acute or chronic liver disease, their concentrations can be decreased concomitantly with the other coagulation factors, but usually not below 20% of normal values.[62] Genetic deficiency of protein C is rare in the general population, but is found in 20% of patients with Budd-Chiari syndrome (BCS). In patients with liver disease who also have genetic deficiency, plasma concentration is often lower than 20%. When there is severe liver disease, it can be difficult to exclude coexistent genetic deficiency because levels may be very low owing to very depressed synthesis.[19] In this situation, a concomitant finding of a normal level of factor II and protein C/factor VII ratio, can help to confirm a coexistent genetic deficit.[63] In acquired deficiency of vitamin K, a defective protein C lacking γ-carboxyl (PIVKA) is produced.[1] Protein C deficiency is not associated with extrahepatic portal vein thrombosis.[64] Genetic deficiency of protein S is rare, yet it accounts for as many as 7% of patients with BCS or portal vein thrombosis (PVT), especially in Asians.[65]

DISORDERS OF THE FIBRINOLYTIC SYSTEM

All the proteins involved in fibrinolysis, except for tPA and PAI-1 are synthesized in the liver, and reduced plasma levels of plasminogen,[66] α_2-plasmin inhibitor, histidine-rich glycoprotein (HRG),[67] factor XIII,[68] and thrombin activatable fibrinolytic inhibitor (TAFI)[66] are documented in patients with liver cirrhosis. Conversely, tPA levels are increased in liver disease owing to decreased clearance, whereas its inhibitor, PAI-1, is normal or only slightly increased in plasma. The inhibitor concentrations are insufficient to counteract the increase in tPA accounting for increased fibrinolysis.[69] In contrast, in patients with acute liver failure, there are high levels of the acute phase reactant PAI-1 leading to a shift toward hypofibrinolysis.[70]

Hyperfibrinolysis is correlated with the severity of liver dysfunction in cirrhosis as assessed by Child-Pugh score.[71] Ascitic fluid has increased fibrinolytic activity: up to 20 liters are reabsorbed daily, with fibrinolysis being correlated with endotoxin levels.[72] Increased levels of D-dimers, prothrombin fragments 1+2 (F1+2) fibrin degradation products, and plasmin:α_2-plasmin inhibitor complexes are found.[73] Many studies using different methodologies demonstrate hyperfibrinolysis (thromboelastography,[74] diluted whole blood clot lysis assay,[75] and euglobin clot lysis time.[76] Recently, TAFI has been evaluated: it is decreased by an average of 26% in cirrhosis and by 50% in acute liver failure.[77,78] However, there is some controversy regarding hyperfibrinolytic activity in cirrhotic patients because not all studies have confirmed this. This may be due to the particular in vitro assay used. In contrast, in vivo correlation between hyperfibrinolysis and an increased risk of variceal bleeding, compatible with the circadian rhythm of the daily hyperfibrinolytic activity has been shown.[79] In addition, increased fibrinolytic activity during liver transplantation and hepatic resection correlates with blood loss.[80]

Interestingly, patients with cholestatic liver disease are characterized by a normal or hypercoagulable state: higher PAI-1 concentrations are seen compared with other etiologies, balancing the increased tPA activity. This results in less hyperfibrinolysis in the reperfusion phase during liver transplantation, and antifibrinolytic therapy is not usually administered.[81] Thus, the clinical issue is whether cirrhotic patients when under "stress" (e.g., during infection, during surgery, or during bleeding) exhibit the increased fibrinolysis, resulting in an increased bleeding tendency, which is not manifest in laboratory terms when patients are stable.

Disseminated Intravascular Coagulation and Accelerated Intravascular Coagulation

Disseminated intravascular coagulation (DIC) is characterized by intravascular fibrin deposition due to activation of the clotting cascade, which overwhelms the anticoagulation pathway. Secondary to the activation of the coagulation pathway, consumption of coagulation factors and platelets begins and secondary fibrinolysis occurs, causing a net increased bleeding tendency.[82]

Low-grade DIC and the hemostatic abnormalities that are present in cirrhotic patients share common laboratory features—a prolonged PT and PTT, low fibrinogen level, elevated fibrin-degradation product and D-dimer, and thrombocytopenia get confused with DIC.[83–85] Thus, diagnosis by laboratory means alone may be confounding. Early reports linked chronic liver disease to low-grade DIC, ascribing the latter to accelerated fibrinolysis. However, the presence of DIC in liver cirrhosis is disputed (see Chapter 12).[86] Although DIC-like laboratory abnormalities (so called "pseudo-DIC") are observed, autopsy studies in cirrhotics have shown little evidence for fibrin deposition and clinically evident DIC is rare.[83]

More highly sensitive tests, quantifying proteolytic cleavage products of the coagulation reaction—that is, fibrinopeptide A, F1+2, and fibrinolysis reactions (fibrin D-dimer, high molecular weight fibrin/fibrinogen complexes, or soluble fibrin), demonstrate an abnormal profile called accelerated intravascular coagulation and fibrinolysis phenomenon (AICF).[86] The studies demonstrate AICF in about 30% of cirrhotics, depending on the severity of liver disease; in two studies, this correlated with a decrease in levels of ATIII, protein C, and protein S.[74]

However, Ben Ari and colleagues analyzed 52 patients with stable liver disease for F1+2, thrombin:antithrombin III complex (TAT) and D-dimer levels which were no different from controls, yet TEG studies were able to detect hyperfibrinolysis. AICF may be important in the portal venous system because this phenomenon is more pronounced there than in systemic blood.[74] This could be related to higher levels of endotoxemia in portal blood, which can trigger the release of IL6 and TNF-α, thereby activating intravascular coagulation.[87]

PROGNOSTIC VALUE OF COAGULATION FACTORS

In cirrhosis, plasma coagulation factor levels are indicators of hepatic synthesis and liver function. A prolonged PT, which is not corrected by intravenous vitamin K administration—10 mg daily for 2 days, helps differentiate vitamin K deficiency from parenchymal liver diseases.[14] PT is part of the Child-Pugh score, which is the most commonly used prognostic score assessing the severity of liver disease.[88] Recently the MELD score, which incorporates INR, has been used to allocate priority for liver transplantation in the United States based on estimated probability of death within 3 months.[89]

Determination of individual coagulation factors adds little prognostic information to measuring PT or INR. Determination of factors V, VII, and VIII are useful indicators of DIC and prognostic indicators in acute liver failure (ALF).[82] The Clichy criteria indicate poor prognosis and need for liver transplantation for ALF, when factor V activity is below 20% in patients ≤30 years of age or below 30% associated with those ≥30 years of age.[90] Factor V activity has less prognostic value in acetaminophen-induced fulminant hepatic failure.[91]

In the King's College criteria in acetaminophen-induced liver failure, PT ≥ 100s is a prognostic indicator on its own for liver transplantation independent of the grade of coma. In patients with non–acetaminophen-induced ALF, PT ≥ 50s together with two of the following criteria: age <10 or >40 years, drug toxicity, interval between jaundice and encephalopathy onset >7 days and serum bilirubin >300 μmol/L are indications of poor prognosis and the need for liver transplantation.[92]

A multivariate analysis of prognostic factors in cirrhotic patients showed that the level of factor VII was an independent predictor factor of survival: factor VII <34% was predictive of a mortality in 93%.[93] Plasma concentration of D-dimer >300 μg/mL has been shown to be correlated with adverse outcome in patients with liver cirrhosis but has only a 20.5% of positive predictive value with a relative risk of 7.5.[94]

ASSESSMENT OF THE RISK OF THROMBOSIS AND ANTICOAGULATION

Thrombotic complications can paradoxically occur in cirrhotic patients even if clinically they are not considered to have hemorrhagic tendencies. Despite prolonged coagulation tests, these patients cannot be viewed as being "auto-anticoagulated." Wanless and associates advocated portal vein and hepatic vein thrombosis as concomitant causes in disease progression in cirrhotic patients. Hepatic vein and portal vein thromboses were found in at least 70% and 36% of explanted livers and were associated with regions of confluent fibrosis (focal parenchymal extinction).[95]

Portal vein thrombosis complicates liver cirrhosis between 0.6% to 15% of cases, leading to worsening of liver function and mesenteric infarction if the mesenteric vein is involved.[96] In these patients, early anticoagulation has been shown to recanalize the splanchnic veins in about 50% of cases and prevent the extension of the thrombus without causing complications.[97]

In BCS, even if a prothrombotic cause is not identified, anticoagulation should be started immediately after this diagnosis because many genetic prothrombic defects remain to be discovered and acquired disorders common in BCS may be elusive, such as polycythemia vera or paroxysmal nocturnal hemoglobinuria (PNH). Early anticoagulation ameliorates prognosis. Anticoagulation therapy should continue even after liver transplantation because of the high rate of recurrence and thrombotic complications after OLT, and also because multiple prothrombotic disorders may exist not limited to protein deficiencies.[19]

The risk of deep vein thrombosis and subsequent complications, such as pulmonary embolism, is not well known in cirrhotic patients, yet is reported in the literature.[98] Patients with cholestatic disease, such as PBC and PSC, who often exhibit a procoagulant state demonstrated by TEG, may be prone to thrombosis, but this is not documented.[51] No guidelines are available for the management of thrombotic complications or for the prevention of embolic phenomena following atrial fibrillation in cirrhotic patients. Patients must be assessed on their own characteristics. An endoscopic screen for varices must be performed and appropriate prophylaxis against variceal bleeding should be instituted, particularly if there has been recent bleeding. Antiplatelet drugs and NSAIDs should be avoided because they may precipitate bleeding and increase fluid retention with increased risk of renal failure. Anticoagulation is not contraindicated; warfarin in cirrhotic patients with PVT does not increase complications.[99,99a]

ASSESSMENT OF THE RISK OF BLEEDING

The role played by coagulation defects in the occurrence of bleeding in cirrhosis is still unclear. This is particularly due to the difficulty (and cost) in measuring static procoagulant and anticoagulant activities, and in formulating the balance between the two (see Table 39-1). In addition, there are very few tests that reflect or predict coagulation in vivo. A recent symposium detailed how little is actually known about hemorrhage in severe liver disease as well as the lack of confidence in routine coagulation tests (PT, PTT) and therapeutic efforts.[99b]

Recently, generation of thrombin has been explored in vitro in patients with liver cirrhosis and found to be normal. In this study, a resetting of the coagulation and anticoagulation system at a lower level was postulated because during liver disease, both procoagulant and anticoagulant pathways are affected in a parallel manner. However, the in vitro technique has some drawbacks, the major one being that platelets are substituted by phospholipids.[3]

Clinical signs of coagulopathy in liver disease depend on the degree of impairment of the hemostatic system. Commonly, minor signs of bleeding tendency are present, such as gum bleeding and epistaxis, but major bleeding can be encountered (Table 39-2). The role of hemostatic abnormalities in the risk of variceal bleeding is not clear. Impaired laboratory studies may indicate worse hepatic synthesis—serving more as a co-marker of disease rather than as a cause of hemorrhage. Hyperfibrinolysis has been shown to be linked to, but not necessarily a cause of, increased risk

Table 39-2 Clinical Hemorrhage in Patients with Liver Cirrhosis

Microvascular Manifestations
Petechiae
Bruising, purpura, bleeding at venipuncture sites or after minor challenges (brushing teeth, shaving)
Epistaxis
Gingival bleeding
DIC versus pseudo-DIC (see text)

Macrovascular Manifestations
Hemorrhage during surgery or invasive procedures (TIPS, ICP monitoring, liver biopsy, paracentesis, thoracentesis)
Variceal hemorrhage
Portal hypertensive gastropathy
Peptic ulcer disease

DIC, disseminated intravascular coagulopathy; ICP, intracranial pressure; TIPS, transjugular intrahepatic portosystemic shunt.

of variceal bleeding in a cohort of 61 cirrhotics. Higher levels of fibrinogen degradation products were associated with a greater risk of variceal bleeding compared with patients without (odds ratio = 8), but Child-Pugh score and endoscopic characteristics of varices remain the most important prognostic factors.[100]

Recently, the roles of infection and endogenous heparin-like substances demonstrated by TEG have been evaluated in variceal bleeding. Infection may be a trigger factor for bleeding[101] and both infection and heparin-like substances may be mechanisms responsible for the persistence of bleeding in some.[102] TEG, which is a quick and reliable method to assess clot formation and lysis,[53] also allows detection of heparin-like substances. Studies from our group have shown data consistent with worsening coagulation during infection due to heparin-like substances detected by TEG (Fig. 39-1).[103]

INVASIVE PROCEDURES

Historically, PT and platelet count have been used to assess the risk of bleeding prior to invasive procedures. Cirrhotic patients have increased mortality and morbidity during surgery[104] mainly due to increased bleeding in 60% of cases.[105,106] Early studies linked PT to this risk during surgery (PT prolongation >1.5 and >2.5 seconds associated with 47% and 87% mortality, respectively),[107] hence platelet count <50,000/μL and PT prolongation of > 3s have been considered relative contraindications to elective surgery.[106] In addition, portal hypertension and collateral veins increase the risk of bleeding during surgical dissection.

Hyperfibrinolysis[108] and clotting activation due to increase tPA levels have been described in patients undergoing liver resection.[109] However, another study performed in patients undergoing laparoscopic liver biopsy failed to demonstrate any correlation between the risk of bleeding evaluated at the hepatic puncture site and coagulation tests, so the degree of injury may be the important factor.[110]

Liver biopsy is widely used diagnostically and to grade the severity of liver disease or fibrosis. Moreover, it is an essential tool after liver transplantation used to diagnose rejection and other causes of graft dysfunction.

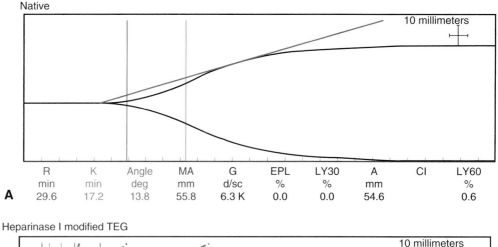

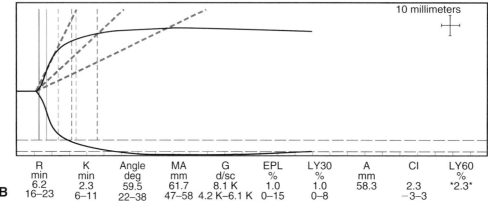

	R min	K min	Angle deg	MA mm	G d/sc	EPL %	LY30 %	A mm	CI	LY60 %
A	29.6	17.2	13.8	55.8	6.3 K	0.0	0.0	54.6		0.6

Heparinase I modified TEG

	R min	K min	Angle deg	MA mm	G d/sc	EPL %	LY30 %	A mm	CI	LY60 %
B	6.2	2.3	59.5	61.7	8.1 K	1.0	1.0	58.3	2.3	*2.3*
	16–23	6–11	22–38	47–58	4.2 K–6.1 K	0–15	0–8		–3–3	

Figure 39-1 Presence of heparin-like effect in a patient with cirrhosis and peritoneal infection. Native-TEG (**A**) and heparinase I-TEG (**B**) on sample collected at the onset of spontaneous bacterial peritonitis in a patient with liver cirrhosis. A significant heparin-like effect was found; the slowed rate of coagulation in **A** compared with **B** is shown by the decrease by slope (lower angle of separation, 13.8 degrees vs 59.5 degrees). Treatment of the sample in **B** with heparinases increases the rate of coagulation, thus implying the presence of heparin-like substances.

Bleeding complications occur in 0.35% to 0.5%, leading to mortality in 0.1%.[111] Despite the evidence that there were no threshold abnormalities of clotting tests associated with risk of bleeding during laparoscopic liver biopsy, INR and platelet count are essential to evaluate the bleeding risk for percutaneous liver biopsy.[112] An audit from the British Society of Gastroenterology (BSG) performed in 1991 showed a doubling of the risk of bleeding in patients with INR ≥ 1.5, but that only 7.1% of the bleeding occurred with INR ≥ 1.5, and 90% occurred with an INR ≤ 1.3.[113] Thus, having a normal INR no more excludes the risk of bleeding than an elevated INR suggests it. A cutoff for platelet count is difficult to justify from the literature. Most textbooks in the United Kingdom and BSG guidelines require (without reporting evidence) a platelet count above 80.000/μL,[14] whereas a survey from the Mayo Clinic suggested 50.000/μL as a reasonable cutoff.[114] Current recommendations state that a percutaneous liver biopsy can be done safely without support with platelet counts above 60.000/μL.[112] Burroughs and coworkers advocated evaluating the use of bleeding time to assess the risk of bleeding for percutaneous liver biopsy,[115] but this is not done in clinical practice. If clotting parameters are outside stipulated ranges, a transjugular liver biopsy can be more safely performed without plasma or platelet therapy.[116] A plugged liver biopsy is also said to be safer, but it may cause a greater risk of bleeding in hypocoagulable patients.[111]

During minor procedures such as thoracentesis, paracentesis, or lumbar puncture performed in patients with liver disease, there are no firm guidelines as to the hemostatic threshold for performing these tests. The largest review on 608 patients who underwent paracentesis or thoracentesis with mild coagulation abnormalities showed 0.2% having excessive bleeding requiring transfusion and 0.02% mortality. There was no correlation with PT, PTT, platelet count, and the risk of bleeding.[117] In another study performed in 200 cirrhotics with INR of 3 and platelet count 19,000/μL who underwent paracentesis, no complications were seen, regardless of baseline INR and platelet count.[118] A contraindication to the procedure is clinically evident DIC or fibrinolysis.[119] It is impossible using evidence-based techniques to establish "safe" coagulation tests for these procedures; it is more important to limit such procedures to circumstances in which the perceived benefit of the procedure is clearly greater than the risk.

COAGULATION DURING INFECTION AND SEPSIS

The overall cumulative incidence of infection in cirrhotic patients is estimated to be at least 30%,[120] and is possibly associated with increased risk of variceal bleeding.[101] Infection is associated with early rebleeding and increased mortality.[121,122] Prophylactic antibiotic therapy has led to earlier rebleeding and better control of bleeding in a randomized study.[123]

Using TEG, 20 cirrhotic patients who experienced early rebleeding were found to have worsening TEG parameters the day before rebleeding.[102] Moreover, patients with bacterial infection have worse TEG parameters, which can be corrected in vitro by heparinase I, which can cleave heparin-like substances (see Fig. 39-1A and B).[103] The presence of heparin-like substances is associated in some patients with increased anti-Xa activity.[124] Heparin-like substances have been detected hours after variceal bleeding in cirrhotic patients.[125] Based on this evidence, it has been postulated that endotoxins and inflammation due to infection can release heparinoids from the endothelium and mast cells.[103] One study, as yet not repeated, showed increased heparan sulfate concentrations in patients with variceal bleeding compared with patients without variceal bleeding.[126] Moreover, sepsis can cause impairment of platelet function, decreasing platelet number and aggregability caused by an increase NO production.[127]

Cytokines, in particular IL6 and TNF-α released during infection, can trigger DIC with hyperfibrinolysis.[128] One study showed a strong association between both fragment F1+2 and D-dimer with endotoxemia. These markers interestingly returned to normal after antibiotic therapy.[84] Another report recently showed decreased platelet count and levels of factors VII, X, V, and II, in cirrhotic patients and severe sepsis, suggesting consumptive coagulopathy,[129] whereas a further study found decreased activity of protein C, which is associated with increased fibrinolysis.[130]

THERAPY OF HEMOSTATIC ABNORMALITIES IN LIVER DISEASE

Usually, hematologic abnormalities in liver disease lead to only mild clinical consequences. However, in particular clinical settings, life-threatening bleeding can occur. Chief among these are the structural bleeds of varices and ulcer disease. Significant microvascular hemorrhage is unusual, despite multiple coagulation test abnormalities. Therapy for hemostatic abnormalities of liver disease is needed only during variceal bleeding, surgery, or before invasive procedures. Intravenous vitamin K injection of 10 mg daily for 24 to 48 hours can reverse vitamin K deficiency.[14]

Fresh frozen plasma (FFP) contains all the clotting factors and can correct the laboratory finding of an elevated PT effectively, but this correction depends on the volume and the baseline abnormality of PT. Whether this correction of the PT results in increased hemostasis has yet to be proved. In addition, the laboratory correction is short term (24 to 48 hours) because it depends on the half-lives of the clotting factors (especially factor VII).[82] A commonly used indication for FFP infusion is the presence of persistent bleeding in patients with INR ≥ 2 or PT prolongation greater than 4s.[131] In surgical or invasive procedures, 50% of the normal PT (i.e., INR of 2) is suggested and should be the aim of replacement therapy. For neurologic procedures such as intracranial pressure monitoring during liver failure, 80% of normal PT range (i.e., an INR of about 1.2 to 1.3) is suggested.[131] During massive blood transfusion, to avoid dilutional decrease of clotting factors for every 2 units of blood, 1 unit of FFP is typically given (See Chapter 46).[132] To increase the activity of clotting factor by 1% to 2%, a dose of 10 mL FFP/kg of body weight is necessary.[133] Because of the high volume required, adequate replacement is difficult in patients with liver cirrhosis, in whom the intravascular plasma volume is already expanded and in whom ascites may be present and in patients with ALF, in whom increasing plasma volume can lead to increases in intracerebral pressure. Moreover, because of the short half-life, infusions every 6 to 12 hours are needed.[11] In patients with INR > 1.5, FFP is typically given at the dose of 12 to 15 mL/kg before liver biopsy, but this practice is not based on evidence. One study showed correction of PT in only 20% of patients receiving such FFP.[112] It is unusual to be able to correct the PT by more than 2 to 3 seconds with less than 500 mL of FFP.[11] Thus, transjugular biopsy should be used in patients with coagulopathy not sufficiently correctable with FFP.

Platelet transfusion is employed, but this practice lacks any evidence-based support. One unit every 10 kg is typically administered, and platelet count should be checked one hour after the infusion.[134] However no correlation between amelioration of bleeding time, increase in platelet count, and enhanced hemostasis has been shown.[112]

Cryoprecipitate contains factors VIII, fibrinogen, VWF, fibronectin, and factor XIII. Because of the small volume (30 to 50mL/U/10 kg) required during infusion,[134] it can be useful in liver cirrhosis and ALF, but it lacks some coagulation factors and may worsen the imbalance already present in patients with liver disease. It is recommended in some patients with DIC and severe (i.e., <50 mg/dL) hypofibrogenemia, otherwise replacement does not correct the underlying hyperfibrinolytic defect.[135] In a recent randomized trial performed in patients with ALF, 5 units of cryoprecipitate were less effective than 4 units of FFP in improving the PTT, but one patient developed pulmonary edema in the FFP group.[136]

Desmopressin (1-deamino-8-D-arginine vasopressin [DDAVP]), an analog of the antidiuretic hormone, increases plasma level of factor VIII and VWF, probably by increasing the release from endothelial storage sites.[137] It can improve bleeding time, enhancing primary hemostasis at the dose of 0.3μg/kg in patients with liver failure.[138] However, a randomized trial associating terlipressin and DDAVP in patients with variceal bleeding, demonstrated no difference in control of bleeding and maybe a worsening of the terlipressin action in the DDAVP group.[139] In a recent randomized trial, DDAVP failed to decrease blood loss during hepatic resection, despite increase of factor VIII and VWF.[140]

ATIII infusion is not routinely recommended, although some studies showed an increase in the fibrinogen concentration during DIC.[141] In liver transplantation, ATIII administration has not been shown to improve blood loss or decrease mortality.[142]

Recombinant activated factor VII (rFVIIa) was first developed for the treatment of patients with hemophilia A or B who developed inhibitors. It may have a promising role in the treatment of coagulation disorders in liver disease.[143] A single dose of rFVIIa has been shown to correct prolonged PT in a dose-dependent manner in non-bleeding cirrhotic patients.[144] The half-life of rFVIIa is 2.3 hours.[145] The median duration of normalization of PT is 2, 6, and 12 hours following single doses of 5, 20, and 80 μg/kg, respectively.[144] A randomized study using rFVIIa in 71 patients undergoing laparoscopic liver biopsy found no differences in liver bleeding time. Two complications occurred in the rFVIIa group (1 DIC and 1 PVT).[146] In ALF, rFVIIa may be useful to normalize PT in the setting of intracranial pressure monitoring because only a small volume of infusion is required. The King's College group reported on seven patients who had normalization of PT after treatment with rFVIIa before ICP monitoring.[147] During variceal bleeding in a randomized trial, a modest reduction of early rebleeding rate was observed in a subgroup of Child B and C patients after rFVIIa infusion, although no difference in control of bleeding or transfusion was shown overall.[148] Another report described initial hemostasis after infusion of rFVIIa in ten patients, but six experienced early rebleeding and all of them died, illustrating the short interval of action of this drug.[149] In a cohort of eight patients with acute variceal bleeding uncontrolled with endoscopic and medical therapy, rFVIIa administration achieved hemostasis in 25% after a single dose.[150]

The efficacy of rFVIIa is limited in patients with low fibrinogen (<100 mg/dL) and concomitant administration of low volumes of plasma is required.[146] Safety, especially concerning the possible prothrombotic effect or triggering of DIC, still has to be assessed in large studies in patients with liver disease.[151] Secondary hyperfibrinolysis due to DIC can occur and DIC should be excluded before administration of antifibrinolytic drugs because these agents can worsen the thrombotic component of DIC.

ORTHOTOPIC LIVER TRANSPLANTATION

Orthotopic liver transplantation (OLT) is the only cure for end stage liver disease. Improvements in operative management, surgical techniques, and graft preservation have contributed to a significant reduction in transfusion requirements during the last decade.[152] However, blood losses are highly variable, and correlate in most studies, but not all, with a higher mortality, poor graft function, and risk of infections.[153] In current practice, a significant proportion of patients receive no blood during surgery. Preoperative identification of patients at high risk of surgical blood loss is of interest, but studies have given contrasting results. Most studies failed to define risks related to bleeding, including preoperative coagulation tests or markers of fibrinolysis during liver transplantation,[154–156] with the exception of the collateral circulation due to portal hypertension and previous abdominal

surgery.[157] Hemostatic abnormalities during liver transplantation are divided according to the surgical phases which are traditionally: pre-anhepatic phase, anhepatic phase and post-reperfusion phase, and postoperative period (Table 39-3).

Pre-Anhepatic Stage

The first operative stage is characterized by extensive surgical trauma, resulting from dissection of adhesions in the abdominal cavity and transection of many collateral vessels. Usually during this phase, mild coagulation abnormalities occur and the blood losses are mainly correlated with the surgical technique and the baseline hypocoagulable state.[157] The etiology of liver disease can influence the blood product requirement in this stage. Hypercoagulability has been demonstrated in patients with hepatocellular carcinoma as well as cholestatic cirrhosis (PBC, PSC). Marked differences have been shown in the pretransplantation coagulation parameters and intraoperative fibrinolytic activity between patients with cholestatic liver diseases (PBC and PSC), and other etiologies.[142] The PBC and PSC patients have a hypercoagulable state by TEG[51] and less fibrinolytic activity during OLT, suggesting that in these patients antifibrinolytic drugs should not be used. Moreover, in pediatric liver transplantation for biliary atresia, plasma studies showed fewer coagulation abnormalities during OLT compared with other etiologies.[158] Enhanced fibrinolytic activity contributes to blood loss in the pre-anhepatic phase in only 10% to 20% of patients.[159]

Anhepatic Phase

During this phase, no important surgical blood loss is seen because appropriate vessels are clamped. However, bleeding can occur owing to hemostatic changes in this phase. Despite impairment of synthetic and clearance function, early studies failed to show dramatic changes in PT and PTT during this stage.[80,160] However, hyperfibrinolysis has been demonstrated in many studies owing to a net increase in tPA derived from endothelial cells; this tPA is not cleared because of the absence of the liver at this time.[161] The presence of an active fibrinolytic process has been demonstrated by simultaneous decrease of α_2-plasmin inhibitor and plasminogen activity, and a concomitant increase in fibrin and fibrinogen degradation products.[162] Use of rFVIIa has been tried in patients with severe coagulopathy (INR 5.7 and 6.9). Moderate bleeding was still reported during surgery, but one patient

Table 39-3 Hemostatic Alterations in Orthotopic Liver Transplantation

	Pre-Anhepatic Phase	Anhepatic Phase	Reperfusion and Post-Reperfusion Phase	Postoperative Period* (Days)
Procoagulant factors	↓	↓↓	↓↓	1–2
Anticoagulant factors	↓	→	→	7–14
Hyperfibrinolysis	↑	↑↑	↑↑↑	1–2
Platelet count	→	→	↓	1–7
Platelet function	→	→	↓	1–2
Heparin-like effect	↑→	↑	↑↑	1–2

*The convalescence period is the time after successful transplantation required to return to normal adult levels.
→, indicates no change; ↑, indicates a mild increase; ↑↑, indicates a significant increase; ↑↑↑, indicates a marked increase.

developed hepatic artery thrombosis after transplant.[163] Studies that evaluated coagulation factors during OLT after rFVIIa infusion showed a sharp increase of thrombin generation, PT, and PTT, but no amelioration of fibrinolysis.[164,165]

Reperfusion and Post-Reperfusion Phase

Reperfusion of the liver is a crucial point of the operation and leads to profound coagulation abnormalities. Within minutes after reperfusion, uncontrollable diffuse bleeding may occur in some patients.[166] The roles of humoral factors such as hypocalcemia, hypothermia, hyperkalemia, metabolic acidosis,[160] and release of proteinases from donor hepatic lysosomes, are all believed to contribute to the blood loss, but these effects are not yet well defined.[167]

Trapping of platelets in the graft may play a role in the bleeding tendency. Experimental studies have shown a 55% gradient in platelet count between arterial and venous blood flow in the new liver. Moreover, some alterations in the bleeding time and platelet function and aggregation have been demonstrated.[168]

Signs of DIC after graft reperfusion have been shown by some investigators, mainly correlated with poor quality of the transplanted organ.[169] During ischemic preservation, damage to vascular endothelial cells may occur. This injured endothelial layer may lead to platelet adhesion and activation of the coagulation system.[170] However both ATIII and heparin administration failed to have any benefit, which suggests DIC is not a major component of the bleeding during the anhepatic phase.[142] Moreover, improvements in the preservation techniques have reduced the frequency of DIC in OLT.

Increase in fibrinolysis has been implicated as the most important and significant phenomenon responsible for bleeding during liver transplantation. Hepatic endothelium is a rich source of plasminogen activators and release and washout of these activators from the transplanted liver have been considered responsible for the increased tPA levels at reperfusion.[171] In pigs, hyperfibrinolysis has been shown to be related to preservation time. It usually subsides within 60 minutes after graft reperfusion, but in donor livers with poor function, a sustained increased fibrinolytic response can be seen.[172]

After reperfusion, release of heparin or heparin-like substances has been shown in 25% to 95% of cases.[173] Protamine sulfate (50 mg) has been used in vivo to antagonize this effect. One study has confirmed the presence of heparin-like compounds using heparinase I-modified TEG, which cleaves heparin and heparan sulfate. Increased blood product requirement was correlated with the presence of heparin-like effects in TEG traces. However a baseline heparin-like effect has recently been found before reperfusion in patients undergoing liver transplantation who had not received heparin.[174]

Antifibrinolytic therapy is used during liver transplantation to reduce blood loss, time of surgery, and fibrinolytic activity. Aprotinin is a serine protease inhibitor that antagonizes various proteases.[175] Some use an initial dose of 2×10^6 KIU/hour followed by 1×10^6 KIU/hour and an additional dose of 1×10^6 KIU before reperfusion.[176] Recent prospective studies have confirmed that this dose is able to reduce blood requirement and fibrinolysis, but

at a lower dose, there was only an effect on the volume of blood products replaced.[177–179] Aprotinin also has anti-inflammatory and antioxidant effects which might also be of benefit. Excessive use of aprotinin is not recommended because of the risks of anaphylactic reactions, renal dysfunction, and stroke.[180]

ε Aminocaproic acid (EACA) interferes with plasminogen binding to fibrin and thus EACA inhibits the conversion of plasminogen to plasmin.[181] In the only prospective randomized trial, an initial dose of 70 mg per kilogram of body weight followed by 16 mg/kg/hour maintenance was shown to reverse TEG fibrinolysis, and reduce blood cell transfusion, without causing thrombotic complications. However this reduction was not statistically significant compared with controls.[182] Similar to EACA, tranexamic acid inhibits fibrinolysis, but it is 6 to 10 times more potent than EACA.[183] It does not have any effect on the bradykinin-kallikrein complex.[184] Recent trials have shown that at a dose of 2 mg/kg/hour, tranexamic acid reduces fibrinolysis and blood loss. However, different doses have been used in other studies without clear-cut effects.[183–186]

The routine use of coagulation monitoring during liver transplantation is established. Usually TEG, a near-site rapid method to globally assess the coagulation process, is used. It provides a rational approach to the use of blood component therapy or pharmacologic intervention, but it does not help in addressing blood transfusion per se.[53] Recently, TEG was used to monitor postoperative coagulation in patients undergoing hepatic resection for living related liver transplantation. In these patients, a hypercoagulable state correlated with the risk of developing thrombotic complications after surgery.[187]

Postoperative Period

Thrombocytopenia is common in the early postoperative period, mainly due to platelet activation and consumption following graft reperfusion.[188] If liver function is restored, thrombocytopenia subsides in a few days after OLT. Following normal synthetic function of the liver, thrombopoietin levels increase significantly on the first day, followed by immature bone marrow megakaryocytes after 3 days, and new circulating platelets after 5 days. Normalization of platelet count is seen after 14 days.[189] The peak TPO levels correlate with the pre-OLT platelet count. Levels of bilirubin, cold ischemia time or episodes of rejection do not influence TPO levels.[190] Persistence of thrombocytopenia can be seen in some patients, which can be ascribed to persistent splenomegaly in some, but not all, patients.[191]

REFERENCES

1. Lisman T, Leebeek FW, de Groot PG: Haemostatic abnormalities in patients with liver disease. J Hepatol 37:280–287, 2002.
2. Rapaport SI: Coagulation problems in liver disease. Blood Coagul Fibrinolysis 11 (suppl 1): S69–S74, 2000.
3. Tripodi A, Salerno F, Chantarangkul V, et al: Evidence of normal thrombin generation in cirrhosis despite abnormal conventional coagulation tests. Hepatology 41:553–558, 2005.
4. Kelly DA, Summerfield JA: Hemostasis in liver disease. Semin Liver Dis 7:182–191, 1987.
5. Ferro D, Quintarelli C, Lattuada A, et al: High plasma levels of von Willebrand factor as a marker of endothelial perturbation in cirrhosis: Relationship to endotoxemia. Hepatology 23:1377–1383, 1996.

6. Wion KL, Kelly D, Summerfield JA, et al: Distribution of factor VIII mRNA and antigen in human liver and other tissues. Nature 317:726–729, 1985.

7. Hollestelle MJ, Geertzen HG, Straatsburg IH, et al: Factor VIII expression in liver disease. Thromb Haemost 91:267–275, 2004.

8. Hollestelle MJ, Thinnes T, Crain K, et al: Tissue distribution of factor VIII gene expression in vivo: A closer look. Thromb Haemost 86:855–861, 2001.

9. Kerr R: New insights into haemostasis in liver failure. Blood Coagul Fibrinolysis 14 (Suppl 1): S43–S45, 2003.

10. Maisonneuve P, Sultan Y: Modification of factor VIII complex properties in patients with liver disease. J Clin Pathol 30:221–227, 1977.

11. Mueller MM, Bomke B, Seifried E: Fresh frozen plasma in patients with disseminated intravascular coagulation or in patients with liver diseases. Thromb Res 107 (Suppl 1): S9–S17, 2002.

12. Blanchard RA, Furie BC, Jorgensen M, et al: Acquired vitamin K-dependent carboxylation deficiency in liver disease. N Engl J Med 305:242–248, 1981.

13. Belle M, Brebant R, Guinet R, et al: Production of a new monoclonal antibody specific to human des-gamma-carboxyprothrombin in the presence of calcium ions: Application to the development of a sensitive ELISA-test. J Immunoassay 16:213–229, 1995.

14. Sherlock S, Dooley J: The haematology of liver disease. In Sherlock S, Dooley J: Diseases of the Liver and Biliary System, Oxford, Blackwell Publishing, 2002, pp 47–64.

15. Pereira SP, Rowbotham D, Fitt S, et al: Pharmacokinetics and efficacy of oral versus intravenous mixed-micellar phylloquinone (vitamin K$_1$) in severe acute liver disease. J Hepatol 42:365–370, 2005.

16. Kerr R, Newsome P, Germain L, et al: Effects of acute liver injury on blood coagulation. J Thromb Haemost 1:754–759, 2003.

17. Weitz IC, Liebman HA: Des-gamma-carboxy (abnormal) prothrombin and hepatocellular carcinoma: A critical review. Hepatology 18:990–997, 1993.

18. Amitrano L, Brancaccio V, Guardascione MA, et al: Inherited coagulation disorders in cirrhotic patients with portal vein thrombosis. Hepatology 31:345–348, 2000.

19. Senzolo M, Cholongitas CE, Patch D, et al: Update on the classification, assessment of prognosis and therapy of Budd-Chiari syndrome. Nat Clin Pract Gastroenterol Hepatol 2:182–190, 2005.

20. Primignani M, Martinelli I, Bucciarelli P, et al: Risk factors for thrombophilia in extrahepatic portal vein obstruction. Hepatology 41:603–608, 2005.

21. Baruch Y, Neubauer K, Ritzel A, et al: Von Willebrand gene expression in damaged human liver. Hepatogastroenterology 51:684–688, 2004.

22. Escolar G, Cases A, Vinas M, et al: Evaluation of acquired platelet dysfunctions in uremic and cirrhotic patients using the platelet function analyzer (PFA-100): Influence of hematocrit elevation. Haematologica 84:614–619, 1999.

23. Kelly DA, Tuddenham EG: Haemostatic problems in liver disease. Gut 27:339–349, 1986.

24. Albornoz L, Alvarez D, Otaso JC, et al: Von Willebrand factor could be an index of endothelial dysfunction in patients with cirrhosis: Relationship to degree of liver failure and nitric oxide levels. J Hepatol 30:451–455, 1999.

25. Lechner K, Niessner H, Thaler E: Coagulation abnormalities in liver disease. Semin Thromb Hemost 4:40–56, 1977.

26. Dymock IW, Tucker JS, Woolf IL, et al: Coagulation studies as a prognostic index in acute liver failure. Br J Haematol 29:385–395, 1975.

27. Francis JL, Armstrong DJ: Fibrinogen-bound sialic acid levels in the dysfibrinogenaemia of liver disease. Haemostasis 11:215–222, 1982.

28. Barr RD, Allardyce M, Brunt PW, et al: Dysfibrinogenaemia and liver cell growth. J Clin Pathol 31:89–92, 1978.

29. Noguchi H, Hirai K, Aoki Y, et al: Changes in platelet kinetics after a partial splenic arterial embolization in cirrhotic patients with hypersplenism. Hepatology 22:1682–1688, 1995.

30. Sohma Y, Akahori H, Seki N, et al: Molecular cloning and chromosomal localization of the human thrombopoietin gene. FEBS Lett 353:57–61, 1994.

31. Yanaga K, Tzakis AG, Shimada M, et al: Reversal of hypersplenism following orthotopic liver transplantation. Ann Surg 210:180–183, 1989.

32. Clavien PA, Camargo CA Jr, Croxford R, et al: Definition and classification of negative outcomes in solid organ transplantation: Application in liver transplantation. Ann Surg 220:109–120, 1994.

33. Giannini E, Botta F, Borro P, et al: Platelet count/spleen diameter ratio: Proposal and validation of a non-invasive parameter to predict the presence of oesophageal varices in patients with liver cirrhosis. Gut 52:1200–1205, 2003.

34. Robson SC, Kahn D, Kruskal J, et al: Disordered hemostasis in extrahepatic portal hypertension. Hepatology 18:853–857, 1993.

35. Panasiuk A, Prokopowicz D, Zak J, et al: Reticulated platelets as a marker of megakaryopoiesis in liver cirrhosis. Relation to thrombopoietin and hepatocyte growth factor serum concentration. Hepatogastroenterology 51:1124–1128, 2004.

36. Jelkmann W: The role of the liver in the production of thrombopoietin compared with erythropoietin. Eur J Gastroenterol Hepatol 13:791–801, 2001.

37. Kitano K, Shimodaira S, Ito T, et al: Liver cirrhosis with marked thrombocytopenia and highly elevated serum thrombopoietin levels. Int J Hematol 70:52–55, 1999.

38. Martin TG 3rd, Somberg KA, Meng YG, et al: Thrombopoietin levels in patients with cirrhosis before and after orthotopic liver transplantation. Ann Intern Med 127:285–288, 1997.

39. Wang GL, Jiang BH, Rue EA, et al: Hypoxia-inducible factor 1 is a basic-helix-loop-helix-PAS heterodimer regulated by cellular O$_2$ tension. Proc Natl Acad Sci USA 92:5510–5514, 1995.

40. Nagamine T, Ohtuka T, Takehara K, et al: Thrombocytopenia associated with hepatitis C viral infection. J Hepatol 24:135–140, 1996.

41. Peck-Radosavljevic M: Thrombocytopenia in liver disease. Can J Gastroenterol 14 (Suppl D): 60D–66D, 2000.

42. Violi F, Leo R, Basili S, et al: Association between prolonged bleeding time and gastrointestinal hemorrhage in 102 patients with liver cirrhosis: Results of a retrospective study. Haematologica 79:61–65, 1994.

43. Violi F, Ferro D, Basili S, et al: Hyperfibrinolysis increases the risk of gastrointestinal hemorrhage in patients with advanced cirrhosis. Hepatology 15:672–676, 1992.

44. Kajihara M, Kato S, Okazaki Y, et al: A role of autoantibody-mediated platelet destruction in thrombocytopenia in patients with cirrhosis. Hepatology 37:1267–1276, 2003.

45. Feistauer SM, Penner E, Mayr WR, et al: Target platelet antigens of autoantibodies in patients with primary biliary cirrhosis. Hepatology 25:1343–1345, 1997.

46. Escolar G, Cases A, Vinas M, et al: Evaluation of acquired platelet dysfunctions in uremic and cirrhotic patients using the platelet function analyzer (PFA-100): Influence of hematocrit elevation. Haematologica 84:614–619, 1999.

47. Laffi G, Marra F, Gresele P, et al: Evidence for a storage pool defect in platelets from cirrhotic patients with defective aggregation. Gastroenterology 103:641–646, 1992.

48. Younger HM, Hadoke PW, Dillon JF, et al: Platelet function in cirrhosis and the role of humoral factors. Eur J Gastroenterol Hepatol 9:989–992, 1997.

49. Owen JS, Hutton RA, Day RC, et al: Platelet lipid composition and platelet aggregation in human liver disease. J Lipid Res 22:423–430, 1981.

50. Riddell DR, Owen JS: Nitric oxide and platelet aggregation. Vitam Horm 57:25–48, 1999.

51. Ben Ari Z, Panagou M, Patch D, et al: Hypercoagulability in patients with primary biliary cirrhosis and primary sclerosing cholangitis evaluated by thrombelastography. J Hepatol 26:554–559, 1997.

52. Pihusch R, Rank A, Gohring P, et al: Platelet function rather than plasmatic coagulation explains hypercoagulable state in cholestatic liver disease. J Hepatol 37:548–555, 2002.

53. Salooja N, Perry DJ: Thrombelastography. Blood Coagul Fibrinolysis 12:327–337, 2001.

54. Bolognesi M, Merkel C, Sacerdoti D, et al: Role of spleen enlargement in cirrhosis with portal hypertension. Dig Liver Dis 34:144–150, 2002.

55. N'Kontchou G, Seror O, Bourcier V, et al: Partial splenic embolization in patients with cirrhosis: Efficacy, tolerance and long-term outcome in 32 patients. Eur J Gastroenterol Hepatol 17:179–184, 2005.

56. Jabbour N, Zajko A, Orons P, et al: Does transjugular intrahepatic portosystemic shunt (TIPS) resolve thrombocytopenia associated with cirrhosis? Dig Dis Sci 43:2459–2462, 1998.

57. Karasu Z, Gurakar A, Kerwin B, et al: Effect of transjugular intrahepatic portosystemic shunt on thrombocytopenia associated with cirrhosis. Dig Dis Sci 45:1971–1976, 2000.

58. Schipper HG, ten Cate JW: Antithrombin III transfusion in patients with hepatic cirrhosis. Br J Haematol 52:25–33, 1982.

59. Liebman HA, McGehee WG, Patch MJ, et al: Severe depression of antithrombin III associated with disseminated intravascular coagulation in women with fatty liver of pregnancy. Ann Intern Med 98:330–333, 1983.

60. Carmassi F, Morale M, De Negri F, et al: Modulation of hemostatic balance with antithrombin III replacement therapy in a case of liver cirrhosis associated with recurrent venous thrombosis. J Mol Med 73:89–93, 1995.

61. Fair DS, Marlar RA: Biosynthesis and secretion of factor VII, protein C, protein S, and the Protein C inhibitor from a human hepatoma cell line. Blood 67:64–70, 1986.

62. Mannucci PM, Vigano S: Deficiencies of protein C, an inhibitor of blood coagulation. Lancet 2:463–467, 1982.

63. Minnema MC, Janssen HL, Niermeijer P, et al: Budd-Chiari syndrome: Combination of genetic defects and the use of oral contraceptives leading to hypercoagulability. J Hepatol 33:509–512, 2000.

64. Primignani M, Martinelli I, Bucciarelli P, et al: Risk factors for thrombophilia in extrahepatic portal vein obstruction. Hepatology 41:603–608, 2005.

65. Bhattacharyya M, Makharia G, Kannan M, et al: Inherited prothrombotic defects in Budd-Chiari syndrome and portal vein thrombosis: A study from North India. Am J Clin Pathol 121:844–847, 2004.

66. Stein SF, Harker LA: Kinetic and functional studies of platelets, fibrinogen, and plasminogen in patients with hepatic cirrhosis. J Lab Clin Med 99:217–230, 1982.

67. Leebeek FW, Kluft C, Knot EA, et al: Histidine-rich glycoprotein is elevated in mild liver cirrhosis and decreased in moderate and severe liver cirrhosis. J Lab Clin Med 113:493–497, 1989.

68. Biland L, Duckert F, Prisender S, et al: Quantitative estimation of coagulation factors in liver disease: The diagnostic and prognostic value of factor XIII, factor V, and plasminogen. Thromb Haemost 39:646–656, 1989.

69. Hersch SL, Kunelis T, Francis RB Jr: The pathogenesis of accelerated fibrinolysis in liver cirrhosis: A critical role for tissue plasminogen activator inhibitor. Blood 69:1315–1319, 1987.

70. Pernambuco JR, Langley PG, Hughes RD, et al: Activation of the fibrinolytic system in patients with fulminant liver failure. Hepatology 18:1350–1356, 1993.

71. Hu KQ, Yu AS, Tiyyagura L, et al: Hyperfibrinolytic activity in hospitalized cirrhotic patients in a referral liver unit. Am J Gastroenterol 96:1581–1586, 2001.

72. Agarwal S, Joyner KA Jr, Swaim MW: Ascites fluid as a possible origin for hyperfibrinolysis in advanced liver disease. Am J Gastroenterol 95:3218–3224, 2000.

73. Paramo JA, Rocha E: Hemostasis in advanced liver disease. Semin Thromb Hemost 19:184–190, 1993.

74. Ben Ari Z, Osman E, Hutton RA, et al: Disseminated intravascular coagulation in liver cirrhosis: Fact or fiction? Am J Gastroenterol 94:2977–2982, 1999.

75. Comp PC, Jacocks RM, Rubenstein C, et al: A lysine-absorbable plasminogen activator is elevated in conditions associated with increased fibrinolytic activity. J Lab Clin Med 97:637–645, 1981.

76. Francis RB Jr, Feinstein DI: Clinical significance of accelerated fibrinolysis in liver disease. Haemostasis 14:460–465, 1984.

77. Lisman T, Leebeek FW, Mosnier LO, et al: Thrombin-activatable fibrinolysis inhibitor deficiency in cirrhosis is not associated with increased plasma fibrinolysis. Gastroenterology 121:131–139, 2001.

78. Colucci M, Binetti BM, Branca MG, et al: Deficiency of thrombin activatable fibrinolysis inhibitor in cirrhosis is associated with increased plasma fibrinolysis. Hepatology 38:230–237, 2003.

79. Piscaglia F, Siringo S, Hermida RC, et al: Diurnal changes of fibrinolysis in patients with liver cirrhosis and esophageal varices. Hepatology 31:349–357, 2000.

80. Lewis JH, Bontempo FA, Awad SA, et al: Liver transplantation: Intraoperative changes in coagulation factors in 100 first transplants. Hepatology 9:710–714, 1989.

81. Segal H, Cottam S, Potter D, et al: Coagulation and fibrinolysis in primary biliary cirrhosis compared with other liver disease and during orthotopic liver transplantation. Hepatology 25:683–688, 1997.

82. Amitrano L, Guardascione MA, Brancaccio V, et al: Coagulation disorders in liver disease. Semin Liver Dis 22:83–96, 2002.

83. Carr JM: Disseminated intravascular coagulation in cirrhosis. Hepatology 10:103–110, 1989.

84. Violi F, Ferro D, Basili S, et al: Association between low-grade disseminated intravascular coagulation and endotoxemia in patients with liver cirrhosis. Gastroenterology 109:531–539, 1995.

85. Kemkes-Matthes B, Bleyl H, Matthes KJ: Coagulation activation in liver diseases. Thromb Res 64:253–261, 1991.

86. Joist JH: AICF and DIC in liver cirrhosis: Expressions of a hypercoagulable state. Am J Gastroenterol 94:2801–2803, 1999.

87. Basili S, Ferro D, Violi F: Endotoxaemia, hyperfibrinolysis, and bleeding in cirrhosis. Lancet 353:1102, 1999.

88. Botero RC, Lucey MR: Organ allocation: model for end-stage liver disease, Child-Turcotte-Pugh, Mayo risk score, or something else. Clin Liver Dis 7:715–727, 2003.

89. Kamath PS, Wiesner RH, Malinchoc M, et al: A model to predict survival in patients with end-stage liver disease. Hepatology 33:464–470, 2001.

90. Bismuth H, Samuel D, Castaing D, et al: Orthotopic liver transplantation in fulminant and subfulminant hepatitis: The Paul Brousse experience. Ann Surg 222:109–119, 1995.

91. Pauwels A, Mostefa-Kara N, Florent C, et al: Emergency liver transplantation for acute liver failure: Evaluation of London and Clichy criteria. J Hepatol 17:124–127, 1993.

92. O'Grady JG, Alexander GJ, Hayllar KM, et al: Early indicators of prognosis in fulminant hepatic failure. Gastroenterology 97:439–445, 1989.

93. Violi F, Ferro D, Basili S, et al: Prognostic value of clotting and fibrinolytic systems in a follow-up of 165 liver cirrhotic patients: CALC Group. Hepatology 22:96–100, 1995.

94. Gutierrez A, Sanchez-Paya J, Marco P, et al: Prognostic value of fibrinolytic tests for hospital outcome in patients with acute upper gastrointestinal hemorrhage. J Clin Gastroenterol 32:315–318, 2001.

95. Wanless IR, Wong F, Blendis LM, et al: Hepatic and portal vein thrombosis in cirrhosis: Possible role in development of parenchymal extinction and portal hypertension. Hepatology 21:1238–1247, 1995.

96. Amitrano L, Guardascione MA, Brancaccio V, et al: Risk factors and clinical presentation of portal vein thrombosis in patients with liver cirrhosis. J Hepatol 40:736–741, 2004.

97. Francoz C, Belghiti J, Vilgrain V, et al: Splanchnic vein thrombosis in candidates for liver transplantation: Usefulness of screening and anticoagulation. Gut 54:691–697, 2005.

98. Espiritu JD: Pulmonary embolism in a patient with coagulopathy from end-stage liver disease. Chest 117:924–925, 2000.

99. Condat B, Pessione F, Helene DM, et al: Recent portal or mesenteric venous thrombosis: Increased recognition and frequent recanalization on anticoagulant therapy. Hepatology 32:466–470, 2000.

99a. Kitchens CS, Weidner MH, Lottenberg R: Chronic oral anticoagulant therapy for extrahepatic visceral thrombosis is safe. J Thromb Thrombolysis 23:223–228, 2007.

99b. Caldwell SH, Hoffman M, Lisman T, et al: Coagulation disorders and hemostasis in liver disease: Pathophysiology and critical assessment of current management. Hepatology 44:1039–1046, 2006.

100. Violi F, Basili S, Ferro D, et al: Association between high values of D-dimer and tissue-plasminogen activator activity and first gastrointestinal bleeding in cirrhotic patients: CALC Group. Thromb Haemost 76:177–183, 1996.

101. Goulis J, Patch D, Burroughs AK: Bacterial infection in the pathogenesis of variceal bleeding. Lancet 353:139–142, 1999.

102. Chau TN, Chan YW, Patch D, et al: Thrombelastographic changes and early rebleeding in cirrhotic patients with variceal bleeding. Gut 43:267–271, 1998.

103. Montalto P, Vlachogiannakos J, Cox DJ, et al: Bacterial infection in cirrhosis impairs coagulation by a heparin effect: A prospective study. J Hepatol 37:463–470, 2002.

104. Perkins L, Jeffries M, Patel T: Utility of preoperative scores for predicting morbidity after cholecystectomy in patients with cirrhosis. Clin Gastroenterol Hepatol 2:1123–1128, 2004.

105. Patel T: Surgery in the patient with liver disease. Mayo Clin Proc 74:593–599, 1999.

106. Friedman LS: The risk of surgery in patients with liver disease. Hepatology 29:1617–1623, 1999.

107. Garrison RN, Cryer HM, Howard DA, et al: Clarification of risk factors for abdominal operations in patients with hepatic cirrhosis. Ann Surg 199:648–655, 1984.

108. Tsuji K, Eguchi Y, Kodama M: Postoperative hypercoagulable state followed by hyperfibrinolysis related to wound healing after hepatic resection. J Am Coll Surg 183:230–238, 1996.

109. Meijer C, Wiezer MJ, Hack CE, et al: Coagulopathy following major liver resection: The effect of rBPI21 and the role of decreased synthesis of regulating proteins by the liver. Shock 15:261–271, 2001.

110. Ewe K: Bleeding after liver biopsy does not correlate with indices of peripheral coagulation. Dig Dis Sci 26:388–393, 1981.

111. Burroughs AK, Dagher L: Liver biopsy. In: Gastroenterological Endoscopy.New York, Thieme, 2002, pp 252–259.

112. Grant A, Neuberger J: Guidelines on the use of liver biopsy in clinical practice. British Society of Gastroenterology. Gut 45 (Suppl 4): IV1–IV11, 1999.

113. Gilmore IT, Burroughs A, Murray-Lyon IM, et al: Indications, methods, and outcomes of percutaneous liver biopsy in England and Wales: An audit by the British Society of Gastroenterology and the Royal College of Physicians of London. Gut 36:437–441, 1995.

114. McGill DB, Rakela J, Zinsmeister AR, et al: A 21-year experience with major hemorrhage after percutaneous liver biopsy. Gastroenterology 99:1396–1400, 1990.

115. Blake JC, Sprengers D, Grech P, et al: Bleeding time in patients with hepatic cirrhosis. BMJ 301:12–15, 1990.

116. Papatheodoridis GV, Patch D, Watkinson A, et al: Transjugular liver biopsy in the 1990s: A 2-year audit. Aliment Pharmacol Ther 13:603–608, 1999.

117. Pache I, Bilodeau M: Severe haemorrhage following abdominal paracentesis for ascites in patients with liver disease. Aliment Pharmacol Ther 21:525–529, 2005.

118. Lin CH, Chen SC, Ko PC: Preprocedure coagulation tests are unnecessary before abdominal paracentesis in emergency departments. Hepatology 41:402–403, 2005.

119. Runyon BA: Paracentesis of ascitic fluid: A safe procedure: Arch Intern Med 146:2259–2261, 1986.

120. Bernard B, Grange JD, Khac EN, et al: Antibiotic prophylaxis for the prevention of bacterial infections in cirrhotic patients with gastrointestinal bleeding: A meta-analysis. Hepatology 29:1655–1661, 1999.

121. Goulis J, Armonis A, Patch D, et al: Bacterial infection is independently associated with failure to control bleeding in cirrhotic patients with gastrointestinal hemorrhage. Hepatology 27:1207–1212, 1998.

122. Bernard B, Cadranel JF, Valla D, et al: Prognostic significance of bacterial infection in bleeding cirrhotic patients: A prospective study. Gastroenterology 108:1828–1834, 1995.

123. Hou MC, Lin HC, Liu TT, et al: Antibiotic prophylaxis after endoscopic therapy prevents rebleeding in acute variceal hemorrhage: A randomized trial. Hepatology 39:746–753, 2004.

124. Zambruni A, Thalheimer U, Coppell J, et al: Endogenous heparin-like activity detected by anti-Xa assay in infected cirrhotic and non-cirrhotic patients. Scand J Gastroenterol 39:830–836, 2004.

125. Thalheimer U, Triantos C, Samonakis D, et al: Endogenous heparinoids in acute variceal bleeding. Gut 54:310–311, 2005.

126. McKee RF, Hodson S, Dawes J, et al: Plasma concentrations of endogenous heparinoids in portal hypertension. Gut 33:1549–1552, 1992.

127. Thalheimer U, Triantos CK, Samonakis DN, et al: Infection, coagulation, and variceal bleeding in cirrhosis. Gut 54:556–563, 2005.

128. Grignani G, Maiolo A: Cytokines and hemostasis. Haematologica 85:967–972, 2000.

129. Plessier A, Denninger MH, Consigny Y, et al: Coagulation disorders in patients with cirrhosis and severe sepsis. Liver Int 23:440–448, 2003.

130. Wong F, Bernardi M, Balk R, et al: Sepsis in cirrhosis: Report on the 7th meeting of the International Ascites Club. Gut 54:718–725, 2005.

131. Everson GT: A hepatologist's perspective on the management of coagulation disorders before liver transplantation. Liver Transpl Surg 3:646–652, 1997.

132. Martin DJ, Lucas CE, Ledgerwood AM, et al: Fresh frozen plasma supplement to massive red blood cell transfusion. Ann Surg 202:505–511, 1985.

133. Maltz GS, Siegel JE, Carson JL: Hematologic management of gastrointestinal bleeding. Gastroenterol Clin North Am 29:169–187, 2000.

134. Gunter P: Practice guidelines for blood component therapy. Anesthesiology 85:1219–1220, 1996.

135. Mammen EF: Disseminated intravascular coagulation (DIC). Clin Lab Sci 13:239–245, 2000.

136. French CJ, Bellomo R, Angus P: Cryoprecipitate for the correction of coagulopathy associated with liver disease. Anaesth Intensive Care 31:357–361, 2003.

137. Mannucci PM, Canciani MT, Rota L, et al: Response of factor VIII/von Willebrand factor to DDAVP in healthy subjects and patients with haemophilia A and von Willebrand's disease. Br J Haematol 47:283–293, 1981.

138. Burroughs AK, Matthews K, Qadiri M, et al: Desmopressin and bleeding time in patients with cirrhosis. Br Med J (Clin Res Ed) 291:1377–1381, 1985.

139. de Franchis R, Arcidiacono PG, Carpinelli L, et al: Randomized controlled trial of desmopressin plus terlipressin vs terlipressin alone for the treatment of acute variceal hemorrhage in cirrhotic patients: A multicenter, double-blind study. New Italian Endoscopic Club. Hepatology 18:1102–1107, 1993.

140. Wong AY, Irwin MG, Hui TW, et al: Desmopressin does not decrease blood loss and transfusion requirements in patients undergoing hepatectomy. Can J Anaesth 50:14–20, 2003.

141. Egbring R, Seitz R, Blanke H, et al: The proteinase inhibitor complexes (antithrombin III-thrombin, alpha 2antiplasmin-plasmin and alpha 1antitrypsin-elastase) in septicemia, fulminant hepatic failure and cardiac shock: Value for diagnosis and therapy control in DIC/F syndrome. Behring Inst Mitt 1986;87–103.

142. Palareti G, Legnani C, Maccaferri M, et al: Coagulation and fibrinolysis in orthotopic liver transplantation: Role of the recipient's disease and use of antithrombin III concentrates S. Orsola Working Group on Liver Transplantation. Haemostasis 21: 68–76, 1991.

143. Caldwell SH, Chang C, Macik BG: Recombinant activated factor VII (rFVIIa) as a hemostatic agent in liver disease: A break from convention in need of controlled trials. Hepatology 39:592–598, 2004.

144. Bernstein DE, Jeffers L, Erhardtsen E, et al: Recombinant factor VIIa corrects prothrombin time in cirrhotic patients: A preliminary study. Gastroenterology 113:1930–1937, 1997.

145. Lindley CM, Sawyer WT, Macik BG, et al: Pharmacokinetics and pharmacodynamics of recombinant factor VIIa. Clin Pharmacol Ther 55:638–648, 1994.

146. Jeffers L, Chalasani N, Balart L, et al: Safety and efficacy of recombinant factor VIIa in patients with liver disease undergoing laparoscopic liver biopsy. Gastroenterology 123:118–126, 2002.

147. Chuansumrit A, Treepongkaruna S, Phuapradit P: Combined fresh frozen plasma with recombinant factor VIIa in restoring hemostasis for invasive procedures in children with liver diseases. Thromb Haemost 85:748–749, 2001.

148. Bosch J, Thabut D, Bendtsen F, et al: Recombinant factor VIIa for upper gastrointestinal bleeding in patients with cirrhosis: A randomized, double-blind trial. Gastroenterology 127:1123–1130, 2004.

149. Ejlersen E, Melsen T, Ingerslev J, et al: Recombinant activated factor VII (rFVIIa) acutely normalizes prothrombin time in patients with cirrhosis during bleeding from oesophageal varices. Scand J Gastroenterol 36:1081–1085, 2001.

150. Romero-Castro R, Jimenez-Saenz M, Pellicer-Bautista F, et al: Recombinant-activated factor VII as hemostatic therapy in eight cases of severe hemorrhage from esophageal varices. Clin Gastroenterol Hepatol 2:78–84, 2004.

151. Shapiro SS: Treating thrombosis in the 21st century. N Engl J Med 349:1762–1764, 2003.

152. Kang YG, Martin DJ, Marquez J, et al: Intraoperative changes in blood coagulation and thrombelastographic monitoring in liver transplantation. Anesth Analg 64:888–896, 1985.

153. Palomo Sanchez JC, Jimenez C, Moreno GE, et al: Effects of intraoperative blood transfusion on postoperative complications and survival after orthotopic liver transplantation. Hepatogastroenterology 45:1026–1033, 1998.

154. Steib A, Freys G, Lehmann C, et al: Intraoperative blood losses and transfusion requirements during adult liver transplantation remain difficult to predict. Can J Anaesth 48:1075–1079, 2001.

155. Steib A, Gengenwin N, Freys G, et al: Predictive factors of hyperfibrinolytic activity during liver transplantation in cirrhotic patients. Br J Anaesth 73:645–648, 1994.

156. Hendriks HG, van der MJ, Klompmaker IJ, et al: Blood loss in orthotopic liver transplantation: A retrospective analysis of transfusion requirements and the effects of autotransfusion of cell saver blood in 164 consecutive patients. Blood Coagul Fibrinolysis 11 (Suppl 1): S87–S93, 2000.

157. Kirby RM, McMaster P, Clements D, et al: Orthotopic liver transplantation: Postoperative complications and their management. Br J Surg 74:3–11, 1987.

158. Carlier M, Van Obbergh LJ, Veyckemans F, et al: Hemostasis in children undergoing liver transplantation. Semin Thromb Hemost 19:218–222, 1993.

159. Kang Y: Coagulation and liver transplantation: Current concepts. Liver Transpl Surg 3:465–467, 1977.

160. Kang YG, Martin DJ, Marquez J, et al: Intraoperative changes in blood coagulation and thrombelastographic monitoring in liver transplantation. Anesth Analg 64:888–896, 1985.

161. Loskutoff DJ, Edgington TE: Synthesis of a fibrinolytic activator and inhibitor by endothelial cells. Proc Natl Acad Sci U S A 74: 3903–3907, 1977.

162. Emeis JJ, van den Hoogen CM, Jense D: Hepatic clearance of tissue-type plasminogen activator in rats. Thromb Haemost 54:661–664, 1985.
163. Kalicinski P, Kaminski A, Drewniak T, et al: Quick correction of hemostasis in two patients with fulminant liver failure undergoing liver transplantation by recombinant activated factor VII. Transplant Proc; 31:378–379, 1999.
164. Hendriks HG, Meijer K, De Wolf JT, et al: Effects of recombinant activated factor VII on coagulation measured by thromboelastography in liver transplantation. Blood Coagul Fibrinolysis 13:309–313, 2002.
165. Meijer K, Hendriks HG, De Wolf JT, et al: Recombinant factor VIIa in orthotopic liver transplantation: Influence on parameters of coagulation and fibrinolysis. Blood Coagul Fibrinolysis 14:169–174, 2003.
166. Porte RJ: Coagulation and fibrinolysis in orthotopic liver transplantation: current views and insights. Semin Thromb Hemost 19:191–196, 1993.
167. Riess H, Jochum M, Machleidt W, et al: Possible role of extracellularly released phagocyte proteinases in coagulation disorder during liver transplantation. Transplantation 52:482–484, 1991.
168. Hutchison DE, Genton E, Porter KA, et al: Platelet changes following clinical and experimental hepatic homotransplantation. Arch Surg 97:27–33, 1968.
169. Porte RJ, Knot EA, Bontempo FA: Hemostasis in liver transplantation. Gastroenterology 97:488–501, 1989.
170. Arnoux D, Boutiere B, Houvenaeghel M, et al: Intraoperative evolution of coagulation parameters and t-PA/PAI balance in orthotopic liver transplantation. Thromb Res 55:319–328, 1989.
171. Porte RJ, Bontempo FA, Knot EA, et al: Systemic effects of tissue plasminogen activator-associated fibrinolysis and its relation to thrombin generation in orthotopic liver transplantation. Transplantation 47:978–984, 1989.
172. Bakker CM, Blankensteijn JD, Schlejen P, et al: The effects of long-term graft preservation on intraoperative hemostatic changes in liver transplantation: A comparison between orthotopic and heterotopic transplantation in the pig. HPB Surg 7:265–280, 1994.
173. Moriau M, Kestens PJ, Masure R: Heparin and antifibrinolytic agents during experimental hepatectomy and liver transplantation. Pathol Eur 4:172–182, 1969.
174. Harding SA, Mallett SV, Peachey TD, et al: Use of heparinase modified thrombelastography in liver transplantation. Br J Anaesth 78:175–179, 1997.
175. Shore-Lesserson L: Point-of-care coagulation monitoring for cardiovascular patients: Past and present. J Cardiothorac Vasc Anesth 16:99–106, 2002.
176. Molenaar IQ, Legnani C, Groenland TH, et al: Aprotinin in orthotopic liver transplantation: Evidence for a prohemostatic, but not a prothrombotic, effect. Liver Transpl 7:896–903, 2001.
177. Findlay JY, Kufner RP: Aprotinin reduces vasoactive medication use during adult liver transplantation. J Clin Anesth 15:19–23, 2003.
178. Marcel RJ, Stegall WC, Suit CT, et al: Continuous small-dose aprotinin controls fibrinolysis during orthotopic liver transplantation. Anesth Analg 82:1122–1125, 1996.
179. Porte RJ, Molenaar IQ, Begliomini B, et al: Aprotinin and transfusion requirements in orthotopic liver transplantation: A multicentre randomised double-blind study. EMSALT Study Group. Lancet 355:1303–1309, 2000.
180. Vater Y, Levy A, Martay K, et al: Adjuvant drugs for end-stage liver failure and transplantation. Med Sci Monit 10:RA77–RA88, 2004.
181. Sopher M, Braunfeld M, Shackleton C, et al: Fatal pulmonary embolism during liver transplantation. Anesthesiology 87:429–432, 1997.
182. Kang Y, Lewis JH, Navalgund A, et al: Epsilon-aminocaproic acid for treatment of fibrinolysis during liver transplantation. Anesthesiology 66:766–773, 1987.
183. Dalmau A, Sabate A, Acosta F, et al: Tranexamic acid reduces red cell transfusion better than epsilon-aminocaproic acid or placebo in liver transplantation. Anesth Analg 91:29–34, 2000.
184. Dalmau A, Sabate A, Koo M, et al: Prophylactic use of tranexamic acid and incidence of arterial thrombosis in liver transplantation. Anesth Analg 93:516, 2001.
185. Dalmau A, Sabate A, Acosta F, et al: Comparative study of antifibrinolytic drugs in orthotopic liver transplantation. Transplant Proc 31:2361–2362, 1999.
186. Dalmau A, Sabate A, Koo M, et al: The prophylactic use of tranexamic acid and aprotinin in orthotopic liver transplantation: A comparative study. Liver Transpl 10:279–284, 2004.
187. Cerutti E, Stratta C, Romagnoli R, et al: Thromboelastogram monitoring in the perioperative period of hepatectomy for adult living liver donation. Liver Transpl 10:289–294, 2004.
188. Richards EM, Alexander GJ, Calne RY, et al: Thrombocytopenia following liver transplantation is associated with platelet consumption and thrombin generation. Br J Haematol 98:315–321, 1997.
189. Faeh M, Hauser SP, Nydegger UE: Transient thrombopoietin peak after liver transplantation for end-stage liver disease. Br J Haematol 112:493–498, 2001.
190. Goulis J, Chau TN, Jordan S, et al: Thrombopoietin concentrations are low in patients with cirrhosis and thrombocytopenia and are restored after orthotopic liver transplantation. Gut 44:754–758, 1999.
191. Sutedja DS, Wai CT, Teoh KF, et al: Persistent thrombocytopenia in liver transplant patients. Transplant Proc 36:2331–2333, 2004.

Chapter 40

Outpatient Anticoagulant Therapy

Jack E. Ansell, MD

The coumarin-type oral anticoagulants have been in use for more than 60 years and are well-established weapons in the armamentarium against thrombotic disease.[1] Their discovery evolved from investigations into a hemorrhagic disease of cattle occurring early in the twentieth century attributed to the consumption of spoiled sweet clover. Karl P. Link,[2] a biochemist at the University of Wisconsin, eventually isolated the responsible agent in spoiled sweet clover, dicumarol (3-3' methyl-*bis*-4-hydroxy coumarin), which quickly entered the clinical arena through work at the Mayo Clinic in 1941. Link subsequently synthesized a related compound (warfarin), initially popularized as a rodenticide in the late 1940s, that entered clinical practice in the 1950s and quickly became the major oral anticoagulant in clinical use. Little has changed in the formulation of the coumarin-type oral anticoagulants. They have remained critically important drugs in the primary and secondary prevention of thromboembolism. In the last 20 years, the use of oral anticoagulants has grown considerably, commensurate with the increased understanding of the important role of thromboembolism in cardiovascular disorders.

MECHANISM OF ACTION

Vitamin K_1 is an essential cofactor in the posttranslational γ-carboxylation of several glutamic acid residues in the vitamin K-dependent coagulation factors II, VII, IX, and X (Fig. 40-1), as well as proteins C and S.[3–5] In the absence of γ-carboxylation, these proteins are unable to bind calcium and phospholipid and, depending on the level of carboxylation, they manifest a reduced coagulant (i.e., enzymatic) potential. Warfarin produces its anticoagulant effect by interfering with the cyclic interconversion and regeneration of reduced vitamin K from its 2,3 epoxide (vitamin K epoxide).[3–5] Warfarin exerts this effect by inhibiting an enzyme, vitamin K oxide reductase complex 1 (VKORC1) responsible for this interconversion (see Fig. 40-1).[6] Dietary vitamin K_1 enters the body in a partially reduced state bypassing the warfarin-sensitive reductase and replenishing fully reduced vitamin K_1 stores in the presence of warfarin therapy.

PHARMACOKINETICS AND PHARMACODYNAMICS

Because of its excellent bioavailability and favorable pharmacokinetics, warfarin is the most commonly used oral anticoagulant in North America. It is highly water soluble and rapidly absorbed from the gastrointestinal tract after oral ingestion.[7,8] Peak absorption occurs in 60 to 90 minutes. Food may delay the rate of absorption but is said not to reduce the extent of absorption.

Warfarin is a racemic mixture of stereoisomers known as the R and S forms; each has distinctive metabolic pathways, half-lives, and potencies. Racemic warfarin has an average plasma half-life of 36 to 42 hours, with ranges from 15 to 60 hours. Variability in warfarin half-life, due either to natural differences in metabolism or to disease and/or drug-induced alterations in metabolic fate, or of the sensitivity of the VKORC1 enzyme to warfarin account for the marked variations in an individual's initial response to, or maintenance requirement for, warfarin. The S enantiomer of warfarin (5 times more potent than the R enantiomer) is metabolized primarily by the CYP2C9 enzyme of the cytochrome P450 system.[9] A number of genetic polymorphisms (single nucleotide polymorphisms [SNPs]) in this enzyme leads to a reduced activity of the enzyme and may influence both the dose required to achieve a therapeutic level and the bleeding risk with warfarin therapy.[10–14] Specifically, the CYP2C9*2 and CYP2C9*3 alleles are associated with lower dose requirements and higher bleeding complication rates compared with the wild-type enzyme CYP2C9*1.[8,10–14] The prevalence of these polymorphisms varies in populations as indicated in Table 40-1.

The recent discovery of a number of SNPs in the VKORC1 gene leading to varying sensitivities of the enzyme to warfarin inhibition has been shown to have a major impact on the pharmacodynamics of warfarin.[15,16] A combination of SNPs leads to various haplotypes of the gene and gene product. Some of these haplotypes result in an enzyme that is sensitive to warfarin inhibition requiring a lower dose of warfarin, whereas others are more resistant, requiring a higher dose (and maintenance dose) of warfarin to achieve a therapeutic International Normalized Ratio.[15,17–20] The prevalence of these haplotypes varies in different populations as indicated in Table 40-1. A combination of genetic alterations in either the CYP2C9 or VKORC1 genes has been shown to account for as much as 20% to 50% of the variability in warfarin maintenance dosing.[14,17,19] The effect of warfarin also varies inversely with the amount of vitamin K_1 absorbed (from the diet and from metabolic by-products of gastrointestinal bacteria) and directly with the amount of warfarin absorbed or available to exert its anticoagulant effect.

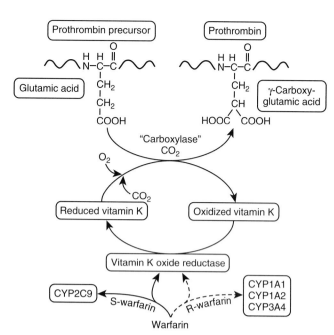

Figure 40-1 Reduced vitamin K is oxidized in the posttranslational modification of prothrombin (and other vitamin K–dependent coagulation factors) introducing carboxyl groups to several glutamic acid moieties in the prothrombin polypeptide, and forming γ-carboxyglutamic acid. The oxidized form of vitamin K is recycled after a reduction mediated by VKORC (vitamin K oxide reductase complex). VKORC is the target enzyme inhibited by the S isomer of warfarin. S-warfarin is the active portion of warfarin, whereas the R isomer has little affect. S-warfarin is metabolized by the cytochrome P450 oxidase enzyme, 2C9.

Table 40-1 Frequency of Genetic Polymorphisms of CYP2C9 and VKORC1 in Different Ethnic Groups

	CYP2C9 Polymorphism*		
	CYP2C9*1 (%)	CYP2C9*2 (%)	CYP2C9*3 (%)
Caucausians	79–89	8–19	6–10
Native Canadians	91	3	6
African Americans	98	1.5–3.6	0.5–1.5
Asians	95–98	0	1.7–5

	VKORC1 Haplotype†	
	H₁H₂(%)	H₈H₉(%)
Euro Americans	37	58
African Americans	14	49
Asian Americans	89	10

*CYP2C9*1 is the wild type (i.e., common genotype) and the *2 and *3 represent polymorphisms that have reduced functional capacity to metabolize the S enantiomer of warfarin.
†H₁H₂ and H₈H₉ represent different haplotypes (combinations of polymorphisms) that are either more sensitive (H₁H₂) or less sensitive (H₈H₉) to warfarin inhibition.
From Takahashi H, Echizen H: Pharmacogenetics of warfarin elimination and its clinical implications. Clin Pharmacokinetics 40:587–603, 2001; and Rieder MJ, Reiner AP, Gage BF, et al: Effect of VKORC1 haplotypes on transcriptional regulation and warfarin dose. N Engl J Med 352:2285–2293, 2005.

WARFARIN AND DRUG INTERACTIONS

Drug interactions commonly occur by affecting the pharmacokinetic or pharmacodynamic behavior of warfarin.[7,21] Drug interactions may interfere with gastrointestinal absorption of warfarin resulting in a reduction in plasma levels, or interfere with the metabolism of warfarin leading to a reduction or increase in clearance, and consequently, higher or lower plasma warfarin levels. The latter effects may be stereospecific in that only one of the enantiomers may be affected or it may be nonspecific in that both enantiomers may be affected. Interference in the metabolism of the S enantiomer, usually by affecting the P450 cytochrome system (CYP2C9 enzyme), is more common and has a greater potential for enhancing the intensity of anticoagulation, because since the S enantiomer is several times more potent than the R enantiomer. Drugs may also decrease plasma warfarin levels by enhancing the metabolic clearance of racemic warfarin.

The pharmacodynamics of warfarin may also be altered when drugs interfere with other aspects of hemostasis or vitamin K₁ homeostasis. Third-generation cephalosporins containing an N-methyl-thiotetrazole side chain are an example in that they interfere with the regeneration of reduced vitamin K₁ from the 2,3 epoxide form. Some drugs or disease states (liver disease, hyperthyroidism) can alter the metabolism of coagulation factors, inhibit coagulation factor interactions by other mechanisms (heparin), or inhibit other aspects of hemostasis (aspirin effect on platelet function) and lead to a greater risk of bleeding. In general, such interactions are most problematic when interacting drugs are added or deleted (or a dose change is made) from a patient's regimen. Once a patient is stabilized on warfarin and an interacting medication, there should be little problem in maintaining stability of warfarin dosing.

Assessing the literature for warfarin-drug interactions is problematic because of the poor quality of the reports. Holbrook and colleagues[22] recently performed a systematic review of warfarin and food interactions and found serious problems of reporting potential interactions. They reviewed 187 separate reports of interactions involving 120 drugs or foods and found that no report met their quality criteria as an excellent study. There were 33 small randomized controlled trials of fair or good quality. There were 148 reports that were rated poor quality and 130 of these were case reports (96% single case reports). Table 40-2 summarizes these interactions and categorizes them by level of cause and effect on INR.

A new problem of recent development is the widespread use of dietary supplements and herbal preparations.[23,24] Unlike drug products, dietary supplements are not tested prior to marketing for safety, efficacy, dosing requirements, or interactions with other medications. They are not required to meet quality standards for labeling, nor are they required to meet United States Pharmacopeia standards for tablet content uniformity (see Chapter 33). Consequently, patients may be exposed to different ingredients as well as different doses of those ingredients among similar products produced by different manufacturers and among batches from the same manufacturer. There is a growing number of case reports describing interactions between warfarin and dietary

Table 40-2 Clinically Significant Interactions with Warfarin by Level of Causation and Drug Group

	Highly Probable	Probable	Possible	Highly Improbable
Potentiation of Warfarin Effect				
Anti-infectives	Ciprofloxacin Cotrimoxazole Erythromycin Fluconazole Isoniazid (600mg/d) Metronidazole Miconazole oral gel Miconazole vaginal suppositories Voriconazole	Amoxicillin/clavulanate Azithromycin Clarithromycin Itraconazole Levofloxacin Ritonavir Tetracycline	Amoxicillin Amoxicillin/ tranexamic rinse Chloramphenicol Gatifloxacin Miconazole topical gel Nalidixic acid Norfloxacin Ofloxacin Saquinavir Terbinafine	Cefamandole Cefazolin Sulfisoxazole
Cardiovascular Drugs	Amiodarone Clofibrate Diltiazem Fenofibrate Propafenone Propranolol Sulfinpyrazone (biphasic with later inhibition)	Acetylsalicylic acid Fluvastatin Quinidine Ropinirole Simvastatin	Amiodarone-induced toxicosis Disopyramide Gemfibrozil Metolazone	Bezafibrate Heparin
Analgesics, Anti-inflammatories, and Immunologics	Phenylbutazone Piroxicam	Acetaminophen Acetylsalicylic acid Celecoxib Dextropropoxyphene Interferon Tramadol	Celecoxib Indomethacin Leflunomide Propoxyphene Rofecoxib Sulindac Tolmetin Topical salicylates	Levamisole Methylprednisolone Nabumetone
CNS Drugs	Alcohol (if concomitant liver disease) Citalopram Entacapone Sertraline	Disulfiram Choral hydrate Fluvoxamine Phenytoin (biphasic with later inhibition	Felbamate	Fluoxetine/diazepam Quetiapine
GI Drugs and Foods	Cimetidine Fish oil Mango Omeprazole	Grapefruit juice	Cranberry juice Orlistat	
Herbal Supplements	Boldo-fenugreek Quilinggao	Danshen Dong quai Lycium barbarum L PC-SPES	Danshen/methyl salicylate	
Other Drugs	Anabolic steroids Zileuton	Fluorouracil Gemcitabine Levamisole/ fluorouracil Paclitaxel Tamoxifen Tolterodine	Acarbose CMF (cyclophosphamide/ methotrexate/ fluorouracil) Carubicin Danazol Ifosphamide Trastuzumab	Etoposide/carboplatin Levonorgestrel
Inhibition of Warfarin Effect				
Anti-infectives	Griseofulvin Nafcillin Ribavirin Rifampin	Dicloxacillin Ritonavir	Terbinafine	Cloxacillin Nafcillin/dicloxacillin Teicoplanin
Cardiovascular Drugs	Cholestyramine	Bosentan	Telmisartan	Furosemide
Analgesics, Anti-inflammatories, and Immunologics	Mesalamine	Azathioprine	Sulfasalazine	
CNS Drugs	Barbiturates Carbamazepine	Chlordiazepoxide		Propofol
GI Drugs and Foods	High vitamin K– content foods/ enteral feeds Avocado (large amounts)	Soy milk Sucralfate	Sushi containing seaweed	
Herbal Supplements		Ginseng		Green tea

(Continued)

40

Table 40-2 Clinically Significant Interactions with Warfarin by Level of Causation and Drug Group (Cont'd)

	Highly Probable	Probable	Possible	Highly Improbable
Other Drugs	Mercaptopurine	Chelation therapy Influenza vaccine Multivitamin supplement Raloxifene hydrochloride	Cyclosporine Etretinate Ubidicarenone	

Adapted from Holbrook AM, Pereira JA, Labiris R, et al: Systematic overview of warfarin and its drug and food interactions. Arch Intern Med 165:1095–1106, 2005.

supplements, but virtually none of these interactions has been systematically substantiated. Because of the uncertainty that exists, it is wise for patients on warfarin to avoid the use of dietary supplements, or at best, to be carefully observed when beginning or stopping a supplement. For a listing of various drug interactions or reported herbal interactions, the reader is referred elsewhere.[21]

THERAPEUTIC RANGE AND MONITORING OF ORAL ANTICOAGULANTS

The concept of a safe and effective therapeutic range evolved largely as a consequence of trial and error and clinical empiricism in the 1940s and 1950s.[1] A prothrombin time (PT) ratio of 2.0 to 2.5 or 3.0, using a human brain thromboplastin reagent sensitive to a reduction in the vitamin K–dependent coagulation factors, was believed to represent this therapeutic range. However, less sensitive rabbit brain thromboplastin reagents came into use in the 1950s and 1960s, resulting in the need for a higher average warfarin dose to achieve the same prolongation of the prothrombin time (PT).[25] Hull and coworkers[26] demonstrated the consequences of this situation in a study of patients with deep venous thrombosis treated with warfarin by documenting a higher incidence of bleeding in those monitored with the less sensitive rabbit brain thromboplastin, yet no increase in recurrent thromboembolism in those monitored by the more sensitive reagent, when both groups were maintained in a similar therapeutic range.

To correct for differences in thromboplastin sensitivity, the World Health Organization recommended the use of an international standard PT.[27] All thromboplastins are equilibrated against a sensitive international reference thromboplastin, and the equilibration factor (the International Sensitivity Index [ISI]) is used to convert PT ratios (PT divided by the mean of the normal range) to an international ratio (the International Normalized Ratio [INR]). The INR is essentially the PT ratio one would obtain if the international reference thromboplastin had been used to measure the PT. Table 40-3 demonstrates how a local PT ratio is converted to an INR, which is now performed automatically by laboratory instrumentation. By converting all PT ratios to INRs one can interpret a patient's PT result

Table 40-3 Use of ISI to Calculate an INR

To convert a prothrombin time (PT) ratio to an INR equivalent:
$INR = PT\ ratio^x\ (x = ISI)$
Example:
PT = 17.9 sec
Mean of normal range = 12.2
ISI of thromboplastin = 2.3
Then:
$17.9 \div 12.3 = 1.47$ PT ratio
$1.47^{2.3} = 2.4$ INR

INR, International Normalized Ratio; a comparative rating of prothrombin time ratios for individuals with stable therapeutic anticoagulation; ISI, International Sensitivity Index; a comparative rating of different thromboplastins.

regardless of where it is performed and then follow the guidelines of international consensus groups for therapeutic effectiveness as outlined in Table 40-4.[28] Use of the INR does not eliminate all discrepancies in PT reporting,[29] but it significantly improves reporting PT results compared with using raw seconds or the PT ratio when monitoring patients on warfarin.

PRACTICAL ASPECTS OF ORAL ANTICOAGULATION MANAGEMENT

Initiation and Maintenance Dosing

The use of a loading dose of warfarin to initiate therapy is of historical interest only. It induces a rapid, but excessive, reduction in factor VII activity, predisposing patients to hemorrhage in the first few days of therapy, while it fails to achieve a more rapid decline of the other vitamin K_1–dependent coagulation factors (II, IX, and X).[30,31] Therapy is properly initiated using an average maintenance dose (~5 mg) for the first 2 or 3 days.[31] When an immediate effect is required, such as in the treatment of acute venous thrombosis, heparin should be given concurrently with warfarin for at least 5 days. Warfarin should overlap with heparin therapy for a period of 4 to 5 days because it takes that long to lower those vitamin K_1–dependent coagulation factors with longer half-lives. Heparin is usually discontinued when the INR has been in the therapeutic range on

Table 40-4 Indications for Oral Anticoagulation and Recommended Intensity of Treatment

Indication	Target INR (Range)
Prophylaxis of venous thrombosis	2.5 (2.0–3.0)
Treatment of venous thrombosis	2.5 (2.0–3.0)
Treatment of pulmonary embolism	2.5 (2.0–3.0)
Prevention of systemic embolism	
Atrial fibrillation	2.5 (2.0–3.0)
Recurrent systemic embolism	2.5 (2.0–3.0)
Postmyocardial infarction*	3.0 (2.5–3.5)
Bioprosthetic heart valves (M or Ao position)†	2.5 (2.0–3.0)
Mechanical prosthetic heart valves	
Bileaflet valve in Ao position	2.5 (2.0–3.0)
Bileaflet or tilting valve in M position	3.0 (2.5–3.5)
Mechanical valve + AF (any position)	3.0 (2.5–3.5)
Mechanical valve + additional risk factors	3.0 (2.5–3.5) + aspirin (81 mg/d)

*For prevention of recurrent MR, an INR of 3.0 (2.5–3.5) is recommended.
†For St. Jude or Carbomedics bileaflet or Medtronic-Hall tilting disc valve.
Ao, aortic valve; M, mitral valve.
From Hirsch J, Dalen JE, Anderson DR, et al: Oral anticoagulants: Mechanism of action, clinical effectiveness, and optimal therapeutic range. Chest 119 (Suppl):8S–21S, 220S–227S, 2001, with permission.

two measurements at least 24 hours apart. If treatment is not urgent (e.g., chronic stable atrial fibrillation), warfarin can be commenced out-of-hospital with an anticipated maintenance dose of ~5 mg/day, which usually achieves a therapeutic anticoagulant effect in about 5 days, although a stable INR may take longer to achieve. A recent study showed that using an initial 10 mg dose of warfarin in outpatients achieved a more rapid therapeutic INR compared with a 5-mg dose without producing a higher rate of excessive anticoagulation.[32] The fear of creating a hypercoagulable state in patients with unrecognized protein C deficiency who are not simultaneously heparinized has not been substantiated. However, in patients with a known protein C deficiency or other thrombophilic state, it would be prudent to begin heparin before, or at the same time as, warfarin. Lower than a 5-mg starting dose might be appropriate in the elderly, in patients with impaired nutrition or liver disease, and in patients at high risk of bleeding. The physician should be aware of variables that influence the response to anticoagulation in the elderly. The dose required to maintain a therapeutic range for patients older than 60 years of age has been shown to decrease with increasing age,[33] and older patients are more likely to have other variables that might influence INR stability or might influence the risk of bleeding—such as a greater number of other medical conditions or concurrent drug use.[33] Consequently, it is advisable to monitor older patients more carefully to maximize their time in therapeutic range.[34]

Estimation of the maintenance dose is often based on observations of the INR response following a fixed dose of warfarin over an interval of a few days. An individual who rapidly achieves a high therapeutic INR (above 2.0) after two doses of warfarin is likely to require a low maintenance dose. The opposite holds for those who show little

elevation of the INR (below 1.5) after two doses. It is now known that a major determinate influencing one's response to initial and maintenance dosing is one's genotype for the principal enzyme that metabolizes warfarin (CYP2C9) and the target enzyme through which warfarin mediates its effect (VKORC1).[10–20] Polymorphisms in these genes account for almost 50% of the variability in dosing requirements. They are also associated with a higher rate of bleeding events. Whether it is cost effective to actually know one's genotype before initiating therapy is currently under scrutiny in randomized controlled trials.[35] Until such information is available, frequent monitoring of the INR response is the best means of predicting and establishing one's maintenance dose requirements.

PT monitoring is usually performed daily in the hospital (somewhat less frequently if initiated as an outpatient) until the therapeutic range has been achieved and maintained for at least 2 consecutive days—then 1 to 2 times weekly for 1 to 2 weeks—then less often, depending on the stability of PT results. Immediately after hospital discharge is often the most unstable and dangerous time for patients. Therefore, monitoring should be performed frequently for the first 1 to 2 weeks after discharge. If the PT response remains stable, the frequency of testing can be reduced to intervals as long as every 4 weeks, although there is growing evidence to suggest that more frequent testing will lead to a greater time in therapeutic range. If adjustments to the dose are required, then the cycle of more frequent monitoring is repeated until a stable dose response is again achieved.

Outpatient management of warfarin therapy should aim for simplicity and clarity to avoid patient confusion, poor compliance, and dosing errors that may result in complications.[1] It is recommended that a limited number of warfarin tablet strengths be used in clinical practice and that patients clearly understand the various dosing patterns that are used, such as alternate-day doses or dosing levels based on days of the week.[1] One must also be aware that there are several different warfarin products on the market that can lead to confusion for the patient. There are generic preparations sold as warfarin, brand preparations sold as Coumadin, and branded generics sold under a different name (e.g., Jantoven). Patients may be given different preparations and be taking both, not knowing that they are the same drug.

Management of Nontherapeutic International Normalized Ratios

Patients receiving long-term warfarin therapy often have unexpected fluctuations in dose response that require careful management. These may be due to inaccuracy in PT testing, changes in vitamin K_1 intake (increased or decreased vitamin K_1 in the diet), changes in vitamin K_1 or warfarin absorption (gastrointestinal factors or drug effects), changes in warfarin metabolism (liver disease or drug effects), changes in vitamin K_1–dependent coagulation factor synthesis or metabolism (liver disease, drug effects, worsening right sided heart failure with increasing hepatic congestion, other medical conditions), or patient compliance issues (surreptitious self-medication, missed doses, miscommunication about dose adjustment, and so on).

A nontherapeutic (e.g., elevated) INR can be managed by briefly discontinuing warfarin, administering vitamin K_1,

40

or infusing fresh frozen plasma (FFP) or a factor concentrate.[36] The choice is based largely on the severity of the clinical situation (e.g., the degree of elevation of the INR or the presence of severe bleeding). Assuming an ongoing normal food intake and reasonable hepatic function, when warfarin administration is interrupted, it takes about 4 to 5 days for the INR to return to the normal range in patients whose INR is between 2.0 and 3.0.[37] Those patients requiring a larger daily maintenance dose will return to normal more quickly than those requiring a lower daily maintenance dose. After treatment with oral vitamin K_1, the INR declines substantially within 24 hours. Because the absolute daily risk of bleeding is low even when the INR is excessively prolonged, many physicians manage patients with INR values of 4.0 to 9.0 by simply holding warfarin and monitoring more frequently,[38] unless the patient is at a higher risk of bleeding or bleeding has already developed. Vitamin K_1 can be administered by the intravenous, subcutaneous, or oral routes. Intravenous injection may rarely be associated with anaphylactic reactions, but it does lead to reversal of the INR more quickly than oral or subcutaneous vitamin K_1.[39] The response to subcutaneous vitamin K_1 may be unpredictable and sometimes delayed.[40] Recent studies confirm earlier reports that oral administration is predictably effective, more so than subcutaneous administration and has the advantages of safety and convenience over parenteral routes. Ideally, vitamin K_1 should be administered in a dose that will quickly lower the INR into a safe, but not subtherapeutic range, without causing resistance when warfarin is reinstated.[41,42] High doses of vitamin K_1, although effective, may lower the INR more than is necessary and lead to warfarin resistance for up to one week.

In the presence of significant bleeding, the INR must be reversed immediately. This can be done by replacing the vitamin K–dependent factors using FFP. At least 15 to 30 mL/kg of FFP should be given to have a significant impact on factor replenishment.[43,44] In the average 70-kg person, this equates to 4 to 8 units of FFP which may take up to 6 to 24 hours to order, thaw, and infuse, and in some patients may put an undue stress on the heart. Additionally, the half-lives of the individual vitamin K–dependent factors govern the durability of any response. More FFP might be required. In a patient with life-threatening bleeding, especially intracranial hemorrhage, maximal factor replacement must be achieved in the shortest interval possible. This can be achieved by using factor concentrates which have high factor concentrations in a small volume.[45] Prothrombin concentrates, containing the vitamin K dependent factors, have traditionally been used, but with the recent development of specific recombinant factors, PT concentrates are less available. Most recently, studies have shown that recombinant factor VIIa (NovoVII) can reverse the coagulopathy and associated bleeding induced by warfarin, as well as in other coagulopathies.[46,47] Given the expense of these agents, one should use the lowest effective dose to control the bleeding. Prothrombin concentrates are often dosed in a range of 25 to 50 IU/kg, but the specific dose will depend on body weight, degree of INR prolongation, and desired level of correction. The same considerations are relevant for the dosing of recombinant rFVIIa, although the range of dosing reported empirically ranges from approximately 20 µg per kilogram body weight to more than 100 µg per kilogram body

weight. Both PT concentrates and rFVIIa have the potential to induce a prothrombotic state, and thromboembolism has occurred as a result of such therapy.[48,49] Table 40-5 outlines the 2004 American College of Chest Physicians (ACCP) recommendations for managing patients on coumarin anticoagulants who need their INR lowered because of actual or potential bleeding.[36]

The decision to cover a patient who presents to one's office with a subtherapeutic INR is similar to a bridging decision. If the thrombogenic risk is so high (such as within the first week or two of treating new DVTs and/or PEs) that even a few days at a subtherapeutic level places the patient at high risk, then treating the patient with LMWH for a few days until a therapeutic INR is achieved with higher doses of warfarin is appropriate. In most cases, this intervention is not needed, and simply raising the dose of warfarin is sufficient to reestablish a therapeutic range in a few days.

Management of Oral Anticoagulation During Invasive Procedures

Clinicians are often confronted with the challenge of managing anticoagulation in individuals requiring noncardiac surgery or other invasive procedures, especially in individuals with prosthetic heart valves who are currently taking warfarin (see Chapter 38). There is a paucity of critical studies examining the alternative choices for anticoagulation (called bridging therapy) in this setting. Physicians must assess the risk of bleeding from a procedure if anticoagulation is continued versus the risk of thrombosis if anticoagulation is discontinued, as well as the cost of alternative anticoagulation options. Recent reviews have addressed the management of these patients and the options available,[50] and the ACCP has made formal recommendations.[36] Historically, full-dose, intravenous unfractionated heparin had been the standard for patients who need full anticoagulant protection that is readily reversible before a procedure. Its major drawbacks are the complexity and cost associated with intravenous heparin therapy and hospitalization. Low molecular weight heparin (LMWH) offers another, less complex alternative in that it requires no monitoring and can be given at home.[51–58] LMWH has been shown to achieve therapeutic anticoagulation more rapidly than UFH and a more consistent therapeutic level during the course of bridging.[58] LMWH is usually given at a therapeutic dose, but in situations where the thrombotic potential is lower, and bridging is still believed to be needed, a prophylactic dose may be suitable. Several recent prospective cohort studies or registries have clarified the risks of bleeding or thrombosis associated with the use of LMWH (Table 40-6).[53–57] What is still unclear, however, is a better understanding of exactly who needs an alternative anticoagulant during the brief period that warfarin is held before and after a procedure.

When bridging therapy is implemented, warfarin is usually discontinued 4 or 5 days before the procedure and the INR is allowed to decline. LMWH is started 2 or 3 days before the procedure, usually at a full treatment dose (100 to 150 anti X_a U/kg subcutaneously) once or twice daily depending on the risk of thrombosis, with the last dose given the morning or night before the procedure (approximately 12 to 24 hours prior to the procedure).

Table 40-5 Recommendations for Managing Elevated INRs or Bleeding in Patients Receiving VKAs*

Condition	Description
INR above therapeutic range but <5.0; no significant bleeding	Lower dose or omit dose, monitor more frequently, and resume at lower dose when INR therapeutic; if only minimally above therapeutic range, no dose reduction may be required (**Grade 2C**)
INR ≥ 5.0 but <9.0; no significant bleeding	Omit next one or two doses, monitor more frequently and resume at lower dose when INR in therapeutic range. Alternatively, omit dose and give vitamin K_1 (≤5 mg orally), particularly if at increased risk of bleeding. If more rapid reversal is required because the patient requires urgent surgery, vitamin K_1 (2 to 4 mg orally) can be given with the expectation that a reduction of the INR will occur in 24 h. If the INR is still high, additional vitamin K_1 (1 to 2 mg orally) can be given (**Grade 2C**)
INR ≥ 9.0: no significant bleeding	Hold warfarin therapy and give higher dose of vitamin K_1 (5–10 mg orally) with the expectation that the INR will be reduced substantially in 24–48 h. Monitor more frequently and use additional vitamin K_1 if necessary. Resume therapy at lower dose when INR is therapeutic (**Grade 2C**)
Serious bleeding at any elevation of INR	Hold warfarin therapy and give vitamin K_1 (10 mg by slow IV infusion), supplemented with fresh plasma or prothrombin complex concentrate, depending on the urgency of the situation; recombinant factor VIIa may be considered as alternative to prothrombin complex concentrate; vitamin K_1 can be repeated every 12 h (**Grade 1C**)
Life-threatening bleeding	Hold warfarin therapy and give prothrombin complex concentrate supplemented with vitamin K_1 (10 mg by slow IV infusion); recombinant factor VIIa may be considered as an alternative to prothrombin complex concentrate; repeat if necessary, depending on INR (**Grade 1C**)

*If continuing warfarin therapy is indicated after high doses of vitamin K_1, then heparin or LMWH can be given until the effects of vitamin K_1 have been reversed and the patient becomes responsive to warfarin therapy. It should be noted that INR values >4.5 are less reliable than values in or near the therapeutic range. Thus, these guidelines represent an approximate guide for high INRs.
INR, International Normalized Ratio; IV, intravenous.

Table 40-6 Recent Studies of LMWH Used as Alternative (Bridging) Therapy in Patients on Warfarin Requiring Invasive Procedures

Study	Patients	Bridging Regimen	Postoperative Follow-up (wks)	Major Bleeding (95% CI)	Thrombosis
Turpie[56]	174	Enoxaparin 1 mg/kg bid	4	2.3% (0.06–5.7)	0.6%
Kovacs[53]	224	Dalteparin 200 IU/kg qd	4	6.7% (4.1–108)	3.6% (1.8–6.9)
Dunn[57]	260	Enoxaparin 1.5 mg/kg qd	2	3.5% (1.6–6.5)	1.5%
Spyropoulos[55]	668	Enoxaparin/dalteparin 1 mg/kg 100 IU/kg bid	4	3.3% (2.0–5.1)	0.9%
Douketis[54]	650	Dalteparin 100 IU/kg bid	1	0.9% (0.4–2.0)	0.3%

bid, Twice daily; qd, every day.

It is then restarted about 12 hours after the procedure along with warfarin. If the risk of postoperative bleeding from the procedure is high, LMWH can be restarted in 24 to 48 hours, rather than 12 hours. When the INR becomes therapeutic, LMWH therapy is stopped. Studies suggest that LMWH is a simple and reasonably inexpensive alternative for full anticoagulation protection,[59] but randomized, controlled trials are still needed to identify the best means of alternative anticoagulation. Table 40-7 summarizes the 2004 ACCP Chest Consensus Conference recommendations for management of oral anticoagulation during invasive procedures.[36]

Dental procedures represent a particularly common intervention for patients on anticoagulants. A recent comprehensive review of the subject indicated that, in most cases, no change in the intensity of anticoagulation is needed.[60] If there is need to control local bleeding, tranexamic acid or ε-aminocaproic acid (EACA) mouthwash have been used successfully without interrupting anticoagulant therapy.[61,62]

Diagnostic Evaluation of Bleeding

When bleeding occurs, especially from the gastrointestinal or urinary tract, it is important to consider the possibility of a serious, underlying occult lesion as the source of bleeding. A number of descriptive studies indicate the probability of finding such a lesion.[63-66] Coon and Willis[64] identified occult lesions responsible for bleeding in 11% of 292 patients with hemorrhage. Jaffin and coworkers[65] found a 12% prevalence of positive stool occult blood tests in 175 patients on warfarin or heparin compared with 3% in 74 controls. There was no difference between the mean PT or PTT in patients with or without lesions. In

Table 40-7 Recommendations for Managing Anticoagulation Therapy in Patients Requiring Invasive Procedures (all Grade 2C)

Condition	Description
Low risk of thromboembolism*	Stop warfarin therapy approximately 4 d before surgery; allow the INR to return to near normal; briefly use postoperative prophylaxis (if the intervention itself creates a higher risk of thrombosis) with a low dose of UFH (5000 U BID SC) or a prophylactic dose of LMWH and simultaneously begin warfarin therapy; alternatively, a low dose of UFH or a prophylactic dose of LMWH can also be used preoperatively.
Intermediate risk of thromboembolism	Stop warfarin approximately 4 d before surgery; allow the INR to fall; cover the patient beginning 2 d preoperatively with a low dose of UFH (5000 U BID SC) or a prophylactic dose of LMWH and then commence therapy with low-dose UFH (or LMWH) and warfarin postoperatively; some individuals would recommend a higher dose of UFH or a full dose LMWH in this setting.
High risk of thromboembolism†	Stop warfarin approximately 4 d before surgery, allow the INR to return to normal; begin therapy with a full dose of UFH or a full dose of LMWH as the INR falls (approximately 2 d preoperatively); UFH can be given as an SC injection as an outpatient, and can then be given as a continuous IV infusion after hospital admission in preparation for surgery and discontinued approximately 5 h before surgery with the expectation that the anticoagulant effect will have worn off at the time of surgery; it is also possible to continue with SC UFH or LMWH and to stop therapy 12–24 h before surgery with the expectation that the anticoagulant effect will be very low or have worn off at the time of surgery.
Low risk of bleeding	Continue warfarin therapy at a lower dose and operate at an INR of 1.3–1.5, an intensity that has been shown to be safe in randomized trials of gynecologic and orthopedic surgical patients; the dose of warfarin can be lowered 4 or 5 d before surgery; warfarin therapy can then be restarted postoperatively, supplemented with a low dose of UFH (5000 U SC) or a prophylactic dose of LMWH, if necessary.

*Low risk of thromboembolism includes no recent (>3 mo) venous thromboembolism, atrial fibrillation without a history of stroke or other risk factors, and bileaflet mechanical cardiac valve in the aortic position.
†Examples of a high risk of thromboembolism include recent (<3 mo) history of venous thromboembolism, mechanical cardiac valve in the mitral position, and old model of cardiac valve (ball/cage).
INR, International Normalized Ratio; LMWH, low molecular weight heparin; SC, subcutaneous; UFH, unfractionated heparin.

16 patients evaluated, 15 had a lesion not previously suspected and 4 had neoplastic disease. Landefeld and coworkers[63] found 14 of 41 patients with gastrointestinal bleeding to have important remediable lesions of which two were malignant. This limited information supports the need for investigation because if occult blood is found in the stool, there may be a 5% to 25% chance of finding a malignant source.

In a randomized controlled study, Culclasure and coworkers[67] found microscopic hematuria at a prevalence of 3.2% in a warfarin-treated group compared with a prevalence of 4.8% in their non-anticoagulated control group. There was no difference in the rate of hematuria with therapeutic or high INRs. Following a second episode of hematuria, 43 patients (32 anticoagulated and 11 control) were investigated; 27 of 32 (84%) of the anticoagulated and 8 of 11 (73%) of the control patients were found to have significant underlying diseases with a total of 3 patients (from both groups) having cancers (7%). These findings are in contrast to results of other case series identifying a much higher likelihood of finding underlying lesions in patients who develop hematuria while receiving anticoagulant therapy.[68–70]

PREDICTING AND MANAGING THE RISKS OF ORAL ANTICOAGULANT THERAPY

Over the last 20 years, several developments have improved the safety and efficacy of oral anticoagulation. These include defining the optimal intensity of therapy by well-designed randomized trials and standardizing the reporting of PTs using the INR, leading to more appropriate and standardized therapy. Identifying the risk factors associated with bleeding has also advanced. Time in therapeutic range (TTR) is an important measure of the quality of anticoagulation care, and a strong relationship exists between TTR and either bleeding or thrombosis rates as demonstrated by Cannegieter and colleagues,[71] Hylek and coworkers,[72,73] and others.[74,75] Besides TTR, a number of patient characteristics serve as risk factors for bleeding. These include age, a history of bleeding (especially gastrointestinal bleeding), a history of stroke, and the presence of a comorbid condition such as renal insufficiency, anemia, or hypertension.[36,76]

Anticoagulation Management Services

A coordinated and focused approach to the management of therapy by specialized programs (anticoagulation clinics) significantly improves clinical outcomes by improving therapeutic control and TTR, lessening the frequency of hemorrhage or thrombosis, and decreasing the use of medical resources, leading to more cost-effective therapy. These programs are characterized by a knowledgeable provider whose primary responsibility is to manage therapy, an organized system of follow-up, rapid and reliable INR monitoring, and good patient communication and education.

Most patients receiving chronic oral anticoagulation today are managed by their personal physician (characterized as usual care) along with all other patients in their physician's practice without an organized program of management, education, or follow-up.[36,77] Studies indicate a rate of major hemorrhage of at least 7% to 8% per patient-year of therapy.[36,78,79] There is a similar rate of recurrent or de novo thromboembolism for an overall serious adverse event rate of at least 15% per patient-year of therapy. These adverse events are generally a consequence of poor therapeutic control with hemorrhage or thrombosis occurring as a consequence of excessive or subtherapeutic anticoagulation. These outcomes can be contrasted to the rates identified in studies of care delivered by an anticoagulation management service (anticoagulation clinic),[36,80-84] which indicate a more than 50% reduction in both major hemorrhage and thrombosis compared with usual care. A few studies also suggest a significant cost benefit to coordinated care compared with usual care by a reduction in adverse events and reduced use of hospital services.

PATIENT SELF-TESTING AND PATIENT SELF-MANAGEMENT

As a result of technological advances in PT measurement, there is potential for further simplifying and improving anticoagulation management by point-of-care (POC) testing.[85] POC testing allows for the determination of a PT from a finger stick sample of whole blood, and consequently, opens the possibility for patient self-testing. Portability of instrumentation means that INR measurements are no longer confined to the physician's office, a private laboratory, or a nearby hospital, but can be moved into the patient's home or even taken with the patient when traveling. Standardization of reagents and instruments, as well as reliance on the INR, further reduce the inaccuracies of multiple reagents and laboratories. In depth discussion of instrumentation for PT monitoring can be found in Chapter 41.

These POC instruments have been tested in a number of different clinical settings and their accuracy and precision are considered to be more than adequate for the monitoring of oral anticoagulant therapy in both adults and children[86-93] and it is possible that this new model of care is significantly more reliable and consistent than the variable and haphazard PT monitoring often employed in the usual care of most patients on oral anticoagulants.[94] Use of these instruments is particularly rational for patients on prolonged or indefinite anticoagulant therapy.

A number of studies have demonstrated the ability of patients to perform self-testing and to obtain an accurate result. Patients can then call their physician and obtain instructions for warfarin dose adjustment, or select patients can manage their own warfarin dosing after proper training.[95-109] Based on the foregoing, POC PT monitors offer the potential to improve the risk:benefit profile of anticoagulant therapy; to improve patient satisfaction, patient involvement, and possibly patient compliance; and by reducing the labor intensity of physician management, to encourage the more widespread use of warfarin. The cost effectiveness of such therapy needs to be studied.

REFERENCES

1. Ansell J: Oral anticoagulant therapy: Fifty years later. Arch Intern Med 153:586–596, 1993.
2. Link KP: The discovery of dicumarol and its sequels. Circulation 19:97–107, 1959.
3. Stenflo J, Fernlund P, Egan W, et al: Vitamin K dependent modifications of glutamic acid residues in prothrombin. Proc Natl Acad Sci USA 71:2730–2733, 1974.
4. Nelsestuen GL, Zytkovicz TH, Howard JB: The mode of action of vitamin K: Identification of gamma carboxyglutamic acid as a component of prothrombin. J Biol Chem 249:6347–6350, 1974.
5. Furie B, Bouchard BA, Furie BC: Vitamin K-dependent biosynthesis of gamma carboxyglutamic acid. Blood 93:1798–1808, 1999.
6. Mukharji I, Silverman RB: Purification of a vitamin K epoxide reductase that catalyzes conversion of vitamin K 2,3-epoxide to 3-hydroxy-2-methyl-3-phytyl-2,3-dihydronaphthoquinone. Proc Natl Acad Sci USA 82:2713–2717, 1985.
7. Hirsh J: Oral anticoagulant drugs. N Engl J Med 324:1865–1875, 1991.
8. Wittkowsky AK: Warfarin pharmacology. In Ansell JE, Oertel LB, Wittkowsky AK (eds): Managing Patients on Oral Anticoagulants: Clinical and Operational Guidelines, 2nd ed. Gaithersburg, Md, Aspen Publishers, 2003, pp 29:1–29:12.
9. Miners JO, Birkett DJ: Cytochrome P4502C9: An enzyme of major importance in human drug metabolism. Br J Clin Pharmacol 45:525–538, 1998.
10. Aithal GP, Day CP, Kesteven PJ, et al: Association of polymorphisms in the cytochrome P450 CYP2C9 with warfarin dose requirement and risk of bleeding complications. Lancet 353:717–719, 1999.
11. Tabrizi AR, Zehnbauer BA, Borecki IB, et al: The frequency and effects of cytochrome P450(CYP)2C9 polymorphisms in patients receiving warfarin. J Am Coll Surg 194:267–273, 2002.
12. Joffe HV, Xu R, Johnson FB, Longtine J, et al: Warfarin dosing and cytochrome P450 2C9 polymorphisms. Thromb Haemost 91:1123–1128, 2004.
13. Visser LE, van Schaik RHN, van Vliet M, et al: The risk of bleeding complications in patients with cytochrome P450 CYP2C9*2 or CYP2C9*3 alleles on acenocoumarol or phenprocoumon. Thromb Haemost 92:61–66, 2004.
14. Gage BF, Eby C, Milligan PE, et al: Use of pharmacogenetics and clinical factors to predict the maintenance dose of warfarin. Thromb Haemost 91:87–94, 2004.
15. Rost S, Fregin A, Ivaskevicius V, et al: Mutations in VKORC1 cause warfarin resistance and multiple coagulation factor deficiency type 2. Nature 427:537–541, 2004.
16. Li T, Chang CY, Jin DY, et al: Identification of the gene for vitamin K epoxide reductase. Nature 427:541–544, 2004.
17. Rieder MJ, Reiner AP, Gage BF, et al: Effect of VKORC1 haplotypes on transcriptional regulation and warfarin dose. N Engl J Med 352:2285–2293, 2005.
18. D'Andrea G, D'Ambrosio RL, Di Perna P, et al: A polymorphism in the VKORC1 gene is associated with an interindividual variability in the dose-anticoagulant effect of warfarin. Blood 105:645–649, 2005.
19. Geisen C, Watzka M, Sittinger K, et al: VKORC1 haplotypes and their impact on the inter-individual and inter-ethnical variability of oral anticoagulation. Thromb Haemost 94:773–779, 2005.
20. Rost S, Fregin A, Hunerberg M, et al: Site-directed mutagenesis of coumarin-type anticoagulant-sensitive VKORC1. Thromb Haemost 94:780–786, 2005.
21. Hansten P, Wittkowsky AK: Warfarin drug interactions. In Ansell JE, Oertel LB, Wittkowsky AK (eds): Managing Patients on Oral Anticoagulants: Clinical Operational Guidelines, 2nd ed. Gaithersburg, Md, Aspen Publishers, 2003, pp 35:1–35:12.
22. Holbrook AM, Pereira JA, Labiris R, et al: Systematic overview of warfarin and its drug and food interactions. Arch Intern Med 165:1095–1106, 2005.
23. Greenblatt DJ, von Moltke LL: Interaction of warfarin with drugs, natural substances, and foods. J Clin Pharmacol 45:127–132, 2005.
24. Ansell J: Effects of dietary supplements on hemostasis. Thromb Res 117:45–47, 65–67, 2005.
25. Hirsh J, Levine MN: The optimal intensity of oral anticoagulant therapy. JAMA 258:2723–2726, 1987.
26. Hull R, Hirsh J, Jay R, et al: Different intensities of anticoagulation in the long-term treatment of proximal venous thrombosis. N Engl J Med 307:1676–1681, 1982.
27. Kirkwood TBL: Calibration of reference thromboplastins and standardization of the prothrombin time ratio. Thromb Haemost 49:238–244, 1983.
28. Hirsh J, Dalen JE, Anderson DR, et al: Oral anticoagulants: Mechanism of action, clinical effectiveness, and optimal therapeutic range. Chest 119 (Suppl): 8S–21S, 2001.

29. Hirsh J, Poller L: The International Normalized Ratio: A guide to understanding and correcting its problems. Arch Intern Med 154:282–288, 1994.

30. O'Reilly RA, Aggeler PM: Studies on coumarin anticoagulant drugs: Initiation of warfarin therapy without a loading dose. Circulation 38:169–177, 1968.

31. Harrison L, Johnston M, Massicotte MP, et al: Comparison of 5 mg and 10 mg loading doses in initiation of warfarin therapy. Ann Intern Med 126:133–136, 1997.

32. Kovacs MJ, Rodger M, Anderson DR, et al: Comparison of 10 mg and 5 mg warfarin initiation nomograms together with low molecular weight heparin for outpatient treatment of acute venous thromboembolism. Ann Intern Med 138:714–719, 2003.

33. Gurwitz JH, Avorn J, Ross-Degnan D, et al: Aging and the anticoagulant response to warfarin therapy. Ann Intern Med 116:901–904, 1992.

34. McCormick D, Gurwitz JH, Goldberg J, et al: Long-term anticoagulation therapy for atrial fibrillation in elderly patients: Efficacy, risk, and current patterns of use. J Thromb Thrombolysis 7:157–163, 1999.

35. You JHS, Chan FWH, Wong RSM, Cheng G: The potential clinical and economic outcomes of pharmacogenetics-oriented management of warfarin therapy: A decision analysis. Thromb Haemost 92:590–597, 2004.

36. Ansell J, Hirsh J, Poller L, et al: Managing oral anticoagulant therapy. Chest 126 (Suppl): 204S–233S, 2004.

37. White RH, McKittrick T, Hutchinson R, et al: Temporary discontinuation of warfarin therapy: Changes in the international normalized ratio. Ann Intern Med 122:40–42, 1995.

38. Lousberg TR, Witt DM, Beall DG, et al: Evaluation of excessive anticoagulation in a group model health maintenance organization. Arch Intern Med 158:528–534, 1998.

39. Watson HG, Baglin T, Laidlaw SL, et al: A comparison of the efficacy and rate of response to oral and intravenous vitamin K in reversal of over-anticoagulation with warfarin. Br J Haematol 115:145–149, 2001.

40. Raj G, Kumar R, McKinney P: Time course of reversal of anticoagulant effect of warfarin by intravenous and subcutaneous phytonadione. Arch Intern Med 159:2721–2724, 1999.

41. Weibert RE, Le DT, Kayser SR, et al: Correction of excessive anticoagulation with low dose oral vitamin K_1. Ann Intern Med 125:959–962, 1997.

42. Crowther MA, Donovan D, Harrison L, et al: Low dose oral vitamin K reliably reverses over anticoagulation due to warfarin. Thromb Haemost 79:1116–1118, 1998.

43. Chowdhury P, Saayman AG, Paulus U, et al: Efficacy of standard dose and 30 ml/kg fresh frozen plasma in correcting laboratory parameters of haemostasis in critically ill patients. Br J Haematol 125:69–73, 2004.

44. Youssef WI, Salazar F, Dasarathy S, et al: Role of fresh frozen plasma infusion in correction of coagulopathy of chronic liver disease: A dual phase study. Am J Gastroent 98:1391–1394, 2003.

45. Hanley JP: Warfarin reversal. J Clin Pathol 57:1132–1139, 2004.

46. Deveras RAE, Kessler CM: Reversal of warfarin-induced excessive anticoagulation with recombinant human factor VIIa concentrate. Ann Intern Med 137:884–888, 2002.

47. Freeman WD, Brott TG, Barrett KM, et al: Recombinant factor VIIa for rapid reversal of warfarin anticoagulation in acute intracranial hemorrhage. Mayo Clin Proc 79:1495–1500, 2004.

48. Mayer SA, Brun MC, Begtrup K, et al: Recombinant activated factor VII for acute intracerebral hemorrhage. N Engl J Med 352:777–785, 2005.

49. Key N: Current insights on the risk of thrombogenicity with off-label use of rFVIIa. Clin Adv Hemat Oncol 4:34–35, 2006.

50. Dunn AS, Turpie AGG: Perioperative management of patients receiving oral anticoagulants: A systematic review. Arch Intern Med 163:901–908, 2003.

51. Tinmouth A, Morrow BH, Cruickshank MK, et al: Dalteparin as periprocedure anticoagulation for patients on warfarin and at high risk of thrombosis. Ann Pharmacother 35:669–674, 2001.

52. Spandorfer JM, Lynch S, Weitz HH, et al: Use of enoxaparin for the chronically anticoagulated patient before and after procedures. Am J Cardiol 84:478–480, 1999.

53. Kovacs MJ, Kearon C, Rodger M, et al: Single-arm study of bridging therapy with low molecular weight heparin for patients at risk of arterial embolism who require temporary interruption of warfarin. Circulation 110:1658–1663, 2004.

54. Douketis JD, Johnson JA, Turpie AG: Low molecular weight heparin as bridging anticoagulation during interruption of warfarin. Arch Intern Med 164:1319–1326, 2004.

55. Spyropoulos AC, Turpie AG, Dunn AS, et al: Clinical outcomes with unfractionated heparin or low molecular weight heparin as bridging therapy in patients on long-term oral anticoagulants: Results from the REGIMEN registry. Blood 104:203a(abstract), 2004.

56. Turpie AG, Douketis AG: Enoxaparin is effective and safe as bridging anticoagulation in patients with mechanical prosthetic heart valve who require temporary interruption of warfarin because of surgery or an invasive procedure. Blood 104:202a(abstract), 2004.

57. Dunn AS, Spyropoulos AC, Sirko SP, Turpie AGG: Perioperative bridging therapy with enoxaparin in patients requiring interruption of long-term oral anticoagulant therapy: A multicenter cohort study. Blood 104:488a(abstract), 2004.

58. Omran H, Hammersting C, Schmidt H, et al: A prospective and randomized comparison of the safety and effects of therapeutic levels of enoxaparin versus unfractionated heparin in chronically anticoagulated patients undergoing elective cardiac catheterization. Blood Coag Fibrinolys Cell Haemost 90:267–271, 2003.

59. Spyropoulos AC, Frost FJ, Hurley JS, Roberts M: Costs and clinical outcomes associated with low molecular weight heparin vs unfractionated heparin for perioperative bridging in patients receiving long-term oral anticoagulant therapy. Chest 125:1642–1650, 2004.

60. Wahl MJ: Dental surgery in anticoagulated patients. Arch Intern Med 158:1610–1616, 1998.

61. Sindet-Pedersen S, Ramstrom G, Bernvil S, et al: Hemostatic effect of tranexamic mouthwash in anticoagulant-treated patients undergoing oral surgery. N Engl J Med 324:840–843, 1989.

62. Soute JC, Oliver A, ZuaZu-Jausoro I, et al: Oral surgery in anticoagulated patients without reducing the dose of oral anticoagulant: A prospective randomized study. J Oral Maxillofac Surg 54:27–32, 1996.

63. Landefeld CS, Rosenblatt MW, Goldman L: Bleeding in outpatients treated with warfarin: Relation to the prothrombin time and important remedial lesions. Am J Med 87:153–159, 1989.

64. Coon WW, Willis PW: Hemorrhagic complications of anticoagulant therapy. Arch Intern Med 133:386–392, 1974.

65. Jaffin BW, Bliss CM, Lamont JT: Significance of occult gastrointestinal bleeding during anticoagulation therapy. Am J Med 83:269–272, 1987.

66. Wilcox CM, Truss CD: Gastrointestinal bleeding in patients receiving long-term anticoagulant therapy. Am J Med 84:683–690, 1988.

67. Culclasure TF, Bray VJ, Hasbargen JA: The significance of hematuria in the anticoagulated patient. Arch Intern Med 154:649–652, 1994.

68. Caralis P, Gelbard M, Washer J, et al: Incidence and etiology of hematuria in patients on anticoagulant therapy. Clin Res 37:791A, 1989.

69. Schuster GA, Lewis GA: Clinical significance of hematuria in patients on anticoagulant therapy. J Urol 137:923–925, 1987.

70. van Savage JG, Fried FA: Anticoagulant associated hematuria: A prospective study. J Urol 153:1594–1596, 1995.

71. Cannegieter SC, Rosendaal FR, Wintzen AR, et al: The optimal intensity of oral anticoagulant therapy in patients with mechanical heart valve prostheses: The Leiden artificial valve and anticoagulation study. N Engl J Med 333:11–17, 1995.

72. Hylek EM, Singer DE: Risk factors for intracranial hemorrhage in outpatients taking warfarin. Ann Intern Med 120:897–902, 1994.

73. Hylek EM, Skates SJ, Sheehan MA, Singer DE: An analysis of the lowest effective intensity of prophylactic anticoagulation for patients with nonrheumatic atrial fibrillation. N Engl J Med 335:540–546, 1996.

74. European Atrial Fibrillation Trial Study Group: Optimal oral anticoagulant therapy in patients with nonrheumatic atrial fibrillation and recent cerebral ischemia. N Engl J Med 333:5–10, 1995.

75. van der Meer FJM, Rosendaal FR, Vandenbroucke JP, et al: Bleeding complications in oral anticoagulant therapy: An analysis of risk factors. Arch Intern Med 153:1557–1562, 1993.

76. Beyth RJ, Quinn LM, Landefeld S: Prospective evaluation of an index for predicting the risk of major bleeding in outpatients treated with warfarin. Am J Med 105:91–99, 1998.

77. Ansell JE, Hughes R: Evolving models of warfarin management: Anticoagulation clinics, patient self-monitoring, and patient self-management. Am Heart J 132:1095–1100, 1996.

78. Landefeld CS, Goldman L: Major bleeding in outpatients treated with warfarin: Incidence and prediction by factors known at the start of outpatient therapy. Am J Med 87:144–152, 1989.

79. Gitter MJ, Jaeger TM, Petterson TM, et al: Bleeding and thromboembolism during anticoagulant therapy: A population based study in Rochester, Minnesota. Mayo Clin Proc 70:725–733, 1995.

80. Forfar JC: Prediction of hemorrhage during long-term oral coumarin anticoagulation by excessive prothrombin ratio. Am Heart J 103:445–446, 1982.

81. Palareti G, Leali N, Coccheri S, et al: Bleeding complications of oral anticoagulant treatment: An inception-cohort, prospective collaborative study (ISCOAT). Lancet 348:423–428, 1996.

82. Palareti G, Manotti C, D'Angelo A, et al: Thrombotic events during anticoagulant treatment: Results of the inception-cohort, prospective, collaborative ISCOAT study. Thromb Haemost 78:1438–1443, 1997.

83. Cortelazzo S, Finazzi G, Viero P, et al: Thrombotic and hemorrhagic complications in patients with mechanical heart value prosthesis attending an anticoagulation clinic. Thromb Haemost 69:316–320, 1993.

84. Chiquette E, Amato MG, Bussey HI: Comparison of an anticoagulation clinic and usual medical care: Anticoagulation control, patient outcomes, and health care costs. Arch Intern Med 158:1641–1647, 1998.

85. Leaning KE, Ansell JE: Advances in the monitoring of oral anticoagulation: Point-of-care testing, patient self-monitoring, and patient self-management. J Thromb Thrombolysis 3:377–383, 1996.

86. Lucas FV, Duncan A, Jay R, et al: A novel whole blood capillary technique for measuring prothrombin time. Am J Clin Pathol 88:442–446, 1987.

87. Weibert RT, Adler DS: Evaluation of a capillary whole blood prothrombin time measurement system. Clin Pharm 8:864–867, 1989.

88. Jennings I, Luddington RJ, Baglin T: Evaluation of the Cibra Corning Biotrack 512 coagulation monitor for the control of oral anticoagulation. J Clin Pathol 44:950–953, 1991.

89. Tripodi A, Arbini AA, Chantarangkul V, et al: Are capillary whole blood coagulation monitors suitable for the control of oral anticoagulant treatment by the international normalized ratio? Thromb Haemost 70:921–924, 1993.

90. McCurdy SA, White RH: Accuracy and precision of a portable anticoagulation monitor in a clinical setting. Arch Intern Med 152:589–592, 1992.

91. Tripodi A, Chantarangkul V, Clerici M, et al: Determination of the international sensitivity index of a new near-patient testing device to monitor oral anticoagulant therapy. Thromb Haemost 78:855–858, 1997.

92. Kaatz AA, White RH, Hill J, et al: Accuracy of laboratory and portable monitor international normalized ratio determinations. Arch Intern Med 155:1861–1867, 1995.

93. Ansell J, Becker D, Andrew M, et al: Accurate and precise prothrombin time measurement in a multicenter anticoagulation trial employing patient self-testing. Blood 86 (Suppl 1): 864a, 1995.

94. Mennenmeyer ST, Winkelman JW: Searching for inaccuracy in clinical laboratory testing using Medicare data: Evidence for prothrombin time. JAMA 269:1030–1033, 1993.

95. White RH, McCurdy A, Marensdorff H, et al: Home prothrombin time monitoring after the initiation of warfarin therapy: A randomized, prospective study. Ann Intern Med 111:730–737, 1989.

96. Anderson D, Harrison L, Hirsh L: Evaluation of a portable prothrombin time monitor for home use by patients who require long-term oral anticoagulant therapy. Arch Intern Med 153:1441–1447, 1993.

97. Beyth RJ, Landefeld CS: Prevention of major bleeding in older patients treated with warfarin: Results of a randomized trial. J Gen Intern Med 12:66(abstract), 1997.

98. Ansell J, Holden A, Knapic N: Patient self-management of oral anticoagulation guided by capillary (fingerstick) whole blood prothrombin times. Arch Intern Med 149:2509–2511, 1989.

99. Ansell J, Patel N, Ostrovsky D, et al: Long-term patient self-management of oral anticoagulation. Arch Intern Med 155: 2185–2189, 1995.

100. Bernardo A: Experience with patient self-management of oral anticoagulation. J Thromb Thrombolysis 2:321–325, 1996.

101. Hasenkam JM, Kimose HH, Knudsen L, et al: Self-management of oral anticoagulant therapy after heart valve replacement. Eur J Cardiothorac Surg 11:935–942, 1997.

102. Sawicki PT: Working Group for the Study of Patient Self-Management of Oral Anticoagulation. A structured teaching and self-management program for patient receiving oral anticoagulation: A randomized controlled trial. JAMA 281:145–150, 1999.

103. Koertke H, Minami K, Breyman K, et al: INR self-management following mechanical heart valve replacement: Are education level and therapeutic compliance connected? J Thromb Thrombolysis 9 (Suppl 1): S41–S46, 2000.

104. Kortke H, Korfer R: International normalized ratio self-management after mechanical heart valve replacement: Is an early start advantageous? Ann Thorac Surg 72:44–48, 2001.

105. Watzke HH, Forberg E, Svolba G, et al: A prospective controlled trial comparing weekly self-testing and self-dosing with the standard management of patients on stable oral anticoagulation. Thromb Haemost 83:661–665, 2000.

106. Cromheecke ME, Levi M, Colly LP, et al: Oral anticoagulation self-management and management by a specialist anticoagulation clinic: A randomized cross-over comparison. Lancet 556:97–101, 2000.

107. Gadisseur APA, Breuking-Engbers WGM, vander Meer FJM, et al: Comparison of the quality of oral anticoagulant therapy through patient self-management versus management by specialized anticoagulation clinics in the Netherlands. Arch Intern Med 163:2639–2646, 2003.

108. Menendez-Jandula B, Souto JC, et al: Comparing self-management of oral anticoagulant therapy with clinic management. Ann Intern Med 142:1–10, 2005.

109. Heneghan C, Alonso-Coello P, Garcia-Alamino JM, et al: Self-monitoring of oral anticoagulation: A systematic review and meta-analysis. Lancet 367:404–411, 2006.

40

Chapter 41

Point-of-Care Testing for Hemostatic Disorders

Kendra Kubiak, MD • B. Gail Macik, MD

With the consolidation of clinical laboratories to buildings often miles away from the patient, the "turn-around time" for a laboratory result is lengthening. For routine tests, consolidation improves cost effectiveness and is unlikely to be detrimental to patient care. However, if the patient is bleeding or is receiving a hemostatic drug, delayed testing cannot accurately monitor the rapidly changing clinical situation. Several coagulation testing systems are available that perform whole-blood prothrombin time (PT), partial thromboplastin time (PTT), heparin monitoring, platelet function studies, and other tests of hemostatic function near the site of patient care.[1] Some point-of-care (POC) technologies offer testing superior to that performed in the centralized laboratory or that is otherwise unavailable. Other technologies are not as precise as those available in the laboratory but provide clinically equivalent results that expedite care.

In 2005, a survey reported the availability of 13 analyzers manufactured by seven companies for measuring hemostasis at the point of patient care.[1] The use of these instruments has become an integral part of patient management. The POC market has grown in response to the demands of cardiologists, interventional radiologists, surgeons, and anesthesiologists whose increasingly complex interventions require a cadre of antiplatelet and anticoagulant drugs. Real-time monitoring of these drugs is a necessary component of care. In order to function as a consultant to the procedure-oriented specialties, the hematologist must be familiar with the technologies that are emerging to monitor hemostasis and drug effect for the best procedural outcome.

In addition to hospital use, POC monitoring of warfarin in the outpatient and home setting is a rapidly growing market. In 2002, Medicare began to cover the home use of POC INR (International Normalized Ratio) monitors for patients with mechanical heart valves on warfarin, a population of almost 600,000 in the United States.[2] The growth of home POC warfarin monitoring is a function of increased patient satisfaction with a technology that saves time and visits to the doctor's office or laboratory. Patients gain a sense of competence in being able to contribute to their own management. In order to support this growing field of POC monitoring, the consultant hematologist must become familiar with the technology that is changing warfarin management.

The practicing hematologist must also be familiar with regulations governing the use of laboratory instruments. The Clinical Laboratories Improvement Act (CLIA) is a set of guidelines outlining the training and regulatory requirements necessary to operate any laboratory instrument. Instruments are rated as low or high complexity depending on the level of expertise required to operate the instrument and interpret the results. A special "waived" category exists for very simplistic tests that require little expertise. Any individual or institution engaged in using laboratory instruments must register for CLIA approval unless the only instruments or tests performed are in the "waived" category.

When is a POC test indicated? The most obvious answer is when the test does not exist in the central laboratory. For example, most centralized laboratories offer no equivalent to the activated clotting time (ACT) for monitoring high-dose heparin during cardiac interventions and surgery. The need for time-sensitive information is another indication for POC testing. On the one hand, if a drug or clinical condition is of brief duration, waiting even 1 or 2 hours for a result from the central laboratory indicates only what *was* happening and not what *is* happening to the patient. On the other hand, obtaining a test result within minutes if no clinical decision will be made for hours is not appropriate use of POC testing. A POC instrument may improve care by enabling patient self-testing and management. For example, monitoring of warfarin by home PT instruments has the potential to improve anticoagulation control.

What are the cost implications and medical-legal implications of POC testing? POC tests usually cost more per test than similar automated batch testing performed in the central laboratory. Cost effectiveness, however, must take into account the effect on all aspects of care. Does rapid testing lead to improved outcome and fewer complications? Does the patient spend less time in the operating room or the hospital? Is the medical professional able to work more efficiently and cost effectively? Is the patient spared unnecessary blood transfusions or medical interventions? Currently, clinical trials are underway to answer the above questions and validate the perceived benefit of POC testing. Because all the POC tests discussed in this chapter have U.S. Food and Drug Administration (FDA) approval, medicolegal questions regarding the use of these instruments have not been an active concern.

OVERVIEW OF HEMOSTATIC POINT-OF-CARE TESTING

Evaluating the array of instruments for POC testing is a daunting experience. Knowing the characteristics and limitations of the technology improves the chance of selecting an appropriate test system.[3] The ideal POC test system is rapid, accurate, easy to use, durable, transportable, and of low cost. Additional desirable features include sample recognition software, continuous electronic monitoring of the system, electronic quality control, a program for transferring results to an information system, and a compact design to compete for space in the crowded workplace.[1,4] Fresh fingerstick samples are popular because of the ease and rapidity of collection, but citrated samples allow repeat testing and addition of other tests to the same sample.

Choice of sample, adaptation of quality-control procedures, correlation to plasma-based assays, and determination of reference ranges are particular challenges for coagulation POC testing systems. New instruments have appeared, and older systems have been given new names as technology and distributors change. All systems in this review are cleared by the FDA for marketing. Other technologies are available for "research use only," but they are "not for use in diagnostic procedures." No specific endorsement or ranking of tests is implied. To expedite inquiries regarding a product, Table 41-1 lists the contact information

Table 41-1 Coagulation Point-of-Care Instruments

Company	Instruments and Tests	Earlier Versions/Alternate Names
Abbott Point of Care Bedford, MA 609-469-0342 www.michael.saperstein@i-stat.com	I-Stat 1—PT/INR, Celite ACT Kaolin ACT I-Stat—PT/INR, Celite ACT, kaolin ACT	
Accumetrics San Diego, CA 800-643-1641 www.accumetrics.com	VerifyNow Assays: monitor platelet inhibition by ASA, clopidogrel, IIb-IIIa inhibitors	Ultegra Rapid Platelet Function Assay
Chrono-log Corporation Havertown, PA 800-247-6665 www.chronolog.com	Whole Blood Aggregometer (WBA): platelet function test	
Dade Behring Deerfield, IL 847-267-5300 www.dadebehring.com	PFA–100: platelet function analyzer	
Haemoscope, Inc. Niles, IL 800-438-2834 www.haemoscope.com	Thromboelastogram (TEG)—platelet function, clot formation and lysis, heparinase cup (to neutralize heparin effect), kits for assessing aspirin and clopidogrel effects on platelets	
Helena Point of Care Beaumont, TX 800-231-5663 www.helena.com	Actalyke XL: MAX-ACT, Celite ACT, Kaolin ACT, glass ACT Actalyke Mini II: Max-ACT, C-ACT, K-ACT, G-ACT	
HemoSense, Inc. San Jose, CA 408-719-1393 www.hemosense.com	INRatio: PT	
Instrumentation Laboratory Lexington, MA 781-861-4165 www.ilus.com	GEM PCL Plus: PT, PTT, ACT, LR-ACT I	
International Technidyne Corp. Edison, NJ 732-548-5700 www.itcmed.com	Pro-Time Microcoagulation System/ Pro-Time 3: PT/INR Hemochron Jr. Signature/Signature⁺: PT/INR, PTT, APTT, LR-ACT, ACT⁺ Hemochron Response: PT, PTT, ACT, HiTT, TT, HNTT, Fib., HRT, KHRT, PRT, PDAO, KPDAO	Pro-Time Micro 1995 Hemochron 401 Hemochron 801 Hemochron 8000
Medtronic Cardiac Surgery Minneapolis, MN 800-328-3320 www.medtronic.com	HMS Plus: ACT, heparin dose response, heparin protamine titration ACT Plus: ACT—high range, low range, high-range heparinase, recalcified	
Roche Diagnostics Corporation Indianapolis, IN 800-852-8766 www.roche.com	CoaguChek S System: PT/INR (professional use only)	CoaguChek Pro/Pro-DM: ACT, PTT, PT CoaguChek Plus
Sienco, Inc. Arvada, CO 800-432-1624 www.sienco.com	SonoClot—global test of platelet function, clot formation and lysis	

for manufacturers and distributors discussed in this chapter. To help follow the course of a technology, earlier generations of the same instruments that have different names than the current model are listed also.

OVERVIEW OF PLATELET FUNCTION ANALYZERS

The surgeon and internist alike dread the management of the patient with an undefined coagulopathy. Common causes of excessive bleeding or oozing at the site of surgical procedures are platelet dysfunction that may be drug induced or congenital or von Willebrand disease (VWD). Traditional laboratory assessment of platelet function is complicated, time consuming, and limited in scope. POC technologies are available that provide global assessment of primary hemostasis. The instruments are easy to use, provide results in less than one hour, and in some cases, provide information not available from larger laboratory instruments. As with most POC, monitoring of therapy (either blood product replacement or antiplatelet drugs) is the most common reason for requesting a platelet analyzer. Table 41-2 lists the platelet monitoring POC analyzers available. The instrument systems differ in the ease of use, parameters tested, and applicability of the test for detecting platelet and/or von Willebrand factor (VWF) abnormalities.[5] Compared with the bleeding time and platelet aggregation studies, the results of POC may prove more clinically relevant than existing test methods.

VerifyNow (Ultegra) Instrument

The VerifyNow Instrument has replaced the Ultegra Rapid Platelet Function Assay (RPFA) (Accumetrics, San Diego, Calif., USA) in the assessment of platelet dysfunction induced by drugs such as inhibitors of the glycoprotein (GP)-IIb/IIa receptor (i.e., abciximab and epifibatide),

as well as by aspirin and clopidogrel. The VerifyNow IIb/IIIa instrument, which measures inhibition of the GP-IIb/IIIa receptor by both abciximab and eptifibatide, performs a semiquantitative, whole-blood platelet function assay.[6–8] During testing, platelets are first activated to express GP-IIb/IIIa receptors that bind to the fibrinogen-coated beads and induce agglutination; however, agglutination is inhibited in the presence of abciximab and epifibitide. The degree of agglutination is detected by a turbidimetric-based optical system, and the result is reported as a platelet aggregation unit (PAU). The assay, which requires 10 minutes to complete, can be used to determine the degree of platelet inhibition in a patient by comparing the PAU measured before and after infusion of the drug.

Similarly, the VerifyNow aspirin assay measures aspirin-induced platelet inhibition. A lyophilized preparation containing human fibrinogen-coated beads and a platelet agonist is added to the patient sample and platelet aggregation is detected as an increase in light transmittance. The Ultegra VerifyNow aspirin test has been demonstrated in the literature to reliably assess patient response to aspirin therapy and has received a CLIA waiver for this use.[9]

The newest assay, the VerifyNow P2Y12 , was cleared by the FDA in August, 2005 for the assessment of the inhibition of the P2Y12 receptor on platelets. The assay does not require a baseline blood sample because the instrument has a second channel in which the platelet inhibition is overcome and a baseline value is calculated. It is the first assay cleared by the FDA to directly quantify platelet inhibition by clopidogrel. The assay is being marketed for the management of patients on chronic clopidogrel therapy; it is also used in the perioperative setting to determine if a patient who has discontinued clopidogrel prior to a procedure continues to exhibit ongoing significant platelet dysfunction.

The VerifyNow assays require a citrated whole blood sample tested within 15 minutes of collection. The evacuated blood-draw tube attaches directly to the instrument. The analyzer automatically dispenses blood into the cartridge.

Table 41-2 Platelet Function Analyzers for Point-of-Care Testing

Company	Instrument	Test Method	Procedure
Accumetrics San Diego, CA 800-643-1641 www.accumetrics.com	VerifyNow Assays	Monitor platelet inhibition by ASA, clopidogrel, IIb/IIIa inhibitors Optical detection of fibrin-coated bead agglutination; drug decreases agglutination	Simple—no pipet sample or sample prep
Chrono-log Corporation Havertown, PA 800-247-6665 www.chronolog.com	Whole Blood Aggregometer (WBA)	Platelet aggregation detected by whole blood electrical impedance Arachidonic acid, collagen, ristocetin, ADP agonists may be used	Moderate—pipet and dilute sample
Dade Behring Deerfield, IL 847-267-5300 www.dadebehring.com	PFA–100	Occlusion of an aperture in a collagen/ADP or collagen/epinephrine cartridge tests platelet adhesion (VWF), activation, aggregation, all in a flow system	Simple—pipet sample
Medtronic Cardiac Surgery Minneapolis, MN 800-328-3320 www.medtronic.com	HMS Plus: ACT, heparin dose response, heparin protamine titration	Indirect test of platelet function related to platelet activating factor (PAF)-induced shortening of the ACT	Simple—requires the HMS system

The result is available in 3 to 5 minutes. Concomitant medications that do not alter results include acetaminophen and other nonsteroidal anti-inflammatory drugs, β-adrenergic blockers, calcium channel blockers, "statins," and nitrates. Variable platelet counts between 100,000 and 350,000/µL, hematocrits between 25% and 45%, and fibrinogen levels between 200 and 600 mg/dL do not affect the assay results. Other GP-IIb/IIIa inhibitors affect the baseline PAU. Previous clinical trials report that the Ultegra RPFA is equivalent to a radiolabeled abciximab receptor blockade assay or platelet aggregometry for monitoring abciximab therapy.[7,8] Data regarding the VerifyNow are currently being collected.

Whole Blood Aggregation

The Whole Blood Aggregometer (WBA) is a modified version of the larger platelet aggregometer manufactured by Chrono-log Corporation (Havertown, Penna., USA). Both systems use electrical impedance to study platelet aggregation in whole blood. An accurate platelet aggregation result can be obtained within 7 minutes of venipuncture. A citrated whole blood sample is diluted with an equivalent volume of isotonic saline and incubated at 37°C. Platelet aggregation is detected by passing a weak electrical current between two electrodes immersed in the sample and measuring the impedance between the electrodes. Platelet aggregation occurs at the electrodes, increasing the impedance. The increase in impedance is directly proportional to the platelet mass deposited on the electrode probe. The final increase in ohms is displayed as a numeric LED readout in a front panel digital display. Analog outputs provide the option to interface a chart recorder for a hard copy record of the aggregation curves.

Measuring 6 × 13 × 9 inches and weighing 10 pounds, the WBA was designed to be smaller, simpler, and more portable.[10] One or two test channels are available. New disposable electrodes simplify testing by eliminating the need to sanitize the electrodes between tests. Automated calibration and readout functions and electronic quality control are provided. An optional printer and data management software are offered. Limitations include the lack of a positive identification system for the patient specimen and the lack of an onboard system for automatic error detection.

The WBA performs all the studies available with the larger instruments, but the smaller design makes it better suited for perioperative or antiplatelet drug monitoring. Like the parent model, the WBA may be used to detect platelet function abnormalities that increase bleeding risk during surgery.[11,12] For drug monitoring, Mascelli and coworkers[10] report that the WBA predicts the amount of GP-IIb/IIIa receptor blockade induced by the drug abciximab.

PFA-100 Platelet Function Analyzer

The PFA-100 Platelet Function Analyzer (Dade-Behring, Deerfield, Ill., USA) is an automated alternative to existing techniques for assessing platelet function.[13–15] The PFA-100 measures platelet function under flow conditions that mimic the process of primary hemostasis in a damaged blood vessel. Whole blood passes through an aperture cut into a membrane coated with collagen and either epineph-

rine or ADP. The system measures the ability of platelets to occlude the aperture and reports the closure time. The biologic stimuli and the high shear rates generated by the standardized flow result in platelet attachment, activation, and aggregation; therefore, the system can detect defects at any stage of platelet function.

The analyzer measures 15.1 × 9 × 14.2 inches, weighs 24 pounds, and is best classified as a bench-top instrument. The disposable test cartridges contain all components for test performance. The collagen/epinephrine (CEPI) cartridge is used first to screen for platelet dysfunction induced by intrinsic platelet defects, VWF defects, or inhibitory drugs or substances. The collagen/ADP (CADP) cartridge is used only if the CEPI cartridge is abnormal. The CADP does not detect aspirin and, therefore, a prolonged CEPI with a normal CAPD suggests an aspirin-like side effect. Citrated whole blood, 800 µL, is transferred into the sample reservoir of the cartridge by pipet. Results are reported as closure times in seconds. Platelet counts of less than 100,000/µL affect the closure time, as does a hematocrit of less than 15% to 20%. Heparin and oral anticoagulants do not affect the closure time, but antiplatelet drugs do.[16–18] Neither electronic nor wet quality-control materials are available, so fresh control blood is required with each new lot of cartridges. Systems for automatic error detection and for identification of patient specimen and reagent are provided. Patient data can be transferred to an information system, but data management capability is lacking. Disadvantages include open sample handling, use of pipet, lack of defined quality controls, and negative effect of moderately decreased platelet counts.

Several studies support the usefulness of the PFA-100 in a variety of clinical settings.[13–23] The instrument can be used to help diagnose VWD,[17,18] monitor antiplatelet drugs including abciximab,[13,16,19] detect aspirin effects,[13–16,20] and uncover congenital[21] and acquired[22] platelet function defects. The instrument has also been used to evaluate platelet-induced hemostasis in the pediatric population.[23] However, data do not support the routine use of the PFA-100 before surgery because the test does not predict surgical bleeding.

In a representative study by Ortel and coworkers,[14] 305 patients from 12 different clinical settings were enrolled in a study to evaluate the PFA-100 in a population typical of a tertiary care practice. Of these patients, 29% reported a previous blood transfusion, 29% reported taking aspirin, and 19% were on oral anticoagulants. Of this population, 37% had a prolongation of the closure time. Isolated prolongation of the CEPI closing time for patients on aspirin was the most common abnormality (69%). Conversely, only 68% of patients who reported taking aspirin had a prolonged closure time. The study was not designed to correlate bleeding risk with closure times, and there was no correlation between results with hemorrhagic symptoms or a history of blood transfusions. In all, 93.5% of the patients with a prolonged closure time were found to have a specific quantitative or qualitative abnormality in platelet or VWF function. Other studies report 88% to 100% sensitivity for uncovering an underlying defect.[13–23] The PFA-100 advantages include its rapidity (results in 5 minutes), simplicity (three-step procedure), and global assessment of primary hemostatic function.

HemoSTATUS Platelet Activated Clotting Test

The HemoSTATUS assay is a family of cartridges used to measure platelet function using the Hepcon HMS analyzer (Medtronic Perfusion Systems, Minneapolis, Minn., USA). The Hepcon HMS platform is discussed subsequently. The system is used during cardiopulmonary bypass to determine pre-, intra-, and postoperative hemostasis. The test is a modified clotting time study that is designed to isolate and test platelet function. Platelet activating factor (PAF) is a potent, endogenous platelet activator that stimulates in vitro clot formation. Increasing concentrations of PAF are present in channels 3 to 6 of the cartridge, whereas channels 1 and 2 serve as controls. A kaolin-activated clotting time (k-ACT) is determined for each channel. Platelet procoagulant activity is determined by measuring the PAF-induced shortening of the k-ACT. A whole blood sample is collected in a 3-mL syringe that is then secured to the Hepcon HMS instrument. The instrument automatically distributes a 0.3 mL volume to each of the six channels in the self-contained test cartridge. Results are shown as a percentage of normal function. Based on these results, the HemoSTATUS test results are interpreted as low incidence of platelet-related bleeding (80% to 120%); moderate incidence of platelet-related bleeding (60% to 80%); and high incidence of platelet-related bleeding (0% to 60%).

The HemoSTATUS test has been reported to correlate with blood loss after cardiac bypass surgery,[24] but other investigators have found no correlation.[25] The test has been used to evaluate the effect of DDAVP during surgery,[26] to detect GP-IIb/IIIa blockade by abciximab,[27,28] and to evaluate the need for platelet transfusion perioperatively.[29] ε-Aminocaproic acid (EACA) and aspirin do not affect the HemoSTATUS test.[27,29] Platelet counts must be above 50,000 to 70,000/μL and the white blood count must be between 4000 and 9000/μL.[28] The controlled, reproducible test procedure is an advantage that is offset by the need for a large, expensive instrument.

OVERVIEW OF CLOT-DETECTION ANALYZERS

When is a second not a second? The answer is when the second is a result of a coagulation assay. Clotting time is determined by assay design, not clinical condition. For example, 200 seconds of actual time may indicate a high heparin concentration for a PTT assay or it may be a normal clotting time for a whole blood ACT system. Simply put, clotting times are "man-made" and there is nothing "physiologic" about a 300-second clotting time. The result of a PT, PTT, or ACT test must be interpreted using the normal and therapeutic ranges determined specifically for the assay method.[30–34] Technology designed for POC testing must provide clinical information equal to that obtained with a standard laboratory method. Equality does not imply identical form or numerical result.[3] However, most manufacturers of POC testing systems succumb to clinical pressure and convert their results to a "plasma equivalent time" to mimic laboratory ranges. Satisfying clinical demand masks the true differences between testing systems. Results differ because of the sample type, reagent, or detection method used by an instrument.[3,30–32] Freshness of the sample may also affect the result because clotting factors degrade and drug effects decay. Mathematical conversion of data cannot correct for all these variables. A new test method is compared with an existing technology to provide a frame of reference. Dissimilar numerical results may correlate better than results altered to give the illusion of being the same number. The take-home message is: look for correlation between methods, but do not expect identical results when comparing different testing systems.

For the PT, the INR improves comparability between results obtained using different reagents and assay systems. However, the INR fails to "normalize" whole blood results reliably, cannot overcome inherent differences in clot detection methods, and cannot completely offset the effect of reagents with markedly different sensitivities (ISI).[30–32] Heparin monitoring with the PTT or ACT test has become an even greater challenge as new reagents and detection methods have entered the market. No INR-like system exists to even attempt to "normalize" differences in heparin response curves observed with different reagents and testing systems.[33,34] Against these obstacles, the following POC instruments are striving to be accepted as accurate and reliable alternatives to standard laboratory testing.

Home PT Testing Systems

Self-testing and self-management of warfarin has emerged as a reliable alternative to traditional provider-based care. In 1999, at the 17th Congress of the International Society on Thrombosis and Hemostasis, several presentations reported that the experience in multiple countries with patient self-monitoring led to improved hemostatic control and increased patient satisfaction. More than 50,000 patients in Germany are currently managing their own anticoagulation using CoaguChek.[35] Several studies report that patients can test, adjust dosage, and achieve therapeutic goals as well as or better than healthcare providers or an anticoagulation clinic.[36–41] Complications of warfarin therapy decrease by as much as 76% if values remain in the therapeutic range.[42] A recent prospective, controlled trial reported by Menedez-Jandula[43] compared both clinical outcomes and the quality of anticoagulation based on self-testing versus management by a conventional anticoagulation clinic in 737 patients. The self-management group ($n = 368$) achieved a 58.6% success rate for keeping the PT in the target range compared with 55.6% for the conventional management group. Both major complications and minor bleeding episodes occurred less frequently in the self-management group (2.2% vs 7.3% and 14.9% vs 36.4 %, respectively). The improved testing outcome is likely due to the increased number of INR determinations and dose adjustments performed, but the impact of patient motivation cannot be ignored. Additionally, less time is spent out of therapeutic range because of the immediate feedback of results. A new trial, known as the INR Study, is currently ongoing through the Veteran's Affairs Hospital System; this trial compares outcomes in patients who are self-testing with those who are being monitored in anticoagulation clinics. The acceptance of home testing grows as studies support improvement in patient care. In the United States, approval by Medicare to fund home monitoring for one subset of patients, mechanical heart valve patients, further opens the door to affordable home testing options. Table 41-3 lists the home PT testing systems. For home testing, the instrument must be extremely easy to use with no pipeting and a limited number of steps. Long-term studies to verify the clinical impact of home management are ongoing, but a new standard for anticoagulation control is on the horizon. Several POC PT/INR systems have been FDA-approved for home testing, but only the Pro-Time (International Technidyne Corp) and the INRatio (HemoSense) are actively marketed.

ProTime Microcoagulation System/ProTime 3 (ProTime Micro 1995; ProTime 3 2001)

The ProTime microcoagulation analyzer is a CLIA-waived home-testing system. (International Technidyne, Edison, NJ, USA). The analyzer is a table-top device measuring 2.5 × 4.5 × 9 inches and weighing 3 pounds. The system uses a fingerstick sample and the sample cup must be completely filled or an error message is generated. There is no electronic control, but the test card has integrated quality-control reaction chambers that allow controls to be run with every patient sample. It takes less than 5 minutes to generate a test result. The instrument sends data to a printer, and automated transfer of data to an information system is available.

The ProTime uses an optical method to detect clot formation. Blood is added to a sample cup on the test cartridge. The sample is drawn into five parallel reaction channels and mixed with the appropriate reagents. A sensitive thromboplastin reagent with an ISI equal to 1.0 is used. When the blood clots, it no longer flows past the optical detector and a clotting time is generated. The result is reported as a plasma equivalent clotting time with calculated INR. The two outside channels serve as high and low controls with appropriate modifiers added to the channels to produce a clotting time within a predetermined value. The three middle reaction channels test the patient's blood in triplicate and a mean value is reported.

The ProTime has been evaluated at many clinical sites and compared in several studies with laboratory and other POC devices.[32,41,44] A representative correlation coefficient compared with a laboratory standard is 0.93 and imprecision studies reveal coefficients of variation of 3% to 6%. As for other POC PT monitors, the INR result shows a positive bias (i.e, overestimation on the lower end of the therapeutic range) when compared with standard laboratory methods.[32,45] Biasiolo and coworkers[41] studied 150 patients presenting to the anticoagulation clinic in a 15-day period. The average difference between the POC and the laboratory method was 0.2 INR. A difference of more than 1.0 INR was obtained in 5 of 150 (3%) patients. In four of five discordant patients, the difference was clinically relevant and in two of five the error was noted to be due to delay in filling the sample chamber. On a smaller number of patients ($n = 30$), Chapman and coworkers[44] reported far more variation between the ProTime and a standard laboratory value, with a mean INR difference of 0.56 and 50% discordance in clinical management prompted by the result. Other studies, however, find the ProTime equivalent to other methods for managing anticoagulation therapy.[46] The integrated high and low controls are a clear advantage for the ProTime.

INRatio

The INRatio is a portable home PT monitor (HemoSense Inc., San Jose, Calif., USA) approved for use in 2002. The hand-held device measures 6.5 ×3 × 2 inches and weighs 10.5 ounces. A fingerstick sample of about 15 uL (an accurate volume is not needed) is applied to the testing strip which contains three channels. The sample is then drawn into three separate testing areas by capillary action where it combines with several reagents. The system uses human recombinant thromboplastin for actual clot detection. Two other areas contain various reagents to create low and high clotting times for normal and therapeutic clotting ranges, respectively. Clot formation is detected by a change in the impedance of the sample and results are available within 2 minutes. Quality control is built into the testing strip and automated high and low quality-control checks are performed with each analysis as mentioned. The testing strips can be stored at room temperature. The machine automatically performs both electronic and procedure self-testing to ensure accurate results and can detect sources of error including strip re-usage, unacceptable temperature ranges, and inadequate blood sample. The meter has memory storage of up to 60 test results which can be downloaded to a computer or a printer. One recent study found good correlation between the results of the INRatio and laboratory testing both in the normal and therapeutic INR ranges.[47]

Table 41-3 PT Home Testing Monitors

Company	Instrument	Testing Method	Procedure
HemoSense, Inc. San Jose, CA 408-719-1393 www.hemosense.com	INRatio	Clot detected by increasing sample impedance; high and low clotting times automatically generated	Simple—fingerstick
International Technidyne Corp. Edison, NJ 732-548-5700 www.itcmed.com	Pro-Time Microcoagulation System/Pro-Time 3: PT/INR	Optical detection of clot formation by interruption of blood flow; high and low controls are included on test cartridge	Simple—fingerstick
Roche Diagnostics Corporation Indianapolis, IN 800-852-8766 www.roche.com	CoaguChek S System: PT/INR (professional use only in the United States, home monitor in Europe)	Optical detection of cessation of movement of paramagnetic iron particles as clot forms	Simple—fingerstick

Table 41-4 Analyzers that Perform Multiple Coagulation Tests

Company	Instruments	Tests Performed and Samples Used
Abbott Point of Care Bedford, MA 609-469-0342 www.michael.saperstein@i-stat.com	I-Stat 1 I-Stat	PT/INR, Celite ACT, kaolin ACT, electrolytes, blood gases Fingerstick or whole blood
Helena Point of Care Beaumont, TX 800-231-5663 www.helena.com	Actalyke XL Actalyke Mini II	MAX-ACT, Celite ACT, kaolin ACT, glass ACT Whole blood
Haemoscope, Inc. Niles, IL 800-438-2834 www.haemoscope.com	Thromboelastogram (TEG)	Platelet function, clot formation, and lysis, heparinase cup (to neutralize heparin effect), kits for assessing aspirin and clopidogrel effects on platelets Whole blood, citrated whole blood or plasma
Instrumentation Laboratory Lexington, MA 781-861-4165 www.ilus.com	GEM PCL Plus	PT, PTT-citrate whole blood ACT, LR-ACT 1-fingerstick or whole blood
International Technidyne Corp. Edison, NJ 732-548-5700 www.itcmed.com	Hemochron Jr. Signature/Signature⁺ Hemochron Response	PT, PTT-citrated or noncitrated whole blood ACT, LR-ACT—fresh whole blood PT, PTT, ACT, HiTT, TT, HNTT, HRT, KHRT, PRT, PDAO, KPDAO fresh or citrated whole blood
Medtronic Cardiac Surgery Minneapolis, MN 800-328-3320 www.medtronic.com	ACT Plus	ACT—high-range, low-range, high-range heparinase, recalcified whole blood
Sienco, Inc. Arvada, CO 800-432-1624 www.sienco.com	SonoClot	Global test of platelet function, clot formation and lysis Whole blood

ACT: activated clotting time; HiTT: high thrombin time; HNTT: heparin neutralizing thrombin time; HRT: heparin response test; KHRT: kaolin-based heparin response test; KPDAO: kaolin-based protamine titration assay; LR-ACT: low-range activated clotting time; MAX-ACT: maximum factor XII activation ACT test; PDAO: celite based protamine titration assay; PRT: protamine response test; TT: thrombin time.

41

CoaguChek S and CoaguChek XS

The CoaguChek PT monitoring system (Roche Diagnostics Corporation, Indianapolis, Ind., USA) is commonly cited in the literature.[37,44,45,48,49] The updated version of the instrument, the CoaguChek S, is approved only for use in a physician's office. Now there is a further update, Coagu-Chek XS, with more quality-control features. Older versions of different POC PT devices known as the CoaguChek DM, PPO, or Plus are no longer being manufactured. The Coagu-Chek S measures 1.8 × 4.9 × 6.8 inches and weighs 1.0 pounds. A fingerstick or venous sample is required. The system has onboard error control and an electronic and liquid quality control feature. The CoaguChek S provides a test result in about one minute. The system does not have data management or download capability. The CoaguChek S information is available in multiple languages and results are reported as an INR, Quick %, or ratio.

Blood (approximately 10 µL) is applied to the sample well on the test strip and drawn by capillary action into a reaction chamber, where it is mixed with a dry PT reagent. Paramagnetic iron particles are present in the reaction chamber and they move in response to a magnetic field. Reflectance photometry detects change in particle movement with clot formation and the time is converted into a plasma equivalent clotting time and INR.

The system is a proven POC device, widely used in clinical trials.[44,45,48,49] Numerous studies have found the imprecision to be between 3% and 6% and the representative correlation coefficients range from 0.9 to 0.97. Chapman and coworkers[44] reported a 0.28 INR average difference between the CoaguChek and the laboratory value, with an 8.3% discordance rate in clinical management decisions. The instrument is reliable and is gaining acceptance in the home market outside the United States. The CoaguChek is not actively marketed but supplies are available.

Multitest Systems: PT, PTT, ACT

Table 41-4 lists the analyzers offering a broader testing menu. These instruments are used primarily for monitoring anticoagulation therapy or for guiding blood product replacement for the perioperative or bleeding patient. Heparin monitoring is a particular strong suit of several of these test systems. Despite the growing use of low molecular weight heparin, unfractionated heparin remains the standard of care for many clinical settings. For high-dose anticoagulation during cardiopulmonary bypass and invasive vascular procedures, heparin has no current rival. These instruments are rated as moderate CLIA complexity and are designed for use by healthcare professionals.

i-STAT and i-STAT 1

The i-STAT and the i-STAT-1 are both portable coagulation analyzers (Abbot Point of Care, East Windsor, NJ, USA). The i-STAT has been extensively documented in the literature to provide reliable results with regard to PT/INR assessment.[50–52] The i-STAT is a bedside instrument that measures 8 × 2.5 × 2 inches and weighs 18 ounces; the i-STAT-1 analyzer measures 9.25 ×3 ×3 inches and also weighs 18 ounces. Both analyzers require either a whole blood or a fingerstick sample which must be added as a fixed volume marked on the cartridge (i-STAT) or cuvette (i-STAT-1). Clot formation is detected by the conversion of a thrombin substrate which is detected by an electrochemical sensor. The devices are FDA-approved to perform PT/INR, Celite, ACT, and Kaolin ACT as well as additional approval for the performance of electrolytes, chemistries, and blood gases. Results are available in two minutes for the PT and slightly longer for the ACT. Both systems will detect error from inadequate sample. Electronic, lyophilized, and liquid quality control are available. Quality control is integrated with each analysis and there is an automatic lockout for QC failure. Data management capability is optional and both machines can transfer the data to an information system.

Actalyke XL/Actalyke Mini II

The Actalyke XL (Helena Point of Care, Beaumont, TX, USA) is another portable coagulation analyzer measuring 5.6 × 10.7 × 10.3 inches and weighing 15 pounds. It requires a whole blood sample of discrete volume entered into a cuvette. The machine uses dual test wells with a two point clot detection mechanism—one at 0 degrees and another at 90 degrees—to determine earliest clot formation. During clot formation, a magnet moves from detector one to detector two, triggering an endpoint when it reaches 46 degrees. It is approved for the evaluation of the ACT, MAX-ACT, celite, kaolin, glass, and maximum factor XII activation. Results are available in five minutes. Electronic, liquid, and lyophilized quality control is available; QC is not performed with each analysis but lockout does occur for QC failure. The system does not have data management capability. The instrument is used primarily during cardiac procedures such as CPB, catheterization, and angioplasty but is also in use for heparin monitoring with dialysis. There is some evidence that the Actalyke will yield shorter ACT values after heparin bolus and during hypothermia.[53]

The Actalyke Mini II is a bench-top version of the XL measuring 6 × 6 × 5 inches and weighing 5.3 pounds. Its mechanism of clot detection is the same as for the XL except that it employs a single testing well. It is approved for the measurement of ACT. MAX-ACT, C-ACT, K-ACT, and G-ACT. Quality-control methods are the same as those for the XL.

GEM Portable Coagulation Laboratory

The GEM Portable Coagulation Laboratory (PCL) is a small, whole blood analyzer that is available free-standing or as a component of the IL Synthesis or IL GEM Premier 3000 comprehensive, compact portable laboratory systems for POC (Instrumentation Laboratory (IL), Lexington, Mass., USA). International Technidyne (ITC) and IL have formed a partnership to co-develop the coagulation component. The GEM PCL offers PT, PTT, ACT (heparin concentration 1.0 to 6.0 U/mL), and low-range ACT (LRACT) (heparin concentration below 2.5 U/mL) tests. The ACT and LRACT report results in "celite-equivalent" clotting times.

The instrument is a portable handheld device measuring 5.5 × 2 × 3.5 inches and weighing 0.75 pounds. The GEM PCL accepts fingerstick or venous whole blood for all tests and citrated whole blood for the PT and PTT. The technology for clot detection is identical to the Hemochron Jr., discussed later, but the software for the clot detection algorithms differs. The analyzer reads the encoded cartridges to determine test type. One drop of blood (approximately 50 µL) is applied to the sample well. The system will display a low sample error if the sample well is not adequately filled. The system is equipped with electronic quality control or wet quality-control material. Outboard error management is present. A comprehensive data management system, downloading, and printing capabilities are available as part of the larger workstation. Results are available in less than five minutes for PT but may require longer for PTT and ACT. Results are stored automatically with time and date. The advantages of the system include the connection to a comprehensive POC testing workstation, the expanded menu of coagulation tests, and a comprehensive onboard data management system. The instrument may be disconnected from the workstation and carried to the bedside.

Hemochron Jr. Signature/Signature⁺

The Hemochron Jr. Signature is the smallest of the line of multitask analyzers manufactured by International Technidyne Corporation (ITC) (Edison, NJ, USA). The system performs the same panel of tests described for the GEM PCL-PT, PTT, ACT (celite), and LRACT—but the reagents and test interpretation may differ. The PT and PTT are available using either citrated or noncitrated whole blood; the ACT and LRACT accept fresh whole blood.

The instrument is a portable, handheld device measuring 2 × 7.5 × 3.75 inches and weighing 12 ounces. The test cartridge is composed of a waste channel and a test channel and is encoded with test type and other parameters. The PT and PTT assays are available in about two minutes, with slightly longer times for ACT. Electronic control and wet quality-control material are available. The Signature package provides a keypad and onboard data management, including the ability to identify, store, date, time stamp, and print patient and quality-control test results. Transfer of the data to an information system is available. No positive identification of patient specimens is available, but the system does have an onboard system for error control.

Blood (approximately 15 µL) is placed in the sample well of the cartridge and a 15-µL aliquot is drawn into the test channel that contains test-specific reagents. Excess blood from the sample well is directed to a waste channel. The test sample is pumped back and forth across a window, blocking light transmission between an LED and a light detector. Clot formation is signaled when the blood ceases to move. Clotting times are converted to test specific results.

The test system compares favorably with the ACT performed on the larger Hemochron instrument and to the laboratory PTT.[54] Correlation of the PT with several other POC instruments found the PT to be adequate, but it had the lowest correlation coefficient with the routine laboratory method ($r = 0.89$) and tended to underestimate INRs above 3.0.[32] This instrument is not approved for home use. The advantages include a variety of test options, and an onboard data management program.

Hemochron Response

A Hemochron analyzer (International Technidyne Corporation, Edison, NJ, USA), which has been used to monitor heparin therapy for the past 30 years, is one of the first portable, rapid, whole blood coagulation analyzers.[55] Several versions of the instrument, including single-well (401), double-well (801), and data management-equipped (8000) models, have been marketed. The newest version, the Hemochron Response, uses fresh or citrated whole blood, offers an expanded test menu, and provides additional software for warfarin, protamine, and heparin management.

The system offers a full package for heparin management. The ACT monitors high-dose heparin therapy (heparin concentration 1.0 to 6.0 U/mL). To supplement the ACT, other heparin tests are available, including a PTT, a thrombin time (TT), the heparin-neutralizing thrombin time (HNTT), the high thrombin time (HiTT), the heparin response test (HRT), and the protamine response test (PRT). The HNTT and HiTT determine circulating heparin effect. The HRT and PRT together with patient-specific determinants (age, weight, baseline ACT) are used by the onboard RxDx management program to determine heparin and protamine dosage.

The instruments vary in size and weight depending on the specific version. A 1.5-mL sample must be accurately pipeted into the sample test tube or an evacuated tube must be used. Test results are available in 1 to 5 minutes depending on the test. Electronic quality control, an onboard system for instrument error detection, and wet quality-control material are available on all instruments. The Hemochron Response offers several features, including quality-control lockout, identification for patient and operator, downloading capabilities, and a bar-code reader to identify reagent tubes.

The technology for clot detection is the same for all versions. Clot formation is detected by a sensitive electromagnetic method. A magnet is located in the sample test tube. The magnet aligns with a magnet detector within the instrument test well. The test well(s) slowly rotates and incubates the test tube during the coagulation test. The magnet and magnet detector remain aligned until the formation of a clot displaces the magnet, signifying test completion. The time to clot formation is converted into a plasma equivalent time for PT, PTT and TT.

A recent study demonstrated coefficients of variation on whole blood for the ACT of 0.6% to 11.2% (celite) and 2.4% to 7.0% (kaolin).[56] Varying results have been reported with the heparin management programs.[57] Many comparison studies are available.[33,42,58–60] The PT and PTT are rarely mentioned in the literature, especially since the arrival of easier-to-use, smaller-volume analyzers. Advantages of the Hemochron include the rapid, easy-to-perform ACT, the heparin package, and the years of testing experience. The need for a measured, large-volume sample is the most important disadvantage as the newer, small-volume instruments gain popularity.

ACT Plus

The ACT Plus Automated Coagulation Timer (Medtronic Perfusion System, Minneapolis, Minn., USA) is another work horse in the operating room and catheterization laboratory. Several different cartridges are available to allow for specific testing scenarios: High Range Activated Clotting Time (HR-ACT) for use with fresh whole blood in cardiovascular or vascular surgery and PTCA; Low Range Activated Clotting Time (LR-ACT) for use with fresh whole blood in dialysis, ECMO and therapeutic heparin monitoring; Heparinase test Cartridge (HTC) for use with fresh whole blood to determine if heparin is present; Recalcified Activated Clotting Time (RACT) for use in citrated whole blood samples; and General Purpose Cartridge (GPC) for use with citrated whole blood or plasma to perform PT/PTT tests. The analyzer measures $11 \times 8 \times 13$ inches, weighs 11.5 pounds, and has two reaction wells that allow for duplicate testing. The test requires at least 15 μL of whole blood, which is added to the cuvette; clot detection is mechanical through impedence of the blood flow. A result is available in up to 12 minutes, slightly longer for high ACT values. The instrument displays the celite-equivalent ACT value. Electronic quality-control and lyophilized quality-control material are available. The system offers data management and a data transfer system. The ACT II, precursor to the ACT Plus, has been compared in numerous studies with other POC heparin monitors.[58,59]

Hepcon HMS Hemostasis Management System

The Hepcon HMS (Medtronic Perfusion System, Minneapolis, Minn., USA) uses the same clot detection method as the ACT Plus; however, the Hepcon is fully automated. The system offers complex testing programs including the HemoStatus platelet function assay (earlier) and a heparin management program. The heparin studies use four- to six-chambered cartridges that contain varying concentrations of heparin or protamine. Patient-specific information (sex, weight, height) and the concentration of heparin desired are entered into the management program and an initial heparin dose is suggested. ACT is followed to monitor the patient's response and to adjust the dose. For heparin reversal, the protamine dose is determined in a similar manner. A protamine assay to determine the concentration of heparin is also possible.

The Hepcon HMS is the largest analyzer in the category of POC instruments and is more transportable than portable. It measures $14.5 \times 16.5 \times 9.5$ inches and weighs 30 pounds. A 3-mL syringe is used to collect a fresh venous sample. The syringe is attached to the instrument and the sample is automatically dispensed to each of the wells within a cartridge. The instrument has electronic quality control and uses a wet quality-control material. A minimum of 12 minutes is required for a test result. The analyzer does not have data management capability and it cannot transfer data to an information system. An onboard error detection system guides the automatic pipeting. The major disadvantages are the size, price, and length of time required for the test to complete. Evaluations of clinical studies have been mixed regarding the usefulness of several of the management programs.[60,61]

GLOBAL ASSESSMENT OF CLOT FORMATION

Other POC instruments are significantly different from extant devises in that they do not mimic existing laboratory tests, but monitor the viscoelastic properties of clot formation. The Thromboelastogram (TEG) has experienced many face-lifts since its debut in the 1940s. The SonoClot Coagulation and Platelet Function Analyzer debuted in the late 1980s. Both of these instruments provide a "clot signature" that traces the progression of clot formation and clot resolution. By analyzing the tracing produced by the instruments, a global assessment can be made of the function of platelets, the soluble clotting proteins, anticoagulants present, and fibrinolysis. The major disadvantages of these systems are the skills required to perform and interpret the test, but newer computerized instruments are entering the market and gaining popularity.

Thromboelastogram (TEG)

The complexity of the Thromboelastogram (Haemoscope, Skokie, Ill., USA) was a major deterrent to routine use of this system for patient monitoring. In recent years, the technology has been automated and computerized to provide more reproducible and interpretable measurements and the instrument has been streamlined into a true POC test. The test is performed by placing a small amount of whole blood (approximately 360 µL) into a cylindrical cup. A pin is suspended in the blood. The cup remains stationary and the pin is rotated though an angle of $4°\ 45'$. As clot forms and viscosity increases, the rotary motion of the pin is progressively inhibited. Characteristic tracings are developed based on the motion of the pin (a tracing is shown in Chapter 39, Fig. 39-1) The components of the tracing have been ascribed to various counterparts of physiologic clot development and dissolution. The "R" value describes the time to clot formation and is prolonged in factor deficiencies or with anticoagulation. The maximal amplitude (MA) of the tracing represents platelet activity and fibrinogen concentration. The time to clot lysis is measured 30 minutes after clot formation. In non-activated blood, more than 30 minutes are required for the generation of the MA; however, an activator (e.g., kaolin) shortens the time to MA by inducing more rapid blood clotting. The major advantage of the TEG is the development of a full clot signature from initial platelet activation to eventual clot lysis. The major disadvantage has been the prolonged time required to see full development of the tracing and interpretation of the data, but computerization is now providing user-friendly clinically applicable results. There is growing literature regarding the clinical applications for the TEG. Perioperative transfusion algorithms based on data generated by the TEG is the most common clinical application.[62] Transfusion, anticoagulant, and antifibrinolytic management for cardiac bypass[63,64] is an active area of investigation and TEG information has long been used during liver transplantation to guide blood product replacement.[65–67] Of interest, the two areas using these devices the most (cardiac surgery and liver transplantation) are also the two characteristically associated with late hyperfibrinolysis (see Chapter 37) underscoring the near monopoly TEG holds on prompt

evaluation of hyperfibrinolysis. Other specific surgical indications including pediatric surgery[68,69] and noncardiac surgery[70] are being investigated.

SonoClot Coagulation and Platelet Function Analyzer

The SonoClot Coagulation Analyzer (Sienco Inc., Wheat Ridge, Colo., USA) differs in design from the TEG, but both systems measure the physical properties of the clot. Whole blood (approximately 400 µL) is placed in a cylindrical cuvette in which a vertically vibrating probe is suspended. The change in mechanical impedance extended on the probe by the viscoelastic properties of the forming clot produces a characteristic clot tracing. Reduced platelet function causes a decreased slope from inflection to peak, a lower peak, and a reduced contraction rate. Several clinical trials have been reported using the SonoClot.[71–74] The advantage of this test is the more rapid completion, usually within 15 minutes, and the global testing of the blood elements of primary hemostasis; however, despite being available for decades, the instrument has yet to make a major impact on the clinical market.

REFERENCES

1. Aller R: Coagulation Analyzers. Survey of the Instruments. CAP Today March 22–31, 2005.
2. Parham S: Shortfall, not windfall, greets PT/INR coverage. CAP Today March 22–4, 2005.
3. Macik BG: Designing a point-of-care program for coagulation testing. Arch Pathol Lab Med 119:929–938, 1995.
4. Jensen R: Near-patient hemostasis testing. Clin Hemost Rev 8:1–4, 1994.
5. McKenzie ME, Gurbel PA, Levine DJ, Serebruany VL: Clinical utility of available methods for determining platelet function. Cardiology 92:240–247, 1999.
6. Smith JW, Steinhubl SR, Lincoff AM, et al: Rapid platelet-function assay an automated and quantitative cartridge-based method. Circulation 99:620–625, 1999.
7. Kereiakes DJ, Mueller M, Howard W, et al: Efficacy of abciximab induced platelet blockade using a rapid point of care assay. J Thromb Thrombolysis 7:265–275, 1999.
8. Steinhubl SR, Kottke-Marchant K, Molitemo DJ, et al: Attainment and maintenance of platelet inhibition through standard dosing of abciximab in diabetic and non-diabetic patients undergoing percutaneous coronary intervention. Circulation 100:1977–1982, 1999.
9. Coleman J, Wang JC, Simon DI: Determination of individual response to aspirin therapy using Accumetrics Ultegra RPFA-ASA System. Point of Care 3:77–82, 2004.
10. Mascelli MA, Worley S, Veriabo NJ, et al: Rapid assessment of platelet function with a modified whole blood aggregometer in percutaneous transluminal coronary angioplasty patients receiving anti-GP IIb/IIIa therapy. Circulation 96:3860–3866, 1997.
11. Kabakibi A, Vamvakas EC, Cannistraro PA, et al: Collagen-induced whole blood platelet aggregation in patients undergoing surgical procedures associated with minimal to moderate blood loss. Am J Clin Pathol 109:392–398, 1998.
12. Ray MJ, Marsh NA, Just SJE, et al: Preoperative platelet dysfunction increases the benefit of aprotinin in cardiopulmonary bypass. Ann Thorac Surg 63:57–63, 1997.
13. Mammen EF, Comp PC, Gosselin R, et al: PFA-100 system: A new method for assessment of platelet dysfunction. Semin Thromb Hemost 24:195–202, 1998.
14. Ortel TL, James AH, Thames EH, et al: Assessment of primary hemostasis by PFA-100® analysis in a tertiary care center. Thromb Haemost 84:94–97, 2000.
15. Harrison P, Robinson MS, Mackie IJ, et al: Performance of the platelet function analyzer PFA-100 in testing abnormalities of primary haemostasis. Blood Coagul Fibrinolysis 10:25–31, 1999.

16. Kottke-Marchant K, Powers JB, Brooks L, et al: The effect of anti-platelet drugs, heparin, and pre-analytical variables on platelet function detected by the platelet function analyzer (PFA-100). Clin Appl Thromb Hemost 5:122–130, 1999.

17. Fressinaud E, Veyradier A, Truchaud F, et al: Screening for von Willebrand disease with a new analyzer using high shear stress: A study of 60 cases. Blood 91:1325–1331, 1998.

18. Cattaneo M, Federici AB, Lecchi A, et al: Evaluation of the PFA-100 system in the diagnosis and therapeutic monitoring of patients with von Willebrand disease. Thromb Haemost 82:35–39, 1999.

19. Hezard N, Metz D, Nazeyrollas P, et al: Use of the PFA-100 apparatus to assess platelet function in patients undergoing PTCA during and after infusion of c7E3 Fab in the presence of other antiplatelet agents. Thromb Haemost 83:540–544, 2000.

20. Homoncik M, Jilma B, Hergovich N, et al: Monitoring of aspirin (ASA) pharmacodynamics with the platelet function analyzer PFA-100. Thromb Haemost 83:316–321, 2000.

21. Cattaneo M, Lecchi A, Agati B, et al: Evaluation of platelet function with the PFA-100 system in patients with congenital defects of platelet secretion. Thromb Res 96:213–217, 1999.

22. Escolar G, Cases A, Vinas M, et al: Evaluation of acquired platelet dysfunction in uremic and cirrhotic patients using the platelet function analyzer (PFA-100): Influence of hematocrit elevation. Haematologica 84:614–619, 1999.

23. Rand ML, Carcao MD, Blanchette VS: Use of the PFA-100 in the assessment of primary, platelet-related hemostasis in a pediatric setting. Semin Thromb Hemost 24:523–529, 1998.

24. Despotis GJ, Levine V, Filos KS, et al: Evaluation of a new point-of-care test that measures PAF-mediated acceleration of coagulation in cardiac surgical patients. Anesthesiology 85:1311–1323, 1996.

25. Ereth MH, Nuttall GA, Santrach PJ, et al: The relation between the platelet-activated clotting test (HemoSTATUS) and blood loss after cardiopulmonary bypass. Anesthesiology 88:962–969, 1998.

26. Despotis GJ, Levine V, Saleem R, et al: Use of point-of-care test in identification of patients who can benefit from desmopressin during cardiac surgery: A randomised controlled trial. Lancet 354:106–110, 1999.

27. Coiffic A, Cazes E, Janvier G, et al: Inhibition of platelet aggregation by abciximab but not by aspirin can be detected by a new point-of-care test, the hemoSTATUS. Thromb Res 95:83–91, 1999.

28. Despotis GJ, Ikonomakiou S, Levine V, et al: Effects of platelets and white blood cells and antiplatelet agent C7E3 (Reopro) on a new test of PAF procoagulant activity of whole blood. Thromb Res 86:205–219, 1997.

29. Saleem R, Bigham M, Spitznagel E, Despotis GJ: The effect of epsilon-aminocaproic acid on HemoSTATUS and kaolin-activated clotting time measurements. Anesth Analg 90:1281–1285, 2000.

30. Becker DM, Humphries JE, Walker FB, et al: Standardizing the prothrombin time: Calibrating coagulation instruments as well as thromboplastin. Arch Pathol Lab Med 117:602–605, 1993.

31. Hirsh J, Dalen JE, Anderson DR, et al: Oral anticoagulants: Mechanism of action, clinical effectiveness, and optimal therapeutic range. Chest 119:22S–38S, 2001.

32. Gosselin R, Owings JT, White RH, et al: A comparison of point-of-care instruments designed for monitoring oral anticoagulation with standard laboratory methods. Thromb Haemost 83:698–703, 2000.

33. Solomon HM, Mullins RE, Lyden P, et al: The diagnostic accuracy of bedside and laboratory coagulation: Procedures used to monitor the anticoagulation status of patients treated with heparin. Am J Clin Pathol 109:371–378, 1998.

34. Brill-Edwards P, Ginsberg JS, Johnston M, Hirsh J: Establishing a therapeutic range for heparin therapy. Ann Intern Med 119:104–109, 1993.

35. Fitzmaurice DA: Recommendations for patients undertaking self management of oral anticoagulation. BMJ 323:985–989, 2001.

36. Ansell JE, Patel N, Ostrovsky D, et al: Long-term patient self-management of oral anticoagulation. Arch Inern Med 155:2185–2189, 1995.

37. Jacobson AK: Patient self-management of oral anticoagulation therapy: An international update. J Thromb Thrombolysis 5:25–28, 1998.

38. Yang DT: Home prothrombin time monitoring: A literature analysis. Am J Hematol 77:177–186, 2004.

39. Oral Anticoagulant Monitoring Study Group: Prothrombin measurement for professional and patient self-testing use: A multicenter clinical experience. Am J Clin Pathol 115:288–296, 2001.

40. Macik BG: New concepts in management of thrombophilia-home PT monitoring. In Schechter GP, Broudy VC, Williams ME (eds): Hematology, 2005. Washington, DC, American Society of Hematology, 2001, pp 330–338.

41. Biasiolo A, Rampazzo P, Furnari O, et al: Comparison between routine laboratory prothrombin time measurements and fingerstick determinations using a near-patient testing device (Pro-Time). Thromb Res 97:495–498, 2000.

42. Bussey H, Chiquette E: Workshop on anticoagulation: Clinic care vs routine medical care: A review and interim report. J Thromb Thrombolysis 2:325–329, 1996.

43. Menedez-Jandula B: Comparing self management of oral anticoagulant therapy with clinic management: A randomized trial. Ann Intern Medicine 142:1–10, 2005.

44. Chapman DC, Stephens MA, Hamann GL, et al: Accuracy, clinical correlation, and patient acceptance of two handheld prothrombin time monitoring devices in the ambulatory setting. Ann Pharmacother 33:775–780, 1999.

45. Murray ET, Fitzmaurice DA, Allan TF, Hobbs FD: A primary care evaluation of three near patient coagulometers. J Clin Pathol 52:842–845, 1999.

46. Nowatzke WL, Landt M, Smith C, et al: Whole blood international normalization ratio measurements in children using near-patient monitors. J Pediat Hematol/Oncol 25:33–37, 2003.

47. Taborski U: Analytical Performance of the new coagulation monitoring system INRatio for the determination of INR compared with the coagulation monitor CoaguChek S and an established laboratory method. J Thromb Thrombolysis 18:103–107, 2004.

48. Van den Besselaar AM, Breddin K, Lutze G, et al: Multicenter evaluation of a new capillary blood prothrombin time monitoring system. Blood Coagul Fibrinolysis 6:726–732, 1995.

49. Douketis JD, Lane A, Milne J, Ginsberg JS: Accuracy of a portable international normalization ratio monitor in outpatients receiving long-term oral anticoagulation therapy: Comparison with a laboratory reference standard using clinically relevant criteria for agreement. Thromb Res 92:11–17, 1998.

50. Schussler J: Comparison of the i-STAT handheld activated clotting time with the Hemochron activated clotting time during and after percutaneous coronary intervention. Am Cardiol 91:464–466, 2003.

51. Paniccia R: Evaluation of a new point of care celite activated clotting time analyzer in different clinical settings: The i-STAT celite activated clotting time test. Anesthesiology 99:54–59, 2003.

52. Schussler J: Validation of the i-STAT handheld activated clotting time for use with bivalirudin. Am J Cardiol 93:1318–1319, 2004.

53. Prisco D, Paniccia R: Point of care testing of hemostasis in cardiac surgery. Thrombos J 1:1–10, 2003.

54. Carter AJ, Hicks K, Heldman AW, et al: Clinical evaluation of a microsample coagulation analyzer, and comparison with existing techniques. Cathet Cardiovasc Diagn 39:97–102, 1996.

55. Esposito RA, Culliford AT, Colvin SB, et al: The role of the activated clotting time in heparin administration and neutralization for cardiopulmonary bypass. J Thorac Cardiovasc Surg 85:174–185, 1983.

56. Zucker ML, Jobes C, Siegel M, et al: Activated clotting time (ACT) testing: Analysis of reproducibility. J Extra Corpor Technol 31:130–134, 1999.

57. Johnson HD, Morgan MS, Koenig GR, et al: Evaluation of the Hemochron 8000 Rx/Dx system for heparin management. J Extra Corpor Technol 29:83–87, 1997.

58. O'Neill AI, McAllister C, Corke CF, Parkin JD: A comparison of five devices for the bedside monitoring of heparin therapy. Anaesth Intensive Care 19:592–596, 1991.

59. Reich DL, Zahl K, Perucho MH, Thys DM: An evaluation of two activated clotting time monitors during cardiac surgery. J Clin Monit 8:33–36, 1992.

60. Murray DJ, Brosnahan WJ, Pennell B, et al: Heparin detection by the activated coagulation time: A comparison of the sensitivity of coagulation tests and heparin assays. J Cardiothorac Vasc Anesth 11:24–28, 1997.

61. Hardy JF, Belisle S, Robitaille D, et al: Measurement of heparin concentration in whole blood with the Hepcon/HMS device does not agree with laboratory determination of plasma heparin concentration using a chromogenic substrate for activated factor X. J Thorac Cardiovasc Surg 112:154–161, 1996.

62. Shore-Lesserson L, Manspeizer HE, DePerio M, et al: Thromboelastography-guided transfusion algorithm reduces transfusions in complex cardiac surgery. Anest Analg 88:312–319, 1999.

63. Stammers AH, Bruda NL, Gonano C, Hartmann T: Point-of-care coagulation monitoring: Applications of the thromboelastograph. Anaesthesia 53 (Suppl 2), 58–59, 1998.

64. Spiess BD, Gillies BSA, Chandler W, Verrier E: Changes in transfusion therapy and reexploration rate after institution of a blood management program in cardiac surgical patients. J Cardiothorac Vasc Anes 9:304–309, 1995.

65. Kang Y: Thromboelastography in liver transplantation. Seminars Thromb Hemost 21 (Suppl4), 34–44, 1995.

66. Gillies BSA: Thromboelastography and liver transplantation. Seminars Thromb Hemost 21 (Supp4), 45–49, 1995.

67. Cerutti E, Stratta C, Romagnoli R, et al: Thromboelastogram monitoring in the perioperative period of hepatectomy for adult living liver donation. Liver Transpl 10:289–294, 2004.

68. Williams JD, Douglas E: Thromboelastography predicts transfusion requirements in kids after heart surgery. Anest News, May 1997;.

69. Miller BE, Guzzetta NA: Rapid evaluation of coagulopathies after cardiopulmonary bypass in children using modified thromboelastography. Anesth Analg 90 (6), 1324–1330, 2000.

70. Burke GW 3rd, Ciancio G, Figueiro J, et al: Hypercoaguable state associated with kidney-pancreas transplantation: Thromboelastogram directed anti-coagulation and implications for future therapy. Clin Transplant 18:423–428, 2004.

71. Miyashita T, Kuro M: Evaluation of platelet function by SonoClot analysis compared with other hemostatic variables in cardiac surgery. Anesth Anal 87:1228–1233, 1998.

72. LaForce WR, Brudno DS, Kanto WP, Karp WB: Evaluation of the SonoClot analyzer for the measurement of platelet function in whole blood. Ann Clin Lab Sci 22:30–33, 1992.

73. Shibata T, Sasaki Y: SonoClot analysis in cardiac surgery in dialysis-dependent patients. Ann Thoracic Surg 77:220–225, 2004.

74. Ganter MT, Dalbert S: Monitoring activated clotting time for combined heparin and aprotinin application: An in vitro evaluation of a new aprotinin-insensitive test using SonoClot. Anesth Analg 101:308–314, 2005.

Chapter 42

Prevention and Treatment of Venous Thromboembolism in Neurologic and Neurosurgical Patients

David Green, MD, PhD

A patient is in a major vehicle accident, sustaining injuries to the brain and spinal cord, requiring immediate surgical intervention. What is the risk of venous thromboembolism (VTE) in the immediate postoperative period? What thromboprophylactic measures should be applied, and for how long? If the patient has a complete motor paralysis, should prophylaxis be continued for days, weeks, months, or indefinitely? Suppose the patient experiences a pulmonary embolism (PE) or deep vein thrombosis (DVT), what treatment would be appropriate, and for how long should it be continued? What is the risk of intracranial or spinal bleeding with anticoagulant therapy? These are some of the difficult questions that confront consultants regarding the care of patients with neurologic illness or injury.

STROKE

Acute Ischemic Stroke: Prophylaxis

Placebo-controlled trials indicate that the frequency of DVT in patients with ischemic stroke not receiving anticoagulant prophylaxis is 22%.[1] The majority of these trials were conducted using a heparinoid[2,3] (danaparoid), which is no longer available in the United States; in only one study was a low molecular weight heparin (LMWH) used.[4] A meta-analysis of all trials showed that the use of heparins achieved an almost twofold reduction in the number of VTEs (from 22% to 13%; $P = 0.002$), and with no increase in bleeding.[1] Based on this analysis, the Seventh American College of Chest Physicians (ACCP) Conference on Antithrombotic and Thrombolytic Therapy recommended that acute stroke patients with restricted mobility receive prophylaxis with low-dose unfractionated heparin (UFH) or LMWHs.[5] They noted that these agents may be safely administered with aspirin, but that they should be withheld for the first 24 hours after thrombolytic therapy is given. Leg compression devices should be used in those patients with strong contraindications to anticoagulants.

Acute Hemorrhagic Stroke: Prophylaxis

Patients with ruptured aneurysms, subarachnoid bleeds, and intraventricular hemorrhage are also at high risk of VTE, but the use of anticoagulants is usually considered to be contraindicated in such persons. Boeer and colleagues[6] observed that giving low dose UFH, 5000 U 3 times daily, lowered the frequency of PE compared with starting heparin 4 or more days later, without an increase in rebleeding in the brain. The ACCP Conference recommends the initial application of compression devices, followed by UFH on the second day after hemorrhage.[5] As a further precaution, one might also repeat central nervous system imaging to confirm the absence of continued bleeding. Because the natural history of each of these three conditions is characterized by spontaneous rebleeding, anticoagulant use cannot be viewed as the sole cause in the event of a rebleed.

Stroke: Chronic Phase

Following recovery from acute stroke, patients are usually transferred to a rehabilitation facility. Studies have shown that the risk of venous thromboembolism persists into the post-stroke period.[7] In a study that randomized post-stroke patients into groups who received either LMWH or compression boots, the frequency of objectively demonstrated DVT was 11.9% in the former and 5% of the latter ($P = $ ns).[8] Only two patients were symptomatic, and there were no PEs. One patient on LMWH had minor bleeding, and six patients assigned to compression boots left the trial early because the devices were too uncomfortable. The conclusion of the study was that use of either compression boots or LMWH is effective for the prevention of thromboembolism after stroke. The LMWH is better accepted, requires less nursing care, and is only marginally more expensive.

Treatment of Venous Thromboembolism in Stroke Patients

In general, the treatment of VTE in patients who have sustained an ischemic stroke is similar to that of most other individuals with PE or DVT, with the exception that there is a danger of converting an ischemic infarct into a hemorrhagic infarct if full doses of anticoagulants are given soon after a stroke. This observation is based on data from the International Stroke Trial,[9] which showed that doses of 12,500 U of UFH twice daily increased the rate of hemorrhagic stroke threefold, and by a trial that administered LMWH (dalteparin, 100 U/kg twice daily) to patients with acute embolic stroke.[10] The frequency of recurrence, progression, death, or symptomatic cerebral hemorrhage within 14 days was significantly increased with LMWH as compared with aspirin. These reports led the ACCP Conference to suggest that patients with acute ischemic stroke not be exposed to full-dose anticoagulation.[5] Unfortunately, there are few data regarding when it is safe to initiate therapeutic anticoagulation in such patients. In the two trials noted earlier, the anticoagulants were initiated within 48 hours of the ictus. Furthermore, large infarct size and elevated blood pressure predict a greater risk of hemorrhagic transformation.[11] Therefore, patients with these risk factors, or patients who sustain a VTE within 48 hours of an acute stroke, should be considered for a vena caval filter to prevent PE. Thought might be given to using a retrievable filter, inasmuch as after 1 to 2 weeks, full-dose anticoagulation would be acceptable and the filter could be removed. A special case pertains to patients with cerebral venous sinus thrombosis. On the basis of limited trial data, the ACCP recommended that heparins be given during the acute phase, even in the presence of hemorrhagic infarction. An alternative treatment in patients not responding to heparin is catheter-directed thrombolysis, which occasionally is successful but carries a greater risk of hemorrhage.[12]

SPINAL CORD INJURY

Prophylaxis

Spinal cord injury poses a great risk for VTE. A recent review of spinal cord injury admissions showed that 51 (21%) of 243 patients undergoing screening tests for VTE had objective evidence of thrombi, despite the use of various methods of thromboprophylaxis.[13] A variety of potential risk factors were examined, including age, sex, weight, location of spinal cord injury, degree of paralysis, and surgical procedures such as spinal fusion. Hierarchical optimal classification tree analysis suggested that patients with concomitant cancer, men with flaccid paralysis, and women between the ages of 36 and 58 years had the highest likelihood of developing DVT or PE. In another study, age greater than 50 years, increased body mass index, and time from injury to initiation of thromboprophylaxis were noted to be weak risk factors for VTE.[14] Because of the high frequency of VTE observed in all studies, the ACCP Conference recommends that all patients with acute spinal cord injury should receive prophylaxis, generally initiated within 24 to 72 hours of injury.[15]

A variety of methods for the prevention of thromboembolism in the spinal injury patient are available (Table 42-1). The use of compression boots alone has been shown to halve the frequency of DVT.[16,17] There have been several theories as to why compression devices are effective. The rhythmic contractions may mechanically improve blood flow. Such a mechanism has been demonstrated for the foot pump, which empties the venous plexus on the sole of the foot, sending pulses of blood up the leg.[18] In addition, stimulation of the vascular endothelium promotes the release of tissue factor pathway inhibitor (TFPI). This potent endogenous anticoagulant blocks the activation of coagulation by inhibiting factor Xa and the tissue factor:factor VIIa complex. A variety of com-

Table 42-1 Methods for the Prevention of Thromboembolism in Spinal Cord Injury
Mechanical Methods
Compression boots, calf and thigh
Foot pump
Graduated compression stockings
Vena caval filter
Pharmacologic Methods
Unfractionated heparin
Low molecular weight heparin
Pentasaccharide (fondaparinux)
Warfarin
Combined Modalities
Compression device plus unfractionated heparin
Graduated compression hose plus low molecular weight heparin
Vena caval filter plus anticoagulants

pression devices have been shown to increase the levels of TFPI and reduce the concentrations of factor VIIa in normal subjects and patients with venous disease.[19] During every nursing shift, the devices should be inspected to confirm that they are in proper position and that the underlying skin is free of abrasions or other damage.

The usefulness of UFH and LMWH has been examined in a number of clinical trials of patients with traumatic spinal cord injury.[15] Several early studies showed that the use of compression boots or UFH alone was inferior to LMWH. Therefore, the Spinal Cord Injury Thromboprophylaxis Investigators[14] randomized patients to receive either UFH (5000 U every 8 hours) plus compression boots or LMWH (enoxaparin, 30 mg every 12 hours). Proximal vein thrombosis or PE was noted in 16% of the former and 12% of the latter (not significant). Also, bleeding complications were similar in the two groups. Therefore, the ACCP Conference recommended either LMWH or UFH plus a compression device in patients with acute spinal injury.[15] The use of compression devices alone is permissible if risk of bleeding contraindicates administration of an anticoagulant. Fondaparinux, a pentasaccharide anticoagulant, is safe and effective in preventing thrombosis in orthopedic and general medical patients,[20,21] but trials in spinal cord injury have not been reported.

Thromboprophylaxis is generally continued during the rehabilitation phase of spinal cord injury. The Spinal Cord Injury Thromboprophylaxis Investigators[22] continued their study of patients free of VTE after 2 weeks in an acute care facility; these patients were then transferred for rehabilitation. Those who had been previously randomized to enoxaparin continued on this agent, and those randomized to UFH and compression boots continued on UFH alone. After 6 weeks of follow-up, 13 of 60 patients on UFH, as compared with 5 of 59 on enoxaparin, developed a new VTE. This difference was of borderline statistical significance ($P = 0.052$). However, because patients were not randomized on admission to rehabilitation, the omission of compression boots from the heparin group could explain the difference in event rates. In a small study, 20 patients admitted to rehabilitation with negative ultrasound studies were randomized to UFH, 5000 U every 12 hours, or LMWH, 5000 U once daily, and a repeat ultrasound examination was performed at the time of discharge (Do V, Green D, unpublished data). There were no symptomatic VTE and no new thrombi on ultrasound. Therefore, it is still unclear whether UFH or LMWH is to be preferred in the rehabilitation setting; only a very large, multicenter study could answer this question. At any rate, it is recommended that thromboprophylaxis be continued in all patients with spinal cord injury until discharge from a rehabilitation facility.

Data on the optimal duration of thromboprophylaxis is fragmentary and anecdotal. The Consensus Conference on Spinal Cord Injury[23,24] reported that thromboembolism occurred 10 weeks or more after injury in an occasional patient whose prophylaxis was stopped at 8 weeks—suggesting that a longer duration of prophylaxis may be appropriate in some patients. One of these late thrombotic episodes was a fatal pulmonary embolism (PE). To examine the risk factors for fatal PE, we reviewed all autopsy-proved cases occurring in our center over a 5-year period.[25] Nine cases were encountered, eight men and one woman, whose ages ranged from 17 to 67 years. Cervical spine fracture with tetraplegia was present in 67%, obesity in 44%, and all had flaccid paralysis. These characteristics were significantly more common in the cases than in a concurrently selected control group. In addition, more of the control subjects than cases had received LMWH (60% vs 22%, $P = 0.07$). It was concluded that thromboprophylaxis needs to be especially aggressive in patients with cervical spine injuries, tetraplegia, and obesity.

Should any studies to detect the presence of thrombosis be performed prior to discontinuing anticoagulant prophylaxis? The experience with routine ultrasound has been disappointing. Ultrasound had a sensitivity of only 62% and a positive predictive value of 66% for detecting proximal thrombi when used to screen for DVT in patients after orthopedic surgery.[26] The D-dimer test may be more helpful in excluding the presence of thrombosis. In 67 patients with either paraplegia or tetraplegia, no patient with DVT had a negative D-dimer test, although 40 patients without thrombosis had positive tests.[27] The D-dimers were detected with either an ELISA test (Asserachrom D-Di) or a rapid automated turbidimetric test (STA-Liatest D-Di); the methods are important because some tests for D-dimer are more sensitive than others.

A reasonable strategy for deciding whether prophylactic anticoagulants should be discontinued is to measure D-dimer by a sensitive method. If the test is negative, prophylaxis is stopped. If the test is positive, prophylaxis should be continued—if clinical suspicion of thromboembolism is high, additional studies such as ultrasound of the legs, ventilation/perfusion lung scans, or other evaluations would be warranted. If a thrombus is detected, full therapeutic doses of anticoagulants should be administered.

Inferior Vena Caval Filters

Inferior vena caval (IVC) filters are devices that can be introduced into the IVC to block the passage of thrombi from the lower extremities and pelvis into the lungs. In recent years, retrievable devices have become available.[28] The largest experience has been with the Günther Tulip filter.[29] These have usually been inserted on admission to the trauma unit to prevent acute VTE in patients considered unsuitable for prophylactic anticoagulation. Such patients might have

intracranial or other active bleeding, coagulopathy, or lower limb fractures not amenable to the use of compression devices. Another potential indication for the use of an IVC filter is the patient with high cervical spinal cord injury who is ventilator dependent; even a small PE in such a patient could prove fatal. The data suggest that filters are effective in preventing PE, but because they do not prevent DVT, anticoagulant prophylaxis should be initiated as soon as feasible. Insertion of the filter requires technical expertise; in less experienced hands, complications such as guidewire entrapment, infection, failure of retrieval, and migration into the right atrium have been reported. Furthermore, the procedure is expensive; in patients receiving appropriate thromboprophylaxis, it is estimated that 100 filters would need to be placed to prevent two nonfatal PEs at a cost of $500,000.[30] Therefore, the ACCP Conference recommended against the use of a filter as primary prophylaxis against PE.[15] See Chapter 31 for a further review of these devices.

Treatment

To date, no studies have compared long-term therapy with warfarin versus LMWH in this patient population. Furthermore, there are no data with regard to the duration of treatment after a patient has experienced a thromboembolic event. Lim and coworkers[31] examined the time to recanalization of thrombus in patients with tetraplegia, paraplegia, hemiplegia, and no paralysis. All patients received at least three months of anticoagulation prior to evaluation. Patients with tetraplegia and paraplegia took significantly longer for recanalization than nonparalyzed controls (54 days vs 33 days, $P = 0.04$); hemiplegic patients were intermediate. If persistent venous obstruction due to residual thrombus represents an ongoing risk factor for recurrent thrombosis,[32] it would seem prudent to continue patients with paralysis on anticoagulant therapy until complete recanalization of veins has been documented by ultrasound or other techniques.

NEUROSURGERY

Prophylaxis

VTE is an important complication in patients undergoing major neurosurgery. Geerts and associates[33] observed that the rate of DVT in patients not receiving thromboprophylaxis was 22%, and the rate of proximal DVT 5%. Turpie and colleagues[34] reported that calf compression decreased the frequency of venous thrombosis from 20.8% in controls to 7.8% in patients given prophylaxis ($P = 0.01$). Subsequently, these investigators examined graduated compression stockings alone or with compression boots in another randomized trial of neurosurgical patients.[35] Again, the frequency of DVT was reduced from 19.8% in patients not receiving prophylaxis to 8.8% in those wearing stockings, and 9% in those with stockings and compression boots. Thus, graduated compression stockings alone or combined with compression devices have been favored by most neurosurgeons because they are efficacious and avoid the risk of inducing hemorrhage.[36]

With the demonstration that LMWH administration was safe and effective thromboprophylaxis for patients undergoing a variety of medical and surgical procedures, researchers became emboldened to evaluate these drugs in neurosurgery. Two clinical trials showed that the addition of LMWH to compression stockings enhanced the protection due to compression stockings alone. In 1996, Nurmohamed and coworkers,[37] using a venographic end point, noted thrombi in 26.3% of stocking-alone patients and 18.7% of stocking plus LMWH patients ($P = 0.065$). Furthermore, the rates for proximal DVT and PE were 10.2% for the stockings and 5.8% for LMWH ($P = 0.036$). Agnelli and colleagues[38] reported that LMWH reduced the frequency of DVT from 32% (stocking group) to 17% (LMWH group), $P = 0.004$. Proximal vein thrombosis was also decreased significantly: from 13% to 5%, $P = 0.04$. Two patients in the placebo group died of proved PE.

In these studies, the frequency of bleeding appeared to be related to the dose and the particular LMWH administered. Nurmohamed and associates[34] gave nadroparin in a dose of 7500 U and reported major bleeding in 6 LMWH versus two stockings-alone patients ($P = 0.87$), whereas Agnelli and coworkers[35] used enoxaparin in a dose of 40 mg daily and observed no difference in the frequency of bleeding (3% of both treated and control patients).

The studies just described, along with two earlier reports, were subjected to a meta-analysis.[39] A total of 187 thrombotic events were recorded in 827 patients (22.6%). Prophylaxis with heparins resulted in a 45% risk reduction for thrombosis. However, there was a twofold increase in overall bleeding rates (5.9% vs 2.9%, $P = 0.02$), but no significant difference in major bleeding events (2.3% vs 1.4%; $P = 0.24$). Thus, there was one major bleed for every seven thrombotic events prevented by heparins. However, it must be recognized that only good-risk patients were selected for these trials; exclusion criteria included patients with abnormal operative bleeding or coagulopathy, multiple cerebral aneurysms or unclipped aneurysm, or renal failure. Patients with these problems are at higher risk for bleeding and probably should not routinely receive anticoagulant prophylaxis. It is recommended that the initial dose of anticoagulant should be given no earlier than 24 hours postoperatively; the patient should be neurologically stable by physical examination and by an imaging study such as CT or MRI; and the surgical lesion should have been well-demarcated. There should have been no blunt dissection, necrotic tissue, or vascular metastasis.[33] In summary, all patients undergoing major neurosurgery should be fitted with compression boots or graduated compression stockings,[15] and if they meet the criteria just indicated, they should receive daily prophylaxis with a LMWH.

Treatment

The management of documented venous thromboembolism in the neurosurgical patient hinges on one key issue: the likelihood of the patient having a hemorrhage when exposed to full therapeutic rather than prophylactic doses of anticoagulants. When does the risk of major intracranial bleeding subside in the patient who has had head trauma or surgery? The answer to this question hinges on several factors including the time and extent of injury, the type of trauma, and the anatomic lesion. For most kinds of

surgery, wounds are well sealed by 24 hours; exceptionally, a ligature will slip after this time and bleeding will recur. Crush injuries with large raw surfaces are more likely to ooze than cleanly severed tissue which has been re-approximated with sutures. Leaking aneurysms that cannot be fully embolized or ablated are another cause of potential bleeding.

The profile of the patient who can tolerate full-dose anticoagulant therapy is an individual who has sustained a well-demarcated wound more than 24 hours earlier and shows no signs of progressive neurologic deficit. A CT scan or MRI of the head should reveal a stable pattern, with no suggestion of continued bleeding. Subarachnoid or subdural hemorrhages should be contained, and multiple metastatic lesions or aneurysms should not be in evidence. If these conditions are met, systemic anticoagulation for newly recognized venous thromboembolism is indicated. LMWH is preferred to UFH for the following reasons:

1. LMWHs have more predictable pharmacokinetics and greater bioavailability than UFH.[40]
2. A meta-analysis of 13 clinical trials has concluded that LMWH is more effective and is associated with less bleeding than UFH when used for the treatment of DVT.[41]
3. LMWH is easier to administer and generally does not require monitoring. However, under special circumstances, measurements of anti-factor Xa levels are suggested to ensure that the doses given are neither excessive nor subtherapeutic. Monitoring is recommended in persons weighing less than 50 kg or more the 120 kg, in children and pregnant women, and in patients with renal failure.[42] Giving very high doses (for subjects weighing more than 110 kg), or treating patients with creatinine clearances of less than 30 mL/minute, may result in anti-factor Xa levels exceeding 1.0 U/mL, and require dose reductions. The half-life of LMWH is only 3 to 4 hours, so it is rarely necessary to try to reverse its action; however, if life-threatening bleeding or surgical intervention is required in a patient who has just received LMWH, efforts to combat its effects are justified. Protamine, in a dose of 50 to 100 mg depending on patient weight, may be given intravenously at a rate not to exceed 5 mg/minute, and with continuous monitoring of blood pressure.
4. An alternative anticoagulant is fondaparinux. This pentasaccharide enhances the activity of antithrombin III and has been effective in the treatment of patients with DVT and PE.[43,44] It compares favorably with intravenous UFH and LMWH, and is given in doses of 7.5 mg subcutaneously daily. It is excreted entirely by the kidney, and is not neutralized by protamine, which are two potential drawbacks to its use.

When there is an absolute contraindication to the use of systemic anticoagulation, IVC filter placement, as previously described, is appropriate. However, anticoagulant therapy should be started as soon as the danger of bleeding has subsided because the filter alone is not an effective treatment of DVT.[37] The neurosurgical patient who has sustained either a DVT or PE is at high risk for a recurrence; long-term anticoagulation is usually necessary. Warfarin is a safe and effective choice for patients who have a stable food intake and are cognitively intact; in such patients, the dose of warfarin can be adjusted to obtain an International Normalized Ratio (INR) in the accepted therapeutic range of 2 to 3. However, if the patient is not eating, having frequent seizures and falls, or cannot be relied on to take the prescribed dose of warfarin, use of the drug is potentially hazardous. Warfarin-induced bleeding is often observed in neurosurgical patients whose food intake is variable, and in those requiring antibiotics for infection control.

Warfarin resistance is found in patients receiving anticonvulsant medications. Therefore, finding a safe and effective dose of warfarin may be challenging in many neurosurgical patients. In these persons, LMWH therapy offers the advantages of safety and simplicity because its effectiveness is not affected by diet or other medications, and it is given once or twice daily subcutaneously without the need for monitoring in most instances. The doses given are based on body weight, either 1.5 mg or 175 to 200 U per kilogram body weight once daily or 1 mg or 100 U per kilogram body weight twice daily, depending on the agent selected.[45,46] The newer long-acting, once-daily pentasaccharide anticoagulants would seem applicable also but have yet to be systematically studied in this situation. Treatment should be continued until the risk of recurrent thromboembolism is low; for patients without filters, this may be 3 to 6 months depending on neurologic recovery, but for those with filters, anticoagulation may be necessary for up to 2 years or more. When the patient is neurologically stable, cognitively intact persons may wish to switch from LMWH to an oral anticoagulant for reasons of convenience and cost.

Cost Containment Issues

Venous thromboembolism in the neurologic and neurosurgical patient is a very costly complication, economically as well as in terms of morbidity and mortality. Although UFH and warfarin are inexpensive medications, giving UFH by continuous intravenous infusion is expensive and prolongs hospitalization. Giving warfarin so that the INR remains within the therapeutic range requires frequent blood tests and dose adjustments; lapses may be penalized by episodes of either thrombosis or bleeding, leading to recurrent hospitalization. LMWH is more expensive but can be given at home and does not require monitoring. Cost-effectiveness analyses of DVT treatment have shown that the use of LMWH compares very favorably with that of UFH.[47]

Medical-Legal Implications

Practicing thromboprophylaxis is good medicine. However, considerable judgment is required for the safe use of anticoagulants in neurologic and neurosurgical patients, and the medical literature is lacking in this regard. Placebo-controlled studies have shown that some patients with neurologic or neurosurgical disease have new intracranial bleeding in the absence of anticoagulants. Nevertheless, when new bleeding occurs, it is invariably attributed to these agents, and there may be litigation. The best defense is that most published reports stress that the benefit of antithrombotics outweighs the risks when the drugs are used in neurologically stable patients.

Role of the Consultant

With regard to the questions posed at the beginning of this chapter, the risk of venous thromboembolism in the immediate postoperative period is 22% and proximal DVT 5%. Graduated compression stockings and leggings should be applied on admission and continued during the perioperative period. The day after surgery, the patient should be evaluated for the use of pharmacologic prophylaxis. The following criteria should be met prior to starting anticoagulants:

- There should be no active bleeding, and the neurosurgeon should confirm that satisfactory hemostasis was achieved at the time of surgery.
- The patient's general condition should be stable; neurologic examination should show no progression of symptoms or signs.
- Laboratory studies should indicate adequate coagulation (platelet count >100,000/μL, prothrombin time <15 seconds, partial thromboplastin time <35 seconds).

If there is any question about neurologic stability, repeat imaging is recommended. LMWH in prophylactic doses is administered daily for at least 6 to 8 weeks. At some centers, patients considered at high risk for thromboembolism at the time of admission will have retrievable vena caval filters inserted and removed two weeks after surgery. Although this may reduce the frequency of PE, the patient is still at risk for DVT, and needs compression devices and anticoagulant prophylaxis. The latter are important not only for prevention of DVT in the lower extremities, but also for preventing thrombi from forming around or above the filter. From the neurosurgeon's point of view, it is certainly preferable to use the lower, prophylactic doses of anticoagulants than the higher doses that would be required if there were a venous thrombotic event.

Should a PE or DVT occur, full-dose anticoagulation should be promptly initiated, preferably with either a LMWH or fondaparinux. If anticoagulants are contraindicated, an IVC filter should be placed and anticoagulant therapy initiated as soon as feasible. Anticoagulants are usually continued for six months, but they may be stopped earlier if the patient becomes fully mobile. The risk of major bleeding with intravenous UFH is <3% in recent trials and between 1.1% and 1.3% in those receiving LMWH or fondaparinux.[48]

REFERENCES

1. Counsell C, Sandercock P: Low-molecular-weight heparins or heparinoids versus standard unfractionated heparin for acute ischemic stroke (Cochrane Review). Stroke 1925–1926, 2002.
2. Turpie AGG, Levine MN, Hirsh J, et al: Double-blind randomised trial of ORG 10172 low-molecular-weight heparinoid in prevention of deep-vein thrombosis in thrombotic stroke. Lancet 1987; i: 523–526.
3. Turpie AGG, Gent M, Cote R, et al: A low-molecular-weight heparinoid compared with unfractionated heparin in the prevention of deep vein thrombosis in patients with acute ischemic stroke. Ann Intern Med 117:353–357, 1992.
4. Hillbom M, Erila T, Sotaniemi K, et al: Enoxaparin vs heparin for prevention of deep-vein thrombosis in acute ischaemic stroke: A randomized, double-blind study. Acta Neurol Scand 106:84–92, 2002.
5. Albers GW, Amarenco P, Easton JD, et al: Antithrombotic and thrombolytic therapy for ischemic stroke. Chest 126:483S–512S, 2004.

6. Boer A, Voth E, Henze T, et al: Early heparin therapy in patients with spontaneous intracerebral hemorrhage. J Neurol Neurosurg Psychiatry 54:466–467, 1991.

7. Brandstater ME, Roth EJ, Siebens HC: Venous thromboembolism in stroke: Literature review and implications for clinical practice. Arch Phys Med Rehabil 73:S379–S391, 1992.

8. Green D, Akuhota V, Eiken M, et al: Prevention of thromboembolism in stroke rehabilitation patients. Topics Stroke Rehabil 5:68–74, 1998.

9. The International Stroke Trial (IST): A randomized trial of aspirin, subcutaneous heparin, both, or neither among 19,435 patients with acute ischaemic stroke. Lancet 349:1569–1581, 1997.

10. Berge E, Abdelnoor M, Nakstad PH, et al: Low molecular weight heparin versus aspirin in patients with acute ischemic stroke and atrial fibrillation: A double-blind randomised study. Heparin in Acute Embolic Stroke Trial. Lancet 355:1205–1210, 2000.

11. Cerebral Embolism Study Group: Immediate anticoagulation of embolic stroke: Brain hemorrhage and management options. Stroke 15:779–789, 1984.

12. Bousser M-G: Cerebral venous thrombosis. Stroke 30:481–483, 1999.

13. Green D, Hartwig D, Chen D, et al: Spinal cord injury risk assessment for thromboembolism (Spirate Study). Am J Phys Med Rehabil 82:950–956, 2003.

14. Spinal Cord Injury Thromboprophylaxis Investigators: Prevention of venous thromboembolism in the acute treatment phase after spinal cord injury: A randomized, multicenter trial comparing low-dose heparin plus intermittent pneumatic compression with enoxaparin. J Trauma 54:1116–1126, 2003.

15. Geerts WH, Pineo GF, Heit JA, et al: Prevention of venous thromboembolism. Chest 126:338S–400S, 2004.

16. Green D, Rossi EC, Yao JST, et al: Deep vein thrombosis in spinal cord injury: Effect of prophylaxis with calf compression, aspirin, and dipyridamole. Paraplegia 20:227–234, 1982.

17. Winemiller MH, Stolp-Smith KA, Silverstein MD, Therneau TM: Prevention of venous thromboembolism in patients with spinal cord injury: Effects of sequential pneumatic compression and heparin. J Spinal Cord Med 22:182–191, 1999.

18. Gardner AMN, Fox RH, Lawrence C, et al: Reduction of post-traumatic swelling and compartment pressure by impulse compression of the foot. J Bone Joint Surg 72-B:810–815, 1990.

19. Chouhan VD, Comerota AJ, Sun L, et al: Inhibition of tissue factor pathway during intermittent pneumatic compression. Arterioscler Thromb Vasc Biol 19:2812–2817, 1999.

20. Turpie AGG, Gallus AS, Hoek JA: A synthetic pentasaccharide for the prevention of deep-vein thrombosis after total hip replacement. N Engl J Med 344:619–625, 2001.

21. Cohen AT, Gallus AS, Lassen MR, et al: Fondaparinux vs placebo for the prevention of venous thromboembolism in acutely ill medical patients (ARTEMIS). Thromb Haemost 1 (suppl): P2046, 2003.

22. Spinal Cord Injury Thromboprophylaxis Investigators: Prevention of venous thromboembolism in the rehabilitation phase after spinal cord injury: Prophylaxis with low-dose heparin or enoxaparin. J Trauma 54:1111–1115, 2003.

23. Green D, Hull RD, Mammen EF, et al: Deep vein thrombosis in spinal cord injury: Summary and recommendations. Chest (suppl): 1992; 102:633S–635S.

24. Green D: Prophylaxis of thromboembolism in spinal cord-injured patients. Chest 102 (suppl): 649S–651S, 1994.

25. Green D, Twardowski P, Wei R, Rademaker AW: Fatal pulmonary embolism in spinal cord injury. Chest 105:853–855, 1994.

26. Wells PS, Lensing AWA, Davidson BL, et al: Accuracy of ultrasound for the diagnosis of deep venous thrombosis in asymptomatic patients after orthopedic surgery. Ann Intern Med 122:47–53, 1995.

27. Roussi J, Bentolila S, Boudaoud L, et al: Contribution of D-dimer determination in the exclusion of deep venous thrombosis in spinal cord injury patients. Spinal Cord 37:548–552, 1999.

28. Offner PJ, Hawkes A, Madayag R, et al: The role of temporary inferior vena cava liters in critically ill surgical patients. Arch Surgery 138:591–594, 2003.

29. Morris CS, Rogers FB, Najarian KE, et al: Current trends in vena caval filtration with the introduction of a retrievable filter at a level I trauma center. J Trauma 57:32–36, 2004.

30. Maxwell RA, Chavarria-Aguilar M, Cockerham WT, et al: Routine prophylatic vena cava filtration is not indicated after acute spinal cord injury. J Trauma 52:902–906, 2002.

31. Lim AC, Roth EJ, Green D: Effect of lower limb paralysis on the recanalization of deep vein thrombosis. Arch Phys Med Rehab 73:331–333, 1992.

32. Prandoni P, Lensing AWA, Prins MH, et al: Residual venous thrombosis as a predictive factor of recurrent venous thromboembolism. Ann Intern Med 87:515–522, 2002.

33. Geerts WH, Heit JA, Clagett GP, et al: Prevention of venous thromboembolism. Chest 119:132S–175S, 2001.

34. Turpie AGG, Delmore T, Hirsh J, et al: Prevention of venous thrombosis by intermittent sequential calf compression in patients with intracranial disease. Thromb Res 15:611–616, 1979.

35. Turpie AGG, Hirsh J, Gent M, et al: Prevention of deep vein thrombosis in potential neurosurgical patients. Arch Intern Med 149:679–681, 1989.

36. Begelman SM, Green D: Patients undergoing surgical resection of primary brain tumors should receive pharmacologic venous thromboprophylaxis (Antagonist's Perspective). Med Clin N Am 87:1179–1187, 2003.

37. Nurmohamed MT, van Riel AM, Henkens CMA, et al: Low molecular weight heparin and compression stockings in the prevention of venous thromboembolism in neurosurgery. Thromb Haemost 75:233–238, 1996.

38. Agnelli G, Piovella F, Buoncristiani P, et al: Enoxaparin plus compression stockings compared with compression stockings alone in the prevention of venous thromboembolism after elective neurosurgery. N Engl J Med 339:80–85, 1998.

39. Iorio A, Agnelli G: Low-molecular-weight and unfractionated heparin for prevention of venous thromboembolism in neurosurgery. Arch Intern Med 160:2327–2332, 2000.

40. Buller HR, Agnelli G, Hull RD, et al: Antithrombotic therapy for venous thromboembolic disease. Chest 126:401S–428S, 2004.

41. Lensing AWA, Prandoni P, Prins MH, Buller HR: Deep-vein thrombosis. Lancet 353:479–485, 1999.

42. Laposata M, Green D, Van Cott EM, et al: The clinical use and laboratory monitoring of low molecular weight heparin, danaparoid, hirudin and related compounds, and argatroban. Arch Path Lab Med 122:799–807, 1998.

43. Buller HR, Davidson BL, Decousus H, et al: Fondaparinux or enoxaparin for the initial treatment of symptomatic deep venous thrombosis: A randomized trial. Ann Intern Med 140:867–873, 2004.

44. Buller HR, Davidson BL, Decousus H, et al: Subcutaneous fondaparinux versus intravenous unfractionated heparin in the initial treatment of pulmonary embolism. N Engl J Med 349:1695–1702, 2003.

45. Merli G, Spiro TE, Olsson C-G, et al: Subcutaneous enoxaparin once or twice daily compared with intravenous unfractionated heparin for treatment of venous thromboembolic disease. Ann Intern Med 134:191–202, 2001.

46. Lensing AWA, Prins MH, Davidson BL, Hirsh J: Treatment of deep venous thrombosis with low-molecular-weight heparins. Arch Intern Med 155:601–607, 1995.

47. Gould MK, Dembitzer AD, Sanders GD, Garber AM: Low-molecular-weight heparins compared with unfractionated heparin for treatment of acute deep venous thrombosis: A cost-effectiveness analysis. Ann Intern Med 130:789–799, 1999.

48. Levine MN, Raskob G, Beyth RJ, et al: Hemorrhagic complications of anticoagulant treatment. Chest 126:287S–310S, 2004.

Chapter 43

Hematologic Interventions for Acute Central Nervous System Disease

Fred Rincon, MD • Andres Fernandez, MD •
Stephan A. Mayer, MD

INTRODUCTION

Acute neurologic emergencies often involve bleeding into the central nervous system (CNS) or occlusion of vessels with resultant ischemia. Thus, the application of hemostatic or antifibrinolytic agents to minimize bleeding—and anticoagulants or fibrinolytic agents to reverse thrombosis and promote perfusion—has been a common clinical challenge that frequently requires hematology expertise. Clinical scenarios involving spontaneous intracerebral hemorrhage (ICH), aneurysmal subarachnoid hemorrhage (SAH), traumatic epidural and subdural hematoma, hemorrhagic infarction, cerebral sinus thrombosis, and brain tumor–related bleeding are among the most frequent issues for the consultant. In this chapter, we review the application of hematologic interventions for a wide variety of acute neurologic conditions.

STROKE

Spontaneous Intracerebral Hemorrhage

Spontaneous intracerebral hemorrhage (ICH) accounts for 10% to 30% of all stroke admissions,[1] leading to catastrophic disability, morbidity, and the highest mortality rates. Depending on the underlying cause of hemorrhage, ICH may be classified as *primary* when it originates from the spontaneous rupture of small vessels damaged by chronic hypertension or amyloid angiopathy, representing 85% of all cases, or *secondary* when bleeding is related to a tumor, vascular malformation, hemorrhagic conversion of an ischemic stroke, abnormal coagulation,[2,3] sympathomimetic agent, trauma, or other cause.[4]

Primary ICH produces devastating neurologic disability and is by far the least treatable form of stroke. Apart from management in a specialized stroke or neurologic intensive care unit, until very recently, no specific therapies had been shown to improve outcome after ICH. ICH continues to be a health problem not only in the United States but also worldwide, with a prevalence of approximately 37,000 to 52,000 cases per year in the United States[5,6]

Differing from ischemic stroke, ICH is accompanied by a unique risk factor profile. Hypertension, particularly if untreated, is the most important risk factor for ICH,[7–9] being present in 50% to 70% of cases.[10,11] Other risk factors include advanced age,[12] male sex, African and Japanese race/ethnicity,[13,14] hypocholesterolemia,[15] high alcohol intake,[16–20] and cocaine use.[21,22] Cerebral amyloid angiopathy (CAA) is an important risk factor for primary lobar ICH in the elderly. CAA is characterized by the deposition of β-amyloid protein in small- to medium-sized blood vessels of the brain and leptomeninges, which may undergo fibrinoid necrosis as seen in chronic hypertension.[3]

Physiopathology and Rationale for Ultra-Early Hemostatic Therapy

What was formerly considered to be a simple and rapid bleeding event is now understood to be a dynamic and complex process that involves several distinct phases. Initially, it was believed that the bleeding associated with ICH was completed within minutes of the ictus, and that the following neurologic derangement observed during the first day after the bleed was attributed to cerebral edema and mass effect around the hemorrhage.[23] However, more recent data from pathologic studies, computed tomography (CT) analysis, and clinical observations suggest that early hematoma growth occurs as a result of "ultra-early rebleeding" during the first 3 to 6 hours after onset (Fig. 43-1). Evidence from studies employing histopathology, CT analysis, single-photon emission computed tomography (SPECT), and both conventional CT and CT angiography (CTA) suggests that secondary multifocal bleeding into the tissue at the periphery of an existing clot as a possible mechanism of early hematoma enlargement. Brain tissue samples from ICH patients have confirmed the presence of microscopic bleeds in brain tissue surrounding the hematoma, representing congested and ruptured venules or arterioles.[24] Other studies employing simultaneous CT and SPECT analysis have shown that in some cases, early hematoma growth relates to secondary bleeding in the periphery of the existing clot into ischemic, congested, peri-lesional tissue.[25] The association between early hematoma growth and irregular clot morphology, which may reflect multifocal bleeding,[26] has been reported by several studies as well. In one study, the frequency of hematoma growth was greater in patients with irregularly shaped hematomas compared with those with round hematomas, and it was postulated that the irregular shape indicated bleeding from multiple arterioles.[26] In studies involving CTA immediately after ICH, active contrast extravasation into the hematoma was detected in more than 30% of

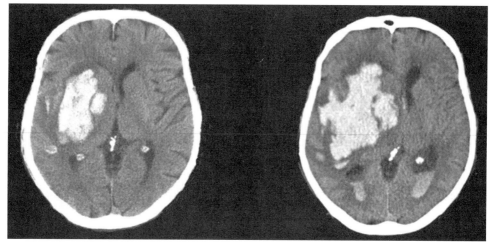

2.0 hours after onset   6.5 hours after onset

Figure 43-1 Early hematoma growth in a patient with a right putaminal intracerebral hemorrhage. The patient was subsequently declared brain dead. (Reproduced with permission from Mayer SA, Rincon F: Treatment of intracerebral haemorrhage. Lancet Neurol 4[10]:662–672, 2005.)

patients, and was associated with subsequent hematoma enlargement[27] and increased mortality.[28] Finally, simultaneous bleeding from multiple, lenticulostriate arteries has been demonstrated angiographically immediately after ICH.[29,30] These data suggest that early hematoma growth occurs because of bleeding into a congested layer of tissue that forms acutely at the periphery of the hematoma.[31]

Frequency of Early Hematoma Growth

Retrospective studies in the late 1980s using CT scan analyses of small numbers of patients[32,33] were the first to describe the phenomenon of early hematoma growth. More recent retrospective studies and a single prospective report involving larger patient populations ($n = 103$ to 627 patients) have provided further support for the occurrence of this early phenomena.[26,34–36] In these studies, patients were scanned within 3 hours of onset of ICH with 18% to 38% of individuals having early hematoma growth as evidenced by subsequent CT scans. Interestingly, the highest rate of early hematoma growth (38%) was documented in the sole prospective study and the investigators concluded that the true frequency of hematoma growth must be higher than this rate, because clinical deterioration and immediate surgical intervention precluded the performance of the follow-up scans in some of the patients.[34]

The only consistently identified predictor of early hematoma growth is the interval from the onset of symptoms to CT; the earlier the first scan is obtained, the more likely subsequent bleeding will be detected on a follow-up scan.[26,36] As a corollary, hematoma growth occurs in only 5% of patients who are initially scanned beyond 6 hours of symptom onset.[26,34,36,37] Early hematoma growth has been consistently associated with poor clinical outcomes[26,34,36,37] and higher mortality rates.[36] Similarly, significantly greater deterioration in the Glasgow Coma Scale (GCS) and National Institute of Health Stroke Scales (NIHSS) has been reported among patients with documented hematoma growth on 1-hour follow-up CT scans, compared with those without growth.[34] Hence, limiting hematoma growth represents a prime target for therapeutic intervention.

Consultation Strategies

Ventilatory support, blood pressure reduction, intracranial pressure monitoring, osmotherapy, fever control, seizure prophylaxis, and nutritional supplementation are the cornerstones of supportive care for ICH in the ICU setting.[38]

Ultra-early hemostatic therapy is a novel approach for treating ICH. When administered alone or in conjunction with surgical or neuroprotective intervention, ultra-early hemostatic therapy may have the potential to become the standard of care for ICH. Ideally, an ultra-early hemostatic medication that inhibits fibrinolysis and activates coagulation at the local level, allowing fast and effective hemostasis but without systemic adverse effects, would be the preferred agent.

Coagulation factor VII (FVII) is a naturally occurring initiator of hemostasis and its activated form (FVIIa) triggers the extrinsic coagulation pathway. Recombinant FVIIa (rFVIIa, NovoSeven; Novo Nordisk, Bagsvaerd, Denmark) is a genetically engineered human protein produced in cultured baby hamster kidney cells that is nearly identical to human plasma-derived FVIIa in structure and function. rFVIIa acts by binding to the surface of activated platelets where, in the presence of tissue factor (TF) generated at the site of the lesion, it accelerates local FXa and thrombin generation.[39] This agent was developed for the treatment of spontaneous and surgical bleeds in patients with hemophilia A or B with inhibitors to factors VIII and IX, respectively.[40] In 1999, a report of its successful use to stop what was deemed to be a lethal hemorrhage after an abdominal gunshot wound in a young soldier with no preexisting coagulopathy has prompted exploration of other uses of rFVIIa.[41] Through its action of enhancing local hemostasis after binding to exposed TF, rFVIIa has been shown recently to be an effective initiator of hemostasis in patients with a normal coagulation system.[42,43] rFVIIa has also been shown to effectively treat CNS bleeds in hemophilic patients. In one study of hemophilic patients with CNS hemorrhages, cessation of bleeding occurred in 84% of CNS bleeding episodes after administration of rFVIIa 80 to 100 µg per kilogram of body weight. Only one patient

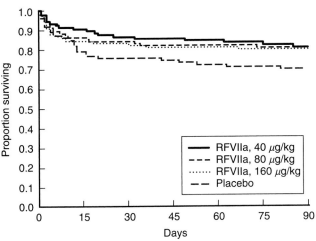

Figure 43-2 Survival at 90 days in the recombinant activated factor VII (rFVIIa) ICH trial according to study group. Survival was significantly improved with treatment ($P = 0.02$, rFVIIa combined versus placebo). (Reproduced with permission from Mayer SA, Brun N, Begtrup K, et al., for the NovoSeven ICH Trial Investigators: Recombinant activated factor VII for acute intracerebral hemorrhage. N Engl J Med 352:777–785, 2005.

died, and there were no adverse events related to rFVIIa administration.[44]

A recent phase IIB, randomized, placebo-controlled, dose-ranging study was conducted with rFVIIa in non-coagulopathic patients with ICH.[45] In that study, 399 patients with primary ICH, diagnosed by CT scan within 3 hours of onset of symptoms, were randomized to receive placebo or one of three doses of rFVIIa (40 μg per kilogram, 80 μg per kilogram, or 160 μg per kilogram body weight) within 1 hour of the baseline CT. The primary outcome of the study was change in hematoma volume at 24 hours. Secondary outcomes included clinical outcome at 3 months as measured by the Modified Rankin Scale, Barthel Index, Extended GCS, and NIHSS. The combined group of patients treated with rFVIIa had nearly 50% less hematoma growth relative to baseline than the placebo group and reduction of mortality by 38% at 3 months (Fig. 43-2). Importantly, there was also significant improvement of clinical outcomes at three months among survivors. This study posed ultra-early hemostatic therapy as a new and promising therapeutic option for ICH.[45] Currently, a phase III multicenter, multinational, randomized, placebo-controlled study, (FAST trial) is being conducted comparing placebo with doses of 20 μg per kilogram body weight and 80 μg per kilogram body weight of rFVIIa within 4 hours of ICH onset. The results of the FAST trial will be available by 2007.[46] Until these data are available, rFVIIa for spontaneous non-coagulopathic ICH should be considered investigational.

Thrombolysis for Intraventricular Hemorrhage. Intraventricular hemorrhage (IVH) commonly results from extension of ICH into the cerebral ventricular system, and is an independent predictor of mortality after ICH.[47] Commonly, hydrocephalus and IVH are managed with an external ventricular drain (EVD), but outcomes remain poor.[38] Intraventricular thrombolysis has recently been advocated for the management of IVH. Several studies have reported successful use of urokinase or tissue plasminogen activator (tPA) for the treatment of IVH, with the goal of accelerating the

clearance of IVH and improving clinical outcome.[48,49] A large multicenter randomized control trial is currently investigating the optimal dose of intravenous tPA for accelerating IVH clot lysis.[49] When used off-label, a dose of 1 mg of tPA every 8 hours (followed by clamping of the EVD for 1 hour) is reasonable until clearance of blood from the third ventricle has been achieved. Doses of 3 mg or more of tPA for IVH thrombolyis have been associated with an unacceptably high bleeding rate (Daniel Hanley, MD, personal communication).

Coagulopathic Intracranial Hemorrhage

A growing source of ICH is vitamin-K inhibitor use, which accounts for approximately 10% to 15% of ICH.[50] Long-term anticoagulation may increase the risk of ICH by tenfold.[51] Antiplatelet agent use has a risk of symptomatic bleeding complications but there is meager evidence implicating the use of single antiplatelet agent as a risk factor for ICH.[52,53] However, a combination of antiplatelet agents such as ASA and ADP-receptor blockers such as clopidogrel, carries a higher incidence of ICH.[54] Other antiplatelet agents such as the glycoprotein receptor blocking agents (GPIIb/IIIa) produce hematologic abnormalities that may put the patient at risk of bleeding as well.[55] Similarly, patients exposed to recombinant tPA for stroke or myocardial infarction have a risk of ICH of 6% to 7%[56] and 0.2% to 1.4%, respectively.[57]

Consultation Strategies

Reversal of Warfarin-Induced Coagulopathy. Warfarin (Coumadin; Bristol-Myers Squibb Co., Princeton, NJ, USA) inhibits vitamin K as a cofactor in the production of coagulation factors II, VII, IX, and X at the hepatic level. Among ICH patients, warfarin therapy doubles the risk of death and increases the risk of progressive bleeding and clinical deterioration.[58] Failure to rapidly normalize the International Normalized Ratio (INR) to below 1.4 further increases these risks.[59] ICH patients receiving warfarin should be reversed immediately with fresh frozen plasma (FFP) or prothrombin-complex concentrates (PCC), and vitamin K (Table 43-1).[60] Treatment should never be delayed in order to check coagulation tests. Unfortunately, normalization of the INR with this approach usually takes several hours, and clinical results are often poor. The associated volume load with FFP may also cause congestive heart failure in the setting of cardiac or renal disease.[61] PCC, a concentrate of the vitamin K-dependent coagulation factors II, VII, IX, and X, normalizes the INR more rapidly than FFP; it can be given in smaller volumes,[59,61] but carries the risk of triggering disseminated intravascular coagulation (DIC) in patients with severe brain injury.

Recent reports have described the off-label use of rFVIIa to speed the reversal of warfarin anticoagulation in ICH patients.[62,63] A single intravenous injection of any dose of rFVIIa can normalize the INR within minutes, with larger doses producing a longer duration of effect (Fig. 43-3).[64] rFVIIa in doses ranging from 10 to 90 μg per kilogram of body weight has been used to reverse the effects of warfarin in acute ICH, primarily to expedite neurosurgical intervention, with good clinical results.[62,64] When this approach is used, rFVIIa should be used as an adjunct to coagulation

Table 43-1 Emergency Management of the Coagulopathic ICH Patient

Scenario	Agent	Dose	Comments	Level of Evidence*
Warfarin	Fresh frozen plasma (FFP) or	15 mL/kg	Usually 4 to 6 U (200 mL) each are given	II
	Prothrombin complex concentrate and	15–30 U/kg	Works faster than FFP, but carries risk of DIC	II
	IV Vitamin K	10 mg	Can take up to 24 hours to normalize INR	II
Warfarin and emergency neurosurgical intervention	Above plus Recombinant factor VIIa	20–80 μg/kg	Contraindicated in acute thromboembolic disease	III
Unfractionated or low molecular weight heparin*	Protamine sulfate	1 mg per 100 U of heparin or 1 mg of enoxaparin	Can cause flushing, bradycardia, or hypotension	III
Platelet dysfunction or thrombocytopenia	Platelet transfusion and/or	6 U	Range 4–8 U based on size; transfuse to >100,000/μL	III
	Desmopressin (DDAVP)	0.3 μg/kg	Single dose required	III

*Class I, based on one or more high-quality randomized controlled trials; Class II, based on two or more high-quality prospective or retrospective cohort studies; Class III, Case reports and series, expert opinion.
†Protamine has minimal efficacy against danaparoid or fondaparinux. DIC, disseminated intravascular coagulation; ICH, intracranial hemorrhage; INR, International Normalized Ratio; IV, intravenous; U, units.
Reproduced with permission from Mayer SA, Rincon F: Treatment of intracerebral hemorrhage. Lancet Neurol 4:662–672, 2005.

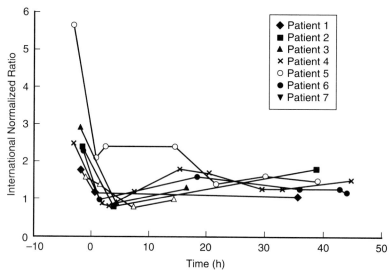

Figure 43-3 International normalized ratios before and as long as 348 hours after treatment with recombinant activated factor VII in anticoagulated patients with intracranial hemorrhage. Time zero is defined as the time of treatment. Patients also received fresh frozen plasma, vitamin K, or both. (Reproduced with permission from Freeman WD, Brott TG, Barrett KM, et al: Recombinant factor VIIa for rapid reversal of warfarin anticoagulation in acute intracranial hemorrhage. Mayo Clin Proc 79:1495–1500, 2004.)

factor replacement and vitamin K because the effect of rFVIIa will last only several hours.[61]

The safety of rFVIIa for warfarin-associated ICH in patients at high risk for thromboembolic complications, such as atrial fibrillation or a mechanical heart valve, has been a matter of intense debate. No definitive data exist on this topic, but several authors have reported the successful use of rFVIIa in this setting.[62,65] The dosages of rFVIIa in these case reports have ranged from 20 to 80 μg per kilogram of body weight. The recently published data from the NovoSeven ICH trial[45] provides some reference data in a moderate-risk population. In this study, the frequency of arterial thromboembolic serious adverse events (SAEs) was 5% in the 303 rFVIIa-treated patients compared with 0% in 96 placebo-treated patients ($P = 0.01$). These SAEs included seven myocardial ischemic events and nine cases of cerebral infarction that typically occurred within 4 days of dosing. However, fatal or disabling thromboembolic SAEs that were considered possibly or probably related to the treatment occurred in exactly 2% of the placebo and rFVIIa-treated patients. Secondary analyses of the trial data revealed that the risk of thromboembolic SAEs is higher when doses exceeding 120 μg per kilogram of body weight are used, but not when patients reported a history of remote thromboembolic disease.[66] Based on these data, it is our opinion that when rFVIIa is used to reverse a coagulopathy in a patient with intracranial bleeding, smaller doses (40 to 80 μg per kilogram body weight) should be used, and a remote history of thromboembolic disease should not be considered an absolute contraindication to its use.

Timing of Reinstitution of Anticoagulation. Patients with ICH receiving long-term anticoagulant therapy for atrial fibrillation (AF) and mechanical valve replacement present a challenging therapeutic scenario because normalizing the INR increases the risk of embolic stroke.[67] Roughly, the incidence of major embolization in otherwise healthy patients with AF is 4% and 15% per patient-year for non-valvular and valvular AF, respectively.[68] It is higher in older or hypertensive patients and especially so in patients with prior embolic stroke. For patients with mechanical valves the incidence of major embolization (resulting in death or a persistent neurologic deficit) is 4% to 20% per patient-year in the absence of antithrombotic therapy. The risk of embolization is increased with mitral-valve prostheses, caged-ball valves, and multiple prosthetic valves.[69] In all of these patients, there is a compelling argument to resume anticoagulation fairly soon after stabilization of a CNS bleed.

Re-initiation of anticoagulation is best performed when clinical and radiologic stability has been achieved, but this approach poses a therapeutic dilemma. In order to clarify both the benefit of anticoagulation after ICH in high-risk patients, Eckman and colleagues developed a decision model to estimate the best clinical decision.[70] For patients with prior lobar ICH suggestive of amyloid angiopathy, withholding anticoagulation therapy indefinitely was the most beneficial strategy for improving quality-adjusted life expectancy. In sensitivity analyses for patients with deep ICH, anticoagulation could be considered if the risk of thromboembolic stroke is particularly high. They concluded that survivors of lobar ICH with AF should not be offered long-term anticoagulation and most patients with deep hemispheric ICH and AF should not receive anticoagulant therapy. However, patients with deep hemispheric ICH at particularly high risk for thromboembolic stroke or low risk of ICH recurrence (i.e., with excellent blood pressure control) might benefit from resuming long-term anticoagulation.[70]

A recent retrospective review investigated the risk of thromboembolism after withholding or reversing the effect of warfarin therapy following a major hemorrhage in patients with prosthetic heart valves. In total, 27 patients were included, 2 patients suffered ICH. The mean time of warfarin withholding was 15 ± 4 days and none of these patients had thromboembolic events during this period.[71] When warfarin is restarted after a major ICH, it can usually safely be started 7 to 14 days after onset.

Heparin-Induced Coagulopathy. Heparin produces an anticoagulant effect by attaching to and upregulating the activity of the plasma protein antithrombin III (ATIII). The ATIII:heparin complex rapidly interacts with circulating thrombin, inhibiting several other circulating coagulation proteases. There may be a slight antiplatelet effect induced by interaction with von Willebrand factor (VWF). Reversal of heparin effect depends on the administered dose.

Normally, the half-life of heparin is 2 hours and in cases of minor non-CNS hemorrhages, the infusion can simply be stopped. In the case of a neurologic or neurosurgical bleeding emergency, use of protamine sulfate is often indicated (see Table 43-1).

Low Molecular Weight Heparin–Induced Coagulopathy. Two commercial low molecular weight heparin (LMWH) preparations are available in the United States: enoxaparin (Lovenox; Rhone-Poulenc Rorer Pharmaceuticals, Collegeville, Pa., USA) and dalteparin (Fragmin; Pharmacia & Upjohn, Kalamazoo, Mich., USA). The mechanism of action of LMWH involves inhibition of activated factor X (Xa) during clot formation. This effect may last 4 to 12 hours after a single dose. Partial reversal of LMWH–induced coagulopathy can be achieved by administration of protamine sulfate at recommended doses (see Table 43-1).

Direct Thrombin Inhibitor–Induced Coagulopathy. Lepidurin (Refludan; Berlex Labs., Inc, Wayne, NJ, USA), argatroban, and bivalidurin (Angiomax; The Medicines Company, Cambridge, Mass., USA) may be used in some patients with allergies or contraindications to standard anticoagulation regimens such as those with heparin-induced thrombocytopenia (HIT). These agents directly inhibit plasma thrombin and, unfortunately, no direct antidote is available for their reversal. The use of rFVIIa to enhance local thrombin production may theoretically be of benefit, but it has not been reported to date.

Acetylsalicylic Acid–and Nonsteroidal Anti-inflammatory Drug–Induced Coagulopathy. Acetylsalicylic acid (ASA) and nonsteroidal anti-inflammatory drugs (NSAIDs) block platelet cyclo-oxygenase, inhibiting production of thromboxane A_2, resulting in inhibition of platelet aggregation for up to 10 days. Theoretically, reversal of the effects of ASA and other platelet antagonists requires stopping the medication and transfusing platelets (see Table 43-1). However, this is not often performed in clinical practice because of lack of evidence that antiplatelet therapy causes a substantially increased risk of uncontrolled intracranial bleeding. A single dose of intravenous desmopressin (DDAVP) might be of benefit by promoting platelet VWF expression, but this remains speculative.

ADP Receptor Blocker–Induced Coagulopathy. Clopidogrel (Plavix) and ticlopidine (Ticlid) alter platelet aggregability by irreversibly inhibiting the surface adenosine diphosphate (ADP) binding site and by reducing ADP release from activated platelets. Similar to the use of ASA, platelet function is permanently impaired and normal platelet production allows platelet function to normalize after 7 days of withholding therapy. As is the case with other antiplatelet agents, treatment of patients with neurologic bleeding emergencies who are taking these agents with platelet transfusion and DDAVP remains untested (see Table 43-1).

GIIb/IIIa–Induced Coagulopathy. Three agents are commerically available in the United States for the management of acute coronary syndromes: abciximab (ReoPro; Eli-Lilly and Co., Indianapolis, Ind., USA), eptifibatide (Integrillin; Cor Therapeutics, San Francisco, Calif., USA), and tirofiban (Aggrastat; Merck, West Point, Pa., USA). Usually, they are administered in combination with ASA, ADP receptor blockers, and LMWH or unfractionated heparin. These

43

agents reversibly bind to the GIIb/IIIa receptor, inhibiting platelet aggregation. Primary intervention GPIIb/IIIa for CNS bleeding emergencies in patients treated with these agents include withholding the medication (which allows platelet function to recover after 48 hours for abciximab and 4 to 8 hours for eptifibatide and tirofiban), and possibly platelet transfusion and DDAVP, which again remains untested (see Table 43-1).

Thrombolytic-Induced Coagulopathy. Several available thrombolytic agents are used by cardiologists and neurologists throughout the world, including alteplase, streptokinase, urokinase, reteplase, and tenecteplase. All agents in this category produce the same anticoagulation effect by directly increasing fibrinolytic activity by the conversion of plasminogen to plasmin. These agents have a prolonged half-life and sometimes are used in association with heparin to extend its therapeutic effect. There are no demonstrated effective treatments available to reverse thrombolytic agents in the setting of CNS bleeding. Guidelines for the management of hemorrhagic complications of thrombolytic therapy published by the Stroke Council of the American Heart Association[72] recommend immediate discontinuation of the agent, coagulation profile and complete blood count testing, and cross-matching for the possible administration of cryoprecipitate, packed red blood cells, FFP, or platelets as appropriate.

Ischemic Stroke with Hemorrhagic Transformation

ICH may occur shortly after ischemic stroke. Hemorrhage into an area of ischemic infarction occurs when vessel walls are damaged by ischemia and blood then extravasates into the brain parenchyma. The transformation requires sufficient time for an ischemic lesion to develop and then partial or total reperfusion with restoration of blood flow through the vessel or by collateralization.[73,74] Large infarct size,[75] older age,[73,74] hyperglycemia,[76] sustained hypertension,[74] thromboembolic mechanism (as opposed to penetrator occlusion),[73–75] and preexisting micro-hemorrhages on magnetic resonance imaging (MRI)[77] have been identified as risk factors for hemorrhagic conversion of an infarct. Small asymptomatic petechiae are less important than frank hematomas, which may be associated with neurologic decline. Early administration of anticoagulants is also associated with an increase in the risk of clinically detectable hemorrhages.[78] In general, spontaneous hemorrhagic conversion after ischemic stroke occurs in 0.6% to 5% of patients admitted to the hospital.[56,79,80] Management of spontaneous hemorrhagic transformations depends on the amount of blood extravasated and clinical symptoms.

Consultation Strategies

Hemorrhagic transformation may be asymptomatic and its management follows similar principles of those for ischemic stroke. Excessive hypertension and hyperglycemia should be avoided and surgical evacuation may be indicated for a life-threatening ICH. When diagnosed by CT or MRI, prompt discontinuation of antiplatelet agents or anticoagulation is indicated. Continuation of anticoagulation in these patients has been proved safe in small case

series when asymptomatic petechial hemorrhage is present,[81,82] but to justify this approach, the indication to continue anticoagulation must be extremely compelling.

Ischemic Stroke after Spontaneous Arterial Dissection

Spontaneous cervicocerebral dissections account for approximately 2% of all ischemic strokes, but may account for more than 20% of strokes in children and young adults. Population-based studies have determined that the incidence of dissections is about 2.6 to 2.9 cases per 100,000 patients per year. The annual incidence of extracranial internal carotid (ICA) dissection is 3.5 cases per 100,000. Extracranial vertebral artery (VA) dissection is less common, accounting for up to 15% of reported cases, whereas intracranial VA dissection accounts for 5% of cases.[83] Observational studies indicate that the risk of recurrent thromboembolism during the first year after symptomatic cervicocranial arterial dissection is approximately 0.9% to 1.8%,[84] and that the greatest risk occurs in the first 30 days.

Consultation Strategies

The treatment of spontaneous extracranial cerebrovascular dissections is controversial and currently there is no controlled clinical trial evaluating the role of anticoagulation for preventing recurrent thromboembolism. In 2003, a Cochrane Review of the use of antithrombotic drugs for carotid artery dissection found no evidence to support routine use of anticoagulation or antiplatelet agents in this setting.[85] Therefore, treatment is based on clinical observations and expert opinions. Acute symptomatic extracranial dissections are commonly managed with full-dose heparin anticoagulant therapy (target PTT 2.0 to 2.5 times normal) and subsequent warfarin therapy (target INR 2.0 to 3.0) for 3 to 6 months. Therapy is monitored in stable patients every 3 months with noninvasive tests such as vascular ultrasound or magnetic resonance angiography (MRA). If at 3 months, noninvasive tests show resolution of dissection, then antiplatelet (usually ASA) therapy is instituted after discontinuation of warfarin. If noninvasive testing shows no reconstitution of the dissection, warfarin is continued for an additional 3 months.[83] At 6 months, new assessment of the involved vessel is performed, if in any circumstance there is persistent filling defect, then lifelong antiplatelet therapy is indicated. Contraindications to the initial anticoagulation include intracranial arterial dissections associated with pseudoaneurysm formation and SAH and the presence of a large infarct with mass effect and/or hemorrhagic transformation. In these patients, a single antiplatelet agent can be used as an alternative.[83]

Cerebral Sinus Venous Thrombosis

Cerebral sinus venous thrombosis (CSVT) is a rare and frequently misdiagnosed entity with an annual incidence of 0.5 cases per 100,000 patients.[86] Acute thrombosis of intracranial venous draining systems may manifest as venous infarcts that tend to become congested and hemorrhagic in about 40% of patients.[87] The clinical presentation depends generally on the venous anatomy, but the subacute onset of headache, abnormal mental status, seizures, and papilledema is suggestive of venous sinus thrombosis.

Superior sagittal sinus thrombosis (SST) is involved in about 70% of the cases. Acute venous sinus thrombosis may be seen in patients with predisposing factors such as dehydration, infection (sepsis), prothrombotic states (hormone related, cancer, and pregnancy), inherited hypercoagulable disorders (activated protein C resistance by factor V Leiden mutation, protein C or S deficiency), inflammatory states, mechanical causes such as cerebrovenous injury such as trauma, and medications (oral contraceptives and asparaginase) (see Chapter 16).[88]

Consultation Strategies

Basic treatment includes rehydration with isotonic intravenous fluid administration, seizure prevention with antiepileptic medications, blood pressure control, and management of symptomatic mass effect and increased intracranial pressure (ICP)[38] with osmotic diuretics. In general, anticoagulation should be performed, even in the presence of hemorrhagic infarction. Small retrospective case series[89,90] and randomized prospective controlled trials[91,92] have demonstrated a nonsignificant beneficial trend toward anticoagulation in patients with CSVT. In the study by Einhaupl and colleagues a nonsignificant benefit of anticoagulation was seen in patients receiving full-dose unfractionated heparin versus placebo.[92] In a prospective randomized controlled study by de Brujin and Stam, the heparinoid nadroparin was compared with placebo in patients with CVT. This study showed a nonsignificant beneficial trend of anticoagulation with LMWH but, importantly, it demonstrated the safety of full anticoagulant therapy even in patients with ICH.[91] A recent meta-analysis involving these studies showed a nonsignificant reduction in the risk of death or dependency.[90] On the basis of these results, we suggest intravenous anticoagulation with heparin with no initial bolus to achieve a minimal but therapeutic heparin level (0.3 to 0.6 U/mL), or standard dosing of low molecular weight heparin to attain full anticoagulation.

Almost all patients with CSVT require long-term oral anticoagulation for a period of at least 3 to 6 months. Duration of long-term anticoagulation depends mainly on whether or not a sustained hypercoagulable state is present. If this is not the case (such as with pregnancy-associated CSVT), then anticoagulation usually can be safely stopped at 6 months.

Endovascular options such as mechanical thrombectomy or thrombolysis are in experimental stages but its use seems attractive and reasonably safe.[93] No randomized prospective control trial has been achieved and its efficacy cannot be assessed based on the current published data. In our opinion, endovascular treatment for CVT should be attempted only at experienced centers when the patient is deteriorating clinically while on intravenous anticoagulant therapy.

Aneurysmal Subarachnoid Hemorrhage

Aneurysmal subarachnoid hemorrhage (SAH) is a complex entity requiring expertise for both recognition and management. Throughout the history of ruptured aneurysm treatment, rebleeding has been identified as a major cause of morbidity and mortality. In past decades, when delayed surgical aneurysm treatment was the norm, a 20% incidence

of rebleeding after 2 weeks and a 30% cumulative risk after 1 month was documented if the aneurysm was left unprotected.[94,95] Currently, early aneurysm repair within 24 hours of diagnosis of SAH is practiced at most centers. However, even with aggressive strategies to clip or coil the aneurysm as soon as possible, rebleeding still occurs in nearly 7% of patients, with the majority of episodes occurring within 72 hours of the index hemorrhage.[96]

Besides rebleeding, early complications of SAH include IVH and vasospasm.[97] IVH occurs in up to 20% of SAH patients and there is strong evidence of its association with increased morbidity, mortality, and poor outcomes.[97] Up to 30% of patients with SAH experienced symptomatic delayed cerebral ischemia, mainly between days 3 to 14 after the initial hemorrhage[97]—a prominent cause of death and disability. The total amount of subarachnoid blood is a strong risk factor for vasospasm.[97] Treatment with *h*ypervolemia, *h*emodilution, and induced *h*ypertension (so called Triple-H therapy) aims to increase cerebral blood flow (CBF) and improve microcirculation by raising systolic blood pressure.

Consultation Strategies

Prevention of Rebleeding. Prevention of rebleeding is the goal before the aneurysm has been secured. This can be achieved by judicious blood pressure control and optimization of coagulopathy or platelet dysfunction if present. For coagulopathic patients, conventional use of FFP, vitamin K and/or platelet transfusions are used (see Table 43-1).

The use of synthetic lysine analogs with antifibrinolytic activity in humans[98] exerting their effect by blocking the lysine-binding site of the plasminogen molecule and displacing plasminogen from fibrin has been studied in SAH patients. In the 1970s and 1980s, before early surgical aneurysm repair was widely prevalent, many neurosurgeons treated SAH patients with antifibrinolytics for up to two weeks during the period of maximal vasospasm to prevent rebleeding prior to performing delayed surgery. Clinical trials and large observational studies indicate that these agents reduced the frequency of rebleeding, but they increased the frequency of delayed cerebral ischemia and other thrombotic complications, resulting in no overall benefit or outcome.[99–101]

More recent evidence suggests that limiting antifibrinolytic therapy to the early period after bleeding onset may be more beneficial. In a large prospective controlled trial, a brief early course of tranexamic acid (1 g every 6 hours up to 72 hours after onset, or until a definitive aneurysm repair procedure was performed) reduced early rebleeding events by 80%.[102] Based on our experience at the Neurological Intensive Care Unit of Columbia University, we give a single intravenous 4 g dose of ε-aminocaproic acid (EACA) (Amicar) followed by an infusion of 1 g per hour until the aneurysm is secured, for up to 72 hours after onset.

A single dose of rFVIIa given at the time of diagnosis of SAH to prevent rebleeding might be considered as well. However, it has not been studied as of yet in a large clinical controlled trial. Pickard and associates[103] performed a pilot study to evaluate the potential use of rFVIIa for the prevention of rebleeding in patients with good grade SAH who were not treated with early surgical repair. The study was suspended after the third rFVIIa-treated patient (who was given an 80 μg per kilogram of body weight loading dose and a 7 μg/kg/hour infusion) developed a complete middle cerebral artery territory infarct after several days of therapy. Presumably the rFVIIa triggered thrombosis in the setting of delayed cerebral vasospasm. For this reason, the use of rFVIIa to prevent aneurysm rebleeding after SAH remains investigational.

Prevention of Symptomatic Vasospasm. Intracisternal fibrinolysis is an experimental approach that aims to decrease the incidence of symptomatic vasospasm by injecting tPA into the basal cisterns to promote the clearance of subarachnoid clot. Several studies have demonstrated that this therapy might decrease the incidence of vasospasm without any change in 3-month outcomes.[104,105] Clinical experience with this technique has been relatively limited over the last decade. To date, no adequately powered randomized prospective controlled trial has evaluated the benefits of this technique over conventional management.

The use of antiplatelet agents or anticoagulants might theoretically reduce the risk of delayed ischemia from vasospasm. A small randomized trial investigating the use of aspirin after SAH has been reported, but definitive data for this approach are lacking.[106]

The presence of large amounts of IVH is a well-established risk factor for poor outcome after SAH as well as ICH. If the third and fourth ventricles are completely filled with blood, the result is acute obstructive hydrocephalus, elevated ICP, and central herniation if a ventricular drain is not placed urgently. As described previously, intraventricular fibrinolysis is an experimental approach that aims to promote the clearance of IVH by injecting tPA via the ventricular drain. This technique is currently being tested on SAH and ICH patients.

BRAIN NEOPLASMS, ANTICOAGULATION, AND CENTRAL NERVOUS SYSTEM BLEEDING DISORDERS

Hemorrhage from a brain tumor comprises 2% to 10% of all cases of secondary ICH. Primary brain tumors with potential bleeding risk include glioblastomas, large schwannomas, and hemangioblastomas. Metastatic tumors can potentially bleed as well. Those that frequently do bleed include melanoma, renal cell carcinoma, choriocarcinomas, and thyroid carcinoma.[107] Nevertheless, bleeding disorders affecting the CNS are more common in patients with hematologic malignancies than those with solid tumors. Hemorrhage into the brain parenchyma, subdural, and subarachnoid spaces may result from DIC in patients with cancer.[108] A high index of suspicion for intracranial bleeding is needed when oncologic patients complain of headaches or sudden onset of neurologic dysfunction.

Venous thromboembolism (VTE) occurs commonly in patients with brain tumors. Symptomatic VTE develops in 19% to 29% of patients with gliomas, the most common type of primary brain tumor.[109,110] Moreover, the incidence of asymptomatic VTE in the glioma population may be as high as 60%.[111] A recognized number of hemostatic and clinical factors contribute to this hypercoagulable state. Concern over the possibility of intracranial bleeding has limited the use of (low dose) prophylactic anticoagulant

therapy in this population yet the specter of requiring (high dose) therapeutic anticoagulant therapy when VTE arises (arguably one of the highest causes of morbidity and mortality in neurosurgical patients) must also be taken into calculating risk:benefit considerations. Probably more than one half of neurosurgeons will still use mechanical methods alone.[112] However, mechanical approaches such as vena caval filters have high complication and treatment failure rates in patients with intracranial malignancies (see Chapter 31). Available data suggest that anticoagulation can be used safely and effectively in most brain tumor patients. The use of LMWH or unfractionated heparin further decreases the rates of VTE as documented by a relative risk reduction of 38% reported in a recent meta-analysis (Figs. 43-4 and 43-5).[113]

For patients requiring craniotomy, the combination of LMWH at prophylactic doses plus mechanical compression devices have been proved superior in the prevention of VTE with nonsignificant risk of bleeding compared with placebo plus mechanical compression even if this approach is started within 24 hours of surgery.[114]

The PRODIGE study (Dalteparin Low Molecular Weight Heparin for Primary Prophylaxis of Venous Thromboembolism in Brain Tumour Patients), an international phase III clinical trial sponsored by the Ontario Clinical Oncology Group, is currently randomly assigning patients with high-grade gliomas to long-term LMWH (dalteparin) versus placebo to evaluate the benefits and risks of primary prophylaxis.

TRAUMA

Traumatic Brain Injury with Coagulopathy

ICH and contusional bleeding may occur after severe head trauma with coup and countre-coup lesions seen in CT scan. Small areas of hemorrhage may occur acutely or delayed at the gray-white matter junction, reflecting axonal disruption due to differential mass density. Pathologic damage of the gray-white matter junction after trauma leads to diffuse axonal injury (DAI), a condition that carries an ominous prognosis. Sometimes, severe traumatic brain injury (TBI) can lead to a systemic coagulopathic state that has been linked to systemic release of TF, resulting in DIC and an enhanced fibrinolytic state.[115,116]

Preinjury warfarin use is associated with an increased risk of morbidity and mortality in traumatized head-injury patients.[117] In a study of 380 anticoagulated patients admitted to a level I trauma service, 37 patients (10%) had intracranial injuries, 12 of whom were receiving warfarin. Mortality in the warfarin group was 33% versus 8% in a matched control group.[117]

Consultation Strategies

FFP, cryoprecipitate, platelet and red blood cell transfusions in conjunction with vitamin K remain the mainstays of therapy for the traumatized patient with coagulopathy. Anecdotal reports of rFVIIa administration suggest that this agent can safely reverse TBI-related coagulopathy and especially serve as an antidote to warfarin-induced coagulopathy in patients with active, life-threatening hemorrhage and a survivable injury. This may facilitate the timely placement of an ICP monitor for management of cerebral edema.

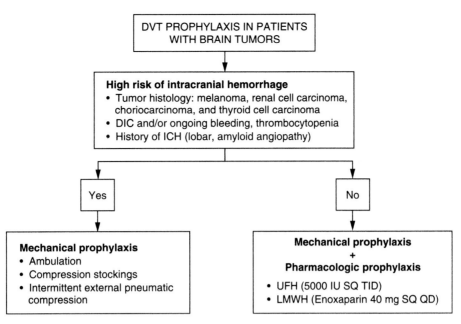

Figure 43-4 Algorithm for the deep vein thrombosis (DVT) prophylaxis in hospitalized brain tumor patients. DIC, disseminated intravascular coagulation; ICH, intracerebral hemorrhage; IU, International Units; LMWH, low molecular weight heparin; SQ, subcutaneously; TID, three times daily; UFH, unfractionated heparin.

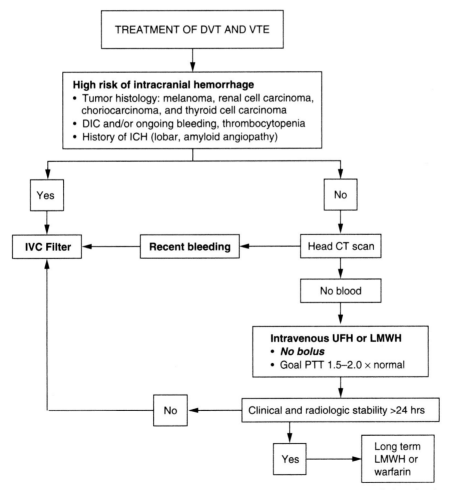

Figure 43-5 Algorithm for the treatment of acute deep vein thrombosis (DVT) or venous thromboembolism (VTE) in brain tumor patients. DIC, disseminated intravascular coagulation; ICH, intracerebral hemorrhage; LMWH, low molecular weight heparin; UFH, unfractionated heparin.

Dutton and coworkers[118] reported a series of 81 traumatized patients who received rFVIIa to stabilize ongoing bleeding. Thirty-one patients had TBI and of this group 20 patients received rFVIIa (dose 41 to 178 μg per kilogram body weight) to control bleeding related to severe TBI or dilutional coagulopathy; eight for correction of warfarin-related coagulopathy; two for multiple organ system failure (MOSF)-related coagulopathy; and one for congenital FVIII deficiency. The majority of the patients with TBI-related coagulopathy also had severe extracranial injuries and were transfused a minimum of 10 U of packed red blood cells and 8 U of FFP prior to rFVIIa treatment. All of the patients in the series had immediate improvement of their PT/INR and 75% achieved clinical hemostasis after rFVIIa administration with an overall survival rate of 42%. In the TBI subgroup, cessation of intracranial hemorrhage occurred in 90% of the patients but long-term outcomes were poor with a mortality rate of 80%. Those authors proposed a possible role of rFVIIa in contributing to inappropriate microvascular thrombosis with subsequent worsening of perfusion, and chose to subsequently limit the use of rFVIIa in this population to patients with severe coagulopathy and early risk of death from exsanguination, or for the support of potential organ donors.[118]

REVERSAL OF COAGULOPATHY BEFORE NEUROSURGICAL INTERVENTIONS

The management of subdural, epidural (intracranial or spinal), and intracerebral hemorrhages requiring rapid surgical evacuation in warfarin-treated patients is a common scenario for the consultant hematologist. By convention, but without study-derived data, most neurosurgeons prefer a documented INR value below 1.4 before they consider proceeding with a craniotomy or placement of an intracranial bolt or ventricular catheter.

Consultation Strategies

The conventional approach of vitamin K and FFP administration is limited by the long time that it takes to order and infuse FFP, and then document normalization of the INR.

Warfarin-Induced Coagulopathy. Several authors have reported on the beneficial effect of rFVIIa for rapid correction of warfarin effect prior to neurosurgical interventions.[62,119–121] rFVIIa has been used successfully in the management of anticoagulated patients with acute intracranial subdural hematomas,[62,122] spinal SAH,[62] and spinal epidural and subdural hematomas.[119,123] All patients were characterized for having a high INR on admission and received intravenous rFVIIa at doses ranging from 10 to 120 μg per kilogram of body weight. In these case reports, rFVIIa was concomitantly used with FFP and vitamin K to achieve and maintain normalization of coagulation parameters.

Miscellaneous Coagulopathic States. Successful treatment of a wide variety of coagulopathies has been reported, including liver failure,[120] dilutional coagulopathy after multiple blood transfusions,[120] DIC,[124] TBI-related coagulopathy,[125] and congenital factor VII deficiency.[124] In these reports, all patients had an elevated INR on admission, received rFVIIa at doses ranging from 10 to 120 μg per

kilogram of body weight, and tolerated the procedure well. There were no thrombotic complications reported. These reports are promising, but because of the potential for publication bias, randomized controlled trials are needed to firmly demonstrate that rFVIIa given in addition to vitamin K and FFP is more effective and as safe as the traditional approach alone, and to identify the optimal dosing regimen for this indication.

In the largest series, Roitberg and colleagues[121] administered rFVIIa to 29 patients as a second-line therapy after initial attempts at reversal with FFP had failed. Twenty-four patients treated with FFP and vitamin K alone before the introduction of rFVIIa were analyzed as control subjects. After initial FFP administration, INR tended to rebound in both groups. In the rFVIIa group, mean INR fell from 2.2 to 1.1 ($P < 0.05$) after an average of 1.4 mg of rFVIIa was given. INR in the rFVIIa group was documented as normalized within 7 hours after admission, compared with 47 hours ($P < 0.0005$) in the control group. The number of patients with good functional outcome was greater among patients treated with rFVIIa compared with those who received only vitamin K and FFP ($P = 0.04$). There were no thrombotic complications reported among the rFVIIa group.

Park and coworkers[120] performed a retrospective review of nine patients with diverse non-hemophilic coagulopathies in which rFVIIa was used in the preoperative period of urgent neurosurgical interventions. The coagulopathies consisted of three patients in anticoagulant therapy for AF, four patients with liver dysfunction, and two patients with dilutional coagulopathy after resuscitation for extensive traumatic hemorrhage. Neurosurgical indications included two patients requiring craniotomy for ICH or epidural hematoma, one patient requiring ventriculostomy for intraventricular hemorrhage, and three patients requiring an ICP monitor for diffuse cerebral edema. All patients, except two, were initially treated with FFP with no effective correction of their coagulopathy. Doses of rFVIIa ranged from 40 to 90 μg per kilogram of body weight; there were no procedure complications or thrombotic events identified. Pre-dose INRs ranged from 1.5 to 3.8, and normalization of the INR was reached in all patients as early as 20 minutes after the infusion of rFVIIa, which allowed for prompt surgical intervention.

Huang and associates[124] report three cases of patients with factor VII deficiency and associated hemorrhages of the CNS. One patient presented with multiple injuries including traumatic SAH and subdural hematoma. He initially received multiple doses of vitamin K and FFP with persistence of coagulopathy and his factor VII level was found to be 21% (reported normal level 50% to 150%). Because of concern about increase in the hematoma and worsening mental status, he was given rFVIIa at an initial dose of 95 μg per kilogram of body weight, and then at lower doses ranging from 10 to 38 μg per kilogram of body weight throughout the next several days. The patient was alert and following commands and discharged at 2 months. The second patient also presented with multiple injuries including contusions, traumatic SAH, and subdural hematoma. On admission, the patient had findings consistent with DIC and received multiple doses of FFP, red blood cells, and platelets, along with antibiotics. After 6 days, the level of factor VII was found to be 40% of normal and rFVIIa therapy was instituted at doses ranging from 45 to 60 μg per kilogram of body weight for the next 12 days.

The patient was discharged after 1 month with slight improvement in neurologic status, but not following commands. The third patient presented 2 weeks after a lumbar laminectomy with a large epidural hematoma which was surgically evacuated. On the second postoperative day from the evacuation, the factor VII level was found to be 27%. Because of continuous bleeding from the incision, rFVIIa therapy was started at 24 μg per kilogram of body weight for the following 3 days. At day 5 after surgery, the mass effect had lessened, but the hematoma persisted.

Liver Disease-Related Coagulopathy. End stage liver disease results in a complex and variably severe failure of hemostasis that predisposes to abnormal bleeding (see Chapter 39). The diverse spectrum of hemostatic defects includes impaired synthesis of clotting factors, excessive fibrinolysis, DIC (and situations mimicking DIC), thrombocytopenia, and platelet dysfunction. Attempts to correct these deficits are required, as much as can be accomplished, in the setting of CNS bleeding emergencies. FFP, cryoprecipitate, and platelet transfusions remain the mainstays of therapy. Anecdotal reports of rFVIIa administration suggest that this agent may safely reverse liver failure-related coagulopathy and facilitate the timely placement of an ICP monitor for management of cerebral edema. Larger trials testing the efficacy and safety of rFVIIa for this indication are ongoing.

REFERENCES

1. Sacco RL, Mayer SA: Epidemiology of intracerebral hemorrhage. In Feldmann E, (ed): Intracerebral Hemorrhage. Armonk, NY, Futura, 1994, pp 3–23.
2. Qureshi AI, Tuhrim S, Broderick JP, et al: Spontaneous intracerebral hemorrhage. N Engl J Med 344:1450–1460, 2001.
3. Skidmore CT, Andrefsky J: Spontaneous intracerebral hemorrhage: Epidemiology, pathophysiology, and medical management. Neurosurg Clin N Am 3:281–288, 2002.
4. Siddique MS, Gregson BA, Fernandes HM, et al: Comparative study of traumatic and spontaneous intracerebral hemorrhage. J Neurosurg 96: 2002;86–89, 2002.
5. Broderick JP, Adams HP, Jr., Barsan W, et al: Guidelines for the management of spontaneous intracerebral hemorrhage: A statement for healthcare professionals from a special writing group of the Stroke Council, American Heart Association. Stroke 30: 1999;905–915, 1999.
6. Taylor TN, Davis PH, Torner JC, et al: Lifetime cost of stroke in the United States. Stroke 27:1459–1466, 1996.
7. Foulkes MA, Wolf PA, Price TR, et al: The Stroke Data Bank: Design, methods, and baseline characteristics. Stroke 19:547–554, 1988.
8. Broderick JP, Brott T, Tomsick T: Importance of hypertension in lobar hemorrhages (Abstract). Neurology 42:181, 1992.
9. Weisberg LA, Stazio A, Shamsnia M, Elliot D: Nontraumatic parenchymal brain hemorrhages. Medicine (Baltimore) 69:277–295, 1990.
10. Wityk RJ, Caplan LR: Hypertensive intracerebral hemorrhage. Epidemiology and clinical pathology. Neurosurg Clin N Am 3: 521–532, 1992.
11. Brott T, Thalinger K, Hertzberg V: Hypertension as a risk factor for spontaneous intracerebral hemorrhage. Stroke 17:1078–1083, 1986.
12. Arboix A, Vall-Llosera A, Garcia-Eroles L, et al: Clinical features and functional outcome of intracerebral hemorrhage in patients aged 85 and older. J Am Geriatr Soc 3:449–454, 2002.
13. Broderick JP, Brott T, Tomsick T, et al: Intracerebral hemorrhage more than twice as common as subarachnoid hemorrhage. J Neurosurg 78:188–191, 1993.
14. Qureshi AI, Mohammad Y, Suri MF, et al: Cocaine use and hypertension are major risk factors for intracerebral hemorrhage in young African Americans. Ethn Dis 11:311–319, 2001.
15. Segal AZ, Chiu RI, Eggleston-Sexton PM, et al: Low cholesterol as a risk factor for primary intracerebral hemorrhage: A case-control study. Neuroepidemiology 18:185–193, 1999.
16. Gill JS, Shipley MJ, Tsementzis SA, et al: Alcohol consumption: A risk factor for hemorrhagic and non-hemorrhagic stroke. Am J Med 90:489–497, 1991.
17. Gill JS, Zezulka AV, Shipley MJ, et al: Stroke and alcohol consumption. N Engl J Med 315:1041–1046, 1986.
18. Gorelick PB: Alcohol and stroke. Stroke 18:268–271, 1987.
19. Klatsky AL, Armstrong MA, Friedman GD: Alcohol use and subsequent cerebrovascular disease hospitalizations. Stroke 6: 741–746, 1989.
20. Thrift AG, Donnan GA, McNeil JJ: Heavy drinking, but not moderate or intermediate drinking, increases the risk of intracerebral hemorrhage. Epidemiology 10:307–312, 1999.
21. Levine SR, Brust JC, Futrell N, et al: Cerebrovascular complications of the use of the "crack" form of alkaloidal cocaine. N Engl J Med 323:699–704, 1990.
22. Ariesen MJ, Claus SP, Rinkel GJ, Algra A: Risk factors for intracerebral hemorrhage in the general population: A systematic review. Stroke 34:2060–2065, 2003.
23. Kase C, Mohr JP: General Features of Intracranial Hemorrhage. New York, Churchill Livingstone, 1986, pp 497–524.
24. Fisher C: Pathological observations in hypertensive intracerebral hemorrhage. J Neuropathol Exp Neurol 30:536–550, 1971.
25. Mayer SA, Lignelli A, Fink ME, et al: Perilesional blood flow and edema formation in acute intracerebral hemorrhage: A SPECT study. Stroke 29:1791–1798, 1988.
26. Fujii Y, Tanaka R, Takeuchi S, et al: Hematoma enlargement in spontaneous intracerebral hemorrhage. J Neurosurg 80:51–57, 1994.
27. Murai Y, Takagi R, Ikeda Y, et al: Three-dimensional computerized tomography angiography in patients with hyperacute intracerebral hemorrhage. J Neurosurg 3:424–431, 1999.
28. Becker KJ, Baxter AB, Bybee HM, et al: Extravasation of radiographic contrast is an independent predictor of death in primary intracerebral hemorrhage. Stroke 10:2025–2032, 1999.
29. Komiyama M, Yasui T, Tamura K, et al: Simultaneous bleeding from multiple lenticulostriate arteries in hypertensive intracerebral haemorrhage. Neuroradiology 2:129–130, 1995.
30. Mizukami M, Araki G, Mihara H, et al: Arteriographically visualized extravasation in hypertensive intracerebral hemorrhage: Report of seven cases. Stroke 3:527–537, 1972.
31. Takasugi S, Ueda S, Matsumoto K: Chronological changes in spontaneous intracerebral hematoma: An experimental and clinical study. Stroke 16:651–658, 1985.
32. Broderick JP, Brott TG, Tomsick T, et al: Ultra-early evaluation of intracerebral hemorrhage. J Neurosurg 72:195–199, 1990.
33. Chen ST, Chen SD, Hsu CY, Hogan EL: Progression of hypertensive intracerebral hemorrhage. Neurology 39:1509–1514, 1989.
34. Brott T, Broderick J, Kothari R, et al: Early hemorrhage growth in patients with intracerebral hemorrhage. Stroke 28:1–5, 1997.
35. Fujitsu K, Muramoto M, Ikeda Y, et al: Indications for surgical treatment of putaminal hemorrhage: Comparative study based on serial CT and time-course analysis. J Neurosurg 73:518–525, 1990.
36. Kazui S, Naritomi H, Yamamoto H, et al: Enlargement of spontaneous intracerebral hemorrhage: Incidence and time course. Stroke 27:1783–1787, 1996.
37. Fujii Y, Takeuchi S, Sasaki O, et al: Multivariate analysis of predictors of hematoma enlargement in spontaneous intracerebral hemorrhage. Stroke 29:1160–1166, 1998.
38. Mayer SA, Rincon F: Treatment of intracerebral haemorrhage. Lancet Neurol 4:662–672, 2005.
39. Monroe DM, Hoffman M, Oliver JA, Roberts HR: Platelet activity of high-dose factor VIIa is independent of tissue factor. Br J Haematol 99:542–547, 1997.
40. Key NS, Aledort LM, Beardsley D, et al: Home treatment of mild to moderate bleeding episodes using recombinant factor VIIa (NovoSeven) in haemophiliacs with inhibitors. Thromb Haemost 80:912–918, 1998.
41. Kenet G, Walden R, Eldad A, Martinowitz U: Treatment of traumatic bleeding with recombinant factor VIIa. Lancet 354:1879, 1999.
42. Hedner U: Recombinant activated factor VII as a universal haemostatic agent. Blood Coagul Fibrinolysis (Suppl 1): 1998;S147–S152.
43. Hedner U, Ingerslev J: Clinical use of recombinant FVIIa (rFVIIa). Transfus Sci 2:163–176, 1998.
44. Rice KM, Savidge GF: NovoSeven (recombinant factor VIIa) in central nervous systems bleeds. Haemostasis 26(Suppl 1):131–144, 1996.
45. Mayer SA, Brun NC, Begtrup K, et al: Recombinant activated factor VII for acute intracerebral hemorrhage. N Engl J Med 352:777–785, 2005.

46. Recombinant Factor VIIa in Acute Intracerebral Hemorrhage. [cited 2005; Available from: *http://www.clinicaltrials.gov/ct/show/NCT00127283? order=1*].

47. Hemphill JC, 3rd, Bonovich DC, Besmertis L, et al: The ICH score: A simple, reliable grading scale for intracerebral hemorrhage. Stroke 32:891–897, 2001.

48. Coplin WM, Vinas FC, Agris JM, et al: A cohort study of the safety and feasibility of intraventricular urokinase for nonaneurysmal spontaneous intraventricular hemorrhage. Stroke 29:1573–1579, 1998.

49. Daniel F, Hanley M Clear IVH Trial. [cited; Available from: *http://www.neuro.jhmi.edu/ivh*].

50. The Stroke Prevention in Reversible Ischemia Trial (SPIRIT) Study Group: A randomized trial of anticoagulants versus aspirin after cerebral ischemia of presumed arterial origin. Ann Neurol 42:857–865, 1997.

51. Wintzen AR, de Jonge H, Loeliger EA, Bots GT: The risk of intracerebral hemorrhage during oral anticoagulant therapy: A population study. Ann Neurol 16:553–558, 1984.

52. Johnsen SP, Pedersen L, Friis S, et al: Nonaspirin nonsteroidal anti-inflammatory drugs and risk of hospitalization for intracerebral hemorrhage: A population-based case-control study. Stroke 34:387–391, 2003.

53. Saloheimo P, Juvela S, Hillbom M: Use of aspirin, epistaxis, and untreated hypertension as risk factors for primary intracerebral hemorrhage in middle-aged and elderly people. Stroke 32:399–404, 2001.

54. Diener HC, Bogousslavsky J, Brass LM, et al: Aspirin and clopidogrel compared with clopidogrel alone after recent ischaemic stroke or transient ischaemic attack in high-risk patients (MATCH): Randomised, double-blind, placebo-controlled trial. Lancet 30;364: 331–337, 2004.

55. Rosove MH: Platelet glycoprotein IIb/IIIa inhibitors. Best Pract Res Clin Haematol 17:65–76, 2004.

56. The National Institute of Neurological Disorders and Stroke rt-PA Stroke Study Group: Tissue plasminogen activator for acute ischemic stroke. N Engl J Med 14; 333:1581–1587, 1995.

57. De Jaegere PP, Arnold AA, Balk AH, Simoons ML: Intracranial hemorrhage in association with thrombolytic therapy: Incidence and clinical predictive factors. J Am Coll Cardiol 2:289–294, 1992.

58. Hart RG, Boop BS, Anderson DC: Oral anticoagulants and intracranial hemorrhage. Facts and hypotheses. Stroke 26:1471–1477, 1995.

59. Fredriksson K, Norrving B, Stromblad LG: Emergency reversal of anticoagulation after intracerebral hemorrhage. Stroke 23:972–977, 1992.

60. Heit JA: Perioperative management of the chronically anticoagulated patient. J Thromb Thrombolysis 12:81–87, 2001.

61. Hart RG: Management of warfarin associated intracerebral hemorrhage. In Rose BD (ed): UpToDate. Wellesley, Mass., UpToDate, 2005.

62. Sorensen B, Johansen P, Nielsen GL, et al: Reversal of the International Normalized Ratio with recombinant activated factor VII in central nervous system bleeding during warfarin thromboprophylaxis: Clinical and biochemical aspects. Blood Coagul Fibrinolysis 14:469–477, 2003.

63. Erhardtsen E, Nony P, Dechavanne M, et al: The effect of recombinant factor VIIa (NovoSeven) in healthy volunteers receiving acenocoumarol to an International Normalized Ratio above 2.0. Blood Coagul Fibrinolysis 9:741–748, 1998.

64. Freeman WD, Brott TG, Barrett KM, et al: Recombinant factor VIIa for rapid reversal of warfarin anticoagulation in acute intracranial hemorrhage. Mayo Clin Proc 79:1495–1500, 2004.

65. Conti S, La Torre D, Gambelunghe G, et al: Successful treatment with rFVIIa of spontaneous intracerebral hemorrhage in a patient with mechanical prosthetic heart valves. Clin Lab Haematol 27:283–285, 2005.

66. Diringer M, Mayer S, Brun N, et al: On behalf of the NovoSeven ICH Trial Investigators: Safety profile of recombinant factor VIIa in patients with intracerebral hemorrhage. Stroke 37:623, 2006.

67. Cannegieter SC, Rosendaal FR, Briet E: Thromboembolic and bleeding complications in patients with mechanical heart valve prostheses. Circulation 89:635–641, 1994.

68. Risk factors for stroke and efficacy of antithrombotic therapy in atrial fibrillation. Analysis of pooled data from five randomized controlled trials. Arch Intern Med 154:1449–1457, 1994.

69. Vongpatanasin W, Hillis LD, Lange RA: Prosthetic heart valves. N Engl J Med 335:407–416, 1996.

70. Eckman MH, Rosand J, Knudsen KA, et al: Can patients be anticoagulated after intracerebral hemorrhage? A decision analysis. Stroke 34:1710–1716, 2003.

71. Ananthasubramaniam K, Beattie JN, Rosman HS, et al: How safely and for how long can warfarin therapy be withheld in prosthetic heart valve patients hospitalized with a major hemorrhage? Chest 119:478–484, 2001.

72. Adams HS, Jr., Brott TG, Furlan AJ, et al: Guidelines for Thrombolytic Therapy for Acute Stroke: A supplement to the guidelines for the management of patients with acute ischemic stroke. A statement for healthcare professionals from a Special Writing Group of the Stroke Council, American Heart Association. Stroke 9:1711–1718, 1996.

73. Hamann GF, del Zoppo GJ, von Kummer R: Hemorrhagic transformation of cerebral infarction: Possible mechanisms. Thromb Haemost 82(Suppl 1):92–94, 1999.

74. Lyden PD, Zivin JA: Hemorrhagic transformation after cerebral ischemia: Mechanisms and incidence. Cerebrovasc Brain Metab Rev 5:1–16, 1993.

75. Hain RF, Westhaysen PV, Swank RL: Hemorrhagic cerebral infarction by arterial occlusion: An experimental study. J Neuropathol Exp Neurol 11:34–43, 1952.

76. Broderick JP, Hagen T, Brott T, Tomsick T: Hyperglycemia and hemorrhagic transformation of cerebral infarcts. Stroke 26:484–487, 1995.

77. Nighoghossian N, Hermier M, Adeleine P, et al: Old microbleeds are a potential risk factor for cerebral bleeding after ischemic stroke: A gradient-echo T2*-weighted brain MRI study. Stroke 33:735–742, 2002.

78. CAST (Chinese Acute Stroke Trial) Collaborative Group: Randomised placebo-controlled trial of early aspirin use in 20,000 patients with acute ischaemic stroke. Lancet 349:1641–1649, 1997.

79. Hacke W, Kaste M, Fieschi C, et al: Randomised double-blind placebo-controlled trial of thrombolytic therapy with intravenous alteplase in acute ischaemic stroke (ECASS II). Second European-Australasian Acute Stroke Study Investigators. Lancet 352: 1245–1251, 1998.

80. Hornig CR, Dorndorf W, Agnoli AL: Hemorrhagic cerebral infarction: A prospective study. Stroke 17(2):179–185, 1986.

81. Ott BR, Zamani A, Kleefield J, Funkenstein HH: The clinical spectrum of hemorrhagic infarction. Stroke 17:630–637, 1986.

82. Pessin MS, Estol CJ, Lafranchise F, Caplan LR: Safety of anticoagulation after hemorrhagic infarction. Neurology 43:1298–1303, 1993.

83. Zweifler RM, Silverboard G: Arterial dissections, 4th ed. Philadelphia, Churchill Livingstone, 2004, pp 549–573.

84. Touze E, Gauvrit JY, Moulin T, et al: Risk of stroke and recurrent dissection after a cervical artery dissection: A multicenter study. Neurology 61:1347–1351, 2003.

85. Lyrer P, Engelter S: Antithrombotic drugs for carotid artery dissection. Cochrane Database Syst Rev (3): CD000255, 2003.

86. Georgiadis D, Schwab S, Hacke W: Critical care of the patient with acute stroke, 4th ed. Philadelphia, Churchill Livingstone, 2005, pp 987–1024.

87. Ferro JM, Canhao P, Stam J, et al: Prognosis of cerebral vein and dural sinus thrombosis: Results of the International Study on Cerebral Vein and Dural Sinus Thrombosis (ISCVT). Stroke 35: 664–670, 2004.

88. Stam J: Thrombosis of the cerebral veins and sinuses. N Engl J Med 352:1791–1798, 2005.

89. Erbguth F, Brenner P, Schuierer G, et al: Diagnosis and treatment of deep cerebral vein thrombosis. Neurosurg Rev 14:145–148, 1991.

90. Stam J, De Bruijn SF, DeVeber G: Anticoagulation for cerebral sinus thrombosis. Cochrane Database Syst Rev (4):CD002005, 2002.

91. de Bruijn SF, Stam J: Randomized, placebo-controlled trial of anticoagulant treatment with low-molecular-weight heparin for cerebral sinus thrombosis. Stroke 30:484–488, 1999.

92. Einhaupl KM, Villringer A, Meister W, et al: Heparin treatment in sinus venous thrombosis. Lancet 338:597–600, 1991.

93. Canhao P, Falcao F, Ferro JM: Thrombolytics for cerebral sinus thrombosis: A systematic review. Cerebrovasc Dis 15:159–166, 2003.

94. Broderick JP, Brott TG, Duldner JE, et al: Initial and recurrent bleeding are the major causes of death following subarachnoid hemorrhage. Stroke 25:1342–1347, 1994.

95. Chyatte D, Fode NC, Sundt TM Jr: Early versus late intracranial aneurysm surgery in subarachnoid hemorrhage. J Neurosurg 69:326–331, 1988.

96. Naidech AM, Janjua N, Kreiter KT, et al: Predictors and impact of aneurysm rebleeding after subarachnoid hemorrhage. Arch Neurol 62:410–416, 2005.

97. Claassen J, Bernardini GL, Kreiter K, et al: Effect of cisternal and ventricular blood on risk of delayed cerebral ischemia after subarachnoid hemorrhage: The Fisher scale revisited. Stroke 32:2012–2020, 2001.

98. Mannucci PM: Hemostatic drugs. N Engl J Med 339:245–253, 1998.

99. Kassell NF, Torner JC, Adams HP, Jr: Antifibrinolytic therapy in the acute period following aneurysmal subarachnoid hemorrhage. Preliminary observations from the Cooperative Aneurysm Study. J Neurosurg 61:225–230, 1984.

100. Tsementzis SA, Hitchcock ER, Meyer CH: Benefits and risks of antifibrinolytic therapy in the management of ruptured intracranial aneurysms: A double-blind placebo-controlled study. Acta Neurochir (Wien) 102:1–10, 1990.

101. Vermeulen M, Lindsay KW, Murray GD, et al: Antifibrinolytic treatment in subarachnoid hemorrhage. N Engl J Med 311:432–437, 1984.

102. Hillman J, Fridriksson S, Nilsson O, et al: Immediate administration of tranexamic acid and reduced incidence of early rebleeding after aneurysmal subarachnoid hemorrhage: A prospective randomized study. J Neurosurg 97:771–778, 2002.

103. Pickard JD, Kirkpatrick PJ, Melsen T, et al: Potential role of NovoSeven in the prevention of rebleeding following aneurysmal subarachnoid haemorrhage. Blood Coagul Fibrinolysis 11(Suppl 1): S117–120, 2000.

104. Findlay JM, Weir BK, Kassell Nf, et al: Intracisternal recombinant tissue plasminogen activator after aneurysmal subarachnoid hemorrhage. J Neurosurg 75:181–188, 1991.

105. Zabramski JM, Spetzler RF, Lee KS, et al: Phase I trial of tissue plasminogen activator for the prevention of vasospasm in patients with aneurysmal subarachnoid hemorrhage. J Neurosurg 75: 189–196, 1991.

106. Hop JW, Rinkel GJ, Algra A, et al: Randomized pilot trial of postoperative aspirin in subarachnoid hemorrhage. Neurology 54:872–878, 2000.

107. Weisberg LA: Hemorrhagic metastatic intracranial neoplasms: Clinical-computed tomographic correlations. Comput Radiol 9: 105–114, 1985.

108. Rogers LR: Cerebrovascular complications in patients with cancer. Semin Neurol 24:453–460, 2004.

109. Quevedo JF, Buckner JC, Schmidt JL, et al: Thromboembolism in patients with high-grade glioma. Mayo Clin Proc 69:329–332, 1994.

110. Ruff RL, Posner JB: Incidence and treatment of peripheral venous thrombosis in patients with glioma. Ann Neurol 13:334–336, 1983.

111. Sawaya R, Zuccarello M, Elkalliny M, Nishiyama H: Postoperative venous thromboembolism and brain tumors: Part I. Clinical profile. J Neurooncol 14:119–125, 1992.

112. Carman TL, Kanner AA, Barnett GH, Deitcher SR: Prevention of thromboembolism after neurosurgery for brain and spinal tumors. South Med J 96:17–22, 2003.

113. Iorio A, Agnelli G: Low-molecular-weight and unfractionated heparin for prevention of venous thromboembolism in neurosurgery: A meta-analysis. Arch Intern Med 160:2327–2332, 2000.

114. Agnelli G, Piovella F, Buoncristiani P, et al: Enoxaparin plus compression stockings compared with compression stockings alone in the prevention of venous thromboembolism after elective neurosurgery. N Engl J Med 339:80–85, 1998.

115. Kaufman HH, Moake JL, Olson JD, et al: Delayed and recurrent intracranial hematomas related to disseminated intravascular clotting and fibrinolysis in head injury. Neurosurgery 7:445–449, 1980.

116. van der Sande JJ, Veltkamp JJ, Boekhout-Mussert RJ, et al: Head injury and coagulation disorders. J Neurosurg 49:357–365, 1978.

117. Mina AA, Bair HA, Howells GA, Bendick PJ: Complications of preinjury warfarin use in the trauma patient. J Trauma 54:842–847, 2003.

118. Dutton RP, McCunn M, Hyder M, et al: Factor VIIa for correction of traumatic coagulopathy. J Trauma 57:709–718, 2004.

119. Lin J, Hanigan WC, Tarantino M, Wang J: The use of recombinant activated factor VII to reverse warfarin-induced anticoagulation in patients with hemorrhages in the central nervous system: Preliminary findings. J Neurosurg 98:737–740, 2003.

120. Park P, Fewel ME, Garton HJ, et al: Recombinant activated factor VII for the rapid correction of coagulopathy in nonhemophilic neurosurgical patients. Neurosurgery 53:34–38, 2003.

121. Roitberg B, Emechebe-Kennedy O, et al: Human recombinant factor VII for emergency reversal of coagulopathy in neurosurgical patients: A retrospective comparative study. Neurosurgery 57:832–836, 2005.

122. Veshchev I, Elran H, Salame K: Recombinant coagulation factor VIIa for rapid preoperative correction of warfarin-related coagulopathy in patients with acute subdural hematoma. Med Sci Monit 8:CS98–100, 2002.

123. Szabo T, Ali S, Camporesi EM: Intraoperative recombinant activated factor VII for emergent epidural hematoma evacuation. Anesth Analg 99:595–597, 2004.

124. Huang WY, Kruskall MS, Bauer KA, et al: The use of recombinant activated factor VII in three patients with central nervous system hemorrhages associated with factor VII deficiency. Transfusion 44:1562–1566, 2004.

125. Morenski JD, Tobias JD, Jimenez DF: Recombinant activated factor VII for cerebral injury-induced coagulopathy in pediatric patients: Report of three cases and review of the literature. J Neurosurg 98:611–616, 2003.

43

Chapter 44

Atrial Septal Abnormalities and Cryptogenic Stroke

Peter C. Block, MD

BACKGROUND

Atrial septal abnormalities (patent foramen ovale [PFO] and/or atrial septal aneurysm [ASA]) occur in up to 20% of the general population, and the link of PFO to patients with cryptogenic stroke may be twice that number. Whether this association has pathophysiologic significance is debated, but most theories suggest a central role for thrombosis and embolization. Thus, aspirin and warfarin are the first line of medical therapy, and a variety of secondary prevention studies have assessed their impact on stroke recurrence. The evaluation of any patient with cryptogenic stroke must rule out other established factors that may cause stroke (carotid stenosis, atrial fibrillation) or contribute to the chance of thromboembolism (hypercoagulable states).

There is no doubt that patients with isolated PFO or atrial septal aneurysm and a first ischemic stroke respond well to either aspirin or warfarin therapy. Aspirin or oral anticoagulation with warfarin is the U.S. Federal Drug Administration (FDA) current recommendation for therapy. PFO closure is FDA indicated only if a second event occurs during adequate anticoagulation or antiplatelet therapy. Despite these guidelines, many patients with a first cryptogenic stroke undergo percutaneous PFO closure. All of these therapies are effective in reducing stroke recurrence, yet all are also associated with some risk. Thus, the correct choice of therapy for individual patients is controversial. In the absence of randomized controlled trials comparing medical therapy and percutaneous closure, the decision for a therapeutic strategy should be done in conjunction with the patient, while considering the individual patient's clinical presentation, risk profile, occupation, choices, and lifestyle.

INTRODUCTION

More than 700,000 new or recurrent stroke cases are diagnosed annually in the United States.[1] Most are ischemic in origin and occur in older patients in association with atrial fibrillation, hypertension, smoking, hyperlipidemia, and diabetes. However, approximately 40% of ischemic strokes are cryptogenic[2] and occur in patients younger than 55 years of age. In such patients, there is frequently an association with atrial septal abnormalities, leading to speculation that there is a causal relationship.

In utero, the cranial remnant of the septum primum covers the foramen ovale and acts as a one-way valve allowing placental, oxygenated blood to flow from the right to left atrium.[3,4] At birth, the lungs expand and pressure in the pulmonary circuit falls. As a consequence, the higher pressure in the left atrium pushes the septum primum against the septum secundum, closing the foramen ovale. The septum primum and the caudal part of the septum secundum then fuse. However, if fusion does not occur or is incomplete, patency of the foramen ovale may persist into adulthood. Transient right-to-left blood flow in such individuals can be induced by a variety of maneuvers and pathologic changes, the most common being a simple Valsalva maneuver. In addition, the cranial portion of the septum primum can be thin and have redundancy and hypermobility. Such an atrial septal aneurysm is identified if septal excursion is >10 mm with a base diameter of more than 15 mm.[5,6] Thrombi might potentially form in the redundant areas of the atrial septal aneurysm or the aneurysm may promote right-to-left blood flow by producing a current effect through the foramen ovale. If the foramen is not overlapped completely or if the septum secundum is incomplete, there is a persistent opening in the atrial septum. Because left atrial pressure normally exceeds right atrial pressure, blood flow is left-to-right through such an atrial septal defect, but may also transiently or permanently become right-to-left if changes in the atrial pressure relationships occur.

STROKE RISK

The potential role of atrial septal abnormalities in the pathogenesis of stroke is supported by an increased prevalence of PFO in patients with cryptogenic stroke compared with controls. In the general population, PFO is present in 9% to 27%.[7–10] In patients with cryptogenic stroke, PFO was found in 42% to 54%, with the strongest association noted in patients ≤55 years of age.[11,12] A meta-analysis of nine case-control studies showed a fivefold increase in the risk of stroke in patients with atrial septal aneurysm, and the strongest correlation was noted with the combination of both PFO and atrial septal aneurysm in patients ≤55 years of age.[5] Mas and colleagues[13] reported an association between interatrial septal abnormalities and stroke recurrence rates in patients (mean age 40 years) with cryptogenic stroke on aspirin, but the risk of recurrent events was only significantly increased in patients with both PFO and atrial septal aneurysm. There is speculation, therefore, that the motion of the aneurysm could favor the movement into the systemic arterial circulation of thrombi formed locally in the PFO or traveling from more distant sites in the venous circulation. The mechanisms remain speculative and appear contradicted in some clinical studies. Homma and colleagues failed to demonstrate an increased risk of recurrence in patients with combined PFO/atrial septal aneurysm compared with those with either abnormality alone.[14] Other studies have shown no association between stroke recurrence and degree of shunting.[15]

Thus, causation of stroke in patients with atrial septal abnormalities remains debatable.[16] Nevertheless, support for the theory of paradoxical embolization of thrombus, air, or fat from the venous system through a PFO, and into the arterial circulation comes from a number of observations (Fig. 44-1).

Right-to-left shunting across a PFO can be induced by transient increases in right atrial pressure. Either deep coughing or the Valsalva maneuver characteristically is used clinically to demonstrate right-to-left shunting by transthoracic or transesophageal echocardiography (TEE) (positive "bubble" study) or transcranial Doppler. Presence of a large remnant eustachian valve can also preferentially direct blood from the inferior vena cava across the PFO and into the left atrium. Strokes may be more common in patients at risk for deep venous thrombosis (cancer, post-immobilization, long travel) or following diving (air accumulation from decompression), although many patients with cryptogenic stroke do not have such predisposing factors. The simultaneous occurrence of right- and left-sided embolic events in the same patient further support this proposed mechanism. The association between PFO and prothrombotic states (mutations in the factor V or prothrombin genes), which result in venous hypercoagulability,[17] may support paradoxical embolization. Alternatively, stroke may occur due to local thrombosis in the cerebral circulation, especially in patients with increased levels of the anticardiolipin antibody, which results in either venous or arterial hypercoagulability. The incidence of deep venous thrombosis (DVT) in patients with cryptogenic stroke and interatrial shunting ranges between 9% and 57%[18,19] making the association

unclear. Further support for the role of paradoxical embolism comes from reports of atrial septal abnormalities associated with PFO.[20–24]

DIAGNOSTIC TESTING

The most sensitive tests for the diagnosis of PFO are a transcranial Doppler of the middle cerebral artery or a transesophageal echocardiography with a "bubble" study[3,4,6] using an intravenous injection of agitated saline. The appearance of bubbles in the left atrium or cerebral circulation within 3 to 5 cardiac cycles of a venous injection of agitated saline identifies PFO with right-to-left shunting. Use of a Valsalva maneuver or cough with injection of the saline into the femoral vein increases the sensitivity of this test.[4,6,25–28] Despite the demonstration of a PFO it is critical to rule out other potential causes of stroke or factors that might contribute to thromboembolism.

Venous hypercoagulable states that may affect therapeutic strategies for care of patients with stroke include positive testing for the factor V Leiden mutation, prothrombin 20210 mutation, antiphospholipid antibodies, hyperhomocysteinemia, protein S deficiency, protein C deficiency, elevated lipoprotein(a), and antithrombin III deficiency. In any patient with cryptogenic stroke, identification of a hypercoagulable state is important because a venous hypercoagulable state may directly impact a decision for or against closure of a PFO and may also affect procedural and periprocedural therapy. Heparin, for example, is usually given during percutaneous closure, but a venous hypercoagulable state increases the risk of venous thrombosis at the femoral vein catheter insertion site, implying prolonged periprocedural heparin use. In such a case should lifelong warfarin be prescribed, and if so, is closure warranted in the first place? If closure is successful, must these patients be treated with lifelong warfarin, or will aspirin be adequate (Table 44-1).

It is also important to screen for arterial hypercoagulable states. Patients with arterial hypercoagulable states and a history of stroke may warrant lifelong oral anticoagulation with warfarin regardless of closure of a PFO. If closure is undertaken, these patients may also require periprocedural heparin therapy. Arterial prothrombotic states that may require indefinite oral anticoagulation with history of stroke are the presence of antiphospholipid antibodies, dysfibrinogenemia, and perhaps protein S and protein C deficiencies.

Thus, the presence or absence of hypercoagulable states should directly affect the decision to either close or not

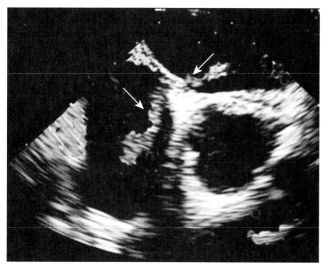

Figure 44-1 Transesophageal echocardiogram showing a long thrombus straddling a patent foramen ovale (*arrows* = thrombus).

Table 44-1 Implications of Results of Screening Tests for Hypercoagulable State

Periprocedural heparin?
  Increased risk of DVT at insertion site?
Postprocedural warfarin?
  Better than aspirin to prevent device thrombosis?
Need for lifelong warfarin anyway?
  Perhaps not, if closed PFO
With a history of stroke, the patient may need lifelong
  anticoagulation regardless of PFO closure

DVT, deep venous thrombosis; PFO, patent foramen ovale.

close a PFO associated with stroke. If a venous hypercoagulable state is present and closure is done, heparin should be used during the procedure and perhaps continued for 12 hours after the venous sheath is removed. Warfarin should probably be used instead of aspirin for at least the first 3 months after closure to minimize thrombus formation on the device. If an arterial hypercoagulable state is present and closure is done, heparin should be used during the procedure, and lifelong warfarin should be prescribed regardless of closure (Table 44-2).

TREATMENT

The best strategy for secondary prevention in patients with cryptogenic stroke is yet to be determined. Randomized trials of medical (antithrombotic) therapy versus anatomic closure have been hampered by slow patient recruitment. Reports of individual site registries are all we have. Medical therapy has centered around the use of antiplatelet agents and warfarin. Aspirin and warfarin have mostly been studied in patients after a first cryptogenic stroke. Here too, the results of retrospective and prospective studies are inconsistent. Daily aspirin use (300 mg/day) was associated with a yearly rate of recurrent stroke/transient ischemic attack (TIA) of 1% in patients with either PFO or atrial septal aneurysm,[13] but recurrence events were 4.7% in patients with coexisting PFO and atrial septal aneurysm.

In the warfarin-aspirin recurrent stroke study (WARSS), comparing warfarin (mean target International Normalized Ratio [INR] 2.1) with aspirin (325 mg/day) in patients with ischemic stroke,[29] recurrent stroke or death occurred in 17.8% of patients assigned to warfarin and in 16% of patients assigned to aspirin ($P = 0.25$) at 2 years. This study may be inadequate owing to the low target INR.

The PFO in cryptogenic stroke study (PICCS) studied 630 WARSS patients who underwent a TEE.[14] Forty percent of the patients had sustained a cryptogenic stroke. The study population was equally divided between aspirin and warfarin therapy. In this substudy, the end point of recurrent stroke or death was similar in patients with ischemic stroke regardless of the presence or absence of a PFO. The size of the foramen (degree of shunting) and the presence of an atrial septal aneurysm did not identify increased risk of events. Whereas data from these studies suggest equal efficacy of aspirin and warfarin in patients with isolated PFO or atrial septal aneurysm manifesting with a first cryptogenic stroke, the best medical therapy for

---

Table 44-2 PFO Closure and Hypercoagulability

No hypercoagulable states: Close
Venous hypercoagulable state: Close, but...
  Periprocedural heparin?
  Warfarin and aspirin for 3 months, then aspirin?
  Probably lifelong warfarin if prior recurrent DVT/PE?
Arterial hypercoagulable state: Close, but...
  Periprocedural heparin?
  Warfarin indefinitely?

DVT/PE, deep venous thrombosis/pulmonary embolism; PFO, patent foramen ovale.

---

patients with the combination of PFO and atrial septal aneurysm remains unclear. The results of the study by Mas[15] showing the inadequacy of aspirin in reducing the risk of stroke in this group of patients are contradicted by the conclusions derived from the PICCS cohort. Some of the discrepancy could be accounted for by the different populations studied. It is possible that in older patients with both PFO and atrial septal aneurysm (mean age 59 years in PICCS) either therapy is effective for secondary prevention, but that younger patients (≤ 55 years) with similar presentation constitute a particularly high-risk group that would benefit most from adequate oral anticoagulation (INR 2 to 3) with warfarin or PFO closure. Strategies for primary prevention still need to be defined. Moreover, the next therapeutic step in patients who fail aspirin, warfarin, or both, has not been established—although PFO closure is currently recommended. Target INRs and especially achieved INRs must be closely considered prior to assigning a patient as a warfarin failure.

Percutaneous PFO closure for patients with cryptogenic stroke is an alternate strategy. Reports of the safety profile and the effect on recurrent stroke rate of percutaneous PFO closure are mostly retrospective. Technical success is excellent with successful closure in more than 90% of patients.[30] At 5-year follow-up,[31] the annual recurrence risk was 3.4% for the combined end point of TIA, stroke, and peripheral embolism. The presence of a postprocedural shunt was the best predictor of recurrent events with a relative risk increase of 4.2 ($P = 0.03$). Hung and colleagues reported their experience using the Clamshell, CardioSEAL, or Sideris buttoned devices.[32] Eighty-six percent of patients had effective closure of the PFO. Stroke recurrences were attributed to suboptimal device performance, including the presence of residual postprocedural shunting. Hong and coworkers reported the experience with the Amplatzer device.[33] Although patients were few, PFO closure was complete in 67% at the end of procedure and 100% at 2 years of follow-up. No recurrent embolic neurologic events were reported.

A larger study using the PFO-STAR device in 276 patients[34] reported implantation success in all patients but periprocedural complications included transient ST-segment elevation (1.8%), and TIA (0.8%). At 15-month follow-up, TIA had occurred in 1.7%. No recurrent stroke or peripheral emboli occurred. Windecker and colleagues[31] provided insight into a potential benefit of endovascular PFO closure over medical therapy in select patients with prior stroke. The study identified 308 patients having had a cryptogenic stroke associated with an atrial septal aneurysm. Of these, 150 patients had percutaneous PFO closure and 158 were treated medically. Patients with residual shunts (17%) or other indication for aspirin continued this therapy indefinitely. In the group receiving medical therapy, one half were prescribed warfarin (target INR 2 to 3), whereas the rest received antiplatelet therapy—mostly in the form of aspirin. PFO closure showed a nonsignificant trend toward a lower risk in the combined end point of death, stroke, or TIA when compared with medical therapy at 4-years follow-up. In a subgroup analysis, percutaneous PFO closure was found to be superior to aspirin but not to warfarin therapy. Importantly, in patients with complete occlusion of their PFO and more than one stroke at baseline had a significantly lower risk of recurrent stroke or TIA after closure compared with medical therapy (7.3% vs 33.2% and 6.5% vs 22.2%, respectively). These results are certainly not conclusive. Medical noncompliance, the long-term use of aspirin in more than one third of patients after closure, and the nonblinded follow-up could have produced bias.

A review of seven reports since 2000 of percutaneous PFO closure[31,32,34,35-38] in a total of 1221 patients with a mean age of 48 years shows a 2.4% weighted recurrence rate of stroke (Table 44-3). It is not statistically valid to compare these results with the recurrence rates of warfarin or aspirin therapy in the Mas[13] and PICCS[14] reports (3.7% and 7.2%, respectively), but it is all that we have.

The lack of randomized studies comparing medical therapy with percutaneous PFO closure thus limits evidence-based recommendations for treatment of patients with cryptogenic stroke and atrial septal abnormalities. Thus, any decision for therapy in patients with cryptogenic stroke must be made on an individual basis using best judgment. Device deployment is not without risks (e.g., bleeding, cardiac tamponade, air embolization, TIA, and stroke) nor is medical treatment (e.g., bleeding, noncompliance with medication). Antiplatelet therapy is a conservative, reasonable first choice in young patients with cryptogenic stroke who have an isolated PFO or atrial septal aneurysm (but **not** the combination). Patients with coexisting PFO and atrial septal aneurysm seem to be better protected from embolic recurrence by warfarin. Warfarin alone or in combination with aspirin could also be considered in patients who failed aspirin therapy alone, although no clear data support such a recommendation. At present, there are no data to support the additional use of clopidogrel or other antiplatelet agents. Importantly, there is little doubt that atrial septal aneurysm with PFO is associated with cryptogenic stroke in patients younger than 55 years of age. Such high-risk patients, those with contraindications for antiplatelet or anticoagulant use, or others at risk (e.g., divers with PFO) should be strongly considered for percutaneous PFO closure.

What should well-informed patients with cryptogenic strokes be told? They should know the following:

1. Young patients with cryptogenic stroke and PFO with atrial septal aneurysm, or others at high risk, should strongly consider percutaneous closure.
2. Patients younger than 55 years of age with cryptogenic stroke and PFO should be told that recurrent risks of CNS events on warfarin or aspirin therapy

range from 3.7%[13] to 7.2%[14] per year and that registry results of PFO closure show slightly lower recurrence rates.

3. For patients older than 55 years of age, the decision is yet to be determined.
4. For patients with associated venous or arterial hypercoagulable states, closure can be performed, but ongoing antithrombotic therapy or antiplatelet therapy will be needed.

REFERENCES

1. Heart Disease and Stroke Statistics—2004 Update. American Heart Assoc.
2. Halperin JL, Fuster V: Patent foramen ovale and recurrent stroke: Another paradoxical twist. Circulation 105:2580–2582, 2002.
3. Horton SC, Bunch TJ: Patent foramen ovale and stroke. Mayo Clin Proc 79:79–88, 2004.
4. Meier B, Lock JE: Contemporary management of patent foramen ovale. Circulation 107:5–9, 2003.
5. Overell JR, Bone I, Lees KR: Interatrial septal abnormalities and stroke: A meta-analysis of case-control studies. Neurology 55: 1172–1179, 2000.
6. Kerut EK, William TN, Plotnick GD, Giles TD: Patent foramen ovale: A review of associated conditions and the impact of physiologic size. J Am Coll Cardiol 38:613–623, 2001.
7. Hagen PT, Scholtz DG, Edwards WD: Incidence and size of patent foramen ovale during the first 10 decades of life: An autopsy study of 965 normal hearts. Mayo Clin Proc 59:17–20, 1984.
8. Schroeckenstein RF, Wanenda GJ, Edwards JE: Valvular competent patent foramen ovale in adults. Minn Med 55:11–13, 1972.
9. Seib GA: Incidence of the patent foramen ovale in adult American whites and American negroes. Am J Anat 55:511–525, 1934.
10. Wright RR, Anson BJ, Clevelend HC: The vestigial valves and interatrial foramen of the adult human heart. Anat Rec 100:331–335, 1948.
11. Lechat P, Mas JL, Lascault G, et al: Prevalence of patent foramen ovale in patients with stroke. N Engl J Med 318:1148–1152, 1988.
12. Di Tullio M, Sacco RL, Gopal A, et al: Patent foramen ovale as a risk factor for cryptogenic stroke. Ann Intern Med 117:461–465, 1992.
13. Mas JL, Arquizan C, Lamy C, et al: Recurrent cerebrovascular events associated with patent foramen ovale, atrial septal aneurysm, or both. N Engl J Med 345:1740–1746, 2001.
14. Homma S, Sacco RL, Di Tullio MR, et al: Effect of medical treatment in stroke patients with patent foramen ovale: PICSS study. Circulation 105:2625–2631, 2002.
15. Mas JL: Patent foramen ovale, atrial septal aneurysm and ischemic stroke in young adults. Eur Heart J 15:446–449, 1994.
16. Ranoux D, Cohen A, Cabanes L: Patent foramen ovale: Is stroke due to paradoxical embolism? Stroke 24:31–34, 1993.
17. Chaturvedi S: Coagulation abnormalities in adults with cryptogenic stroke and patent foramen ovale. J Neurol Sci 160:158–160, 1998.
18. Lethen H, Flachskampf FA, Schneider R, et al: Frequency of deep vein thrombosis in patients with patent foramen ovale and ischemic stroke or transient ischemic attack. Am J Cardiol 80:1066–1069, 1997.
19. Stollerberger C, Slany J, Schuster I, et al: The prevalence of deep venous thrombosis in patients with suspected paradoxical embolism. Ann Intern Med 19:461–465, 1993.
20. Silver MD, Dorsey JS: Aneurysms of the septum primum in adults. Arch Pathol Lab Med 102:62–65, 1978.
21. Schneider B, Hanrath P, Vogel P, Meinertz T: Improved morphological characterization of atrial septal aneurysm by transesophageal echocardiography: Relation to cerebrovascular events. J Am Coll Cardiol 16:1000–1009, 1990.
22. Mugge A, Daniel WG, Angermann C, et al: Atrial septal aneurysm in adults patients: A multicenter study using transthoracic and transesophageal echocardiography. Circulation 91:2785–2792, 1995.
23. Berthet K, Lavergne T, Cohen A, et al: Significant association of atrial vulnerability with atrial septal abnormalities in young patients with ischemic stroke of unknown cause. Stroke 31:398–403, 2003.
24. Lamy C, Giannesini C, Zuber M, et al: Clinical and imaging findings in cryptogenic stroke patients with and without patent foramen ovale. The PFO-ASA Study. Stroke 33:706–711, 2002.

Table 44-3 Combined Results of Recent Percutaneous Closure Registries

Study (number)	CNS Recurrence Rates/Yr (%)
Hung[32] (63)	3.2
Windecker[31] (80)	3.4
Sievert[34] (281)	3.1
Wahl[35] (152)	4.9
Martin[36] (110)	0.9
Braun[37] (276)	1.7
Sommer[38] (259)	1.2
Total number = 1221 patients (mean age, 48 years)	Weighted average of recurrence of CNS events = 2.4%/yr

25. Gin KG, Huckell VF, Pollick C: Femoral vein delivery of contrast medium enhances transthoracic echocardiographic detection of patent foramen ovale. J Am Coll Cardiol 22:1994–2000, 1993.

26. Hamann GF, Schatzer-Clotz D, Frohlig G, et al: Femoral vein delivery of echo contrast may increase the sensitivty of testing for a patent foramen ovale. Neurology 50:1423–1428, 1998.

27. Heckman JG, Niedermeirer W, Brandt-Pohlmann W, et al: Detektion Eines Offenen Foramen Ovale: Transosophageale Echokardiographie and Transkranielle Doppler-Sonographie mit Ultraschallkontrastmittel Sind"Erganzende, Nicht Konkurrierende Methoden." Med Klin (Munich). 94:367–370, 1999.

28. Karttunen V, Markku V, Markku I, et al: Ear oximetry: A noninvasive method for detection of patent foramen ovale. Stroke 32:448–453, 2001.

29. Mohr JP, Thompson JLP, Lazar RM, et al: A Comparison of aspirin and warfarin for the prevention of recurrent ischemic stroke. N Engl J Med 345:1444–1451, 2001.

30. Windecker S, Meier B: Percutaneous patent foramen ovale (PFO) closure: It can be done but should it? Catheter Cardiovasc Interv 47:377–380, 1999.

31. Windecker S, Wahl A, Chatterjee T, et al: Percutaneous closure of patent foramen ovale in patients with paradoxical embolism: Long-term risk of recurrent thromboembolic events. Circulation 101:893–898, 2000.

32. Hung J, Landzberg MJ, Jenkins KJ, et al: Closure of patent foramen ovale for paradoxical emboli: Intermediate-term risk of recurrent neurological events following transcatheter device placement. J Am Coll Cardiol 35:1311–1326, 2000.

33. Hong TE, Thaler D, Brorson J, et al: Amplatzer PFO Investigators: Transcatheter closure of patent foramen ovale associated with paradoxical embolism using the Amplatzer PFO occluder: Initial and intermediate-term results of the U.S. multicenter clinical trial. Catheter Cardiovasc Interv 60:524–528, 2003.

34. Sievert H, Horvath K, Zadan E, et al: Patent foramen ovale closure in patients with transient ischemia attack/stroke. J Intervent Cardiol 14:261–266, 2001.

35. Wahl A, Windecker S, Eberli FR, et al: Percutaneous closure of patent foramen ovale in symptomatic patients. J Intervent Cardiol 14:203–210, 2001.

36. Martin F, Sanchez PL, Doherty E, et al: Percutaneous transcatheter closure of patent foramen ovale in patients with paradoxical embolism. Circulation 106:1121–1126, 2002.

37. Braun MU, Fassbender D, Schoen SP, et al: Transcatheter closure of patent foramen ovale in patients with cerebral ischemia. J Am Coll Cardiol 39:2019–2025, 2002.

38. Sommer RJ, Kramer PH, Sorensen PH, et al: Transcatheter closure of patent foramen ovale with the CardioSEAL® Septal Occluder: Late neurologic sequelae. Presented at TCT 2002, Washington, D.C.

Chapter 45

Pulmonary Hypertension: Thrombotic and Nonthrombotic in Origin

Lewis J. Rubin, MD

INTRODUCTION

Pulmonary arterial hypertension (PAH), defined as a mean pulmonary arterial pressure greater than 25 mm Hg at rest or 30 mm Hg with exercise with a normal left heart filling pressure (<15 mm Hg), is increasingly recognized as a source of major morbidity and mortality. A revised classification system for pulmonary hypertension has recently been proposed that highlights the heterogeneous nature of this condition.[1] Pulmonary hypertension can be classified into the following four broad categories (Table 45-1): (1) pulmonary arterial hypertension (PAH); (2) pulmonary venous hypertension (e.g., left ventricular dysfunction, mitral valve disease); (3) pulmonary hypertension due to chronic thrombotic or embolic disease; and (4) pulmonary hypertension associated with disorders of the respiratory system, usually with hypoxemia (e.g., chronic obstructive or restrictive lung disease).

Although therapy for PAH has evolved dramatically over the past decade, including the development of new potent pulmonary vasodilator and antiproliferative agents,[2] the optimal implementation of treatment strategies is contingent on establishing the diagnosis and defining its etiology. When medical therapy fails, lung transplantation provides a surgical option, with pulmonary hypertension from all causes accounting for approximately one third of all lung transplants performed. However, this surgical therapy carries a significant operative risk, and its effectiveness is limited in the long term by the side effects of immunosuppressive therapy and allograft rejection.[3]

As awareness of pulmonary hypertension has increased, it has become apparent that chronic thromboembolic pulmonary hypertension (CTEPH) as a cause of chronic pulmonary hypertension is a more prevalent condition than had been previously considered.[4] With the development and acceptance of pulmonary endarterectomy as a definitive surgical therapy for these patients, recognition and identification of CTEPH as the cause of unexplained dyspnea or pulmonary hypertension is critical.

PATHOGENESIS

The pathogenesis of PAH is complex and our understanding of the interplay between a variety of pathogenic mechanisms is evolving.[5] Simply put, pulmonary hypertension can be caused by narrowing of the precapillary vessels,

loss of vascular surface area, or passive back pressure from the postcapillary vessels.

Precapillary pulmonary hypertension can be produced by several mechanisms. Embolic material, such as venous thrombi, can lodge in the pulmonary artery, producing acute obstruction or, if unresolved and organized into the vessel wall, chronic obstruction. In situ thrombosis can also occur. Chronically increased blood flow, as seen in large left-to-right intracardiac shunts, is associated with remodeling of the pulmonary arterial walls into vessels that resemble systemic arteries. Remodeling of the pulmonary arterial and arteriolar walls as a result of inflammation or endothelial dysfunction can also occur, for example, in idiopathic pulmonary artery hypertension (IPAH) or PAH due to connective tissue diseases. Loss of the pulmonary vascular bed as a result of destructive processes such as emphysema or interstitial fibrotic disease will increase resistance to blood flow and produce pulmonary hypertension. Hypoxia-induced pulmonary vasoconstriction and vascular remodeling further augment the degree of pulmonary hypertension in this setting. Processes that increase left atrial or left ventricular end-diastolic pressures will also increase pulmonary arterial pressure, with less dramatic increases in intrinsic pulmonary vascular resistance.

Regardless of the etiology, when pulmonary hypertension occurs, the vasculature responds by undergoing changes that further increase its resistance. The patterns of histopathologic change seen in pulmonary hypertension, including medial hypertrophy, intimal thickening, plexogenic pulmonary arteriopathy, and thrombotic pulmonary arteriopathy likely represent a final common pathway of response to pulmonary vascular injury and persistent pulmonary hypertension.

ENDOTHELIAL INJURY

The lungs contain the largest expanse of endothelium in the body. In addition to its role as a semipermeable barrier between blood and interstitium, the endothelium serves a wide array of biologically important functions. Among these functions are the synthesis, uptake, storage, release, and metabolism of vasoactive substances; transduction of blood-borne signals; modulation of coagulation and thrombolysis; regulation of cell proliferation; engagement in the local inflammatory and proliferative reactions to injury; involvement in immune reactions; and angiogenesis.

Table 45-1 Nomenclature and Classification of Pulmonary Hypertension

Pulmonary Arterial Hypertension (PAH)
Sporadic (intermittent) (IPAH)
Familial (FPAH)
Related to
 Collagen vascular disease
 Congenital systemic to pulmonary shunts (large, small, repaired, or nonrepaired)
 Portal hypertension
 HIV infection
 Drugs and toxins
 Other (glycogen storage disease, Gaucher disease, hereditary hemorrhagic telangiectasia, hemoglobinopathies, myeloproliferative disorders, splenectomy).
Associated with significant venous or capillary involvement
 Pulmonary veno-occlusive disease
 Pulmonary capillary hemangiomatosis

Pulmonary Venous Hypertension
Left-sided atrial or ventricular heart disease
Left-sided valvular heart disease

Pulmonary Hypertension Associated with Hypoxemia
Chronic obstructive pulmonary disease
Interstitial lung disease
Sleep disordered breathing
Alveolar hypoventilation disorders
Chronic exposure to high altitude

Pulmonary Hypertension due to Chronic Thrombotic and/or Embolic Disease
Thromboembolic obstruction of proximal pulmonary arteries
Thromboembolic obstruction of distal pulmonary arteries
Pulmonary embolism (tumor, parasites, foreign material)

Miscellaneous
Sarcoidosis, histiocytosis X, lymphangiomatosis, compression of pulmonary vessels (adenopathy, tumor, fibrosing mediastinitis)

The cells that compose the monolayered endothelial lining communicate not only with each other by anatomic junctions and bridges but also with the underlying smooth muscle by way of biologically active substances. This interaction participates in regulating normal vasomotor tone as well as in response to the administration of vasoactive substances. It is not difficult to imagine that damage to the lining cells, proliferation of the intima, or hypertrophy of the smooth muscle will upset the normal interplay. Endothelial injury is a central process in the pathogenesis or progression of the pulmonary vasculopathy that characterizes many forms of PAH. This injury results in impaired production of vasodilator, antiproliferative and antithrombotic substances such as prostacyclin and nitric oxide, as well as excessive production of vasoconstrictive and angiogenic substances such as endothelin. Furthermore, the injured endothelium is more susceptible to thrombotic influences, predisposing to in situ thrombosis as a contributory factor in the pathogenesis of pulmonary vascular disease.

THROMBOSIS

Although most patients who experience an acute pulmonary embolism manifest resolution of the emboli with no physiologic or functional sequelae, both acute and chronic

thromboembolism can result in pulmonary hypertension. Patients with sufficient clot burden to result in acute pulmonary hypertension usually experience prompt and dramatic hemodynamic improvement or resolution of cardiopulmonary compromise with thrombolytic therapy; rarely is acute surgical embolectomy indicated in the modern era. Although a clinical history of acute pulmonary embolism is absent in half or more of all patients who develop chronic thromboembolic pulmonary hypertension (CTEPH), it is likely that most of these patients have experienced one or more clinically silent episodes of acute venous thromboembolism in the past.[6] Thrombotic material will proceed along large vessels until it reaches a bifurcation where the luminal diameter is less than the diameter of the material resulting in occlusion. At this point, the blood in the distal vessel will demonstrate stasis, with in situ thrombosis leading to the development of propagated thrombus, as originally described by Virchow.[7] In addition, the proximal blood flow becomes turbulent with associated development of laminar thrombus. The original occlusive material may now change in one of two ways: First, the organized thrombus may recanalize, producing a variable number of endothelialized channels, which may also demonstrate internal elastic laminae. These channels remain separated by fibrous septa. Second, the clot may undergo complete fibrinous organization without canalization, which in turn becomes continuous with the propagated thrombus, forming dense plugs that completely occlude the arterial lumen. In these patients, failure to resolve these thromboemboli is the presumed cause of the disease, although the exact mechanism responsible for failure of the normal fibrinolytic pathway is unclear.

Although the prevalence of CTEPH is unknown, a recent report of patients followed after an initial episode of pulmonary embolism found an incidence of 3.8% at 2 years.[4] However, this may be an underestimation of the true prevalence because many patients with CTEPH have not experienced a clinically recognized prior episode of venous thromboembolism.

Approximately 20% of patients with CTEPH have an identifiable prothrombotic predisposition, including antithrombin III, protein C or S deficiencies, lupus anticoagulant, or antiphospholipid antibodies.[6] Recent evidence suggests that some patients with CTEPH have elevations in factor VIII that may also be responsible.[8]

Patients with predisposing factors to the development of pulmonary hypertension may also develop in situ thrombosis;[5,9] in these cases, differentiation between thrombosis as the primary, and, therefore, potential reversible, process from a secondary complication can be challenging. Other conditions mimicking CTEPH include patients with embolizing myxomas, tumor emboli, and emboli from indwelling prostheses such as ventriculoatrial shunts or pacing systems. In addition, pulmonary artery sarcomas may also manifest with the features of CTEPH.[10]

Although loss of up to one half of the pulmonary vascular bed (for example, with a surgical pneumonectomy) does not result in the development of PH, pulmonary hypertension is present in many cases of CTEPH in which less than one half of the pulmonary vascular bed is obstructed. It has been suggested that the nonobstructed pulmonary capillary beds develop a vasculopathy similar to that seen in other forms of pulmonary hypertension.

These changes may persist even after surgical clearance of occlusive material and result in persistent PH.

The factors responsible for this small-vessel arteriopathy remain unknown, although it has been suggested that a variety of locally produced mitogens or vasoactive mediators may be responsible.[9] These findings support early intervention—before the vascular changes in other parts of the lung have become established.

DIAGNOSIS

The diagnosis of pulmonary vascular disease may be difficult to establish because its clinical presentation is often insidious and it is often confused with other conditions.[11] Pulmonary arterial hypertension occurs at all ages, but it is most common between the ages of 30 and 50 years; overall, there is no substantial difference in distribution between the sexes.

The most frequent early symptom is progressive exertional dyspnea, which will be present before the development of pulmonary hypertension at rest. Dyspnea is often initially attributed to other conditions such as airway disease, cardiac disease, or physical deconditioning. Indeed, the average delay from the onset of cardiopulmonary symptoms to the establishment of the correct diagnosis is typically several years.[8] More advanced symptoms include exertional chest pain, a chronic nonproductive cough, hemoptysis, palpitations, and exertional dizziness or syncope.

Signs

As with the symptoms, the physical signs seen in patients with PH are often relatively nonspecific and may become apparent only as right-sided heart failure ensues. Peripheral cyanosis may occur with severe reduction in cardiac output, and central cyanosis may be present if there is a significant intracardiac right-to-left shunt, for example, through a patent foramen ovale. Examination of the legs may reveal signs of chronic venous stasis and skin discoloration, gross varicose veins or even varicose ulceration. Peripheral edema is usually present as right heart failure develops.

Auscultation of the chest is often unremarkable, although in later stages of the disease the murmur of tricuspid regurgitation may be audible. Auscultation may also reveal the presence of intrapulmonary systolic bruits in patients with CTEPH.[6] These bruits resemble those encountered in congenital pulmonary branch stenosis and are assumed to result from turbulent blood flow past a segmental narrowing. These bruits have not been described in patients with other forms of pulmonary arterial hypertension.

Investigations

Complete blood count and biochemical studies are standard but are rarely disordered. Hematologic abnormalities that may predispose to pulmonary hypertension, such as sickle cell disease or previous splenectomy, may be identified. Secondary erythrocytosis may develop in cases of longstanding low cardiac output and hypoxemia. Liver function tests may be disordered as a result of hepatic congestion or intrinsic liver disease with portal-pulmonary hypertension. Additionally, low cardiac output states may produce prerenal

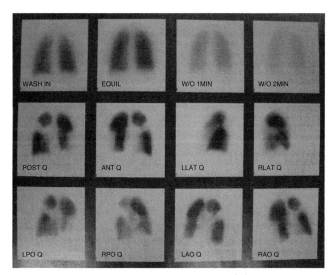

Figure 45-1 Ventilation/perfusion lung scan ($\dot{V}/\dot{Q}$) from a patient with chronic thromboembolic pulmonary hypertension (CTEPH) demonstrating multiple mismatched perfusion defects.

impairment with elevation of serum creatinine levels. Chest radiograph, electrocardiogram, and pulmonary function tests are useful investigations to exclude other conditions, but they have little value in differentiating thromboembolic pulmonary hypertension from other forms of pulmonary hypertension.

Two-dimensional transthoracic echocardiography is a useful investigation because this helps to define the presence of pulmonary hypertension and excludes underlying cardiac conditions. The typical findings are of right-sided dilatation and right ventricular hypertrophy. The main pulmonary trunk is also enlarged. Interventricular septal motion is paradoxical and the septum may appear flattened, with encroachment of the right ventricle into the left ventricular cavity. Tricuspid regurgitation is usually present to varying degrees. It is unusual to identify pulmonary arterial obstructive material echocardiographically.

Radioisotope perfusion scanning is a critical screening investigation. In chronic thromboembolic disease, discrete lower or segmental defects are normally seen (Fig. 45-1)—in contrast to the appearance of primary pulmonary hypertension in which the scan is either normal or has a patchy and mottled appearance.[12,13] The presence of an equivocal scan in patients with other features suggestive of chronic thromboembolic disease should always prompt additional investigation.[13]

CT scanning has also proved very useful in helping to identify patients with parenchymal lung disease or CTEPH (Fig. 45-2).[14] The imaging can confirm occlusion in the main and lobar pulmonary arteries and, on occasion, it may be possible to follow thrombotic material into segmental vessels. Occlusion of the main pulmonary arteries is relatively uncommon and its presence suggests a pulmonary artery tumor. When viewed on lung settings, a mosaic pattern of lung attenuation on the CT scan represents regional perfusion inhomogeneities that may be suggestive of chronic pulmonary thromboembolism. The standard for the diagnosis and planning of surgery, however, remains the standard pulmonary angiogram.[15] The combination of right heart catheterization and selective pulmonary artery angiography allows accurate assessment of

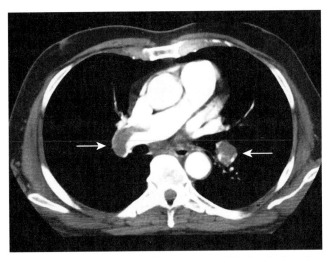

Figure 45-2 Helical CT scan from a patient with chronic thromboembolic pulmonary hypertension (CTEPH) demonstrating organized thrombotic material in the proximal vasculature (*arrows*).

the level of pulmonary hypertension, permits an assessment of surgical accessibility, and excludes other diagnoses.[15,16] When the pulmonary vascular resistance appears to be higher than expected based on the degree of vascular occlusion, the presence of underlying small vessel arteriopathic changes should be considered. These patients will carry a higher perioperative risk and their long-term benefit is unlikely to be as great.[16]

Pulmonary angiography has been reported as being a high-risk procedure for patients with pulmonary hypertension, but in our experience this investigation can be performed safely and is performed on an almost daily basis at our centers. We have performed more than 3000 angiograms in CTEPH patients without a death and with minimal morbidity using selective injections with nonionic contrast agents.

The classic signs visible on pulmonary angiography are dilated proximal and main pulmonary arteries with irregular lumens, indicating the attachment of thrombus to the

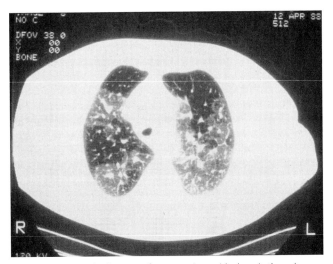

Figure 45-3 Helical CT scan from a patient with chronic thromboembolic pulmonary hypertension (CTEPH) showing a mosaic-like perfusion pattern.

vessel wall.[6] Bands or webs may be seen crossing the vascular lumen, sometimes with a post-stenotic dilatation, and with failure of filling of branch vessels to the periphery. In addition, there may be abrupt termination of pulmonary vessels with a pouch-like appearance (Fig. 45-3).

MEDICAL THERAPY

Several detailed discussions of medical therapy have been recently published.[11,17] Most of the newer treatments have been shown to produce benefit in a broad array of conditions causing pulmonary hypertension, largely through their antiproliferative effects. Among the most potent therapies used for PAH, the prostacyclins also exert antiplatelet effects that may account for part of their potency in these conditions.

Although not supported by results from randomized, controlled clinical trials, chronic anticoagulant therapy has become a mainstay of medical management for many forms of PAH, as well as CTEPH. The rationale for anticoagulation in PAH is based on the increased risk of thromboembolic events due to physical inactivity, venous stasis, dilated right heart chambers, and sluggish pulmonary blood flow. Additionally, sudden death occurs in approximately 10% of PAH patients and may be due to venous thromboembolism, in addition to other potential causes such as arrhythmia. The pathologic demonstration of organized thrombus in the small vessels of patients with PAH suggests a contributing role in its pathogenesis. Several uncontrolled studies have suggested improved survival in PAH patients treated with oral anticoagulants. Accordingly, consensus has been that patients with PAH should be treated indefinitely with warfarin to achieve an International Normalized Ratio (INR) between 2.0 and 2.5.[17] Patients with CTEPH are similarly treated unless specific thrombotic predispositions, such as the antiphospholipid antibody syndrome, warrant a more intense degree of anticoagulation.

Pulmonary Thromboendarterectomy for CTEPH

Patients suspected of having CTEPH should be referred to a center experienced with this condition to determine candidacy for pulmonary thromboendarterectomy (PTE). A detailed discussion is beyond the scope of this chapter, and the reader is referred to descriptions of the procedure published elsewhere.[6,18,19] It should be emphasized, however, that this procedure is a true endarterectomy, not embolectomy: the organized, fibrothrombotic material is adherent to the vessel wall and must be dissected off the wall, much like removing an orange from the peel without destroying the orange or the peel.

The majority of patients undergoing PTE will experience near normalization of their pulmonary hemodynamic derangement.[6,18,19] Even patients with severe right heart failure exhibit normalization of right heart function once right ventricular afterload is reduced. Further improvement is often observed over the first year after surgery. For the majority of patients, surgery results in effective and complete treatment of their pulmonary hypertension, although some patients require medical therapy for persistent pulmonary hypertension.[20] These patients, who are both high-risk candidates for surgery and are the least likely to benefit from PTE, may now be identifiable preoperatively using novel techniques to differentiate those with proximal (and operable) vascular obstruction from those with distal (inoperable) disease.[16] Because more than one third of perioperative deaths and nearly one half of long-term deaths are attributed to persistent pulmonary hypertension,[20] implementation of these novel diagnostic techniques will hopefully lead to improved patient selection and reduced operative morbidity and mortality.

Special Circumstances for the Consulting Hematologist

Patients with severe pulmonary hypertension may develop thrombocytopenia, which has been attributed to increased intrapulmonary platelet destruction due to shear stress. Epoprostenol therapy has also been suggested as a cause of thrombocytopenia, although it is unclear whether it is the cause, because this therapy is reserved for patients with the most advanced disease. Patients with portal pulmonary hypertension may develop thrombocytopenia due to hypersplenism.

Bosentan may cause a mild anemia that is believed to be due to hemodilution. Patients with hereditary hemorrhagic telangiectasia who carry the *Alk-1* gene mutation are at risk for developing pulmonary artery hypertension.[21] As with any patient with impaired cardiopulmonary function, anemia can compromise tissue oxygen delivery in PAH and its cause should be sought and treated aggressively.

CONCLUSIONS

Pulmonary hypertension remains an underdiagnosed condition. Many patients receive inappropriate therapy in the belief that they have some other underlying condition such as asthma or heart failure of unclear origin. Until recently, the only effective therapy was lung or heart-lung transplantation, but with the associated perioperative mortality and the long-term complications of immunosuppressive therapy, this is now unnecessary for the majority of patients.

With the advent of effective medical and surgical treatment options, the responsibility must lie with physicians to recognize this condition. There are now options for patients that will allow their return to normal levels of activity, with improved life expectancy. The hematologist may play a critical role in assisting in the diagnostic approach of patients with unexplained pulmonary hypertension and with the management of these patients once a diagnosis has been established.

REFERENCES

1. Simonneau G, Galie N, Rubin LJ, et al: Clinical classification of pulmonary hypertension. J Am Coll Cardiol 43:5S–12S, 2004.
2. Galie N, Seeger W, Naeije R, et al: Comparative analysis of clinical trials and evidence-based treatment algorithm in pulmonary arterial hypertension. J Am Coll Cardiol 43:81S–88S, 2004.
3. Hertz MI, Taylor DO, Trulock EP, et al: The registry of the International Society for Heart and Lung Transplantation: Nineteenth Official Report 2002. J Heart Lung Transplant 21:950–970, 2002.
4. Pengo V, Lensing AWA, Prins MH, et al: Incidence of chronic thromboembolic pulmonary hypertension after pulmonary embolism. N Engl J Med 350:2257–2264, 2004.
5. Humbert M, Morrell NW, Archer SL, et al: Cellular and molecular pathobiology of pulmonary arterial hypertension. J Am Coll Cardiol 43:13S–24S, 2004.
6. Fedullo PF, Auger WR, Kerr KM, Rubin LJ: Chronic thromboembolic pulmonary hypertension. N Engl J Med 345:1465–1472, 2001.
7. Phlogose und thrombose in Gefassystem. In Virchow R, Gesammelteandlungen zur Wissenschaftlichen Medecin. Berlin, Verlag von Max Hirsch, 1862, p 458.
8. Bonderman D, Turecek PL, Jakowitsch J, et al: High prevalence of elevated clotting factor VIII in chronic thromboembolic pulmonary hypertension. Thromb Haemost 90:372–376, 2003.
9. Lang IM: Chronic thromboembolic pulmonary hypertension—not so rare after all. N Engl J Med 350:2236–2238, 2004.
10. Kerr KM: Pulmonary vascular tumors. In Peacock AJ, Rubin LJ (eds): The Pulmonary Circulation. Oxford, Oxford University Press, 2004.
11. Rubin LJ, Badesch DB: Evaluation and management of the patient with pulmonary arterial hypertension. Ann Intern Med 143:282–292, 2005.
12. Ryan KL, Fedullo PF, Davis GB, et al: Perfusion scan findings understate the severity of angiographic and hemodynamic compromise in chronic thromboembolic pulmonary hypertension. Chest 93:1180–1185, 1998.
13. Moser KM, Page GT, Ashburn WL, et al: Perfusion lung scans provide a guide to which patients with apparent primary pulmonary hypertension merit angiography. West J Med 148:167–170, 1998.
14. Bergin CJ, Sirlin CB, Hauschildt JP, et al: Chronic thromboembolism: Diagnosis with helical CT and MR imaging with angiographic and surgical correlation. Radiology 204:695–702, 1997.
15. Doyle RL, McCrory D, Channick RN, et al: Surgical treatments/interventions for pulmonary arterial hypertension: An ACCP evidence-based clinical practice guideline. Chest 126:63S–71S, 2004.
16. Kim NHS, Fesler P, Channick RN, et al: Pre-operative partitioning of pulmonary vascular resistance correlates with early outcome following thromboendarterectomy for chronic thromboembolic pulmonary hypertension. Circulation 109:18–22, 2004.
17. Badesch DB, Abman SH, Ahearn GS, et al: Medical therapy for pulmonary arterial hypertension: ACCP Evidence-Based Clinical Practice Guidelines. Chest 126:35S–62S, 2004.
18. Jamieson SW, Kapelanski DP, Sakakibara N, et al: Pulmonary thromboendarterectomy: Experience and lessons learned in 1,500 cases. Ann Thorac Surg 76:1457–1464, 2003.
19. Klepetko W, Mayer E, Sandoval J, et al: Interventional and surgical modalities of treatment for pulmonary arterial hypertension. J Am Coll Cardiol 43:73S–80S, 2004.
20. Archibald CJ, Auger WR, Fedullo PF, et al: Long-term outcome after pulmonary thromboendarterectomy. Am J Resp Crit Care Med 160:523–528, 1999.
21. Trembath RC, Thomson JR, Machado RD, et al: Clinical and molecular genetic features of pulmonary hypertension in patients with hereditary hemorrhagic telangiectasia. N Engl J Med 345:325–334, 2001.

Chapter 46

Hemorrhage Control and Thrombosis Following Severe Injury

Ann B. Zimrin, MD • John B. Holcomb, MD • John R. Hess, MD

INTRODUCTION

Injury is common. Small hospitals have emergency rooms, which deal with a spectrum of injuries, but intensive care of the most severely injured is a highly centralized endeavor, taking place chiefly in regional trauma centers. It has been estimated that in the United States, 36 million people (one in every seven members of the population) are significantly injured each year. Three quarters of the injured seek medical care, leading to 27 million doctor or hospital visits annually.[1] About 1 in 10 of the injured who are medically evaluated is hospitalized, leading to 2.7 million admissions each year. About 1 million of the more severely injured are directly admitted or transferred to one of the nation's 1200 Level I, II, or III trauma centers. Altogether, about 93,000 individuals die each year as a result of their injuries, with fully one half dying before they reach the hospital. Of those who will die, but reach the hospital alive, the great majority die of brain injury or uncontrolled hemorrhage within the first 24 hours of hospitalization.[2] Of those admitted to a hospital, about 250,000 receive blood products. From these numbers, it can be further estimated that perhaps 20,000 times each year, an injured patient will be admitted to a trauma center with massive uncontrolled hemorrhage and will be transfused acutely with more than 10 units of red blood cells (RBCs) in the first 24 hours of care. Such patients stand an approximately 40% chance of dying and an equivalent chance of developing thrombotic complications if they survive the first day.[3] They are cared for by trauma and critical care surgeons, trauma anesthesiologists, intensivists, trauma orthopedists, and neurosurgeons. The hematologic questions that lead to consultation in this environment can be as broad as the background population that sustains injury and/or as restricted as the blood products available for their treatment. The common element is urgency.

Appropriate disaster preparedness suggests that hematologists who work in acute care hospitals should be able to address the basic issues that are likely to arise after massive injury. Determining the extent of injury is facilitated now with 13-second whole body CT scans and focused abdominal sonography for trauma (FAST). At the extreme end of the survivable injury spectrum are the patients with devastating injuries for whom immediate hemorrhage control is not always possible. These patients require large amounts of blood while surgeons work to limit hemorrhage, control gut contamination of body cavities, and shunt blood, bypassing disruptions of the largest vessels, in a process called "damage control" that emphasizes reestablishing normal physiology at the expense of normal anatomy.[3a] This chapter deals with the hematologic issues that arise during this process, as well as later in the course of care of the severely injured trauma patient.

As the consulting hematologist arrives on the trauma floor, operating room, or section of the emergency department, a sense of culture shock might be the prevailing emotion. In short supply are thoughtful, deliberative internists, replaced by fast-moving figures in scrubs who must make life-changing decisions with insufficient data and expect quick answers from consultants for problems involving patients who are unresponsive, have "too many" IVs, and injuries which threaten to become lethal in the immediate future. A familiarity with the pathophysiology of the hematologic abnormalities involved, preplanned approaches, and the presence of a well-prepared blood bank will stand the hematologist in good stead.

MASSIVE TRANSFUSION AND THE COAGULOPATHY OF TRAUMA

Pathogenesis

Exsanguinating hemorrhage is second only to head trauma as the most common cause of death among injured patients who reach the hospital alive.[2] Although disruption of the integrity of the vasculature is the proximate cause of the bleeding, the primary injury, the body's response, and therapeutic interventions can combine to produce a secondary coagulopathy that complicates efforts to both evaluate and control bleeding. This coagulopathy of trauma is a combination of the effects of blood loss, physiologic and therapeutic hemodilution, coagulation factor and platelet consumption, acidosis, hypothermia, and inappropriate fibrinolysis.

Loss of clotting activity occurs early in massive hemorrhage. The entire store of clotting activity for a healthy 70 kg man is 10 grams of fibrinogen and 15 mL of platelets. One half of that fibrinogen and one third of those platelets can be lost in massive hemorrhage or hematomas even before the treatment of injury begins. Therapies aimed at increasing vascular volume also increase blood pressure and drive more blood loss.

Dilution of remaining blood by physiologic vascular refill and from the administration of asanguinous fluid or plasma-poor RBCs further reduces coagulation factor activity and platelet concentration. This therapeutic dilution is considered standard of care. Emergency medical technicians and paramedics administer intravenous (IV) fluids in the field. Larger IV lines are placed on arrival at the trauma center and vascular access is tested with fluid boluses. Hypotension that threatens tissue perfusion is treated aggressively with volume. In the early phases of trauma care, before a blood type is available, volume is provided with crystalloid fluids and uncross-matched blood group O packed red blood cells (pRBC). Because blood volume is reduced, the combination of ongoing loss and dilute replacement leads to accelerated whole-body washout of clotting activity.

Consumption of plasma coagulation factors and especially platelets leads to significant decreases in their concentrations in the circulating blood, especially after blunt trauma, ballistic wounds, or high-energy-transfer injuries. These injuries typically cause millions of endothelial microtears, each exposing subendothelial tissue factor and collagen, which then serve as sites for local activation of coagulation factors and platelet adhesion. Moderate injury can largely deplete the platelet pool, which in aggregate can cover only a very small fraction of the total endothelial surface. The lung capillary bed, as an example, has a surface area similar in size to a football field, whereas the circulating blood contains enough platelets to cover 5 square meters. Moreover, certain injuries, such as head injury with brain tissue embolization, large bone fractures with fat embolization, or amniotic fluid embolization can cause acute disseminated intravascular coagulation (DIC) with defibrination.

Hypothermia occurs when the injured suffer exposure in the prehospital and assessment phases, are resuscitated with cold fluids, or sustain evaporative and conductive heat loss in the operating room.[4] Hypothermia slows the rates of all the enzymatic plasma coagulation reactions,[5,6] but has its greatest effect on the activation of platelets. Platelet activation from torsion on the GP-Ib-IX-V complex by von Willebrand factor is largely abolished at 30° C.[7] This acquired Bernard-Soulier–like platelet dysfunction results in platelets in the wound that do not secrete, aggregate, or provide active surfaces for coagulation factor complex assembly. At core temperatures between 32° C and 34° C, platelet activities are present but reduced.

Acidosis occurs when hypotension leads to loss of critical oxygen delivery to tissues. Acidosis interferes with plasma coagulation by reducing the activity of the vitamin K–dependent factor complexes on negatively charged cell surfaces.[8] These complexes are held together by the γ-carboxyglutamic diacids complexing calcium ions against negatively charged phospholipid rafts on activated platelet surfaces. Increased proton concentrations partially destabilize and markedly reduce the activity of these coagulation factor complexes.

Thrombolysis is activated at the same time as the coagulation cascade, but is normally inhibited by the thrombin-activated fibrinolysis inhibitor (TAFI). However, when thrombin activity is reduced by low concentrations of prothrombin and low activity of the activating complexes, TAFI is not released.[9] Fibrin strands, normally thick when

Table 46-1 Probability of Life-Threatening Coagulopathy Increases with Shock, Acidosis, and Hypothermia*

Clinical Status	Conditional Probability of Developing Coagulopathy (%)
No risk factor	1
ISS > 25	10
ISS > 25 + SBP < 70 mm Hg	39
ISS > 25 + pH < 7.1	58
ISS > 25 + temperature < 34° C	49
ISS > 25 + SBP < 70 mm Hg + temperature < 34° C	85
ISS > 25 + SBP < 70 mm Hg + temperature < 34° C + pH < 7.1	98

*The risk factors for developing coagulopathy in the early phases of trauma care include severe injury, shock, and hypothermia. When patients have all of the risk factors, they are almost universally coagulopathic.
ISS, Injury Severity Score; SBP, systolic blood pressure.
From Cosgriff N, Moore EE, Sauaia A, et al: Predicting life-threatening coagulopathy in the massively transfused trauma patient: Hypothermia and acidoses revisited. J Trauma 42:857–862, 1997.

produced by high local activities of thrombin acting on normal concentrations of fibrinogen, are thin with high surface-to-volume ratios when laid down in the presence of reduced thrombin activity or low concentrations of fibrinogen. The high surface-to-volume ratio makes the fibrin strands more susceptible than usual to enzymatic lysis.

The interactions of these pathophysiologic mechanisms are at least additive and in many cases multiplicative (Table 46-1).[10] Loss, dilution, and consumption all contribute to reduce the concentrations of plasma coagulation factors and platelets. Hypothermia and acidosis reduce the activities of those factors and platelets that remain. Uninhibited thrombolysis reduces the effect of the limited clotting activity available and contributes fibrin breakdown products, which interfere with further coagulation. The ongoing result of all of these mechanisms is the coagulopathy of trauma.

The coagulopathy of trauma bears a strong resemblance to, and is sometimes indistinguishable from, DIC.[11] As noted earlier, in the presence of brain, fat, or amniotic fluid embolization, coagulation with marked consumption of coagulation factors and platelets can occur in the intravascular space at sites remote from initial injury. This is classic DIC. However, in the usual situation in severe trauma, consumption of coagulation factors and platelets is largely restricted to sites of injury, but is made ineffective because of concurrent loss, dilution, hypothermia, acidosis, and thrombolysis (Fig. 46-1).

Clinical Presentation

The disturbance in the coagulation system caused by the initial physiologic response, and the subsequent complications of hypothermia and acidosis, are demonstrated in clinical studies of patients arriving in emergency departments, in whom abnormal coagulation parameters were common and unrelated to dilution. The presence of an abnormal coagulation test on arrival in the emergency

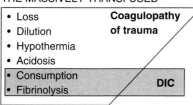

CAUSES OF COAGULOPATHY IN
THE MASSIVELY TRANSFUSED

- Loss
- Dilution
- Hypothermia
- Acidosis
- Consumption
- Fibrinolysis

Coagulopathy
of trauma

DIC

Figure 46-1 The causes of coagulopathy in severely injured patients are multifactorial. DIC, disseminated intravascular coagulation.

department increased with the severity of the injury, and predicted an increased mortality rate.[12,13] An elevation in the prothrombin time was a particularly ominous sign, correlating with a 326% increase in all-cause mortality.[13]

The initial treatment of the severely injured, hypotensive patient results in an exacerbation of the coagulopathy in several different ways. Infusion of crystalloid or colloid solutions dilutes the clotting factors and platelets remaining within the vasculature.[14–18] Although it is not intuitively obvious, massive transfusion of rapidly hemorrhaging patients, using a unit-for-unit ratio of RBCs, plasma, and platelets, will inevitably result in a coagulation defect. Because the processing of 500 mL of donated red cells involves the addition of 180 mL of anticoagulant and additive solutions and results in the loss of some of the cellular components as the blood is processed, when recombined the resulting product has a hematocrit of 29%, coagulation factor levels of approximately 60% of their normal levels, and a platelet count of 90,000/μL.[19] Any increase in the relative amount of plasma or platelets transfused to correct the coagulopathy will decrease the effective hematocrit of the material infused. In addition, transfusion of RBCs, which are stored at 4° C, worsens hypothermia if blood is not warmed; older RBC, units have a decreased pH, which exacerbates the acidosis that may already be present.

Although considerable individual variability is seen, dilutional coagulopathy generally becomes a problem when approximately one blood volume has been transfused (10 to 12 U in the average patient). The clinical manifestations of this dilutional coagulopathy are a diffuse bleeding diathesis, with oozing from surgical incisions, mucous membranes, and venipuncture sites, as well as difficulty controlling the bleeding in the traumatized region.

Patients with injury to the brain are at particularly high risk for the development of bleeding problems. The brain is rich in tissue thromboplastin which, when exposed to circulating blood, activates the extrinsic arm of the clotting cascade. Traumatic brain injury is commonly associated with thrombocytopenia and coagulopathy, with the incidence increasing with the severity of the insult. DIC can be seen, although its incidence is variably reported. The incidence of abnormal coagulation tests increases in the population of patients with moderate or severe traumatic brain injury over the 3 days following the insult, so repeat laboratory evaluation is warranted.[20]

Treatment of Post-injury Coagulopathy

The treatment of the coagulopathy seen after major trauma is multifaceted—only a small portion of which is within

the purview of the consulting hematologist. A resuscitation effort with a blood pressure target that is appropriately low will minimize the crystalloid dilution of the patient's blood and decrease the rebleeding risk.[21,22] Aggressive rewarming efforts will reverse the coagulopathy and platelet dysfunction associated with hypothermia.[8,23] Damage control surgery, an approach to intra-abdominal trauma that involves surgical control of the hemorrhage and intra-abdominal packing, with definitive repair of the injuries deferred until the patient has been stabilized, has been shown in retrospective studies to result in a decreased mortality rate in the most severely injured patients.[24]

In patients who are bleeding steadily but not to a degree to cause hemodynamic instability, replacement should be guided by frequent CBCs and coagulation testing, addressing prothrombin or partial thromboplastin times greater than 1.5 times normal with thawed plasma, platelets less than 50,000/μL with platelet concentrates, and fibrinogen levels less than 0.8 mg/dL with cryoprecipitate.[25] These end points are somewhat arbitrary—not derived from prospective studies—but do reflect consensus.

In patients who are exsanguinating, resuscitation should be started with uncross-matched group O red blood cell transfusions. Patients in this group usually are bleeding fast enough that it is impossible and inappropriate to rely on laboratory values as a guide to transfusion. If bleeding persists beyond 6 U of RBC and the stability of the patient and speed of the clinical laboratory do not allow decisions regarding the use of plasma and platelets to be based on test results, empiric plasma transfusions (2 to 6 U for each 6 U of red cells), although not proved useful in prospective clinical trials, will provide fluid, colloid, and coagulation factor support and is a rational choice for the patient in extremis. In these patients, it is deemed appropriate to stay out of trouble, rather than get out of trouble. By the time 12 U of RBC in additive solution have been given without plasma support, frank coagulopathy will have developed. Higher ratios of numbers of units of plasma to units of RBC, up to 1:1, appear desirable in mathematical models, in retrospective series, and from the practical standpoint of ease of administration.[26] A recent international consensus conference on massive transfusion for trauma has recommended this ratio.[27] Platelet concentrates should also be added empirically before 20 U of RBC have been given, and again mathematical considerations and retrospective series suggest that massively transfused patients who receive more platelets fare better.[28] Maintaining thawed plasma in the blood bank allows the issue of plasma as soon as an ABO type is known.

Use of Factor VIIa for Post-injury Coagulopathy

Since the first report of the successful use of recombinant factor VIIa (rFVIIa) in a patient with life-threatening bleeding after a gunshot wound lacerated his inferior vena cava, there have been many reports of its use in post-injury coagulopathy. Case reports and series of patients have shown that rFVIIa is often effective in stopping the hemorrhage.[29] A single randomized trial comparing three doses of rFVIIa with placebo showed that when early deaths were excluded, there was a decrease in the number of RBC transfusions in patients with blunt trauma in patients treated with rFVIIa, but no survival advantage.[30] rFVIIa appears to be less effective at very low pH (<7.10)[31,32] which may account for the rare clinical failures. For rFVIIa to work, platelets and fibrinogen must be present in quantities sufficient to form a viable clot. The optimal dose has not been determined; doses of 70 to 100 µg per kilogram of body weight have been recommended, based on the available empiric evidence.[27,33] Controlled clinical trials are necessary to definitively determine the role of rFVIIa in the care of trauma patients.

Patients with Congenital Bleeding Diatheses

Patients with preexisting bleeding diatheses are particularly problematic. Because the physiologic response to trauma can cause abnormalities in the coagulation profile,[12] the diagnosis of a preexisting coagulopathy can be difficult in a patient with severe trauma who is unable to give a history. In patients with a known preexisting coagulopathy and severe trauma, treatment should be aimed at providing 100% correction using standard guidelines for 3 days or until clinical stability is achieved. In patients with hemophilia A, a bolus dose of factor VIII of 25 to 50 u per kilogram of body weight followed by a continuous infusion at 4u/kilogram/hour has been shown to be effective in maintaining hemostasis,[34,35] and could be considered an alternative to the more standard bolus dosing. If signs of head trauma are present or its presence is suspected by the history, 100% replacement should be sought and maintained while confirmatory scans are being performed. With lesser injuries, infusions at a rate of 2u/kilogram/hour or bolus doses of factor VIII to maintain 50% levels may be adequate. In patients with known inhibitors to factor VIII, rFVIIa should be administered at doses ranging from 90 to 200 µg per kilogram of body weight, depending on the severity of the injury.

Patients with Acquired Bleeding Diatheses and Comorbid Conditions

As the population of the industrialized countries ages, the elderly are increasingly represented in the population presenting to trauma centers. Patients in this age group are more likely to have comorbid conditions, and are more likely to be on anticoagulant and platelet-inhibiting drugs. Preinjury warfarin use has been shown to be associated with more severe brain bleeding and a higher likelihood of death.[36,37] In patients with minor head injury and normal neurologic examination on presentation, neurologic deterioration occurred within 6 hours of the injury in those patients who developed significant intracranial hemorrhage.[38] However, several studies suggest that when patients with head injury are excluded, patients taking warfarin are not at higher risk for in-hospital complications and have similar mortality rates to case-matched controls.[39,40]

In anticoagulated patients with prolonged prothrombin times who have severe injuries, the warfarin effect may need to be reversed quickly with rFVIIa followed by infusions of fresh frozen plasma and intravenous vitamin K, 5 to 10 mg. rFVIIa at doses of 15 to 90 µg per kilogram of body weight, have been shown to be effective in antico-

agulated patients with intracranial hemorrhage or in need of invasive procedures,[41] but it should be kept in mind that the duration of action of rFVIIa is short (2 to 3 hours), and further therapeutic intervention with repeat dosing or plasma may be necessary. The immediate post-injury state is often characterized by a hypercoagulability (discussed in more detail subsequently), and anticoagulation should be re-instituted as soon as the stability of the patient permits.

The data regarding aspirin use and risk of intracranial bleeding is conflicting, with studies showing an increase in mortality[42] and no increase in bleeding.[43] In patients without head trauma, there is no conclusive evidence for an increased bleeding risk, although patients taking aspirin were more likely to be anemic on presentation.[44,45]

Other comorbid conditions can affect the patient's bleeding risk. Renal dysfunction can cause a platelet function disorder,[46] which is difficult to quantitate. Patients with end-stage renal disease on chronic hemodialysis have an increased rate of complications and an increased mortality rate following major trauma,[47,48] but this seems to be secondary to ongoing metabolic disturbances and an increased incidence of coexisting medical problems, such as diabetes, hypertension, and cardiac disease.

Hepatic cirrhosis, with its myriad of concomitant hemostatic alterations (discussed in Chapter 39), poses a more formidable challenge. In a retrospective analysis of the effect of preexisting medical conditions on mortality, cirrhosis was most strongly associated with a higher mortality rate.[49] Specific factors that appear to play a role in the pathophysiology of the poor outcome include the increased risk of bleeding, decreased hepatic blood flow in conditions of low perfusion pressure secondary to the increased dependence on the arterial blood supply, and increased risk of other organ failure, such as renal failure and acute respiratory distress syndrome. Mortality in cirrhotic trauma patients undergoing laparotomy approaches 50%[50,51] and is high even in patients with minor or moderate injuries.[50] Close monitoring and aggressive intervention to correct coagulopathy is suggested to improve the outcome in this very high risk group. rFVIIa has been shown to control bleeding in patients with upper gastrointestinal hemorrhage and Child B-C cirrhosis, but was not successful in decreasing transfusion requirements in a trial of patients undergoing liver transplantation.[52] Its use in patients with liver disease and trauma has not been investigated.

Thrombocytopenia

Thrombocytopenia is common in victims of severe trauma, more so even than in the population of critically ill patients as a whole.[46,53] The fall in the platelet counts seen in the first 3 to 4 days appears to be secondary to dilution and consumption (see earlier). Causes of thrombocytopenia occurring later in the patient's course include the usual etiologic factors found in critically ill patients: sepsis/infection causing increased consumption and/or bone marrow suppression; medication-induced thrombocytopenia, including heparin-induced thrombocytopenia, more rarely EDTA-dependent pseudothrombocytopenia,[54] and post-transfusion purpura. This subject is discussed in more detail in Chapters 9, 10, 12, and 25.

THROMBOSIS IN TRAUMA PATIENTS

Although excessive bleeding is often the first manifest challenge to confront the consulting hematologist, hypercoagulability soon supersedes coagulopathy as a source of morbidity and mortality. Tissue factor is released after major trauma and the concentration of fibrinogen increases as an acute phase reactant causing a hypercoagulable state; this combines with the other two components of the Virchow triad, stasis and vascular injury, to cause a thrombotic diathesis. In a study of untreated trauma patients who underwent serial impedance plethysmography and lower-extremity contrast venography, 58% were found to have deep venous thrombosis, with the vast majority of those being unsuspected on clinical grounds.[55] Risk factors can be identified to delineate the patients at highest risk—age, lower extremity fractures, spinal cord injury, head injury, high injury severity score, more than 3 ventilator days, venous injury, and the need for a major operative procedure.[56,57] However, there is no group of patients who have sustained major trauma whose risk is low enough that thromboprophylaxis is not necessary.

Given the obvious risk of anticoagulation in patients who have recently had the integrity of their vasculature interrupted, thromboprophylaxis in trauma patients presents a challenging problem. Lower extremity compression devices can be applied very early in the hospital course, although they are not feasible in many patients with lower extremity injuries—a group at high risk for thrombotic disease. Although the notion of heparin prophylaxis in the acute trauma patient seems initially uncomfortable, it must be recalled that prophylactic doses are considerably lower than therapeutic doses, especially considering the very high rate of thromboses in trauma patients surviving the first few days. Because prophylaxis is effective, fewer patients will need the higher therapeutic doses of anticoagulants if prophylaxis is generally employed. Although the data from prospective randomized clinical trials are limited, the available information suggests that low molecular weight heparin is the most efficacious method of reducing the risk of thromboembolic events.[52,57,58] The timing of the initiation of therapy needs to be carefully judged, given the risk of bleeding, particularly at sites that are difficult to detect. More information about thrombosis and thromboprophylaxis is available in Chapters 14 and 15 of this text. Briefly, many critical care providers wait 72 hours before starting DVT prophylaxis in the head and spine injured patient and wait until the prothrombin time is approaching normal before starting anticoagulation in the massively transfused.

Thrombocytosis in Trauma Patients

Although a fall in the platelet count during the first week following the injury is common in trauma patients, the second week is often accompanied by a rise in platelet counts to supra-normal levels, with one quarter of trauma patients in the ICU developing levels above the normal range.[53,59] This increase is caused by increased production of thrombopoietin in response to inflammatory factors, such as IL-6, and is not associated with an increased risk of thromboembolic events or increased mortality.[60] The inflammatory stimuli that provoke the thrombocytosis can include the injury itself, particularly in the case of crush injuries with massive tissue damage, infection, and acute respiratory distress syndrome. Thrombocytosis can also be seen in the postsplenectomy state, beginning 2 to 10 days after the surgery and continuing for 2 weeks to several months. There does not appear to be a need for treatment in this situation, even when platelet counts exceed 1,000,000/μL.

REFERENCES

1. Trunkey DD: Trauma in modern society: Major challenges and solutions. Surgeon 3:165–170, 2005.
2. Sauaia A, Moore FA, Moore II, et al: Epidemiology of trauma deaths: A reassessment. J Trauma 38:185–193, 1995.
3. Como JJ, Dutton RP, Scalea TM, et al: Blood transfusion rates in the care of acute trauma. Transfusion 44:809–813, 2004.
3a. Holcomb JB, Jenkins D, Rhee P, et al: Damage control resuscitation: Directly addressing the early coagulopathy of trauma. J Trauma 62:307–310, 2007.
4. Patt A, McCroskey BL, Moore EE: Hypothermia-induced coagulopathies in trauma. Surg Clin North Am 68:775–785, 1988.
5. Rohrer MJ, Natale AM: Effect of hypothermia on the coagulation cascade. Crit Care Med 20:1402–1405, 1992.
6. Wolberg AS, Meng ZH, Monroe DM, et al: A systematic evaluation of the effect of temperature on coagulation enzyme activity and platelet function. J Trauma 56:1221–1228, 2004.
7. Kermode JC, Zheng Q, Milner EP: Marked temperature dependence of the platelet calcium signal induced by human von Willebrand factor. Blood 94:199–207, 1999.
8. Petrone P, Kuncir EJ, Asemsoa JA: Surgical management and strategies in the treatment of hypothermia and cold injury. Emerg Med Clin N Am 21:1165–1178, 2003.
9. Bouma BN, Meijers JC: New insights into factors affecting clot stability: A role for thrombin activatable fibrinolysis inhibitor. Semin Hematol 41:13–19, 2004.
10. Cosgriff N, Moore EE, Sauaia A, et al: Predicting life-threatening coagulopathy in the massively transfused trauma patient: Hypothermia and acidoses revisited. J Trauma 42:857–862, 1997.
11. Hess JR, Lawson JH: The coagulopathy of trauma versus disseminated intravascular coagulation. J Trauma 60(6 Suppl): S12–S19, 2006.
12. Brohi K, Singh J, Heron M, et al: Acute traumatic coagulopathy. J Trauma 54:1127–1130, 2003.
13. MacLeod JBA, Lynn M, McKenney MG, et al: Early coagulopathy predicts mortality in trauma. J Trauma 55:39–44, 2003.
14. Hardy J-F, de Moerloose P, Samama M: Massive transfusion and coagulopathy: Pathophysiology and implications for clinical management. Can J Anesth 51:293–310, 2004.
15. Kuitunen AH, Hynynen MJ, Vahtera E, et al: Hydroxyethyl starch as a priming solution for cardiopulmonary bypass impairs hemostasis after cardiac surgery. Anesth Analg 98:291–297, 2004.
16. Lim RC Jr, Oclott C 4th, Robinson AJ, et al: Platelet response and coagulation changes following massive blood replacement. J Trauma 13:577–582, 1973.
17. Valeri CR, Cassidy G, Pivaced LE, et al: Anemia-induced increase in the bleeding time: Implications for treatment of nonsurgical blood loss. Transfusion 41:977–983, 2001.
18. Wilson RF, Mammen E, Walt AF: Eight years of experience with massive blood transfusions. J Trauma 11:275–285, 1971.
19. Armand R, Hess JR: Treating coagulopathy in trauma patients. Transfus Med Rev 17:223–231, 2003.
20. Carrick MM, Tyroch AH, Youens CA, et al: Subsequent development of thrombocytopenia and coagulopathy in moderate and severe head injury: Support for serial laboratory examination. J Trauma 58: 725–730, 2005.
21. Dutton RP: Low-pressure resuscitation from hemorrhagic shock. Int Anesthesiol Clin 40:19–30, 2002.
22. Sondeen JL, Coppes VG, Holcomb JB: Blood pressure at which rebleeding occurs after resuscitation in swine with aortic injury. J Trauma 54 (5 Suppl): S110–117, 2003.
23. Lapointe LA, Von Rueden KT: Coagulopathies in trauma patients. AACN Clin Issues 13:192–203, 2002.
24. Schreiber MA: Damage control surgery. Crit Care Clin 20:101–118, 2004.
25. British Committee for Standards in Haematology, Blood Transfusion Task Force: Guidelines for the use of fresh frozen plasma, cryoprecipitate and cryosupernatant. Br J Haematol 126:11–28, 2004.

26. Malone DL, Hess JR, Fingerhut A: Massive transfusion practices around the globe and a suggestion for a common massive transfusion protocol. J Trauma 60 (6 Suppl): S91–S96, 2006.

27. Holcomb JB, Hess, JR: Early massive transfusion for trauma: State of the Art: Editor's Introduction. J Trauma 60 (6 Suppl): S1–S2, 2006.

28. Ketchum L, Hess JR, Hiippala S: Indications for early fresh frozen plasma, cryoprecipitate, and platelet transfusion in trauma. J Trauma 60 (6 Suppl): S51–S58, 2006.

29. Dutton RP, McCunn M, Hyder M, et al: Factor VIIa for correction of traumatic coagulopathy. J Trauma 57:709–719, 2004.

30. Boffard KD, Riou B, Warren B, et al: NovoSeven Trauma Study Group. Recombinant factor VIIa as adjunctive therapy for bleeding control in severely injured trauma patients: Two parallel randomized, placebo-controlled, double-blind clinical trials. J Trauma 59:8–15, 2005.

31. Martini WZ, Pusateri AE, Uscilowicz JM, et al: Independent contributions of hypothermia and acidosis to coagulopathy in swine. J Trauma 58:1002–1010, 2005.

32. Meng ZH, Wolberg AS, Monroe DM, et al: The effect of temperature and pH on the activity of factor VIIa: Implications for the efficacy of high-dose factor VIIa in hypothermic and acidotic patients. J Trauma 55:886–891, 2003.

33. Barletta JF, Ahrens CL, Tyburski JG, et al: A review of recombinant factor VII for refractory bleeding in nonhemophilic trauma patients. J Trauma 58:646–651, 2005.

34. Batorova A, Martinowitz U: Continuous infusion of coagulation factors. Haemophilia 8:170–177, 2002.

35. Dingli D, Gastineau DA, Gilchrist GS: Continuous factor VIII infusion therapy in patients with haemophilia A undergoing surgical procedures with plasma-derived or recombinant factor VIII concentrates. Haemophilia 8:629–634, 2002.

36. Lavoie A, Ratte S, Clas D, et al: Preinjury warfarin use among elderly patients with closed head injuries in a trauma center. J Trauma 56:802–807, 2004.

37. Mina AA, Knipfer JF, Park DY, et al: Intracranial complications of pre-injury anticoagulation in trauma patients with head injury. J Trauma 53:668–672, 2002.

38. Reynolds FD, Dietz PA, Higgins D, et al: Time to deterioration of the elderly, anticoagulated, minor head injury patient who presents without evidence of neurologic abnormality. J Trauma 54:492–496, 2003.

39. Kirsch MJ, Vrabec GA, Marley RA, et al: Preinjury warfarin and geriatric orthopedic trauma patients: A case-matched study. J Trauma 57:1230–1233, 2004.

40. Wojcik R, Cipolle MD, Seislove E, et al: Preinjury warfarin does not impact outcome in trauma patients. J Trauma 51:1147–1152, 2001.

41. Levi M, Peters M, Bueller HR: Efficacy and safety of recombinant factor VIIa for treatment of severe bleeding: A systematic review. Crit Care Med 33:883–890, 2005.

42. Ohm C, Mina A, Howells G, et al: Effects of antiplatelet agents on outcomes for elderly patients with traumatic intracranial hemorrhage. J Trauma 58:518–522, 2005.

43. Spektor S, Agus S, Merkin V, et al: Low-dose aspirin prophylaxis and risk of intracranial hemorrhage in patients older than 60 years of age with mild or moderate head injury: A prospective study. J Neurosurg 99:661–665, 2003.

44. Manning BJ, O'Brien N, Aravindan S, et al: The effect of aspirin on blood loss and transfusion requirements in patients with femoral neck fractures. Injury 35:121–124, 2004.

45. Schafer AI: Effects of nonsteroidal anti-inflammatory therapy on platelets. Am J Med 106:25S–36S, 1999.

46. George JN, Shattil SJ: The clinical importance of acquired abnormalities of platelet function. N Engl J Med 324:27–39, 1991.

47. Blake A-M, Toker SI, Dickerman R, et al: Trauma management in the end-stage renal disease patient. Am Surg 68:425–429, 2002.

48. Lorelli DR, Kralovich KA, Seguin C: The impact of pre-existing end-stage renal disease on survival in acutely injured trauma patients. Am Surg 67:693–696, 2001.

49. Morris JA, MacKenzie EJ, Edelstein SL: The effect of preexisting conditions on mortality in trauma patients. JAMA 263:1942–1946, 1990.

50. Demetriades D, Constantinou C, Salim A, et al: Liver cirrhosis in patients undergoing laparotomy for trauma: Effect on outcomes. J Am Coll Surg 199:538–542, 2004.

51. Wahlstrom K, Ney AL, Jacobson S, et al: Trauma in cirrhosis: Survival and hospital sequelae in patients requiring abdominal exploration. Am Surg 66:1071–1076, 2000.

52. Roger FB, Cipolle MD, Velmahos G, et al: Management of venous thromboembolism in trauma patients. Available at: *http://www.east.org/tpg/dvt.pdf*

53. Akca S, Haji-Michael P, de Mendonca A, et al: Time course of platelet counts in critically ill patients. Crit Care Med 30:753–756, 2002.

54. Edelman B, Kickler T: Sequential measurement of anti-platelet antibodies in a patient who developed EDTA-dependent pseudothrombocytopenia. Am J Clin Pathol 99:87–89, 1993.

55. Geerts WH, Code KI, Jay RM, et al: A prospective study of venous thromboembolism after major trauma. N Engl J Med 331:1601–1606, 1994.

56. Geerts WH, Pineo GF, Heit JA, et al: Prevention of venous thromboembolism: The Seventh ACCP Conference on Antithrombotic and Thrombolytic Therapy. Chest 126 (3 Suppl): 338S–400S, 2004.

57. Knudson MM, Morabito D, Paiement GD, et al: Use of low molecular weight heparin in preventing thromboembolism in trauma patients. J Trauma 41:446–459, 1996.

58. Geerts WH, Jay RM, Code KI, et al: A comparison of low-dose heparin with low-molecular-weight heparin as prophylaxis against venous thromboembolism after major trauma. N Engl J Med 335:701–707, 1996.

59. Gurung AM, Carr B, Smith I: Thrombocytosis in intensive care. Br J Anaesth 87:926–928, 2001.

60. Kaser A, Brandacher G, Steurer W, et al: Interleukin-6 stimulates thrombopoiesis through thrombopoietin: Role in inflammatory thrombocytosis. Blood 98:2720–2725, 2001.

Additional References (Not Cited)

Goodnough LT, Lublin DM, Zhang L, et al: Transfusion medicine service policies for recombinant factor VIIa administration. Transfusion 44:1325–1331, 2004.

Hanes SD, Quarles DA, Boucher BA: Incidence and risk factors of thrombocytopenia in critically ill trauma patients. Ann Pharmacother 31:285–289, 1997.

Knudson MM, Ikossi DG, Khaw L, et al: Thromboembolism after trauma: An analysis of 1602 episodes from the American College of Surgeons National Trauma Data Bank. Ann Surg 240:490–496, 2004.

Zimrin AB, Dutton RP, McCunn M, et al: Management of post-injury coagulopathy. Transfus Altern Transfus Med 6:37–41, 2005.

Chapter 47

Hemostatic Aspects of Sickle Cell Disease

Kenneth Ataga, MD • Richard Lottenberg, MD

HISTORICAL PERSPECTIVE

The seminal work of Pauling and colleagues on the properties of hemoglobin S provided the basis for a hypothesis that heralded the concept of "molecular medicine."[1] Indeed, sickle cell anemia (SCA*) is touted to be the prototypic example of a single gene disorder. Although a single gene mutation is responsible for the sickle hemoglobin abnormality, inter-individual variability is observed in clinical manifestations and laboratory findings that cannot be accounted for simply by the hemoglobin genotype (e.g., Hb SS, S/ß thalassemia, or Hb SC). It is now appreciated that there are multiple genetic determinants interacting with environmental factors contributing to the occurrence of painful crises and other complications of sickle cell disease (SCD).[2,2a]

Remarkable improvement in the survival of patients with SCD has occurred over the past 25 years. The use of prophylactic penicillin therapy and administration of effective vaccines in infancy have resulted in a dramatic reduction in life-threatening pneumococcal infections.[3] Additional preventive measures, as well as ongoing care provided by comprehensive pediatric sickle cell disease programs, have provided the opportunity for the majority of such patients to reach the age of 18.[4] A prospective 10-year cohort study initiated in the late 1970s revealed a median survival of 42 to 48 years for patients with Hb SS and 60 to 68 years for patients with Hb SC.[5] It can be anticipated that continuing improvement in survival for patients with SCD will be observed as hydroxyurea therapy for symptomatic patients becomes more widely adopted and more effective strategies to prevent end-organ complications become available.

PATHOGENESIS

Red Blood Cell and Hemoglobin S Polymerization

Sickle hemoglobin (HbS) results when the normal β^6 glutamic acid residue is replaced by valine (GAG to GTG mutation at codon β^6). The polymerization that occurs when homozygous HbS ($\alpha_2\beta_2^S$) is deoxygenated is the primary event in the pathophysiology of SCD and results in damage

to erythrocytes, tissues, and organs.[6] Notwithstanding this straightforward molecular basis, the pathophysiology of clinical disease is exceedingly complicated. The rate and extent of HbS polymer formation is dependent on the intraerythrocytic HbS concentration, the degree of hemoglobin deoxygenation, and the intracellular concentration of fetal hemoglobin (HbF).[6] The HbS polymer is a twisted, rope-like structure composed of 14 strands[6] that distorts the red blood cell into the classic sickle shape. The Hb tetramer is oriented such that in one of the two β subunits, β^6 valine forms a hydrophobic contact with a complementary site on a β subunit of the partner strand. There is evidence that the polymerization of HbS is extremely cooperative and can be regarded as a simple crystal-solution equilibrium.[7] The lag period required for the concerted formation of polymer is referred to as the delay time. Because the range of transit times in the microcirculation is short relative to the range of delay times of sickle red blood cells (sRBCs), polymers do not form in most of the cells.[8] If, however, the sRBCs are subjected to prolonged transit times, then HbS polymer would form in almost all the cells as a result of equilibration at the lower oxygen tension. Hb F inhibits the polymerization of HbS, primarily owing to the glutamine residue at codon $\gamma87$,[9] which prevents a critical lateral contact in the double strand of the sickle fiber.

The density distribution of sRBC is unusually broad, due mainly to the high number of reticulocytes with a relatively low intracellular hemoglobin concentration, and the presence of a high number of very dense cells. These dense cells occur due to enhanced cellular dehydration following polymerization-induced damage to the cell membrane.[6] Because the rate of HbS polymerization is strongly dependent on the intracellular hemoglobin concentration,[7] dense sRBC are more likely to polymerize and contribute to the hemolytic and vaso-occlusive aspects of SCD than less dehydrated cells.

Leukocytes

The important contribution of leukocytes to the pathogenesis of the sickle hemoglobinopathies is illustrated by the clinical findings that elevation of the leukocyte count is now recognized as a risk for early death,[5] acute chest syndrome,[10] and hemorrhagic stroke[11] in patients with SCA. Episodes of severe vaso-occlusive crisis and acute chest syndrome have occurred following administration of granulocyte colony-stimulating factor (G-CSF) to patients with SCD in their steady state.[12,13] Leukocytes interact with sickle cells and vascular endothelium and are stimulated to release injurious cytokines.[14,15] The

---

*SCA refers to a specific disease, namely, homozygosity for hemoglobin S (i.e., Hb SS); SCD is the more generic term referring to any sickling syndrome that is composed, at least in part, of Hb S and includes Hb SS as well as double heterozygous genotypes (e.g., Hb S/ß+ thalassemia, Hb SC).

adhesion of leukocytes to vascular endothelium is mediated by several adhesion molecules.[16] In addition to the adhesion to vascular endothelium, leukocytes interact with platelets and erythrocytes to form cell aggregates, stabilized via CD36-TSP, CD31-CD31, and CD62L-CD162 bonds.[16] In patients with SCD, these cell aggregates could more effectively occlude the microvasculature than single cells. Activated neutrophils also contribute to endothelial damage. During episodes of infection, increased numbers of activated neutrophils secrete inflammatory cytokines that activate the vascular endothelium.[16] In addition, these activated leukocytes express increased levels of adhesion molecules and attach more readily to activated endothelium.

Monocytes may enhance vaso-occlusion in SCD by contributing to endothelial activation. Monocytes from patients with SCA are activated and can enhance vaso-occlusion through an endothelial inflammatory response promoted by the nuclear factor-kappa B-mediated upregulation of adhesion molecules and tissue factor.[17] The activation of endothelial cells by monocytes from patients with SSD appears to be mediated by tumor necrosis factor-α and interleukin-1β, both markers of monocyte activation. The activated endothelial cells increase their expression of ligands for adhesion molecules on leukocytes (WBCs) and RBCs, thereby promoting vaso-occlusion.

Platelets

Older children and adults with SCD typically exhibit moderate degrees of thrombocytosis.[18] These patients also exhibit increased numbers of young, metabolically active platelets (megathrombocytes), a finding that is attributed to a loss of splenic sequestration following the functional asplenia observed in SCA patients. Although there are conflicting reports regarding platelet survival in SCD,[19,20] platelet aggregation does appear to be enhanced in adult patients in the non-crisis, steady state possibly due to an increase in the number of megathrombocytes in the peripheral circulation.[18,21,22] The enhanced platelet aggregation could also reflect increases in the circulating levels of such platelet agonists as thrombin, ADP, or epinephrine. In children however, platelet aggregation is normal or reduced, a finding attributed to preservation of some of their splenic function and/or to fewer circulating megathrombocytes.[23–25] The reduced platelet responsiveness to aggregating agents observed in children with SCD may be a result of ongoing, platelet activation and secretion in vivo, changes that could, in turn, cause depletion of platelet granule stores.

There is evidence of increased platelet activation in the non-crisis, steady state.[26–33] Patients with SCD have decreased platelet thrombospondin-1 (TSP-1) content when compared with normal controls,[27] suggesting a state of ongoing release and depletion of TSP-1 from activated platelets in these SCD patients. Platelet expression of CD62, CD63, and PAC-1 antigen in SCD patients are significantly increased compared with ethnically-matched and nonmatched controls.[33] The expression of both P-selectin (CD62P) and CD40 ligand (CD40L) is substantially higher in children with SCD than in healthy control subjects.[29] Plasma from patients with SCD in the non-crisis, steady state exhibits significantly higher levels of platelet factor 4 and β thromboglobulin.[26] In addition,

platelet procoagulant activity demonstrated by binding of annexin V to phosphatidylserine(PS)-rich membrane domains, is increased when compared with platelets from normal control individuals.[26]

Endothelium

Because the potential for sRBCs to initiate a vaso-occlusive event is dependent on whether the rate of polymer formation is within the range of the capillary transit time,[34] any event that slows the transit of sRBCs through the microcirculation could be expected to have an effect on the pathogenesis of vaso-occlusion. The degree of adherence of sRBCs to vascular endothelium strongly correlates with the severity of disease.[35] Multiple studies in static and dynamic conditions demonstrate that sRBCs attach more readily to cultured endothelial cells than do normal RBCs.[35–38]

These adhesion reactions are mediated mainly by interactions between receptors on sRBCs and endothelial cells or subendothelial matrix proteins (Fig. 47-1). The plasma ligand thrombospondin (TSP) provides a bridge between the RBC receptor CD36 and several constitutively expressed endothelial receptors.[39,40] As TSP is composed of a number of heterogeneously distinct domains, vascular adhesion to TSP depends on several endothelial sites, including the vitronectin receptor ($\alpha_v\beta_3$), the transmembrane glycoprotein CD36, and endothelial cell surface heparan sulfate proteoglycans, Sickle RBCs also interact with immobilized TSP via the integrin-associated protein, CD47, a molecule that is associated with the Rhesus membrane complex.[41] Interactions occur between the integrin complex, $\alpha_4\beta_1$ (VLA-4), expressed on reticulocytes, and both endothelial vascular-cell adhesion molecule 1 (VCAM-1),[42–45] a molecule expressed on the surface of endothelial cells (especially following activation by inflammatory cytokines and hypoxia) and fibronectin.[46] High molecular weight multimers of von Willebrand factor (VWF)[47,48] promote red cell adhesion to endothelial vitronectin receptor $\alpha_v\beta_3$ and the GP-Ib-IX-V complex. Interactions also occur between sRBCs and subendothelial immobilized matrix proteins, including laminin, TSP, VWF, and fibronectin, proteins also present in plasma in a soluble form.[49] Laminin binds avidly to sRBCs via the erythrocyte basal cell adhesion molecule-Lutheran protein receptor (B-CAM/LU), the protein that carries Lutheran blood-group antigens.[50] Non–receptor-mediated adhesive mechanisms include a role for RBC sulfated glycolipids and PS.[51–53]

Inflammation

SCD is often referred to as a chronic inflammatory state owing to the presence of a chronic elevation in leukocyte counts, shortened leukocyte half-life, and abnormal activation of neutrophils and monocytes.[54,55] The circulating endothelial cells in patients with SCD are activated, with pro-adhesive and procoagulant properties, and exhibit evidence of oxidative stress.[54] In addition, there is activation of the coagulation system,[56] increased circulating platelets, and increased number of microparticles (MPs) derived from monocytes and endothelial cells.

In addition to these observations, SCD patients, even in the non-crisis, steady state exhibit elevated levels of inflammatory mediators (such as interleukin-6, tumor necrosis

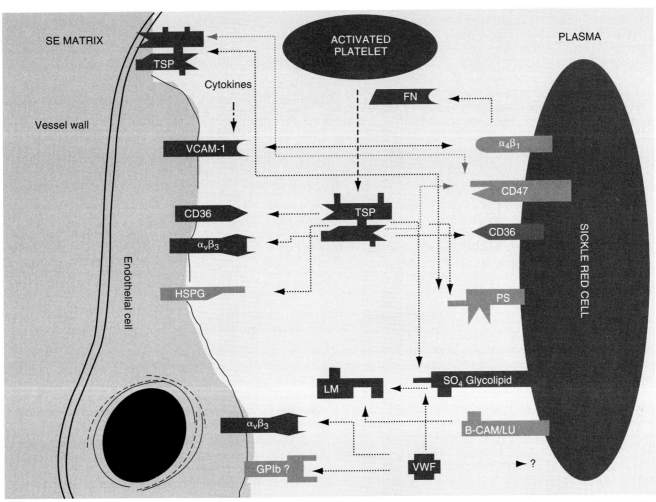

Figure 47-1 Adhesive interactions between sickle RBCs and endothelium or plasma proteins. $\alpha_4\beta_1$, integrin receptor VLA-4; $\alpha_V\beta_3$, integrin vitronectin receptor; B-CAM/LU, basal cell adhesion molecule/Lutheran protein; FN, fibronectin; GP-1b, glycoprotein 1b; HSPG, heparan sulfate proteoglycan; LM, laminin; PS, phosphatidylserine; SE matrix, subendothelial matrix; SO$_4$ glycolipid, sulfated glycolipid; TSP, thrombospondin; VCAM-1, vascular cell adhesion molecule-1; VWF, von Willebrand factor. CD47 is also known as the integrin-associated protein or IAP. (From Setty BNY, Kulkarni S, Stuart MJ: Role of erythrocyte phosphatidylserine in sickle red cell-endothelial adhesion. Blood 99:1564–1571, 2002.)

factor α, and interleukin-1), acute phase reactants (such as C-reactive protein, secretory phospholipase A2, and G-CSF), and markers of endothelial cell injury (such as soluble VCAM).[54] The inflammatory biology in patients with SCD appears to result from infection, as well as iron replete (or overloaded) states, sRBC adhesion to endothelium, and the reperfusion-injury physiology observed in these patients.[54]

Hemostatic Changes

Multiple studies show that SCD patients exhibit increased thrombin generation, abnormal activation of fibrinolysis, decreased levels of anticoagulant proteins, activation of platelets, as well as increased circulating levels of soluble tissue factor (TF)[56] in the non-crisis, steady state (Table 47-1). As a result of these findings, SCD has been referred to as a "hypercoagulable state." There, however, remain conflicting data as to whether further activation of coagulation and platelets occur coincident with the development of vaso-occlusive crises.

TF, a transmembrane protein that provides for calcium-dependent binding of coagulation factor VII and its activated form, factor VIIa[57,58] is abnormally expressed on circulating endothelial cells in patients with SCD and its expression is increased further during pain crises.[59] In addition, TF levels, as well as TF procoagulant activity are elevated in the plasma of patients with SCD when compared with normal controls,[60,61] although no difference in TF procoagulant activity was observed when patients with SCD in steady state were compared with those patients with a pain crisis.[60]

MPs, which are small, membrane-derived vesicles released by cells on activation or during apoptosis, are TF positive. MPs in circulating blood are derived from RBCs and platelets as well as endothelial cells and monocytes.[62] Both total MPs, as well as TF-positive MPs are significantly elevated in SCD patients in steady state compared with normal controls and are further increased during pain crises.[62] The TF-positive MPs appear to be derived from endothelial cells and monocytes, but not from RBCs or platelets.

Patients with SCD have elevated levels of prothrombin fragment 1.2 (F1.2) and thrombin:antithrombin III complexes (TAT), both markers of thrombin generation.[63–66] Along with this, they have reduced plasma levels of factors V and XIII in the steady state, findings that are consistent with ongoing generation of thrombin

47

Table 47-1 Evidence for Increased Coagulation and Platelet Activation in Sickle Cell Disease Patients in the Steady, Non-Crisis State

Coagulation/Platelet Parameter	Increased (↑) or Decreased (↓)	References (First Author Only)
Tissue factor (TF)	↑	Solovey[59]; Key[60]; Mohan[61]
Prothrombin fragment 1.2 (F1.2)	↑	Westerman[63]; Peters[65]; Tomer[68]
Thrombin-antithrombin III complex (TAT)	↑	Westerman[63]; Green & Scott[64]; Peters[65]; Kurantsin-Mills[65]; Tomer[68]
Fibrinopeptide A (FPA)	↑	Westerman[63]; Green & Scott[64]; Kurantsin-Mills[66]
β-dimer	↑	Westerman[63]; Kurantsin-Mills[66]; Tomer[68]; Francis[69]
Fibrin-fibrinogen fragment E	↑	Leslie[67]
Factor V	↓	Leslie[67]
Plasmin-antiplasmin (PAP)	↑	Tomer[68]
Platelet factor 4 (PF4)	↑	Tomer[68]; Adamides[31]
Plasma β-thromboglobulin (βTG)	↑	Green & Scott[64]; Tomer[68]; Mehta[30]; Adamides[31]
CD62P (P-selectin) expression	↑	Tomer[68]; Inwald[29]
Platelet thrombospondin content	↓	Browne[27]
CD40-ligand expression	↑	Inwald[29]

activity.[67] Plasmin-antiplasmin complexes (PAP), D-dimers, fibrinopeptide A, and fibrin-fibrinogen fragment E are elevated when plasma samples from SCD patients in the steady state are compared with those of normal individuals,[63,64,66–69] suggesting enhanced thrombin formation, fibrinogen proteolysis, and subsequent fibrin degradation. There is a significant correlation between markers of coagulation activation (D-dimer, F1.2, and TAT) and total MPs, total TF-positive MPs, monocyte-derived TF-positive MPs, and RBC-derived MPs.[62] In addition, a significant correlation exists between the frequency of pain episodes and the extent of plasma fibrinolytic activity, assessed by D-dimer levels, when SCD patients are in the non-crisis, steady state.[68]

In addition to the increased thrombin generation and abnormal fibrinolysis, both protein C activity and protein S antigen and activity levels are decreased in plasma from patients with SCD.[63,70] Decreased protein C and S activity levels are also observed in plasma from SCA patients who have experienced thrombotic strokes when compared with SCA patients who have not experienced similar events.[71,72] Investigators disagree on the activity of antithrombin III (ATIII) in SCD patients both in the non-crisis, steady state and during vaso-occlusive crises.[73–75]

Pathogenesis

The pathogenesis of the hemostatic changes in SCD is likely secondary to multiple factors. In the steady state, the choline-containing phospholipids, phosphatidylcholine and sphingomyelin are located in the outer monolayer of the RBC plasma membrane, whereas phosphatidylserine (PS) is exclusively and phosphatidylethanolamine (PE) is primarily found in the inner monolayer.[76] In normal erythrocytes, maintenance of membrane phospholipid asymmetry is provided by the action of an ATP-dependent aminophospholipid translocase (or flipase), that transports PS and PE from the outer to the inner membrane surface,[77,78] and a nonspecific flopase that transports phospholipids from the inner to the outer monolayer.[79] In addition, scramblase, when activated, results in the movement of all phospholipids in both directions to achieve

rapid PS exposure.[76] Loss of normal phospholipid asymmetry is present in SCD, occurring in mature erythrocytes, RNA-containing reticulocytes, and transferrin receptor-positive "stress" erythrocytes.[80–85] The abnormal PS exposure is believed to occur due to sickling-induced membrane damage,[86] inactivation of the ATP-dependent translocase and premature activation of apoptosis in bone marrow cells. The abnormal phospholipid asymmetry and the resulting adherence of sRBCs to the vascular endothelium both appear to be involved in the hemostatic changes observed in SCD.[35,87,88] Several factors provide evidence for a relationship between the sRBC membrane abnormalities and the hypercoagulable state in patients with SCD. Plasma prothrombin F1.2 levels are significantly associated with the quantity of PS-positive RBCs.[85] Furthermore, there is a significant correlation between PS-positive sRBCs and F1.2, D-dimer, and PAP complexes.[89] However, no correlation was found between PS-positive platelets and any hemostatic markers,[89] suggesting that sRBC, and not platelets, are responsible for the hypercoagulable state observed in SCD. Finally, sRBCs containing high amounts of HbF are associated with decreases in MP formation, PS exposure, and thrombin generation,[85] suggesting a protective effect of HbF on membrane bilayer flip-flop and PS exposure.

Circulating endothelial cells are identified in patients with SCD.[90–92] The surface expression of endothelial adhesion molecules[90,91] plays a significant role in the recruitment of leukocytes[93,94] and the promotion of thrombosis[95] at sites of vascular inflammation. The expression of adhesion molecules (VCAM-1, intercellular adhesion molecule [ICAM-1], E-selectin, and P-selectin), elevated plasma levels of inflammatory mediators (interleukin-6, monocyte chemotactic protein-1, platelet activating factor), and the increased procoagulant phenotype (decreased thrombomodulin and increased VWF and TF phenotype) are characteristic of endothelial activation or injury and have been implicated in the vascular biology of SCD.[36]

The inflammatory state present in SCD may also contribute to its hypercoagulability. Studies in transgenic mouse models show that exposure of NY1DD mice (a mild sickle cell phenotype) to hypoxia-reoxygenation (H/R) results in increased TF expression in the pulmonary veins of the mice following placement in a hypoxic environment for 3 hours followed by a return to ambient air for 18 hours, suggesting a role for ischemia-reperfusion injury.[96]

CLINICAL CONSIDERATIONS

The Role of Hemostatic Abnormalities in Vaso-occlusion

Despite the plethora of evidence supporting activation of coagulation and platelets in the non-crisis, steady state in patients with SCD, there are conflicting data as to whether further increases occur during vaso-occlusive crises.[90,97–106] This apparent conflict may be a result of the somewhat artificial distinction between steady state and pain crisis.

The supporting evidence for a role of activation of the coagulation system in the pathophysiology of SCD remains weak. Activation of the coagulation system and/or platelets may be secondary to, rather than causative of, the ongoing vascular occlusion and/or end-organ damage that characterizes this clinical disorder. Furthermore, the published clinical studies of either anticoagulants or antiplatelet agents in SCD have been small, poorly controlled, and of relatively low quality (Table 47-2).[103,107–115] However, the majority of these studies, which have focused on pain crisis as a clinical outcome, report that treatment with antiplatelet agents or anticoagulants results in only modest clinical benefit at best.

A demonstration of the etiologic relationship between activated platelet and blood coagulation and SCD will come only from well-designed, adequately-powered studies employing anticoagulant and/or antiplatelet therapy, employing both clinical end points of vaso-occlusion and suitable laboratory markers.

By reducing TF activity at sites of mechanical vascular injury, dietary n-3 fatty acids appear to abolish vascular thrombosis in experimental animals without significantly impairing their hemostatic function.[116] A controlled study of dietary n-3 fatty acids in SCD patients demonstrated a significant reduction in the frequency of pain episodes along with decreased markers of thrombin generation and fibrinolysis.[116] Whether the observed reduction in pain episodes was a consequence of this reduction in prothrombotic activity still needs confirmation.

Although the majority of studies have failed to assess the in vivo effect of antiplatelet agents on platelet activation, it remains possible that newer antiplatelet agents such as glycoprotein-IIb/IIIa inhibitors, some of which may have anti-adhesion effects,[117] when administered at doses sufficient to inhibit platelet activation, could have important therapeutic benefits in SCD.

Thrombophilic DNA Mutations

With the evidence of clinical thrombosis and increased thrombin generation in SCD, multiple studies have evaluated the roles of various inherited thrombophilic mutations.

Table 47-2 Published Reports of Anticoagulants and Antiplatelet Agents in Patients with Sickle Cell Disease

Study (First Author)	Genotype	No. of Subjects	Therapy	Randomized	Duration	Efficacy Outcome Measure
Salvaggio[107]	Hb SS	12	Warfarin	No	12–34 Months	Frequency and severity of VOEs
Chaplin[110]	Hb SS	4	Heparin	No	2–6 Years	Frequency and severity of VOEs
Wolters[108]	Hb SS Hb SC	6 1	Acenocoumarol	No	2 Months	Prothrombin fragment 1.2
Schnog[109]	Hb SS Hb SC	14 8	Acenocoumarol vs placebo	Yes	14 Weeks	Frequency of VOEs, Markers of coagulation activation
Chaplin[114]	Hb SS	3	ASA/dipyridamole	No	104 Weeks	Frequency/severity of VOEs, platelets, fibrinogen level
Osamo[111]	Hb SS	100	ASA	Yes	6 Weeks	Total Hb, pO₂ and O₂ Sat, 2,3 BPG level
Greenberg[112]	Hb SS Hb SC Hb SO^Arab	40 8 1	ASA vs placebo	Yes	21 Months	Frequency/severity of VOEs
Semple[103]	Hb SS Hb Sβ Thal	8 1	Ticlopidine vs placebo	Yes	4 weeks	Platelet survival and platelet release products
Cabannes[115]	Hb SS	140	Ticlopidine vs placebo	Yes	6 Months	Frequency/severity of VOEs and CBCs
Zago[113]	Hb SS Hb Sβ Thal	25 4	ASA vs placebo	Yes	5 Months	Frequency/severity of VOEs CBCs, ISCs, and Hb F level

2,3 BPG, 2,3 bisphosphoglycerate; ASA, aspirin; CBC, complete blood count; Hb F, fetal hemoglobin; Hb, hemoglobin; ISC, irreversible sickle cell; O₂ Sat, oxygen saturation; pO₂, partial pressure of oxygen; VOE, vaso-occlusive episode.

Although SCD patients are resistant to activated protein C (APC) when they were compared with normal control subjects,[118] there have, to date, been no reported relationships between either the factor V Leiden (i.e., G1691A) or the prothrombin gene (i.e., G20210A) mutation and the subsequent development of complications in patients with SCD.[119,120]

Plasma homocysteine levels obtained from children with SCD are similar to those obtained from healthy children,[121] although higher homocysteine levels were reported in SCD patients who have experienced one or more ischemic strokes compared with SCD patients who have not had ischemic strokes.[122] Finally, although the methylenetetrahydrofolate reductase (MTHFR) mutation was identified as a risk factor for the development of avascular necrosis among SCD patients,[123] multiple other studies do not show a significant association between the MTHFR mutation and a variety of thrombotic complications in patients with SCD.[119,124–126]

RED BLOOD CELL TRANSFUSION

Transfusion remains a mainstay in the treatment of SCD. Patients experiencing symptomatic anemia benefit from the simple transfusion of packed RBCs. Alternatively, blood transfusion is used to dilute the concentration of red cells containing Hb S to ameliorate or prevent vaso-occlusive events. Although beyond the scope of this chapter, specific indications for transfusion have been addressed and the reader is referred to the monograph by Rosse and colleagues[127] and the NIH publication on the Management of Sickle Cell Disease for a comprehensive review.[128]

In direct contrast to transfusion therapy for patients without SCD, strict attention to avoiding hyperviscosity is necessary to minimize complications. In the acute setting, the posttransfusion total Hb levels should not exceed the 10 to 11 g/dL range. Depending on the baseline Hb level or the posttransfusion Hb S target, it is often necessary to use exchange transfusion to accomplish this goal. Manual or automated techniques can be used depending on the urgency of transfusion and/or availability of erythrocytapheresis equipment (see Chapter 30). Patients with SCD are at a particular high risk of alloimmunization, which can be reduced by leukodepletion and selecting units that are phenotypically matched for the C, E, and Kell in addition to ABO and D antigens.[129]

HYDROXYUREA THERAPY

Hydroxyurea (HU) is currently the only drug approved by the U.S. Food and Drug Administration to treat SCD. Hydroxyurea inhibits DNA synthesis by targeting ribonucleotide reductase, the enzyme responsible for the conversion of ribonucleotide diphosphates to the corresponding deoxyribose forms.[130] Its exact mechanism of action in SCD is unknown. Although it is generally assumed that the benefit of HU is due to an increase in Hb F levels, a multivariable analysis of data from the Multicenter Study of Hydroxyurea in Sickle Cell Anemia (MSH) showed that the percentage of F cells was inversely correlated with the rate of painful crises only during the first three months of therapy.[131] However, there was a strong correlation

between the neutrophil count and the rate of pain crises throughout the treatment period. As a result, the observed neutropenia may not only contribute to, but also be necessary for the effectiveness of the drug. HU has also been reported to decrease the expression of PS on the surface of RBCs and platelets in patients with SCD, an effect that may contribute to its therapeutic benefit.[132] The RBCs from those patients receiving HU adhere less avidly to thrombospondin,[133] and in preliminary studies, treatment with HU resulted in a decrease in the level of D-dimer in the peripheral circulation.[134] Finally, the ability of HU to decrease vaso-occlusive phenomena may, in part, be attributed to vasodilation and/or decreased platelet activation induced by HU-derived nitric oxide.[135,136]

Treatment with HU results in a significant decrease in the frequency and severity of painful crises, a reduction in the incidence of acute chest syndrome, and a reduction in the need for blood transfusions.[131] HU treatment also results in substantial reduction in clinical events requiring hospitalization.[137] Furthermore, HU has been reported to result in reduced mortality in adults with severe SCA.[138]

ACUTE CHEST SYNDROME

Acute chest syndrome (ACS) is the second most common cause of hospitalization and a leading cause of death in patients with SCD.[5,10] It is defined by the presence on a chest radiograph of a new pulmonary infiltrate and respiratory symptoms that include cough, tachypnea, and chest pain.[139–141] The symptoms at presentation are age-dependent, with fever, wheezing, and cough being predominant in children younger than 10 years.[142] Adults, on the other hand, typically present with shortness of breath, chills, and severe pain, with multilobe and lower lobe involvement on chest radiograph.[142] Nearly one half of the patients are admitted with a diagnosis other than ACS (usually pain), with the syndrome being defined after about 2.5 days of hospitalization.[143]

The incidence of ACS is higher in patients with Hb SS [12.8/100 patient-years] and in patients with Hb Sβ0 thalassemia (9.4/100 patient-years), and lower in patients with Hb SC (5.2/100 patient-years) and patients with Hb Sβ+thalassemia (3.9/100 patient-years). ACS occurs more commonly in young children, patients with low levels of Hb F, and patients with higher steady state WBC counts and hemoglobin levels.[10]

Etiology and Pathophysiology

In a study using rigorous methods, including bronchoscopy, deep sputum cultures, and extensive serologic evaluations, a specific etiology (pulmonary fat embolism or an infectious agent) was identified in 70% of cases of ACS with complete data.[143] Pulmonary infarction was presumed to be the cause in 16% of episodes in those subjects with complete data for whom no etiology was identified. Of the multiple isolated pathogens, *Chlamydia pneumoniae* and *Mycoplasma pneumoniae* were the most frequently identified. Patients with pulmonary fat embolism as the cause of ACS were older, had lower oxygen saturation, and were more likely to have upper lobe infiltrates compared with those patients with infection or infarction as the cause.[143]

However, the overall complication rates, with the exception of incidence of pain events, were similar in all three groups.

The pathogenesis of ACS appears to be due to hypoxia-enhanced in vivo sRBC adhesion to pulmonary microvasculature.[144] Hypoxia has been shown to enhance the adhesion of RBCs to endothelial cells, an interaction mediated by the binding of VCAM-1, expressed on endothelial cells, to $\alpha_4\beta_1$ on red cells.[45] Plasma concentrations of soluble VCAM-1 are elevated in patients with ACS, and this increase is inversely related to plasma concentrations of nitric oxide (NO) metabolites.[144] In accompanying in vitro experiments, exposure to both hypoxia and oleic acid increased the expression of VCAM-1 in pulmonary endothelial cells and resulted in increased adherence of sRBCs to these endothelial cells. However, exposure to NO donors resulted in reduced adhesion of sRBCs to endothelial cells following exposure to hypoxia and oleic acid.[144] These findings suggest that increased expression of adhesion molecules as a result of hypoxia, fat embolization, and cytokines in the setting of decreased NO production observed in sickle cell pain crises and ACS contributes to systemic and pulmonary RBC sequestration.[145]

Clinical Management

The routine use of invasive procedures, such as bronchoscopy, is not required in the evaluation of patients with ACS (Table 47-3). However, routine serologic tests for *Chlamydia*, *Mycoplasma*, and *Legionella* may be incorporated (when available) with routine cultures in the overall management strategy. Prophylactic measures such as incentive spirometry for SCD patients hospitalized for vaso-occlusive episodes[146] and judicious use of analgesics to avoid excessive sedation are especially important.[147] Once patients develop ACS, the use of antibiotics, such as newer fluoroquinolones or macrolide and a cephalosporin, with coverage against *Chlamydia* and *Mycoplasma* are recommended. Oxygen therapy is indicated for hypoxia, and strict attention to fluid balance to avoid overhydration is necessary.

Blood transfusion improves oxygenation, as well as the clinical status of patients with ACS.[143,148] Its use may be especially important in those patients with radiographic evidence of extensive lobar involvement, thrombocytopenia, and a history of cardiac disease (all predictors of respiratory failure),[143] as well as neurologic abnormalities. Either simple or exchange transfusion appears to result in similar improvements in oxygenation.[143] There are no strict criteria for choosing between the techniques, but exchange transfusion to reduce the Hb S level below 30% should be considered if there is respiratory failure. However, during transfusion of these patients, it is important not to exceed a hemoglobin concentration of 10 to 11 g/dL. In those instances when patients develop respiratory failure, mechanical ventilation, as well other modalities such as extracorporeal membrane oxygenation (ECMO), may be helpful.[149]

There are several reports of the pharmacologic use of NO in mechanically ventilated patients with respiratory failure.[150,151] A short course of steroid therapy was shown to reduce the length of hospital stay in children with ACS, although a rebound effect with increased patient readmission was observed.[152] Additional rigorous studies of both steroid and NO administration in ACS are required before they are recommended for routine use.

PULMONARY HYPERTENSION IN SICKLE CELL DISEASE

Pulmonary hypertension (PHT) (see Chapter 45), usually defined as a sustained elevation of the mean pulmonary arterial pressure to more than 25 mm Hg at rest or to more than 30 mm Hg with exercise,[153] is recognized as a common complication in patients with SCD. Multiple reports suggest a high occurrence of PHT in these patients, with recent cross-sectional studies reporting a prevalence of 20% to 35%.[154–157] Furthermore, SCD patients with PHT have a significantly increased mortality rate compared with those SCD patients without PHT.[154,156,158–160] In the study by Castro and coworkers, SCD patients with PHT confirmed by right heart catheterization had a 50% 2-year mortality rate compared with a survival greater than 70% at the end of a 119-month observation period in SCD patients without PHT.[160]

Pathophysiology

The pathogenesis of PHT in SCD is likely multifactorial. Chronic intravascular hemolysis, with resultant scavenging of NO and development of NO resistance, appears to play a prominent role in the development of PHT.[156,161–166] As a result of this NO resistance, vascular smooth muscle guanylyl cyclase is not activated and vasodilation is

---

Table 47-3 Management of Acute Chest Syndrome

Prophylaxis
Close monitoring of oxygen saturation during hospitalization
Aggressive incentive spirometry and ambulation as tolerated
Judicious use of opioid analgesics to avoid oversedation
Avoidance of overhydration—encourage oral hydration if patient is able to drink adequately
Adequate immunization—pneumococcal, influenza, and possibly parvovirus B19
Hydroxyurea in patients with frequent pain episodes or history of severe/recurrent acute chest syndrome

Diagnostic Testing
Blood cultures and serologies for *Chlamydia*, *Mycoplasma* (if available)
Deep sputum for bacterial culture
Chest radiograph
Arterial blood gas for changes in oxygen saturation

Treatment
Supplemental oxygen for hypoxia (oxygen saturation <92%)
Judicious fluid management
Optimal pain control
Incentive spirometry and chest physical therapy (unless chest pain is present)
Empiric antibiotics to cover community-acquired pneumonia (levofloxacin or azithromycin + cephalosporin)
Bronchodilator therapy (even in the absence of obvious wheezing)
Blood transfusion therapy (simple or exchange) with leukocyte-reduced phenotypically compatible red cells keeping total hemoglobin ≤10–11 g/dL
Mechanical ventilation or extracorporeal membrane oxygenation, if necessary

inhibited. Hemolysis also results in the release of arginase, which converts L-arginine (the substrate for NO synthesis) to ornithine.[167] Elevated arginase activity, with resultant decrease in arginine/ornithine ratio is associated with elevated pulmonary pressures.[156,168] Furthermore, lower arginine/ornithine ratio is independently associated with increased mortality in patients with SCD.[168]

PHT may also result from recurrent vaso-occlusion and ACS leading to parenchymal lung injury,[169,170] although recent studies[156,157] did not find any association between PHT and a previous history of ACS. Pulmonary thromboembolism[171–174] and progressive endothelial damage with concentric pulmonary vascular intimal hyperplasia and in situ thrombosis[174,175] may contribute to the pathogenesis of PHT in SCD. Other mechanisms that may contribute to the development of PHT in SCD include chronic and recurrent acute hypoxemia, possibly exacerbated by hypoventilation during sleep;[176] elevated pulmonary capillary wedge pressure due, in large part, to left ventricular diastolic dysfunction[160]; and functional asplenia, present in most adult patients with SCA.[177]

Clinical Management

The symptoms of PHT in patients with SCD are nonspecific in the early stages.[169] Patients may present with increasing shortness of breath after physical exertion, chest pain, near-syncope or syncope, and peripheral edema in more advanced stages. With the nonspecific nature of symptoms at the early stages and recognition of increased mortality, many experts now advocate periodic screening of SCD patients with transthoracic echocardiography, at least every 2 to 3 years.[178,179]

Despite the increased recognition of PHT in patients with SCD, there is no consensus in the management of these patients. There are conflicting reports on the effect of HU in PHT.[156,157] However, a recent report suggests a lower prevalence of PHT in those SCD patients on HU therapy.[157] The role of transfusion therapy in the treatment of patients in this setting remains controversial. Although some preliminary studies suggest that PHT may be ameliorated or even partially reversible with transfusion therapy,[180] others have reported no benefit with RBC transfusion.[159] Hypoxia is known to result in vasoconstriction of the pulmonary vessels[181] and as a result, supplemental oxygen would be expected to be of benefit in hypoxic patients with PHT. Those with disorders of breathing during sleep should be assessed for response to nocturnal oxygen or continuous positive airway pressure (CPAP).

A short course of oral arginine given to 10 SCD patients with PHT led to a significant decline in the pulmonary artery systolic pressure (PASP) (63.9 ± 13 to 54.2 ± 12 mm Hg, $P = 0.002$).[182] However, adequately powered, controlled studies are required to confirm the efficacy of arginine in these patients. With the possibility that thrombosis contributes to the pathogenesis of PHT in SCD, clinical trials evaluating the effect of anticoagulant therapy are needed. This is especially in view of reports that anticoagulation provides a survival benefit for patients with idiopathic pulmonary arterial hypertension.[183] The prostacyclin analog, epoprostenol, known to prolong survival in patients with primary PHT,[184] and other prostacyclin analogs have been used in SCD patients with PHT,[160] although their usefulness has

yet to be confirmed in controlled trials. Treatment with sildenafil, a phosphodiesterase type 5 inhibitor, for at least 3 months results in improved PASP and functional capacity, as assessed by a 6-minute walk test.[185] Most of the patients in this preliminary study were women (of the three male subjects, two were receiving chronic RBC transfusion and one had erectile dysfunction); there remains concern regarding the risk of priapism in male SCD patients on sildenafil therapy.

With the increased mortality associated with PHT in patients with SCD, it is imperative that patients are aggressively evaluated and treated. They should be evaluated in their non-crisis, steady state, as increases in the PASP are known to occur during vaso-occlusive episodes[186] and during ACS. In the absence of proved therapies from adequately controlled studies, newly diagnosed patients should be enrolled in clinical trials evaluating the effects of different treatments on PHT in SCD.

STROKE

The overall reported prevalence of overt stroke in children with SCA is approximately 10%. These events are predominantly ischemic in etiology. In addition to the clinically identified events, MRI scans of the brain of apparently unaffected children reveal a 15% to 20% incidence of silent infarction.[187,188] The pathogenesis of cerebral infarction in children with SCD is not simply sickling of RBCs in the microcirculation. Endothelial injury as described earlier for vaso-occlusive events is likely a major contributor to the pathophysiology.[189] Prior transient ischemic attack, anemia, recent or frequent ACS episodes, and hypertension have been identified as risk factors.[190] The majority of children presenting with stroke symptoms corresponding to a specific arterial distribution demonstrate stenosis or occlusion of major intracranial arteries. In a subset of patients with such abnormalities of the internal carotid arteries, a network of collateral vessels develop (moyamoya syndrome) which appears to confer an increased risk for recurrent cerebrovascular events.[191]

The Stroke Prevention Trial in Sickle Cell Anemia (STOP) addressed the use of prophylactic RBC transfusion in children 2 to 16 years of age with SCA who were at high risk for an initial stroke based on transcranial Doppler ultrasonography (TCD).[192] There was a significant reduction in the incidence of strokes in patients randomized to receive prophylactic transfusions to reduce the hemoglobin S level to below 30% (1 of 63) compared with patients receiving standard care (11 of 67). The optimum duration of chronic transfusion necessary to provide protection from a cerebrovascular event is not known. However, the results of the Optimizing Primary Stroke Prevention in Sickle Cell Anemia (STOP 2) trial addressing this issue have recently been reported.[193] Seventy-nine patients with abnormal TCD before transfusion and who had received at least 30 months of RBC transfusion were randomized to stop or continue transfusions. Of the 41 patients randomized to discontinue transfusion, 16 reached the primary end point events (14 patients with reversion to high-risk TCD and 2 patients with ischemic strokes) compared with neither of these events in the 38 patients continuing to receive transfusions. These results indicate that discontinuation of chronic transfusion after 30 months cannot be recommended. Primary prevention of cerebrovascular events in patients older than 16 years of age has not been addressed in clinical trials and TCD screening for adults cannot be recommended for routine use at this time.

The differential diagnosis of a child with SCD presenting with new neurologic deficits includes infection, ischemic stroke, and intracranial hemorrhage. The initial evaluation should include a non-contrast CT scan. For the patient with apparent evolving or completed ischemic stroke, emergent transfusion is indicated. Although simple transfusion can be considered if the Hb level is below 10 g/dL, exchange transfusion is recommended to more promptly reduce the Hb S level to below 30%. MR imaging including MRA will assist in providing essential information concerning the presence of arterial vasculopathy. Hemorrhagic stroke occurs more commonly in young adults.[190] Subarachnoid hemorrhage may be due to rupture of a cerebral aneurysm (which may be multiple in SCD) or the moyamoya collaterals. Conventional angiography may be necessary to identify arteriovenous malformations or aneurysms.

The recurrence rate of stroke in children with ischemic events not receiving subsequent treatment was found to be 66%.[194] Two case series demonstrated that long-term blood transfusion substantially reduced the risk of recurrence.[195,196] Current clinical practice is to begin a chronic transfusion program to maintain the Hb S level below 30%. After 3 to 4 years, a decrease in frequency of transfusion to allow the target value to rise to 50% may be considered.[197] Randomized clinical trials addressing the duration of transfusion for secondary stroke prevention have not been conducted. Children stopping transfusion after 5 to 12 years experienced a 50% recurrence rate.[198] The current standard of care is to continue a chronic transfusion program indefinitely. Recurrent events are observed for patients continuing on a chronic transfusion program. The largest published experience is a retrospective multicenter study of 137 children with stroke maintained on chronic transfusion for at least 5 years revealing a recurrence rate of 2.2 per 100 patient-years.[199]

HU therapy combined with phlebotomy has been evaluated in 35 children as an alternative to chronic transfusion.[200] Patients received transfusions for approximately 4 years prior to being switched to HU, which was titrated to maximally tolerated doses. The recurrence rate was 5.7 events per 100 patient-years with a mean duration of 3.5 years follow-up. The protocol was modified to overlap HU rather than to abruptly discontinue transfusions and resulted in a reduced recurrence rate of 3.6 events per 100 patient-years. A multicenter randomized controlled trial examining HU therapy as an alternative to transfusion is planned. HU therapy should be considered for patients who wish to discontinue transfusion or have such problems as extensive alloimmunization preventing maintenance transfusions.

For adolescents and adults, the evaluation of acute stroke should also address etiologies relevant to patients without SCD (e.g., hypertension, embolism, arterial dissection, atrial fibrillation, and infection). There are no clinical trials addressing the use of recombinant tissue plasminogen activator or the role of antiplatelet agents in SCD patients with acute ischemic events. The role of chronic transfusion for the patient with the initial event as an adult has not been defined.

REFERENCES

1. Pauling L, Itano HA: Sickle cell anemia: A molecular disease. Science 110(2865): 543–548, 1949.
2. Steinberg MH: Predicting clinical severity in sickle cell anaemia. Br J Haematol 129(4): 465–481, 2005.
2a. Frenette PS, Atweh GF: Science in Medicine. Sickle cell disease: Old discoveries, new concepts, and future promise. J Clin Invest 117:850–858, 2007.
3. Gaston MH, Verter JI, Woods G, et al: Prophylaxis with oral penicillin in children with sickle cell anemia: A randomized trial. N Engl J Med 314:1593–1599, 1986.
4. Quinn CT, Rogers ZR, Buchanan GR: Survival of children with sickle cell disease. Blood 103(11): 4023–4027, 2004.
5. Platt OS, Brambilla DJ, Rosse WF, et al: Mortality in sickle cell disease: Life expectancy and risk factors for early death. N Engl J Med 330(23): 1639–1644, 1994.
6. Bunn HF: Pathogenesis and treatment of sickle cell disease. N Engl J Med 337(11): 762–769, 1997.
7. Hofrichter J, Ross PD, Eaton WA: Supersaturation in sickle cell hemoglobin solutions. Proc Natl Acad Sci USA 73:3035–3039, 1976.
8. Mozzarelli A, Hofrichter J, Eaton WA: Delay time of hemoglobin S polymerization prevents most cells from sickling in vivo. Science 237:500–506, 1987.
9. Nagel RL, Bookchin RM, Johnson J, et al: Structural bases of the inhibitory effects of hemoglobin F and hemoglobin A2 on the polymerization of hemoglobin S. Proc Natl Acad Sci USA 76:670–672, 1979.
10. Castro O, Brambilla DJ, Thorington B, et al: The acute chest syndrome of sickle cell disease: Incidence and risk factors. The Cooperative Study of Sickle Cell Disease. Blood 84:643–649, 1994.
11. Ohene-Frempong K, Weiner SJ, Sleeper LA, et al: Cerebrovascular accidents in sickle cell disease: Rates and risk factors. Blood 91:288–294, 1998.
12. Abboud M, Laver J, Blau CA: Granulocytosis causing sickle cell crisis. Lancet 351:959, 1998.
13. Alder BK, Satzman DE, Carabasi MH, et al: Fatal sickle cell crisis after granulocyte colony-stimulating factor administration. Blood 97:3313–3314, 2001.
14. Dias-da-Motta PM, Arruda VR, Muscara MN, et al: The release of nitric oxide and superoxide anion by neutrophils and mononuclear cells from patients with sickle cell anaemia. Br J Haematol 93:333–340, 1996.
15. Hofstra TC, Kalra VK, Meiselman HJ, et al: Sickle erythrocytes adhere to polymorphonuclear neutrophils and activate the neutrophil respiratory burst. Blood 87:4440–4447, 1996.
16. Okpala I: The intriguing contribution of white blood cells to sickle cell disease: A red cell disorder. Blood Reviews 18:65–73, 2004.
17. Belcher JD, Marker PH, Weber JP, et al: Activated monocytes in sickle cell disease: Potential role in the activation of vascular endothelium and vaso-occlusion. Blood 96:2451–2459, 2000.
18. Francis RB: Platelets, coagulation, and fibrinolysis in sickle cell disease: Their possible role in vascular occlusion. Blood Coagul Fibrinolysis 2:341–353, 1991.
19. Haut MJ, Cowan DH, Harris JW: Platelet function and survival in sickle cell disease. J Lab Clin Med 82:44–53, 1973.
20. Semple MJ, Al-Hasani SF, Kioy P, et al: A double-blind trial of ticlopidine in sickle cell disease. Thromb Haemostas 51:303–306, 1984.
21. Kenny MW, George AJ, Stuart J: Platelet hyperactivity in sickle cell disease: A consequence of hyposplenism. J Clin Pathol 33:622–625, 1980.
22. Westwick J, Watson-Williams EJ, Krishnamurthi S, et al: Platelet activation during steady state sickle cell disease. J Med 14:17–36, 1983.
23. Mehta P, Mehta J: Abnormalities of platelet aggregation in sickle cell disease. J Peds 96:209–213, 1980.
24. Gruppo RA, Glueck HI, Granger SM, et al: Platelet function in sickle cell anemia. Thromb Res 10:325–335, 1977.
25. Stuart MJ, Stockman JA, Oski FA: Abnormalities of platelet aggregation in the vaso-occlusive crises of sickle cell anaemia. J Peds 85:629–632, 1974.
26. Tomer A, Harker LA, Kasey S, et al: Thrombogenesis in sickle cell disease. J Lab Clin Med 137:398–407, 2001.
27. Browne PV, Mosher DF, Steinberg MH, Hebbel RP: Disturbance of plasma and platelet thrombospondin levels in sickle cell disease. Am J Hematol 51:296–301, 1996.

28. Wun T, Paglieroni T, Tablin F, et al: Platelet activation and platelet-erythrocyte aggregates in patients with sickle cell anemia. J Clin Lab Med 129:507–516, 1997.

29. Inwald DP, Kirkham FJ, Peters MJ, et al: Platelet and leucocyte activation in childhood sickle cell disease: Association with nocturnal hypoxaemia. Br J Haematol 111:474–481, 2000.

30. Mehta P: Significance of plasma β-thromboglobulin in patients with sickle cell disease. J Pediatrics 97:941–944, 1980.

31. Adamides S, Konstantopuoulos K, Toumbis M, et al: A study of β-thromboglobulin and platelet factor-4 levels in steady state sickle cell patients. Blut 61:245–247, 1990.

32. Buerling-Harbury C, Schade SG: Platelet activation during crisis in sickle cell anemia patients. Am J Hematol 31:237–241, 1989.

33. Wun T, Paglieroni T, Rangaswami A, et al: Platelet activation in patients with sickle cell disease. Br J Haematol 100:741–749, 1998.

34. Eaton WA, Hofrichter J: Hemoglobin S gelation and sickle cell disease. Blood 70:1245–1266, 1987.

35. Hebbel RP, Boogaerts MAB, Eaton JW, et al: Erythrocyte adherence to endothelium in sickle cell anemia: A possible determinant of disease severity. N Engl J Med 302:992–995, 1980.

36. Hebbel RP, Yamada O, Moldow CF, et al: Abnormal adherence of sickle erythrocytes to cultured vascular endothelium: Possible mechanism for microvascular occlusion in sickle cell disease. J Clin Invest 65:154–160, 1980.

37. Hoover R, Rubin R, Wise G, et al: Adhesion of normal and sickle erythrocytes to endothelial monolayer cultures. Blood 54:872–876, 1979.

38. Barabino GA, McIntire LV, Eskin SG, et al: Endothelial cell interactions with sickle cell, sickle trait, mechanically injured, and normal erythrocytes under controlled flow. Blood 70:152–157, 1987.

39. Brittain HA, Eckman JR, Swerlick RA, et al: Thrombospondin from activated platelets promotes sickle erythrocyte adherence to human microvascular endothelium under physiologic flow: A potential role for platelet activation in sickle cell vaso-occlusion. Blood 81:2137–2143, 1993.

40. Gupta K, Gupta P, Solovey A, et al: Mechanism of interaction of thrombospondin with human endothelium and inhibition of sickle erythrocyte adhesion to human endothelial cells by heparin. Biochim Biophys Acta 453:63–73, 1999.

41. Brittain JE, Milner KJ, Anderson CS, et al: Integrin-associated protein is an adhesion receptor on sickle red blood cells for immobilized thrombospondin. Blood 97:2159–2164, 2001.

42. Swerlick RA, Eckman JR, Kumar A, et al: $\alpha_4\beta_1$ Integrin expression on sickle erythrocytes: Vascular cell adhesion molecule-1 dependent binding to endothelium. Blood 82:1891–1899, 1993.

43. Joneckis CC, Ackley RL, Orringer EP, et al: Integrin $\alpha_4\beta_1$ and glycoprotein IV (CD36) are expressed on circulating reticulocytes in sickle cell anemia. Blood 82:3548–3555, 1993.

44. Gee BE, Platt OS: Sickle reticulocytes adhere to VCAM-1. Blood 85:268–274, 1995.

45. Setty BNY, Stuart MJ: Vascular cell adhesion molecule-1 is involved in mediating hypoxia-induced sickle red cell adherence to endothelium: Potential role in sickle cell disease. Blood 88:2311–2320, 1996.

46. Kumar A, Eckmann JR, Swerlick RA, et al: Phorbol ester stimulation increases sickle erythrocyte adherence to endothelium: A novel pathway involving alpha 4 beta 1 integrin receptors on sickle reticulocytes and fibronectin. Blood 88:4348–4358, 1996.

47. Kaul DK, Tsai HM, Liu D, et al: Monoclonal antibodies to alpha V beta3 7E3 and LM609) inhibit sickle red blood cell-endothelium interactions induced by platelet-activating factor. Blood 95:368–374, 2000.

48. Wick TM, Moake JL, Udden MM, et al: Unusually large vWF multimers increase adhesion of sickle erythrocytes to human endothelial cells under controlled flow. J Clin Invest 80:905–910, 1987.

49. Harlan JM: Introduction: Anti-adhesion therapy in sickle cell disease. Blood 95:365–367, 2000.

50. Udani M, Zen O, Cottman M: Basal cell adhesion molecule/Lutheran protein: The receptor critical for sickle cell adhesion to laminin. J Clin Invest 101:2550–2558, 1998.

51. Hillery CE, Du MC, Montgomery RR, et al: Increased adhesion of erythrocytes to components of the extracellular matrix: Isolation and characterization of a red blood cell ligand that binds thrombospondin and laminin. Blood 87:4879–4886, 1996.

52. Manodori AB, Barabino GA, Lubin BH, et al: Adherence of phosphatidylserine—exposing erythrocytes to endothelial matrix thrombospondin. Blood 95:1293–1300, 2000.

53. Setty BNY, Kulkarni S, Stuart MJ: Role of erythrocyte phosphatidylserine in sickle red cell-endothelial adhesion. Blood 99:1564–1571, 2002.

54. Hebbel RP, Osarogiagbon R, Kaul D: The endothelial biology of sickle cell disease: Inflammation and a chronic vasculopathy. Microcirculation 11:129–151, 2004.

55. Platt OS: Sickle cell anemia as an inflammatory disease. J Clin Invest 106:337–338, 2000.

56. Ataga KI, Orringer EP: Hypercoagulability in sickle cell disease: A curious paradox. Am J Med 15:721–728, 2003.

57. Edgington TS, Mackman N, Brand K, et al: The structural biology of expression and function of tissue factor. Thromb Haemost 66:67–79, 1991.

58. Nemersom Y: The tissue factor pathway of blood coagulation. Semin Hematol 29:170–176, 1992.

59. Solovey A, Gui L, Key NS, Hebbel RP: Tissue factor expression by endothelial cells in sickle cell anemia. J Clin Invest 101:1899–1904, 1998.

60. Key NS, Slungaard A, Dandelet L, et al: Whole blood tissue factor procoagulant activity is elevated in patients with sickle cell disease. Blood 91:4216–4223, 1998.

61. Mohan JS, Lip GYH, Wright J, et al: Plasma levels of tissue factor and soluble E-selectin in sickle cell disease: Relationship to genotype and to inflammation. Blood Coagul Fibrinolysis 16:209–214, 2005.

62. Shet AS, Aras O, Gupta K, et al: Sickle blood contains tissue factor-positive microparticles derived from endothelial cells and monocytes. Blood 102:2678–2683, 2003.

63. Westerman MP, Green D, Gilman-Sachs A, et al: Antiphospholipid antibodies, protein C and S, and coagulation changes in sickle cell disease. J Lab Clin Med 134:352–362, 1999.

64. Green D, Scott JP: Is sickle cell crisis a thrombotic event? Am J Hematol 23:317–321, 1986.

65. Peters M, Plaat BEC, ten Cate H, et al: Enhanced thrombin generation in children with sickle cell disease. Thromb Haemost 71:169–172, 1994.

66. Kurantsin-Mills J, Ofosu FA, Safa TK, et al: Plasma factor VII and thrombin-antithrombin III levels indicate increased tissue factor activity in sickle cell patients. Br J Haematol 81:539–544, 1992.

67. Leslie J, Langler D, Serjeant GR, et al: Coagulation changes during the steady state in homozygous sickle-cell disease in Jamaica. Br J Haematol 30:159–166, 1975.

68. Tomer A, Harker LA, Kasey S, et al: Thrombogenesis in sickle cell disease. J Lab Clin Med 137:398–407, 2001.

69. Francis RB Jr: Elevated fibrin D-dimer fragment in sickle cell anemia: Evidence for activation of coagulation during the steady state as well as in painful crisis. Haemostasis 19:105–111, 1989.

70. Wright JG, Malia R, Cooper P, et al: Protein C and S in homozygous sickle cell disease: Does hepatic dysfunction contribute to low levels? Br J Haematol 98:627–631, 1997.

71. Tam DA: Protein C and S activity in sickle cell disease and stroke. J Child Neurol 12:19–21, 1997.

72. Khanduri U, Gravell D, Christie BS, et al: Reduced protein C levels: A contributory factory for stroke in sickle cell disease [letter]. Thromb Haemost 79:879–880, 1998.

73. Richardson SGN, Matthews KB, Stuart J, et al: Serial changes in coagulation and viscosity during sickle-cell crisis. Br J Haematol 41:95–103, 1979.

74. Porter JB, Young L, Mackie IJ, et al: Sickle cell disorders and chronic intravascular haemolysis are associated with low plasma heparin cofactor II. Br J Haematol 83:459–465, 1993.

75. Karayalcin G, Chung D, Pinto P, et al: Plasma antithrombin III levels in children with homozygous sickle cell disease (SCD). Pediatr Res 18:242A, 1984.

76. Zwaal RFA, Schroit AJ: Pathophysiologic implications of membrane phospholipids asymmetry in blood cells: A review. Blood 89:1121–1132, 1997.

77. Koopman G, Reutelingsperger CP, Kuijten GA, et al: Annexin V for flow cytometric detection of phosphatidylserine expression on B cells undergoing apoptosis. Blood 84:1415–1420, 1994.

78. Seigneuuret M, Devaux PF: Asymmetric distribution of spin-labeled phospholipids in the erythrocyte membrane: Relation to shape changes. Proc Natl Acad Sci USA 81:3751, 1984.

79. Bitbol M, Devaux PF: Measurement of outward translocation of phospholipids across human erythrocyte membrane. Proc Natl Acad Sci USA 85:6783, 1988.

80. Kuypers F, Lewis RA, Ernst JD, et al: Detection of altered membrane phospholipid asymmetry in subpopulations of human red blood cells using fluorescently labeled annexin V. Blood 87:1179–1187, 1996.

81. Chiu D, Lubin B, Shohet SB: Erythrocyte membrane lipid reorganization during the sickling process. Br J Haematol 41:223–234, 1979.

82. Franck PF, Chiu DT, Op Den Kamp JA, et al: Accelerated transbilayer movement of phosphatidylcholine in sickled erythrocytes: A reversible process. J Biol Chem 258:8436–8442, 1983.

83. Tait JF, Gibson D: Measurement of membrane phospholipid asymmetry in normal and sickle-cell erythrocytes by means of annexin V binding. J Lab Clin Med 123:741–748, 1994.

84. Helley D, Eldor A, Girot R, et al: Increased procoagulant activity of red blood cells from patients with homozygous sickle cell disease and β-thalassemia. Thromb Haemost 76:322–327, 1996.

85. Setty BNY, Kulkarni S, Rao AK, et al: Fetal hemoglobin in sickle cell disease: Relationship to erythrocyte phosphatidylserine exposure and coagulation activation. Blood 96:1119–1124, 2000.

86. De Jong K, Larkin SK, Styles LA, et al: Characterization of the phosphatidylserine-exposing subpopulation of sickle cells. Blood 98:860–867, 2001.

87. Schroit AJ, Zwaal RFA: Transbilayer movement of phospholipids in red cell and platelet membranes. Biochim Biophys Acta 1071:313–329, 1991.

88. Chiu D, Lubin B, Roelofsen B, Van Deenen LL: Sickled erythrocytes accelerate clotting in vitro: An effect of abnormal membrane lipid asymmetry. Blood 58:398–401, 1981.

89. Setty BNY, Rao AK, Stuart MJ: Thrombophilia in sickle cell disease: The red cell connection. Blood 98:3228–3233, 2001.

90. Solovey A, Gui L, Key NS, et al: Tissue factor expression by endothelial cells in sickle cell anemia. J Clin Invest 101:1899–1904, 1998.

91. Solovey A, Lin Y, Browne P, et al: Circulating activated endothelial cells in sickle cell anemia. N Engl J Med 337:1584–1590, 1997.

92. Solovey A, Gui L, Ramakrishnan S, et al: Sickle cell anemia as a possible state of enhanced anti-apoptotic tone: Survival effect of vascular endothelial growth factor on circulating and unanchored endothelial cells. Blood 93:3824–3830, 1999.

93. Springer T: Traffic signals for lymphocyte recirculation and leukocyte emigration: The multistep paradigm. Cell 76:301–314, 1994.

94. Carlos TM, Harlan JM: Leukocyte-endothelial adhesion molecules. Blood 84:2068–2101, 1994.

95. Mann KG, van't Veer C, Cawthern K, et al: The role of the tissue factor pathway in initiation of coagulation. Blood Coagul Fibrinolysis 9 (Suppl 1):S3–S7, 1998.

96. Solovey A, Kollander R, Shet A, et al: Endothelial cell expression of tissue factor in sickle mice is augmented by hypoxia/reoxygenation and inhibited by lovastatin. Blood 104:840–846, 2004.

97. Key NS, Slungaard A, Dandelet L, et al: Whole blood tissue factor procoagulant activity is elevated in patients with sickle cell disease. Blood 91:4216–4223, 1998.

98. Westerman MP, Green D, Gilman-Sachs A, et al: Antiphospholipid antibodies, protein C and S, and coagulation changes in sickle cell disease. J Lab Clin Med 134:352–362, 1999.

99. Green D, Scott JP: Is sickle cell crisis a thrombotic event? Am J Hematol 23:317–321, 1986.

100. Tomer A, Harker LA, Kasey S, et al: Thrombogenesis in sickle cell disease. J Lab Clin Med 137:398–407, 2001.

101. Francis RB Jr: Elevated fibrin D-dimer fragment in sickle cell anemia: Evidence for activation of coagulation during the steady state as well as in painful crisis. Haemostasis 19:105–111, 1989.

102. Haut MJ, Cowan DH, Harris JW: Platelet function and survival in sickle cell disease. J Lab Clin Med 82:44–53, 1973.

103. Semple MJ, Al-Hasani SF, Kioy P, et al: A double-blind trial of ticlopidine in sickle cell disease. Thromb Haemostas 51:303–306, 1984.

104. Browne PV, Mosher DF, Steinberg MH, et al: Disturbance of plasma and platelet thrombospondin levels in sickle cell disease. Am J Hematol 51:296–301, 1996.

105. Freedman ML, Karpatikin S: Short Communication: Elevated platelet count and megathrombocyte number in sickle cell anemia. Blood 46:579–582, 1975.

106. Alkjaersig N, Fletcher A, Joist H, et al: Haemostatic alterations accompanying sickle cell pain crisis. J Lab Clin Med 88:440–449, 1976.

107. Salvaggio JE, Arnold CA, Banov CH: Long-term anticoagulation in sickle cell disease. N Engl J Med 1963 269:182–186, 1963.

108. Wolters HJ, Ten Cate H, Thomas LLM, et al: Low-intensity oral anticoagulation in sickle-cell disease reverses the prethrombotic state: Promises for treatment? Br J Haematol 90:715–717, 1995.

109. Schnog JB, Kater AP, MacGillavry MR, et al: Low adjusted dose acenocoumarol therapy in sickle cell disease: A pilot study. Am J Hematol 68:179–183, 2001.

110. Chaplin MR Jr., Monroe MC, Malecek MC, et al: Preliminary trial of minidose heparin prophylaxis for painful sickle cell crises. East Afri Med J 66:574–584, 1989.

111. Osamo NO, Photiades DP, Famodu AA: Therapeutic effect of aspirin in sickle cell anaemia. Acta Haematol 66:102–107, 1981.

112. Greenberg J, Ohene-Frempong K, Halus J, et al: Trial of low doses of aspirin as prophylaxis in sickle cell disease. J Pediatr 102:781–784, 1983.

113. Zago MA, Costa FF, Ismael SJ, et al: Treatment of sickle cell diseases with aspirin. Acta Haematol 72:61–64, 1984.

114. Chaplin H, Alkjaersig N, Fletcher AP, et al: Aspirin-dipyridamole prophylaxis of sickle cell pain crises. Thromb Haemostas 43:218–221, 1980.

115. Cabannes R, Lonsdorfer J, Castaigne JP, et al: Clinical and biological double-blind study of ticlopidine in preventive treatment of sickle-cell disease crises. Agents Actions Suppl 15:199–212, 1984.

116. Tomer A, Kasey S, Connor WE, et al: Reduction of pain episodes and prothrombotic activity in sickle cell disease by dietary n-3 fatty acids. Thromb Haemost 85:966–974, 2001.

117. Lele M, Sajid M, Wajih N, et al: Eptifibatide and 7E3, but not tirofiban, inhibit $\alpha_v\beta_3$ integrin-mediated binding of smooth muscle cells to thrombospondin and prothrombin. Circulation 104:582–587, 2001.

118. Wright JG, Cooper P, Malia RG, et al: Activated protein C resistance in homozygous sickle cell disease. Br J Haematol 96:854–856, 1997.

119. Andrade FL, Annichino-Bizzacchi JM, Saad STO, et al: Prothrombin mutant, factor V Leiden, and thermolabile variant of methylenetetrahydrofolate reductase among patients with sickle cell disease in Brazil. Am J Hematol 59:46–50, 1998.

120. Kahn MJ, Scher C, Rozans M, et al: Factor V Leiden is not responsible for stroke in patients with sickling disorders and is uncommon in African Americans with sickle cell disease. Am J Hematol 54:12–15, 1997.

121. Balasa VV, Gruppo RA, Gartside PS, et al: Correlation of the C677T MTHFR genotype with homocysteine levels in children with sickle cell disease. J Ped Hematol/Oncol 21:397–400, 1999.

122. Houston PE, Rana S, Sekhsaria S, et al: Homocysteine in sickle cell disease: Relationship to stroke. Am J Med 103:192–196, 1997.

123. Kutlar F, Tural C, Park D, et al: MTHFR (5,10-methylenetetrahydrofolate reductase) 677 C→T mutation as a candidate risk factor for avascular necrosis (AVN) in patients with sickle cell disease. Blood 82:695a, 1998.

124. Adekile AD, Kutlar F, Haider MZ, et al: Frequency of the 677 C→T mutation of the methylenetetrahydrofolate reductase gene among Kuwaiti sickle cell disease patients. Am J Hematol. 66:263–266, 2001.

125. Cumming AM, Olujohungbe A, Keeney S, et al: The methylenetetrahydrofolate reductase gene C677T polymorphism in patients with homozygous sickle cell disease and stroke. Br J Haematol 107:569–571, 1999.

126. Zimmerman SA, Ware RE: Inherited DNA mutations contributing to thrombotic complications in patients with sickle cell disease. Am J Hematol 59:267–272, 1998.

127. Rosse WF, Telen M, Ware R: Transfusion Support for Patients with Sickle Cell Disease. Bethesda, Md: American Association of Blood Banks; 1998.

128. Management of sickle cell disease. NIH Publication No. 02–2117, 4th Ed. NIH, NHLBI, Monograph, 2002.

129. Vichinsky EP, Luban NL, Wright E, et al: Stroke prevention trial in sickle cell anemia. Transfusion 41:1086–1092, 2001.

130. Thelander L, Reichard P: Reduction of ribonucleotides. Ann Rev Biochem 48:133, 1979.

131. Charache S, Terrin ML, Moore RD, et al: Multicenter study of hydroxyurea in sickle cell anemia: Effect of hydroxyurea on the frequency of painful crises in sickle cell anemia. N Engl J Med 332:1317–1322, 1995.

132. Covas DT, Angulo I, Palma PVB, et al: Effects of hydroxyurea on the membrane of erythrocytes and platelets in the sickle cell anemia. Haematologica 89:273–280, 2004.

133. Hillery CA, Du MC, Wang WC, et al: Hydroxyurea therapy decreases the in vitro adhesion of sickle erythrocytes to thrombospondin and laminin. Br J Haematol 109:322–327, 2000.

134. Orringer EP, Jones S, Strayhorn D, et al: The effect of hydroxyurea (hu) administration on circulating D-dimer levels in patients with sickle cell anemia. Blood 88:496A, 1996.

135. Glover RE, Ivy ED, Orringer EP, et al: Detection of nitrosyl hemoglobin in venous blood in the treatment of sickle cell anemia with hydroxyurea. Molecular Pharmacol 55:1006–1010, 1999.

136. Gladwin MT, Shelhamer JH, Ognibene FP, et al: Nitric oxide donor properties of hydroxyurea in patients with sickle cell disease. Br J Haematol 116:436–444, 2002.

137. Ferster A, Vermylen C, Cornu G, et al: Hydroxyurea for treatment of severe sickle cell anemia: A pediatric clinical trial. Blood 88:1960–1964, 1996.

47

138. Steinberg MH, Barton F, Castro O, et al: Effect of hydroxyurea on mortality and morbidity in sickle cell anemia: Risks and benefits up to 9 years of treatment. JAMA 289:1645–1651, 2003.

139. Davis SC, Luce PJ, Winn AA, et al: Acute chest syndrome in sickle cell disease. Lancet. 1:36–38, 1984.

140. DeCeulaer K, McMullen KW, Maude GH, et al: Pneumonia in young children with homozygous sickle cell disease: Risk and clinical features. Eur J Pediatr 144:255–258, 1985.

141. Poncz M, Kane E, Gill F: Acute chest syndrome in sickle cell disease. Etiology and clinical correlates. J Pediatr 107:861–866, 1965.

142. Vichinsky EP, Styles LA, Colangelo LH, et al: Acute chest syndrome in sickle cell disease: Clinical presentation and course. Blood 89:1787–1792, 1997.

143. Vichinsky EP, Neumayr LD, Earles AN, et al: Causes and outcomes of the acute chest syndrome in sickle cell disease. N Engl J Med 342:1855–1865, 2000.

144. Stuart MJ, Setty BNY: Sickle cell acute chest syndrome: Pathogenesis and rationale for treatment. Blood 94:1555–1560, 1999.

145. Gladwin MT, Rodgers GP: Pathogenesis and treatment of acute chest syndrome of sickle cell anaemia. Lancet 355:1476–1478, 2000.

146. Bellet PS, Kalinyak KA, Shukla R, et al: Incentive spirometry to prevent acute pulmonary complications in sickle cell diseases. N Engl J Med 333:699–703, 1995.

147. Stuart MJ, Setty BNY: Acute chest syndrome of sickle cell disease: New light on an old problem. Current Opin Hematol 8:111–122, 2001.

148. Emre U, Miller ST, Gutierez M, et al: Effect of transfusion in acute chest syndrome of sickle cell disease. J Pediatr 127:901–904, 1995.

149. Pelidis MA, Kato GJ, Resar LMS, et al: Successful treatment of life-threatening acute chest syndrome of sickle cell disease with venovenous extracorporeal membrane oxygenation. J Pediatr Hematol/Oncol 19:459–461, 1997.

150. Alz AM, Wessel DL: Inhaled nitric oxide in sickle cell disease with acute chest syndrome. Anesthesiology 87:988–990, 1997.

151. Sullivan KJ, Goodwin SR, Evangelist J, et al: Nitric oxide successfully used to treat acute chest syndrome of sickle cell disease in a young adolescent. Crit Care Med 27:2563–2568, 1999.

152. Bernini JC, Rogers ZR, Sandler LS, et al: Beneficial effect of intravenous dexamethasone in children with mild to moderately severe acute chest syndrome complicating sickle cell disease. Blood 92:3082–3089, 1998.

153. Farber HW, Loscalzo J: Pulmonary arterial hypertension. N Engl J Med 351:1655–1665, 2004.

154. Sutton LL, Castro O, Cross DT, et al: Pulmonary hypertension in sickle cell disease. Am J Cardiol 74:626, 1994.

155. Simons BE, Santhanam V, Castaner AJ, et al: Two-dimensional echo and Doppler ultrasonographic findings in the hearts of adults with sickle cell anemia. Arch Intern Med 148:1526, 1988.

156. Gladwin MT, Sachdev V, Jison ML, et al: Pulmonary hypertension as a risk factor for death in patients with sickle cell disease. N Engl J Med 350:886–895, 2004.

157. Ataga KI, Sood N, De Gent G, et al: Pulmonary hypertension in sickle cell disease. Am J Med 117:665–669, 2004.

158. Ataga KI, Jones S, Olajide O, et al: The relationship of pulmonary hypertension and survival in sickle cell disease. Blood 104:1665a, 2004.

159. Collins FS, Orringer EP: Pulmonary hypertension and cor pulmonale in the sickle hemoglobinopathies. Am J Med 73:814–821, 1982.

160. Castro O, Hoque M, Brown BD: Pumonary hypertension in sickle cell disease: Cardiac catheterization results and survival. Blood 15:1257–1261, 2003.

161. Aslan M, Ryan TM, Adler B, et al: Oxygen radical inhibition of nitric oxide-dependent vascular function in sickle cell disease. Proc Nat Acad Sci 98:15215–15220, 2001.

162. Reiter CD, Wang X, Tanus-Santos JE, et al: Cell-free hemoglobin limits nitric oxide bioavailability in sickle cell disease. Nat Med 8:1383–1389, 2002.

163. De Franceschi L, Baron A, Scarpa A, et al: Inhaled nitric oxide protects transgenic SAD mice from sickle cell disease-specific lung injury induced by hypoxia/reoxygenation. Blood 102:1087–1096, 2003.

164. Jison ML, Gladwin MT: Hemolytic anemia-associated pulmonary hypertension of sickle cell disease and the nitric oxide/arginine pathway. Am J Respir Crit Care Med 168:3–4, 2003.

165. Krasuski RA, Warner JJ, Wang A, et al: Inhaled nitric oxide selectively dilates pulmonary vasculature in adult patients with pulmonary hypertension, irrespective of etiology. J Am Coll Cardiol 36:2204–2211, 2000.

166. Martinez-Ruiz R, Montero-Huerta P, Hromi J, et al: Inhaled nitric oxide improves survival rates during hypoxia in a sickle cell (SAD) mouse model. Anesthesiology 94:1113–1118, 2001.

167. Morris CR, Morris SM, Hagar W, et al: Arginine therapy: A new treatment for pulmonary hypertension in sickle cell disease? Am J Respir Crit Care Med 168:63–69, 2003.

168. Morris CR, Kato GJ, Poljakovic M, et al: Dysregulated arginine metabolism, hemolysis-associated pulmonary hypertension, and mortality in sickle cell disease. JAMA 294:81–90, 2005.

169. Castro O: Systemic fat embolism and pulmonary hypertension in sickle cell disease. Heme/Oncol Clin N Am 10:1289–1303, 1996.

170. Aquino SL, Gamsu G, Fahy JV, et al: Chronic pulmonary disorders in sickle cell disease: Findings at thin-section CT. Radiology 193:807–811, 1994.

171. Yung GL, Channick RN, Fedullo PF, et al: Successful pulmonary thromboendarterectomy in two patients with sickle cell disease. Am J Respir Crit Care Med 157:1690–1693, 1998.

172. Manci EA, Culberson DE, Yang YM, et al: Investigators of the cooperative study of sickle cell disease: Causes of death in sickle cell disease: An autopsy study. Br J Haematol 123:359–365, 2003.

173. Beuzard Y: Transgenic mouse models of sickle cell disease. Curr Op Hematol 3:150–155, 1996.

174. Adedeji MO, Cespedes J, Allen K, et al: Pulmonary thrombotic arteriopathy in patients with sickle cell disease. Arch Pathol Lab Med 125:1436–1441, 2001.

175. Oppenheimer EH, Esterly JR: Pulmonary changes in sickle cell disease. Am Rev Respir Dis 103:858–859, 1971.

176. Samuels MP, Stebbens VA, Davis SC, et al: Sleep related upper airway obstruction and hypoxaemia in sickle cell disease. Arch Dis Child 67:925–929, 1992.

177. Machado RF, Gladwin MT: Chronic sickle cell lung disease: New insights into the diagnosis, pathogenesis and treatment of pulmonary hypertension. Br J Haematol 129:449–464, 2005.

178. Ataga KI, Moore CG, Jones S, et al: Pulmonary hypertension in patients with sickle cell disease: A longitudinal study. Br J Haematol 134:109–115, 2006.

179. Castro O, Kato G, Sachdev V, et al: The sickle cell-pulmonary hypertension screening study: Echo findings at two-years of follow-up. Blood 106:314A, 2005.

180. Claster S, Hammer M, Hagar W, et al: Treatment of pulmonary hypertension in sickle cell disease with transfusion. Blood 94:420A, 1999.

181. Strange JW, Wharton J, Phillips PG, et al: Recent insights into the pathogenesis and therapeutics of pulmonary hypertension. Clin Sci 102:253–268, 2002.

182. Morris CR, Morris SM, Hagar W, et al: Arginine therapy: A new treatment for pulmonary hypertension in sickle cell disease? Am J Respir Crit Care Med 168:63–69, 2003.

183. Fuster V, Steele PM, Edwards WD, et al: Primary pulmonary hypertension: Natural history and the importance of thrombosis. Circulation 70:580–587, 1984.

184. Barst RJ, Rubin LJ, Long WA, et al: A comparison of continuous epoprostenol (prostacyclin) with conventional therapy for primary pulmonary hypertension. N Engl J Med 334:296–302, 1996.

185. Machado RF, Martyr SE, Anthi A, et al: Pulmonary hypertension in sickle cell disease: Cardiopulmonary evaluation and response to chronic phosphodiesterase 5 inhibitor therapy. Blood 104:235A, 2004.

186. Kato GJ, Martyr S, Machado R, et al: Acute on chronic pulmonary hypertension in patients with sickle cell disease. Blood 104:1669A, 2004.

187. Pegelow CH, Macklin EA, Moser FG, et al: Longitudinal changes in brain magnetic resonance imaging findings in children with sickle cell disease. Blood 99:3014–3018, 2002.

188. Bermaudin F, Verlhac S, Freard F, et al: Multicenter prospective study of children with sickle cell disease: Radiographic and psychometric correlation. J Child Neurol 15:333–343, 2000.

189. Hoppe C: Defining stroke risk in children with sickle cell anaemia. Br J Haematol 128:751–766, 2005.

190. Ohene-Frempong K, Weiner SJ, Sleeper LA, et al: Cerebrovascular accidents in sickle cell disease: Rates and risk factors. Blood 91:288–294, 1998.

191. Dobson SR, Holden KR, Nietert PJ, et al: Moyamoya syndrome in childhood sickle cell disease: A predictive factor for recurrent cerebrovascular events. Blood 99:3144–3150, 2002.

192. Adams RJ, McKie VC, Hsu L, et al: Prevention of a first stroke by transfusions in children with sickle cell anemia and abnormal results on transcranial Doppler ultrasonography. N Engl J Med 339:5–11, 1998.

193. Adams RJ, Brambilla D: Optimizing primary stroke prevention in sickle cell anemia (STOP 2) Trial Investigators. Discontinuing prophylactic transfusions used to prevent stroke in sickle cell disease. N Engl J Med 353:2769–2778, 2005.

194. Powars D, Wilson B, Imbus C, et al: The natural history of stroke in sickle cell disease. Am J Med 65:461–471, 1978.

195. Sarniak S, Soorya D, Kim J, et al: Periodic transfusions for sickle cell anemia and CNS infarction. Am J Dis Child 133:1254–1257, 1979.

196. Pegelow CH, Adams RJ, McKie V, et al: Risk of recurrent stroke in patients with sickle cell disease treated with erythrocyte transfusions. J Pediatr 126:896–899, 1995.

197. Cohen AR, Martin MB, Silber JH, et al: A modified transfusion program for prevention of stroke in sickle cell disease. Blood 79:1657–1661, 1992.

198. Wang WC, Kovnar EH, Tonkin IL, et al: High risk of recurrent stroke after discontinuance of five to twelve years of transfusion therapy in patients with sickle cell disease. J Pediatr 118:377–382, 1991.

199. Scothorn DJ, Price C, Schwartz D, et al: Risk of recurrent stroke in children with sickle cell disease receiving blood transfusion therapy for at least five years after initial stroke. J Pediatr 140:348–354, 2002.

200. Ware RE, Zimmerman SA, Sylvestre PB, et al: Prevention of secondary stroke and resolution of transfusional iron overload in children with sickle cell anemia using hydroxyurea and phlebotomy. J Pediatr 145:346–352, 2004.

Chapter 48

Anticoagulation for Atrial Fibrillation and Prosthetic Cardiac Valves

Thomas G. DeLoughery, MD

OVERVIEW

The most common indications for chronic anticoagulation therapy are stroke prevention for patients with atrial fibrillation and embolism prevention for those with prosthetic cardiac valves. However, many patients have risk factors for bleeding or other comorbid conditions that can make anticoagulation challenging. This chapter will review the data supporting antithrombotic therapy. Most attention will be spent on discussing challenging patients—older patients, those with risk factors for bleeding, those difficult to anticoagulate, and pregnant patients—the very patients most likely to generate consultation.

Atrial Fibrillation

Atrial fibrillation is the most common cardiac condition leading to embolism. The risk of stroke due to embolism in patients with atrial fibrillation is 3% to 7% per year. It is estimated that 15% of all strokes can be attributed to atrial fibrillation. The incidence of atrial fibrillation is age dependent and ranges from 0.5% for people younger than age 55 to 9% for people older than age 80.[1]

In the past 15 years, well-designed studies have clarified the role of antithrombotic therapy for stroke prevention in patients with nonvalvular atrial fibrillation.[2] Robust data support the effectiveness of warfarin. Five randomized clinical trials have shown that warfarin anticoagulation reduces the risk of first stroke from 5% per year down to 1% per year.[3–5] Warfarin is the only effective therapy that prevents disabling and fatal strokes.[6–8] There is evidence that results of these trials can be replicated in clinical practice.[9,10] In addition, the EAFT study demonstrated the effectiveness of warfarin in secondary prevention of stroke with a reduction from 16.5 to 8.5 strokes per year.[11]

An International Normalized Ratio (INR) range of 2 to 3 is most effective for stroke prevention. Stroke risk rises with INRs of less than 1.9 and is no different than no therapy at INRs below 1.5.[9,12,13] Conversely, the risk of excessive bleeding does not fall to baseline risk until INRs are 1.5 and below. These data refute the common practice of using a lower INR target in patients at high risk for bleeding (1.5 to 1.9); such practice does not reduce the risk of bleeding yet will increase the risk of stroke. The INR range of 2 to 3 has been supported by studies showing that, even when patients have strokes, those in the therapeutic range have smaller strokes and better outcomes.[14,15,15a]

The issue of antiplatelet therapy for stroke prevention in atrial fibrillation remains contentious.[2] The AFASAK trial showed 75 mg of aspirin (ASA) to be of no benefit in the prevention of embolism. SPAF showed 325 mg of aspirin was effective but only in patients younger than 75 years of age.[3,4,16] SPAF III demonstrated that in patients believed to be at low risk of stroke, aspirin was effective in preventing embolism.[17] However, the effect of aspirin is modest, with meta-analysis showing only a 22% risk reduction.[18–20] Head-to-head studies of aspirin versus warfarin *strongly* favor warfarin.[8] Finally, aspirin has no effect on preventing disabling or fatal strokes. It may be that in patients who have no other risk factors for stroke, the presence of atrial fibrillation acts as a marker for cerebrovascular disease for which aspirin might offer protection.[21,22]

It seemed intuitive to think that converting patients' cardiac rhythm from atrial fibrillation to sinus rhythm would reduce the risk of stroke, but two randomized trials have shown that rhythm control without anticoagulant therapy offers no advantage in reducing strokes over rate control.[23–26] These findings support the notion that having or having had atrial fibrillation serves as a marker, more than a cause, for cardiovascular disease sufficient to be associated with cardioembolism.

Prediction rules now exist to risk-stratify patients and help the clinician choose between warfarin and aspirin therapy. Data have been pooled from multiple clinical trials to make a variety of these prediction rules. Clinically the most useful appears to be the CHADS2 rule (Table 48-1).[27,28,160] In the CHADS2 system, one point is assessed for presence of Congestive heart failure, Hypertension, Age greater than 75 years, and Diabetes, respectively, and two points for history of Stroke. For the average patient, a CHADS2 score of 0 to 2 would suggest low risk of stroke and aspirin therapy, whereas a higher score would support the use of warfarin.

Given the practical difficulties in using warfarin, the appeal is great for new antithrombotic agents that would be easier to use. The oral direct thrombin inhibitor ximelagantran appeared in two randomized trials to offer the same antithrombotic protection as warfarin without need for dose adjustment or interactions with other medications.[29] Unfortunately, the rates of liver toxicity were deemed unacceptable and at the time of this writing, no new agents have advanced into the late clinical testing phase.

Table 48-1 CHADS2 Scoring System*

CHADS2 Score	Yearly Risk of Stroke	Therapy
0	1.9	Aspirin
1	2.8	Aspirin
2	4.0	Warfarin
3	5.9	Warfarin
4	8.5	Warfarin
5	12.5	Warfarin
6	18.2	Warfarin

*One point each for recent heart failure, hypertension, age >75 years, and diabetes. Two points assigned for history of stroke. CHADS2: Congestive heart failure, Hypertension, Age >75 years, Diabetes, history of Strokes (two).
Data from Gage BF, Waterman AD, Shannon W, et al: Validation of clinical classification schemes for predicting stroke: Results from the National Registry of Atrial Fibrillation. JAMA 285(22):2864–2870, 2001.

Table 48-2 Outpatient Bleeding Index

Assign one point for:
- Age ≥65
- History of stroke
- History of gastrointestinal bleeding
- Recent myocardial infarction, hematocrit <30%, creatinine >1.5 mg/dL, or diabetes (one point maximum)

Score	Risk Group	Yearly Risk of Major Bleeding
0	Low	0%–1.1%
1–2	Intermediate	2.5%–4.9%
3–4	High	8.8%–10.6%

Data from references 28, 57, and 58.

Risk of Bleeding with Warfarin

The use of warfarin is increasing markedly due to data indicating that warfarin is the most effective agent for stroke prevention in atrial fibrillation. Accompanying the increased use is a higher rate of patients bleeding due to warfarin.[30] The annual risk of fatal bleeding is 0.6% to 1% and the risk of major bleeding is 3%.[31,32]

Risk factors for bleeding on warfarin therapy have been studied many times, but most reports agree on several basic factors. The first is supratherapeutic INRs.[33–37] The two-week bleeding risk for an INR greater than 6 is 4.4%.[38] The risk of bleeding and of intracranial hemorrhage (ICH) rises dramatically with increasing INRs.[34,39] The odds ratio for ICH with an INR greater than 4.5 is from 8 to 11.[36,40] Duration of therapy is also a reproducible risk factor with patients just starting therapy being at highest risk of bleeding.[31,32,36] Concomitant use of antiplatelet agents increases the risk of bleeding by 20% to 100%.[41–44] History of gastrointestinal bleeding, poor compliance, stroke, low vitamin K intake, and alcohol abuse are also risk factors for bleeding.[31,35,41,45–49]

Recent research has focused on variations in cytochrome 2C9 (CYP2C9) and the VKORC1 gene affecting warfarin metabolism.[50,50–56] Patients with polymorphisms that predict a lower maintenance dose of warfarin have a higher risk of bleeding. However, until rapid assays are available for these polymorphisms, the usefulness of prospectively knowing these genotypes to predict bleeding in an individual patient will remain limited.

There is increasing evidence that assessing a limited set of pretreatment variables can help predict the risk of bleeding. The best studied is the outpatient bleeding index (Table 48-2).[28,57,58] In several studies, the risk of bleeding has ranged from 0% to 2% per year for low-risk patients to 10% per year for high-risk patients. Although further validation is needed for a broad range of patients, the outpatient bleeding index can be helpful for anticoagulation decision making.

Atrial Fibrillation—Special Situations

Patients with atrial fibrillation undergoing cardioversion have up to a 5% incidence of embolism at or near the time of cardioversion. Consequently, patients with atrial fibrillation for more than 2 days typically receive warfarin to achieve a documented INR of 2.0 to 3.0 for a duration of 3 weeks prior to cardioversion. This should allow any thrombus present to organize. Because mechanical activity of the atria may not fully resume until some time after resumption of normal sinus rhythm, patients should remain anticoagulated for at least 4 weeks if not indefinitely after cardioversion. The same procedure should be followed for patients undergoing chemical cardioversion for atrial fibrillation. Atrial fibrillation in thyrotoxic heart disease is associated with a high rate of embolic phenomena. Therefore, these patients should receive warfarin to maintain an INR of 2.0 to 3.0 until 4 weeks after the resumption of normal sinus rhythm.

CARDIAC VALVES

Mechanical Prosthetic Heart Valves

Patients with mechanical heart valves have an extremely high risk for embolization, and continuous anticoagulation is strongly recommended.[59–61] It is estimated that the risk of thrombosis without anticoagulant ranges from 12% to 30% per year. It does appear that the newer generation of mechanical valves is less thrombogenic than the older ball-cage valves. Even with anticoagulation, the yearly rate of thrombosis ranges from 2.5% with ball-cage to 0.5% with bileaflet valves.[59] Patients with mechanical aortic valves are at lesser risk of thrombosis than those with mechanical mitral valves. However, the rates of embolism and valve thrombosis are still substantial with newer valves, and anticoagulation is still recommended.

For all valve types and positions, the addition of antiplatelet therapy is useful for additional protection.[62] The effect of antiplatelet therapy is most important for "high-risk" situations—older valves in the mitral position. The risk of bleeding is increased but is outweighed by the benefit of therapy. The addition of proton-pump inhibitor therapy to aspirin therapy will reduce the risk of gastrointestinal bleeding.

Patients with mechanical prosthetic valves can be stratified by assessing (1) type of valve; (2) valve position; (3) history of stroke; and (4) presence of atrial fibrillation. Using these four clinical factors to risk stratify patients[62–64] one can select an antithrombotic strategy as follows:

- Bi-leaflet valve in aortic position: INR 2 to 3
- Ball-cage valve: INR 2.5 to 3.5 with 80 to 100 mg/day aspirin

- Others: INR 2.5 to 3.5, or INR 2 to 3 with 80 to 100 mg/day aspirin
- Patients with risk factors such as atrial fibrillation, previous embolism, or coronary artery disease should be considered for combined therapy.

Bioprosthetic Heart Valves

Although the risk is lower, bioprosthetic heart valves still have a definite risk of associated embolization. This is highest immediately after surgery and in patients with bioprosthetic valves who have other risk factors such as atrial fibrillation. In the past, it was recommended that patients with a newly placed bioprosthetic valve should be anticoagulated with warfarin for 3 months after surgery to an INR of 2.0 to 3.0. Recent data and clinical trials do not support this recommendation; for most patients, aspirin suffices for antithrombotic therapy.[65] Patients with atrial fibrillation, history of embolism, or those with left atrial thrombi should be anticoagulated indefinitely with warfarin.

WHO SHOULD NOT RECEIVE ANTICOAGULANT THERAPY

Although there is much discussion in the literature regarding who should be administered oral anticoagulants, there are some patients for whom the risk of therapy is so substantial that they are judged to be safer with no therapy; if such is determined, that decision should be documented in the patient's chart. Patients with severe underlying bleeding diathesis are not candidates for antithrombotic therapy. An example of this would be a patient with classic hemophilia A or B. In patients with type 1 von Willebrand disease, decision making is harder. One strategy is to approach the risk of warfarin therapy in these patients in a manner similar to the risk of combined warfarin-antiplatelet therapy because, in effect, von Willebrand disease results in platelet function similar to the platelet defect from aspirin administration. When risk of thrombosis is high, use of warfarin would be justified. Severe thrombocytopenia is also a contraindication to warfarin. Based on the data showing that hemophiliacs encounter a higher rate of intracranial bleeding with platelet counts below 50,000/μL, this count might be a reasonable cutoff for use of warfarin.

Dialysis patients are especially challenging to anticoagulate. The rate of bleeding in the dialysis patient even without anticoagulation is substantial—as high as 11% per year in one study.[66] This complication rate doubles with use of warfarin. Uremia slows the metabolism of warfarin and the bleeding defects of uremia are well known. However, dialysis patients are also at much higher risk for thrombotic complications. In one study, atrial fibrillation was a predictor of both stroke (35%) and increased risk of death.[67,68] Dialysis patients with mechanical valves or atrial fibrillation with high CHADS2 scores (≥4) should be strongly considered for warfarin therapy.

If warfarin is used, scrupulous attention must be paid to control of the INR. Erratic drug metabolism can result in unstable INRs. Despite its renal clearance, we have had good outcomes with using renal dose-adjusted low molecular weight heparin in dialysis patients who had complications stemming from erratic INRs.

Management of High INRs and Bleeding

The risk of bleeding with an elevated INR depends on the degree of elevation of the INR and on the reason for anticoagulation therapy. An older patient being anticoagulated for an arterial reason (stroke, valve, and so on) is at higher risk for bleeding than a younger patient being anticoagulated for a venous indication. The rate and route of therapeutic intervention to address the INR correction depend on whether the patient is bleeding.

For modest INR elevations (4.5 to 10) in a nonbleeding patient, the goal is to return the INR to the 2 to 3 range. The choice is between oral vitamin K versus holding the warfarin for one or more doses. One study clearly shows faster INR correction and a lesser incidence of long-term bleeding with 1 mg of oral vitamin K. For patients at increased risk for bleeding, oral vitamin K is recommended. For higher INRs (>10), 2.5 to 5 mg of oral vitamin K is needed.

In the bleeding patient, use of vitamin K is mandatory. Oral vitamin K acts within 12 hours. For faster onset, intravenous vitamin K will take effect in 4 to 6 hours. If given slowly over 1 hour, the risk of anaphylaxis with vitamin K is 1 in 3300.[69–73] In multiple studies, subcutaneous vitamin K administration has been shown to be less reliable than oral vitamin K and should not be used for this indication.[73–77] Fresh frozen plasma can be used to supplement the vitamin K effect, but large amounts are needed— 15 mL per kilogram of body weight—which is 4 to 5 units for the average patient. It is important to supplement the plasma with vitamin K because the effect of plasma is brief; the patient may have a rebound rise in the INR within several hours if vitamin K is not given owing to the short half-lives of some transfused factors.

In the patient with intracranial or other life-threatening hemorrhage, correction of the INR with vitamin K and plasma is too slow; faster modalities are needed. The use of prothrombin concentrates (which contain all the vitamin K–dependent clotting factors) results in a more rapid correction of coagulation than does plasma.[78–80] Patients suffering life-threatening hemorrhage should be considered to receive prothrombin concentrates such as Konyne or Profilnine at a dose of 50 U per kilogram of body weight.[79,81–83] Unfortunately, these products are not often readily available. There are some recent data showing that the use of recombinant factor VIIa (rFVIIa) can reverse warfarin-induced bleeding.[84,85] The exact dose of rFVIIa is uncertain; given a need for prompt and complete reversal, our approach has been to err on the side of using a larger dose of 40 μg per kilogram of body weight.

When is it Appropriate to Restart Anticoagulation after Serious Bleeding?

A common dilemma concerns the timing of resumption of anticoagulation after a serious bleeding episode. Although people are more fearful about resuming anticoagulation after a cerebral bleeding event, data show that gastrointestinal bleeding has the higher rate of recurrence. Rebleeding after intracranial hemorrhage is low—perhaps 1% to 2%

over the next few years. For most patients this risk is outweighed by the benefits of anticoagulation. The exception to this is the patient with evidence of cerebral amyloid angiopathy who should probably never be re-anticoagulated given their very high (>30%) risk of rebleeding even independent of warfarin resumption. The timing of resumption of anticoagulation is also not settled. Studies do indicate that with intracranial hemorrhage, only a short period off anticoagulation is needed. There are even two reports of patients continuing to receive heparin at therapeutic doses despite the presence of an intracranial hemorrhage. There are enough data to suggest that once the INR is normal, a period of only 24 to 48 hours without anticoagulant therapy is necessary before resumption of warfarin therapy.

In summary, when a patient presents with bleeding, one should rapidly normalize the INR. For intracranial hemorrhage, heparin can be started within 1 to 2 days if the patient's INR is corrected. For life-threatening gastrointestinal or genitourinary bleeding, the patient should have a vigorous evaluation for any underlying lesions.

Temporary Cessation of Warfarin for Procedures

As more and more patients are receiving chronic anticoagulant therapy, management around the time of medical procedures or operations has become more of an issue.[86,87] The risk of thrombosis or embolism needs to be balanced by the risk of surgical bleeding. The approach needs to take into account the reason the patient is being anticoagulated (extremely variable risks) and the risk of bleeding (nearly always overestimated) with a given procedure.

In theory, the risk of thrombosis with holding anticoagulation should be low. For example, if the 1-year risk of thrombosis/embolism with a mitral ball-cage valve is 30%, then simple math yields a daily risk of 0.08% and a 2-week risk of 1.15%. For less thrombogenic valves, presumably the risk would be lower. However, this calculation does not take into account the considerable enhancement of hypercoagulability induced by the surgery, which itself appears to significantly increase the risk of thrombosis. Retrospective data suggest an overall risk as high as 1% to 2% of thrombotic arterial events in patients if their anticoagulation is held before surgery.[87]

One can approach perioperative anticoagulation in several ways. The simplest is to continue the warfarin and perform the procedure with the patient anticoagulated. This is the standard approach for dental procedures, cataract surgery, and endoscopy. A recent pilot study also showed this method to be a safe and effective approach even for complex surgeries.[88] This approach is associated with the lowest risk of strokes (0.4%) but does carry the risk of increased bleeding.[87]

The next simplest approach would be to stop the warfarin 4 to 5 days before surgery, allow the INR to drift back to normal, and then restart oral anticoagulation after surgery. This would expose the patient to a thrombotic risk for up to 4 to 8 days.

In recent years the concept of "bridging" therapy has been proposed with the idea of using low molecular weight heparin (LMWH) to "bridge" the patient when the warfarin effect is gone.[89–91] This presumably would have the lowest risk of thrombosis but may expose the patient to

Table 48-3	Bridging Therapy

Consider bridging for patients with mechanical cardiac valves, bioprosthetic valve with history of thrombosis, and patients with atrial fibrillation who have suffered a stroke or have a high CHADS2 score.

Method

Day–5: Stop warfarin 5 days before procedure.
Day–3: Start therapeutic LMWH every 12–24 hours
Day–1: If on q day LMWH therapy, give last dose in AM. If on q12-hour therapy, give last dose evening before surgery unless patient is to receive an epidural; then only the AM dose is given.
Day–0: Check PT/INR/PTT morning of surgery. For most procedures restart warfarin the night of surgery. If very minor procedure, restart therapeutic LMWH; otherwise start prophylactic dose and change to therapeutic dose when risk-to-benefit ratio is favorable.

PT/INR/PTT, prothrombin/International Normalized Ratio/prothrombin time; LMWH, low molecular weight heparin.

bleeding, especially postoperatively. Previous fears about reduced effectiveness of LMWH with prosthetic valves have proved unfounded with the risk of embolism estimated at 0.4% when used as bridging therapy.[90,92] The newer pentasaccharide anticoagulant agent may have a yet-to-be confirmed role in this area.

Analysis of published studies suggests the following approach: for low bleeding risk procedures (and modest risk ones—if the surgeon agrees) warfarin is continued with an INR goal in the 2 to 2.5 range. For patients with low risk of thrombosis—that is, primary stroke prevention in atrial fibrillation—the warfarin can be held before surgery and restarted afterward. For patients at higher risk of bleeding, bridging therapy such as suggested in Table 48-3 can be used.

Epidural Hematomas

The increasing use of LMWHs for both therapy and prophylaxis has lead to concerns about the risk of epidural hematomas. With unfractionated heparin prophylaxis (most often starting 2 hours before surgery), epidural hematomas were rare. Large case series have reported that patients who received epidural anesthesia during full anticoagulation with unfractionated heparin suffered a low incidence of complications (1:22,000). Early European use of LMWH was associated with rare bleeding complications in case series involving more than 23,000 cases.[93,94] However, with the introduction in the United States of LMWH, multiple case reports of epidural hematomas were reported. The exact reason for the disparity between Europe and the United States is unknown. One major factor that has been cited is differences in dosing. European dosing practice is a single daily dose of the agent (most often enoxaparin 40 mg every day) versus 30 mg twice daily in the United States. The twice a day dose is associated with high trough levels of LMWH which may predispose to bleeding. However, European patients also received a dose of LMWH 2 hours before surgery, which intuitively would seem to have increased the risk of bleeding. Another major factor is that all patients reported to the FDA had additional risk factors for bleeding—such as concomitant use of antiplatelet agents, early administration of LMWH, and difficulty with the epidural procedure.[95]

The absolute magnitude of risk of epidural hematoma with spinal anesthesia is unknown, with estimates ranging from 1:10,000 to 1:3000 for patients receiving LMWH.[95] Risk of hematoma with standard heparin ranges from 0% to 0.2%.[93] This risk must be balanced by the fact that without prophylaxis, up to 1 in 250 patients receiving lower-extremity orthopedic procedures will die of pulmonary embolism.

Current guidelines suggest that, if LMWH is used for prophylaxis, the first dose should be given 10 to 12 hours after placement of the epidural catheter and LMWH should be held 12 hours before removal of the catheter. Given the longer half-life of fondaparinux, epidural catheters are contraindicated in patients receiving this agent unless the drug is held for 48 hours before catheter insertion.

The Patient with an Erratic INR

Rarely the clinician is faced with the patient who requires massive doses of warfarin for adequate anticoagulation or the patient who seems to be resistant to even large doses of warfarin. In these patients, a careful evaluation is needed to determine the cause of the warfarin resistance. True genetic warfarin resistance is extremely rare, with only four kindreds reported.[96] The patients are always difficult to anticoagulate and may respond to only very large doses (i.e., 150 milligrams) of warfarin. More common is acquired resistance to warfarin. The three major causes of acquired resistance are medications, concurrent ingestion of vitamin K, and noncompliance.[97]

It is less common for medicines to inhibit rather than to potentiate the action of warfarin. Common drugs that inhibit warfarin action are barbiturates, rifampin, and nafcillin.[98] Patients on these medications may require 20 mg of warfarin per day to maintain a therapeutic INR. Because most drug–warfarin interactions are mediated through induction of liver enzymes, it may take several days for the warfarin resistance to be noticed after starting the drug. Cholestyramine uniquely interferes with warfarin absorption.

Vitamin K is found in several nutritional supplements and use of these products can result in warfarin resistance (see Chapter 33). For example, Ensure contains 80 μg of vitamin K per 1000 kcal and Sustacal 230 μg per 1000 kcal.[96] In patients who depend solely on these products for nutrition, large doses of warfarin or anticoagulation with heparin may be required. If the patient changes supplements or starts ingesting regular food, warfarin requirements often change dramatically. Even 1 or 2 days of high intake of vitamin K–rich food can dramatically lower INRs.[97]

Some patients who present with warfarin resistance are simply not compliant. These patients initially require the usual doses of warfarin therapy but then present with normal INRs despite increasing warfarin dosage. Measuring serum warfarin levels is useful in patients suspected of non-compliance.[99] Patients with undetectable warfarin levels, despite allegedly being on large doses of warfarin are most likely not taking the drug. In the patient who has nondetectable warfarin, a level should be repeated after the patient is witnessed taking the drug to ensure that the patient is not suffering from rare malabsorption of warfarin. One case has been described of a patient who could not absorb

warfarin but could absorb phenindione, a non-coumarin vitamin K inhibitor.[100] Curiously, this malabsorption occurred after 2 years of stable warfarin therapy.

Anticoagulation in the Elderly Patient

Age alone remains controversial as a risk for bleeding.[40,101,102] Older patients are more sensitive to warfarin, tend to be on more medications that may interact with warfarin, and have more comorbid illnesses.[103,104] Patients who are older require less warfarin, with patients older than age 65 requiring one half to one third of the warfarin doses of younger patients.[105,106] Another difficulty in older patients is poor nutrition. Low or irregular intake of vitamin K can lead to unstable INRs.[47,107] Older patients are more likely to be suffering from cerebral amyloid angiopathy, which is a potent risk factor for bleeding.[108,109] Unfortunately, older patients are also at higher risk for embolic events and should not be denied warfarin unless other major bleeding risk factors are present.[102,110]

Despite years of robust trials demonstrating that warfarin is effective in atrial fibrillation, only 50% of patients eligible for therapy receive warfarin, with older patients being less likely to be anticoagulated.[111,112] More disturbing are data showing that known risk factors for stroke do not seem to play a role in physician decision making about antiplatelet or warfarin therapy for stroke. Physicians tend to overestimate the risk of bleeding with warfarin and underestimate the benefits.[113] Patients, in contrast, fear stroke more than death and are more willing than physicians to accept the risk of serious or fatal bleeding to prevent strokes.[114]

One common but unsubstantiated reason for denying older patients warfarin therapy is the fear of bleeds with falls. The incidence of intracerebral hemorrhage (ICH) with falling is very low; it has been estimated that there will be one ICH for every 254 ground level falls.[115] In addition, the patient who falls is also the patient at risk for stroke. Instead of denying a beneficial therapy, the patient who falls and also needs warfarin should receive it along with efforts made to address risk factors for falling.

Pregnancy and Valves

A growing number of pregnant women need anticoagulant therapy (see Chapter 36). Once rare, increasing experience is being gained in the management of anticoagulants during pregnancy. However, the lack of clinical trials in this population has made this area contentious. The use of warfarin is now considered contraindicated during pregnancy by the manufacturer.[116] Warfarin use significantly increases the rate of fetal loss.[117] Warfarin crosses the placenta, rendering the fetus unable to synthesize vitamin K–dependent proteins. From gestational week 6 to 12, synthesis of proteins crucial for bone and cartilage formation is impaired by warfarin and its ingestion results in a condition known as warfarin embryopathy.[118] Babies affected with this condition will have nasal and limb hypoplasia and stippling of the cartilage. The incidence of children with warfarin embryopathy born from mothers exposed to warfarin is estimated in large series to be 5% to 10%.[119] The incidence of the embryopathy appears to be dose dependent with low rates reported with average daily doses under 5 mg.[120,121] Later in pregnancy, the fetus itself becomes anticoagulated, resulting in a higher incidence of intracranial hemorrhage and fetal loss. In addition, a variety of central nervous system abnormalities involving midline structures have been reported.[119]

Because of these concerns about warfarin, heparin has become the anticoagulant of choice for pregnant women, despite concerns about its effectiveness in women with mechanical heart valves. Advantages of heparin are that it does not cross the placenta and has not been associated with teratogenic effects.[119,122] However, standard heparin has several disadvantages for it use in pregnancy. One is that the partial thromboplastin time (PTT) can be unreliable for monitoring, especially as the pregnancy progresses; therefore, specific heparin assays should be used.[119,123] Second, at the time of delivery there may be a sudden prolongation of the half-life of heparin leading to persistent anticoagulation of the mother.[124]

The major concern with the long-term use of standard heparin is the development of osteoporosis.[125] The risk of osteoporosis varies with different studies but evidence of bone loss can be seen in up to 20% of women on therapeutic standard heparin for more than 6 weeks with 2% of women having fractures.[119,125] In two prospective cohort studies, 28% to 36% of pregnant women experienced a significant decline in bone density while receiving heparin.[125,126] Surprisingly, neither of these studies demonstrated greater osteoporosis with increasing heparin dosage. Pregnant women on standard heparin should receive calcium and vitamin D, although there is no evidence this will prevent bone loss.[127] Bone loss is greatest during the time of breastfeeding.[128] Warfarin is secreted in an inactive form in the breast milk, so there is no contraindication to initiation of warfarin therapy after birth to lessen time of heparin exposure.[116]

For these reasons, LMWH is now considered the antithrombotic therapy of choice in pregnant women.[119,129,130] Multiple studies have demonstrated that LMWHs do not cross the placenta. LMWHs have multiple pharmacokinetic advantages over standard heparin and display consistently more reliable dosages.[131,132] Dosing of LMWH appears to remain stable throughout the duration of the pregnancy.[119,133] LMWHs are associated with a lower incidence of osteoporosis than standard heparin—with several trials showing no difference in bone density compared with a control group of pregnant women.[127,129,134,135]

Although poor results have been reported with the use of standard heparin in women with mechanical heart valves,[136] many of these patients receive only 5000 to 10,000 U of heparin twice a day or, if higher doses were used, a target PTT ratio of 1.5 to 2.0 was selected.[118] This dose would be subtherapeutic in most patients—predisposing them to thrombosis. A review of reports concerning valve thrombosis in pregnant woman receiving LMWH also demonstrates that most women were not receiving adequate doses of LMWH.[137] In these studies, the thrombosis rate appears higher with heparin than with warfarin. This is in contrast to other situations where heparin is superior to warfarin and can "salvage" warfarin failures.[138,139] In reviewing these early studies, none appeared to use heparin levels or PTT calibrated against heparin levels. In a recent study of 54 women (37 with prosthetic valves), heparin dosage was guided by heparin levels.[140] Only one valve thrombosis was

reported in a woman who was initially treated at another center with low dose heparin (15,000 U per day).

In the patient with a mechanical prosthetic valve, one should use either standard heparin or LMWH.[116,119,140] It is uncertain but highly likely that the new pentasaccharide agent will also be useful in this situation. Some articles recommend using heparin only during weeks 6 to 12 and then after week 32,[141] but it is unclear whether this approach entirely eliminates the risk of fetal malformation and still places the fetus at risk of warfarin-induced intracranial hemorrhage. Standard heparin should be started at a dose of 17,500 to 20,000 U every 12 hours to achieve a goal PTT that corresponds to an anti-Xa level of 0.3 to 0.7 U/mL.[118,142,143] If LMWH is used, one should start with a dose of enoxaparin 1 mg per kilogram of body weight every 12 hours and monitor anti-Xa levels. A level should be performed every 2 to 4 weeks, 4 to 6 hours after the injection—aiming for an enoxaparin level between 0.9 and 1.1 anti-Xa units.[131,137,144]

When the patient goes into labor, further doses of heparin should be held. If the labor is prolonged, one might start a lower dose of heparin (400 U/hour) to provide prophylaxis or 40 mg of enoxaparin can be used.[130]

Women of childbearing age who require prosthetic cardiac valves might consider having a bioprosthesis placed to minimize the concerns about pregnancy and anticoagulation.[145–147] Reported thromboembolism rates of bioprosthetic valves range from 0.5% to 3% per year without the use of anticoagulants.[148,149] This thromboembolism rate is comparable with that of anticoagulated patients with mechanical valves. However, the life span of bioprosthetic valves in young women is considerably shorter than in older patients.[150] In a recent study by Salazar and colleagues the failure rate was 3.5% per year.[151] Also disturbing is the mortality rate of reoperation that ranged from 5% to 11%.[136,151,152] Given the improved results seen with appropriate monitoring of women with mechanical valves, it is not clear that placement of a bioprosthesis with the need for eventual reoperations is safer than a mechanical valve.[119]

The Patient on Warfarin Who Desires to Become Pregnant

There are several treatment options for the patient on warfarin who is seeking pregnancy.[116] One is simply to stop the anticoagulation. This is obviously the least desirable option, but this may be a useful time to review the indications for the patient being on anticoagulant therapy.

Another option is to change the patient to heparin while the couple is trying to conceive. This is the most "desirable" as far as risk to the child but carries the highest risk of osteoporosis. Using LMWH instead of standard heparin simplifies monitoring and lessens the risk of osteoporosis, but this option could result in very long-term heparin exposure if there is difficulty conceiving. Patients will need heparin monitored periodically to ensure that heparin levels are in the therapeutic range.

The final option would be frequent pregnancy tests and immediate conversion to heparin when the test becomes positive. This reduces the risk during the most dangerous time of warfarin therapy for the 6- to 12-week-old fetus. Couples who pursue this option need to be facile and compliant with pregnancy testing.

Endocarditis and Anticoagulation

Embolic events are frequent complications of endocarditis.[153,154] Despite the fact that infectious vegetations are rich in fibrin and platelets, the use of anticoagulants in native valve endocarditis is associated with an increased rate of hemorrhage.[155,156] Therefore, anticoagulation should be limited to patients with clear indications such as venous thrombosis or severe heart failure with emboli. However, for most prosthetic valve endocarditis the continuation of anticoagulation is indicated to prevent embolic events, although clearance of the infection is crucial.[157] Exceptions to this are patients with left-side prosthetic valves who are bacteremic with *Staphylococcus aureus* endocarditis. These patients have a high rate (>50%) of fatal central nervous system hemorrhage and should have anticoagulants held until the bacteremia has resolved.[59,158] Kupferwasser and coworkers reported that patients with endocarditis who have antiphospholipid antibodies have a dramatically higher rate of embolism (61.5% vs 23.1%).[159] If these findings are confirmed, this may lead to trials of "targeted" anticoagulation therapy. For patients with intracranial hemorrhage, anticoagulation should be held for 1 week before restarting.

REFERENCES

1. Go AS, Hylek EM, Phillips KA, et al: Prevalence of diagnosed atrial fibrillation in adults: National implications for rhythm management and stroke prevention: The AnTicoagulation and Risk Factors in Atrial Fibrillation (ATRIA) Study. JAMA 285:2370–2375, 2001.
2. Singer DE, Albers GW, Dalen JE, et al: Antithrombotic therapy in atrial fibrillation: The Seventh ACCP Conference on Antithrombotic and Thrombolytic Therapy. Chest 126(3 Suppl):429S–456S, 2004.
3. Stroke Prevention in Atrial Fibrillation Investigators. Stroke prevention in Atrial Fibrillation Study: Final results. Circulation 84:527–539, 1991.
4. Stroke Prevention in Atrial Fibrillation Study Group: Preliminary report of the stroke prevention in atrial fibrillation study. N Engl J Med 322:863–868, 1990.
5. Singer DE, Hughes RA, Gress DR, et al: The effect of aspirin on the risk of stroke in patients with nonrheumatic atrial fibrillation: The BAATAF study. Am Heart J 124:1567–1573, 1992.
6. Aguilar MI, Hart R: Oral anticoagulants for preventing stroke in patients with non-valvular atrial fibrillation and no previous history of stroke or transient ischemic attacks. Cochrane Database Syst Rev (3): CD001927, 2005.
7. Currie CJ, Jones M, Goodfellow J, et al: Evaluation of survival and ischaemic and thromboembolic event rates in patients with nonvalvular atrial fibrillation in the general population when treated and untreated with warfarin. Heart 92:196–200, 2006.
8. van WC, Hart RG, Singer DE, et al: Oral anticoagulants vs aspirin in nonvalvular atrial fibrillation: An individual patient meta-analysis. JAMA 288:2441–2448, 2002.
9. Go AS, Hylek EM, Chang Y, et al: Anticoagulation therapy for stroke prevention in atrial fibrillation: How well do randomized trials translate into clinical practice? JAMA 290:2685–2692, 2003.
10. Poli D, Antonucci E, Lombardi A, et al: Management of oral anticoagulant therapy in the real practice of an anticoagulation clinic: Focus on atrial fibrillation. Blood Coagul Fibrinolysis 16:491–494, 2005.
11. EAFT (European Atrial Fibrillation Trial) Study Group: Secondary prevention in non-rheumatic atrial fibrillation after transient ischaemic attack or minor stroke. Lancet 342:1255–1262, 1993.
12. Reynolds MW, Fahrbach K, Hauch O, et al: Warfarin anticoagulation and outcomes in patients with atrial fibrillation: A systematic review and meta-analysis. Chest 126:1938–1945, 2004.
13. Jones M, McEwan P, Morgan CL, et al: Evaluation of the pattern of treatment, level of anticoagulation control, and outcome of treatment with warfarin in patients with non-valvar atrial fibrillation: A record linkage study in a large British population. Heart 91:472–477, 2005.
14. Hylek EM, Go AS, Chang Y, et al: Effect of intensity of oral anticoagulation on stroke severity and mortality in atrial fibrillation. N Engl J Med 349:1019–1026, 2003.
15. Indredavik B, Rohweder G, Lydersen S: Frequency and effect of optimal anticoagulation before onset of ischaemic stroke in patients with known atrial fibrillation. J Intern Med 258:133–144, 2005.
15a. White HD, Gruber M, Feyzi J, et al: Comparison of outcomes among patients randomized to warfarin therapy according to anticoagulant control: Results from SPORTIF III and V. Arch Intern Med 167:239–245, 2007.
16. The Stroke Prevention in Atrial Fibrillation Investigators: A differential effect of aspirin on prevention of stroke in atrial fibrillation. J Stroke Cerebrovasc Dis 3:181–188, 1993.
17. Stroke Prevention in Atrial Fibrillation Investigators: Adjusted-dose warfarin versus low-intensity, fixed-dose warfarin plus aspirin for high-risk patients with atrial fibrillation: Stroke prevention in atrial fibrillation II randomised clinical trial. Lancet 348:633–638, 1996.
18. Segal JB, McNamara RL, Miller MR, et al: Prevention of thromboembolism in atrial fibrillation: A meta-analysis of trials of anticoagulants and antiplatelet drugs. J Gen Intern Med 15:56–67, 2000.
19. Hart RG, Benavente O, McBride R, Pearce LA: Antithrombotic therapy to prevent stroke in patients with atrial fibrillation: A meta-analysis. Ann Intern Med 131:492–501, 1999.
20. The Atrial Fibrillation Investigators. The efficacy of aspirin in patients with atrial fibrillation: Analysis of pooled data from 3 randomized trials. Arch Intern Med 157:1237–1240, 1997.
21. Miller VT, Pearce LA, Feinberg WM, et al: Differential effect of aspirin versus warfarin on clinical stroke types in patients with atrial fibrillation. Neurology 46:238–240, 1996.
22. Hart RG, Pearce LA, Miller VT, et al: Cardioembolic vs noncardioembolic strokes in atrial fibrillation: Frequency and effect of antithrombotic agents in the stroke prevention in atrial fibrillation studies. Cerebrovasc Dis 10:39–43, 2000.
23. de Denus S, Sanoski CA, Carlsson J, et al: Rate vs rhythm control in patients with atrial fibrillation: A meta-analysis. Arch Intern Med 165:258–262, 2005.
24. Sherman DG, Kim SG, Boop BS, et al: Occurrence and characteristics of stroke events in the Atrial Fibrillation Follow-up Investigation of Sinus Rhythm Management (AFFIRM) study. Arch Intern Med 165:1185–1191, 2005.
25. Pelargonio G, Prystowsky EN: Rate versus rhythm control in the management of patients with atrial fibrillation. Nat Clin Pract Cardiovasc Med 2:514–521, 2005.
26. Corley SD, Epstein AE, DiMarco JP, et al: Relationships between sinus rhythm, treatment, and survival in the Atrial Fibrillation Follow-Up Investigation of Rhythm Management (AFFIRM) Study. Circulation 109:1509–1513, 2004.
27. Wittkowsky AK, Whitely KS, Devine EB, Nutescu E: Effect of age on international normalized ratio at the time of major bleeding in patients treated with warfarin. Pharmacotherapy 24:600–605, 2004.
28. Aspinall SL, DeSanzo BE, Trilli LE, Good CB: Bleeding Risk Index in an anticoagulation clinic: Assessment by indication and implications for care. J Gen Intern Med 20:1008–1013, 2005.
29. Petersen P: New approaches to anticoagulation in atrial fibrillation. Curr Cardiol Rep 6:354–364, 2004.
30. Hirsh J, Raschke R: Heparin and low-molecular-weight heparin: The Seventh ACCP Conference on Antithrombotic and Thrombolytic Therapy. Chest 126(Suppl 3):188S–203S, 2004.
31. Landefeld CS, Beyth RJ: Anticoagulant-related bleeding: Clinical epidemiology, prediction, and prevention. Am J Med 95:315–328, 1993.
32. Linkins LA, Choi PT, Douketis JD: Clinical impact of bleeding in patients taking oral anticoagulant therapy for venous thromboembolism: A meta-analysis. Ann Intern Med 139:893–900, 2003.
33. Landefeld CS, Rosenblatt MW, Goldman L: Bleeding in outpatients treated with warfarin: Relation to the prothrombin time and important remediable lesions. Am J Med 87:153–159, 1989.
34. Poli D, Antonucci E, Lombardi A, et al: Low rate of bleeding and thrombotic complications of oral anticoagulant therapy independent of age in the real-practice of an anticoagulation clinic. Blood Coagul Fibrinolysis 14:269–275, 2003.
35. Palareti G: Hemorrhagic complications of oral anticoagulants. Haematologica 88(Suppl. 6):72–76, 2003.
36. Torn M, van der Meer FJ, Rosendaal FR: Lowering the intensity of oral anticoagulant therapy: Effects on the risk of hemorrhage and thromboembolism. Arch Intern Med 164:668–673, 2004.

37. The Stroke Prevention in Atrial Fibrillation Investigators: Bleeding during antithrombotic therapy in patients with atrial fibrillation. Arch Intern Med 156:409–416, 1996.

38. Hylek EM, Chang YC, Skates SJ, et al: Prospective study of the outcomes of ambulatory patients with excessive warfarin anticoagulation. Arch Intern Med 160:1612–1617, 2000.

39. Oden A, Fahlen M: Oral anticoagulation and risk of death: A medical record linkage study. BMJ 325:1073–1075, 2002.

40. Fang MC, Chang Y, Hylek EM, et al: Advanced age, anticoagulation intensity, and risk for intracranial hemorrhage among patients taking warfarin for atrial fibrillation. Ann Intern Med 141:745–752, 2004.

41. Levine MN, Raskob G, Beyth RJ, et al: Hemorrhagic complications of anticoagulant treatment: The Seventh ACCP Conference on Antithrombotic and Thrombolytic Therapy. Chest 126(3Suppl):287S–310S, 2004.

42. Rothberg MB, Celestin C, Fiore LD, et al: Warfarin plus aspirin after myocardial infarction or the acute coronary syndrome: Meta-analysis with estimates of risk and benefit. Ann Intern Med 143:241–250, 2005.

43. Hurlen M, Abdelnoor M, Smith P, et al: Warfarin, aspirin, or both after myocardial infarction. N Engl J Med 347:969–974, 2002.

44. Hurlen M, Erikssen J, Smith P, et al: Comparison of bleeding complications of warfarin and warfarin plus acetylsalicylic acid: A study in 3166 outpatients. J Intern Med 236:299–304, 1994.

45. Beyth RJ, Milligan PE, Gage BF: Risk factors for bleeding in patients taking coumarins. Curr Hematol Rep 1:41–49, 2002.

46. Berwaerts J, Webster J: Analysis of risk factors involved in oral-anticoagulant-related intracranial haemorrhages. QJM 93:513–521, 2000.

47. Sconce E, Khan T, Mason J, et al: Patients with unstable control have a poorer dietary intake of vitamin K compared to patients with stable control of anticoagulation. Thromb Haemost 93:872–875, 2005.

48. McMahan DA, Smith DM, Carey MA, Zhou XH: Risk of major hemorrhage for outpatients treated with warfarin. J Gen Intern Med 13:311–316, 1998.

49. Sanderson S, Emery J, Higgins J, et al: CYP2C9 gene variants, drug dose, and bleeding risk in warfarin-treated patients: A HuGEnet systematic review and meta-analysis. Genet Med 7:97–104, 2005.

50. Sconce EA, Khan TI, Wynne HA, et al: The impact of CYP2C9 and VKORC1 genetic polymorphism and patient characteristics upon warfarin dose requirements: Proposal for a new dosing regimen. Blood 106:2329–2333, 2005.

51. Rieder MJ, Reiner AP, Gage BF, et al: Effect of VKORC1 haplotypes on transcriptional regulation and warfarin dose. N Engl J Med 352:2285–2293, 2005.

52. Bodin L, Verstuyft C, Tregouet DA, et al: Cytochrome P450 2C9 (CYP2C9) and vitamin K epoxide reductase (VKORC1) genotypes as determinants of acenocoumarol sensitivity. Blood 106:135–140, 2005.

53. Wadelius M, Chen LY, Downes K, et al: Common VKORC1 and GGCX polymorphisms associated with warfarin dose. Pharmacogenomics J 5:262–270, 2005.

54. Gage BF: Pharmacogenetics-based coumarin therapy. Hematology (Am Soc Hematol Educ Program). 467–473, 2006.

55. Geisen C, Watzka M, Sittinger K, et al: VKORC1 haplotypes and their impact on the inter-individual and inter-ethnical variability of oral anticoagulation. Thromb Haemost 94:773–779, 2005.

56. Higashi MK, Veenstra DL, Kondo LM, et al: Association between CYP2C9 genetic variants and anticoagulation-related outcomes during warfarin therapy. JAMA 287:1690–1698, 2002.

57. Beyth RJ, Quinn LM, Landefeld CS: Prospective evaluation of an index for predicting the risk of major bleeding in outpatients treated with warfarin. Am J Med 105:91–99, 1998.

58. Wells PS, Forgie MA, Simms M, et al: The outpatient bleeding risk index: Validation of a tool for predicting bleeding rates in patients treated for deep venous thrombosis and pulmonary embolism. Arch Intern Med 163:917–920, 2003.

59. Seiler C: Management and follow up of prosthetic heart valves. Heart 90:818–824, 2004.

60. Vongpatanasin W, Hillis LD, Lange RA: Prosthetic heart valves. N Engl J Med 335:407–416, 1996.

61. Vink R, Kraaijenhagen RA, Hutten BA, et al: The optimal intensity of vitamin K antagonists in patients with mechanical heart valves: A meta-analysis. J Am Coll Cardiol 42:2042–2048, 2003.

62. Salem DN, Stein PD, Al-Ahmad A, et al: Antithrombotic therapy in valvular heart disease—native and prosthetic: The Seventh ACCP Conference on Antithrombotic and Thrombolytic Therapy. Chest 126(3 Suppl):457S–482S, 2004.

63. Mauri L, O'Gara PT: Valvular heart disease in the pregnant patient. Curr Treat Options Cardiovasc Med 3:7–14, 2001.

64. Hering D, Piper C, Horstkotte D: Drug insight: An overview of current anticoagulation therapy after heart valve replacement. Nat Clin Pract Cardiovasc Med 2:415–422, 2005.

65. Gherli T, Colli A, Fragnito C, et al: Comparing warfarin with aspirin after biological aortic valve replacement: A prospective study. Circulation 110:496–500, 2004.

66. Vazquez E, Sanchez-Perales C, Garcia-Cortes MJ, et al: Ought dialysis patients with atrial fibrillation be treated with oral anticoagulants? Int J Cardiol 87:135–139, 2003.

67. Vazquez E, Sanchez-Perales C, Borrego F, et al: Influence of atrial fibrillation on the morbido-mortality of patients on hemodialysis. Am Heart J 140:886–890, 2000.

68. Vazquez E, Sanchez-Perales C, Lozano C, et al: Comparison of prognostic value of atrial fibrillation versus sinus rhythm in patients on long-term hemodialysis. Am J Cardiol 92:868–871, 2003.

69. Riegert-Johnson DL, Volcheck GW: The incidence of anaphylaxis following intravenous phytonadione (vitamin K_1): A 5-year retrospective review. Ann Allergy Asthma Immunol 89:400–406, 2002.

70. Watson HG, Baglin T, Laidlaw SL, et al: A comparison of the efficacy and rate of response to oral and intravenous Vitamin K in reversal of over-anticoagulation with warfarin. Br J Haematol 115:145–149, 2001.

71. Shields RC, McBane RD, Kuiper JD, et al: Efficacy and safety of intravenous phytonadione (vitamin K1) in patients on long-term oral anticoagulant therapy. Mayo Clin Proc 76:260–266, 2001.

72. Raj G, Kumar R, McKinney WP: Time course of reversal of anticoagulant effect of warfarin by intravenous and subcutaneous phytonadione. [erratum appears in Arch Intern Med 2000. Apr 10; 160(7):986]. Arch Intern Med 159:2721–2724, 1999.

73. Makris M, Watson HG: The management of coumarin-induced over-anticoagulation Annotation. Br J Haematol 114:271–280, 2001.

74. Nee R, Doppenschmidt D, Donovan DJ, Andrews TC: Intravenous versus subcutaneous vitamin K_1 in reversing excessive oral anticoagulation. Am J Cardiol 83:286–288, 1999.

75. Whitling AM, Bussey HI, Lyons RM: Comparing different routes and doses of phytonadione for reversing excessive anticoagulation. Arch Intern Med 158:2136–2140, 1988.

76. Taylor CT, Chester EA, Byrd DC, Stephens MA: Vitamin K to reverse excessive anticoagulation: A review of the literature. Pharmacotherapy 19:1415–1425, 1999.

77. Wilson SE, Watson HG, Crowther MA: Low-dose oral vitamin K therapy for the management of asymptomatic patients with elevated international normalized ratios: A brief review. CMAJ 170:821–824, 2004.

78. Nitu IC, Perry DJ, Lee CA: Clinical experience with the use of clotting factor concentrates in oral anticoagulation reversal. Clin Lab Haematol 20:363–367, 1998.

79. Cartmill M, Dolan G, Byrne JL, Byrne PO: Prothrombin complex concentrate for oral anticoagulant reversal in neurosurgical emergencies. Br J Neurosurg 14:458–461, 2000.

80. Aguilar MI, Hart RG, Kase CS, et al: Treatment of warfarin-associated intracerebral hemorrhage: Literature review and expert opinion. Mayo Clin Proc 82:82–92, 2007.

81. Taberner DA, Thomson JM, Poller L: Comparison of prothrombin complex concentrate and vitamin K1 in oral anticoagulant reversal. BMJ 2:83–85, 1976.

82. Makris M, Greaves M, Phillips WS, et al: Emergency oral anticoagulant reversal: The relative efficacy of infusions of fresh frozen plasma and clotting factor concentrate on correction of the coagulopathy. Thromb Haemost 77:477–480, 1997.

83. Warkentin TE, Crowther MA: Reversing anticoagulants both old and new. Can J Anaesth 49:S11–S25, 2002.

84. Deveras RA, Kessler CM: Reversal of warfarin-induced excessive anticoagulation with recombinant human factor VIIa concentrate. Ann Intern Med 137:884–888, 2002.

85. Berntorp E: Recombinant FVIIa in the treatment of warfarin bleeding. Sem Thromb Hemost 26:433–435, 2000.

86. Spyropoulos AC, Bauersachs RM, Omran H, et al: Periprocedural bridging therapy in patients receiving chronic oral anticoagulation therapy. Curr Med Res Opin 22:1109–1122, 2006.

87. Dunn AS, Turpie AG: Perioperative management of patients receiving oral anticoagulants: A systematic review. Arch Intern Med 163:901–908, 2003.

88. Larson BJ, Zumberg MS, Kitchens CS: A feasibility study of continuing dose-reduced warfarin for invasive procedures in patients with high thromboembolic risk. Chest 127:922–927, 2005.

89. Douketis JD, Johnson JA, Turpie AG: Low-molecular-weight heparin as bridging anticoagulation during interruption of warfarin: Assessment of a standardized periprocedural anticoagulation regimen. Perspect Vasc Surg Endovasc Ther 17:176, 2005.

90. Spyropoulos AC: Bridging of oral anticoagulation therapy for invasive procedures. Curr Hematol Rep 4:405–413, 2005.

91. Kovacs MJ, Kearon C, Rodger M, et al: Single-arm study of bridging therapy with low-molecular-weight heparin for patients at risk of arterial embolism who require temporary interruption of warfarin. Circulation 110:1658–1663, 2004.

92. Seshadri N, Goldhaber SZ, Elkayam U, et al: The clinical challenge of bridging anticoagulation with low-molecular-weight heparin in patients with mechanical prosthetic heart valves: An evidence-based comparative review focusing on anticoagulation options in pregnant and nonpregnant patients. Am Heart J 150:27–34, 2005.

93. Tyagi A, Bhattacharya A: Central neuraxial blocks and anticoagulation: A review of current trends. Eur J Anaesthesiol 19:317–329, 2002.

94. De Tommaso O, Caporuscio A, Tagariello V: Neurological complications following central neuraxial blocks: Are there predictive factors? Eur J Anaesthesiol 19:705–716, 2002.

95. Horlocker TT: Low molecular weight heparin and neuraxial anesthesia. Thromb Res 101:V141–V154, 2001.

96. Hulse ML: Warfarin resistance: Diagnosis and therapeutic alternatives. Pharmacotherapy 16:1009–1017, 1996.

97. Pedersen FM, Hamberg O, Hess K, Ovesen L: The effect of dietary vitamin K on warfarin-induced anticoagulation. J Int Med 229:517–520, 1991.

98. Tiede DJ, Nishimura RA, Gastineau DA, et al: Modern management of prosthetic valve anticoagulation. Mayo Clin Proc 73:665–680, 1998.

99. Bentley DP, Backhouse G, Hutchings A, et al: Investigation of patients with abnormal response to warfarin. Br J Clin Pharmacol 22:37–41, 1986.

100. Talstad I, Gamst ON: Warfarin resistance due to malabsorption. J Intern Med 236:465–467, 1994.

101. Fihn SD, Callahan CM, Martin DC, et al: The risk for and severity of bleeding complications in elderly patients treated with warfarin. Ann Intern Med 124:970–979, 1996.

102. Torn M, Bollen WL, van der Meer FJ, et al: Risks of oral anticoagulant therapy with increasing age. Arch Intern Med 165:1527–1532, 2005.

103. Sebastian JL, Tresch DD: Use of oral anticoagulants in older patients. Drugs and Aging 16:409–435, 2000.

104. Fitzmaurice DA, Blann AD, Lip GY: Bleeding risks of antithrombotic therapy. BMJ 325:828–831, 2002.

105. Pautas E, Gouin-Thibault I, Debray M, et al: Haemorrhagic complications of vitamin K antagonists in the elderly: Risk factors and management. Drugs Aging 23:13–25, 2006.

106. Singla DL, Morrill GB: Warfarin maintenance dosages in the very elderly. Am J Health Syst Pharm 62:1062–1066, 2005.

107. Oldenburg J: Vitamin K intake and stability of oral anticoagulant treatment. Thromb Haemost 93:799–800, 2005.

108. Rosand J, Hylek EM, O'Donnell HC, Greenberg SM: Warfarin-associated hemorrhage and cerebral amyloid angiopathy: A genetic and pathologic study. Neurology 55:947–951, 2000.

109. Attems J: Sporadic cerebral amyloid angiopathy: Pathology, clinical implications, and possible pathomechanisms. Acta Neuropathol (Berl) 110:345–359, 2005.

110. Man-Son-Hing M, Laupacis A: Anticoagulant-related bleeding in older persons with atrial fibrillation: Physicians' fears often unfounded. Arch Intern Med 163:1580–1586, 2003.

111. Tapson VF, Hyers TM, Waldo AL, et al: Antithrombotic therapy practices in U.S. hospitals in an era of practice guidelines. Arch Intern Med 165:1458–1464, 2005.

112. Brophy MT, Snyder KE, Gaehde S, et al: Anticoagulant use for atrial fibrillation in the elderly. J Am Geriatr Soc 52:1151–1156, 2004.

113. Bungard TJ, Ghali WA, McAlister FA, et al: Physicians' perceptions of the benefits and risks of warfarin for patients with nonvalvular atrial fibrillation. CMAJ 165:301–302, 2001.

114. Man-Son-Hing M, Gage BF, Montgomery AA, et al: Preference-based antithrombotic therapy in atrial fibrillation: Implications for clinical decision making. Med Decis Making 25:548–559, 2005.

115. Bond AJ, Molnar FJ, Li M, et al: The risk of hemorrhagic complications in hospital in-patients who fall while receiving antithrombotic therapy. Thromb J 3:1, 2005.

116. Bates SM, Greer IA, Hirsh J, et al: Use of antithrombotic agents during pregnancy: The Seventh ACCP Conference on Antithrombotic and Thrombolytic Therapy. Chest 126(3 Suppl):627S–644S, 2004.

117. Blickstein D, Blickstein I: The risk of fetal loss associated with Warfarin anticoagulation. Int J Gynaecol Obstet 78:221–225, 2002.

118. Danik S, Fuster V: The obstetrical patient with a prosthetic heart valve. Obstet Gynecol Clin North Am 33:481–491, 2006.

119. Barbour LA: Current concepts of anticoagulant therapy in pregnancy. Obstet Gynecol Clin North Am 24:499–521, 1997.

120. Cotrufo M, de FM, De Santo LS, et al: Risk of warfarin during pregnancy with mechanical valve prostheses. Obstet Gynecol 99:35–40, 2002.

121. Vitale N, de FM, De Santo LS, et al: Dose-dependent fetal complications of warfarin in pregnant women with mechanical heart valves. J Am Coll Cardiol 33:1637–1641, 1999.

122. Ginsberg JS, Hirsh J, Turner DC, et al: Risks to the fetus of anticoagulant therapy during pregnancy. Thromb Haemost 61:197–203, 1989.

123. Barbour LA, Smith JM, Marlar RA: Heparin levels to guide thromboembolism prophylaxis during pregnancy. Am J Obstet Gynecol 173:1869–1873, 1995.

124. Anderson DR, Ginsberg JS, Burrows R, Brill-Edwards P: Subcutaneous heparin therapy during pregnancy: A need for concern at the time of delivery. Thromb Haemost 65:248–250, 1991.

125. Douketis JD, Ginsberg JS, Burrows RF, et al: The effects of long-term heparin therapy during pregnancy on bone density: A prospective matched cohort study. Thromb Haemost 75:254–257, 1996.

126. Barbour LA, Kick SD, Steiner JF, et al: A prospective study of heparin-induced osteoporosis in pregnancy using bone densitometry. Am J Obstet Gynecol 170:862–869, 1994.

127. Nelson-Piercy C: Heparin-induced osteoporosis. Scand J Rheumatol (Suppl) 107:68–71, 1998.

128. Shefras J, Farquharson RG: Bone density studies in pregnant women receiving heparin. Eur J Obstet Gynecol Reprod Biol 65:171–174, 1996.

129. Sanson BJ, Lensing AWA, Prins MH, et al: Safety of low-molecular weight heparin in pregnancy: A systematic review. Thromb Haemost 81:668–672, 1999.

130. Nelson-Piercy C, Letsky EA, De Sweit M: Low-molecular weight heparin for obstetric thromboprophylaxis: Experience of sixty-nine pregnancies in sixty-one women at high risk. Am J Obstet Gynecol 176:1062–1068, 1997.

131. Laposata M, Green D, Van Cott EM, et al: College of American Pathologists Conference XXXI on laboratory monitoring of anticoagulant therapy: The clinical use and laboratory monitoring of low-molecular-weight heparin, danaparoid, hirudin and related compounds, and argatroban. Arch Pathol Lab Med 122:799–807, 1998.

132. Hirsh J, Raschke R: Heparin and low-molecular-weight heparin: The Seventh ACCP Conference on Antithrombotic and Thrombolytic Therapy. Chest 126(3 Suppl):188S–203S, 2004.

133. Brennand JE, Walker ID, Greer IA: Anti-activated factor X profiles in pregnant women receiving antenatal thromboprophylaxis with enoxaparin. Acta Haematologica 101:53–55, 1999.

134. Collins JJ: Risks of valve replacements in young women. Circulation 99:2613, 1999.

135. Casele HL: The use of unfractionated heparin and low molecular weight heparins in pregnancy. Clin Obstet Gynecol 49:895–905, 2006.

136. Sbarouni E, Oakley CM: Outcome of pregnancy in women with valve prostheses. Br Heart J 71:196–201, 1994.

137. Elkayam U, Singh H, Irani A, Akhter MW: Anticoagulation in pregnant women with prosthetic heart valves. J Cardiovasc Pharmacol Ther 9:107–115, 2004.

138. Alderman CP, McClure AF, Jersmann HP, Scott SD: Continuous subcutaneous heparin infusion for treatment of Trousseau's syndrome. Ann Pharmacother 29:710–713, 1995.

139. Callander N, Rapaport SI: Trousseau's syndrome. West J Med 158:364–371, 1993.

140. Lecuru, Desnos M, Taurelle R: Anticoagulant therapy in pregnancy: Report of 54 cases. Acta Obstet Gynecol Scand 75:217–221, 1996.

141. Oakley CM: Anticoagulants in pregnancy. Br Heart J 74:107–111, 1995.

142. Olson JD, Arkin CF, Brandt JT, et al: College of American Pathologists Conference XXXI on laboratory monitoring of anticoagulant therapy: Laboratory monitoring of unfractionated heparin therapy. Arch Pathol Lab Med 122:782–798, 1998.

143. Frewin R, Chisholm M: Anticoagulation of women with prosthetic heart valves during pregnancy. Br J Obstet Gynaecol 105:683–686, 1998.

144. Oran B, Lee-Parritz A, Ansell J: Low molecular weight heparin for the prophylaxis of thromboembolism in women with prosthetic mechanical heart valves during pregnancy. Thromb Haemost 92:747–751, 2004.

145. Glower DD: Does pregnancy affect the durability of valvular bioprostheses? [editorial; comment]Am Heart J 137:t-1, 1999.

146. Elkayam U, Bitar F: Valvular heart disease and pregnancy: Part II: Prosthetic valves. J Am Coll Cardiol 46:403–410, 2005.

147. Hung L, Rahimtoola SH: Prosthetic heart valves and pregnancy. Circulation 107:1240–1246, 2003.

148. Coulshed DS, Fitzpatrick MA, Lee CH: Drug treatment associated with heart valve replacement. Drugs 49:897–911, 1995.

149. Kulik A, Bedard P, Lam BK, et al: Mechanical versus bioprosthetic valve replacement in middle-aged patients. Eur J Cardiothorac Surg 30:485–491, 2006.

150. Mihaljevic T, Paul S, Leacche M, et al: Valve replacement in women of childbearing age: Influences on mother, fetus, and neonate. J Heart Valve Dis 14:151–157, 2005.

151. Salazar E, Espinola N, Roman L, Casanova JM: Effect of pregnancy on the duration of bovine pericardial bioprostheses. Am Heart J 1999; 137:t-20, 1990.

152. Hanania G, Thomas D, Michel PL, et al: Pregnancy and prosthetic heart valves: A French cooperative retrospective study of 155 cases. Eur Heart J 15:1651–1658, 1994.

153. Fabri J, Jr., Issa VS, Pomerantzeff PM, et al: Time-related distribution, risk factors and prognostic influence of embolism in patients with left-sided infective endocarditis. Int J Cardiol 110:334–339, 2006.

154. Tunkel AR, Kaye D: Neurologic complications of infective endocarditis. Neur Clin 11:419–440, 1993.

155. Delahaye JP, Poncet P, Malquarti V, et al: Cerebrovascular accidents in infective endocarditis: Role of anticoagulation. Eur Heart J 11:1074–1078, 1990.

156. Carpenter JL, McAllister CK: Anticoagulation in prosthetic valve endocarditis. South Med J 76:1372–1375, 1983.

157. Davenport J, Hart RG: Prosthetic valve endocarditis 1976–1987. Antibiotics, anticoagulation, and stroke. Stroke 21:993–999, 1990.

158. Tornos P, Almirante B, Mirabet S, et al: Infective endocarditis due to *Staphylococcus aureus:* Deleterious effect of anticoagulant therapy. Arch Intern Med 159:473–475, 1999.

159. Kupferwasser LI, Hafner G, Mohr-Kahaly S, et al: The presence of infection-related antiphospholipid antibodies in infective endocarditis determines a major risk factor for embolic events. J Am Coll Cardiol 33:1365–1371, 1999.

160. Gage BF, Waterman AD, Shannon W, et al: Validation of clinical classification schemes for predicting stroke: Results from the National Registry of Atrial Fibrillation. JAMA 285:2864–2870, 2001.

Index

Note: Page numbers followed by f and t indicate figures and tables, respectively.